NURSING CARE OF THE CHILDBEARING FAMILY

Laurie N. Sherwen, PhD, RN
Nurse Researcher/Associate Professor
Department of Nursing
College of Allied Health Sciences
Thomas Jefferson University
Philadelphia, Pennsylvania

Mary Ann Scoloveno, EdD, RN
Associate Professor
Rutgers, The State University of New Jersey
College of Nursing
Newark, New Jersey

Carol Toussie Weingarten, PhD, RN
Associate Professor
College of Nursing
Villanova University
Villanova, Pennsylvania

APPLETON & LANGE
Norwalk, Connecticut/San Mateo, California

0-8385-7011-9

91 92 93 94 95 / 10 9 8 7 6 5 4 3 2 1

Prentice Hall International (UK) Limited, *London*
Prentice Hall of Australia Pty. Limited, *Sydney*
Prentice Hall Canada, Inc., *Toronto*
Prentice Hall Hispanoamericana, S.A., *Mexico*
Prentice Hall of India Private Limited, *New Delhi*
Prentice Hall of Japan, Inc., *Tokyo*
Simon & Schuster Asia Pte. Ltd., *Singapore*
Editora Prentice Hall do Brasil Ltda., *Rio de Janeiro*
Prentice Hall, *Englewood Cliffs, New Jersey*

Library of Congress Cataloging-in-Publication Data

Sherwen, Laurie Nehls, 1947–
Nursing care of the childbearing family / Laurie N. Sherwen, Mary Ann Scoloveno, Carol Toussie Weingarten.
p. cm.
Includes bibliographical references.
ISBN 0-8385-7011-9
1. Obstetrical nursing. 2. Family nursing. I. Scoloveno, Mary Ann. II. Toussie-Weingarten, Carol, 1949– III. Title.
[DNLM: 1. Obstetrical Nursing. 2. Patient Care Planning—nurses' instruction. 3. Pediatric Nursing. 4. Perinatology—nurses' instruction. 5. Pregnancy—nurses' instruction. WY 157.3 S554n]
RG951.S473 1991
610.73'678—dc20
DNLM/DLC 90-14508
for Library of Congress

Executive Editor, Nursing: William Brottmiller
Senior Development Editor: Donna Frassetto
Developmental Assistant: Trisha Foldeak
Managing Editor: John Williams
Editorial Assistant: Sasha Kintzler
Art Director: Steven M. Byrum
Designers: Michael J. Kelly, Janice Barsevich
Manufacturing Buyer: Alexis Heydt

Most of the original photographs in this text were taken by Carol Toussie Weingarten. The authors would also like to acknowledge the following individuals who supplied additional photographs:
James Bowns: 30–7
John DePalma: 8–opener, 37–2
Susan K. Fabry: 33–21A
Robert Gomberg: 25–opener
Barbara S. Kiernan: 4–1, 11–opener, 32–6, 33–opener, 33–3, 33–4, 33–6, 33–7, 33–8, 33–12, 33–15, 33–16, 33–17, 33–18, 33–19, 33–20A, 33–21B, 33–22(L), 33–22(R), 33–23, 33–24, 33–25, 33–26, 33–27, 33–28, 33–30, 33–31, 34–2, 34–6A, 34–13
Marilyn Rogers: 34–16
Mary Ann Scoloveno: 3–1A, 3–1B, 24–9, 34–9, 34–15, 37–1, 43–2
John D. Sherwen, Jr.: 30–3, 30–6
Ellen Solomon: 22–opener, 24–1
Joan Weiss: 32–5, 34–opener
44–opener, courtesy of Thomas Jefferson University Medical Center

PRINTED IN THE UNITED STATES OF AMERICA

To Douglas . . .
my husband and best friend for all times
and
To the Nehls and Sherwen clans . . .
who taught me to appreciate families.

Laurie Nehls Sherwen

To my husband Red . . .
the wind beneath my wings
To Bobby and Michael . . .
a source of unending love and devotion
and
To my parents, Michael and Lee DePalma . . .
for their love and belief in me.

Mary Ann Scoloveno

To my husband Michael . . .
ever my North Star
To my daughter Robin . . .
for her courage, patience, and love
and
To Jeanne Toussie Jacobwitz . . .
my sister, colleague, and friend.

Carol Toussie Weingarten

We also dedicate this book to the nursing students and faculty at
Thomas Jefferson University,
Rutgers University,
and
Villanova University.

Reviewers

Gary Boyce, RN
College of Nursing, University of Florida, Gainesville, Florida

Linda Curry, PhD, RN
Assistant Professor, Harris College of Nursing, Texas Christian University, Fort Worth, Texas

Margaret Dick, PhD, RN
Associate Professor, School of Nursing, University of North Carolina at Greensboro, Greensboro, North Carolina

Marilyn Evans, PhD, RN
Associate Professor, Parent–Child Division, University of North Carolina at Greensboro, Greensboro, North Carolina

Martha Sue Forsbrey, MSN, RN
Doctoral Student, Associate Professor of Nursing, College of Health Sciences, University of Charleston, Charleston, West Virginia

Robert C. Goodlin, MD
Clinical Professor of Obstetrics and Gynecology, University of Colorado, Denver, Colorado

Mary Gottesman, PhD, RN
Assistant Professor, Maternal–Child Health, School of Nursing, University of California, Los Angeles, California

Brett B. Gutsche, MD
Professor of Anesthesia and Professor of Obstetrics and Gynecology, Hospital of the University of Pennsylvania, Philadelphia, Pennsylvania

Carol Howe, DNSc, CNM
Associate Professor, Department of Family Nursing and Department of Obstetrics and Gynecology, Director, Nurse Midwifery Program, Oregon Health Sciences University, Portland, Oregon

Jane M. Kirkpatrick, MSN, RN
Associate Professor, School of Nursing, Purdue University, West Lafayette, Indiana

Amy Levi, MSN, CNM
Director, Nurse Midwifery Services, The Birth Center, Bryn Mawr, Pennsylvania

Elizabeth Libby, RN
Associate Professor of Nursing Education, School of Nursing, University of Augusta, Augusta, Maine

Linda Lutz, MS, CNM
Assistant Professor, Family Nursing Department, Oregon Health Sciences University, Portland, Oregon

Gail McDonald, MS, RN
Assistant Professor, Maternal–Child Health, Massachusetts College of Pharmacy and Allied Health Sciences, Boston, Massachusetts

Vincent F. Mileto, MD, FACOG
Somerset Ob/Gyn Associates, Somerville, New Jersey

Sharon Pontious, PhD, RN
Senior Clinical Nurse Specialist, Department of Nursing, St. Louis Children's Hospital, Adjunct Assistant Professor, Department of Nursing, University of Missouri, St. Louis, Missouri

Ronnie Remsburg, MS, RN
School of Nursing, University of North Carolina at Greensboro, Greensboro, North Carolina

Karen Stevens, MSN, FNP
Associate Professor, School of Nursing, The Catholic University of America, Washington, DC

Deborah Sweeney, MS, CNM
Associate Professor, School of Nursing, Medical College of Georgia, Athens, Georgia

Meredith Taylor, MS, RN
Professor, School of Nursing, University of Oklahoma Health Science Center, Oklahoma City, Oklahoma

Celesta Warner, MS, RN
Instructor, School of Nursing, Wright State University, Miami Valley, Dayton, Ohio

Francene Weatherby, DSN, RNC
Assistant Professor, College of Nursing, University of Oklahoma Health Sciences Center, Oklahoma City, Oklahoma

Michael S. Weingarten, MD, FACS
Chief, Division of Vascular Surgery, The Graduate Hospital, Clinical Assistant Professor of Surgery, University of Pennsylvania, Philadelphia, Pennsylvania

Contributors

Patricia Cramer Arentsen, MSN, RN
Formerly, Undergraduate Faculty
Health Care of Women
University of Pennsylvania
School of Nursing
Philadelphia, Pennsylvania
(*Chapter 18*)

Lauren S. Arnold, MSN, RN
Doctoral Candidate
Graduate Faculty, Perinatal Nursing
University of Pennsylvania
School of Nursing
Philadelphia, Pennsylvania
(*Chapter 18*)

Sandra Goodman Brown, MS, RN
Assistant Professor
Medical University of South Carolina
Charleston, South Carolina
(*Chapter 37*)

Pamela Chally, PhD, RN
Assistant Professor
Northern Illinois University
School of Nursing
DeKalb, Illinois
(*Chapter 38*)

Mary Ann Blum Condon, MS, RN
Assistant Professor
Austin Peay State University
Clarksville, Tennessee
(*Contributed to Chapter 14*)

Marcia Cauley Costello, MS, RD
Assistant Professor
College of Nursing
Villanova University
Villanova, Pennsylvania
(*Chapter 10; nutrition consultant to Chapters 34, 38, and 39*)

Nancy Sharts Engel, PhD, RN, FAAN
Associate Professor
College of Nursing
Villanova University
Villanova, Pennsylvania
(*Chapter 39*)

Gloria C. Essoka, PhD, RN
Associate Professor, Nursing
Hunter Bellevue School of Nursing
New York, New York
(*Chapter 34*)

Susan K. Fabry, MS, PNP, RNC
Nurse Practitioner
Pediatrics Inc.
Huntington, West Virginia
(*Chapter 33*)

Judy Garbinski, MS, RN
Doctoral Candidate
Kent State University
Kent, Ohio
Director, Nursing and Allied Health Sciences
Community College of Beaver County
Monaca, Pennsylvania
(*Chapter 40*)

Sandra Myers Gomberg, MSN, RNC
Nurse Manager, Pediatrics
Albert Einstein Medical Center, Northern Division
Philadelphia, Pennsylvania
(*Chapter 42; consultant to Chapter 43; Glossary*)

Cynthia B. Hughes, EdD, CPNP, RN
Associate Professor
Seton Hall University
College of Nursing
South Orange, New Jersey
(*Chapter 8*)

Barbara S. Kiernan, MSN, PNP, RNC
Doctoral Candidate
University of Kentucky
Lexington, Kentucky
Nurse Practitioner, Valley Health Systems
Huntington, West Virginia
(*Chapter 33*)

Susan M. Lisby-Sutch, PharmD
Rutgers College of Pharmacy
Busche Campus
Piscataway, New Jersey
(*Pharmacology Boxes; Appendices A, B, and G*)

Dianne S. Moore, MPH, CNM, PhD
President
*MOORE*INFO, Inc.
Irvington, New York
(*Chapter 27*)

Karen H. Morin, DSN, RN
Assistant Professor
Widener University
School of Nursing
Newark, Delaware
(*Chapter 9*)

Rosanne Perez-Woods, EdD, RN
Niehoff Chair and Professor
Maternal Child Nursing
Loyola University of Chicago
Chicago, Illinois
(*Chapter 35*)

Virginia Prout, MS, RN
Doctoral Candidate
Adjunct Faculty, Maternal–Child Health Department
Boston College
School of Nursing
Chestnut Hill, Massachusetts
(*Chapter 42*)

Carmen Ramirez, PhD, RN
Assistant Professor
University of Maryland
College of Nursing
Baltimore, Maryland
(*Chapter 34*)

Cathy Kahn Recht, RN, MS
Director of Maternal–Infant Nursing
Medical Center of Central Massachusetts
Worcester, Massachusetts
(*Chapter 43*)

Christine Schifiliti, RN, MS
Medical Center of Central Massachusetts
Worcester, Massachusetts
(*Chapter 43*)

Ellen Shuzman, MSN, RN
Doctoral Student
New York University
New York, New York
Assistant Professor
Rutgers, The State University of New Jersey
College of Nursing
Newark, New Jersey
(*Chapters 29 and 31*)

Elizabeth Thomson, MS, RN
Genetic Counselor
Department of Pediatrics
University of Iowa Hospitals and Clinics
Iowa City, Iowa
Special Assistant to the Director
National Institutes of Child Health
and Human Development
Washington, DC
(*Chapter 9; contributed to Chapters 6 and 7*)

Julia Van Muiswinkel, PhD, RN
Associate Professor
Department of Nursing Care of Children
University of Pittsburgh
School of Nursing
Pittsburgh, Pennsylvania
(*Chapter 26*)

Katherine Wiley, PhD, RN
Assistant Professor
Maternal Child Nursing
Loyola University of Chicago
Chicago, Illinois
(*Chapter 35*)

Caryle G. Wolahan, EdD, RN
Associate Dean and Associate Professor
State University of New York
Health Science Center at Brooklyn
Brooklyn, New York
(*Chapter 11*)

Marion Zimmerman, EdD, RN
Assistant Professor
Rutgers, The State University of New Jersey
College of Nursing
Newark, New Jersey
(*Chapter 25*)

Preface

This is a book about the beginning of life, childbearing, and the unique nursing care needs of families during the reproductive years. Our goal as authors has been to develop a comprehensive textbook to serve as a foundation for nurses and nursing students caring for childbearing families. The family-centered approach to the content, topics selected, scope of each chapter, visual presentation, and accompanying pedagogy have been carefully designed to meet this goal. We hope this textbook will foster excellence in nursing practice, stimulate research related to parent–newborn health, encourage thoughtful consideration of ethical issues related to childbearing, and promote appreciation for culturally sensitive nursing care based on the unique needs of each family.

APPROACH

The outline, approach, and content for this text evolved from the results of the Maternal Infant Core Competency (MICC) Project. Laurie N. Sherwen was Project Director for this large national project, sponsored by the March of Dimes Birth Defects Foundation, the American Association of Colleges of Nursing, the American Nurses' Association, and the Organization for Obstetric, Gynecologic, and Neonatal Nurses. Funding for the MICC was provided by the Division of Maternal–Child Health, Public Health Service, of the United States Department of Health and Human Services.

The MICC Project involved a large national survey of maternity faculty and nurses in clinical practice in nearly every state. Findings from the study provided essential information to us about what nursing experts believe students need to learn about parent–infant nursing. Our own experiences as educators led us to refine, organize, and present this information in a manner that enhances student learning.

Although pregnancy necessarily entails processes of continual change, there are specific characteristics of early, middle, and late pregnancy. By tradition, pregnancy is described by trimester. From our years in clinical nursing education, we have found that students consistently have difficulty in identifying processes of early, middle, and late pregnancy when this content is presented in chapters dealing with the entirety of pregnancy. Students then have problems applying theory to actual pregnant clients. For this reason, we have taken a trimester approach in the discussion of low- and high-risk pregnancy. This comprehensive trimester approach facilitates classroom reading assignments, clinical reference, and application of the nursing process to real families.

Nursing Care of the Childbearing Family emphasizes the importance of wellness, as well as the perinatal perspective. Indeed, a nurse must thoroughly understand variations of normal to care effectively for clients at risk. Throughout the textbook, psychosocial perspectives are featured and ways in which nurses can provide emotional support to clients during situations ranging from wellness to catastrophic loss are discussed. The importance of designing care based on each family's cultural background is emphasized, particularly in those chapters dealing with psychosocial and cultural aspects related to childbearing.

Scientific advances have made a vast store of obstetric and neonatal technology available; however, technology provides tools to be used judiciously by practitioners. Although technologic advances are discussed throughout the textbook, nurses are also challenged to consider risks, as well as benefits, and to use technology both thoughtfully and appropriately.

Care of the childbearing family has become too complex for any one discipline. Effective health care requires collaboration among nurses, among nurses and other health care providers, and among nurses and the family. For this reason, collaborative aspects of care of the childbearing family are integrated throughout the textbook, along with unique nursing implications.

ORGANIZATION

Nursing Care of the Childbearing Family is organized into 12 units. Units 1 through 9 focus on the low-risk childbearing family from pregnancy through the end of the infant's first year after birth. Units 10 through 12 discuss the high-risk family during the same time period. This organization highlights the importance of both wellness and the perinatal perspective.

Chapter 1 introduces the text and presents current perspectives on parent–newborn care. Unit 1 contains chapters related to theoretical and preconceptional content about the reproductive family. A theoretical background for the approach to childbearing families is discussed in Chapters 2 through 4 to illustrate the importance of developing theory-based nursing care.

The importance of preconceptional health for childbearing has been receiving increased emphasis in current practice. Chapter 5 discusses the normal health maintenance and health promotion topics related to gynecologic health and the well woman during her reproductive years. Gynecologic pathology requires a depth of discussion beyond the scope of most undergraduate courses about the childbearing family and is therefore not a focus of this textbook. Preconceptional health and related issues are further addressed in Chapters 6 through 9. These chapters discuss basic anatomy and the physiology of human reproduction, reproductive problems, such as genetic structural chromosome abnormalities and infertility, sexuality across the lifespan, and planning a family.

Unit 2 includes chapters on nutrition during pregnancy and fetal development. These chapters provide information that students will use as a basis for care throughout pregnancy. Units 3, 4, and 5 then focus on physiologic and psychosocial dimensions, assessment, and care of the childbearing family during the first, second, and third trimesters. In each unit, chapters on physiologic changes and psychosocial aspects provide the theoretical foundation for subsequent chapters describing prenatal assessment and management for that trimester. Trimester-specific management strategies are addressed according to nursing care goals, and these strategies are further illustrated with case study/care plan examples.

Unit 6 addresses teaching–learning concepts and presents information necessary for educational preparation during childbearing.

Units 7 through 9, on the intrapartum, postpartum, and infant, continue the nursing process format of the earlier trimester units with specific chapters on physiologic and psychosocial aspects of care. These chapters reinforce the focus on the whole person and family during childbearing that is basic to our philosophy.

Unit 10 deals with high-risk maternal–fetal nursing. The perinatal perspective is discussed in Chapter 35, which emphasizes collaboration as a basis for perinatal care. Chapter 36 addresses psychosocial concerns of the high-risk childbearing family. The special concerns related to care of pregnant adolescents and clients who delay childbearing are detailed in Chapter 37. Chapters 38 through 41 discuss high-risk maternal conditions during the first, second, and third trimesters and the intrapartum and postpartum periods.

Unit 11 covers high-risk neonatal nursing. Chapter 42 addresses alterations in neonatal functioning, whereas Chapter 43 focuses specifically on problems related to preterm birth, gestational age, and birth weight. Unit 12 concludes the textbook with a focus on societal trends in care of the childbearing family and discusses home care of the low- and high-risk childbearing family.

NOTEWORTHY FEATURES

Several chapters provide special dimensions to this text:

- Chapter 28 specifically deals with issues, needs, and care related to the cesarean birth experience.

- Nurses caring for the childbearing family often must provide anticipatory guidance on infant care topics that extend beyond the neonatal period. Chapter 34 provides a foundation for this teaching by discussing the neonate and infant through the end of the first year after birth.
- During the 1990s, home care for high-risk childbearing families will be an increasingly used alternative to hospitalization. Chapter 44 specifically discusses home health care services and nursing implications for care of the childbearing family. The infant and home health care chapters also help students prepare clients for discharge and follow-up.

LEARNING AIDS

The chapters in this textbook have been carefully developed and designed to aid student learning and facilitate review of information. Each chapter begins with a *chapter outline* and list of *key terms*. These features enable the reader to preview chapter content and reinforce important vocabulary. Key terms are highlighted by boldface type where defined within the chapter, and terms with definitions are included in the glossary at the end of the textbook.

Each chapter ends with a *summary* of key content to reinforce learning and aid the student in reviewing essential chapter content. Several *review questions*, designed to stimulate thought about essential points covered in the narrative, are also included. Extensive *references* are provided, highlighting nursing research and classic sources; these provide a resource for further exploration of topics discussed in each chapter.

Several additional features included throughout the textbook also enhance students' learning:

- *Case Study/Care Plans*. Twenty-seven care plans based on case studies illustrate ways in which the nursing process can be applied to clinical situations for low-risk, healthy clients as well as high-risk clients.
- *Nursing Research, Research Abstracts*. Research abstract boxes, included throughout the text, summarize relevant clinical studies and provide a comment section discussing the application to practice. Current research findings are integrated throughout the book and form the basis for discussion of clinical content. Readers are encouraged to appreciate, critique, use, and develop clinical research related to parent–infant nursing.
- *Issues and Controversies*. Probably no other health care area raises as many strong issues and controversies as childbearing, and nurses must be aware of these topics. Boxes included throughout the text identify issues and controversies and encourage readers to think about ways in which they have an impact on the health care childbearing clients seek and receive.
- *Pharmacology Highlights*. Seventeen boxes highlight pharmacologic agents and their nursing implications for childbearing clients or infants.
- *Numerous Tables and Boxes*. Key points are summarized and highlighted in tables and boxes. Unique tables of commonly asked questions supplement the preconceptional and prenatal chapters, providing students with answers to clients' most frequently expressed concerns.
- *Original Photographs and Drawings*. Numerous original photographs have been taken specifically for this text to illustrate specific teaching points and to portray the human aspects of nursing care. Black-and-white and two-color drawings are used extensively throughout the text to enhance student understanding.

TEACHING–LEARNING PACKAGE

Educational companions to this textbook include:

- An *Instructor's Manual*, written by Karen H. Morin, DSN, RN, supplements the text chapter by chapter and provides teaching strategies, audio-visual listing, additional references, and research problems correlated with the text chapters.
- A *Testbank*, available in book form or as computer software, tests students' knowledge of essential chapter content.
- A *Study Guide* for students, written by Francene Weatherby, PhD, RNC, provides content overview, learning objectives, study questions, and a post-study quiz with answers, for each chapter.
- A set of two-color *Transparencies* selected from the text illustrations aids in classroom instruction.

These resources enhance the teaching–learning experience for faculty and students using this text.

As practicing nurses, researchers, and educators, we are committed to family-centered care for all childbearing families. We believe that nurses have a crucial role in ensuring that compassionate, expert care is delivered to clients regardless of their risk or socioeconomic status. Over the years, we have seen first-hand many changes in parent–newborn nursing, among them the development of family-centered care, and both the benefits and dilemmas presented by evolving technology. With satisfaction we have seen how persistent struggles, such as the efforts to establish childbirth education programs or the right of a father to be present at the birth of his child, have resulted in practices that are now considered commonplace. Yet there is so much more to do and fewer financial resources to meet increasing costs. Each day we see how lack of funds brings hardships to childbearing families and cripples organizations trying to provide care. It seems appropriate, therefore, that we, the authors, designate part of our proceeds from *Nursing Care of the Childbearing Family* to non-profit charities giving direct assistance to individuals and families in need.

Laurie N. Sherwen
Mary Ann Scoloveno
Carol Toussie Weingarten

Acknowledgments

In the preparation of this book, we were fortunate to rely on some very special people. Several colleagues generously and graciously provided valuable consultation. Kathleen Baker, MS, RN, Denise Braun, MS, RN, Marcia Cauley Costello, MS, RD, Ninetta Dickerson, BSN, RN, Maureen Esteves, PhD, RN, Steven Golden, MD, MBA, Sandra Myers Gomberg, MSN, RNC, David E. Jacobwitz, MD, FACOG, Michael Ross, MD, Ellen Shuzman, MSN, RN, Hester M. Sonder, MD, FACOG, and Alan B. Zubrow, MD, FAAP, always made time in their extremely busy schedules to answer our questions, no matter how basic or complex. Our expert group of nurse, certified nurse-midwife, and physician reviewers offered comments that strengthened the manuscript. Our enthusiasm for this project was also encouraged by Dorothy DeMaio, EdD, RN, FAAN, M. Louise Fitzpatrick, EdD, RN, FAAN, Beverly Raff, PhD, RN, FAAN, and Pamela Watson, ScD, RN. We greatly appreciate the reference consultation, so competently given by Jacqueline H. Mirabile, MLS. Mark Pappiani supplied computer consultation, and Red Scoloveno donated his time in artistic assistance.

As practicing nurses, we have often been impressed by the creativity, competence, and compassion of colleagues. This book presented the opportunity to record some of these dimensions of care through original photographs of staff in action. The photo opportunities for this book would not have been possible without help from Kathleen Baker, MS, RN, Denise Braun, MS, RN, Regina Scharle Catalano, BSN, RN, Ninetta Dickerson, BSN, RN, Elise Dormand, Sandra Myers Gomberg, MSN, RNC, Amy Levi, MSN, CNM, Wilma Manning, RNC, Ellen Zangaro, RN, the staffs of the obstetric and neonatal units of The Albert Einstein Medical Center, Northern Division, Thomas Jefferson University Medical Center, the Medical College of Pennsylvania, the Northeastern Hospital, all in Philadelphia, Morristown Memorial Hospital in Morristown, New Jersey, and the staff of the pediatric office of John B. Lewy, MD. We are also grateful to the many clients who allowed us to share in the joy or, at times, the sorrow of their childbearing experiences. Their commitment to helping others by sharing their own situations was inspiring.

Certified nurse-midwives currently deliver expert primary care to well women and to low-risk childbearing clients. In their daily activities, Amy Levi, MSN, CNM, Laura Barbour, MSN, CNM, and Barbara Harris, MSN, CNM, of The Birth Center in Bryn Mawr, Pennsylvania, exemplify the highest standards of care for the childbearing family. Amy Levi, Director of Midwifery Services, spent hours consulting with us about well-woman care, delivery alternatives, and care of the low-risk childbearing family. The certified nurse-midwives and staff of The Birth Center allowed us to photograph them just as they practice. Many of the wellness photographs in this book were taken there.

The process of bringing a major core textbook

from beginning ideas to finished pages is at times exciting, often difficult, and always enormously challenging. We were energized and encouraged by wonderful friends and family members who let us know they would wait for us until the day we were really, really done with the first edition. We are especially grateful to our parents, Lee and Michael DePalma, Gladys (Toussie) and Marty Markuson, and Marjory and William Nehls, and to Robert Blitzer, DDS, Nancy and Ian Clelland, Bruce Cohen, MD, Susan Zwerling Cohen, Donald and Geysah DePalma, John and Rosemary DePalma, Michael and Kathleen DiChiara, Pamela W. Fox, Michael J. Fox, MD, MBA, Jane and Bud Fried, Robert Gomberg, Sally and William Henrickson, Phyllis Jacobwitz, John B. Lewy, MD, Catherine Hill, Noreen Mahon, PhD, RN, Jacqueline Mileto, Vincent F. Mileto, MD, FACOG, Patricia Murphy, PhD, RN, Georgia and William Nehls, Jr., Lisa and David Nehls, David Price, PhD, Maryanne Rose, RN, Benita Ross, Delores Scoloveno, Grace Sherwen, Patricia Sherwen, Sam R. Toussie, PhD, Theresa M. Valiga, EdD, RN, Adela Yarcheski, PhD, RN, Alice Sheflin Zal, DO, and H. Michael Zal, DO, FACN.

We thank Barbara Johnson, Doreen Formisano Lockwood, Patricia Pump, Maria Ricciardi, Ann Marie Vendemia, and Denise Zielinski, whose fine typing skills enabled us to meet our deadlines in a legible format. W. Robert Schwartz of The Camera Shop in Bryn Mawr, Pennsylvania, helped us with processing the many photographs taken for this book.

We appreciate the opportunity to work with the excellent and committed staff at Appleton & Lange. At the beginning of the project, David Gordon assisted us in refining our plans for *Nursing Care of the Childbearing Family*. Executive Editor Marion Kalstein Welch provided valuable guidance as the project evolved. John Williams was integral to the process of steering the book through the production process. Donna Frassetto, our development editor, truly became an adopted member of our families, as she worked closely with us in the development of this book from first draft through final page proofs. To Donna, expert editor and best of the best, we offer our respect, admiration, friendship, and thanks.

Contents in Brief

Contents in Detail

NURSING CARE
OF THE
CHILDBEARING FAMILY

Issues and Trends in Nursing Care of the Childbearing Family

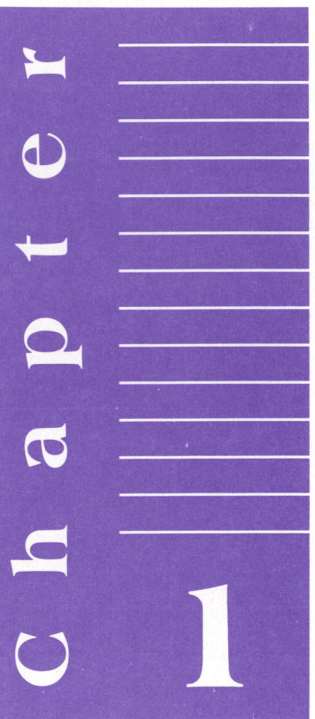

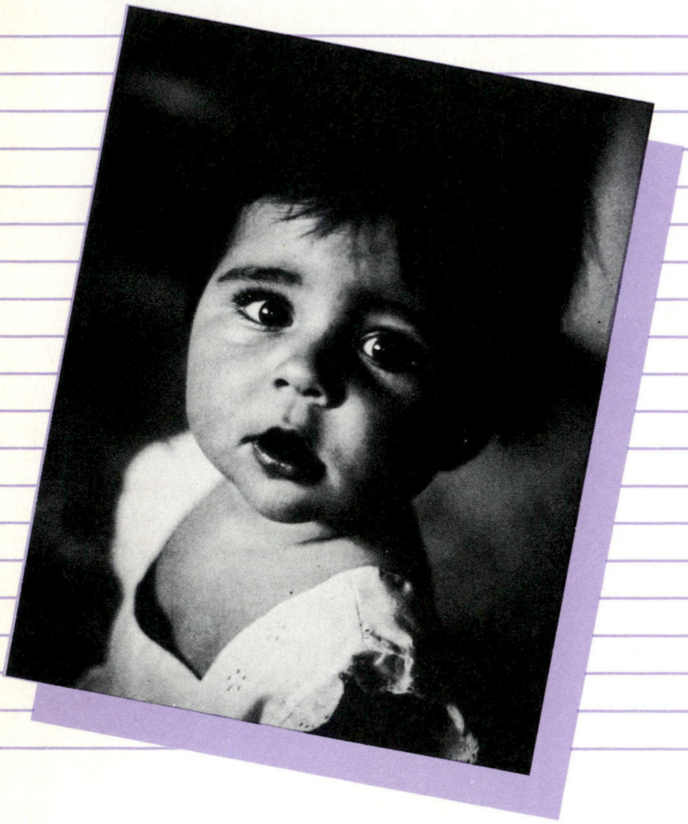

Chapter 1

Key Terms

abortus
birth rate
direct maternal death
indirect maternal death
infant mortality rate
live birth
maternal mortality rate
maternity care
midwife
midwifery
neonatal mortality rate
obstetrics
perinatal mortality rate
stillbirth

The technologic innovations available in the 1990s enable health care providers to ensure the survival of many low-birth-weight infants and many sick infants who would have died even 10 years ago. But while health care providers can do much for many people in our society, there are many more who live with impairments or don't live because of barriers restricting their access to care.

Morbidity and mortality associated with childbearing have improved dramatically in the past 50 years in the United States, but the United States still lags far behind other Western nations in overall maternal and infant mortality statistics. Adequate prenatal care is seen as essential in improving pregnancy outcomes for both mother and neonate.

The challenge to nurses and other health professionals in the final decade of the 20th century will be to improve access to care for all individuals in our society, and in particular to ensure appropriate prenatal care to childbearing women. Through education, practice, and research, nurses can and must play an important role in helping to achieve these health care objectives in the coming decade and into the 21st century.

HISTORICAL TRENDS

The provision of care to childbearing families has evolved over the course of many centuries. The evolution of this care can be identified through the changing terms used to describe the provider and recipient of care. The earliest term used to refer to providers of care to childbearing women was that of **midwife.** This term was derived from *mid,* meaning "with" and *wif,* meaning "wife" or "woman." It was used as early as the Middle Ages, around 1303.[1] Noble women were responsible for the delivery of infants for the serfs on their estates. Hence, they served as the midwives during the Middle Ages.

The branch of medicine that dealt with childbearing was known as **midwifery** until the latter part of the 19th century in the United States and Great Britain. At that time, the term "obstetrics" was introduced. The word is derived from the Latin *obstetrix*, meaning "midwife," and is also related to the Latin *obstare*, meaning "to stand by or in front of."

Obstetrics is currently defined as that branch of medicine that deals with the phenomena and management of pregnancy, labor, and the postpartum in low- and high-risk circumstances. Midwifery is still the term used to delineate the practice of a nurse who is responsible for management of childbearing women—an alternate-care provider for families today.

An important phase in the provision of care to childbearing families occurred after World War II, when the focus of care shifted from the provider of care to the recipient. **Maternity care** was the term used to denote a broader focus to health care, involving psychosocial and cultural aspects of the woman as well as physiologic aspects.

Today, the focus of practice has expanded to encompass the childbearing family as a whole, as well as the woman. Health care providers recognize that when one member of the family system is affected by pregnancy and birth, all other members are also affected and the family structure changes.

The evolution of concepts, definitions, and terms related to care of the childbearing family demonstrates a broadening perspective. The focus has shifted from the provider to the woman as recipient of care and finally to the entire family unit as recipient of care. The evolving concept also demonstrates the importance of nurses as an integral part of the health care team.

CONTEMPORARY ISSUES AND TRENDS

Among the most notable trends in care of the childbearing family has been the improvement in maternal and infant outcomes that has occurred worldwide over the past half century. In contrast to this trend, however, the ranking of the United States relative to other industrialized nations has actually worsened in recent decades. This has led many health care providers and policy makers in the United States to question aspects of the current health care delivery system for mothers and infants. A review of current US vital statistics illustrates both of these trends.

Current Vital Statistics

There has been a dramatic decrease in the maternal, neonatal, and infant mortality rates over the past 35 to 37 years. See Table 1–1 for a summary of these rates.

TABLE 1–1. MATERNAL AND INFANT MORTALITY STATISTICS FOR THE UNITED STATES, 1960–1985

	1960	1970	1975	1980	1985
Birth Rate					
(Number of live births per 1000 in population)					
Total	23.7	18.4	14.6	15.9	15.8
White	22.7	17.4	13.8	14.9	14.8
Black	31.9	25.3	20.7	22.1	21.1
Maternal Mortality					
(Maternal deaths per 100,000 live births from complications of pregnancy, childbirth, and the puerperium)					
Total	37.1	21.5	12.8	9.2	7.9
White	26.0	14.4	9.1	6.7	5.1
Black	103.6	59.8	31.3	21.5	22.2
Neonatal Mortality					
(Infant deaths per 1000 live births before 28 days old, exclusive of fetal deaths [20 weeks of gestation to delivery])					
Total	18.7	15.1	11.6	8.5	7.0
White	17.2	13.8	10.4	7.5	6.1
Black	27.8	22.8	18.3	14.1	12.1
Infant Mortality					
(Infant deaths from birth to 1 year of age per 1000 live births)					
Total	26.0	20.0	16.1	12.6	10.6
White	22.9	17.8	14.2	11.0	9.3
Black	44.3	32.6	26.2	21.4	18.2

From US National Center for Health Statistics: Health—United States, 1987. Government Printing Office, 1987.

Data on which vital statistics are based are collected periodically. Analysis of these statistics is time consuming; thus, statistics for a year may not be reported until several years later. The National Center for Health Statistics, located in the US Department of Health and Human Services, is a resource for the most current statistics available.

Definitions. Definitions of vital statistics related to the childbearing cycle are necessary to ensure a standard method for reporting births and maternal and infant mortality and morbidity rates across the United States. The following definitions are important in understanding the meaning of reports of vital statistics:

- **Birth rate:** The number of live births per 1000 population. The birth rate in the United States for the year ending February, 1988, was 15.7 births per 100 population.[2]
- **Live birth:** An infant who, at birth, demonstrates signs of life such as breathing, heartbeat, or voluntary muscle movements.
- **Stillbirth:** An infant past the point of viability who is born dead.

- **Abortus:** A fetus or embryo removed or expelled from the uterus at 20 weeks or less, or weighing less than 500 grams or measuring less than 25 centimeters.
- **Neonatal mortality rate:** The number of infant deaths occurring in the first 28 days of life per 1000 live births.
- **Perinatal mortality rate:** The number of stillbirths plus the number of neonatal deaths per 1000 live births.
- **Infant mortality rate:** The number of deaths of infants under 12 months of age per 1000 live births.
- **Maternal mortality rate:** The number of maternal deaths resulting from the reproductive process per 100,000 live births. This rate is further broken down into two categories. **Direct maternal deaths:** Death of the mother resulting from reproductive complications of pregnancy, labor, postpartum, or interventions. An example is maternal death from hemorrhage as a result of cervical lacerations of labor. **Indirect maternal death:** Death of a mother not directly related to the childbearing cycle but resulting from a previously existing disease or a disease not related to reproduction that developed during the childbearing cycle and that was aggravated by the pregnancy. An example is maternal death from mitral valve disease during childbearing.

Infant Mortality. The infant mortality rate is often cited as the gauge of the health of a nation. The lowest infant mortality rate ever recorded in the United States (10.1 infant deaths per 1000 live births) was recorded in the year 1987. Among white infants, the rate was 8.6, demonstrating a decline of 3 percent from 1986 (8.9). The rate for black infants, however, was 17.9 in 1987, compared with 18.0 in 1986. Although rates for both black and white infants continue to decline at approximately the same rates per year, the rate for black infants continues to remain twice as high as the rate for white infants.[3] Figure 1–1 illustrates the declining rates and the difference between black and white infant deaths. Clearly, segments of the US population have health needs that still go unmet.

Maternal Mortality. In 1987, 251 women were reported to have died in the United States from complications of pregnancy, childbirth, and the postpartum. The maternal mortality rate was 6.6 deaths per 100,000 live births in 1987. Similar to the statistics for black and white infant deaths, black women were 2.8 times more likely to die of complications related to pregnancy than were white women.[3]

International Infant Mortality Rates. In 1985, the United States ranked 19th among industrialized nations in infant mortality rates, behind such countries as Finland, Sweden, and the United Kingdom. Table 1–2 illustrates the comparisons in ranking for selected countries for 1985. Despite a continued decline in the infant mortality rate, the United States is losing ground in comparison with other industrialized countries. Current statistics report that the United States now ranks 21 among industrialized countries.

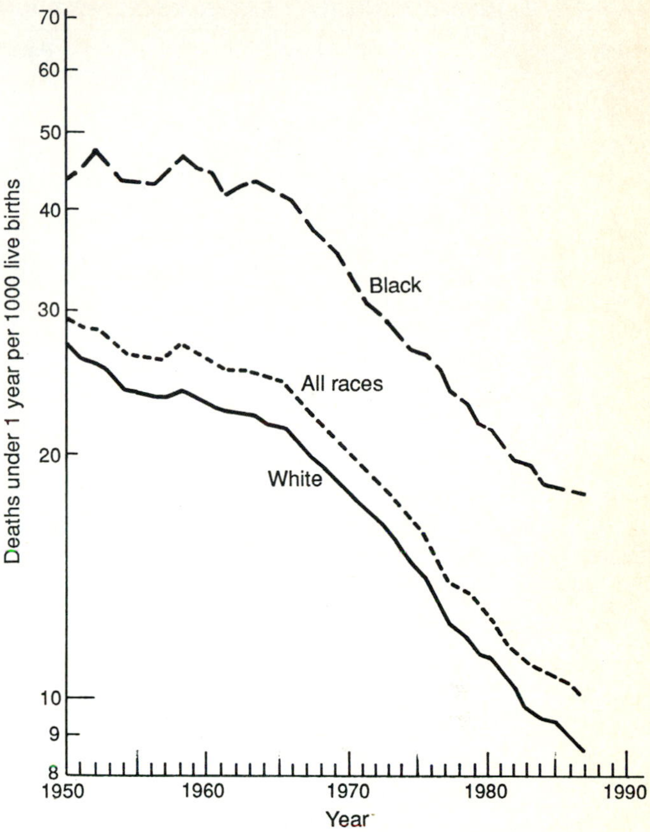

Figure 1–1. Infant mortality rates by race: United States 1950–1987. (*From National Center for Health Statistics.* Monthly Vital Statistics Report. *1989;38 (September 26) (suppl):9.*)

A study conducted by Miller reported by the National Center for Clinical Infant Programs[4] focused on the possible reasons for the discrepancy between the United States and other developed countries. Miller reports that the other countries do a better job of ensuring infant survival than the United States by:

1. Having readily available, easily understood provider systems for prenatal care
2. Removing economic barriers to access to prenatal care
3. Linking prenatal care to comprehensive social and financial benefits that support the optimal health and well-being of mothers and infants

These findings and suggestions may have relevance for policy development in the United States.

TABLE 1–2. INFANT MORTALITY RATES, SELECTED COUNTRIES, 1985

Rank	Country	Rate[a]	Rank	Country	Rate[a]
1	Finland	6	14	Spain	10
1	Japan	6	14	United Kingdom	10
1	Sweden	6		*US (White)*	10
4	France	8	19	Austria	11
4	Denmark	8	19	Italy	11
4	Netherlands	8	19	United States (*Total*)	11
4	Norway	8	22	New Zealand	12
4	Switzerland	8	23	Israel	13
9	Australia	9	24	Greece	14
9	Belgium	9	25	Cuba	15
9	Canada	9	25	Czechoslovakia	15
9	Hong Kong	9	27	Bulgaria	16
9	Singapore	9	28	Costa Rica	19
14	German Democratic Republic	10	28	Poland	19
14	Germany, Federal Republic	10	28	Portugal	19
14	Ireland	10		*US (Black)*	19

[a] Deaths per 1000 live births

Information from UNICEF as reported to the Children's Defense Fund, Washington, D.C. Used by permission.

Access to Prenatal Care

Several national commissions, including the Institute of Medicine, the Consensus Conference on Access to Prenatal Care, and the National Center for Clinical Infant Program study have indicated that one of the primary factors related to infant mortality in the United States is the increase in delivery of low-birth-weight infants. Low birth weight has been linked, in turn, to the lack of prenatal care. The commissions identified the following barriers to a woman's access to prenatal care in the United States[5, 6]:

1. Limited financial resources
2. Uncoordinated service systems
3. Individual behaviors and beliefs concerning health care
4. Bureaucratic obstacles, such as complicated, lengthy application forms for Medicaid
5. Unavailability of maternal services in certain parts of the country
6. Underfunded and overcrowded publicly supervised clinics
7. Difficulty in recruiting and retaining health care providers in publicly subsidized clinics
8. Lack of coordination among services for needy individuals
9. Inaccessible prenatal care services because of transportation, location, and lack of child-care facilities

The commissions also recommend the following maternal-infant health care objectives:

1. Every pregnant woman and every infant should receive appropriate and adequate care
2. Health and welfare of mothers and infants should become a national priority
3. All sectors of society should develop strategies regarding infant mortality; these sectors include: government, business, industry, communities, health professionals, and consumers

Strategies to achieve these recommendations include: broadening private and health insurance coverage for childbearing women and infants; improving coordination and funding of public programs; simplifying bureaucratic procedures; increasing the number of maternal care providers; establishing a national council on children and health; and raising public awareness throughout the country. Further, Congress should extend Medicaid coverage to all pregnant women and infants at or below 200 percent of the US poverty level, and various means should be taken to retain maternal health care providers, such as solving the medical and nursing malpractice issues in maternity care. Finally, funding should be increased for the maternal and child health block grants, community and migrant health centers programs, the Women-Infant-Children Supplemental Food Program (WIC), the federal Family Planning Program (Title X), and the National Service Corps.[5, 6]

Issues in the Delivery of Care

Contemporary issues that affect the care delivered to the childbearing family may be divided into four major areas: economic, social, legal, and technologic. Although these four areas are discussed briefly below, because of their importance, the issues identified will be elaborated on throughout the text.

Economic Issues. Shifting demographics and an increased emphasis on costly technologic interventions have created a crisis in the health care system today.[7] As the US population grows older and experiences more health problems, the emphasis of care delivery and funds are being drawn away from pregnant women and children. At the same time, technologic advances are enabling health care providers to keep preterm infants alive, but at great costs to society. The lifetime cost of caring for a low-birth-weight infant can reach as high as $400,000.[8] Paradoxically, the cost of prenatal care that may prevent low birth weight can be as low as $400. Surely, society must recognize that prenatal care is more cost-effective than intensive, highly technologic care of sick infants.

Because of these issues, there will be a continuing need to deliver care in a cost-effective manner. Diagnostic Related Groupings (DRGs) are currently being used in most areas of health care to control costs (*see* Chapter 44 for an in-depth discussion of DRGs). While DRGs are far from perfect, they do represent an organized effort of the health care industry to scrutinize some of these issues. Whether or not DRGs continue to play a role in care delivery, it is likely that some form of cost-containment effort will affect care delivered to childbearing families now and in the future.

Social Issues. Infant mortality statistics do not reflect the current increase in drug abuse by pregnant women and the numbers of infants born addicted. Punitive actions taken against pregnant addicts do little to encourage early and consistent prenatal care among these women.

Compounding this problem is the close relationship between women and infants infected with human immunodeficiency virus (HIV) and the drug culture. Both HIV infection and drug use occur frequently in urban, minority, poor women—those already at risk for adverse pregnancy outcomes. The demand and need for services for these individuals cannot be met by current funding levels.

Legal Issues. Issues of malpractice for providers of care to childbearing families affect not only the nature of care delivered but also the recruitment and retention of health care professionals in this specialty. Escalating malpractice premiums among physicians, certified nurse-midwives, and clinical nurse specialists in maternity have curtailed services to recipients of public programs who are at high risk for problems.[9]

Malpractice issues have not only created a shortage of providers for the childbearing family, they have also increased tension among members of the interdisciplinary team, including consumers. Further, providers of care may often use all available technology, even among low-risk populations, to protect themselves against malpractice suits. Providers may perform certain procedures routinely even though they may be neither necessary nor useful.

Technologic Issues. Technology today is a double-edged sword. On the one hand, technologic advances have greatly improved the outcome of pregnancy for high-risk pregnant women and have facilitated survival of infants who would have died 10 years ago. On the other hand, increased technology has contributed to the burdensome cost of neonatal and maternal care and the rate of cesarean deliveries. The rate of cesarean deliveries has increased from 4.5 percent in 1965 to 23 percent in 1985. This means that nearly one in four infants is born by cesarean delivery.[1]

Computer systems are also technologies whose uses have increased significantly in care of childbearing families. Although they have been very beneficial in coordinating data bases and in transferring information between sites around the country, they do have a potential to dehumanize care. For example, when computers are placed at the mother's bedside, nurses may spend a large part of the mother's stay in the unit inputting data into the computer instead of interacting with the mother.

Trends in Nursing Care

Trends in nursing care of the childbearing family are reflected in nursing practice, nursing education, and nursing research.

Nursing Practice. Trends in nursing practice include the development of standards of care by the profession; use of the nursing process, which includes development of nursing diagnoses; increase in specialization and certification of nurses; movement of nursing care into the home health environment; and consumer involvement in childbearing care.

Standards. The profession of nursing has an obligation to the public to deliver high-quality nursing care. In an effort to meet this obligation, nursing standards have been developed by several nursing organizations,[10] among them the American Nurses' Association (ANA), the ANA Council of Maternal-Child Nursing, and the Organization for Obstetric, Gynecologic and Neonatal Nurses (NAACOG). The standards for maternity nursing practice apply to homes, alternate birthing centers, hospitals, and ambulatory care settings.

Because standards reflect current knowledge in the field, they are dynamic and subject to change; however, they always represent levels of practice agreed on by leaders in the profession or specialty.

Nursing Diagnosis. Maternity specialty organizations, such as NAACOG, are focusing on nursing diagnoses, an integral component of the nursing process. The North American Nursing Diagnosis Association (NANDA) and other groups studying diagnoses are working to expand the taxonomy of diagnoses that nurses use in delivery of care to clients. Nursing organizations such as NAACOG and others concerned with childbearing families have encouraged NANDA to explore mechanisms for incorporating diagnoses relevant to the healthy childbearing family into the current taxonomy.[11]

Increased Specialization and Certification of Nurses. The increased complexity of care to childbearing families has created increased specialization of maternity nurses. For example, a maternity nurse may specialize solely in the care of the well neonate. Further, nurses are gaining in-depth knowledge through advanced degrees and seeking recognition and credibility through certification mechanisms. Both NAACOG and ANA offer a variety of certifications in maternal-newborn nursing.

Home Health Care. The practice setting for nurses who care for childbearing families has also begun to shift from acute care institutions to the home. Even high-risk maternity and neonatal clients are being cared for at home. Technologies that were formerly available only in the hospital are now found in the home as well. Nurses who practice in the community have had to change the focus of their practice to incorporate skills that were once needed only in hospitals. (*See* Chapter 44 for a discussion of home health maternity and neonatal care).

Consumer Involvement in Childbearing Care. The current involvement of the consumer in all aspects of daily life has affected delivery of care to childbearing families. Examples of the effects of consumer involvement include: preparation for client involvement in childbirth; the Vaginal Birth After Cesarean (VBAC) movement; decisions not to circumcise newborns; alternative childbirth settings; and the family-centered maternity care movement. These consumer-fostered trends are discussed throughout the text.

Family-centered maternity care deserves particular mention here. This concept of care, perhaps more than any other philosophy that has affected the health care industry, has had a major impact on the manner in which nurses deliver care to childbearing families. The emphasis of family-centered maternity care is not only on the delivery of safe, quality care to the mother and neonate, but also on care that will foster family unity. The concept of family-centered maternity care includes several components:

1. Childbirth preparation for both partners (and for siblings as well)
2. Father involvement in the entire birthing process
3. Choice of birthing environment alternatives when possible (all hospitals should have a birthing room as an alternative to traditional labor and delivery suites)
4. Sibling visitation
5. Early discharge programs for mothers and infants when possible
6. Strategies to foster family members' attachment to the newborn

Each of these components is discussed in detail elsewhere in the text. In addition, nursing management for families throughout the childbearing cycle is based on a family-centered care philosophy and is detailed in Chapters 15, 19, 23, 27, and 30.

Nursing Education. Many nursing leaders have become concerned with the manner in which schools of nursing educate future nurses to practice with childbearing families. It has been suggested that health professionals, including nurses, should be prepared to provide sensitive care that incorporates health education and counseling. For the nurse to successfully implement the components of care for childbearing families identified by national commissions such as the Institute of Medicine (IOM), nursing education must reflect appropriate curricular content.[6]

To this end, the former Division of Maternal-Child Health of the Public Health Service funded the March of Dimes Birth Defects Foundation to investigate and develop the core competencies in maternal-infant health that should be included in a nurse's basic education program. Table 1–3 is a summary of the competencies identified by this project.[12]

On the graduate level, programs are available for nurses to gain in-depth knowledge in specialized areas of advanced maternal-newborn nursing. Some of these areas include perinatal nursing, neonatal nursing, and home health care of childbearing families.

In addition, at both the undergraduate and graduate level, technical equipment used in maternity care settings must be understood by the nurse. The educational process must include coverage of advanced technology, so nurses are comfortable with these advances and can explain use of such technology to their clients.

Nursing Research. Nursing research concerned with the childbearing family attempts to explain vari-

TABLE 1–3. MATERNAL-INFANT PRACTICE COMPETENCIES FOR GRADUATES OF NURSING PROGRAMS

1. The graduate of a program in nursing will practice maternal-infant nursing based on theoretic and empiric knowledge of normal and selected abnormal patterns of biophysic and psychosocial growth and development of the pregnant woman, fetus, newborn, and family.
2. The graduate of a program in nursing uses the nursing process to assess, diagnose, implement, evaluate, and revise a safe plan of nursing care based on standards of practice to achieve mutually agreed on priorities and goals with the healthy childbearing family.
3. The graduate of a program in nursing assists families in understanding and coping with normal developmental and common situational crises during childbearing.
4. The graduate of a program in nursing promotes the maintenance and restoration of the reproductive health of individuals and families during the preconceptional and interconceptional phase, and of individuals who decide not to bear or cannot bear children.
5. The graduate of a program in nursing is expected to maintain and upgrade his or her knowledge, develop proficiency in psychomotor skills, and re-evaluate appropriateness of affective behaviors required for maternal-infant nursing practice.
6. The graduate of a program in nursing collaborates with nurses and others in using community resources to provide care to childbearing families.
7. The graduate of a program in nursing improves maternal-infant-nursing practice through use of research findings and evaluation of current practice.

From Sherwen LN. MICC: The Maternal-Infant Core Competency Project. *White Plains, NY: March of Dimes Birth Defects Foundation, 1987.*

ables concerned with childbearing phenomena and to shed light on problems relating to clinical practice. Thus, research in this area tends to focus on current priorities in delivery of health care to childbearing families.

Nursing research that will answer some of the questions related to childbearing will be both quantitative and qualitative. Quantitative research is rigorously designed and controlled to develop and test theories by focusing on the relationships among variables identified as important to care of childbearing families and individuals. Qualitative research focuses on describing phenomena and evolving theories of importance to nursing and uses more naturalistic, less controlled research methods. Both types of research are necessary to expand our understanding of the childbearing family. Later chapters in this text contain research abstracts that describe and comment on both quantitative and qualitative studies concerned with childbearing.

Priorities for federal and private funding of nursing research in the area of childbearing often parallel major national concerns. For example, at this time, the highest research priority identified by the National Center for Nursing Research at the National Institutes of Health (NIH) is research dealing with low-birth-weight infants.[13] Similarly, one of the highest priorities for the nation's health is lowering the infant mortality and morbidity rates. In addition, NAACOG, a private organization, has identified research priorities in the areas of maternity nursing, women's health, and neonatal nursing. Table 1–4 summarizes these priorities.[14]

TABLE 1–4. NAACOG RESEARCH PRIORITIES

Research in obstetric, gynecologic, and neonatal nursing, especially studies of the nursing process and interventions and outcomes of care. Areas of high priority are:

Maternity Nursing
- Prenatal Care
- Low birth weight
- Mothers and infants positive for HIV
- Adolescent pregnancy and prepregnancy counseling or care
- Drug and other substance abuse during pregnancy
- Stressors and their effects during pregnancy
- Use of care by pregnant population

Women's Health Nursing
- Prevention of sexually transmitted diseases (STDs) in women, particularly the prevention of HIV infection, and care and support of women and families with STDs
- Psychosocial and physical experience of women in midlife and later years
- Behavioral and environmental factors influencing the health of minority women, including ethnic and cultural minorities and social minorities such as the homeless and other vulnerable groups
- Women's adaptations to multiple roles and related health outcomes
- Impact of reproductive technology and reproductive pharmacology on women's health over the life span

Neonatal Nursing
- Low-birth-weight infants and infants in families known to experience high rates of disease, dysfunction, and death
- Promotion of growth and development in all settings, including the hospital and the home
- Short- and long-term consequences of care and parenting
- Evaluation of current and evolving models of home care in terms of quality of patient outcomes and cost of care

Research on the professional role of maternity, women's health, and neonatal nurses in delivery of care
- Context of nursing practice, including constraints and support in the professional environment and effects of malpractice
- Factors affecting recruitment, retention, and attrition
- Alternative educational pathways and new roles for nurses providing care
- Description of role and scope of current nursing practice in various settings
- Dissemination and use of research findings

Nursing research about childbearing families is important to develop knowledge on which to base practice with the childbearing family.[15] Nurses need to incorporate research findings into their practice.

Future Trends in Delivery of Care

Several issues will affect the future of health care services for the childbearing family. First, the health care industry in general will reflect changes in society. This, in turn, will alter care delivered to childbearing families. Nornhold[16] delineates several changes that will occur in the health care industry in the decade of the 1990s. Among them are:

1. The health care industry may be dominated by cost-conscious outsiders, not health care professionals.
2. Hospitals may resort to rationing health care.
3. One out of every ten hospitals (most in inner cities) may close by the end of the decade.
4. More hospitals may band together to form health-care-delivery coalitions.
5. There may be a strain in professional relations, which may be exacerbated by the nursing shortage.
6. More clients might be transferred from one hospital to another.
7. Nurses are likely to become more and more specialized.
8. State nurse practice acts will need to be changed to reflect expanding nursing practice.
9. Specialty organizations for nursing, such as NAACOG, will most likely become more involved in political issues.

Nornhold also makes specific predictions for the future of maternal-newborn care[16]:

1. Most uncomplicated births may take place in the home.
2. Nursing care and new technology will probably further increase survival rates among high-risk neonates.
3. Neonatal care will likely become more and more complex.
4. The number of infants born with health problems related to maternal substance abuse during pregnancy is likely to increase. This will include a growing number of infants infected with HIV.

Other groups have looked at prenatal care in the 1990s. In a controversial report by an expert government panel on prenatal care, a recommendation was made as to the content and timing of prenatal visits. The panel recommended that prenatal clients receive prenatal care according to their risk status. In essence, low-risk women would receive fewer prenatal visits than high-risk women.[17] Controversy surrounds this report because the recommendations, if adopted, might have the effect of reducing funding for health-oriented prenatal care.

Because of the potential consequences to childbearing families, nurses who practice with this population will need to understand both societal and health care trends and their implications for health care delivery. In addition, nurses will need to assume active roles in policy decisions to ensure that adequate resources are allocated to mothers, infants, and their families. Nurses can be instrumental in advocating health-related prenatal care as well as care for high-risk childbearing families.

SUMMARY

Historical trends in care of the childbearing family are illustrated by the changing terms used to refer to this care. The first term related to such care was *midwife*, used as early as the Middle Ages. The concept of obstetric care was introduced in the 19th century. *Obstetrics* currently refers to the branch of medicine that deals with the reproductive cycle. The term *maternity care* began to be used after World War II, reflecting a change in focus from the provider to the recipient of care and an expanded focus on the psychologic and cultural, as well as physiologic, aspects of childbearing. Today, the focus of practice has expanded further to include the childbearing family as a whole. Family-centered maternity care thus looks at childbearing as it affects all members of the family system.

Increased knowledge and improvements in technology over the past 50 years have greatly improved the outcomes for mothers and infants in US society; however, maternal and infant mortality statistics reveal that many women and children in the United States do not benefit from these improvements in care. An important priority for the nation is to reduce the infant mortality rate, which demonstrates a significant discrepancy in outcomes for white and black populations. Ensuring prenatal care to childbearing women is essential if this goal is to be met.

Contemporary socioeconomic and technolegal trends provide a context for viewing the nature of care delivered to childbearing families. These trends are further discussed in the chapters that follow. By understanding current issues and trends, nurses are better able to formulate and implement strategies that contribute to the well-being and care of childbearing families. Nursing practice, education, and research will continue to change in response to the evolving needs of this childbearing population.

REFERENCES

1. Cunningham FG, et al. *Williams Obstetrics.* 18th ed. Norwalk, Conn: Appleton & Lange, 1989.
2. National Center for Health Statistics. *Births, Marriage, Divorces and Deaths for February, 1988.* 37(3).
3. National Center for Health Statistics. *Monthly Vital Statistics Report, 1989.* 38(September 26).
4. Miller A. *Maternal Health and Infant Survival.* Washington, DC: National Center for Clinical Infant Programs, July 1987.
5. Institute of Medicine. *Preventing Low Birthweight.* Washington, DC: National Academy Press, 1985.
6. American Nurses' Association. *Access to Prenatal Care.* Kansas City, Mo: American Nurses' Association, 1987.
7. Joel L. Nursing's role in the changing health scene. *Proceedings of the Elizabeth Sterling Soule Lecture.* Seattle, Wash. 1987.
8. The National Commission to Prevent Infant Mortality. *Death before Life: The Tragedy of Infant Mortality.* Washington, DC: 1988.
9. Brecht MC. The tragedy of infant mortality. *Nursing Outlook.* 1989; 37:18–22.
10. Gillies DA. *Nursing Management: A Systems Approach.* 2nd ed. Philadelphia: Saunders, 1989.
11. Organization for Obstetric, Gynecologic, and Neonatal Nurses (NAACOG). *OGN Nursing Practice Resource, Nursing Diagnosis.* Washington, DC: NAACOG, 1989.
12. Sherwen LN. *MICC: The Maternal Infant Core Competency Project.* White Plains, NY: March of Dimes Birth Defects Foundation, 1987.
13. *Facts about Funding.* US Dept of Health and Human Resources, National Center for Nursing Research (in-house publication), 1989.
14. Organization for Obstetric, Gynecologic, and Neonatal Nurses. New NAACOG research priorities define further research agenda. *NAACOG Newsletter.* August 1988.
15. Sherwen LN. *Psychosocial Dimensions of the Pregnant Family.* New York: Springer, 1987.
16. Nornhold P. Predictions for the 90's. *Nursing 90.* January 1990, 34–41.
17. Expert Panel on the Content of Prenatal Care. *Caring for Our Future: The Content of Prenatal Care.* US Public Health Service, 1989.

Prepregnancy Phase

unit

1

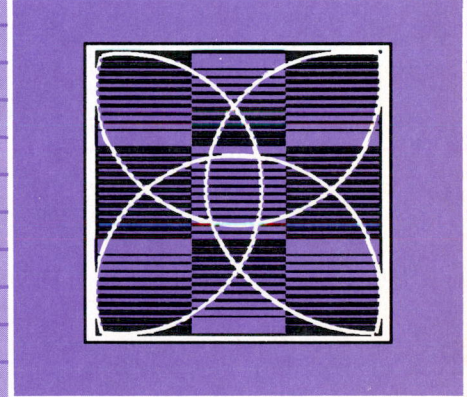

Nursing Process and the Childbearing Family

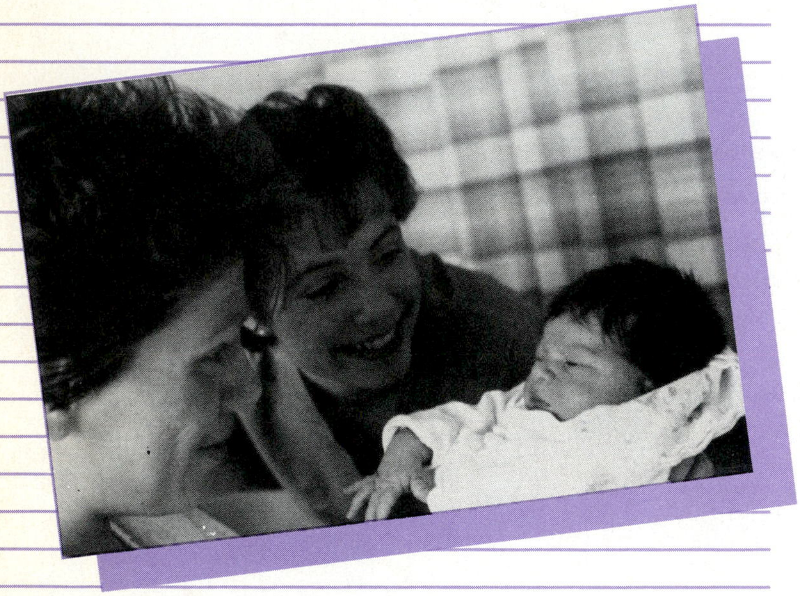

Chapter 2

Key Terms

assessment	nursing diagnosis
conceptual model	nursing process
evaluation	outcome criteria
implementation	planning

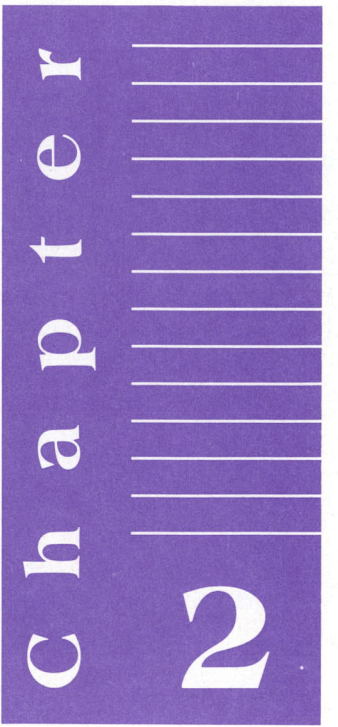

Students learning how to deliver nursing care to childbearing families are faced with a complex task. There are many facts, skills, and pieces of knowledge to master. In addition, the student must decide *what* facts, skills, and knowledge *should* be mastered, and how they can be used in caring for the childbearing family. In the past, this task may have seemed simple. Nursing students learned what was necessary to practice in the medical care delivery system (obstetric medicine), along with the obstetrician. Because the physician "delivered" obstetric and medical care to pregnant clients, the nurse learned what was necessary to assist in this endeavor. Thus, nurses were structuring their professional world, their practice, and their education according to a medical model of health care of pregnant women.

In the past 20 years, nursing has made great strides in defining itself as a profession separate from medicine. Nursing has its own unique perspective of models of care. Nursing invents and develops its own theories, discovers its own knowledge through research, designs practice and care delivery specific to nursing, and educates future nurses within a nursing framework.

Students today and in the future will learn about care of families from a nursing perspective, based on a nursing conceptual model. A **conceptual model** is a type of world view, a way of looking at and organizing objects and occurrences to make them meaningful. Without a conceptual model, observations have no meaning and carry no information by which the nurse can plan care. Students will also practice nursing according to the **nursing process,** an organized, systematic way of delivering care.

This chapter discusses the method by which nursing care of the pregnant family is delivered: the nursing process. It also discusses the concept of conceptual models of nursing and how they are used to deliver care to the childbearing family.

NURSING PROCESS

The nursing process is the "action component" of theory-based nursing practice. To put nursing conceptual models and theories into practice, the nurse must use the nursing process as an organizing principle.

Nursing process is not a theory in itself. It is defined by Yura and Walsh as: ". . . an orderly, systematic manner of determining the client's problems, making plans to solve them, initiating the plan or assigning others to implement it, and evaluating the extent to which the plan was effective in resolving the problems identified."[1]

Process implies control and change over time through a specific set of steps. Deliberate effort is necessary in carrying out the process to reach a goal. Without substance or content, however, process is meaningless—that is, process indicates the way, step by step, to solve problems and reach goals defined within a theory. Nursing process is the means to "do" nursing as conceptualized by the particular nursing conceptual model or theory the nurse chooses.

One basic idea of process is that it is a unit, consisting of phases. Each phase is dependent on the phases that precede and follow it and in actual practice cannot be separated from them; however, for purpose of analysis, we do study each phase of nursing process: assessment, diagnosis, planning, implementation, and evaluation.

Preprocess Goals

The following preprocess goals need to be achieved before the nursing process begins[1]:

1. Establishment of a degree of trust between client and nurse
2. Definition of the nurse's and client's respective roles in the nursing care situation
3. Establishment of a degree of client comfort in the chosen role
4. Establishment of a positive environment to pursue the nursing process

Assessment

This is the first phase of the nursing process, in which the situation is reviewed for the purpose of diagnosing the client's problems. **Assessment** consists of several subphases[1]:

1. Examining the client through history taking and inspection. This includes physical, psychologic, and social examination techniques, and communication with the client to validate data.
2. Collecting and analyzing data by arranging and summarizing it so conclusions can be drawn.
3. Reaching conclusions, or defining and stating the nursing diagnosis. Yura and Walsh indicate that nursing diagnosis is the end product of assessment, reflecting the nurse's conclusions and judgments about data obtained from the client. Others view nursing diagnosis as a separate step; this is the way it is conceptualized for the purpose of this text.

Diagnosis

Stating Nursing Diagnoses. Yura and Walsh define **nursing diagnosis** as the "judgment or conclusion reached by the nurse based on assessment data that indicates the potential for or actual human fulfillment or alteration viewed as an excess, disturbed pattern of expression or a deficit, lack, or limitation for the client as person, family, or community."[1] Nursing diagnosis provides the basis for the continuation of the nursing process. Without it, there would be no need to plan, intervene, or evaluate judgments about the client's state.

Nursing diagnoses related to nursing care of the childbearing family are, however, somewhat problematic. Childbearing is basically a healthy, normal process for family members, although things can go wrong. For maternity nurses who are dealing primarily with health maintenance of pregnant clients, or whose client goals are to remain well, a negative problem statement that focuses on *actual* or *potential* problems is not appropriate. Insufficient emphasis is placed on planning nursing care to enhance strengths and assets of the client when health care plans are developed solely around actual or potential problems. Thus there is a need to develop positive nursing diagnoses. Stolte gives some examples of such positive diagnoses[2]:

1. Joy related to birth of a healthy baby
2. Successful, rapid convalescence related to philosophy of positive thinking

It is likely that future efforts at establishing nursing diagnoses will consider this need.

In this textbook, examples of positive or strength-oriented diagnoses such as these will be found along with NANDA-format problem-oriented diagnoses. Both strength- and problem-oriented diagnoses will also be included in the nursing care plans found throughout the text.

Writing the Statement of Diagnosis. Guidelines for writing the nursing diagnosis include[3,4]:

1. Keep the process simple
2. Cite problems or strengths that the nurse can do something about
3. Make clear and concise statements of problems or strengths and diagnoses
4. Describe the etiology clearly and concisely
5. Differentiate the problem or strength and the etiology clearly
6. Use the diagnostic statement as the basis for the next step in client care and planning

Nursing diagnoses may be further qualified by prefixing the diagnosis with such adjectives as *acute, chronic, full, complete, partial, intermittent, internally induced* or *externally induced*.[1] Statements of nursing diagnoses are also followed by the identified supporting evidence (both objective and subjective data) and the selected reason(s), or cause(s) or etiology.[1] The usual linking words between the diagnosis and its etiology are *due to* or *related to*. Yura and Walsh categorize some of the reasons behind or causes of nursing diagnoses[1]:

1. Personal and situational occurrences
2. Environmental influences
3. Medical, dental, pharmacologic, and nursing therapies (commissions and omission)
4. Pathophysiologic states
5. Psychologic states
6. Legal states and occurrences
7. Physiologic occurrences
8. Congenital situations
9. Philosophic, ethical, and religious considerations
10. Social and economic situations
11. Education, knowledge, or informational states
12. Growth and developmental states
13. Heredity and genetic impacts
14. Cultural states
15. Geographic and climatic occurrences
16. Functional role structure
17. Political impacts
18. Communication patterns

Use of the described format will assist the nurse to determine the appropriate goal and select nursing strageties.

Establishing Data-based Nursing Diagnoses. Much concern has been directed toward formally identifying, classifying, and cataloguing nursing diagnoses.[5–8] Two major nursing groups, the National Conferences on Classification of Nursing Diagnoses, and the North American Nursing Diagnosis Association (NANDA), have been very active in this endeavor.[9] There are, however, still many concerns about the form and language of the nursing diagnostic statements. Further concern is expressed over the fact that many client experiences of importance to nurses simply do not fit into the currently identified categories.[4, 10] (*See* the earlier discussion of strength-oriented, positive diagnoses.)

The form and language of the diagnostic statement as well as the client experiences or problems that are identified as diagnoses will come from the conceptual model or theory used by the nurse making the assessment. The data collected will be based on the concepts of people and health specified by the chosen conceptual model. What is considered a problem or a strength is also based on the concepts of the model or theory. Finally, the form and language of the diagnostic statement will evolve from the nursing conceptual model or theory used by the nurse—be it the medical model, Roger's Life Processes Model, or Attachment Theory. Nursing process, including the making of a diagnosis, remains a systematic way to "do" the nursing specified by the model and theory. Like nursing process, nursing diagnosis has no meaning without a knowledge of the model on which it is based.

ISSUES AND CONTROVERSIES

In an effort to achieve the status of a profession, nurses have attempted to state and categorize nursing diagnoses (or the phenomena nurses can treat as independent caregivers). Not all nurse leaders believe that nursing diagnoses developed by NANDA are appropriate, however, or that the process of attempting to state in diagnosis form all the phenomena of interest to nursing is worthwhile. There are several issues, including:

1. What are the pros and cons of establishing a listing or taxonomy of nursing diagnoses that would be used by all nurses in planning client care? For example, communication between nurses would be improved; however, nursing interventions might become more rigid and limited by the diagnosis.
2. How might this movement toward establishing nursing diagnoses affect maternity nursing? Childbearing is largely a healthy phenomenon, yet most currently accepted diagnoses deal with problems. How will strength-oriented diagnoses be most expediently incorporated into the taxonomy?

Planning

The third phase of the nursing process, **planning,** involves the determination of what can be done to assess the client.[1] It involves setting goals, deciding the priorities of the goals, and designing methods to resolve problems and reach goals. As Yura and Walsh indicate, "the essence of planning includes a deliberate approach to setting precise goals, both ultimate and proximate, continually validating the data obtained by assessing the client's problems, establishing priorities, and making decisions about specific measures to be used to resolve . . . problems."[1] The nurse and client need to determine both long-term (ultimate) and short-term, immediate (proximate) goals. These goals provide the blueprint for the rest of the phases of the nursing process and the basis for determining the best way to achieve goals.

Implementation

The fourth phase of nursing process, **implementation,** is the start and completion of the actions necessary to accomplish the previously defined goals.[1] This is the action phase of the nursing process. The nurse may carry out the actions her- or himself or may coordinate the therapeutic actions of others.

Independent nursing interventions are those nursing actions that fall under the scope of a nurse practice act and that the nurse performs independently. *Interdependent* nursing interventions are those therapeutic actions that the nurse performs in collaboration with other health professionals, such as physicians, physical therapists, nutritionists, and so on. In this textbook, there will be a focus on *collaborative care* or management and the health care team approach. Health care of childbearing families is a highly complex endeavor, requiring the combined efforts of nurses and many other health professionals.

Evaluation

Evaluation, the last phase, is the appraisal of the changes experienced by the client as a result of the actions of the nurse.[1] The nurse must compare pre-set goals, also called **outcome criteria,** to the actual attainment or progress toward attainment of the goals in the real care situation. Data on whether goals are reached or not will provide feedback by which the original planning for the client may be altered or revised. Perhaps the goals set were inappropriate, or the actions and methods designed to reach them were inadequate. The evaluation component of nursing process will allow for needed revisions in the plan of care.

The nursing care plan is the written version of the nursing process, usually in outline form. In this text, the emphasis is on nursing process, or the cognitive and action-oriented steps that are taken to develop nursing care plans. Rather than expecting a student to memorize an outline, a more important emphasis is the manner in which data can be collected, judgments made, and actions designed to solve problems and reach goals in a specific clinical situation. Thus, in this textbook, nursing care plans have been developed based on specific case studies depicting "real" clinical situations. In this manner, the student can become aware of the thought process in using the nursing process as it relates to a clinical problem involving childbearing families and individuals. The student can then better understand how to write a nursing care plan, an essential means of transmitting nursing process method to colleagues. In particular, the reader is referred to Chapters 15, 19, and 23 as examples of the nursing process used in care of the family during each trimester of pregnancy.

CONCEPTUAL MODELS

Fawcett and Downs[11] define a conceptual model as a set of abstract and general concepts and propositions that provides a frame of reference for the phenomena of interest to a profession. A conceptual model further performs the function of identifying certain things as important, while classifying other things as irrelevant to the conceptual model.

The term *conceptual model* is synonymous with the term **paradigm,** and is used interchangeably with such terms as **conceptual framework** and **theoretical model.** A conceptual model reflects the beliefs, philosophies, and values of a *group* of individuals in a discipline—not necessarily all of the members of that discipline.[12] Thus, the development of several conceptual models is common in many disciplines, including nursing. According to Fawcett and Downs,[11] nursing has at least seven conceptual models: Johnson's Behavioral System Model, King's Open Systems Model, Levine's Conservation Model, Neuman's Systems Model, Orem's Self-care Model, Roger's Life Processes Model, and Roy's Adaptation Model. Each of these models has its own vocabulary and meanings for terms, as well as its own assumptions. Each looks at the world in a slightly different way, within certain limits.

A conceptual model simplifies reality—all that is "out there"—narrowing attention to specific concerns, for example, concerns related to maternity nursing. A conceptual model in nursing has been described as a map, and reality as geographic territory.[12,13] There are many different types of maps that can be used to describe any one piece of geographic territory. For example, there are road maps, which emphasize highways; there are weather maps, which indicate atmospheric weather patterns; and there are maps of air-traffic patterns, which indicate major airplane routes. All of these maps may deal with the same spot on earth. They *look* very different to the map user, however, because they emphasize and highlight very different aspects of reality concerning that spot on earth. All these things (that is, highways, air routes) are present all the time at this geographic locale. A motorist, however, relies on a road map whereas a jet pilot uses a map of airplane routes. Thus, the purpose that an individual has for using a map will determine which map he or she will choose. It is important to remember that many different maps may be "true" or correct. There are simply "best" maps for particular purposes. Maps are *invented* to represent an aspect of reality, they are not reality themselves. In summary, maps, like conceptual models, are invented for particular purposes, give specific information for those purposes, and omit information that is not relevant.

The purpose of a profession determines the conceptual models it develops or creates. Individuals within a profession may have different purposes and belief systems; even within a profession there may be various conceptual models—each providing a specific map that emphasizes certain aspects of reality and omits others. Nursing has several conceptual models, and each emphasizes some different and some similar aspects of reality. The choice of which model to use is determined by the user and depends on his or her purpose and belief. In learning about the nursing profession, a student masters a "map," or conceptual model. The student then comes to know what questions to ask, what observations to make, what the appropriate focus is, and is therefore guided by that map (conceptual model). Conceptual models (and maps) allow the student to focus on the "essential" aspects of a nursing care situation and ignore the nonessential aspects.

Specifically, a conceptual model guides the nurse working with the childbearing family in developing appropriate observations, judgments concerning health, and care strategies. Childbearing is a major phenomenon in the life of individuals and families. Many different disciplines, such as anthropology, nursing, and medicine, consider it so. According to their different conceptual models, however, each discipline focuses on something different in the pregnancy experience. The anthropologist may focus on cross-cultural birth practices, the nurse on family coping strategies as they relate to pregnancy wellness, and the physician on nutrition as it relates to pathophysiology of the fetus. Each profession has its own "map" that emphasizes observations with which it is concerned.

Within nursing, different nursing conceptual models, which share some common beliefs on what is the appropriate focus for nursing, concentrate attention on certain different aspects of the phenomenon called pregnancy. One example is a nurse viewing the pregnancy experience through Roger's conceptual model. Using this model, the nurse might focus on the repatterning of the dynamic family energy field as it incorporates the fetus/newborn. Another nurse viewing the pregnancy experience through Orem's conceptual model might focus on the pregnant woman's ability to function as a self-care agency. The reader is encouraged to consult specific texts concerned with nursing theory for further discussion of these theories.

Many nursing programs have curricula that are structured according to a nursing conceptual model—either one described formally in the literature by a nurse theorist or one developed by the faculty of the program. Thus, students in a nursing program may have the phenomenon of pregnancy and the childbearing family interpreted according to the specific "map" chosen to structure the "world view" of the program. The information on childbearing given in this text will be molded by the faculty to fit the world view determined by the nursing conceptual model of the student's program. Not all information given in this text will fit in all conceptual models in the same manner; however, the conceptual model evident in the program curriculum will allow the student to structure this information—the "raw data"—and the observations made in practice in a unique manner.

Conceptual Models and Theories

Perhaps one of the greatest confusions in nursing is the distinction between conceptual models and theories. Often these terms are mistakenly used interchangeably. They do not, however, mean the same thing. A **theory** is defined as a statement that accounts for or characterizes some phenomenon.[14] Theories differ from conceptual models because they address phenomena with much greater specificity than do conceptual models,[15] and are tied more closely to particular individuals (the laboring mother), groups (the pregnant family), situations (maternal-newborn interaction in the hospital), or events (the birthing experience).

Many theories are necessary to describe all phenomena included in a conceptual model and each theory deals with only a portion of the model. Although nursing's conceptual models provide the focus and direction for developing new nursing theories, existing theories may be linked to a conceptual model. This is done when the conceptual model and theory are compatible in terms of their world view and beliefs concerning the phenomenon: the existing theory provides the necessary specificity of the conceptual model's concepts and their relationships for a particular situation.[15] This is more than merely "borrowing" theories from other disciplines. By visualizing these theories through a nursing conceptual model and adapting them to a nursing problem or situation, the theories evolve into theories that nursing shares equally, and in its own way, with other professions.[16] For example, in caring for parents of an infant in special care (*see* Chapters 42 and 43), nurses and physicians may use Stress Theory. However, the physician might focus on pathophysiologic aspects of stress, while the nurse may focus more on stress as a precipitator of family crisis or on strategies to alleviate stress.

Chapter 3 will discuss in some depth theories concerning the family and family development. Chapter 4 will describe theories that have often been applied during pregnancy and childbearing. They are: Crisis Theory, Stress Theory, Attachment/Bonding Theory, Separation-Individuation Theory, and Transcultural Care Theories. In addition, some theories that have been developed about pregnant individuals and families specifically will be explored. Some of these include maternal and paternal role attainment theories, theories concerning the role of fantasy during pregnancy, theories about maternal body image during pregnancy, paternal couvade theories, theories concerned with paternal style during pregnancy, and theories about the siblings' and grandparents' experiences during childbearing.

Some of these theories will be relevant for the conceptual model of the student's program and some may not fit as well. Student and faculty must decide on the "fit" of theory and conceptual model and the theory's relevance for practice under the program's model.

Conceptual Models and the Nursing Metaparadigm

Thus far, we have emphasized the *differences* between conceptual models, even those models within the nursing profession. Despite differences, nursing's conceptual models do share much common ground. Nurses are therefore able to work together effectively regardless of the conceptual model they select to guide practice. Fawcett describes this "common ground" as the **metaparadigm of nursing.**[15]

The metaparadigm consists of the central concepts of the discipline of nursing which are person, environment, health, and nursing.[15, 17–19] *Person* refers to the individual(s) who receive nursing care because of his or her state of *health.* Interactions between the person and nurse occur within a particular *environment,* and involve *nursing* actions. It is important to remember the "person" can be the individual, family, community, society, and so on; environment can be anything that surrounds the person; health includes wellness or illness; and nursing includes all nursing activities.

Each conceptual model of nursing speaks to these four major concepts in some way. Some conceptual models have developed certain concepts more fully than others. All concepts are present in nursing conceptual models, however. The fact that nursing models deal with the four concepts of person, environment, health, and nursing allows for communication between groups using different conceptual models.

In this text, the student will be presented with information and theories that fit into the four concepts of nursing's metaparadigm: person (eg, the pregnant mother, father, childbearing family), environment (eg, the health care delivery system for mothers and infants), health (eg, normal and deviant physiology of labor and delivery, stress and pregnancy) and nursing (eg, nursing management of the pregnant adolescent).

Conceptual Models and Practice in Maternal-Infant Nursing

Nursing conceptual models and related theories provide a structure, discipline, focus, direction, or goal for nursing practice.[20, 21] Nurses have a style of thinking about situations that uses concepts to sort out events.[22] These concepts and their underlying assumptions (the elements of which models are composed) provide shorthand ways of describing what nurses observe and experience in a clinical situation. Conceptual models and theories relate to nursing practice in two ways.[21] First, they help the nurse understand nursing behaviors and the client. Second, they assist the nurse in predicting client needs and behaviors.

By using a conceptual model, nurses become at once the observer, analyzer, and modifier of the conceptual model and theories they are using; in this way nurses increase their competency in their nursing roles.[23] Professional nurses also have a responsibility to test conceptual models and theories that may be useful in practice.[20] By scrutinizing use of conceptual models and theories in practice situations, nurses can identify new relationships and ideas for testing, can determine which conceptual models and theories work best in certain clinical situations, and can identify those models and theories that professionals can feel most confident in using.

The process of nursing will differ according to the conceptual model and theory used to guide practice. The conceptual model used will identify the boundaries of nursing in a clinical situation.[24] Further, the conceptual model will become a framework for knowledge that serves as a basis of professional accountability in clinical nursing practice.

The use of nursing conceptual models to guide nursing practice is a relatively new phenomenon. Until recently, nursing practice (as well as education) was strongly influenced by the "medical model," or a focus on diseases or organ pathophysiology. This model continues to be a useful conceptual model in the realm of nursing's interdependent collaborative responsibilities—when the nurse works with the physician in the diagnosis and treatment of pathophysiology. It is important, however, that nurses also develop and value their own conceptual models and theories if nursing is to advance as a profession. Nurses in clinical practice need a nursing conceptual model to focus attention on, guide assessments of, and develop treatments for core nursing concerns[25]—for example, a woman's progress in attainment of the maternal role. A nursing conceptual model can direct the nurse's assessment of the client by determining areas in which questions can be asked and observations made. Further, a nursing conceptual model can determine the nature of the nursing diagnosis, the type of nursing interventions planned, and the criteria to be used for evaluating client outcome.

Choosing a Conceptual Model in Nursing

How does a nurse choose a conceptual model for practice? As established earlier in this chapter, the *purpose* for using a conceptual model is one major contributing factor in making this choice. In addition, a student generally learns nursing under the conceptual model of her or his nursing program. After graduation, however, the nurse has more than likely become aware of several nursing conceptual models and will need to determine which model (or combination of models) will guide his or her practice. Because the underpinnings of conceptual models derive from beliefs about people and life, before adopting one model over another to direct practice, a nurse must explore her or his personal philosophy about the essential units of nursing and their relationships (that is, person, environment, health, and nursing, and how they interact). The nurse must next determine whether congruence exists between his or her personal values and assumptions and those of the model. If the nurse finds congruence between personal beliefs concerning person, environment, health, and nursing and the model, he or she may use it as a valuable tool to guide daily nursing practice. The choice of nursing conceptual model is, first of all, one based on personal and professional values, beliefs in what "works" for the individual in one's own delivery of nursing care.[23]

SUMMARY

Nursing process is an orderly, systematic method by which to provide nursing care of the childbearing family. Its major phases are: assessment, diagnosis, planning, implementation, and evaluation. Conceptual models are the "road maps" that enable the nurse to observe and focus on certain facts of importance to childbearing and ignore other facts that are not considered important in the conceptual model. Theories are seen as specific ideas and concepts about the childbearing individuals and family that allow the nurse to give care to them or to do research on the phenomena of childbearing. Theories "fit into" or emerge from conceptual models.

All phases of the nursing process, including nursing diagnosis, will be affected by the theory or conceptual model used by the nurse. The conceptual model or theory will determine what is to be assessed, what is an appropriate nursing diagnosis, what are the valued client goals, what are relevant nursing actions, and what constitutes an evaluation.

The metaparadigm of nursing is the "umbrella" that describes the limits of all the nursing conceptual models; that is, the concepts with which the nursing profession is concerned. There are four concepts in nursing's metaparadigm: person, environment, health, and nursing. Each conceptual model in nursing describes these concepts in a unique fashion. The metaparadigm, however, also ensures that nurses can communicate with each other about clients regardless of the conceptual model they use.

REVIEW QUESTIONS

1. Describe each phase of the nursing process.
2. Differentiate among the terms metaparadigm, conceptual model, and theory, and describe each as it relates to nursing.
3. Describe how a conceptual model in nursing can be used to understand the childbearing family.
4. Describe how use of one nursing conceptual model or nursing theory will affect (a) the nurse's research and (b) the nurse's clinical practice.
5. List four factors that would influence your choice of a conceptual model in nursing practice with the childbearing family.

REFERENCES

1. Yura H, Walsh MB. *The Nursing Process: Assessing, Planning, Implementing, Evaluating.* 5th ed. Norwalk, Conn: Appleton & Lange, 1988.
2. Stolte K. A complementary view of nursing diagnoses. *Public Health Nurs.* 1986;3(1):23–28.
3. Dossey B, Guzzette C. Nursing diagnosis. *Nursing 81.* 1981;11:34–38.
4. Gorrie TM. *Clinical Nursing Diagnosis Series: A Guide to the Nursing of Childbearing Families.* Baltimore: Williams & Wilkins, 1989.
5. Gebbie KM. *Classification of Nursing Diagnoses: Summary of the Second National Conference.* St. Louis: CV Mosby, 1976.
6. Gebbie KM. *Classification of Nursing Diagnoses: Proceedings of the First National Conference.* St. Louis: CV Mosby, 1975.
7. Kim MH, Moritz DA. *Classification of Nursing Diagnoses: Proceedings of the Third and Fourth National Conferences.* New York: McGraw-Hill, 1982.
8. Kim MH, et al. *Classification of Nursing Diagnoses: Proceedings of the Fifth National Conference.* St. Louis: CV Mosby, 1984.
9. Pridham K, Schutz M. Rationale for a language for naming problems from a nursing perspective. *Image.* 1985;17:122–127.
10. Shamansky S, Yanni CR. In opposition to nursing diagnosis: a minority opinion. *Image.* 1983;25:47–50.
11. Fawcett J, Downs F. *The Relationship of Theory and Research.* Norwalk, Conn: Appleton-Century-Crofts, 1986.
12. Field L, Winslow EH. Moving to a nursing model. *AJN.* 1985; 85:1100–1102
13. Visintaniner M. The nature of knowledge and theory in nursing. *Image.* 1986;18:32–38.
14. Stevens BJ. *Nursing Theory. Analysis, Application, Evaluation,* 2nd ed. Boston: Little, Brown, 1984.
15. Fawcett J. *Analysis and Evaluation of Conceptual Models of Nursing.* Philadelphia: FA Davis, 1984.
16. Beck CT. Theoretical frameworks cited in *Nursing Research* from January 1974–June 1985. *Nurse Educ.* 1985;10: 36–38.
17. Flaskerud JH, Halloran EJ. Areas of agreement in nursing theory development. *ANS.* 1980;1:1–7.
18. Newman MA. The continuing revolution: a history of nursing science. In Chaska NL, ed. *The Nursing Profession: A Time to Speak.* New York: McGraw-Hill, 1983.
19. Torres G. The place of concepts and theories within nursing. In George J, ed. *Nursing Theories: The Base for Professional Nursing Practice,* 3rd ed. Norwalk, Conn: Appleton & Lange, 1990.
20. Stanton M. Nursing theories and the nursing process. In George J, ed. *Nursing Theories: The Base for Professional Nursing Practice,* 3rd ed. Norwalk, Conn: Appleton & Lange, 1990.
21. Roberts KL. Theory of nursing as curriculum content. *JA Nurs.* 1985;10:209–215.
22. Chin P, Jacobs M. *Theory and Nursing: A Systematic Approach.* Toronto: CV Mosby, 1983.
23. Ross MM, Bourbonnais FF. The Betty Neuman Systems Model in nursing practice: a case study approach. *JA Nurs.* 1985;10:199–207.
24. McKay R. Theories, models and system for nursing. *NR.* 1979;18:393–399.
25. Levine ME. Holistic nursing. *Nurs Clin North Am.* 1971;6: 253–264.

Family Theory and the Childbearing Family

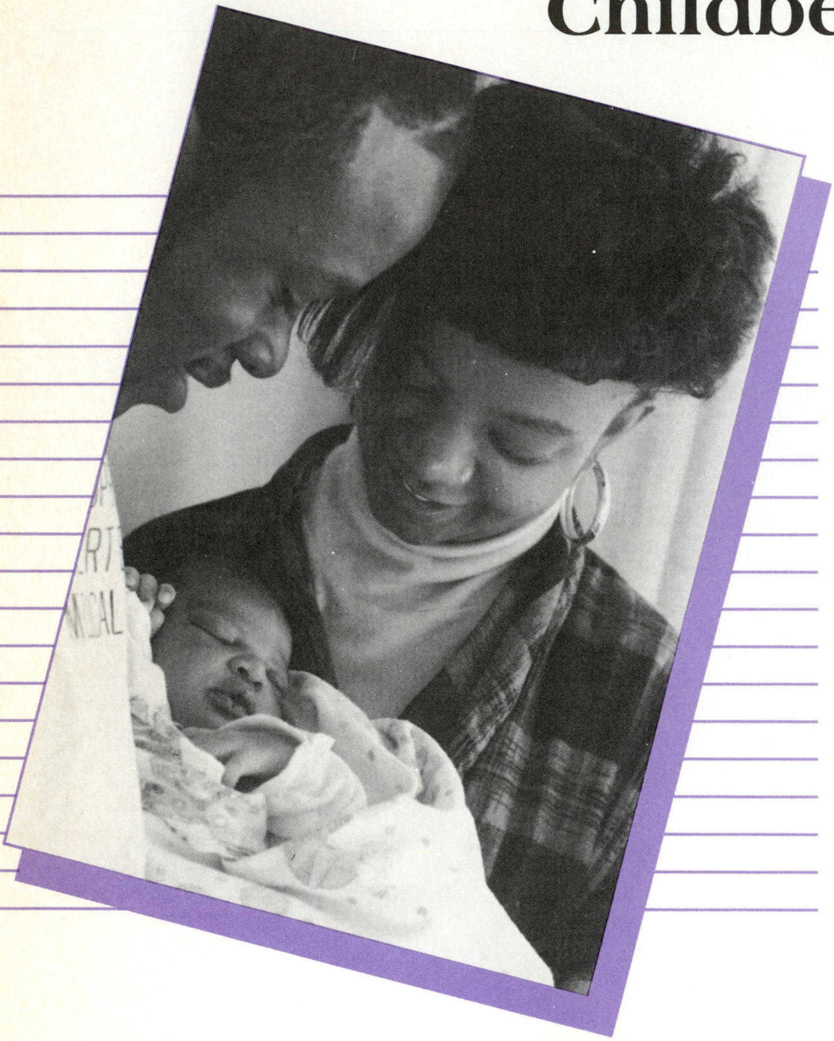

Chapter 3

Key Terms

extended family
family
family developmental tasks
family health
family of orientation
family of procreation
nuclear family
system

Chapter 2 introduced the concept of theories and how they may relate to the childbearing family. Family theory provides an organizing framework for interpreting and understanding many events that occur during pregnancy. These theories describe and explain the family unit as a whole or a unified system that is more than the sum of its parts. The focus is not on an individual member of a family, such as the mother or newborn, but on the interactions and relationships among all members. The way family members relate to each other is important in determining the way the family, as a whole, will adjust to pregnancy, childbirth, and addition of a neonate.

In this theoretical perspective, the family, in total, becomes the client and the recipient of nursing interventions. Interventions are not directed toward the pregnant woman alone, because she will be affected by and, in turn, affect her entire family unit. Family theory provides a nursing approach that acknowledges the importance of all members of the family in the process of childbirth.

This chapter introduces the family systems theory, the family developmental cycle, the notion of "family health," and specific phenomena of importance in the family unit that forms a base for nursing assessments. Family concepts are applied specifically to the expectant family, and possible nursing interventions are summarized. Finally, a case study and related care plan provide a "real life" illustration of the nursing process viewed from a family theory perspective.

FAMILY STRUCTURE AND FUNCTION

The family unit is probably one of the most vital considerations of the maternity nurse. Regardless of the form in which it occurs, the family is the basic unit of our society and, as such, is the social institution that has the greatest effect on individuals and how they develop. It has been called the "primary group," because of its importance in the life of an individual.

Family is defined as a small social system made up of individuals related to each other by reason of strong reciprocal ties and constituting a permanent household (or cluster of households) that persists over years.[1] Members usually enter through birth, adoption, or marriage and leave only by death. Even divorce or abandonment cannot totally remove a person from his or her family, although they will dramatically alter the nature of the relationships within the family system.

The United States stereotype of a family is still that of two parents and their children, with grandparents who do not reside in the same household. The concept of family has expanded over time, however, to include groups of unrelated people living and caring for each other as well as blood relatives.

Different terms describe types of families usually found in our society (Figure 3–1). Most individuals belong to one of these families at some point in their life cycle. The United States stereotype constitutes a unit that is generally called a **nuclear family** (or more simply, a family). There are two subtypes of nuclear families: (1) the group into which a person is born, called the **family of orientation;** and (2) the group into which people enter as adults and in which they usually appear in the positions of husband and wife or mother and father. This second type of family is called the **family of procreation.** The family is considered to have flexible boundaries delineating who is included in the family and who is excluded. This is especially so in families from certain cultural groups. The term **extended family** refers to any grouping related in some manner that is broader than the nuclear family.[2,3]

Friedman believes that the family unit occupies a vital position between the individual and society and has two functions or roles. These functions are: (1) to meet the needs of the individuals who constitute the family unit; and (2) to meet the needs of the society of which it is a part.[4] These functions for society and the individual can only be met by the family unit.

Childbearing and rearing are two of the primary tasks the family fulfills for society. The family unit provides a stable, recognized, legitimate unit for bringing new members into a society and for socializing those new members so that they can function in society.

The function of the family as concerns the individual is also important during the phase of childbearing. The family provides for survival and ensures development of the newborn infant and dependent child. For adults, it meets affectional, socioeconomic, and sexual needs. For all members, it serves as a buffer between the individual and society.[4,5] Thus, family theory, of all theories relating to childbearing, deserves attention as a basis for understanding client behaviors during pregnancy.

FAMILY SYSTEMS THEORY

Family systems theory is an umbrella theory that allows for a comprehensive understanding of the family. Family systems theory will be the approach used to view the family in this text. It evolves from general systems theory, developed in 1946 by Von Bertalanffy.

Systems theory is simply the study of the relationships of interactional parts in the context of a whole unit.[6] One definition of a **system** is: a set of different things or parts that meet two requirements:

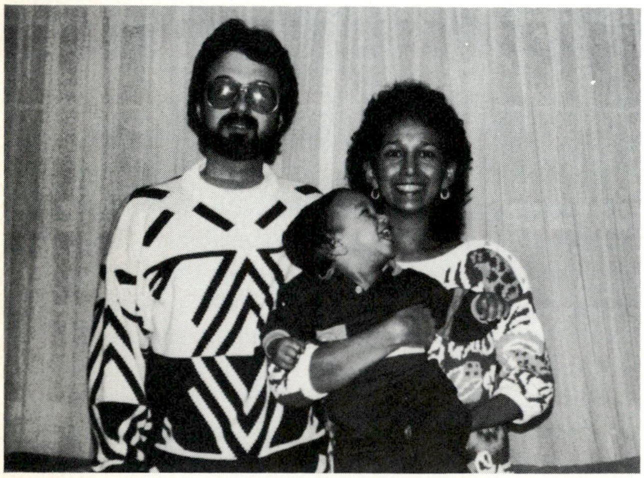

A

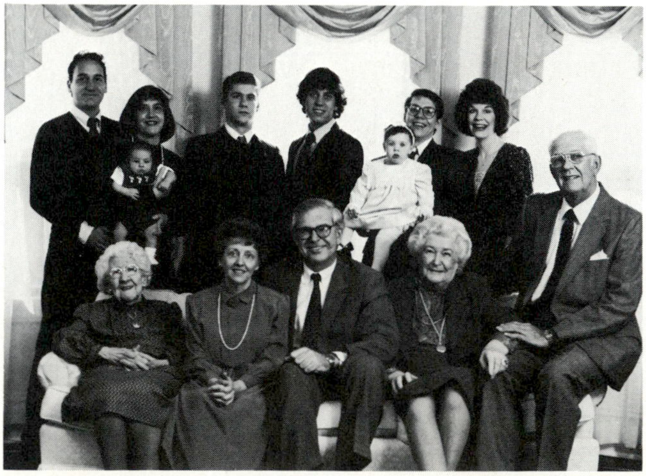

B

Figure 3–1. A. A nuclear family, consisting of mother, father, and child. **B.** A multigenerational, extended family.

(1) the parts are directly or indirectly related to one another in a network of reciprocal causal effects; and (2) each component part is related to one or more parts of that set in a stable but dynamically changing manner during any point in time.[7,8]

The system and its environment make up a universe—the totality of what should be studied in a given situation.[4] This situation is similar to the old cliché: "You can't see the forest for the trees." When you look at *parts* of a system (the trees), the totality of the whole system (the forest) is missed. Conversely, when you look at the whole forest, the trees are not visible as single units, they constitute the forest. When you observe a system as a complete unit, the functions of the parts are not important except in how they interact. Behaviors or functions of the system as a whole are different from behaviors or functions of one part acting by itself. For example, a pregnant woman's behavior cannot simply be explained by the function of her uterus. The totality of behaviors of the person evolves from an interaction of *all* the parts of the person acting together, including psychologic, physical, social, cultural, spiritual components, and so on. Furthermore, change in one part of a system would produce change in the entire system because of the inseparable interrelationships. Thus, a change in the reproductive subsystem of a woman would produce change in all other subsystems, and thus new behaviors of the woman (system) as a whole.

The family in this framework is a network or system of relationships. It can be described as an integrated system of interdependent structures and functions that consists of people who must relate and interact with each other.[9] The individuals who are organized into this single family unit must attain specific purposes—the family functions and goals. As in general systems theory, interrelationships of family members in the family system are so tied together that a change in any one part of the system invariably results in changes in the entire system.[4] Thus a woman's pregnancy (change in one part, the woman) does not affect only her. Her partner is also affected, even though he does not physically carry a fetus. He now must alter his life to become a father. He must attain and complete certain preparatory tasks for fatherhood; he must reconsider his economic status, his time commitments, and so on. Similarly, the children in the family must adjust to their mother's pregnancy. Their mother may be too tired to play with them as she did in her nonpregnant state. They also may have to deal with an alteration in their space or territory to accommodate a new baby.

Concepts of Importance in the Family System

Several concepts are basic to an understanding of family systems theory. These concepts are of concern to this book, because they change during childbearing. Table 3–1 lists and describes these concepts.

THE CONCEPT OF FAMILY HEALTH

Family health may be defined as a state of integrated dynamic functioning of the total human family within the internal and external environment directed toward a higher level of functioning.[16] Family health is not based on the individual alone, because the family is the source of health care, health beliefs, and health values. Such input from the family will affect an individual's perceptions of health and hence individual health care behaviors. Some characteristics of the healthy family have been defined. They include: functional communication among members, parental unity, flexibility of roles, the ability to function during periods of stress, and the ability to function during physical illness of a member.[17]

Family function, in terms of family health, refers to interaction and cohesion within the family; the ability of the family to satisfy physical, psychologic, and social needs of members; the capacity to cope with stress; participation in community life; the ability to fill assigned roles competently; and members' responsibility concerning self and family.[17] Reidy and Thibedeau suggest nine dimensions to be assessed in making a determination of family health. These include[17]:

1. The family's knowledge of health and illness
2. The family's ability to solve health problems and deal with complications
3. Existing health habits in the family
4. The family's attitudes toward health and health services
5. The family's ability to cope with stressful situations
6. Family life patterns
7. Family action on and interaction with the environment
8. The family's knowledge and use of community and health resources
9. The family's participation in community life

Families have a level of health that is more than the composite of the health of its members. Family health must be assessed by looking at the family as a whole, not just at members as individuals.

TABLE 3–1. CONCEPTS IMPORTANT TO FAMILY SYSTEMS THEORY

Concept	Description
Structure	
Family Subsystem	System made up of sets of relationships involving 2 or more members.[4] Subsystems inherent to nuclear and extended families include spouse, parent–child, sibling, and grandparent–grandchild subsystems.[10,11]
Triangle	Subsystem of 2 interacting individuals and one person treated as an outsider. Can be very unstable and set up negative effects in family system. An example of a triangle pattern is the birth of a first baby; usually the father, but at times the mother, may feel like an outsider as attention focuses on the infant.
Pattern of Closeness	Linked to how clearly family members see themselves as individuals and the amount of sharing and intimacy in the family interaction. The family establishes patterns of separateness and connectedness between members. In healthy families where members have a clear sense of personal boundaries, intimacy and individuality exist together.
Power	
Style of Power	How a family uses power; may be chaotic, held by one "leader", or egalitarian (distributed among members).[12]
Interpersonal Power	Who holds power in a family;[12] may be overt (openly acknowledged by the group) or covert (not sanctioned by the group). An example of covert power is the family in which an infant "runs the show".
Boundaries	Crucial means by which families adapt to outside demands and internal needs. Families may be viewed as "open" or "closed". Closed families view change as threatening. Healthy families are open, welcoming input from the environment that will aid system changes. Boundary ambiguity exists when families are uncertain of who is in or out of the family system or who performs what tasks.[13] A family with ambiguous boundaries will have difficulty altering family patterns, as in the birth of an infant.
Affect or Feelings	
Expressiveness	Healthy families have few rules against members expressing a range of feelings; problem families have many, as expression might disrupt the family's weak control.[12]
Mood and Feeling Tone	Healthy families project positive feelings, eg, joy and comfort; problem families project negative feelings, eg, unresolved anger or depression.[12]
Empathy	Refers to the capacity to experience another member's feelings, wishes, or ideas, eg, a mother's ability to sense and respond to an infant's nonverbal cues.[12]
Conflict	Present to some degree in all families; indicates functioning difficulty only when chronically unresolved.[12]
Intergenerational Patterns and Networks	Patterns of interactions that a family system, or an individual member, has with members of the extended family; may be positive and supportive or negative and disruptive.[13,14]
Roles	Roles can be general (eg, mother, father), specific (eg, mother of Johnny), ascribed by society (mother or father), or acquired (President of the United States). All roles are learned. Children learn social role behavior through imitation, identification, and reciprocal transactions with parents and other family members. Individuals in particular roles are expected to follow norms or rules with individual variation. Role conflict can arise, however, when role partners do not meet each other's expectations of appropriate behaviors. This can produce tension, anxiety, and hostility.
Communication Patterns	Refers to patterns of verbal and nonverbal behavior that occur within a social context.[15] Functional communications are complete messages without ambiguity, and have "channels" that are kept open between the sender and receiver. Dysfunctional communications are ambiguous and incomplete messages, which may lead the 2 parties to misunderstand each other.
Cultural Background	Each cultural group develops value orientations that are transmitted by the family system to its members. Individuals who come from families with different value orientations often have very different philosophies of life, which will affect behavior. A family made up of individuals from different cultural backgrounds thus has the potential for conflict when members' expectations of others' behavior are not met.
Rituals	Symbolic forms of communication, acted out in a systematic fashion over time, that help to establish and preserve a family's identity or sense of "self" (Figure 3–2), and to stabilize family identity by clarifying expected roles, delineating boundaries, and defining rules.
Celebrations	Holidays and occasions that are considered special and are widely practiced throughout the family's cultural group; examples are rites of passage (weddings, bar mitzvahs), annual religious holidays (Christmas, Passover), and secular holidays (Thanksgiving).
Traditions	Less culture-specific and more likely to be unique to each family; examples include birthday customs, vacations. Each family chooses which occasions will become traditions in its life.
Patterned Family Interactions	The least deliberate, most casual family rituals; most frequently enacted but least consciously planned by members, examples include dinnertime and bedtime routines, discipline of children, leisure activities in the evenings and weekends, and everyday greetings and goodbyes.

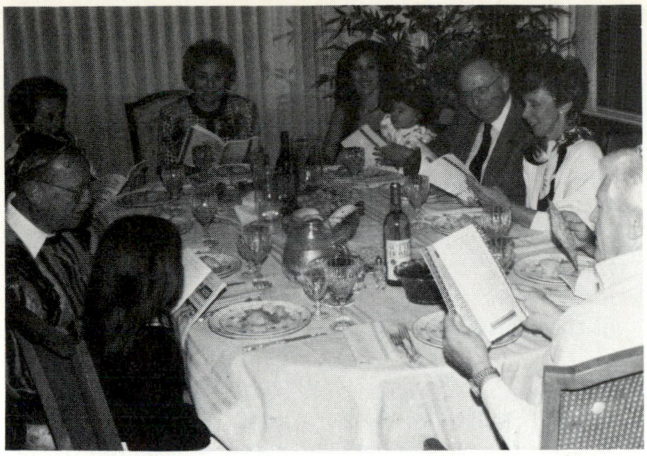

Figure 3–2. Family celebrations: a Jewish family celebrates a Seder together.

THE FAMILY DEVELOPMENTAL CYCLE

The family system, as an integrated entity, may grow and develop in a sequential fashion, much in the manner that an individual person develops. This section focuses on family growth and development through one of the most important phases of the family cycle, that of childbearing. Childbearing entails a major reorganization of family structure and function. Such major reorganization of a system may produce a crisis state (here, a developmental crisis). (*See* Chapter 4 for an in-depth discussion of crisis.) This section will discuss the childbearing family in the developmental crisis of reorganizing to incorporate a new member and nursing interventions to assist the family.

Family System Development

In 1974, Minuchin described the family developmental cycle as a key component in any framework that views the family as a system.[18] Such a concept originated in the 1950s with Duvall, who also saw the family itself as a basic unit of development. The family system, like the individual system, grows and changes and, as a whole, has its own developmental tasks.[19]

The life cycle of the family is described as a dynamic process that has a beginning, middle, and end phase. During the beginning phase, the major theme of family function and of the developmental tasks is establishment. The middle phase has a theme of expansion, extension, maintenance, and continuation. Finally, the end phase has a theme of and tasks related to transition, contraction, and completions.[20,21] Each of the above stages can be identified, success at achieving developmental tasks can be assessed, and diagnosis concerned with family needs, strengths, and weaknesses can be formulated.

Family Developmental Tasks

Family developmental tasks are those basic family tasks that are specific to a given stage of development in the family life cycle. They are directed toward maintaining family well-being and continuation at any particular period during that life cycle. Family developmental tasks are seen by Duvall as the growth responsibilities a family must accomplish at its stage of development to (1) satisfy its biologic requirements; (2) meet its cultural imperatives; and (3) satisfy its own aspirations and values. Family developmental tasks will shift with each stage of the family life cycle.[22]

Like an individual, a family can achieve success or failure in meeting tasks or growth responsibilities that arise at various stages in the life cycle. Family success in mastering current tasks leads to success in mastering subsequent tasks that will arise in new developmental phases. Failure, however, will lead to difficulty with later family developmental tasks and disapproval from society.[22,23]

Family developmental tasks arise when the needs of one or more family members converge with the expectations of society in terms of family performance. Internal (subsystem) tension and pressure combine with societal expectations (input) to produce a necessity for family system change. The need for change (which can be viewed as a developmental crisis for the family) engenders new tasks, which must be mastered by the family to resolve the crisis, restore homeostasis, and become ready for the next stages of development.

Duvall and others have identified critical stages in the family life cycle at which the above conditions will exist, and the family must solve stage-critical developmental tasks. Duvall's focus is primarily on childrearing. Thus critical events that will require the family to accomplish developmental stages are such family-related phenomena as getting married, giving birth, launching young adults, and adjusting to the "empty nest." Stress on the family system is inevitable during these stages of growth over the life cycle, and this stress gives impetus to family solution of developmental tasks. This picture may be complicated, however, by unpredictable events during the life cycle, such as birth of a defective child, untimely death of a member, or natural disasters. Thus family systems, as well as individual systems, may have situational crises as well as normal, expected developmental crises where family developmental tasks are expected and predictable.[19]

RESEARCH ABSTRACT

Loveland CC, et al. A psychometric analysis of the family environment scale. Nurs Res. *1989;5:38.*

This study presents a psychometric analysis of Moos's Family Environment Scale (FES), a tool that is used extensively in family research. This questionnaire was designed to explore three dimensions of the family environment: interpersonal relationships among family members, directions of personal growth emphasized in the family, and the organizational structure of the family. Although many studies have used the FES, information concerning the reliability and validity of the instrument is lacking. The investigators attempted to determine reliability and validity concerning the tool with data from their own sample.

Analyses for this study were based on data from a convenience sample of 257 individuals from 73 two-parent and 19 single-parent families. Mothers, fathers and one child completed the FES questionnaire during an interview conducted in the home.

On analysis, investigators found that the reliability of the scales was below that reported by Moos. Furthermore, when reliability scores were examined for mothers, fathers, and children separately, it was found that children's scores were consistently lower than those of their parents. The investigators noted that children demonstrated indecision and difficulty with interpretation of items during the interview.

A statistical analysis was done to test if Moos's model (the dimensions of the family) adequately represented structure for groups in this study. The investigators concluded that none of the confirmatory factor analyses, including an analysis of the data published by Moos himself, support the hypothesized dimensions of the family (the model).

Comment:
Although it is theoretically possible that findings in this study might be aberrations related specifically to the sample used, it points up an important consideration for nurse researchers who use already established instruments. Few other investigators had made their own reliability checks of the scales, relying instead on the statistics published by Moos. Furthermore, no one questioned the validity of the model on which the subscales were based. This study puts the believeability of this tool as a measure of the family environment in some question. Nurses should not assume that all published instruments are "good" instruments, or that they measure what they are supposed to measure.

Duvall's Eight-Stage Family Life Cycle

Duvall identifies eight stages of family development.[22] Other theoreticians have elaborated on this scheme, but it remains the predominant mode of viewing the life cycle.

Duvall's Family Stages

- *Stage 1* Beginning: married couple without children
- *Stage 2* Childbearing: oldest child under 30 months
- *Stage 3* Preschool: oldest child 30 months to 6 years
- *Stage 4* School: oldest child 6–13 years
- *Stage 5* Teenage: oldest child 13–20
- *Stage 6* Launching: period between the leaving of the oldest child and the youngest child
- *Stage 7* Middle: "empty nest" until retirement
- *Stage 8* Aging: retirement to death of both spouses

Developmental Tasks of the Early Family

The stage-specific basic family system tasks in the establishment phase of marriage (dependent on the couple's social status, ethnic and racial group, and family background) are[22]:

1. Finding, furnishing, and maintaining a first home
2. Establishing mutually satisfactory means of support
3. Allocating responsibilities
4. Establishing mutually acceptable personal, emotional, and sexual roles
5. Interacting with in-laws, relatives, and community
6. Planning for possible children (including contraceptive use, decision to have children, and dealing with pregnancy)
7. Maintaining couple motivation and morale

Developmental Tasks of the Childbearing Family

The childbearing stage of the family life cycle begins with the birth of the first child and continues until the firstborn is in preschool. During this phase, husband and wife must make the difficult transition to parenthood, a process that will be a focus of later chapters in this book. Tasks for the childbearing family include[22]:

1. Arranging space (territory) for a child
2. Financing childbearing and childrearing

3. Assuming mutual responsibility for childcare and nurturing
4. Facilitating role learning of family members (that is, assuming the maternal and paternal roles)
5. Adjusting to changed communication patterns in the family to accommodate a newborn and young child
6. Planning for subsequent children
7. Realigning intergenerational patterns (that is, establishment of grandparent-grandchild subsystems)
8. Maintaining family members' motivation and morale
9. Establishing family rituals and routines

As with individual systems, growth and development through the stages of the life cycle may produce a crisis (maturational or developmental) for the family system. One of the first individuals to suggest that parenthood is a crisis was LeMasters. He reasoned that, because a family is a small social system, the adding of a new member will force a reorganization of the system as dramatic as the removal of a member.[24] Although this reorganization and subsequent crisis is most profound with the first child, all subsequent births will produce the necessity to reorganize, and hence, a variant of the first developmental crisis of childbearing.

Based on his studies and clinical work, LeMasters draws several conclusions concerning parenthood as a crisis state:

1. Parenthood (and not marriage) is the real "romantic complex" in our culture. Middle-class couples often find their new parental roles in conflict with other socioeconomic roles.
2. Couples are seldom trained in parenthood. Society has few means to prepare husbands and wives to become fathers and mothers.
3. Birth of an infant forces immediate reorganization of the two-person (dyadic) pattern of group interaction into a triangle pattern. This is painful, especially if one member of the previous pair (often the father) is forced into the position of semi-isolate.
4. Parenthood marks the final transition to maturity and adult responsibility in our society. The couple now has achieved a certain equality with their own parents.[24]

Since LeMasters developed his theory, several investigators and theorists have challenged this notion of pregnancy as a crisis.[25, 26] Lederman indicates that it seems more appropriate to "conceptualize the normal course of childbearing as a test which comes as part of growth, and as a challenge rather than a crisis."[26] This view, however, is not at all inconsistent with the view of a normal developmental crisis discussed in Chapter 4. Crisis, especially a developmental crisis, is not inherently a positive or negative event. It is a period of great physical, psychologic, and social change in wihch certain tasks must be faced and mastered by the system. The challenge comes in the successful mastering of these developmental tasks, leading the family to a higher level of function. Crisis, therefore, is neither a negative nor a positive entity, but has the potential for a positive or negative outcome based on the manner in which it is resolved.

The Life Cycle of Poor Families

Being poor in and of itself does not make a family dysfunctional. Many families can fulfill developmental needs of members. Poverty is still a very powerful negative force on a family, however, especially as many poor families in the United States are also made up of minority individuals.[27] Some major stressors on poor families have been described[27]:

1. Ongoing intrusion of a variety of agencies and officials in the family's daily life
2. Discriminatory societal attitudes, especially if the family is also not of the dominant cultural group
3. Constant bombardment with complex, extreme, and unrelenting situations over which the family has little control
4. Great interdependence of family members financially and emotionally; survival for one member often depends on survival of other members
5. Continual stress and change; the family is at a great disadvantage in dealing with normal developmental stressors over time

It is important for the nurse to recognize, however, that families often do learn a variety of creative responses to deal with an impoverished and hostile environment. Not everything the family does is maladaptive—behaviors must be assessed in the context of the family's specific situation.[27]

The life cycle of poor black families has been described.[27] Many observations are relevant to families of various ethnic groups who live in poverty. Several patterns are evident:

1. The life cycle is punctuated by many unpredictable life events and stresses (situational crises)

2. The family has few resources available to cope with crises
3. Life cycle stages are shortened, with blurred transitions between stages
4. Black and other cultural groups living in poverty are often headed by females and are often extended family types

The Family Life Cycle. Shortened life cycle events mean that there is often less calendar time in poor families to complete developmental stages. Further, at each stage with its "normal" maturational crises, there are often several unpredictable situational crises. Members of poor families often are hampered in solving developmental tasks of each stage, making it more and more difficult to meet the tasks of subsequent stages. Hines describes three stages[27]:

Stage 1: Adolescence or Unattached Young Adulthood. During this stage, three tasks face the young person:

1. Establishing the self as a person. Children are either pushed out of the home early or are seen as an important source of support for the family. Peer groups often attain major importance in the young person's life, for example, attaining membership in a gang.
2. Attempting to find work. This is often difficult for poor minority youths. The "underground" economy has great appeal.
3. Developing intimate heterosexual peer relationships. There is much sexual experimentation among young people. Girls may see pregnancy and motherhood as their only chance at having an identity; boys, because there are few economic opportunities, often become transients in heterosexual relationships.

Stage 2: The Family With Children. Three tasks are accomplished by poor families during this stage:

1. Forming a marital system. This is again difficult because of chronic stress and conflicts over use of time and money.
2. Taking on parental roles. Young parents often still identify with single peers and avoid the parental role. If the mother accepts Aid to Families with Dependent Children (often called "welfare"), the father is often pushed into the role of the "peripheral male."
3. Realigning relations with the extended family. Because extended family boundaries may be more flexible among poor ethnic groups, young parent(s) may be easily accepted into the extended family hierarchy.

Stage 3: The Family in Later Life. The task of this stage, becoming a grandparent and turning over the reins to the next generation, is difficult for the elderly poor. Generally, there is no "empty nest" and older family members must still contribute to make financial ends meet. Poor individuals are often grandparents by midlife and may find themselves rearing a young parent and his or her child as "siblings." In black families, Hines describes the woman who cannot move out of the child care role and who becomes the "nonevolved grandmother."[27]

The life cycle described above may be more relevant for some groups of poor families than others. Culture will affect to some extent how poverty shapes the family life cycle. Yet it is most likely that the life cycle will be shortened in some manner for all families living in poverty. This, as well as the necessity to deal with continual situational crises, will make achievement of developmental tasks difficult for family members.

OVERVIEW OF THE CHILDBEARING FAMILY

Childbearing can be seen as a developmental crisis and a developmental challenge for the family system. Within the system, a variety of changes in structure, function, and existing subsystems will occur. Pregnancy and the perinatal period initiate such reorganization of the family system—indeed, many of the changes must be completed before the infant is actually on the family scene. The chapters in this book will focus in depth on changes that will occur in the family system and its members during pregnancy and childbirth. The following section will give a brief overview of some of these changes.

Changes in Family Patterns During Childbearing

For the family unit as a whole, and for the expectant woman and man as individuals, childbearing represents both a developmental crisis and developmental opportunity for maturation and growth. The family and family members will change in irreversible ways. As a result, they may experience internal family stress. Prior to birth of an infant, the man and woman may function as relatively independent individuals.

After pregnancy occurs, however, the couple participates in the creation and shaping of a new human being who will, to some extent, reflect each of them and their relationship. Thus, during childbearing, the expectant woman and man will experience major and important shifts in themselves in their relationship with each other and with others outside the nuclear family, and in the patterns of their family as a whole.[28]

Changes that occur in the psychologic makeup of the expectant woman are now fairly well recognized, and changes that occur in the expectant man are becoming a current focus of interest. Little emphasis has been placed on the couple as a unit, however, and the changes that will inevitably occur in their patterns of interacting and the changes in the family as a whole. Table 3–2 outlines some of the changes that may occur in the family system during the childbearing cycle.[29]

Effects of Pregnancy on the Marital Relationship

Lederman's research indicates that pregnancy and addition of a child to the marriage is one event that will change the nature of the bond between husband and wife.[26] This change will signify a developmental challenge for both husband and wife and add a new dimension in the way they relate to one another. In Lederman's study, some women felt that pregnancy brought the couple closer together. This was due to their sharing of the pregnancy and of their maturing and moving into new parental roles together. Furthermore, the marital bond itself was found to be relatively conflict-free when the man and woman agreed on value systems, areas of responsibility, sex roles, and child care.[30]

Not all couples, however, grow closer as a result of pregnancy. In fact, some women in Lederman's study initially expressed anxiety that the pregnancy might disrupt the relationship. Some factors that might interfere with strengthening the marital bond during pregnancy are the lack of caring or empathy and an inability to share, communicate, and trust on the part of either the man or woman, or both.[26] Further, the marriage can be affected by the maturity of the husband and wife and by the father's acceptance of the pregnancy and fatherhood role. Lederman's research affirms an old

TABLE 3–2. CHANGES IN THE FAMILY SYSTEM DURING THE CHILDBEARING CYCLE

Family System Component	Change During Childbearing
Structure	First pregnancy involves shift from stable dyad to a volatile triangle. Subsequent pregnancies involve development of several complex, shifting triangular structures. Family members must occasionally cope with being the "isolate" in a triangle. Stress and tension may increase.
	Additional subsystems must be established: mother-child; father-child; sibling; grandparent-grandchild.
Power	Patterns often alter; egalitarian power patterns often become more "traditional" with father as decision-maker. Fetus and newborn may become very powerful in family system, producing major changes in parents' behavior and family patterns.
Boundaries	Mother's boundary incorporates another human within, the embryo-fetus. Becomes a "protective" container for fetus, progressively closing in and focusing her attention inward.
	Father's boundary must expand to give support and become empathetic with mother.
	Family boundary must become highly permeable to selected input, for example, health care and education.
Affect or Feelings	Stress arising from structural change may alter feeling tone in family system. Danger signs are perception of hidden anger and hostility; pervasive depression; and apathy, unresponsiveness, or "flat" emotion.
Intergenerational Patterns	Parents' parents must "move up" a generation to become grandparents.
Roles	Each member of the family system (both nuclear and extended) must assume new roles—whether this is a first or subsequent pregnancy (*see* Chapters 13, 17, and 21).
Communication Patterns	Family members must learn to communicate as a triangle. One member needs to learn to be a temporary outsider or "isolate" left out of communications, since only two people can communicate at one time.
Cultural Background and Rituals	Family members from different cultural backgrounds may have different values concerning pregnancy and childbearing, may perceive new roles differently, and may have different practices and rituals for this event. Differences can produce family conflict and stress.

TABLE 3–3. NURSING INTERVENTIONS FOR THE THREE PHASES OF CRISIS

Goal of Nursing Intervention:
Assist the client (pregnant family) to capitalize on the growth potential inherent in this crisis.

Level	Nursing Interventions
Precrisis: Predictable risks and development events in the life cycle (childbearing)	Anticipatory guidance; discuss changes in family structure concerned with adding a new member. Assessment of risk factors, potential family strengths and weaknesses, past coping and problem solving, resources. Health teaching Health promotion or maintenance strategies.[a]
Crisis: Coping strategies not sufficient to deal with changes in family structure and problems in development (pregnancy, birth, the newborn)	Clarification of the problem(s)[b] Assistance for the family in gaining an understanding of the situation.[32] Acceptance of the family.[b] Use of appropriate interpersonal and institutional resources.[b] Assistance for the family to express feelings.[c,d] Assistance for the family to explore alternative means of problem solving.[c] Assistance for the family to use new resources and strategies.[c]
Postcrisis: Crisis has been resolved leading to a higher, the same, or lower level of family function	Support for the family in its new strategies of resolution. Emphasis on growth potential in solutions. Attempt to reverse or lessen effects of maladaption through appropriate rehabilitative effort or therapy.[a]

[a] Thibedeau J, Hawkins J. *Primary Care Nursing: Crisis Model in Client Management.* Monterey, Calif: Wadsworth Health Science Division, 1982, p 81.
[b] Rapport L. The state of crisis: some theoretical considerations. In Parad H, ed. *Crisis Intervention: Selected Readings.* New York: Family Services Association of America, 1969, p 22.
[c] Aquilera D. *Crisis Intervention: Theory and Methodology.* St Louis: CV Mosby, 1982, p 55.
[d] *Family: A Critical Factor in Prevention.* Washington, DC: National Center for Education in Maternal and Child Health, 1983.

cliché: pregnancy and parenthood do not generally help to resolve conflicts and are not a remedy for marital problems.

The Family System and Its Environment

As a system that is rearing and socializing children, the family will receive input from many other systems in its environment, such as the health care system, schools, and so on. Because the family has a mandate to develop individuals who will fit into society, a given culture, and a given extended family, many institutions and systems have a stake in how the family rears its children. Society's expectations of parental roles and functions may be in conflict with family expectations. Input from the environment can produce stress and tension (as well as be supportive) for the childbearing and childrearing family, especially if social institutions see family roles differently from members of the family. For example, schools see the educational system as a proper source for sex education for children. Many parents see sex education of children as a task belonging to the parental roles.

Nursing Interventions

The structural change and accompanying stress of childbearing produce a developmental crisis (or challenge) for the family. This crisis requires the family to master several developmental tasks in order to attain a higher level of growth and complexity. New coping strategies must evolve for the family to master these tasks. It is not surprising, then, that a model for nursing interventions with the childbearing family comes from crisis theory. Table 3–3, based on the work of Thibedeau and Hawkins, and others, provides a framework for nursing interventions during the three phases of crisis: the precrisis; the crisis state, and the postcrisis state. (*See* Chapter 4 for a more in-depth discussion of crisis).

The nursing interventions outlined in Table 3–3 for the family in crisis are, necessarily, broad and general. The nurse needs to assess each pregnant family and adapt such interventions to the family's unique needs and attributes. Later chapters will give more insight into specific forms of intervention, dependent on unique aspects and needs of the childbearing family.

CASE STUDY/CARE PLAN: FAMILY DEVELOPMENTAL CRISIS

Sara S., age 21, met Mike P., age 22, at a friend's party and began dating. After a 3-month romance, they decided to get married. Mike's salary from his job as a sports equipment salesman and Sara's salary from her job as a receptionist for an insurance company would allow them to maintain Mike's studio apartment.

For the first 2 months after their wedding, Sara and Mike had an active social life. In the third month of their marriage, Sara missed her menstrual period. A home pregnancy test indicated that she was pregnant. Both Sara and Mike were surprised but pleased by the pregnancy.

Sara's parents began to pressure the couple to move into the four-room upstairs apartment in their two-family house in the suburbs. Mr. and Mrs. S reasoned that the couple could save money, have more room for the baby, and Sara could get prenatal care from Mrs. S's obstetrician-gynecologist. Mike was not in favor of the move because he felt uncomfortable living so close to Sara's parents and would have to commute to work.

For the first month of Sara's pregnancy the couple continued to live in their city apartment. Sara was bothered with "morning sickness" and numerous other discomforts of pregnancy and received prenatal care from a public hospital's clinic to save money. Their social life had ceased, and Mr. and Mrs. S constantly voiced their disapproval of the situation. Finally, Mike reluctantly agreed to move to the S's upstairs apartment. Sara resigned from her job at the insurance company because she did not feel well enough to take the long trip into her job. With only one salary coming in, Mike and Sara became dependent on financial support from Mr. and Mrs. S. They lived rent-free, and Sara's parents agreed to pay for her prenatal care and delivery at their local hospital.

As the pregnancy progressed, Mike and Sara found that they had little to talk about and almost no interests in common. Sara spent her days with her mother. Mike found Sara's expanding body unattractive. Commuting to work was tiring, and he began to stay after work to socialize with his friends. Mike began to be more and more concerned with his ability to support a wife and baby on his salary. Whenever he went home, he seemed to fight with Sara, and he knew Mr. and Mrs. S thought he was "no good."

Supporting Assessment Data	Expected Client Outcome	Nursing Actions/ Intervention	Rationale	Criteria for Evaluation
Nursing Diagnosis: Inability of family to meet family developmental tasks of childbearing family because of poor resolution of earlier tasks.				
■ **Family Developmental Status** Have not established tasks of early family: living arrangements, finances, roles, interactions with extended family, planning a family, maintaining motivation and morale.	The nuclear family will regain a stable, workable, positive structure and function	■ **Crisis intervention strageties** Help nuclear family understand crisis Assist nuclear family to express feelings openly Assist nuclear family to explore alternative means of problem solving and coping	The family, as a unit, undergoes development as does the individual. Family development occurs in stages, each with tasks that must be mastered. Families experience developmental crises. Thus crisis intervention strageties are appropriate here.	The nuclear family reorganizes structure and function in a positive manner.

(continued)

CASE STUDY/CARE PLAN: Family Developmental Crisis *(continued)*

Supporting Assessment Data	Expected Client Outcome	Nursing Actions Intervention	Rationale	Criteria for Evaluation
■ **Family Structure and Function** *Structure:* No spouse subsystem, difficulty in transition from dyad to triangle during pregnancy *Power:* Couple has turned over power to extended family. *Goal:* No long-term nuclear family goals established. *Boundaries:* Ambiguous. Husband is withdrawing from nuclear family. Extended family intruding into boundaries. *Feeling tone:* Hostility, anger, unresolved conflict. *Intergenerational pattern:* Disordered. Neither spouse function as adults. *Family roles:* Spouses have not assumed adult family roles. *Communication:* Dysfunctional	The nuclear family will successfully master the developmental tasks of early family (thus providing a strong base for mastering the next stage's tasks).			The nuclear family accomplishes necessary developmental tasks.

SUMMARY

Family theory is one of the most important of the theories that describe phenomena during childbearing. The family systems approach, which looks at the family as a network of relationships, provides the most comprehensive picture of the childbearing family. Concepts of importance in the family systems approach include: structure, power, boundaries, affect or feeling tone, intergenerational networks, roles, communication patterns, cultural value orientation, family rituals, and family health.

The family may also be seen as a system that undergoes phases of development, that is, has a developmental cycle like the individual. During this cycle, the family must accomplish several developmental tasks. For the family system, childbearing can be seen as both a developmental crisis and challenge. Changes in family patterns of interacting occur as the fetus and, later, infant is integrated into the family system.

REVIEW QUESTIONS

1. Describe how the structure of the family will alter with the birth of the first child.
2. List four reasons for role conflict in the family. Describe situations where these role conflicts might arise during pregnancy.
3. Discuss the similarities and differences between the individual's developmental cycle and the family's developmental cycle.
4. List five tasks that the childbearing family must accomplish.
5. Discuss three changes that occur in the family system during pregnancy.

REFERENCES

1. Terkelson K. Toward a theory of the family life cycle. In Carter E, McGoldrick M, eds. *The Family Life Cycle: A Framework for Family Therapy.* New York: Gardner Press, 1980, pp 21–52.
2. Bell N, Vogel E. Toward a framework for functional analysis of family behavior. In Bell N, Vogel E, eds. *A Modern Introduction to the Family.* New York: Free Press, 1968, pp 1–36.
3. Figley C. *Treating Stress in Families.* New York: Brunner/Mazel Inc, 1988.
4. Friedman M. *Family Nursing: Theory and Assessment,* 2nd ed. Norwalk, Conn: Appleton-Century-Crofts, 1986.
5. Thibedeau J, Hawkins J. *Primary Care Nursing: Crisis Model in Client Management.* Monterey, Calif: Wadsworth Health Science Division, 1982, p 81.
6. Von Bertalanffy L. Systems, symbols and the image of man. In Galdston I, ed. *The Interface Between Psychiatry and Anthropology.* New York: Brunner/Mazel Inc, 1971, p 15.
7. Kanter D, Lehr W. *Inside the Family.* New York: Harper & Row, 1975, p 120.
8. Sherman R, Dinkmeyer D. *Systems of Family Therapy.* New York: Brunner/Mazel Inc, 1987.
9. Sedgewick R. The family as a system: a network of relationships. In Backer B, et al, eds. *Psychiatric/Mental Health Nursing: Contemporary Readings.* New York: D. Van Nostrand Co, 1978, p 31.
10. Handel G. *The Psychosocial Interior of the Family.* Chicago: Aldine Publishing Co, 1967, p 84.
11. *Proceedings: Social Factors in the Health of Families.* Washington, DC: National Center for Education in Maternal and Child Health, 1986.
12. Beavers WR. *Psychotherapy and Growth: A Family Systems Perspective.* New York: Brunner/Mazel Inc, 1977, p 29.
13. Boss P, Greenberg J. Family boundary ambiguity: a new variable in family stress theory. *Fam Process.* 1984;23:535–546.
14. Boszormeyi-Nagy I, Spark G. *Invisible Loyalties.* New York: Harper & Row, 1973, pp 1–18.
15. Satir V. *Conjoint Family Therapy.* Palo Alto, Calif: Science and Behavior Books, Inc, 1967, pp 1–55.
16. Blume N. The role of the family nurse clinician in family health care. *Home Healthcare Nurse.* 1985;3:35–38.
17. Reidy M, Thibedeau M. Evaluation of family functioning: development of a scale which measures family competence in matters of health. *Nurs Papers.* 1984;16:42–56.
18. Minuchin S. *Families and Family Therapy.* Cambridge, Mass: Harvard University Press, 1974, p 58.
19. Carter E, McGoldrick M. The family life cycle and family therapy: an overview. In Carter E, McGoldrick M, eds. *The Family Life Cycle.* New York: Gardner Press, 1980, pp 3–20.
20. Blair C, Salerno E. *The Expanding Family: Childbearing.* Boston, Mass: Little, Brown & Co, 1976, pp 35–45.
21. Lewis J. *The Birth of the Family: An Empirical Inquiry.* New York: Brunner/Mazel Inc, 1989.
22. Duvall E. *Marriage and Family Development,* 5th ed. Philadelphia: J B Lippincott Co, 1977, p 20.
23. Group for the Advancement of Psychiatry: Psychiatric Prevention and the Family Life Cycle. New York: Group for the Advancement of Psychiatry, 1986.
24. LeMasters B. Parenthood as crisis. In Parad G, ed. *Crisis Intervention: Selected Readings.* New York: Family Service Association of America, 1969, p 111.
25. Grossman F, et al. *Pregnancy, Birth and Parenthood.* San Francisco, Calif: Jossey-Bass Inc, 1980.
26. Lederman R. *Psychosocial Adaptation in Pregnancy.* Englewood Cliffs, NJ: Prentice Hall Inc, 1984.
27. Hines PM. The family life cycle of poor black families. In Carter B, McGoldrick M, eds. *The Changing Family Life Cycle,* 2nd ed. New York: Gardner Press, 1988.
28. Osofsky H, Osofsky J. Normal adaptation to pregnancy and new parenthood. In Taylor PM, ed. *Parent-Infant Relationships.* New York: Grune & Stratton Inc, 1980.
29. Sherwen LN. *Psychosocial Dimensions of the Pregnant Family.* New York: Springer Publishing Co, 1987.
30. Lederman R, et al. Relationship of psychological factors in pregnancy to progress in labor. *Nurs Res.* 1979;28:94–97.

Theoretical Basis for Nursing Care of the Childbearing Family

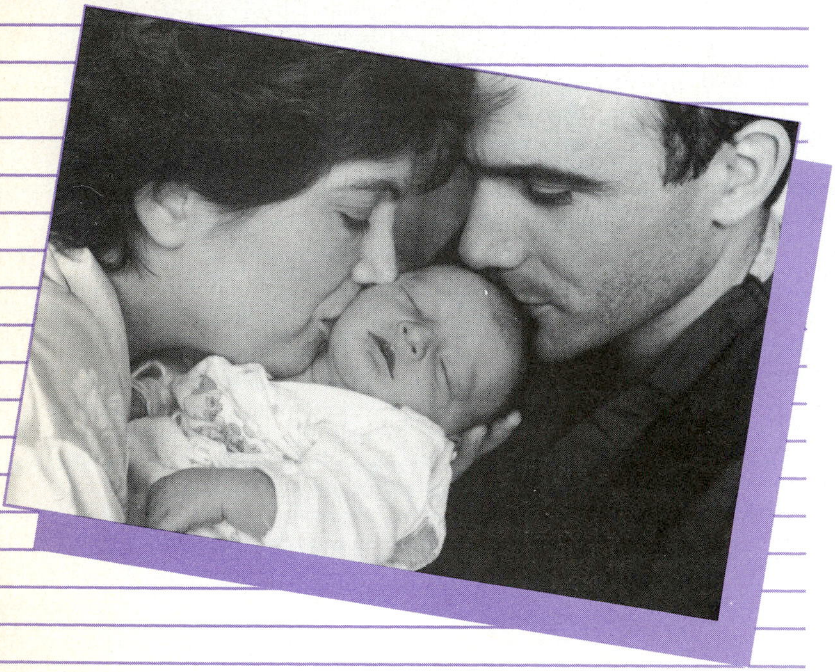

Chapter 4

Key Terms

attachment relationship
body boundary
bonding
couvade syndrome
crisis
dedifferentiation
fantasy
folk health system
maternal sensitive period
maturational (developmental) crisis
mimicry
physiologic stress
professional health care system
psychologic stress
replication
role playing
separation-individuation
situational (accidental) crisis
stress
symbiotic unity
transcultural nursing

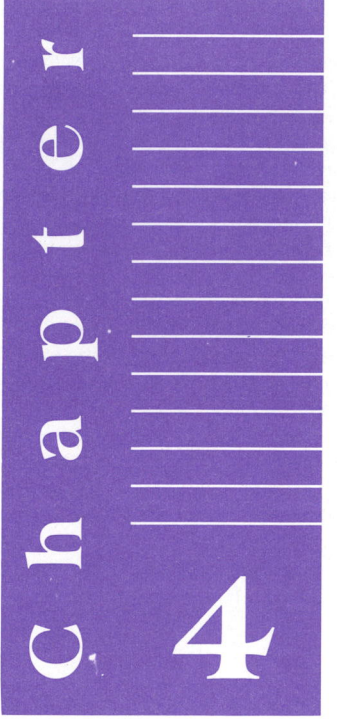

Chapter 2 highlighted the importance of nursing process and conceptual models in care of childbearing families. The childbearing phenomenon may be seen differently in each conceptual model developed by nurses and other professionals. However, all conceptual models provide general concepts and, therefore, require more specific theories concerning pregnancy and childbearing. Specific theories make it possible for the nurse to deliver care to the mothers, infants and families in the real world.

Many existing theories already relate to the pregnancy cycle as well as to other aspects of life and seem to be applicable and relevant within the "umbrella" of many nursing conceptual models. These theories are frequently used by nurses to form the basis or rationale for nursing practice with childbearing families, infants, and mothers and are discussed in some depth in this chapter. Included are such theories as: Crisis Theory, Stress-Adaptation-Coping Theory, Attachment Theory, Separation-Individuation Theory, and Transcultural Care Theory.

Many of these theories, although they usefully explain the phenomenon of childbearing, were not developed specifically for understanding childbearing families. Nurse investigators and others have, however, developed theories that do relate specifically to childbearing families through research on pregnant clients. Some major pregnancy-related theories that the student will need to understand to deliver care to childbearing families are discussed in the later part of this chapter.

THEORIES FOR UNDERSTANDING THE CHILDBEARING FAMILY

Crisis Theory

Crisis is defined as the impact of an event that challenges the assumed state of an individual and forces that individual to change his or her view of, or readapt to, the world, to himself or herself, or to both.[1] Crisis has commonly been used as a theoretical base for intervention in nursing. Although it can be used for assessing individuals, it is also highly useful for analyzing the family system. Furthermore, it is based on the developmental stage concept because it includes the idea of developmental crisis. Because pregnancy and childbearing are often considered developmental events, crisis theory is a very useful theory for understanding the childbearing family.

The concept of crisis contains both positive and negative aspects. When crisis is handled well by the person or family, it results in a higher, more complex level of functioning through the development of new coping strategies. However, when crisis is handled poorly, it can lead to a decline in the level of system functioning.[2]

When a crisis occurs, there is a period of disequilibrium that overpowers the individual's or the family's homeostatic mechanisms.[1] The family or individual is then faced with problems that are of basic importance, because they are linked with inherent needs. Conversely, these problems cannot be solved quickly by means of the person's or family's normal range of problem-solving mechanisms. Life events likely to induce a crisis have two broad criteria—they are of basic importance to the system and resist solutions by familiar methods. Pregnancy, birth, and role transitions are examples of such events.[1]

A crisis situation or event passes through sequential stages. In stage I, the precrisis period, the individual or family is faced with an event or stressor that threatens and disrupts the equilibrium and requires a system change. The person or family unit experiences a rise in tension with the disruption and prepares to deal with the problem. If past coping strategies are adequate to deal with the demand to change posed by the problem (stressor), the person or family deals with the stressor, evolves a new structure, and grows from the experience.[2] If, however, the person or family does not have adequate resources to meet the challenge of the stressor, the unit will experience a further increase in tensions and must develop new resources and coping strategies to deal with the stressful event. This stage is called crisis, or stage II.

Stage II, or crisis itself, is a self-limiting state, because the person or family cannot remain in a stage of disequilibrium for more than 6 weeks. During this time, the crisis will either be resolved successfully and appropriate changes in the system made or major disorganization will occur. This disorganized stage of the person or family is called postcrisis, or stage III. The disorganized unit now functions at a lower or less healthy level than it did before the impact of the stressor event.[2]

There is some question as to whether a process that is successfully resolved by the person or family in stage I, precrisis, can actually be considered to have produced a crisis situation. Individuals who view crisis as a negative event would indicate that preventive interventions might avoid the crisis. One could prevent the crisis stage with a normative or developmental stress event such as childbearing through primary health care. It is likely that some events, however, especially some normative or developmental ones, will produce the need for structural changes in the family (or individual). When a person or family must make structural changes, new behaviors and functions must be developed (as well as new coping strategies). Theoretically, crisis is neither positive nor negative but an open, unstructured stage, full of potential. The restructuring will lead to higher or lower levels of function, depending on many factors in the person or family and the resources available. No matter what the stage is called, however, the crisis model is the same, and the same nursing interactions are relevant.

There are two types of crises: **maturational** (or **developmental**), and **situational** (or **accidental**).[1] A situational crisis is an unexpected, stressful external event and may or may not coincide with a developmental crisis.[3] (*See* Chapter 36 for a description of a situational crisis: a high-risk pregnancy.) A maturational or developmental crisis, with which this chapter is concerned, is somewhat different. It is seen as "normal," because most persons and families experience such crises routinely in the process of growth and development. These crises are generally viewed as periods of marked physical, psychologic, and social change that are characterized by disturbances in life's pattern. During these periods, a complex of biopsychosocial stimuli poses certain tasks that must be faced and mastered by the person or family with a reasonable degree of effectiveness if the next maturational stage is to yield its full potential for further growth and development.[1]

The "normal stages of transition" in human development are[4]:

- Prenatal to infancy
- Infancy to childhood
- Childhood to puberty and adolescence
- Adolescence to adulthood/maturity
- Maturity to middle age
- Middle age to old age
- Old age to death

Similar transitions are also experienced by families.

During each phase, the person (or family) is subject to unique stresses different from previous phases. Each is faced with developmental tasks that are specific for that phase. Accompanying the phases are high levels of anxiety, because major changes must be made in the human or family system and in functions and behaviors. For example, a person might be expected to evolve new roles, a new body image, a new manner of interacting and behaving in the world, and so on. If the person fails to cope with changes and master tasks, the failure will stunt human growth and development. The individual may then fail to meet his or her potential.[4] The pattern is similar for families as units.

With appropriate support from others, however, the person or family normally can meet the challenges posed by growth and development. Thus, developmental crises are seen as normal, providing a new sense of self-mastery for an individual or family who successfully completes the development tasks posed by the transitions.[5,6]

To summarize, crisis is dependent on a variety of factors including: (1) the nature of the crisis event; (2) the state of organization or disorganization of the person or family at the point of impact; (3) the resource of the person or family; and (4) the person's or family's experience with crisis.[7] The system, be it a family or individual, will resolve the crisis in a positive or negative manner.

Stress Theory

Stress is defined as an emotional–psycho-physiologic state of the organism that occurs in a situational context involving stimuli that serve as cues to elicit anxiety or fear responses;[8] however, the term often is used to refer both to the stressor and the effects of the stressor.[8,9] Stress differs in its duration and intensity and is also unique to each person. What one individual finds stressful, another may not. Stress that affects the individual may be classified as either physiologic stress or psychologic stress.

Physiologic stress refers to the disturbances or functions of body systems and tissue as a result of insult by a dangerous stimulus. The manner in which the body responds to dangerous stimuli is the way it defends itself against the damage the stimuli may cause and returns itself to normal. The body's reaction to physiologic stress occurs in stages: (1) the alarm stage, which acts as a call to all defensive body forces; (2) the resistance (or adaptation) stage, in which the body returns to a normal stage; and (3) the exhaustion stage, which is also called the "disease of adaptation."[8] A familiar example of such a disease state is a gastrointestinal ulcer. If the stressor persists too long, disease and death of the organism may occur.[8]

Psychologic stress, refers to the purely psychologic aspects of the problem. Although the stimulus in physiologic stress consists of physical injuries to or physical changes occurring in the individual, psychologic stress is different. In psychologic stress, both psychologic and physical changes can be brought about by stimuli that never actually come in contact with body tissues but whose psychologic meanings are threatening or frustrating to the individual.[9]

The tissues, in psychologic stress, are not directly assaulted. Some stressor event threatens the individual because of the way it is interpreted and judged to be harmful. The individual then attempts, through behavioral means, to cope with the stressor event. Interestingly enough, the physiologic effects of the psychologic stress processes are similar to those processes that occur in response to physically dangerous stimuli that actually assault body tissue.[9] Physiologic stress reactions or responses can be brought about by the anticipation of a harmful experience as interpreted by the individual.

Stress can have an impact on the family unit as well as an individual. In this case, a stressor is seen as a life event that has an impact on the family unit and produces, or has the potential of producing, change in the family social system.[10,11] Included in the stress event for the family are hardships or demands placed on the family as part of the stressor event. For example, childbirth may be a stressor event that forces the family to make changes in its structure. Associated hardships may be lack of personal time for parents because of demands of child care.

Potential stressors for the family include[12]:

1. Accession or changed family structure by addition of a new member (eg, birth or adoption of a child)
2. Dismemberment or changed family structure by loss of a member (eg, through death of a parent)
3. Loss of family morale and unity (eg, through alcoholism)
4. Changed structure and morale (eg, through divorce)

All these situations produce the need for major structural alterations in the family unit. Normative transitions such as birth produce some of these stressor events.

How Stress, Crisis, Adaptation, and Coping Interact in the Family

Crisis and stress fit together with the concepts of coping and adaptation to explain how the family adjusts to the transition to childbearing. One problem with using crisis or crisis intervention theory to look at a

RESEARCH ABSTRACT

Tilden VP. The relation of life stress and social support to emotional disequilibrium during pregnancy. Res Nurs Health. *1983;6:167–174.*

Believing that pregnancy is a life-cycle event that may serve as context for high rates of emotional distress, Dr. Tilden focused her study on life stress and social support as contributors to emotional disequilibrium during normal pregnancy. One hypothesis was tested: "High life stress (as measured by the Sarason Life Experience Survey) and low social support (as measured by the Social Support Questionnaire) are related to high emotional disequilibrium (scores of anxiety, depression, and self-esteem) during pregnancy, beyond any variance in emotional disequilibrium due to women's marital or partner status."

A convenience sample of 141 medically normal adult women was recruited from a prenatal clinic in an urban health center. Women were over 20 years of age, in their second trimester, and were various ethnic backgrounds, marital and partner status, and socioeconomic and education status. The women were tested during a routine prenatal visit. Instruments used were the Sarason Life Experience Survey, the Social Support Questionnaire, and three instruments indicative of "emotional disequilibrium" (the Spielberger State-Trait Anxiety Scale, the Lubin Depression Adjective Checklist, and the Rosenberg Self-Esteem Scale). These last three instruments collected data that were subjected to a factor analysis, which produced one construct—emotional disequilibrium. All instruments had reported reliability and validity data.

Data were analyzed by a hierarchical multiple regression technique, which allowed the investigator to know how much of the variance in the emotional equilibrium was due to life stress or social support separately and in interaction with each other. Life stress and social support separately accounted for a significant percent of the variance in emotional disequilibrium. There was no effect due to their interaction. These effects were also separate from the effect on emotional disequilibrium of subjects' marital and partner status. The investigator concluded that emotional disequilibrium in pregnancy decreased as a function of decreasing life stress and increasing social support.

Comment:
This study is very important, because it provides statistical documentation of long-standing clinical observations. It is also a well-constructed study using a fairly large sample. Thus the practicing nurse may have some confidence in its findings. The study also provides the basis for further investigations. One question that immediately comes to mind is: How would these findings dealing with pregnant women compare to the same data collected on nonpregnant women? Such an extension of the current study may give more insight into the nature of pregnancy as a life event per se, and its relations with life stress and social support.

family unit is that it does not explain why crisis is a unique experience for each family. Why is it that some first-time parents seem to move easily from being a two-person unit to being a three-person family unit, whereas others seem to have much difficulty and unhappiness in the process of transition? For one couple, tasks of this transition are easily met, and a crisis (in the sense of disorganization of the family unit) does not really occur. For a second family, however, a full-blown crisis situation exists in which neither mother nor father can master the tasks of parenthood, in which family coping strategies are inappropriate, and in which the family unit begins to break down. Clearly, a single developmental situation such as childbirth can produce different reactions in families, ranging from equilibrium to complete disorganization.

There is evidence that many characteristics of the family itself and the nature of the stressor event will interact to determine the extent of a crisis situation.[10, 12] These factors include:

1. The nature of the stressor (that is, is it expected and desired, as in the birth of a planned-for child, or is it unexpected and feared, such as a high-risk pregnancy?)
2. The number of crisis events facing the family at the same time (for example, the birth of a first child coupled with loss of a parent's job or death of an extended-family member)
3. The way the family defines and gives meaning to the crisis event (that is, is the event seen as a challenge, where everyone has the opportunity to grow, or is it seen as inflicting unwanted change on the family?)
4. The internal resources a family has for dealing with crisis (such as individual member strengths, affection between members, flexible role patterns in the family, and so forth)
5. The external resources a family has for dealing with crises (such as social support networks—extended family, parent groups, friend networks—and so on)

6. The ability of the family to change and adapt to the crisis event through development of short- and long-term coping strategies

All these factors will interact and determine a family's ability to "weather" a crisis. Because each factor may be different in each family, it may be expected that each family will react to the same potential crisis event, such as birth of an infant, in a unique manner.

Attachment and Bonding Theory

Considerable confusion surrounds the similar theories of bonding and attachment: how they relate, their differences, and the importance of the two theories during the phase of childbearing. These two theories will be discussed together because they relate closely and are often used interchangeably.

ISSUES AND CONTROVERSIES

"Bonding" is a theoretical concept that has been highly popularized in both the professional and popular media. Birthing institutions give much thought to promotion of "bonding" among family members and the neonate. Bonding (or attachment) is, however, a difficult concept to measure scientifically. To date, no reliable and valid measurement instrument has been developed to quantify this phenomenon. Yet nurses continue to rate maternal-infant bonding using a variety of instruments and checklists of dubious value. Issues are:

1. Should nurses make judgments about and interventions concerning bonding (and the future parent-child relationship that bonding is said to affect) based on unvalidated assessment tools?
2. Conversely, should the nurse not assess the process and risk missing a truly disturbed (or potentially disturbed) maternal-infant interaction?

Bonding Theory. Bonding theory has recently received a large amount of attention from the mass media, and many parents are familiar with the term. A bond is defined as ". . . a unique relationship between two people that is specific and endures over time."[13] The term **bonding** is used most often to refer to a rapid process, occurring immediately after birth, that reflects mother-to-infant attachment (not the infant's attachment to the mother).[14,15] This process of establishing a bond between mother and newborn is seen as being facilitated by physical and skin-to-skin contact between mother and newborn. Infant suckling, visual contact between mother and infant, and the mother's fondling and touching the infant are involved. Similar behaviors on the part of the father and infant are said to result in a bond as well.

Two major factors said to influence bond formation between parent and infant are: (1) parental background; and (2) care practices (that is, at the location of the birthing). Parental background includes: the care the parents received from their own parents; parents' genetic and other inborn endowments; parents' culture; relationships in the family; and parents' experiences with previous pregnancies.[13,14] Care practices refer primarily to the interventions of caregivers during the birthing process, along with the institutional practices concerning birth. These include: behavior of physicians, nurses, and other hospital personnel; the care and support parents receive during labor and delivery; the course of events during the first days of the postpartum period and newborn life (especially the amount of separation of mother and infant); and the rules of the hospital.[13]

Because health care personnel cannot really hope to change parental background to improve bonding, much of the focus of nursing intervention is on the birthing period. A major point in bonding theory is the concept of a sensitive period for the mother (and to some extent the father) immediately following birth. This is called the **maternal sensitive period.**[13] During this time, complex interactions between mother and infant occur and help to lock the two together. Although some researchers and practitioners support the idea of a sensitive period, others have taken issue with this concept, which is borrowed from animal research.[16]

During the so-called maternal sensitive period, which includes the first days of life—usually the time spent in the hospital for most mothers and infants—the mother is particularly sensitive and open to becoming involved and forming a bond with the infant. Bond formation involves many interrelated processes, which are actually reciprocal interactions between mother and infant (that is, both mother and infant contribute to bond formation through their actions). The bonding actions will be discussed in more detail in Chapter 30.

Bonding and Separation. One of the major outgrowths of bonding theory was the belief that separation of the mother and infant immediately after birth might impede the bonding process. Much concern with separation had emerged from studies of sick or premature infants who were removed from their mother for high-risk caretaking purposes. Some of these infants were subsequently abused by parents. It was feared that separation of sick infants from their mothers interfered with bonding and thus negatively affected the emerging parent-child relationship.

The notion that any separation of normal infants and their mothers immediately postpartum may hurt the future mother-infant relationship was an easy theoretic step. The media presented sensationalized concepts of bonding to susceptible parents, who came to believe that unless they bonded immediately to their newborn, their relationship to their child would be ruined forever. Parents who were separated from their newborn after birth were upset and concerned and even felt guilty.

Problems with Bonding Theory. As often happens when a theory gains such popularity, critics emerged and attempted to point out flaws in the ideal of bonding. The criticisms took two basic tacks. First, formation of a relationship (ie, parent-infant relationship) evolves out of many experiences rather than one specific "event," such as the immediate postpartum period in the hospital.[17] This criticism points to the complexity of human behavior and the numerous factors that shape the person.

Second, several investigators have challenged the idea that there is a sensitive period in humans.[15,16] They believe that the transfer of the theory that concerns animal attachment to offspring does not apply to humans, who are infinitely more complex than animals.

Regardless of the justification of these criticisms, another factor should be considered in attempting to arrive at a more flexible concept of bonding for the nurse and other professionals working with childbearing families. A danger in the idea that early separation can lead to permanent damage to the mother-infant relationship is the real distress and unhappiness (and even guilt) it can cause to those parents who are aware of this theory and who are separated from their infants. They may come to believe that irreparable damage has been done to the present and future relationship and nothing they can do afterwards can "fix" it. Other parents who cannot be present at a birth—for example, adoptive parents—are discouraged in their efforts to relate to their adoptive children from the start. In addition, professionals may begin to treat all parents the same way. If a mother chooses not to be with her infant, she may be seen as a candidate for a parenting disorder, with little consideration given to other factors that might be present (for example, fatigue!).[18] One way to look more flexibly at bonding is to consider this in relation to the process of attachment.

Attachment Theory. Attachment theory, developed by Bowlby[19] and Ainsworth,[20] proposes that the affectional tie between mother, father, and infant develops out of response patterns that ensure that infants will be cared for during their years of dependency. This **attachment relationship** is said to develop over the first year of life, with the quality of attachment between mother and infant at 1 year relating to later social and cognitive development of the child. Early attachment behaviors coming from the infant are specific to humans and are elicited by any human adult. As the infant grows and develops, the responses become increasingly complex and directed to particular others in the infant's environment.[16] The nature of the relation is mutual—affection grows in *both* the mother (or father) and the infant, over time (Figure 4–1). Secure attachment between mother and infant is the basis for trust, which allows the infant to function eventually as an independent individual apart from parents.

If early maternal-infant contact increases maternal feelings of affection and sensitivity to the infant's individual response style, this should be reflected in the patterns of caregiving that influence the quality of attachment at 1 year.[15,16] In other words, bonding may set the stage, in a positive direction, for the developing patterns of interactions between mother and infant during the first year and help ensure the attainment of secure attachment between both mother

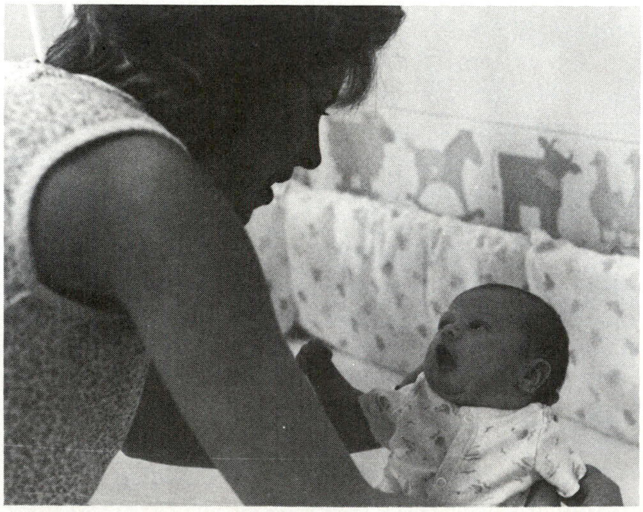

Figure 4–1. Mother-infant attachment develops mutually over the first year of life.

and infant at 1 year and after. Separation during this time, however, does not prevent subsequent positive patterns of interaction between mother and infant and the development of affectional ties over the first year of the infant's life.

Separation-Individuation Theory

Bonding and attachment are only half of the process necessary for the evolution of a positive mother-child-family relationship. There is a complementary process that must occur—the process of separation, or more accurately, separation-individuation. As noted in the previous discussion of theories of bonding and attachment, separation has acquired a somewhat negative connotation. Many believe that the separation of the mother and infant will interfere with bonding and the evolving mother-child relationship; however, the lack of separation-individuation experience will also be detrimental to the evolution of a healthy mother-child relationship.

The term separation is defined as the infant's psychologic development track of differentiation, distancing, boundary-formation, and disengagement from the mother.[21] Individuation is the infant's development of psychologic autonomy—that is, the development of his or her own unique personality characteristics.[21] The theory of separation-individuation was first developed by Mahler, who spoke of the process as the psychologic birth of the human infant.[22] Psychologic birth is the outcome of specific age-related subphases, which occur gradually. Table 4–1 summarizes these subphases.

Separation-individuation is a sort of second birth experience, or a psychologic "hatching" from the maternal-infant common boundary. The mother and infant are said to occupy the same "field" during pregnancy, having a common boundary. This state is said to continue for a time after birth.[22] The theoretical focus of separation-individuation theory is the means by which the infant separates out from the common boundary with the mother and becomes an autonomous, independent individual.

Both total attachment and separation can be viewed as potentially helpful and harmful phases of the developmental process. Both must be present in interrelations between mother, infant, and other family members for normal growth and development to occur; problems seem to arise when there is

TABLE 4–1. SUBPHASES OF SEPARATION–INDIVIDUATION

Subphase	Description
Symbiotic unity (birth–4 months)	Before separation-individuation process begins, infant is in a state of "fusion," merged with mother.[22]
Differentiation (4–8 months)	Infant "hatches" in a psychologic sense, begins to have some awareness of self and mother as separate individuals, and begins to develop a body image. Objects and individuals "other than mother" are identified. Infant begins to use vision to gain distance from mother and also to bridge the gap to her.
Practicing (8–18 months) Early practicing period (8–11 months)	Infant's ability and inclination to move away physically from mother increases through crawling, paddling, and climbing. Infant demonstrates growing interest in inanimate objects (eg, blanket or toy), and in exercise of autonomous functions, especially mobility. It is common for infant to forget mother for periods of time; however, he or she returns to mother frequently for emotional refueling.[23]
Practicing period (10–12 through 16–18 months)	Toddler begins to walk and shows great pleasure in practicing this and other motor skills. Toddler can now substitute other familiar adults for mother.
Rapprochement (18–24 months)	This is a period of crisis in separation-individuation process. Child is aware of growing separation and autonomy and begins to fear loss of mother.[22] In this phase, child is easily frustrated and in conflict concerning amount of maternal attention he or she desires. Child may have dramatic fights with mother, is highly sensitive to disapproval, and defends his or her autonomy and separateness by saying "no." This subphrase marks increasing use of symbolic communication and play, which develop mastery of developmental tasks. Conscience emerges as child demonstrates internalization of parental rules and demands.
Individuality (24–36 months)	As crisis of rapprochement subphase is resolved, consolidation of individuality and beginning of emotional object constancy emerges. Child now achieves tasks of establishment of individuality and of object constancy, which refers to a stable internal image of significant others (eg, mother) that allows child to function separately in their absence.[22]

too much attachment or separation, or both. The responsibility of the nurse and others working with parents and children may be not so much ensuring that bonding occurs for all time, but instead assessing the progressive change in proportions of attachment and separation-individuation at various phases of the life cycle.[23]

Transcultural Care Theory

The idea of **transcultural nursing** and transcultural care was proposed by Leininger in the mid 1960s. She has since developed the idea into a theory of nursing that she calls Transcultural Care Diversity and Universality.[24] This theory of care is highly relevant to nursing, "because it gets to the heart and nature of nursing, and [it] . . . has the greatest potential to explain nursing phenomena and actions."[24]

Leininger's theory states that different cultures perceive, know, and practice care in different ways. Yet there are some commonalities about care among all cultures in the world. Identifying the differences and similarities among cultures can provide a basis for nursing knowledge that can be used to guide nursing care decisions and actions to benefit clients.[24]

The nursing profession, as the profession most interested in providing holistic care to individuals, must be knowledgeable about and skilled in values, beliefs, and health-illness practices of different cultures. Without this knowledge and skill, a gap in provision of competent nursing care will occur. Because cultural factors are one major force that will influence the quality of health and nursing care given to people, omission of cultural factors is a major obstacle to providing care.[25]

Some common transcultural concepts are important to understanding transcultural nursing care. These are:

- *Ethnocentrism.* This is the assumption that one's own beliefs and ways of doing things are the best, superior, or preferred way of function. Such an assumption is often rigidly ingrained in an individual.[25] For example, for many years, the nursing subculture has viewed strict asepsis during labor and delivery as essential to well-being of mother and infant. Other cultures' birth practices that do not occur in sterile environments may be seen by many nurses as "barbaric."
- *Cultural imposition.* One's values, beliefs, and practices are imposed on the client, family, or community. This is usually done in the belief that one's own lifeways are "best," and from ignorance of others' cultural practices. In the health care area, however, cultural imposition can lead to serious conflicts and interpersonal difficulties that are obstacles to delivering quality care.[25] An example may be seen in nursing's value on father participation in the birth process, which ignores cultural variation in perception of appropriate masculine roles.
- *Cultural exclusion.* This is the conscious or unconscious avoidance or omission of cultural values and practices (and other cultural groups) in nursing and health care. This occurs often, as these cultural values and practices are seen as inferior, incompetent, too difficult to work with, and so forth. Individuals whose cultural practices differ from the dominant culture's are excluded or not treated like individuals. The excluded person, in turn, feels left out, demeaned, and in a position of great disadvantage.[25]
- *Cultural accommodation.* This occurs when health personnel are sensitive to the cultural values and practices of the client. This allows the client's needs to be met appropriately, respects his or her cultural practices, and recognizes his or her lifeways. One way nurses can do this is through use of folk health practices in addition to professional health ideas in the delivery of care.[25]

Health Systems. Two other related aspects of transcultural nursing and care concern the folk health system and the professional health system, and the differences between the two. These two systems of health care currently exist in the United States and in all other cultures (and countries) of the world.[25] It is vital that nurses understand the two systems in order to promote cultural accommodation and provide therapeutic, culturally sensitive care.

The **professional health care system** consists of the group of health care personnel who assume health care roles serving clients and who have been educated through formal programs of professional education. These individuals include nurses, physicians, social workers, pharmacists, physical and occupational therapists, and others. In the United States, formal education consists of Western ideologies of health care.[25]

In contrast, the **folk** (local, indigenous) **health system** is the group of people who have local beliefs and values and have assumed service roles to help people in their own community. These folk health–caregivers are prepared through informal experiential methods and reflect local cultural health beliefs and practices. Folk practices develop through daily life experiences in each culture and are related to the group's social structure. They are generally known and recognized by members of the particular community or cultural groups.[25]

Most individuals in the professional health system fail to recognize the folk health system, or if they are aware of it, they usually belittle it as "nonscientific," "superstition," "quackery," and so on. Until health professionals recognize and respect the folk system along with the professional health system, conflicts with clients from different cultures and gaps in health care services will result. Leininger states ". . . the two systems complement each other and need to be blended together to provide therapeutic and meaningful health services to people."[25]

Many studies document the effects of clashes between the professional health care system and professional caregivers and the client's cultural beliefs and the folk health–care system. Often this results in great stress for the client and perhaps even the client's ignoring the prescription for care offered by the professional health-care system.[26–29] In most studies, flexibility, understanding, and the respecting and incorporation of the client's culture and cultural practices facilitate acceptance of the professional and his or her health ideas by the client and reduce client stress.[26–29]

Developing Cultural Awareness. How can a nurse develop the ability to give culturally appropriate health care to clients from different cultures? The primary way is through the education system. Transcultural nursing is a specialty area in nursing, just as maternal-infant nursing is a specialty. Transcultural care concepts should, however, be considered in all phases of the nursing curriculum and in continuing education.

There are several strategies that can help develop cultural awareness[30]:

1. The student may explore his or her own cultural background.
2. The student may then learn about a different culture through reading literature, seminars, formal courses, and so forth.
3. The student may conduct a small-scale cultural profile of a community and attend cultural events in a community.
4. The student may direct study to learning cultural norms of the people met in nursing practice.

Of course, major anthropologic and ethnographic study is necessary before one can gain a true understanding of cultural groups.[31] Many individuals actually live and participate in a culture to gain understanding of that group. The enormous variety of cultural groups makes it impossible for the nurse to be a universal expert. It is, however, vital that nurses recognize culture as one of the most important considerations in care delivery. If care practices suggested to the pregnant woman of a particular cultural group are in conflict with her practices, beliefs, and values, they will not be carried out, no matter how good they are.

Finally, the student must realize that nursing itself is a culture. When viewed from a different perspective, nursing's practices might seem barbaric or inappropriate. The student needs to keep an open, flexible mind concerning health care and other culturally based beliefs, as well as remaining aware of culture as a major factor in a person's beliefs and practices about health and other behaviors.

The Culture of Poverty. The concept of poverty as a culture, in and of itself, was developed by Lewis in 1966.[32] Poverty may be seen as a culture in the traditional anthropologic sense. Like other cultures, it provides human beings with a design for living, a set of solutions for human problems, and attitudes and values that will allow an individual to adapt and survive within the culture. Victims of poverty may suffer from a set of cultural and personality handicaps that tend to persist and perpetuate their lifestyle.

Some characteristics of individuals growing up in the culture of poverty include[32]:

1. Feelings of fatalism
2. Feelings of helplessness
3. Feelings of dependency
4. Feelings of inferiority
5. Present time orientation
6. Inability to delay gratification
7. Inability to plan for the future

Further, Lewis believes that the culture of poverty is basically similar in whatever society it is found. Thus, the lifestyle of poverty may transcend national boundaries and geographic regions. Victims of poverty may show similar patterns in the way they live their lives and order their families regardless of where they are or in which dominant cultural group they find themselves.[27]

Although Lewis' view presents a very stereotypic picture of the poor and has been often criticized, it does make the point that the lifestyles and belief systems of people living in poverty may be quite different from those of their largely middle class caregivers. Attitudes and beliefs of individuals vary, not only as a result of ethnicity, but also as a result of a client's economic level. Care delivery must be tailored accordingly.

One area that has been recently documented to differentiate the poor from other groups is family life cycle.[33] This altered cycle of family development was discussed in Chapter 3.

THEORIES CONCERNING PSYCHOSOCIAL ASPECTS OF CHILDBEARING

The theories that will be discussed in this section differ from those in the previous section in a very important way. Theories discussed in the first section were not necessarily developed from research or observations on pregnant women, newborns, or families. Although they are useful in explaining phenomena that occur in childbearing families, they also explain phenomena in other situations that have nothing to do with pregnancy.

The theories to be discussed in this section were developed specifically from research and observations on childbearing families. Thus, they relate specifically to pregnancy and help flesh out the picture of individuals and families experiencing pregnancy. Concepts introduced in these theories, such as role development or fantasy during pregnancy, will be elaborated on in future chapters discussing psychosocial changes during each trimester. The specific theoretic concepts to be introduced here include psychosocial changes in the mother during pregnancy (including pregnancy acceptance, symbolic meanings of the pregnancy, maternal role assumption, establishing a relationship to the fetus, fantasy during pregnancy, self and body image during pregnancy, and perception of time and space during pregnancy), psychosocial changes in the father during pregnancy (including paternal role assumption and paternal pregnancy experiences—especially paternal style and the couvade syndrome), experiences of siblings during pregnancy, and experiences of grandparents during pregnancy.

Psychologic Changes in the Mother: An Overview

Pregnancy and bearing a child represent major changes in the life of a woman. It has been theorized that pregnancy represents a period of transition between two completely different lifestyles—that of woman-without-a-child and woman-and-child.[34] Although this shift in lifestyle is most dramatic with a first child, lifestyle also must change with additional births. Life with one child is certainly different from life with two or three children. Lederman sees the lifestyle shift as a shift in the constellation of a woman's self-image, beliefs, values, priorities, behavior patterns, relationships with others, and problem-solving (coping) skills.[7] Coleman states that included in the psychologic dynamics of change during pregnancy are the woman's characteristic coping mechanisms, stage of pregnancy, her current life stresses, stage in the life cycle, the symbolic meaning of the pregnancy for the woman, and her relationship to her family.[35] In other words, the woman will gain a completely new perceptual framework by which to interpret her world. Although this transition might seem an enormous endeavor, the mother-to-be usually has 40 weeks to make all necessary changes. Coleman reminds us that the psychologic work of pregnancy is for the woman to prepare for parenthood, to get herself ready to accept a child (or additional child) into the family, and in essence, to transform her deepest sense of self and work out new patterns to replace old ones that are no longer relevant.[35]

This and subsequent chapters take a closer look at the changes occurring in each trimester that will essentially result in a complete lifestyle change for the woman.

Accepting the Pregnancy. Accepting the pregnancy is one of the first changes a woman must make for a successful transition in lifestyle. This acceptance refers to a woman's adaptive responses to all of the changes inherent in prenatal growth and development.[34] If the woman cannot come to accept the pregnancy, it will be very difficult for her to accept the other changes necessitated by pregnancy, childbirth, and interaction with the newborn.

Lederman's research indicated that low acceptance of pregnancy was generally associated with unplanned pregnancy, greater conflicts and fears, many physical discomforts during pregnancy, and depression. Acceptance of pregnancy, on the other hand, was linked to feelings of happiness and enjoyment of the pregnancy, little physical discomfort, moderate mood swings, and relatively little reported ambivalence during the first trimester. Actually, complete acceptance of pregnancy was found to be a rare occurrence in Lederman's sample of pregnant women. Some ambivalence was felt to be "normal" (Figure 4–2). Most ambivalence concerned two areas: financial security and changed lifestyle (including the motherhood-career conflict).[34]

Other researchers confirm the fact that complete acceptance is rare and perhaps even has some negative impact on the outcome of pregnancy. One researcher, who attempted to identify factors occurring during pregnancy that are associated with obstetric complications, found that behaviors and attitudes that reflect a denial of difficulties that occur frequently during pregnancy may be associated with obstetric complications. Further, an acknowledgment of some of the negative aspects of pregnancy appeared, in this study, to be less strongly related to subsequent obstetric difficulties.[36] Thus acceptance of the reality of pregnancy coupled with overall general acceptance of

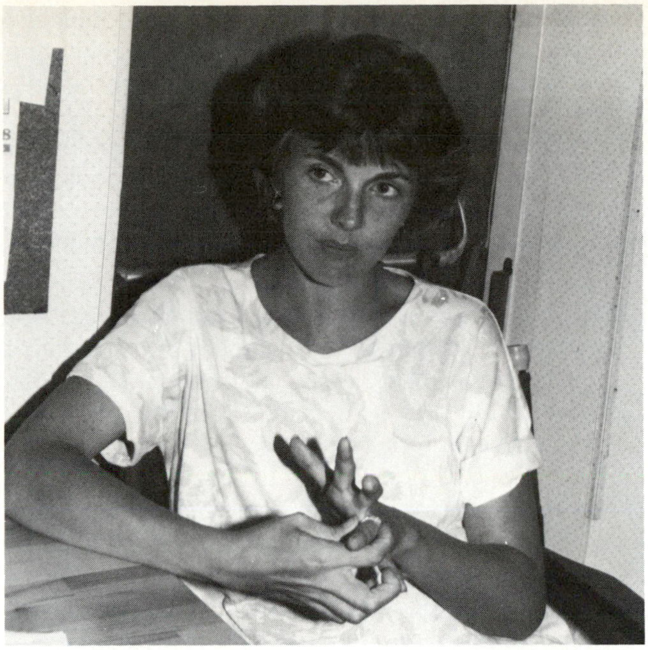

Figure 4–2. Ambivalence may normally recur at times during pregnancy.

the pregnancy may be the best indicator of healthy change in the pregnant woman.

Particular areas to be assessed concerning a woman's acceptance of pregnancy include[34]:

1. The extent to which the pregnancy was planned and wanted by the woman and her partner
2. The amount of time the woman is happy versus depressed during the pregnancy (this may have different meanings depending on the woman's trimester of pregnancy)
3. The amount of reported discomfort during pregnancy and how the woman responds to the discomfort
4. The extent to which the woman accepts or rejects changes in her body
5. The amount of ambivalence or experienced conflict concerning the pregnancy expressed by the woman near term

The Symbolic Meaning of the Pregnancy. Another factor influencing how a woman accomplishes the transition to a different lifestyle is the symbolic meaning of the pregnancy for the woman. This symbolic meaning is both a product of a woman's specific culture and of her own unique personality structure. The meaning that pregnancy holds for a woman may greatly shape the pregnancy experience and the manner in which the woman moves through transition to the new lifestyle of woman-and-child. Coleman describes some of the more common meanings that pregnancy and birth can hold for a woman in the predominant Western culture.[35] These are summarized in Table 4–2. When the nurse has an understanding of the symbolic meaning of the pregnancy for the client, the nature of the transition during pregnancy will be more evident.

Role Assumption and Maternal Adaptation: Becoming a Mother. Assuming and adapting to the role of "mother" is part of a long-term process. Although the expectant woman must undergo major

TABLE 4–2. COMMON MEANINGS OF PREGNANCY AND BIRTH

1. *The ultimate creative act:* The ultimate symbol and concrete example of all creative acts.
2. *Birth and rebirth:* A time of "rebirth" for all family members. Pregnancy is often linked with a woman's and family's desire for change or new beginning in their lives. Birth of an infant, however, does not always accomplish the change for which the woman and family hope.
3. *A rite of passage into adulthood:* The ultimate movement into womanhood and adulthood, carrying with it true adult responsibilities. The woman may seek or avoid it as the act of becoming a "true adult."
4. *Proof of womanhood:* The ultimate proof that one is a woman. The course of the pregnancy also can serve as an evaluation of how adequate one is at being a woman. For example, a woman who has complications during labor that necessitate a cesarean delivery may feel that she has "failed childbirth" and is not adequate as a "real woman."
5. *A symbol of sexuality:* May reflect a woman's need to demonstrate her fertility; the ultimate and concrete expression of sexuality and sexual activity. It has been suggested that before infertile couples can move on to adoption, they must come to terms with and mourn their inability to reproduce a child.[37]
6. *An expression of relationship with the woman's mother:* Women may become pregnant in response to unconscious feelings about their own mothers. Many clinicians and researchers have noted the importance of the mother-daughter link during pregnancy and its effect on the mother-to-be's psychologic adjustment.
7. *An expression of relationship with the baby's father:* Can be the healthy expression of the union of man and woman in the creation of new life. Some women, however, get pregnant "for" their men—most commonly in an attempt to cement the relationship.
8. *A trap:* Some women, especially those who see mothering behaviors as representing something negative, may see pregnancy as a trap. They may perceive that pregnancy will curtail their hard-won freedom and push them into a role of a self-sacrificing dependent, housewife-mother. Pregnancy may also be viewed as the end or interruption of a promising career. Coupled with this feeling may be the real threat to a couple's economic lifestyle.

changes to assume this role in time to nurture her newborn, the alterations that occur during the 9 months of pregnancy actually build on a lifelong process of learning a feminine identity. Rubin defines "feminine identity" as the woman's orientation and definition of herself and of the outside world.[38] Feminine identity begins as early as there is a sense of self—sometime around 2 years of age. A little girl may develop an identity of what it means to be female through playing with dolls, wearing ruffled dresses, and interacting with people who expect her to act like a "little lady." A girl may also develop a feminine identity through engaging in "gender-free" activities and playing with toys not deemed to be specific for girls or boys. She may also develop her identity through associating with and playing with little boys.

The feminine identity undergoes development at various phases of the woman's life—during the preschool period, school age period, puberty, adolescence, childbirth, and menopause. As long as there is a life and a self, there is a developing identity of the self as a woman.[38, 39]

Feminine identity is especially affected by periods in the life cycle in which there is marked physical, physiologic and psychologic change—such as puberty, pregnancy, and menopause. During the time of the massive changes that occur during pregnancy, many factors will affect the evolution of feminine identity into a sense of being a mother.

Osofsky and Osofsky indicate that many of the woman's personality traits (for example, her temperament, belief system, or level of assertiveness) will determine how well she adapts to the maternal role.[40] The expectant woman's perception of and relationship with her own mother are seen as key in the process of adapting to the maternal role. Furthermore, the extent of stress (including marital disharmony) will affect the woman's attainment of the maternal role and identity.

During this movement toward a maternal identity, emotional disturbances can occur. These disturbances seem to be related to psychologic readiness for the process of pregnancy, emotional stability or instability at the time pregnancy occurs, the woman's early life experiences, her overall social situation, and the physiologic and hormonal shifts that occur during pregnancy.[40–42]

The assistance of the expectant woman in attaining a maternal role has been studied by many nurse researchers and clinicians. Reva Rubin and Regina Lederman are two prominent nurses who have described the process of maternal role attainment and adaptation. Rubin began developing her clinically based theories concerning the psychologic changes of pregnancy in the early 1960s. Some of her writings have had a profound influence on thought about a woman's movement into motherhood.

Lederman has emerged as a prominent nurse-researcher in the area of pregnancy. Her book, *Psychosocial Adaptation in Pregnancy,* was based on extensive research concerning maternal development.

Rubin's Conceptual Framework for Maternal Role Assumption. Rubin sees movement into a maternal role as a process that occurs not only with the first pregnancy but also with each successive pregnancy. It is an active, voluntary process in which the woman moves closer to her "ideal" in terms of desired attributes and performance as a mother.

The development of the maternal role (or, as Rubin describes it, a maternal identity for this child) is effected in a progressive series of cognitive operations. Furthermore, the maternal role is linked to achievement of certain "maternal tasks." It is the involvement in the continuous and increasingly more complex maternal tasks that allows the mother to bind into the maternal identity in relation to this child.[38] Again, the tasks are self-imposed and motivated by the desire to have *this* child and be competent as a mother to the child. The cognitive operations of maternal role attainment are discussed here; because maternal tasks occur predominantly in the second trimester, they will be discussed in Chapter 17.

Cognitive Operations. Rubin originally formulated a framework for maternal role assumption involving four cognitive operations: mimicry or role play, fantasy, introjection/projection/rejection, and grief work. These original operations have been reformulated into three operations: replication, fantasy, and dedifferentiation.

Replication. Rubin describes **replication** as the voluntary search for and trying on of separate valued elements in behavior and attitude that are esteemed by society and constitute the primary method of incorporation of "binding in" of the maternal role. Replication is a self-initiated activity. The woman actively searches out new desired elements of the maternal role to be replicated or taken on by the self. For example, a newly pregnant woman may observe the behaviors of women more advanced in pregnancy in her obstetrician's or midwife's offices. When she leaves, she may try to copy some of the observed behaviors. In this early phase, most replicative behavior is not integrated into the personality.

Mimicry and role playing are seen as the two forms of replicative behaviors. **Mimicry** is the first suboperation and constitutes literal "copying" of the practices and customs of other women who are or have been pregnant. For example, a woman may copy the ways in which other pregnant women walk, even though physiologically there is no reason for it.

The second form of replication is role playing. **Role playing** is a trying on of the maternal role. Instead of just modeling behaviors, there is now a partner with whom to practice role behaviors. For example, the woman may "practice" being a mother with a pet or niece. While role playing is seen more frequently in primiparas, multiparas role play with their husbands and children "as if" the new infant were born and present.

Fantasy. Fantasy state during pregnancy as a specific psychosocial entity on its own will be discussed separately in this and later chapters. Rubin and others believe, however, that fantasy is an intrinsic component of maternal role-taking. Thus the discussion here will be limited to the role of fantasy as a cognitive operation in assumption of maternal role or identity.

Rubin sees the process of role assumption moving inside the woman through fantasy. **Fantasy** is defined as the projection in imagery of the mother and her child-to-be into the future. Stimulus for fantasy is said to originate in models and situations of replication. In fantasy, there is no third person, however—there is just the mother and her fantasy child. In fantasy, the mother can cognitively explore a variety of situations and experiences she will find herself in with her future infant.

Grief work is incorporated into the cognitive operation of fantasy. As the woman binds in fantasy about future life with the infant, there is a loosening and realigning of bonds to other persons in her "old" life. There is also a loosening of parts of her own personality, aspirations, activities, lifestyle, and life space that she will no longer need for her new life. At first, the woman may resist giving up these facets of life, but as she binds in to the child in fantasies and to her role in mothering this child, she is able to disengage and distance herself from other roles, commitments, aspirations, and involvements. Part of this function of fantasy in resolving grief involves review in memory of past stages of life no longer compatible with the evolving future with a child.

Dedifferentiation. The final phase in maternal role assumption, which incorporates the activities of introjection, projection, and rejection, is dedifferentiation. In reaching this last operation, past operations have greatly changed the woman. Accommodations made in the wish for replication, felt experiences in fantasy, and preparatory relinquishment and reorganization of bonds to self and to others now form a substantive core of maternal identity. With this core, the woman is still receptive to elements for replication of her ideal. Now, however, there is no longer a taking on in mimicry. Instead, the operation available to the mother is dedifferentiation. **Dedifferentiation** refers to the woman's examination and evaluation of the attitudes and behaviors of a model to determine how well these fit with her current self-image as mother. There is a trying on, an introjection of a new modeled element, then a projection of the mental image of the self with that new element in action or in appearance, and the decision to accept or to reject the new element as a congruent part of the self.[38] For example, the mother may have established an attitude about breastfeeding her infant. She may seek out other pregnant women and discuss feeding practices with them. She will then imagine their applicability to her situation. If they do not "fit" her attitudes toward breastfeeding, she will reject them.

The complete attainment of the maternal role or identity, although much of the process has occurred in pregnancy, awaits birth of the infant and an identification of the child in reality.[35]

Lederman's Conceptual Framework for Maternal Role Assumption. Lederman saw maternal assumption, or as she described it, identification with a motherhood role, as part of the larger process of psychosocial development in pregnancy. Lederman's work evolved from a research project that investigated the relationship of maternal psychosocial adaptation in pregnancy to maternal anxiety and labor progress during childbirth.[34]

Lederman described the goal of identification with a motherhood role as a "developmental step of the woman-without-child to be woman-with-child"[34] and indicated that it could be thought of as a process characterized by progressive emphasis in the mother's thinking away from the single self and toward the mother-infant unit. Identification of the motherhood role involved two important factors: how motivated the woman was to assume that role and the extent to which the woman had prepared for a motherhood role. Furthermore, Lederman found identification of the role to be closely related to the woman's relationship with her own mother. These three areas will be discussed in the following section.[34]

Motivation for Motherhood. Motivation for motherhood included concepts of how much a woman wanted to become a mother—her interest and ability to nurture and empathize with a child. In addition, motivation for motherhood included the woman's perception of motherhood as a fulfilling or important event in life. Motivation was questioned if a woman's thoughts about a child were infrequent, aversive, avoided, or denied; or if the woman seemed to desire the pregnancy and not the child.[34]

Preparation for Motherhood. Lederman believed that it was not enough for a woman only to want to be a mother. She also needed to prepare for her new role by envisioning herself as a mother and contemplating her life as a woman with a child. Lederman viewed this as happening mainly through fantasy (both daydreams and night dreams).[16,17] Preparation also includes a woman's life experiences, the degree of conflict resolution a woman attains, and the need to attach to the infant.

Fantasy (Day Dreams). Fantasizing is made up of three processes: envisioning oneself as a mother, thinking about characteristics one would like to have as a mother, and anticipating future life changes that will be necessary with a child. Blocks to these processes were seen as excessive doubts and fears; the inability to accept life change and find compensation in the infant-to-be; and an inability to engage in abstract thought.[34]

Dreaming (Night Dreams). Lederman found dreaming to be important in identifying the motherhood role because dream content tended to parallel a woman's actual concern in waking life. Lederman identified five categories of dreams: reliving childhood, school dreams, motherhood-career conflict dreams, confidence in maternal skill dreams, and food and infant intactness dreams.

Life Experience. Lederman found that a woman's ability to fantasize depended on her life experiences, especially how she was nurtured. If the woman was well nurtured, she generally had a good role model to emulate for mothering. Positive experience with and the ability to identify with other women also were seen as positive factors in assuming the role of mother.[34]

Conflict Resolution. Every woman in Lederman's study brought some conflicts to the pregnancy. If a woman's doubts were not overwhelming, however, conflicts were worked out over the course of the pregnancy, allowing the woman to reach an appropriate level of preparedness and confidence. One conflict reported by Lederman's sample was the need to be a mother and the need to identify oneself as a career woman. If either of these needs was amenable to adjustment, the conflict could be resolved. Sustained motherhood-career conflicts, caused by the mother's unwillingness to let go of parts of her career role or perception of the motherhood role as unrewarding, were, however, seen to raise feelings of inadequacy regarding mothering.[34]

Maternal Attachment Behavior. Attachment behavior includes recognition of the individuality and attributes of the fetus-child, imaginative role rehearsal, thoughts about giving oneself to the child, and fantasy about interacting with the child. Maternal attachment behavior, in Lederman's study, was associated with future acceptance, nurturance and protection of the child, and was seen as a process that begins well before the birth of the infant. Behaviors associated with attachment, according to Lederman, include selection of names, evaluation of feeding methods, talking to the fetus, and touching or stroking fetal parts.

Relationship with the Mother. Although Lederman's study did not include the pregnant woman's relationship with her own mother as a factor in woman's identification with a motherhood role, it indicated that this variable did appear to greatly influence the gravida's identification with the role.[34]

Four components were found to be important in the gravida's relationship with her mother[34]: (1) availability of the grandmother (gravida's mother) to the woman in the past and during pregnancy; (2) the grandmother's reaction to the pregnancy, especially her acceptance of the grandchild-to-be and her acknowledgment of her daughter as a mother; (3) the grandmother's respect for her daughter's autonomy, as demonstrated by relating to the gravida as a mature adult rather than a child; and (4) the grandmother's willingness to reminisce with her daughter about her own childbearing and childrearing experiences.

On the opposite side of the coin, Lederman discerned that the daughter (the gravida) also contributed to the quality of the relationship with her mother (the grandmother). Her ability to empathize with her mother's experiences as a parent and with the changes her mother must go through in transition to her new role as grandparent were seen as important in the mother-daughter relationship.[34]

Lederman indicated that if the gravida's mother is available to her and their relationship is a mutual one the mother will be supportive to the woman during pregnancy and childbirth. The gravida's mother, then, will serve as a constructive role model and can help the gravida establish an identification with the motherhood role.[34]

Role Conflict and Attainment of the Maternal Role. Assumption of a role does not always proceed smoothly. For several reasons, a person may not "fit" into a particular role. These situations are commonly labeled role conflicts, and they evolve continually for individuals who must function in a complex social structure.[44] Role conflicts may develop in several ways. For example, there may be major discrepancies between the anticipated role and the actual, experienced role. Large shifts from familiar to unfamiliar roles, or roles that have conflicting but desired goals may also produce role conflict. Furthermore, inadequate preparation for the role or vague and ambiguous role definitions may also produce role conflict in the individual.[44]

Another potential source of role conflict stems from an individual's membership in multiple groups. It is likely that at least one role necessary for social interactions in one group will be incompatible with a role necessary for interactions in a second group. The necessity to give up or alter one or both roles may produce conflict for the individual.

Several potential situations may directly produce conflict in a woman attempting to move into the maternal role, among them: inability to achieve the "good mother" role; lack of knowledge and preparation for the maternal role; career conflicts; and conflicts in disengaging from past life roles.

Inability to Achieve the "Good Mother" Role. Role conflict will increase if the mother believes that she cannot imitate the "good mother" of her childhood or has unrealistic expectations of the behaviors she will perform as the "good mother." If perceptions of her own mother are unrealistic and idealistic, the woman may fear her perceived inability, or be unable to emulate the desired behaviors. She then sees herself as functioning in the role of the "bad mother."[45]

Lack of Knowledge and Preparation for the Maternal Role. In his now classic work on parenting, LeMasters describes the lack of preparation that individuals in modern society have for assuming roles of mother and father. In a "modern" nuclear family, guidelines for parenting are ambiguous and role models less apparent than in some other family types. Stressors include the rapid necessity to redesign old roles; adapt to new ones; reassess goals, values, and priorities associated with new roles; and determine alternative means of gratification from the new roles.[7] Other investigators have also pointed to the lack of guidelines for successful parenting and the abruptness of the transition to parenthood at the birth of the child.[46,47]

Some of this source of conflict may be alleviated by childbirth preparation during pregnancy and by family living courses in high school. This problem in role assumption, however, will probably continue as society becomes more complex and mobile and the role of parent becomes more and more ambiguous and unclear.

Career Conflicts. Lederman clearly identifies the maternal-role–career-role conflict in her discussion of maternal dreams during pregnancy. Women in Lederman's study equated loss of the career role as loss of self.[34] Kutzner and Toussie-Weingarten identify three factors that prompt the woman with children to work outside the home or pursue a career: economic factors, societal factors (the blurring of traditional roles of mother and father and emergence of androgynous roles), and personal factors.[48] These personal factors include self-respect, self-confidence, and independence gained from a career.[49] The crucial question is whether a woman can successfully integrate career roles and family roles.[50]

Conflicts in Disengaging From Past Life Roles. Rubin's discussion of the grief work that must occur as a woman gives up her previous life to accept a new life with an infant encompasses career conflicts but tends to broaden to the whole of the woman's past life space and lifestyle.[38] Binding in to the fantasy child is viewed as promoting loosening and distancing from other roles, all replete with their commitments, aspirations, and involvements. A key to giving up past roles is the woman's acceptance of new roles involved with the infant-to-be and the feeling that the child compensates for what is given up. If the woman does not perceive compensation as adequate, role conflict may occur.

Establishing a Relationship to the Fetus. During the course of pregnancy, and the transition to a new lifestyle and the maternal role, the mother needs to establish a relationship with the infant-to-be (the fetus). This relationship to the fetus is thought to be a first stage of the establishing of a relationship with the newborn and then the child. Many clinicians have sought ways to foster maternal attachment or "bonding" to the fetus in utero.[51]

Believing that the fetus and then the child actualize the process of becoming a "mother," Rubin sees that the previously mentioned maternal "tasks" must be accomplished to solidify the relationship. The fetus (unless the woman has ultrasound) is only a reality, however, during the second trimester, when fetal movements can be felt. The abstraction of a child is then transformed into the "real" child. Maternal tasks and other aspects of relating to the fetus will therefore be discussed in Chapter 17, concerned with psychosocial changes during the second trimester.

Fantasy During Pregnancy: An Overview. Fantasy is an important factor in assumption of the maternal role and moving into the lifestyle of woman-and-child. Fantasies during pregnancy also have an important role in and of themselves, in allowing the woman to have a "dress rehearsal" in fantasy of labor and delivery and of "mothering" an infant. Further, fantasy allows the pregnant woman to do "the work of worry"[52] that must be done during pregnancy. Realistic fantasies of potential problems that might occur during pregnancy and labor and delivery can help the woman prepare herself to cope with these problems or complications, if they really do occur. Finally, fantasies, especially during the third trimester, may give the nurse clues to concerns the woman may have about pregnancy, birth, and mothering the child.

Fantasies during pregnancy are most vivid (and disturbing) during the third trimester (although they are present to a lesser extent during the first and second trimesters as well). Thus, a more in-depth discussion will appear in Chapter 21 dealing with psychosocial changes during the third trimester.

View of the Self and Body Image During Pregnancy. Another aspect of the psychologic change that the woman undergoes during pregnancy concerns her self and body image. Evolution of a new view of the self is an essential component of the new, altered lifestyle. The self and body image will be different, depending on the woman's trimester of pregnancy. Rubin indicates that there are three spheres of self that are affected and altered by pregnancy: the ideal self, the self image, and the body image.[38]

Ideal Self. The ideal self is composed of all the attributes, qualities, and images that a person would like to have and aspires to include in the self. For the pregnant woman, the ideal self represents her image of the "ideal mother" she would like to become.

Self-Image. Self-image refers to the more reality-oriented, active self. It is the self that will interact with the real world, here and now. It incorporates both the ideal self and the body image, holding the desirable aspects of the ideal self as a standard of behavior to be attained by the woman. As such, it is an evaluation of what the person really is in the real world. This "self" of the expectant mother will evaluate how successfully or unsuccessfully she will be at attaining maternal behaviors.

Body Image. Body image is a view of the self that is critical in the structure and function of the self-image.[53] Body image during pregnancy has to do with a woman's perception of her size, how she moves, and her perceptions of her own physical beauty or ugliness. One vital component of body image that plays a role during pregnancy is body boundary. **Body boundary** separates self from nonself, or the surrounding environment. Body boundary during pregnancy becomes an important protector of the fetus; it literally keeps the fetus inside the woman's protective container of a body.

Mercer found, in her study, that, as pregnancy progresses, the body boundary progressively contracts around the woman and her pregnant self.[54] Fawcett found that women perceive an increase in body boundary as the pregnancy cycle progresses—over and above the actual physical size of the pregnant body and the actual weight gain.[55]

Perceptions of Time and Space During Childbearing. The final aspect that alters during childbearing to allow the mother-to-be to move into a changed lifestyle of woman-and-child is the subjective experience of time and space. The human moves through space over time.[56] Rubin believes that during pregnancy the woman's experience of time and physical and social space changes as extensively as does her pregnant body.[38,57] In each trimester, the woman subjectively experiences the passage of time and her body's movement through her surrounding space very differently. Experiences of time and space during pregnancy will be discussed in subsequent chapters.

Psychologic Changes in the Father: An Overview

Until recently, almost nothing was known about the father's experience of pregnancy and his evolution into the paternal role. Nurses and other health professionals treated fathers as though they had no part in the pregnancy and birth and would have no role in raising the child.

With the advent of family-centered maternity care, however, nurses found themselves caring for the whole family, not just the maternal-infant dyad. Suddenly, what the father and siblings felt and did was of importance, and this knowledge was necessary for delivery of nursing care to the childbearing family unit. Knowledge concerning fathering and the father's experience during pregnancy and childbirth still lags well behind knowledge concerning the mother; however, a beginning in understanding fathering has been made.

Fathers, as well as mothers, must make a major lifestyle change during the childbearing cycle. The man must gain a new perceptual framework, that of man-and-child, to be able to father his infant. Changes that the father must undergo to make the necessary lifestyle shift can, at present, be grouped into two categories:

1. Changes concerned with development of the role of father
2. Changes in the man's experiences that occur during his partner's pregnancy[43]

Development of the Father Role. The role of father can be seen to develop in three interdependent ways:

1. Through personal and environmental factors that occur during the man's course of development
2. Through participation in the childbearing cycle
3. Through interactions with the newborn infant[43]

Developmental Factors. Generally in the course of growing up in a family, the young boy identifies with both his mother and father. Thus, to some extent his adult personality and attitudes will retain some nurturing (mothering) aspects as well as the more traditional, and heavily emphasized, instrumental (fathering) aspects.[58] In many men, then, there is the desire to "create life" like their mothers, and to nurture.

Researchers have identified some other developmental factors associated with the father role.[59] These include the man's childhood experience with his own father, marital satisfaction, and experience with infants.

Participating in the Childbearing Cycle. The father's active participation and involvement in pregnancy, labor, and delivery fosters his perception of himelf in the father role (Fig. 4–3). This involvement also will assist his partner in seeing him as a father.[35, 60, 61] Participation in the childbearing cycle also seems to have an influence on the evolving father-infant relationship and on paternal attachment.[62]

Father-Infant Interactions and the Father Role. Many studies document that the father's interaction with the newborn infant ushers in bond formation between the father and infant and solidifies the father role.[43, 63–67] Fathers have been shown to be able to nurture the newborn as efficiently as mothers and to function as competent infant caregivers.

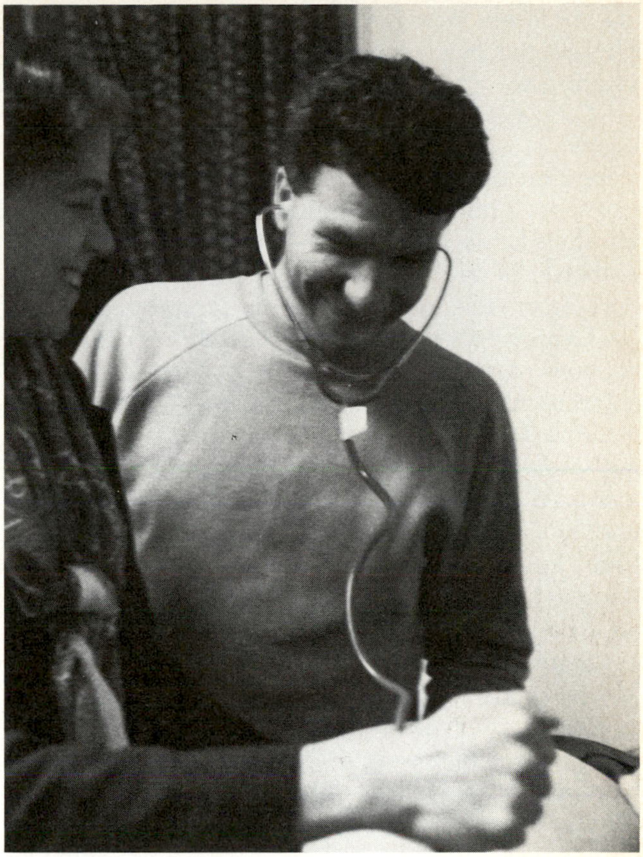

Figure 4–3. Paternal role attainment: a father takes joy in the fetus prenatally.

The Father's Psychologic Experiences During Pregnancy

The Couvade. "Couvade" is an anthropologic term designating a set of rituals or behaviors in certain cultures that regulate paternal actions during childbirth. It is derived from the French verb *couver*, which means "to brood" or "to hatch." In the cultural groups in which couvade is practiced, the man is assisted, by performing certain rituals activities and behaviors, to gain entry into the role of father and to gain acknowledgment of this major transition from his partner and his society.

Interestingly enough, some men in the predominant Western cultures go through what has been called the **couvade syndrome.**[68] This syndrome consists of bodily symptoms experienced by the father during the course of his partner's pregnancy. Symptoms can include gastrointestinal disorders, nausea and vomiting, increased or decreased appetite, backache, toothaches, syncope, fatigue, leg cramps, and weight gain.

Couvade phenomena have had several interpretations. Most commonly, they are believed to be an expression of the father-to-be's involvement in the pregnancy and identification with his partner. Theoretically, the more the father-to-be identifies with the mother-to-be and is involved in the pregnancy, the more he experiences the couvade symptoms.

Clinton followed 81 expectant fathers throughout their partner's pregnancy and postpartum in order to identify factors that might predict those men prone to develop the couvade syndrome. She found that six factors partially explained health events experienced by expectant fathers: effective involvement in the pregnancy, the number of previous children, low socioeconomic status, ethnic identity, perceived stress, and recent health before expectant fatherhood.[69]

In another study, Fawcett demonstrated that the father's body boundaries altered throughout the course of pregnancy and the puerperium, even though his actual weight did not.[55] Thus, involved expectant fathers can and do experience bodily sensations, even though they do not actually carry a fetus.

Stages of the Pregnancy Experience for Men. Although much is still unknown about the progression of the pregnancy experience for an expectant father, at least one study has identified stages through which men involved in the pregnancy (those who are attuned to the pregnancy and their feelings about it) pass. These stages are[70]:

1. The getting ready period (when the couple attempts to create a pregnancy)
2. The stage of conception (when conception is medically confirmed)
3. The end of the first trimester
4. Midpregnancy
5. The stage of turning toward father and fathering (between 15 to 25 weeks of pregnancy)
6. The end of pregnancy (26 weeks to end of pregnancy)

The father-to-be's concerns in each of the stages will be discussed in the later chapters dealing with each specific trimester.

Paternal Fantasies During Pregnancy. Expectant fathers also experience fantasies about the course of the pregnancy and the infant-to-be during pregnancy. It may be that fantasy performs a similar function during pregnancy for the expectant man as it does for the expectant woman.[71] Like those of the expectant mother, an expectant father's fantasies become more vivid toward the end of pregnancy, although some might be present in the first two trimesters as well. In general, however, men seem to be more reluctant to admit to having fantasies (both day and night dreams) during pregnancy than are their partners.

Styles of Paternal Involvement in Pregnancy. Some fathers are "attuned" to their pregnancy experiences and some are not. Fathers who are attuned are able to describe their inner experiences concerning the pregnancy.[70] May studied the experiences of 20 first-time expectant fathers in order to develop a theory that describes a typology of styles adopted by fathers during pregnancy. This theory explains, in part, the phenomenon of an expectant father's involvement (or noninvolvement) in the partner's pregnancy. A man's involvement can be seen on a continuum between two opposing dimensions: he can be either detached from the pregnancy or involved in the pregnancy, or somewhere between the two. The varying level of detachment and involvement characterizes three styles of paternal pregnancy involvement.[72] These are:

- *Observer style.* The man reports certain emotional distance from the pregnancy and sees himself largely as a bystander. This style is the most detached of the three, involes little decision making in the pregnancy, and can have either a happy or unhappy affective state associated with it.
- *Expressive style.* The man reports a highly emotional response to pregnancy and sees himself as a full partner in it. This style allows for more involvement in the pregnancy, and fathers adopting this style often have a high incidence of pregnancy symptoms. These fathers also expect to actively parent their children.
- *Instrumental style.* The man reports an emphasis on tasks to be accomplished and sees himself largely as a caretaker or manager of the pregnancy. These fathers downplay the emotional impact of the pregnancy and pride themselves in carrying out traditional functions central to their role as husband and father. They "take care of business," often making appointments for their wives, keeping wives on diets, and making major purchases and decisions concerning the infant. This style represents a midpoint along the detachment-involvement continuum.

The Sibling's Experience: An Overview

Very little is known about how children in a family adapt to pregnancy and a new infant. Even more baffling is the manner in which a first-born child moves into the new role of brother or sister with the birth of a new infant. It has been estimated, however, that some 80 percent of children in the United States grow up with siblings. Furthermore, the patterns of sibling interactions seem to be established during infancy of the later-born child and continue throughout childhood. These interactions may influence the nature of later relationships between the siblings and may even have an influence on the personality development of each child.[73] Thus it is an area of concern for the nurse delivering family-centered care.

Studies have shown that the relationships between parents and children in a family also may alter during pregnancy and after birth of a new infant. There generally seems to be an increase in confrontation between mothers and first-born children and a decrease in maternal availability to the first-born child.[74,75] Even during pregnancy, the anticipation of the expected birth may affect the parent-child relationship and parental availability to the first-born child.[76]

Kutzner, in an extensive review of the literature, cites many studies that document changes in sibling behavior with birth of a new infant.[77] Withdrawal and antagonism, especially in relation to the new baby, are common. This phenomenon is well known as "sibling rivalry." Current child preparation programs offered by hospitals during pregnancy and sibling visitation, sibling bonding, or sibling presence at the birth are all seen as ways to improve relationships and foster attachment between older children and the new infant.[78] There is, however, little documentation as yet to indicate that these programs actually do improve behaviors of older children. This is an area that requires extensive nursing research.

There is indication that some factors that cannot be altered may play a role in an older child's adaptation to a new baby. The child's age may be a factor, as children younger than five are more likely to become upset by a sibling's birth. In addition, the child's existing personality and the nature and stability of the parent-child relationship may be the most important factor in sibling adjustment.[79] Nurses have a major role in helping the family develop an individualized strategy to support and prepare a child for the mother's pregnancy, labor and delivery, and introduction of the new sibling.[77] They may also need to support the family throughout the older child's course of adjustment to a new sibling.

The Grandparents' Experience: An Overview

To date, there has been almost no research into the psychosocial aspects of becoming a grandparent. This is unfortunate, as we do know how important the grandparents are to the childbearing couple. Furthermore, grandparents may form vital support structures for parents after the birth of the infant. Conversely, grandparents may produce many conflicts for the childbearing family. Subsequent chapters will give some of the scant information that exists about how individuals "move up a generation," graduating from the role of "parent" to that of "grandparent."

SUMMARY

This chapter discusses some theories that allow the nurse to understand the phenomenon of pregnancy and to plan specific care strategies for the family. Some theories do not specifically concern childbearing families but relate closely to events that occur in the families. Other theories relate specifically to childbearing families and were developed through research on pregnant women, their partners, and neonates.

Pregnancy and birth may be seen as a potential crisis situation for families, with all the inherent challenges and opportunities for family growth. Similarly, pregnancy may act as a stressor for individuals and the family as a whole, requiring all members to develop new coping strategies.

Attachment and its component, bonding, are seen as a more comprehensive process of attachment and separation-individuation. These processes describe how family members develop necessary affectional ties to each other, and in addition, function as separate, autonomous individuals.

Transcultural care theory takes the perspective that culture is a vital aspect of each individual's makeup and that care delivered must be culturally relevant and sensitive. Economic status further complicates the picture and has been seen as influencing culturally related behaviors. It is important for the nurse to remember that nursing is also a culture that will shape her or his world view.

Theories that relate specifically to pregnancy or childbearing include theories concerning psychosocial changes in the mother, father, siblings, and grandparents. These changes are discussed in a general overview in this chapter. They will be discussed in more detail in Chapters 13, 17, 21, 26, and 30, which focus on each trimester, the intrapartum period, and the postpartum period.

REVIEW QUESTIONS

1. Discuss at least one of the following theories: Crisis Theory, Stress-Adaptation Theory, Attachment Theory, Separation-Individuation Theory. How do these theories relate to the childbearing cycle?
2. Explain why nursing is considered a "culture."
3. Compare the maternal role assumption theories of Rubin and Lederman. Specify both similarities and differences.
4. Relate each of the three paternal styles during pregnancy to the level of paternal involvement observed.
5. Discuss three characteristics of the sibling experience of pregnancy in the family.

REFERENCES

1. Parad H, Caplan G. A framework for studying families in crisis. In Parad H, ed. *Crisis Intervention: Selected Readings.* New York: Family Services Association of America, 1969.
2. Thibedeau J, Hawkins J. *Primary Care Nursing: Crisis Model in Client Management.* Monterey Calif: Wadsworth Health Science Division, 1982.
3. Hayes G, et al. After disaster: a crisis support team at work. *AJN.* 1990;90(2):61–65.
4. Hoff LA. *People in Crisis: Understanding and Helping.* Menlo Park, Calif: Addison-Wesley Publishing Co., 1978.
5. Fawcett J. *Analysis and Evaluation of Conceptual Models of Nursing.* Philadelphia: FA Davis, 1984.
6. Fawcett J. Conceptual models and theory development. *J Obstet Gynecol Neonatal Nurs.* 1988;17:400–403.
7. LeMasters BE. Parenthood as crisis. In Parad H, ed. *Crisis Intervention: Selected Readings.* New York: Family Services Association of America, 1969.
8. Selye H. *The Stress of Life.* New York: McGraw-Hill Book Co, 1956.
9. Lazarus R. *Patterns of Adjustment and Human Effectiveness.* New York: McGraw-Hill Book Co, 1969.
10. McCubbin H, Patterson JM. Family transitions: adaptation to stress. In McCubbin H, Figley C, eds. *Stress and the Family.* New York: Brunner/Mazel Publishers, 1983, vol 1.
11. Austin MJ. Assessment of coping mechanisms used by parents and children with chronic illness. *J Mat Child Nurs.* 1990;15:98–103.
12. Hill R. Generic features of families under stress. *Soc Casework.* 1958;49:139–150.
13. Klaus M, Kennel J. *Parent-Infant Bonding.* 2nd ed. St. Louis: C.V. Mosby Co, 1982.
14. Tomlinson PS. Verbal behavior associated with indicators of maternal attachment with the neonate. *J Obstet Gynecol Neonatal Nurs.* 1990;19:76–77.
15. Campbell S, Taylor P. Bonding and attachment: theoretical issues. In Taylor PM, ed. *Parent-Infant Relationships.* New York: Grune & Stratton, 1980.
16. Nelson S. Attachment theory. *Nurse Pract.* 1985;10:34–36.
17. Richards MPM. Bonding babies. *Arch Dis Child.* 1985;60: 293–294.
18. Klaus M, Kennell J. Bonding—another view. *Perinatol/Neonatol.* 1984;8:72–73.
19. Bowlby J. *Attachment and Loss.* New York: Basic Books, 1969, vol 1.
20. Ainsworth M. Object relations, dependency, and attachment: a theoretical review of the infant-mother relationship. *Child Dev.* 1969;40:969–1025.
21. Edward J, Ruskin N, Turrini P. *Separation-Individuation: Theory and Application.* New York: Gardner Press Inc, 1981.
22. Mahler, M Pine, F, Bergman A. *The Pyschological Birth of the Human Infant.* New York: Basic Books, 1975.
23. Sherwen L. Separation: the forgotten phenomenon of child development. *TCN.* 1983;3:1–11.
24. Leininger M. Transcultural care diversity and universality: a theory of nursing. *Nurs Health Care.* 1985;6:209–212.
25. Leininger M. Transcultural nursing: its progress and its future. *Nurs Health Care.* 1981;2:365–371.
26. Scott MD, Stern PN. The ethno-market theory: factors influencing childbearing health practices in northern Louisiana black women. *Health Care Women Int.* 1985;6:45–60.
27. Stern PN, Tilden VP, Maxwell EK. Culturally induced stress during childbearing: the Filipino-American experience. *Health Care Women Int.* 1985;6:105–121.
28. Lawson LV. Culturally sensitive support for grieving parents. *MCN.* 1990;15:76–81.
29. Harris C, Stern PN. Women's health and the self-care paradox: case study and analysis. *Health Care Women Int.* 1985;6:165–174.
30. Walker R. Developing cultural awareness. *AORN J.* 1978; 27:1302–1304.
31. Jordan B. *Birth in Four Cultures.* Montreal: Eden Press, 1983.
32. Lewis O. The culture of poverty. *Sci Am.* 1966;7: pp 19–25.
33. Hines PM. The family life cycle of poor Black families. In Carter B, McGoldrick M, eds. *The Changing Family Life Cycle.* 2nd ed. New York: Gardner Press, 1988.
34. Lederman RP. *Psychosocial Adaptation in Pregnancy.* Englewood Cliffs, NJ: Prentice-Hall, 1984.
35. Coleman LL. Psychology of pregnancy. In Sonstegard L, et al, eds. *Women's Health. II: Childbearing.* New York: Grune & Stratton, 1983, pp 3–16.
36. Chalmers B. Behavioral associations of pregnancy complications. *J Psychosom Obstet Gynecol.* 1984;3:27–35.
37. Sherwen LN, et al. Common concerns of adoptive mothers. *Pediatr Nurs.* 1984;10:127–134.
38. Rubin R. *Maternal Identity and the Maternal Experience.* New York: Springer Publishing Co, 1984.
39. Gay JT, et al. Reva Rubin revisisted. *J Obstet Gynecol Neonatal Nurs.* 1988;17:394–399.
40. Osofsky H, Osofsky J. Normal adaptation to pregnancy and

new parenthood. In Taylor PM, ed. *Parent-Infant Relationships.* New York: Grune & Stratton, 1980, pp 25–48.
41. Majewski JL. Conflicts, satisfactions, and attitudes during transition to the maternal role. *Nurs Res.* 1986;31:10–14.
42. Humenick SS, Bugen LA. Parenting roles: expectation versus reality. *MCN.* 1987;12:36–39.
43. Pedersen R, Robson KS. Father participation in infancy. *Am J Orthopsychiatry.* 1969;19:466–472.
44. Minkler M, Biller R. Role shock: a tool for conceptualizing stresses accompanying descriptive role transitions. *Hum Relations.* 1979;32:125–140.
45. Jessner, L, et al. The developing of parental attitudes in pregnancy. In Anthony EJ, Benedek T, eds. *Parenthood: Its Psychology and Psychopathology.* Boston: Little, Brown, 1970.
46. Rossi A. Transition to parenthood. *J Marriage Fam.* 1968; 30:26–39.
47. Bee HL, et al. The impact of parental life and change on the early development of children. *Res Nurs Health.* 1986;9: 65–74.
48. Kutzner S, Toussie-Weingarten C. Working parents. the dilemma of childrearing and career. *Top Clin Nurs.* 1984;6: 30–37.
49. Lancaster J. Coping mechanisms for the working mother. *AJN.* 1975;75:1322–1323.
50. Collins C, Tiedje LB. A program for women returning to work after childbirth. *J Obstet Gynecol Neonatal Nurs.* 1988;17: 246–254.
51. Carlson D, Labarba C. Maternal emotionality during pregnancy and reproductive outcome: a review of the literature. *Int J Behav Dev.* 1979;2:343–376.
52. Levy J, McGee R. Childbirth as a crisis: a test of Janis' theory of communication and stress resolution. *J Pers Soc Psychol.* 1975;31:171–179.
53. Schilder P. *The Image and Appearance of the Human Body.* New York: International Universities Press, 1970.
54. Mercer R. *First Time Motherhood.* New York: Springer, 1986, pp 52–57.
55. Fawcett J. Body image and the pregnant couple. MCN. 1978;4:227–233.
56. Rogers M. *Theoretical Basis of Nursing.* Philadelphia: FA Davis, 1970.
57. Rubin R. Fantasy and object constancy in maternal relations. *Matern Child Nurs J.* 1977;6:67–75.
58. Furlong R, Berkowitz R. Intrauterine treatment: meeting the psychosocial needs of the family. *Health Soc Work.* 1985; 3:55–62.
59. Soule B, et al. Father identity. *Psychiatry.* 1979;42:255–263.
60. Tanzer D, Block J. *Why Natural Childbirth?* New York: Shocken Books, 1976.
61. Porter L, Demeuth B. The impact of marital adjustment on pregnancy acceptance. *MCN.* 1979;8:103–112.
62. Bowen SM, Miller BC. Paternal attachment behavior as related to presence at delivery and preparenthood classes: a pilot study. In Sherwen LN, Weingarten C, eds. *Analysis and Application of Nursing Research: Parent-Neonate Studies.* Monterey, Calif: Wadsworth, 1983.
63. Parke RD. The father's role in infancy: a re-evaluation. *Birth Fam J,* 1975;5:211–213.
64. Kestenberg J, et al. The development of paternal attitudes. In Cath S, et al, eds. *Father and Child.* Boston: Little, Brown, 1982.
65. Ferketich SL, Mercer RT. Men's health status during pregnancy and early fatherhood. *Res Nurs Health.* 1989;12: 137–148.
66. Jones LC, Lenz ER. Father-newborn interaction: effects of social competence and infant state. *Nurs Res.* 1986;35: 149–153.
67. Earls F. The fathers (not mothers): their importance and influence with infants and young children. In Chess S, Thomas A, eds. *Annual Progress in Child Psychiatry and Child Development.* 10th ed. New York: Brunner/Mazel, 1977.
68. Trethoivan WH, Conlon MF. The couvade syndrome. *Br J Psychol.* 1965;3:57–60.
69. Clinton J. Expectant fathers at risk for couvade. *Nurs Res.* 1986;35:290–295.
70. Herzog JM. Patterns of expectant fatherhood: a study of the fathers of a group of premature infants. In Cath S, et al, eds. *Father and Child.* Boston: Little, Brown, 1982.
71. Sherwen LN. Third trimester fantasies of first-time expectant fathers. *Matern Child Nurs J.* 1986;15:153–170.
72. May KA. A typology of detachment/involvement styles adopted during pregnancy by first-time fathers. *West J Nurs Res.* 1980;2:445–453.
73. Dunn J. *Sisters and Brothers.* Cambridge, Mass: Harvard University Press, 1985.
74. Dunn J, Kendrick C. The arrival of a sibling: changes in patterns of interactions between mother and firstborn child. *J Child Psychol. Psychiatry.* 1980;21:119–132.
75. Dunn J, Kendrick C. Interaction between young siblings in the context of family relationships. In Lewis M, Rosenblum LA, eds. *The Child and Its Family.* New York: Plenum Press, 1979.
76. Nedelman L, Begun A. The effect of the newborn on the older sibling: mother's questionnaires. In Lamb ME, Sutton-Smith B, eds. *Sibling Relationships: Their Nature and Significance Across the Lifespan.* Hillsdale, NJ: Lawrence Erlbaum Associates, 1982.
77. Kutzner S. Responses of siblings to pregnancy. In Sherwen LN: *Psychosocial Dimensions of the Pregnant Family.* New York: Springer, 1987.
78. Spadt SK, et al. Experiential classes for siblings to be. *MCN.* 1990;15:184–186.
79. Hines PM, Boyd-Franklin N. Black families. In McGoldrick M, et al, eds. *Ethnicity and Family Therapy.* New York: Guilford Press, 1982.

The Well Woman of Childbearing Age

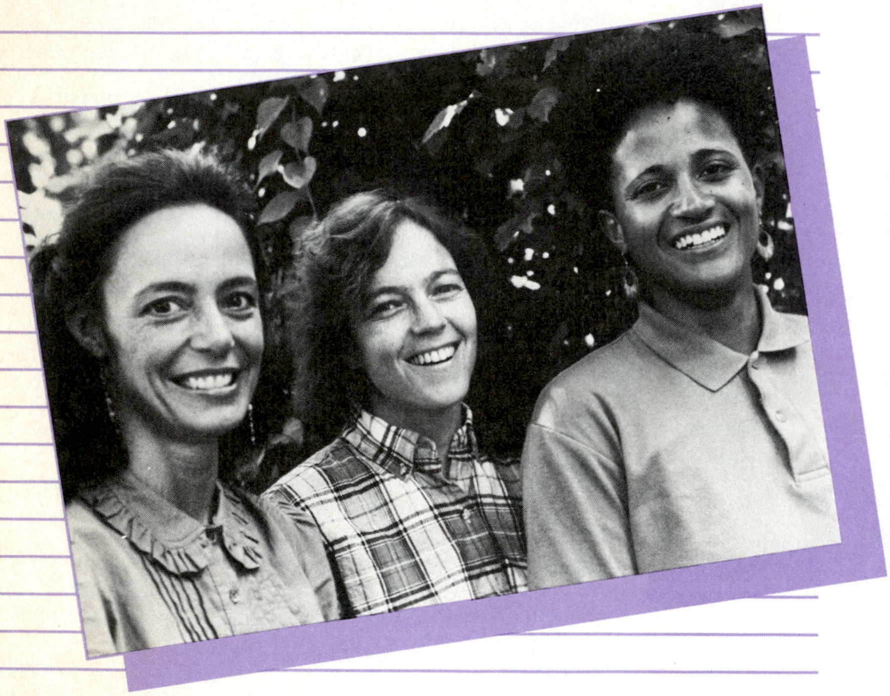

Chapter 5

Key Terms

climacteric
dysmenorrhea
endometriosis
gynecology
mammography
menarche
menopause
menstruation
Papanicolaou (Pap) smear
postmenopausal period
premenopause
premenstrual syndrome
puberty
tampons
toxic shock syndrome

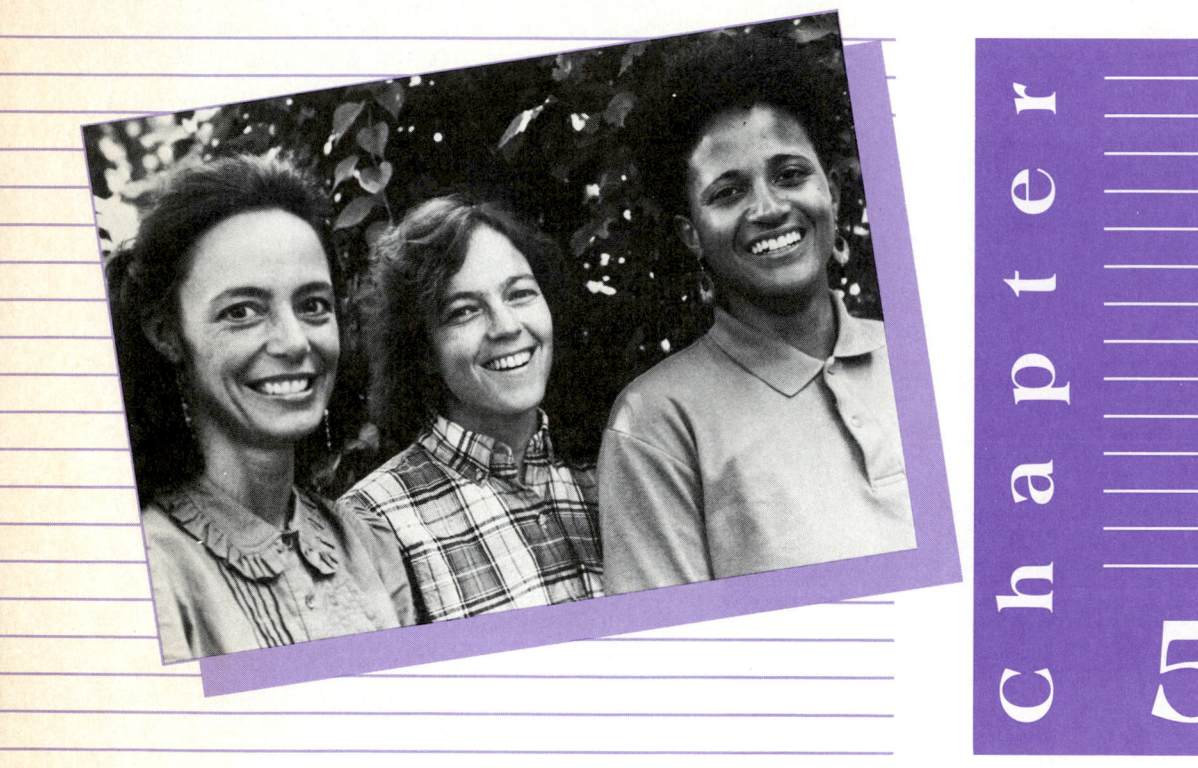

Reproductive health care for the well woman of childbearing age is a major nursing focus. Indeed, the well woman often has initial and ongoing contact with health care providers because of services related to reproductive care. Nurses specializing in health care of women need to develop excellent overall assessment, communication, and teaching skills. In addition to provision of gender-related care, nurses serve as important sources of information and referral for follow-up of physical, emotional, and social problems experienced by the woman client and her family.

Traditionally, health care of women was classified as part of **gynecology**, the branch of medicine dealing with the physiology and the pathology of the female reproductive organs in the nonpregnant state, or obstetrics, which deals with the physiology and pathology of the female reproductive organs during and related to pregnancy.[1] Gynecology is, however, only one aspect of the care of women. Health care providers need to regard women clients as more than the sum of their reproductive organs.[2] To deliver optimal care to women, nurses need to understand the physical, psychologic, sociocultural, historic, and political factors related to being female. Women's health care focuses not only on illness, but on wellness and on health promotion. Issues such as exercise, nutrition, employment, daycare, hazards in the workplace, mental health, and victimization are examples of topics related to women's health.

The purpose of this chapter is to address reproductive health and the well woman of childbearing age; however, complete coverage of women's health is beyond the scope of this book. The nurse working with women clients is therefore referred to the extensive literature that exists on women's health.

SOCIAL TRENDS AND WOMEN'S HEALTH CARE

Historically, health care for women has been directed toward gynecologic and reproductive concerns and has reflected the views of society as a whole toward women. Throughout history there have been examples of outstanding women who have forged leadership or otherwise unique roles for themselves. Most American females were, however, raised to be the "woman behind the man." An economically good marriage and children to provide a man with heirs were, for a daughter, basic lifetime hopes. Education in the domestic arts and at times elaborate social rituals, such as "coming out" parties, were employed to make girls more marketable to eligible men. Marriages were frequently arranged to unite families. The roles of wives and mothers were women's primary ones in the United States, where women did not have the basic right to vote confirmed until the nineteenth amendment to the US Constitution was ratified in 1920. Indeed, women were traditionally considered as existing primarily to continue the species and were regarded as property of their fathers and husbands, although in rural agricultural areas women necessarily assumed more of a partnership type of role in marriage. Nevertheless, in many states, on marriage, men gained complete control of their wives' property.

During periods of national stress, such as war, women effectively pitched in and competently attended to jobs in industry and business. When the men were again available, women tended to return to the home, which was considered their natural environment.[3] Women who sought a career were frequently regarded as eccentric, unmarriageable, or as having to work because of unfortunate circumstances. Female physiology was also frequently cited as a reason to bar women from careers. For example, monthly changes associated with normal body functions, such as menstruation, were used as excuses to keep women away from decision-making jobs.[2]

The women's movement, which had roots in the late nineteenth- and early twentieth-century women's suffrage activities, and which gained momentum during the 1960s and 1970s, had far-reaching effects on the expectations and roles of women. Women began to organize, to question female stereotypes, to push against restrictive roles, to identify womanhood as special, and to reinforce the idea that women are different from, but not inferior to, men. A major belief of the women's movement was that women needed to be educated about their own bodies.[4] Well-woman care became a major priority, linked to the overall status of women in American society.

Women and Health Care

Unfortunately, women's reproductive functions have traditionally been viewed from an illness or paternalistic (father or physician knows best) perspective. The treating of women in gynecologic settings, rather than comprehensive women's health facilities, highlights this pathologic orientation. In such settings, the woman client was often treated like a child and the (usually) male physician as the parent who made important decisions for her about topics such as childbearing and contraception. Such an approach was fostered to some degree by compliance on the part of the woman herself. This may have reflected such factors as the role of women in society or, generally, the passive and vulnerable role of clients in the health care system.

The women's movement, as well as other social trends in the 1960s, 1970s, and 1980s, has begun to change the focus of health care toward a more self-care–focused model. The woman client is becoming more widely regarded as an active participant and decision maker in the health care process. Littlefield noted that health education assumes great importance for women, because women tend to consider health a significant aspect of life, are more likely than men to pursue health as a goal, and are frequently responsible for the health of others such as their husbands, children, and relatives.[5] She suggested that health education strategies that focus on women and include lifestyle and behaviors might have the related benefit of improving the health of the population in general.

Currently there is wide variation in accessibility, quality, and approach to health care for the well woman of childbearing age. Although the professional and lay literature consistently encourages assessment of the whole client and family, in reality women's health care often remains fragmented. Most reproductive health care is given in gynecologic settings where heavy client loads limit the amount of time caregivers spend with the client. The focus of care may be only on the reproductive organs. The scheduling of appointments for well women several months after requests are made, or the request that women "call back next month when the schedules are available," serve as deterrents to wellness-oriented care. In addition, high liability for obstetrics and gynecology for both physicians and nurse practitioners has detracted from the recruitment appeal of this once-popular specialty. This has a potential long-term effect of limiting the availability of health care professionals specializing in reproductive care.

From their initial contacts with clients in office and clinic settings, nurses have important roles in assessment and intervention. Much of the nursing care for the well woman of childbearing age involves teaching directed toward health maintenance and health promotion. In addition, nurses can do much to support women receiving wellness care and to ensure appropriate referrals whenever appropriate.

Providers of Well-Woman Health Care

In some settings, wellness care is planned and implemented by nurses who refer clients to physicians when medical problems are identified. Health assessment, including complete physical examinations, may be done by nurse specialists such as certified nurse-midwives, nurse practitioners, or nurses with other advanced specialty credentials. Nurse specialists work in health clinics and in private practices under several types of practice arrangements. For example, nurse specialists may be in independent practice, group practice with other nurse specialists, or group practice with physicians and other health care providers. When standing orders have been provided by a physician, nurse specialists may also dispense medications such as birth control pills. In the United States, however, there are many more physicians than nurse-midwives or nurse practitioners. Therefore, most physical assessment of the well woman is done by physicians (usually gynecologists) in private offices or in clinics.

Although the staff nurse in a well-woman setting usually does not perform certain physical assessment procedures such as vaginal examinations, he or she has a major role in other aspects of assessment, intervention, and education. The staff nurse's role may encompass most of the teaching that clients receive. Indeed, the nurse can take the opportunity to identify a unique professional role in the care of the well woman client. As in any setting, an interdisciplinary approach that involves all members of the wellness team and that focuses on accomplishing client- and family-centered goals is essential.

Settings for Well-Woman Health Care

Well-woman health care may be delivered in a variety of settings. These include clinics in hospitals, schools, or community settings, private offices run by physicians or nurse specialists, and health maintenance organizations. In addition to providing prenatal care, birth centers may offer wellness care for the nonpregnant woman.

Some settings for well-woman health care may be lavishly decorated, while others may have only the most basic equipment. In certain poverty areas or places where there are no established health care facilities, well-woman care may be provided wherever an examining area can be devised. Regardless of the setting, the philosophy of the caregivers, their expertise, and their commitment to thorough assessment and understanding of the client are critical to ensuring quality care.

THE WELL-WOMAN HEALTH VISIT

Goals

The goals of the well-woman health visit focus on primary prevention, secondary prevention, and health promotion.

Primary prevention involves specific protection against disease to prevent its occurrence.[6] Examples of primary prevention include rubella immunization for nonpregnant women. Although pregnancy certainly is not a disease state, family planning counseling may be considered primary prevention.

According to Pender, secondary prevention includes "organized, direct screening efforts or education of the public to promote early case finding of individuals with disease, so that prompt intervention can . . . halt pathologic processes and limit disability."[6] A major goal of the history, physical, and laboratory assessment is the identification of abnormalities. For example, cancer of the cervix has a nearly 100 percent cure rate if detected early. Early detection of breast cancer and the stage of the disease at diagnosis seem to affect a woman's survival more than any type or types of treatment.[7]

Health promotion focuses on activities that raise the level of well-being and help clients actualize their health.[6] Primary and secondary prevention are disease- or problem-specific and help thwart the occurrence of an undesirable condition. Health promotion helps or encourages certain behaviors. Client history, physical, and laboratory evaluation assist the nurse in identifying client and family strengths so that health promotion goals can be planned. Health promotion activities for the well woman might include learning about dietary planning for optimal health.

During the well-woman visit, the nurse conducts and participates in client assessment to evaluate the woman's overall level of wellness, her knowledge of her own body and health-promoting behaviors, and the presence of abnormal conditions. The nurse has a major role as a facilitator who teaches clients how to assess themselves, decide on wellness goals, develop strategies to meet those goals, and evaluate their success.[8]

Beginning the Visit

The wellness health visit actually begins with the scheduling of the appointment, usually initiated by the client. In some settings, a nurse speaks to each client by telephone prior to the first visit, particularly if the client is coming because of a specific problem. In many settings, the actual scheduling is done by the secretarial staff. The nurse and physician need to ensure, however, that accurate information is given in a courteous manner, and that appropriate referral is made whenever clients have questions. At the time of the initial contact, several goals need to be accomplished:

- *To welcome the client into the health care system.* Most established health care systems operate on an advance appointment basis, although some, especially in school or college settings, may have "walk in" hours for well-woman care. A welcoming, friendly approach that encourages wellness assessment is important. Many clients need courage simply to call.
- *To identify the reason for the visit.* While every attempt should be made to avoid delays in any client's visits, clients who have possible pathologic conditions (eg, breast lump) or who have discomfort (eg, vaginal infections) need to be seen without delay. Clients with certain pathologic conditions can be directly referred elsewhere, if necessary, thereby sparing them delays and appointment fees. Waiting several months for an appointment may deter a client from even coming for care; therefore, practitioners in clinic and private settings should have referral sources accessible. No client should ever be turned away without appropriate referral.
- *To identify who will examine the client at the time of the visit.* This is especially important in clinic or group practice situations where the client is likely to see any of several health care providers. Knowing which person will attend her visit promotes a feeling of personalized care. Clients scheduling return visits should be asked whom they had seen previously and whether they would like their appointment scheduled with the same person. Staff who work in clinics where clients are seen by resident physicians or rotating midwives can post rotation schedules if possible and inform clients over the telephone of the name of the health care provider they may expect to see. In this way, clinic clients can receive the same courtesy and information as private clients.
- *To outline briefly what can be expected at the visit.* Although this can be discussed over the telephone, staff can develop a pamphlet that can be mailed to the client in advance of the visit.

Well-woman health care, like any aspect of client care, is based on subjective and objective assessment, diagnosis, goals, interventions, and evaluation, the steps of the nursing process. For the well woman, much of the focus of the health visit is primary prevention——that is, providing immunizations and education for promotion of health—and secondary prevention—that is, screening for abnormalities. Nurses have important roles in both aspects of care.

Nurses should welcome the client and provide basic anticipatory guidance about the visit. This information could include:

1. The name and status of health care personnel who will work with the client that day. For example, after introducing herself or himself, the nurse could inform the client that the nurse practitioner, "Ms Jones,"will perform the examination.
2. Information about what will happen during the visit. The client should be aware that a history will first be taken, certain laboratory specimens, such as blood and urine samples, will be obtained, and that a physical examination, including a pelvic examination, will be performed.
3. Whether the physician or nurse practitioner will speak with them in the examining room or in a conference room after they are dressed and whether the nurse will provide specific teaching. Speaking with the client after she is dressed promotes a sense of dignity for the client and facilitates an atmosphere in which discussion can take place.

Assessment

Well-woman assessment includes a history, a physical examination, and laboratory data. The history is a thorough report of the client's current and past health. From the recorded history alone, the reader should be able to have a distinct picture of the client's health status and concerns.[9] The history provides background information that directs health care providers during the physical examination and identifies areas for special focus. Figure 5–1 provides a sample outline for a well-woman health history.

The well-woman history may be obtained from the client (and her significant others, when appropriate) through individual interviews or a combination of interviews, questionnaires, and previous records. Obviously, questionnaires or other written methods of history taking should be avoided if clients are not able to read or write. Interpreters should be used whenever the examiner or staff nurse does not speak the same language as the client. Attention needs to be given to any questionnaires translated into another language, because one language does not translate into another word for word. Attempts to make literal (word-for-word) translations can have inaccurate or insulting results.

The usual interval between well-woman health visits is about 1 year, although some women may come more frequently (eg, for weight management programs or because they are at higher risk for breast cancer). A comprehensive history therefore needs to be taken because of the long interval between visits.

The history provides subjective data, ie, informa-

Goals: to gather data from which a care plan can be developed
to identify woman's perception of her own needs
to recognize potential problems and strengths
to identify educational needs

Background Information

Full name
Address, accessible telephone; length of time at address
Date and place of birth
Primary language spoken; other languages spoken
Educational background; student status; last year of school completed, particular learning difficulties
Usual occupation; past employment if relevant; hours of work
Financial status (client's perception of whether or not income meets basic needs, eg, food, shelter, clothing)
Health insurance; insurance for wellness and illness
Other source(s) of health care (present and past, also includes herbalists and other alternative sources of health care)
Overall satisfaction with lifestyle

Marital status (married, single, widowed, divorced):
- Partner's name
- Partner's occupation
- Partner's address, if different from client
- Partner's overall health; client's identification of any health problems (including drug or alcohol abuse)
- Overall evaluation of relationship with spouse (include incidents or fear of abuse)

Children:
- Ages, health status
- Children's addresses (if different from client's address)
- Children's health status
- Child care arrangements
- Perceived personal problems related to parenting

Significant others:
- Relationships, ages, addresses if appropriate
- Dependents
- Substance abuse or other problems in any members of household (includes cigarettes, alcohol, drugs, and so forth)
- Perceived personal problems related to significant others

Cultural history; includes cultural beliefs related to wellness, diet, reproduction, family planning, examination of breasts or genitals by self or others, preventive practices, culturally prescribed treatments, visits to culturally identified healers and others

Religious background

Racial background

Current visit
- Reason for current visit
- Client's stated goals for current visit
- Client's concerns related to current visit

Current and past state of health
- History of present state of health
  - Client's perception of usual state of health
  - Client's perception of being at risk for any health problem
  - Allergies (foods, medications, and so forth)
  - Medications
  - Special health requirements
- Past health history
  - Previous wellness visits
  - Previous illnesses (hospitalizations, surgery, childhood illnesses, and so forth)
  - Accidents and injuries
  - Immunizations (type, dates)
  - Medications
- Family history
  - Acute or chronic illnesses in any family members (especially client's parents, grandparents, siblings)
  - Date and reason for death of family members, if appropriate
  - Congenital problems in family members
  - Family attitudes and practices related to wellness

Review of Systems

General: Overall feelings of wellness; fatigue, chills, fever, weakness, night sweats; unexplained feelings of illness

Integument:

Skin: Intact, scaling, changes in pigmentation, presence of warts, moles, birthmarks; changes in moles; lesions, acne, dryness, rashes, bruising, swelling

Hair: Any change in pattern of hair growth or loss; chemical treatments (coloring, depilatories, and so forth)

Nails (hands and feet): Any changes in color, shape, or condition of nails; nail biting; infections around or under nails

HEENT:

Head: Headaches (location, duration, frequency, treatments, perception of cause), dizziness, loss of consciousness, injury related to any cause

Eyes: Problems seeing (for any reason, specify), eyeglasses or contact lenses (corrective or cosmetic purposes), eye infections, tearing, pain, previous surgery or injury, discharge, date of last eye examination; family history of eye disease

Ears: Tinnitus, discharge, pain, history of infections, vertigo, hearing aids, history of hearing impairment, date of last hearing examination

Nose and sinuses: Nasal discharge, bleeding (frequency, amount, client's perception of cause), sinus problems, frequent colds, loss of smell, nasal obstructions, drug use ("snorting"), smoking, treatments (prescribed by self or others)

Mouth: Type of oral hygiene; knowledge and regularity of oral hygiene practices; prosthetics (dentures, braces, other corrective applicances), lesions on lips or anywhere in mouth, "cold" sores (frequency, severity), excessive salivation, problems with teeth, lumps in mouth, difficulty speaking, change in taste of foods, sore or bleeding gums, discoloration in mouth (mucosa or teeth), last dental examination, regularity of dental evaluation

Throat: Difficulty swallowing, soreness, infections, hoarseness, irritations, coughing, treatments (prescribed by self or others)

Neck: Swelling, soreness, stiffness, lumps, thyroid problems

Cardiovascular: Chest pain, palpitations, claudication, varicosities, edema, shortness of breath; number of pillows used for sleeping; mottling of skin; hypertension; history of heart murmur, rheumatic fever, congenital heart problems; any type of cardiac disease; smoking, exercise patterns; exercise tolerance

Respiratory: Shortness of breath; difficult or painful breathing; cyanosis; cough (productive, nature of secretions, presence of blood); allergies, wheezing, history of respiratory infections (type; treatments), night sweats; history of emphysema, asthma, tuberculosis, bronchitis; date and results of chest x-rays; tuberculin tests; smoking habits; respiratory medications taken

Figure 5–1. Sample outline for a well-woman health history. (*Figure continues.*) (*Reproduced, with permission, from Block GJ, Nolan JW.* Health Assessment for Professional Nursing. *2nd ed. Norwalk, Conn: Appleton-Century-Crofts, 1986.*

Gastrointestinal: Appetite, difficulty swallowing, bowel patterns, changes in bowel or stool patterns, diarrhea, constipation, hemorrhoids, rectal bleeding or blood in stool (frank blood or "tarry" stools), jaundice, history of ulcers; nausea, vomiting, gallbladder disease, hepatitis; anorexic or bulemic behaviors; use of antacids, laxatives, or other drugs for gastrointestinal purposes; history of enteric infections or parasites (dates, type of treatment and success)

Urinary: Frequency, polyuria, urgency, pain, burning, itching, pyuria, hematuria, nocturia, color change in urine, foul odor, hesitancy, incontinence, leakage, history of urinary tract infection or trauma (dates and treatment), use of diuretics or other drugs

Reproductive:

Breasts: Pain, lumps, lesions, nipple discharge, history of breast disease of any kind (including types and dates of treatment), understanding of breast self-examination, regularity of breast self-examinations, etc), client's perceptions of own risks for breast disease

Menstrual history: date of beginning of last menstrual period, age at menarche, length of cycles, duration of menses, regularity, character of menses, menorrhagia, metrorrhagia, dysmenorrhea, premenstrual symptoms, current or previous treatments for menstrual problems

Family planning history: Birth control practices (attitude toward birth control, types of methods used at present and in past, level of understanding of methods, satisfaction with methods, problems related to methods)

Obstetric history: Current possibility of pregnancy; previous pregnancies (planned, unplanned), outcome of previous pregnancies, dates and types of deliveries, infant's birth weight and status, obstetric or neonatal complications and treatments; infertility problems and treatments.

Gynecologic history: Vaginal discharge (nature, amount, duration, foul odor), itching, burning, lesions, past vaginal infections (type, dates, treatments); gynecologic problems of infectious (eg, sexually transmitted diseases) or noninfectious origins (eg, endometriosis, fibroids, surgery), including dates and treatments. Date of last Pap test; understanding and practice of genital self-examination.

Sexual history: Frequency of sexual relations; sexual orientation (homosexual, heterosexual, bisexual); satisfaction with the sexual relationship; client's perception of problems or concerns related to own sexuality or sexual relationship; understanding of risk for sexually transmitted diseases; history of multiple sexual partners

Musculoskeletal: Pain, stiffness, limited movement, history of injury or disease, redness, swelling, deformities of joints; skeletal deformities (eg, scoliosis); vigorous activity (regular practice or recent undertaking)

Neurologic: Seizures (type, onset, treatment, level of control), tremors, problems with balance, speech, weakness or paralysis (transient or permanent), problems with gait, paresthesias, loss of consciousness, loss of memory, mood swings, depression, anxiety or other mental symptoms, drug use and effects

Hematopoietic: Current or past anemia (type and treatment), sickle-cell (trait or disease), bleeding or other blood disorders, including frequent unexplained bruising, transfusions (dates, reasons, reactions), history of hemophilia in family

Lymphatic: Pain, tenderness, swelling, infections of any nodes

Endocrine: Change in glove or shoe size, hirsutism, excessive sweating, excess thirst, polyuria, polyphasia, goiter, other endocrine problems and treatments; heat or cold intolerance; unexplained weight change

Lifestyle

Nutritional history: Access to adequate foods; location of meals; food preparation (self or others); typical 24-hour or weekly diet; vitamin and mineral supplements; types of foods preferred; snacking patterns; fluids (type, amount, including alcoholic beverages); allergies to foods (specify allergy and type of reaction); dietary supplements (type, amount, duration) recent weight gain or loss; salt intake; caffeine intake; ingestion of nonfood items. Client's perception of being overweight, underweight, or normal weight; weight control practices; satisfaction with current nutritional status and weight; weight fluctuations; use of diet aids

Smoking: Nonsmoker, current smoker (specify type); length of time smoking; amount smoked; brand; level of understanding of effects of smoking; desire to quit; attempts to quit; history of smoking-related illnesses; smokers in home or work environment

Drug use: Present or past use of drugs (prescription or recreational, type, and route of administration), history of intravenous drug use. History of sharing needles or other drug equipment; drug treatment programs (date and effects of treatment); illnesses related to drug use (cellulitis, hepatitis, human immunodeficiency virus seroconversion, HIV infection, and so forth)

Alcohol intake: Current intake (amount, type, frequency); previous or current intake of history of alcohol treatment; alcohol-related illnesses (physical, mental, social)

Occupational history: Type of present or past jobs (includes work for monetary or nonmonetary pay and includes occupations of housewives and househusbands); job satisfaction; description of the physical work environment, including size of work area, ventilation, noise levels, safety measures, exposure to chemical or other potentially hazardous conditions (eg, asbestos, benzene, oils), stress (means of relieving stress, support from others, occupational transitions, and client's reactions), exposure to heat or cold, protective devices available and used; client's perceptions of specific present or past occupational hazards

Exposure to infectious diseases: Known exposure, (eg, from known contacts at home, work, or during travel); contact with animals or animal excrement, especially cat feces

Sleep, rest, exercise and activity patterns: Amount and pattern of sleep and rest; amount and type of exercise; regularity of exercise programs; client's reaction to exercise; level of exercise; client's perception of own activities

Stress patterns: Client's perception of acute or chronic stress; reactions to stress; ways of coping with stress; effectiveness of coping strategies; individuals who assist client in dealing with stress

Threats to safety: History of trauma; history of current or past mental or physical abuse (client as victim of abuse)

Interpersonal relationships: Presence of support system; resource people available; degree of social isolation

Concluding impression

Figure 5–1. *(continued)* Sample outline for a well-woman health history.

tion that the client reports. The physical examination, measurement of physical parameters such as blood pressure, and laboratory data provide objective data, ie, information the health care provider identifies through his or her own senses or information contributed by specific tests.[9] All three are necessary for complete health assessment of any client. The client history for the well woman is taken first; the physical examination is then performed. As summarized in Table 5–1, a variety of screening tests may be performed during a well-woman visit. Relevant specimens for laboratory analysis are obtained before physical examination (eg, urine sample), during the physical examination (eg, cervical specimens), or after the physical examination (eg, blood specimens, although in some places these may be drawn at other times). History, physical examination, and laboratory values are recorded in this order.

Nursing diagnoses and client care goals are developed from all the assessment information. Comprehensive assessment is not only necessary to provide high-quality wellness care, but is also a standard to which nurses may be legally held. In addition, understanding of wellness is necessary in order to identify pathologic conditions.

TABLE 5–1. SCREENING TESTS PERFORMED DURING A WELL-WOMAN VISIT

Blood pressure
Pulse
Temperature
Respirations
Height
Weight
Blood tests during gynecologic visit: hemoglobin and hematocrit rubella titer (unless recently documented as immune) blood glucose
Blood tests during comprehensive examination: complete blood count electrolytes cholesterol and complete lipid profile blood type and antibody screen
Optional screening blood tests for clients at risk: HIV, hepatitis B, toxoplasmosis, syphilis, other
Stool hematest; stool analysis for ova and parasites for individuals from areas where parasitic diseases are problems
Urine (protein, glucose, acetone, blood)
Cytology specimen, eg, Pap test
Specimens for gonorrhea, chlamydia, herpes, or other sexually transmitted diseases, as indicated
Tine test/PPD screening for tuberculosis
Mammogram (depending on woman's age, history, and risk factors)

HIV = human immunodeficiency virus, PPD = purified protein derivative.

Important components of the well-woman history are: background information, including demographic, socioeconomic, and cultural data; the client's reason for her visit; current and past state of health; review of systems with respect to symptoms; and history related to other lifestyle factors affecting health, such as sexual history, smoking, drug and alcohol patterns, and occupational history (*see* Figure 5–1).[9,10] In women's health settings, special attention is given to reproductive history, ie, menstrual history, family planning history, obstetric history, and sexual history. A complete physical may be done if the well-woman visit involves comprehensive assessment. Figure 5–2 provides a sample outline for a well-woman physical examination. In gynecologic settings, the physical examination is frequently modified to focus on the reproductive system, including the breasts. Constraints, such as lack of time or the nature of the setting, may make the outlines unworkable in certain situations. The reader is therefore encouraged to adapt the outlines provided to meet the needs of individual clinical circumstances or clients.

The well woman often uses a gynecologic health care provider as her only source of wellness assessment.[10] Therefore, gynecologists, nurse midwives and other gynecologic nurse specialists may be placed in a role of primary care provider, rather than as an expert referral who focuses only on gynecologic assessment. Women's health care providers must be able to identify potential nongynecologic problems and be able to refer clients appropriately, especially in settings in which only gynecologic management can be performed. For example, a woman who reports persistent headaches may be referred to an internist or neurologist; a woman with a breast lump found on physical examination may be referred to a surgeon; a woman who is identified as being abused may be referred to emergency assistance services.

Strategies to Ensure Comprehensive Wellness Evaluation

Health care providers can use several strategies to ensure that the client receives a comprehensive wellness evaluation. These include:

1. Provision of sufficient time for wellness evaluation. The initial wellness visit is time-consuming and may require about an hour and a half for the history and physical. Return visits normally take less than an hour, because the history only needs to be updated rather than re-created. Additional time may be required for all wellness clients if screening tests such as mammograms or blood profiles are performed. Wellness visits are elective

Name
Age
Sex
Height
Weight

Vital signs:
Temperature
Pulse
Respirations
Blood pressure (both arms; sitting, standing, supine)

General impression

Neurologic status: Mental status; motor function; reflexes

Integument: Skin color, texture, lesions, (breaks, bruising, rashes, sores, pigmented areas, moles or warts, infected areas); hair (skin or hair parasites); nails (fingernails, toenails)

HEENT:

Head: Size; lesions, lumps, scaling, parasites; facial symmetry; edema

Eyes: Alignment; lids; lacrimal apparatus; conjuctiva; cornea; sclera; irises; pupils; lenses; ophthalmoscopic; presence of infection; pupils equal and react to light and accomodation (PEARLA)

Ears: Hearing; external ear; otoscopic (ear canals, tympanic membranes)

Nose and sinuses: Nasal septum; mucosa; presence of inflammation, discharge, lesions, polyps; pain or tenderness

Oral cavity: Condition of mouth; lesions or bleeding of lips, gums, tongue or oral cavity; condition of teeth (obvious decay, missing teeth; oral appliances), condition of tongue, pharynx, and tonsils; pain or soreness

Neck: Masses, edema, tenderness; position of trachea; nonpalpable thyroid, lymph nodes

Chest: Character and rate of respirations; symmetry of chest expansion; lungs clear; masses or tenderness; presence of infections

Breast: See Table 5–2

Cardiac and peripheral vascular: Presence, rate, and regularity of cardiac and peripheral pulses; no carotid bruits; no heart murmurs; color and temperature of extremities; any evidence of varicosities or phlebitis; any evidence of needle tracks, shunts, or other vascular invasions

Abdomen: Symmetry; muscle tone; presence of masses; tenderness; scars; bowel sounds; aortic size; nonpalpable and nontender spleen and kidneys; no liver enlargement or tenderness; presence of hernias; no lymph node enlargement or tenderness

Genitalia and anal area: See Table 5–2

Musculoskeletal:

Neck: pain, condition of temporomandibular joint

Back: posture, pain or tenderness, deformity or curvature

Extremities: symmetry of arms and legs; pain in joints, muscles or bones; redness, swelling; restricted movement

Concluding impression

Figure 5–2. Sample outline for a well-woman physical examination.

visits and therefore should be scheduled when health care providers will have ample time to devote to the client. In some settings, only a few "first time" clients are scheduled per client care session. "Squeezing" a client in may be more of a disservice than a courtesy, as staff may be rushed and the quality of care may be compromised.

2. Communication of time requirements to staff and to clients. During an initial wellness visit, the woman may be seen by several health care providers, including a staff nurse and nurse practitioner or physician. Although actual time spent with a client is based on the woman's unique needs, staff need to have a general time plan for initial and follow-up visits. Clients should also be informed about the expected length of the visit so that arrangements for child care, time away from home or work, and parking can be made.
3. Creation of an environment conducive to client assessment. Client evaluation should be done in a setting that affords privacy. When separate rooms are not available, screens or curtains may be used. Voice tones need to be kept low enough so that conversations cannot be overheard. The client needs to be reassured that confidentiality will be maintained.
4. Understanding that many women may dread or fear aspects of physical assessment such as breast, pelvic, and rectal examinations. Anticipatory guidance, a supportive attitude, and the use of relaxation techniques during the examination (see later discussion) can do much to foster a therapeutic working relationship. Understanding various cultural reactions to gynecologic assessment is also essential.
5. A nonjudgmental, interested professional approach. Proper introduction of all health care providers is essential. A nonjudgmental attitude, good listening and observation skills, the ability to ask questions in a nonthreatening manner, and the ability to convey genuine interest in the client are qualities that foster the client-nurse relationship and therefore contribute to client assessment.
6. A focus on women's health, as well as on gynecologic topics.
7. A collaborative approach toward the wellness history. Traditionally, separate histories have been taken by health care professionals from different disciplines. At times, health care providers focus only on their specialty and do not read what others have written. This results in fragmented care, although the staff may take the histories within minutes of each other in the same facility. Although health care disciplines each have a unique

body of knowledge, there are many overlapping areas of information. In reality, clients are often asked many of the same background questions by nurses, physicians, dietitians, and others. This approach wastes time for everyone, detracts from rapport between clients and health care providers, and can limit the opportunities for interventions such as client teaching. When staff all focus on the same questions at the beginning of the outline, information dealing with topics toward the end may not be obtained. Through advance collaboration with each other, health care providers can develop a comprehensive history-taking approach that obtains necessary information without duplication and that makes best use of the expertise of various health care professionals. An efficient and comprehensive approach to history taking demonstrates respect for clients and encourages health care providers to work together.

8. Use of a topic-oriented outline for client assessment (*see* Figure 5–2).

Gynecologic Assessment

The gynecologic physical examination (Table 5–2) includes evaluation of the breast and related structures (Figure 5–3),[11] the external genitalia, vagina, cervix, uterus and adnexa, and rectum. Regular gynecologic examination is important for primary and secondary prevention and health promotion. The gynecologic physical examination is performed by a nurse specialist, such as a certified nurse-midwife, or by a physician. To protect both the client and examiner against misunderstandings, misconduct, or charges of misconduct, a female staff member remains during the physical examination. To promote the client's comfort, a partner, friend, or relative may be invited to accompany the client during the physical examination, if the client so desires. The history may be taken with only one health care specialist present. In many instances, clients appreciate having a significant other with them during health visits; however, an opportunity for the client to speak privately with the health care provider should be ensured. Clients may hold

TABLE 5–2. COMPONENTS OF THE GYNECOLOGIC PHYSICAL EXAMINATION

BREAST EXAMINATION (done by physician or nurse practitioner)	
Technique:	
Inspection	
Sitting:	Arms at side for inspection Arms raised overhead for inspection of breasts Hands placed firmly on hips, elbows brought forward for chest muscle flexion during inspection
Palpation	
Sitting:	Examination begins with palpation of lymph nodes (axillary, subscapular, pectoral, clavicular, and lateral; *see* Figure 5–3.
Lying down:	The breast is flattened, facilitating lump detection. The woman lies on her back on a firm surface (examining table), a small folded towel or wedge positioned under her shoulder on the side being examined; this facilitates palpation by distributing the breast tissue more evenly. The woman raises her arm on the side to be examined, placing her hand behind her head. Another approach is to have the woman lie on the hip opposite to the breast being examined. She then rotates her shoulders so they are flat against the examining table and places the hand on the side to be examined against her forehead. This position also flattens the breast tissue for examination.
Method:	Palpating for lumps: The examiner palpates with the pads of the middle three fingers. The tips of the fingers are not used. Light, medium, firm pressure is applied to detect abnormalities throughout the breast. The examiner's fingers make small circles and palpate all areas of the breast, including the tail of Spence in the upper, outer breast quadrant. A vertical stripping or circular search pattern may be used.
Identifying breast discharge:	Using both hands, the examiner uses a "milking" technique, beginning with the outer portion of the breast and moving toward the nipple that is lifted upward. Another approach is to squeeze each nipple for discharge. (The "milking" technique may, however, be more effective in identifying breast discharge).
Breasts are examined for:	Size, symmetry, dimpling, lesions, masses, areas of thickening, tenderness, areas of inflammation Presence of breast implants Nipples (everted or inverted), discharge, crusting, presence of scars on breasts or nipples Lymph nodes assessed for size, condition, tenderness

(*continued*)

TABLE 5–2. COMPONENTS OF THE GYNECOLOGIC PHYSICAL EXAMINATION (continued)

Breast Examination (*continued*)	
Client education:	Teach and evaluate client's mastery of breast self-examination (importance and technique) Teaching done by staff nurse, nurse practitioner, or physician (who teaches varies among settings and should be the result of a collaborative decision among nurses and physicians)
GENITALIA EXAMINATION	
External technique:	
Inspection	
Lithotomy position:	
External genitalia are examined for:	Hair distribution Color and condition of vulva and perineum Presence of lesions, rashes, masses, swelling, varicosities, parasites, discharge Bruising or trauma Scars Needle track marks in groin or elsewhere Unnatural odor
Internal technique:	
Inspection (after speculum insertion)	Specimens from vagina and cervix obtained during speculum examination (the speculum may be lubricated with a small amount of warm water, used sparingly to avoid interfering with specimen results)
Vagina examined for:	Condition and color of mucosa Lacerations, lesions, discharge, cystocele or rectocele, muscle tone, unnatural odor, signs of bruising or trauma
Cervix examined for:	Color and condition Erosions, cysts, lesions, discharge from os, signs of trauma, string indicating presence of intrauterine device Speculum removed, examining glove lubricated, and uterus, ovaries, and adnexa manual palpated
Uterus examined by palpation for:	Size, shape, masses, tenderness
Adnexa examined by palpation for:	Masses, tenderness
Comfort promoted by:	Elevation of head and shoulders to a semisitting position while in lithotomy position Adjusting stirrups to a comfortable length for the woman's height in order to prevent excess hip abduction Speculum neither too warm nor too cold Well-lubricated glove Relaxation techniques, such as deep-breathing or assisting client to "follow" examination through use of hand mirror Positioning client's hands at her sides, over her chest, or holding mirror at her knee or vulva to promote abdominal muscle relaxation Avoiding placement of hands over head, which tightens abdominal muscles
Client education:	Using mirror, teach client to perform vulvar self-examination or assess client's technique in performing vulvar self-examination
RECTAL EXAMINATION	
External technique:	
Inspection *Lithotomy position*	Inspect for inflammation, visible hemmorhoids
Internal technique:	Digital palpation with well-lubricated glove
Anal and rectal areas examined for:	Hemorrhoids, lesions, masses in rectum or adnexa palpated through rectovaginal wall, sphincter tone, bleeding, signs of trauma, positive hematest, pain
Comfort promoted by:	Having client bear down gently at beginning of rectal examination Well-lubricated glove
OVERALL IMPRESSION	

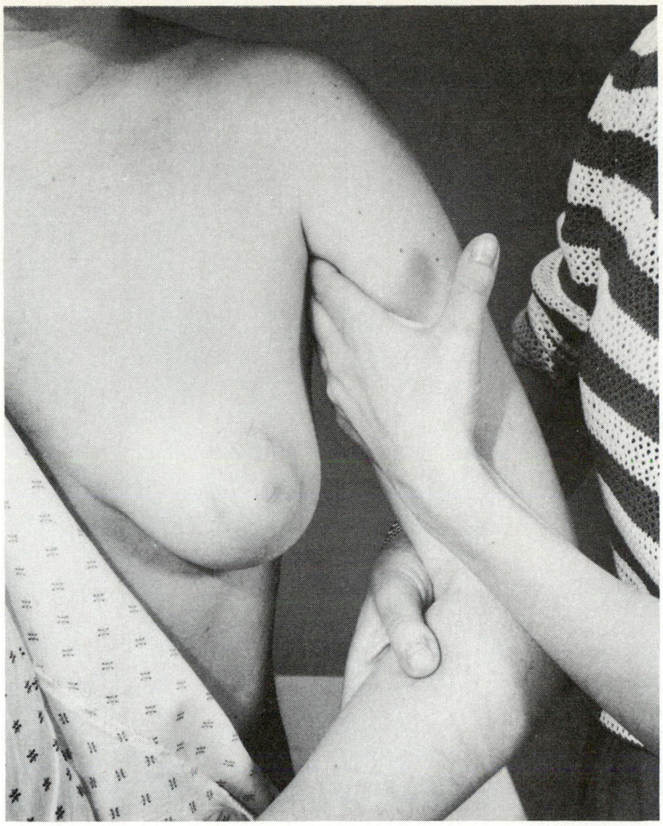

A

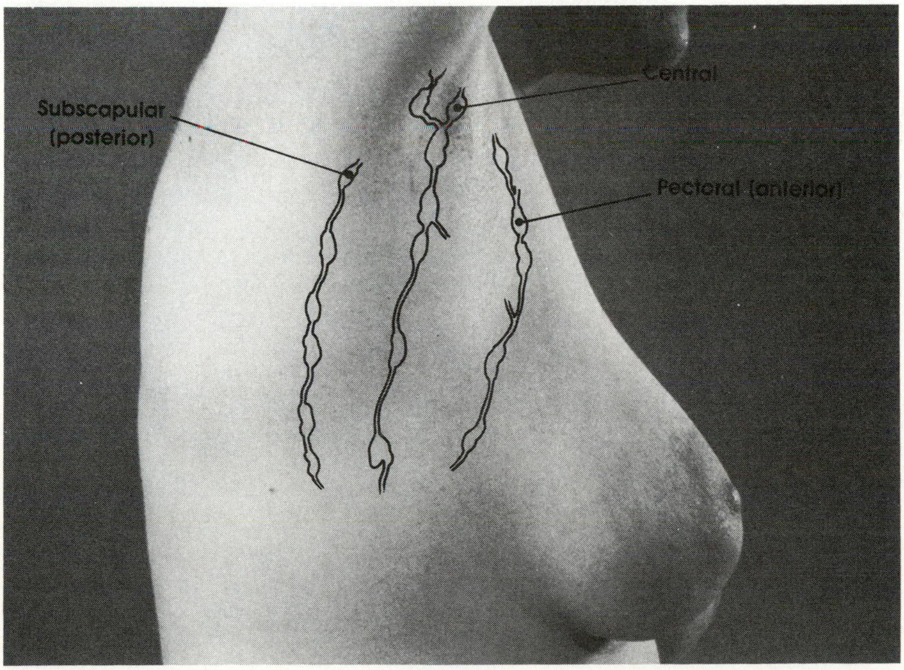

B

Figure 5–3. Breast examination. **A.** Positioning for palpation of the axilla. **B.** Location of the subscapular, central axillary, and anterior pectoral nodes. (*Figure continues.*) (*Reproduced, with permission, from Block GJ, Nolan JW.* Health Assessment for Professional Nursing. *2nd ed. Norwalk, Conn: Appleton-Century-Crofts, 1986, pp. 267–269.*)

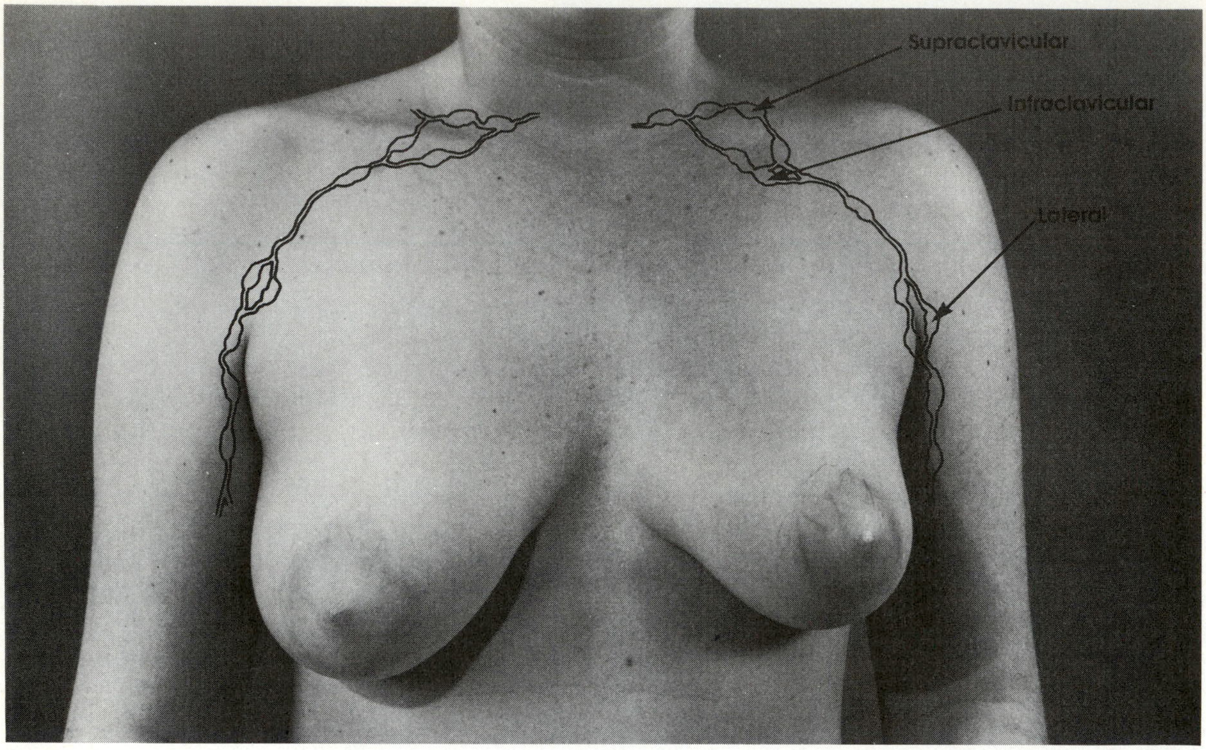

C

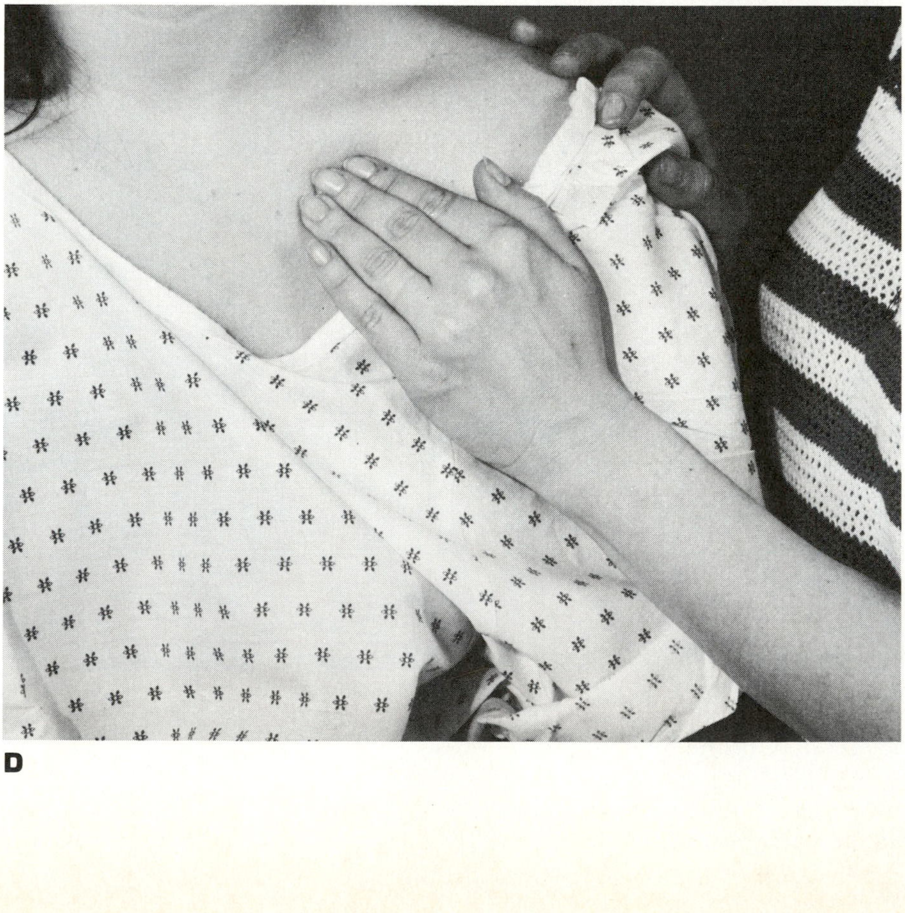

D

Figure 5–3. (*Continued.*) Breast examination. **C.** Location of the clavicular and lateral axillary nodes. Also note difference in size that can normally occur between breasts. **D.** Palpation of the infraclavicular nodes. (*Figure continues.*) (*Reproduced, with permission, from Block GJ, Nolan JW.* Health Assessment for Professional Nursing. *2nd ed. Norwalk, Conn: Appleton-Century-Crofts, 1986, pp 267–269.*)

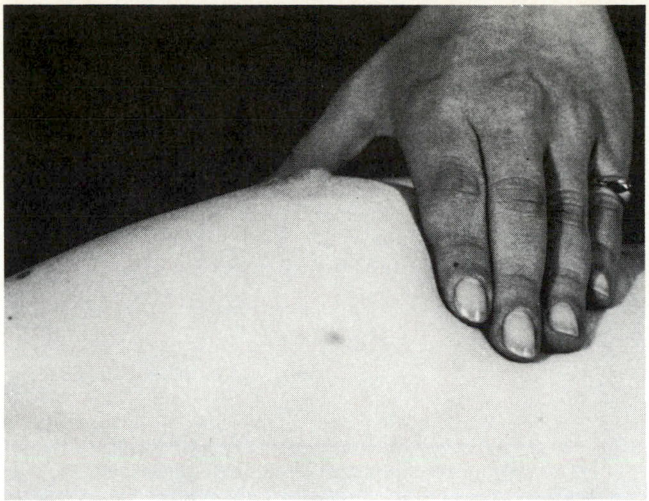

E

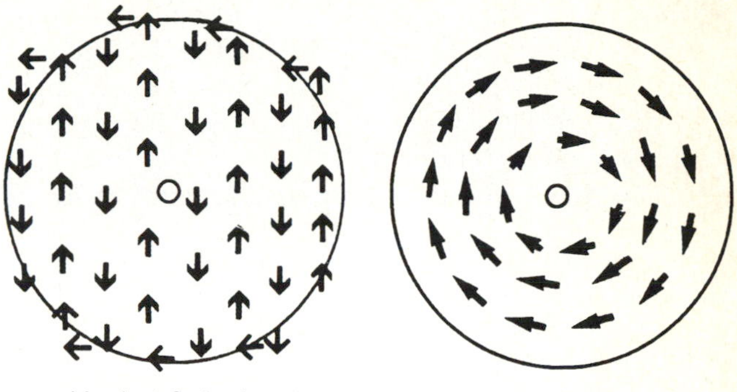

F

Figure 5–3. (*Continued.*) Breast examination. **E.** Palpating the breast. **F.** Search patterns for examination of the breast. (**E.** *Reproduced, with permission, from Block GJ, Nolan JW.* Health Assessment for Professional Nursing. *2nd ed. Norwalk, Conn: Appleton-Century-Crofts, 1986, pp 267–269.* **F.** *Reproduced, with permission, from Nettles-Calson B. Early detection of breast cancer.* J Obstet Gynecol Neonatal Nurs. *1989;18:378.*)

back certain important health information, such as abuse, when in the presence of relatives or friends, especially if they have been accompanied to the visit by their abuser.

After completion of the client's history, the client's vital signs are taken, and she is requested to empty her bladder. A full bladder can alter the position of the uterus, cloud the interpretation of normal findings, and add to the discomfort of the procedure. At this time a urine specimen can be obtained. In many settings, the nurse tests the urine with a "dipstick" chemical test method. The urine is screened for the presence of protein, glucose, blood, leukocytes, and acetone.

Blood may also be drawn for testing during the wellness visit. Wellness settings vary as to when the blood is drawn, who draws it (technician, nurse, physician), and what tests are actually performed (*see* Table 5–1). Tests for sexually transmitted diseases or antibodies for the human immunodeficiency virus (HIV) may be offered to clients. HIV testing is not routinely done for all well clients, however, and may not be performed without the permission of the well woman.

In a clinic or office setting, the client changes into a dressing gown open to the front to allow breast and abdominal assessment. When such facilities are not available, staff need to improvise. For example, the client may first remove her shirt and bra for examination of her upper body, including breasts. She may put them on again to cover herself during the examination of her lower body.

In preparing the client for the physical examination, the nurse or examiner helps her onto the examining table. The heart, lungs, and abdomen are examined first. As noted in Table 5–2, assessment of the breast and lymph nodes is begun with the client in the sitting position. The client then lies on her back for completion of the breast examination and palpation of the abdomen. A light drape is used so that only the parts of the client's body being examined are exposed. For examination of the external and internal genitalia, the client is instructed to move her hips

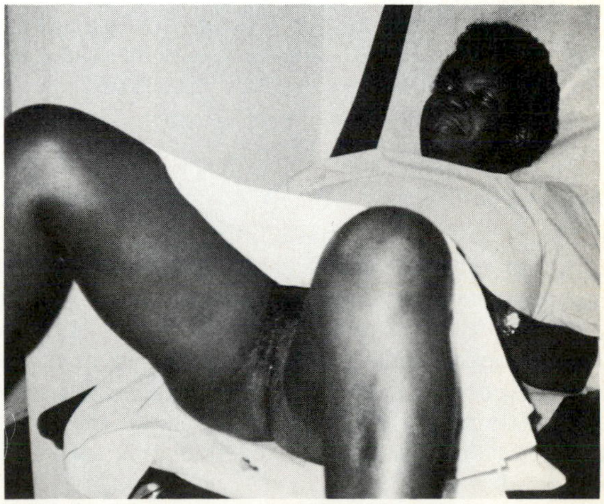

Figure 5–4. Client in lithotomy position during the educational gynecologic examination. (*Reproduced, with permission, from Lichtman R, Papera S.* Gynecology: Well Woman Care. *Norwalk, Conn: Appleton & Lange, 1989, p 33.*)

toward the bottom of the examining table and is assisted into the lithotomy position (Figure 5–4). The client is placed in a semisitting position, and is offered the use of a hand mirror, so that she can observe the examination. Table 5–2 presents an outline for examination of the genitalia; Figure 5–5 pictures equipment needed for the gynecologic examination, and Figure 5–6 illustrates technique used for insertion of the vaginal speculum.

The nurse provides support and comfort to the client during the examination and also assists the examiner with obtaining vaginal or cervical specimens. Specimens for cytologic analysis are routinely taken during the speculum examination (*see* box on Pap smear). In areas where sexually transmitted diseases are prevalent, tests for organisms such as chlamydia and gonorrhea also may be done routinely. In other settings, however, tests for these and other organisms are done only when indicated by history or direct physical observations. The person who does the

THE PAPANICOLAOU (PAP) SMEAR

The **Papanicolaou (Pap) smear** is usually used to screen for precancerous and cancerous conditions of the vagina, cervix, and endometrium.[a] Pap testing can also be done for hormonal evaluation (smear taken from the vagina), for identification of inflammatory diseases, or for diagnosis of some vaginal infections. The Pap test is based on the idea that cells from genital cancers are easily shed or scraped off. When diagnosed early, certain cancers, such as cervical cancers, can be effectively treated. The Pap test can be a reliable, inexpensive screening method when specimens are sampled and analyzed accurately.

The American College of Obstetricians and Gynecologists recommends annual cervical cytologic screening for women over the age of 18, or for younger sexually active women. Women at risk include those who have had: a positive test for the human papilloma virus; more than one sexual partner; one sexual partner at a time, but different partners over a course of time; a personal or family history of cervical or vaginal abnormalities; coitus before age twenty; a history of other sexually transmitted diseases in self or partner; or a history of exposure to diethylstilbestrol (DES). A woman who has had a hysterectomy still needs Pap testing, because the same factors that activate cancer in the cervix also can affect the vagina.

Procedure

During the pelvic examination, with the speculum in place, the examiner takes an endocervical and ectocervical smear for microscopic examination. A vaginal smear from the posterior fornix may also be obtained. A cotton-tipped applicator and spatula are commonly used for specimen collection.[b] Each laboratory has different slide preparation requirements. All use a fixative to prevent cellular changes that may take place through air drying.

Classification and Description of Results

Originally Papanicolaou smear results were reported according to a five-point scale to which some clients may still refer:

I. No atypical or abnormal cells; a negative result
II. Atypical cytologic findings, dysplastic, questionable, but not malignant
III. Cytologic findings suggesting, but not conclusive for malignancy
IV. Cytologic findings, strongly indicative of malignancy
V. Cytologic findings, definitive of malignancy; cancer cells noted

A newer system (Bethesda Reporting System) describes test results in a more narrative form, as[c]:

- Within normal limits
- Reactive and reparative changes
- Atypical squamous or glandular cells of undetermined significance
- Low-grade squamous intraepithelial lesions (human papillomavirus infection or mild squamous dysplasia/cervical intraepithelial neoplasia [CIN 1])
- High-grade squamous epithelial lesions (moderate to severe squamous dysplasia, carcinoma in situ [CIN 2–3]
- Suspicious squamous or glandular cells
- Squamous cell carcinoma
- Adenocarcinoma

Client Instructions

The client should be advised to avoid vaginal medications, tampons, contraceptives, douche-type products, or intercourse for three days before sampling. These factors may influence the specimen collection or results of the Pap test. Also, Pap testing is not recommended during menstruation or if the client has an infection, because these conditions can interfere with evaluation of cells.[d]

[a] *Baldwin K, Goodwin K. The Papanicolaou smear.* J Nurse Midwifery. *1985;30:327–332.*

[b] *Shen J, et al. Efficacy of cotton-tipped applicators for obtaining cells from the uterine cervix for Papanicolaou smears.* Obstet Gynecol Surv. *1985;40:312–313.*

[c] *National Cancer Institute Workshop: The 1988 Bethesda system for reporting vaginal cytologic diagnoses. Acta Cytol.* 1989;33:567–574.

[d] *Murphy PA. Laboratory testing. In Lichtman R, Papera S.* Gynecology: Well Woman Care. *Norwalk, Conn: Appleton & Lange, 1990.*

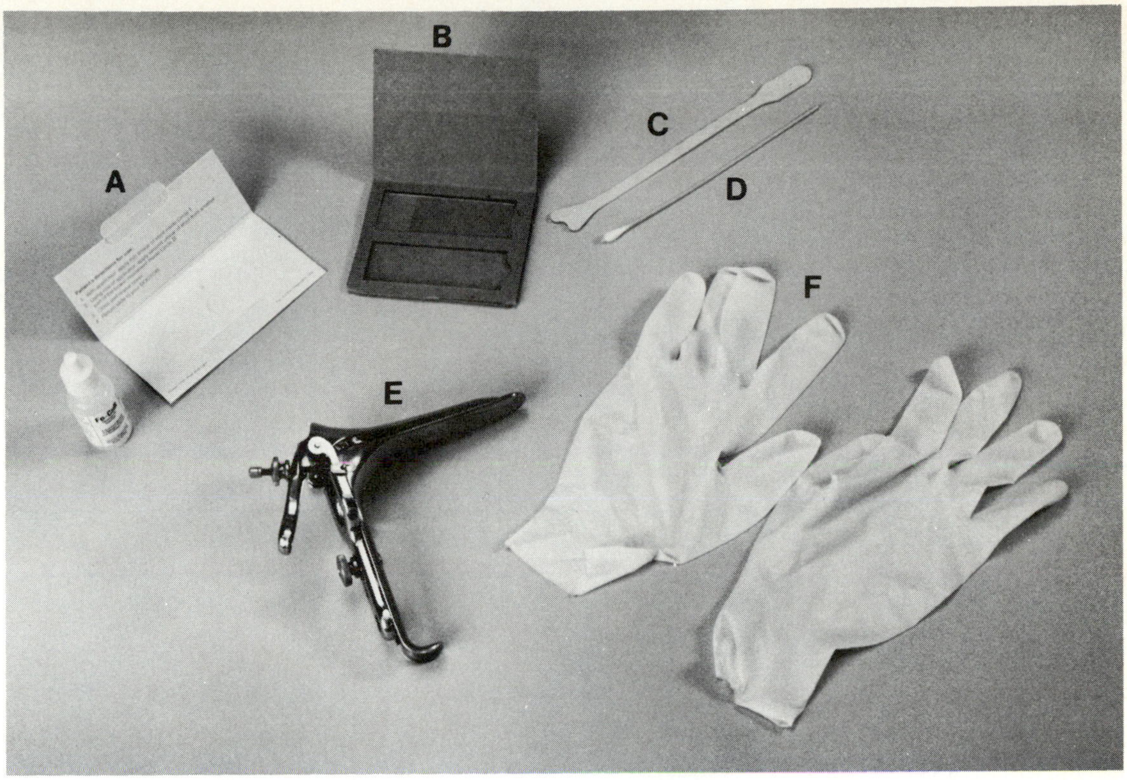

Figure 5–5. Equipment for pelvic and rectal examination. **A.** Stool guaiac slide test. **B.** Pap slide. **C.** Ayre spatula. **D.** Swab. **E.** Speculum. **F.** Gloves. (*Reproduced, with permission, from Block GJ, Nolan JW.* Health Assessment for Professional Nursing. *2nd ed. Norwalk, Conn: Appleton-Century-Crofts, 1986, p 309.*)

gynecologic examination provides explanations as the physical assessment progresses; this is an important part of the practitioner-client relationship.

Client Participation and the Educational Gynecologic Examination. Traditionally the examiner performed the physical assessment as the client lay back on the table. The client often could not see the examiner's face because of drapes placed over her. Although this procedure is still widely used in the United States, the educational gynecologic examination has been employed, especially by nurse practitioners and certified nurse-midwives. With this approach, the client is encouraged to participate and to learn about herself during the examination.[12] Few clients independently ask for a mirror; therefore, the health care provider should offer the use of a mirror. Approaches such as, "If you hold the mirror like this, I can show you what I am doing during the examination and answer any questions," convey the expectation of the woman's interest and participation. Through the use of a hand mirror, the client can watch the examination. Raising the head of the table and modifying drapes promotes anatomic visibility as well as eye contact with the examiner. Reasons for educational gynecologic assessment include:

- Helping the client to get to know her own anatomy and physiology.
- Providing opportunities for discussion of issues related to reproductive and sexual expression.[12]
- Instructing the client in the importance and technique of vulvar self-examination. The widespsread occurrence of pathologic conditions such as condyloma acuminatum (venereal warts), and the increasing incidence of vulvar carcinoma, especially among younger women, make early detection very important. Clients with a history of vulvar condyloma or vulvar pathology should be advised to self-examine on a monthly basis; those without such a history may self-examine every 3 to 4 months.[13]
- Helping women to relax during the examination.
- Making the gynecologic examination less threatening and thereby promoting the client's health-care–seeking behavior.[12] Being examined on a regular basis promotes early detection and possible cure of conditions such as cervical carcinoma.

Post-Examination Interventions. After the examination, the client is assisted to a sitting position. Whether results are discussed with her at that time or whether she dresses and then meets with the health care providers varies according to practitioner and

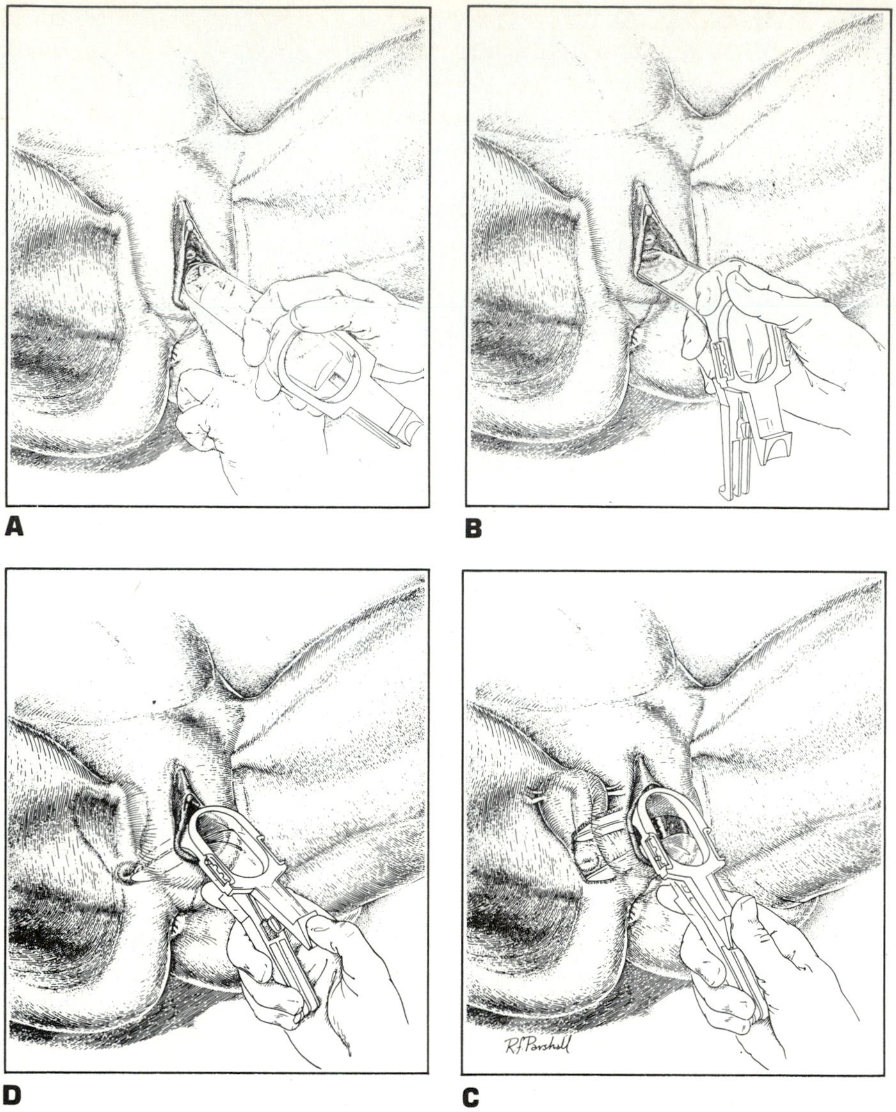

Figure 5–6. Procedure for insertion of the vaginal speculum. **A.** Opening the introitus and oblique insertion of the speculum blades. **B.** Speculum blades parallel to the table. **C.** Speculum blades directed at a 45-degree angle into the vagina. **D.** Opening the speculum blades. (*Reproduced, with permission, from Block GJ, Nolan JW.* Health Assessment for Professional Nursing. *2nd ed. Norwalk, Conn: Appleton-Century-Crofts, 1986, p 315.*)

facility. Ideally, the client dresses after the examination and then meets with the examiner in a consultation-type manner; this approach promotes the client's dignity. The client needs to be told of the procedure, so that she simply does not get dressed and leave uninformed and with staff waiting for her in another room. The examiner may discuss findings with the client, and the staff nurse may then focus on specific teaching needs. Coordinated, collaborative care planning is therefore necessary to ensure that the client receives interventions based on needs identified during the history and physical.

Goals and Interventions for Care

Nursing and medical diagnoses, goals, and plans for intervention need to be formed efficiently and promptly, because the well client may not return to the office for a year or more. For the well woman, nursing goals usually focus on the teaching-learning process, as described in the beginning of Chapter 24.

Client Reaction to Gynecologic Examination. Many women regard gynecologic examinations with negative feelings such as dread, embarrassment, fear, and high-level anxiety.[14–17] There are many factors that may account for this. For example, the breasts and genitalia have been regarded as "private" body parts, to be touched by another person only within a sexual relationship. While media images place great emphasis on reproductive anatomy and its mystique, the taboos against touch remain. In addition, gynecologic assessment includes a physically invasive, intimate examination that requires the client to assume a lithotomy position. This awkward position in itself can be distressing. As one client reported, "I felt so open, undignified, and vulnerable . . . almost like a chicken waiting to be stuffed."

Gynecologic examination is done to screen for potential pathologic conditions. Some clients may fear that abnormalities will be found, especially if they are considered at risk. Among some groups in the general population, gynecologic examination may be incorrectly regarded as appropriate only for married or sexually experienced women. In this sense, women may worry about being stigmatized if their friends or family learn about their gynecologic visit. Some clients may mistakenly fear they will lose their virginity if they have a vaginal examination.

Willard and colleagues studied attitudes of 213 women toward pelvic examination.[12] The clients were selected from the practices of physicians and nurses and assigned at random to traditional or educational examination groups. The women completed questionnaires before and after their examinations. Before the examination, the two groups of women did not differ from each other in their attitudes toward pelvic examination. After the examination, the women in the educational examination group reported being significantly more comfortable physically, felt they had learned more from the examination, and found the examination to be a better experience than expected. In addition, the educational group was more positive toward the examination and had a greater total improvement in attitude toward pelvic examination (from pretest to posttest) than did the traditional group. Over half (54.7 percent) of all the women in the sample reported dreading the first pelvic examination they ever had, and 44 percent felt that the experience was what they had expected or worse, despite the professional interest of their examiners. Willard and colleagues suggested that something more than interest and explanations was essential in order to address the problem of women's negative reactions to pelvic examination. From their study, they concluded that the educational, or "mirror" examination, along with modification in the use of drapes, might offer one solution.

Pain During Gynecologic Examination. Gynecologic assessment for the well woman should not be more than mildly uncomfortable. The breast examination should be painless, although women being examined during the latter part of the menstrual cycle may have generalized breast tenderness. (Pain in a discrete part of the breast is not a normal finding).

Muscle tension, related to anxiety, can produce pain for women during manual and speculum examination and difficulty in maintaining the lithotomy position during examination. A stinging, stretching type of pain, related to snugness of the hymen, may be experienced by clients who are virgins and who do not regularly use tampons.

Several strategies may promote client comfort during physical gynecologic examination. A collaborative approach is used, although the actual physical examination is done by a nurse specialist or physician. Strategies to promote comfort include:

- Establishing a professional rapport with the client.
- Ensuring privacy during the examination.
- Covering the woman's breasts and shoulders with her gown or a drape before proceeding to the pelvic examination. (This also provides warmth in cool examining rooms.)
- Providing comfort measures such as: adjusting room temperature when possible; raising the head of the examining table to elevate the woman's head and shoulders; pulling out the stirrups attached to the table to avoid painful abduction of the woman's hips[16]; and making sure the speculum is at a comfortable temperature.
- Providing anticipatory guidance and explaining every step of the examination; maintaining eye contact as appropriate[16]; and using an educational gynecologic approach as described above.
- Stirrup modification (padded foot supports, cloth-covered foot supports) to reduce discomfort of the cold metal stirrups.[18]
- Techniques to promote relaxation. For example, the client can be encouraged to breathe in through the nose and out through the mouth. She should be advised to avoid clenching her fists or squeezing her eyes shut, because these activities can lead to general muscle tightness, which in turn can make the examination harder to perform. Distraction techniques, such as conversation during the educational examination, can also be helpful.

Client Safety During Gynecologic Examination. Client safety during gynecologic examinations refers to protection against infection and injury. Proper hand-washing techniques should be used before and after the examination. Gloves should be used and changed between vaginal and rectal examinations. This decreases the likelihood that organisms will be spread from the vagina to the rectum in situations in which vaginal infections are present. Gloves should be well-lubricated with a water-soluble preparation after specimens are taken in order to minimize injury to delicate tissues and discomfort to the client. Occasionally a client may be allergic to substances in the lubricant and may then experience burning and itching related to the development of an allergic rash in the vagina or rectum. The client should therefore be asked about any known allergies before the examination. In cases where commercially prepared lubricants cannot be used, a small amount of warm water on the examining glove and a gentle approach can facilitate examination. Examiners can prevent gloves from tearing and thereby decrease risks for themselves and their clients by keeping nails short and not wearing jewelry beneath gloves.

Falls from the examining table present a potential threat to safety, especially when clients leave the lithotomy position. Primrose described a situation in which a woman fell seat first from the examining table because she was not reminded to slide her hips back from the edge.[16] Indeed, anxiety related to the examination and relief when it is over may make some clients "absentminded," and possibly liable to injury. Hamilton and Dodge suggested several steps the nurse could use to help clients safely off an examining table[14]:

1. The nurse stands at the side of the table with her left shoulder at the client's right shoulder (or vice versa).
2. The nurse puts her right hand over the client's symphysis.
3. The nurse puts her left hand on the back of the client's neck; the nurse's lower two fingers spread to the client's upper back, and the upper fingers are on the base of the client's head.
4. The client is asked to sit up and remove her feet from the stirrups at the same time.

By acting as a pivot to provide support and guidance as the client rises, the nurse can avoid strain on herself and assist the client safely off the table.

Protective Measures for Staff During Gynecologic Examination. Concerns for safety and well-being apply to staff as well as to clients. Universal precautions are used by the examiner and by anyone else who may be likely to come into contact with body fluids. Nurses should wear gloves when drawing blood or testing urine specimens. In addition, moistureproof barriers need to be placed beneath open specimens; spills should be cleaned with a fresh solution of 10-percent sodium hypochlorite (bleach). Food items, such as staff lunches, should *never* be stored in a refrigerator with specimens of body fluids.

Lifting an adult well client on or off an examining table can result in musculoskeletal injury to the nurse. While the steps noted above are of help, the reader also needs to review fundamental body mechanics. As previously discussed, other protective measures for staff include the presence of a female associate during the client's physical examination.

THE MENSTRUAL EXPERIENCE

Normal Menstruation

Menstruation is a normal, cyclic physiologic event signifying the reproductive years in the human female (*see* Chapter 6). The nurse must realize, however, that menstruation is a physiologic process surrounded by myth, secrecy, and ceremony. The nature and extent of menstruation-related practices vary according to individual religions and cultural beliefs. For example, some societies segregate menstruating women in special menstrual huts. The Hasidim (members of an extremely orthodox branch of Judaism) consider a menstruating or postpartum woman "unclean." The Hasidic husband may not directly touch his wife while she is bleeding. For fear of contaminating her husband through accidental touch, the Hasidic wife might request that the nurse transfer her newborn from her own arms to her husband's arms; she might also put her baby down for her husband to lift by himself. At the end of the menstrual flow, or postpartum, the Hasidic woman might attend a mikvah, or special bath, where she would undertake a ritual cleansing.

Historically, in the United States, menstruation was treated as a "delicate," difficult subject that was not discussed in polite company. Even the term *menstruation* is often not used directly but has been referred to by such terms as "period," "friend," "flux," or "the curse." Production of feminine hygiene products constitutes a gigantic corporate industry and they are widely advertised. The advertising itself, however, is couched in indirect phrases such as "feeling fresh" and "feminine protection."

ISSUES AND CONTROVERSIES

Several issues surround myths related to the menstrual cycle. Traditionally, emotional changes linked to the menstrual cycle have been used as barriers to hiring and promoting women to decision-making positions. Attempts have been made to place the effects of the menstrual cycle in proper perspective; however, attention to conditions such as premenstrual syndrome and dysmenorrhea have seemed at times to work at cross-purposes with women's career efforts. Does establishing PMS as a type of chronic illness, albeit a wellness-oriented one, detract from the advancement potential of women?

TABLE 5–3. ANSWERS TO QUESTIONS COMMONLY ASKED ABOUT MENSTRUATION

What is a normal menstrual period?

A normal menstrual period represents the shedding of the lining of the uterus. Menstrual flow includes substances such as blood, some endometrial tissue, white blood cells, and mucus.

How long should menstrual periods last?

There is considerable variation among the length of menstrual periods among women. Menstrual periods can last from 2 to 8 days.

How often does menstruation occur?

Although the menstrual cycle has traditionally been described as being about 28 days in length, cycles vary greatly among women. Menstrual cycles also vary within the same woman by about 5 to 10 days. Menstruation reflects complex physical, psychologic, and environmental interactions; factors such as extreme weight loss, vigorous physical activity, and emotional stress can affect menstrual patterns.

How much blood is lost?

About 30–100 mL of blood is lost during menstruation. The amount of flow depends on factors like the thickness of the endometrium and certain medications.[a]

Are clots abnormal?

Because of the presence of fibrinolysin, which breaks down clots, menstrual flow does not tend to clot. Clots may represent heavy bleeding related to a variety of pathologic causes (*see* Table 5–6). Clots also occur, however, in normal, healthy women. A study of hemoglobin or hematocrit should be routine at gynecologic visits and can indicate whether excessive bleeding is taking place during menstruation.

How much iron do women lose during menstruation?

Women can loose about 0.5 to 1 mg of iron daily in menstrual flow.

Should exercise be restricted during mensturation?

There is no reason why a woman cannot continue with her usual pattern of activities. Indeed, exercises such as brisk walking or tennis may promote feelings of well-being and reduce menstrual discomforts.

Should vaginal sprays or douches be used to prevent menstrual odor?

No. Despite vigorous advertising campaigns, vaginal sprays or douches should not be used by the healthy woman; these preparations can cause problems such as rashes, itching, and burning. Showering, bathing, or external cleansing with water or water and gentle soap, as well as regular changing of pads or tampons, is sufficient. Normal menstrual flow has a mild "fleshy" odor. Foul-smelling discharge could indicate abnormal conditions such as infection and should be reported to the health care provider without delay.

Can a woman get pregnant during her period?

Although the menstrual phase is the least fertile time during a woman's cycle, pregnancy could, in theory, occur. It is important to remember that the graafian follicle begins to mature in the ovary while menstruation is taking place in the uterus. Considering that sperm can live up to six days, unprotected intercourse toward the end of menstruation (eg, day 8) increases the chances of pregnancy.

Is it all right for a woman to have intercourse during menstruation?

The healthy woman does not have to refrain from intercourse on the basis of menstruation alone. Religious, cultural or other personal beliefs do, however, affect sexual behavior during menstruation. Women need to be informed about the risk of pregnancy with unprotected intercourse at any time during the menstrual cycle. Although contact with vaginal secretions is an important source of transmission of certain diseases, menstruation can bring the male into direct contact with his partner's blood. This may be a concern for some couples.

[a] Ganong WF. Physiology of reproduction. In Perroll ML, Benson RC. *Current Obstetric and Gynecologic Diagnosis and Treatment.* 6th ed. Norwalk, Conn: Appleton & Lange, 1987, pp 109–126.

Although women experiencing menstrual problems may seek care or offer reports of symptoms during wellness visits, some women may be too embarrassed to discuss this topic openly. The nurse should anticipate client difficulties and initiate discussion of menstrual concerns. Table 5–3 presents answers to questions women frequently ask related to menstruation.

Menarche: The Adolescent Experience

Menarche, the first menstrual period at puberty, can take place in girls as young as 9 or as old as 17. Most girls begin menstruating between 11 and 13 years of age. Referral for endocrinologic assessment usually is not made unless the girl is 16 and has not been showing signs of pubertal development. In the United States, many girls and their mothers become unduly worried if menarche has not taken place by age 13. In most cases, reassurance and anticipatory guidance are the only necessary interventions.

The average age of menarche in the United States is 12.5 years, however, puberty actually begins before this. The term **puberty** refers to the period when the endocrine and gametogenic functions of the ovaries first develop to the point at which reproduction can take place. It is theoretically possible for a girl who has entered puberty, but who has never menstruated, to become pregnant. According to Ganong, the age at which girls enter puberty has been declining at the rate of 1 to 3 months per decade over the past 175 years.[19] Girls in the United States currently enter puberty beween the ages of 8 and 13.

Ideally, all girls would be well prepared for menarche and menstruation. However, the nature, extent, and accuracy of information girls receive varies widely. Although some girls look forward to menarche with excitement, others experience menarche with surprise and fear. Developmentally, pubescent girls are concerned about topics such as body integrity, being accepted, and being normal. Worries about their own body changes and physical health assume great importance.

Educational Preparation for Menarche. A girl's positive response to menarche and her adaptation to menstruation are related to the prior preparation and the quality of support she receives at this time.[20–22] Preparation for menarche should begin before the first menstrual period, around age 10. Content should be spread over more than one session. Teaching should be done in a manner that fosters questions and discussion and should include attitudes and beliefs as well as physical information. Preparation for menarche might include the following topics:

- Anatomy and physiology of the reproductive system
- Definition of menarche and menstruation
- Body changes related to puberty and menstruation
- Cultural and religious beliefs about menstruation
- Family beliefs about menstruation; information and attitudes of relatives and friends
- Fears, embarrassment, and other personal feelings related to menstruation
- What menstruation may actually feel like
- How to perform self-care during menstruation (personal cleanliness; how to select, use, and dispose of products available, eg, sanitary napkins and tampons)
- Ways of coping with discomforts related to menstruation
- The importance of regarding menstruation and the reproductive system as normal, healthy parts of being a woman
- The irregular nature of menstruation in teenagers (factors affecting menstruation should be addressed; for example, active, ongoing participation in heavy exercise, as expected for track and gymnastics teams, may delay menarche or account for menstrual variations such as amenorrhea or irregular menstrual periods)
- Reproductive capability and reproductive responsibility
- Sources of referral for questions or problems related to menarche and menstruation

Sources and Settings for Teaching About Menstruation. Traditionally, education about menstruation and puberty was considered part of the maternal role, although some fathers were also involved in the educational process. This provided an opportunity for the mother to share with her daughter the realization of the girl's evolving physical maturity. Such discussions could potentially strengthen the mother-daughter relationship. Not all parents however, were able to do this. Factors such as lack of parental knowledge, inability of parents to feel comfortable talking about puberty with their child, and beliefs that menstruation is "sinful" or "dirty" had negative effects on girls. Many a school nurse can recall situations in which terrified adolescent girls came to them shocked by the unexplained bleeding of menarche.

In recent years, education about puberty has been included in many elementary school curricula. Educational programs are usually begun around fourth or fifth grade. Consideration needs to be given to actual ages of the children. In some school districts, there is a tendency for children to start school later and therefore to be 10 years old in fourth grade.

Teaching about changes related to puberty and about reproductive function has frequently been controversial. Issues such as parental versus school control of "sensitive" information and the rights and responsibilities of parents to provide any direct reproductive teaching to their children have brought various community and religious groups into heated quarrels and even legal conflict with school boards.

Nursing Roles in Educational Preparation for Menstruation. Nurses have broad health-promotion teaching roles in the educational preparation of young people about menstruation and reproductive maturity. As experts on subjects of menstruation and puberty, nurses need to accept responsibility for making certain that accurate and appropriate health education takes place. Nursing roles include:

1. Teaching boys and girls directly. School nurses frequently lead class presentations on topics related to puberty and counsel students on an individual basis. Serving as guest speakers, nurses can

also present programs on menstruation through schools or organizations such as Girl or Boy Scouts, Campfire Girls, or various types of summer camps. Nurses at overnight camps need to be prepared to work with girls undergoing a "crisis" of menarche in a communal setting away from home. Nurses who work in outpatient pediatric settings have opportunities during well-child checkups to provide direct teaching on menstruation to girls, boys, and parents.

2. Teaching parents and helping parents teach their children about menstruation. Educational programs can be prepared for parents on subjects such as "The Latest Information about Menstruation" and "How to Talk to Your Child about Menstruation." Nurses can therefore help parents clarify information, dispel misconceptions about menstruation, and indirectly, promote communication between parents and children.
3. Ensuring that content on menstruation is appropriately and sensitively addressed in school curricula. Through roles as advocates and social activists nurses can affect the nature and scope of information about menstruation presented to students.
4. Working as authors, producers, and consultants for the development of learning materials on this topic.

As part of an educational approach focusing on sexual development and responsibility, information about menstruation needs to be made available to both boys and girls. Nurses, however, need to be sensitive to feelings of embarrassment characteristic of coed groups of budding adolescents.

In a descriptive study, Havens and Swenson found that 89 percent of 74 eighth- and tenth-grade girls wanted boys to be told about menstruation.[22] Nevertheless, 65 percent of the girls preferred menstrual education to be provided separately to boys and to girls in order for them to feel more comfortable in open discussion. These findings are consistent with the traditional cultural belief of menstruation as a topic for presentation to girls-only or boys-only groups. On the other hand, coed sessions run in a compassionate, professional manner could potentially foster thoughtful, open communication about an important bodily function.

Premenstrual Syndrome

Premenstrual syndrome (PMS) refers to a variety of physical and emotional symptoms that can occur 1 to 2 weeks before the start of menstruation and that disappear at the start, or shortly after the start, of menstruation (Table 5–4).[23] Although symptoms vary among women, each woman tends to have a consistent pattern of symptoms. The symptom-free phase occurs postmenstruation and should last a minimum of seven days. PMS tends to be most acute in women in their thirties but may occur sooner or later. Menstruation is often pain-free.[23]

TABLE 5–4. SYMPTOMS OF PREMENSTRUAL SYNDROME

Behavioral	Tension, depression, irritability, sleep disturbances, fatigue, lethargy, alcoholic bouts, panics, suicide, homicide, assaults, child abuse
Neurologic	Headaches, aggravation of epilepsy, vertigo, syncope, fainting, migraine, paresthesias of hands or feet
Respiratory	Colds, hoarseness, rhinitis, asthma, sinusitis, sore throat
Gastrointestinal	Abdominal bloating, nausea, vomiting, constipation, food cravings (especially for sweets), compulsive eating
Dermatologic	Acne, boils, urticaria, easy bruising, recurrence of herpes
Urologic	Cystitis, urethritis, oliguria, enuresis
Ophthalmologic	Styes, conjunctivitis, visual change
Mammologic	Breast tenderness, engorgement, enlargement, heaviness
Miscellaneous	Backache, joint pain, edema, weight gain, palpitations

Reproduced, with permission, from Wilson MA, Menstrual disorders: premenstral syndrome, dysmenorrhea, amenorrhea. J Obstet Gynecol Neonatal Nurs. *1984; 13 (suppl):135.*

Premenstrual syndrome has been noted to occur worldwide, although the major complaint may be affected by each culture.[24] Estimates of the incidence of PMS have ranged from a conservative 25 percent[20] to a sweeping 70 to 90 percent of menstruating women.[25, 26] Five percent to 15 percent of women are thought to experience severe symptoms.[18]

Brown and Zimmer referred to PMS as a "unique type of chronic illness."[25] In the extreme, the emotional and behavioral changes of severe PMS have been accepted by courts in the United Kingdom and France as grounds for a plea of temporary insanity.[27] Despite some dramatic reports linking PMS to severe physical, psychologic, and behavioral problems among a small number of women, however, current evidence indicates that mild to moderate PMS symptoms do not impair most women.[28] Rapkin and colleagues compared women with PMS with women who were clinically depressed. Women with PMS did report subjective symptoms such as depression, anxiety, and fatigue. Unlike the clinically depressed women, however, they did not have objective changes in information processing or performance, as tested by measures of cognitive functioning.[29]

It is difficult to identify the actual incidence of PMS for the following reasons:

- Many women who experience mild or moderate symptoms do not seek assistance from health care workers. Indeed, they may simply regard their symptoms as part of being female or initiate self-care practices learned from friends, the media, or devised from their own home remedies.
- PMS tends to be diagnosed in women whose symptoms are severe enough to seek help from health professionals.[30]
- There is a wide diversity of symptoms used to identify PMS, with up to 150 different symptoms linked to the menstrual cycle.[31]
- No uniform, accepted, operational definition of PMS exists.[31]

The cause of PMS is not known, although many theories have been suggested. These theories focus on such factors as estrogen-progesterone imbalance, excess aldosterone, vitamin deficiencies, and psychologic factors. Excess or abnormal prostaglandin function has also been suggested because nonsteroidal anti-inflammatory drugs often relieve symptoms.[30] Thorough assessment of psychosocial factors is always essential, because PMS has also been regarded as a physiologic response to psychosocial stress. For example, 57 percent (139) of clients who completed base-line assessment for PMS at the Duke University PMS Clinic did not respond to dietary, exercise, or vitamin therapy and eventually required referral for mental health care, individual psychotherapy, or marital therapy.[32] PMS seems to illustrate the complex interaction among physical, psychosocial, and environmental factors.

Impact of PMS on Male Partners. The discomforts and behavioral changes related to PMS may be expected to have an effect on the woman's interactions with her significant others, particularly her husband or male partner. For example, Cortese and Brown found that men actively responded to their partners' premenstrual symptoms.[33] Men in their study used a wide variety of coping strategies, such as telling themselves the woman had no control over the symptoms, seeking more information about PMS, getting angry with the woman, and providing reassurance and support.

PMS Management and Nursing Implications. Management of PMS depends on accurate diagnosis, client interest in relieving PMS symptoms, and a col-

RESEARCH ABSTRACT

Cortese J, Brown MA. Coping responses of men whose partners experience premenstrual symptomatology. J Obstet Gynecol Neonatal Nurs. *1989;18:405–412.*

The purpose of this study was to investigate ways in which men cope with partners who experience premenstrual syndrome. Eighty-six healthy couples, recruited from a variety of sources, such as advertisements, community information seminars on PMS, and announcements in the media, were interviewed separately in their homes. Interviews were scheduled to immediately precede the woman's next expected period. The two research instruments used had an interview format and were developed for the purposes of the study. Couples were identified as being part of the high- or low-PMS-symptom group, as a result of the woman's premenstrual intensity scores. The high-symptom group had more children and a lower level of education than the low-symptom group, indicating potentially more stress in the group. Study results did not identify any groupings of coping strategies on the part of the men. Results of the study indicated, however, that men actively responded to their partners' PMS and used a large variety and combination of coping responses, such as telling themselves that the woman's words and actions were not intentional, seeking more information about PMS, becoming angry at their partner, providing reassurance and support, and reminding themselves of the temporary nature of PMS.

Comment:

Little research has been done with partners of women experiencing PMS. This study highlights the importance of this topic for both men and women and demonstrates that PMS affects not only the woman, but her partner. By identifying the men's need for information and attempts to seek outside assistance, the investigators underscore the importance of health promotion teaching, directed toward both men and women, about PMS. They further identify the premenstrual period as a time of potential risk for disruptions in the couple's relationship and suggest that couples experiencing severe PMS might avoid discussion of sensitive issues during this difficult time. The study also points to the importance of identifying men who use health-damaging behaviors, such as verbal or physical violence, in response to PMS. Cortese's and Brown's study clearly provides a foundation for further research about the impact of PMS on men.

laborative relationship between client and health care professionals. The health care team may routinely include a nurse, gynecologist, and nutritionist, with consultation as necessary from specialists in endocrinology, psychology, neurology, and social work. Unfortunately, there is no magical cure or method to relieve all symptoms of PMS. PMS is a complex phenomenon. Whereas many women can experience excellent results from therapy, some do not respond at all or respond to varying degrees. Successful therapy may result over time from behavioral and lifestyle changes. Using a supportive-educative role based on a self-care model, nurses work closely with clients in the diagnosis and treatment of PMS. While pharmacologic therapy is prescribed by the physician or nurse practitioner using standing orders, nurses frequently manage nonpharmacologic approaches to PMS treatment.

Careful history and physical examination are necessary to make certain that client symptoms are due to PMS and not to some other physical or psychologic condition. Marked change in intensity of symptoms measured on postmenstrual and premenstrual days and identification of changes for at least two cycles are necessary for diagnosis.[34] Laboratory tests (eg, for plasma hormones such as progesterone or prolactin) are not useful in the diagnosis of PMS and are usually done only to rule out other endocrine problems.[24, 35]

Wilhelm-Hass recommended the use of a menstrual diary in which the client rates her daily experiences of symptoms according to whether they: do not occur; occur in a mild form but do not interfere with activities; are moderate, interfere with activities, but are not disabling; or are severe and disabling.[24] In addition, the client's recording of her basal body temperature before rising, eating, or smoking each morning can be compared with the menstrual diary. This can be used to demonstrate the absence of symptoms in the follicular phase of the menstrual cycle and to support the diagnosis of PMS. Ideally the client troubled by PMS should be seen during the follicular phase and the luteal phase of her cycle. In this way, the client can be evaluated during times when symptoms are and are not present. Other pathologic conditions, which would be likely to persist throughout the woman's cycle, could then be diagnosed. Table 5–5 outlines an example of a general PMS nursing protocol.

Interventions for PMS depend on correct identification of the syndrome and upon the nature and severity of symptoms. Controlled clinical studies do not, however, support the effectiveness of any particular therapy for all women. Nevertheless, the nonpharmacologic recommendations represent healthy lifestyle practices. The potential effectiveness of nonpharmacologic approaches was illustrated by a study conducted in the Duke University PMS clinic. A study of the first 350 patients at the clinic brought a response rate of 70 percent; 1 in 6 (ie, 36) of these women reported needing no further treatment after making dietary, lifestyle, and behavioral changes. Nonpharmacologic interventions used in current practice include:

- Validation that PMS is a real and legitimate concern.
- Communicating the importance of client responsibility for self-care, especially during the 1 to 3 months necessary for dietary or lifestyle changes to show results.[24]
- Nutritional counseling. Reduction of intake of caffeine, refined sugars, red meat, and salt; cessation of smoking[24, 32]; a well-balanced daily diet rich in green, leafy vegetables, complex carbohydrates, legumes, whole grains, cereals, and nuts[36]; adequate intake particularly of vitamin E (up to 800 units). Vitamin supplements must always be given with caution and counseling to avoid excessive intake. Eating nutritious foods at regular intervals, rather than skipping meals, should be advised.
- Moderate exercise.
- Stress reduction; relaxation techniques; adequate rest and sleep.
- Alteration in lifestyle practices.
- Individual psychotherapy or marital counseling if necessary.
- Referral to PMS support groups. Such groups provide benefits that include increased knowledge about PMS, confirmation of PMS as a chronic disease that can be coped with, comfort in sharing the PMS experience with others having similar experiences, validation of PMS symptoms, discussion of therapies and lifestyle changes to relieve symptoms, and help in self-awareness and understanding.[26]

Pharmacologic Interventions for PMS. At times pharmacologic agents may be used to reduce uncomfortable symptoms related to PMS. Pharmacologic therapies have been controversial, as the cause of PMS is unknown and no specific therapy is universally successful. Pharmacologic therapies have included vitamin and mineral supplements to physiologically relieve such symptoms as fluid retention, diuretics to relieve swelling, and psychotropic drugs to relieve depression and other emotional symptoms. Progesterone vaginal suppositories, prolactin inhibitors such as bromocriptine mesylate, and cortisol have also been used. One study of 17 women

TABLE 5–5. PMS CLINIC NURSING PROTOCOL

Evaluation: The Initial Menstrual Cycle

Tools

Menstrual symptomatology diary, as developed by Abraham,[a] every evening; basal body temperature chart every morning.

Self-assessment scales for anxiety and depression (an easy-to-score tool administered during the client's visit; questionnaires should not be completed retrospectively because of the possibility of inaccurate recall).

Menstrual symptomatology questionnaire[a]

History

General and gynecologic assessment as well as data on social supports; suicidal risk; weight gain in kg for vitamin B_6 regimen; smoking; intake of caffeine, red meat, fats, complex carbohydrates, vitamins and dairy products; number of meals per day; weekly aerobic activity; prior therapies; self-education to date; coping habits and lifestyle data.

Intervention: Nonpharmacologic Strategies

Appointments

Follicular phase (ideally the initial appointment): features literature distribution, client education, history, and tool administration.

Luteal phase: follow-up of client education and evaluation; tool administration. Correlate all tool and historical findings; conference with client. Develop client-centered, goal-oriented, self-management strategies and nursing interventions.

Provide written guidelines for client with every appointment.

Evaluation, examination, and laboratory work as indicated by reproductive endocrinologist (ob-gyn) physician at second appointment. Pharmacologic therapy as directed (frequently progesterone suppositories: obtain consent, teach drug protocol featuring luteal self-administration, signs or symptoms for which to notify clinic, usual nursing drug education.)

[a]Abraham GE. *Premenstrual Blues.* Los Angeles: Porter & Griffin, 1982.
Adapted from Wilhelm-Hass E. Premenstrual Syndrome: its nature, evaluation and management. J Obstet Gynecol Neonatal Nurs. *1984;13: 223–229.*

with mood disorders related to PMS and 9 women without PMS found no difference, however, between the groups in blood levels or patterns of secretions of progesterone, cortisol, and other substances often thought to be related to PMS. Based on the study's results, the researchers could find no physiologic basis for the use of bromocriptine, progesterone, or cortisol in the treatment of PMS.[35] Clearly, PMS is a controversial subject in need of further research.

Alterations in Patterns of Uterine Bleeding

Well-woman assessment includes questions directed toward the nature of menstruation along with physician referral, as appropriate, of those women who do experience patterns of abnormal bleeding. Abnormal menstrual patterns are not diseases in themselves but signs of other conditions that range from benign to malignant. Specific questions about uterine bleeding patterns provide an opportunity for identification of gynecologic problems. Actual management depends on the reason for the abnormal bleeding.[37–39]

Women often do not know what normal menstruation is; they may need reassurance that their menstrual flow is normal (*see* Table 5–3) or prompt follow-up if the reported flow pattern is abnormal. Table 5–6 summarizes patterns of abnormal and normal uterine bleeding.[30,37,38] In-depth discussion of gynecologic pathology is, however, beyond the scope of this textbook.

Dysmenorrhea

Dysmenorrhea, pain during menstruation, is the most common complaint of gynecologic clients.[30] Although many adolescents and adult women have mild discomfort during menstruation, only a small number are incapacitated by menstrual pain. According to Gerbie, "dysmenorrhea is present if pain prevents normal activity and requires medication, whether over-the-counter drugs or those prescribed. . . ."[30] The nurse should realize that dysmenorrhea is a real physical condition experienced by psychologically healthy women from various backgrounds and socioeconomic groups.[40]

Dysmenorrhea is a symptom that can be attributed to several possible causes (Table 5–7).[23,30,40] Reasons for pain can be attributed to increased prostaglandin activity with no organic pathology (primary dysmenorrhea) or to various acquired uterine and pelvic abnormalities (secondary dysmenorrhea). On rare occasion, extreme cramping pain may be experienced if the whole endometrial lining is sloughed intact through the undilated cervix. Cramping pain during menstruation, along with heavier bleeding, may be an expected side effect of intrauterine devices (IUD). Pain is a subjective and personal experience. A client's culture and psychosocial background, as well as the reactions to menstruation on the part of close female family members, may affect her experience of dysmenorrhea.

Management of Dysmenorrhea. A careful history and physical need to be performed in order to establish whether the client's pain is related to pathologic conditions. Questions about the pain should include[30]:

- What is the pain like?
- How severe is the pain?

TABLE 5–6. PATTERNS OF ABNORMAL AND NORMAL UTERINE BLEEDING

Pattern	Type of Bleeding	Possible Cause
Menorrhagia (Hypermenorrhea)	Heavy bleeding with or without clots; may be "gushing" or like an "open faucet" Occurs at regular intervals Usually greater than 100 mL	Adenomyosis Submucous myoma Endometrial hyperplasia Tumors Dysfunctional bleeding
Hypomenorrhea	Very light flow; "spotting"	Oral contraceptives Asherman's syndrome (amenorrhea and secondary sterility caused by intrauterine adhesions and uterine synechiae) May be normal for some women
Cryptomenorrhea	Bleeding occurs but does not show externally	Obstruction of lower vaginal canal (eg, hymenal or cervical stenosis)
Metrorrhagia	Bleeding between menstrual periods	Ovulation (spotting at midcycle) Endometrial polyps; endometrial and cervical carcinoma Estrogen administration
Polymenorrhea	Periods occur too often	Associated with anovulation
Menometrorrhagia	Bleeding at irregular intervals Variable amount and length of bleeding	Any condition causing bleeding between periods; sudden onset may indicate malignancy
Oligomenorrhea	Bleeding more than 35 days apart; decreased amount of bleeding Usually irregular periods every 2–5 months	Associated with anovulation, eg, from endocrine conditions (menopause), systemic conditions (large weight loss), estrogen-secreting tumors
Amenorrhea		
Primary	Absence of menarche by age 16 with absence of secondary sexual development	Associated with low estrogen production or other endocrine abnormalities, severe nutritional deprivation Severe stress Congenital disorders, anovulation
Secondary	Absence of menses longer than 6 months in a woman who had previously menstruated	Associated with numerous factors, such as: Nutritional alterations (obesity, weight loss, malnutrition); Hypothalamic, pituitary, or endocrine disorders; vigorous exercise, severe stress, or psychogenic factors; Chronic illness Drug use
Physiologic	Absence of menses as a result of normal bodily processes	Pregnancy, lactation, menopause
Contact bleeding	Bleeding after vaginal intercourse	Associated with cervical cancer, cervical polyps, cervical or vaginal infections May be normal in pregnancy, as a result of softening of cervix Rarely normal in nonpregnant woman

- In what ways has the pain interfered with or prevented usual activities?
- When does the pain start?
- What makes the pain worse?
- How long has this type of pain existed?
- How long does the pain last?
- Has the pain been getting better, worse, or staying the same over time?
- Are any other symptoms present?
- What has the client done to relieve the pain?
- Have these remedies helped?
- Has the client been worried about the pain?
- If the client has taken oral contraceptives, has the pain been better or worse?

Several interventions may be helpful in providing relief for dysmenorrhea. Primary dysmenorrhea may be relieved by nonpharmacologic strategies alone or in combination with certain medications. Nonpharmacologic strategies include: heat (warm showers, heating pad to abdomen or back, warm beverages), massage (back rub or abdominal massage), mild exercise, stress reduction and relaxation techniques, education and reassurance, and teaching

TABLE 5–7. TYPES OF DYSMENORRHEA

Type	Cause	Characteristics
Primary	No organic disease Pain related to prostaglandin activity and to uterine ischemia	Begins with onset of regular ovulation (1–3 years after menarche) Associated with ovulatory cycles More common in women never pregnant May decrease after childbirth More common in obesity Less common in athletes Less common in women with irregular menses Pain most severe on first or second day of flow Cramping (low, midline) May have pain in back or thighs May have nausea, vomiting, diarrhea, headache General pelvic tenderness on examination during menses
Secondary	Pain a result of pelvic pathologic condition	Begins after age 20 Pain may be one-sided
	Pelvic inflammatory disease	Acute onset Painful intercourse Tenderness on examination May have adnexal mass Confirmed by cervical culture, CBC, eosinophile sedimentation rate
	Endometriosis	Cyclic pain on intercourse Pain increases throughout menses Steady, rather than crampy pain Pain may be in one site Nodules may be felt on pelvic exam; diagnosis confirmed by laparoscopy
	Uterine prolapse	Most common in multiparas Occurs later in reproductive years Painful intercourse Backache, beginning premenstrually, lasting through menses Pelvic pain, more severe premenstrually Pain may be relieved by lying down or knee-chest position May also have cystocele or urinary stress incontinence
	Fibroids or polyps	Pain in later reproductive years Associated with changes in flow pattern Cramping type pain Fibroids may be felt on pelvic exam Fibroids confirmed by ultrasound Polyps not easily felt
Membranous	Passage of intact endometrial lining through undilated cervix (rare occurrence)	Intense cramping
Intrauterine device	Presence of IUD	Cramping during menses Heavier bleeding

strategies focusing on development of positive attitudes toward menstruation.[40]

Medications that block prostaglandin synthesis have been useful in relieving dysmenorrhea. Traditionally, aspirin was used for its mild antiprostaglandin effect, anti-inflammatory actions, and analgesic properties. Currently medications such as ibuprofen and naproxen sodium have been successfully used. Antiprostaglandins prevent prostaglandin synthesis and should be given before pain is severe.[30]

Relief of secondary dysmenorrhea depends mostly on treatment of the pathologic condition. Management may include specific pharmacologic or surgical interventions, as well as symptomatic relief strategies used for primary dysmenorrhea.

Occasionally, dysmenorrhea related to IUD use

is severe enough for a woman to elect another form of contraception. Once the IUD is removed, related menstrual cramping is relieved.

Endometriosis. Endometriosis is a condition characterized by ectopic growth of endometrial-like tissue in locations outside the uterus. Dysmenorrhea and dyspareunia are clinical symptoms. Endometriosis is frequently associated with infertility and for this reason is discussed in Chapter 7.

Menstrual Hygiene

Sanitary Pads or Napkins. Sanitary pads or napkins have been the most widely used method of containing menstrual flow. Pads have been made from a variety of synthetic and natural fabrics. Many women purchase disposable sanitary pads in supermarkets, pharmacies, and other convenience stores. Some women, however, particularly those who cannot afford the purchase price or who live in areas where these products are not accessible, use homemade pads, made from a variety of fabrics. Cotton is the most absorbent. These menstrual "rags" are then laundered and reused.

Sanitary pads may be held in place by a belt or by adhesive strips that attach to the crotch of the woman's undergarment. (The adhesive strips are never applied to the skin.) The menstrual flow leaves the body and collects on the menstrual pad. For this reason, women using pads are at lower risk for infections such as toxic shock syndrome than women who use tampons. The pad is replaced when it becomes moderately saturated. Disposable sanitary pads are not flushable. Women need to protect others from contact with bloody body fluids and should take care to wrap soiled pads and discard them in a closed container. Regular changing of the pads, daily showering, and cleansing bloody flow from the perineum with mild soap and water are adequate to control any menstrual odor.

Commercial sanitary pads are marketed in a variety of sizes and thicknesses, ranging from thin "mini" pads to superabsorbent "maxi" pads for heavy flow days. The thicker pads are usually more expensive. Selection of type of pad is determined by flow patterns, personal choice, and also by the impact of advertising campaigns. Some women use sanitary pads along with tampons to prevent leakage onto their clothing during days of heaviest flow.

Sanitary pads are available in deodorant and nondeodorant varieties. Deodorant pads are not recommended, as some women may find the perfumes irritating.

Advantages of pads include ease in use, no need for internal application, wide accessibility, greater cultural acceptance, and decreased risk of infection. Disadvantages of pads include less comfort than tampons, presence of external menstrual flow, and "bulkiness."

Tampons. Tampons are plugs inserted into the vagina for the purpose of absorbing menstrual flow. It has been estimated that 70 percent of the 30,000,000 menstruating women in the United States use tampons.[41] In the United States, tampons are commercially made from a combination of cotton and rayon and from polyacrylate fibers. Some tampons also contain deodorant perfumes to alter menstrual odor, although these can be irritating to some women. Tampons can be used by almost any menstruating woman or girl. Slight stretching related to insertion of the first tampon may be mildly uncomfortable for the woman who has never before used tampons or who has never had a vaginal examination. Tampon insertion should not, however, be painful after the first time. After proper insertion, the tampon should be so comfortable that the woman should be unaware of its presence (Figure 5–7). By absorbing menstrual flow before it leaves the vagina, tampons minimize the chance of bloody soiling of clothing and are therefore often selected over external menstrual pads, which may be bulky, irritating, and uncomfortable.

Selection of Tampons. The choice of tampons or pads is a personal decision made by the client. Nurses working with adolescent and adult females, however, have important teaching roles regarding menstrual hygiene. Some girls or women mistakenly fear that

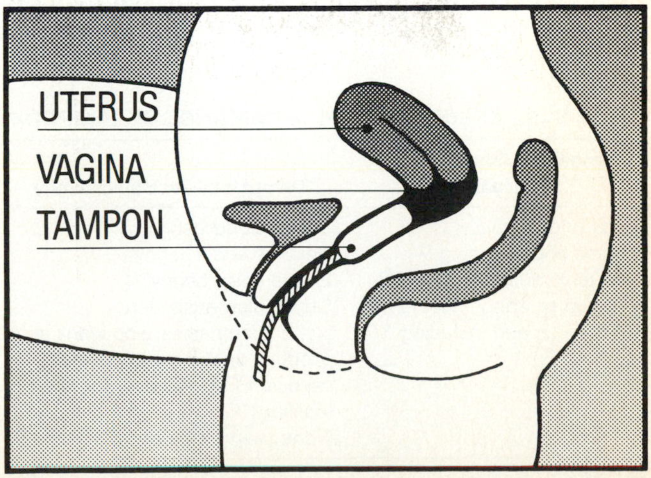

Figure 5–7. Tampon in proper position.

use of tampons will indicate they are no longer virgins. Mothers of young teenagers often need to be reassured that tampons do not cause hymenal tearing and do not predispose their daughters to sexually promiscuous behavior.

Tampons are an excellent choice for most women, but they are not acceptable to every woman. To use tampons successfully, a woman needs to want to use tampons, be willing and able to assume self-care practices involving touching of her genitalia, have access to a clean water supply for hand-washing, be able to afford or have access to an adequate supply of tampons (so that prolonging time between changing is not done to save money), and have access to a health care provider in case infection develops.

Tampons are marketed in a variety of absorbency sizes. Most companies produce "junior" sizes for young or first-time users of tampons. Other sizes range from "regular" to "super" and "super plus" absorbency. In accordance with a final rule issued by the U S Food and Drug Administration (FDA), terms used to describe tampon absorbency are now standardized.[42] In the past, considerable variation in absorbency existed between brands using the same terms. As of March 1, 1990, tampon manufacturers must label their products using the term corresponding to the absorbency of their tampons, as determined by a specified FDA test method (Table 5–8). Labeling tampons now permits consumers to compare the absorbency of different brands, to know the absorbency they are buying, and to get similar absorbency when they change brands. The lowest absorbency required to control menstrual flow is recommended, as the chance of toxic shock syndrome, described below, rises with each additional gram of tampon absorbency.

Selection of brand depends on personal choice and is affected by factors such as advertising, brands used by family and friends, brands stocked by local stores, presence or absence of tampon applicator, and type of applicator. Selection of tampon requires thoughtful evaluation of the menstrual flow, identification of times of heaviest bleeding, purchase of more than one absorbency size or a combination of tampons and sanitary pads, and consideration of risk of toxic shock syndrome. Table 5–9 provides answers to commonly asked questions about tampon use.

TABLE 5–8. ABSORBENCY PERFORMANCE OF TAMPONS

Ranges of Absorbency (in grams)	Term Used for Absorbency
6 and under	Junior absorbency
6 up to and including 9	Regular absorbency
> 9 up to and including 12	Super absorbency
> 12 up to and including 15	Super plus absorbency
> 15 up to and including 18	None (companies who want to produce these tampons must receive FDA approval for their labeling)
> 18	None (same rule as > 15 to 18)

Ranges and terms according to US Food and Drug Administration ruling.

Toxic Shock Syndrome

Toxic shock syndrome (TSS) is a rare but potentially life-threatening condition, thought to be caused by toxins produced by the *Staphylococcus aureus* bacterium. The onset of TSS is sudden; the syndrome can produce severe illness. Three to 6 percent of women who develop TSS die.[41] Death results from such complications as adult respiratory distress syndrome, persistent hypotension, and excessive bleeding related to disseminated intravascular coagulopathy. Toxic shock syndrome occurs mostly in menstruating women under age 30 who use tampons and especially in young women 15 to 19 years of age.[42] The syndrome has been associated with use of tampons, particularly superabsorbent tampons, and other devices (such as the contraceptive sponge or diaphragm) that allow for pooling of fluid in the vagina and the growth of bacteria. Toxic shock syndrome also occurs in men, women, and children who are not menstruating or using the diaphragm or sponge, although the highest incidence is in menstruating women using tampons.[40]

Tampons provide an internal pooling place for blood and an excellent site for bacterial growth. Women who use more absorbent tampons do not have to change as frequently and therefore are at greater risk for TSS than women who use minimally absorbent tampons or who use external pads. The risk of TSS has been noted to increase 37 percent for every 1 gram increase in absorbency[44] (*see* Table 5–8). Hemsell and associates estimated that superabsorbent tampons are used by more than half of women in the United States who use tampons; therefore, a large number of women are at risk.[41]

Toxic shock syndrome tends to recur in about 30 percent of women who develop this condition. The largest risk for recurrent TSS is during the first three menstrual periods after treatment, and the syndrome may recur with greater or lesser intensity. It has been recommended that women not resume tampon use until two cervicovaginal and throat cultures, taken 4 weeks apart, have been negative for *S. aureus*. Women with a history of TSS may also be advised to avoid use of tampons, especially superabsorbent tampons.

TABLE 5–9. ANSWERS TO QUESTIONS COMMONLY ASKED ABOUT TAMPONS

Can tampons be used by girls or women who are not sexually experienced?

Yes. Tampons can be used by menstruating girls or women regardless of sexual experience.

Will a girl or woman still be a virgin if she uses tampons?

Yes. A virgin is a female who has never had sexual intercourse. Tampons do not break the hymen within the vagina nor do they in any way indicate whether or not a girl or woman is a virgin.

Should deodorant tampons be used to "feel fresher?"

No. Tampons containing deodorants or perfumes are not recommended, because some women may experience allergic reactions to these additives. Regular changing and daily external cleansing of the perineum with water or mild soap and water should be adequate. If a foul menstrual odor persists despite these measures, the health care provider should be contacted.

How often should tampons be changed?

About every 4 hours. Many women prefer to switch to pads for sleep. Although the risk of infection is very low, use of pads during long sleep periods further decreases chance of infection.

How should tampons and tampon applicators be discarded?

In areas where sewers are in use and plumbing works well, tampons can be flushed through the toilet. The paper applicator tubes that encase some tampon brands may be flushed; however, plastic tubes that are used by certain brands are not biodegradable and cannot be flushed without causing plumbing problems. Neither tampons nor paper tubes should be flushed into septic systems.

For the protection of others, care needs to be taken when any product soaked with blood or body fluids is discarded. Tampons and applicators should be wrapped and discarded in a manner that will not bring others into direct contact with body fluids.

Should douching be done regularly following tampon changes or after the last tampon is used?

No. Douching is never routinely recommended for the well woman. Indeed, complications of douching, such as allergic reactions to the solutions or overgrowth of certain microorganisms related to the douching solution's changing of the vaginal flora can result.

Are there any girls or women who should not use tampons?

Yes. Safe use of tampons depends on the ability of clients to follow directions properly, and to afford the cost of fresh tampons, the client's access to water and hygienic facilities, and the client's access to health care should tampon-related infection (toxic shock syndrome) occur. Clients who cannot assume responsibility for a basic self-care practice, clients who live in extreme poverty, clients who do not have access to bathroom facilities (homeless, and so forth), and clients who will have no access to health care (professionals doing field work in remote areas, individuals who live in poverty areas with little transportation, knowledge, or trust in health care facilities, and so on) should be advised to use external pads. Tampons are not recommended for any woman with a history of toxic shock syndrome.

Why should women care about the absorbency size of tampons?

The risk for toxic shock syndrome increases substantially for each gram increase in absorbency.[a] Therefore, women should use the lowest absorbency that will work for them. Whereas a higher absorbency tampon may be used during waking hours during the day(s) of heaviest flow, smaller or "regular" sizes should be used during times of lighter flow, eg, the first and last days of menstruation.

Should tampons be used between menstrual periods during times when vaginal discharge is heavier, for example at ovulation?

No. The healthy girl or woman should only use tampons during menstruation so as to minimize the possibility of tampon-related infection. In the absence of menstrual flow, the tampon can absorb so much moisture from the vaginal walls that tissue injury can occur when the tampon is removed in a dry, expanded state. External mini pads, along with regular daily cleansing with mild soap and plain water, are recommended. Any girl or woman having "very heavy" vaginal discharge between periods should be examined by a gynecologist or gynecologic nurse specialist.

Can tampons, inserted after intercourse, be used for contraception?

No. Tampons are not contraceptives. (Tampons must also be removed prior to intercourse to prevent trauma).

[a]Hemsell DL, et al. Pelvic infections and sexually transmitted diseases. In Pernoll ML, Benson RC, eds. *Current Obstetric & Gynecologic Diagnosis & Treatment.* 6th ed. Norwalk, Conn: Appleton & Lange, 1987, pp 715–741.

Toxic shock syndrome is a fairly "new" pathologic syndrome, as it was first identified in children in 1978. Incidence of TSS in menstruating women peaked in 1980 when 90 percent of cases occurred in menstruating women, but has declined steadily since. Currently about 55 percent of cases are related to menstruation and 45 percent occur in nonmenstruating individuals.[43] Public education, media attention, tampon labeling, lowering of tampon absorbency by manufacturers, and inclusion of literature about TSS in tampon boxes may have contributed to this decline.

In addition to absorbency labeling, the FDA requires tampon manufacturers to provide legible and clear information with all tampon packages about the following topics related to TSS: the risk of TSS to women using tampons, particularly the reported higher risks to teens and women under age 30; the estimated incidence of TSS of 1 to 17 per 100,000 menstruating women and girls per year; the possibility of death from TSS; the advice to use the lowest absorbency required to control menstrual flow to lower the risk of TSS; the ability to avoid tampon-associated TSS by not using tampons; and the advice to tampon users to decrease the risk of TSS by alternating tampons with sanitary pads during menstruation.[43] Nevertheless, TSS still occurs in menstruating women, and it remains a potential health threat to the well woman of childbearing age.[41,42]

Nursing Strategies and Toxic Shock Syndrome. The topic of TSS should be routinely discussed with all clients at well-woman health visits. Women educated about TSS are then prepared to make personal lifestyle choices that may affect their risk of TSS, such as use and selection of tampons and contraceptive methods. Although treatment of acute TSS is initiated by the physician, nurses have major health promotion roles in education about TSS. Nursing strategies could include:

- Assisting the client to identify the pattern of her menstrual flow
- Helping the client to identify the type of tampons best suited to her needs
- Assisting the client to identify other lifestyle practices (such as use of contraceptive sponge or diaphragm) that may increase the risk of TSS by providing a way for fluid to pool in the vagina and foster the growth of pathogenic bacteria
- Teaching clients about the syndrome and the signs and symptoms of TSS (Table 5–10)
- Providing written information about TSS and encouraging clients to read literature included in tampon packages by manufacturers
- Advising the client to remove the tampon, diaphragm, or sponge she is using if signs or symptoms occur
- Helping the client identify the importance of contacting her physician promptly if she develops signs or symptoms of TSS

The nurse's health promotion role also extends to public education. For example, through individual efforts or through such nursing organizations as the Organization for Obstetric, Gynecologic, and Neonatal Nurses (NAACOG), nurses could serve as authors or consultants in the development of public education packages.

Although TSS is a severe illness that may result in death, TSS affects only a small portion of the population. Tampons or contraceptive products such as the diaphragm or sponge work effectively throughout the reproductive lives of millions of women. With a few exceptions, such as clients who have a history of TSS, women need not be discouraged from using these products. Rather, they can be counseled on their selection and safe use.

TABLE 5–10. SIGNS AND SYMPTOMS OF TOXIC SHOCK SYNDROME

Sudden fever (102° F or higher)
Client feels very ill (may have headache or sore throat)
Diffuse "sunburn" type rash, especially on face and trunk
Hypotension (systolic < 90 for adults), which may progress to shock within 48 hours
Fainting or fainting on standing (orthostatic syncope)
Vomiting or watery diarrhea
Lesions on the vaginal mucosa; presence of *Stapholococcus aureus* demonstrated on cultures
Sloughing of skin, especially on soles of feet and palms of hands (this may happen 1–2 weeks after the onset of TSS)
Symptoms related to involvement of several organ systems (nervous [nuchal rigidity, other central nervous system signs], gastrointestinal [as above, also abdominal tenderness], muscular [muscle tenderness], mucous membrane [conjunctivitis, erythema of nasopharynx], renal, hepatic, cardiovascular)

Data from Hemsell DL, et al. Pelvic infections and sexually transmitted diseases. In Pernoll ML, Benson RC, eds. Current Obstetric & Gynecologic Diagnosis & Treatment. *6th ed. Norwalk, Conn: Appleton & Lange, 1987, pp. 715–741.*

The Climacteric: Reproductive Concerns

The **climacteric** is the process through which the reproductive ability of the woman ends. Like puberty, the climacteric represents a reproductive transition in a female's life and occurs over a period of years. The climacteric includes the premenopause, and the **menopause,** which technically refers to the last menstrual period. The term can also refer to the **postmenopausal period,** during which "change of life" symptoms continue to occur, although "postmenopause" is commonly used to refer to the rest of a woman's life after menopause.[45] The climacteric lasts from about age 40 through age 60, thus spanning about 15 to 20 years, although there is wide variation among women.[46,47] In the United States, the average age for physiologic menopause is 50 to 51 years.[48,49]

Although the term **premenopause** can refer to any woman still menstruating, the premenopausal part of the climacteric is a time of decreased ovarian reproductive activity. During this period, the menstrual cycle may change. Irregularly spaced anovulatory cycles may occur. The menstrual period itself may vary or it may stay the same; some periods may produce heavy bleeding, while others have scant flow. Shortening of the follicular phase of the cycle may result in periods that occur at shorter intervals than during the earlier reproductive years.[45] For example, a woman whose menstrual cycle at age 25 was 30 days might experience a menstrual cycle of 28 days by the time she is 35. The actual transition from regular cycles to the permanent absence of menstruation may be accompanied by a series of irregular menstrual periods; however, as evidenced by couples who have had "bonus babies" or "change-of-life" babies, ovulation may still take place. Women in the climacteric should continue to use birth control until at least 1 year after their last menstrual period. The menstrual changes of the climacteric make natural family planning methods especially unreliable. This presents problems for the woman who finds other methods of fertility control unacceptable and who may therefore be faced with a choice between abstinence and unintended pregnancy.

In recent years there has been a trend among career couples toward later childbearing. Starting a family has frequently been delayed until the partners have become established in their careers; second marriages and second families are also more common. Whereas age 30 used to be considered "old" for a first baby, more women are now attempting to start families after age 35 or 40.

Although by the time of the climacteric the woman may be emotionally and financially ready for childbearing, reproductively she is at a disadvantage. Anovulatory cycles may make infertility a major problem during this time. After being concerned about not getting pregnant for so many years, the woman may experience a personal crisis related to inability to conceive. While various strategies to promote conception may be used (*see* Chapter 9), the client and her partner benefit greatly from the nurse's support and knowledgeable encouragement.

BREAST CARE

Changes that occur within the breast can produce a variety of benign or malignant conditions. These abnormalities may be detected by women themselves or by health care providers during the assessment process. Nurses working with well women must be knowledgeable about breast assessment and must be prepared to provide appropriate referrals should breast abnormalities be detected.

Benign Breast Conditions

The female breast from puberty to menopause is in a constant state of change. These changes in the breast tissue are for the most part due to the effects of estrogen and progesterone on the breast tissue itself. Estrogen stimulation during puberty causes proliferation of the vascular, glandular, fatty, and connective tissues of the breast. Breast tissue during menses undergoes cyclic changes, once again in response to increasing and decreasing levels of estrogen and progesterone.[50,51]

Breast tissue may also respond in abnormal ways to hormonal changes, with fibrosis of the tissue, cyst formation, or abnormal proliferation (growth) of cells. The changes that take place in these conditions may be due to the direct effect of hormones or to an abnormal responsiveness of the breast tissue itself to normal levels of hormones.[51]

Benign breast disease is extremely common and affects all women at one time or another.[50] Fibrosis of the breast tissue and cyst formation are the most common form of benign breast disease, so-called fibrocystic disease. These findings are so prevalent in women that the American Cancer Society has suggested that fibrocystic *disease* be called fibrocystic *change*.[52] Women with fibrocystic changes have tender nodular areas, particularly in the upper outer quadrants of the breasts. These areas may change in size during the menstrual cycle. Tenderness may increase just before menstruation.[50] Treatment of fibrocystic change with vitamin E, avoidance of caffeine, and vitamin A, have had mixed results.[50] Hormonal manipulation with danazol and tamoxifen has also been recommended.[50] Fibrocystic changes in the breast are not associated with an increased incidence of breast cancer.[53] Fibrocystic disease presenting with cysts or solid, discrete masses may mimic breast cancer, however.

Isolated cysts may be treated with aspiration. The fluid should be sent for cytologic examination. If the cyst does not disappear after aspiration, if the fluid reaccumulates, or the fluid is bloody or analyzed as being suspicious for cancer, an excisional biopsy should be done. Solid, discrete masses must be biopsied to rule out malignancy.

Fibroadenomas are another type of benign breast lesion. Fibroadenomas are discrete, rubbery nontender masses. They are found most often in the upper outer quadrant of the breast. They are the most common breast tumor in adolescents, with a peak incidence at age 17 to 20 years.[54] Fibroadenomas tend to be more common in blacks. These masses are slow-growing, often increase in size during pregnancy, and decrease in size after delivery. A finding of a fibroadenoma is not associated with an increased incidence of breast cancer. Surgical excision is, however, generally advised.

Duct ectasia, another type of benign breast disease, occurs when stasis and obstruction occur in the breast ducts, leading to inflammation of the area. The ducts involved are usually under the nipple. Women present with a mass under the nipple or in the areola and a sticky nipple discharge. The discharge may be greenish, greenish-brown, or bloodstained. The inflammation may progress to abscess formation. Duct ectasia is not associated with an increased risk of breast cancer.[51] A subareolar mass, however, especially when associated with a bloody nipple discharge, may mimic breast cancer.[50]

Intraductal papillomas are growths of the linings of the mammary ducts; the growths project into the walls of the ducts. Intraductal papillomas are very fragile, bleed easily, and also obstruct the duct. These growths account for the majority of cases of spontaneous nipple discharge in the nonlactating female.[50] Solitary papillomas are not associated with an increased risk of malignancy. Multiple intraductal papillomas, however, are associated with an increased risk of breast cancer.[51]

Growths of the breast ductal or lobular cells may occur and may present as discrete breast masses. These growths may have different pathologic diagnoses and include apocrine metaplasia, adenosis, and epitheliosis or papillomatosis.[51] Benign breast tumors associated with growth of the cells of the breast (proliferation), and atypia of these cells, have been associated with an increased risk of breast cancer.[53]

Breast Cancer and the Well Woman

Breast cancer is the most common malignancy in women. It is estimated that approximately one in ten women in the United States will develop cancer of the breast, up from an estimate of one in fifteen in 1975.[55] Lung cancer is the leading cause of female cancer deaths in the United States; however, more women are diagnosed with breast cancer than any other kind of cancer.[56] In North America, the incidence of breast cancer rises with age, although breast cancer occurs in all age groups of women. By age 50, there are estimated to be 180 cases per 100,000 women.[57]

The cause of breast cancer is unknown. Breast cancer in a particular client may be due to a combination of genetic, environmental, hormonal, nutritional, and environmental factors, although to date no direct cause-effect relationship from these factors has been proven. The most important risk factor appears to be a family history of the disease. If a woman's mother had breast cancer, the incidence of breast malignancy in the daughter increases by 1.6 times the incidence in the general population. If a woman's sister develops breast cancer, the incidence increases by 1.4 times the incidence in the general population. Only 10 percent of clients who develop breast cancer, however, have a mother or sister with breast cancer; most women diagnosed with breast cancer do not have maternal relatives who had the disease.[58] Therefore, every woman in the United States may be considered at risk for breast cancer and in need of information about early detection.

It has been suggested that increased dietary fat may lead to a higher incidence of breast cancer. There is no conclusive evidence, however, that dietary fat directly causes breast cancer, although further research on this topic is underway.[59–61] Likewise, cigarette smoking, alcohol consumption, and environmental factors have not been proven to significantly increase the risk of breast cancer, although they do increase the risk of other types of pathologic conditions.[62–64] Controversy exists over whether or not or to what extent oral contraceptive use is linked to breast cancer. For example, in a review of studies on hormones and breast cancer, Wile and Disaia found no conclusive evidence linking oral contraceptives with the onset or worsening of breast cancer.[65] In a study of British women who were diagnosed with breast cancer before age 36, the United Kingdom National Case Control Study Group, however, did find a relationship between the risk of breast cancer at an early age and the use of oral contraceptives.[66]

Currently, there is no known way to prevent breast cancer. Survival therefore depends largely on early detection. Early detection is made possible by a three-point program that includes clinical examination, breast self-examination, and radiographic screening through use of mammography. Breast cancer screening is a method of secondary prevention, because the goal is to detect disease in its earliest stages. Deaths from breast cancer have been shown to be reduced substantially through careful screening that makes early detection possible.[67]

Clinical Breast Examination and Breast Self-Examination

Clinical breast examination is performed by a physician or nurse skilled in breast examination. The frequency of clinical breast examination varies, according to the client's age and risk factors such as family history or history of breast disease. For example, a healthy 30-year-old woman whose mother developed breast cancer before menopause might be examined every 6 months. A healthy 30-year-old woman with no known risk factors might be examined annually. Table 5–2 outlines techniques recommended for clinical breast examination.[7,11]

The smallest palpable breast cancer detected on physical examination by the experienced examiner is about 1 cm. It is estimated that by the time a breast cancer is palpable it has been present for 2 years or more. At this stage, some 20 to 33 percent of clients already have tumor metastases to the axillary lymph nodes or other areas of the body.[68,69] Women who practice routine breast self-examination tend to find masses sooner, however, and at a time when the masses are smaller than do women who do not routinely self-examine. A study by Foster and Costanza found that the long-term mortality rate was lower in women who practiced breast self-examination.[70]

Mammography in Breast Screening

Long-term survival has been further increased by detection of breast tumors before they are palpable. **Mammography,** a type of x-ray examination of the breast, is a mass screening technique that is about 90 percent accurate in detecting the presence of breast abnormalities (Figure 5–8).[69] In one study, 49 (32 percent) of 151 breast cancers were diagnosed as a result of mammography, because they were as yet too small to feel.[71] In reports of clients who had tumors that were detected by mammography only, the incidence of metastases decreased and survival increased.[69,72] Actual survival, however, depends on such factors as whether the cancer has spread. Currently, mammography units (called "dedicated" units) use lower radiation doses than did units in the past, and modern mammography is considered safe. The dose of radiation to the breast during one mammographic study is 0.1 to 0.2 rads.[51] It would take approximately 26 to 40 mammograms per year to cause a 1 percent increase in breast cancer in a given client.[73]

A negative mammogram does not exclude cancer. Although a mammogram can indicate whether a lump is malignant, it cannot with certainty identify

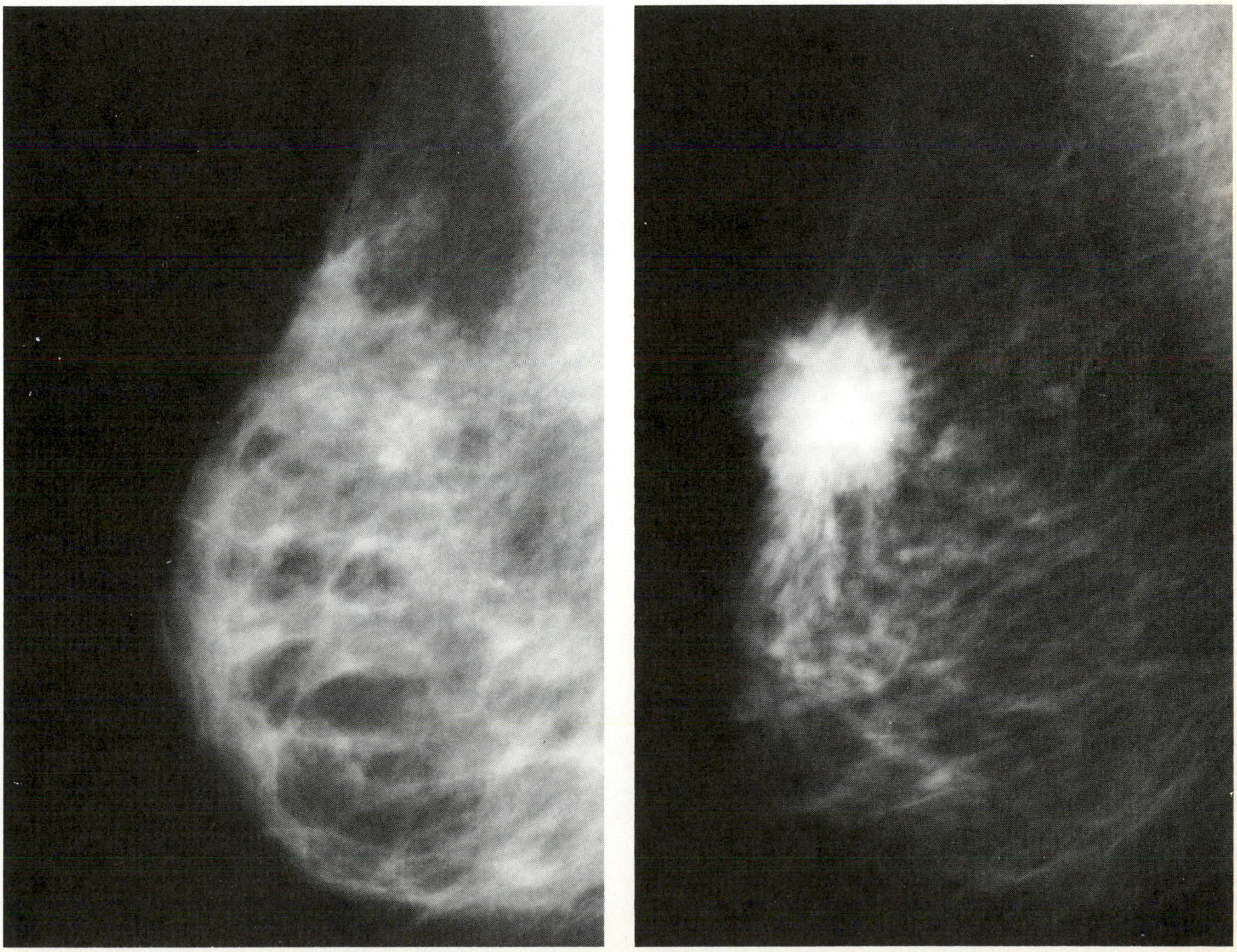

A **B**

Figure 5–8. A. Normal mammogram. **B.** Abnormal mammogram.

whether or not a mass is benign. For this reason, a discrete breast lump must be biopsied, ie, surgically sampled for direct microscopic examination.[74]

Several barriers have prevented mammography from being put into general use. These barriers have included[7]:

- Health care providers' lack of understanding of the value of mammography in screening women who do not have identifiable pathologic conditions of the breast; erroneous beliefs that mammography is unnecessary.
- Mistaken beliefs about radiation risks related to mammography.
- Cost of mammography. Many insurance plans will cover the cost of mammography only if done for diagnostic, rather than routine screening purposes. The well client must then pay for the mammogram herself. While free screening programs do exist, they are not widely available or may be available only on a limited basis.
- Client's lack of knowledge about mammography as a part of routine screening for the well woman. Clients themselves can do much to inspire health care providers to investigate the benefits of mammography.

Other screening techniques such as thermography, diaphanography (transillumination), ultrasonography, and computerized tomography (CT scan) have not been shown to be as useful as mammography in screening for lesions too small to palpate. Nuclear magnetic resonance imaging may be an important screening device; however, the costs remain too high for MRI to be widely available.[51, 75]

Recommendations for Breast Cancer Screening

The nurse will find that various recommendations for breast cancer screening exist and depend on the group issuing the guidelines. The American Cancer Society, for example, recommends that[55]:

1. Breast self-examination should be done each month beginning at age 20, regardless of whether a woman is examined annually or more often by a health care provider
2. Between the ages of 20 and 40, women should have a clinical breast examination at least every 3 years
3. All women with signs or symptoms of breast disease should have a clinical breast examination and mammography (further management is based on the woman's unique situation)
4. All women should have a base-line mammogram between the ages of 35 and 40, whether symptomatic or not
5. All women over 40 should have a clinical breast examination annually; mammograms are recommended yearly or every other year until age 49
6. All women over 50 should have a physical examination and mammography every year

Educating the Well Woman About Breast Self-Examination

It is not possible for women to be examined often enough by health professionals for the earliest detection of breast cancer. Most breast lumps are discovered by women themselves. Therefore, women need to be taught to develop skill in breast self-examination (Table 5–11 and Figure 5–3 E and F). Nurses, nurse specialists, and physicians have important roles in providing education about the importance of breast self-examination (BSE), in teaching the technique of BSE, in providing information about breast care, and in ensuring that accurate information is conveyed to all women through public education campaigns.

Teaching Strategies for Breast Self-Examination

A variety of teaching strategies for BSE have been used and have included pamphlets, videotapes, slide-tape programs, films, lecture, group discussion, and one-to-one breast instruction. Successful BSE is a self-care, wellness practice that incorporates accurate, adequate information, a positive, willing attitude to perform BSE effectively and regularly, and the skill to do BSE well. Lump detection requires a degree of skill that can be assessed through return demonstration.

Passive methods, such as pamphlets or videotapes alone, are not as effective as hands-on one-to-one teaching that requires return demonstrations by the client. Assaf and associates studied women who were given BSE pamphlets, women who viewed a BSE videotape, and women who practiced BSE on a lifelike breast model.[76] Three months after the training, lump detection performance was significantly higher among those women who were given the chance to practice BSE on a model with corrective feedback given by an instructor. The investigators concluded that the opportunity to practice BSE with guided feedback was crucial to the development of women's skill in BSE.

McLendon and colleagues worked with a disadvantaged group of women from low socioeconomic-class backgrounds.[77] Their study findings showed

TABLE 5–11. TECHNIQUE OF BREAST SELF-EXAMINATION

Goals

To identify the presence of any abnormality in the breast and to obtain treatment without delay. Women should not focus on making their own diagnoses of whether or not a lump is malignant.

Timing

Monthly. For the premenopausal woman, about seven days after the onset of menstruation, when breasts are at the softest. On the same date each month for women who are not menstruating, for example during pregnancy, before menstruation resumes after childbirth, and after menopause.

Sequence

Similar to breast examination performed by a physician or nurse skilled in clinical examination of the breast. The intent of breast examination is to inspect and to palpate all areas of the breast and lymph nodes.

Step 1: Stand or sit in front of a mirror. First look at breasts carefully with arms at side, then with arms raised overhead, and finally with hands on hips and elbows moved forward to flex the chest muscles. Observe for *changes* in breast size, shape, skin texture; for areas of dimpling in the skin, flattening, broadening or retraction of the nipples, or discharge or crusting on the nipple surface.

Normal Observations: In most women, one breast is larger than the other and should cause no alarm. Women who are pregnant, have recently given birth, or who are breast-feeding will normally have a clear or milky discharge from the nipple.

Step 2: Feel for lumps in the armpit. Begin with arms at side; with the right hand reach across and feel the left armpit area. Repeat on the opposite side (*see* Figure 5–3,A–D).

Step 3: Palpation of the breast for lumps (*see* Figure 5–3E). Lie on the back on a firm surface, such as a firm bed or the floor. Put a small pillow or folded towel under the right shoulder and place the right hand behind the head. (This stretches and flattens the breast and makes self-examination easier).

Procedure: Using the flat part of the fingers of the left hand, feel every part of the breast, nipple, and chest area toward the shoulder and armpit. A circular or vertical pattern, as shown in Figure 5–3F, can be used. Repeat this procedure on the opposite side.

Normal Finding: A firm ridge of tissue in the lower curve of the breast.

Guidelines: As long as all areas of the breast are felt, it does not matter which pattern for palpation is chosen. Be careful not to "skip around" while palpating.

Step 4: Check nipples for discharge. Starting at the outside of each breast, use both hands in a "milking" motion that moves toward the nipple in order to express any discharge present. Another approach is to squeeze each nipple to check for discharge.

Step 5: Repeat the pattern while in the shower.

Step 6: If any abnormality is found, call a health care provider. Although most breast abnormalities are not cancer, do not wait to see if any changes take place.

that women who received one-to-one BSE instruction demonstrated a significantly greater increase in BSE knowledge and performed BSE with greater accuracy than women who did not receive this type of instruction. Difficulty with extended follow-up of the population in the study highlighted the importance of providing the most effective instructional program possible on initial contact with clients.

Breast self-evaluation can be taught to adolescent and adult females. Indeed, a goal is for BSE to be regarded as a natural, self-care practice. A woman's long-term familiarity with her normal breast places her in a better position to identify abnormalities at a future date. A financially cost-free technique, BSE can be performed easily within the privacy of a woman's home at her convenience. The nurse should realize that BSE can be taught to all women, regardless of their socioeconomic background. The nurse needs to understand and to be sensitive to the client's cultural background and reactions to touching herself, however.

Some clients are terrified of self-examination and may fear the possibility of breast cancer. For many women, BSE requires a certain degree of courage.[78] The nurse needs to reassure the client that BSE should be performed monthly, not daily. Teaching strategies that allow for discussion of feelings and fears are necessary, as well as ample opportunity for guided practice and for the woman to provide a return demonstration of her own BSE. The nurse should emphasize that the woman need only to identify normal and abnormal variations in her own breasts and to contact her health care provider without delay if she discovers any abnormality. Trying to diagnose the nature of her own breast lumps is not part of her tasks in BSE.[7] The woman's partner can be taught the technique of breast examination in cases in which the woman is unable to perform BSE independently.

Providing Support for the Woman Undergoing Routine Breast Screening

Providing a calm, welcoming approach and addressing emotional concerns related to assessment can do much to ease the emotional stress related to routine breast screening. In some places, mammography is done in breast imaging units, separate from other diagnostic radiologic areas. In this way the special needs of the woman undergoing breast screening can be addressed without the emotional pressure inherent in units where clients are being evaluated for various other problems. In some units, the radiologist reads the mammogram immediately, so the woman is spared the strain of waiting to hear of her results. Before leaving, the well woman may also meet with a nurse specialist who provides an educational session related to breast self-examination and screening.

Nursing Strategies for Care of the Woman with a Breast Lump

Nurses in wellness settings may frequently work with women who have breast lumps discovered during routine office examination or by BSE. Although most breast lumps are not malignant, many women respond to this finding with fear and anxiety. Nursing strategies to assist the client include:

- Provision of emotional support to the client. There is a natural tendency to want to comfort clients with the reassurance that the lump is benign. The nurse needs to remember, however, that a definitive diagnosis of a discrete lump can be made only with a biopsy. Remaining with the client and encouraging her to express her feelings are ways to demonstrate support.
- Providing anticipatory guidance about procedures to follow. All women with breast lumps should be referred for a mammogram. Whereas this study can provide some information about the mass (eg, whether or not it is suggestive of malignancy), its greatest use is in detection of other breast lumps too small to feel. As noted, the mammogram cannot be used to tell with certainty whether or not a lump is cancerous. If the breast lump is suspicious clinically or by mammography, the woman will be scheduled for a biopsy. If a breast lesion is detected by mammography only on screening but cannot be felt by the examiner, a needle is placed in the suspicious area immediately before the biopsy. This procedure is done by the radiologist in the mammography unit under local anesthesia and is termed *needle localization*. The woman is then taken to the operating suite where the surgeon biopsies the area around the needle. The specimen may be sent for repeat mammography to make certain the suspicious area has been removed. When breast lumps are removed, results of a "frozen" section of the specimen will often be given at the time of the procedure. The definitive final analysis of the specimen takes a few days to complete, however. If the lump is benign, no further treatment, other than suture removal and then regular breast evaluation will be necessary. If the lump is malignant, a variety of treatment options will be considered. Detailed discussion of treatment of benign and malignant disorders of the breast is beyond the scope of this chapter. The reader is referred to the vast nursing and medical literature on breast pathology.
- "Protection" of the client. The occurrence of a breast lump is often of clinical interest to medical and nursing staff. In the interest of client health, manipulation of the mass should be kept to a minimum.
- Referral of the client for surgical follow-up. Identification of a breast mass is usually made by the nurse practitioner or gynecologist in the wellness setting or by the client herself. Treatment of the mass is currently done by surgeons, particularly those skilled in treating diseases of the breast. An essential strategy is prompt referral to the appropriate resource. The nurse or physician in the wellness setting should never simply "follow" a lump over time, as there is no way to feel or "just intuitively know" whether a lump is benign. Although treatment of a breast lump needs to be done without delay, it is not an emergency. Mammography and biopsy may be scheduled within a few days of the wellness visit, but the client should not leave the office or clinic without a definite return appointment. In addition, health care professionals need to be certain that the client is not too distraught. If necessary, the client should be asked to remain until she calms or until a relative, friend, or other means of safe transportation home can be found.

Current Therapies for Breast Cancer

Currently there are a variety of therapeutic alternatives available to the woman diagnosed with breast cancer. The therapy actually selected depends on several factors, such as the size of the tumor, the type of tumor, whether or not the tumor has spread beyond the breast, the age of the client, and the client's personal choice. The nurse should be prepared to reinforce or explain the various treatment options in order to assist the client in making her own decisions. Examples of current therapeutic approaches include:

1. Lumpectomy and axillary lymph node dissection, radiation to the affected breast, and additional chemotherapy or hormonal therapy, depending on factors such as the woman's age, the status of the lymph nodes, and whether or not the tumor is estrogen- or progesterone-receptor positive
2. Modified radical mastectomy; in addition, chemotherapy or hormonal manipulation therapy

Choice of medical therapy following mastectomy depends on factors such as the woman's age, type of tumor, lymph node status, and estrogen- or progesterone-receptor status.

CASE STUDY/CARE PLAN: TEACHING BREAST SELF-EXAMINATION

Erma James, 24 years old, comes to the health center for a well-woman checkup and to learn about breast self-examination (BSE), which she heard about on television. She has no family history of breast cancer. Thorough assessment confirms that she is currently in good health.

Supporting Assessment Data	Expected Client/Family Outcome	Nursing Action/ Intervention	Rationale	Criteria for Evaluation
Nursing Diagnosis: Potential asset in self-care practices, related to desire to learn self-screening techniques				
24-year old woman seeks teaching about the correct technique for breast self-examination (BSE)	After completion of the visit, client will continue self-screening practices	Recognize and support client's initiative and positive self-care practices.	Rewarding positive self-care practices helps build confidence and reinforces continuation of these practices.	Client continues to practice self-screening techniques. Client continues to seek well-woman care.
Nursing Diagnosis: Knowledge deficit, related to BSE				
Client states desire to learn because of emphasis on BSE in a television program	After completion of the visit, client will:			
Current clinical examination is normal; client has had no breast pathology to date	Identify the importance and timing of monthly BSE	Discuss the importance of BSE for all women.	One in 10 women in the United States develops breast cancer in her lifetime. Most breast cancers are diagnosed in women without risk factors. Early detection improves survival and depends on BSE along with clinical examinations. BSE should be a life-long practice for all women. Knowing what is normal helps women identify any abnormalities.	When asked, client is able to state the importance and timing of BSE.
	Demonstrate ability to perform BSE independently	Identify knowledge deficits by having client demonstrate BSE	Teaching is based on assessment of existing knowledge.	
		Demonstrate how to perform BSE. Models, pamphlets, and audiovisual aids can be used		Client is able to see correct technique and practice on models.
		Have client perform return demonstration	Return demonstration of BSE allows for assessment of client's technique of BSE.	Client demonstrates correct technique for BSE.
	State her intention to perform BSE monthly	Discuss client's feelings about the value of BSE	Attitude about BSE affects actual performance of technique.	On future visits, client reports performing BSE each month after her menstrual period.
	Identify importance of contacting health care providers without delay if abnormalities are detected during BSE	Discuss the importance of prompt reporting of breast abnormalities	Reporting abnormalities promptly leads to earlier diagnosis and potentially more effective treatment.	Client returns promptly for follow-up if she discovers any abnormality during BSE.

SUMMARY

The goals of health care for the well woman of childbearing age encompass primary prevention, secondary prevention, and health promotion. Nurses have major assessment and teaching roles in well-woman care. Well-woman care extends beyond gynecology to encompass the total health needs of the woman. Many women come to gynecologic settings for their primary health care as well, therefore increasing the importance of a comprehensive approach. Effectiveness of well-woman health care is impeded by such factors as variation in assessibility, affordability, and quality of care available.

Well-woman health care includes a history, physical examination, and appropriate diagnostic tests. Health care providers must also pay attention to factors such as the client's comfort and privacy during the visit and the safety of both the client and staff examiners.

Nurses frequently teach female and male clients about menstruation and answer questions girls and women have about their own bodies. Attitudes toward menstruation are influenced by many factors, such as the client's cultural background and personal experiences. Nurses must be knowledgeable about subjects such as: normal menstruation; abnormal menstrual patterns; menstrual hygiene issues, such as the use of tampons and pads; toxic shock syndrome; dysmenorrhea; premenstrual syndrome; and reproductive transitions, such as menarche and the climacteric.

One in ten women develops breast cancer during her lifetime. Early detection is crucial to successful management. Therefore, breast screening programs are based on breast self-examination performed monthly by the client, clinical breast examination at every well-woman visit, and screening tests such as mammography, ordered as appropriate. Nurses working with well women need to be aware of various types of breast abnormalities. In one-to-one or group sessions at well-woman visits and through roles in the development and implementation of public health education, nurses teach teenagers and women about the importance and technique of breast self-examination and provide referrals whenever indicated. Specially educated nurses may also perform breast screening.

REVIEW QUESTIONS

1. Describe ways in which well-woman assessment differs from gynecologic assessment.
2. Describe components of a well-woman visit.
3. Describe premenstrual syndrome and several strategies to deal with this condition.
4. Describe how tampons should be used; discuss ways in which complications related to tampon use may be avoided.
5. Discuss the importance of clinical examination, breast self-examination, and mammography in screening for breast disease.

REFERENCES

1. Cunningham FG, et al. *Williams Obstetrics.* 18th ed. Norwalk, Conn: Appleton & Lange, 1989.
2. Abrums M: Health care for women. *J Obstet Gynecol Neonatal Nurs.* 1986; 15:250–255.
3. Kutzner SK, Toussie-Weingarten C. Working parents: the dilemma of childrearing and career. *Top Clin Nurs.* 1984; 6:30–37.
4. Boston Women's Collective. *Our Bodies, Ourselves.* 2nd ed. New York: Simon & Schuster, 1986.
5. Littlefield VM. Health education for women: why? In Littlefield VM (ed). *Health Education for Women.* Norwalk, Conn: Appleton-Century-Crofts, 1986, pp 3–13.
6. Pender N. *Health Promotion in Nursing Practice.* 2nd ed. Norwalk, Conn: Appleton & Lange, 1987.
7. Nettles-Carlson B. Early detection of breast cancer. *J Obstet Gynecol Neonatal Nurs.* 1989;18:373–384.
8. Clark CC. *Wellness Nursing: Concepts, Theory, Research and Practice.* New York: Springer, 1986, pp 1–4.
9. Block GJ, Nolan JW. *Health Assessment for Professional Nursing: A Developmental Approach.* 2nd ed. Norwalk, Conn: Appleton-Century-Crofts, 1986.
10. Burnett LS. Gynecologic history, examination, and operations. In Jones HW III, et al, eds. *Novak's Textbook of Gynecology.* 11th ed. Baltimore: Williams & Wilkins, 1988, pp 3–39.
11. Winfield AC, Page DL. The breast. In Jones HW III, et al, eds. *Novak's Textbook of Gynecology.* 11th ed. Baltimore: Williams & Wilkins, 1988, pp 534–556.
12. Willard MD, et al. The educational pelvic examination: women's responses to a new approach. *J Obstet Gynecol Neonatal Nurs.* 1986;15:135–141.
13. Lawhead, RA. Vulvar self-examination (correspondence). *Am J Obstet Gynecol.* 1988;158:1238.
14. Hamilton MS, Dodge, EF. Pelvic examination: patient safety and comfort. *J Obstet Gynecol Neonatal Nurs.* 1981;10: 344–345.
15. Latta W, Weismeier E. Effects of an educational gynecological exam on women's attitudes. *J Obstet Gynecol Neonatal Nurs.* 1982;11:242–245.
16. Primrose RB. Taking the tension out of pelvic exams. *AM J Nurs.* 1984;84:72–74.

17. Areskog-Wigma B. The gynaecological examination: women's experiences and preferences and the role of the gynaecologist. *J Psychosom Obstet Gynaecol.* 1987;6:59–69.
18. Olson K. Patient comfort during pelvic examination: new foot supports vs metal stirrups. *J Obstet Gynecol Neonatal Nurs.* 1981;10:104–107.
19. Ganong WF. Physiology of reproduction. In Pernoll ML, Benson, RC. *Current Obstetric & Gynecologic Diagnosis & Treatment.* 6th ed. Norwalk, Conn: Appleton & Lange, 1987, pp 109–126.
20. Benson RC. Psychologic aspects of obstetrics & gynecology. In Pernoll ML, Benson, RC. *Current Obstetric & Gynecologic Diagnosis & Treatment,* 6th ed. Norwalk, Conn: Appleton & Lange, 1987, pp 1032–1065.
21. Grief E, Ulman K. The psychological impact of menarche on adolescent females: a review of the literature. *Child Dev.* 1982;53:1413–30.
22. Havens B, Swensen I. Menstrual perceptions and preparation among female adolescents. *J Obstet Gynecol Neonatal Nurs.* 1986;15:406–411.
23. Wilson MA. Menstrual disorders: premenstrual syndrome, dysmenorrhea, amenorrhea. *J Obstet Gynecol Neonatal Nurs.* 1984;13 (suppl.): 11S–19S.
24. Wilhelm-Hass E. Premenstrual syndrome: its nature, evaluation and management. *J Obstet Gynecol Neonatal Nurs.* 1984;13:223–229.
25. Brown MA, Zimmer PA. Personal and family impact of premenstrual symptoms. *J Obstet Gynecol Neonatal Nurs.* 1986;15:31–38.
26. Walton J, Youngkin E. The effect of a support group on self-esteem of women with premenstrual syndrome. *J Obstet Gynecol Neonatal Nurs.* 1987;16:174–78.
27. Goldstein S, et al. Premenstrual hostility, impulsivity, and impaired social functioning. *J Psychosom Obstet Gynecol* 1986;5:33–38.
28. Johnson SR, et al. Epidemiology of premenstrual symptoms in a nonclinical sample. *J Reprod Med.* 1988;33: 340–346.
29. Rapkin AJ, et al. Mood and cognitive style in premenstrual syndrome. *Obstet Gynecol.* 1989;74:644–49.
30. Gerbie MD. Complications of menstruation: abnormal uterine bleeding. In Pernoll ML, Benson RC. *Current Obstetric and Gynecologic Diagnosis and Treatment.* 6th ed. Norwalk, Conn: Appleton & Lange, 1987, pp 612–617.
31. York R, et al. Characteristics of premenstrual syndrome. *Obstet Gynecol.* 1989;73:601–605.
32. Frank EP. What are nurses doing to help PMS patients? *Am J Nurs* 1986;86:137–140.
33. Cortese J, Brown MA. Coping responses of men whose partners experience premenstrual symptomatology. *J Obstet Gynecol Neonatal Nurs* 1989;18:405–412.
34. Freeman EW, et al. Evaluating premenstrual symptoms in medical practice. *Obstet Gynecol* 1985;65:500–505.
35. Rubinow D, et al. Changes in plasma hormones across the menstrual cycle in patients with menstrually related mood disorder and in control subjects. *Am J Obstet Gynecol* 1988;158:5–11.
36. Abraham GE. Premenstrual tension. *Curr Probl Obstet Gynecol* 1980;3:1–38.
37. Wentz AC. Amenorrhea: evaluation and treatment. In Jones HW III, et al, eds. *Novak's Textbook of Gynecology.* 11th ed. Baltimore: Williams & Wilkins, 1988, pp 351–377.
38. Wentz AC. Abnormal uterine bleeding. In Jones HW III, et al, eds. *Novak's Textbook of Gynecology.* 11th ed. Baltimore: Williams & Wilkins, 1988, pp 378–396.
39. Muratta JM. Abnormal genital bleeding and secondary amenorrhea: common gynecological problems. *J Obstet Gynecol Neonatal Nurs.* 1990;19:26–36.
40. Brown MA, Woods NF. Correlates of dysmenorrhea: a challenge to past stereotypes. *J Obstet Gynecol Neonatal Nurs.* 1984;13:259–266.
41. Hemsell DL, et al. Pelvic infections and sexually transmitted diseases. In Pernoll ML, Benson RC, ed. *Current Obstetric & Gynecologic Diagnosis & Treatment.* 6th ed. Norwalk, Conn: Appleton & Lange, 1987, pp 715–741.
42. Food and Drug Administration, U.S. Dept. of Health and Human Services. Medical devices; labeling for menstrual tampons; ranges of absorbency; final rule. *Federal Register.* 1989;54:43766–43775.
43. Faley D. Preventing TSS: new tampon labeling lets women compare absorbencies. *FDA Consumer.* 1990;24:6–9.
44. Berkeley SF, et al. The relationship of tampon characteristics to menstrual toxic shock syndrome. *JAMA.* 1987;258–917–920.
45. Judd HL. Menopause and postmenopause. In Pernoll ML, Benson, RC. *Current Obstetric & Gynecologic Diagnosis & Treatment.* 6th ed. Norwalk, Conn: Appleton & Lange, 1987, pp 959–978.
46. Cutick R. Special needs of perimenopausal and menopausal women. *J Obstet Gynecol Neonatal Nurs.* 1984;13 (suppl): 68–73.
47. Cobb JO. Demystifying menopause. *Can Nurse.* 1987;83: 17–20.
48. Wentz AC. Management of the menopause. In Jones HW III, et al, eds. *Novak's Textbook of Gynecology.* 11th ed. Baltimore: Williams & Wilkins, 1988, pp 397–442.
49. Engel NS. *Menopausal Stage, Current Life Change, Attitude Toward Women's Roles and Perceived Health Status in Middle-Aged Women.* Thesis. New York University, School of Education, Health, Nursing, and Arts Professions, New York, 1983.
50. Ellerhorst-Ryan JM, et al. Evaluating benign breast disease. *Nurse Pract.* 1989;13:13–28.
51. Hendler FJ. Southwestern internal medicine conference: breast diseases and the internist. *Am J Med Sci.* 1987; 293:332–347.
52. Hutter RUP. Goodby to fibrocystic disease. *N Engl J Med.* 1985;312:179–181.
53. Spratt JS, et al. Breast cancer risk: a review of definitions and assessments of risk. *J Surg Oncol.* 1989;41:42–46.
54. Greydanus DE, et al. Breast disorders in children and adolescents. *Pediatr Clin North Am.* 1989;36:601–638.
55. American Cancer Society. *Cancer Facts and Figures: 1989.* New York: American Cancer Society, Inc, 1989.
56. Tapley DF, ed. The specter of breast cancer. *J Coll Physician Surg Columbia Univ.* 1989;9:6–21.
57. United States Preventive Services Task Force. Screening for breast cancer. *Am Fam Physician.* 1989;39:89–96.
58. Bodian C, Haagensen CD. Family history of breast cancer predisposing to the disease. In CD Haagenson, ed. *Diseases of the Breast.* 3rd ed. Philadelphia: W.B. Saunders, 1986, pp 408–423.
59. Wynder EL. Dietary factors related to breast cancer. *Cancer.* 1980;46:899–904.
60. Mettlin C. Diet and the epidemiology of human breast cancer. *Cancer.* 1984;53:605.

61. Schatzkin A, et al. The dietary fat—breast cancer hypothesis is alive. *JAMA.* 1989;261:3284–3287.
62. Rosenberg L, et al. Breast cancer and cigarette smoking. *N Engl J Med.* 1984;310:92–94.
63. Webster LA, et al. Alcohol consumption and risk of breast cancer. *Lancet.* 1983;2;724–726.
64. Lowenfeis AB, Zevola SF. Alcohol and breast cancer: an overview. *Alcoholism (NY).* 1989;13:109–111.
65. Wile AG, Disaia J. Hormones and breast cancer. *Am J Surg.* 1989;157:438–442.
66. United Kingdom National Case Control Study Group. Oral contraceptive use and breast cancer risk in young women. *Lancet.* 1989;1:973–982.
67. Shapiro S. The status of breast cancer screening: a quarter century of research. *World J Surg.* 1989;13:9–18.
68. Cooperman AM, Hermann R. Breast cancer: an overview. In *Surgical Clinics of North America: Symposium on Breast Cancer, 64.* Philadelphia: W.B. Saunders, 1984.
69. Holmberg, L, et al. The biology and natural history of breast cancer from the screening perspective. *World J Surg.* 1989;13:25–30.
70. Foster RS, Costanza MC. Breast self-examination practices and breast cancer survival. *Cancer.* 1984;53:999–1005.
71. Goodno JA. Breast cancer detection: experience in a suburban community. *Am J Obstet and Gynecol.* 1990;162:1393–1396.
72. Shapiro S. Evidence on screening for breast cancer from a randomized trial. *Cancer.* 1977;39:2772–82.
73. Dodd GD. Present status of thermography, ultrasound and mammography in breast cancer detection. *Cancer.* 1977; 2796–2805.
74. Mann BD, et al. Delayed diagnosis of breast cancer as a result of normal mammograms. *Arch Surg.* 1983;16:23–24.
75. El Yousef SJ, et al. Magnetic resonance imaging of the breast. *Radiology.* 1984;150:761–766.
76. Assaf AR, et al. Comparison of three methods of teaching women how to perform breast self-examination. *Health Educ Q.* 1985;12:259–272.
77. McLendon MS, et al. Effectiveness of BSE teaching to women of low socioeconomic class. *J Obstet Gynecol Neonatal Nurs.* 1982;11:7–14.
78. Haagenson CD. Women's role in recognizing the symptoms of breast disease. In Haagenson CD. *Diseases of the Breast.* 3rd ed. Philadelphia: W.B.Saunders, 1986, pp 501–515.

Human Reproduction

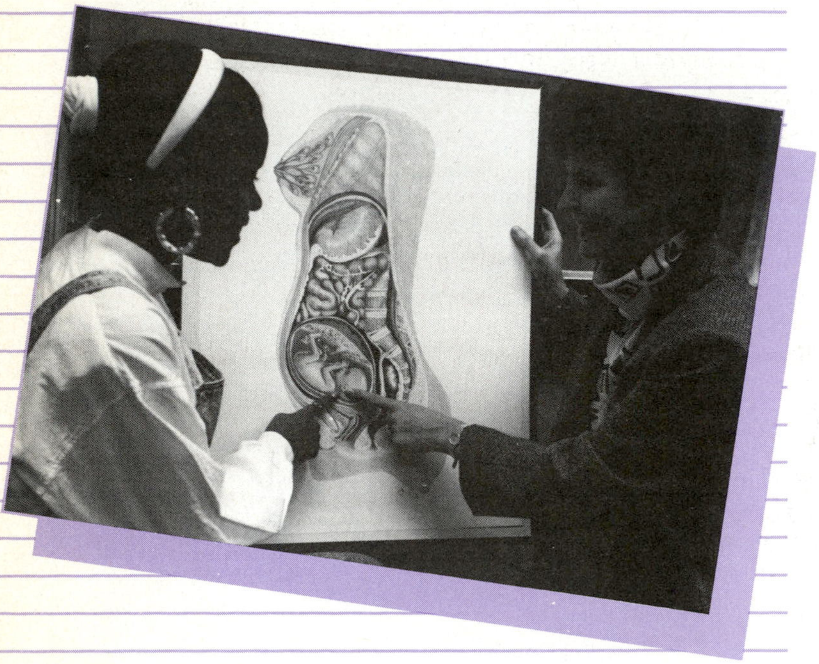

Chapter 6

Key Terms

- android (male) pelvis
- anteflexion
- anthropoid pelvis
- autosomes
- endometrial cycle
- ferning
- fertilization
- gametogenesis
- gynecoid (female) pelvis
- imperforate hymen
- meiosis
- menstrual cycle
- mitosis
- mittelschmerz
- oogenesis
- ovarian cycle
- ovulation
- playtypelloid pelvis
- retrocession
- retroflexion
- retroversion
- spermatogenesis
- spinnbarkeit
- uterine cycle

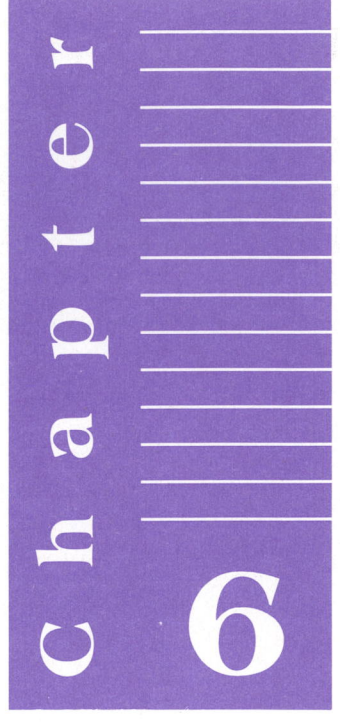

At no other time in the life cycle of a human being is the interplay of genetics and environment so apparent as when the sperm fertilizes the ovum to begin the development of a unique individual. Growth and development of the resulting individual will be influenced by the transmission of genetic material and by the presence of a healthy uterine environment. The ovum and sperm each carry to the union a half share of genetic information so that the united cell receives the full amount of genetic information required for directing the growth and development of the new individual. The reproductive system in both the male and the female is designed to ensure the successful union of the sperm and the ovum.[1]

This chapter describes the genetic aspects of human reproduction, the anatomy of the male and female reproductive systems, and the processes of spermatogenesis and oogenesis. The chapter concludes with a description of the phases of the menstrual cycle, including the ovarian and endometrial cycles. A thorough knowledge of this content is required by the nurse who cares for the woman and her partner prior to and during pregnancy.

GENETIC ASPECTS OF HUMAN REPRODUCTION

Each human being has unique hereditary characteristics that are the result of contributions of genetic material by the ovum and sperm at conception. Hereditary characteristics are determined by genes that appear in pairs (alleles) on the chromosomes within the human cell nucleus. It is estimated that there are between 30,000 and 50,000 gene pairs in each human cell nucleus.

Genes are the basic units of inheritance and are composed of deoxyribonucleic acid (DNA). A double-stranded molecule in the shape of a coiled ladder, DNA is present in the nucleus of each human cell.

The genes in each cell nucleus are tightly intertwined in the DNA of the chromosomes. The several functions of DNA include: replication during cell division, coding for the production of structural proteins and enzymes, and regulating the rate of synthesis of these proteins and enzymes.

Chromosomes are the threadlike structures within the nucleus of the cell that carry the genes. They are formed by DNA molecules winding themselves around protein molecules like thread around a spool. Genes are arranged linearly along the chromosomes, with each gene having a particular location (locus). A gene locus on one chromosome has a matching gene locus on its paired chromosome.

The human cell has 23 pairs of chromosomes (46 total) in its nucleus, half donated by the mother and half by the father. Twenty-two pairs (n = 44) of chromosomes are identical in males and females; they are called **autosomes.** The remaining two chromosomes, called sex chromosomes, are alike in the female (*XX*) and different in the male (*XY*) (Figure 6–1).

Cell Division

There are two methods of human cell division, mitosis and meiosis. **Mitosis** is the process by which body cells are duplicated for growth in the developing fetus and the child and damaged or dead cells are replaced in the adult. This growth process occurs as a result of replicative division in which a parent cell having 46 chromosomes forms two daughter cells, each having 46 chromosomes identical to the parent cell (*see* Figure 6–3). The second method of cell division, **meiosis,** is a special type of cell division that occurs in ovum and sperm cell formation (gametogenesis). Meiosis is the process of reduction division, during which the parent cell with 46 paired chromosomes forms four daughter cells (called gametes), each with 23 unpaired chromosomes (*see* Figure 6–4). In other words, the total number of chromosomes in an ovum or sperm are reduced by half, so that when the gametes unite during fertilization, the resulting one-celled human organism contains the necessary 46 chromosomes.

Before cells divide, DNA replication must occur. The double strand of DNA must unwind and sepa-

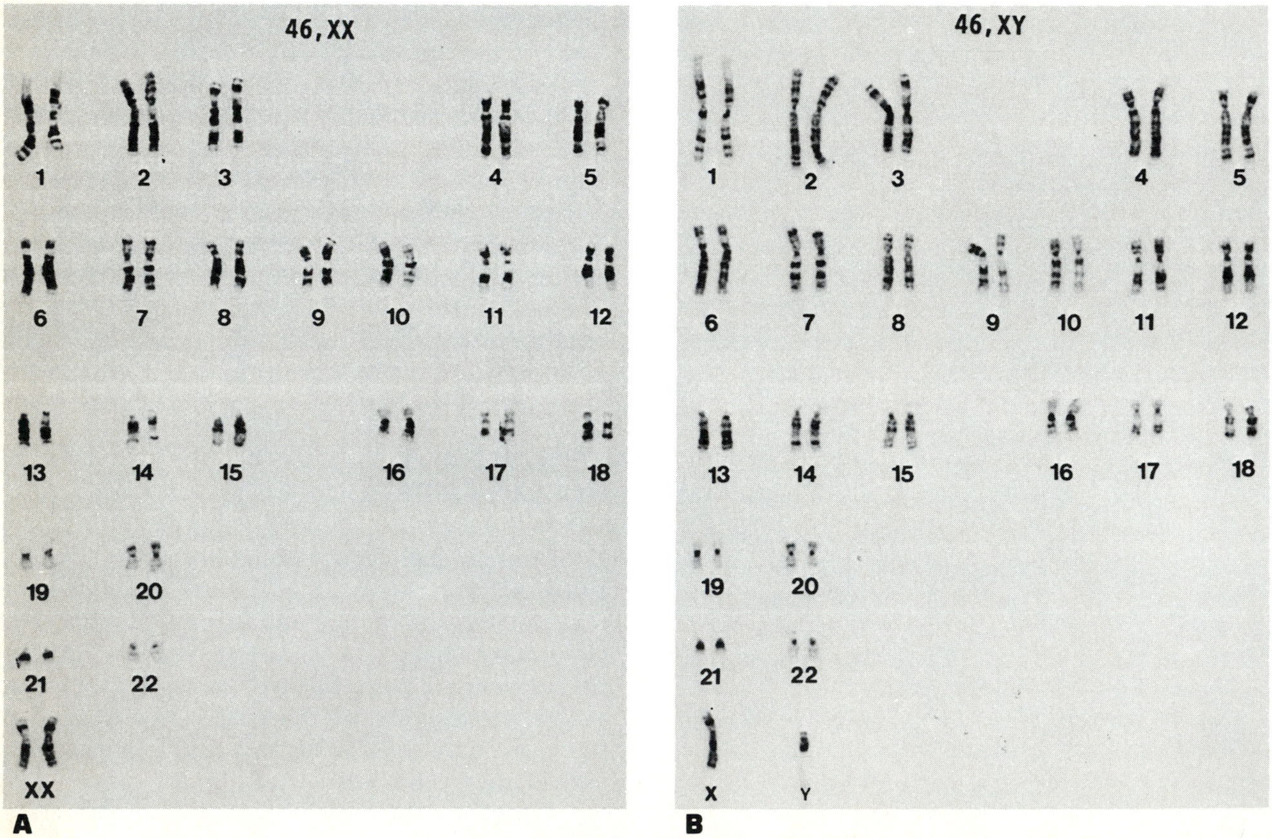

Figure 6–1. Normal chromosomes at metaphase. **A.** Female karyotype. **B.** Male karyotype.

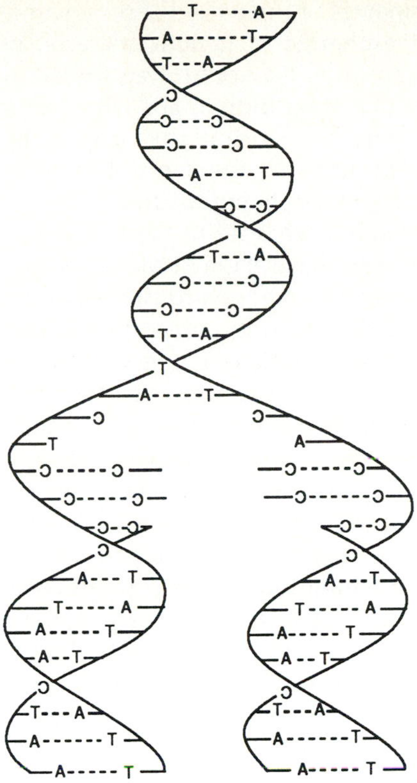

Figure 6–2. DNA replication resulting in two strands of DNA identical to the parent DNA.

rate. The individual strands then serve as a model for a new strand of DNA to be formed (*see* Figure 6–2). The result is two new strands of DNA that are genetically identical to the original DNA strands. Genetic mutations can occur during cell division if the DNA strand is not replicated exactly, causing a permanent change in the genetic material. An example of a genetic mutation during meiosis is trisomy 21, or Down's syndrome, which results in an extra chromosome in each cell. An example of a genetic mutation during mitosis is mosaicism, an unequal number of chromosomes in the cells; for example some cells may have 46 chromosomes whereas others have 47.

Mitosis. There are five stages of mitotic division: interphase, prophase, metaphase, anaphase, and telophase.

Interphase I, the stage before cell division occurs, is sometimes called the "resting stage" of cell division. During this phase, no chromosomal activity can be observed under the microscope (*see* Figure 6–2A). It is thought, however, that the strands of DNA are not actually "resting" during this stage and that DNA replication actually occurs near the end of interphase.

Protein synthesis, which is required before a cell can begin mitosis and actually divide, also is thought to occur during interphase. During protein synthesis, one strand of DNA serves as the model for the formation of messenger ribonucleic acid (mRNA). This process, called transcription, takes place in the nucleus of the cell. The transcribed mRNA transports the DNA code for individual genes. Once formed, mRNA travels from the cell nucleus to the cytoplasm, where translation occurs. During translation, amino acids are brought into place in an ordered sequence to form a polypeptide chain resulting in the final gene product. If the exact message of the DNA is not transcribed and translated, the result may be an altered gene product (eg, a structural protein or enzyme) that does not adequately carry out its function.

During prophase, cell division begins. The chromosomes begin to coil and condense and develop a definite configuration, appearing as two duplicated longitudinal halves called chromatids. The two halves, or chromatids, are held together in a constricted area called the centromere. If the centromere is located in the center, the chromosome has an X-shaped appearance; if it is located at a terminal location on the chromosome, the chromosome has a wishbone or Y-shaped appearance.

During prophase, two centrioles (cytoplasmic structures) can be seen at one side of the nucleus (*see*

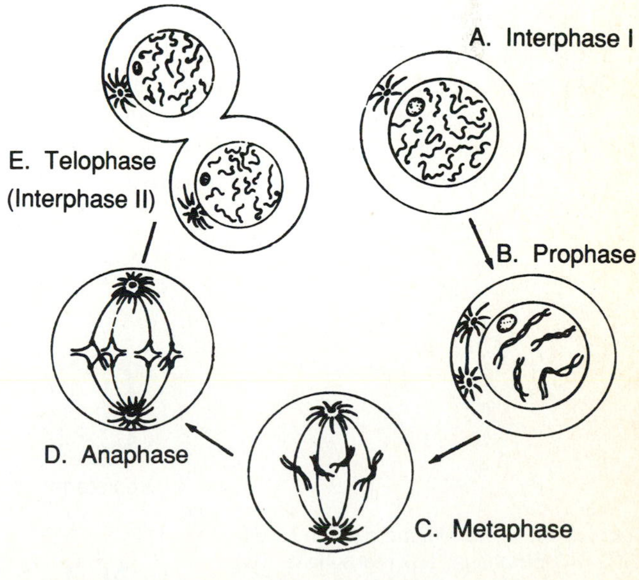

Figure 6–3. Mitosis. (Reproduced, with permission, from Hathaway WE, et. al. *Current Pediatric Diagnosis & Treatment.* 10th ed. Norwalk, Conn: Appleton & Lange, 1991, p. 1017.

Figure 6–3B). By the end of prophase, the centrioles begin moving apart and are separated by spindle fibers made up of protein. The nuclear membrane disappears during this phase.

During early metaphase, the centrioles are pulled to opposite poles of the cell (*see* Figure 6–3C). The chromatid pairs move back and forth within the spindle fibers as they are tugged toward first one pole and then the other. Finally, they line up along the equator of the cell (middle of the cell), marking the end of metaphase (*see* Figure 6–3C).

At the beginning of anaphase, the centromeres separate simultaneously in all the chromatid pairs. The spindle fibers contract and draw the chromatids of each pair apart toward the centrioles at the opposite poles of the cell (*see* Figure 6–3D). Each chromatid then becomes a separate chromosome.

During early telophase (also called interphase II), the chromosomes have reached the opposite poles. The spindle fibers disperse and the cytoplasm divides. The nuclear membrane reforms, separating each newly formed nucleus from the cytoplasm. The sister chromatids unwind and uncoil and are no longer visible under the microscope. At the end of telophase, the parent cell is divided into two daughter cells that are genetically identical to the original cell (*see* Figure 6–3E). The two cells are exactly alike in genetic material and each has 46 chromosomes. The cells then again enter interphase I.

Meiosis. Meiosis consists of two successive cell divisions, resulting in the formation of four daughter cells, each with a haploid (or halved) number of chromosomes (that is, 23 chromosomes).

During the first cell division (meiosis I), the chromosomes coil and condense. They have already duplicated and formed four sister chromatids. During prophase I, there is a close association of the four sister chromatids of the paired chromosomes. In fact, a physical exchange of genetic material occurs between the chromatids, accounting for the wide variation of traits among individuals who are children of the same parents. During this stage, the nuclear membrane disappears, the centriole duplicates, and the centriole pairs each migrate toward opposite poles of the cell (*see* Figure 6–4A).

In the metaphase stage of meiosis I, the four sister chromatids migrate toward the equator of the cell (*see* Figure 6–4B). During the anaphase stage of meiosis I, the first meiotic division occurs with paired sister chromatids separating and migrating toward opposite poles (*see* Figure 6–4C). During the telophase stage, the nuclear membrane reforms and division of cytoplasm occurs (*see* Figure 6–4D).

The first cell division in meiosis differs from mitotic division. The chromosome pairs separate intact instead of the longitudinal splitting of each chromosome found in mitosis. One intact member of each chromosome pair goes to each of the newly formed daughter cells by the end of meiosis I.

In meiosis II, the pattern of cell division is the same as that found in mitotic cell division. The second meiotic division occurs immediately after meiosis I without a resting phase or further DNA replication. During the prophase stage of meiosis II, the chromatids continue to be coiled and condensed and the nuclear membrane again disappears (*see* Figure 6–3A, mitosis). In metaphase II, the chromatids migrate toward the equator of the cell (Figure 6-5A). During anaphase II, the centromere splits and the spindle fibers contract pulling the individual sister chromatids toward opposite poles of the cell (Figure 6–5B). At telophase II, the cytoplasm again divides. The result of the meiotic division is four daughter cells, each with 23 chromosomes present (Figure 6–5C), or half as many chromosomes as the original cell. One of

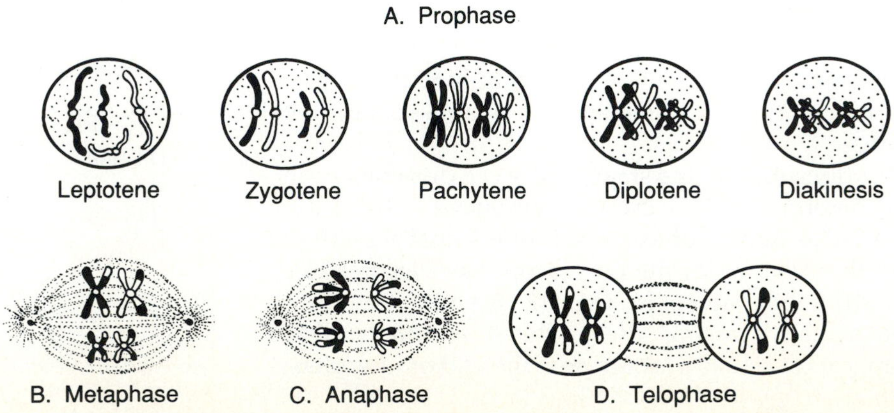

Figure 6–4. First meiotic division (meiosis I): (A) prophase, (B) metaphase, (C) anaphase, (D) telophase. (*Reproduced, with permission, from Stenchever MA.* Human Cytogenics: A Workbook in Reproductive Biology. *The Press of Case Western Reserve University, 1972.*)

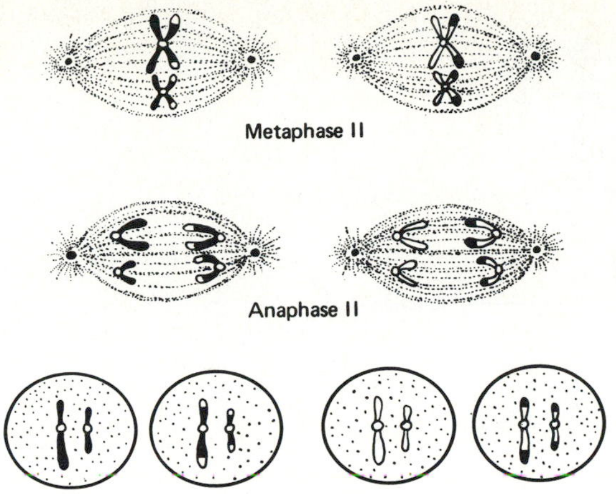

Figure 6–5. Second meiotic division (meiosis II). (*Reproduced, with permission, from Stenchever MA.* Human Cytogenics: A Workbook in Reproductive Biology. *The Press of Case Western Reserve University, 1972.*)

these 23 chromosomes is a sex chromosome. If the parent cell is an ovum, each of the four resulting daughter cells will contain one *X* sex chromosome; but if the parent cell is a sperm, two of the daughter cells will contain *X* chromosomes and two will contain *Y* chromosomes.

Gametogenesis

Gametogenesis is the process by which the sperm and ovum are produced. During gametogenesis, meiotic reduction cell division occurs, resulting in a haploid number of chromosomes (23) in the daughter cells, or gametes. Sperm cell formation is referred to as spermatogenesis and ovum cell formation as oogenesis. (These processes will be described later in the chapter.)

Fertilization

Fertilization occurs when a sperm penetrates the outer layer of the ovum, setting off a chain of events that will result in the development of the human embryo. At fertilization, the ovum and sperm cells unite to form the single-celled human organism (called a zygote), containing 46 chromosomes (22 pairs of autosomes and 1 pair of sex chromosomes [XX resulting in a female; XY in a male]). The single-celled fertilized zygote then begins to undergo mitotic cell division, which initiates embryonic and subsequent fetal development. (*See* Chapter 11, Growth and Development of the Embryo/Fetus.)

EMBRYOLOGIC DEVELOPMENT OF THE MALE AND FEMALE REPRODUCTIVE SYSTEMS

The male and female reproductive systems begin development during the embryologic period (the first 5 weeks of intrauterine development). The structure and function of the reproductive organs in both sexes follow an organized and complex pattern of development.

The sex of the embryo is determined at fertilization by the genetic makeup of the sperm that fertilizes the ovum. If the X-bearing sperm unites with the X-bearing ovum, the resulting sex chromosome complex will be XX and the genetic sex of the embryo female. If the Y-bearing sperm unites with the X-bearing ovum, the sex chromosome complex will be XY and the genetic sex male.

Although the genetic sex of the embryo is determined at fertilization, the reproductive organs initially begin to develop in the same way in both sexes. In fact, there is no difference in the appearance of the reproductive organs of males or females until about the seventh week of gestation. The period in which the female and the male internal reproductive organs and external genitalia are similar is referred to as the indifferent or undifferentiated stage of development.

Development of the Internal Reproductive Systems

The immature gonads are first seen during the fifth week of embryologic development when thickened epithelial cells form gonadal ridges. Fingerlike epithelial cords soon grow from the gonadal ridge of each gonad. Each indifferent gonad now consists of an outer cortex and an inner medulla.[1] In embryos with an XX sex chromosome complex, the cortex differentiates into an ovary, and the medulla regresses. In embryos with an XY sex chromosome complex, the medulla differentiates into a testis and the cortex regresses.[2]

Two pairs of genital ducts also develop in both sexes, mesonephric (wolffian duct) and paramesonephric (mullerian duct). The ducts come together in the median plane in both sexes and fuse into a Y-shaped uterovaginal canal, which opens into the urogenital sinus.

The mesonephric ducts play an essential role in the development of the male reproductive system. They form the epididymides, the ductus deferens, the ejaculatory ducts, and the efferent ductules. The lateral portion of the duct forms into the seminal vesicle. The remainder of the male genital system con-

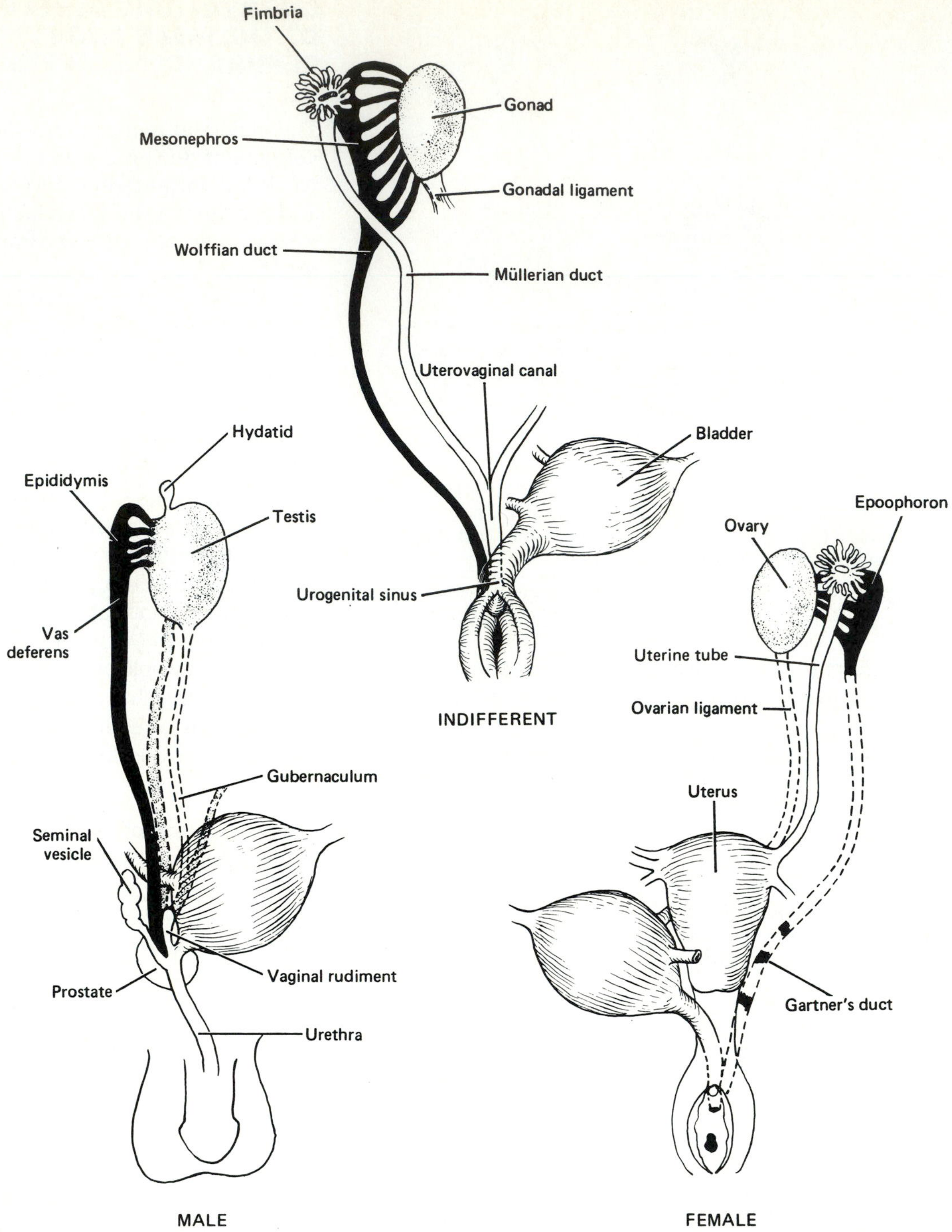

Figure 6–6. Development of the internal reproductive structures, male and female. (*After Corning HK, Wilkins L. Redrawn and reproduced, with permission, from Van Wyk J, Grumbach M. In Withaus RH, ed.* Textbook of Endocrinology. *5th ed. Philadelphia: WB Saunders, 1974.*)

sists of the urethra, which gives rise to the prostate gland.[2]

In female embryos, the mesonephric ducts regress and the paramesonephric ducts develop into the female reproductive tract. The unfused portions of paramesonephric ducts develop into the uterine tubes. The fused portions form the uterovaginal primordium, which develops into the epithelium and glands of the uterus and the fibromuscular vaginal wall. Fusion of the paramesonephric ducts brings together two peritoneal folds, forming right and left broad ligaments.[2] (Figure 6–6).

In genetic males, primitive sperm (called spermatogonia) are formed during fetal life. Beginning during puberty, formation of spermatogonia again occurs; these primitive sperm cells will continue to form and mature into spermatozoa throughout the male's fertile years.

In genetic females, the primitive ova (called oogonia) are formed during fetal life. Through mitosis, thousands of oogonia are formed. Because no oogonia are formed postnatally, females are born with the primary oocytes that they will have throughout their reproductive years.

The fetal testes produce two hormones: a nonsteroidal inducer substance and androgens. The inducer substance stimulates the development of the mesonephric ducts into the male genital tract. It also suppresses the development of the mullerian glands. In female embryos, the mesonephric ducts regress and the paramesonephric ducts develop into the female genital tract. Unlike the testes, which produce hormones to stimulate male development, the ovaries are not needed to stimulate primary sexual female development. It is most likely the absence of testicular hormone that stimulates primary sexual development in the female.[2]

Development of the External Reproductive Systems

The development of the external genitalia in males and females also begins with an undifferentiated stage for about the first 7 weeks of development. A genital tubercle develops in both sexes in the fourth week of development. On either side of a cloacal membrane, labioscrotal swellings and urethral folds develop. The genital tubercle becomes longer and is called a phallus.

By the tenth week of development, the male testes secrete fetal androgen (testosterone) hormone. Under the influence of testosterone, the anterior part of the genital tubercle develops into the penis. The urethral folds fuse together to form the spongy urethra; the external opening of the urethra moves to the glans penis and an opening is evident at the tip of

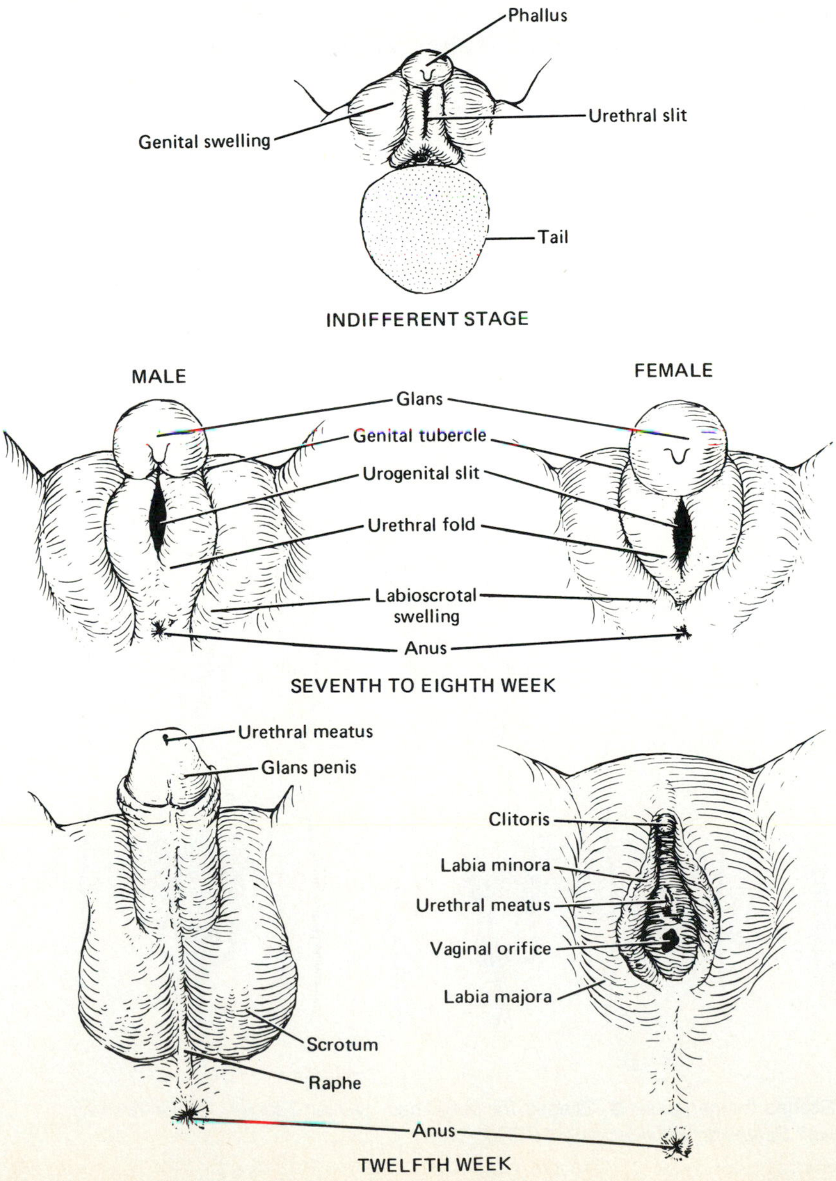

Figure 6–7. Development of the external reproductive structures. (*Reproduced, with permission, from Ganong, WF:* Review of Medical Physiology. *14th ed. Norwalk, Conn: Appleton & Lange,* 1989, *p 356*)

the penis. The labioscrotal swellings become larger, fuse and develop into the scrotum (Figure 6–7).

In the absence of fetal testosterone, the female clitoris is formed from the genital tubercle or phallus. In the female, the urethral folds do not fuse, giving rise to the labia minora. The labioscrotal swellings become the labia majora. Two openings, the urethral and vaginal openings, are formed between the labia minora (*see* Figure 6-7).

PUBERTY

Puberty is defined as the developmental phase in males and females that results in physical maturity and the capacity to reproduce. The changes that occur are hormonally mediated and take place over a period of several years. The rate at which physical maturity takes place is highly variable among individuals, but the sequence of events is very predictable. Secondary sex characteristics, those that distinguish the sexes, are used to identify the pattern of events.[3,4] The sequence of events for females includes the appearance of breast buds, appearance of pubic hair (about 16 percent develop pubic hair prior to breast enlargement), change in vaginal secretions, linear growth acceleration, appearance of axillary hair, and lastly, ovulation. For boys, the usual pattern of events begins with testicular enlargement and is followed by appearance of pubic hair, increased growth of the penis, first ejaculation, peak height growth, axillary hair, beginning facial hair, and lastly, voice deepening.[3,5]

Tanner divides the period of puberty into five stages based on secondary sex characteristics.[3] The secondary sex characteristics assessed in boys include the size of the male genitals and the development of pubic hair. For girls, pubertal development is assessed by the size of the breasts and the development of pubic hair. The rate at which adolescents proceed through the stages is variable.

Stages of Pubertal Development in Boys

In males, pubertal development of the genitals progresses from the childhood size of the penis, tes-

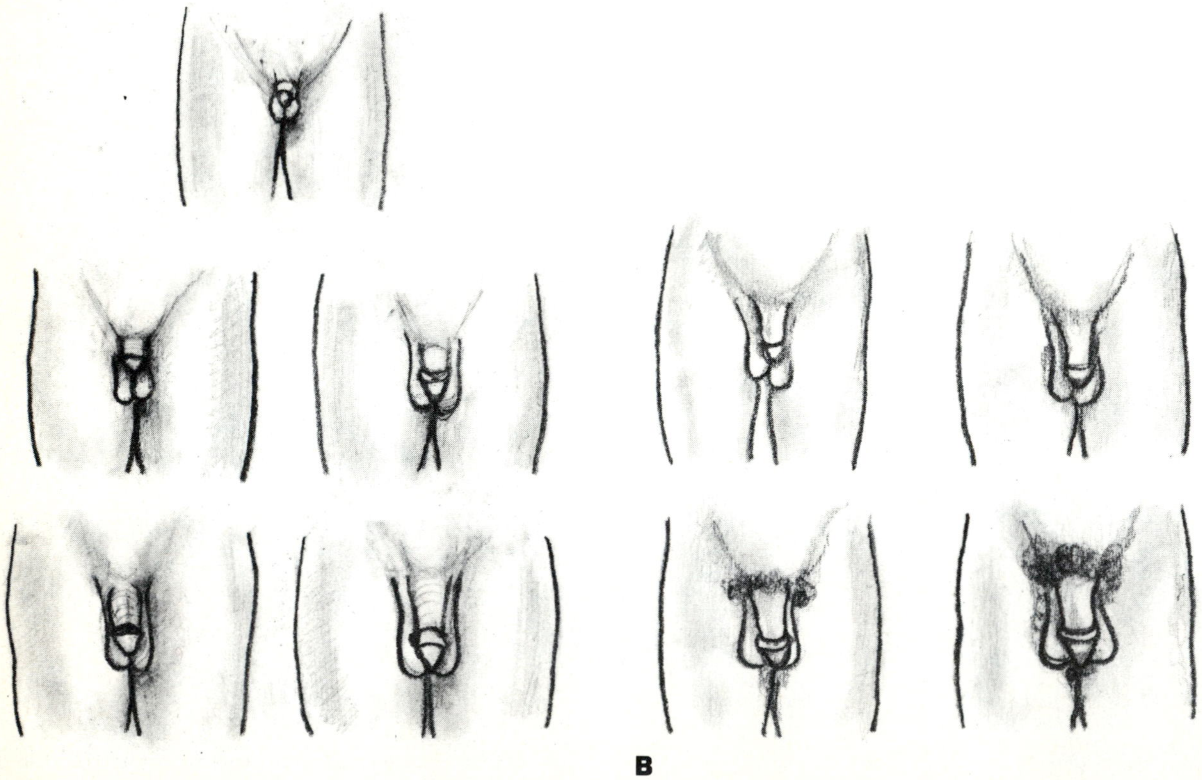

A **B**

Figure 6–8. Male pubertal development. **A.** Stages for genitalia. **B.** Stages for pubic hair. (*After Tanner JM.* Growth at Adolescence, *2nd ed. Oxford, England: Blackwell Scientific Publications, 1962.*)

tes, and scrotum (stage 1), to the enlargement of the testes and scrotum (stage 2), to enlargement of the penis (stage 3). Stage 4 demonstrates further growth of the testes, scrotum, and penis. In stage 5, the male genitals are adult in size and shape (Figure 6–8A).

Pubertal development of pubic hair in boys progresses from no pubic hair (stage 1), to sparse growth of slightly pigmented hair at the base of the penis (stage 2), to dark, coarse hair, sparsely spread over the junction of the pubis (stage 3). Stage 4 demonstrates hair that is adult in type, and in stage 5, pubic hair is adult in type and quantity, extending to the thighs (Figure 6–8B).[3,6]

The adolescent growth spurt in boys occurs on the average between the ages of 12 and 16 years, coinciding with Tanner's stages 3 and 4. Ejaculation of semen usually occurs before the growth spurt, whereas the androgen-induced enlargement of the larynx (which stimulates voice changes) corresponds with the growth spurt.[3,6] Axillary hair appears during stage 4, and facial hair develops slightly after the appearance of axillary hair.

Stages in Pubertal Development in Girls

Breast and pubic hair development are used as assessment parameters for pubertal development in females (Figure 6–9). The development of the female breasts progresses from the preadolescent phase, in which there is only development of papillae (stage 1), to the breast bud stage, in which a mound of breast and papilla is formed, with areolar enlargement (stage 2). In stage 3, there is additional enlargement of the breasts and areola, without separation of their contours. Stage 4 is delineated by a secondary mound above the level of the breasts, and stage 5 is characterized by areolar recession and appearance of ma-

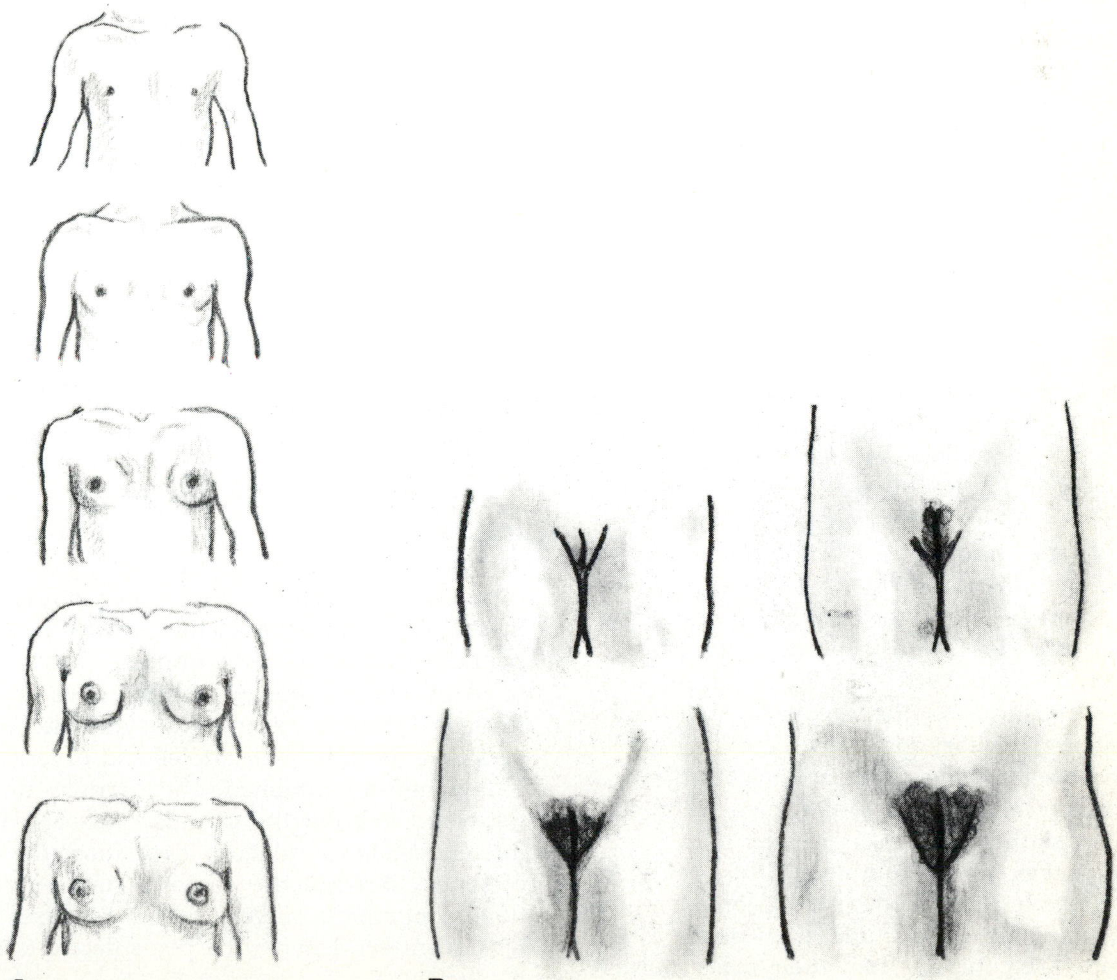

A B

Figure 6–9. Female pubertal development. **A.** Breast stages. **B.** Stages for genitalia. (*After Tanner JM.* Growth at Adolescence, *2nd ed. Oxford, England: Blackwell Scientific Publications, 1962.*)

ture breasts. The breasts do not develop symmetrically, one being slightly larger than the other.[7–9]

The female pubertal growth spurt begins earlier than in boys, usually between the ages of 10 and 14 years. The female growth acceleration begins in stage 2 and reaches a peak in stage 3. Voice changes also occur in girls but are not as pronounced as those found in boys. The appearance of axillary hair occurs on the average of 2 years after the onset of pubic hair development. The onset of the first menstrual period occurs during stage 4 of female breast development and follows the growth spurt.[3,9] In stage 5, ovulation occurs.

Hormonal Influences on Puberty

The changes at puberty are influenced by hormones that are secreted by the anterior pituitary gland. These hormones are called gonadotropins and include follicle-stimulating hormone (FSH) and luteinizing hormone (LH), also referred to as interstitial cell-stimulating hormone (ICSH) in the male.

During puberty, the hypothalamus secretes gonadotropin-releasing factor (GnRF), which stimulates the anterior pituitary gland to release the gonadotropin hormones, FSH and LH. Follicle-stimulating hormone stimulates the growth of the ova in the ovary and sperm-producing cells in the male testis. The cells in the ovary and testis in turn produce female and male sex hormones (estrogen in the female and testosterone in the male). These sex hormones are responsible for the development of the secondary sex characteristics.

The regulatory mechanisms for the onset of puberty are not fully understood. The hormones produced by the anterior pituitary gland are thought to be controlled by a feedback mechanism from the hypothalamus. One theory suggests that prior to puberty, small amounts of hormones are secreted by the immature ovaries and testes. The hypothalamus is sensitive to the inhibiting effect of these small quantities of hormones. The anterior pituitary gland, therefore, is not stimulated to produce gonadoatropin hormones. At puberty, the hypothalamus becomes less sensitive to the feedback and begins stimulating the pituitary gland to secrete the gonadotropin hormones in increasing amounts until a new equilibrium is reached in late adolescence, when maturation has occurred.[10,11]

When puberty is complete, the estrogen-dominated females have wider hips, a broader skeleton, and more fat distribution, particularly in the breasts, hips, and thighs, than their male counterparts. Testosterone-dominated males have larger skeletons, greater muscle mass, and broader shoulders than females.

THE MALE REPRODUCTIVE SYSTEM

The mature male reproductive system consists of internal and external genital organs. The external organs are the penis and the scrotum; the internal organs are the testes, epididymides, ductus deferens, ejaculatory ducts, and urethra. Accessory glands of the male reproductive system include the seminal vesicles, the prostate gland, and the bulbourethral glands (Cowper's glands) (Figure 6–10).

External Genital Organs

Penis. The **penis** functions in both the reproductive and urinary systems. It is called the male organ of copulation because it deposits sperm in the female vagina during sexual intercourse. The penis also conducts urine from the body through the urethral meatus, which is located at the tip of the penis.

The penis consists of a body, or the shaft, and a cone-shaped end, or glans. The shaft contains three cylindrical masses of erectile tissue, two dorsal corpora cavernosa and one ventral corpus spongiosum. These bodies are surrounded by the tunica albuginea, a layer of dense fibrous connective tissue that helps control the distension of the erectile tissue.

The corpus spongiosum contains the urethra and becomes enlarged at the distal end of the penis to form the **glans penis.** The penis is covered by loose skin. The skin covering the glans penis is called the foreskin, or prepuce. Surgical removal of the foreskin is referred to as circumcision.

The blood supply to the penis is mainly through the internal and external pudendal arteries and veins. The penis is innervated by sympathetic and parasympathetic nerve fibers.

The cavernous bodies of erectile tissue contain spaces (venous sinusoids), which become engorged during sexual arousal, causing the penis to become rigid and erect. The erection of the penis is caused by mechanical stimulation of the glans. When the glans penis is stimulated, nerve impulses travel to the spinal cord, where parasympathetic nerve fibers are activated. At the same time the sympathetic nerve fibers that control the arterioles and cavernous tissue of the penis are inhibited. The arterioles dilate, causing blood to enter the venous sinusoids. If there is intense sexual stimulation, ejaculation, the expulsion of semen through the penis, occurs. After ejaculation, sympathetic nerve stimulation causes the arteries to contract, leaving the penis flaccid (*see* Chapter 8, Sexuality).

Scrotum. The **scrotum** is a pouchlike structure, divided in the middle by a septum (raphe), forming

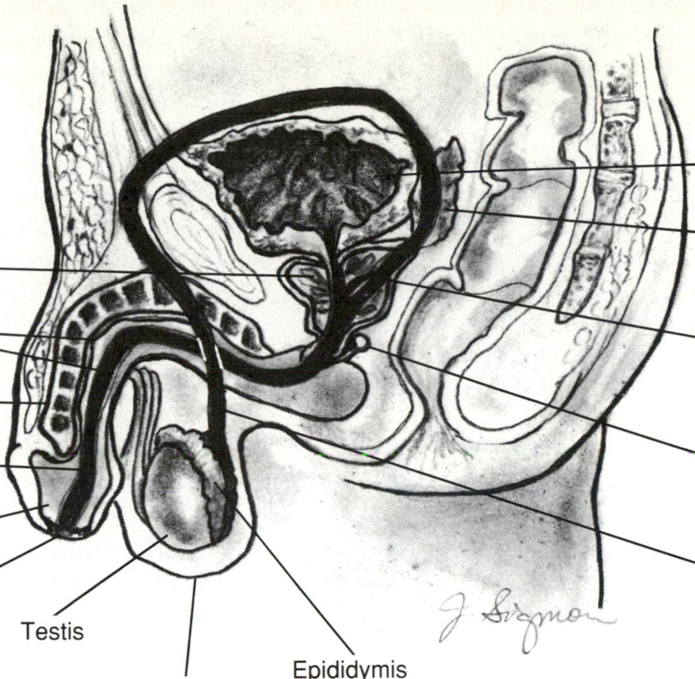

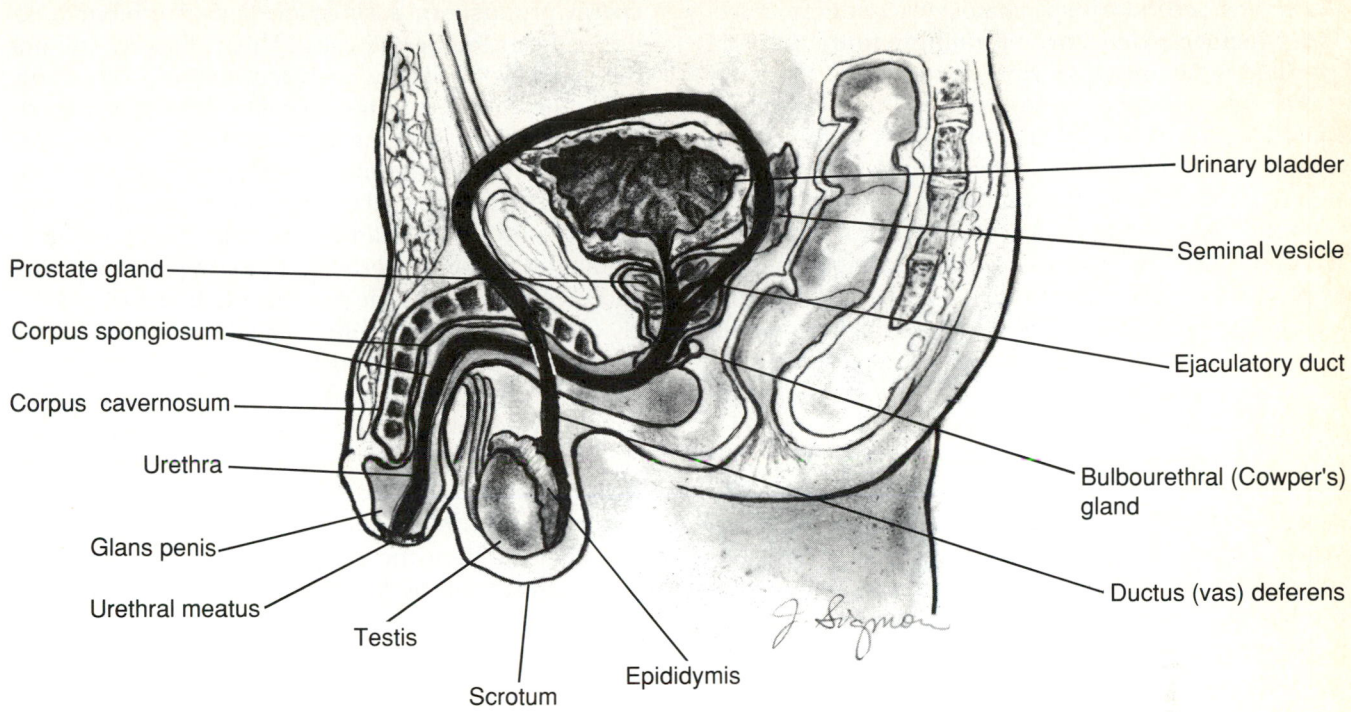

Figure 6–10. The male reproductive organs, showing pathway of the sperm.

two scrotal sacs. Each scrotal sac contains one testis, one epididymis, and parts of the spermatic cords. The left scrotal sac is usually longer than the right because the left spermatic cord is longer.

The scrotum is made up of fascia and smooth muscle, together called the tunica dartos. When exposed to cold, the dartos muscle and cremaster muscle of the spermatic cords contract, causing the scrotum to appear wrinkled. This mechanism draws the scrotum closer to the body for warmth.

The scrotal temperature is 2°C lower than the internal body temperature and provides the ideal temperature for spermatogenesis, which occurs in the testes. If, during development, the testes do not descend into the scrotum, the temperature of the body will inhibit spermatogenesis.

Internal Genital Organs

Testes. The **testes** are two oval-shaped organs located in the scrotum. Each testis is approximately 4 to 5 cm long, 2 to 3 cm in diameter, and 10 g in weight. A single testis is located in each of the scrotal sacs. The testes are suspended on each side by **spermatic cords.** The spermatic cords, which begin slightly above the inguinal canal, pass through the canal into the scrotum.

The testes are surrounded by a membrane called the tunica vaginalis and by fibrous connective tissue called the tunica albuginea. The tunica albuginea projects inside each testis and forms septa, which divide the testis into about 250 lobules. Each lobule contains one to three convoluted (coiled and folded) tubules referred to as the **seminiferous tubules.**

The seminiferous tubules come together to form thin-walled spaces, the rete testis, which in turn form efferent ducts, which go through the tunica albuginea and empty into the epididymis.

The seminiferous tubules contain two types of cells: (1) Sertoli cells; and (2) interstitial cells of Leydig. The Sertoli cells provide nutrients and enzymes to the immature spermatocytes during the maturation process. The interstitial cells of Leydig produce testosterone, the main male sex hormone.

Spermatogenesis. **Spermatogenesis** is the process by which spermatogonia, the fetal sperm cells, are transformed into mature sperm. The spermatogonia remain dormant in the seminiferous tubules of the testes until they begin to increase in number at puberty. Mitotic divisions allow the spermatogonia to grow and transform into primary spermatocytes, the largest sperm cells in the tubules.[1]

The primary spermatocytes undergo the first meiotic division, forming two secondary spermatocytes about half the size of the primary spermatocytes. The secondary spermatocytes undergo a second meiotic division, forming four haploid spermatids having 23 chromosomes each; the spermatids are about half the size of the secondary spermatocytes.[1] The spermatids attach to the Sertoli cells, found in the lining of the seminiferous tubules, and are transformed into four mature **sperm cells** or **spermatozoa** after several weeks in the epididymis.

A mature sperm consists of a head, neck, middle piece, and a tail (Figure 6–11). The head forms the bulk of the sperm and consists of the nucleus, which is covered by a membrane called the acrosome. The acrosome contains enzymes that assist in the penetration of the ovum by the sperm (*see* Chapter 11). The neck of the sperm contains centrioles, which carry the chromosomal material of the sperm. The middle piece of the sperm contains mitochondria, arranged in a coil, which provide the sperm with energy. The tail, or flagellum, is long and propels the sperm through the female reproductive tract.

Spermatogenesis is hormonally mediated in the male. During puberty, the hypothalamus secretes releasing hormones, which stimulate the anterior pituitary gland to secrete FSH and ICSH.

FSH stimulates the production of sperm by the seminiferous tubules; ICSH stimulates the interstitial cells of Leydig to secrete testosterone. When the testosterone levels in the blood are elevated during sperm production, a substance called inhibin is released from the Sertoli cells. This substance inhibits the release of FSH by the anterior pituitary gland. Also, the elevated testosterone levels inhibit the release of ICSH so that the interstitial cells of Leydig do not produce testosterone. As the blood levels of testosterone drop, the inhibitory effects of inhibin and testosterone on FSH and ICSH are lost; FSH again stimulates the seminiferous tubules to produce sperm and ICSH stimulates the production of testosterone.[12]

Testosterone and other male hormones secreted by the testes, as well as steroids secreted by the adrenal cortex, are called androgens. Testosterone, the most prevalent and potent of the testicular hormones, stimulates the development of the secondary sex characteristics in the male and is needed for the production of mature sperm and seminal fluid. It is produced throughout the life of a man, although secretions of testosterone begin diminishing after the age of 40.

Epididymis. The **epididymis** is a duct consisting of a coiled tubule that is located above and behind each testis. If stretched the tubule would measure about 20 feet, or 6 meters, in length. Each epididymis extends from the efferent duct at the top of each testis to the ductus deferens. The purpose of the epididymis is to store sperm received from the seminiferous tubules.

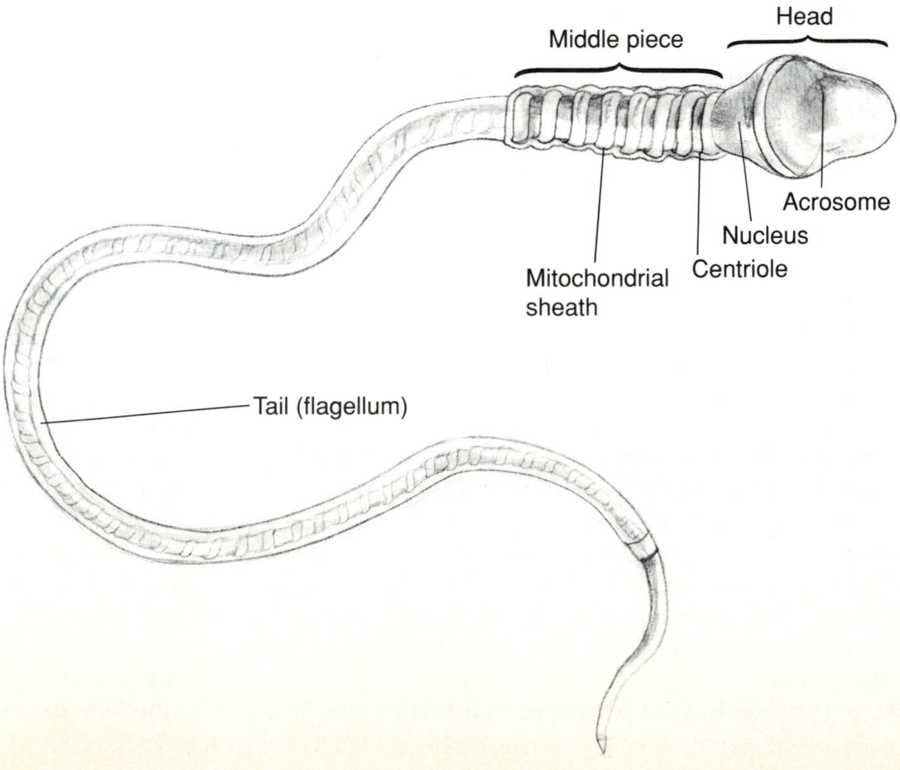

Figure 6–11. Structure of the sperm.

When the sperm enter the epididymis, they are immotile. After 2 to 3 weeks in the epididymis, the sperm become relatively motile and their maturation becomes complete. The wall of the epididymis consists of smooth muscle, which contracts during ejaculation, pushing the sperm into the ductus deferens.

Ductus Deferens (Vas Deferens). The **ductus deferens (vas deferens)** is continuous with the duct of the epididymis and is approximately 18 inches (46 cm) in length. A ductus deferens arises from the posterior wall of each testis and joins the spermatic cord. After joining with the spermatic cord, each ductus deferens passes through the inguinal canal, enters the pelvic cavity, and passes downward to the posterior wall of the urinary bladder. Before reaching the entrance to the bladder, the ductus deferens enlarges. The enlargement, called the ampulla, is a place where sperm can be stored. Each ampulla joins with a duct from the seminal vesicle and becomes known as the ejaculatory duct. The ductus deferens is made up of layers of smooth muscle, which contract during ejaculation and push sperm from the epididymis to the ejaculatory duct.

Ejaculatory Ducts. The **ejaculatory duct** is continuous with the ductus deferens and is formed by the union of the seminal vesicle and the ductus deferens. The ejaculatory ducts extend through the prostate gland and end at the prostatic urethra. Each duct ejects sperm received from one of the testes into the prostatic urethra.

Urethra. The **urethra,** the passageway for both sperm and urine in the male, extends from the neck of the bladder to the glans penis. It is surrounded by the prostate gland and consists of three sections: the prostatic, membranous, and cavernous urethra.

The prostatic urethra extends from the bladder through the prostate gland, where the ejaculatory ducts join it to the membranous urethra. The membranous urethra extends from the prostastic urethra through the urogenital diaphragm, the floor of the pelvic cavity, where it forms the urethral sphincter. The membranous urethra becomes the cavernous urethra, which is made up of spongy erectile tissue and extends through the penis. The reproductive purpose of the urethra is to eject semen containing mature sperm (spermatozoa) outside the body.

Accessory Glands

The **accessory glands** of the male reproductive system consist of the seminal vesicles, the prostate gland, and the bulbourethral glands (Cowper's glands). The male accessory glands secrete materials into the fluid ejaculated with the sperm (semen). The purpose of these secretions is to provide nutrients to the sperm and to increase the fluid in which the sperm are transported.

Seminal Vesicles. The **seminal vesicles** are two pouch-like structures that join the end of each ductus deferens to become the ejaculatory ducts. The seminal vesicles secrete a viscous fluid that contains fructose, fibrinogen, proteins, and prostaglandins. During ejaculation, the fructose provides energy to the sperm, increasing the motility and fertilizing ability of the sperm. Fibrinogen, a plasma protein, adds to the viscosity of the seminal fluid. Proteins provide nutrients to the sperm, while prostaglandins may assist the movement of the sperm to the female fallopian tubes by stimulating uterine contractions.

Prostate Gland. The **prostate gland** is a single gland located beneath the bladder. It surrounds the base of the urethra and adds to the semen by secreting a milky fluid. The fluid assists in the motility of the sperm and contributes to the alkalinity of the semen because it contains bicarbonate ions. The prostatic secretions also contain small amounts of lipids, enzymes, and citric acid.

The prostate gland has several lobes, and the gland can be palpated during rectal examination for size and congestion. It measures approximately 4 cm in diameter and is made up of both glandular and muscular tissue. When the muscular tissue contracts, the milky fluid is secreted into the urethra.

Bulbourethral Glands. The **bulbourethral glands (Cowper's glands)** are located in the floor of the pelvic cavity (urogenital diaphragm) on either side of the membranous urethra. These glands secrete a lubricating mucinous substance that coats the surface of the urethra. The fluid secreted by the bulbourethral glands is alkaline and assists in neutralizing the acidic environment of the male urethra and female vagina. This increases the viability of sperm, which need an alkaline environment for survival.

Semen

Semen, or **seminal fluid,** is ejaculated with the sperm from an erect penis. It consists of the secretions of the accessory glands and the epididymis. Each ejaculate contains 2 to 6 ml of fluid with a pH of 7.35 to 7.50. The alkalinity of the fluid buffers the sperm from the acidity of the vaginal secretions. Each mililiter of semen contains from about 50 to 150 million sperm. In addition to other substances, the seminal fluid contains the enzyme hyaluronidase, which helps the sperm penetrate the ovum.

Transport of Spermatozoa

The spermatozoa are produced from the fetal spermatogenic cells that lie dormant in the male testes until they begin increasing in number during puberty. In the seminiferous tubules of the testes, several mitotic divisions occur, transforming the immature sperm cells into primary spermatocytes. Meiotic divisions then occur, forming secondary spermatocytes and, subsequently, spermatids. The spermatids are pushed into the epididymis, which stores the sperm and contributes secretions to the seminal fluid. The sperm obtain the capability for some movement in the epididymis. Through muscular contraction, the sperm are transported from the epididymis to the ductus deferens, which is made up of layers of smooth muscle. When the smooth muscle contracts, the sperm are transported to the duct of the seminal vesicle. The seminal vesicle adds nutrients to the seminal fluid and joins the ejaculatory duct. The ejaculatory duct transports the sperm through the prostate gland to the prostatic urethra where the sperm exit the body through the penis at the external urethral opening (*see* Figure 6–10).

There is no cyclic nature to the production and transport of sperm. The sperm are viable in the male reproductive tract for several weeks. When the mature sperm are ejaculated, they can live for 48 to 72 hours in the female reproductive tract. When the sperm are not ejaculated, they dissolve and are reabsorbed.

THE FEMALE REPRODUCTIVE SYSTEM

The female reproductive system consists of external and internal genitalia. The structures of the female reproductive tract are needed for copulation, fertilization, implantation of the fertilized ovum, and development and birth of the fetus.[11]

External Genitalia

The external genitalia of the female reproductive system are called the **vulva** or **pudendum.** They include the mons veneris, the labia majora, the labia minora, the clitoris, the vaginal vestibule, urethral meatus, introitus and hymen, the openings of the Skene's and Bartholin's glands, and the perineum (Figure 6–12).

Mons Veneris (Mons Pubis). The **mons veneris,** also known as the **mons pubis,** is a fatty pad that covers the anterior portion of the symphysis pubis. After puberty, the female mons veneris is covered by curly hair distributed in a triangular pattern. The base of the triangle is formed at the upper margin of the symphysis pubis. The apex of the triangle of hair growth is found over the labia majora. This triangular distribution of hair is referred to as the escutcheon and may differ in women of varying ethnic backgrounds. The mons veneris acts as a cushion for the pelvic bones.

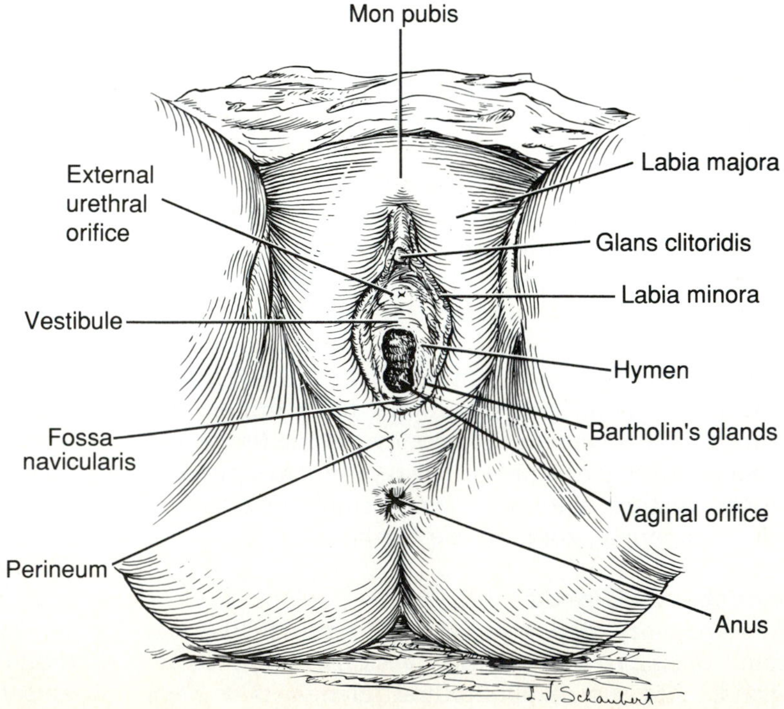

Figure 6–12. The female external genitalia (adult parous female). (*Reproduced, with permission, from Pernoll ML, Benson RC.* Current Obstetric & Gynecologic Diagnosis and Treatment. *6th ed. Norwalk, Conn: Appleton & Lange, 1987, p 12.*)

Labia Majora. The **labia majora** are two lateral folds of adipose tissue covered by skin and hair. They extend posteriorly from the mons veneris to the anterior border of the perineum, where they merge to form the posterior commissure. The labia majora are 7 to 8 cm in length, 2 to 3 cm in width, and 1 to 1.5 cm in thickness.

The labia majora are covered with stratified squamous epithelium that is richly supplied with sebaceous glands. Beneath the skin, there is a layer of thin, poorly developed muscle called the tunica dartos labialis, and a mass of adipose tissue. In nulliparous women, the inner surface of the labia majora looks like a mucous membrane, whereas in multiparous women, it appears more skinlike. After repeated childbearing, the labia majora are less prominent and with menopause they begin to shrink.[11]

The arterial blood supply to the labia majora is from the internal and external pudendal arteries. The labia majora have extensive venous drainage. The veins communicate with the dorsal vein of the clitoris, the veins of the labia minora, and the perineal veins. This extensive plexus of veins can result in varicosities during pregnancy and hematomas during labor and delivery.[10,11]

The labia majora also have an extensive lymphatic system both under the skin and deeper within the subcutaneous tissue. Innervation is also extensive, involving the anterior hypogastric nerves, which supply the superior portion of the labia majora, and the posterior iliac nerves, which innervate the gluteal area. The nerve supply makes the labia majora sensitive to painful stimuli, pressure, and temperature.

Labia Minora. The **labia minora** are two thin, pink folds of tissue located on the inner surface of the labia majora. They extend dorsally on either side of the vaginal orifice and are not covered with hair. The labia minora are covered with stratified squamous epithelial cells, which are continuous with the mucous membrane of the vagina. The tissues of the labia minora unite to form two thin plates of skin: the lower plate forms the frenulum of the clitoris, and the upper plate forms the prepuce of the clitoris. Inferiorly, the labia minora extend toward the perineum and fuse to form the fourchette. The fourchette, the posterior ring of the vaginal introitus (opening), is easily visible in nulliparous women. In multiparas, the labia minora usually appear as if they are part of the labia majora.[11]

The interior folds of the labia minora consist of erectile tissue containing many blood vessels. The main arteries supplying the labia minora come from the superficial perineal artery and from the rete of the labia majora. Venous drainage is by way of the perineal and vaginal veins. The labia minora are supplied by many nerve endings, making them very sensitive to stimuli such as touch.

Clitoris. The **clitoris** is a small structure found posterior to the mons veneris. It is homologous to the penis in the male because it is made up of erectile tissue that is highly sensitive to sexual arousal. The clitoris has a richer nerve supply than the male penis, being innervated primarily through the terminal branch of the pudendal nerve.

The clitoris consists of a glans, a corpus (body), and two crura. The glans contains spindle-shaped cells, which are highly sensitive to stimuli. It is covered by the prepuce, a hoodlike structure formed by the labia minora. The body is made up of two corpora cavernosa, homologous to the corpus spongiosum in the male penis. The crura extend laterally and are attached to the inferior rami of the pubis to form the central body of the clitoris.

The blood supply to the clitoris is from the pudendal artery. The nerve supply is mainly found within the prepuce. The clitoris is one of the principal erogenous organs of women; it rarely exceeds 2 cm in length even in a state of erection.[11]

Vaginal Vestibule. The **vaginal vestibule** is an almond-shaped area extending from the clitoris to the fourchette. The urinary meatus (the opening of the urethra), the introitus (the opening of the vagina), and the openings of the ducts of the Bartholin's and Skene's glands are found in the vestibule.

Urethral Meatus. The **urethral meatus** is in the middle of the vestibule, 1 to 1.5 cm below the clitoris. It is located above the vaginal opening and appears slitlike and puckered.

The **paraurethral glands (Skene's glands)** usually open on either side of the urethra. The openings are small, each measuring about 0.5 mm in diameter. The Skene's glands secrete a lubricating substance into the vaginal vestibule.

Vaginal Opening and Hymen. The vaginal opening, or **introitus,** is located in the lower portion of the vestibule and differs in size and shape among women. The introitus may be partially covered by a thin, connective tissue membrane called the **hymen.** The hymen may be ruptured through sexual intercourse, physical activity, or use of tampons. The idea that virginity can be established by an intact hymen is false, although some cultures may still adhere to this belief. Once the hymen is ruptured, hymenal tags called hymenal caruncles or carunculae myrtiformes remain. In rare instances, the hymen completely occludes the vaginal opening, resulting in retained menstrual flow. This condition is called **imperforate hymen** and can be treated by surgical removal of the hymen.

Bartholin's glands open on either side of the vaginal orifice at approximately 5 and 7 o'clock above the bulbocavernous muscles of the vagina. They are a pair of glands, measuring 0.5 to 1 cm in diameter. The ducts are 1.5 to 2.0 cm long and transport a secretion originating in the glands.

The glands lubricate the introitus with a clear, viscous secretion, particularly at the time of sexual arousal. The ducts of Bartholin's glands may harbor bacteria, such as *Neisseria gonorrhoeae*, that may gain access to the gland and cause a Bartholin's gland abscess.[11]

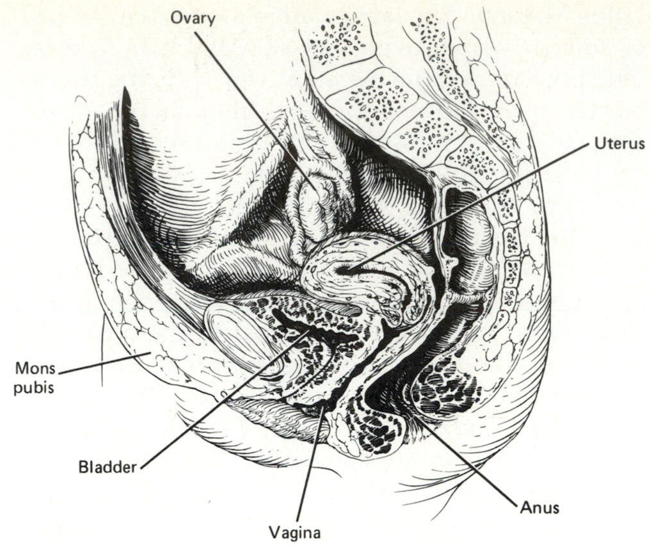

Figure 6–13. The internal female reproductive organs. (*Reproduced, with permission, from Benson RC.* Handbook of Obstetrics & Gynecology. *8th ed. Los Altos, Calif: Lange Medical Publications, 1983.*)

Perineum. The **perineum** is the area between the vagina and the anus. It is made up of connective tissue, muscles, fascia, and adipose tissue. The pelvic diaphragm and the urogenital diaphragm support the perineum. The pelvic diaphragm consists of the levator ani and coccygeous muscles, which support the pelvic structures. Between the levator muscles pass the vagina, urethra, and rectum. The urogenital diaphragm, which is found below the pelvic diaphragm, consists of deep transverse perineal muscles, the sphincter of the membranous urethra, and internal and external fascial coverings. It helps support the external genitalia and the vagina. The blood supply to the perineum comes from the internal pudendal artery and vein.

The area that lies between the lower one third of the posterior vaginal wall and the anal canal is referred to as the perineal body. The bulbocavernous muscles, the transverse muscles of the perineum, and the external sphincter ani muscles reinforce the perineal body and support the perineal floor.

Internal Genitalia

The internal genitalia of the female reproductive system consist of the ovaries, the fallopian tubes (oviducts or uterine tubes), the uterus, and the vagina (Figure 6–13). These organs have specialized functions in the female reproductive cycle.

Ovaries. The **ovaries** are two almond-shaped organs, measuring 2 to 5 cm in length, 1.5 cm in breadth, and 0.6 to 1.5 cm in width. They are located in the upper pelvic cavity near the ends of the fallopian tubes.

Each ovary is covered by germinal epithelium and consists of an outer cortex and an inner medulla. The cortex contains epithelial cells, within which are ova in various stages of development. The outer layer of the cortex is made up of dense connective tissue called the tunica albuginea. The medulla consists of loose connective tissue, numerous arteries and veins, some smooth muscle fibers, nerves, and lymphatic vessels.

The ovaries are supported by the utero-ovarian ligaments, mesovarium, and infundibulopelvic ligaments. The utero-ovarian ligaments are made up of connective tissue and muscle fibers. They extend from the cornua of the uterus to the lower pole of the ovary, anchoring the ovary to the uterus.

The mesovarium is a short tissue, consisting of two layers of peritoneum, which connect the ovary to the posterior portion of the broad ligament. The mesovarium contains branches of the ovarian and uterine arteries.

The infundibulopelvic ligament is the suspensory ligament of the ovary. It consists of a fold of peritoneum arising from the upper, outer pole of the broad ligament and extending to the pelvic wall. The infundibulopelvic ligament supports and suspends the ovary. It attaches to the mesovarium and contains the ovarian artery, veins, and nerves, which branch off into the mesovarium.

The functions of the ovary are the development and expulsion of ova and the secretion of the female hormones, estrogen and progesterone. The process by which the mature ova are formed is called oogenesis.

Oogenesis. In the female, ovum cell formation is called **oogenesis.** During early fetal life primitive ova (oogonia) are formed through a process of meiosis, which arrests at prophase I (meiosis I). The primitive oogonia enlarge to form primary oocytes before birth. Each of the primary oocytes is contained in a cavity referred to as the primitive or primordial follicle. At birth, the woman has all the oocytes that she will have for a lifetime (about 400,000). These cells then become dormant until the time of puberty, when the female begins to ovulate. Shortly before ovulation, a primary oocyte completes meiosis I, or the first meiotic division, resulting in a haploid number of chromosomes (23). At the completion of meiosis I, two cells are produced, the secondary oocyte and the first polar body. The secondary oocyte matures into the **ovum,** receiving almost all of the cytoplasm from the parent cell; the first polar body receives little cytoplasm and begins to degenerate (*see* Chapter 11).[2]

After the onset of puberty, one of the primordial follicles matures each month and ruptures, releasing the mature ovum into the fallopian tube (ovulation). At ovulation the secondary oocyte begins the second meiotic division (meiosis II) but progresses only to metaphase, where division is arrested. When the secondary oocyte is penetrated by a sperm, the second meiotic division is completed. (*see* Chapter 11).[2] Usually one mature ovum is formed each month throughout the female's fertile life (30 to 40 years).

Fallopian Tubes (Oviducts). The two **fallopian tubes,** also referred to as oviducts and uterine tubes, extend laterally from the uterine cornua (part of the uterus where the fallopian tubes open) to the ovaries. Each measures approximately 8 to 14 cm in length and each is divided into four areas: (1) the interstitial portion; (2) isthmus; (3) ampulla; and (4) infundibulum. The interstitial portion is found within the uterine musculature and extends upward and outward from the uterine cavity. The isthmus is the narrow, straight portion of the tube that adjoins the uterus. The isthmus passes into the wider, more tortuous portion called the ampulla. The ampulla ends in the funnel-shaped infundibulum, which is covered with projections called **fimbriae.** The fimbriated end of the tubes opens into the peritoneal cavity. The longest of the fimbriae is called the fimbria ovarica, which forms a shallow gutter that reaches the ovary.

The wall of the tube is made up of serous (or peritoneal), subserous (or adventitial), muscular, and mucous tissue layers. The serous layer completely covers the tube except for a small portion at the lower border. The subserous layer contains the blood and nerve supply to the tube.

The muscular layer has an inner, circular and an outer, longitudinal arrangement, which is more prominent at the uterine end of the tube. The musculature of the tube is responsible for the continuous rhythmic tubal contractions which become more intense at the time of ovulation.

The mucous membrane that lines the fallopian tube contains ciliated epithelial cells, which are found most abundantly at the fimbriated end of the tube. At the time of ovulation, the cilia at the fimbriated end of the tube assist in directing the ovum into the tube; the cilia in the rest of the tube propel the ovum toward the uterus.

The blood supply for the fallopian tubes comes from the ovarian and uterine arteries. The nerves that supply the tubes are derived from the parasympathetic and sympathetic nervous systems.

Fertilization occurs in the distal third of the fallopian tube, and the fertilized ovum is transported through the tube to the uterus (*see* Chapter 11). The environment in the tube assists in the nourishment of the fertilized ovum before it reaches the protection of the uterus.

Uterus. The **uterus** is a pear-shaped, muscular organ, which in the nonpregnant woman is situated between the urinary bladder and the rectum. It varies in size and shape according to the age and number of pregnancies that the woman has had. In the prepubertal girl, the uterus measures from 2.5 to 3.5 cm. Before the first pregnancy, the uterus of the adult woman measures approximately 5.5 to 8 cm and weighs from 50 to 60 g. In women who have been pregnant the uterus measures 9 to 10 cm in length and weighs about 80 g (Figure 6–14).

The uterus is divided into two major parts, the corpus or upper two thirds, and the cervix, or lower third. The upper portion of the corpus, extending above the attachment of the fallopian tubes, is called the fundus.

Corpus. The **corpus,** or body, of the uterus is made up of three layers: the perimetrium, or outer serous layer; the myometrium, or muscular middle layer; and the endometrium, or innermost layer.

The outermost serous layer, the **perimetrium,** is formed by peritoneum, extending from the anterior wall of the uterus to the surface of the bladder. It also covers the surface of the superior vaginal fornix and forms the anterior wall of the pouch of Douglas. At the lateral margins of the uterus, the peritoneum forms the broad ligaments.

The **myometrium,** the middle layer of the corpus, is continuous with the muscular layer of the fallopian tubes and the vagina. The smooth muscle fibers of this layer extend into the round, cardinal, and

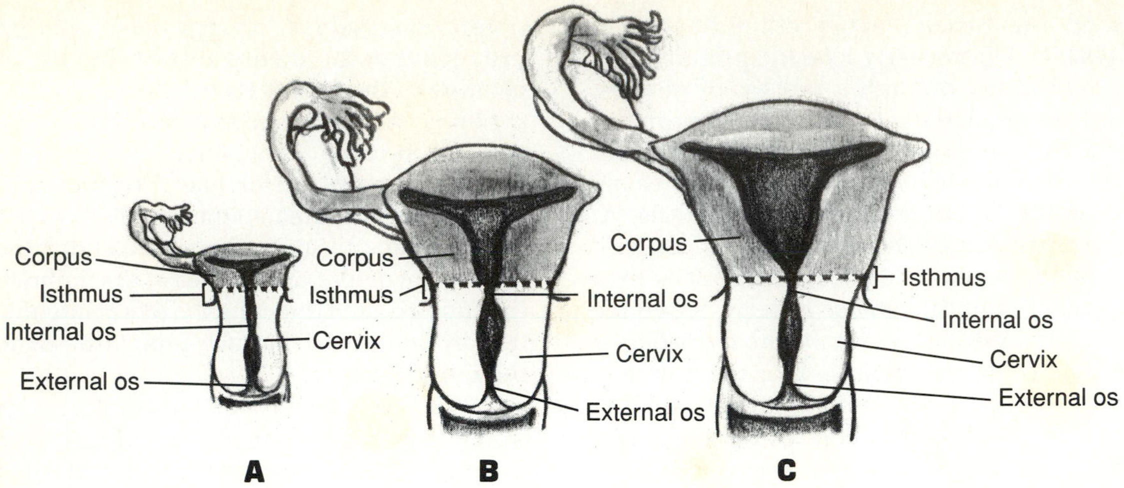

Figure 6–14. Comparative sizes of uteri. **A.** Prepubertal. **B.** Adult nonparous. **C.** Multiparous.

ovarian ligaments. There are three layers of muscles that make up the myometrium. The outer layer is composed of longitudinal fibers found mostly around the fundus; these help expel the fetus during labor. The middle layer is made up of interlacing muscle fibers, which run in various directions. The inner layer is composed of circular muscle fibers, which hypertrophy forming a sphincter at the internal os of the cervix (Figure 6–15). The bundles of smooth muscle of the myometrium are united by connective tissue.

The **endometrium** of the uterus, or the innermost mucous layer, is made up of a single layer of ciliated columnar epithelium, glands, and stroma. The thickness of the endometrial lining depends on the stage of the menstrual cycle, and ranges from 0.5 to 5 mm.

Late in the menstrual cycle, under the influence of estrogen and progesterone, the endometrial layer is composed of two layers, the surface layer or zona functionalis and deep layer, the zona basalis. The zona functionalis is expelled during menstruation, whereas the zona basalis remains.

The glands extend through the whole surface of the endometrium. They secrete a thin alkaline fluid that keeps the uterus moist, assists in the transport of sperm, and nourishes the fertilized ovum before its implantation in the uterus.

The endometrial lining also has coiled or spiral arteries, which respond to hormonal influence during the menstrual cycle and pregnancy. During pregnancy, these arteries contribute to the blood supply of the placenta (*see* Chapter 11).

Isthmus. The isthmus of the uterus is located between the corpus and the cervix. It measures 5 to 7 mm and is significant during pregnancy because it is necessary to the formation of the lower uterine segment (*see* Chapter 12).[11]

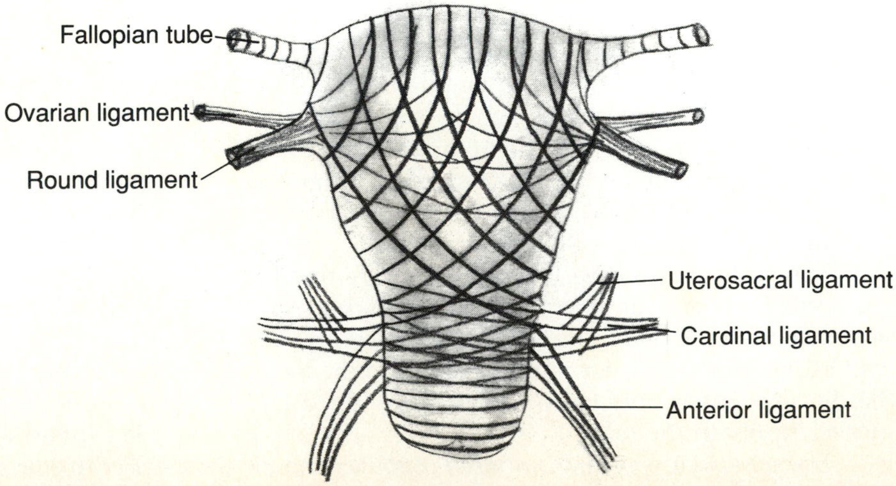

Figure 6–15. Schematic arrangement of directions of muscles of the myometrium.

Cervix. The lowest portion of the uterus, or the neck, is called the **cervix.** The cervix is 2 to 3 cm in length. The **internal os** of the cervix divides the uterine cavity (corpus) and the cervical canal. The **external os** of the cervix opens into the vagina.

The cervix is divided into a vaginal and a supravaginal portion. The lower area of the vaginal portion of the cervix is referred to as the portico vaginalis, or ectocervix. At the lower extremity of the ectocervix is the external cervical os. On speculum examination, the external os varies in appearance. Before childbirth it is regular and spherical in appearance; after childbirth it appears like a transverse slit that divides the external os into anterior and posterior lips. If trauma has occurred during delivery, the external os of the cervix may appear irregular, nodular, or stellate.

The muscular wall of the cervix is not as thick as that of the corpus of the uterus. It is composed mainly of collagenous and elastic tissue, which gives the cervix the ability to stretch during the labor and delivery process.

The cervical canal is also lined with columnar ciliated epithelium, containing mucus-secreting glands. The cervical mucosa provides an alkaline environment for the sperm during ovulation and lubrication for the vaginal canal.

The ectocervix or vaginal portion is lined with squamous stratified epithelium, which is continuous with the squamous epithelium of the vagina. The point at which the squamous epithelium and the columnar epithelium meet is called the **squamocolumnar junction.** The location of the squamocolumnar junction differs according to age and number of deliveries (Figure 6–16). In women who have given birth one or more times, the squamous epithelium may extend up the cervical canal, lining up to one half of the canal. The lips of the cervix in a woman who has given birth may also appear everted (ectropian). The squamocolumnar junction is important as a component of the female reproductive system assessment because it is in this area that cervical cancer may develop. Cells from the squamocolumnar junction are obtained during Pap smears (*see* Chapter 5).

The supravaginal segment of the cervix is covered with peritoneum on its posterior surface. It is surrounded by the pubocervical, uterosacral, and transverse cervical ligaments, which provide stability to the uterus.

Ligaments of the Uterus. The uterus is supported in the pelvic cavity by ligaments, which include the broad, round, and sacrouterine ligaments (Figure 6–17).

Broad Ligaments. The **broad ligaments** extend on either side of the uterus to the pelvic floor, dividing the pelvic cavity into an anterior and posterior compartment. Each broad ligament consists of folds of peritoneum, continuous with those of the abdominal

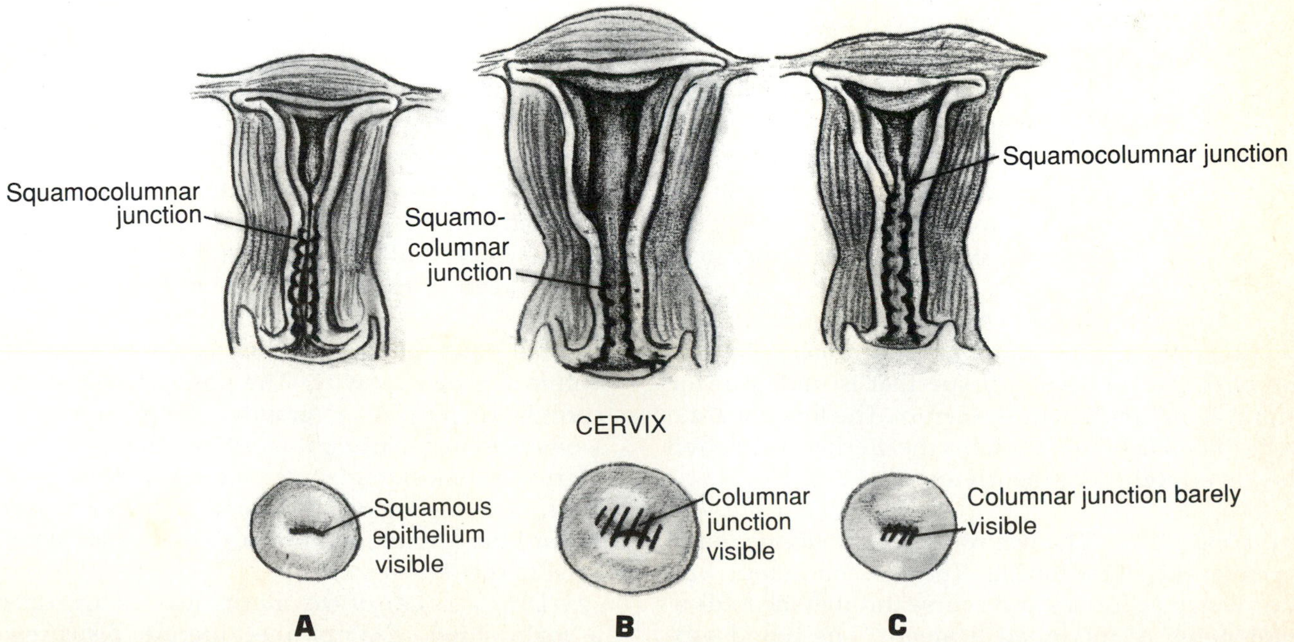

Figure 6–16. The squamocolumnar junction across the lifespan. **A.** Childhood. **B.** Reproductive years. **C.** Postmenopausal.

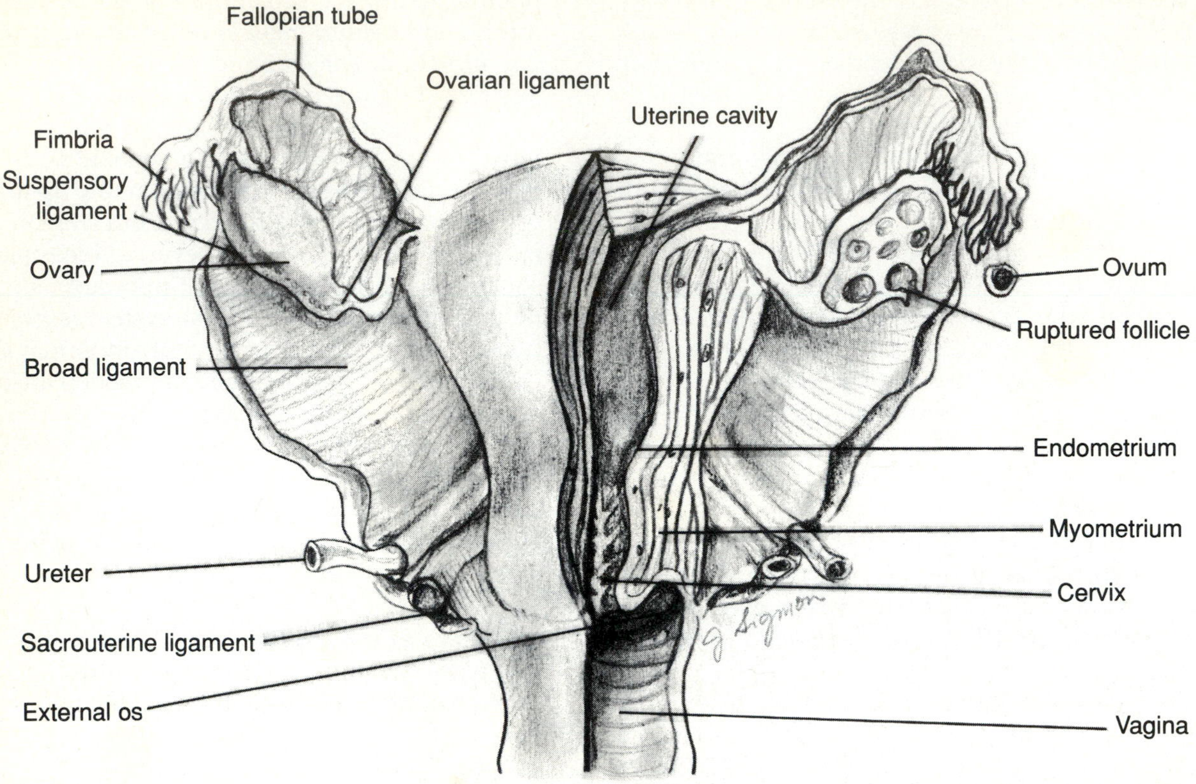

Figure 6–17. Organs of the female reproductive system and their supporting structures.

peritoneum. The folds of peritoneum are divided into upper and lower borders.

At the upper, outer border, the broad ligaments enfold the fallopian tubes and the ovarian and round ligaments. At this point, the broad ligament forms the infundibulopelvic (or suspensory) ligament, which extends from the fimbriated end of the fallopian tube to the lateral pelvic wall. The infundibulopelvic ligament serves to suspend the ovaries; the ovarian vessels pass through this structure. The fallopian tubes are attached to the broad ligament at the mesosalpinx, the inner two thirds of the upper margin of the broad ligament.

At the lower border, each broad ligament forms the cardinal ligament and anterior ligament, consisting of dense connective tissue that is united to the supravaginal portion of the cervix. The lower margin of the broad ligament contains the uterine vessels and the lower portion of the ureter.

Round Ligaments. The two **round ligaments** are found on either side of the fundus. They are continuous with the ovarian ligaments and course through the folds of peritoneum of the broad ligament. The round ligaments extend through the inguinal canal to the labia majora, attaching the uterus to the external genitalia. These ligaments consist of smooth muscle cells, connective tissue, blood vessels, and nerves. The round ligaments provide support to the uterus, especially during pregnancy when they enlarge considerably.

Sacrouterine Ligaments. The two **sacrouterine ligaments** extend from the supravaginal portion of the cervix to the sacrum. They insert on the lateral borders of the first and second sacral vertebrae. The sacrouterine ligaments are covered with peritoneum and consist of connective tissue and some smooth muscle, blood vessels, and nerves. They serve to support the corpus and cervix, keeping the uterus in the anterior position.

Uterine Positions. The uterine position is not fixed within the pelvic cavity. The position may vary according to posture or gravity. If the nonpregnant woman is in an upright position, the body of the uterus is almost horizontal, flexed anteriorly, with the fundus resting on the bladder. The cervix is back toward the sacrum, with the external os at about the level of the ischial spines.[11]

Displacement of the uterus may occur, causing a malposition. Examples of uterine displacement include: (1) retroflexion; (2) retrocession; (3) anteflexion; and (4) retroversion (Figure 6–18).

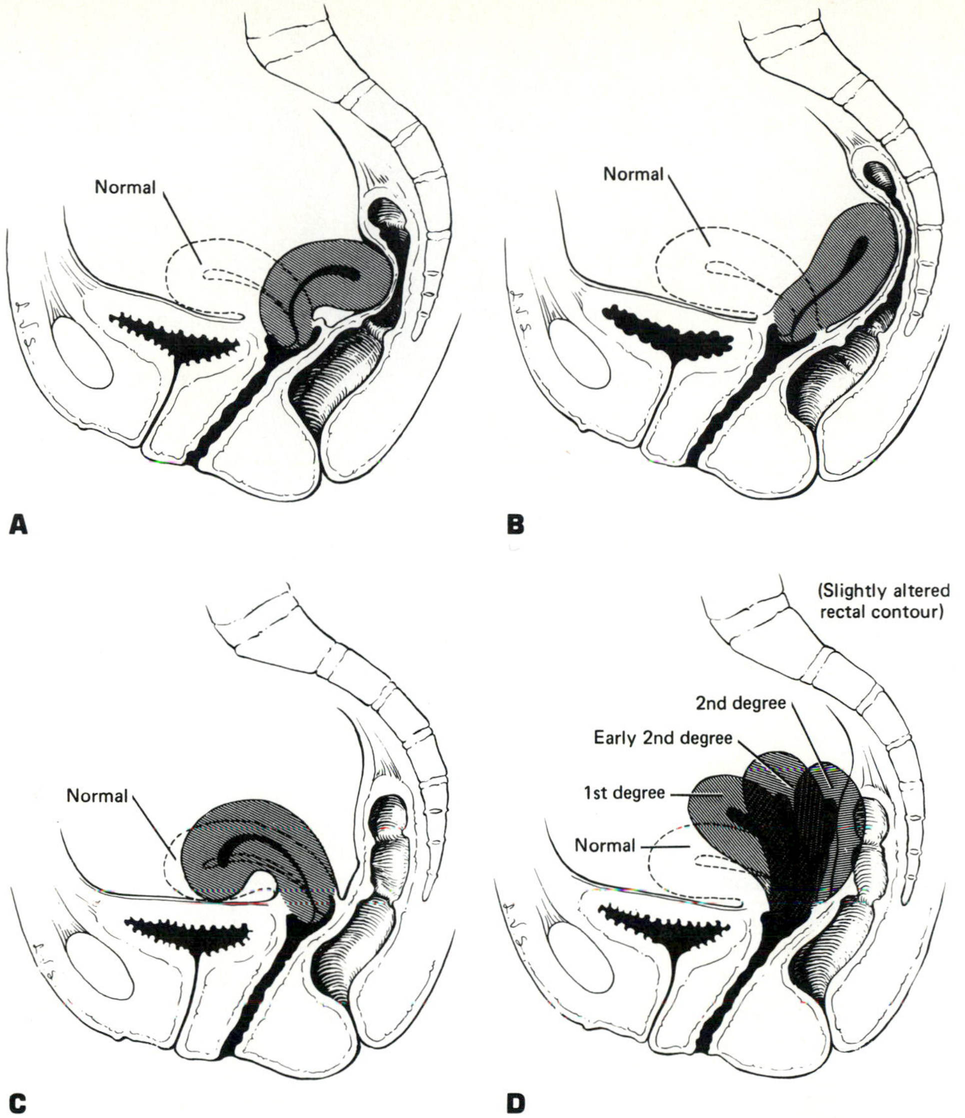

Figure 6–18. Uterine malpositions. **A.** Retroflexion. **B.** Retrocession. **C.** Anteflexion. **D.** Retroversion. (*Reproduced, with permission, from Pernoll ML, Benson RC.* Current Obstetric & Gynecologic Diagnosis & Treatment. *6th ed. Norwalk, Conn: Appleton & Lange, 1987, p 764.*)

Retroflexion of the uterus is the term used when the corpus of the uterus bends back toward the cervix, resulting in a sharp angle. Persistent retroflexion of the uterus during pregnancy is usually incompatible with the advancement of pregnancy.[11] **Retrocession** refers to displacement of the uterus when both the cervix and the corpus bend backward toward the sacrum. In **anteflexion,** the uterus bends forward on itself. **Retroversion** of the uterus may occur with or without retroflexion. A retroverted uterus turns backward, with the uterine fundus lying in the pouch of Douglas instead of anteriorly on the bladder.

Women with malpositions of the uterus may complain of symptoms such as back pain and dysmenorrhea. If the malposition is severe, the pregnant uterus may become incarcerated, preventing uterofetal growth and may cause urinary retention and abortion.[10]

The blood supply for the uterus comes from the uterine and ovarian arteries. The uterine artery, the terminal branch of the hypogastric arteries, is the principal source of blood to the uterus. The ovarian artery, a branch of the aorta, divides into small branches as it extends to the ovary. The main stem of the ovarian artery anastomoses to the ovarian branch of the uterine artery (Figure 6–19). Both the uterine and ovarian arteries enter the uterus via the broad ligament. The return of blood from the uterus and vagina is made through a venous plexus, the uterovaginal plexus, which is located in the uterine muscle. The uterovaginal plexus joins the uterine vein, and empties into the hypogastric vein.

The nerve supply for the uterus is derived from the sympathetic and parasympathetic nervous systems. The sympathetic nervous system causes muscular contraction, whereas the parasympathetic ner-

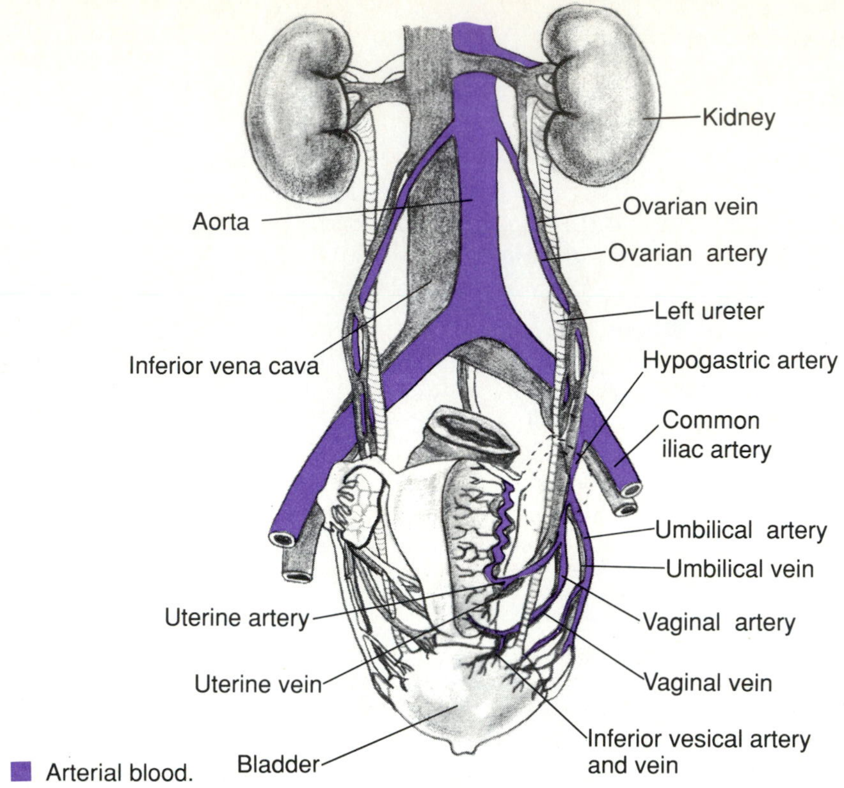

Figure 6–19. Blood supply to the internal female reproductive organs.

vous system inhibits uterine muscular contraction.

The uterus has the ability to increase to 500 times its capacity during pregnancy. It provides a safe, nourishing environment for the fertilized ovum to grow and develop. During labor, the muscular contractions of the uterus facilitate the descent and expulsion of the products of conception.

The Vagina. The **vagina** is a musculomembranous tube, extending from the uterus to the vulva and measuring an average 10 cm in length. It is located between the bladder and rectum. Anteriorly, the vagina comes in contact with the bladder and urethra. The connective tissue separating the vagina from the bladder and urethra is called the vesicovaginal septum. Posteriorly, between the lower portion of the vagina and rectum, the connective tissue separating the vagina from the rectum is called the rectovaginal septum. If overdistension of the vagina occurs during childbirth, the vesicovaginal and rectovaginal septa may tear, causing a prolapse of the bladder (cystocele), the urethra (urethrocele), or the rectum (rectocele).

The vaginal canal has many elastic folds or rugae in its muscular walls, allowing the canal to expand during intercourse and childbirth. Mucous membranes line the vaginal canal and a membrane, the hymen, may partially cover the vaginal orifice. The mucosa of the vagina is made up of stratified squamous epithelium.

The lower portion of the cervix projects into the upper 1 to 2 cm of the vagina. A blind vault or recess surrounds this area, which is divided into the anterior, the posterior, and two lateral fornices. The posterior fornix is deeper than the anterior and lateral fornices because the vagina is attached higher on the posterior wall of the cervix than on the lateral or anterior walls. The walls of the fornices are thin, facilitating the palpation of the internal pelvic organs on vaginal examination. The anterior wall of the vagina measures 6 to 8 cm in length; the posterior wall measures 7 to 10 cm in length.

The environment of the vaginal canal is acidic and responds to hormonal levels throughout the menstrual cycle. When stimulated by estrogen, the vaginal mucosa metabolizes glycogen. Glycogen metabolism is promoted by lactobacilli, normal bacterial inhabitants of the vagina. As a result of glycogen metabolism, lactic acid is produced, causing the pH of the vagina to become acidic, ranging from 4.0 to 5.0 in an adult woman in the reproductive years. The acidic environment of the vagina minimizes the possibility of vaginal infection.

The vagina receives its blood supply from

branches of the uterine, inferior vesicle, and internal pudendal arteries. The network of veins follows the path of the arteries. Venous return of blood from the vagina is made through the uterovaginal venous plexus, which empties into the hypogastric veins.

The vagina functions as the female organ of copulation and the passage for the menstrual flow. It also forms part of the birth canal and it is capable of significant distension during labor and delivery.

Musculoskeletal Supports for the Genitalia

The female reproductive organs are supported by the bony pelvis. In addition, fibromuscular structures support the external and internal genitalia.

Bony Pelvis. The **bony pelvis** consists of four bones that are joined together by ligaments. The four bones include the paired innominate bones, the sacrum, and the coccyx. Each innominate (hip) bone is composed of the fusion of the ilium, the ischium, and the pubis. Anteriorly, the paired innominate bones are joined at the symphysis pubis and posteriorly they are joined to the sacrum, forming the sacroiliac joints.

The sacrum is a heavy bone that is formed by the union of five sacral vertebrae. The superior border of the sacrum is prominent because the sacrum is directed downward and backward. The sacral prominence is referred to as the sacral promontory, an important landmark when assessing the size of the female pelvis. The coccyx is loosely articulated with the lower border of the sacrum, making the coccyx moveable. In some women the coccyx may be fused to the sacrum.

The pelvis is divided into two parts, the false pelvis and the true pelvis. The line that demarcates the false pelvis from the true pelvis is called the iliopectineal line, which is part of the linea terminalis. Above the iliopectineal line is the false pelvis, which is bounded posteriorly by the lumbar vertebrae, anteriorly by the abdominal wall, and laterally by the iliac fossae. The false pelvis has little significance in maternity care.

Below the iliopectineal line lies the true pelvis, which is significant in maternity care. The true pelvis may be divided into the pelvic inlet, midpelvis, and pelvic outlet, the dimensions of which are important to the passage of the fetus during labor and delivery. (*See* Chapter 14 for a complete discussion of the true pelvis.)

The true pelvis is classified according to the shape of the pelvis, using the Caldwell-Moloy classification system. The pure types of pelvic shapes include: (1) gynecoid; (2) android; (3) anthropoid; and (4) platypelloid.

The **gynecoid pelvis** has a slightly oval inlet with the anteroposterior diameter of the inlet being slightly less than the transverse diameter. The sides of the posterior segment of the pelvis are spacious and well-rounded. The ischial spines are not prominent and the pubic arch is wide. The sacrum is somewhat hollow and the sacrosciatic notch is well rounded (Figure 6–20A). This type of pelvis is also called the **female pelvis.** Its structure facilitates the passage of the fetus during labor and delivery. This type of pelvis is found in 50 to 55 percent of women.

The **android pelvis,** also known as the **male pel-**

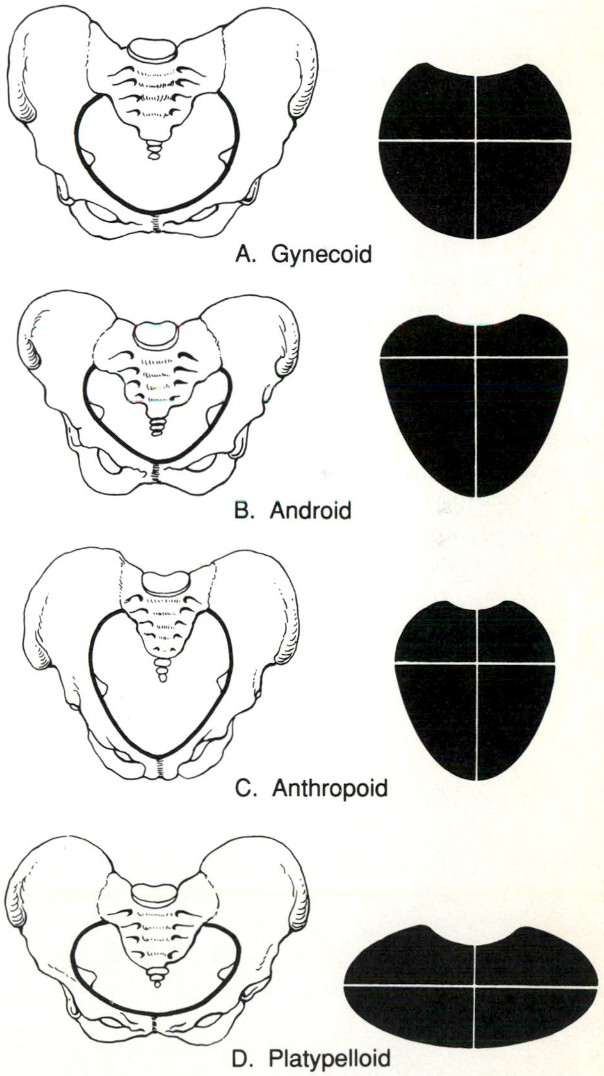

A. Gynecoid

B. Android

C. Anthropoid

D. Platypelloid

Figure 6–20. Variations of female pelves. White lines in diagrams at right (after Steele) show the greatest diameters of the pelves at left. (*Reproduced, with permission, from Benson RC.* Handbook of Obstetrics & Gynecology. *8th ed. Los Altos, Calif: Large Medical, 1983.*)

vis, has a heart-shaped outline. This type of pelvis has a wedge-shaped inlet because the sides of the posterior segment tend to form a wedge at the juncture with the anterior segment. The anterior pelvis and the subpubic arch are narrow and the ischial spines are prominent. The sacrum inclines forward in the pelvis with little or no curvature, and the sacrosciatic notch is narrow (Figure 6–20B). Women with android pelves (about 20 percent) usually need cesarean deliveries. The **anthropoid** (or apelike) **pelvis** is oval in shape, with the largest diameter of the inlet running anterior-posteriorly. The anterior and posterior segments are narrow and pointed and the walls are straight. The side walls converge and the sacrum is straight, making this type of pelvis deep. The interspinous diameter and the subpubic arch are wide and the ischial spines are prominent. The anthropoid pelvis is more common in nonwhite than in white women, making up about one fourth of the pure variety of pelves in white women and nearly one half of those in nonwhite women (Figure 6–20C).[11]

The **platypelloid pelvis** has a flattened gynecoid shape. The inlet is oval with a wide transverse diameter and a short anteroposterior diameter. The posterior segment is flat and the angle of the anterior pelvis is wide. The interspinous diameter is also wide. In this type of pelvis, the sacrum is well-curved and rotated backward, making the sacrum short and the pelvis shallow and the sacrosciatic notch narrow. The platypelloid pelvis is rare in comparison to other pure pelvic varieties and is found in less than 3 percent of women (Figure 6–20D).

Women's pelves may be one of the four pure types described above or may be one of the intermediate or mixed types. When describing the intermediate pelvis, the posterior segment is described first and the anterior segment is described next (eg, android-anthropoid).[10]

Pelvic Muscles. The pelvic structures are supported by the muscles of the pelvic floor, which insert at various points around the bony pelvis (Figure 6–21). The pelvic floor consists of the muscular pelvic diaphragm, which separates the pelvic cavity from the perineal space. The levator ani muscles and the coccygeus muscle make up the pelvic diaphragm. Each of the levator ani muscles is, in turn, composed of pubococcygeus and iliococcygeus muscles. The pubococcygeus muscle is the most specialized of the muscles of the pelvic floor, expanding to allow delivery of the newborn and contracting to support the pelvic structures. The iliococcygeus muscles join the pubococcygeus muscle proper and insert into the lateral margins of the coccyx. These muscles act like a musculofascial layer.[13]

The ischiococcygeus or coccygeus muscles occupy most of the posterior portion of the pelvic floor. They originate from the ischial spines and insert into the coccyx and the fifth sacral vertebra. These muscles supplement the levator ani muscles in supporting the pelvic contents.[13] The obdurator internus muscles form the lateral walls of the pelvis.

The perineum lies below the pelvic diaphragm, bounded superiorly by the levator ani muscles and the coccygei. The central portion of the perineum, called the perineal body, is formed by the anal

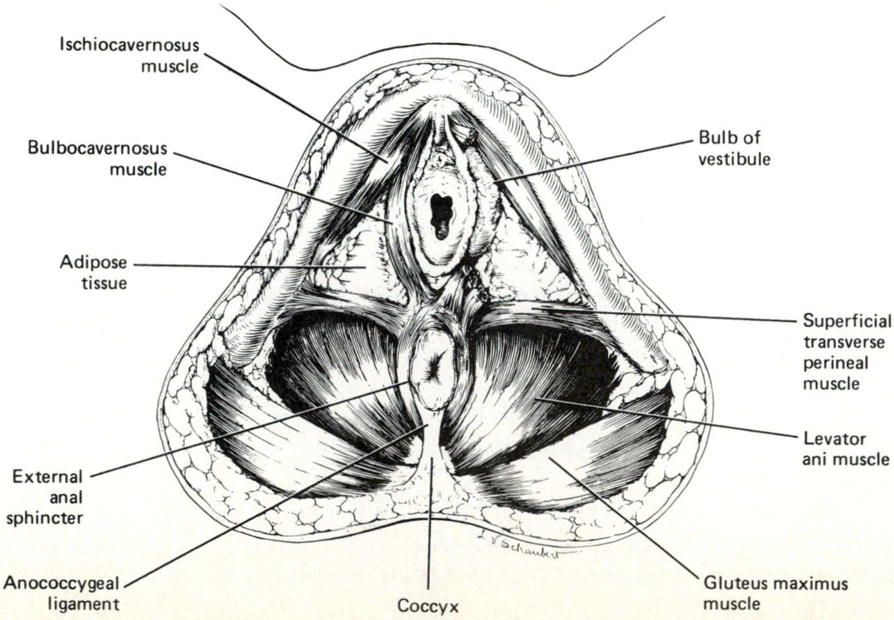

Figure 6–21. Pelvic musculature (inferior view). *(Reproduced with permission from Pernoll ML, Benson RC.* Current Obstetric & Gynecologic Diagnosis & Treatment, *6th ed. Norwalk, Conn: Appleton & Lange, 1987, p 16.)*

sphinter, two levator ani muscles, the superficial and deep transverse perineal muscles, and the bulbocavernosus muscles. These muscles reinforce the perineum and support the perineal floor.

Collectively the muscles of the pelvic floor are referred to as the circumvaginal muscles. Childbearing may weaken the tone of pelvic floor muscles, causing problems later in life, such as lack of urinary control. Research has demonstrated that exercise of these muscles before and during pregnancy improves the strength and tone of the circumvaginal muscles. (*See* Chapters 24 and 31).[14–16]

Mammary Glands (Breasts)

The **mammary glands** or **breasts** are considered accessory glands of the female reproductive system because of their role in lactation. The breasts, which are modified sebaceous glands, are located over the pectoral muscles on either side of the anterior wall of the chest. During puberty the female breasts respond to stimulation of estradiol and other hormones and they begin to develop.

Externally, each breast is covered with skin and has an areola and a nipple. The **areola** is pigmented and contains modified sebaceous glands referred to as **Montgomery's glands.** Montgomery's glands make the surface of the areola rough. In the center of the areola is the nipple, which consists of erectile tissue. Milk ducts drain milk into the nipple during lactation.

Internally, each breast is divided into 15 to 20 lobes. Each lobe is further divided into lobules consisting of glandular tissue within adipose tissue. The size of the breasts is determined by the amount of adipose tissue they contain and has no relationship to the ability to lactate. The lobules contain acinic cells, which are composed of connective tissue and capillaries. The milk is secreted from the acini cells into the mammary ducts. The mammary ducts dilate as they reach the nipple to form ampullae, where the milk is stored. They narrow as they approach the nipple and are known as **lactiferous ducts.** The lactiferous ducts transport the milk from the ampullae to the nipple (Figure 6–22).

The blood supply for the breasts comes from the intercostal and internal mammary arteries. The venous return of blood from the mammary glands is made through the mammary veins.

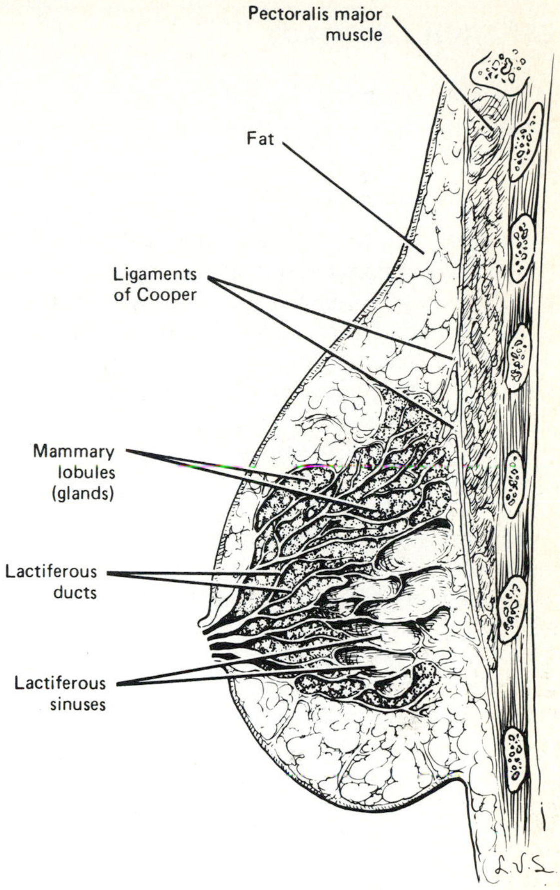

Figure 6–22. Anatomy of the mammary gland. (*Reproduced, with permission, from Lindner HH.* Clinical Anatomy. *Norwalk, Conn: Appleton & Lange, 1989, p 202.*)

THE MENSTRUAL CYCLE

The **menstrual cycle** occurs cyclically in the sexually mature female throughout the reproductive years. It includes two interrelated cycles, the ovarian and the endometrial, which occur continuously and influence the ability of the woman to reproduce. The menstrual cycle begins with the first day of menstruation and ends with the onset of menses the following month. The length of the cycle may vary from about 24 to 35 days, averaging 28 days. Ovulation occurs about 14 days prior to the next menses. The duration of the menstrual flow is variable, lasting anywhere from two to eight days.

Ovarian Cycle

The **ovarian cycle** may be divided into four parts for descriptive purposes. These are the follicular phase, ovulation, the luteal phase, and the premenstrual phase.

Follicular Phase. The follicular phase begins about the third to the fifth day of the cycle, and there is great variability in its length. During this phase, FSH secreted by the anterior pituitary gland stimulates a number of primitive or primordial follicles to develop. Each of the follicles contains an immature ovum. A proliferation of cells occurs within the follicles, stim-

RESEARCH ABSTRACT

Schaver JF, Woods NF. Concordance of perimenstrual symptons across two cycles. Res Nurs Health. *1985; 8:313–319.*

This study investigated perimenstrual symptoms reported by women during two menstrual cycles.

The sample consisted of 63 women between the ages of 18 and 36 years who were not pregnant, and the women varied in racial composition as well as socioeconomic status. Symptoms associated with the menstrual cycle included somatic complaints such as weight gain, back pain, headache, skin disorders, cramps, and painful breasts as well as cognitive or affective symptoms such as anxiety, irritability, depression, and tension.

The women completed a health diary, and their symptoms were compared to the recordings in the diary. In the diary the women were asked to describe their daily experience and any health problems. Single words or short phrases such as "headache" or "swelling of abdomen" were listed. The only reference to menstruation was an item asking the woman to mark an *X* if she was menstruating.

The responses were coded in cycle phases, which were defined as premenstruum, including the week prior to the last menstrual period, and menstruum, including the time during the most recent menstrual flow. The remainder of the cycle was coded as residual days.

Women in the sample reported nine symptoms for either of the two cycles during the premenstrual phase. Only the symptoms of backache, cold sweats, fatigue, depression, and tension, however, were reported across the two cycles. Nine symptoms also were mentioned for either of the two cycles in the menstrual phase. Again, only three, headache, backache, and cramps, were reported across both cycles.

The investigators concluded that reliance on symptoms identified using only one menstrual cycle may be inaccurate and inadequate for therapeutic intervention. Because the prevalence of symptoms changes over two menstrual cycles, data is needed to determine which clusters of symptoms are experienced by menstruating women.

Comment:

This study demonstrates the importance of evaluating perimenstrual systems over more than one cycle. Further research is needed with similar and differing groups to determine which perimenstrual symptoms are common. It would also be interesting to note differences in reported symptoms of women from various cultural groups.

ulated by FSH, with follicular fluid developing between the cells. The hormone estrogen is secreted by all of the developing follicles, but secretion is greatest in the dominant follicle that will reach maturity. As the estrogen secretion increases, it triggers a negative feedback mechanism in the hypothalamus and anterior pituitary gland so that the secretion of FSH is inhibited. When the ovum in the dominant follicle reaches maturity, the follicle ruptures and the ovum is expelled during ovulation. Only the dominant follicle matures to this point; the other follicles are pushed aside and degenerate. The length of the follicular phase varies so that it is difficult to predict ovulation from one cycle to the next based on the follicular phase.

Ovulation. Ovulation usually occurs 14 days before the next menstrual period. If sperm are present, fertilization will occur 24 to 48 hours after ovulation. Because there is a brief period when fertilization can occur, it is important to have some idea of the timing of ovulation when planning a pregnancy. Women can be taught the subjective signs that sometimes accompany ovulation. These signs include ovulatory cervical muccorrhea and ovulatory pain called mittelschmerz.

Ovulatory muccorrhea occurs for one to three days around the time of ovulation. The woman can be taught to be alert to the increased slippery vaginal discharge, which resembles the uncooked white of an egg. Cervical muccorrhea is "runny" in consistency, and the woman will have a slippery sensation as she wipes her vulva after urination.

A second sign of ovulation, ovulatory pain or **mittelschmerz,** occurs in approximately 25 percent of women. The pain occurs at the time of ovulation in either lower quadrant, although it is more frequent in the lower right quadrant. Ovulatory pain may also alternate regularly from one side to the other in successive cycles. The pain is located over the ovarian region, suprapubic, and is frequently accompanied with pressure and ache in the rectum and a feeling of gaseous distension. The duration of the pain varies from one to three days, with the peak of the discomfort at the estimated time of ovulation.

There are also objective signs of ovulation. These include changes in the basal body temperature, spinnbarkeit, and the fern pattern of the cervical mucus. The basal body temperature for the female varies according to the phase of the menstrual cycle. In the follicular phase, the basal body temperature is usually below 98°F (36.7°C). As the estrogen secretion of the ovary reaches its peak just prior to ovulation, a drop in the basal temperature occurs. When ovulation occurs, there is a rise in basal temperatue of 0.5° to 1°F (0.3° to 0.6°C). This rise in basal body temperature is thought to be due to the secretion of progesterone by the corpus luteum. The temperature continues to stay elevated until the premenstrual phase of the cycle, when there is a decline in progesterone. Women can take their basal body temperature daily before arising in the morning. A special basal body thermometer, calibrated by tenths of a degree, can be purchased. The woman is taught to plot her basal body temperatures for the month, noting onset of menses and other factors such as illness that may interfere with the accuracy of the temperature. Although the basal body temperature chart cannot predict ovulation, it can provide information to the woman regarding the actual occurrence of ovulation and the approximate length of the cycle (*see* Chapter 7).

Spinnbarkeit, or elasticity of the ovulatory cervical mucus, is a helpful guide in predicting the day of ovulation. There is maximal activity of the endocervical glands at the time of ovulation because of the increase in secretion of estrogen by the ovary. Within two to three days before ovulation, there is a dramatic change in the cervical mucus, from no elasticity of the cervical mucus to the ability to stretch the cervical mucus an average of 10 to 20 centimeters. There is a rapid decrease in this ability after ovulation (Figure 6–23). The spinnbarkeit is also a sign that the quality of the cervical mucus is such to permit penetration of the sperm.

Another objective sign of ovulation is the absence of **ferning,** which refers to the fernlike pattern of the cervical mucus under microscopic examination. About the time of ovulation, ferning reaches its maximum profusion because of the high estrogen levels. After ovulation, the cervical mucus no longer takes on this pattern because progesterone is present. The degree of fern pattern is usually directly related to the degree of muccorrhea and spinnbarkeit.

Luteal Phase. After ovulation, the cells in the ruptured follicle increase in size and fill with a yellow material called lutein. The follicle is now called the corpus luteum, or yellow body. Luteinizing hormone is secreted by the anterior pituitary gland and stimulates the corpus luteum to secrete progesterone. During the luteal phase, both estrogen and progesterone are secreted by the follicle. If fertilization does not occur, the corpus luteum reaches full development in 8 to 10 days and begins retrogressing. Concentrations of LH become low and the production of estrogen and progesterone declines rapidly. The decline in circulating estrogen and progesterone triggers a positive feedback mechanism to the hypothalamus, which stimulates the anterior pituitary gland to begin secreting FSH in preparation for a new cycle.

Premenstrual Phase. The premenstrual phase occurs two to three days before menstruation. The cor-

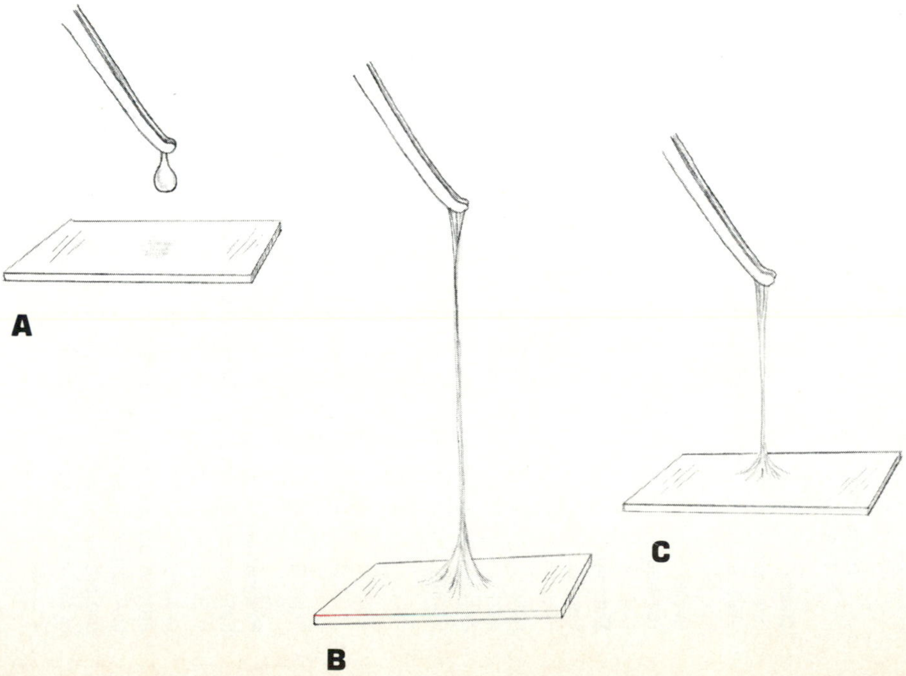

Figure 6–23. Criteria of ovulation: spinnbarkeit. **A.** Three days before ovulation. **B.** Day of ovulation. **C.** Day after ovulation.

TABLE 6–1. IMPORTANT MILESTONES IN THE CORRELATION OF OVARIAN AND ENDOMETRIAL (MENSTRUAL) CYCLES

Phase						
Menstrual 1–5 Days	**Early Follicular 6–8 Days**	**Advanced Follicular 9–13 Days**	**Ovulation 14 Days**	**Early Luteal 15–19 Days**	**Advanced Luteal 20–25 Days**	**Premenstrual 26–28 Days**
Ovary						
Formation of corpus albicans from corpus luteum of preceding cycle. Recruitment of follicles.	Folicular maturation and development of the chosen or dominant follicle.		Ovulation and luteinization of granulosa cells in the ruptured follicle.	Vascularization of granulosa lutein cells and formation of corpus luteum. Follicular atresia.	Mature corpus luteum and continued follicular atresia.	Involution of corpus luteum and initiation of follicular recruitment for the next cycle.
Estrogen						
Low; derived principally from extraglandularly produced estrone; little estradiol-17β secretion by the ovary.	Estradiol-17β secretion, principally by granulosa cells of the dominant follicle, increases strikingly, maximal rates being attained just prior to the LH surge.		Immediately after, or coincident with, ovulation, there is an abrupt, indeed, precipitous decline in estradiol-17β secretion.	Gradual and progressive postovulatory rise in estradiol-17β secretion by the corpus luteum.	Maximal rates of postovulatory estradiol-17β secretion are attained; luteal phase estradiol-17β secretion rates, however, are not nearly as great as those observed in the immediate preovulatory phase.	Estradiol-17β secretion declines precipitously and, as during menstruation, the principal estrogen produced is estrone, which is formed in extraglandular sites.
Progesterone						
Low secretion; there is little secretion of progesterone by the adrenal cortex, and the corpus luteum of the preceding ovarian cycle has regressed.	During the follicular phase of the ovarian cycle, progesterone levels remain low. This is because human granulosa cells cannot synthesize cholesterol, the obligate precursor of progesterone, but are dependent on LDL-cholesterol that can be obtained only from the blood after vascularization of the granulosa cells after ovulation.		Progesterone secretion increases steadily as the consequence of the availability of LDL and LH action to effect cholesterol side-chain cleavage.	Progesterone secretion remains high until the end of the advanced luteal phase.		Precipitous decline in progesterone secretion.

Endometrium						
Menstrual desquamation and early reorganization of endometrial glandular epithelium.	Proliferation of glandular epithelium with many mitoses.	Pseudostratification of nuclei—no secretion, early stromal changes.	Appearance of subnuclear vacuoles that are rich in glycogen.	Migration of vacuoles to the luminal surface; cessation of mitosis. The endometrial glands become very tortuous.	Vacuoles have been secreted and decidualization commences. Stromal edema and enlargement of stromal cells is prominent.	Disruption and disintegration of stromal cells. Leukocyte infiltration and interstitial hemorrhage.
Pituitary Secretion: FSH						
Continuing decline in FSH levels that had become modestly increased coincident with the decline in steroid secretion by the regressing corpus luteum of the preceding cycle.	FSH secretion is at all times pulsatile in nature but during the proliferative phase of the ovarian cycle, prior to the time of the LH surge at midcycle, FSH levels remain low.		There is a significant surge of FSH secretion, albeit less prominent than that of LH, that heralds the commencement of the ovulatory process.	After the midcycle gonadotropin surge, FSH levels fall abruptly to levels similar to those found during the preovulatory phase of the cycle.		As steroid secretion by the regressing corpus luteum diminishes, there is a modest but significant increase in FSH.
LH						
The levels of LH are low and reasonably constant until just prior to ovulation.			Coincident with, or just after, the striking increase in estradiol-17β secretion by the dominant follicle, there is a striking increase in LH secretion—the LH "surge."	The levels of LH decline if fertilization does not occur.		

LDL = low-density lipoprotein.

Adapted with permission, from Cunningham FG, et al. Williams Obstetrics. *18th ed. Norwalk, Conn: Appleton & Lange, 1989, p 31.*

pus luteum retrogresses, with a concomittant decline in estrogen and progesterone levels. These changes in hormone levels are followed by the endometrium shedding its lining during menstruation.

Endometrial Cycle

In all stages of the ovarian cycle the endometrium of the uterus demonstrates changes in response to hormone levels. The **endometrial cycle,** sometimes referred to as the **uterine cycle,** includes changes in the uterus that are stimulated by hormones during the ovarian cycle. The endometrial cycle may be divided into three phases: proliferative, secretory, and menstrual. It is significant to note that there is individual variation in the activity of the ovary and the effect on the uterus. The changes in the ovarian and uterine cycles are not coincident in time. In other words, the follicular phase of the ovarian cycle is not absolutely parallel to the proliferative phase of the endometrial cycle. The changes are continuous throughout the cycle and the phases are artificial, used for descriptive purposes only.[11]

Proliferative Phase. In the early part of the proliferative phase of the endometrial cycle, immediately after menstruation, the endometrium is very thin and the endometrial glands are narrow. Under the influence of estrogen that is secreted by the ovary, the cells of the endometrium become thicker and multiply by mitosis. As the proliferative phase progresses, the endometrium becomes even thicker as a result of glandular hyperplasia and growth of the stroma. The stroma becomes edematous as a result of stimulation of estrogen and increases in ions, water, and amino acids. During this phase, the endometrium proliferates from approximately 0.5 mm to 5 mm in height and increases approximately eightfold in thickness. This proliferation of cells serves to prepare the uterus for implantation of the fertilized ovum. The proliferative phase of the endometrial cycle varies in length among women. For example, a 28-day menstrual cycle has a shorter proliferative phase than a 32-day cycle. Unlike the proliferative phase, the secretory or postovulatory phase of the cycle is fairly consistent so that it can be predicted that ovulation will occur about 14 days prior to menstruation.

Secretory Phase. After ovulation, under the influence of estrogen supplemented by progesterone secreted by the ovary, the endometrial glands become increasingly tortuous. There is increased edema of the stroma and dense coiling of the spiral vessels. The endometrium during the secretory phase is succulent and rich in glycogen, preparing for implantation of the fertilized ovum and growth of the embryo. The endometrial changes that occur during this phase are precise and must be mediated by progesterone, which is secreted by the ovary during the luteal phase of the ovarian cycle. If a biopsy of the endometrium is done during this phase and demonstrates changes in the endometrium consistent with the secretory phase, it can be said that ovulation has taken place. The secretory phase of the menstrual cycle will last about 14 days. About two or three days before menstruation, in response to the decline in levels of estrogen and progesterone, there is a reduction in endometrial tissue fluid, a decrease in blood flow, and a disintegration of the stromal cells.

Menstrual Phase. The cellular debris, blood, and mucus that are found with degeneration of the endometrium are discharged through the cervix to the vagina and out of the body via the vaginal orifice. Other materials in the menstrual flow include prostaglandins, a unique class of tissue hormones, which have a role in the initiation of menstruation and possibly contribute to the menstrual discomfort that some women experience.[11] The menstrual phase lasts from about the first to the fifth day of the menstrual cycle. Toward the end of this phase FSH, secreted by the anterior pituitary gland, stimulates the secretion of estrogen by the ovarian follicles and the endometrial lining is reconstructed in a new cycle.

Hormonal Activity During the Menstrual Cycle

The menstrual cycle is hormonally mediated through the activity of the hypothalamus, anterior pituitary gland, and the ovary. When stimulated by the hypothalamus, the anterior pituitary gland produces gonadotropin hormones. One of these hormones, FSH, stimulates the growth and development of the graafian follicle. The follicle secretes estrogen, which stimulates proliferation of the endometrial lining of the uterus. When ovulation occurs, the anterior pituitary gland secretes LH, which stimulates the development of the corpus luteum. The corpus luteum secretes progesterone, which further develops the lining of the uterus in preparation for the fertilized ovum. In the absence of pregnancy, the corpus luteum degenerates, decreasing the levels of estrogen and progesterone, and causing the lining of the uterus to shed during menstruation. The decline in estrogen and progesterone triggers a positive feedback to the hypothalamus, which stimulates the anterior pituitary gland to se-

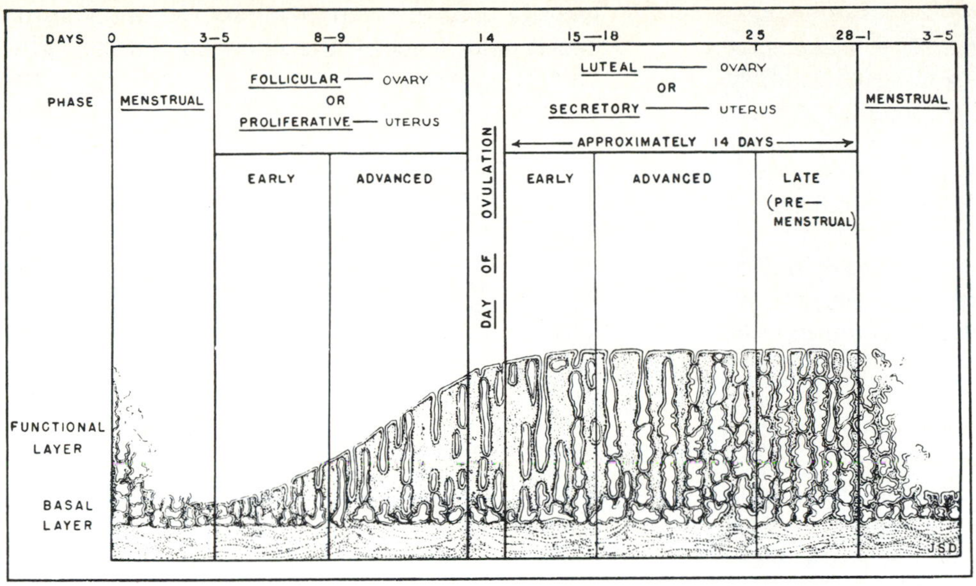

Figure 6–24. Cyclic changes in thickness and form of glands and arteries of the endometrium during the ovarian cycle. (*Reproduced, with permission, from Cunningham FG,* et. al. Williams Obstetrics. *18th ed. Norwalk, Conn: Appleton & Lange, 1989, p 32.*)

crete FSH once again. Summaries of the hormones of the ovarian cycle and the action of the pituitary gonadotropin hormones are found in Table 6–1 and in Figure 6–24.

SUMMARY

Human reproduction is dependent on the transmission of genetic material via the ovum and sperm at conception. These specialized cells each contribute half of the chromosomes containing the hereditary characteristics for the new individual. Genes, the basic units of inheritance, are composed of deoxyribonucleic acid (DNA). Chromosomes, the threadlike structures within the nucleus of the cell, carry the genes. There are 23 pairs of chromosomes (or 46, total) in the human cell nucleus.

Human cell division is an essential component of the reproductive process. The two types of cell division are mitosis and meiosis. Mitosis occurs as a result of replicative division in which a cell having 46 chromosomes divides to form two identical daughter cells, each having 46 chromosomes. Meiosis is a process of reduction division in which the number of chromosomes in an ovum or sperm is reduced by half. After fertilization, the resulting zygote will have a full complement of 46 chromosomes, half contributed by the mother and half by the father.

The development of the male and female reproductive systems occurs during fetal life. Final maturation of the male and female reproductive systems occurs during puberty in a predictable fashion. The rate of maturation may be variable among adolescents. During puberty, the male and female develop secondary sex characteristics that distinguish the sexes, and they develop the capacity to reproduce.

The male reproductive system is made up of external and internal organs. The external organs are the penis and the scrotum. The internal organs consist of the testes, epididymides, ductus deferens, ejaculatory ducts, and urethra. The accessory organs to the male reproductive tract include the seminal vesicles, prostate gland, and bulbourethral glands.

The process of spermatogenesis, the production of mature sperm, is mediated by hormones. Mature sperm consist of a head, neck, middle piece, and tail. They are ejaculated from the male urethra during sexual stimulation along with seminal fluid. The seminal fluid contains materials that assist in the transportation and viability of the sperm.

The female reproductive system also consists of external and internal genitalia. The external genitalia are the vulva, labia majora, labia minora, vestibule, and perineum. The internal genitalia include the vagina, uterus, fallopian tubes, and ovaries. The supporting structures of the female reproductive tract include the bony pelvis, pelvic muscles, and ligaments. The breasts, or mammary glands, are considered accessory to the reproductive system in the female because of their role in lactation. Internally each breast consists of glandular and adipose tissue. Milk is manufactured and stored in each breast during lactation.

Oogenesis refers to the production of mature ova. Oogenesis begins before birth and is completed during puberty. Puberty in females also marks the onset of menstruation. Menstruation is cyclic in nature and is mediated by hormones.

The menstrual cycle consists of the ovarian and endometrial cycles. The ovarian cycle may be divided into four parts: the follicular phase, ovulation, the luteal phase, and the premenstrual phase. Concurrent with the ovarian cycle is the endometrial cycle, which may be divided into three phases: the proliferative, secretory, and menstrual. In all stages of the ovarian cycle, the endometrium changes in response to hormone levels.

Nurses need to have a thorough knowledge of human genetics and the anatomy and physiology of the male and female reproductive systems when caring for couples who are planning or experiencing a pregnancy. This knowledge will guide the nurse in assessing the client and family and in planning care for family members.

REVIEW QUESTIONS

1. List the stages in mitosis and meiosis.
2. Identify and describe the changes that occur in the stages of puberty in the male and female.
3. Describe each of the phases and structures involved in transportation of mature sperm.
4. Describe the structure and function of the uterus with its musculoskeletal supports.
5. Identify phases of the ovarian and endometrial cycles and describe the changes that occur in each.

REFERENCES

1. Moore KL. *Before We Are Born: Basic Embryology and Birth Defects*. 3rd ed. Philadelphia: W.B. Saunders, 1989.
2. Moore KL. *The Developing Human: Clinically Oriented Embryology*. 4th ed. Philadelphia: W.B. Saunders, 1988.
3. Tanner JM. *Growth at Adolescence*. 2nd ed. Oxford, England: Blackwell Scientific Publications, 1962.
4. Lee PA. Normal ages of pubertal events among American males and females. *J Adolesc Health Care*. 1980; 1:26–29.
5. Tanner JM. *Into Man: Physical Growth from Conception to Maturity*. Cambridge, Mass: Harvard University Press, 1978.
6. Copeland K., et al. Assessment of pubertal development. Columbus, Ohio: Ross Laboratories: *Pediatrics in Review*. 1986; 8(2):21–25.
7. Job JC, Canlorbe P. The sex glands. In Job JC, Pierson M, eds. *Pediatric Endocrinology*. New York: John Wiley & Sons, 1981.
8. Tanner JM. Growth and endocrinology of the adolescent In Gardner LI, ed. *Endocrine and Genetic Diseases of Childhood and Adolescence*, 2nd ed. Philadelphia: W.B. Saunders, 1975.
9. Marshall WA, Tanner JM. Variations in pattern of pubertal changes in girls. *Arch Dis Child*. 1969; 44:291.
10. Pernoll ML, Benson RC. Current Obstetric & Gynecologic Diagnosis & Treatment. Norwalk, Conn: Appleton & Lange, 1987.
11. Cunningham FG, et al. *Williams Obstetrics*. 18th ed. Norwalk, Conn: Appleton & Lange, 1989.
12. Creager JG. *Human Anatomy and Physiology*. Belmont, Calif: Wadsworth Publishing, 1983.
13. Oxorn H. *Human Labor and Birth*. 5th ed. Norwalk, Conn: Appleton-Century-Crofts, 1986.
14. Dougherty M, et al. The effect of circumvaginal muscle (CVM) exercise. *Nurs Res*. 1989;38(6):331–335.
15. Sampsells CM, et al. Digital measurement of pelvic muscle strength in childbearing women. *Nurs Res*. 1989;38(3): 134–138.
16. Samples JT, et al. The dynamic characteristics of the circumvaginal muscles. *J Obstet Gynecol Neonatal Nurs*. 1988;17(3):194–201.

Problems in Human Reproduction

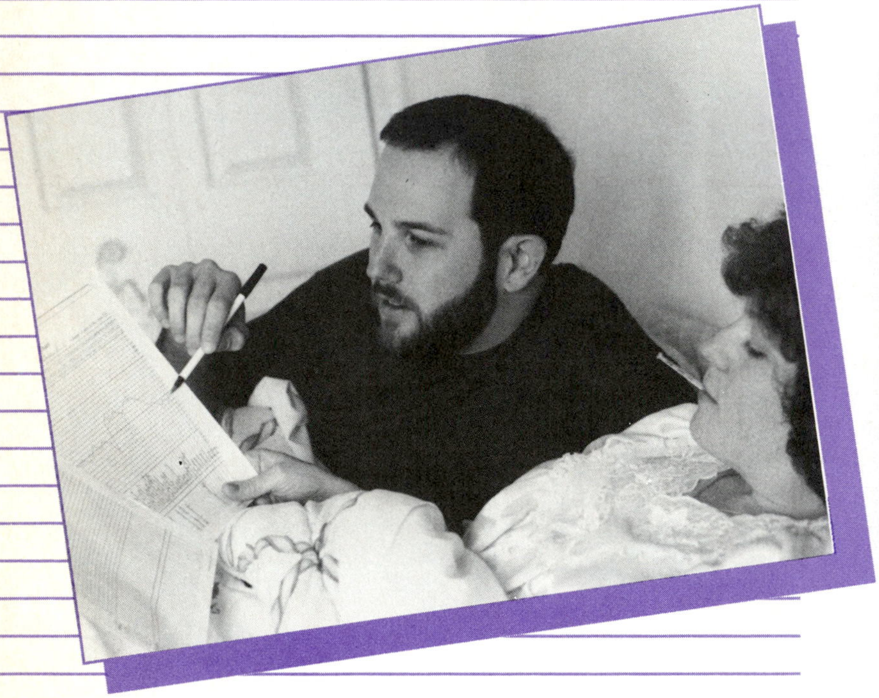

Chapter 7

Key Terms

balanced translocation carrier
Barr body
bicornate (septate) uterus
dominant
endometriosis
genotype
GIFT procedure
heterozygous
homozygous
hysterosalpingogram
in vitro fertilization
isochromosome
karyotype
laparoscopy
monosomy
mosaicism
multifactorial (non-Mendelian) inheritance
phenotype
primary infertility
recessive
retrograde ejaculation
sex chromatin
single-gene (Mendelian) inheritance
sterility
trisomy

A complex interplay of genetics and reproductive physiology is required for the creation of new human life. This process is usually successful, resulting in the development of a viable, healthy embryo and fetus. In some instances, however, problems can occur, creating situational crises for the family and individual family members. Examples are genetic abnormalities of the offspring and the family crisis of infertility.

Genetic problems include autosomal chromosomal abnormalities, which are those abnormalities involving the first 22 pairs of chromosomes, and sex chromosomal abnormalities, which are abnormalities involving the pair of sex chromosomes. Genetic problems can be further classified according to the modes of inheritance, single-gene inheritance or multifactorial inheritance. The multifactorial pattern of inheritance is a result of the interaction of genetic and environmental influences. This mode of inheritance causes the largest number of birth defects in humans.

Other problems of human reproduction center on the inability of the couple to conceive or produce a viable offspring. Infertility can be related to problems specific to the female or male partner, to a combination of female and male problems, or to unexplained causes.

Genetic abnormalities and infertility represent major life crises for the family. In each case, family members experience a loss. Families who give birth to a child with a genetic abnormality grieve for the loss of the perfect child; families facing infertility grieve over the loss of the children they never had. Families experiencing problems in human reproductive physiology, such as genetic abnormalities and infertility, therefore require comprehensive nursing and collaborative care to help them to cope with these problems and reach a healthy resolution to the crises.

GENETIC AND STRUCTURAL CHROMOSOMAL ABNORMALITIES

Genetic disorders represent the major causes of congenital malformations in children. Chromosomal abnormalities are thought to be present in 6 percent of all fertilized ova, but many of these embryos abort spontaneously during the first three weeks of pregnancy.[1]

Normal human body cells have a complement of 46 chromosomes: 22 pairs of autosomes and 1 pair of sex chromosomes. The gene complement of the individual is referred to as the **genotype;** the characteristics or appearance of the individual as a result of the genotype is called the **phenotype.** Individuals with genetic abnormalities will usually have characteristic genotypes as well as phenotypes.

Chromosomal abnormalities that occur in the first 22 pairs of chromosomes are called autosomal chromosomal abnormalities. Abnormalities may also occur in the pair of sex chromosomes. Such abnormalities are thus called sex chromosomal abnormalities. Chromosomal abnormalities may be further classified into numerical chromosomal abnormalities, resulting in an individual who has too many or too few chromosomes, and structural chromosomal abnormalities, in which an individual usually has the complement of 46 chromosomes present, but a piece of a chromosome may be missing or an extra piece of chromosomal material may be attached. In either case the individual has too many or too few genes present, resulting in abnormalities in both growth and development.

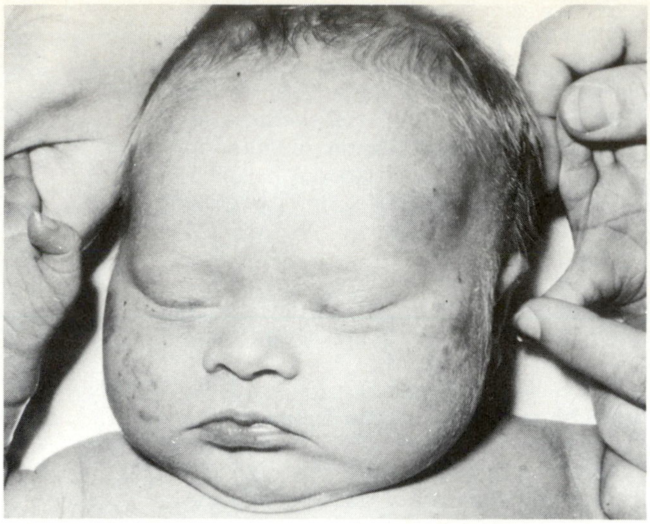

Figure 7–1. An infant with Down's syndrome as a result of trisomy 21. Note the low nasal bridge, upward slanted palpebral fissures on the face, and simian creases on the palms. (*Reproduced, with permission, from Rudolph AM.* Pediatrics. *18th ed. Norwalk, Conn: Appleton & Lange, 1987, p 113.*)

Numerical Chromosomal Abnormalities

Numerical chromosomal abnormalities are usually a result of nondisjunction, an error in cell division in which the paired chromosomes fail to separate at anaphase. This error may occur during mitotic cell division or during the first or second meiotic divisions.[1,2] (For a detailed discussion of cell division, *see* Chapter 6.) Numerical chromosomal abnormalities also may occur in either the autosomes or in the sex chromosomes. When a chromosome is missing, so that the human body cells contain one less than the normal complement of 46 chromosomes, the numerical abnormality is called a **monosomy.** When human body cells have an extra chromosome along a pair, the abnormality is called a **trisomy.**

Numerical Autosomal Abnormalities. Numerical autosomal abnormalities involve the first 22 pairs of chromosomes, or autosomes. A monosomy of the autosomes is very rare in living persons because this abnormality is usually not compatible with life.[1]

Trisomies of the autosomes are the result of nondisjunction in the ovum or sperm in which either germ cell has 24 instead of 23 chromosomes. When fertilization occurs, the new individual has a complement of 47 chromosomes instead of the normal 46 chromosomes. The most common numerical autosomal abnormality is **Down's syndrome** or **trisomy 21,** in which there are three number 21 chromosomes instead of two. Children with this syndrome have characteristic features or phenotypes that distinguish them from other members of the same family (Figure 7–1). Other examples of trisomies of the autosomes include trisomy 18 (Edwards's syndrome) and trisomy 13 (Patau's syndrome). These autosomal trisomies are less common than trisomy 21, and children with these conditions usually die during infancy. (Table 7–1).[1] Autosomal trisomies occur with increasing frequency as maternal age increases and are usually due to nondisjunction in oogenesis. This is particularly true of trisomy 21, which is found in 1 in 1550 births in mothers under the age of 25, but once in about 25 births in mothers over the age of 45.[1]

Numerical Abnormalities of the Sex Chromosomes. Numerical abnormalities of the sex chromosomes are relatively common and may result in monosomies and trisomies.[3] In the vast majority of cases, these abnormalities do not produce the severe handicaps that are present with autosomal numerical abnormalities. The reason for this stems from the unique characteristics of the X chromosome.

During early divisions of the fertilized ovum, only one X chromosome is biologically active; the other or others are inactivated. The number of inactivated X chromosomes is one less than the total number of X chromosomes found in the nucleus of the cell.[4] The inactivated X chromosome is one of the last chromosomes to replicate its DNA. The **Barr body** or **sex chromatin** is thought to represent this genetically inactive, late-replicating X chromosome.

TABLE 7–1. EXAMPLES OF NUMERICAL CHROMOSOMAL ABNORMALITIES

Chromosomal Disorder	Average Incidence	Characteristics
Autosomal Disorders		
Trisomy 21 (Down's syndrome)	1 : 700	Mental retardation; flat occiput; upper slant to palpebral fissures; protruding tongue; broad, short hands with simian creases; possible congenital heart defects
Trisomy 18 (Edwards' syndrome)	1 : 5000	Mental retardation; low-set malformed ears; prominent occiput; congenital heart defects; failure to thrive; usually death in infancy
Trisomy 13 (Patau's syndrome)	1 : 7000	Mental retardation; bilateral cleft lip and palate; polydactyly; malformed ears; death early in infancy
Sex Chromosome Disorders		
Turner's syndrome (45 total chromosomes; XO sex chromosomes)	1 : 2500	Female; short stature; webbed neck; negative sex chromatin test; absence of sexual maturation at puberty; amenorrhea; broad chest with widely spaced nipples; sterile
Klinefelter's syndrome (47 chromosomes; XXY sex chromosomes)	1 : 1000	Male; tall, long legs in relation to trunk; mental deficiency of varying degree; small testes; absence of sperm or oligospermia; 80% are sex-chromatin–positive
Triple X syndrome (47 chromosomes; XXX sex chromosomes)	1 : 1000	Female; normal in appearance; two sex chromatin bodies; may be mentally retarded; fertile
XYY syndrome (47 chromosomes; XYY sex chromosomes)	1 : 1000	Male; tall, long head; may display antisocial behavior; normal appearance and sexual development

Normal female body cells have one active and one inactivated X chromosome; thus, females are sex-chromatin–positive. The normal male body cells have one active and no inactivated X chromosomes; thus, males are sex-chromatin–negative. Whenever an increased number of X chromosomes exists, all but one of the X chromosomes replicate late; and when one of the two X chromosomes has a structural abnormality, it often replicates late. X chromosome abnormalities (in number or structure) are more compatible with life and cause less profound effects than those of the autosomes because the genetic material that causes the abnormality is found in the inactive, late-replicating X chromosome.[3]

The Barr test has become an effective test for screening sex chromosomal abnormalities. The test can be done rapidly by microscopic analysis of cells scraped from the buccal mucosa under the microscope. The inactivated X chromosome (the Barr body) can be seen as a dark-staining mass on the periphery of the cell nucleus. (Figure 7–2).[4]

Most monosomies of the sex chromosomes result in death of the embryo. It is estimated that 20 percent of early spontaneous abortions are the result of sex chromosome monosomies.[5] **Turner's syndrome,** a genetic abnormality affecting females, is an example of a monosomy of the sex chromosomes in which the child survives. This syndrome occurs when nondisjunction during spermatogenesis results in the absence of the paternal X chromosome. Female children with Turner's syndrome have 45 chromosomes: 44 autosomes and one X chromosome.

Trisomies of the sex chromosomes may also be found; however, the characteristic physical features of these abnormalities usually do not appear until adolescence (*see* Table 7–1). Sex chromatin patterns

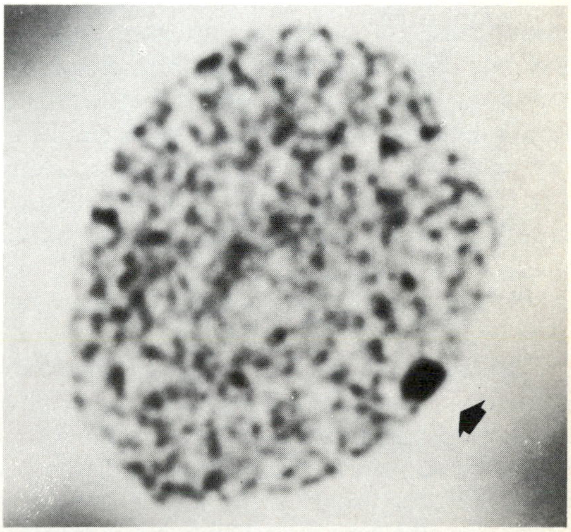

Figure 7–2. Nucleus of a cell showing the Barr body (arrow points to the densely stained Barr body). (*Reproduced, with permission, from Kempe CH, et al.* Current Pediatric Diagnosis & Treatment. *9th ed. Norwalk, Conn: Appleton & Lange, 1987, p 1011.*)

are used to detect some of the trisomies of the sex chromosomes. For example, when their cells are examined microscopically, females who have an XXX sex chromosome complement will have two masses of sex chromatin; males who have an XXY sex chromosome complement will usually have one mass of sex chromatin.[2]

Mosaicism

Mosaicism is a genetic mutation that results in an unequal number of chromosomes in the cells. Mosaic individuals thus have cells with varying genetic constitutions or genotypes; some of the body cells have one number of chromosomes (eg, 47 or 45), while others have another number of chromosomes (eg, 46). Most individuals who are diagnosed as mosaic have a mixture of normal cells with 46 chromosomes and trisomic cells with 47 chromosomes. The usual cause of mosaicism is nondisjunction during early cell division of the fertilized ovum. Mosaic individuals may display handicaps such as mental deficiencies, but these handicaps are usually less serious than those of persons with trisomies or monosomies.[1]

Structural Chromosomal Abnormalities

Abnormalities in the structure of the chromosomes usually occur when a piece of a chromosome breaks and is missing or transfers from one chromosome to another chromosome. Most of these abnormalities are caused by environmental factors such as exposure to radiation and drugs. The type of abnormality that the individual develops depends on what happens to the pieces of chromosomes that are broken.[1,2]

Translocation. Translocations are the transfer of a piece of one chromosome to a nonhomologous chromosome (one that is not part of the transferring chromosome's matched pair). They can occur between any two chromosomes in the genotype during the process of meiosis or mitosis.[6] If two chromosomes undergo breaks and exchange pieces, the individual will have no missing or extra chromosomes and is said to be a **balanced translocation carrier.** The balanced translocation carrier may produce germ cells (ovum or sperm) with the abnormal translocation chromosome, causing his or her offspring to have an abnormal extra chromosome. For example, a woman with a balanced translocation between chromosome number 21 and chromosome number 14 or number 15 may produce offspring with Down's syndrome. The syndrome in this case is caused by a translocation trisomy instead of an autosomal trisomy; the fertilized ovum has two normal number 21 chromosomes (one from the mother and one from the father), and an extra piece of number 21 chromosome attached to chromosome 14 or 15. Offspring that are affected with this syndrome have an extra chromosome even though their body cell chromosome count is 46. Three to 4 percent of individuals with Down's syndrome have translocation trisomies. These are not related to increasing maternal age.[1] Either mother or father can be a carrier of the translocation, with the chances of an affected offspring being 1:5 if the mother is a carrier and 1:20 if the father is a carrier.

Deletions. Deletions occur when a chromosome breaks and a portion of the chromosome is lost.[1] An example of a chromosomal structural abnormality caused by a deletion is the **cri du chat syndrome.** In this syndrome, there is a deletion of the short arm of the number 5 chromosome. Infants with this syndrome display a characteristic weak, high-pitched, catlike cry. They also have small heads (microcephaly), severe mental retardation, failure to thrive, and congenital heart disease.

Structural Abnormalities of the Sex Chromosomes. The most common structural abnormality of the sex chromosomes is **isochromosome.** This abnormality is caused by an injury to the X chromosome during meiosis, resulting in a loss of the short arm of one X chromosome. The cell in this abnormality divides transversely instead of longitudinally. After the arm breaks, rehealing occurs, forming the isochromosome, both arms of which originate from the chromatids of a single arm of the original chromosome. Individuals with this abnormality, therefore, will lack the genes that are normally found on the other arm of the chromosome.[3] Individuals affected by this abnormality are usually short in stature and display some of the same characteristics as those who have Turner's syndrome.[1]

Patterns of Inheritance and Abnormalities

Patterns of inheritance may be classified as **single-gene inheritance** or **Mendelian inheritance,** and **multifactorial inheritance** or **non-Mendelian inheritance.** The genes found along the chromosomes determine the structure and function of the proteins and enzymes of the human body. These genes determine the eye color, hair color, blood and tissue type, and whether an individual has a genetic disorder such as phenylketonuria (PKU), cystic fibrosis, or sickle cell anemia.

Single-Gene Inheritance. Genes, like the chromosomes, come in pairs, half received from the mother and half received from the father. The gene that is expressed by the individual is referred to as **dominant;** the gene that is present but not expressed by the individual is called **recessive.** When individuals have one dominant and one recessive gene for a trait, they are called **heterozygous** for that trait. Conversely, when individuals have identical genes in a pair, they are called **homozygous** for that trait. A recessive trait may be expressed by the individual if there is no dominant gene on either chromosome of the pair. There are four types of single-gene patterns of inheritance including: autosomal dominant, autosomal recessive, X-linked dominant, and X-linked recessive.

Autosomal Dominant Disorders. Autosomal dominant disorders are caused by a single altered gene along one of the autosomes. The disease trait is a heterozygous trait in which one gene in the pair is normal and the other gene in the pair is abnormal. The single altered gene is dominant, thus causing the individual to express the abnormal trait. These disorders may occur as the result of a new mutation (change in genetic material) in an individual ovum or sperm cell, or they may be inherited from one parent or the other who is affected by the disorder. An individual who has an autosomal dominant disorder has a 50 percent risk of passing the gene to each of his or her offspring. In other words, each offspring of an affected parent has a 1 in 2 chance of demonstrating the disorder. If the parent does not transmit the abnormal gene to the offspring, the child will be normal and his or her offspring will be normal. Males and females are equally likely to be affected because the gene does not involve the sex chromosomes. Figure 7–3 illustrates the pattern of autosomal dominant inheritance; Table 7–2 lists some common autosomal dominant disorders.

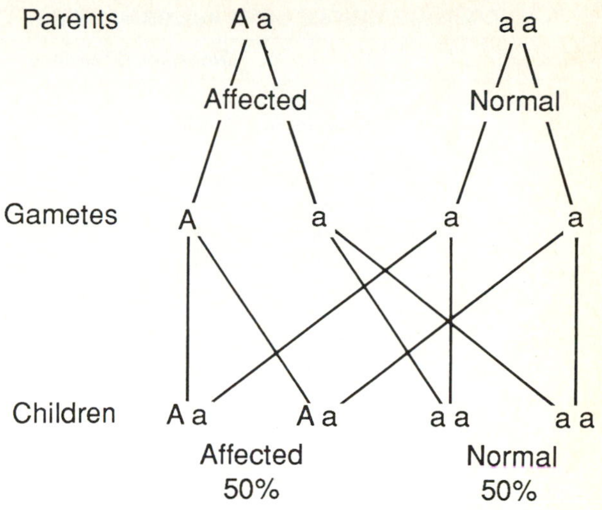

Figure 7–3. Diagram illustrating autosomal dominant inheritance. (*Reprinted, with permission, from Blackman J.* Medical Aspects of Developmental Disabilities in Children Birth to Three. *2nd ed. Rockville, Md: Aspen Systems, 1984, pp 152–153.*)

Autosomal Recessive Disorders. Autosomal recessive disorders are expressed in an individual when both members of an autosomal gene pair are altered. Although both parents carry the recessive altered genes, they are not affected by the disorder because they are heterozygous for the trait and the altered gene does not express itself. When two individuals carrying the same recessive altered gene reproduce, however, they may both pass the altered gene to their offspring, who will then have no normal gene to carry out the necessary function. Both parents are called carriers of the autosomal recessive disorder, and they have a 25 percent risk of passing the disorder to each of their offspring. That is, each offspring has a 1 in 4 chance of demonstrating the disorder. Moreover, each offspring has a 1 in 2, or 50 percent chance of being a carrier of the recessive trait even though the offspring is normal and does not express the disorder; each child also has a 25 percent chance of not having the disease and not being a carrier.

Because parents must pass the same altered gene for expression of the disorder to occur in their children, parents who are closely related (consanguinous matings) are more likely to produce offspring with the recessive disorder than parents who are unrelated. Again males and females are equally likely to be affected, because the genes are not present in the sex chromosomes. Moreover, specific populations may have a higher frequency of recessive disorders than other populations. For example, sickle cell anemia is found more frequently in black populations than in Caucasian populations. Figure 7–4 illustrates the pattern of autosomal recessive inheritance; Table 7–2 lists examples of these disorders.

X-linked Dominant Disorders. X-linked dominant disorders are extremely rare in humans. They are the result of an alteration in a gene located along an X chromosome. Because females have two X chromosomes present, these disorders will occur twice as often in females as in males. X-linked dominant disorders will be passed from an affected male to all of his daughters, because the daughters receive the father's altered X chromosome. None of his sons will be affected, because they receive their father's Y chromosome.

TABLE 7–2. COMMON SINGLE GENE ABNORMALITIES

	Dominant Disorders	Recessive Disorders
Autosomal disorders	Achondroplasia Huntington's disease Tuberous sclerosis Marfan syndrome Neurofibromatosis Stickler syndrome Myotonic dystrophy	Cystic fibrosis Glactosemia Glycogen storage disease Hurler syndrome Limb-girdle muscular dystrophy Maple syrup urine disease Phenylketonuria Sickle cell anemia Tay-Sachs disease
X-linked disorders	Hypophosphatemia (vitamin D-resistant rickets) Cervico-oculo-acoustic syndrome	Duchenne muscular, and Becker muscular dystrophies Hemophilia A Hemophilia B Hunter's syndrome Color blindness Lesch-Nyhan syndrome G6PD

A female with an X-linked dominant disorder has a 50 percent chance of passing the altered genes to her daughters and sons. Each child of a female with the X-linked dominant disorder will then have a 1 in 2 chance of expressing the disorder. Figure 7–5 illustrates the pattern of X-linked dominant inheritance; Table 7–2 lists X-linked dominant disorders.

X-linked Recessive Disorders. X-linked recessive disorders are much more common than X-linked dominant disorders. They occur more frequently in males than in females, because males have a single X chromosome and the single X chromosome carries the altered gene. When males receive a "single dose" of the altered gene, therefore, they express the disorder. Females, on the other hand, have two X chromosomes, one that carries the abnormal gene for the trait and one with a normal gene to carry out the function of the trait. Females with two X chromosomes present must have the gene present in a "double dose" or in both X chromosomes in order to be affected. On rare occasions, however, females will manifest some characteristics of the disorder because the X chromosome carrying the normal trait is randomly inactivated, allowing the abnormal trait to express itself.

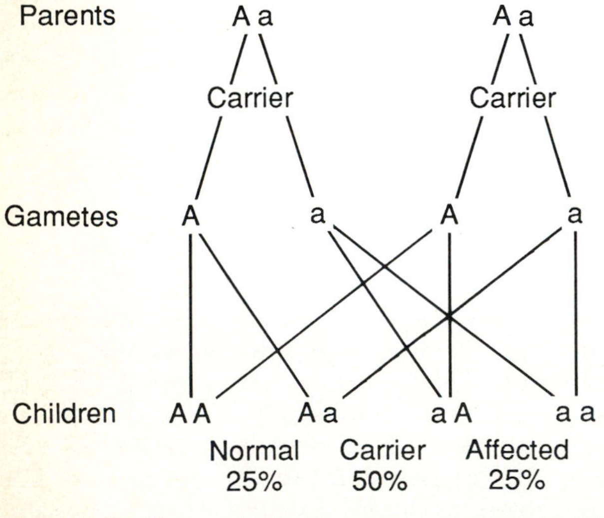

Figure 7–4. Diagram illustrating autosomal recessive inheritance. (*Reprinted, with permission, from Blackman J.* Medical Aspects of Developmental Disabilities in Children Birth to Three. *2nd ed. Rockville, Md: Aspen Systems, 1984, pp 152–153.*)

A female who is a carrier of a gene that causes an X-linked recessive disorder has a 50 percent risk of passing the abnormal gene to her sons. Each son will have a 1 in 2 chance of demonstrating the disorder. The female carrier also has a 50 percent chance of passing the altered gene to her daughters, who will then have a 1 in 2 chance of becoming carriers of the altered gene. The son who is affected by the X-linked disorder has a 50 percent chance of passing the gene to his daughters, who will become carriers of the altered gene. Fathers cannot transmit the altered gene to their sons because they transmit the Y instead of the X chromosome to their sons. Figure 7–6 illustrates the pattern of X-linked recessive inheritance; Table 7–2 lists some common X-linked recessive disorders.

Multifactorial Inheritance and Abnormalities

Multifactorial inheritance occurs as a result of the interaction of several genes and environmental influ-

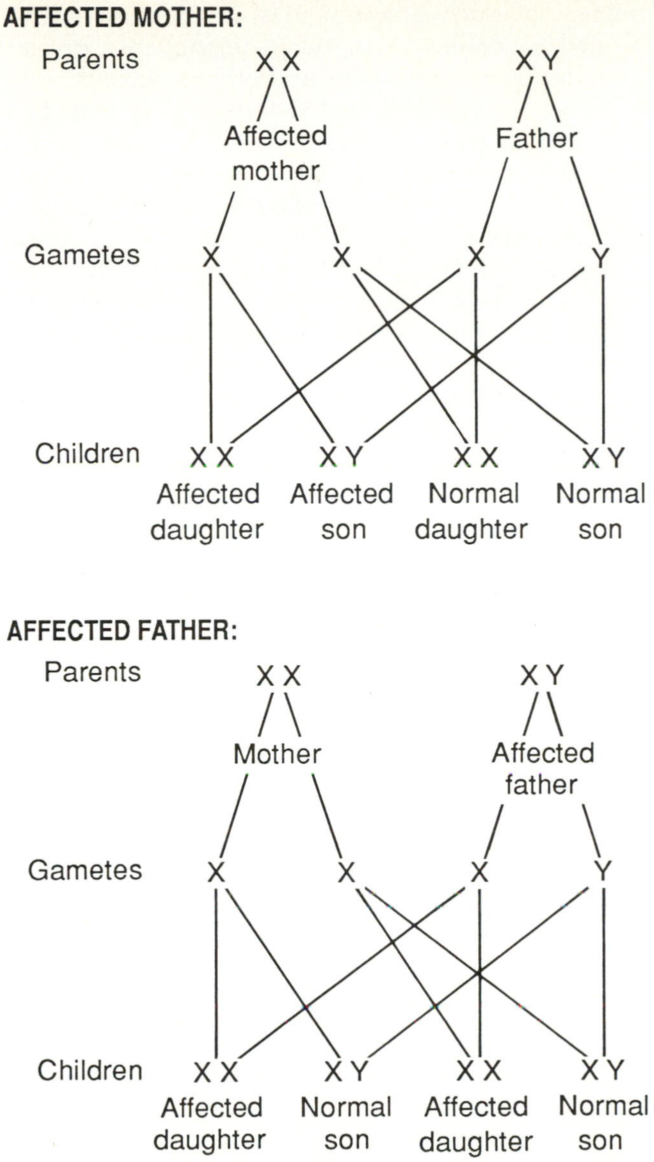

Figure 7–5. Diagram illustrating X-linked dominant inheritance. (*Reprinted, with permission, from Blackman J.* Medical Aspects of Developmental Disabilities in Children Birth to Three. *2nd ed. Rockville, Md: Aspen Systems, 1984, pp 152–153.*)

ences. Many human characteristics are determined by multifactorial inheritance, accounting for the wide variation seen among normal humans in such areas as size, intelligence, blood pressure, and probably the susceptibility to some diseases.[5,6]

Birth defects that are multifactorial in origin are by far the largest group of birth defects that occur in humans. Common congenital malformations with an incidence at birth of at least 1 in 1,000 are inherited and are modified by environmental influences.[5] These defects include cleft lip, pyloric stenosis, spina bifida, and others (Table 7–3). Multifactorial birth defects have a polygenic component in which the cumulative effect of many genes produces the expression of the disorder. Many theories have been proposed regarding the mechanisms of multifactorial inheritance. None of these theories, however, has been readily accepted by all scientists and clinicians.

Some facts are known. For example, multifacto-

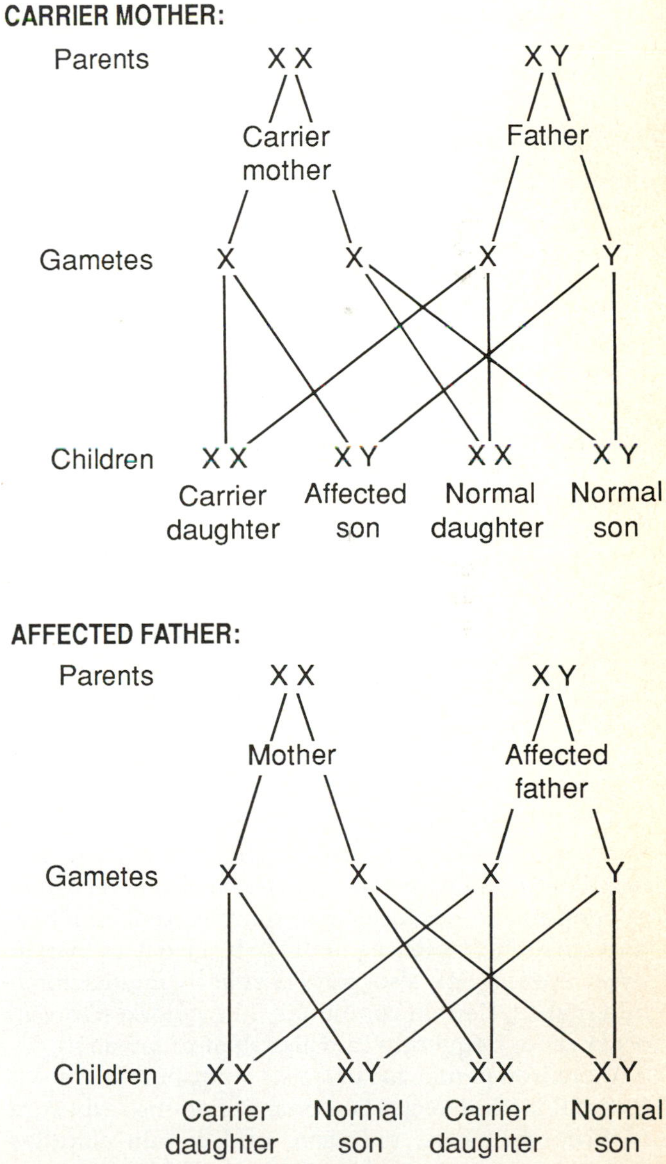

Figure 7–6. Diagram illustrating X-linked recessive inheritance. (*Reprinted, with permission, from Blackman J.* Medical Aspects of Developmental Disabilities in Children Birth to Three. *2nd ed. Rockville, Md: Aspen Systems, 1984, pp 152–153.*)

TABLE 7–3. EXAMPLES OF MULTIFACTORIAL BIRTH DEFECTS

Neural tube defects
Anencephaly (absence of cerebral hemispheres)
Myelomeningocele (opening in the lumbosacral vertebrae through which the meningeal sac and spinal cord protrudes)
Spina bifida (opening in the lumbosacral vertebrae; may be slight or may be associated with protrusion of the meningeal sac or spinal cord)
Congenital heart disease (may include patent ductus arteriosis, septal defects, pulmonary stenosis, tetralogy of Fallot)
Cleft lip or cleft palate
Orthopedic defects
Talipes equinovarus (clubfoot)
Congenital hip dislocation
Umbilical hernia and inguinal hernia

rial disorders tend to cluster in families and are found more frequently among relatives than in the general population. Unlike the risk of single-gene disorders, which remains the same with each pregnancy, the risk of multifactorial disorders increases when more than one member of the family has the disorder. For example, the risk for the single-gene disorder sickle cell anemia is 25 percent or 1 in 4 for each pregnancy if both parents carry the recessive gene for the trait, regardless of the number of children in the family who have the disorder. In contrast, a family who has a child with the multifactorial birth defect spina bifida has a greatly increased risk of having a subsequent child with the disorder (from 1 in 2000 before the birth of the first affected child to 1 in 40 after the birth of the affected child).[7] Moreover, the more severe the defect the more likely the risk of recurrence in subsequent siblings. For example, the risk of recurrence is greater for future siblings of a child with bilateral cleft lip (5.6 percent) as opposed to one who has a unilateral cleft lip (2.6 percent).[3]

Multifactorial birth defects also vary among races, so that there may be a higher incidence of certain defects among persons of one particular race than in persons of other races. For example, umbilical hernias are found more frequently in black babies than in white babies. Sex also plays a role in multifactorial inheritance. Certain conditions, like pyloric stenosis, occur more frequently in males than in females.

Environmental factors also contribute to multifactorial birth defects. Seasonal variations, exposure to toxic chemicals, radiation, and certain altitudes seem to contribute to these defects. There also seem to be variations in occurrence from place to place in the world. Interestingly, not all of these defects appear to be environmentally induced, because the frequency of such abnormalities in identical twins, termed concordance, is four to eight times greater than in nonidentical twins and other siblings.[6]

Overall, multifactorial defects are identified in about 1 percent of newborn infants. In most cases, a simple pattern of inheritance cannot be demonstrated, and risk rates are difficult to estimate. In general, the risk of significant malformation in any pregnancy is approximately 1 to 2 percent. The risk of a second malformed child is about 5 percent, with the risk increasing with subsequent malformed children.[5] Even with the difficulty in providing accurate risk rates for multifactorial birth defects, the risk for these defects is still much lower than for single gene defects.[3]

THE FAMILY AT RISK FOR GENETIC AND CHROMOSOMAL ABNORMALITIES

Nursing and Collaborative Assessment

Nursing and collaborative assessment for potential or actual genetic disorders focuses on counseling and support of the family. A comprehensive family history and genogram will provide the nurse with information about the family pedigree. This information includes health and illness data as well as information about psychologic factors, racial and ethnic background, parental age, maternal health history, reproductive history, and history of present pregnancy, when applicable (*see* Chapter 9). History regarding family members includes the health status of first-degree relatives (eg, mother, father, siblings) as well as second-degree relatives (eg, aunts, uncles, cousins, grandparents). The child who is born with a suspected or actual genetic abnormality is given a complete physical examination to determine the extent of the disability caused by the defect.

To determine risk status for genetic abnormalities, the constitution of the chromosomes in number and structure is assessed by obtaining a photomicrograph of the chromosomes and arranging them in numerical order. This arrangement, called the **karyotype,** is used by the geneticist and other members of the health team to assess alterations in chromosome number and structure and risk of abnormalities to present or future offspring. The karyotypic assessment of individuals is done by analysis of 20 to 50 chromosome spreads for chromosome number. Several spreads are required to determine whether the cells have different chromosome counts (eg, mosaicism). Photographs are taken of representative chromosome spreads and karyotypes are constructed.

Banding techniques also are used to determine numerical counts of chromosomes. In this technique, the cells are stained at metaphase to determine the banding patterns of each chromosome. It is thus possible to identify every chromosome in the karyotype and clearly identify translocations and trisomies. Sex chromatin (Barr body) analysis also may be done to determine the number of X chromosomes present in the cells. The number of X chromosomes is the number of Barr bodies plus one.

Nursing and Collaborative Management

Risk determination for genetic disorders or birth defects allows the couple to become involved in reproductive decision making (*see* Chapter 9). Nurses, in collaboration with other health team members, support the couple through the decision-making process. If the woman is pregnant, several antenatal tests can be done to assess for genetic disorders (*see* Chapters 14, 18, 22). The nurse needs to provide the couple with factual information about the tests and the risks and benefits of the testing procedures. Emotional support for the couple and other family members is important because of the anxiety-producing nature of the testing procedures and the possibility of actual genetic problems.

The couple may be referred to a geneticist for genetic screening. Some nurses intervene as genetic counselors for the family, whereas others provide support to the family during and after the genetic counseling session. The purpose of genetic counseling is to provide the family with information about the risk of occurrence of a genetic disorder in their offspring. Genetic screening for genetic disorders or the potential risks of disorders is done as part of the counseling.

Faced with the risk of having a child with a genetic abnormality, the couple will need to engage in reproductive decision making regarding the present pregnancy, if applicable, or future pregnancies. For example, a couple who is presented with the risks of having a child with Down's syndrome may decide that they will take the risk; and that if, through antenatal testing, the fetus is found to have Down's syndrome, they will carry the pregnancy to term and care for the child. The nurse should never attempt to influence a couple with regard to their present or future childbearing decisions. Rather, the couple should be supported through the decision-making process in a nonjudgmental manner. The nurse assists the couple by providing them with information; however, the decision must be made by the couple.

If a child is born with a genetic disorder, the family will need a great deal of emotional support from the nurse and other members of the health care team. The family must be allowed to grieve for the loss of the "perfect" child that they had imagined during the pregnancy. The family will also need information regarding support services for follow-up care of the child, such as developmental centers and foundations that are specifically dedicated to the child's disorder. The nurse can help to promote family coping by coordinating the services of a variety of resources for families who are confronted with children who have genetic disorders or who are at risk for genetic disorders.

THE INFERTILE COUPLE

Infertility represents a major life crisis to more than 15 percent of couples of childbearing age in the United States. About 2.5 million American couples are infertile. At least one out of six couples will experience this crisis during their lifetime, with some indication that the incidence is on the rise.[5,6,8]

The increased incidence of infertility may be related to the postponement of childbearing until after the optimum age of fertility (ie, age 24 to 30), the increased prevalence of venereal diseases, and the side effects associated with some contraceptive methods, such as the complication of infections with the intrauterine device (IUD). Environmental hazards and stress also are thought to contribute to the problem. Further, the higher incidence may reflect the greater number of people currently seeking help for this problem.

Definition

Infertility is generally defined as the inability to conceive after 1 year of regular sexual intercourse without contraception or to carry a pregnancy to a live birth.[8] **Primary infertility** is defined as the inability to conceive or carry a pregnancy to a live birth with no previous history of pregnancy. **Secondary infertility** refers to an inability to conceive or carry a pregnancy to viability after one or more successful pregnancies. **Sterility** is the term used when there is an absolute inability to conceive.

The criterion of 1 year in the definition is based on statistics for a normal population of couples who are not using contraception; these statistics show that approximately 25 percent of all sexually active couples will conceive in the first month, 63 percent in 6 months, and 80 percent in 1 year. In the second year, another 5 to 10 percent will achieve a pregnancy. The remaining 15 percent will have a diminished chance of becoming pregnant without treatment.[8] Some health care practitioners will not initiate an infertility work-up until the 1-year criterion is met. Waiting 1 year for treatment can, however, be problematic for the couple who wishes to initiate an infertility work-up sooner. The wait may add to the individual couple's problems and needs.[9] It has been suggested that infertility is collaboratively determined by the couple and the health care provider, taking into account the health history, family history, risk factors, and the perception of the couple's fertility status over time. These factors should be taken into consideration, along with the couple's desires regarding the initial work-up.[9,10]

Etiology

The etiology of infertility can be identified in 80 to 90 percent of the couples investigated. Factors related to the female partner account for 40 to 50 percent of the infertility problems; factors related to the male partner for an additional 40 percent; and a combination of factors related to both male and female partners account for another 10 to 20 percent. Approximately 50 percent of those couples who seek treatment will conceive, although those who conceive are at greater risk than the general population for poor pregnancy outcome.[11,12]

Problems Related to the Female Partner

It is assumed that the prerequisites for fertility in the female include the ability to produce a normal ovum capable of fertilization in the fallopian tube and a healthy endometrium in which the fertilized ovum implants and which is capable of nourishing the embryo-fetus.[13] Problems with fertility associated with the female can be grouped according to mechanical barriers, endocrine disorders, and structural disorders of the reproductive tract.

Mechanical Barriers. Mechanical barriers contributing to infertility in the female include infection of the pelvic organs, cervical problems, and endometriosis. These problems can affect fertilization or implantation of the fertilized ovum into the uterus.

Infections. Vaginitis (inflammation of the vagina) and cervicitis (inflammation of the cervix) may be caused by infections. These infections can interfere with the viability of the sperm by making the environment of the cervix and vagina hostile to the sperm. Infections of the endometrial lining of the uterus may contribute to difficulty in implantation and survival of the fertilized ovum. Adhesions within the uterus, referred to as **Asherman's syndrome,** may result from inflammation and infection of the pelvic organs. Asherman's syndrome also may be a relatively frequent sequel of curettage.[14] Because of the increased incidence of pelvic inflammatory disease, partly as a result of the rising incidence of venereal disease, infections of the fallopian tubes are also becoming more common. Adhesions and scar tissue in the tubes interfere with fertilization and transportation of the fertilized ovum to the uterus. Infections may also interfere with the healthy functioning of the ovaries.

Cervical Problems. Cervical factors contributing to infertility in the female include a cervical environment that affects the survival and motility of sperm. Physiologically the cervical mucus should change under the influence of estrogen and luteinizing hormone (LH) at the time of ovulation. If the production of these hormones is low or if cervicitis is present, sperm may be impeded or destroyed by a hostile cervical mucus.[15,16]

Endometriosis. **Endometriosis,** a condition in which endometrial tissue grows outside the uterine cavity, may also contribute to female infertility. Endometriosis is an important health problem of women, and is estimated to be present in 15 percent of women in the reproductive years. The prevalence of this condition doubles to 30 percent among infertile women.[6] It is thought that endometriosis has a polygenic or multifactorial etiology because it is found more frequently in women whose mothers and sisters are affected.[17]

Endometriosis is diagnosed when functional endometrium or tissue resembling the uterine lining is found implanted outside the uterus. Although endometriosis may be found in other areas of the body, it is found most frequently on the ovaries and in the cul-de-sac, particularly on the uterosacral ligament and on the peritoneum of the broad ligaments (Figure 7–7).[17]

Women with endometriosis have a progressive disease that may cause pelvic pain and infertility. The mechanisms by which endometriosis cause these problems are only partially understood. It is thought that premenstrual and menstrual pelvic pain occurs in some women with endometriosis because the endometrial implants respond to the stimulation of progesterone and estrogen by the ovary, not unlike normal endometrial uterine tissue. The implants enlarge and undergo secretory changes and bleed during menses. The tissues surrounding the implants, however, prevent the escape of the blood. The implants may spill their contents within the pelvis, resulting in

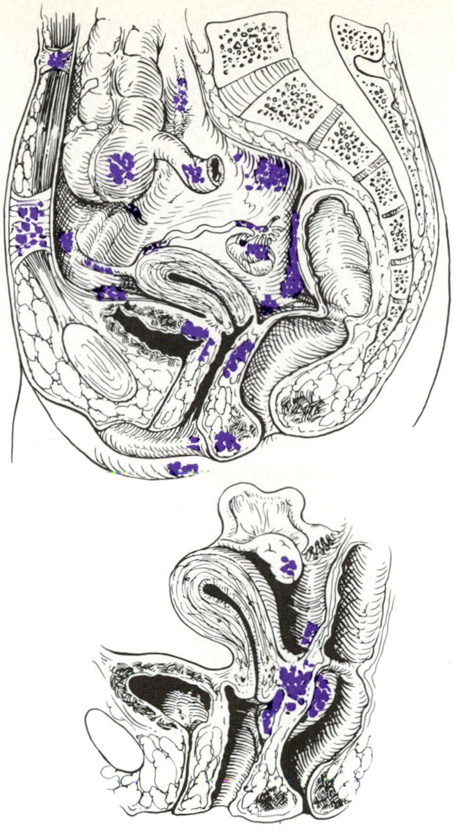

Figure 7–7. Common sites for endometriosis. (*Reproduced, with permission, from Way LW, ed.* Current Surgical Diagnosis & Treatment. *9th ed. Norwalk, Conn: Appleton & Lange, 1990 p 961.*)

reimplantation of the endometrial tissue. With subsequent menstrual cycles, the process repeats itself. Pain occurs as the result of pressure and inflammation around the implants, adhesions associated with the implants, and the implants' proximity to nerves.[6] Pain is not a consistent symptom and is not always proportional to the extent of the endometriosis.[16]

The relationship between endometriosis and infertility has been extensively investigated. Moderate and severe endometriosis is related to pelvic adhesions. Implants involving the ovaries, the most common site of endometriosis, may impair ovulation, while implants involving the fallopian tubes may interfere with transportation of the fertilized ovum through the tube. Adhesions in the cul-de-sac caused by endometriosis may cause a noncongenitally retroverted uterus. Moreover, endometrial implants may secrete prostaglandins that possibly interfere with ovulation and tubal function.[17] Mild endometriosis as well as advanced disease can cause infertility, although the mechanism by which this occurs is unknown.[6]

Endocrine Problems. Hormone activity is important to the processes of ovulation and development of a healthy endometrium, capable of nourishing the fertilized ovum. Problems arising from dysfunction of the pituitary, thyroid, or adrenal glands, or the ovaries may impede these processes. Anovulation may be related to increased levels of prolactin, secreted by the anterior pituitary gland. It is thought that prolactin may cause anovulation by blocking the action of gonadotropins on the ovaries.[6] Significant increases in prolactin may indicate the presence of a pituitary adenoma, a prolactin-secreting tumor, causing ovulatory failure and amenorrhea. Women experiencing hypothyroidism may also be anovulatory; hyperthyroidism may contribute to amenorrhea. Elevated steroid hormones secreted by the adrenal glands may also affect ovulation because the increased androgen production blocks the action of the female hormones estrogen and progesterone.

Estrogen and progesterone secretion by the ovary may also be inadequate. If the secretion of estrogens is inadequate during the follicular phase of the menstrual cycle, the woman may not ovulate. If on the other hand, progesterone production during the luteal phase is inadequate, the woman may ovulate, but may abort the fetus. Luteal-phase inadequacy is characterized by a defective endometrial response caused by insufficient progesterone output from a poorly developed corpus luteum.[18]

Polycystic ovaries, a condition in which the ovaries have a thick, fibrous surface with multiple cysts, also may impede ovulation. Women with polycystic ovaries may have increased testosterone levels because of the androgen-secreting tissue of the multiple cysts found on the ovary.[6]

Structural Disorders. Structural disorders that may be associated with infertility in the woman include malformation of the uterus and fibroid tumors. Malformation of the uterus is a congenital phenomenon. The uterus may be completely or partially Y-shaped (bicornuate or septate). A **bicornuate** or **septate uterus** may have a complete septum that extends to the external os, creating a double uterus with two separate uterine cavities; or the bicornuate uterus may have a partial septum that does not extend to the internal or external os (Figure 7–8). Large uterine fibroid tumors may also impede implantation or cause habitual spontaneous abortions.

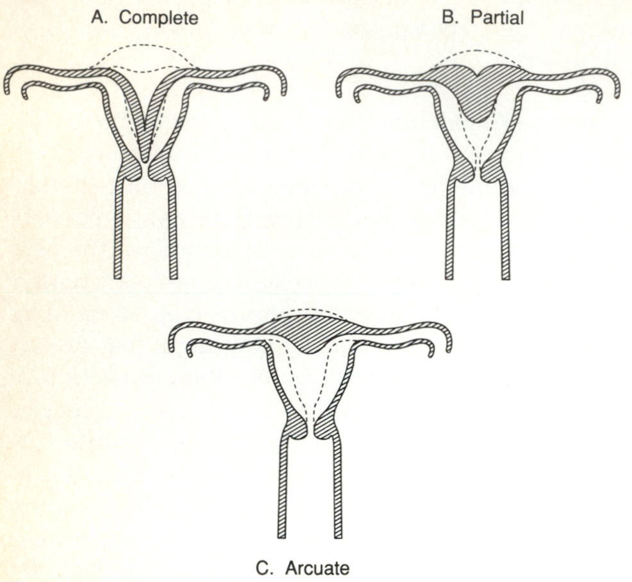

Figure 7–8. Septate uteri. (*Reproduced, with permission, from Cunningham FG, et al.* Williams Obstetrics. *18th ed. Norwalk, Conn: Appleton & Lange, 1989, p 733.*)

Problems Related to the Male Partner

It is assumed that the prerequisites for fertility in the male include production of sufficient numbers of mature sperm that are motile and are able to be transported through the male reproductive tract. Problems related to fertility in the male may thus be grouped into problems in sperm production, motility, and transport.

Problems in Sperm Production. The average number of sperm deposited in the vagina is 70 million/mL of semen, with a semen volume of 2 to 6 mL. A sperm count of 20 million or below in 2 to 6 mL of semen is suggestive of inadequate sperm production. Factors that may influence adequate sperm production may be grouped into infections, mechanical problems, and environmental influences.

Infections. Infections of the reproductive organs that affect sperm production include gonorrhea and chlamydia. Testicular inflammation (orchitis) caused by mumps in adulthood may also be associated with low sperm production. A high fever in the male, causing prolonged elevation of temperature in the scrotum, will also affect the quantity and quality of sperm ejaculated.

Mechanical Factors. Mechanical factors related to low sperm production include varicocele, a varicose vein in a spermatic cord. It is usually found in the left spermatic cord because the left spermatic cord is longer than the right spermatic cord. A varicocele causes an increase in spermatic cord temperature and poor spermatogenesis.[19] Undescended testicles (cryptorchism) in the reproductive male leads to irreversible inability to produce sperm. Failure to correct cryptorchism in the young child will cause the testicles to remain in the abdominal cavity. During puberty and thereafter, the increased temperature of the abdominal cavity as compared to the cooler environment of the scrotum will impede spermatogenesis.

Environmental Influences. Environmental influences on sperm production include exposure to radiation and industrial chemicals, which may injure the testicles. Excessive smoking and alcohol intake may also lower sperm production by decreasing testosterone levels. Intake of certain drugs such as antihypertensives and marijuana may also cause hypospermatogenesis. Moreover, in utero exposure to diethylstilbestrol (DES) has been linked to inadequate sperm production.[20] Finally, malnutrition, stress, and the use of hot tubs may also be related to the inadequate production of sperm.

Problems in Sperm Motility. Problems in sperm production are interrelated with problems in sperm motility. Motility of the sperm is caused by flagellar action and is necessary for the maintenance and transport of sperm. Greater than 60 percent of the sperm per ejaculate should be motile for effective fertility in the male. Factors that may affect the motility of the sperm include decreased levels of testosterone, which may lower the level of seminal plasma needed for motility and transport of sperm. Infection and prostate disease may also contribute to decreased sperm motility.

Problems in Sperm Transport. Problems that affect the ability of the male to transport the sperm through his reproductive tract and deposit the sperm in the female may also occur. The male reproductive tract may be obstructed by scar tissue formation as a result of infections. An injury to the vas deferens or a vasectomy will also impede the transport of the sperm.

The adequacy of deposition of sperm in the female is dependent on the ability of the male to ejaculate. Problems with ejaculation may be the result of impotence (the inability of the male to achieve or maintain erection), premature ejaculation, or **retrograde ejaculation,** a condition in which the sperm flows backward into the bladder instead of out of the penis. The latter problem may be caused by diabetes mellitus, surgical trauma, or neurologic damage.[8] Hypospadias, a congenital abnormality in which the male urethra opens on the shaft of the penis instead of the glans, may also cause problems in ejaculating sperm high in the vagina.

Combined Problems

Combined problems, those that are attributed to both partners, include problems with sexual technique and sexual timing, as well as with immunologic responses to sperm.

Sexual Technique and Timing. Certain positions during sexual intercourse favor transport of the sperm to the cervical opening (eg, woman on her back with knees flexed). Another technique that enhances the delivery of sperm to the cervical opening is the woman remaining on her back with her knees flexed for 10 to 15 minutes after intercourse.

Another problem that can be categorized as a combined problem is the couple's lack of knowledge regarding the timing of intercourse during the fertile period and the life span of the sperm and ovum. Fertility is favored when intercourse is timed around ovulation, which occurs approximately 14 days prior to the onset of menses. The life span of the sperm is approximately 48 to 72 hours, while the life span of the ovum is about 12 to 24 hours. Infrequent intercourse also may affect fertility by diminishing the motility of the sperm, while too frequent intercourse may lower the number of sperm, especially mature sperm.

Immunologic Factors. A relatively new theory of the etiology of infertility focuses on immunologic factors involving the female or male partner. For example, some women develop antibodies against their partners' sperm, with the result that healthy sperm do not survive the hostile cervical environment. The male partner also may have an autoimmune response to his own sperm. In this condition, the male makes antibodies against and destroys his otherwise healthy sperm.[21] Antibodies to sperm may be found in the blood as well as in the genital secretions.

Unexplained Infertility

Although the etiology of infertility can be explained in 80 to 90 percent of infertile couples, at times, even after careful investigation, the cause of infertility remains unexplained. Factors that have been implicated in unexplained infertility include ovum entrapment, occult spontaneous abortion, and defects in the ability of the sperm to penetrate and fertilize the ovum. There is a high spontaneous pregnancy rate among couples with unexplained infertility. Because many of these couples will achieve a pregnancy without treatment, causation and treatment methods for unexplained infertility remain unproven.[22]

INFERTILITY STUDY OF THE COUPLE

Infertility represents a life crisis to couples. Olshansky suggests that people who are distressed by their infertility "take on" a central identity of self as infertile.[23] For these couples, infertility becomes the central focus of their lives as they actively attempt to intervene in the problem. Identities such as "career person," "spouse," and "friend" become less important than the identity as an infertile couple. Infertility investigation and treatment may be threatening and uncomfortable for the couple, but because infertility is central to their lives, they will actively seek such investigations and treatment in an effort to solve the problem.

The focus of the infertility investigation should be on the couple because, too often, the woman is made to feel that she is the sole cause of the problem.[13] Nurses and other members of the health team should begin the infertility investigation in a supportive atmosphere for the couple. The goals of the initial steps of the work-up include performing a health assessment of the couple, determining possible etiologies, providing correct advice and support, and facilitating referrals.[9]

Nursing and Collaborative Assessment

Health History. Both partners should be seen early in the investigation so that a complete history of each partner can be obtained and assistance can be provided in creating an atmosphere in which the partners can support each other. A detailed history includes present and past health status, family, social, sexual, and reproductive data. At the outset, the couple should be asked if the infertility is primary or secondary in nature and the length of time they have been attempting a pregnancy. The health history includes data regarding childhood illnesses, immunizations, allergies, hospitalizations and serious illnesses, accidents and injuries, medications, and habits. Social data includes information related to family relationships and support systems, as well as ethnic and religious affiliations. Occupational, educational, and financial status are important parts of the social data base. The couple's patterns of health care and of daily living are also considered in this portion of the history.[24] A review of systems will provide the nurse with significant data regarding the health of the partners in general and the problem of infertility specifically.

The sexual history includes pertinent data related to the couple's sexual practices and perceptions of their sexuality. This part of the history can be threatening to an infertile couple, who may view having children as an important aspect of their sexuality. The history should be approached in a supportive and nonthreatening manner so that the couple feel comfortable in discussing such sexual functions as frequency of intercourse and techniques used during intercourse.

The reproductive history also may be anxiety-provoking to the couple because it focuses attention on possible perceived inadequacies. A history of pregnancies, abortions, live births and stillbirths is elicited, as well as any surgical interventions, such as tubal ligation or vasectomy.

For the woman, a detailed menstrual history is obtained, including onset, duration, frequency, regularity, and problems of menstruation, as well as a history of premenstrual symptoms and dysmenorrhea. A history of infections of the pelvic organs, including pelvic inflammatory disease, vaginitis, and cervicitis, may be significant to the problem of infertility. Additional important problems include a history of endometriosis, and disorders of the pituitary, thyroid, or adrenals, which may indicate problems in hormonal activity. Any history of structural disorders such as congenital malformation of the uterus and fibroid tumors also is significant. A contraceptive history also is taken and any information regarding systemic or chronic illness or past surgeries is recorded.

For the man, significant factors in the health history include infections of the reproductive organs, orchitis (inflammation of the testes), mumps in adulthood, and prostatitis (inflammation of the prostate). Any history of factors that may cause prolonged elevation of temperature in the scrotum should also be assessed. These factors may include high fevers, exposure to heat from the environment, the wearing of tight underclothes, excessive exercise, and the use of hot tubs. A history of surgery, such as herniorrhaphy or vasectomy reversal surgery, may also be significant. The male may also have had a problem with varicocele or hydrocele (fluid in the scrotum) in the past, as well as endocrine disorders involving the pituitary and thyroid glands.

There are certain factors that are found in the history that may be significant for both the male and female partner. These include such environmental factors as exposure to radiation or toxic substances such as lead. The use of drugs such as alcohol or marijuana should also be assessed as well as medications that may affect sexual functioning (eg, some antihypertensive drugs).

Both partners are also asked about a history of venereal disease and their mothers' use of DES. Occupational data that may provide information regarding work-related stress, as well as occupational hazards, is also obtained. The couple are asked questions pertaining to the frequency of coitus, premature ejaculation, and the use of lubricants that may be spermicidal.

The complete health history is an important assessment tool for the nurse and other members of the health team. It provides information regarding general health, as well as relevant data specific to the problem of infertility. It also enables the nurse to determine the way the couple defines the problem, how they have coped with problems in the past, and who is identified as their support network. The infertility study is tedious and sometimes fraught with disappointment. It also assumes that the couple will take part in the testing and intervention procedures. It is during the initial health history that the nurse can provide a supportive atmosphere for the couple and information to the couple regarding the work-up.

Physical Examination. The next step in the infertility investigation is a complete physical examination. Included in the examination is a pelvic examination for the female. The structure of the vagina is carefully assessed, as well as the shape and size of the cervix, uterus, and ovaries. Any signs of pelvic inflammatory disease or palpable tubal or ovarian masses should be noted. An enlarged uterus may indicate the presence of fibroid tumors, which may impede the implantation of the fertilized ovum. The cervix is also assessed to determine if production of clear, copious, acellular mucus is evident. Cervical and vaginal specimens are taken to determine the possibility of infection.[9,19]

As part of the complete assessment of the male, an examination of the male genitalia is performed. The structure, size, and shape of the penis, scrotum, testes, and prostate are assessed, and the scrotum is palpated for varicocele. Any abnormal discharge from the penis also is assessed.

The physical examination also affords the nurse or other health care practitioner an opportunity to assess secondary sex characteristics of the partners. Absent or minimal secondary sex characteristics may indicate reproductive immaturity and endocrine problems. During the physical examination, the nurse has an opportunity to educate the partners regarding anatomy and physiology and reproductive function. An assessment of each partner's feelings also may be made at this time.[9]

Diagnostic Tests. Diagnostic testing during the infertility assessment focuses on adequacy of ova and sperm production and possible impediments to fertilization. The most frequently conducted tests are: semen analysis, basal body temperature analysis, postcoital test, sperm penetration assay, endometrial biopsy, hysterosalpingogram, and laparoscopy. Culdoscopy occasionally is performed. Other tests that may be performed include thyroid function tests, complete blood count, and urinalysis.

Semen Analysis. The semen analysis provides information regarding the number, structure, and motility of the sperm. It also determines the volume and viscosity of the semen, as well as the presence of infection or agglutination of the sperm. The male partner is instructed to abstain from ejaculation for 48 to 72 hours prior to the collection of the specimen. The specimen may be obtained through masturbation, coitus interruptus, or by use of a special condom called a seminal pouch. Regular condoms should be avoided as they contain spermicides. The semen analysis is repeated several times at greater than 70-day intervals to allow further spermatogenesis to occur.[9] A sperm count below 20 million in 2 mL of semen with less than 60 percent motility two hours after ejaculation is suggestive of an infertility problem.

The semen analysis should be done early in the infertility investigation. It provides needed information and is noninvasive in nature.

Basal Body Temperature Chart. The purpose of the basal body temperature (BBT) chart is to determine if ovulation has occurred. The woman is instructed to take her temperature on awakening each morning. In the first half of the menstrual cycle, prior to ovulation, the BBT is usually below 98°F (36.7°C). Just prior to ovulation, when estrogen level has reached a peak, a drop in the BBT occurs. Following ovulation, there is a rise in BBT of 0.5° to 1°F (0.3° to 0.6°C). This rise in temperature is due to the surge of LH and the secretion of progesterone. The temperature continues to remain higher until the premenstrual phase of the cycle, with a decline in progesterone. The woman should chart the BBT on a graph for three consecutive cycles, noting the onset of menses, illness, or other factors that may interfere with the readings. She should also indicate times when intercourse has occurred. Figure 7–9A is a graph of an anovulatory cycle; Figure 7–9B demonstrates an ovulatory chart.

Basal body temperature charting is a relatively simple procedure. Like the semen analysis, however, it can be anxiety-laden, reminding the partners that a problem exists and placing a burden on the couple to have scheduled sexual relations.

Postcoital Test. The postcoital (or Sims-Huhner) test is performed late in the follicular phase of the menstrual cycle. The purpose of this test is to determine

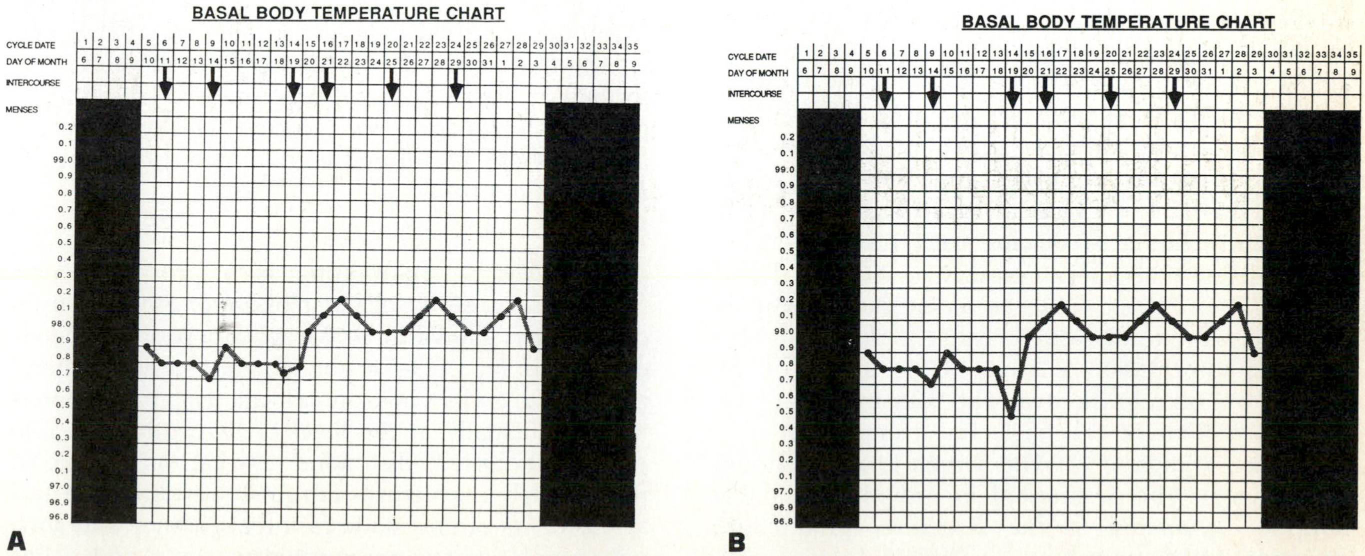

Figure 7–9. Basal body temperature chart. **A.** Anovulatory cycle. **B.** Ovulatory cycle.

the clarity and consistency of the cervical mucus and the viability and motility of the sperm in the cervical environment. The couple is instructed to have intercourse within 8 hours of the examination, after abstaining from intercourse for 48 hours.

The optimal time for performing the test is one to two days prior to expected ovulation, when the cervical mucus normally undergoes characteristic changes consistent with peak estrogen secretion by the ovary. At this time, the cervical mucus is at its most elastic, demonstrating spinnbarkeit (the ability to stretch to 10 to 20 cm). (For further discussion of cervical mucus changes, *see* Chapter 6.) The presence of sodium chloride precipitation in the cervical mucus at this time results in a ferning pattern when the mucus is viewed under a microscope. The presence of sperm also is assessed, as well as sperm motility. There is evidence that postcoital sperm motility in cervical mucus is strongly associated with total sperm count per ejaculate.[25]

If the results of the postcoital test reveal cervical mucus that is cloudy and cellular, a less than optimum environment for sperm survival, or few viable and motile sperm, the test should be repeated. The test is usually repeated within the same menstrual cycle or during the next menstrual cycle. In some settings, the postcoital examination is done prior to the semen analysis, but usually before any further rigorous or invasive infertility testing is done.[19]

Sperm Penetration Assay. The sperm penetration assay (SPA) is a relatively new procedure that tests the functional capacity of sperm to penetrate and fertilize the ovum. It is based on the ability of human sperm to penetrate zona-free hamster eggs in the laboratory. There is a good correlation between the ability of ejaculated sperm to penetrate zona-free hamster eggs and to fertilize human ova. There is also a significant relationship between the ability of the sperm to penetrate the zona-free hamster eggs and sperm count, motility, and structure. Mean penetration rates for hamster ova are shown to be significantly higher in males with proven fertility than in those who are categorized as infertile. These infertile men may not be identified routinely through semen analysis because semen analysis gives no information relative to the ability of the sperm to penetrate the ova. The SPA may therefore better complement the postcoital examination than the semen analysis.[26–30] The semen analysis should not, however, be discounted in providing valuable information related to the structure, production, and motility of sperm.

Endometrial Biopsy. The endometrial biopsy is performed during the luteal phase of the menstrual cycle to determine if ovulation has occurred and to provide information related to the condition of the endometrium. It is generally agreed that although plasma progesterone levels and BBT charts are useful in the detection of ovulation, a properly obtained endometrial biopsy is necessary to diagnose a luteal phase defect.[18] The test is done 5 to 7 days prior to the onset of menses. A sample of endometrial tissue is taken with a currette after the cervix is gently dilated. The endometrium at this time should be secretory in nature because of the influence of progesterone after ovulation. A proliferative endometrium indicates that ovulation has not taken place or that a luteal phase deficiency may be present. Progesterone assays may be done to complement the endometrial biopsy. A plasma progesterone level of greater than 4 ng per mL and a urinary pregnandiol level of at least 2 mg per 24 hours are indicative of ovulation.

Hysterosalpingogram. The **hysterosalpingogram** usually follows the previously mentioned tests. This test is done in the early proliferative phase of the cycle to avoid interfering with ovulation or an early pregnancy. A radiopaque dye is instilled in the uterine cavity via the cervix. Through fluoroscopy and x-ray techinques the tubes are visualized for patency. When the tubes are patent, the radiopaque substance will enter the peritoneal cavity. If the tubes are not patent, the substance will not enter the cavity and a diagnosis of tubal occlusion is made.

The hysterosalpingogram may be therapeutic as well as diagnostic in that previously occluded tubes may be opened through the insertion of the dye. Other tests for tubal patency, such as the laparoscopy or, less frequently, the culdoscopy, are therefore performed at least 6 months after the hysterosalpingogram to allow conception to occur. Hysterosalpingograms may be performed without anesthesia and on an outpatient basis.[6]

Laparoscopy. A **laparoscopy** is a procedure performed in the early follicular phase of the menstrual cycle which allows direct visualization of the pelvic organs (*see* Figure 9–5). The woman is given general anesthesia, and an instrument called a laparoscope is inserted, usually at the level of the umbilicus. The peritoneal cavity is distended with carbon dioxide so that the pelvic structures can easily be visualized and assessments can be made for tubal patency and such pelvic pathology as endometriosis, cysts, and pelvic inflammatory disease. There are some minor postoperative discomforts associated with insertion of the laparoscope and the distension of the peritoneal cavity with carbon dioxide. The woman can, however, be assured that normal activity can be resumed in 1 to 2 days after the procedure.

Culdoscopy. The culdoscopy procedure is used less frequently today because of the advent of laparoscopy. It is also performed early in the follicular phase of the cycle and its purpose is consistent with that of laparoscopy. The woman is placed in a knee-chest position and the posterior cul-de-sac is entered with an instrument called a trocar. Tubal patency is assessed and the pelvic structures are visualized for pathology.

Other Tests. Other tests may be ordered when specific problems are suspected. These include hormonal assays, hysteroscopy, and immunologic tests. Hormonal studies such as LH, estrogen, and progesterone assays are sometimes performed.

Hysteroscopy is also sometimes used as an adjunct to the endometrial biopsy, hysterosalpingography, and laparoscopy. This procedure is performed concurrently with laparoscopy. A hysteroscope is placed into the uterine cavity for direct visualization of the uterus for such uterine pathology as intrauterine adhesions and fibroid tumors.[31]

An additional test, the echohysteroscopy, combines ultrasonography with hysteroscopy. It also provides information about the structure of the internal genitals and abnormalities that might be present. The echohysteroscopy is a relatively new procedure that, with time and experience, will provide still another useful diagnostic tool.[32]

The detection of sperm antibodies is the basis for immunologic testing in the infertility workup. Screening tests for antisperm antibodies in either partner can be done.

Immunologic tests that can be applied to the cervical mucus of females include the sperm toxicity test (STT) and the sperm immobilization test (SIT).[33] Another test that may be performed is the leukocyte migration inhibition test (LMIT), which detects female cell-mediated immunity against sperm.

In males, a blood test may reveal the presence of antisperm antibodies in the blood; this indicates that antibodies also exist in the seminal fluid.[34] Another test for antisperm antibodies is the mixed erythrocyte-spermatozoa antiglobulin reactions (MAR test), which can be done as part of the semen analysis to detect antibodies on spermatozoa.[35,36]

Immunologic testing is often done when the infertility is unexplained. Its role has become more useful as the impact of immunologic reactions on infertility has become more apparent.

Nursing Role in Care of the Infertile Couple

The nursing role in care of the infertile couple is varied. In collaboration with other health team members, nurses act as counselors and advocates for the infertile couple. Nurses often begin the infertility investigation through history and physical examination of both partners. Through this initial assessment, problems and strengths can be identified, nursing diagnoses formulated (*see* box), and interventions, based on scientific rationale, planned.

The nursing role includes providing the couple with anticipatory guidance about testing and possible treatments. As an advocate, the nurse ensures that both partners understand the risks, as well as benefits, of the various treatment modalities. Success rates should always be given to the couple so that they have a clear understanding of the possibility of pregnancy with various treatments. The nurse also provides unbiased support to the couple throughout the decision-making process.

Nursing and Collaborative Management

Management of the Female Partner. Management of female infertility is based on the diagnosis of the

NURSING DIAGNOSES FOR THE INFERTILE COUPLE

Problem-Oriented

Self-esteem disturbance, related to diagnosis of infertility

Personal identity disturbance, related to unsuccessful infertility treatment

Ineffective family coping: compromised, related to infertility study of the couple

Strength-Oriented

Positive self-concept, related to positive coping behaviors during infertility study

Positive individual coping, related to social support of the infertile couple

Effective family coping, related to positive family adaptation throughout infertility study of the couple problem(s). For example, infections of the reproductive tract are treated with antibiotics.

Management of infertility caused by endometriosis may be medical, surgical, or a combination of treatments, reflecting the needs of the woman and the extent of the problem. Medical treatment most often involves danazol (Danocrine) therapy, in an attempt to inactivate the ectopic endometrial tissue. Danazol, a synthetic androgen, suppresses ovulation and FSH and LH secretion, as well as menstruation. It is given orally, 200 mg four times daily for 6 to 12 months, depending on the severity of the problem (refer to the case study/care plan for the infertile couple later in the chapter). Side effects of danazol therapy include weight gain, hot flashes, decreased breast size, and vaginitis.[17] After the drug is discontinued, menstruation usually recurs in 1 to 6 weeks. Continuous oral contraceptives have also been used to decrease FSH and LH activity and suppress ovulation and menstruation in an effort to heal endometriosis. In women with moderate to severe disease, surgical resection of the endometriosis implants is accomplished during laparoscopy. During surgery it is important to preserve fertility by avoiding any risk to vital reproductive organs.[17]

If the cause of infertility is determined to be cervical, estrogen therapy may be used prior to anticipated ovulation for several months. Estrogen is thought to enhance the quantity and quality of the cervical mucus and make it more receptive to the sperm. Cryosurgery, a simple procedure to freeze the surface of the cervix, may also be used in the treatment of cervicitis or problems with cervical mucus.

Treatment of endocrine disorders is based on their etiologies. For example, treatment for thyroid disease may include replacement therapy for hypothyroidism, and medications, radioiodine, or surgery for the treatment of hyperthyroidism.

Problems related to ovulation or the follicular and luteal phases of the menstrual cycle also may be managed pharmacologically. In anovulatory women, clomiphene citrate (Clomid) may be given to induce ovulation (*see* Box 7–1). This compound promotes the secretion of the gonadotropins FSH and LH by the anterior pituitary gland, which, in turn, stimulates the development of the follicle and induces ovulation. The drug is given in the absence of pathologic conditions of the ovary and pituitary, and the woman is carefully monitored for ovulation and side effects. The woman is instructed on when to take the medication in relation to the menstrual cycle. She is also instructed to chart her BBT to determine if ovulation has occurred. Plasma progesterone levels may also be assessed as an indication of ovulation. Clomiphene citrate gives some evidence of being antiestrogenic, which may affect the cervical mucus. For this reason, small doses of estrogen may be administered concurrently with clomiphene. Ovulation usually occurs on the 14th to 20th day of the menstrual cycle. Clomiphene therapy is usually discontinued if there are enlargement of the ovary or any visual symptoms, or if after three ovulatory cycles the woman does not become pregnant.[37]

Another agent that is used to stimulate follicular growth is human menopausal gonadotropin (hMG). This drug is a purified preparation of FSH and LH, extracted from the urine of postmenopausal women. The drug stimulates ovarian follicular growth and maturation. To induce ovulation, human chorionic gonadotropin (hCG) must be given after the administration of hMG and when assessment of the woman indicates that sufficient follicular maturation has occurred, coinciding with the LH surge. Follicular maturity is measured by estrogen levels and the quality and quantity of cervical mucus. Estrogen levels may be obtained by determining plasma estradiol levels and obtaining a 24-hour urine sample for urinary excretion of estrogen. The appearance and volume of the cervical mucus, spinnbarkeit, and ferning patterns also will help to identify the LH surge. Side effects of hCG therapy include ovarian enlargement and ovarian hyperstimulation syndrome. The incidence of multiple fetuses following this type of therapy is 20 to 40 percent.[38] Like other forms of treatment for infertility, therapy is expensive and requires commitment on the part of the couple and health care provider so that timing of needed tests for LH surge and intercourse can be optimal. It is imperative, as with any type of therapy, that the couple make an educated choice as to the acceptance or rejection of treatment.

Infertility associated with luteal phase inadequacy may be caused by increased prolactin secretion by the anterior pituitary gland (hyperprolactinemia). Elevated prolactin levels inhibit FSH and LH secretion and their actions on the ovary so that ovulation does not occur. Bromocriptine mesylate may be prescribed to inhibit prolactin secretion by the anterior pituitary gland. It is a nonhormonal, nonestrogenic agent, which modulates the secretion of a prolactin inhibitory factor, with little or no effect on other pituitary hormones. If production of prolactin is decreased, secretion of FSH and LH will be enhanced and ovulation will occur. The basal metabolic temperature demonstrates a biphasic pattern, indicating ovulation, when the drug is therapeutic. The woman

BOX 7–1 CLOMIPHENE CITRATE

Proprietary Names
Clomid (Merrell Dow); Serophene (Serono)

Classification
Nonhormonal fertility agent

Action
Precise mechanism not determined. Appears to stimulate release of FSH and LH from pituitary, resulting in development of ovarian follicle, with subsequent development of corpus luteum in anovulatory females.

Indications
Induces ovulation in anovulatory women desiring pregnancy. Ineffective in women with primary pituitary or ovarian failure.

Dosing
Administered orally only. If induced or spontaneous uterine bleeding occurs prior to therapy, the regimen should start on the fifth day of the cycle. Starting dose: 50 mg once daily for five days. If ovulation does not occur, 100 mg once daily for five days can be tried during the next cycle. Higher doses may be needed but are associated with more side effects. Therapy should not generally extend beyond three to four cycles.

Pharmacokinetics
(Data are limited). *Absorption:* Readily absorbed from GI tract. *Elimination:* Metabolized in liver and excreted in feces via biliary elmination, with half-life of about five days.

Contraindications and Precautions
Contraindicated in women with ovarian cysts, uterine bleeding of undetermined origin, liver disease, and in pregnancy. Use with caution in clients with polycystic ovary syndrome.

Adverse Reactions
Most common: ovarian hyperstimulation resulting in ovarian enlargement and midcycle ovarian pain, ovarian cysts, vasomotor symptoms (ie, hot flashes), bloating.
Less common:
CNS: fatigue, dizziness, depression.
GI: nausea, vomiting, increased appetite, weight gain.
Dermatologic: urticaria, rash, allergic dermatitis.
Ophthalmic: transient blurred vision, diplopia, photophobia, decreased visual acuity.
Reproductive: heavier menses, multiple gestations (twins most common), spontaneous abortion. Decrease in production of cervical mucous.
Other: breast discomfort, reversible hair loss.
Fetal: incidence of major congenital anomalies; however no specific malformations have been related to clomiphene.

Drug Interactions

- Danazol: may inhibit response to clomiphene
- Ethinyl estradiol: may suppress response to ethinyl estradiol

Nursing Implications

1. Teach client to begin taking medication on fifth day of cycle and take drug at the same time each day.
2. Reinforce teaching about drug and potential risks and benefits.
3. Teach client to report symptoms of hot flashes, nausea, vomiting, headache, visual symptoms.
4. Instruct woman to stop taking drug if pregnancy is suspected.

is given 2.5 mg of bromocriptine mesylate per day for several months or until pregnancy occurs. The drug should be discontinued when ovulation is suspected and during the luteal phase to prevent complications to the fetus. Prolactin levels are assessed periodically to determine the effectiveness of the drug, and the cervical mucus is assessed to determine if ovulation has occurred. Side effects of this therapy include dizziness, fainting, nausea, vomiting, insomnia, and headache.

Luteal phase inadequacy also may be managed with progesterone therapy. While some authorities recommend the use of other therapies, such as clomiphene citrate, most agree that to improve pregnancy outcome in women with a luteal phase defect, supplementation with natural progesterone is needed. Therapy consists of progesterone suppositories, administered either vaginally or rectally twice daily from the time of ovulation until the next menses. If menses do not occur on the 16th or 17th day after ovulation, a pregnancy test is performed. If pregnancy occurs, progesterone therapy is continued for 8 to 12 weeks, at which time the placenta begins to secrete progesterone in quantities capable of retaining the pregnancy. Progesterone therapy is thus used to increase the luteal phase so that a pregnancy can be maintained.[18] Again, it is important that assessment of ovulation be made by the woman as well as by the health care practitioner. Observation of the pattern of the BBT and the quality and consistency of the cervical mucus can provide evidence of ovulation.

Progesterone therapy, as well as other pharmacologic therapies for infertility, may extend the menstrual cycle, thus delaying the onset of menses. The nurse should prepare the couple for this prospect so that they do not experience false hope that a pregnancy has occurred, compounding their disappointment if it has not.

Infertility associated with the fallopian tubes may be caused by infections, adhesions, or endometriosis. As stated previously, tubal blockage is sometimes resolved by a hysterosalpingogram which may clear the tubes of remnants of mucus. This occurs in about 3 percent of the women undergoing the procedure.[6] Lysis and excision of adhesions are sometimes accomplished through microsurgery. A carbon dioxide laser method for reconstructive pelvic surgery has also been attempted in women with tubal occlusion.[39]

Structural defects related to the uterus may also be treated with surgical intervention. Myomectomies, removal of uterine fibroids, and reconstructive surgery for congenital malformation of the uterus have been performed in an attempt to enhance fertility. In an effort to divide the intrauterine adhesions of Asherman's syndrome, concurrent hysteroscopy and hysterography may be performed. This can be done through a one-stage method, in which lysis of adhesions is accomplished by hysteroscopy and is followed by immediate hysterography. If adhesions are still present, a second hysteroscopic division of adhesions is done. This is followed by cyclic hormonal treatment in an effort to maintain a normal uterine lining.[40]

Management of the female partner is dependent on the etiology(ies) of the problem(s) and the commitment of the couple. The treatments for mechanical, endocrine, and structural factors can be tedious, time-consuming, and costly. They may also be physically and emotionally taxing for the individual and the couple. It is thus important that the couple make an informed decision regarding testing and therapies.

Management of the Male Partner Management of male infertility focuses on the adequacy of production, number, motility, and structure of sperm. Treatment is based on the ability of the sperm to survive the cervical environment and penetrate the ovum.

If the cause of infertility is oligospermia (few sperm), changes in lifestyle may help to correct it. The man should be advised to avoid prolonged exposure to heat sources, such as hot tubs, and restrictive clothing, which may interfere with sperm production and viability. Sources of radiation and chemical hazards should be assessed, as well as the use of alcohol, drugs, and tobacco. Hormone therapy consisting of clomiphene or testosterone also may be used to increase sperm count. There is some evidence to suggest that poor ovulation is an added problem in infertile couples with oligospermia; thus simultaneous treatment of both partners is recommended.[41]

If after treatment the sperm count remains low, or if the volume of semen is low, artificial insemination of the woman with her partner's sperm may be considered. Because sperm occur in highest concentration and are most motile in the first few drops of semen, the ejaculate is split and the first fraction saved. This may be done several times, and the resulting first-fraction-split ejaculates combined and inseminated into the female partner. The use of split ejaculates enhances cervical mucus penetrability and sperm characteristics.[42]

Artificial insemination with the partner's sperm is also considered when the cervical environment is hostile to the sperm. In some couples, a combination of sperm washing and intrauterine insemination is used. The semen is washed with a medium to obtain a seminal plasma-free, highly concentrated sperm suspension for intrauterine insemination. This method appears to be most successful with couples who exhibit a poor postcoital test, especially if the male partner's fertilizing ability, as measured by the sperm penetration test, appears normal.[43]

If insemination using the male partner's sperm is ineffective, or azoospermia (no sperm) or severe oligospermia are present, donor insemination may be presented to the couple as an option.

If the cause of the male infertility is related to problems in ejaculation, several treatments may be pursued. Retrograde ejaculation, as previously described, is a relatively rare occurence, but it is the most common cause of absence of ejaculate at orgasm. Infertility caused by this condition is sometimes treated by retrieving semen from postcoital voiding specimens or from the bladder through catheterization. The specimen is then buffered and artificially inseminated into the uterus.[44] Problems related to ejaculation may also be caused by impotency, especially during the infertility study itself when the man feels the need to perform. A supportive, nonjudgmental atmosphere is needed for the couple, along with reassurance that this may be a transient problem.[19] Sexual counseling also may be needed.

If a varicocele is diagnosed, surgery to ligate the

spermatic vein is sometimes performed. Varicocele ligation has demonstrated improvement in sperm motility and morphology.[19] This procedure has, however, been of little benefit to men whose sperm count is below 10 million/mL.[45]

Management of male infertility is varied, and the benefits of therapies aimed at improving sperm production, motility, viability, and structure are inconclusive. Ideally, management is directed to specific causation, as nonspecific therapies have produced disappointing results.[46] *See* the case study/care plan detailing nursing care of an infertile couple for problems involving both female and male partners.

Management of Combined Problems. When the infertility results from a combined problem, such as faulty sexual technique or lack of knowledge related to timing of sexual relations, sexual counseling is warranted. The need for counseling also should be assessed throughout the infertility workup because the procedures and the perception of the couple of the need to perform may interfere with sexual functioning.

If the combined problem is immunologic, treatment aimed at reduction of sperm antibodies is sometimes implemented. Sperm autoimmunity in men may be treated by immunosuppression with glucocorticoid therapy. The man may be instructed to take prednisolone (0.5 to 0.75 mg/kg of body weight) for seven days each month for 4 to 7 months in an effort to increase sperm concentration, motility, and mucus penetration, and to decrease sperm immobilization titres. The man's semen and serum, as well as the woman's cervical mucus, are monitored for antibody titres to evaluate the effectiveness of the therapy. The side effects of prednisolone treatment include fluid and electrolyte disturbances, Cushing's syndrome, glycosuria, nervousness, insomnia, and changes in mood.

If it is found that the woman has antibodies to her partner's sperm, condom therapy is usually recommended. The couple is instructed to use condoms during intercourse for a period of 6 months; this reduces exposure to sperm and may decrease the female partner's sensitivity. Sperm antibody titres are retested after the therapy and the couple is encouraged to attempt conception.

Management of Unexplained Infertility When investigations fail to reveal a cause for infertility, management may then be based on possible causes. Because of the high spontaneous pregnancy rate in unexplained infertility, however, the effectiveness of the various treatments is difficult to assess. Treatments have included correction of anatomic problems and the use of hormonal manipulation during the follicular and luteal phases of the cycle. Treatment for immunologic factors also has been attempted to decrease sperm antibodies, with few conclusive results. It is difficult to assess whether treatments aimed at improving cervical mucus or the use of antibiotics for infections have more than a placebo effect.[22] The choice of no treatment and the hope for spontaneous pregnancy may be a better option than trials of treatment that have not been proven.

The management of infertility is most effective when a causative factor is identified. Diagnosis and management of ovulatory disorders have demonstrated relatively good results, and tubal infertility may be treated effectively with microsurgery. Treatment of male infertility is, however, often ineffective and largely empirical. Although new techniques have been developed in the treatment of infertility, any treatment should be based on the decision of the couple themselves after they have received a full and unbiased appraisal of their problem and the probability of successful managment.[47]

New Techniques in Management of Infertility. In vitro fertilization (IVF) is a newer technique used in the management of infertile couples. The procedure encompasses the fertilization of a mature ovum outside the mother in a laboratory setting. In vitro fertilization is often referred to as test-tube fertilization, and infants conceived through such a procedure have been termed "test-tube babies" in the popular press. The procedure for IVF involves the removal of a mature ovum from the ovary of a woman whose fallopian tubes are occluded, followed by fertilization with sperm in a petri dish, and reimplantation of the embryo into the uterine cavity.[48] Criteria for selection for IVF treatment include a normal semen sample and ovarian accessibility at laparoscopy.

In preparation for IVF, the female partner is treated with FSH to encourage the development of numerous ova. The drugs are taken on cycle days 3 through 7 to produce a number of ovarian follicles. The maturity of the follicles is usually monitored, using ultrasound and measuring serum estradiol levels, on a daily basis beginning on cycle days 8 through 10.[48] When the largest follicle reaches a diameter of approximately 20 mm, the mature ova are recovered through follicular aspiration during laparoscopy. The extracted ova are placed in a simple culture medium and sperm in a concentrated suspension are added (100,000 of the most active sperm per oocyte). Following fertilization, the zygote is allowed to develop to the 8- to 16-cell (blastocyst) stage (*see* Chapter 11), about 45 to 69 hours after insemination, when embryo transfer is made to the uterine cavity of the mother. Often several embryos are transferred in order to increase the chances of pregnancy. Some of the fertilized ova are sometimes frozen to be used in additional cycles if pregnancy is not sustained. The success rate of pregnancy and delivery of a healthy newborn by means of in vitro fertilization is reported to be approximately 20 percent.[48–52] The procedure is controversial and requires a substantial investment of personal and monetary resources with a low chance of success.[53]

The most recent procedure to be used in the treatment of infertility is the gamete intrafallopian transfer (GIFT) procedure. This approach, developed in 1984, involves the direct transfer of preovulatory oocytes and washed sperm into the fallopian tubes after aspiration of the ovarian follicles at laparoscopy. The technique attempts to mimic the early physiologic processes that lead to pregnancy in the human by placing both the male and female gametes at the normal site of fertilization.[54] Like in vitro fertilization, mature oocytes are aspirated from the female client after she has been treated with FSH. These oocytes are evaluated and then loaded into a catheter for transfer. The catheter is also loaded with a sperm preparation containing 100,000 sperm. The catheter tip is guided approximately 1.5 cm into the fimbriated end of the fallopian tube and the contents of the catheter are gently discharged.[55]

The GIFT procedure can only be used with women who have at least one intact, functional fallopian tube, because after fertilization occurs, the zygote must be able to travel through the tube to the uterus for implantation. The woman must also have one accessible ovary on which to perform the follicular aspiration.[56] The success rate for GIFT in these early reports is between 20 and 27 percent.[55]

An advantage of GIFT over IVF is that the entire procedure is performed during the laparoscopy procedure, thereby eliminating the two-day laboratory incubation period and subsequent introduction of the embryo into the uterine cavity required postlaparoscopy in IVF. The disadvantage of the GIFT procedure is the speed with which laboratory personnel must work while the client is under anesthesia.[54,55]

When male infertility is a problem, the couple may choose a combination IVF and GIFT procedure. The ova are fertilized in the laboratory during the IVF procedure and then transported to the fallopian tube for development and transport to the uterus. If fertilization does not occur in the laboratory and the woman does not achieve a pregnancy from the GIFT attempt, this combination is contraindicated for future attempts.[56]

Psychologic Aspects of Infertility

Infertility is a major life crisis for many couples. Menning describes a predictable sequence in the couple's response to infertility. This includes surprise, stemming from the couple's assumption that they are fertile and the fact that typically they have practiced birth control to await the right time to have children. Denial of the problem also is common and acts as a protective mechanism for the couple. It should, however, be short-term so that the couple may gain realistic awareness and acceptance of the problem.[8]

Grief is the most common response to infertility. Even when the diagnosis is tentative, the couple will experience a period of grief for the children they never had. In fact, the couple with an inconclusive diagnosis of infertility may have profound cyclic feelings of hope and despair and may have great difficulty in acknowledging the loss.[8]

Isolation is another common response, which may be a result of lack of social support. Well-meaning friends, who may suggest solutions to the problem such as "relax and you'll get pregnant," instead may cause the couple to further isolate themselves from support systems. This isolation delays the grief process and places strains on marital relationships and friendships.[8,57] It has been documented that infertile individuals feel greater dissatisfaction with themselves and their marriages than couples who are not infertile, and women experience greater discontent over time and have greater emotional investment than males.[57] Ambiguity, or uncertainty regarding infertility, was found to be the most prevalent emotional experience among infertile women.[58]

Physical inability to have a child may be perceived as personal inadequacy and social failure. The infertile couple often feel helpless. Having made the decision to have children, the couple may perceive that their options have been taken away. The couple may respond with anger toward family members or health care providers who delve into intimate details of their lives. The perception that testing and sexual relations must be programmed also may cause anger, directed at those who place them in uncomfortable situations. Old marital conflicts may be reawakened and the couple may feel that they are losing control of their life plans.

Guilt is also a common feeling among infertile

RESEARCH ABSTRACT

Olshansky EF. Identity of self as infertile: an example of theory-generating research. Adv Nurs Sci. *1987; 9:54–63.*

The purpose of this qualitative study was to gain an understanding of human responses to infertility. A grounded-theory methodology was used to explore the meaning of infertility to those persons experiencing it. Thirty-two individuals were interviewed, including 15 married couples and two married women. The sample was recruited from a university infertility clinic as well as from RESOLVE, an infertility support organization.

A series of interview questions were used in an attempt to generate a theory that explained human responses to infertility. The findings of this study suggest that infertile persons who are distressed by their infertility take on an identity of self as infertile. Other important identities such as career identity become less important than the identity of an infertile person. Once the person has taken on the formal identity of being infertile, he or she must manage the identity of infertility. The research suggests that some people overcome the identity by becoming pregnant. This may occur through medical intervention. Others manage infertility through technologic means such as in vitro fertilization; whereas still others choose alternative measures such as adoption. The investigator found that still another group remains "in limbo," as the individuals try unsuccessfully to conceive.

The investigator concludes that a theory about the work of taking on and managing a self-identity as infertile was generated from the data.

Comment:
This research is an important step in understanding the human response to infertility. It should be repeated using persons from various ethnic and socioeconomic groups. A testing of the theory is also needed with populations who do not conceive and who remain infertile.

couples and may stem from a prior history of premarital sex, use of birth control, extramarital sex, or abortion. The nurse may, therefore, wish to interview the partners alone, as well as together, in order to ensure privacy for discussion of details of their lives that each does not wish the other to know.[9]

The longer the couple remain infertile, the less likely they are to feel in control of their lives. In order to regain control, both partners must work through the grief process to reach a sense of resolution. Nurses and other health team members often can provide the support necessary for the couple to resolve the crisis of infertility in a positive manner. In addition, the couple may be referred to RESOLVE, the support organization founded in 1973 by a nurse, Barbara Eck Menning. This organization disseminates educational information and also provides needed referral services for infertile couples.

As various treatments for infertility are pursued and found unsuccessful, the couple are faced with several choices. They may discontinue further treatment, with the possibility of remaining childless. Adoption may be another option that the couple will pursue. It is, however, important that the couple resolve their loss of biologic parenting so that parenting of an adopted child can be a positive experience. The options of artificial insemination by the partner or a donor, IVF, and the GIFT procedure may also be suggested to the couple. It is imperative that the nurse understand the couple's feelings regarding these technologies. Sometimes the zeal of health professionals for new procedures leads them to ignore the couple's reasons for finding such procedures unacceptable. It is important that the couple be supported through their infertility investigation and treatment. Regardless of whether couples choose to continue or terminate the treatment, their wishes should be respected by the health care staff.

CASE STUDY/CARE PLAN: THE INFERTILE COUPLE

David and Susan Weiss, 31 and 30 years old respectively, have been married for 5 years. After 1 1/2 years of attempting to become pregnant, the couple has sought medical help from an infertility center for possible infertility.

The gynecologist suggests that David be tested first to determine sperm production. David is found to have a low sperm count with low motility (18 million/2 mL semen and 40 percent motility). David is treated with clomiphene and antibiotics, and after the initial therapy, his sperm count improves to 30 million/2 mL semen with 70 percent motility. After progressive infertility testing (eg, BMT to laparoscopy), Susan is found to have endometriosis with endometrial implants on the right ovary and along the right fallopian tube. Susan is placed on a regimen of danazol therapy for 6 months. After this time period, the couple again attempt to become pregnant.

After one additional year of unsuccessful attempts to become pregnant, the couple are again tested. David's sperm count is found to be 40 million/2 mL semen and 70 percent motility. Susan's BMT indicates an ovulatory pattern suggesting that the danazol therapy has helped; however, endometriosis can still be found on the right ovary and fallopian tube. Options are discussed with the couple: artificial insemination using the husband's sperm, IVF, and GIFT.

Supporting Assessment Data	Expected Client/Family Outcome	Nursing Action/ Intervention	Rationale	Criteria for Evaluation
Nursing Diagnosis: Knowledge deficit, related to treatments for infertility				
Clients state "we don't understand how treatments for infertility work" Couple wants to know success rates for each treatment	By the end of the visit, the couple will: Describe each of the potential treatment modalities Identify the risks and benefits of each treatment Discuss the success rate of each treatment By the next visit, couple will make an informed decision as to subsequent treatment	Teach clients procedure used for: *Insemination using man's sperm:* Sperm is washed Highly concentrated sperm suspension is used Inseminated at time of ovulation into cervix Success rate greater than 30% reported *In vitro fertilization:* Multiple mature ova recovered via laparoscopy after woman is treated with FSH Woman monitored for mature follicles by ultrasound and estrogen levels prior to procedure Extracted ova placed in a petri dish with man's concentrated sperm suspension Fertilization takes place 45–69 hours after placement in petri dish Embryo(s) transfer made into uterine cavity 20% reported success rate	Infertility treatment requires decision making on the part of the couple. Realistic decision making requires knowledge of alternatives, risks, and benefits.	When asked, clients: Discuss each of the treatment alternatives and procedures involved. List risks and benefits associated with each treatment. Discuss the chances of success or failure of each treatment. Clients make a knowledgeable decision about treatment or decision not to pursue treatment.

Supporting Assessment Data	Expected Client/Family Outcome	Nursing Action/ Intervention	Rationale	Criteria for Evaluation
		GIFT procedure: Direct transfer of ova and washed sperm into fallopian tubes A combination of GIFT and in vitro fertilization may be used 27% success rate reported		
Nursing Diagnosis: Self-esteem disturbance, related to guilt about possibly contributing to infertility				
Couple states "We shouldn't have used birth control for so long. Do you think we made ourselves infertile?"	By the end of the first visit, the couple will: Identify their feelings related to their infertility	Listen and offer support in a nonjudgmental manner Acknowledge the clients' feelings of hope and despair Answer questions concerning infertility and their feelings of causation	Guilt is a salient feature of infertility. Infertility represents the loss of the fantasized child.	Couple relate their feelings freely to nurse Couple will realistically relate their infertility problem. Couple will discuss their future plans concerning infertility.
	Focus on making decisions about treatment	Give unbiased support to couple through their decision-making processes Give couple realistic explanations about their condition	Support of the couple in a nonjudgmental manner will foster resolution of grief.	
		Refer to RESOLVE	Support organizations such as RESOLVE assist the couple to cope with the infertility and work through their grief.	

SUMMARY

Problems in human reproductive physiology include genetic disorders and infertility.

Genetic disorders represent the major causes of congenital malformations in children and include disorders of the autosomes (the first 22 pairs of chromosomes), and disorders of the pair of sex chromosomes. Chromosomal abnormalities also may be classified as numerical chromosomal abnormalities (too many or too few chromosomes), and structural abnormalities (a piece of a chromosome is transferred to another chromosome or missing).

Some individuals demonstrate mosaicism (cells with differing genetic constitutions). Most mosaic individuals have a mixture of normal cells with 46 chromosomes and trisomic cells with 47 chromosomes and usually have less severe handicaps than individuals with numerical chromosomal abnormalities. Structural abnormalities include translocations and deletions. Translocations occur when a piece of one chromosome transfers to a chromosome other than the one found in the pair. If two chromosomes break and exchange pieces, the individual is said to be a balanced translocation carrier. Deletions occur when a chromosome breaks and a portion of the chromosome is lost.

Patterns of inheritance are important in understanding genetic disorders and may be classified either as single-gene or multifactorial inheritance. In single-gene inheritance, the gene that expresses itself is referred to as dominant; the gene that is present but does not express itselfis called recessive. Thus, single-gene disorders are autosomal dominant, autosomal recessive, X-linked dominant, or X-linked recessive disorders. Multifactorial disorders occur as a result of the interaction of several genes and environmental influences.

Nursing care of families at risk for genetic disorders begins with a comprehensive data base, including history and physical examination. Management of these families includes risk determination and genetic counseling. If the child is born with a genetic disorder, the family will need support and guidance by the nurse and other members of the health team.

Other problems of human reproduction include infertility. Infertility may be a result of problems of the female partner, male partner, or a combination of both. Problems related to the female partner include mechanical barriers, endocrine problems, and structural disorders. Problems related to the male partner are those of sperm production, motility, and transport. Infertility associated with both partners may be caused by problems with sexual technique and timing, as well as immunologic responses to sperm. Occasionally the cause of infertility remains unexplained.

The infertility study begins with a comprehensive history and physical examination. Diagnostic tests are performed as indicated by the suspected problems, the most frequent being those that determine ovulation in the female and sperm quality and quantity in the male. Tests that assess ovulation include the basal body temperature chart (BBT) and the endometrial biopsy. A postcoital examination will also provide information regarding the quality of the cervical mucus immediately prior to ovulation and the ability of the sperm to survive the cervical mucus. To gain information about sperm production, structure, and motility, a semen analysis is performed.

If the tests for ovulation and sperm production and motility are normal, other tests are done to determine tubal patency (including the hysterosalpingogram), pelvic pathology, and the ability of the sperm to penetrate the ovum (assessed through the sperm penetration test). Depending on the nature of the problem, other tests may be ordered, including hormonal assays, hysteroscopy, and immunologic tests. Laparoscopy also may be performed to visualize the female pelvic organs directly.

Management of infertility is based on the etiology or etiologies of the problem and may be medical, surgical, or a combination of both. Newer techniques in the treatment of infertility are in vitro fertilization (IVF) and the gamete intrafallopian transfer (GIFT) procedures.

Infertility is a major life crisis for families. Couples respond to the loss of the children they will not have in ways that resemble the grieving process. In addition, the infertility study is taxing, expensive, and often uncomfortable emotionally for the couple. Nurses can provide needed support to the couple during the infertility study, as well as referral to support groups such as RESOLVE.

REVIEW QUESTIONS

1. Define the following terms: (a) autosomal chromosomal abnormalities; (b) sex chromosomal abnormalities; (c) genotype; (d) phenotype; (e) karyotype; (f) single-gene inheritance; and (g) multifactorial in heritance.
2. Identify the risk probabilities of autosomal dominant and autosomal recessive inheritance. Give two examples of disorders that are autosomal dominant and autosomal recessive.
3. Describe the Barr body. Briefly explain why sex chromosomal abnormalities cause less severe handicaps than autosomal abnormalities.
4. Identify at least two factors that can be attributed to infertility in the female and the male.
5. Briefly describe two tests that are specific to the female and the male in the study of infertility.

REFERENCES

1. Moore KL. *Before We Are Born: Basic Embryology and Birth Defects*. 3rd ed. Philadelphia: W.B. Saunders, 1989.
2. Moore KL. *The Developing Human: Clinically Oriented Embryology*. 4th ed. Philadelphia: W.B. Saunders, 1988.
3. Kempe CH, et al, eds. *Current Pediatric Diagnosis & Treatment*. 9th ed. Norwalk, Conn: Appleton & Lange, 1987.
4. Whaley LF, Wong DL. *Nursing Care of Infants and Children*. 3rd ed. St. Louis: CV Mosby, 1987.
5. Cunningham FG, et al. *Williams Obstetrics*. 18th ed. Norwalk, Conn, Appleton & Lange, 1989.
6. Pernoll ML, Benson RC, eds. *Current Obstetric & Gynecologic Diagnosis & Treatment*. Norwalk, Conn: Appleton & Lange, 1987.

7. March of Dimes. *Spina Bifida*, pamphlet. White Plains, NY: March of Dimes Birth Defects Foundation, 1985.
8. Menning BE. The psychosocial impact of infertility. *Nurs Clin North Am.* 1982;17:155–63.
9. Draye MA. An approach to infertility investigation. *Nurse Pract.* 1985;16:21–22.
10. Camillo P. Infertility: education for understanding well-being and alternatives. In Littlefield V (ed). *Health Education for Women.* Norwalk, Conn: Appleton-Century-Crofts, 1986.
11. Hatcher R, et al, eds. *Contraceptive Technology 1988-1989.* 14th ed. New York: Irvington Publishers, 1988.
12. Kraft A, et al. The psychosocial dimensions of infertility. *Am J Orthopsychiatry.* 1980;50:620–624.
13. Lindell S, Dineen K. The stress of infertility. In Kjervik DK, Martinson IM. *Women in Health and Illness: Life Experiences and Crises.* Philadelphia; W.B. Saunders, 1986.
14. Lanat M, Mass N. Concomitant hysteroscopy and hysterography in Asherman's syndrome. *Int J Fertil.* 1981;26: 267–272.
15. DeCecco L, et al. The cervical factor of sterility: clinical and diagnostic problems. *Eur Fertil.* 1983;14:163–171.
16. Shulman S. Cervical factors and immunological problems: diagnosis and treatment. *Eur Fertil.* 1983;14:101–105.
17. Wedell MA, et al. Endometriosis and the infertile client. *J Obstet Gynecol Neonatal Nurs.* 1985;14:280–283.
18. Darland NW. Infertility associated with luteal phase defect. *J Obstet Gynecol Neonatal Nurs.* 1985;14:212–21.
19. Friedman BM. Infertility workup. *Am J Nurs.* 1981;81: 2041–2046.
20. Stenchever MA, et al. Possible relationship between in utero diethystilbestrol exposure and male fertility. *Am J Obstet Gynecol.* 1981;140:186–193.
21. Jones WR. Immunologic infertility—fact or fiction? *Fertil Steril.* 1980;33:577.
22. Pepperell RJ, McBain JC. Unexplained infertility: a review. *Br J Obstet Gynecol.* 1985;92:569–580.
23. Olshansky EF. Identity of self as infertile: an example of theory-generating research. *Adv Nurs Sci.* 1987; 9:54–63.
24. Block G, Nolan JE. *Health Assessment for Professional Nursing: A Developmental Approach. 2nd ed.* Norwalk, Conn: Appleton-Century-Crofts, 1986; 4–57.
25. Collins JA, et al. The post-coital test as a predictor of pregnancy among 355 infertile couples. *Fertil Steril.* 1984; 41: 703–08.
26. Campana A, et al. Relationship between fertility, semen analysis, and human sperm penetration of zona-free hamster eggs. *Eur Fertil.* 1983;14:331–336.
27. Stenchever, MA, et al. Benefits of the sperm (hamster ova) penetration assay in the evaluation of the infertile couple. *Am J Obstet Gynecol.* 1982;143:91–96.
28. Martin RH, Taylor PJ. Reliability and accuracy of the zona-free hamster ova assay in assessment of male infertility. *Br J Obstet Gynecol* 1982;89:951–956.
29. Sutherland PD, et al. Clinical evaluation of the heterologous oocyte penetration test. *Br J Urol.* 1985;57:233–236.
30. Ausmanas M, et al. The zona-free hamster egg penetration assay as a prognositic indication in human in vitro fertilization program. *Fertil Steril.* 1985; 43:433–437.
31. Valle RF. Hysteroscopy in the evaluation of female infertility. *Am J Obstet Gynecol.* 1980;137:425–431.
32. Nannini R, et al. Dynamic echohysteroscopy: new perspectives for diagnostic sonography in female infertility. *Eur Fertil.* 1984;15:141–143.
33. Dor J, et al. Cell-mediated and local immunity to spermatozoa in infertility. *Int J Fertil* 1979;24:94–100.
34. Baker HW, et al. Treatment of sperm autoimmunity in men. *Clin Reprod Fertil.* 1983;2:55–71.
35. Scarselli G, et al. The MAR test as immunologic screening of male infertility. *Euro Fertil.* 1985;16:187–190.
36. Stedronska J, Hendry WF. The value of the mixed antiglobulin reaction (MAR test) as an addition to routine seminal analysis in the evaluation of the subfertile couple. *Am J Reprod Immunol.* 1983;3:89–90.
37. Cantor B. Induction of ovulation with clomiphene citrate. In Sciarra JJ, et al (eds). *Gynecology and Obstetrics.* Hagerstown, Md: Harper & Row, 1982, vol. 5.
38. Smith P. Ovulation induction. *J Obstet Gynecol Neonatal Nurs.* 1985;14:(suppl):37–39.
39. Bellina JH. Microsurgery of the fallopian tube with carbon dioxide laser. *Surg Med.* 1982;2:129–136.
40. Lancet M, Mass N. Concomitant hysteroscopy and hysterography in Asherman's syndrome. *Int J Fertil.* 1981;26: 267–272.
41. Silber SJ, Cohen R. Simultaneous treatment of the wife in infertile couples with oligospermia. *Fertil Steril.* 1983;40: 505–511.
42. Kotoulas IG, et al. Clinical studies II: Use of split-ejaculates. *Fertil Steril.* 1984;42:268–273.
43. Wiltbank MC, et al. Treatment of infertile patients by intrauterine insemination of washed spermatzoa. *Andrologia.* 1985;17:22–30.
44. Zavoa PM, Wilson EA. Retrograde ejaculation: etiology and treatment via the use of a noninvasive method. *Fertil Steril.* 1984;42:627–632.
45. Smith KD. Endocrine problems and treatment. *Clin Obstet Gynecol* 1982;25:483–493.
46. Swerdloff RS, et al. UCLA conference: infertility in the male. *Ann Intern Med.* 1985;103:906–919.
47. Leeton J. The management of infertility: where to stop. *Clin Reprod Fertil.* 1982;1:249–259.
48. Pace-Owens S. In vitro fertilization and embryo transfer. *J Obstet Gynecol Neonatal Nurs.* 1985;14:44–48.
49. Langman J. *Medical Embryology.* Baltimore; Williams & Wilkens, 1985.
50. Andrews LB. Legal and ethical aspects of new reproductive technologies. *Clin Obstet Gynecol.* 1986;68:190–204.
51. Asch RH, et al. Gamete intrafallopian transfer (GIFT): a new treatment for infertility. *Int J Fertil.* 1985;30:41–45.
52. Molloy D, et al. A laparoscopic approach to a program of gamete intrafallopian transfer. *Fertil Steril.* 1987;47:289–294.
53. Milne BJ. Couples' experiences with in vitro fertilization. *J Obstet Gynecol Neonatal Nurs.* 1988;17(5):347–352.
54. Asch RH, et al. Preliminary experiences with gamete intrafallopian transfer (GIFT). *Fertil Steril.* 1985;43:335–336.
55. Asch RH, et al. Pregnancy after translaparoscopic gamete intrafallopian transfer. *Lancet.* 1984;2:1034–1035.
56. Pace-Owens S. Gamete intrafallopian transfer (GIFT). *J Obstet Gynecol Neonatal Nurs.* 1989;18:93–97.
57. Hirsch AM, Hirsch SM. The effect of infertility on marriage and self-concept. *J Obstet Gynecol Neonatal Nurs.* 1989; 18:13–20.
58. Sandelowski M. The color gray: ambiguity and infertility. *Image.* 1987; 19(2)70–74.

Sexuality

Chapter 8

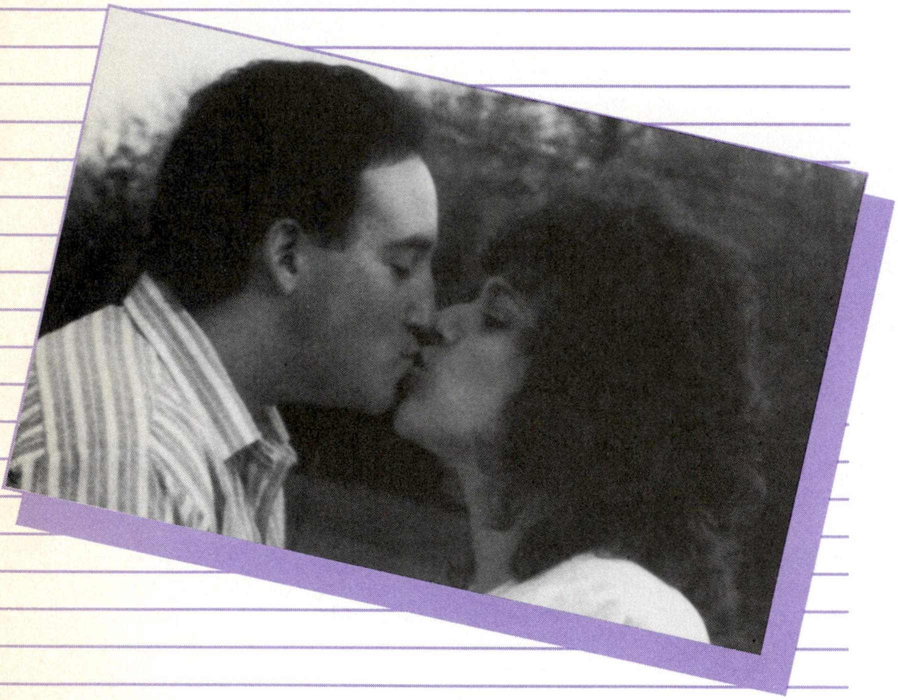

Key Terms

androgynous
coitus
femininity
foreplay
gender
masculinity
myotonia
sex role behaviors
sexuality
sexually transmitted disease
perinatal transmission
vasocongestion

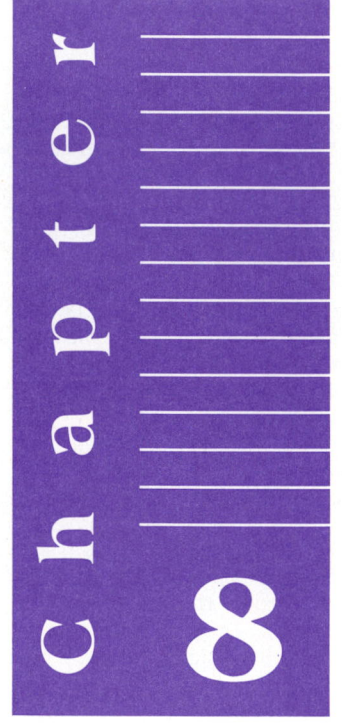

Sexuality has been defined as the part of life that has to do with being male or female. Sexuality in an individual evolves and matures as an interactional process in a biologic environment influenced by family members, friends, church, culture, social, and school factors.

The World Health Organization defines sexual health as "the positive integration of somatic, emotional, intellectual, and social aspects of sexual being in ways that are positively enriching and that enhance personality, communication, and love."[1] Woods suggests that sexual health consists of sexual function, sexual self-concept, and sexual relationship, which are interrelated over the life span.[2]

Issues related to sexuality are at the forefront of health concerns today. Unplanned pregnancy, particularly in adolescents, is an important and serious concern. Furthermore, sexually transmitted diseases, among them the life-threatening HIV infection, have stimulated parents, health professionals, and educators to support dissemination of information about protective behaviors related to sexuality. The increased awareness of sexual abuse of children has led to aggressive measures to assure protective sexual education of children.

This chapter provides an overview of sexuality throughout the life span: its biologic and developmental components, its cultural and behavioral expression. Sexuality during the childbearing phase of family life is highlighted as one life-cycle phase. Nursing implications for the human sexuality process are woven throughout the narrative.

SEXUAL SELF-CONCEPT

How individuals perceive themselves in terms of gender, masculinity or femininity, and their adoption of effective sex-role behaviors will have an effect on their relationships with peers, adults, and members of the opposite sex; on play and work choices; and on their developmental expression of human sexuality. This interrelationship of biology, psychology, sociology, and culture is basic to the individual's sexual self-concept.

Gender is a biologic concept that refers simply to an individual's sex, male or female. Children's idea of their gender is usually fixed by 3 years of age. Biologic differences between males and females include (as discussed in Chapter 6) primarily chromosomal and anatomic differences and physiologic differences in the endocrine and genitourinary systems.

Nonbiologic concepts also are important for an understanding of sexuality. **Masculinity** and **femininity** are culturally prescribed; reinforced characteristics of the sexes are independent of gender. **Sex-role behaviors** are behaviors commonly assigned to men and women; these are more likely to change in response to situational demands. Sex-role attributes are elements of culturally accepted characteristics of masculinity and femininity that are more stable over time.[3] Thus, biologic gender, ideas of masculinity and femininity, and appropriate sex-role behaviors all affect one's developing sexuality.

Theories about sex-role development and sex-role behaviors have varied. Freud's theory of biologic determinism suggested that sexuality is instinctively patterned; he based his sexual development theories primarily on the male. Social learning theory postulated that sex-role behaviors are learned the way other behaviors are learned—through reward, punishment, and observation of behaviors that are congruent with family, social, and cultural groups.[4] A third model—the cognitive developmental model—portrayed the child as actively structuring his or her own experience. The child from the age of 1½ to 3 years categorizes himself or herself as a male or female and then, in light of this definition, begins the process of "cognitive rehearsal" in which the appropriate sex roles are acted out.[4]

Sex-Role Behaviors

Regardless of how children learn sex-role behaviors, it is clear that development of sex-role behaviors begins in infancy. A classic study by Money of individuals with physical abnormalities of the genital tract supports this view.[5] Money found that the psychologic aspects of sexuality are independent of the biologic aspects, ie, that a sexually ambiguous individual at birth, if labeled a female and socialized as a female, will comfortably take on the psychologic identity of a female.

In an early but authoritative review of sex-role research, Maccoby and Jacklin examined differences between boys and girls.[6] They concluded that intelligence was equal between the sexes; however, there were fairly well-established differences between the sexes in the areas of verbal skills (girls), visual-spatial ability (boys), mathematical ability (boys), and aggressiveness (boys). Other studies disagree with these conclusions, which support biologically based differences in cognition and sex-role behavior. Fausto-Sterling contends that although there may be a biologic origin for such differences, the actual differences are very small.[7] Furthermore, there are differences among individuals within each sex that, in certain instances, would be as great as the differences between the sexes. Fausto-Sterling concludes that definitive statements about biologically based sex-role differences cannot be made until research methods improve.

Femininity, Masculinity, and Androgyny

Femininity and masculinity are concepts that take on meaning in the context of the sociocultural environment of the individual. As any child grows up in a community, he or she receives messages about what masculinity and femininity mean.

Traditionally, the role of female in the United States has been that a woman be popular, desirable, marriageable, and able and willing to bear children. Feminists have aimed to incorporate the characteristics of activity, assertiveness, and achievement as part of the feminine perception. Jean Baker Miller notes that while our fundamental sense of identity is linked very early to a sense of being male or female, the concepts of "femaleness" and "maleness" do not require all of the meanings we now give them.[8] Miller points out that women hold many strengths that are essential for a society to meet human needs.[8] Society has not, however, been willing to identify these characteristics as strengths and therefore to benefit from women's skills. For example, Miller cites women's skills in affiliation and attachment as essential for social advancement. Yet paradoxically these skills are a source of women's current problems because women do not cherish these skills and because affiliation and attachment may lead them into subservience.[8]

Other characteristics that have traditionally been viewed as feminine include being affectionate, nurturant, yielding, and understanding—a predominance of expressive behaviors. Characteristics that have traditionally been viewed as masculine include being aggressive, independent, analytic, and competitive.

Individuals who incorporate both feminine and masculine characteristics are termed **androgynous.** Androgynous individuals have been characterized by certain researchers as having greater behavioral flexibility, which may be related to increased mental health and personal competence.[9] Other researchers have found that males and females with a masculine sex-role orientation have higher self-esteem.[10]

Cultural Factors

An understanding of sexuality today requires a look across cultures. Cross-cultural studies have supported the existence of sex differences in the areas of aggressiveness and dominance.[11] The expression of

RESEARCH ABSTRACT

Schuster E, et al. A theory of protection: parents as sex educators. ANS. *1985;7:36–42.*

This study investigated what occurs as parents engage in activities related to the sex education of their children. The researchers performed a qualitative appraisal of parental ideas, experiences, convictions, and concerns and used the grounded theory method to analyze the data that they acquired through interviews with parents.

The sample consisted of 16 volunteer mothers of children who were enrolled in a Head Start daycare center. The sample varied as to age, marital status, presence of biologic father in the home, employment status, and educational level. Subject interviews were conducted using a semi-structured questionnaire and were tape-recorded by three interviewers on a one-time basis.

The interview data were coded according to the various educational processes that were used by parents that were evident in the interviews such as teaching, learning, correcting behavior, and questioning. These data were then grouped into clusters or categories. Six final categories emerged: learning, mutuality, protecting, valuing, boundaries, controlling, and knowledge. From these categories, the researchers developed a theory of protection. The theory postulated that parents interacting with their children in matters relating to sexuality are engaged in protective behaviors, which are formed through their own values and are moderated by knowledge.

The principal means through which parents provided protection was through the assignment, establishment, and maintenance of a psychologic or physical limit or boundary. In practical terms this meant that families established ground rules about sexual behavior that determined what was in or out of bounds. Parents' greatest concerns about boundary maintenance were related to their ability to institute and maintain a boundary or boundary control. Parents were also concerned about the adequacy and accuracy of their knowledge and wanted their children to be taught facts earlier and more thoroughly. Finally mutuality was identified as the level of congruence between the parents' and child's understanding, values, and expectations.

Comment:

Although the researchers do report variability in income and education among subjects, the site of parental recruitment, a Head Start daycare center, does connote certain homogenous demographic characteristics that may limit generalizability to only that population.

An omission of the semi-structured questionnaire may be information related to children's actual sexual behavior—their activities, language, and questions, and parents' responses. Though some of the anecdotal data implied parents may have provided this information, the instrument did not, as published, directly address this area of concern.

The goal of grounded theory research is to generate key variables, identify links, and suggest hypotheses. The researchers accomplished this and began to suggest how predictions could be made based on their theoretic findings. This study did not describe specific deficiencies in parental sexual knowledge, or what strategies of boundary control parents found effective, or what were commonly held values, or when children should learn about sexuality.

The theoretic framework does have interesting implications. If protection is thought of as an essentially defensive and "negative" concept, the reader could ask how this compares to sex education in other cultures and how it relates to our difficulties with sexuality and our lack of contraceptive sophistication. In conclusion, this study points the way to future research and breaks ground by finding out what is relevant about sex education, rather than simply prescribing sex education.

sexual behaviors and the characteristics of masculinity and femininity differ across cultures.[12] Thus, although most cultures subscribe to sex-role stereotypes, these stereotypes differ among cultures. Not all cultures expect women to be passive, dependent, and gentle. In some cultures sexual expression differs; eg, sexual stimulation has been used as a pacifier for newborns and as an aid in weaning older infants. In other cultures, children play at intercourse during childhood; and real intercourse may begin as early as the age of 8 or 10.

The American cultural attitude toward sexuality has been described as paradoxical. Parents and adults have been described as protective or prohibitive concerning sexual behavior. They discourage the expression of sexual behaviors such as masturbation and sex play between children and adolescents. Yet society has titillated youth with media images of youthful sensuality and sexuality. Superficial communications, which glamorize sexual behavior but lack meaningful knowledgeable information, have been linked to the high adolescent pregnancy rate in the United States. Adults in our society have also been reluctant to take on the role of sex educators. Our culture has been contrasted with European cultures, which have encouraged more open communication and expression of sexuality and hence more responsible sexual behavior.

SEXUAL RESPONSE CYCLE

The sexual response cycle is the physiologic manifestation of the interplay of sexual interest, culture, and psychology. This cycle has been studied and reported in detail largely as a result of the pioneering work of Masters and Johnson.[13,14] It can be initiated by an individual alone as in masturbation or through a relationship with another person.

Masters and Johnson emphasized that the entire human body, including the nervous system, is involved in sexual arousal.[13,14] Two particular responses are important during the sexual response cycle, myotonia and vasocongestion.

Myotonia, or muscle tension, increases throughout the body during sexual stimulation and is controlled by the peripheral nervous system (PNS). During sexual arousal, there are links between the sense organs (input) of the PNS, the central nervous system, and the output branches, the somatic and autonomic branches. The facial, abdominal, pelvic, back, leg, and arm muscles, which are controlled by the somatic branch of the PNS, all show increased activity and tension during the sexual response cycle.

In the circulatory system, **vasocongestion,** or blood pooling, increases the size of many parts of the body. One type of vasocongestion occurs in erectile tissue; here the blood fills specially constructed spaces, the nipples, clitoris, and penis. The shaft of the penis is made up of spaces and cavities like a sponge. The blood vessels leading into the tissue dilate, permitting an increased inflow of blood, thereby filling the spaces in the erectile tissue with blood. The fibrous tissue surrounding the erectile tissue limits the expansion; and the pressure maintains a rigid structure.

A second type of vasocongestion occurs when existing blood vessels engorge with blood; this results in the increased size of breasts and labia and the color changes noted in certain organs during sexual arousal. Vaginal lubrication is a byproduct of vasocongestion. As the vaginal capillaries increase in size, the fluid pressures are altered in the walls of the vagina, and increased fluid passes into the vagina. Each capillary is surrounded by smooth muscle; when the smooth muscles are stimulated by the sympathetic branch of the autonomic nervous system they contract and the vessel shrinks. When sympathetic stimulation *decreases,* as during sexual arousal, the blood pressure in the vessels causes them to expand because of the relaxed smooth muscle. The expansion of many vessels at one time causes vasocongestion in nonerectile tissue.

Different organ systems are innervated by the sympathetic and parasympathetic branches of the PNS. While most organs are dominated by one or the other branch, the sex organs receive messages from both branches. Two centers in the spinal cord (S-2, S-3, and S-4, and T-11 to L-2) cause the arteries to dilate. In females, vasocongestion and orgasm appear to be under sympathetic control. Orgasm is a genital reflex consisting of contractions of certain genital muscles governed by spinal neural centers. On the other hand, penile erection is primarily a parasympathetic response, and ejaculation is a sympathetic response.

In addition to Masters and Johnson's model of the sexual response cycle, discussed in depth here, Kinsey[15] and Kaplan[16] also described models of the sexual response cycle. Table 8–1 contrasts these models. Basically, the models differ in the inclusion or omission of a phase. All the models have an excitement phase and an orgasm phase; but although each researcher observed the process of resolution or the return of the body to prestimulation levels, Kaplan did not label this as a separate phase, minimizing its importance.[16]

Four similar phases of the sexual response cycle have been described for both males and females by Masters and Johnson:[13,17] the excitement phase, the plateau phase, the orgasmic phase, and the resolution phase. The same sexual response cycle is initiated regardless of the type of sexual stimulation, be it masturbatory, mechanical, coital, or fantasy, although the response varies in intensity and duration.

TABLE 8–1. THEORETICAL MODELS OF THE SEXUAL RESPONSE CYCLE

Theorist:	Kinsey (1948; 1953)	Masters & Johnson (1966)	Kaplan (1979)
Phases:	—	—	Desire
	Buildup	Excitement	Excitement
	—	Plateau	—
	Orgasm	Orgasm	Orgasm
	Aftereffects	Resolution	—

Kaplan H. Disorders of Sexual Desire. *New York: Brunner/Mazel, 1979; Kinsey AC, et al.* Sexual Behavior in the Human Male. *Philadelphia: WB Saunders, 1948; Kinsey AC, et al.* Sexual Behavior in the Human Female. *Philadelphia: WB Saunders, 1953; Masters WH, Johnson VE.* Human Sexual Response, *Boston: Little, Brown, 1966* .

Masters and Johnson reported the most intense orgasmic response from masturbation.

Kaplan's modification of the human sexual response cycle included principally the addition of the desire phase, and the concept that each phase is governed by a separate neuro-physiologic system.[16] Sexual desire or sexual appetite is promoted by the hormone testosterone in both sexes; and two neurotransmitters, serotonin and dopamine. These are important in mediating sexual desire. External stimuli, such as an emotional bond to another person, sensory cues, such as erotic media, or smells may act as stimuli to sexual desire. During the excitement phase, vasodilation occurs as a result of activation of the two spinal centers mentioned previously. The orgasm phase is a genital reflex resulting from the sympathetic nervous system and the higher brain.

Tables 8–2 and 8–3 depict the physiologic sexual response of females and males according to Masters and Johnson's phases in the sexual response cycle. These tables detail the particular responses noted in the various organ systems.

Subjectively, the orgasmic phase is the peak pleasurable experience in both sexes. Women have the potential for multiple orgasms and may experience the second or third orgasm as the most pleasurable. In men, the orgasm with the largest ejaculate is experienced as the most pleasurable and this is usually the first orgasm. The orgasms of women have been described as twice as long as men's with a greater inten-

TABLE 8–2. PHYSIOLOGIC SEXUAL RESPONSE: WOMEN

Excitement	Vagina	Vaginal lubrication occurs Inner ⅔ of vagina lengthens and distends, color changes to dark purple Outer ⅓ of vagina fills with blood
	Labia	Labia minora enlarge, become more deeply colored Labia majora, flatten and thin, move away from midline
	Uterus	Uterus elevates, pulling on vagina making a tent or open area at inner ⅓ of vagina
	Breasts	Breasts increase in size Nipples become erect
	Cardiovascular/respiratory	Heart rate slows early, then increases in rate Breathing may increase in rate BP elevates as phase progresses
	Skin	Sex flush, measles-like rash occurs on chest or upper abdomen
Plateau	Vagina	Vaginal opening decreased in size by ⅓
	Labia	Sex skin reaction of labia minora from pink to bright red in nulliparous women and red to deep wine in multiparous women
	Clitoris	Retracts from unstimulated position to inaccessible place under clitoral hood
	Skin	Sex flush spreads to all areas of breast, chest, and abdomen
Orgasmic	Vagina	Contractions begin in outer ⅓ of vagina; begin at 0.8 second intervals and recur from 3 to 15 times. Time between contractions becomes longer and the strength of the contractions decreases
	Uterus	Uterus contracts, similar to labor
	Rectum	Rectal contractions linked in time with vaginal contractions
	Muscular	Release of muscular spasm, some loss of voluntary control, with spasms and contractions of many muscle groups
	Cardiovascular	Heart rate two times normal Blood pressure increases by ⅓
	Respiratory	Breathing rate three times normal
Resolution	Breasts	Loss of nipple erection, slower loss of breast volume Sex flush and swelling around nipples disappear
	Skin	Film of perspiration covers body
	Vagina	Within 5 to 10 seconds clitoris returns to normal position, loss of vasocongestion slower Congestion in outer ⅓ of vagina disappears Congestion in vaginal walls disappears in 15 minutes or more
	Labia	Labia majora return to unstimulated size Labia minora, prestimulation color returns in 15 seconds, size returns more slowly Cervix descends to unstimulated position
	Respiratory/cardiovascular	Breathing, heart rate, and blood pressure return to prestimulation condition
	Urinary	Urge to urinate, particularly in nulliparas

Reproduced, with permission, from Masters WH, Johnson VE. Human Sexual Response. *Boston: Little, Brown, 1966.*

TABLE 8–3. PHYSIOLOGIC SEXUAL RESPONSE: MEN

Excitement	Penis	Penile erection caused by blood engorgement, penile size increases
	Scrotum/testes	Skin of scrotum tenses, becomes congested and thick
		Testes rise higher in scrotum, increase in size as much as 50%
	Breast	Nipple erection and swelling
	Muscular	Increasing spasm of long muscles of legs and arms and abdomen muscles
	Rectum	Some voluntary contractions late in phase
	Respiratory	Breathing may increase late in phase
	Cardiovascular	Heart rate slows initially then quickens
Plateau	Skin	Sex flush occurs (not as frequent as in women) over chest, neck, and face
	Muscular	Increased muscular tension of face, neck, abdomen, and limbs
	Penis	Penile glans enlarges
	Testes	Testicular size increase from 50–100%
		Elevation of testes fully accomplished
	Blood pressure	Elevates as phase progresses
Orgasmic	Respiratory/cardiovascular	Breathing, heart rate, and blood pressure increase—generally higher than women
	Testes	Contractions of testes, prostate gland, and seminal vesicles as they collect sperm and seminal fluid and expel them into the entrance of the urethra
	Muscular	Release of muscular spasm, some loss of voluntary control with spasms and contractions of many muscle groups
	Penis	Penile muscle contraction and urethral contractions result in actual ejaculation of the seminal fluid out of the penis
	Rectum	Contractions linked to genital contractions
Resolution	Penis	After ejaculation ½ erection is lost quickly. Second stage is slower
	Testes/scrotum	Scrotal wall reverts to uncongested state
		Testes descend rapidly in most men, loss of swelling
	Skin	Skin flush disappears
		Perspiration usually confined to palms and soles of feet, but sometimes widespread
	Nipple	Nipple erection lost
	Muscular	Loss of muscle tension over a 5-minute period
	Cardiovascular/respiratory	Heart rate, breathing, and blood pressure return to prestimulation state

Reproduced, with permission, from Masters WH, Johnson VE: Human Sexual Response. *Boston: Little, Brown, 1966.*

sity. Individual variations, of course, do result in differences from these generalizations. The vasocongestion of the female is more generalized to the entire pelvic area in contrast to the male's more localized congestion and there is more total blood volume to be removed by muscle contraction in the female.[18]

Another unique feature of the female sexual response is that the uterine contractions in women during orgasm have the same recorded pattern as the first stage of labor; they differ only in amplitude. Women with hysterectomies also experience intense orgasms. The sexual arousal of women occurs more readily during the luteal phase or the last 14 days of the menstrual cycle. This is a result of increased pelvic congestion, increased vaginal fluid, and subsequent increased "interest."

The source of the orgasm in terms of its link to a certain organ has received a lot of attention in the literature. Freud thought the vaginal orgasm was the truly mature orgasm; Masters and Johnson emphasized the importance of the clitoral orgasm, or the tenting type of orgasm (erectile tissue contracts like a tent), which is a result of clitoral stimulation. Most recently, an extremely sensitive area on the anterior wall of the vagina 1 or 2 inches above the vaginal orifice was discovered. This was dubbed the "G" spot or the Grafenberg spot.[19] Stimulation of this spot results in a uterine orgasm.

Singer and Singer described the vulval, uterine and blended orgasms.[20] The vulval orgasm involves involuntary contractions of the vascular tissue at the outer third of the women's vagina and the labia minora. Uterine orgasm involves stimulation of the cervix, which in turn stimulates the peritoneum. Blended orgasm involves a combination of both sensations. For the clinician, the important issue is the client's and her partner's satisfaction with the sexual response.

Masters and Johnson interpreted sexual functioning as an interaction between the biophysic and psychosocial systems.[13] These systems could reinforce each other positively or inhibit one another. If positive attitudes and values have been acquired about gender, sex role, and characteristics of masculinity and femininity, and one has a positive image as a sexual being, the biologic and sexual response cycle will be enhanced.

Certain cultural characteristics of femininity and masculinity may inhibit or enhance the biophysic response cycle. Feminine characteristics of affection and affiliation may enhance the sexual relationship, whereas passivity and submissiveness may contribute to a denial and suppression of individual sex needs. Similarly, a masculine identity of assertiveness and activity may contribute to a healthy acknowledgement and pursuit of a sexual relationship, but competitiveness and independence may inhibit the affectionate relationship underlying the sexual relationship.

SEXUALITY OVER THE LIFE SPAN

The individual's experience and understanding of sexuality over the life span change as a function of cognitive, psychosocial, cultural, and physiologic maturation. Masters and Johnson's important documentation and research on the human sexual response point out that the physiologic experience of sexual arousal and consummation shows little variation over the life span.[13] The physiologic phenomena are only one component of human sexuality; the behavorial, social, and psychologic expressions of sexuality in the developing individual do vary over the life span.

Calderone and Johnson emphasized that sexuality is a characteristic of *all* children and that evidence of the functioning of the human sexual response cycle is demonstrated in infancy when an infant boy has an erection and an infant girl has signs of fluid in her vagina.[21] When the infant a few months later discovers his or her genital organs through touch, the infant is initiating the sexual response cycle. The behaviors associated with unfolding sexuality include looking at and touching the genitalia in the first year of life. These early experiences of touching accompany the feeling of pleasure associated with the genitalia.

Gesell and others have summarized the usual stages of sexual awareness and sex play in the young child.[22] They describe 2½-year-olds as showing interest in urination and the different postures boys and girls assume as well as their genital differences; 3-year-olds will verbalize interest in gender differences; 4-year-olds will play games of "show" and continue verbal play and names related to elimination and other people's bathrooms; 5-year-olds will be more modest, and engage in less bathroom play; 6-year-olds will participate in mild sex play or exhibitionism, and playing hospital, giggling, and toilet talk will continue. Less interest occurs at 7 years, but at 8 years interest in sex is rather high and includes peeping, smutty jokes, and whispering. Nine-year-olds are interested in the details of their own organs and may begin sex swearing and reciting sex poems. Ten-year-olds like smutty jokes, although the peak interest may be at 11 to 12. Within these stages there are periods of intense interest in sex interwoven with periods of less interest. Many individual children will progress through these stages exhibiting a wide range of individual variations. Gesell and colleagues describe "twosomes" occurring at 6, 7, and 8 and then not so much a latency period but an interest in the opposite sex that is expressed as a movement away, a dislike of "jerkos" and "nerds."[22] Exploratory behaviors resulting in pleasure in the preschool and older child include mutual touching between boys and girls, simulated sexual games, and repetitive self-stimulation of genitalia, or masturbation. The response of peers, siblings, parents, or other adults to this behavior will affect its development.

In the psychoanalytic view of childhood sexuality, the parents are the primary love objects of a child's sexual hugs and longings. Continuing maturity demands that the child relinquish these desires and replace parents with love objects outside the family.[23] Congruent with this perspective of sexuality are childhood behaviors that depict the child as close to mother, then the opposite sex parent, then peers. The child may exhibit intrusiveness and jealousy of the marital relationship at certain stages. The child may also talk of marrying the parent of the opposite sex and physical embraces of the loved parent may mimic more adult sexual embraces.

During adolescence the individual experiences dramatic physiologic, cognitive, psychologic, social, and sexual development. At the onset of puberty, the hormonal changes and subsequent physical changes will have an effect on an individual's self-image, self-esteem, and social relationships with same sex and opposite sex peers.

Developmental tasks of adolescence have been described by such noted theorists as Havinghurst[24] and Erikson.[25] Kriepe views adolescent sexual expression as dependent on four dynamic forces: (1) acceptance of physical maturation; (2) attainment of adult thinking skills; (3) achievement of independence; and (4) an adult identity.[26] Physically mature adolescents may not be emotionally mature, and early sexual development is not necessarily accompanied by early achievement of independence or attainment of adult thinking skills.[26]

The adolescent does not focus on the consequences of behavior or the alternatives of behavior; thinking is limited to the here and now. Adult thinking skills, on the other hand, reflect planning for the future and recognition of the long-range consequences of behavior. Attainment of these skills will be an important factor in the adolescent's ability to make responsible sexual decisions.

Identity formation is another important aspect of adolescent development. The influence of the peer group is important to sexual activity in the phase of identity formation. The peer group is often the standard against which many adolescent behaviors are measured; familial values are sometimes rejected to attain peer approval. This is especially true in early and mid-adolescence.[26] The attainment of mature adulthood finds the adolescent realigning himself or herself with family and adult values. Sexual expression, during this phase, is similar to that found in adult development.

Adolescence is usually identified in age with the onset of puberty. Because the normal range of the onset of puberty varies widely—ie, 9 years to 16 years—it is hard to pinpoint exact ages. The age of onset of puberty may have genetic familial determinants and in addition is affected by culture, economy, and habitat as well as psychologic and emotional factors.

The secretion of pituitary and gonadal hormones results in the obvious physical changes in the girl of breast development, pubic and axillary hair, height spurt, and the onset of menarche. In the boy, there is penile and testicular growth, axillary, facial, and pubic hair growth, along with the first ejaculation and voice change. Along with these physiologic changes comes an increased interest in the opposite sex. Males often focus on the size and growth of their penises as an indication of their sexuality. Females, because of the internal nature of their organs, focus on breast size and the onset of menarche as an indication of their sexual maturity.

The adolescent years are an incredibly needy period in terms of sexuality. Adolescents are immature in knowledge, impulse control, relationships, self-esteem, and identity, but have strong feelings of sexuality. This combination requires guidance and maturity from parents and other adults. Furthermore, for sexually active teenagers, the multiple partners experienced during adolescence, anxiety about performance, and societal taboos against open sexual expression result in teenagers participating in "fast sex in awkward places." A general lack of adequate information can lead to a high-risk climate for sexually transmitted diseases and impotence or premature ejaculation in men or early pregnancy or orgasmic dysfunction in women.

Sarrel and Sarrel describe various phases in sexual development over the life span.[27] Underlying this approach to sexual development is the awareness of sexuality blossoming over time and then being affected by and changing as a result of developmental life cycles and situational occurrences. The act of first intercourse, then, is not an end but an incident occurring at some point during the sexual process. The sexual unfolding stage will begin in adolescence for most individuals but is not limited to these chronologic years. Some individuals may be dealing with the challenges of sexual unfolding at a much later age.

During the childrearing phase, couples must adapt their needs for marital intimacy and privacy to the changes of pregnancy, lactation, and the needs of their children. Frequently it is the parents' private time that is diminished and sacrificed, to the detriment of their sexual relationship. Sexuality becomes a family process as parents recognize their children's developing sexuality and create a family environment in which they can grow and flourish.

The end of the reproductive years—voluntarily through tubal ligation or vasectomy or through menopause—means that sexuality is distinct from the procreative period. This stage may be welcomed as a period of freedom from early childrearing cares or there may be a feeling of loss and aging associated with it.

Masters and Johnson[13] in their study of middle-aged and elderly men and women established several important points: people of all ages respond sexually past menopause.[13] There is no definitive age of cessation of sexuality. However, several changes do occur in the sexual response cycle as an individual ages. In the aging female, sex flush occurs less frequently, labia majora do not move away from the midline, labia minora lose the response of enlargement, vaginal lubrication occurs at a slower rate, the vagina's ability to increase in width and depth decreases, and the subjective experience of orgasm diminishes.

In the aging male, the amount of time necessary to attain an erection is lengthened, but the erection is maintained for longer periods. The loss of erection is more rapid and the force of ejaculation and the intensity of contractions is reduced. The scrotum has reduced vasocongestion; there is less elevation of the testes and the increase in the size of the testes is not evident.

SEXUALITY AND THE CHILDBEARING COUPLE

Pregnancy

Much of the knowledge about the sexual response cycle during pregnancy again comes from the early work of Masters and Johnson.[13] Later researchers have supplemented this work. Findings are not always consistent and, although researchers report on group findings, it is clear that individual variations and responses to sexuality need to be respected throughout the pregnancy cycle.

Table 8–4 summarizes alterations in the sexual response cycle occurring during pregnancy.

Certain physiologic changes related to the breast tissue and pelvic viscera affect the sexual response cycle in pregnant women. Enlargement of glandular tissue and increased vascularity of the breasts often lead to breast tenderness in early pregnancy. This can decrease a woman's interest in having her breasts stimulated during foreplay. This breast tenderness tends to decrease in the second and third trimester.

Increased pelvic vascularity occurring during pregnancy can lead to changes in sexual interest and increased orgasmic experiences, as well as some signs of uterine irritability such as abdominal cramping, aching, and low backache. Masters and Johnson reported that during the excitement phase, pregnant women experienced increased engorgement of the labia majora.[13] The labia minora enlarged two to three times their unstimulated size, and, in the third trimester were chronically congested. Near the end of the first trimester vaginal lubrication increased during the excitement phase.

In general, the increased vascularity of the entire pelvis with resulting vasocongestion facilitates coital orgasm in the pregnant woman. For this reason women who have not achieved orgasm prior to conception may well experience orgasm for the first time during pregnancy. In general, the increased volume of the pelvic venous bed during pregnancy will enhance the capacity for sexual tension and improve orgasmic intensity, frequency, and pleasure.[18] Other authors have attributed increased orgasmic competency during pregnancy to the psychologic factors of improved "relaxation related to sexuality" and "affirmation of womanliness." During the resolution phase orgasm during pregnancy frequently does not relieve pelvic vasocongestion; therefore, a sustained feeling of sexual tension often persists.

TABLE 8–4. CHANGES IN SEXUAL RESPONSE CYCLE DURING PREGNANCY

Excitement	Labia	Increased engorgement of labia majora Labia minora increase 2–3 times unstimulated size
	Vagina	Increased vaginal lubrication
	Breast	Increased enlargement and congestion of breast tissue
Plateau	Increased pelvic congestion	
Orgasm	Increased orgasmic intensity, duration, and frequency	
Resolution	Sustained pelvic congestion; therefore, may be sustained sexual tension	

In addition to the general changes in the sexual response cycle described above, other researchers have looked at factors affecting sexual interest during pregnancy. The complexity of the concept of sexual drive and interest is not altered by pregnancy. Additional factors influencing the pregnant couple can, however, result in increased or decreased interest in sexuality. General factors affecting sexual activity during pregnancy, other than the pregnancy itself, include the age of the mother, length of marriage, quality of the marital relationship, and the preexisting sexual relationship. Sexual frequency during pregnancy seems to be increased in younger mothers and younger marriages.

Research findings can be summarized as portraying three desire phase patterns for pregnant women: (1) women whose sexual activity and desire remain constant throughout pregnancy; (2) women who, as in the study by Solberg and colleagues,[28] show a steady decline in sexual activity over the pregnancy; and (3) women who, as reflected in Masters and Johnson's[17] group, show a decline in the first and third trimester but an increase in sexual activity and interest during the second trimester.

Factors in early pregnancy other than breast tenderness that can inhibit sexual interest are the symptoms of early pregnancy—fatigue, nausea, and vomiting. Research has indicated that there is a decrease in sexual interest and functioning as a result of first trimester changes.[13,29,30] On the other hand, satisfaction stemming from the knowledge that the couple has been able to conceive, freedom from having to use contraceptives, and increasing pelvic congestion may contribute to a woman's or couple's increased interest in sexuality. The woman or couple who will be experiencing sexuality for its own sake may find this stressful; others may experience it as joyous.

During the second trimester, Masters and Johnson reported a marked increase in eroticism and effectiveness of sexual performance.[13] In fact, as mentioned previously, sexual performance surpassed that in the nonpregnant state.[29,30] Many of the "nuisance" symptoms of the first trimester have disappeared. The pregnant woman's body has changed. These changes may be perceived as very attractive and sensual or as unappealing to the pregnant woman and her spouse, affecting sexual interest accordingly.

During the third trimester Masters and Johnson[13] and Solberg and colleagues[28] reported a decrease in sexual interest. A variety of reasons have been put forth to explain this. Women during the third trimester report more physical complaints, such as pelvic tension and backaches. Discomfort with increased body weight and body shape and difficulty in finding comfortable sexual positions are also a factor cited in decreasing sexual activity. Medical advice or medical contraindications account for another factor in the decrease of sexual activity during the third trimester. Marital partners also are concerned about the safety of the fetus and frequently opt to decrease sexual activity during the last trimester for this reason. Solberg and colleagues described 25 percent of their sample as ceasing sexual activity in the eighth month, and 60 percent of the sample ceasing sexual activity in the ninth month.[28]

Two specific concerns underlie the couples' general concern for fetal safety and influence their decision to persist or abstain from intercourse: the first is the precipitation of premature labor; the second, the introduction of infection or air embolism into the uterine cavity.

Although hypotheses have suggested a relationship among prostaglandins, semen, increased oxytocin levels and uterine contractions (*see* Chapter 25), there is a lack of clinical evidence to connect orgasm to the onset of premature labor.[31–33]

In Klebanoff and associates' study of 32,217 women, increasing coital frequency was associated with increasing length of gestation in blacks, whites, and Puerto Ricans.[33] Neither clinical nor research evidence upholds a relationship between premature labor and intercourse late in pregnancy for normal women without a high-risk history. A relationship may exist between these factors for those women who have a known history of premature onset of labor.

Oral-genital sexual activity has been associated with air embolism late in pregnancy. For this reason, blowing into the vaginal area during late pregnancy has been advised against.[34]

Childbirth

Oxytocin is a hormone produced by the pituitary gland that initiates uterine contractions, triggers milk let-down for breastfeeding mothers, and is found in the bloodstream during vaginal dilation. This hormone appears to link the three experiences of birth, lactation, and orgasm, and may account in part for the sensual or erotic feelings experienced by some women when giving birth or breastfeeding. Orgasms have been reported by some women during the second stage of labor as a result of increased vasocongestion when the clitoris is engorged and the woman is bearing down. Not all women perceive the delivery or breastfeeding experience with this degree of sensuality and the health care professional must be sensitive to the range of normal experiences for individual women.

Postpartum Period

Because sexuality is not simply a function of biologic or physiologic changes, the postpartum period reflects the contradictions and complexities of the childbearing period. Physiologically, pelvic vasocongestion and hence enhanced sexuality has dissipated with the delivery of the infant. Perineal irritation or pain secondary to tears, episiotomy repairs, or rectal hemorrhoids may occur in the early postpartum period. Fatigue, anxiety, vaginal discharge, or breast soreness may result in decreased sexual interest during the postpartum period. Furthermore, negative feelings about body image, lack of privacy, and appropriate timing for marital intimacy may also contribute to women's diminished sense of sexuality in the postpartum period.

On the other hand, breastfeeding mothers continue to experience enlargement and engorgement of the breasts, which in some women has resulted in a feeling of enhanced sexual stimulation to the plateau or orgasmic levels. An enhanced sense of femininity or womanliness as a result of the birthing experience may also contribute to a positive interest in sexuality.

Labor and breastfeeding both have physiologic similarities to the orgasmic experience, and some women have subjectively noted this and described this response. The association of breastfeeding and sexuality has been accepted by some women and enjoyed, whereas other women have felt anxious and guilty. Conversely, body contact and fatigue secondary to the breastfeeding experience may result in diminished sexual interest and drive and temporary loss of the breast as an erogenous zone. Sexual excitement may stimulate the milk let-down reflex, which may also alter the woman's or couple's sexual enjoyment.

Some research indicates that sexual intimacy returns to prepregnancy levels as early as 6 weeks postpartum. In some couples an interest in and desire for sex comes even earlier. Other researchers report fatigue, anxiety, and preoccupation with the infant as factors that affect the marital relationship negatively for up to a year. Some women experience an enhanced sexuality and enhanced womanliness during the postpartal period as a result of the breastfeeding relationship.[3] Levels of estrogen drop after delivery, causing decreased lubrication and a tighter, more sensitive vagina. Until ovulation occurs, both breastfeeding and non-breastfeeding mothers can be considered to be "estrogen starved." Vulvar and vaginal tissues may be more sensitive or sore during intercourse or genital manipulation. Monilial infections may flare during the postpartum period, causing uncomfortable sex.

Obstetric tears or a torn or stretched perineal body may inhibit sexual satisfaction or delay this process further in other couples. If an episiotomy was performed after delivery, intercourse can be resumed in 2 weeks. Positive aspects of episiotomy repair may include heightened sensitivity over the repair area or a tighter vagina. Extremely stretched tissues or poorly repaired tears or episiotomies, however, may lead to changes in vaginal muscles or the size of the vaginal orifice, thus altering the tone of the vagina. This may change the man's or the woman's sensation of the penis in the vagina and alter the sexual response cycle. Postpartal exercises (Kegels) may be encouraged to increase and maintain perineal and vaginal tone. It is important to note that a loose vagina, occurring after a precipitous delivery, closely spaced pregnancies, or large babies is balanced by the vasocongestion that occurs during sexual stimulation. The vasocongestion, which is often increased after childbirth, makes the vagina very snug.[27]

Lochia may continue up to 6 weeks after delivery. Intercourse may be resumed during the alba, or whitish, phase. Its normal odor or presence, though, may be a barrier for some couples over a longer period. Open communications between partners and a health provider are important to identify any sexual alterations as a result of the pregnancy or postpartum process.

The literature has often emphasized women's sexual responsiveness during the childbearing year. In fact, theorists have related a woman's comfort with her own sexuality to her ease in adaptation to the parenthood role.[35] Furthermore, Sherfey felt that high estrogen and progesterone levels during pregnancy increased the vascular bed in the pelvis, contributing to long-range improvements in sexual arousal and potential for orgasm.[18]

May reviewed research summarizing the father's sexual response to the childbearing year.[36] The identified changes discussed in the woman's sexual patterns may be congruent with the man's changes (the man may also experience decreased sexual interest in the last trimester) or incongruent (the man or woman may have sustained interest in sex throughout the pregnancy). These disruptions require adaptation by the sexual couple. Fein reported fathers particularly being unprepared for a sustained interruption of sexual relations in the postpartum period.[37] Fathers' sense of well-being was found by Wandersman to be most closely related to their perception of the quality of the marital relationship.[38] The quality of sexual functioning is an important aspect of marital satisfaction and is an important component of the male's concept of self. Alterations in sexuality for fathers may more directly affect their self-concept and marital functioning. May suggested that nurses be aware that childbearing may affect sexual responsiveness of the marital partners differentially and that men, in particular, may need assistance in adapting to the inevitability of change in their sexual partners.[36]

Nursing Implications: Sexuality and Childbearing

Nursing care of the childbearing couple includes obtaining a complete data base. This includes a complete sexual history (see later section on taking a sexual history). Ideally, the history taking should include both partners. If the father cannot be physically present at some point for interviewing, careful attention should be given to eliciting information about his perspective; for example, the interviewer might ask, "Did your partner want this pregnancy?" "Does your partner have any feelings about sex possibly hurting the baby?" A complete data base will provide knowledge of common areas of need for childbearing couples as well as specific problem identification.

Sexuality is often considered a secret and taboo subject. However, sexual attitudes and values are formed over a lifetime, and these attitudes must be considered and respected. All couples can benefit from simple factual information about factors affecting sexuality during pregnancy and postpartum, safe sexual practices during childbearing, and common problems and concerns (eg, comfortable sexual positions).

As in other aspects of intimate relationships, the couple's ability to communicate openly, identify and articulate concerns, be open to new information, be flexible, and adapt to ways of problem solving are all strengths that will enhance sexual functioning. These aspects of a relationship, particularly in young marriages, may need reinforcing or development. A sexual relationship between partners that already included a variety of methods of stimulating each other, use of different positions for intercourse, and orgasmic competence, is different from one in which partners are just beginning to explore their sexual selves and only achieve satisfaction infrequently. Sensitivity to these relationship differences and the ability to communicate information in a nonjudgmental manner are critical to the success of sexual education and counseling.

The nurse can provide simple, factual information, such as: (1) grooming and hygiene may need to be modified during pregnancy to enhance the sexual self; (2) increased vaginal discharge, heat sensitivity, nausea, and vomiting may contribute to a need for increased baths, mouth care, and deodorant; (3) attractive feminine clothes can highlight a woman's increased voluptuousness and yet accommodate the pregnant or nursing mother's body shape (many women with small breasts enjoy their breast development during this period).

Timing for intimacy may have to be reevaluated during the childbearing cycle as fatigue, gastrointestinal disturbances, or demands from the new infant or siblings may render previous rituals of sexual intimacy inappropriate. The late-night sexual contact may now be a time when the woman experiences great fatigue or complains of sore nipples because of frequent nursings.

Anticipation by the couple about changing time and relationship demands can help the couple to think about the need to set up time for themselves as a couple alone and schedule childcare support.

The nurse can communicate that penile-vaginal intercourse can be considered safe for pregnant couples except in the following situations:

- History of repeated early miscarriage
- History of uterine abnormalities or cervical incompetence (if cervical banding has taken place, couples may have intercourse)
- History of premature onset of labor (women should avoid orgasm but not necessarily intercourse)
- History of premature rupture of the membranes because of the risk of introduction of bacterial infection
- Unexplained vaginal bleeding
- Unexplained abdominal pain

The techniques of intercourse may change for pregnant couples as pregnancy progresses. Manual fondling or mouth stimulation may be suggested as alternatives to penile-vaginal intercourse. The side-by-side, rear entry, or female superior positions may be suggested as alternatives to the male upright (missionary) position. Deep penetration may be uncomfortable during periods of pelvic vasocongestion, and these alternate positions may control the rate and depth of penetration. Rear entry when the women is in the knee-chest position will also aid in shifting pelvic contents upward. This avoids direct pressure on the abdomen and allows freedom of hands for manual stimulation.

Touching, caressing, and holding are important alternatives if orgasm and intercourse are contraindicated. Back rubs, full-body massage, sensual stroking, hugging, or use of vibrators may be an important form of sexual communication suggested by the nurse. The nurse encourages the couple to communicate about changing erogenous zones during the childbearing cycle (eg, nipple soreness, episiotomy scar sensitivity).

During the postpartum period, decreased vaginal lubrication may result in the need for a water-soluble lubricant or, if need be, a prescription for an estrogen-based vaginal cream.

SEXUALLY TRANSMITTED DISEASE

There are more than 50 diseases and syndromes currently classified as sexually transmitted diseases. They account for 13 million cases and 7000 deaths annually. Recently, increased incidences have been reported in many of the principal sexually transmitted diseases as well as in several previously obscure sexually transmitted diseases.[39]

Sexually transmitted disease (STD) is a category of diseases that are transmitted through sexual intercourse and intimate sexual contact with the genitals, mouth, or rectum. This does not mean that sex is the exclusive mode of transmission. Some STDs (HIV, syphilis, gonorrhea) may be transmitted perinatally from the mother to the fetus; other STDs, such as moniliasis, may result from changes in host factors, such as diabetes; still others (HIV, hepatitis B) occur as a result of blood-to-blood contact from means such as shared contaminated needles. Nevertheless, they all share the definition of STD in that a principal means of transmission is through sexual contact.

Perinatal Transmission

Some STDs pose a health risk both to the mother and the fetus. **Perinatal transmission,** or infection from the mother to the fetus, involves several possible routes. Transplacental transmission occurs when the infected maternal blood results in placentitis, which then spreads to the fetus. This is one way in which cytomegalovirus and syphilis are thought to be transmitted from the mother to the fetus. Transmembranous infection results when cervical infection or endometrial infection spreads to the membranes and hence to the fetus. Perinatal transmission may also occur as a result of exposure to infected cervical or vaginal secretions at the time of delivery—so-called vertical transmission. Herpes simplex virus 2 (HSV-2) is predominantly transmitted this way. Finally, breast milk may be the reservoir for the organism. For example, some cases of HIV infection in infants have been attributed to breast-milk transmission.[40]

Several factors in today's society have contributed to the magnitude of sexually transmitted diseases. They are:

- *The large number of high-risk young adults.* (The maturing "baby boomers:" 49 million Americans in 1985 were between the ages of 18 and 29.)
- *Changing sexual behaviors.* (Earlier sexual intercourse among women aged 15 to 19 years; increasing numbers of individuals in the single-adult category either because of postponement of marriage, divorce, or widowhood, resulting in an increased multiplicity of sexual partners.)
- *A higher proportion of infections with multiple modes of transmission that are being transmitted sexually.* (For example, hepatitis A and B, HIV, group B streptococcus.)[41,42]
- *Increasing incidences of diseases associated with sex-for-drugs prostitution.*
- *The diversion of local venereal disease control efforts to combat the threat of HIV infection.*[39]

STDs are important health concerns for several reasons other than the discomfort of the acute symptoms of the diseases themselves. The sequelae of untreated STDs can lead to pelvic inflammatory disease in women or other types of irreversible organ damage. This damage to the genital area leads to scarring and adhesions within the reproductive tract, ultimately contributing to increasing rates of infertility, ectopic pregnancies, reproductive loss, and neoplasms. Another important concern is the transmission of certain organisms from the pregnant mother to her fetus. In pregnant women STDs can have life-threatening implications for the fetus. In addition, the risk of the mother's contracting STDs is increased during pregnancy.

Finally, HIV infection, an internationally acknowledged STD with exceedingly high mortality rates at present, has alerted everyone to the life-threatening consequences of STDs and the financial and human cost to society in general.

Some of the common STDs that will be discussed briefly here are summarized in Table 8–5. In the 1960s and 1970s the two major "venereal diseases," as they were called, were syphilis and gonorrhea, and the three minor diseases were chancroid, lymphogranuloma venereum, and granuloma inguinale. Recently there has been a rise in the incidence of these three formerly minor diseases, although the incidence is far less than for the major STDs. The greatly expanded list in the 1980s includes over 20 organisms that spread disease person to person during sexual contact, such as *Chlamydia trachomatis*, genital herpes, cytomegalovirus, hepatitis, vaginitis including *Candida albicans* and *Trichomonas vaginalis*, enteric infections, ectoparasitic diseases, and HIV (human immunodeficiency virus).[42]

Women are alerted to the possibility of infectious disease in the reproductive tract principally by the symptoms of discharge and pain and itching. Not all STDs result in clear symptoms, thus making diagnosis and treatment difficult for both the client and the health care practitioner.

Chlamydia trachomatis

In the United States, *Chlamydia trachomatis* has replaced *Neisseria gonorrhoea* as the most frequently contracted STD.

There are 4 million new infections reported annually.[39] Chlamydia are small intracellular parasites with two nucleic acids; they infect the mucosa and are susceptible to antibiotics. In women, the principal signs of infection are vaginal discharge or pruritus, although an infection may be asymptomatic. Clinically these symptoms are not distinctive and cannot be differentiated from gonorrhea. In fact, chlamydia are frequently found in mixed infections, such as with gonorrhea, monilia, or *Trichomonas vaginalis*. Chlamydia can be diagnosed by isolation and growth of the organism after culture or through serologic tests. The usual drug of choice in *non-pregnant* women is tetracycline. For pregnant women erythromycin is the drug of choice. Neonates born of mothers with a genital chlamydia infection have a 40 percent chance of developing chlamydial conjunctivitis and a 10 to 20 percent chance of developing chlamydial pneumonia. *See* Chapter 39 for further discussion of *Chlamydia trachomatis* infection during pregnancy.

Gonorrhea

Gonorrhea is the second most frequently occurring STD in listings of annual new infections by the Centers for Disease Control. It is also identified as a serious infectious disease in terms of its sequelae: pelvic inflammatory disease, or pelvic abscess, with resulting infertility. The initial site is the lower reproductive tract and, if untreated, the organisms ascend to produce upper reproductive tract illness. Irritation, discharge (yellow and purulent), and painful, frequent urination are symptoms, but it is estimated that at least 50 percent of women with gonorrhea are asymptomatic.[43] Symptoms, if present, usually occur two to five days after exposure.

Most clients who contract gonorrhea are single and under 25. Women with decreased levels of estrogen are at a greater risk for developing gonorrheal

TABLE 8–5. SUMMARY OF THE PRINCIPAL SEXUALLY TRANSMITTED DISEASES

Disease and Etiologic Agents	Typical Clinical Presentation	Presumptive Diagnosis (Warrants full treatment and followup)	Therapy	Complications and Sequelae
Nongonococcal Urethritis (NGU)				
Chlamydia trachomatis: A human mycoplasma of the T-strain. Other sexually transmissible agents can cause NGU; these include: *Ureaplasma urealyticum, Trichomonas vaginalis, Candida albicans,* Herpes simplex virus.	Men usually have dysuria, frequency, and mucoid to purulent urethral discharge. Some men have asymptomatic infections. Steady female sexual partners of men with chlamydial NGU are likely to have chlamydial endocervicitis.	Men with typical clinical symptoms are presumed to have NGU when their gonorrhea tests are negative and they have either WBCs on Gram's stain of urethral discharge or sexual exposure to an agent known to cause NGU. Asymptomatic men with negative gonorrhea tests are also presumed to have NGU if they have at least 4 WBCs per oil immersion field on an intraurethral smear.	Tetracycline hydrochloride (HCl) 500 mg, PO, 4 times daily for 7 days; or doxycyline 100 mg, PO, 2 times daily for 7 days.	Urethral strictures. Prostatitis. Epididymitis. Chlamydial NGU may be transmitted to female sexual partners, resulting in mucopurulent endocervicitis, PID, and other adverse outcomes (see below).
Mucopurulent Cervicitis (MPC)				
Chlamydia trachomatis is the principal pathogen, although *Neisseria gonorrhoeae,* herpes simplex virus, *Candida albicans,* and *Trichomonas vaginalis* can also produce cervicitis (see relevant panels).	The client may be symptomatic or asymptomatic, and a yellow mucopurulent endocervical exudate may be present. Cervical ectopy appears to correlate with cervical infection with this agent.	The presence of yellow mucopurulent endocervical exudate or the finding of this exudate on a white cotton-tipped swab of endocervical secretions suggests infection with *Chlamydia trachomatis.* In women without visible exudate, the presence of greater than or equal to 10 polymorphonuclear leukocytes per x 1000 field on a Gram-stained specimen of endocervical mucus (without contamination by vaginal cells) also allows a presumptive diagnosis.	If *N. gonorrhoea* is not found, treatment should be given as noted above for NGU. Special considerations should be given to: *Treatment during pregnancy:* Erythromycin base or stearate: 500 mg, PO, 4 times daily for 7 days; or erythromycin base 250mg PO, 4 times daily for 14 days.	Ascending infections may lead to symptomatic or asymptomatic endometritis and salpingitis and subsequent infertility. Ascending infection during pregnancy may lead to adverse obstetric outcomes, conjunctivitis or pneumonia in the infant, and puerperal infection.
Gonorrhea				
Neisseria gonorrhoea: A gram-negative diplococcus.	When symptomatic, men usually have dysuria, frequency, and purulent urethral discharge. Women may have muccopurient endocervical exudate, abnormal menses, dysuria, or be asymptomatic.	Microscopic identification of typical gram-negative intracellular diplococci on smear of urethral exudate (men) or endocervical material (women). Cervical specimens that are Gram-stain-tested should also be cultured for *N. gonorrhoeae.*	A wide range of antimicrobial therapy ia available. For example, for uncomplicated urethral, endocervical, or rectal infection: ceftriaxone 250 mg IM once plus doxycycline 100 mg, PO, 2 times daily for 7 days; or spectinomycin 2g IM in a single dose plus doxycycline as above.	10–20 percent of women develop PID and are at risk for its sequelae Men are at risk for epididymitis, sterility, urethral stricture, and infertility. Newborns are at risk for ophthalmia neonatorum, scalp abscess at

TABLE 8–5. SUMMARY OF THE PRINCIPAL SEXUALLY TRANSMITTED DISEASES (*continued*)

Disease and Etiologic Agents	Typical Clinical Presentation	Presumptive Diagnosis (Warrants full treatment and followup)	Therapy	Complications and Sequelae
Gonorrhea (*continued*)				
	Anorectal and pharyngeal infections are common. These may be symptomatic or asymptomatic.	or Growth on selective medium demonstrating typical colonial morphology, positive oxidase reaction, and typical Gram's stain morphology.	In clients in whom tetracyclines are contraindicated or not tolerated, the single-dose regimen may be followed by: erythromycin base or stearate: 500 mg, PO, 4 times daily for 7 days; or erythromycin ethylsuccinate 800 mg, PO, 4 times daily for 7 days. *Treatment during pregnancy:* ceftriaxone 250 mg IM, once, plus erythromycin base, 500 mg, PO, 4 times daily for 7 days.	the site of fetal monitors, rhinitis, pneumonia, or anorectal infections. All infected, untreated persons are at risk for disseminated gonococcal infection (includes septicemia, arthritis, dermatitis, meningitis, and endocarditis).
Vaginitis				
Trichomonas vaginalis vaginitis: A motile protozoan with an undulating membrane and four flagella.	Presentations vary from no signs or symptoms to erythema, edema, and pruritus of the external genitalia. Excessive and malodorous discharge are common findings.	*Trichomonas vaginalis vaginitis:* There are no presumptive criteria for this diagnosis.	*Trichomonas vaginalis vaginitis:* Metronidazole 2.0 g, PO, in a single dose.	Secondary excoriations. Recurrent infections are common.
Bacterial vaginiosis (predominantly *Gardnerella vaginalis*)		*Bacterial vaginosis:* The presumptive criteria include three of the following: ▪ a homogenous gray or white, adherent discharge; ▪ vaginal pH greater than 4.5; ▪ release of a fishy-smelling amine mixed with 10% KOH; and, ▪ presence of "clue cells."	*Bacterial vaginosis:* Metronidazole 500 mg, PO, 2 times daily for 7 days or clindamycin, 300 mg, PO, 2 times daily for 7 days. *Treatment during pregnancy:* Clindamycin, 300 mg, PO, 2 times a day for 7 days.	*Bacterial vaginosis:* May be associated with infectious complications of pregnancy, such as chorioamnionitis and puerperal infection, and with polymicrotract infections in nonpregnant women, such as endometritis and salpingitis.
Fungal vaginitis (predominantly *Candida albicans*): Dimorphic fungi, which grow as oval budding yeast cells and as chains of cells (hyphae).	Male sexual partners may develop urethritis, balanitis, or cutaneous lesions on penis.	*Fungal vaginitis:* The presumptive criteria are the typical symptoms of vaginitis or vulvitis and microscopic identification of yeast (budding cells or hyphae) in Gram's stain.	*Fungal vaginitis:* Miconazole nitrate or clotrimazole 100 mg intravaginally daily for 7 days. The medication is available as cream or tablets, and the forms are equally effective; or miconazole nitrate or clotrimazole daily for 3 days; clotrimazole 500 mg tablet intravaginally as a single dose; or	Fungal vaginitis in pregnancy increases the risk of neonatal oral thrush.

(*continued*)

TABLE 8–5. SUMMARY OF THE PRINCIPAL SEXUALLY TRANSMITTED DISEASES *(continued)*

Disease and Etiologic Agents	Typical Clinical Presentation	Presumptive Diagnosis (Warrants full treatment and followup)	Therapy	Complications and Sequelae
Vaginitis *(continued)*			nystatin 100,000-unit tablets, 1 tablet intravaginally daily for 2 weeks.	
Herpes Genitalis *Herpes simplex virus (HSV) types 1 and 2:* DNA viruses that cannot be distinguished clinically.	Single or multiple vesicles appear anywhere on the genitalia. Vesicles spontaneously rupture to form shallow ulcers, which may be very painful. They resolve spontaneously without scarring. The first occurrence is termed *initial infection* (mean duration 12 days). Subsequent, usually milder, occurrences are termed *recurrent infections* (mean duration 4.5 days). The interval between clinical episodes is termed *latency.* Viral shedding occurs intermittently during latency.	When typical genital lesions are present or a pattern of recurrence has developed, herpes infection is likely. A presumptive diagnosis is further supported by direct identification of multinucleated giant cells with intranuclear inclusions in a clinical specimen prepared by Papanicolaou or other histochemical stain; or typical HSV morphology by electron microscopy; or detection of HSV antigens by monoclonal or polyclonal antibody detection systems. (*Note:* Antibody detection systems may detect biologically inactive viral particles.) Primary HSV infection is presumed, if any initially negative serologic titer becomes significantly detectable in convalescent serum.	*First clinical episode:* To reduce the signs and symptoms, use acyclovir 200 mg, PO, 5 times daily for 7 to 10 days, initiated within 6 days of onset of lesions. For clients who have severe symptoms or complications that necessitate hospitalization, an alternative regimen is acyclovir 5 mg/kg of body weight IV every 8 hours for 5 to 7 days. *Recurrent genital herpes:* Acyclovir 200 mg, PO, 5 times daily for 5 days initiated within 2 days of onset. Treatment during pregnancy: Systemic acyolovir should be avoided in pregnant women without life-threatening (disseminated) infection.	*Males and females:* Neuralgia, meningitis ascending myelitis, urethral strictures, and lymphatic suppuration may occur. *Females:* There is possibly an increased risk for cervical cancer and fetal wastage. *Neonates:* Virus from an active genital infection may be transmitted during vaginal delivery causing neonatal herpes infection. Neonatal herpes ranges in severity from clinically inapparent infections to local infections of the eyes, skin, or mucous membranes to severe disseminated infection that may involve the central nervous system. The infection has a high case fatality rate and many survivors have ocular or neurologic sequelae.
Syphilis *Treponema pallidum* spirochete with regular spirals and characteristic motility.	*Primary:* The classical chancre is located at the site of exposure. All genital lesions should be suspected to be syphilitic. *Secondary:* Clients may have a highly variable skin rash, mucous patches, condylomata lata, lymphadenopathy, or other signs. *Latent:* Clients are without clinical signs.	*Primary:* Clients have typical lesion(s) and positive serologic test for syphilis (STS) or their present titer is at least fourfold greater than the last, or there has been syphilis exposure within 90 days of lesion onset. *Secondary:* Clients have the typical clinical presentation and a strongly reactive STS. *Latent:* Clients have serologic evidence of untreated syphilis without clinical signs.	Primary and secondary, or early syphilis treated with benzathine penicillin G, 2.4 million units IM in one dose. Syphilis of indeterminate length or of more than one year's duration: benzathine penicillin G, 7.2 million units total; 2.4 million units IM, weekly, for 3 consecutive wk.	Both late syphilis and congenital syphilis are preventable with prompt diagnosis and treatment of early syphilis. Sequelae of late syphilis includes neurosyphilis (general paresis, tabes dorsalis, and focal neurologic signs), cardiovascular syphilis (thoracic aortic aneuryism, aortic insufficiency), and localized gumma formation.
Human Immunodeficiency Virus (HIV) Infection Also referred to as *acquired immunodeficiency syndrome* (AIDS),	The range of symptoms associated with HIV may extend from mini-	Presumptive diagnosis of HIV infection is usually made on clinical evi-	To date, no treatment has been identified to eradicate the virus or	The outcome in clients with HIV infection is not completely under-

TABLE 8–5. SUMMARY OF THE PRINCIPAL SEXUALLY TRANSMITTED DISEASES (*continued*)

Disease and Etiologic Agents	Typical Clinical Presentation	Presumptive Diagnosis (Warrants full treatment and followup)	Therapy	Complications and Sequelae
Human Immunodeficiency Virus (HIV) (*continued*)				
lymphadenopathy associated virus, and AIDS-related retrovirus. (All are agreed to be the same virus, which contains RNA and is in the retrovirus family.)	mal to the full clinical syndrome of HIV infection. Clients with the clinical syndrome of HIV infection often give a history of nonspecific symptoms for months prior to diagnosis. These symptoms may include easy fatigue, poor appetite, weight loss, lymphadenopathy, diarrhea, fever, and night sweats. Other symptoms specific to opportunistic diseases occur in clients with HIV infection, such as purple to bluish skin lesions associated with Kaposi's sarcoma (KS) or shortness of breath and nonproductive cough resulting from *Pneumocystis carinii* pneumonia (PCP). Symptoms for infants include failure to thrive, lymphadenopathy, hepatosplenomegaly, encephalopathy, pneumocystis carinii pneumonia (PCP), lymphocystic interstitial pneumonia (LIP), recurrent bacterial infection, recurrent diarrhea, kidney and heart failure.	dence, supported by serologic tests for antibodies to HIV. Once an individual is infected, current research suggests the individual remains infected indefinitely and may transmit the infection to others. As yet unidentified factors may influence which infected individuals develop HIV disease and which particular opportunistic illness may occur.	reverse the immunologic dysfunction associated with HIV infection. Standard therapy consists of treating opportunistic diseases aggressively as they occur. AZT suppresses HIV replication and is FDA approved for adults and children. It may slow progress of the disease. Research protocols for experimental drugs such as ddl are being used across the country.	stood. Studies in a cohort of gay men whose serum contained antibodies to HIV showed about 5-10% of these clients were subsequently diagnosed with the clinical syndrome AIDS within 2-5 yr, and another 25% had generalized lymphadenopathy or other HIV-related conditions. The other two thirds of the men were clinically well after 5 yr, although still HIV positive.

PID = pelvic inflammatory disease.
Adapted from Sexually Transmitted Disease Summary 1986. *Washington, D.C.: US Government Printing Office, US Department of Health & Human Services.*

vulvovaginitis; thus women who are premenstrual, in the postpartum period, or who are postmenopausal are also at a higher risk. Gonorrhea is caused by a gram-negative diplococcus and can be diagnosed by history and by microscopic examination after culturing of the organism. Cultures can be taken from the endocervical canal, the rectal area, and the pharyngeal area. Simple treatment with aqueous procaine penicillin and probenecid or its alternatives has been complicated by the growth of penicillin-resistant organisms. Medications such as spectinomycin or cefoxitin are currently used to treat these gonorrheal infections.

Condyloma Acuminatum

One million new infections of the virus-caused genital warts (condyloma acuminatum) are diagnosed annually.[39] These warts are found on the genitalia or the rectum and can be painful. The initial therapy of choice remains the topical application of podophyllin. Surgical removal of the warts is also an option.

Herpes Simplex Virus 2

Genital herpes caused by the herpes simplex virus 2 (HSV-2) accounts for up to 500,000 new cases of sexually transmitted diseases per year and is said to affect 15 percent of American adults.[39] The highest incidence of HSV-2 infection is in adolescent women. The initial infection usually occurs three to seven days after exposure to the virus. The primary infection (the initial illness after exposure) can include diverse symptoms such as fever, headache, malaise, chills, anorexia, or painful urination. The typical lesions of HSV-2 are found on the labia, the perineum, the vulva, the vagina, and the bladder and are initially heralded by burning and numbness. This sensation is followed by vesicles, which rupture and result in shallow, painful ulcers. These initial lesions can last 3 to 6 weeks. The first episode of this chronic illness is generally more severe and longer lasting than recurrences.

After the initial illness, the HSV-2 virus is thought to lie dormant in sensory nerve ganglia and thus can recur throughout the lifetime. Triggers for recurrence have been identified, including menstruation, fever, stress, and infectious illness. There is increased risk for HSV-2 for both the mother and fetus during pregnancy and the neonatal period. The frequency of HSV-2 infections in pregnant women is three times that of nonpregnant women.[44] *See* Chapter 39 for additional discussion of HSV-2 infection during pregnancy.

Finally, women with HSV-2 seem to be at a greater risk for cervical cancer. The symptoms of HSV-2 can be suppressed by acyclovir in oral or systemic form. There is no known cure for HSV-2.

Because of the painful and recurring nature of the disease, and the risk to the mother and fetus during pregnancy, a great deal of publicity about this disease was generated during the early and mid-1980s. Anxiety and stress about the symptoms and sequelae of this STD warrant a great deal of psychosocial support from a caring, sensitive nurse. More positively, for many women who pay attention to lifestyle factors and maintain a healthy therapeutic regimen, many of the symptoms of HSV-2 can be controlled during recurrences.

Cytomegalovirus

Cytomegalovirus (CMV) is transmitted through various routes including both sexual contact and perinatal transmission. It is found in saliva, respiratory secretions, breast milk, cervical secretions, and semen. Many children secrete CMV in their urine. There are 1 million new cases identified annually according to the Centers for Disease Control.[39] Further, 55 percent of young adults have CMV antibodies in their blood. In adults, CMV is thought to pattern itself after HSV-2 in that it probably lies dormant in host tissue indefinitely and is reactivated periodically, and particularly during pregnancy. For adults, even the primary infection is largely asymptomatic. Certain blood and liver function tests mirror mononucleosis infection in the adult, but there is a lack of throat, tonsil, or lymph symptomatology. The transmission of the infection to the fetus, however, results in possible defects in every organ system and subsequent central nervous system dysfunction. The greatest risk to the fetus is from mothers who have a primary infection with CMV. Chapter 39 discusses effects of CMV on the pregnancy and fetus.

Some antiviral chemotherapeutic agents have been evaluated for treatment. Although these drugs show promise, they are highly toxic.

Syphilis

Syphilis accounts for 85,000 new cases of sexually transmitted diseases annually.[39] This represents a 30 percent increase from 1985 to 1987. Over 50 percent of the increases in syphilis were reported from South Florida, California, and New York City.[39] Although increases have occurred in all groups, the greatest increases in syphilis and other diseases are among *young* women and heterosexual men in inner-city black and Hispanic populations.

The *Treponema pallidum* spirochete is transmitted by sexual contact, blood transfusion, or accidental inoculation to the adult, and transplacentally to the fetus. In the adult, depending on the type of sexual contact experienced, the painless ulcer or chancre (the initial sign of syphilis) may be found on the lip, tongue, nipple, fingers, anus, or genital area 10 to 90 days after exposure. Many syphilitic ulcers are atypical, so genital lesions should be considered suspicious.[43]

Six weeks after the primary chancre the secondary stage occurs and frequently includes a generalized rash. For the first 2 to 4 years after initial exposure there may be recurrences. During this time, the so-called early latency period, the individual is infectious to other individuals and to the fetus. The later stages present a much lowered risk of communicability. Syphilis is diagnosed through the screening blood tests, such as Venereal Disease Research Laboratories (VDRL), or rapid plasma reagent (RPR), followed by a confirmatory Fluorescent Treponemal Antibody Absorption (FTA) test. Syphilis is treated with benzathine penicillen G, aqueous procaine penicillin, tetracycline, or erythromycin. Untreated congenital syphilis in the infant results in high mortality rates and in multiple body system pathology.

Vaginitis

Several types of vaginitis are included as STDs. They are those caused by *Trichomonas vaginalis* and *Hemophilis vaginalis* (now known as *Gardnerella vaginalis*), and candidal vulvovaginitis. Trichomonas infection is caused by a unicellular protozoan and results in vaginal discharge (30 percent of women have this complaint).[43] The vaginal discharge has been described as profuse, frothy, and malodorous. Small hemorrhages of the cervix give the cervix the classical "strawberry" appearance. Pruritus and dysuria may also be symptoms resulting from infection with this organism, which frequently resides in the vagina, the urethra, the bladder, and Skene's glands. As many as 60 percent of women who have gonorrhea are also found to have trichomoniasis. Women presenting with symptoms of either infection should be evaluated for both. The usual diagnosis of *Trichomonas vaginalis* infection is made by microscopic examination of a saline wet-mount in which motile trichomonads are seen. The recommended treatment is 2 g (in a single dose) of metronidazole therapy. This is *not* recommended during pregnancy—particularly, the first 20 weeks of pregnancy. Alternative iodine preparations also pose a risk to the fetus because excessive absorption of iodine may result in suppression of the fetal thyroid. Metronidazole therapy is also controversial because of a possible link to cancers.

Candidiasis actually results from an overgrowth of organisms present in 25 percent of women's normal vaginal flora. *Candida albicans*, a saprophytic fungus, causes 90 percent of yeast infections. It frequently coexists with trichomoniasis. Symptoms in some women include intense pruritus, and a cheesy-white curd-like discharge. Many women do not have this discharge. Often, but not always, the vagina will be bright red with white plaques. The overgrowth of *Candida* is attributed to changes in host factors. Frequent triggers, which alter host resistance and thus result in infection, include pregnancy, diabetes, use of broad spectrum antibiotics, and HIV infection. Diagnosis of monilial infection is by Gram's stain or by wet-mount examination under the microscope. The treatment of choice is local vaginal therapy, particularly miconazole nitrate and clotrimazole. There is a possibility of fetal teratology, even though limited absorption occurs, so this medication is not advised during the first 20 weeks of pregnancy.

Bacterial vaginosis results from the overgrowth of the organism *Gardnerella vaginalis* (formerly called *Hemophilis vaginalis*). This infection is typically identified by its fishy foul odor and a yellow-gray vaginal discharge. The vaginal wall appears normal. It is diagnosed by the presence of "clue cells" under the microscope, a pH greater than 4.5, and its fishy odor. Clue cells are vaginal epithelial cells to which gram-negative organisms are attached. The most effective treatment is metronidazole.

Human Immunodeficiency Virus

An in-depth discussion of infection with HIV (human immunodeficiency virus) is inappropriate in this chapter; however, it is a life-threatening STD affecting the mother, infant, family, and society. Infection with HIV causes HIV disease, the terminal phase of which is acquired immunodeficiency syndrome (AIDS). As with the epidemiology of other STDs, a high-risk group for infection with HIV is the inner-city, disadvantaged minority population, primarily black and Hispanic. Intravenous drug use or homosexuality are critical lifestyle factors contributing to the increased likelihood of HIV infection.

To be considered HIV-positive, an individual must test positive for the HIV antibody three times (twice with the ELISA screening test and once with the more specific, and expensive, Western blot test). A positive result means that an individual is considered infected for life and can transmit the virus to

ISSUES AND CONTROVERSIES

Several controversial issues concern sexuality. Some of these focus on preventive programs for sexually transmitted diseases, such as HIV infection. Questions are asked as to when children should be taught about sexually transmitted diseases, and by whom. Is sex education the responsibility of the parents, the school, or a combination of both? Should condoms be distributed to teenagers in school? What is the responsibility of personnel in family planning clinics concerning prevention of sexually transmitted diseases?

The AIDS epidemic has ushered in many ethical and moral issues, especially in the area of sexuality and reproduction. (1) Should all pregnant women be tested for the HIV antibody? Currently, such testing is voluntary. (2) What responsibility do health care workers have to inform partners of clients who test positive for HIV? (3) Who should be informed if an individual tests positive for the HIV antibody? (4) Should health care workers be required to care for clients who test positive for the HIV antibody, or have HIV infection? Nurses who work with childbearing families at risk for HIV infection need to take leadership roles in coordinating care and educating support people in the community. They also must serve as advocates for these clients. Facts should substitute for myths. These facts can be found in several publications from the Surgeon General's office.

others, even if he or she has no symptoms. If the individual tests negative, there is still the possibility that he or she will convert to an antibody-positive status. The time lag between when a person is exposed to the virus and develops antibodies may be as long as 6 months.

For the childbearing family, fetal infection can be the result of maternal transmission from an infected mother who was infected through her own intravenous drug use or through heterosexual contact with an intravenous drug user.[46]

Heterosexual transmission from an IV-drug–using male partner to a non-IV-drug–using sexual partner occurs in about 40 percent of cases. Transmission can occur after only one at-risk sexual encounter or after repeated contact over several years. There is a likelihood of increased risk of infection in conditions in which blood is present or tissue is damaged such as cervicitis, vaginitis, or menstruation.[47]

A large percentage (52 percent) of women with HIV infection are intravenous drug users themselves. Because intravenous-drug-using women may have limited social or economic resources, prostitution may be a means of support for the drug habit and family, thus, contributing to the double risk of infection from contaminated needles or heterosexual transmission. It is estimated that three quarters of the HIV-infected children were infected through perinatal transmission. Perinatal transmission is as of yet poorly understood. Three typical models are suggested: transplacental passage, contact with maternal blood or vaginal secretions during labor and delivery, and postpartum ingestion of breast milk.

The frequency of perinatal transmission when the mother is HIV positive is considered to be approximately 50 percent, although a range of 20 to 60 percent has been found. Both symptomatic and asymptomatic infected mothers can transmit HIV to their infants; HIV can be transmitted in more than one pregnancy; and each infant is at risk of developing HIV infection.[47] *See* Chapter 39 for additional information on HIV infection during pregnancy.

For nurses, information regarding HIV infection and other STDs cannot be separated from the emotional response evoked by individuals concerned about HIV or AIDS. One report concluded that even considering whether to be tested constitutes a crisis in a person's life—a crisis that is exacerbated if the results are positive and by no means ended if the results are negative.[46]

Many of the individuals confronted by HIV infection have already experienced social isolation and rejection because of a deviant lifestyle, poverty, or minority status. Their social, economic, and educational resources are limited. This is the background from which they face another crisis. Denial, anger, fear, somatization, sexual dysfunction, depression, and thoughts of suicide are a range of anticipated emotional responses to the possibility of HIV infection. Mothers who give birth to children infected with HIV experience guilt and grief. A sophisticated complex assessment and management plan for this illness is a challenge for all health professionals and warrants in-depth attention.

According to Siegel, education regarding means of transmission remains the most important public health strategy for controlling the spread of HIV.[48] These educational efforts should be particularly targeted at groups with high-risk behaviors for whom the message should be simple, direct, clear, and culturally specific. It has been suggested that if childbearing-age women who are at high risk for HIV infection would avoid pregnancy, there would eventually be no new cases of pediatric HIV[49]; however, advising these women not to become pregnant is controversial and may reflect the caregiver's bias. HIV is associated with high-risk behaviors, not with specific groups or individuals.

The Surgeon General's Workshop Report recommended vigorous expansion of HIV antibody testing and counseling to all pregnant women as early in pregnancy as possible.[46] Because of the delay in seroconversion and also the possibility of new exposure to an HIV-infected individual, some authorities suggest that testing should be repeated in the third trimester of pregnancy.

Particular education, counseling, and intervention programs should be aimed at substance abusers, who are projected to account for a substantially rising proportion of new cases of HIV infection, certainly affecting women and children with HIV.

Health Education and Sexually Transmitted Diseases

The Surgeon General has identified STDs as one of 15 health priority areas for national prevention and control. The following important priorities are: (1) to reduce the incidence of gonorrhea, syphilis, and gonococcal pelvic inflammatory disease; (2) to provide accurate and timely education about STDs to every junior and senior high school student; and, (3) to train health care providers so that 95 percent will be capable of diagnosing and treating all currently recognized STDs.[42]

Some of the key activities identified by a World Health Organization/Pan American Health Organization Scientific Group include (1) health education; (2) disease detection; (3) appropriate treatment; (4) partner tracing and client counseling; (5) clinical service evaluation; (6) training; and (7) research.

Though nurses should be involved in all of these activities, it is clear from past experience that one professional or one strategy alone will not solve the problem of HIV infection, STDs, or drug abuse. Instead, multifaceted, multisensorial, and multidisciplinary approaches have the greatest hopes for success. The "Just Say No" campaign has not been a successful strategy to contain drug-related AIDS.

Health education is a broad mandate to be implemented at the primary, secondary, or tertiary level of prevention. Health education at the primary prevention level includes providing information about STDs, the mode of transmission, and healthy protective behaviors aimed at reducing the incidence of such diseases. Health education strategies need to be creative and developmentally, culturally, educationally, and linguistically appropriate: posters, brochures, telephone audiotapes, ads in school newspapers, films, classes led by peer educators, classes using a variety of techniques such as role playing, group discussions, one-to-one teaching contacts, and an essay assignment in which drugs or AIDS is the topic are all examples of the ways that health education may be implemented. Education is aimed at multiple target populations and should be appropriate for low-risk groups, high-risk groups, and parents or spouses of high- or low-risk groups. In particular, educational strategies must be devised to reach adolescents, who because of their developmental stage are seen as the "next wave" of the HIV epidemic.

Professional nurses, through careful history taking, symptom analysis, observation and recording of physical findings, and referral contribute to disease detection. Nurses facilitate treatment through the education, monitoring, and follow-up of clients' cooperation with the medical regimen, addressing supportive measures that will facilitate treatment, (such as fluid intake and hygiene practices), and fostering healthy lifestyle behaviors. These are traditional nursing roles. Nurses will broaden their role by carefully investigating treatment cooperation issues, modifying regimens accordingly, and evaluating new approaches that enhance treatment cooperation and ensure the practice of safe sex in the future. The contacting and treatment of sexual partners is an important adjunct to treatment. The nurse focuses on the responses of the client to treatment as well as on monitoring the response of the client's support system or family to the detection and treatment regimen. Pregnancy poses a particular health risk to the mother because of increased susceptibility to disease and contraindications to certain drug therapies. It is also a substantial health risk to the fetus. Active anticipatory education and counseling related to this lifecycle phase is warranted.

Furthermore, the nurse has a responsibility to influence policy making through such community roles as parent, politically involved voter and lobbyist, PTA member, member of community organizations, and Girl Scout or Boy Scout leader. The problem of HIV infections or STDs or drug abuse will not be solved by a superlative 20-minute presentation by a nurse but by a widespread distribution of information and acknowledgement by all of society that this is a problem our adult members and children must address. Certainly nursing, together with other groups and individuals, has a key role to play in this endeavor.

TAKING A SEXUAL HISTORY

Taking a sexual history is a skill that the nurse develops with experience. Acquiring the ability to gather the most relevant information in a timely manner in the context of a warm, open, trusting relationship is indeed a valued achievement. Taking a sexual history incorporates all the skills necessary for taking a nursing history along with additional sensitivity. In our culture, for the most part, sexual information is private; there is an unwillingness to share and trust this information to others. Our sexual self-esteem is closely related to some of our core self-concepts: male, female, masculinity, femininity. The sharing of problems and conflicts in this area should be valued and treated as confidential. The individual's need for self-worth must be respected.

If a sexual problem is suspected or identified, a more thorough sexual history is warranted for the purpose of identifying a long-term or situational problem. Focusing on the whole picture aids the nurse in deciding if external stress, such as financial worries, may be spilling over to affect the sexual relationship or if the primary problem resides in the sexual relationship. More appropriate consultation or referral can be made with this complete information. Achieving openness in communication between nurse and client about sexual matters is aided by the health professional's awareness of her or his own self on the sexual continuum, comfort with his or her unfolding or maturing sexuality, and the resulting ability to learn to communicate with others in this area.

Pomeroy suggested other specific strategies when taking a sex history.[50] Assume everyone does everything; give positive feedback to the individual; and follow the lead of the respondent, that is, listen carefully to the client's messages about what concerns her or him. Though a skilled interviewer avoids using ambiguous euphemisms like "making love" for vaginal intercourse, it is important to be familiar with and use when appropriate the special vocabularies of cultural or economic groups like "prick" (for penis) or "cunt" (for vagina). It is also important to know what particular sexual customs and norms predominate in these special groups. For example, in some Hispanic cultures, it is essential that a woman be a virgin when she marries. Thus, before she is married, she may engage in anal rather than vaginal intercourse.

Other suggestions include validating the client's responses by clarifying and restating the question or response and avoiding statements such as "everyone does that."

Depending on the setting, checklists and standard forms can aid in sexual history taking (Table 8–6). This base-line data gathered from standard forms can open doors for more deeply probing questions. A Planned Parenthood agency will have such a form; a postpartum unit may need to add sexuality as an assessment or educational area to the history form.

Important general categories for a nurse to assess include any change in the individual's experience of sexuality. Evaluating the biologic health of the individual's genitourinary tract will include assessment of appropriate variations as a result of developmental differences. Information in this category includes menstrual regularity or symptoms of infections or normal states of postpartum changes in the genitourinary tract. Information related to means of sexual expression includes type of sexual behavior (masturbation, vaginal intercourse), sexual orientation, frequency, and number of partners. Satisfaction with sexual expression and past and current biologic health is another important area to assess. Assessment of prevention and STD protective behaviors, where appropriate, are also important.

TABLE 8–6. SEXUAL HISTORY COMPONENTS

General physical, developmental, and lifestyle factors
Past history of systemic illness, eg, diabetes
History of sexually transmitted diseases, eg, vaginitis
Progression of physical sexual maturity (eg, onset of menarche, regularity of menses)
Past history of contraceptives, abortions, losses
Current review of symptoms
Nutrition, drugs, and alcohol use
Psychosocial factors
Progression through and accomplishment of age-appropriate psychosocial tasks
Body image, satisfaction with physical appearance
Self-concept, self-evaluations re: gender, femininity or masculinity, etc
Past parent-child relationship, attitudes and values conveyed toward sex
Quality of current intimate relationships
Past sexual activity
Age of first intercourse
Frequency
Types of sexual contact
Partners, number, ages, sex
Problems and satisfaction and orgasmic competency
Current sexuality related to childbearing
Attitudes or myths or knowledge related to sexuality and childbearing
Change in frequency
Change in sexual interest
Techniques of intercourse
Satisfaction and problems
Spouse agreements or differences

SUMMARY

Sexuality is an integral aspect of human functioning across the life span. Concepts such as masculinity, femininity, androgyny, biologic gender, and sex-role behaviors are important in an understanding of sexuality. Research on sexuality has added to knowledge of the human sexual response cycle in both men and women and has shed light on the changes in sexual response during pregnancy.

Societal and cultural changes over the past two decades have led to a growing incidence of sexually transmitted diseases, such as *Chlamydia trachomatis*, gonorrhea, condyloma acuminatum, genital herpes, cytomegalovirus, syphilis, and vaginitis. The most dramatic example of an STD is the current HIV epidemic.

Nursing responsibilities related to sexuality include taking a sexual history, counseling clients concerning sexual expression and safe sex practices, and planning consumer programs concerned with prevention of sexually transmitted diseases. Nurses also can be instrumental in determining policies on the institutional, local, and national level related to sexuality.

REVIEW QUESTIONS

1. Compare and contrast the following concepts: gender, masculinity, femininity, sex role, and sex-role behaviors.
2. Describe the physiological changes during pregnancy that have contributed to a variation in human sexual responsiveness.
3. Identify the principal sexually transmitted diseases.
4. Discuss the role of nurses in preventing and treating sexually transmitted diseases.
5. Outline key aspects of a sexual history.

REFERENCES

1. World Health Organization. Education and treatment in Human Sexuality: The Training of Health Professionals, report of a World Health Organization meeting. Technical Report Series, No. 372. Geneva: World Health Organization, 1975.
2. Woods NF. Towards a holistic perspective of human sexuality: alterations in sexual health and nursing diagnosis. *Holistic Nurs Prac.* 1987;1:1–11.
3. Lenz E, et al. Sex role attributes, gender, and postpartal perceptions of the marital relationship. *ANS.* 1987;7:49–62.
4. Skolnick A. *The Intimate Environment Exploring Marriage and the Family.* Boston: Little, Brown, 1973;158–175.
5. Money J. *Sex role learning in childhood and adolescence.* Read before the American Association for Advancement of Science meetings, Washington DC, 1972.
6. Maccoby E, Jacklin C. *The Psychology of Sex Differences.* Stanford, Cal.; Stanford University Press, 1974.
7. Fausto-Sterling A. *Myths of Gender.* New York: Basic Books, 1985.
8. Miller J. *Toward a New Psychology of Women.* Boston: Beacon Press, 1989.
9. Wiggins J, Holzmuller A. Further evidence on adrongeny and interpersonal flexibility. *J Res Pers* 1981;15:67–80.
10. Whitney B. Sex role orientation and self-esteem: a critical meta-analytic review. *J Pers Soc Psychol.* 1983;44:765–778.
11. Whiting BB, Whiting IWN. *Children of Six Cultures.* Cambridge, Mass: Harvard University Press, 1975.
12. Stephens WN. *The Family in Cross-Cultural Perspective.* New York: Holt, Reinhart, and Winston, 1963.
13. Masters WH, Johnson VE. *Human Sexual Response.* Boston: Little, Brown, 1966.
14. Masters WH, Johnson VE. *Human Sexual Inadquacy.* Boston: Little, Brown, 1970.
15. Kinsey AC, et al. *Sexual Behavior in the Human Male.* Philadelphia: WB Saunders, 1948.
16. Kaplan H. *Disorders of Sexual Desire.* New York: Brunner/Mazel, 1979.
17. Masters WH, et al. *Human Sexuality.* Boston: Little, Brown, 1982.
18. Sherfey MJ. *The Nature and Evaluation of Human Sexuality.* New York: Random House, 1973.
19. Perry JD, Whipple B. Pelvic muscle strength of female ejaculators: evidence in support of a new theory of orgasm. *J Sex Res.* 1981;17:22–39.
20. Singer J, Singer I. Types of female orgasm. *J Sex Res.* 1973;8:255–267.
21. Calderone M, Johnson E. *The Family Book About Sexuality.* New York: Bantam Books, 1983.
22. Gesell, et al. *Infant and Child in the Culture of Today.* New York: Harper & Row, 1974.
23. Kaplan L. *Adolescence: The Farewell to Childhood.* New York: Simon & Schuster, 1984.
24. Havinghurst RJ. *Developmental Tasks and Education.* New York: Longmans, Green, 1972.
25. Erikson EH. *Childhood and Society.* 2nd ed. New York: WW Norton, 1963.
26. Kriepe RE. Prevention of adolescent pregnancy: a developmental approach. In McAnarney ER: *Premature Adolescent Pregnancy and Parenthood.* New York: Grune & Stratton, 1983, p 37–59.
27. Sarrel L, Sarrel P. *Sexual Turning Points.* New York: Macmillan Co, 1984.
28. Solberg, et al. Sexual behavior in pregnancy. *N Engl J Med.* 1973;288:1098–1102.
29. Battacchi M. Personality and stress factors in women's sexuality in pregnancy. In Carenzo L, et al. eds: *Clinical Psychoneuroendocrinology in Reproduction.* New York: Academic Press, 1978.
30. Robson K, et al. Maternal sexuality during first pregnancy and after childbirth. *Br J Obstet Gynecol* 1981;88:882–889.
31. Goodlin RC, et al. Orgasm during late pregnancy: possible deleterious effects. *Obstet Gynecol.* 1971;38:916.
32. Goodlin RC, et al. Uterine tension and fetal heart rate during maternal orgasm. *Obstet Gynecol.* 1972;39:148–153.
33. Klebanoff, et al. Coitus during pregnancy: is it safe? *Lancet.* 1984;10:914–916.
34. Aronson ME, Nelson PK. Fetal air embolism in pregnancy resulting from an unusual sex act. *Obstet Gynecol.* 1967; 30:127–131.
35. Wolkind S, Zajicek E. *Pregnancy: A Psychological and Social Study.* New York: Grune & Stratton, 1981.
36. May K. Men's sexuality during the childbearing year: implications of recent research findings. *Holistic Nurs Prac.* 1987;1:60–66.
37. Fein R. The first weeks of fathering: the important choices and supports for new parents. *Birth Fam J.* 1976;3:53–57.
38. Wandersman L. The adjustment of fathers to their first baby: the roles of parenting groups and marital relationship. *Birth Fam J.* 1980;3:151–161.
39. Leary W. Rare venereal diseases increase sharply. *New York Times.* July 13, 1988, p 35.
40. Rogers M. *Pediatric HIV infection: epidemiology, etiopathogenesis and transmission. Pediatr Ann.* 1988;17:324–331.
41. US Department of Health and Human Services. 1989 sexually transmitted diseases treatment guidelines. *MMWR.* 1989;38:S8.
42. Cates W, Holme K. *Public Health and Preventive Medicine.* 12th ed. 1986, 257–295.
43. Eschenback D. Pelvic infections. In Danford D, Scott J (eds): *Obstetrics and Gynecology.* 5th ed. Philadelphia: J.B. Lippincott Co, 1986.
44. Edwards MS. Venereal herpes: a nursing overview. *J Obstet Gynecol Nurs.* 1978;7(S):7–15.
45. Fogel C. The gynecologic triad: discharge, pain, bleeding. In Fogel C, Words N (eds): *Health Care of Women.* St Louis: C.V. Mosby 1981.
46. First Interdisciplinary conference on HIV Antibody Testing and Counseling. *Report of the Surgeon General's Workshop,* 1987.
47. Rogers M. Transmission of human immunodeficiency virus infection. In the *Report of the US Surgeon General's Workshop.* Washington, D.C.: US Government Printing Office, 1987, 17–19.
48. Siegel K. Education to prevent HIV infection. In *Report of the Surgeon General's Workshop.* Washington, D.C.: US Government Printing Office, 1987, 35–40.
49. Oleske J, et al. A perspective on pediatric AIDS. *Pediatr Ann.* 1988;17:319–323.
50. Pomeroy W, et al. *Taking a Sex History.* New York: Free Press, 1982; pp 9–23.

Planning a Family

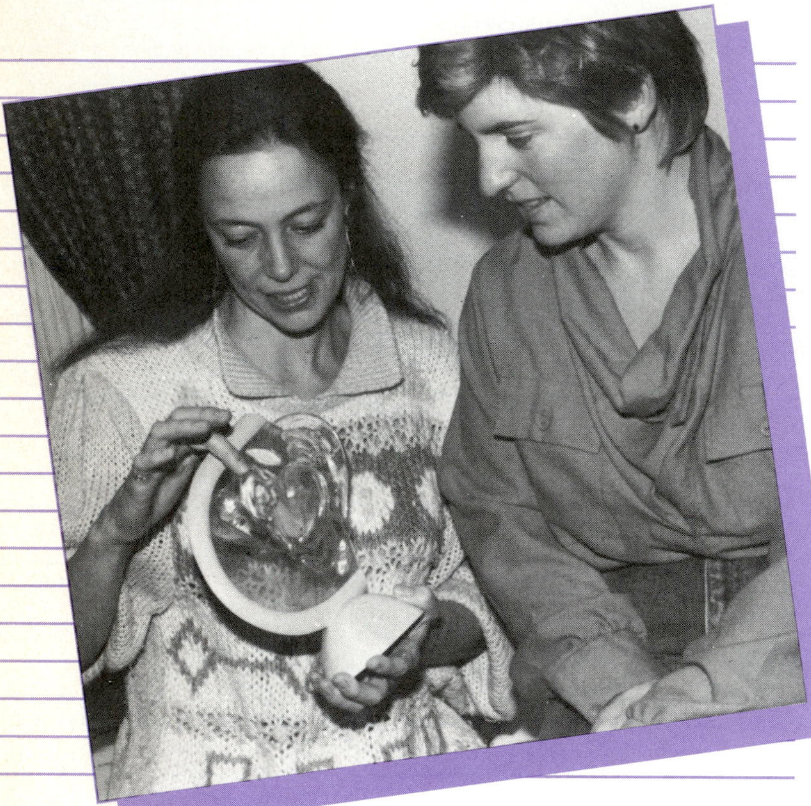

Chapter 9

Key Terms

bilateral tubal ligation
calendar method
cervical cap
coitus interruptus
condom
diaphragm
dilation and curettage
dilation and evacuation
douching
hysterotomy
intrauterine device
menstrual extraction
minipill
morning-after pill
oral contraceptives
postovulation method
prostaglandin instillation
saline termination
spermicidal agents
sympto-thermal method
thermal (cervical mucus) method
vacuum aspiration
vaginal sponge
vasectomy

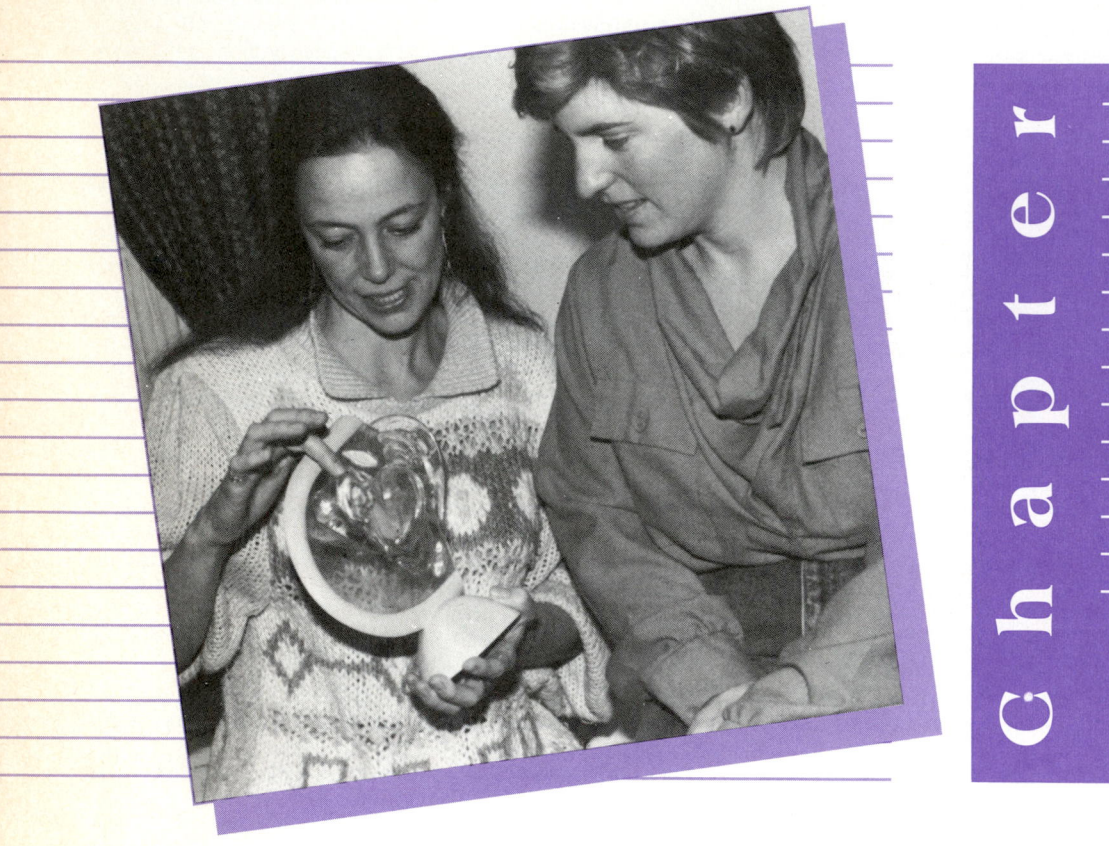

There has been a tremendous growth in world population in the 20th century. In 1900, world population was 1.5 billion people. Current estimates suggest that in the year 2000, the population will have quadrupled to 6 billion people.[1] In 1985 the population growth rate was 1.69 percent per year. If the current growth rate continues or declines only slightly, 100 years from now the world's population will quadruple again to almost 26 billion people.[2] Such continued growth will certainly stretch the earth's carrying capacity to its limits.

Most individuals or couples considering reproduction are not aware of these statistics. They are primarily interested in achieving their reproductive goals and not concerned about world population. It is important, however, for all members of society to be familiar with the overpopulation problem, especially as it affects the health and well-being of all humankind.

Conception control is not a new concept. Both women and men have been concerned for some time about controlling their own reproduction. Attempts at conception control date back at least 5000 years. Poisonous, deadly, often ineffective substances were used orally by both men and women and vaginally by women to prevent pregnancy from occurring or continuing. Most couples have at some time during their lives sought freedom from the risk of pregnancy. It was not until the late 1800s and early 1900s, however, that women themselves became active in the birth control movement. It was not until the 1960s that birth control methods were openly discussed with women in health care settings.[3]

The concept of the two-child family has had increasing support among women of childbearing age in the United States.[4] The United States fertility rate (number of children per woman) has dropped below replacement levels, declining from a high of 3.68 in 1957 to 1.80 in 1983.[5] There is a changing social value system that encourages smaller family size. Other factors that may be influencing this trend include changing lifestyles, economic factors, improved contraceptive technology, and better methods of communicating information about contraceptive methods to the total population. Thus people are more likely to demand access to information about contraceptive technologies as a part of their health care services.

The terms "birth control," "contraception," and "family planning" have often been used interchangeably. The term "family planning" or more recently the term "planning a family" encompasses the broadest concepts. It includes assessing the genetic, physical, psychosocial, and theological concerns of individuals or couples considering reproduction. It also involves seeking solutions to infertility, controlling when a pregnancy occurs, and voluntary interruption of pregnancy. The terms "birth control" and "contraception" generally refer to the methods employed to avoid or space pregnancies. "Planning a family" is a relatively new concept. It is one, however, that should be incorporated into each nurse's practice.

REPRODUCTIVE DECISION MAKING

"It used to be so simple: women and men married and engaged in sexual intercourse, which usually resulted in pregnancy."[6] Human reproduction was characterized primarily by one feature—chance. Today, however, human reproduction is quite different. The primary characteristic at this time is not chance, but choice. Today couples may choose to become parents without choosing to marry or they may choose to be sexually active and avoid unintended pregnancies or births.[6]

Despite the reproductive options available to people today, analysis of survey data from both 1975 and 1980 provides continuing evidence that the majority of women can still be expected to have a first child eventually. The data continue to show that most women in the United States will probably have two children in their lifetime and that their childbearing will be compressed into an ever-narrowing span of time. Thus there is strong evidence that family size in the United States is becoming increasingly limited to no, one, or two children.[7]

Reproductive decisions today are based on complex value systems in which alternatives are considered, each having its own risks, benefits, and uncertainties.[8] Procreative drive, intelligence, educational background, career goals, financial considerations, and ethical, moral, and religious beliefs are all factors considered in reproductive decision making. Many women who practice contraception continue to regard the possibility of getting pregnant and having a baby with some positive feelings. Some women also associate the practice of contraception with some negative feelings. Thus many women have to maintain a balance of conflicting emotions that on any given occasion may determine the use or nonuse of their contraceptive method.[9] At any one time there may be the motivation to avoid conception being weighed against the perceived risk of conception occurring. Other factors that may influence a woman's use or nonuse of a contraceptive method are the attitudes of her partner or even of extended community members, such as close friends and other family members.

Procreative drive is the innate desire for children. This desire may be predetermined by cultural and personal influences and may be fixed in early childhood. It is determined by both individual experience in the family and by more widespread cultural influences of society and the individual's specific ethnic or religious group. The desire for children may vary with time, place, socioeconomics, race, and religious beliefs.[8]

Financial considerations are becoming increasingly significant in today's reproductive decision making. The cost of raising a single child in an affluent society is considered prohibitive by some. Raising two or three children is more than many are willing to undertake financially.

Reproductive Decision Making for Couples Identified To Be at Risk

When a coupled is identified to have an increased risk of having a child with a birth defect or genetic disorder, this risk becomes an important factor that influences their reproductive decision-making process. Past experience with a disorder and subjective interpretation of risk are two factors that highly influence such a couple's reproductive decision making.

Subjective interpretation of risk by a couple is influenced by many factors. The same objective risk may mean different things to different people and in fact may mean different things to the same person at different times in his or her life.[8] What one person considers a high risk may be a low or acceptable risk to another.

One factor that may influence risk perception is past experience with the "odds." Many couples believe that a 1 percent risk of having a child with Down's syndrome is low. But a 20-year old couple's risk of having a child with Down's syndrome is approximately 1 in 2000; if they happen to be the 1 in 2000 that has already had one affected child, they may not feel reassured that their risk of having another affected child is less than 1 percent. In fact, if either parent is a translocation carrier, the chances of having another affected child is increased significantly (1 in 5 if the mother is a carrier and 1 in 20 if the father is a carrier). In this case, the couple's risk is higher than it was before their first affected child was born, because having one Down's child increases the chance of having a second affected child.

A second factor that may influence risk interpretation is the nature and severity of the disorder for which the family is at risk. A 50 percent risk of having a child with extra fingers would not likely have the impact on a couple's reproductive decision making that a 2 to 3 percent risk of having a child with a neural tube defect might have. A 5 percent risk of having a child who will survive for many years with severe mental retardation may have much more significance for a couple than a 25 percent risk of having a child who will die shortly after birth.

Past experience with the disorder may also have a significant impact on the couple's subjective interpretation of risk. If a woman herself has lived with a cleft of the lip and palate, how she felt about her own birth defect while growing up may directly influence how she perceives a 3 percent risk of her having a similarly affected child. A woman who is identified to be a carrier of Duchenne muscular dystrophy who has watched her brother die with this disorder will be directly influenced by how her parents and other family members dealt with her brother's degenerative condition.

It is important for nurses to be aware that their own interpretation of risk may also influence a couple's reproductive decision making. The manner in which risk figures are expressed is important and may influence a couple's reproductive choices. A risk may be presented as a 1 in 4 risk, a 25 percent risk, or a 3 to 1 chance against having an affected child. When presenting risk figures to families it may be helpful to present both absolute and relative risk figures. In communicating to a couple that their risk of having a child with a birth defect is 1 percent, it should be remembered that the same couple's risk may be one hundred times greater than the general population risk; thus it may be important for them to hear this risk figure in more than one way. It is also important for the nurse to inform the couple that their specific risk must be added to the 3 percent general population risk that any reproducing couple faces of having a child with a birth defect.

In counseling families who are at risk of having children with birth defects or genetic disorders, it should be kept in mind that a decision regarding reproductive behavior must not be unduly influenced by the health care provider. It is important for nurses to be supportive, nonjudgmental, and nondirective in the counseling that they provide. Nurses are responsible for ensuring that the information a couple receives is factually correct and presented in a sensitive manner. It is also important to allow adequate time for questions and discussion when a couple receives this information. Follow-up supportive counseling should be offered to the family as well. Nurses can help couples sort through the information available to them and support them in the reproductive decisions that they make.

ASSESSMENT OF RISK IN THE REPRODUCING COUPLE

A pregnancy at risk is one in which there is an increased chance of morbidity or mortality for the mother, fetus, or infant. A pregnancy is also considered high-risk when a pregnancy is unplanned or undesired or the individual or couple is unable to adequately care for the child economically, socially, or psychologically.[10]

Provider Responsibilities

Identification of families at risk and the communication of this risk are expected behaviors in the provision of health care today. There have been a number of court cases in which health care providers have been held liable for not identifying families at risk.[11] Courts now recognize wrongful conception claims of parents who seek damages after the birth of a healthy but unplanned child born as a result of a failed sterilization or abortion or the improper filling of a birth control prescription.[12] Thus there is legal precedent that health care providers have responsibility to ensure access to competent and comprehensive family planning services. They also have the responsibility to assess common risk factors and to provide correct information about reproductive risks that are identified. Nurses must be able to provide specific, accurate, and understandable information to clients so that they may make informed reproductive decisions. Nurses should not attempt to influence reproductive decisions according to their own values or desires. Information should be provided regarding reproductive alternatives in an environment that is as value-free as possible.

Approaches to Risk Assessment

There are a number of approaches that are useful in identifying individuals or couples at risk. These include obtaining a thorough family history, assessing psychosocial factors, identifying parental age and racial and ethnic background, and discussing of maternal health history, past reproductive history, and when applicable, a history of the present pregnancy.

Family Health History. When an individual or couple considering reproduction seeks care, it is important to obtain a thorough family history, which may give clues to their risk status. Specific questions about individual family members should be asked regarding the health status of all first-degree (parent, child, and siblings) and second-degree (half-siblings, grandparent, aunt, uncle, niece) relatives. Of concern would be the identification of a history of multiple miscarriages, stillbirths, children who are born with birth defects or who have died at a young age, any pathologic condition that occurred more than once in a family, or any known genetic disorders. If the family history reveals that this pregnancy is the result of a consanguineous mating (mating between individuals related by blood), the risk of having a child with a genetic disorder may be increased.

Psychosocial Factors. Low level of education, low socioeconomic status, and associated poor nutrition and limited access to prenatal care increase a couple's risk of having a low birth weight child. Occupation is often related to socioeconomic status. The highest incidence of perinatal loss, in families in which the father is present, occurs when the father is in semiskilled labor or a manual occupation. The lowest loss rate occurs when the father is a professional or a farmer. The highest incidence of perinatal loss, however, occurs in families in which the father is absent.[10]

Racial and Ethnic Background. It is also important to identify both racial and ethnic background, because perinatal risk is increased in specific groups (*see* Chapters 37, 38, and 39). In addition, some genetic disorders are associated with a specific ethnic group. These are included in Table 9–1.

Parental Age. Advancing maternal age is associated with an increasing risk of having children with chromosome abnormalities (*see* discussion in Chapter 7). Recent studies, however, suggest that there is a small but increasing risk for single-gene abnormalities associated with advancing paternal age. Maternal age of less than 17 is a risk factor associated with low birth weight. An adolescent father often provides a poor or even no support system for the mother or the child.

Maternal Health History. Women who have low weight for height or chronic hypertension are at risk of having children with low birth weight.[13] Maternal metabolic disorders such as juvenile onset insulin-dependent diabetes increase a woman's risk two- to threefold of having a child with a birth defect. Genetic disorders such as maternal myotonic dystrophy or maternal phenylketonuria (PKU) can result in the birth of an infant with significant health or learning problems.

Intake of prescription drugs such as certain anticoagulants, anticonvulsants, and antineoplastic agents have been shown to damage the developing baby. Nonprescription drugs such as alcohol and cigarettes can be harmful as well. Table 9–2 summarizes some of the drugs known to be teratogenic. (Fetal teratogens are described in detail in Chapter 11.)

TABLE 9–1. GENETIC DISORDERS ASSOCIATED WITH SPECIFIC RACIAL AND ETHNIC GROUPS

Genetic Disorder	Racial or Ethnic Group	Carrier Frequency	Incidence
Cystic fibrosis	Caucasians	1 in 20	1 in 600
Tay-Sachs disease	Ashkenazi Jews	1 in 25	1 in 2500
Sickle cell anemia	Blacks	1 in 10	1 in 400
Thalassemia	Mediterraneans	1 in 25	1 in 2500

Reproductive History. An individual or couple's past reproductive history should be reviewed, including information about reproduction with other partners. Of specific concern is the identification of recurrent fetal wastage, previous children who were born preterm or with low birth weight, stillborn, malformed, or who have since died.

History of the Present Pregnancy. An interpregnancy interval of less than 6 months increases a woman's risk of having a baby with low birth weight. Poor nutrition and poor weight gain are other crucial risk factors that have been identified, along with multiple gestation, preeclampsia, eclampsia, oligohydramnios or polyhydramnios, and bleeding during pregnancy.[13]

Assessment of exposure to potential teratogens is important. Women who during their pregnancy have had infectious diseases such as rubella are at risk of having a child with major birth defect problems including cataracts, congenital blindness, microcephaly, hearing loss, spasticity, mental retardation,

TABLE 9–2. EXAMPLES OF DRUGS KNOWN TO BE TERATOGENIC

Alcohol
Anticancer drugs (e.g., methotrexate)
Coumarin derivatives (e.g., Coumadin)
Diethylstilbestrol
Isotretinoin (i.e., retinoic acid)
Phenytoin (e.g., Dilantin)
Oxazolidinediones (e.g., trimethadione)
Sodium valproate (i.e., valproic acid)

and major heart malformations. Other health problems, such as prolonged high fevers during the early part of pregnancy, have been associated with an increased risk for neural tube defects and possible other central nervous system abnormalities.[14] Chapter 11 discusses effects of potential teratogens on the developing embryo.

Nursing Diagnosis and the Nursing Process

Many nursing diagnoses may be derived from data obtained during the assessment. Table 9–3 gives some examples of nursing diagnoses for the couple who are at reproductive risk. Figure 9–1 depicts nursing process for this couple.

GENETIC EVALUATION AND COUNSELING

When an individual or a couple is identified to have an increased reproductive risk, they should be referred for genetic evaluation and counseling, and if necessary, prenatal diagnosis and high-risk obstetric care. Genetic counseling refers to the problem-solving process concerning the occurrence or risk of genetic disorders in the family.[15] The goals of the genetic counseling process are: (1) to provide the family with a better understanding of the medical facts, prognosis, management, inheritance, risk of recurrence, and alternatives for dealing with the risk; (2) to make the family aware of the educational, health care, and reproductive options available; and (3) to help them to make the best possible adjustment to the disorder's presence or to its risk.

The genetic counseling process has evolved over time, and though it may have started as a service to produce primarily reproductive information and options, most genetic counseling services today provide diagnostic consultation and confirmatory testing and use a case-management approach for providing information, support, and follow-up to families and to individuals affected with genetic disorders.

If an individual or couple is believed to be "at risk," either preconceptionally or prenatally, the nurse should initiate a referral for genetic evaluation and counseling. A genetic counselor or a genetic nurse specialist will then contact the family to arrange their visit to the genetic counseling clinic. The genetic specialist will review the family and other history, pertinent records, and the health care provider's evaluation, and construct an in-depth pedigree. The risk factors identified will be carefully considered.

The individual or couple will then be scheduled for a genetic counseling visit. If indicated, diagnostic tests, such as chromosome analysis, will be carried out (*see* Chapter 7). If a specific diagnosis can be confirmed, informative and supportive counseling will be provided in the clinic. A plan will then be determined for follow-up counseling, and if necessary, referrals for prenatal diagnostic testing or high-risk obstetric care will be initiated.

PRENATAL DIAGNOSIS

Several methods of prenatal screening and diagnosis have been developed. Some of the more common include maternal serum alpha-fetoprotein (MSAFP), amniocentesis, chorionic villus sampling, cordocen-

TABLE 9–3. CONTRIBUTING FACTORS FOR A NURSING DIAGNOSIS WITH A COUPLE IDENTIFIED TO BE "AT RISK"

Nursing Diagnosis	Examples of Contributing Factors
Potential for reproductive anxiety	Related to: • Family history of birth defects or genetic disorders • Ashkenazi Jewish background • Advancing maternal age • Maternal diabetes • Maternal drug or alcohol use • Viral illness or high fever during pregnancy
Body image disturbance	Related to: • One member of the couple identified to be a "carrier" of a genetic disorder (e.g., female a carrier of the gene for Duchenne muscular dystrophy or male identified to carry the gene for Huntington's disease) • One member of the couple identified to be infertile (e.g., female with 45,XO or 46,XY r with 47,XXY)
Anticipatory grieving	Related to: • Couple identified to be at risk of having child with birth defect or genetic disor • Previous pregnancy losses including miscarriage, pregnancy termination, st child who has since died

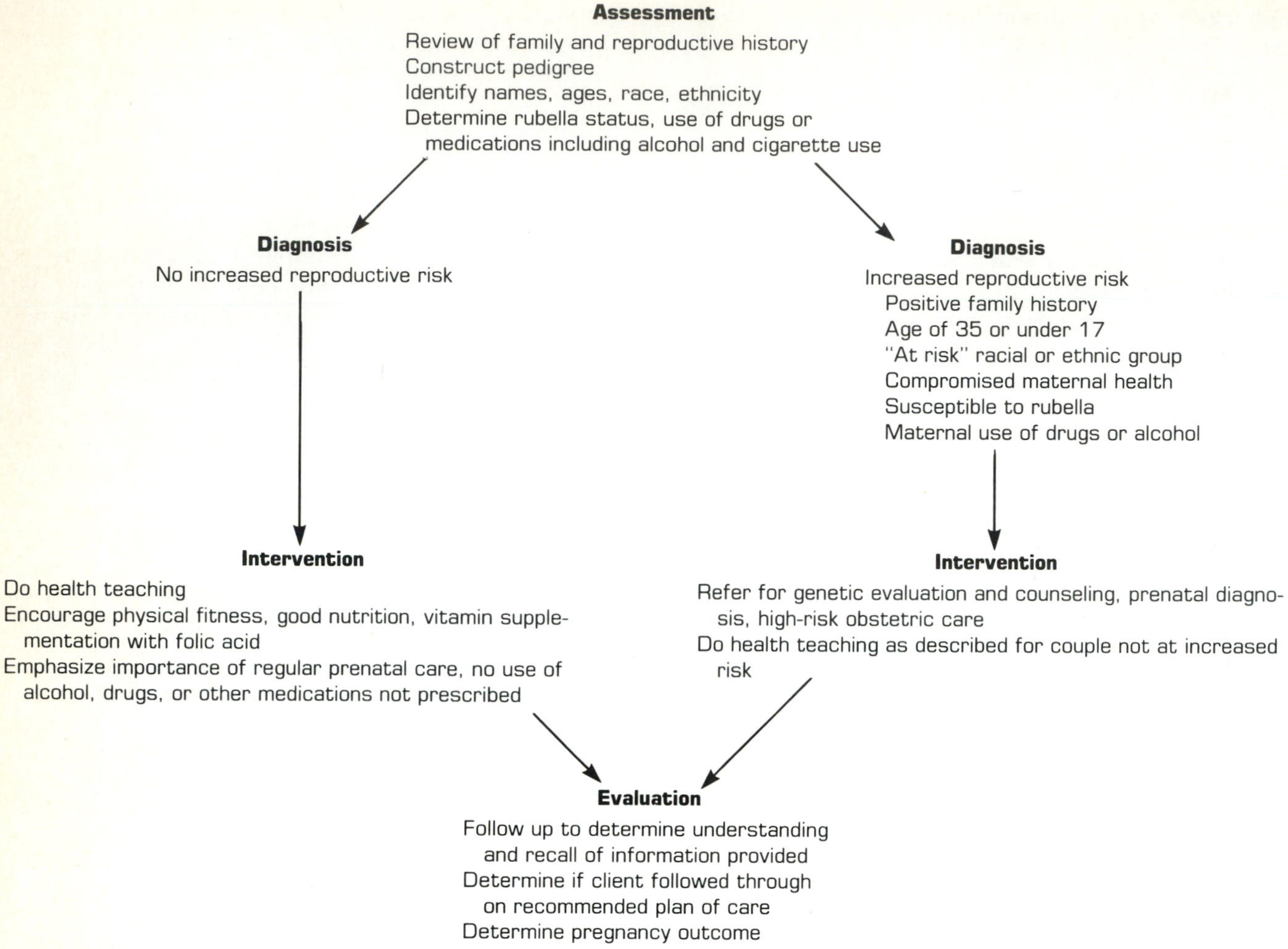
Assessment
Review of family and reproductive history
Construct pedigree
Identify names, ages, race, ethnicity
Determine rubella status, use of drugs or medications including alcohol and cigarette use
Diagnosis
No increased reproductive risk
Diagnosis
Increased reproductive risk
Positive family history
Age of 35 or under 17
"At risk" racial or ethnic group
Compromised maternal health
Susceptible to rubella
Maternal use of drugs or alcohol
Intervention
Do health teaching
Encourage physical fitness, good nutrition, vitamin supplementation with folic acid
Emphasize importance of regular prenatal care, no use of alcohol, drugs, or other medications not prescribed
Intervention
Refer for genetic evaluation and counseling, prenatal diagnosis, high-risk obstetric care
Do health teaching as described for couple not at increased risk
Evaluation
Follow up to determine understanding and recall of information provided
Determine if client followed through on recommended plan of care
Determine pregnancy outcome

Figure 9–1. Nursing process: preconception risk assessment.

tesis, ultrasonography, magnetic resonance imaging (MRI), fetoscopy, and roentgenograms (x-rays). Many birth defects or genetic disorders are diagnosable prenatally by more than one of these methods. Often several methods are employed together to more carefully delineate or monitor the birth defect or genetic disorder present in the fetus.

Chapters 14, 18, and 22, which describe assessment techniques in each trimester, discuss these methods in greater depth. Table 9–4 provides a summary of defects that may be identified by prenatal diagnostic screening. The usual outcome of prenatal diagnostic evaluation is reassurance; that is, the couple is informed that the disorder being investigated is, in fact, not present in their expected child. The small percentage of couples in which the abnormality is identified, however, are faced with the decision of whether to continue or terminate the pregnancy. The issue of pregnancy termination when a birth defect has been identified is addressed later in this chapter.

CONTRACEPTIVE COUNSELING

The majority of American women and couples, regardless of their religious affiliation and racial or ethnic background, approve of and use contraception. The motives for contraceptive use are unique, and the choice of method and its meaning to the couple are highly individual. Thus the full range of contraceptive alternatives must be discussed with the client, so that a fully informed and satisfactory choice can be made. Individual differences must be respected by the nurse.

Maternity and community health nurses play an important role in the care of a client seeking information about planning a family or pregnancy avoidance. The professional nurse must ensure that information, guidance, and methods are available to all clients. If the nurse feels unqualified or uncomfortable giving such information, she or he should state this to the client and provide an appropriate referral.

Every nurse who provides information about

TABLE 9–4. FETAL ABNORMALITIES THAT MAY BE IDENTIFIED BY PRENATAL DIAGNOSTIC SCREENING

Fetal Abnormalities	Prenatal Diagnostic Screening Test						
	Amniocentesis	CVS	Cordocentesis	Ultrasonography	MRI	Fetoscopy	X-Ray
Chromosomal abnormalities	+	+	+	−	−	−	−
Neural tube defects	+	−	−	+	+/−	+/−	+/−
Biochemical defects	+	+	+	−	−	−	−
Molecular defects	+	+	+	−	−	−	−
Skeletal anomalies	−	−	−	+	+	+/−	+/−
Soft-tissue anomalies	−	−	−	+	+	−	−
Prenatal infections	+	−	+	−	−	−	−
Hemolytic disease	+	−	+	−	−	−	−

+ = method can be used; − = method not useful; +/− = method may be useful, but is usually not used for this purpose.

contraception or assists individuals or couples to plan their families should be aware of all available methods of contraception, their advantages and disadvantages, both at the functional and psychologic level. The individual or couple's contraceptive choice may vary throughout their life span depending on many factors. Factors that influence the choice of a method include: personal values, religious beliefs, family traditions, and cultural practices. Other factors include: expense, availability of bathroom facilities, frequency of intercourse, number of children, the risk of pregnancy the couple wishes to accept, the presence of illness or physical problems, the level of comfort with the body and its functions, and the self-image of the individual client or couple.

An important point to remember when assisting clients to select a suitable contraceptive method is that choice may involve the *couple's* decision. Unlike most health measures, pregnancy prevention ideally involves the participation of both male and female partners. Optimally nurses should encourage the man's participation and provide an opportunity for him to share in the selection of the method and ultimately share the responsibility for fertility control. In some ethnic/cultural groups, if the woman chooses a method of contraception that her partner disapproves of, the couple will most likely not use the method.

Planning a family deals with the client's sexuality; therefore, a private setting should always be provided for the counseling session. The client's feelings about family plans should be explored in a nonjudgmental way. All contraceptive methods should be discussed and summarized in order to allow an informed decision to be made by the client(s). There is no single "best method" of contraception, only the method that works best for the individual client or couple.

Informed Consent

The issue of informed consent is particularly important in the area of contraceptive counseling. Usually it is healthy clients who are requesting information about contraceptive methods. The information is often sought without specific health indications. The nurse has the responsibility to ascertain that the client has sufficient information about the proposed method to make a sound decision and give truly informed consent. Also, it must be determined that the client is competent to consent on her or his own behalf. The key factors to providing sufficient information include a discussion of the methods available, their benefits, risks, rate of effectiveness, contraindications, and alternatives to the method chosen.

Risks. There are certain risks related to every contraceptive method. These risks may be associated with the method itself or the risk of pregnancy as a result of contraceptive failure or misuse. The nurse must discuss how often the method is associated with mortality, hospitalization, hysterectomy, infection, loss of fertility, pain, or nuisance side effects. It should be noted that the maternal mortality associated with pregnancy is far greater than mortality associated with any commonly used contraceptive.

There are also inconvenience risks such as making sexual intercourse less pleasant. Partner dissatisfaction or embarrassment associated with the method may also occur. Finally, the risk of pregnancy, should the method fail, must be discussed, including how often a pregnancy occurs (Table 9–5), what the dangers of pregnancy to this woman are, and what major life disruptions would occur should a pregnancy occur.

Benefits. The nurse should explain the noncontraceptive as well as contraceptive benefits to the client. There are therapeutic effects associated with many of the methods of contraception (for example, reducing the risk of pelvic inflammatory disease). The noncontraceptive benefits may influence an individual or

TABLE 9–5. FIRST-YEAR EXPECTED AND TYPICAL FAILURE RATES OF CONTRACEPTIVE METHODS

Method	Lowest Expected (%)	Typical[a] (%)
Male sterilization: vasectomy	0.1	0.15
Female sterilization: tubal ligation	0.2	0.4
Implants[b]		
Rods	0.2	0.2
Capsules	0.3	0.3
Injectable progestogen		
DMPA (Depo-Provera)	0.3	0.3
NET[b] (Noristerat)	0.4	0.4
Oral contraceptive agents	—	3
Combined	0.1	—
Progestogen only	0.5	—
Intrauterine device (IUD)		
Medicated	1	6
Nonmedicated	2	6
Condom (without spermicides)	2	12
Diaphragm (with spermicidal agent)	3	18
Sponge: nullipara	5	18
multipara	8	28
Cervical cap (with spermicidal agent)	5	18
Coitus interruptus (withdrawal)	4	18
Periodic abstinence	—	20
Postovulation	2	—
Symptothermal	6	—
Ovulation method	8	—
Calendar	10	—
Spermicidal agents (foams, jellies, creams, vaginal suppositories)	3	21
Chance	89	89

[a] Percentage of women experiencing an accidental pregnancy during first year of method usage.
[b] Not available in the United States.
Adapted with permission from Hatcher RA, et al. Contraceptive Technology, 1988–*1989. 14th ed. New York: Irvington Publishers, 1988.*

couple's decision regarding which method of birth control to choose.

Effectiveness. Effectiveness is likely the primary concern of clients seeking contraception. When counseling clients about effectiveness, nurses must be familiar with two types of effectiveness rates: theoretical effectiveness rates and use effectiveness rates. The theoretical effectiveness rate is the method's effectiveness in preventing pregnancy under ideal conditions (when it is completely understood and used correctly at all times). This is the method's maximum rate of effectiveness. If a pregnancy occurs, it is then due to a failure of the method itself and not how it is being used. The use effectiveness rate takes into consideration the method's effectiveness with actual use, in which some people use the method correctly and others use it carelessly or incorrectly. Use effectiveness rates are lower because of human error.

Cost. Contraceptive information should include information about method cost. An individual or couple must be informed about what their ongoing associated expenses will be. If cost imposes a hardship for the individual or couple, alternative contraception or a means of obtaining the desired method less expensively should be offered.

The Ideal Contraceptive

All fertile couples who are sexually active must use some form of birth control or anticipate a pregnancy to occur in 6 months to 1 year. All birth control methods have advantages and disadvantages. No one method is perfect in every way. The ideal contraceptive would, however:

1. Be easy to use
2. Have no side effects
3. Be available to everyone
4. Be instantly reversible
5. Be 100 percent safe
6. Be independent from intercourse
7. Be 100 percent effective
8. Be nonsexist in its use
9. Require minimum input from health care providers

It is not likely that an ideal contraceptive will be available for every individual or couple in the near future. The optimum birth control method for an individual or couple is one that makes them feel in control of their reproductive lives. It also makes them feel the most natural and comfortable with its use.

Contraceptive Counseling with Teenagers

The number of sexually active teenagers has increased substantially over the past two decades. Concommittantly, the age at which teenagers report their first experience with sexual intercourse has also declined. In 1981, pregnancy occurred in 1.4 percent of 14-year-old girls. This percentage continues to rise throughout the teen years with 15 percent of 19-year-olds becoming pregnant. At least four out of five pregnancies occurring in the teen years are unintended.[16] The reasons cited for this high unintended pregnancy rate include poor education in areas of family living, sexuality, and contraception, not only by the schools but also by the family and church, and the lack of access to both contraceptive information and contraceptive methods. In addition, there seems to be a "double standard" regarding sexuality that is ever present in a teenager's daily life. Sex is portrayed in books, magazines, and on television and radio as something wonderful and desirable. Very early, however, many teens have received the message regarding the taboos associated with sex outside of marriage. *See* Chapters 8 and 37 for additional discussion of teenage sexuality.

There is a great need to promote awareness regarding responsible sexuality among teenagers. Some parents and adults believe that teenagers should be taught only that sex outside of marriage is bad. Others believe that whatever is taught to teenagers should only be that which is taught in the home and perhaps at church. Still others believe that there is a need to promote an increase in awareness regarding sexuality and contraception. They feel that the needs are not being met in the home or in the church and, therefore, it is the responsibility of society to provide this information, both in schools and in family planning centers. They believe that to provide this information and service well, more school-based programs should be initiated. They also feel there should be improved access to family planning clinics away from the home or school. To provide these services well, they believe that confidentiality should be ensured in education, counseling, and in the actual provision of contraceptive methods. These suggestions are considered by some to be extremely controversial. Nonetheless, the teenage pregnancy rate continues to speak in favor of such programs.

The legal rights of minors to obtain contraceptive services without parental consent is an area of concern to all health professionals involved in providing family planning services. The laws related to minors' rights to contraception vary from state to state. In 1977, the United States Supreme Court ruled that minors do have a right to contraceptives. To date, there have been no rulings on the rights of minors to prescriptive contraceptives. Nurses must remain informed regarding the current legal statutes in the state in which they practice. Providing adequate information is one way to increase optimum contraceptive use. When a couple or an individual have weighed the benefits and risks of the methods available, have made a choice based on which method best meets their needs, and fully understand how to use the method, the likelihood of discontinuation and misuse is substantially reduced. The following sections discuss methods currently available to prevent pregnancy.

PREGNANCY PREVENTION METHODS

Various approaches can be adopted to organize information about the many pregnancy prevention methods. Frequently, contraceptive choices are categorized according to method of action. The approach adopted in this text, however, is to discuss pregnancy prevention methods in descending order of effectiveness (*see* Table 9–5).

Sterilization

Effectiveness and Action. As Table 9–5 indicates, both male and female methods of sterilization are extremely efficient in the prevention of pregnancy. The typical failure rate after a vasectomy is 0.15 percent; after a tubal ligation the typical failure rate is 0.4 percent. Consequently, for individuals who no longer wish to have children, sterilization is an effective, safe choice.[17,18] In fact, by 1982, sterilization was the contraceptive method of choice among married women.[17–21]

Sterilization is accomplished by means of the creation of an artificial obstruction in either the vas deferens (**vasectomy**) or the fallopian tubes (**bilateral tubal ligation**). Vasectomy is a relatively simple procedure during which both vasa are isolated, cut, and tied (Figure 9–2). Coagulation may also be employed to create the obstruction in the vas. Given the nature of the procedure, a vasectomy can be performed in the physician's office under either local or spinal anesthesia.[22] Consequently, the client may go home as early as 15 to 20 minutes after the procedure has been completed.[19] Sterility is achieved after a vasectomy when "a minimum of 16 ejaculations with 2 sperm-free ejaculations have been produced."[23] In order to ensure sterility, a period of 4 months should elapse between vasectomy and last sperm-free specimen.

A vaginal or abdominal route may be taken to obtain access to the fallopian tubes (Figure 9–3). The tubes are obstructed by means of rings, bands, ligation, or coagulation.[19] Unless ovulation occurred within 48 hours before the surgical procedure, sterility is immediate.

Minilaparotomy and laparoscopy (Figures 9–4, 9–5) are two methods frequently employed to effect tubal sterilization. Of the two methods, the former is the easier. A feature of both procedures is that they can be performed under local anesthesia; consequently, these procedures are frequently done on an outpatient basis.

Historically, hysterectomy, not tubal ligation,

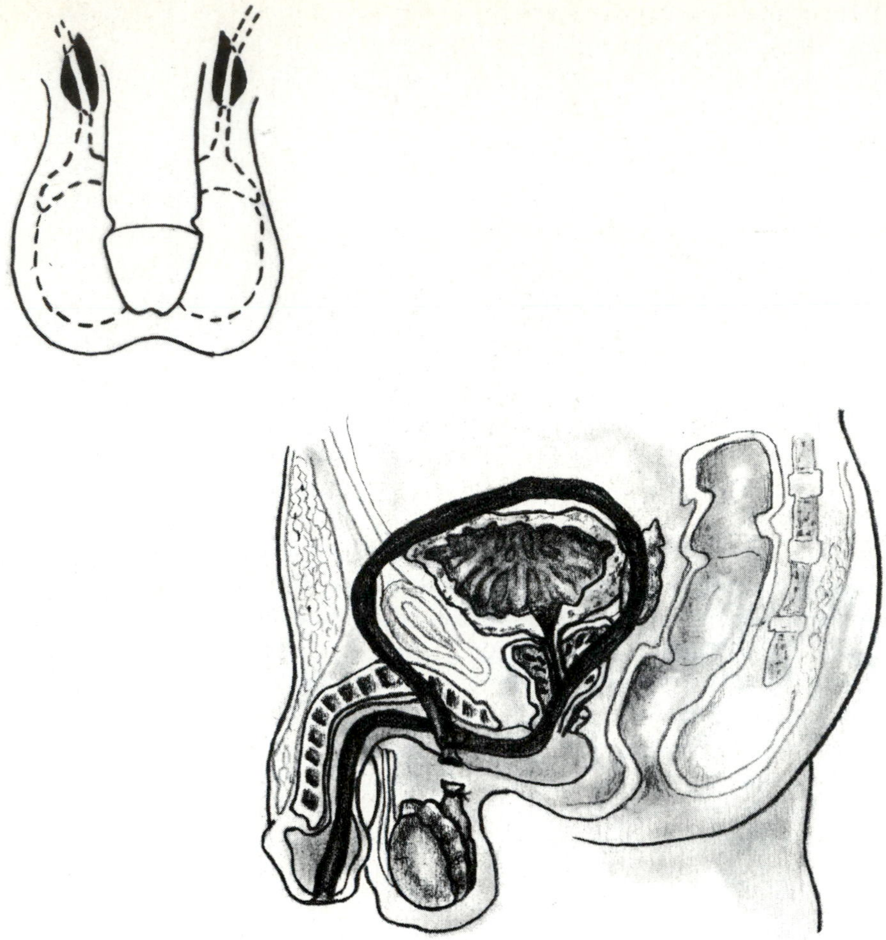

Figure 9–2. Vasectomy.

was the most frequent method of sterilization. Because of the increased toll in terms of cost, recovery time, and physical and emotional impact, however, hysterectomies are no longer justified solely for the purpose of sterilization.[19]

Informed Consent. Because of the nature and permanency of the procedure, an informed consent should be obtained. The general irreversibility of the procedure should be stressed, the procedure simply but accurately explained, and risks and benefits clearly stipulated by the physician in terms that are easily understood by the client. An additional consent may be required for the type of anesthesia to be employed. Currently, spousal consent is not required.

Benefits. All methods of sterilization are considered permanent and consequently are extremely effective. In addition, when compared with other pregnancy prevention options, sterilization is an inexpensive procedure because the financial outlay occurs once rather than on a monthly or more frequent basis. Another benefit is the singular nature of the sterilization procedure, which frees the client from having to make repeated contraceptive decisions. Lastly, sterilization provides a pregnancy prevention option that is independent of coitus, a desirable attribute for any contraceptive method.

Risks and Contraindications. As with any operative procedure there are associated risks. Complications consequent to vasectomy or tubal ligation include infection, bowel perforation, hemorrhage, and incisional pain as well as those potential complications associated with the type of anesthesia. For instance, an individual is more susceptible to pulmonary complications after the use of general anesthesia. Furthermore, the type of surgery and the methods used in the sterilization procedure will influence the complications seen.

Vasectomy clients may also experience epididymitis and sperm granulomas.[19] Approximately 30 percent of those undergoing vasectomy will develop antibodies to sperm antigens.[19] Fortunately there are no

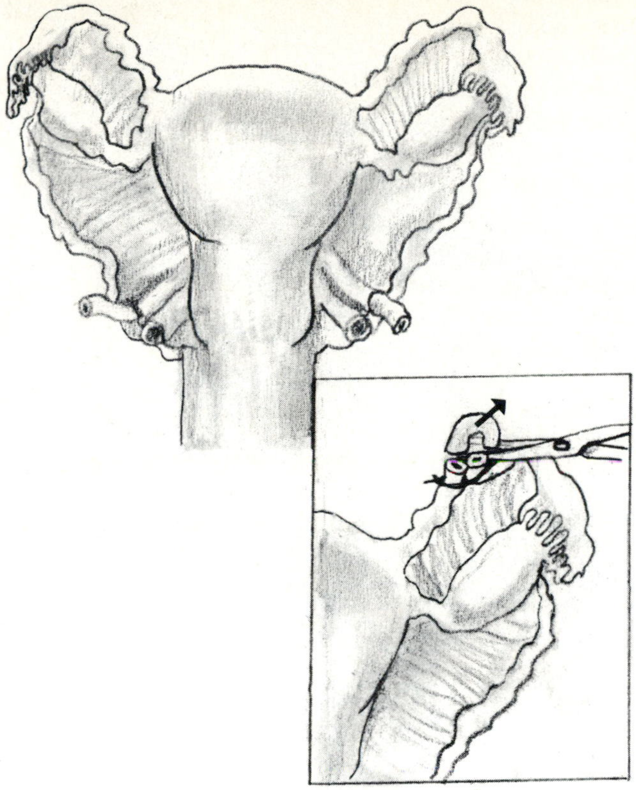

Figure 9–3. One method of tubal ligation.

pathologic changes associated with this antibody development, a fact that may need to be reinforced when a client is contemplating this option. Vasectomy has also been implicated with heart disease. Although atherosclerotic plaques were shown to develop in monkeys consequent to vasectomy, however, no cardiovascular complications have been evident in long-term human studies.[19]

Women undergoing sterilization occasionally experience a change in menstrual patterns. This is thought to be due to the change in pregnancy prevention method rather than to the procedure itself: frequently, an intrauterine device is removed or consumption of the pill is stopped shortly before the procedure. Consequently an increased menstrual flow could be attributed to these factors rather than to the sterilization procedure itself. Although tubal sterilization has been implicated in breast cancer, a recent study found that breast-cancer risk was not significantly altered.[24] Sterilization does *not* protect against sexually transmitted diseases.

Occasionally, both men and women may wish to have the sterilization procedure reversed. For either sex, reversal success is dependent on the initial surgical procedure;[19,25,26] that is, such factors as the amount of tube (vas or fallopian) removed and the use of coagulation as the ligation method influence the success of the reversal procedure. Sperm will be found in the ejaculate of 67 to 100 percent of men undergoing a vasectomy reversal procedure, however, "only 29 to 85 percent are able to impregnate their female partner."[19] The success rate for tubal ligation reversal is 40 to 75 percent.[19,26]

Teaching Needs. Information needs for those undergoing either sterilization procedure are addressed prior to the procedure and again before the client goes home. They include the following:

- *Rest.* Clients should be instructed to rest for about two days before resuming normal activities.
- *Activity.* Strenuous exercise should be avoided for about 1 week in order to prevent undue pressure to the excision area.
- *Complications.* Danger signs should be explained; they include: bleeding from the incision site, excessive pain, and temperature greater than 100.4° F.[19]
- *Resumption of sexual activity.* Sexual intercourse may be resumed between three and seven days after the procedure. The client should be counseled to stop if discomfort is experienced.
- *Pain.* A mild analgesic, such as codeine or aspirin, may be taken for incision pain. Appropriate interval times for these medications should be explained to avoid oversedation or undersedation.

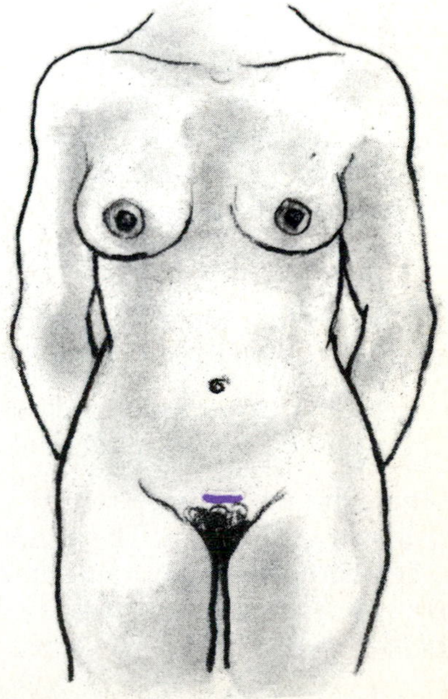

Figure 9–4. Minilaparotomy incision. (*Redrawn, with permission, from Hatcher RA, et al.* Contraceptive Technology, 1988–1989. *14th ed. New York: Irvington Publishers, 1988.*)

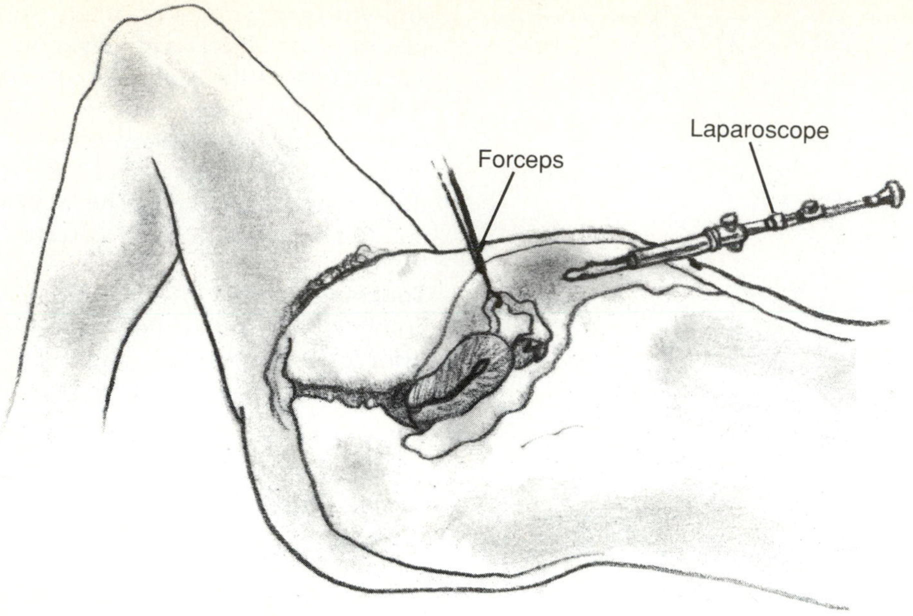

Figure 9–5. Laparoscopy. (*Redrawn, with permission, from Hatcher RA, et al.* Contraceptive Technology, 1988–1989. *14th ed. New York: Irvington Publishers, 1988.*)

Specific teaching needs for the client experiencing a vasectomy are related to comfort, hygiene, and contraception.

- *Comfort.* The client should be instructed to purchase and wear a good scrotal support continuously for the first two days. Application of an ice pack to the scrotum for at least 4 hours immediately after the procedure will also lessen the discomfort.[19]
- *Hygiene.* The client should be instructed to take a sponge bath, not a shower or tub bath, for the first 48 hours after the vasectomy. Sitz baths can be started after 48 hours. The client should be instructed to take sitz baths at least once daily, with the goal being four times a day.
- *Contraception.* Because sterility is not achieved immediately, the client should be instructed to use another pregnancy prevention method.

Specific teaching needs for the client having a tubal ligation relate to hygiene and contraception.

- *Hygiene.* There are no bathing restrictions. The client may shower or bathe at liberty. She should, however, be instructed to pat, rather than rub, the incision dry. Furthermore, she should avoid irritating the incision; wearing loose undergarments will help.
- *Contraception.* If other contraceptive measures have been employed before the surgical procedure, no preventive measures need be taken after the surgical procedure. Should this not be the case, however, the client should be instructed to employ other pregnancy prevention measures if intercourse occurs within the first few days after the procedure (although this is unlikely, given the comfort level immediately following surgery).

Injectable Progestogen

Effectiveness and Action. Both medroxyprogesterone acetate (Depo-Provera), sometimes called depomedroxyprogesterone (DMPA), and norethindrone exanthane (Noristerat or NET) are highly effective pregnancy prevention agents, with typical failure rates of 0.3 and 0.4 percent, respectively. Both agents are approved for use in 90 countries. Five million women in 40 countries have used these agents to prevent pregnancy. Both are long-acting progestins administered intramuscularly: once every 7 to 10 weeks for norethindrone exanthane; once every three months for medroxyprogesterone.[19] As both are hormonal preparations, they exert their contraceptive action by disrupting the normal hormonal balance of the menstrual cycle. Medroxyprogesterone's ultimate result is suppression of graafian follicle development.

Informed Consent. There is considerable controversy in the United States over the use of medroxyprogesterone as a contraceptive agent. In fact, its use as a means of pregnancy prevention is not approved, even though its efficacy is well recognized, especially for those women for whom other methods are not acceptable.[27] To date norethindrone exanthane has not been released for use in the United States.[28]

Benefits. Use of long-acting injectable progestins has been associated with significant pelvic inflammatory disease (PID) protection, the prevention of anemia, and a reduction in the risk for the development of ovarian and endometrial carcinoma.[19] Client privacy can also be maintained more effectively.[27]

Risks. The woman's menstrual pattern is altered, usually becoming minimal or absent. Rarely does heavy bleeding occur. Although ovulation may be delayed after discontinuation of either drug, 90 percent of women can expect to conceive within 24 months.

Oral Contraceptive Agents (Combined Pills)

Effectiveness and Action. **Oral contraceptive** pills (OCPs) are the most effective method of reversible pregnancy prevention.[29] In the United States alone, the pill is used by approximately 10 million women.[19] Combined oral contraceptive agents have a lowest expected failure rate of 0.1 percent, comparable to that of male sterilization. Typical failure rate, however, is 3 percent and is attributed to high rate of discontinuation by users for nonmedical reasons.[19] In other words, pregnancy may result because an individual stopped taking the pill because of inconvenience or expense, rather than because the pill was not exerting its pregnancy prevention action.

Combined oral contraceptive agents are hormonal in nature, consisting of an estrogen and progestin preparation. These hormonal preparations exert their pregnancy preventive effects by:

1. Suppressing hormonal reproduction in the hypothalamus and the anterior pituitary, resulting in the inhibition of ovulation[19]
2. Altering the endometrial surface so that it is unfavorable for implantation
3. Altering peristalsis and secretions within the fallopian tubes, thereby interfering with sperm, ovum, and gamete movement
4. Accelerating the degeneration of the corpus luteum, removing the source of needed hormones for the continuation of pregnancy
5. Changing the consistency of cervical mucus, creating a hostile environment

There are many different preparations currently available in the United States: the difference among products is reflected by differences in the amount of estrogen and progestin.[30–35] Table 9–6 summarizes oral contraceptives and amounts of estrogen and progestin in each. The pill is available in either 21-day or 28-day packages. Because risks associated with oral contraceptive agents increase as hormonal concentrations increase "the most prudent course in oral contraceptive therapy is to select a formulation containing a low dose of estrogen; for example, less than 50 μg, plus a low dose of progestin."[36]

Informed Consent. Figure 9–6 presents one institution's efforts to provide comprehensive information and documentation of receipt of information. Having the client sign this consent form reinforces the seriousness of the decision.

The client choosing OCPs should be well-versed in the early identification of potential problems (*see* Figure 9–6). The health care provider is encouraged to assess the client's level of understanding of the written and verbal information presented. Appropriate changes in level of instruction should be made to ensure client understanding of the ramifications of her decision.

Benefits. Many noncontraceptive benefits are associated with OCP consumption. Women experience a decrease in amount and length of menstrual flow, a lessening of menstrual cramps, and a greater regularity of menstrual cycles. Because of the decrease in menstrual flow, pill users are less susceptible to iron-deficiency anemia.[19] Although the mechanisms are not fully known, OCP may offer the user protection against PID. There is currently no evidence, however, to indicate that there is the same protection against HIV. Furthermore, evidence indicates that chlamydial growth is enhanced by oral contraceptive pills. Consequently, if the client is exposed to multiple sexual partners, she should be encouraged to use a method more effective in preventing infection, such as a condom or vaginal sponge as added protection.

There is evidence that OCPs exert a protective action against both endometrial and ovarian cancer.[37] Furthermore, those at greatest risk for these two conditions, that is, those women who have born few or no children, receive the most protection.[19,37]

Other conditions that appear to benefit from OCP administration include endometriosis and fibrocystic breast disease. Both are diminished. Furthermore, bone density is increased and persists after menopause. Consequently, some believe postmenopausal osteoporosis may be prevented by ingestion of OCPs.[37]

Risks and Contraindications. Oral contraceptive pills have been associated with an increased incidence of cardiovascular complications, specifically stroke,

TABLE 9–6. ORAL CONTRACEPTIVES CURRENTLY AVAILABLE IN THE UNITED STATES

MONOPHASIC ORAL CONTRACEPTIVES

Product name (Distributor)	Estrogen (μg)	Progestin (mg)
Loestrin 1/20[a] (Parke-Davis)	20 ethinyl estradiol	1.0 norethindrone acetate
Loestrin 1.5/30[a] (Parke-Davis)	30 ethinyl estradiol	1.5 norethindrone acetate
Lo/Ovral (Wyeth)	30 ethinyl estradiol	0.3 norgestrel
Levlen (Berlex)	30 ethinyl estradiol	0.15 levonorgestrel
Nordette (Wyeth)	30 ethinyl estradiol	0.15 levonorgestrel
Demulen 1/35 (Searle)	35 ethinyl estradiol	1.0 ethynodiol diacetate
Ovcon-35 (Mead Johnson)	35 ethinyl estradiol	0.4 norethindrone
Brevicon (Syntex)	35 ethinyl estradiol	0.5 norethindrone
Gynex 0.5/35E (Searle)	35 ethinyl estradiol	0.5 norethindrone
Modicon (Ortho)	35 ethinyl estradiol	0.5 norethindrone
Genora 1/35 (Rugby)	35 ethinyl estradiol	1.0 norethindrone
Gyntex 1/35E (Searle)	35 ethinyl estradiol	1.0 norethindrone
Norinyl 1+35 (Syntex)	35 ethinyl estradiol	1.0 norethindrone
Ortho-Novum 1/35 (Ortho)	35 ethinyl estradiol	1.0 norethindrone
Ovral (Wyeth)	50 ethinyl estradiol	0.5 norgestrel
Norlestrin 2.5/50[a] (Parke-Davis)	50 ethinyl estradiol	2.5 norethindrone acetate
Demulen 1/50 (Searle)	50 ethinyl estradiol	1.0 ethynodiol diacetate
Norlestrin 1/50[a] (Parke-Davis)	50 ethinyl estradiol	1.0 norethindrone acetate
Genora 1/50 (Rugby)	50 mestranol	1.0 norethindrone
Norinyl 1+50 (Syntex)	50 mestranol	1.0 norethindrone
Ortho-Novum 1/50 (Ortho)	50 mestranol	1.0 norethindrone
Ovcon-50 (Mead-Johnson)	50 mestranol	1.0 norethindrone
Enovid 5 mg (Searle)	75 mestranol	5.0 norethynodrel
Norinyl 1+80 (Syntex)	80 mestranol	1.0 norethindrone
Ortho-Novum 1/80 (Ortho)	80 mestranol	1.0 norethindrone
Ovulen (Searle)	100 mestranol	1.0 ethynodiol diacetate
Norinyl 2 mg (Syntex)	100 mestranol	2.0 norethindrone
Ortho-Novum 2 mg (Ortho)	100 mestranol	2.0 norethindrone
Enovid-E (Searle)	100 mestranol	2.5 norethynodrel

TABLE 9–6. ORAL CONTRACEPTIVES CURRENTLY AVAILABLE IN THE UNITED STATES (*continued*)

TRIPHASIC ORAL CONTRACEPTIVES

Product name (Distributor)	Estrogen and Progestin Contents		
	Phase I	**Phase 2**	**Phase 3**
Ortho Novum 7/7/7 (Ortho)	0.5 mg norethindrone 35 μg ethinyl estradiol (7 tabs)	0.75 mg norethindrone 35 μg ethinyl estradiol (7 tabs)	1 mg norethindrone 35 μg ethinyl estradiol (7 tabs)
Tri-Norinyl (Syntex)	0.5 mg norethindrone 35 μg ethinyl estradiol (7 tabs)	1 mg norethindrone 35 μg ethinyl estradiol (9 tabs)	0.5 mg norethindrone 35 μg ethinyl estradiol (5 tabs)
Tri-Levlen (Berlex) Triphasil (Wyeth)	0.05 mg levonorgestrel 30 μg ethinyl estradiol (6 tabs)	0.075 mg levonorgestrel 40 μg ethinyl estradiol (5 tabs)	0.125 mg levonorgestrel 30 μg ethinyl estradiol (10 tabs)

BIPHASIC ORAL CONTRACEPTIVES

Product name (Distributor)	Estrogen and Progestin Contents	
	Phase I	**Phase 2**
Ortho Novum 10/11 (Ortho)	0.5 mg norethindrone 35 μg ethinyl estradiol (10 tabs)	1 mg norethindrone 35 μg ethinyl estradiol (11 tabs)

PROGESTIN-ONLY PRODUCTS

Product name (Distributor)	Progestin
Micronor (Ortho)	0.35 mg norethindrone
Nor-Q.D. (Syntex)	0.35 mg norethindrone
Ovrette (Wyeth)	0.075 mg norgestrel

[a] Product also available with addition of 75 mg ferrous fumarate

hypertension, clot formation, and heart attack.[19] Current literature, however, implicates the concentration of hormones in combination oral contraceptive agents; that is, the risk is lower for medium- and low-fixed-dose preparations.[38–43] Furthermore, the occurrence of cardiovascular risks has been demonstrated in a select group of women:

- Women who smoke
- Women who are over 35 years of age
- Women who have other health problems such as hypertension, diabetes, a history of heart or vascular disease
- Women who have a family history of diabetes or a heart attack in a person under the age of 50 (particularly heart attack in a female family member)[19]

On the other hand, recent studies indicate that healthy, nonsmoking women up to the age of 45 are at no greater risk of serious cardiovascular disease when taking oral contraceptive preparations containing less than 50 μg of estrogen.[37,38] Although oral contraceptive pills alter lipid metabolism, the major cardiovascular risks are associated not with atherosclerosis but with thrombus formation.[36,39,40] Counseling with regard to signs and symptoms of clot formation is of paramount importance.

OCPs exert both negative and positive effects on lipid metabolism, a noteworthy characteristic given our society's preoccupation with cholesterol levels and efforts to lower them. Estrogenic effects are HDL and HDL_2 increase, LDL decrease, and triglycerides increase.[36] Opposite effects are true for progestin; that is, they tend to decrease HDL and HDL_2, increase LDL, and decrease triglycerides.[36] Consequently, it is recommended that a lipoprotein profile consisting of total cholesterol, HDL-C, and total triglycerides be

ORAL CONTRACEPTIVE CONSENT FORM

I agree that I am receiving birth control Pills of my own free will. Pills are the method of family planning which I have chosen from all the methods that have been explained to me. The advantages and disadvantages of the other methods of birth control have been explained to me.

BENEFITS: I am aware that oral contraceptives are *not* guaranteed to be 100% effective. It is my understanding that combined birth control Pills can be 99% effective if I take them exactly according to instructions. I understand that progestin-only Pills (Mini-Pills) are slightly less effective even if I follow the instructions. I understand that some women experience the following *benefits* from using birth control Pills:

- Decreased menstrual cramps
- Decreased menstrual bleeding
- More regular menstrual bleeding
- Decreased pain at the time of ovulation
- Less risk of acute gonococcal pelvic inflammatory disease (gonorrhea infection in the tubes)
- Improvement in acne
- Less risk of cancer of the uterus or ovary
- Less risk of benign breast tumors and/or ovarian cysts

RISKS: I have been told to watch out for the following danger signals and to return to the clinic or make contact with my clinician at once if I develop one of these problems. These could be warnings of serious or even life-threatening illness.

EARLY PILL DANGER SIGNS

caution

- A ■ Abdominal pain (severe)
- C ■ Chest pain (severe), cough, shortness of breath
- H ■ Headache (severe), dizziness, weakness, or numbness
- E ■ Eye problems (vision loss or blurring), speech problems
- S ■ Severe leg pain (calf or thigh)

See your clinician if you have any of these problems, or if you develop depression, yellow jaundice or a breast lump.

I am aware that while using oral contraceptives, I could have the following side effects, many of which can be temporary:

Major Problems

- Blood clot of the leg or the lung
- Stroke or heart attack
- Gallbladder disease
- One type of liver tumor
- Death

Minor Problems

- Nausea
- Spotting between periods
- Less menstrual bleeding
- Breast tenderness
- Weight gain
- Headache
- Depression
- High blood pressure
- Splotchy darkening of the skin on my face
- Worsening of acne
- Infections in the vagina

I have been told that most of the serious problems in Pill users happen to women over 30 who are heavy smokers (15 or more cigarettes a day).

STOPPING PILLS: I have been told that I may stop using the Pills *at any time*. I have been told I should use another means of birth control until I have had three regular periods before attempting to become pregnant. I have also been informed that if my periods were very irregular, very heavy, and/or very painful before taking Pills, they may return to this pattern when I stop taking Pills.

INSTRUCTIONS for the use of birth control Pills have been given to me in writing and I have been given a patient package insert for my specific brand of Pill.

QUESTIONS: I have been given the chance to ask questions about all forms of birth control and about the Pill in particular. My questions have been answered to my satisfaction.

____

Signature

Figure 9–6. Informed consent form for oral contraceptive counseling. (*Adapted, with permission, from Hatcher RA, et al.* Contraceptive Technology, 1988–1989. *14th ed. New York: Irvington Publishers, 1988.*)

obtained before initiation of either OCPs or hormone replacement therapy.[44–46]

Breast cancer has also been associated with OCPs. Data have failed to validate this association.[19,47,48] Other data, however, have implicated parity and age with an increased risk of breast cancer, specifically nulliparity and age at onset of menarche.[49] The relationship between OCPs and other types of cancer (cervical, skin, and liver) remains unclear.[19]

Minor risks associated with OCPs include the development of oily skin or acne, absence of menses, midcycle spotting or break-through bleeding, breast discomfort or fullness, and possibly depression. Women may also experience persistent nausea, morning sickness, or a weight gain while taking OCPs.

Contraindications to combined OCPs vary. Table 9–7 lists absolute and relative contraindications.

Teaching Needs. Teaching about benefits and risks should be reinforced; the fact that no protection is provided against human immunodeficiency virus (HIV) should be stressed. Information about the pill's action should be reinforced and the method of taking the pill should be clearly explained (21-day versus 28-day preparations). Measures should be taught that will facilitate adherence to the regimen, for example, taking the pill before going to bed or on rising. (*See* box on page 206 for more client instructions.)

Oral Contraceptive Pills—Progestogen Only (Minipill)

Effectiveness and Action. The progestins found in the **minipill** are the same as those found in combined oral contraceptives, except that they are present in smaller doses.[19] They are an effective pregnancy prevention option with a lowest expected failure rate of 0.5 percent. Progestogen-only pills exert their effect by altering the endometrial surface of the uterus as well as the consistency of cervical mucus. Suppression of ovulation occurs in less than 40 percent of cycles.[19]

The minipill is an alternative hormonal agent for those women with histories of mild hypertension, headaches, or who experienced some of the less pleasant effects of combined oral contraceptive pills (morning sickness, persistent nausea, weight gain).

Informed Consent. As with combined oral contraceptives, the client needs to be aware of the benefits and risks associated with progestogen-only pills. Af

TABLE 9–7. CONTRAINDICATIONS TO COMBINED BIRTH CONTROL PILLS

Below are some of the contraindications to pill use.
When considering use of the pill for women with strong relative contraindications, it is extremely important to weigh the risks and benefits of the pill and to consider carefully alternatives to its use.

In some settings, the contraceptive options available to a woman are limited. When a wide range of choices is not available, the pill may become a more attractive choice.

Client concerns regarding an unplanned pregnancy due to use of a less effective contraceptive may be a factor in the woman's decision to use pills.

It is strongly suggested that you not consider the relative contraindications as categorical prohibitions against a specific method for a specific client.

Absolute contraindications:

1. Thrombophlebitis or thromboembolic disorder (or history thereof)
2. Cerebrovascular disorders (or history thereof)
3. Ischemic heart disease or coronary artery disease (or history thereof)
4. Known or suspected carcinoma of the breast (or history thereof)
5. Known or suspected estrogen-dependent neoplasia (or history thereof)
6. Pregnancy, known or suspected
7. Benign or malignant liver tumor (or history thereof)
8. Undiagnosed abnormal genital bleeding

Strong relative contraindications:

9. Severe headaches, particularly vascular or migraine
10. Hypertension with resting diastolic BP of 90 or greater, or a resting systolic BP of 140 or greater on three or more separate visits, or an accurate measurement of 110 diastolic or more on a single visit
11. Diabetes
12. Active gallbladder disease
13. Mononucleosis, acute phase
14. Sickle cell disease (SS) or sickle C disease (SC)
15. Elective major surgery planned in next 4 weeks or major surgery requiring immobilization
16. Long-leg cast or major injury to lower leg
17. 40 years of age or older, accompanied by a second risk factor for the development of cardiovascular disease
18. 35 years of age or older and currently a heavy smoker (15 or more cigarettes a day)

Other possible relative contraindications:

19. Prediabetes or a strong family history of diabetes
20. Previous cholestasis during pregnancy, congenital hyperbilirubinemia (Gilbert's disease)
21. Known impaired liver function at present time
22. Impaired liver function within past year
23. 45 years of age or older
24. Completion of term pregnancy within past 10–14 days
25. Weight gain of 10 pounds or more while on the pill
26. Failure to have established regular menstrual cycles

Reproduced with permission from Hatcher RA, et al. Contraceptive Technology, 1988–1989. *14th ed. New York: Irvington Publishers, 1988.*

CLIENT INSTRUCTIONS: COMBINED ORAL CONTRACEPTIVE PILLS

1. Establish a pattern for taking the pill.
2. As there are a variety of ways to initiate taking the pill, follow the approach presented by your health care provider.
3. The package insert should be read before you start the pill.
4. You may experience some bleeding between periods. Taking the pill at the same time every day may alleviate this.
5. Certain drugs, such as phenytoin (Dilantin), affect the protective level of the pill. You may need to employ an additional contraceptive method.
6. A good way to prevent overlooking a missed pill is to check your pack daily.
7. A missed pill should be taken as soon as you remember. Two missed pills should be taken as soon as you remember. You should also take two pills the next day.
8. Whether one or two pills are missed, some other contraceptive measure should be employed until the next period occurs.
9. Become very familiar with an alternative form of pregnancy prevention.
10. Know the early danger signs associated with the pill (*see* Figure 9–6).

Adapted, with permission, from Hatcher RA, et al. Contraceptive Technology, 1988–1989. *14th ed. New York: Irvington Publishers, 1989, p. 216.*

ter a thorough explanation a consent form should be signed (*see* Figure 9–6).

Benefits. Dysmenorrhea is lessened,but not to the extent obtained by combined oral contraceptives. Although two possible major benefits of combined oral contraceptives—protection against both endometrial cancer and PID—are influenced by progestin, no data are currently available to suggest that similar protection exists when progestogen-only contraceptive pills are taken.[19] Both headaches and hypertension do occur less frequently.

Risks and Contraindications. Irregular bleeding is more common with this form of contraceptive pill. The same absolute contraindications that apply for combined oral contraceptives are applicable for the progestogen-only preparation (*see* Table 9–7). Should pregnancy occur, the likelihood of an ectopic pregnancy is greater when the minipill is being taken.

Teaching Needs. Teaching needs are similar to those identified for the combined oral contraceptive. Often a woman who is initiating oral contraceptive use for the first time is given a three-month supply of pills. This procedure ensures that the client will return to the health care facility to receive her additional prescription. In this manner health care providers can assess the client's possible side effects, level of knowledge, and use patterns of the oral contraceptive method.

Intrauterine Devices

Effectiveness and Action. Of the methods currently used to prevent pregnancy, the **intrauterine device** (IUD) ranks third in effectiveness (*see* Table 9–5). Medicated IUDs have a lowest expected failure rate of 1 percent; the lowest expected failure rate for nonmedicated IUDs is 2 percent. Typical failure rate is 6 percent.

Intrauterine devices are thought to exert their pregnancy preventive action in a variety of ways: (1) creation of a hostile uterine environment (inflammatory response); (2) destruction of sperm or blastocyst; (3) prevention of implantation; and (4) increased production of thick cervical mucus.[19]

There are two IUDs currently available. The Progestasert releases progesterone into the uterine cavity from a storage area on the device (Figure 9–7). The increased levels of progesterone alter the uterine environment. Should fertilization occur, implantation is prevented. Because the Progestasert has a monofilamented tail, the incidence of infection is decreased. The Progestasert needs to be replaced after 1 year: this is a positive attribute because an opportunity is provided for the health care provider to reassess the client and to perform an annual breast examination and Pap smear.[50]

The other IUD currently available is the ParaGard, Model T380A. This IUD is the most effective device to date, with a "cumulative net pregnancy rate of 0.5 per 100 women years."[37] Approved by the Food and Drug Administration (FDA) in 1984, the ParaGard was released for use in May 1988. This T-shaped device has both copper wire wrapped around its stem and copper collars on its horizontal arms.[50] It, too, has a monofilamented tail. The exact mechanism of action is not currently known. It is thought, however, that "copper acts primarily to prevent fertilization of the egg, and that this action takes place before implantation in the uterus."[50] Unlike the Progestasert, the ParaGard can remain in place for 4 years before being replaced. Good preventive health habits should be fostered in the recipients of this IUD

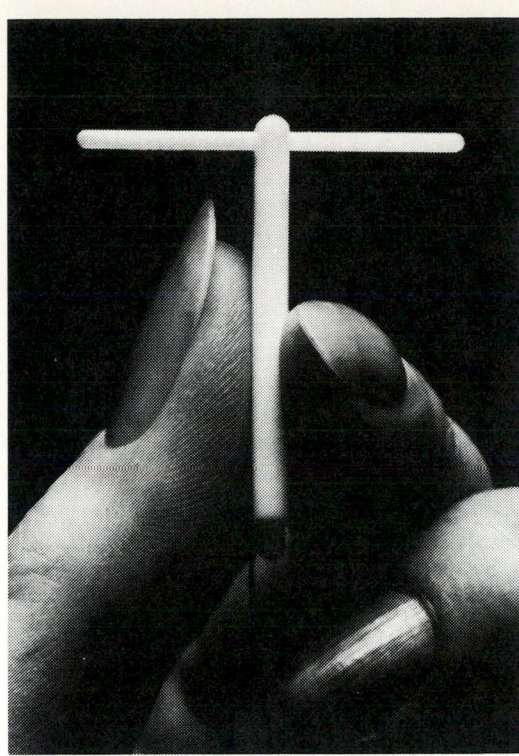

Figure 9–7. The Progestasert IUD. (Progestasert® Intrauterine Progesterone Contraceptive System, Oct, 1989; Patient Information, Dec, 1989. Reproduced, with permission, of ALZA Corporation, Palo Alto, California.)

so that clients will continue to have annual Pap smears and breast examinations.

Informed Consent. The IUD received significant negative publicity in the 1980s, particularly with regard to one product, the Dalkon shield. Women with these devices in place developed serious pelvic infections. In fact, the Dalkon shield was implicated in 10 to 15 deaths.[50] The design of the Dalkon shield was such that bacterial entry into the uterus was enhanced. Its tail consisted of hundreds of fibers encased in a sheath. The sheath isolated the fibers from the bacteria-destroying cervical mucus, thereby providing bacteria with direct access to the uterus and fallopian tubes. As a result of litigation, production of the Dalkon shield was discontinued. Furthermore, between 1984 and 1986, production of three other devices was discontinued.[50]

Current manufacturers are very aware of the legal aspects of their product. Progestasert manufacturers have developed a seven-page leaflet in which the mechanisms of action and effectiveness are explained. The leaflet also contains information about side effects, risk factors, and warning signs.[51] Both physician and client are encouraged to sign it. Furthermore, each section is to be initialed by the client.[51]

ParaGard manufacturers have developed a similar pamphlet that is 10 pages in length. The client's initials are required after each major section of the document (12 in all). In addition, both client's and physician's signatures are required at the end of the document. Information within the document is comprehensive.

The IUD has never had its approval for use withdrawn by the FDA, even during the tumultuous portion of its history. Health care providers may wish to point out this little-known fact when discussing various pregnancy prevention methods with clients.

Benefits. The major benefit of the IUD is that compliance is not an issue. In fact the highest continuation rates for a pregnancy prevention method are associated with IUD users. Candidates for the IUD are those women who are in a monogamous relationship and have had at least one child.[52,53]

Risks and Contraindications. As with any contraceptive agent there are certain risks associated with the IUD. Furthermore, the type of risk depends on the type of IUD (*see* Informed Consent).[54]

Pelvic inflammatory disease is increased when the IUD is used, particularly within the initial 4-month period following insertion.[37,54] Pelvic inflammatory disease that occurs after this time is associated with sexually transmitted pathogens.[37] Consequently, meticulous aseptic technique should be used to decrease the introduction of bacteria during insertion of the IUD.[37] The risk of PID is increased in nulliparous women and in those having multiple sexual partners. The incidence of tubal infertility among nulliparous women has been intimated to be approximately twice that of nonusers. No change in fertility rates, however, has been reported in the literature.[54]

Uterine perforation has been associated with the IUD. This risk is rare, with an occurrence of 1:1000 to 1:5000 insertions.[54] Its occurrence is confirmed by ultrasound or x-ray.

One of the more common problems is a tendency for increased uterine cramping. This discomfort is influenced by the shape and size of the IUD as well as the obstetric history and physical status of the uterus. Increased bleeding is also associated with an IUD in place. Alterations in bleeding may be manifested by increased amount of bleeding, increased number of menstrual days, and intermittent spotting. This increased blood loss may also result in a decrease in hematocrit, overtly demonstrated by weakness and pallor.[19] Spontaneous expulsion of the IUD occurs in

EARLY IUD DANGER SIGNS

caution

- P ■ Period late (pregnancy), abnormal spotting or bleeding
- A ■ Abdominal pain, pain with intercourse
- I ■ Infection exposure (such as Gonorrhea), abnormal discharge
- N ■ Not feeling well, fever, chills
- S ■ String missing, shorter or longer

Figure 9–8. Early IUD danger signs. (*Reproduced, with permission, from Hatcher RA, et al.* Contraceptive Technology, 1988–1989. *14th ed. New York: Irvington Publishers, 1988.*)

5 to 20 percent of users within the first year. Symptoms range from cramping to actually feeling the device in the vagina.[19]

Contraindications to the use of the IUD as a pregnancy prevention option include suspected or known pregnancy, presence of an acute pelvic infection or a history of PID, presence of uterine anomalies, and suspected or known malignancies. Women who have a history of PID, who have multiple sexual partners, who have never had a child, and who are less than 25 years old should be offered another pregnancy prevention option rather than the IUD.[53]

Should pregnancy occur with an IUD in place and it not be removed, there is a 50 percent chance of spontaneously aborting the fetus. The risk is lower if the device is removed. The risk of ectopic pregnancy is increased when the Progestasert fails.[37]

CLIENT INSTRUCTIONS: INTRAUTERINE DEVICE (IUD)

1. Be knowledgeable about how your IUD works and what its side effects are. Read the insert that comes with your IUD before it is inserted.
2. You will need to feel the IUD string in your vagina after it is inserted. Feel the back of your vagina before the IUD is inserted. That will help you become more familiar with your body and make finding the IUD string easier.
3. After IUD insertion, the strings will need to be checked frequently for the first few months. Make a special effort to check string placement before having sex during those first few months.
4. Check string placement when you finish your period.
5. Check string placement if you have unusual cramping during your period.
6. You may expel the IUD and not be aware of it. Because IUDs tend to be expelled during menses, make a habit of checking tampons or pads.
7. Use an additional pregnancy prevention method for the first 3 months.
8. Know the danger signs associated with IUD use (*see* Figure 9–8).

Adapted, with permission, from Hatcher RA, et al. Contraceptive Technology, 1988–1989. *14th ed. New York: Irvington Publishers, 1989, pp. 291–292.*

Teaching Needs. Clients choosing to employ IUDs as their pregnancy prevention methods need to be informed about the associated risks. Furthermore, clients need to be comfortable touching their body, as assessment of IUD placement will be their responsibility. Sufficient time should be allocated to this issue at the time of IUD insertion. Nutritional habits should be assessed and plans identified to increase daily iron intake. It may be necessary to review basic nutritional information with the client. Should iron be prescribed, methods of counteracting some of the side effects should be addressed. Figure 9–8 provides further educational information. The box presents client instructions.

Condoms (Without Spermicides)

Effectiveness and Action. The **condom** (Figure 9–9) is the most reversible form of male pregnancy prevention options, with the exception of coitus interruptus.[19] Made of either a latex rubber (basic or thin)[55] or skin (collagen tissue that has been processed)[19] and placed over the erect penis, the condom acts as a barrier to the transmission of semen into the vagina. Condom production must adhere to stringent FDA standards.[56]

Although the lowest expected failure rate is 2 percent, typical failure rate for the condom is 12 percent. Efficacy of this method appears to be inversely influenced by age: the younger the user, the higher the failure rate.[37]

Benefits. A major benefit is the protection that the condom affords against sexually transmitted diseases (STDs) and HIV.[55–57] Furthermore, a recent study suggests that use of nonoxynol 9 may provide even greater, though not absolute, protection against HIV.[57] Latex rather than skin condoms provide the best protection against STDs.

Another benefit is the increased level of male participation in pregnancy prevention. Condoms may be the couple's primary preventive method or their back-

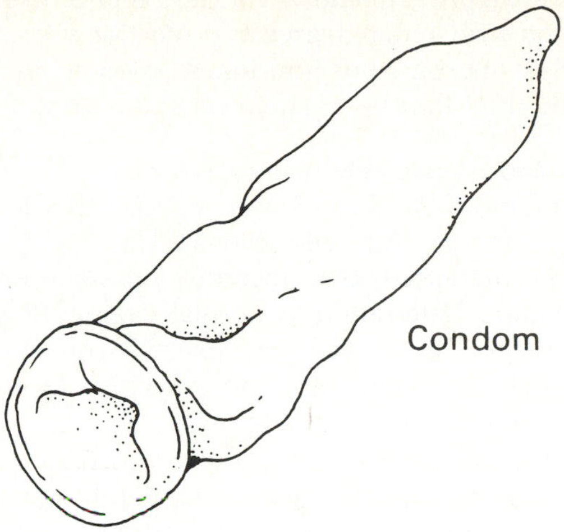

Figure 9–9. Unrolled condom with reservoir tip. *(Reproduced, with permission, from Lichtman R, Papera S.* Gynecology: Well-Woman Care. *Norwalk, Conn: Appleton & Lange, 1990, p 80.)*

up method. Condom use can enhance sexual intimacy by involving both partners in its application.

Although length and width remain relatively constant, the client has a variety of options when choosing a condom. Condoms can be smooth or ribbed. They may be lubricated or not lubricated, have spermicidal agents on the inside and outside of the sheath, and be tapered. Some condoms have sperm reservoirs at the tip, others do not. Hatcher and colleagues present a comprehensive guide to condoms that considers these characteristics.[19]

Condoms are readily accessible. They may be purchased over the counter in any pharmacy at very little cost. Furthermore, the client has a choice of quantity to purchase. The client may purchase one condom or many condoms. The decision rests with the client.

Risks and Contraindications. Glans sensitivity is reduced by the condom. This fact makes many men reluctant to use it. Use of a thinner condom that is lubricated and textured may, however, enhance sensitivity.

Foreplay is interrupted during the application of the condom, making condom use objectionable. Encouraging partner participation in the application of the condom may contribute to a more mutually positive experience. Finally, men in certain ethnic or cultural groups may reject the use of condoms. Generally, other options should be suggested for these couples.

Teaching Needs. The client should be well informed about the benefits of condom use. The client should also be made aware of the characteristics that are perceived as less attractive. It is imperative that the client understand how the condom is applied (*see* box).

Diaphragm (with Spermicidal Agents)

Effectiveness and Action. Like the condom, the **diaphragm** is a physical barrier between cervix and sperm. As is evident from Table 9–5, although the lowest expected failure rate is 3 percent, the typical failure rate for diaphragm users is 18 percent, three times that of the IUD, and 1.5 times that of the condom. There are at least four different styles of diaphragm (Figure 9–10). All have a flexible rim and a rubber cup that is shaped like a dome. The dome is the portion that covers the cervix. An additional pregnancy prevention action is that spermicidal jelly is placed in the dome and around the rim of the diaphragm (Figure. 9–11). Because diaphragms need to be fitted on an individual basis, there are a variety of sizes available. The largest rim size that will fit the client comfortably is selected. The diaphragm should stay in place for six to eight hours after intercourse to achieve maximum pregnancy prevention action.

Benefits. A major benefit of diaphragm (and spermicidal agent) use is the protection it offers against

CLIENT INSTRUCTIONS: CONDOM USE

1. Use a condom every time you have intercourse.
2. Put on a condom before entering the vagina.
3. Apply the condom by rolling it over your erect penis, right to the base of the penis.
4. Make sure that there is a place at the tip to hold the semen.
5. Use of spermicidal latex condoms or spermicidal foams adds more protection against infection.
6. Contraceptive foams, water, or K-Y jelly are excellent lubricants. Do *not* use petroleum jelly (such as Vaseline).
7. Enlist the help of your partner. The application of the condom can be pleasurable for both of you.
8. If possible, use another form of pregnancy prevention with the condom.
9. When withdrawing the penis from the vagina, hold the rim of the condom. This will prevent spillage.
10. Check the condom for tears before throwing it away.
11. Use a condom only once.

Adapted, with permission, from Hatcher RA, et al. Contraceptive Technology, 1988–1989. *14th ed. New York: Irvington Publishers, 1989, pp. 349–352.*

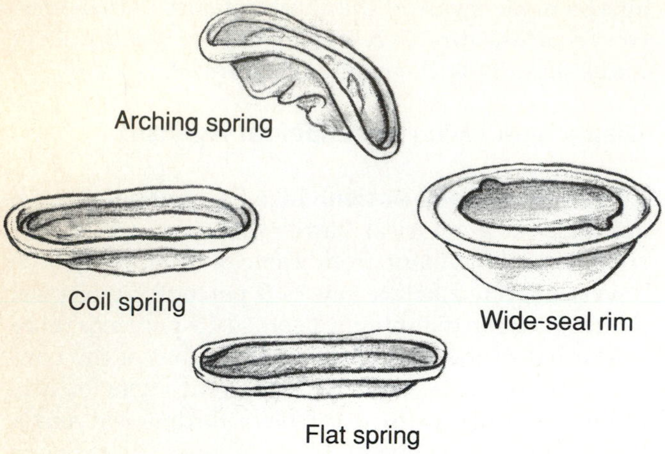

Figure 9–10. Types of diaphragms. (*Redrawn, with permission, from Hatcher RA, et al.* Contraceptive Technology, 1988–1989. *14th ed. New York: Irvington Publishers, 1988.*)

such STDs as gonorrhea. The diaphragm's protective action against the HIV or chlamydia is not known at present. There is a decreased incidence of cervical neoplasia with diaphragm use. This finding is thought to be caused by the decreased transmission of human papilloma virus (HPV).[37]

The diaphragm allows for flexibility of use in association with a high degree of protection without the influence of exogenous hormones. Many women prefer a method that helps them retain control.

Risks and Contraindications. Women who use the diaphragm are at an increased risk for the development of urinary tract infections (UTIs).[58–61] Reasons for this increased risk include: possible urethral obstruction,[58] alteration in normal vaginal flora as a consequence of diaphragm use,[58,60] questionable postcoital voiding habits, and possibly the bactericidal effects of spermicidal jelly.[58]

Women may develop an allergy to either the rubber used in the construction of the diaphragm or the spermicidal agent used in its application. In addition, both partners can develop an irritation as a result of the spermicidal agent.

The risk of the development of toxic shock syndrome (TSS) as a result of diaphragm use is under study, with conflicting results being demonstrated. Nonetheless, the health care provider should provide explicit directions that decrease the likelihood that TSS will occur (*see* box). Minor risks include the development of a foul-smelling vaginal discharge, pelvic discomfort, and possible vaginal trauma as a result of prolonged wear or diaphragm rim pressure.[19]

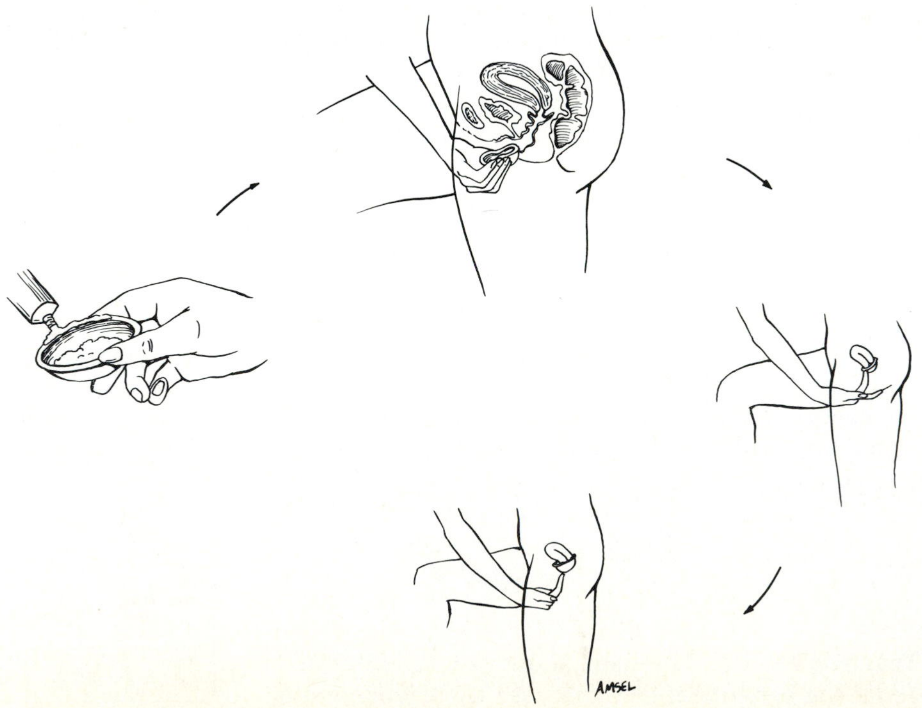

Figure 9–11. Placement of diaphragm.

CLIENT INSTRUCTIONS: DIAPHRAGM USE

1. Leave the diaphragm (with spermicidal agent) in place every time you have intercourse.
2. Leave the diaphragm in for 6 to 8 hours after intercourse; use more spermicidal cream or jelly if you have intercourse more than once during this time.
3. Remove your diaphragm at least once in a 24-hour period. This decreases the chance of developing toxic shock syndrome (TSS).
4. Be aware of the TSS danger signs:
   - Fever
   - Diarrhea
   - Vomiting
   - Muscle aches
   - Rash (like sunburn)

Adapted, with permission, from Hatcher RA, et al. Contraceptive Technology, 1988–1989. *14th ed. New York: Irvington Publishers, 1988, p. 309.*

A disadvantage is that intercourse must be planned with this method of pregnancy prevention. Couples may find that use of the diaphragm interferes with spontaneity of intercourse and may not use it, thereby increasing the chance of conception.

Women who have had a history of UTIs or TSS, who are allergic to rubber, have abnormal vaginal anatomy, or who cannot learn the proper method of inserting the diaphragm should consider another form of pregnancy prevention.

Teaching Needs. The client will need to have a good understanding of and be comfortable with her body. In addition, the client will need to know how to insert the diaphragm (*see* Figure 9–11), what discomforts may occur, and the signs and symptoms of TSS. Care of the diaphragm should also be shown, including washing it with mild soap and water, placing it in a case after it is dry, keeping it away from heat, and inspecting it for damage. The box presents more specific teaching instructions.

Vaginal Sponge

Effectiveness and Action. Lowest expected failure rates (5 to 8 percent) and typical failure rates (18 to 28 percent) for the vaginal sponge are presented in Table 9–5. As is reflected in that table, failure rates appear to be dependent on reproductive status, with more pregnancies occurring in those who have had children. Parity was not found, however, to be a significant factor in sponge effectiveness by Edelman and North.[62]

The **vaginal sponge** is a pliable round device made of polyurethane and containing nonoxynol-9. It is approximately 6 cm in diameter and 1.5 cm thick, with an attached loop to facilitate removal (Figure 9–12). The sponge's pregnancy prevention action occurs in three ways. Like the diaphragm and the condom, the sponge acts as a barrier between the cervix and sperm. In addition, spermicides contained within the sponge are released, immobilizing the sperm. Lastly, the sponge entraps the sperm.

Benefits. The vaginal sponge is readily available, relatively inexpensive, and may be purchased over the counter. This accessibility makes it very attractive as a pregnancy prevention method. Unlike the diaphragm, no fitting is required. The sponge can be inserted just prior to intercourse and remains effective for 24 hours. It must remain in place for at least 6 hours after the last act of intercourse for a maximum 30-hour wear time.

Risks and Contraindications. Many of the risks and discomforts seen with diaphragm use are also seen with sponge use. The client may develop an allergy or intolerance to the spermicidal agent. The sponge may also become difficult to remove.

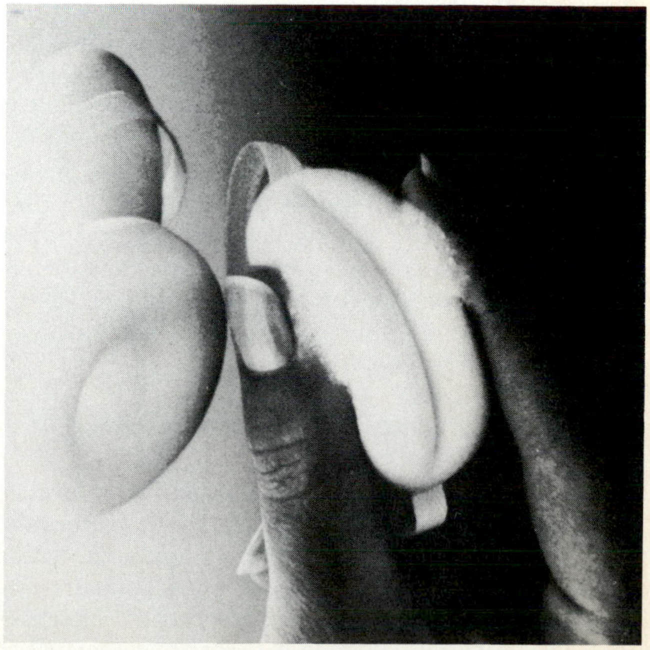

Figure 9–12. Vaginal contraceptive sponge. (*Courtesy of Whitehall Labs.*)

RESEARCH ABSTRACT

Loucks A. A comparison of satisfaction with types of diaphragms among women in a college population. J Obstet Gynecol Neonatal Nurs. *1989;18:194–200.*

The major purpose of this exploratory study was to examine the effects of three different types of diaphragms on consumer satisfaction. Specifically, the author investigated differences between the wide-seal arching diaphragm, the arching spring diaphragm, and the coil spring diaphragm with regard to discomfort, ease of insertion, and overall satisfaction. The sample (n = 38 at 1 year) consisted of female college students, ranging in age from 18 to 25 years, who were first-time diaphragm users. The author reported that the majority of the study participants were Caucasian. Subjects were fitted first with either an arching spring or a coil spring diaphragm, then with the wide seal diaphragm. They were then instructed to alternate diaphragms on a weekly basis for the first 2 to 4 weeks. Alternate diaphragms were then to be used on a monthly basis. Total time of the study was 1 year, with follow-up visits scheduled at 2 to 4 weeks, 4 to 6 months, and 1 year after initial fitting. Continued use of any diaphragm was a substantial problem. Factors such as menstruation, discomfort, not planning ahead, and difficulty in removing the diaphragm contributed to nonuse. Analysis of the 1-year findings indicated that comfort or ease of insertion were not influenced by the type of diaphragm. Overall satisfaction was greater for users of the coil spring diaphragm than for users of the other two diaphragms. An additional finding was that women recommended the diaphragm as a pregnancy prevention method to their friends.

Comment:
The author presents a timely piece of research. The findings, although not statistically significant, provide information upon which further research can be based. Several appropriate methodologic limitations are identified by the investigator: small sample size; frequency of intercourse not controlled; use of a recall questionnaire that was not pretested; and the collection of minimal demographic data.

Despite limitations, factors that contribute to the high discontinuation rate may warrant consideration in one's practice. The nurse may wish to present a thorough discussion of these factors at the time of the initial fitting for a diaphragm. In this manner, measures can be identified that will foster the continued use of the diaphragm. Furthermore, as the type of diaphragm does not seem to alter the continuation rates, every measure should be taken to fit the client with the type most comfortable for her. The favorable reception that the diaphragm received when initially used also deserves mention. Nurses responsible for family planning may wish to offer the diaphragm as an initial means of pregnancy prevention.

Teaching Needs. Teaching needs are similar to those for diaphragm users for duration of insertion and TSS (*see* box on page 211). In addition, the client should be instructed to use two tablespoons of tap water to thoroughly wet the sponge prior to insertion. The sponge should be inserted with the dimple toward the cervix. The client removes the sponge by grasping the loop and gently pulling it. The client should be instructed to inspect the sponge for intactness before discarding it. Like the condom, the sponge is *not* reusable. Repeated intercourse can occur, however, once a sponge has been inserted.

Cervical Cap (with Spermicidal Agents)

Effectiveness and Action. As Table 9–5 indicates, the effectiveness of the cervical cap (with spermicidal agent) is comparable to that of the diaphragm, with a typical failure rate of 18 percent. Typical failure rate may, however, be as low as 6.4 percent.[63] Effectiveness of the cervical cap as a pregnancy prevention method is dependent on consistency of use.[63]

The **cervical cap** exerts its pregnancy prevention action in the same manner as the diaphragm. That is, as the rubber cap is fitted over the cervix, it serves as a physical barrier preventing contact between sperm and cervix (Figure 9–13). The cap can be compared to a thimble, with the portion that would cover the finger being the portion inserted over the cervix.

The Prentif Cavity Rim cervical cap received FDA approval for national use in May 1988. The Prentif cervical cap is the only cap available for contraceptive use in the United States. As with diaphragm use, the cervical cap must be fitted to the individual wearer; it is available in four sizes.

Benefits. The cervical cap provides another method of pregnancy prevention for diaphragm users who wish to continue using barrier methods but are unable to do so because of recurrent urinary infections associated with diaphragm use. The cervical cap is also an alternative for women who are unable to use birth control pills.[63]

The cervical cap provides more flexibility in that

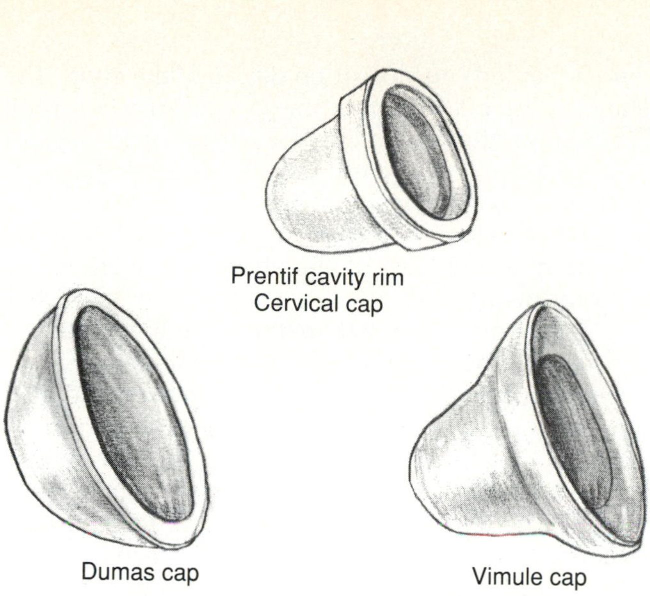

Figure 9–13. Three types of cervical caps. (*Redrawn, with permission, from Hatcher RA, et al.* Contraceptive Technology, 1988–1989. *14th ed. New York: Irvington Publishers, 1988.*)

it can be worn for up to 48 hours and does not require either as much spermicide as the diaphragm or additional spermicide applications with repeated acts of intercourse. Furthermore, no additional spermicidal agents are required when the cervical cap is inserted several hours prior to coitus.

Because of the cervical cap's similarity to the diaphragm, a protective action against STDs may exist. No data currently exists, however, to support this belief.

Risks and Contraindications. Conversion of normal to abnormal Pap tests have been documented for both cervical cap and diaphragm users. The rates are, however, significantly different: 4 percent for the cervical cap versus 1.7 percent for the diaphragm. Consequently, the cervical cap should only be prescribed for women with normal Pap tests.[63] Furthermore, women who choose to use the cervical cap should return for a Pap test after using the cap for 3 months.

Allergic reactions to either the rubber cap or to the spermicidal agent is a possibility, as with diaphragm use. Another possibility is the occurrence of TSS, particularly when the cap is worn for extended periods of time.

Other risks include unpleasant vaginal odor, difficulty in inserting and removing the cap, and discomfort or trauma when the cervical cap is used.[64] The cervical cap is not the pregnancy prevention method of choice for those women who have (1) allergies to rubber or spermicide; (2) history of TSS, cervical cell changes (dysplagias), or UTIs; (3) vaginal or pelvic infections; or (4) a history of HPV.[19]

Teaching Needs. The time required to be fitted with the cervical cap is between a half to one and a half hours. The client needs to be aware of this in order to make appropriate arrangements (work, child care, transportation). The client should be encouraged to remove the cap after 24 hours of use, as cap wear, vaginal odor, and incidence of TSS increase with length of time in place.[63,64] The client should be instructed in the proper care of the cap (*see* teaching needs of diaphragm users).

Coitus Interruptus

Effectiveness and Action. **Coitus interruptus** occurs when, during intercourse, the man withdraws his penis from his partner's vagina and ejaculates external to the woman's external genitalia. Penile withdrawal has a typical failure rate of 18 percent, comparable to diaphragm, sponge, and cervical cap failure rates. Although employed by few couples in the United States, this method of pregnancy prevention is popular in such countries as Poland, Italy, and France.

Coitus interruptus is a pregnancy preventive method in that ejaculation occurs away from the female's external genitalia. Theoretically, then, sperm do not come in contact with the cervix and pregnancy is prevented. There are, however, many practical considerations that make this method difficult to use effectively.

Benefits. Coitus interruptus is always available. Furthermore, its use requires neither devices nor chemicals. There is no cost associated with coitus interruptus. Use of this method of pregnancy prevention may enhance a couple's ability to communicate and to explore other means of sexual satisfaction.

Risks and Contraindications. Many couples consider withdrawal as very effective in preventing pregnancy in that ejaculation occurs outside the woman's body; however, excellent self-control is required with this method. Consequently, in the excitement of impending orgasm, the male partner may not be able to exert sufficient control to withdraw prior to ejaculation (nor may the female partner wish him to do so).

The incidence of conception is related to the number of orgasms. Multiple orgasms occurring over a short time period increase sperm concentration in preejaculation fluid. Therefore, even if the male partner withdraws prior to ejaculation, the female partner may be exposed to a sufficient number of sperm to result in conception.

The sex act is interrupted at a crucial moment with this method. Consequently, a factor to consider is that the sexual pleasure of both partners may be diminished when coitus interruptus is employed.

Teaching Needs. The couple should be encouraged to wipe off the tip of the penis before insertion, thereby decreasing the chance of unknowingly introducing sperm in to the vagina.[19] Risks should be emphasized and alternative contraceptive methods discussed. The couple may wish to use a spermicide should ejaculation occur while the penis is in the vagina. If coitus interruptus is the method adopted, the couple's decision should be reinforced, given that some method is better than no method.

Furthermore, the health care provider should make every effort to provide information about alternative methods of achieving orgasm, especially when the possibility of decreased sexual pleasure is very real. Mutual masturbation is one example of an alternative method. In addition the health care provider will need to keep in mind the religious and cultural beliefs of the couple, as these factors can influence the reception of the information given.[19]

Periodic Abstinence (Natural Family Planning)

Effectiveness and Action. Four methods of periodic abstinence, also called natural family planning, are identified in Table 9–5. Lowest expected failure rates range from 2 to 10 percent. The typical failure rate for all methods is 20 percent. Effectiveness is contingent on the accurate definition of the fertile period that is to be avoided.[65] Although methods of assessment vary, all periodic abstinence options are based on "voluntary avoidance of intercourse by a couple during the fertile phase of the menstrual cycle to avoid pregnancy."[65] All methods require extensive instruction for maximum effectiveness.

Using the **postovulation method,** the couple may have intercourse only after the occurrence of ovulation has been determined. Sufficient time, generally at least three days, should have passed between ovulation and intercourse. For example, if a woman's normal cycle is 30 days, ovulation (*see* discussion of calendar method) may occur on day 16 of the cycle. The couple abstains from the time of menstruation until three days after ovulation, for a total of 19 days of abstinence. Consequently, for this example the couple has 11 "safe" days during a 30-day cycle in which to have intercourse. This method is hypothesized to be the most effective of the abstinence methods to prevent pregnancy.

The **sympto-thermal method** combines the assessment of body symptoms with temperature readings. Basal body temperature (BBT) is taken and documented on a daily basis, as are cervical mucus changes. In addition, women employing this method observe for such other signs and symptoms as spotting, breast tenderness, and mid-cycle pain (mittelschmerz). A cervical palpation is sometimes employed with the sympto-thermal method. By using her middle finger, a woman can assess the consistency of the cervix: the cervix becomes softer, more open, and "moves up and away from the vaginal opening" during ovulation.[66]

Both the **thermal method** and the **cervical mucus** method are forms of the **ovulation method.** The thermal method assesses changes in the BBT. Employing an expanded-scale thermometer, the woman takes her temperature (usually oral) every morning on awakening, before any activity is undertaken. To facilitate this, the thermometer can be shaken down before going to bed the previous night. Temperature readings are then recorded and inspected for an elevation (*see* Figure 7–9). When the temperature remains elevated for three days, ovulation is thought to have occurred.[66] Intercourse is then considered safe and can occur after this time. When used in conjunction with other methods, the thermal method helps predict ovulation. Hatcher and colleagues provide very comprehensive instructions on this method.[19]

The cervical mucus method assesses changes in cervical mucus as a result of hormonal fluctuations associated with the normal menstrual cycle.[66] As ovulation approaches or occurs, the characteristics of cervical mucus change. It becomes more abundant and stretchy, thin, clear, and slippery. Table 9–8 presents a summary of cervical mucus changes during the menstrual cycle. Interestingly, most users of this method rely on bodily sensations of lubrication, moisture, and stickiness rather than the actual characteristics.[66]

The **calendar method** provides the individual or couple with opportunity to determine when intercourse should be avoided because of the presence of an ovum. This method identifies the couple's fertile

TABLE 9–8. CYCLIC CHARACTERISTICS OF THE CERVIX AND CERVICAL MUCUS

Time of Cycle	Amount	Viscosity	Appearance	Spinnbarkeit	Ferning	Cervix
Postmenstruation	Moderate	Thick	Cloudy	None	None	Firm, closed
Nearing ovulation	Increasing	Somewhat thick to thin	Mixed/cloudy and clear	Moderate	Moderate	Firm, closed
Ovulation	Maximum	Very thin and slippery	Clear	Maximum 2–3 or more inches	Well developed	Soft, open
Post-ovulation (about 3 days)	Decreasing	Thin	Mixed cloudy and clear	Minimal or none	Minimal or none	Firm, closed
Nearing menstruation	Minimal	Thick	Cloudy	None	None	Firm, closed

Reprinted with permission, from Hatcher RA, et al. Contraceptive Technology, 1988–1989. *14th ed. New York: Irvington Publishers, 1988. Adapted from Health Education Bulletin, July 1979, by the National Clearinghouse for Family Planning Information DHEW, Bureau of Community Health Services.*

period and is based on three assumptions: (1) ovulation occurs on day 14 (plus or minus two days) before the onset of the next menses; (2) sperm remain viable for two to three days; and (3) the ovum survives for 24 hours.[19]

In order to enhance its predictive abilities, and before using this method, the client must maintain a menstrual calendar documenting the length of her menstrual cycle for an 8-month period. The period of abstinence can be determined once the pattern of the cycle is apparent; the earliest fertile day is then calculated by subtracting 18 days from the length of the shortest cycle.[19] Subtracting 11 days from the woman's longest cycle will identify the woman's latest fertile day. Because truly regular cycles are experienced by few women, and because an abnormal cycle is not unusual over a single year, this method is now generally supplemented by more reliable assessment methods.[66]

An alternative to periodic abstinence, with well-defined assessment measures, is **total abstinence.** This form of pregnancy prevention is very acceptable and should be recognized and accepted by health care professionals. Other forms of expressing the individual's sexuality bear exploration when total abstinence is chosen.

Benefits. Many benefits are associated with periodic abstinence methods. They are (1) always available; (2) inexpensive; (3) always reversible; and (4) have no side effects.[66] They provide a pregnancy prevention method for those for whom other methods are unacceptable, whether for physical, ethical, or religious reasons. Furthermore, periodic abstinence methods increase the woman's understanding of her body and the couple's awareness of their fertility. Certainly communication between partners is encouraged through the use of such a pregnancy prevention method.

Risks and Contraindications. Although not risks, there are several disadvantages associated with abstinence methods. Meticulous record keeping is required for all methods. Participation in the chosen method is on a daily basis. Motivation must remain high for both partners. Extensive training, over several months, is required to enhance effectiveness. Sexual spontaneity may be stifled. Breastfeeding mothers may be unable to determine accurately safe or infertile periods, so this method is not recommended for them.

There are no absolute contraindications. Such factors as irregular menstrual cycles and irregular temperature charts, however, may impede the use of this method as a method of pregnancy prevention.

Teaching Needs. Couples choosing periodic abstinence methods will require extensive education with regard to accurate documentation and accurate assessment. If a combination of methods is used, all components must be addressed. Hatcher and colleagues present a comprehensive discussion of needed instruction.[19]

Spermicidal Agents

Effectiveness and Action. As Table 9–5 indicates, the lowest expected failure rate of spermicidal agents is 3 percent; typical failure rate is 21 percent, and may even be as high as 30 percent.[19] Rate of effectiveness is related to accessibility. Spermicidal agents can be readily obtained in pharmacies. Rate of effectiveness is also enhanced when spermicidal agents are combined with a second method, such as the condom or diaphragm.

Spermicidal agents consist of an inert substance that holds the spermicidal chemical in place. The spermicidal chemical is usually nonoxynol-9, the same chemical that is used in certain condoms (*see* section on condoms). Pregnancy is prevented by means of active destruction of sperm by the chemical.

Another over-the-counter product, recently made available and comparable in action and rate of effectiveness to the sponge, is a spermicidal film called Vaginal Contraceptive Film (VCF). Measuring only 2 inches by 2 inches, this translucent paper-thin square dissolves into a cohesive gel when inserted into the vagina. Insertion time is 15 minutes before intercourse. Effectiveness is maintained for up to two hours after insertion.[67,68] If used correctly with a condom the VCF is 100 percent effective.[67]

Benefits. There are a variety of spermicidal agents: foams, jellies, film, suppositories.[19] Consequently, the client has considerable flexibility in choosing the agent most suitable to meet his or her needs. Many forms are individually packaged, adding even greater user appeal. Spermicidal agents are also readily accessible, making them an attractive method. Spermicidal agents may provide some protection against STDs, reflected by the decreased incidence of PID in women who use spermicides.

Risks and Contraindications. Occasionally an allergic response may occur, or suppositories may not melt or foam when placed in the vagina. An unpleasant taste may be noted by couples having oral-genital sex. The possibility that spermicidal agents may have teratogenic effects has been studied and although results do not support an association, controversy continues.[19]

Teaching Needs. Clients need to be informed about proper insertion techniques and signs and symptoms of an allergic response. Insertion times should be clearly understood. Table 9–9 presents a comprehensive review of pertinent client informational needs.

Ineffective Methods

Despite the wide variety of contraceptive methods available, some individuals still practice methods that are ineffective in preventing conception. Among these are douching and breastfeeding.

Douching. **Douching,** or cleansing of the vagina to rid it of sperm, has been used as a contraceptive method for centuries. Agents such as citrus, herbs, cola, and lye have been used with poor or even lethal results. The use effectiveness rate of douching is less than 60 percent. When vaginal spermicides are used, it is especially important not to douche for at least six hours after intercourse because the spermicide will be rendered ineffective.

Breastfeeding. Breastfeeding is not a reliable method of birth control because there is no way to determine when ovulation and subsequent menstruation will first occur after birth. All women have postpartum amenorrhea for a time. Breastfeeding mothers experience a longer period of amenorrhea and anovulation than bottlefeeding mothers. Prolactin, the hormone that stimulates milk production, also decreases the level of luteinizing hormone necessary for maintaining the menstrual cycle, thus delaying the onset of menses. Women who breastfeed on demand for long periods of time have more contraceptive benefits. Women in the United States, however, tend to supplement feedings and often nurse on a schedule and for a shorter period of time, thus creating the increased chance that ovulation will occur.

Future Trends in Pregnancy Prevention Methods

Currently, options for pregnancy prevention include those listed in Table 9–5 as well as the morning-after pill. The trend will be toward making more options available to all individuals desiring pregnancy prevention.

A new product, undergoing clinical trials since March 1988, is a female condom. Known as the WPC-33, "the device consists of a soft, loose-fitting polyurethane sheath and two flexible polyurethane rings."[53] One ring anchors the device, the other remains outside the vagina.[53] Unlike the male condom, this device can be lubricated and inserted any time before intercourse.

Extensive work is currently in progress to develop and refine hormonal contraceptive devices that are long-acting in nature.[69–73] Pregnancy prevention action could then be provided for a period of several weeks to perhaps 5 years. For example, estrogen-releasing skin patches are currently in use with gynecologic clients. Their use as a pregnancy prevention method is being considered.[69]

Subdermal implants, whether in the form of silastic tubes, biodegradable capsules, pellets, or mi-

TABLE 9–9. VAGINAL SPERMICIDES FOR USE ALONE OR WITH A VAGINAL DIAPHRAGM[a]

	How many applicators-full in one application?	How long before this spermicide will be effective?	How far in advance of intercourse can this spermicide be inserted?[b]	How long after intercourse before douching?
Foams				
Delfen	2	0	30–60 min	8 hr
Emko	1	0	30–60 min	8 hr
Emko Because	1	0	30–60 min	8 hr
Emko Pre-Fil	1	0	30–60 min	8 hr
Koromex	2	0	30–60 min	8 hr
Jellies				
Conceptrol gel	1	0	30–60 min	8 hr
Ramses Contraceptive Vaginal jelly	1	0	30–60 min	8 hr
Creams				
Conceptrol Birth Control Cream	1	0	30–60 min	8 hr
Koromex IIA	1	0	30–60 min	8 hr
Suppositories				
Encare Oval	1 pellet	10 min	30–60 min	8 hr
Intercept	1 pellet	10 min	30–60 min	8 hr
Semicid	1 pellet	15 min	30–60 min	8 hr
Jellies				
Gynol II	1	0	6–8 hr	8 hr
Koromex II	1	0	6–8 hr	8 hr
Koromex Crystal Clear gel	1	0	6–8 hr	8 hr
Ortho-Gynol Contraceptive Jelly	1	0	6–8 hr	8 hr
Creams				
Koromex Contraceptive Cream	1	0	6–8 hr	8 hr
Ortho-Creme Contraceptive Cream	1	0	6–8 hr	8 hr

[a] Any of the spermicidal creams or jellies listed may be used with the cervical cap.
[b] Although some manufacturers of spermicides suggest that vaginal spermicides used without a diaphragm may be inserted up to 1 hour before intercourse, we recommend that these spermicides be inserted no more than 30 minutes before intercourse to ensure maximum effectiveness. Likewise, we recommend inserting the diaphragm with spermicidal cream or jelly no more than 6 hours before intercourse.
Reprinted, with permission, from Hatcher RA, et al. Contraceptive Technology, 1988–1989. *14th ed. New York: Irvington Publishers, 1988.*

crospheres, are under investigation as other methods of pregnancy prevention. The Norplant silastic tube is a pregnancy prevention method already available in 12 countries.[69] The FDA is currently considering its use in the United States. Although a surgical incision is required for insertion and removal of the implant, Norplant has been received favorably by those using it, primarily because the implant removes the need for regular or intermittent occasional pregnancy prevention methods.[70]

Silastic implants can be removed at any time either because of side effects or the desire to conceive. Consequently, they deliver the hormonal preparation over a period of years. On the other hand injectable microspheres, because they dissolve and are therefore not retrievable, have a limited period of action: 1 to 6 months.[70]

Biodegradable implants, placed under the skin, dissolve over a period of time. Capronor, a biodegradable implant, is anticipated to be active for at least 18 months.[19] Capronor is not currently available in the United States.

Another option available outside the United States is monthly hormonal injections.[19] The woman's menstrual cycle undergoes minimal disruption with this combination hormonal preparation. Levonorgestrel-releasing vaginal rings and intracervical devices are also being investigated.[74]

A birth control vaccine may be available in the future.[75–77] Its action may be to prevent either fertilization or implantation.[75]

Other future pregnancy prevention methods include postcoital contraceptives and luteinizing hormone–releasing hormone (LH-RH) antagonists. A progesterone antagonist, RU 486, has recently received considerable attention.[19,78–80] Because some consider RU 486 an abortifacient, its use as a pregnancy prevention method remains controversial.

The preceding discussion has presented potential alternatives for women. Research efforts have, however, also recently been directed toward the development of male pregnancy prevention methods. Blocking the vas deferens by the injection of a polymer has been shown to lower the pH in the vas of monkeys.[19] No data are currently available assessing this technique in humans. Other forms of male contraception that hold promise for the future include the use of ultrasound to suppress spermatogenesis and LH-RH analogues with androgens.[19] Both of these have been demonstrated to suppress spermatogenesis in humans. A male pill, gossypol, has also been investigated.[19,81] Although its effectiveness in the prevention of pregnancy has been ascertained, the toxic effects associated with its use remain of grave concern. Both the irreversibility of the pill and the hypokalemia that occurs consequent to gossypol usage bear further investigation.

As is evident, the future holds many alternatives for individuals and couples seeking to prevent pregnancy. Certainly, as many choices as possible should be made available to meet individual and couple needs. Inherent in the increased number of options is the responsibility of the health care professional to provide comprehensive and complete information on which the client can make a knowledgeable choice.

PREGNANCY TERMINATION

Approximately half of all pregnancies are unintended; however, many women decide to continue their pregnancy. The decision-making process regarding whether to continue or terminate a pregnancy begins when a woman first suspects she is pregnant. This decision-making process may be brief or a woman may take weeks or even months to come to a decision. During this time a woman should have an opportunity to discuss openly with a nurse or other health professional whether or not she wishes to continue her pregnancy. The discussion should include a review of the woman's situation, her age, marital status, family stability, socioeconomic status, personal goals and values, religious beliefs, and many other social and psychologic factors. A pregnancy risk assessment should be carried out by the nurse so that identified risk factors and reproductive options may be weighed in her decision.

Women have terminated undesired pregnancies for many generations. This has been true whether their culture approved or disapproved. Accurate statistics regarding pregnancy termination are difficult to ascertain, especially in countries where the procedure is not legal. Statistics in the United States indicate that the pregnancy termination rate steadily increased in the 1970s. It began to level off around 1979. In 1984 there were slightly more than 1.5 million pregnancy terminations. This number is lower than that observed in the late 1970s.[82] The decline in the pregnancy termination rate does not appear to be due to women being more likely to carry an unintended pregnancy to term, because there was no corresponding increase in the number of live births. Thus it is believed that the decline in the termination rate reflects the lower pregnancy rate.[82]

Despite the slight decline in the pregnancy termination rate, the majority of United States adults continue to approve of legal pregnancy termination. In 1980 a survey showed that 90 percent of the adults

ISSUES AND CONTROVERSIES

In the 1990s there will be no more controversial area in health care than that concerned with reproductive and fertility control (and methods of doing so). Two major issues include:

1. What will be the impact of the July 1989 Supreme Court ruling described in this chapter? Throughout the 1990s, many issues concerning rights of women and rights of fetuses will continue to be the bases of heated controversy on a state and national basis. These issues will be intensified should future Supreme Court rulings overturn *Roe v Wade*.
2. What rights and options for reproduction are available for homosexuals? For individuals with HIV infection? For individuals who are very likely to pass on severe genetic problems to offspring? For individuals who are mentally retarded? Over the years some segments of the population have favored mandatory sterilization of certain individuals, a highly controversial sentiment that still exists today.

in the United States approved of legal termination if a woman's health were endangered by the pregnancy; 83 percent approved if the woman became pregnant as a result of rape; 83 percent approved if there was a strong chance that the fetus had a serious birth defect; 52 percent approved if the family could not afford the child; 48 percent approved if the woman was not married and did not wish to marry; 47 percent approved if a woman was married but did not desire the child; 41 percent approved for "any reason."[83]

Legal Status of Pregnancy Termination in the United States

On January 22, 1973, the United States Supreme Court announced the decision of two landmark cases (*Roe v Wade* and *Doe v Bolton*) related to pregnancy termination. A summary of the decision follows[19]:

1. In the first trimester, the termination decision and its performance must be left to the judgment of the pregnant woman and her physician.
2. In the second trimester, the state, in prompting its interest in the health of the pregnant woman, may choose to regulate the termination decision in ways that are reasonably related to her health.
3. Subsequent to viability, the state, in promoting its interest and the interest in the potentiality of human life, may, if it chooses, regulate and even prohibit termination except where it is necessary, according to appropriate medical judgment, for the preservation of the life or health of the pregnant woman.

On July 1, 1976, the Supreme Court held that the state cannot impose the requirement of consent by a third party on a woman's right to abortion. This "veto" power cannot be exercised by a spouse or a parent (Supreme Court). Despite strong antitermination sentiments in some populations, the Supreme Court repeatedly upheld the woman's right to a pregnancy termination, until July 3, 1989. At this time, the Supreme Court, in *Webster v Reproductive Health Services*, upheld a Missouri law that in effect gave individual states a much greater ability to restrict pregnancy termination. In this ruling, a law banning use of state facilities, and prohibiting state employees from performing abortions was upheld. Furthermore, a provision requiring physicians to perform tests to determine whether a 20-week-old fetus could survive outside the uterus was also upheld on the grounds that such testing furthered the state's interest in protecting potential human life. While the Supreme Court decision stopped short of reversing *Roe v Wade*, other tests cases that are pending in the Supreme Court might result in its overthrow. Health care professionals must remain aware of the possible impact of the July 3, 1989, Supreme Court ruling on current and future contraceptive technology. As individual states make decisions concerning the beginnings of life and their responsibility in that area, certain contraceptive methods (for instance, the morning-after pill) also may be called into question.

Since 1977 Congress and state legislatures have imposed many restrictions related to federal and state funding of pregnancy terminations. While the federal government (as of 1981) provides funding for terminations only in the case of a threat of death to the mother should she carry the pregnancy, some states have chosen to provide funding for these services for welfare-eligible clients.[19]

In 1985, 14 states had no public funding limitations for pregnancy terminations, five because of court order. Thirty states were limiting the funding of pregnancy termination to cases where the woman's life was threatened. The remaining six states allowed public-funded termination if the woman was a victim of rape or incest, if her life was endangered by the pregnancy, or in some cases if the fetus was abnormal.[84] With the new ruling, however, it is likely that state legislatures will be reconsidering their roles in pregnancy termination.

The availability of legal pregnancy terminations has dramatically decreased the maternal mortality and morbidity previously associated with illegal, criminal terminations.[82] Prior to legalization, terminations were responsible for the majority of maternal deaths in urban areas, with estimates of 800 to 5000 maternal deaths per year.[82]

Psychosocial Factors Affecting Pregnancy Termination

In most societies there is a high value placed on women in their role as mothers, and powerful systems of reinforcement operate to make motherhood central to women's lives. A decision to terminate a pregnancy is rarely made without some conflict of emotions because of the complex values associated with womanhood and motherhood. Even if the child is unwanted, the woman may on some levels desire to remain pregnant as a symbol of potency, vitality, or reconnection with inner wishes and desires. Though some unintended pregnancies can be completely accidental and the result of a contraceptive method failure, many result from contraceptive misuse or nonuse. An "accidental" pregnancy sometimes is a mechanism used to affect relations with important people in a woman's life, such as a husband, lover, or parents.

Some teenagers become pregnant to demonstrate

their sexuality and maturity, and to bolster their self-concept. An infant may be desired, in some instances, as someone to love them. The use of contraceptive methods may be avoided because it represents premeditation regarding sexual activity, which they feel is taboo. On finding she is pregnant, the teenager may decide that she cannot face the responsibilities of caring for and raising a child and thus elects abortion.

A woman may become pregnant to force a lover into marriage or salvage a troubled marriage or other relationship. She may then find that the pregnancy did not produce the desired result and elect to terminate the pregnancy.

Poor physical or mental health can result in pregnancy termination. A woman to whom the pregnancy poses a risk to her physical or mental health may choose a termination.

Termination may be chosen if a pregnancy is untimely. Finishing an education, reaching a personal or professional goal, recent marriage, recent childbirth, and income collapse are reasons that some women elect a pregnancy termination.

Sociocultural factors can also play an important role in a decision to seek pregnancy termination. If termination is illegal, a woman may risk minimal prosecution to terminate her pregnancy. If social values condemn terminations, she faces disapproval by peers, family members, and members of her community. When pregnancy terminations are legal and societal values are more accepting, deciding to have a termination may be less traumatic.

Although at this time the United States places no legal restrictions on early pregnancy terminations and very few requirements on later ones, this does not mean that every woman who desires to terminate a pregnancy has equal access. The ability to obtain a termination is greatly influenced by such factors as the availability and accessibility of facilities providing these services, methods of financing health care services, and personal and economic resources.

For women with health insurance or adequate means to pay for a termination, lack of facilities providing this service can be a problem. Eight of every ten counties in the United States have no facility providing these services. It is estimated that one fourth of the women in need of this service live in these counties.

The situation for poor women has become particularly difficult in the last several years. Since the enactment of the Hyde Amendment, which restricted federal funds for pregnancy termination, funding has dropped 99 percent for Medicaid patients.[85] Many states have even chosen not to fund the terminations the federal government left to state control. The new Supreme Court ruling, which resulted in the closing of publicly subsidized facilities in Missouri, will exacerbate this situation as other states follow suit.

The impact of this decrease in publicly funded pregnancy terminations is felt in many ways. Women with no or low income who are intent on having a termination often delay their procedure while seeking the necessary funds. This leads to an increase in the complication rate because the pregnancy termination takes place at a later gestational age. It often also results in the need for a more costly procedure for a second-trimester abortion. Women with low income who are able to raise the money for their own terminations may do so at the expense of their rent or utility bills, food, clothing, or by fraudulent use of relatives' insurance policies. Extreme desperation may lead to self-induced abortion or even suicide.

In the United States, termination of pregnancy is, like all health care, usually an option dependent on adequate income.

Counseling Regarding Pregnancy Termination

The nurse is often a key professional in providing counseling to women considering a pregnancy termination. The need to make responsible decisions about an unwanted or problem pregnancy may become apparent in a prenatal or family planning clinic or in another health care setting. The nurse may institute initial discussion and assistance in beginning to solve problems with women or couples facing an unintended pregnancy.

Many women need to think beyond their initial reaction to the unintended pregnancy. They need to be encouraged to consider all options available to them. It is important for the nurse to encourage the woman to make the decision herself, even though she may feel confused and ambivalent, because of pressure from her partner, other family members, or peers. Regret and emotional sequelae will be minimized when the choice is not perceived as being forced by others. Exploring alternatives helps to realistically clarify the situation. Thinking through each choice should include not only exploring present feelings and relationships, but also future circumstances, goals, and needs.

The nurse or counselor should also explain the abortion procedure required for the client's stage of gestation, how it is done, its discomforts, safety, risks, duration, cost, and follow-up care instructions. Written information summarizing this discussion should be provided to the client to ensure informed choice or consent.

Many psychosocial factors are weighed in the decision to continue or terminate a pregnancy. If the woman is involved in a stable relationship she may wish to include her partner in the decision-making process. It is important, however, for the woman's desires to be respected in this regard.

As prenatal diagnostic techniques have become more sophisticated and accessible, more women are choosing to determine if the child they are carrying has a birth defect or genetic disorder. The decision to terminate a pregnancy because of an abnormality in the fetus presents additional psychosocial factors that complicate the woman or couple's decision-making process and thus will be dealt with separately in this chapter.

Termination Procedures

Pregnancy terminations may be carried out during the first trimester (during the first 13 weeks after the beginning of the last menstrual period) or the second trimester (from 14 to 24 weeks of gestation). If a woman suspects that she may be pregnant but no positive diagnosis has been made, a menstrual extraction or a vacuum aspiration of uterine contents can be carried out before the woman's first missed period.

First Trimester Pregnancy Terminations

The Morning-After Pill. The **morning-after pill** requires the administration of a high dose of synthetic estrogen during the first days after possible conception. This high level of estrogen intake causes the endometrial lining to shed. At the present time a combined oral contraceptive is more frequently used than the morning-after pill. Two combined oral contraceptive pills (usually Ovral) are taken within 72 hours of intercourse. Two more combined oral contraceptive pills are taken 12 hours later.

Menstrual Extraction. **Menstrual extraction** may be performed if the client's menstrual period is less than 2 weeks late. Some clients choose not to confirm the presence of the pregnancy so they can avoid the ethical dilemma of continuing or terminating the pregnancy.

Menstrual extraction is performed by inserting a sterile plastic cannula into the endometrial cavity. Suction is then applied with a large syringe to withdraw the uterine contents. This procedure is performed on an outpatient basis, requires no anesthesia, no cervical dilation, and takes only a few minutes to complete. It is also low in cost.

Vaccum Aspiration. Pregnancies that are less than 12 to 13 weeks of gestation may be terminated by **vacuum aspiration** using a cannula and suction. For this procedure to be carried out, the cervix must be dilated. The amount of dilation required is determined by the gestation of the pregnancy. After cervical dilation, the cannula is introduced into the uterus and a small suction pump is used to remove the products of conception. The procedure takes less than ten minutes to complete and is usually performed under local anesthesia to the cervix and on an outpatient basis. The client is allowed to go home within one to four hours after the procedure.

Dilation and Curettage. The **dilation and curettage** (D and C) procedure is similar to a vacuum aspiration except that the uterine walls are scraped with a curet instead of using a cannula and suction.

Second Trimester Pregnancy Terminations

Dilation and Evacuation. A **dilation and evacuation** (D and E) procedure is very similar to a D and C. It can be used for pregnancy termination between 13 and 24 weeks of gestation. With a D and E the cervix requires substantially more dilation, because the products of conception are much larger. Local anesthesia is used for this procedure and the woman is usually allowed to go home on the same day as the procedure.

Prostaglandin Instillation. **Prostaglandin instillation** may be used to terminate a pregnancy around 15 weeks of gestation. Prostaglandin can be inserted vaginally as a suppository into the cul-de-sac or administered intra-abdominally into the amniotic sac. It is used to induce uterine contractions. After instillation of prostaglandin, uterine contractions usually begin within a few hours. Uterine contractions continue until the fetus is delivered. Hospitalization is required for this method and the woman should be observed for nausea, vomiting, cervical lacerations, and tissue reactions. The major disadvantage to the use of this method late in pregnancy is the possibility that a live fetus may be delivered.

Saline Induction. A **saline termination** of pregnancy is a method that may be used after 16 weeks of gestation. An amniocentesis is performed to remove some of the amniotic fluid. After the amniotic fluid is removed, a hypertonic saline solution is introduced into the amniotic sac. Uterine contractions usually begin within 12 to 24 hours. The labor may last 10 to 24 hours. The woman will need to be hospitalized and must be treated similarly to other women in labor. Sometimes, prostaglandin instillation and saline induction are used in combination for pregnancy termination.

Hysterotomy. Hysterotomy is the removal of the products of conception through an incision in the uterine and abdominal walls. It is rarely used for pregnancy termination. It may be a method chosen when other termination methods are contraindicated. It might be chosen as the method when a woman desires a sterilization procedure at the same time.

Risk Factors and Complications

The risks associated with pregnancy terminations since terminations have become legal are minimal. The potential complications that have been observed are less likely if: the pregnancy is terminated early; the client is healthy; the clinician performing the procedure is well trained and experienced; the uterus is not severely anteverted or retroverted; the client understands the warning signs for post-termination complications; prompt follow-up care is immediately accessible; careful examination of the products of conception is carried out to ensure complete termination and to rule out the possibility of a molar or ectopic pregnancy; Rh immune globulin is given to Rh-negative women; the client does not have infection such as gonorrhea or chlamydia; and the client is not ambivalent about having the termination or believes that she can cope with the ambivalent feeling she may be experiencing. Local anesthesia is used rather than regional or general anesthesia and *Laminaria digitata* is used to soften the cervix.[19]

The five most common post-termination physical problems observed include: bleeding, infection, retained products of conception or uterine blood clots, continuing pregnancy, and cervical or uterine trauma.[19] The woman should be instructed verbally and given written instructions to contact the clinic or physician if any of the following physical signs occur: fever and chills, foul smelling discharge, heavy bleeding, severe abdominal pain, and nausea and vomiting. The woman should be informed that she should avoid intercourse, use of tampons, and douching for approximately 2 weeks to reduce the risk of introducing bacteria that may cause infection. A discussion should take place regarding the woman's plans for further reproduction. If a woman desires a contraceptive method, she should be provided with this method and instructed on its use.

The woman who has terminated a pregnancy early for psychosocial indications should be informed that she may anticipate a possible grief reaction that may last several months. She should be informed that this is common among women who have terminated pregnancies. The women should be evaluated 2 weeks after the termination for both physical and emotional adjustment to the procedure. At that time a decision about further follow-up evaluation or counseling may be made.

Termination of Pregnancy for a Birth Defect or Genetic Indication

Terminating a pregnancy for a birth defect or a genetic indication is an area that has only been recently studied. Donnai and colleagues reported that grief after such a termination is significant and can be long-lasting.[86] The results of a follow-up investigation in Iowa confirmed the Donnai findings.[87]

In the Iowa study 13 women who had previously terminated their pregnancies in a two-and-a-half-year period were interviewed. Two of the 13 women continued to express a significant grief reaction after their termination. They had experienced major physical changes such as weight loss, the need for medication to sleep, and a change in behavior, particularly exhaustion. They expressed a significant amount of anger and guilt about their termination. They stated that they had withdrawn from their previous activities and felt that they had little or no support from family and friends. One of the two women sobbed throughout the interview.

Four women continued to express a moderate grief reaction. They had difficulty maintaining their activity level and continued to feel quite angry about their loss. They expressed hostility directed at their physicians, their spouse, and other individuals who were able to have normal children. All four cried at their interview.

Two women continued to express a mild grief reaction after their termination. They became tearful during the interview and expressed significant sadness about their loss. They expressed that they believed they had begun to look ahead in their lives. They were eating well, sleeping without difficulty, and they felt they were meeting all of their prior responsibilities.

Five women of the 13 interviewed appeared to have a well-resolved grief process. They did not cry during the interview. They did, however, express a sadness about their loss. They did not express anger or guilt about their termination experience.

These differences in grief resolution were compared to the length of time since the women's pregnancy termination. No major differences were observed in the groups of women who terminated their pregnancies during the year prior to the interview compared to the group of women who had terminated 1 to 2 years before and the group who had terminated more than 2 years before the interview.

The one factor identified that might be associated with the women's resolution of their grief was that of other children being born or adopted into the family subsequent to their termination. It was noted that, of the five women who appeared to be coping well, three of them had given birth to or adopted children since their pregnancy terminations. One woman was currently pregnant and had already received normal prenatal diagnostic results. One of the five women with a well-resolved grief process had made a firm decision not to have further children.

In the group of women who were having difficulty coping, four of the eight women were planning no further children because of their increased age, their risk, or their past experience. Two of the eight women were facing a significant risk of recurrence (25 percent) and had not yet decided about future children. Two of the eight women were planning pregnancies "at some time in the future."

There are many factors that may complicate the grief process associated with a termination of pregnancy because of a birth defect or genetic disorder, among them:

1. Often, few people may know about the pregnancy. The individual or couple may have chosen to keep it private until they received the results of the prenatal diagnostic testing. The pregnancy may have been kept a secret so that if an abnormality was identified and the pregnancy was terminated, there would be fewer people to explain to. This means, however, that there are also fewer people to provide support.
2. Some women have not yet resolved their ambivalent feelings about the pregnancy. The pregnancy may have been untimed or undesired, but the fact that the woman undertook prenatal diagnostic testing was a statement that she intended to continue the pregnancy.
3. An individual or couple who receives abnormal prenatal diagnostic results has little time for anticipatory grief. The couple may be given information about the abnormality present in the fetus on one day and the termination of pregnancy may occur the next.
4. A termination of pregnancy late in the second trimester causes substantial physical pain. There will be cramping and blood loss along with emotional anguish, all of which will magnify a woman's vulnerability.
5. Guilt is a feeling expressed by almost all couples who have a child with a birth defect or genetic disorder. Most individuals or couples believe that it must be something they did or did not do to cause their child to have this problem. Thus the guilt may add to the already complicated grief process.
6. Couples who terminate their pregnancy may not have an opportunity to see or hold their lost baby. They can only fantasize about how their baby might have looked and what he or she would have become. There is also usually no funeral or memorial service. The baby is not given a name. There may be no birth or death certificate. Nothing of the pregnancy remains. The couple has experienced a significant loss and yet it is not acknowledged by many friends, family members, or most of society.
7. Many women who have had prenatal diagnostic tests are nearing the end of their reproductive life. They may have other children who are young adults and leaving home and they may be at an age where they are beginning to be concerned about menopause. These factors too can complicate the grief process the woman is experiencing.
8. Caregivers, friends, and family may have difficulty recognizing or acknowledging that the loss of this pregnancy is significant. Many health care providers have trouble understanding why a woman would be so upset about her pregnancy termination when this is the course of action that she has chosen. It is difficult for health care providers to understand that in this situation, a couple is forced to choose between two difficult alternatives, to terminate the pregnancy or to continue the pregnancy and have a child with a birth defect or genetic disorder.

Because there is significant grief associated with a pregnancy termination for a birth defect or genetic indication, it is important that these families receive ongoing follow-up care after this event.

Whenever possible a couple terminating a pregnancy for a genetic indication should be seen at the time of their termination by a health care provider equipped to provide support and follow-up counseling. At the time of the termination, supportive grief counseling should be initiated. The significance of the loss should be acknowledged and the couple should be encouraged to express their sadness. At that time a plan should be made for follow-up counseling.

Two to 6 weeks after the loss, the woman should have a postpregnancy evaluation. At the time of that visit, the results of any evaluation done on the fetus should be discussed with the couple. Their level of

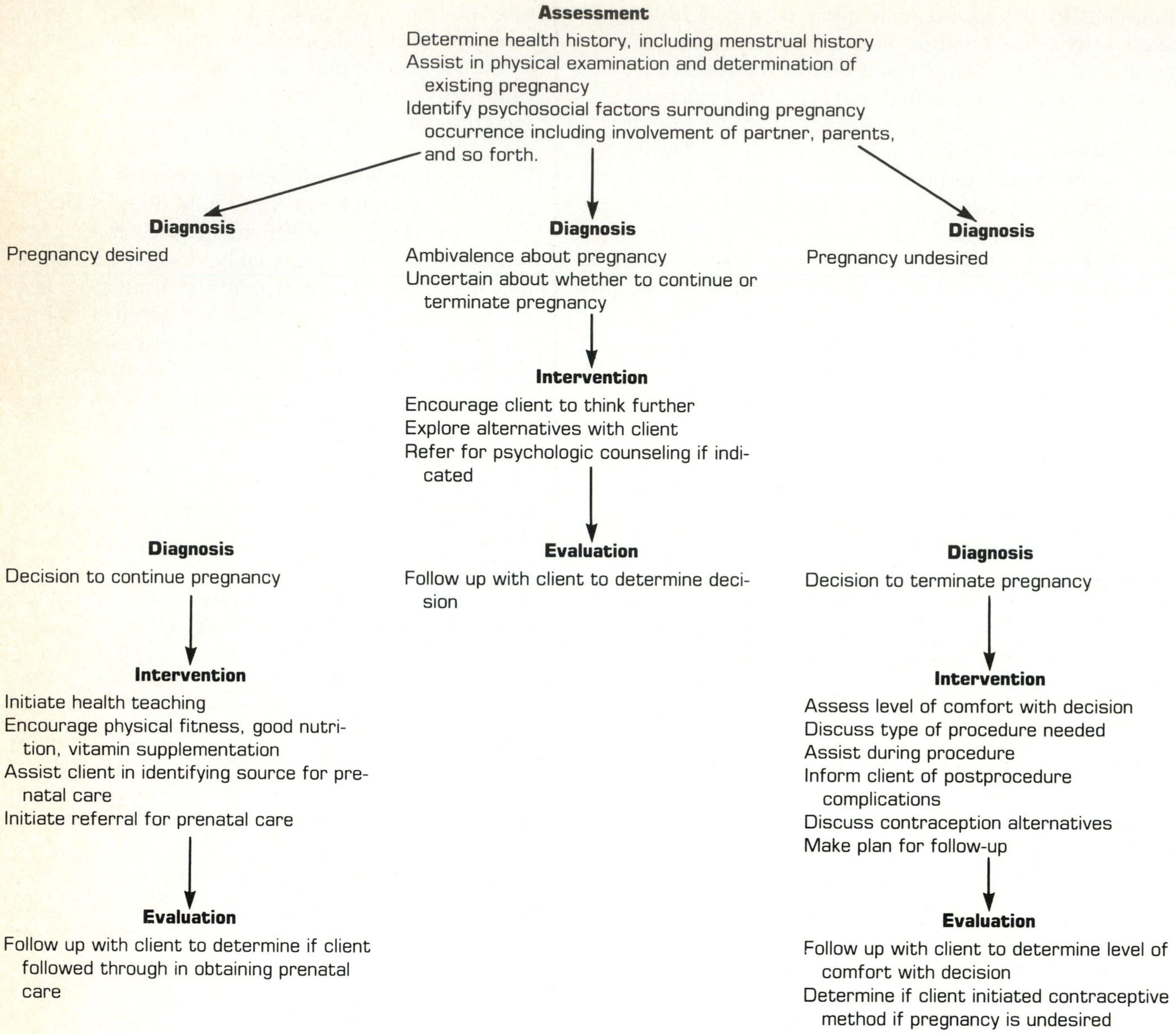

Figure 9–14. Nursing process: pregnancy termination.

grief and support systems available to them should be assessed. A discussion should also take place regarding future reproductive plans and methods of contraception if the couple desires.

Four to 6 months after the loss, a second visit with the couple should take place. This will occur at about the time of the estimated due date. This date may be very important for this couple. It is a date that the couple will have on their minds, perhaps for many years. Again the couple's level of grief and support systems available should be assessed. Further discussion regarding reproduction should take place.

Depending on how the couple is coping, a third visit may be scheduled. This visit should take place 6 to 12 months after the due date. By this time the couple's grief should be fairly well resolved. They should now be looking ahead toward the future rather than back at their loss. If a delayed or distorted grief reaction is identified at this time or at any time during this process, a referral for more in-depth psychological counseling should be considered.

Pregnancy termination for a birth defect or a genetic disorder can have a tremendous impact on a couple. Support and intervention is needed to help the couple in this time of crisis. Figure 9–14 provides a diagram of nursing process for a client with a pregnancy termination.

CASE STUDY/CARE PLAN: SUPPORTING THE COUPLE IN CONTRACEPTIVE DECISION MAKING

Alice and Joe Pulaski have just delivered their fifth baby, a healthy eight-pound girl. Mother, father, and siblings are attaching well to the new baby.

Alice and Joe have been married for 6 years. Their other children are ages 5, 3, 2 and 1 years. When the nurse assesses the couple for discharge planning, Alice confides in her that although she is very happy with this baby, she hopes it will be her last. She states "We just can't afford any more children and it's so hard to take care of so many little ones."

Alice and Joe also confide that their religious beliefs prevent use of the pill, barrier methods, or sterilization. They have been using the rhythm and coitus interruptus methods, which have not been effective, as their last three children were unplanned. After reviewing with the couple the various methods of contraception, the couple decides to use the sympto-thermal method to control their fertility.

Supporting Assessment Data	Expected Client/Family Outcome	Nursing Action/ Intervention	Rationale	Criteria for Evaluation
Nursing Diagnosis: Potential for compromised family coping, related to needed family planning				
Couple indicates that they would like to use a more effective contraceptive method Have five children ages 5, 3, 2, 1, and newborn State that last 3 were unplanned State that they have used "rhythm and coitus interruptus" unsuccessfully Have religious beliefs that preclude use of certain contraceptives	The couple will agree on a method that is compatible with their needs and beliefs before discharge The couple will relate reduced anxiety in use of the chosen method at the 6-week visit Concerns about limiting the family size will not interfere with attachment behaviors in the immediate puerperium	Discuss advantages and disadvantages of available contraceptive methods. Support the couple in choosing a contraceptive method that is compatible with their religious and cultural beliefs and family needs and life-style. Discuss past contraceptive history with couple and identify why they feel it was not effective.	Discussing contraceptives in a nonjudgmental manner will alleviate anxiety and motivate clients to proper use of the method. Anxiety can interfere with attachment behaviors; alleviation of anxiety will foster family attachment. Considering the culture and religious beliefs will foster comfort with use of contraception.	Couple identify a method for planning their family at the end of the discharge planning session. At the 6-week visit, couple relates confidence in using chosen method. At the 6-week visit, family relates and demonstrates appropriate attachment behaviors.
Nursing Diagnosis: Knowledge deficit, related to selected family planning method				
Couple states that they would like to use the sympto-thermal method	On discharge, the couple will discuss: the effectiveness the use advantages and disadvantages of the chosen method During the 6-week postpartum visit, the couple will demonstrate effective use of chosen contraceptive method	Demonstrate the use of the basal thermometer, use of the chart, and methods of interpretation to couple Teach changes in cervical mucus in relation to ovulation (Spinnbarkeit). Teach couple about subjective signs of ovulation such as Mittelschmerz. Teach couple procedure for taking basal temperature and evaluating the temperature in relation to the menstrual cycle. Refer couple to classes on natural family planning.	Knowledge about usage and effectiveness of contraceptive methods will foster proper and effective use. Demonstration reinforces learning. Referral to support groups enhances learning.	Couple is able to discuss the effectiveness, procedure, and evaluation criteria for chosen method. During 6-week visit, couple will give a demonstration of the use of the basal temperature and interpret chart that they have kept. The couple will describe the objective and subjective signs of ovulation. The couple informs the nurse at the 6-week visit that they have attended a natural family planning support group.

SUMMARY

Although some individuals and couples choose to remain childless, for the majority of people, having a child may be one of the most significant life events that they experience. It is an event that may be anticipated with great joy, if planned and desired, or it may be an event that is dreaded, if the pregnancy is unplanned and the child is undesired.

The nurse plays an important role in assisting individuals to plan their families. Nurses may serve as teachers, counselors, and as support and resource persons regarding contraceptive choices. They can bring understanding and empathy to client care. Nurses should be equipped to discuss reproductive goals and alternatives available to individuals and couples. They should be able to assess reproductive risks and support individuals or couples in following through with the reproductive decisions that they make.

A variety of contraceptive methods is available and described in this chapter. From the most effective to the least effective, they include sterilization, injectable progestogen, oral contraceptive agents, intrauterine devices, condoms, diaphragms, sponges, cervical caps, coitus interruptus, periodic abstinence, and spermicidal agents. Each method has advantages and disadvantages; however, a major factor in effectiveness is proper use of whichever method is chosen. Experimental methods that will likely be available in the future also are discussed.

While not a contraceptive method, pregnancy termination is one means by which couples regulate their families. Pregnancy termination requires complex decision making, and the nurse supports the client throughout the process. Of particular difficulty is the decision to terminate a pregnancy because of a prenatally diagnosed birth defect or genetic abnormality.

Today human reproduction is not a matter of chance but of choice. It is a choice that will not only have an impact on an individual or couple, but also on society as a whole and, as such, should be a planned and desired event.

REVIEW QUESTIONS

1. List four factors that influence reproductive choices.
2. Discuss components of preconception risk assessment.
3. Identify four goals of genetic counseling.
4. List benefits and risks of two of the *most* effective and two of the *least* effective pregnancy prevention methods.
5. Describe nursing interventions for a couple whose pregnancy was terminated because of the presence of a birth defect.
6. Describe how planning a family affects maternal and infant morbidity and mortality and the quality of human life.

REFERENCES

1. Loraine J A. Family planning: the global challenge. *Practitioner.* 1985;229:407–412.
2. Kent M, Haub C. *World Population Data Sheet.* Washington, DC: Population Reference Bureau, 1985.
3. Finch BE, Green H. *Contraception Through the Ages.* Springfield, Ill: Charles C. Thomas, 1963.
4. Birth expectation among U.S wives. *Fam Plann Perspect.* 1975;7:5–6.
5. National Center for Health Statistics. Advance report: a final natality statistic. *Monthly Vital Statistic Report.* 1985; 34(Suppl).
6. Cushner IM. Reproductive technologies: new choices, new hopes, new dilemmas. *Fam Plann Perspect.* 1986;18:129–132.
7. Tsui AO, Bogue BJ. Declining world fertility: trends, causes and implications. *Population Bulletin.* 1978;33:26–33.
8. Pearn J. Decision-making and the reproductive choice. *Counsel Genetics.* 1979;15:223–238.
9. Miller WB. Why some women fail to use their contraceptive method: a psychological investigation. *Fam Plann Perspect.* 1986;18:27–32.
10. Sherwen LN, Miele N. Assessing and identifying the high-risk pregnancy: a holistic approach. *Top Clin Nurs.* 1986;8: 33–34.
11. Coplan J. Wrongful life. *Pediatr.* 1985;75:65–72.
12. Donovan P. Wrongful birth and wrongful conception: the legal and moral issues. *Fam Plann Perspect.* 1984;16:64–69.
13. Brown S. Can low birth weight be prevented? *Fam Plann Perspect.* 1985;17:112–118.
14. Hanson JW. Teratogenic agents. In Emery A, Rimoin E, eds. *Principles and Practice in Medical Genetics.* Edinburgh: Churchill Livingstone, 1983.
15. Fraser FC. Genetic counseling. *Am J Hum Genet.* 1974;26: 637.
16. Forrest J: United States. In *Teenage Pregnancy in Developed Countries.* New York: Alan Guttmacher Institute, 1985.
17. Queenan JT. Editorial. *Fertil.* (Contemporary Ob/Gyn special issue), 1988;32:7–8.
18. Forrest JD. Contraceptive needs through stages of women's reproductive lives. *Fertil.* (Contemporary Ob/Gyn special issue), 1988;32:12–22.
19. Hatcher RA, et al. *Contraceptive Technology, 1988–1989.* 14th ed. New York: Irvington Publishers, 1988.

20. Kendrick JS, et al. Complications of vasectomies in the United States. *J Fam Prac.* 1987;25:245–248.
21. Shain RN, et al. Married women's dissatisfaction with tubal sterilization and vasectomy at first-year follow-up: effects of perceived spousal dominance. *Fertil Steril.* 1986;45: 808–819.
22. Loughlin KR. Complications of vasovasostomy. *Urol Clin North Am.* 1988;15:243–248.
23. Marshall S. Common misconceptions about vasectomy. *Med Aspects Hum Sex.* 1988;11:105–107.
24. Irwin KL, et al. Hysterectomy, tubal sterilization, and the risk of breast cancer. *Am J Epidemiol.* 1988;127:1192–1201.
25. Rock JA, et al. Tubal anastomosis: pregnancy success following reversal of fallopian ring or monopolar cautery sterilization. *Fertil Steril.* 1987;48:13–17.
26. Siegler A, et al. Reversibility of female sterilization. *Fertil Steril.* 1985;43:499–510.
27. Richard BW, Lasagna L. Drug regulation in the United States and the United Kingdom: the Depo-Provera study. *Ann Int Med.* 1987;106:886–891.
28. Dickey RP. *Managing Contraceptive Pill Patients.* 5th ed. Durant, Okla: Creative Informatics, 1987.
29. Grimes DA. Reversible contraception for the 1980's. *JAMA.* 1986;255:69–75.
30. Woutersz TB, et al. A low-dose triphasic oral contraceptive. *Fertil Steril.* 1980;47:425–430.
31. Speroff L, et al. Multiphasic and monophasic OCs: is there a difference? *Fertil.* (Contemporary Ob/Gyn special issue), 1988;32:124–145.
32. Grimes, DA. Multiphasic Ocs and functional ovarian cysts. *Fertil.* (Contemporary Ob/Gyn special issue), 1988;32: 103–112.
33. Ellsworth H. Focus on triphasil. *J Reprod Med.* 1986; 31(suppl):559–564.
34. Gillmer MD. Progestogen potency in oral contraceptive pills. *Am J Obstet Gynecol.* 1987;157:1048–1051.
35. Runnebaum B, Rabe T: New progestogens in oral contraceptives. *Am J Obstet Gynecol.* 1987;157:1059–1063.
36. Knopp RH, Mishell DR. Introduction. *Am J Obstet Gynecol.* 1988;128:1551–1552.
37. Mishell DR. Contraception. *N Engl J Med.* 1989;320:777–784.
38. Mishell DR. Use of oral contraceptives in women of older reproductive age. *Am J Obstet Gynecol.* 1988;158:1612–1619.
39. Crook D, et al. Oral contraceptives and coronary heart disease: modulation of glucose tolerance and plasma lipid risk factors by progestins. *Am J Obstet Gynecol.* 1988; 158:1612–1619.
40. Gaspard UJ. Metabolic effects of oral contraceptives. *Am J Obstet Gynecol.* 1989;127:1029–1041.
41. Meade TW. Risks and mechanisms of cardiovascular events in users of oral contraceptives. *Am J Obstet Gynecol.* 1988; 158:1646–1652.
42. Roy S. Effects of oral contraceptives on cholesterol. *J Reprod Med.* 1986;31:546–547.
43. Bonnar J, Sabra AM. Oral contraceptives and blood coagulation. *J Reprod Med.* 1986;31(suppl):551–555.
44. Krauss RM. Effects of oral contraceptives on lipid metabolism. *J Reprod Med.* 1986;31(suppl):549–550.
45. LaRosa C. The varying effects of progestins on lipid levels and cardiovascular disease. *Am J Obstet Gynecol.* 1988; 158:1621–1629.
46. Grimes DA. Prevention of cardiovascular disease in women: role of the obstetrician–gynecologist. *Am J Obstet Gynecol.* 1988;158:1662–1668.
47. Schlesselman JJ, et al. Breast cancer risk in relation to type of estrogen contained in oral contraceptives. *Contraception.* 1987;36:595–611.
48. Webster L. Epidemiology of oral contraceptives and the risk of breast cancer. *J Reprod Med.* 1986;31(suppl):540–545.
49. Stadel BV, Lai S. Oral contraceptives and the risk of breast cancer in nulliparous women. *Contraception.* 1988;38:287–299.
50. Tatum HJ. A new IUD offering more copper, better results. *Fertil.* (Contemporary Ob/Gyn special issue), 1988;32(2): 36–47.
51. Soderstrom R. IUD's now require patients' informed consent. *Fertil.* (Contemporary Ob/Gyn special issue), 1988; 32(2):115–123.
52. Sivin I, Schmidt R. Effectiveness of IUDs: a review. *Contraception.* 1987;36:55–57.
53. Connell EB. Reevaluating women's contraceptive needs. *Fertil.* (Contemporary Ob/Gyn special issue), 1988;32(2): 27–34.
54. Edelman DA. IUD complications in perspective. *Contraception.* 1987;36:159–166.
55. Dirubbi N. The condom barrier. *Am J Nurs.* 1987;11:1306–1309.
56. Condoms for prevention of sexually transmitted disease. *MMWR.* 1988;37:133–137.
57. Rietmeijer CA, et al. Condoms as physical and chemical barriers against human immunodeficiency virus. *JAMA.* 1988; 259:1851–1853.
58. Fihn SD, et al. Association between diaphragm use and urinary tract infection. *JAMA.* 1985;254:240–245.
59. Foxman B, Fredricks RR. Epidemiology of urinary tract infection: 1. Diaphragm use and sexual intercourse. *Am J Public Health.* 1985;75:1308–1313.
60. Wagner C, et al. Diaphragm insertion increases human vaginal oxygen tension. *Am J Obstet Gynecol.* 1988;158: 1040–1043.
61. Stott P. Rediscovering the diaphragm. *Br Med J.* 1988; 296:377–378.
62. Edelman DA, North BB. Updated pregnancy rates for the today contraceptive sponge. *Am J Obstet Gynecol.* 1987; 157:1164–1165.
63. Cervical cap enters North American market. *NAACOG Newsl.* 1988;15:1–6.
64. Powell MG, et al. Contraception with the cervical cap: effectiveness, safety, continuity of use, and user satisfaction. *Contraception.* 1986;23:215–231.
65. Brown JB, et al. Natural family planning. *Am J Obstet Gynecol.* 1987;157:1082–1089.
66. Zinaman MJ. Why you should know about natural family planning. *Fertil.* (Contemporary Ob/Gyn special issue), 1988; 32(2):69–86.
67. Contraceptive film comes to the United States. *NAACOG Newsl.* 1988;15:11.
68. Frank ME. Ask the experts. *NAACOG Newsl.* 1988;15:8.
69. Darney PD. Long-acting hormonal contraception. *Fertil.* (Contemporary Ob/Gyn special issue), 1988;32(2):90, 97–100.
70. Segal S. A new delivery system for contraceptive steroids. *Am J Obstet Gynecol.* 1987;157:1090–1092.
71. Olsson S-E, et al. Contraception with Norplant Implants and

Norplants-2 Implants (Two covered rods). *Contraception.* 1988;37:61–73.
72. Fakeye O, Balogh S. Effects of Norplant contraceptive use on hemoglobin, packed cell volume and menstrual bleeding patterns. *Contraception.* 1989;39:265–274.
73. Sitruk-Ware R. Transdermal delivery of steroids. *Contraception.* 1989;39:1–17.
74. Ratsula K, et al. Plasma levonorgestrel levels and ovarian function during the use of a levonorgestrel-releasing intracervical contraceptive device. *Contraception.* 1989;39: 195–203.
75. Jonis WR, et al: Phase I clinical trial of a world health organization birth control vaccine. *Lancet.* 1988;8598:1295–1298.
76. Aitken RJ, Paterson M. New horizons in contraception. *Nature.* 1988;335:492–493.
77. Talwar GP, Gaur A. Recent developments in immunocontraception. *Am J Obstet Gynecol.* 1989;157:1075–1078.
78. Hodgen GD. Progesterone antagonists: useful for contraception. *Fertil.* (Contemporary Ob/Gyn special issue), 1988; 32(2):65–66.
79. Baulieu E-E. Contraception by the progesterone antagonist RU 486: a novel approach to human fertility control. *Contraception.* 1989;36(Suppl):1–5.
80. Lähteemäki P., et al. Late postcoital treatment against pregnancy with antiprogesterone RU 486. *Fertil Steril.* 1988;50:36–38.
81. Liu GA, et al. Experiences with gossypol as a male pill. *Am J Obstet Gynecol.* 1987;14:1079–1081.
82. Henshaw S. Trends in abortions 1982–1984. *Fam Plann Perspect.* 1986;18:34.
83. Granberg D, Granberg B. Abortion attitudes 1965–1980: trends and determinants. *Fam Plann Perspect.* 1980;12: 250–261.
84. Sollum T, Donavan P. State laws and the provision of family planning and abortion services in 1985. *Fam Plann Perspect.* 1985;17:262–266.
85. Gold RB. After the Hyde amendment: public funding for abortion in F.Y. 1978. *Fam Plann Perspect.* 1980;12:131–134.
86. Donnai P, et al. Attitudes of patients after "genetic" termination of pregnancy. *Br Med J.* 1981;282:621–622.
87. Thomson E. Early pregnancy loss. March of Dimes/Birth Defects Foundation, Original Article Series, Strategies in Genetic Counseling. 1985;23:37–44.

Establishment Phase

unit 2

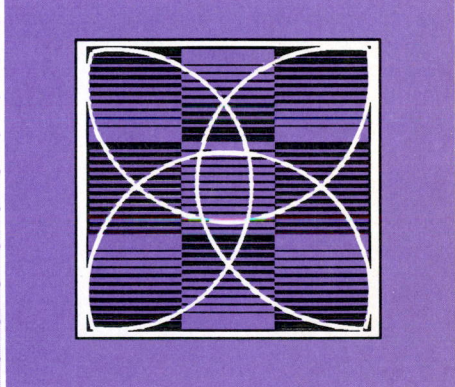

Nutrition During Pregnancy

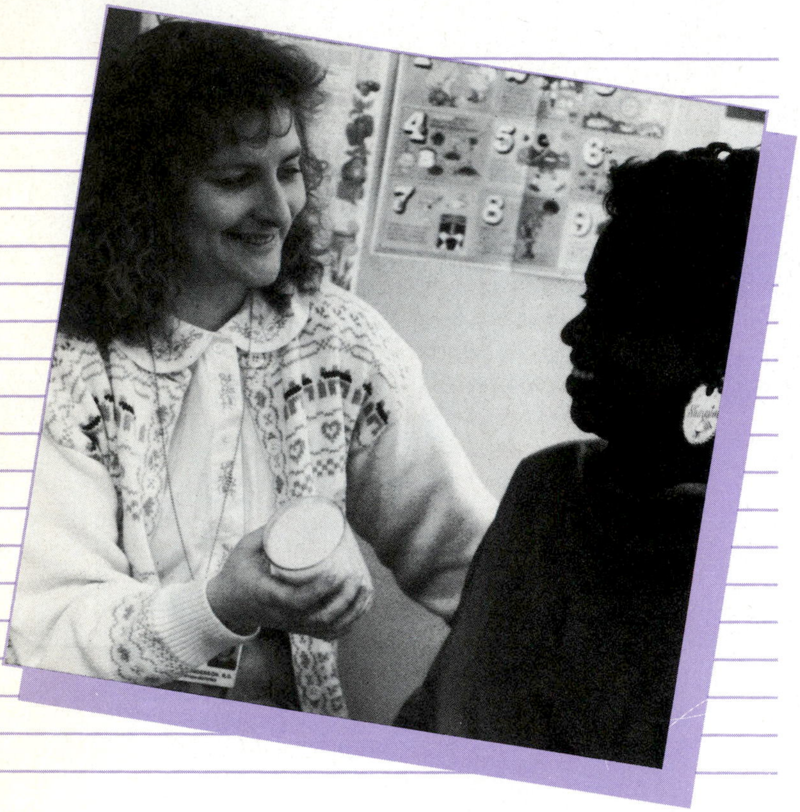

Chapter 10

Key Terms

anorexia nervosa
anthropometry
bulimia
morbid obesity
obesity
pica
underweight

Research in the last several decades has identified the important role of nutrition during pregnancy in influencing maternal and fetal health. The deleterious effects of inadequate maternal nutrition are well recognized by health professionals. The importance of the nutritional health of pregnant women has led to a greater nursing emphasis on obtaining a thorough nutrition assessment, monitoring nutritional status, and promoting nutrition education.

The nurse plays a vital role in obtaining the nutrition assessment and acting as a nutrition educator. The frequent personal and physical contacts nurses have with clients are opportunities to gather pertinent information about food practices, lifestyle, and physical signs; to observe clinical signs and symptoms that may reflect nutritional health; to communicate to the client the importance of a healthy diet during pregnancy; and to respond to the client's particular needs or concerns regarding her eating habits.

Nutrition during pregnancy is a complex subject. This chapter focuses on the specific nutritional requirements of a normal healthy pregnant woman, with emphasis on providing nutritional counseling. The collaboration with nutritionists and other members of the interdisciplinary team is also emphasized as a means to ensure comprehensive care of the childbearing woman.

WEIGHT GAIN DURING PREGNANCY

Satisfactory weight gain during pregnancy is necessary for maternal health and normal fetal growth and development. The pattern of this weight gain is particularly important.

The National Academy of Sciences Institute of Medicine recommends that pregnant women gain between 25 and 35 pounds (11.4 to 16 kg) over the course of pregnancy.[1] These recommendations were developed to reduce the risk of interuterine growth retardation. Postpartum maternal weight retention and fetal macrosomia are both recognized as a possible outcome of weight gain in the higher range of the recommendations. Because desirable weight gain for

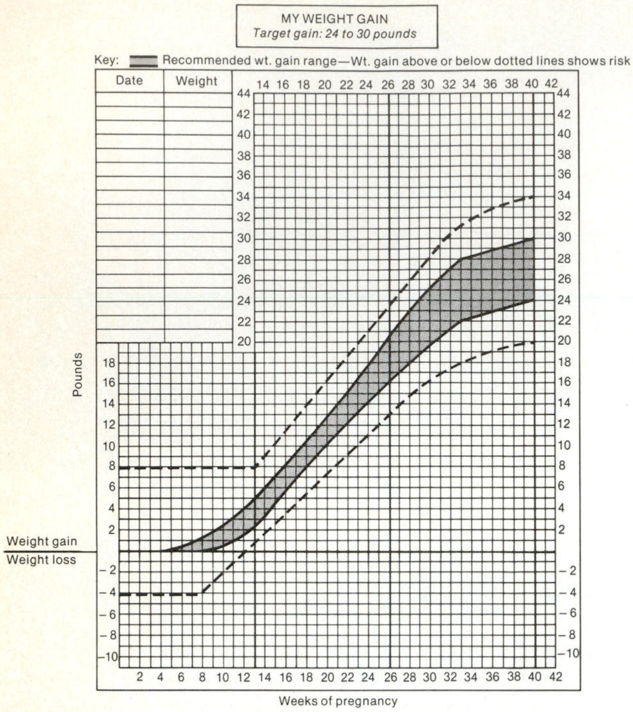

Figure 10–1. Optimal weight gain for normal weight women, as illustrated on a prenatal weight grid. (*Developed by the 1987 Idaho* WIC *program; reproduced, with permission, from Worthington-Roberts BS, Williams SR.* Nutrition in Pregnancy and Lactation. *St. Louis: Times Mirror/Mosby; 1989:114.*)

vided. Figure 10–1 illustrates the pattern of normal weight gain during pregnancy. The recommended pattern of weight gain is 3 pounds (1.36 kg) for the first trimester, or 1 pound (0.45 kg) per month; and 1 pound (0.45 kg) per week for the second and third trimesters for a total of 29 pounds (13.18 kg).

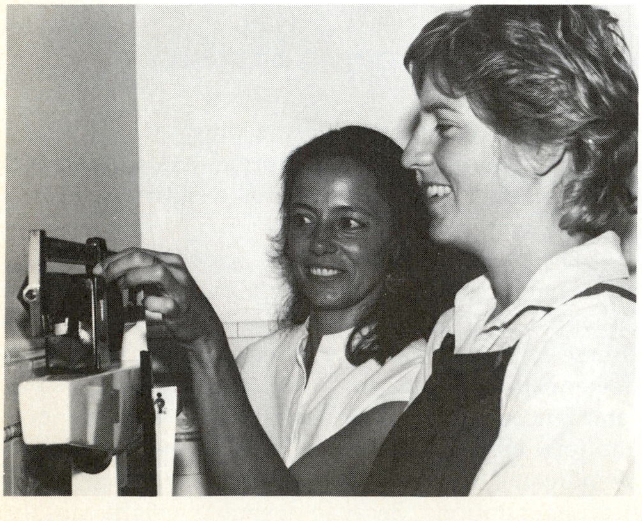

Figure 10–2. The client is weighed at each prenatal visit.

Many practitioners use a prenatal growth grid to monitor changes in body weight. The client's preconception weight is compared with her weight at the first prenatal visit, and weights are recorded at each subsequent visit (Figure 10–2). The prenatal growth grid can be used as a teaching tool in emphasizing the importance of a steady, gradual weight gain.

Major gains in maternal and fetal organ development and fluid volume do not begin until approximately the 12th week of gestation. The weight gain in the first trimester is due primarily to the growth of the uterus and the increase in the mother's blood volume. At the end of the first trimester, the fetus weighs only about 5 g (0.18 oz). After the first trimester, maternal weight gain increases significantly, as a result of growth and development of the fetus, placenta, uterus, breasts, and increase in maternal blood volume.

The components of weight gain are listed in Table 10–1. As shown, only 7 pounds of the total weight gained during pregnancy is body fat. The remaining distribution of body weight is composed of placental, uterine, fetal, and breast tissue, and blood and fluid volume. The increased store of body fat serves primarily as a reserve for energy needs during lactation.

Any rapid changes in body weight should be closely evaluated, as they may indicate a problem. Recommended weight gains for obese and underweight clients are discussed later in this chapter. Many women do gain more than the recommended amount simply because they eat too much. That the pregnant woman should be "eating for two," however, is a myth. Remember that the second person, the fetus, weighs, on average, only 3.18 kg, or 7 pounds, at birth. Dietary assessment can identify excesses in intake, and nutritional counseling can help the client to select foods that will meet pregnancy needs and prevent excess weight gain. The client should be counseled not to skip meals or undertake vigorous exercise programs to lose the excess weight. Rather, the practitioner should advise the client to limit her intake of excess fats and sugar to maintain a conditioned, but slowed, pattern of weight gain.

NUTRIENT REQUIREMENTS

Kilocalories

To achieve the current recommended rate of weight gain, the Food and Nutrition Board of the National Research Council recommends an intake of an additional 300 kcal per day above normal nonpregnant requirements. Total kilocalorie intake should not be below 36 kcal/kg body weight in adult pregnant women. Recommended total kilocalorie intake should be approximately 2200 kcal per day, or an increase of

TABLE 10–1. COMPONENTS OF THE AVERAGE WEIGHT GAINED IN NORMAL PREGNANCY

	Amount Gained (g)			
Component	**10 Weeks**	**20 Weeks**	**30 Weeks**	**40 Weeks**
Total body weight gain	650 (1.5 lb)	4000 (9.0 lb)	8500 (19.0 lb)	12,500 (27.5 lb)
Fetus	5	300	1500	3300
Placenta	20	170	430	650
Amniotic fluid	30	250	600	800
Increase in uterus	135	585	819	900
Increase in mammary glands	34	180	360	405
Increase in maternal blood	100	600	1300	1250
Total (rounded)	320	2100	5000	7300
Weight not accounted for	330	1900	3500	5200

From the Committee on Maternal Nutrition, Food and Nutrition Board, National Research Council, National Academy of Sciences. Maternal Nutrition and the Course of Pregnancy. *Washington, DC: US Government Printing Office; 1980.*

about 15 percent above normal requirements. Individual energy needs, however, reflect basal body requirements, which are dependent on body and muscle size and fat, composition, and physical activity level. Therefore, a woman who has a large body mass and engages in regular physical exercise may require more than 2400 kcal. To obtain the most accurate estimation of energy needs, a thorough nutrition assessment should be conducted (*see* "Nutrition Assessment" under "Nutritional Care During Childbearing").

Because nutrient requirements are elevated during pregnancy, the extra 300 kcal should come from foods that contribute needed nutrients, such as protein and calcium. The recommended dietary pattern is described in Table 10–2. This is only a guideline to the recommended minimum intake. Individual needs may vary according to the client's specific nutrient requirements and cultural dietary practices (*see* "Cultural Food Practices").

The energy nutrients—protein, carbohydrates, and fat—are essential in meeting the body's requirements for kilocalories and in performing other vital functions in the body.

Protein

Protein requirements are based on the nutrient needs for synthesis of maternal and fetal tissue and the increase in blood volume that occurs during pregnancy. Approximately one kilogram of protein is stored during pregnancy. More specifically, protein is needed for development of the placenta, enlargement of the uterus, growth of the fetus, formation of the amniotic fluid, increase in maternal tissue, and increased supply of serum proteins such as hemoglobin and serum albumin. The mother's body builds a reserve of protein during the luteal phase of pregnancy (when the corpus luteum supplies estrogen and progesterone). These stores are later mobilized during the placental phase (that is, when the placenta produces estrogen and progesterone).

The Recommended Dietary Allowance for protein is 60 g of protein per day. Equally as important as the total protein requirements is the need for high-quality protein that contains all the essential amino acids in adequate proportions. Animal products such as meats, fish, poultry, dairy foods, and eggs all contain sufficient amounts of the essential amino acids. Milk is a good source of protein, as well as calcium and vitamin D, and the pregnant woman is encouraged to drink up to 4 glasses per day as part of her

TABLE 10–2. RECOMMENDED DIETARY PATTERN DURING PREGNANCY

Food	Number of Servings	Serving Size
Dairy Products	4	
Milk		8 oz
Cheese		1 oz
Yogurt		8 oz
Meat	4	2 oz
Lean meat, fish, poultry, cheese; eggs		
Breads and cereals		
Bread		1 slice
Cereal	4 or more	½ cup
Rice		½ cup
Pasta		½ cup
Vegetables		
Dark green or orange-yellow vegetable	1	½ cup
Other vegetables	2 or more	½
Fruits		
Citrus fruit or juice, cantaloupe, strawberries	1	½ cup
Other fruits or juices	2 or more	½ cup

fluid intake. If the client chooses to follow a vegetarian diet and avoid all animal products, it is important that she obtain proper amounts of amino acids from plant foods. Plant foods such as dried beans, nuts, grains, and seeds, if consumed in appropriate combinations, can supply adequate amounts of protein. To ensure that her protein intake is adequate, a pregnant vegetarian should receive nutritional counseling from a nutritionist.

For protein to perform its vital function in promoting the building of tissue, a sufficient supply of calories in the form of carbohydrate and fat must be available. If kilocalorie intake is inadequate (that is, inadequate intake of carbohydrates and fats for energy) protein will not be used for growth and development of new tissue but will instead be used for energy. A reduction in dietary protein in experimental animals has been associated with low-birth-weight offspring. Results of experiments in humans involving the effects of protein supplementation versus deprivation have been conflicting[2,3]; however, fasting during pregnancy has been demonstrated to cause catabolism of muscle protein and gluconeogenesis from amino acids.[4]

Carbohydrates

The fetus is entirely dependent on the mother for meeting its glucose needs. A fetus requires approximately 30 g of glucose a day, which acts as its primary fuel source. The serum glucose level in the fetus' circulation is approximately 10 to 20 mg/100 mL lower than that in the maternal circulation. Glucose travels across the placental membrane via simple diffusion and active transport. Maternal insulin is unavailable to the fetus; therefore, the fetus is dependent on its own supply, which is first produced at 12 weeks of gestation. Glucagon is present in the fetal circulation at 8 weeks of gestation.

As a result of hormonal changes, there are various alterations in carbohydrate metabolism during pregnancy. During the first trimester, the maternal fasting blood glucose level decreases slightly to approximately 75 mg/100 mL of blood because of the increase in glucose supplied to the fetus and the accompanying decrease in insulin production.

During the second half of pregnancy, placental hormones have a diabetogenic effect (producing a diabetic-like state). Estrogen decreases insulin's effectiveness, and cortisol increases the production of glucose from gluconeogenesis. There is also maternal peripheral tissue resistance to insulin. During pregnancy, insulin requirements are increased up to 70 percent. Because of these changes there is a greater risk of starvation ketosis, which is characterized by hypoglycemia, increased nitrogen excretion, raised plasma levels of free fatty acids, and elevated plasma and urinary ketones. This is particularly common when the mother skips meals, especially if she omits breakfast after an overnight fast. Pregnant women should be encouraged to consume three meals a day with nutritious snacks between meals to promote normal blood glucose levels. A minimum intake of 150 g of carbohydrate per day is also advised, but to meet actual kilocalorie requirements during pregnancy, a larger intake of carbohydrate is required. After delivery, insulin requirements return to normal as a result of the excretion of placental anti-insulin hormones.

Carbohydrates should be provided primarily in the form of complex carbohydrates, such as enriched and whole grain breads and cereals, vegetables, and fruits. Simple carbohydrates or sugars in the diet should be provided mostly from naturally occurring sources, such as fruits and fruit juices. Simple carbohydrates found in such foods as cakes, pies, cookies, candy, and soda should be minimized in the diet, as these foods provide few vitamins and minerals and are high in kilocalories. Total carbohydrate intake should be approximately 50 to 55 percent of total kilocalorie intake.

Fats

Fats are required in the diet to provide a concentrated source of energy and essential fatty acids. Maternal fatty acids enter the fetal circulation but are not considered to be a major fuel source for the fetus, as the enzymes required to metabolize fat are present in small amounts. Fatty acids are valuable for myelinization of nerves and membrane synthesis that occurs in utero; therefore, fat is an essential nutrient for fetal development.

Fats should be primarily high in polyunsaturated and monounsaturated fatty acids, such as vegetable oils; less emphasis should be placed on foods high in saturated fatty acids such as red meats with a high fat content. The client should choose such foods as lean meats, skinless poultry products, and fish, which are high in protein and low in saturated fat. Total fat intake should be approximately 30 percent of the total kilocalorie intake.

Vitamins and Minerals

Vitamins and minerals are essential in the diet to promote the use of energy from carbohydrates, fat, and protein; to build new tissue; and to act as regulating agents in many metabolic processes in the body. To meet vitamin and mineral requirements, pregnant women, in addition to eating a healthy diet, are often advised to take a multivitamin and multimineral preparation. With the exception of the nutrients iron and folic acid, adequate amounts of vitamins and minerals can be provided in a healthy, well-balanced diet; however, supplements are sometimes recommended as a precautionary measure to ensure adequate vitamin and mineral intake.

Table 10–3 provides a comparison of commonly used prenatal vitamins. Pregnant women should take only those supplements designed for prenatal needs and should avoid any preparation that contains nutrients in higher dosages that may be unsafe. Table 10–4 lists the 1989 Recommended Dietary Allowances (RDAs) for all vitamins and minerals during pregnancy. Table 10–5 summarizes the physiological functions of vitamins and minerals and common food sources.

Fat-Soluble Vitamins. The fat-soluble vitamins A, D, E, and K are stored in the body; therefore, any excess intake can be extremely toxic. Consumption of megadoses of vitamin A during pregnancy have been reported to cause teratogenic effects.[5] Vitamin D has also been shown to be teratogenic when consumed in megadose amounts.

Vitamin A is essential for normal bone development and growth and for growth and maintenance of normal epithelial tissue. Vitamin D is required for normal mineralization of the fetal skeletal system. Vitamin D is a unique nutrient because it is produced in the body by exposure to sunlight of 7-dehydrocholesterol, which is found in the skin. Brief periods of sunlight exposure can provide adequate supplies of the vitamin, which is also supplied by dietary sources such as fish and vitamin-fortified milk.

Protection of the integrity of the cellular membrane and intracellular structures are principal functions of vitamin E. Vitamin K functions in promoting normal blood clot formation, by acting as a cofactor for an enzyme required for the clotting mechanism. Because this vitamin is produced by the microflora of the lower intestinal tract, there is no established RDA.

Water-Soluble Vitamins. Vitamins C and the B-complex vitamins—folacin, niacin, riboflavin (B_2), thiamine (B_1), vitamin B_6, and vitamin B_{12}—make up the water-soluble vitamins. Toxic effects from excessive intake of water soluable vitamins are generally not considered as likely as for the fat-soluble vitamins because excess amounts are excreted in the urine. Pregnant women should take vitamin and mineral supplements only as prescribed by their health care provider. Indeed, in high doses, vitamin B_6 can be

TABLE 10–3. COMPARISON OF PRENATAL VITAMINS

	Ca (mg)	Fe (mg)	A (IU)	D (IU)	E (mg)	B_1 (mg)	B_2 (mg)	B_3 (mg)	B_5 (mg)	B_6 (mg)	B_{12} (μg)	C (mg)	FA (mg)	Other
Pramet FA Filmtabs (Ross)	250	60	4000	400		3	2	10	0.9	5	3	100	1	Cu,I
Natabec Rx Kapseals (Parke-Davis)	240	30	4000	400		3	2	10		3	5	50	1	
Prenatal-1 tabs (Major)	200	65	8000	400	30	2.5	3	20		10	12	90	1	I,Mg
Stuartnatal 1 + 1 tabs (Stuart)	200	65	8000	400	30	2.5	3	20		10	12	90	1	I, Mg, 25 mg Zn
Natalins Rx tablets (Mead Johnson)	200	60	8000	400	30	2.5	3	20	15	10	8	90	1	Cu,I,Mg,15 mg Zn, 500 g biotin
Natalins tablets (otc) (Mead Johnson)	200	45	8000	400	30	1.7	2	20		4	8	90	0.8	1,Mg
Stuart Prenatal (otc) (Stuart)	200	60	8000	400	30	1.7	2	20		4	8	60	0.8	I,Mg,25 mg Zn
Prenatal with Folic Acid (otc) (Geneva Generics)	200	60	8000	400	30	1.7	2	20		4	8	60	0.8	I,Mg
Prenavite Tabs (otc) (sugar-free) (Rugby)	200	60	8000	400	30	1.7	2	20		4	8	60	0.8	1,Mg

Ca = calcium, Fe = iron, B_3 = niacin, B_5 = pantothenic acid, FA = folic acid, Cu = copper, I = iodine, Mg = magnesium, Zn = zinc, otc = over the counter.

TABLE 10–4. 1989 RECOMMENDED DIETARY ALLOWANCES FOR ADULT PREGNANT WOMEN

Nutrient	Non-pregnant	Pregnant	Lactating: First 6 months	Lactating: Second 6 months
Protein (g)	46–50	60	65	62
Fat-Soluble Vitamins				
Vitamin A (μg RE)	800	800	1300	1200
Vitamin D (μg)	5–10	10	10	10
Vitamin E (mg TE)	8	10	12	11
Water-Soluble Vitamins				
Vitamin C (mg)	60	70	95	90
Folacin (μg)	180	400	280	260
Niacin (mg NE)	15	17	20	20
Riboflavin (B_2) (mg)	1.3	1.6	1.8	1.7
Thiamine (B_1) (mg)	1.5	1.1	1.6	1.6
Vitamin B_6 (mg)	1.6	2.2	2.1	2.1
Vitamin B_{12} (mg)	2.0	2.2	2.6	2.6
Minerals				
Calcium (mg)	1200	1200	1200	1200
Phosphorus (mg)	800	1200	1200	1200
Iodine (mg)	150	175	200	200
Iron (mg)[a]	15	30	15	15
Magnesium (mg)	280	320	355	340
Zinc (mg)	12	15	16	16
Energy (kcal)	2200	+ 300[b]	+ 500[b]	+ 500[b]

[a] Supplemental iron 30–60 mg/day is recommended.

Reproduced, with permission, from the Food and Nutrition Board, National Research Council, National Academy of Sciences. Recommended Dietary Allowances. *10th ed. Washington, DC: Government Printing Office, 1989.*

[b] Energy requirements for pregnancy and lactation are additional to normal requirements for kcal.

very toxic. Adequate daily intake is essential, however, because the body stores only small amounts of these vitamins.

Vitamin C is required for promoting blood clot and collagen formation. A deficiency of vitamin C has not been shown to affect adversely the course or outcome of pregnancy, but some research has associated low plasma levels of vitamin C with premature rupture of the membranes and pre-eclampsia. Excessive supplemental use of vitamin C has been demonstrated to cause a "rebound scurvy" effect: neonates exposed to high levels of vitamin C in utero develop symptoms of scurvy after birth; therefore, large doses of supplemental vitamin C during pregnancy should be avoided.

The B-complex vitamins serve chiefly as coenzymes (substances that work along with other enzymes) in the various metabolic pathways of the body. Thiamine functions in carbohydrate metabolism, and riboflavin and niacin in the metabolism of all three energy nutrients.

Folacin needs are increased during pregnancy because of the large increase in maternal erythropoiesis and fetal and placental growth. Folacin is essential for the synthesis of purines and pyrimidines such as DNA and RNA. (Chapter 38 discusses the assessment and management of folacin deficiency.) Vitamin B_{12} (cobalamin) requirements are also related to the development of maternal and fetal tissue. Vitamin B_{12} works together with folacin to promote the transfer of methyl groups in the synthesis of nucleic acids and purines and pyrimidines.

Vitamin B_6 (pyridoxine) functions as a coenzyme in amino acid metabolism; therefore, as protein requirements increase during pregnancy, B_6 needs are also elevated. Vitamin B_6 supplements have been used to treat nausea and vomiting during pregnancy, but research has indicated mixed results.[6] A previously prescribed antiemetic containing vitamin B_6 was removed from the market because of concerns related to its possible teratogenic effects.

Minerals. Minerals are essential in the diet during pregnancy. Many contribute to cell and tissue formation in the body and work with enzymes to stimulate biochemical reactions. The increase in mineral re-

TABLE 10–5. VITAMINS AND MINERALS AND THEIR PHYSIOLOGIC FUNCTIONS DURING PREGNANCY

Nutrient	Physiologic Function	Food Source
Fat-Soluble Vitamins		
Vitamin A	Maintenance of normal epithelial cells, bone growth, and tooth formation	Beef liver, butter, margarine, whole milk, supplemented nonfat milk, dark green leafy vegetables, dark yellow-orange vegetables
Vitamin D	Increased absorption of calcium and phosphorus from maternal gastrointestinal tract, mineralization of fetal bones and teeth	Fortified milk, margarine, fish, liver oils (also supplied via nondietary source through exposure to sunlight)
Vitamin E	Protection of integrity of cellular and intracellular structures, maintenance of red blood cells	Vegetable and seed oils, green leafy vegetables, liver, wheat germ oil
Vitamin K	Promotion of normal blood clot formation by acting as cofactor with enzyme in clotting mechanism	Green leafy vegetables, egg yolk, liver (also produced by microflora of gastrointestinal tract, therefore no established RDA)
Water-Soluble Vitamins		
Vitamin C (ascorbic acid)	Promotion of blood clot and collagen formation, enhancement of absorption of iron, conversion of inactive folic acid to active form	Citrus fruits and juices, green peppers, potatoes, tomatoes, broccoli, cabbage, cantaloupe, strawberries
B-Complex Vitamins		
Folacin	Production of hemes for hemoglobin, prevention of megaloblastic anemia	Liver, green leafy vegetables, kidney beans, lean beef, whole wheat bread, yeast (vitamin's activity lost with cooking; supplementation of 200 to 400 μg recommended in latter part of pregnancy)
Niacin	Coenzyme in the metabolism of carbohydrates, fats, proteins	Organ meat, lean meats, poultry, fish, peanuts, vegetables, dry beans, pears
Riboflavin (B_2)	Coenzyme in the metabolism of carbohydrates, fats, proteins	Milk, eggs, organ meats, veal, beef, cheddar cheese, green leafy vegetables
Thiamine (B_1)	Coenzyme in carbohydrate metabolism	Pork products, organ meats especially liver, nuts, dried beans, brewer's yeast, wheat germ, whole grain and enriched breads and cereals
Vitamin B_6 (pyridoxine)	Coenzyme in amino acid metabolism	Meat, poultry, fish, eggs, dairy products, wheat
Vitamin B_{12} (cobalamin)	Maintenance of the myelin sheath of nerve and epithelial cells, maintenance of red and white blood cell formation	Animal proteins, seaweed
Minerals		
Iron	Manufacture of maternal and fetal hemoglobin, increased maternal blood volume (storage of iron compensates for loss of blood during delivery)	Egg yolks, red meats, organ meats, especially liver (Other sources include poultry, fish, dried beans, green leafy vegetables, prunes, but iron in these foods is less efficiently absorbed. Because iron-rich foods may be limited in diet, supplementation with 30–60 mg of ferrous salts is recommended, beginning in the second trimester.)
Calcium and phosphorus	Formation of fetal skeleton and teeth, maternal calcium absorption	Calcium: whole milk, nonfat milk, buttermilk, yogurt, hard cheese, green leafy vegetables, sardines, nuts, dried beans Phosphorus: nearly all foods, animal proteins, nuts, dried beans, as a food additive in cola drinks and processed foods
Iodine	Synthesis of T_3 and T_4[a]	Iodized salt, saltwater fish, produce grown in iodine-rich soil
Sodium	Normal body metabolism	A variety of fresh and processed foods, especially cured meats, and salty foods such as potato chips pretzels, salted nuts, and popcorn, salted pickles, olives, and relishes
Magnesium	Activation of enzyme systems in energy-producing reactions, synthesis of proteins, nucleic acids, fats	Dark green leafy vegetables, dried beans, nuts, soybeans, whole grain cereals, milk, meat, seafood
Zinc	Synthesis of DNA and RNA, role in metabolism and maintenance of acid-base balance	Animal proteins, shellfish especially Atlantic oysters (also found in moderate amounts in eggs, milk, and cheese, and in smaller amounts in legumes, nuts, and whole grains, but zinc from these sources may not be well absorbed)

[a] T_3 = triiodothyronine, T_4 = 3,5,3′,5′-tetraiodothyronine-thyroxine.

quirements during pregnancy is based on the normal physiological changes associated with pregnancy.

Iron. The large increases in iron in maternal blood volume, fetal iron stores, placental iron content, and blood losses during delivery emphasize the need for increased iron requirements during pregnancy. In the normal nonpregnant woman, iron stores average 3500 mg. The total iron needed during pregnancy is about 1000 mg: 300 mg for the needs of the placenta and fetus, 570 mg for the increase in maternal total erythrocyte volume, and 130 mg for normal blood losses during gestation and labor and delivery. Iron stores in the newborn average 275 mg/kg. These stores are formed primarily during the last trimester of pregnancy and serve to provide sufficient amounts of iron to last approximately 6 months.

Maternal absorption of iron is estimated to be 30 percent above nonpregnant levels; however, to meet iron needs and prevent iron deficiency anemia, iron supplementation is usually advised during pregnancy. (Chapter 38 presents information on the assessment and management of iron deficiency anemia.) In addition to the RDA of 15 mg, an additional daily supplement of 30 to 60 mg of ferrous salts is recommended.

There are conflicting reports as to the effects of iron deficiency on pregnancy outcome.[7,8] Infants born to anemic mothers may have reduced iron stores at birth. Because of iron's role in promoting normal hemoglobin production, iron deficiency can lead to excess demands on cardiac output. A low maternal hemoglobin level can also cause complications if hemorrhaging should occur during delivery.

Calcium and Phosphorus. Calcium and phosphorus act synergistically to promote fetal skeletal development. Approximately 30 g of calcium is stored in the mother and fetus during pregnancy. The fetus accumulates 25 g of calcium by the time of birth. The majority of calcium and phosphorus is supplied from the mother to the fetus during the last 4 weeks of pregnancy; however, it is important that the mother consume adequate amounts of calcium and phosphorus throughout pregnancy to build up sufficient stores. If calcium supplies are inadequate, maternal bones will be demineralized in an attempt to provide adequate supplies of calcium to the fetus. This demineralization of bones can lead to the development of osteoporosis during later life. Because excessive phosphorus may impede calcium absorption, it is recommended that individuals have a one-to-one ratio of calcium to phosphorus in their diet.

Iodine. Iodine is a vital component of the thyroid hormones, which regulate the body's growth, reproduction, and metabolism. An iodine deficiency during pregnancy can result in insufficient fetal production of the thyroid hormones, leading to physical and mental retardation.

Sodium. In pregnancy, approximately 950 mEq of sodium is retained. This additional supply of sodium can be found in the fetus (290 mEq), the placenta (57 mEq), the amniotic fluid (100 mEq), the maternal extracellular volume including the uterus (80 mEq), the breasts (35 mEq), the plasma (140 mEq), and the edema fluid (240 mEq). Because of the extra requirements for sodium storage in the body, sodium intake should not be restricted during pregnancy. Rigid sodium restriction during pregnancy has been observed to lead to neonatal hyponatremia. Sodium intake should be no less than 2 to 3 g per day. This level can be achieved by the consumption of moderate amounts of sodium in processed foods, with a variety of fresh foods in the diet.

Magnesium. Magnesium functions as a cofactor (a mineral that works with an enzyme) in stimulating the biochemical reactions involved in the metabolism of carbohydrates, fats, and proteins. Magnesium deficiency can lead to neuromuscular dysfunctions.

Zinc. The mineral zinc is thought to be important for normal growth of tissues. An adequate zinc intake is achieved by a diet high in both proteins and calories. There is no evidence that well-chosen diets are inadequate in meeting maternal and fetal needs even though these diets furnish less than half of the recommended dietary allowance.

Water

Water is frequently overlooked as a nutrient. Its role in promoting a healthy pregnancy is equally important as that of vitamins and minerals. Water functions in the processes of digestion, absorption, excretion, and circulation. It acts as the body's solvent and transport medium for nutrients and body substances. Water also assists in maintaining a homeostatic body temperature. Because of the increases in blood and fluid volume, it is recommended that pregnant women drink eight glasses of fluids per day.

SUBSTANCES TO AVOID DURING PREGNANCY

Many clinicians and practitioners believe that certain substances should be avoided during pregnancy.

These include caffeine, saccharine and aspartame, and alcohol. The nurse, when taking a health history, assesses the client's use of these substances. Through teaching and counseling, the nurse provides the pregnant woman and family members with information that will allow them to make decisions concerning positive health care practices.

Caffeine

Caffeine is a stimulant present in a wide variety of beverages, foods, and medications. Sources of caffeine are listed in Table 10–6. Questions regarding safe intake of caffeine during pregnancy are focused primarily on its ability to cross the placenta and enter the fetal circulation. Common anomalies observed in the offspring of rodents exposed to high doses of caffeine include facial cleft, limb anomalies, low birth weights, small litters, and fetal death.[9] The teratogenicity of caffeine in humans has not, however, been clearly demonstrated.

In a Harvard University study involving 12,000 pregnant women, those who consumed four or more cups of coffee or tea per day were not at greater risk of delivering a child with congenital abnormalities. Measurement of caffeine consumption was determined by a self-administered questionnaire asking how many cups of coffee or tea per day were consumed.[10] Critics of the study contend that this form of caffeine intake assessment is inadequate in determining accurate caffeine content of a diet as it neglects other caffeine-containing foods and medications.[11] The relationship between birth weight and caffeine intake was studied by Martin and Bracken.[12] Of the 3841 full-term infants examined, maternal caffeine consumption did not influence the infants' risk of weighing less than 2.5 kg at birth.

Despite the many studies that have failed to show any hazardous effects of moderate amounts of caffeine in pregnancy, the Food and Drug Administration (FDA) in 1981 issued a warning concerning caffeine use in pregnancy. Until further research is conducted pregnant women should avoid excessive daily intake (more than 500 mg) of caffeine during pregnancy. When conducting a nutrition assessment, the nurse should question the client about her caffeine consumption and recommend caffeine-free beverages.

TABLE 10–6. COMMON SOURCES OF CAFFEINE

Beverage or Food	Caffeine (mg)[a]
Coffee	
Drip (5 oz)	146
Percolated (5 oz)	110
Instant, regular (5 oz)	53
Decaffeinated (5 oz)	2
Tea	
1-minute brew (5 oz)	9–33
3-minute brew (5 oz)	20–46
5-minute brew (5 oz)	20–50
Canned iced tea (12 oz)	22–36
Cola drinks (12 oz)	
Coca-Cola	65
Pepsi-Cola	43
Tab	50
Cocoa and chocolate	
Cocoa drink (6 oz)	10
Milk chocolate (1 oz)	6
Baking chocolate (1 oz)	35

[a] Strength of the brew and length of brewing time for hot beverages influence caffeine content; additionally, caffeine content of domestic teas is less than that of imported black teas.

Saccharin and Aspartame

Saccharin and aspartame are additives used as sugar substitutes. Saccharin is derived from naphtha or naphthalene and is 300 times sweeter than sucrose. On the basis of a Canadian research study implicating its role in the development of bladder tumors in the offspring of rodents fed saccharin, the FDA in 1977 passed the Saccharin Study and Labeling Act. This legislation requires a warning label on all saccharin-containing products. To meet consumer demands, Congress placed a moratorium on the ban until further research is conducted. Saccharin is reported to cross the human placenta.[13] Animal studies have demonstrated that saccharin tends to clear the fetal circulation very slowly; saccharin is still present in the fetus after maternal levels are negligible. The Council on Scientific Affairs of the American Medical Association advised, in a report that reviewed current research, "careful consideration of saccharin use by young children and pregnant women."[14] On the basis of the data available it would be prudent for mothers to avoid use of saccharin during pregnancy.

Aspartame, which is marketed under the trademarks Nutrasweet and Equal, is composed of a methyl ester of the amino acid L-phenylalanine and aspartic acid, and is 180 to 200 times sweeter than sucrose. Because it is composed of two amino acids, it provides 4 kcal/g. Aspartame is hydrolyzed to phenylalanine, aspartate, and methanol by the intestinal luminal cells and enzymes. After absorption into the portal circulation all three compounds are either metabolized or excreted. Aspartic acid has not been shown to cross the placenta, but it is unclear if methanol reaches fetal circulation.[13]

Phenylalanine is one of the eight essential amino acids required for protein synthesis. Individuals with the genetic disorder phenylketonuria (PKU) have a deficiency of the enzyme phenylalanine hydroxylase, which converts phenylalanine to tyrosine in the liver, resulting in high levels of phenylalanine and its metabolites in the blood and tissues. If untreated, the accumulation of the amino acid can result in mental retardation and developmental delays. All infants are screened at birth for PKU. Approximately 1 in 15,000 neonates is diagnosed with the disease and treated with a low phenylalanine diet. All aspartame products contain a warning label for phenylketonurics.

Several studies have indicated that peak plasma levels achieved in normal nonpregnant women exposed to high dosages of aspartame are far below what would be considered dangerous to fetal health.[15] Despite this, the nurse should avoid recommending a liberal intake of aspartame during pregnancy until further research on its safety is established.

Alcohol

Because of the devastating effects of alcohol on fetal growth and development, total abstinence should be recommended during pregnancy. Even the consumption of a healthy diet cannot prevent the teratogenic effects of ethanol in pregnancy. (*See* Chapter 42 for further discussion of fetal alcohol syndrome.)

CULTURAL FOOD PRACTICES

Cultural food practices can influence food consumption during pregnancy in a variety of ways. Beliefs and behaviors that are culturally related can affect the way in which foods are cultivated, distributed, purchased, prepared, served, and consumed, or avoided.[16] A pregnant client's ethnic and geographic heritage can determine not only the actual foods she consumes but also the manner in which and occasions on which she eats them.

Many cultures have certain food taboos that restrict consumption of particular foods, such as pork products by Jews who follow Kosher dietary laws. Cultural health beliefs can also strongly influence food practices. During childbearing, in particular, pregnant and lactating women may have strict rules on acceptable food intake. For example, some Puerto Rican families classify foods, health states, and medicines according to a therapeutic system called the hot-cold theory of disease.[17,18] According to this theory, bodily humors, such as bile and blood, vary in both temperature and moistness. Health is perceived as a balance between these humors, whereas illnesses are classified as hot or cold. Foods that have the opposite classification of the illness state are needed to return the body to its natural balance. During pregnancy, a woman adhering to this theory is careful to eliminate "hot" foods and medications from her diet, because pregnancy is considered to be a "hot" condition. The belief is that the elimination of "hot" substances will prevent the infant from being born with such conditions as a rash. Because iron tablets and

RESEARCH ABSTRACT

Gulick E, et al. Elinson M. Food beliefs and food behaviors among minority pregnant women. J Perinatol. *1987; 6:197–202*

This study examined food beliefs influencing food behavior among black, Puerto Rican, and Haitian women during pregnancy. An understanding of food beliefs could assist health professionals to encourage health-promoting food behavior among various cultural groups.

The sample for the study consisted of 15 black, 20 Puerto Rican, and 21 Haitian pregnant women who were attending an urban prenatal clinic. The investigators used the 24-hour dietary recall to determine food beliefs and behavior. They attempted to minimize error in reporting by taking the average of the 24-hour dietary score and the 24-hour food record. Women were interviewed during the first, second, and third trimesters. A follow-up dietary record was to be completed by the participants after the clinic visit and returned to the primary investigator. Although the return rate for the Haitian group was 100 percent, more than half of the Puerto Rican and black women failed to respond. This low return rate limited the use of the 24-hour food record as a method of analysis.

The investigators found that a common cultural belief was that eating certain foods would make the women and their infants healthy. Also, each cultural group had low intakes of milk and cheese in each trimester. There were marked cultural differences in the foods that were eaten and in the beliefs regarding certain foods.

Comment:

The investigators recognized several study limitations, including the small sample size, the 24-hour dietary method of reporting food intake, and the missed prenatal appointments. This study, however, helps to identify attitudes, beliefs, and food behaviors among various cultures. In addition, it highlights the cultural importance of food beliefs during pregnancy. To be successful, nutritional counseling should be based on understanding of cultural influences. The study should be replicated, using a larger sample size with similar and different populations of pregnant women.

vitamins are also considered "hot," they are avoided, unless taken with herb tea or fruit juice, which help to "neutralize" them. Foods considered "hot" include chili peppers and some salty, fatty, or sweet foods. "Cold" foods include fresh lemon, tomatoes, and watermelon. It should be emphasized that not all Puerto Rican families adhere to these practices and that nutritional beliefs vary among Hispanic cultural groups. The nurse should determine if the client follows any cultural dietary practices before initiating diet counseling.

Many cultures use diet therapy for health restoration and maintenance. For example, diet therapy is considered an integral component of traditional Chinese medicine.[19] According to the ancient philosophy of Tao, to maintain harmony with the universe a balance of the elements yin and yang must first be achieved. Body organs, diseases, and stages of the life cycle are characterized as yin or yang. An imbalance in these two elements is believed to result in disease. Yin conditions such as pregnancy must be balanced with yang foods. A fever is considered to be a yang condition and must be counteracted with yin foods. "Neutral" foods such as soft rice, sugars, sweets, or noodles may be used in either condition. Yin conditions such as pregnancy are believed to weaken the body; therefore, yang foods that are purported to "build the blood," such as fatty meats, chicken, ginger root, eggs, and garlic, are recommended. Although some Asian-Americans do practice food-related health beliefs, the extent to which they adhere to the traditional diet may vary greatly.

Many cultural food patterns do not follow what is commonly known as the "basic four food groups": meats, dairy products, fruits and vegetables, and breads and cereals. Certain cultures lack certain food groups as a result of the agricultural capabilities of the particular country. Nurses should not assume that an individual's diet is unbalanced because it does not meet the "basic four." Many Asians have lactose intolerance and avoid dairy products but are able to obtain adequate dietary calcium from tofu, fish paste made from small whole fish, and soups made from fish bones. Table 10–7 presents food plans for selected cultural groups.

Pica

Pica, the unusual craving for non-food items, may begin during the first trimester of pregnancy. Substances ingested by pregnant women practicing pica include dirt or clay, starch, ice or refrigerator frost, wall plaster, cigarette ashes, coffee grounds, and burnt matches. Several theories exist to explain this behavior, which is also observed during other stages of the life cycle, such as childhood. Some theories associate pica with sociocultural beliefs; others hypothesize that the non-food item is believed to help meet iron or calcium needs. Potential complications associated with pica include maternal malnutrition due to displacement of nutritious foods in the diet, decreased bioavailability of essential nutrients, parasitic infections from contaminated clay, congenital lead poisoning due to maternal consumption of wall plaster, and dystocia from fecal impaction as a result of clay ingestion.

All pregnant clients should be screened for pica during initial assessment. Because of the high rate of iron deficiency among individuals practicing pica, screening for pica is recommended if the woman is anemic; screening for anemia is recommended if the woman practices pica. Other tests, such as serum lead levels, may be performed according to hazards related to substances ingested. Clients should be counseled on the dangers associated with potentially harmful pica practices.

Fast Foods and Pregnancy

Fast foods have become an integral part of the culture in the United States. Many families incorporate a variety of fast foods into their daily diets. It is unlikely that families will eliminate these food items from their diets when the mother is pregnant. Pregnant adolescents in particular are likely to continue to consume fast foods. It is unrealistic for nurses and other health professionals to expect pregnant clients to change these ingrained food patterns completely.

A realistic way for nurses to ensure that pregnant clients who consume fast foods maintain a healthy diet is to become familiar with the nutrient values of these food items. With this knowledge the nurse can suggest substitution of more nutritious fast foods for less nutritious foods. For example, chicken that is not fried, salad, and a milk shake can be substituted for hamburgers, french fries, and a coke. Figure 10–3 illustrates several fast food alternatives that can provide a more nutritious diet.

Nursing Strategies Related to Cultural Food Practices

Nurses should become familiar with the cultural food practices of the community in which they work. Knowledge of ethnic and other food habits will facilitate better communication between the caregiver and the client. Cross-cultural and subcultural nutrition counseling can be challenging because it requires that counselors be accepting of values, customs, and behaviors of a culture or subculture that may be very different from their own. When recommending di-

TABLE 10–7. SELECTED CULTURAL FOOD PLANS

A. Vietnamese Food Plan

Foods	Preparation
Meats: Pork, beef, chicken, sausage, chicken feet, ox tails, liver, stomach.	Pork is most common. Chicken is consumed only on special occasions. Meats are usually cut into small pieces and fried, boiled, or steamed.
Fish: Numerous types of freshwater and saltwater fish and shellfish.	Eaten fresh, dried, salted, or fermented. Chinese like to steam fish, while Vietnamese like it fried and dipped in fish sauce.
Other proteins: Eggs, soybeans, peanuts, other legumes.	Soybeans eaten in processed forms such as soy sauce and soybean milk and curd (tofu). Peanuts eaten in soups or as a snack. Legumes eaten in desserts (Chinese influence) or in soups.
Vegetables: Wide variety of vegetables, including bamboo shoots, bok choy, broccoli, carrots, cauliflower, napa cabbage, mustard greens, bittermelon, wintermelon, green beans, eggplant, corn, water chestnut.	Eaten fresh, dried, or pickled. Usually eaten with meat or fish. Vietnamese eat raw vegetables more often than Chinese-Vietnamese.
Fruits: Wide variety of fruits, including bananas, mangoes, papayas, pineapples, melons, oranges, pears, grapefruit, longans, and tamarinds.	Usually eaten fresh. Sometimes cook pear or papaya to make a sweet soup for dessert.
Cereals and breads: Short-grain, long-grain, and glutinous rice, bean thread, wheat and rice noodles, French bread.	Rice is often eaten with every meal. It is rinsed several times before steaming. Bread eaten plain or with pork, paté, or sweetened condensed milk.
Milk: Sweetened condensed milk.	Served in coffee, with hot water or on bread. Also sometimes used as infant formula.
Fats: Lard, peanut oil.	
Seasonings: Oyster sauce, soy sauce, monosodium glutamate, black pepper, ginger, garlic, green onion, coriander, sesame oil (Chinese influence), curry (Indian influence), mint, dill, red pepper, lemon grass, vinegar, lemon, *nuoc mam* sauce.	Vietnamese food tends to be hotter than Chinese food. *Nuoc mam* sauce is a fish sauce, a thin extract made from fermented fish and salt.
Beverages: Tea, coffee, soft drinks, soybean milk, sugar-cane drink, beer, and wine.	Tea is the most common beverage. Beer and wine are only for the men.

B. Japanese Food Plan

Foods	Preparation
Meats: The Buddhist tradition of not eating meat conforms with the physical necessities of agriculture. The Japanese consume very little meat, except beef. Since World War II, however, protein intake has increased; from 1950 to 1960 it increased 10% and animal protein almost doubled.	Quantity is small. Usually cut into small pieces and served mixed with vegetables and cereal products.
Fish: Liked and one of the staple foods.	Prefer fish, shellfish, and other marine life to meats of all types. Certain kinds of raw fish are considered great delicacies. Others cooked or dried.
Other proteins: Soybean preparations used freely. Eggs used when available.	Variety of soybean preparations.
Vegetables: Prefer plants such as seaweed, bamboo shoots, onions, large radishes, dried mushrooms (*shitake*), beans. Potatoes and others when available.	Pickled is the favorite form. Others cooked with meat or fish.
Fruits: Principal fruit is *nasi* (tastes somewhat like pear, shaped like an apple; yellow, rough skin). Some persimmons and mulberries. Tangerines in mountain regions. Postwar increase in variety.	Dessert.
Cereals and breads: Rice is main food. Some barley, oats, and rye.	Rice is mixed with barley by farmers and the poorer classes. Wheat bread, especially in urban communities.
Milk: Enjoy when available; mainly import evaporated or dry milk powder.	Mostly for children.
Cheese: Very little.	
Fats: Soy oil. Rice oil. Suet when available. Practically no butter and cream.	Used in cooking.
Seasoning: Salt, *sake* (liquor distilled from rice).	
Beverages: Tea, *sake.*	Tea freely used when afforded.

TABLE 10–7. SELECTED CULTURAL FOOD PLANS *(continued)*

C. Hispanic-American-Mexican Food Plan

Foods	Preparation
Meats: Chicken, pork chops, weiners, cold cuts, and hamburger.	Used only once or twice a week.
Other proteins: Eggs, beans.	Eggs used frequently and usually fried. In rural areas, chickens are kept for their eggs. Beans usually eaten mashed and refried with lard.
Vegetables: Potatoes, red and green chiles, fresh and canned tomatoes, pumpkin, corn, field greens, onions, carrots.	Potatoes are basic item, usually fried; may be used three times a day. Chiles are popular at each meal and are a good source of vitamin A even when dried. Fresh tomatoes are very popular. Other vegetables used frequently.
Fruits: Bananas, melons, peaches, canned fruit cocktail, oranges, apples.	Oranges, apples used occasionally as snacks. Others are the more popular fruits.
Cereals and breads: Oatmeal, enriched white flour, packaged breakfast cereals, macaroni, white bread, tortillas, sweet rolls.	Sugar-coated packaged cereals are popular; oatmeal used occasionally. Macaroni is fried and served with beans and potatoes. Tortillas are homemade daily. Both purchased and homemade breads are used frequently. Purchased sandwich bread is a status symbol.
Milk: Limited availability, expensive.	
Cheese: Limited amounts used.	
Fats: Lard, salt pork, bacon fat.	Used liberally. Most foods are fried.
Beverages: Soft drinks; other sweets very popular.	

A and B: Developed by Andrea Carlson, MS, Rd. C. Adapted from *Cultural Food Patterns in the USA*. Chicago: American Dietetic Association; 1976. Reprinted from Krause M, Maha K. *Food, Nutrition, and Diet Therapy*, Philadelphia: WB Saunders, 1984.

etary changes, consider advising only those that are essential to good health.[20] Cultural and other food practices that are neutral or beneficial to the client's health should be praised and supported. For example, the client's consulting a folk healer about diet or maintaining good nutrition through use of culturally specific or more nutritious fast food items should be encouraged. The degree of dietary adherence in cross-cultural or subcultural counseling may be less than optimal if the client's values conflict with the underlying rationale for the recommended change. By studying cultural and other health benefits and food practices, the nurse can be more successful in promoting healthy behaviors.

POSTPARTUM NEEDS

The nutrient needs of the postpartum woman depend on whether or not she is breastfeeding her infant. For the woman who is not lactating, a healthy diet is still important. Fatigue, weight loss, and changes in appetite are all areas that need to be addressed when providing dietary counseling during the postpartum period.

To help cope with problems of fatigue, it is essential that the postpartum woman consume adequate kilocalories. An infant's irregular eating and sleeping schedule may interfere with the family's meal times, so it is best to have available food items that can be simply prepared.

Women who are concerned about weight loss should be provided with sensible weight loss plans that promote a gradual reduction in weight. As with pregnancy, the postpartum period is not a time for fad or unhealthy diets. To prevent iron deficiency anemia, clients are generally advised to continue to take iron supplements up to 6 weeks postpartum or while lactating.

Nutrition and Lactation

To provide sufficient quantities of nutritionally sound breast milk, the lactating mother needs a diet higher in calories and fluids than that of a nonpregnant, nonlactating woman. Production of 850 mL of breast milk each day requires about 600 to 800 kcal per day of energy.[21] As fat storage during pregnancy provides between 200 and 300 kcal/day for the first three postpartum months, an increase of 500 kcal/day over nonpregnant intake is required for lactation. Caloric intake frequently needs to be further adjusted when the mother breastfeeds the infant more than 3 months, when there is more than one infant, and when the mother is below her ideal weight.

Lactating women need approximately 2500 to 3000 mL of fluid each day to produce a sufficient

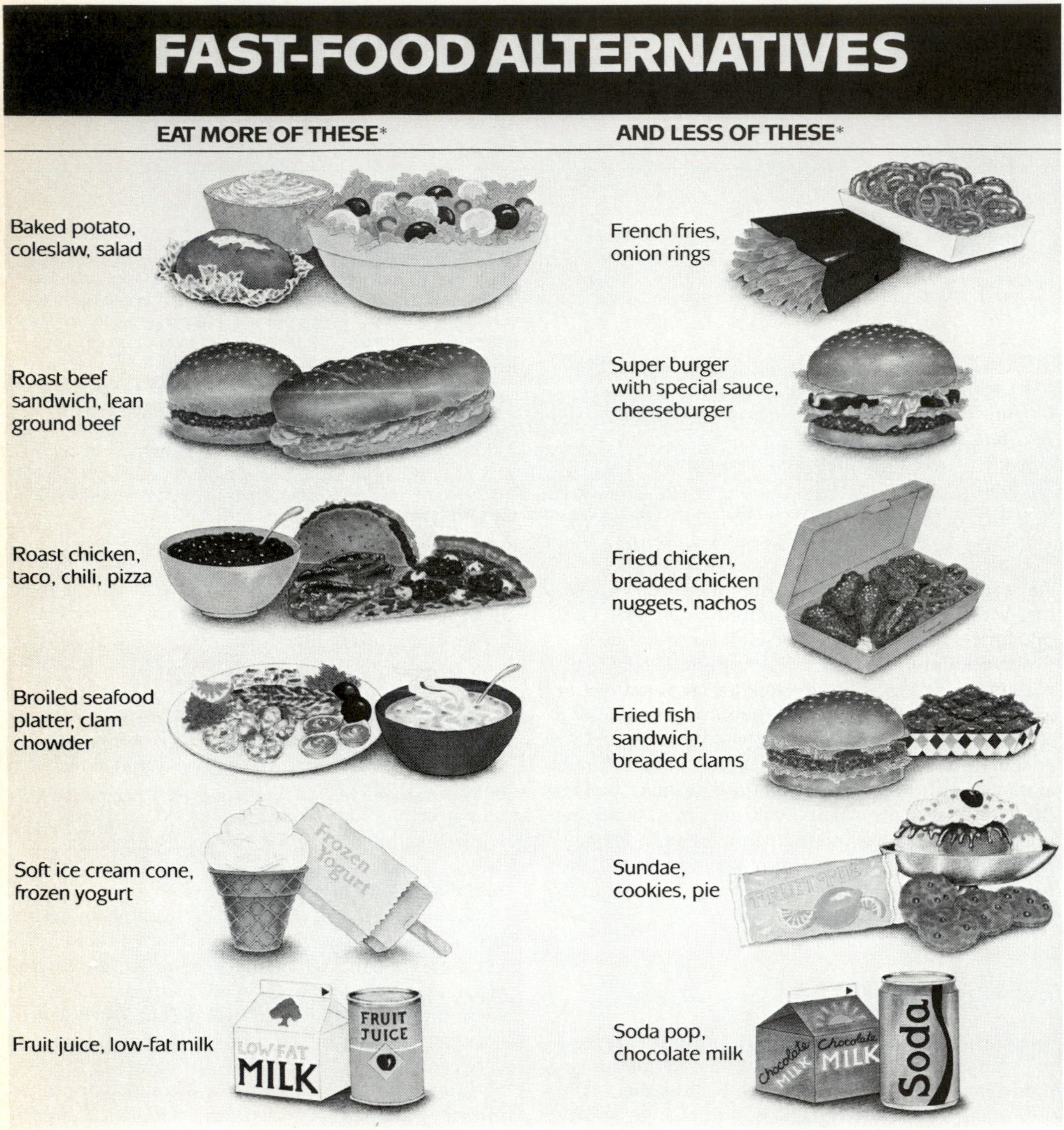
FAST-FOOD ALTERNATIVES
EAT MORE OF THESE*
AND LESS OF THESE*
Baked potato, coleslaw, salad
French fries, onion rings
Roast beef sandwich, lean ground beef
Super burger with special sauce, cheeseburger
Roast chicken, taco, chili, pizza
Fried chicken, breaded chicken nuggets, nachos
Broiled seafood platter, clam chowder
Fried fish sandwich, breaded clams
Soft ice cream cone, frozen yogurt
Frozen Yogurt
Sundae, cookies, pie
FRUIT PIE
Fruit juice, low-fat milk
LOW FAT MILK
FRUIT JUICE
Soda pop, chocolate milk
Chocolate MILK
Chocolate MILK
Soda

Figure 10–3. Fast food alternatives. (*Adapted from the* American Diabetes Association/American Diatetic Association Family Cookbook, *Vol. II. Copyright © 1984 by The American Diabetes Association/American Diatetic Association. Used, with permission, of the publisher, Prentice-Hall, Englewood Cliffs, NJ. Copyright © 1987, Wyeth Laboratories, Philadelphia, Penn.*)

quantity of breast milk. The breastfeeding woman should therefore be encouraged to consume up to 8 glasses of fluids per day. Excessive maternal diaphoresis and thirst during hot weather and strenuous activity are indications that fluid intake needs to be increased. Additionally, the infant may demand more breast milk during growth spurts and in hot weather, requiring that the mother in turn increase her fluid intake.

The increased calories and fluids should provide the nutrients required for breast milk production, as well as provide nutritionally sound breast milk. Several nutrients are needed in greater amounts during lactation: protein, riboflavin, niacin, vitamin A, vitamin C, calcium, and phosphorus (*see* Table 10–4). A total daily protein intake of 62 to 65 g per day is required to sufficiently support the energy and nutritional needs of lactation. Lactating women are advised to continue to consume at least 1200 mg of calcium per day. Phosphorus, which is also needed for infant skeletal development, should be increased by 400 mg over the non-pregnant level. If too much phosphorus is ingested, calcium absorption will be diminished; if not enough calcium is ingested and absorbed, calcium deposited in maternal bones will be depleted. Approximately 1.8 mg of riboflavin and 20 mg of niacin are needed daily. Both riboflavin and niacin are concerned with energy production and also help to remove nitrogen from amino acids when protein must be used for energy. Increased amounts of vitamins A, C, and E are needed to promote functional and structural properties of cells.[21]

A healthy diet during lactation is just as important as it was during pregnancy. Breastfeeding women should receive dietary counseling to assist them in making the proper food choices. Because of the increased need for vitamins, lactating women also are advised to take vitamin supplements. Without vitamin supplements, lactating women are prone to vitamin deficiencies in biotin, B_{12}, B_6, C, A, folic acid, B_1, and B_2.[22]

NUTRITIONAL CARE DURING CHILDBEARING

Nutrition services in a perinatal clinic should be provided according to written policies and procedures that establish protocols for nutritional screening, assessment, planning, implementation, and evaluation of care. The development of protocols and the services delivered should involve the entire perinatal interdisciplinary team: nurse, physician, nutritionist, social worker, and any other personnel involved in the provision of health services.

Nutrition assessment and management serves several purposes: it allows for early detection and correction of nutrition-related abnormalities or disorders; it establishes baseline data for further evaluation of the client's health status; and it allows the health professional to formulate and implement plans for intervention. The nursing process in management of nutritional problems utilizes the following steps:

1. Assessment of nutritional status
2. Formulation of nursing diagnosis
3. Design of a plan for intervention to improve nutritional status
4. Implementation of strategies of meet identified goals and objectives
5. Evaluation of the effectiveness of the plan with appropriate recommendations

Nutrition Assessment

The purpose of the initial nutrition screening is to elicit data about the client's nutritional status. This information is usually obtained during the first prenatal visit, when a physical examination is performed, anthropometric measurements such as height and body weight are obtained, and laboratory studies are conducted. The data obtained at this screening will verify the existence of any nutritional risk factors and help prioritize the mother's health care needs. Table 10–8 lists maternal risk factors that may be present at the onset of pregnancy or may develop during pregnancy. The identification of risk factors helps the nurse formulate the plans for nutrition intervention and refer the appropriate clients to the nutritionist for further assessment of nutritional status.

In many health care settings, registered dietitians are available to conduct the assessment, but in most facilities, the collection of data requires the collaboration of the entire health care team. There are four components of the assessment process: dietary data, anthropometric measurements, biochemical indexes, and physical examination. A diagnosis or plan should not be based on one component alone but should instead evolve from assessment of all four components. The assessment data can be recorded on a separate form for prenatal nutrition history (Figure 10–4) or can be integrated into the health assessment form, depending on the protocol of the health care facility.

Dietary Data. The nurse may use the health history, 24-hour dietary recall, or food diary to elicit information about the client's diet. The health history provides information about the type of diet being followed, who does the shopping and cooking, and any cultural practices related to diet. Of particular importance are the following:

TABLE 10–8. MATERNAL NUTRITIONAL RISK FACTORS

At the Onset of Pregnancy

Adolescence: less than 3 years postmenarche

Three or more pregnancies within 2 years

Past reproductive performance characterized by abortions, pregnancy complications, low-birth-weight infants, or perinatal loss

Economic deprivation

Unusual dietary practices

Heavy smoker (more than 20 cigarettes per day)

Excessive alcohol intake (chronic use of more than 5 oz whiskey per day or its equivalent in beer or wine) or history of binge drinking

Drug addiction

Chronic systemic diseases

Prepregnant weight below 85 percent standard height and weight (less than 60 in. in height and 100 lb in weight) or obesity above 120% of standard weight and height

During Pregnancy

Hemoglobin below 11 g/dL or hematocrit below 33 percent

Inadequate weight gain (less than 1 kg per month)

Excessive weight gain (3 kg per month) possibly associated with fluid retention

Following Pregnancy

Nutritional demands of lactation

Reproduced, with permission, from National Academy of Sciences, Nutrition Services in Perinatal Care. *Washington, DC: National Academy Press, 1981.*

1. Factors that affect eating patterns, especially
   a. Nausea
   b. Vomiting
   c. Constipation
   d. Pica
2. Effect of pregnancy on eating patterns
3. Socioeconomic factors relevant to food intake
   a. Family size
   b. Education
   c. Income
   d. Occupation
   e. Activity level
4. Type of diet being followed (any cultural biases to the diet)
5. Sources of food: Who purchases the food? Where is it purchased? Is any food produced in home? Does the family have or need assistance with food purchasing (e.g., food stamps, WIC program)?
6. Food preparation: How and where is food prepared? Who prepares the food? What cooking and storage facilities are available?
7. Amounts and types of fluid consumed with and between meals
8. Consumption of substances detrimental to maternal and fetal health (e.g., alcohol)
9. Relationship, as viewed by the pregnant client, between food intake and health of the fetus and herself

The 24-hour dietary recall is the method most frequently used to estimate the client's nutrient intake, because it is simple to administer. In this method, the client recalls her food intake of the previous day. The nurse or nutritionist acquires the information during an interview with the client, or the client reports it on a self-assessment form. To improve the reliability of the recall, the interviewer should carefully review that day's intake with the client, with particular attention to items that are frequently omitted, such as condiments, dressings, butter, margarine, gravies, and snacks. If a food group such as milk is omitted, the interviewer should ask the client if these items are normally found in her diet. This may be accomplished by using an abbreviated form of a food tool that asks specifically how many times per day, per week, or per month the client consumes a particular food.

Another dietary evaluation method is the food diary. The client keeps a record for at least 4 days (preferably one weekend and two weekdays) listing every food item she consumes. The diary may also provide information related to the client's lifestyle, such as the location and time of meals and with whom the client ate.

Using the information acquired with the dietary assessment tools, the nutrient content of the diet can be calculated by hand or by use of a computer program with a nutrient data bank. To evaluate nutrient intake accurately, the diet should be compared with the RDAs for women during pregnancy (*see* Table 10–4). From these results, dietary interventions can be planned.

Anthropometric Measurements. Anthropometry is the measurement of physical characteristics of the body. These physical findings can be used to assess a client's growth and development by comparison with a standard, or to evaluate individual fluctuations in body composition. Height and body weight measurements are most commonly obtained during pregnancy. To assess the pattern of weight gain, the preconception weight and the body weight are recorded at all prenatal visits.

The pattern of weight gain during pregnancy should be followed closely to monitor rapid fluctuations in body weight. A sudden increase in weight gain could indicate excessive calorie intake or edema.

Biochemical Indexes. Biochemical data can be used to detect a nutrient deficiency before clinical signs

Name:	Age:	Date:
Height:	Present weight:	Preconceptual weight:
Weight history:		
Dietary modifications (eg, low sodium):		
Food allergies/intolerances:		
Prescribed medications:		
Vitamin/mineral supplements:		
Medical history:		
Obstetric history:		
Social history:		
Dental history:		
Physical activity:		
Education:	Occupation:	
Marital status:	Number in household:	
Person responsible for food shopping/cooking:		
Unusual/fad dietary habits (eg, pica):		
Cultural/ethnic food practices:		
Number of meals/snacks per day:		
Alcohol intake:		
Caffeine intake:		
Federal assistance (eg, Food Stamp Program, WIC):		
Biochemical indices:		
Clinical data:		

Figure 10–4. Sample prenatal nutritional assessment tool.

become apparent. Many tests can be influenced by the client's gender, age, nutritional status, or disease state. These factors should therefore be considered in the interpretation of the results. Routine nutrition-related laboratory tests conducted during prenatal visits include urinary analysis for the presence of glucose, ketones, and protein and a complete blood count, which includes measures of iron status such as hemoglobin and hematocrit. The hemoglobin level and hematocrit are obtained on the first prenatal visit and, if within normal limits, again in the third trimester. Pregnant women may develop a physiologic anemia in the second trimester and need supplementary iron and folacin. If the mother is found to be anemic, hemoglobin levels and hematocrits are obtained more frequently. In some instances where nutritional deficiency is suspected, serum iron studies or other more sophisticated blood tests are also done.

Physical Examination. Nursing assessment can identify clinical signs of a nutrient deficiency. Special attention is given to the skin, gums, tongue, eyes, and hair because these parts of the body have the most rapid cell turnover (mucosal and epithelial tissue) and therefore are most susceptible to changes in nutritional status. For example, skin pallor during pregnancy may be related to an iron deficiency. Table 10–9 describes physical signs of good and poor nutritional status.

Nursing Diagnosis

Once a complete assessment of dietary, anthropometric, biochemical, and clinical data is conducted, nursing diagnoses are developed, and a plan for intervention can then be initiated. (*See* the box for nursing diagnoses that may be related to nutritional status during pregnancy.)

Nursing and Collaborative Management

Planning nutritional interventions involves the pregnant woman, her family, and the nurse. Another

NURSING DIAGNOSES RELATED TO NUTRITION DURING PREGNANCY

Problem-Oriented

Alteration in nutrition, related to nausea and vomiting

Alteration in nutrition, related to inappropriate dieting behavior during pregnancy

Alteration in nutrition, related to pica practices during pregnancy

Strength-Oriented

Asset in nutrition, related to knowledgeable consumption of food

Asset in nutrition, related to knowledgeable habits about foods and eating behaviors

TABLE 10–9. PHYSICAL SIGNS OF GOOD AND POOR NUTRITIONAL STATUS

Tissue	Normal Appearance	Signs Associated with Malnutrition
Eyes	Bright, clear, moist, and shiny with pink membranes; no prominent blood vessels or mound of tissue on sclera	Membranes pale or red; drying of eye, eyelids, cornea; increased vascularization of the cornea (bloodshot eyes); increased sensitivity to bright light, burning, itching, soreness; poor vision in dim light following exposure to bright light (night blindness)
Hair	Shiny, lustrous, and not easily pulled out; healthy scalp	Dull, dry, brittle, thin, depigmented, easily pulled out
Skin	Smooth, slightly moist, good color; no signs of rashes, swellings, dark or light spots	Skin pallor; dermatitis; rough, dry, scaly skin with hardness of papillae at base of hair follicles; sores that fail to heal; petechiae, bruises; depigmentation or hyperpigmentation of the skin
Teeth and gums	Bright, straight teeth without crowding in well-shaped jaw; no evidence of caries (cavities); firm, reddish pink gums with no evidence of swelling or bleeding	Caries present; missing teeth; malposition or abnormal eruption of teeth; worn or mottled tooth surfaces; soft, spongy, bleeding gums
Mucous membranes, mouth, lips, and tongue	Reddish pink color to lips, tongue, mucous membranes; absence of lesions; adequately moist; surface papillae present on tongue	Pale mucous membranes; purplish red to scarlet-red tongue, fissures of the lips and/or corners of mouth; sore mouth and sore, swollen tongue; tongue smooth due to atrophy of surface papillae
Skeleton	Good posture; no malformation present	Poor posture; malformations such as beading of the ribs, bowlegs, or knock-knees
Nails	Firm, pink	Spoon-shaped, brittle, and ridged nails
Muscles	Well-developed, firm	Flaccid, undeveloped, or wasted appearance; tender
Abdomen and lower extremities	No tenderness, weaknesses, or swelling of feet and legs	Abdomen swollen (abdominal swelling unrelated to pregnancy); weakness, tenderness, or tingling in feet or legs; edema
Thyroid gland	No enlargement	Enlarged (simple goiter)

Adapted, with permission, from Lewis CM. Basic and Family Nutrition. A Self-Instructional Approach. *2nd ed. Philadelphia: FA Davis; 1984:119, 120, 122.*

member of the interdisciplinary team who is particularly important in nutritional planning is the nutritionist. Collaboration will help to ensure that a realistic plan for the pregnant client and her family is developed.

Dietary Counseling. Dietary counseling should be directed toward the needs identified during screening and assessment. On the basis of this information, short-term objectives and long-term goals that represent input from the client and health care team members can be developed. Specific goals and objectives should reflect a realistic assessment of the client's needs and abilities based on a thorough review of the health, social, and dietary data. These goals and objectives should be stated clearly in the health record to provide a means of evaluating the client's progress, and as a channel of communication among health professionals to ensure continuity of care.

The nurse should emphasize the positive aspects of the mother's diet and help her to correct any nutritional deficiencies. Nutritional counseling should incorporate any assessed nutritional deficiencies, income of the family, and cultural food preferences. Parents should be given information about the dietary requirements of pregnancy. If supplementation is required (e.g., iron and folacin), the woman should be informed of the rationale for the supplementation and any discomforts that might occur, such as constipation. The nurse monitors nutritional intake throughout pregnancy, facilitates appropriate dietary planning, assists the mother in planning her own diet, and fosters positive self-care practices. Moreover, referral to such programs as WIC assists the low-income family to obtain the food needed for good nutrition for pregnant and lactating women, infants, and young children (*see* later section).

TABLE 10–10. NUTRITION EDUCATION TOPICS FOR PRENATAL CLIENTS

Recommendations for weight gain during pregnancy
Vitamin and mineral supplementation
Control of common gastrointestinal problems, i.e., nausea, vomiting, constipation
Preparation of easy, nutritious snack foods
Increasing calcium, iron, and folic acid in the diet
Breastfeeding
Formula feeding
Introduction of solid foods into infant's diet
Food assistance programs

Nutrition Education. Nutrition education involves teaching clients to make knowledgeable decisions about their nutritional health. It may occur on an individual basis or among groups. Many perinatal clinics provide nutrition education classes targeted toward the needs of the prenatal client. Potential nutrition education topics are listed in Table 10–10. Group classes are often popular because they allow mothers an opportunity to share information and ask questions in a supportive atmosphere. Nutrition education programs are also an effective use of the nurse's and nutritionist's time, as many clients have similar needs that can be discussed in a group rather than focused on individually.

Evaluation

Nutritional assessment and management is an ongoing process that requires continuous reassessment of the client's nutritional status, redefinition of goals and objectives, and evaluation of the changes implemented. Good nutritional practices during pregnancy help to ensure a healthy newborn and an uncomplicated postpartum recovery. There is little question that nutrition profoundly affects pregnancy and the fetus. The objective of nursing management is to promote the best possible level of health for the childbearing individual and family through positive nutritional practices. These practices motivate the family to maintain a healthy diet throughout the family life span.

MANAGEMENT OF NUTRITIONAL RISK FACTORS DURING PREGNANCY

Management of individuals who are at risk for nutritional problems during pregnancy is the joint responsibility of the interdisciplinary perinatal team. Important members of this team are nurses and nutritionists, who collaborate to provide comprehensive nutritional care to the high-risk mother and her family.

Later chapters of this text will discuss nutritional management of clients with diabetes mellitus (Chapter 39), hypertension (Chapter 39), and anemia during pregnancy (Chapter 38). This section briefly describes care of the woman who is at risk because of her weight, and nutritional considerations in care of the pregnant adolescent.

Obesity, Underweight, and Low Weight Gain

Obesity. Nutritional management of obese women during pregnancy has historically been an area of controversy, particularly in regard to recommended weight gain. Obesity during pregnancy is associated with both increased maternal mortality and morbidity and increased fetal morbidity.[23] The complications related to obesity (Table 10–11) are of critical importance in determining the principles of prenatal care. **Obesity** is generally defined as a weight 20 percent above ideal body weight, and **morbid obesity** is described as a weight 100 percent above ideal body weight. An estimated 6 to 10 percent of women who are pregnant are considered to be morbidly obese.

The Collaborative Perinatal Project of the National Institute of Neurological and Communicative Disorders and Stroke conducted a prospective study on the relationship of weight gain to the outcome of pregnancy.[24] The study followed 53,518 subjects during an 8-year period and recorded the events of gestation, labor, and delivery and the health history of the offspring until 8 years of age. The results demonstrated that the optimal weight gain during pregnancy was dependent on the mother's weight. The lowest fetal and neonatal mortality rates were associ-

TABLE 10–11. RISKS ASSOCIATED WITH OBESITY DURING PREGNANCY

Gestational diabetes
Urinary tract infections
Inadequate weight gain
Wound infection
Thromboembolism
Pregnancy-induced hypertension
Fetal monitoring difficulties
Prolonged labor
Fetal macrosomia
Birth trauma

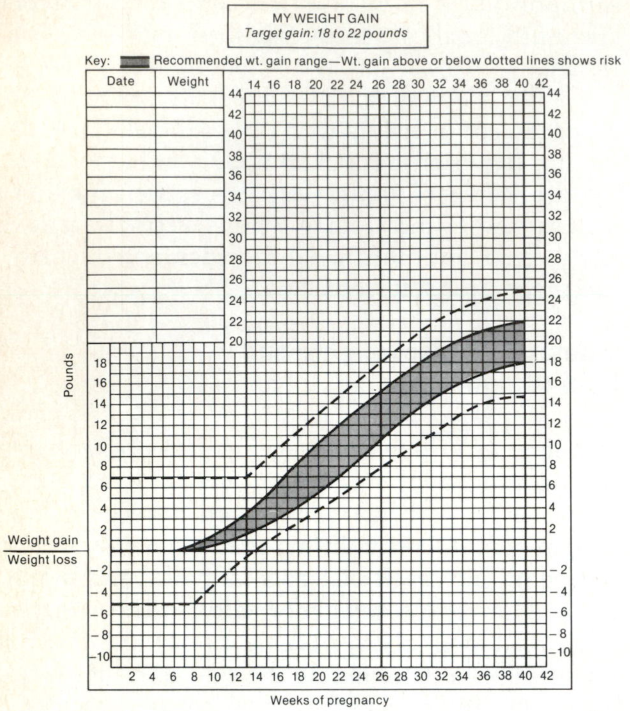

Figure 10–5. Optimal weight gain for overweight women, as illustrated on a prenatal weight grid. (*Developed by the 1987 Idaho* WIC *program; reproduced, with permission, from the Worthington-Roberts BS, Williams SR.* Nutrition in Pregnancy and Lactation. *St. Louis Times Mirror/Mosby; 1989:116.*)

ated with a 15- to 16-pound weight gain among obese women. (Figure 10–5). Overweight women who gained less than 15 pounds had a perinatal mortality rate two times higher than that of normal-weight women with similar low weight gain.

Some researchers support the belief that the recommended 7-pound increase in maternal fat stores in preparation for the last trimester may be unnecessary in obese women who already have sufficient fat stores. Thus far, though, no research has clearly demonstrated that fat deposition among obese women during pregnancy is unnecessary. Although the ideal weight gain for obese pregnant women appears to be less than that recommended for normal-weight women, pregnancy is not the time to diet or lose weight. When kilocalorie intake is less than the body's requirements, ketones become the chief energy substrate. The long-term effect of maternal ketosis on fetal development is unknown, but there is some evidence it may lead to neurologic damage to the fetus. Ketones do cross the placental barrier and will be utilized for energy by the fetus who is not receiving adequate supplies of glucose and amino acids. In addition, insufficient caloric intake can also lead to inadequate intake of essential vitamins and minerals.

Nutritional management of obese pregnant women requires special considerations. Many women, particularly those who were dieting, are reluctant to accept the recommendation for a 15- to 20-pound weight gain. In addition, the mother may experience lack of support by family members who fail to understand the need for weight gain in an obese person. Before providing nutrition education it is valuable to assess the client's attitudes and beliefs about weight gain. During the initial assessment, the nurse or nutritionist should also inquire about the client's weight and diet history. Such information as recent weight loss or weight gain prior to conception, or fad diets currently or previously followed, aids in the development of an appropriate nutritional care plan. The client is also advised that liquid diets and diet pills are unsafe during pregnancy.

To aid the client and family in understanding nutrient and kilocalorie needs during pregnancy, a diagram illustrating the components of weight gain is helpful. The obese client is then able to visualize that the recommended 20-pound weight gain does not accumulate into 20 pounds of body fat, but is used in normal maternal and fetal growth and development. The pattern of weight gain recommended is as follows: no weight gain during the first trimester (as opposed to a 3-pound weight gain in a normal-weight woman) and an approximately half-pound increase in weight each week during the second and third trimesters. To promote adequate weight gain, total kilocalorie intake should be 300 kcal per day above the level that would otherwise maintain the client's present body weight. In general, pregnancy is not the time to diet, but obese women may need strong support and close supervision to achieve the recommended weight gain.

Underweight Before Pregnancy. Underweight for height is defined as less than 90 percent of ideal body weight. Several complications are associated with the pregnancies of underweight women, such as low birth weight, prematurity, low Apgar scores, and iron deficiency anemia in the mother.[25] To offset the potential adverse effects of being underweight during pregnancy, the recommended amount of weight gain is 28–40 pounds.[1] Like the obese mother, the underweight woman may be reluctant to increase her body weight, preferring a slim body profile. Attitudes toward weight gain should be explored during the initial nutrition assessment to identify women who are at risk for poor weight gain or who are at risk for eating disorders. Under ideal conditions, underweight women should achieve an ideal body weight prior to conception to ensure the availability of optimal nutrient stores.

Eating Disorders. Anorexia nervosa and bulimia are examples of eating disorders that can lead to poor nutrition, fetal growth retardation, and life-threatening maternal and fetal conditions such as electrolyte imbalance and organ damage. **Anorexia nervosa** is a condition in which the client has an extreme fear of becoming fat and refuses to maintain a minimal normal body weight.[26] Drastic methods of weight loss, such as excessive dieting and exercise or use of laxatives, diuretics, or self-induced vomiting may be employed in an effort to "stay slim." Anorexia nervosa often is associated with amenorrhea and infertility; however, women who have a body fat percentage of at least 22 percent or women who have been able to recover their weight may become pregnant. **Bulimia** is an abnormal behavioral pattern in which binge eating is followed by repeated attempts at weight loss using self-prescribed techniques such as fasting or intense dieting, self-induced vomiting, and use of diuretics, laxatives, and enemas.

The client should be asked about present and past practices used to control weight, although many clients may be reluctant to admit to these problems. Being underweight prior to pregnancy or a history of large weight fluctuations may indicate an eating disorder. Clients with eating disorders, however, may or may not be underweight. Clients routinely should be advised against practices such as self-induced vomiting and use of enemas or any unprescribed medications during pregnancy. Eating disorders are complex problems that should not be ignored. Clients with eating disorders should be referred to health professionals specializing in their treatment.

Low Weight Gain. Low weight gain during pregnancy can occur among women who are considered to be of normal weight, obese, or underweight before conception. Low weight gain has been associated with prematurity and low infant birth weight. In a study of 2,163 women, Abrams and colleagues found that women with a low rate of weight gain were more than twice as likely to deliver prematurely than were women with a high weight gain (> 0.52 kg/wk).[27]

Mothers who are exhibiting low weight gain during pregnancy should be monitored very closely and referred to the nutritionist for periodic evaluation of the diet. There may be several different reasons for the lack of adequate weight gain and these should all be explored: Does kilocaloric expenditure exceed kilocaloric intake because of vigorous physical exercise during work or recreation? Is kilocaloric intake appropriate for kilocalorie needs during pregnancy? Are adequate food resources available? Is there evidence of alcohol or drug abuse? Does the client find weight gain during pregnancy undesirable? Are gastrointestinal problems (nausea, vomiting, constipation, heartburn) interfering with normal food intake? Once the underlying problem related to poor weight gain has been recognized, strategies toward improving nutrient intake can be implemented.

Adolescent Pregnancy

Adolescence is a period of the human life cycle in which rapid physical growth occurs and nutrient requirements increase. A teenager who conceives within 4 years of menarche (average onset: 12.5 to 13 years of age) is considered to be at high nutritional risk, as she must meet not only her own nutrient needs but also those of the developing fetus.

Many other factors may place a pregnant teenager at nutritional risk. One example is related to weight gain during pregnancy. Teenagers frequently have a low prepregnancy weight and a gain of less than 16 pounds during their pregnancy. Poor weight gain during pregnancy is positively associated with low-birth-weight infants. Nineteen percent of the offspring of teens weigh less than 2000 g.[28] The incidence of low-birth-weight infants decreases to 7.4 percent when weight gain improves to 21 to 25 pounds, and to 6.3 percent when weight gain increases to 26 to 35 pounds.[28] Adequate weight gain also lowers fetal mortality rates. As weight gain in pregnant teenagers increases from 16 to 26 to 35 pounds, the fetal mortality rate is reduced by half, from 8.0 to 3.9 deaths per 1000 live births.[28]

Research studies have indicated that the energy needs of the pregnant teenager vary between 38 and 50 kcal/kg per day. Different patterns of physical activity can influence the variation in energy requirements. Because of the extensive tissue growth and development that occur during pregnancy, high protein intake is advised. For 15- to 18-year-olds, the RDA for protein is 1.5 g of protein per kilogram of body weight, and for younger females, 1.7 g of protein per kilogram of body weight.

In addition to the physiologic and nutritional demands of pregnancy, the erratic eating habits of pregnant teenagers also contribute to their nutritional risk. Food patterns commonly observed include frequent meal skipping (particularly breakfast) and consumption of foods high in salt and sugar and low in vitamins and minerals. Limited financial resources to purchase healthy foods may also have detrimental effects on the diet. Lack of knowledge concerning the diet may make it difficult for the individual to make healthy food choices. Pregnant teenagers who are financially eligible will benefit by being referred to the WIC program, which provides nutritional counseling and food vouchers that allow the individual to purchase nutritious foods.

To reduce perinatal risks, pregnant teenagers should receive early and ongoing nutrition assessment and intervention. Attention should be focused on promoting healthy eating habits and preventing consumption of harmful substances (Figure 10–6). For example, if snacking is a predominant feature of the diet, the nurse should emphasize nutritious snack foods. Nutritious snack foods that might appeal to a teenager include fresh fruits, cheese, fresh vegetables with yogurt dip, granola bars, and peanut butter.

PREVENTING LOW-BIRTH-WEIGHT INFANTS

Low birth weight in infants is identified as an unfavorable outcome of pregnancy because of the associated health risks, particularly in terms of perinatal mortality. Maternal age, parity, prior obstetric performance, race, and social class all influence infant birth weight. Although most of these factors are not amenable to change, one influence on birth weight is controllable: the nutritional health of the mother.

There have been several initiatives in both the private and the public health sectors to reduce the incidence of low birth weight among infants by improving the quality of the mother's diet. For example, the March of Dimes Birth Defects Foundation, a private foundation, has made reduction of low-birth-weight infants a priority, and funds a variety of projects and research studies related to maternal and fetal nutrition. Well-known public initiatives, such as WIC, are discussed here.

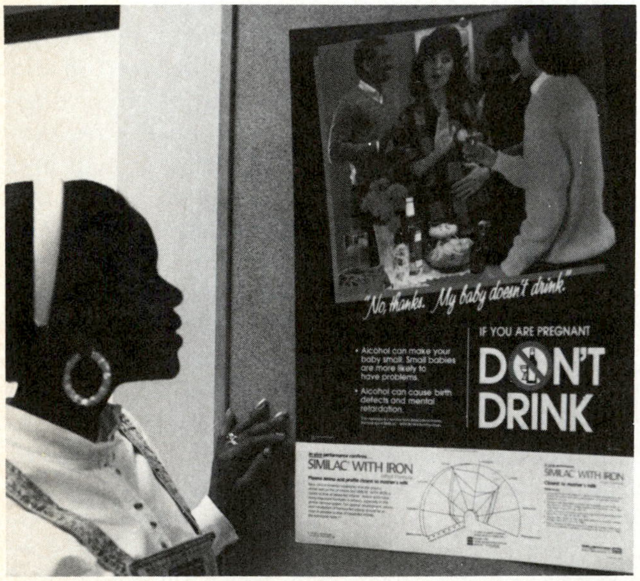
"No thanks. My baby doesn't drink."
Alcohol can make your baby small. Small babies are more likely to have problems.
Alcohol can cause birth defects and mental retardation.
IF YOU ARE PREGNANT
DON'T DRINK
SIMILAC WITH IRON
SIMILAC WITH IRON

Figure 10–6. Visual aids such as posters help educate pregnant adolescents.

Public Health Nutrition Programs

Women of low socioeconomic status are at high risk for delivering premature and low-birth-weight infants as a result of several factors, including inadequate health care, poor sanitation and housing, and inadequate diet. Brennan examined the diets of 22 low-income pregnant women in a 24-hour period.[29] The mean kilocalorie intake was 72% of the RDA, and the mean intakes of zinc, magnesium, and folic acid were less than 50% of the RDAs. These findings are supported in earlier work by Snowman, who found the diets of low-income women to be particularly low in energy, calcium, and iron.[30]

Special Supplemental Food Program for Women, Infants, and Children. To improve the nutritional status of low-income women and therefore help to reduce infant mortality and morbidity, and to promote good health from conception through early childhood, the federally funded Special Supplemental Food Program for Women, Infants, and Children (WIC) was established in 1973. The program, funded by the US Department of Agriculture (USDA), serves to provide food and nutrition education to low-income pregnant women classified as being at medical or nutritional risk. Also eligible are lactating women, infants, and children up to 5 years of age who meet the medical and financial criteria. The monthly food package for pregnant women includes vouchers to purchase such foods as milk, cheese, eggs, vitamin- and mineral-fortified cereals, fruit juice, dried peas and beans, and peanut butter. To be eligible to receive the food package, the applicant must first meet financial eligibility guidelines as determined by the annual federal poverty income guidelines. Screening also requires a physical examination by a private or clinic physician and a nutrition assessment by a WIC nurse or nutritionist. Examples of factors indicating nutritional risk include nutritional anemia, age (less than 18 or greater than 35), short interconceptional period, and previous history of delivering a premature or low-birth-weight infant. Once the applicant is certified, she must receive regular medical checkups and attend nutrition education classes given by the WIC nurse or nutritionist. The food package is designed to serve as a supplement to foods already in the diet, with an emphasis on increasing the intake of both energy and the essential nutrients during pregnancy.

Endes and coworkers analyzed the nutrient intake of pregnant women enrolled in WIC programs and compared it with the diets of non-WIC participants by using a 24-hour dietary recall.[31] Clients enrolled in WIC had a greater intake of milk, juice, and fortified cereal than non-WIC clients. The WIC participants met 77% of the RDA for energy, as compared with the reported 68% for non-WIC clients. WIC participants met or exceeded 100% of the RDAs for thiamine, riboflavin, niacin, vitamins A and C, and protein. The non-WIC group exceeded 100% of the RDAs for riboflavin and vitamin C only. The researchers were able to demonstrate a significant difference between the dietary intakes of pregnant WIC and non-WIC women.

Expanded Food and Nutrition Education Program. In addition to WIC, other federally funded nutrition programs are available. The Expanded Food and Nutrition Education Program (EFNEP) established in 1968 by USDA provides nutrition education in the home by paraprofessional nutrition aides. The nutrition aides, trained by nutritionists from the Cooperative Extension Service, conduct home visits to assess their clients' diets and to provide nutrition education on such topics as shopping for economical food and preparing nutritious meals. The success of the program is related to the fact that the aides reside in the same community and therefore are familiar with the local resources and community needs.

Food Stamp Program. The Food Stamp Program is available to low-income individuals who meet financial guidelines determined by the federal poverty level. Each month, eligible participants receive food stamps (coupons) with which they purchase food. The value of the stamps depends on the size of the family and the available income. Food stamps can be used to purchase any food except pet food and any beverages except alcoholic beverages.

The Food Stamp Program, WIC, EFNEP, and other such programs, allow the health professional to refer clients to other agencies for food assistance. Many public health clinics employ social workers who refer clients to the appropriate programs. The initial nutrition assessment should include questions related to the economic resources available for food purchases, to identify those individuals eligible for food assistance. Many prenatal clinics routinely screen for eligibility for the WIC program. By establishing a system of referral to local agencies that provide food and nutrition services, the health care center can provide more comprehensive health services.

CASE STUDY/CARE PLAN: INADEQUATE NUTRITION RESULTING FROM NAUSEA AND VOMITING IN EARLY PREGNANCY

Barbara Tate is a 28-year-old primipara who is 8 weeks pregnant. During the assessment, Barbara tells the nurse that she is experiencing nausea and vomiting throughout the day. She states, "I know what food I should eat for the baby, but most foods make me sick."

Barbara indicates that she is able to "keep down" plain spaghetti, crackers, and broiled chicken without the skin. Further, she states her husband is getting annoyed that she does not cook other food.

Physical examination reveals that Barbara has lost 2 pounds since her last visit 1 month ago. Hemoglobin and hematocrit levels are normal and urine is negative for protein and acetone. Prior to becoming pregnant, Barbara's weight (130 pounds) was appropriate for her height (5 ft 7 in.).

(continued)

CASE STUDY/CARE PLAN: Inadequate Nutrition Resulting from Nausea and Vomiting in Early Pregnancy (*continued*)

Supporting Assessment Data	Expected Client/Family Outcome	Nursing Action/ Intervention	Rationale	Criteria for Evaluation
Nursing Diagnosis: Alteration in nutrition: potential for lack of nutrients and fluids, related to nausea and vomiting during the first trimester				
First trimester of pregnancy—8 weeks pregnant—and experiencing nausea and vomiting throughout the day.	By the end of the visit, client will: Identify nausea and some vomiting as a common occurence during the first trimester	Explain causes of nausea and vomiting during the first trimester.	The discomfort of nausea and vomiting may be related to hormone levels and altered carbohydrate metabolism during the first trimester. These symptoms usually decline after the first trimester.	When asked, client is able to identify nausea and vomiting as a common occurence.
Lost 2 pounds in 1 month.	Identify nutritious foods that she will be able to tolerate	Identify foods from necessary food groups that are acceptable to client and ways to prepare them.		When aksed by a nurse or a nutritionist, client will identify foods that she can tolerate from each food group.
States "I know what food I should eat for the baby, but most foods make me sick." Can tolerate plain spaghetti, crackers, and broiled chicken	By the end of the first visit, client agrees to attempt self-care practices to reduce nausea and vomiting	Instruct client to eat smaller meals, to eat dry crackers before rising, to avoid odors, and to call if the self-care measures do not help.	Self-care practices such as eating dry crackers and small meals may alleviate symptoms and allow client to eat nutritious food.	Client relates during next visit the self-care practices she has attempted and how they worked.
Hgb = 13 g/dL, Hct = 39% Weight = 130 pounds Height = 5 ft 7 in Urine = negative for protein and acetone	Throughout first trimester, client will maintain nutrient and fluid needs	Assess nutritional intake through 24-hour dietary recall, weight, condition of skin, blood work, mucous membranes.		On next visit, client maintains or increases her weight; Hbg, Hct, and urinalysis are normal.
	Client will report any increase in vomiting that prevents fluid and food intake	Advise client to contact health care provider for persistent vomiting. Refer client to nutritionist as necessary.	Referral to a nutritionist provides comprehensive health care to client.	Client reports by phone any changes in nausea and vomiting. client visits nutritionalist.
Nursing Diagnosis: Potential for compromised family functioning, related to marital conflict over food and food preparation				
Client states that husband is unhappy that she is no longer cooking	By next visit: Husband will be encouraged to call nurse and discuss nausea and nutrition during pregnancy, if necessary Couple will relate a dietary plan acceptable to both	Provide client with written information about nausea and vomiting and dietary intake during pregnancy, which she can review with husband.		
		Provide client with telephone number so that husband can call if he wants more information.	Involving family members in the planning of care will facilitate fulfillment of individual members' health care needs.	Before next visit, client's husband calls nurse and discusses nutrition and diet during pregnancy. By next visit, client will complete a weekly menu developed by her and her husband.

Supporting Assessment Data	Expected Client/Family Outcome	Nursing Action/ Intervention	Rationale	Criteria for Evaluation
	Couple will relate that husband assists in food preparation when client is nauseated	Discuss with husband possible alternatives in selecting and preparing foods; encourage him to assist in preparation when client is nauseated.		Client relates that her husband helps her prepare meals if she is nauseated.

SUMMARY

Research confirms that nutrition plays an important role in maternal and fetal health. Weight gain during pregnancy is a result of growth of the fetus, placenta, amniotic fluid, uterus, and breasts and increase in maternal blood volume. It is important for the nurse to know the recommended weight gain and pattern of weight gain during pregnancy. Currently, the recommended weight gain for adult women of normal weight is 25 to 35 pounds over the course of pregnancy.

Nutrient requirements during pregnancy are based on the increased needs of the mother and fetus. Kilocalories provide the mother and fetus with the necessary energy requirements. Proteins, carbohydrates, and fats are essential in meeting the body's requirements for kilocalories. In addition, vitamins and minerals play an essential role in promoting the utilization of energy from carbohydrates, fats, and proteins. With the exception of iron and folacin, the needed vitamins can be obtained from a well-balanced diet.

The nurse uses the nursing process to assess the nutritional status of the pregnant woman and plan appropriate care. Special attention should be given to practices that may be detrimental to the health of the mother and the fetus, such as alcohol use or poor food habits. Cultural food practices, including the ingestion of fast foods, should be considered. Nutrition assessment should be continued after delivery, as postpartum and lactating mothers also have increased nutrient and energy demands related to healing and lactation. Collaboration with a nutritionist assists the family in obtaining comprehensive care.

Management of nutritional risk factors during pregnancy involves all members of the perinatal team. Specific concerns include problems of overweight, underweight, low birth weight, and adolescent pregnancy. The nutritional health of the mother is an important factor in preventing low-birth-weight infants. Studies have shown the desirable effects of food supplementation during pregnancy on neonatal health. Referral of the pregnant client to WIC, EFNEP, the Food Stamp Program, or other such programs can improve both maternal and fetal outcome.

REVIEW QUESTIONS

1. Describe the recommended pattern of weight gain during pregnancy.
2. Discuss how a nonpregnant diet should be modified to meet the nutritional requirements of normal pregnancy.
3. Describe the components of a nutrition history.
4. Discuss ways in which cultural beliefs affect nutrition during pregnancy.
5. Discuss the effects of an expectant mother's preconceptional body weight has on pregnancy outcome.

REFERENCES

1. National Academy of Sciences Institute of Medicine, Subcommittee on Nutritional Status Weight Gain During Pregnancy. Nutrition During Pregnancy. Washington. D.C; National Academy Press; 1990.
2. Lechtig A, et al. Effect of moderate maternal malnutrition upon the placenta. *Am J Obstet Gynecol.* 1975;123:191–201.
3. Tontisirin D, et al. Formulation and evaluation of supplementary foods for Thai pregnant women. *Am J Clin Nutr.* 1986; 43:931–939.
4. Metzger B, et al. Accelerated starvation and the skipped breakfast in late normal pregnancy. *Lancet.* 1982;1:588–592.
5. Krause M, Mahan L. *Food, Nutrition and Diet Therapy.* 7th ed. Philadelphia: WB Saunders: 1984;246.
6. Wheatley D. Treatment of pregnancy sickness. *Br J Obstet Gynecol.* 1977;84:444–447.

7. Dawson E, McGanity W. Protection of maternal iron stores in pregnancy. *J Reprod Med.* 1987;32(suppl):478–487.
8. Wallenburg H, van Eijk H. Effect of oral iron supplementation during pregnancy on maternal and fetal iron status. *J Perinatol Med.* 1984;12:7–12.
9. Leviton A. Caffeine consumption and the risk of reproductive hazards. *J Reprod Med.* 1988;33:175–178.
10. Linn S, et al. No association between coffee consumption and adverse outcomes of pregnancy. *N Engl J Med.* 1982; 306:141–145.
11. Bracken M, Bryce-Bukchanan C, Silten R, et al. Coffee consumption during pregnancy. *N Engl J Med.* 1982;306:1548.
12. Martin T, Bracken M. Association of low birth weight with passive smoke exposure in pregnancy. *Am J Epidemiol.* 1986;124:633–642.
13. London R. Saccharin and aspartame: are they safe to consume during pregnancy? *J Reprod Health.* 1988;33:17–21.
14. American Medical Association, Council on Scientific Affairs. Saccharin: Review of safety issues. *JAMA.* 1985;254: 2622–2624.
15. Stegink L. Aspartame metabolism in humans: acute dosing studies. In: *Aspartame Physiology and Biochemistry.* New York: Marcel Dekker; 1984:509–553.
16. Kaufman-Kurzock DL. Cultural aspects of nutrition. *Topics in Clinical Nutrition.* 1989;4:1–6.
17. Gulick E, et al. Food beliefs and food behaviors among minority women. *J Perinatol.* 1987;6:197–202.
18. Harwood A. The hot-cold theory of disease. *JAMA.* 1971; 216:1153–1158.
19. Ludman E, Newman J. Yin and yang in the health related food practices of three Chinese groups. *J Nutr Educ.* 1984; 16:3–5.
20. Mansfield PK. Teenage and midlife childbearing update: implications for health educators. *Health Educ.* 1987;18:18–23.
21. Worthington RB, et al. *Nutrition in Pregnancy and Lactation.* St. Louis: Times Mirror/Mosby; 1989.
22. Dostalova L. Vitamin status during puerperium and lactation. *Ann Nutr Metab.* 1984;28:385–408.
23. Phillips C, Johnson N. The impact of diet and other factors on birth weight of infants. *Am J Clin Nutr.* 1977;30:214–225.
24. Naeye R. Weight gain and the outcome of pregnancy. *Am J Obstet Gynecol.* 1979;135:3–9.
25. Edwards L, et al. Pregnancy in the underweight woman: course, outcome, and growth patterns of the infant. *Am J Obstet Gynecol.* 1979;135:297–302.
26. Bowles BC, Williamson BP. Pregnancy and lactation following anorexia and bulimia. *J Obstet Gynecol Neonatal Nurs.* 1990;19:243–248.
27. Abrams B, et al. Maternal weight gain and preterm delivery. *Obstet Gynecol.* 1989;74:577–583.
28. American Dietetic Association. Position of the American Dietetic: nutrition management of adolescent pregnancy. *Journal of the Am Diet Assoc.* 1989;89:104–109.
29. Brennan R. Nutrient intake of low-income pregnant women: laboratory analysis of foods consumed. *Am Diet Assoc.* 1983;83:546–550.
30. Snowman M. Nutrition component in a comprehensive child development program, II: Nutrient intake of low-income pregnant women and the outcome of pregnancy. *J Am Diet Assoc.* 1979;74:124–129.
31. Endes J, et al. Dietary assessment of pregnant women in a supplemental food program. *J Am Diet Assoc.* 1981;79: 121–126.

Growth and Development of the Embryo/Fetus

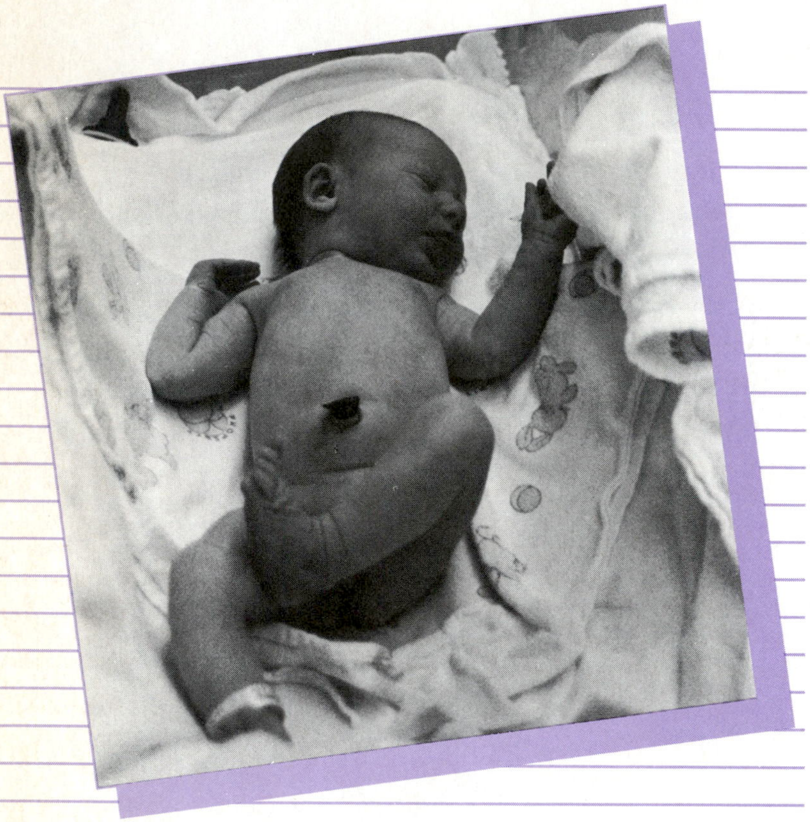

Chapter 11

Key Terms

acrosome reaction
amnion
blastocyst
brown fat
capacitation
chorion
chorionic villi
cleavage
conception
decidua
decidua basalis
decidua capsularis
decidua vera
dizygotic twins
embryonic disc
embryonic period
fertilization
fetal alcohol syndrome
fetal period
implantation
lanugo
mesoderm
monozygotic twins
morula
organogenesis
placental membrane
pre-embryonic period
primitive streak
quickening
surfactant
syncytial membrane
trophoblast
vernix caseosa
Wharton's jelly
yolk sac
zygote

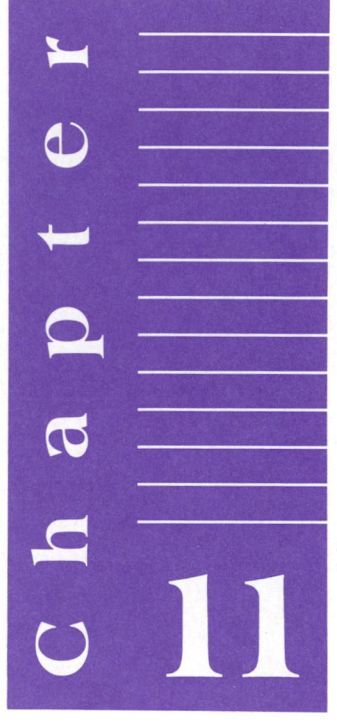

Over the centuries many theories have been put forth to explain fertilization and reproduction. These include the familiar "old wives' tales," which attempted to tell us where babies came from and how they were delivered. Some of these tales had their origins in folk medicine, prior to the advent of scientific research into reproduction. In modern times, talented researchers have labored diligently to define the molecular events essential to successful reproduction.[1] Their research has resulted in improved pregnancy outcomes, genetic advances, advances in the treatment of infertility, and development of safe and effective birth control methods. Despite the breakthroughs in research contributing to the knowledge of reproductive mechanisms, fertilization and reproduction remains a wondrous process through which a single human egg develops into a 7½-pound infant.

During the first month of pregnancy, often before a woman knows that she is pregnant, the embryo increases about 40-fold in size, and almost 3000-fold in weight. A single cell grows into an embryo with a head, a trunk, the rudiments of organs, in close association with the body of the mother. Blood cells begin to form at 17 days, and the heart as early as 18 days, after fertilization.[2] The heart will go on to beat more than 100,000 times each day for the individual's lifetime, which may be 90 to 100 years.

The nurse's role during development of the embryo and fetus is one of advocate and counselor. Early in the pregnancy, the mother may not know what to expect; indeed, she may be unaware that she is pregnant and thus unlikely to seek health care. Anticipatory guidance for this period should be provided to women of childbearing age at their regular checkups, in school health classes, in community groups, and through educational materials that are readily available to women of all economic and social groups. This anticipatory guidance should include planning for pregnancy, genetic counseling (if indicated), nutritional counseling, general health counseling, and teaching and counseling regarding embryonic and fetal development. As an advocate, the nurse assists the client in negotiating the health care system during pregnancy, plans for delivery and ongoing care for the mother and her family, coordinates interagency activities, and prepares the family for the new member. The importance of the nurse's role during this period cannot be overemphasized. This role will be discussed throughout this chapter and the remaining text.

DEVELOPMENT

Conception

The time span during which **conception,** or **fertilization,** can take place is quite limited in the usual 28-day menstrual cycle. The oocyte, or ovum, is thought to survive only 12 to 24 hours after ovulation. It is now believed that sperm may remain alive in the female reproductive tract up to 72 hours.[3]

Fertilization usually occurs in the wide lateral portion, or ampulla, of the fallopian tube. Contractility of the fallopian tube is increased as a result of high estrogen levels at the time of ovulation. This heightened contractility serves to propel the ovum through the fallopian tube. The high estrogen levels also cause an increase in the amount of cervical mucus, which is less viscous and more easily penetrated by spermatozoa. Spermatozoa move through the cervix, the body of the uterus, and into the fallopian tubes by using their flagella (tails) and through uterine contractions. The total critical time span during which fertilization may occur is 24 to 48 hours. This includes the 12 to 24 hours preceding ovulation and the 12 to 24 hours following ovulation; fertilization usually occurs within 24 hours after ovulation. Spermatozoa must remain in the female genital tract 4 to 6 hours before they are capable of fertilizing the ovum.

The mature ovum is surrounded by two plasma membranes, the zona pellucida and the corona radiata. The zona pellucida is the clear, gelatinous, noncellular layer closest to the cell membrane; its function is not known. The corona radiata is a ring of elongated cells that radiate from the ovum like the gaseous corona around the sun. These layers are held together by hyaluronic acid; they are the two layers the sperm must penetrate to achieve fertilization.

The mature sperm consists of a head and a tail, the head forming most of the bulk of the sperm. The anterior two thirds of the nucleus in the head of the sperm is covered by the acrosome, which contains enzymes that are believed to facilitate sperm penetration through the corona radiata and zona pellucida of the ovum.[4]

Before a mature sperm can penetrate the corona radiata and zona pellucida, it must undergo **capacitation.** Capacitation is an enzymatic process that results in the removal of plasma protein over the acrosome. After capacitation, the acrosome of the sperm undergoes a sequence of events termed the **acrosome reaction.** During this reaction, the acrosome undergoes structural changes; the outer membrane fuses with the overlying cell membrane of the sperm head, and the fused membranes rupture, producing multiple perforations.[4] During the acrosome reaction, the enzymes hyaluronidase and proteinase are secreted by the acrosome. They are released through the perforations in the acrosome of the sperm, and help to dissolve the membranes of the ovum. Progesterone, secreted by the ovum, also seems to stimulate the acrosomal process in the sperm (Figure 11–1).

Fertilization

As the spermatozoa surround the ovum they deposit minute amounts of hyaluronidase, which break down enough hyaluronic acid in the outer layer to allow one sperm to penetrate the ovum. The head and neck of the sperm enter the ovum and the two plasma membranes fuse.[3] Once the sperm has entered the ovum, the egg responds in three ways: (1) cortical and zona reactions, (2) resumption of the second meiotic division, and (3) metabolic activation.

Cortical and Zona Reactions. The ovum membrane becomes impenetrable to other spermatozoa and the zona pellucida alters its structure and composition, thus preventing more than one sperm from penetrating the ovum.

Resumption of the Second Meiotic Division. The second maturational division occurs, resulting in a second polar body which, along with the first polar body from the first maturational division, is discarded (*see* Chapter 6). The ovum is now mature and the remaining nucleus is called the female pronucleus. The female pronucleus contains 22 autosomes and an X sex chromosome. The sperm head enlarges, forming the male pronucleus, which contains 22 autosomes and an X or Y sex chromosome. The tail of the sperm is detached from the head and degenerates. The male pronucleus now lies in close proximity to the female pronucleus. The male and female pronuclei lose their nuclear membranes, fuse, and randomly intermingle their chromosomes, forming a one-celled animal, the **zygote.** The zygote has 46 chromosomes (23 pairs): 22 autosomes from the mother, 22 autosomes from the father, and a pair of sex chromosomes, one from each parent.

Metabolic Activation of the Egg. Postfusion activation occurs, encompassing the initial cellular and molecular events associated with early embryogenesis.[3] Fertilization is dependent on three factors: (1) maturation of the ovum and sperm, (2) motility of the sperm or ability of the sperm to reach the ovum, and (3) ability of the sperm to penetrate the zona pellucida and cell membrane to achieve active fertilization. The product of fertilization, called the zygote, contains a new combination of genetic material that will

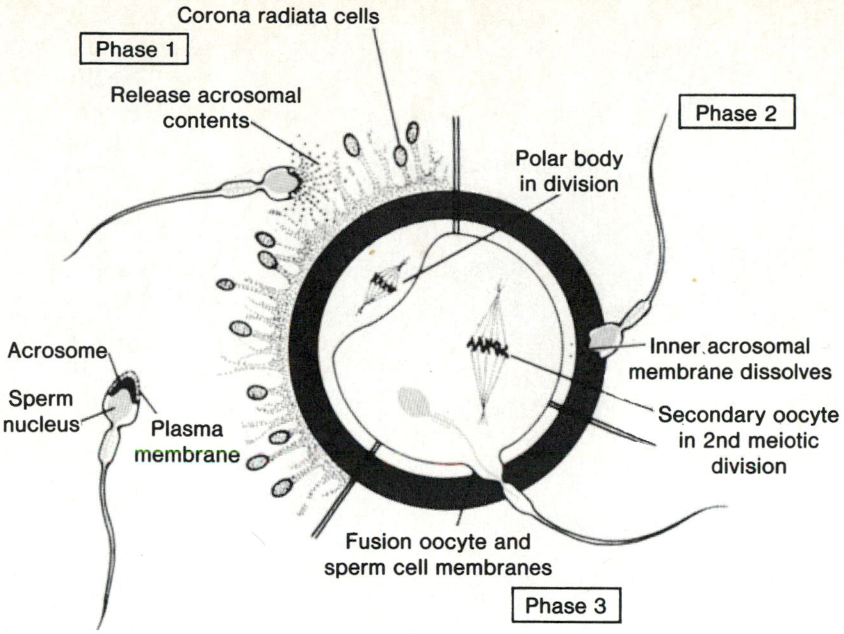

Figure 11–1. Acrosome reaction and sperm penetration of an oocyte. (*Reproduced, with permission, from Sadler TW.* Langman's Medical Embryology. *5th ed. Baltimore: Williams & Wilkins; 1985:25.*)

develop into a new individual, different from anyone else in the world. The zygote will form the embryo and fetus as well as the structures needed to support the fetus during intrauterine life, such as the placenta, the fetal membranes, the amniotic fluid, and the umbilical cord.

Pre-embryonic Period

The first 14 days of development, referred to as the **pre-embryonic period,** is characterized by rapid cellular multiplication and differentiation, establishment of embryonic membranes, and development of the primary germ layers. At the same time these changes are occurring, the placenta is developing.

Days 1 to 3: Cleavage. Immediately after fertilization, rapid cell division of the zygote begins as the fertilized ovum is transported through the fallopian tube. This early cell division is called **cleavage.** The first cleavage is completed in about 36 hours, each successive division taking slightly less time. Although the number of cells in the zygote increases, the size of the developing organism does not increase at this time.[5] The process of cleavage, which occurs in the fallopian tube and takes about 3 days, creates smaller cells with each division (Figure 11–2). These smaller cells are known as blastomeres.[1,3]

By the third day, a mulberry-like mass of cells (12–16 blastomeres) known as the **morula** has formed. The morula is thought to reach the uterine cavity at about the 12- to 16-cell stage, approximately 60 hours after fertilization.

When the morula enters the uterus, it is filled with fluid, pushing the blastomeres out to the periphery in two layers: the outer layer of cells forms the **trophoblast,** and the inner layer of cells differentiates into the embryo. The morula, now known as the **blastocyst,** contains fluid-filled spaces and two layers of cells (Figure 11–2).

Days 4 to 6. By the fourth day, the fluid-filled spaces in the blastocyst form one large central space, called the blastocyst cavity. The two layers of cells in the blastocyst are called the embryoblast (inner layer) and the trophoblast (outer layer). By day 6 the cells of the inner cell mass, or embryoblast, are located at one pole of the blastocyst. These cells will eventually form the embryo and amnion. The cells of the outer cell mass, or trophoblast, flatten and form the epithelial wall of the blastocyst, which eventually develops into the chorion[3,6] (Figures 11–2 and 11–3).

Days 7 to 9: Implantation. Implantation occurs 7 to 9 days after fertilization, when the blastocyst attaches itself to the endometrium. Prior to implantation, while the blastocyst is floating freely in the uterine cavity, the fertilized ovum receives its nutrition from the uterine glands, which secrete a mixture of mucopolysaccharides, lipids,and glycogen. Implantation must occur for nourishment to continue.

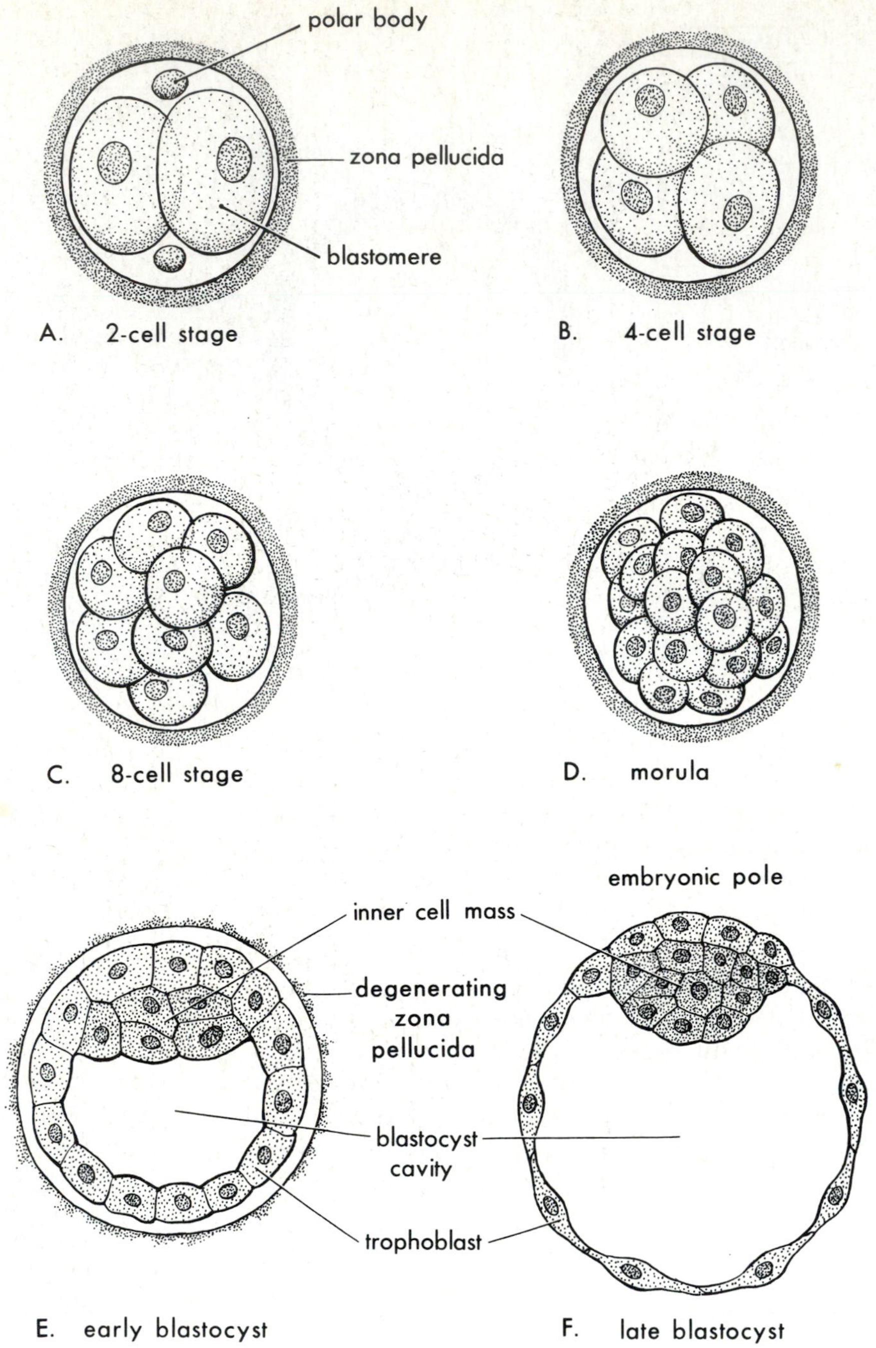

Figure 11–2. Cleavage of the zygote and formation of the blastocyst. (*Reproduced, with permission, from Moore KL.* Before We Are Born. *3rd ed. Philadelphia: WB Saunders; 1989:29.*)

At the time of implantation, the mucosa of the uterus is in the secretory (progestational) phase of the menstrual cycle. The arteries that supply the layers of the uterus become tortuous, forming a dense capillary bed just beneath the uterine epithelium. The endometrium becomes highly edematous and the uterine mucosa prepares to receive the blastocyst. Implantation occurs often along either the posterior or anterior walls of the body of the uterus. The trophoblastic layer of cells in the blastocyst contacts the endometrium. When this occurs, the trophoblast differentiates into two layers: the cytotrophoblast, which is composed of cells, and the syncytiotrophoblast, a protoplasmic mass.[4]

Spaces called lacunae appear in the syncytiotrophoblast; these are filled with blood from the ruptured maternal capillaries in the endometrium. The syncytiotrophoblastic lacunae fuse and form lacunar networks; maternal blood flows slowly through these networks and a primitive uteroplacental circulation is established. Oxygenated blood passes into the lacunae from spiral arteries, and deoxygenated blood is removed from them by way of the veins of the uterus.[4]

The blastocyst, now about 1/100th of an inch in diameter, becomes oriented so that the embryonic mass of cells is directed toward the endometrium, which is now known as the **decidua.** (*See* "Second Week: Preplacental Phase.") The decidua basalis, which contains a large number of blood vessels, is that portion of the decidua beneath the implanted blastocyst and from which the maternal portion of the placenta develops. Implantation enables the blastocyst to absorb nutrients from the glands and blood vessels of the endometrium (decidua) for its subsequent growth and development[3,6] (Figure 11–3).

Second Week: Preplacental Phase

Decidua. The endometrium undergoes changes in response to the action of progesterone to prepare for implantation and nutrition of the fertilized ovum. After implantation, the decidua undergoes several rapid changes. The portion of the decidua directly beneath the site of implantation forms the **decidua basalis.** The portion that overlies the developing ovum and separates it from the rest of the uterine cavity is the **decidua capsularis.** The remaining area of the uterus is lined by the **decidua vera.**[3]

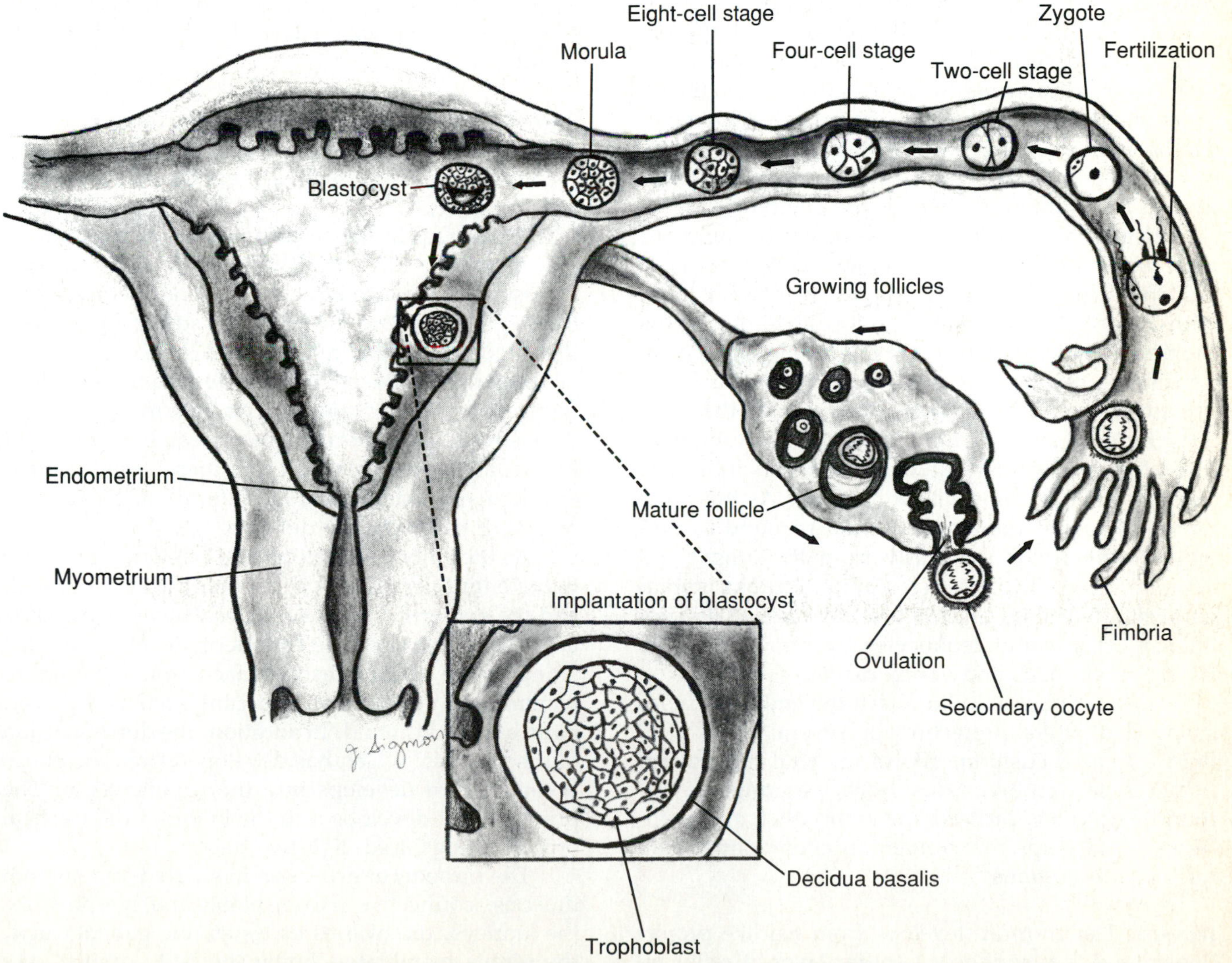

Figure 11–3. Sequence of implantation of the blastocyst.

Embryonic Layer of Cells. Implantation of the blastocyst in the decidua of the uterus is completed by the second week of development. Simultaneously, the embryonic layer of cells becomes the **embryonic disc,** which forms two basic layers: the ectoderm and the endoderm. The ectoderm gives rise to the amnion, and the endoderm to the primitive yolk sac.

Yolk Sac. The **yolk sac** arises from the endoderm of the embryonic disc. Unlike yolks of other eggs, it does not provide direct nutrition for the developing embryo/fetus; however, it does have several important functions.[4] Two are its role in the transfer of nutrients to the embryo while the uteroplacental circulation is being established, and its role in providing blood cells until embryonic/fetal hemopoiesis begins. In addition, cells of the yolk sac become incorporated into embryonic/fetal organs.

Amnion and Amniotic Cavity. As the decidua is differentiating, a fluid-filled space develops around the embryo. This space is lined with a smooth, glistening membrane, the **amnion,** which originates from the ectoderm in the early stages of embryonic development. As the amnion enlarges, the growing embryo gradually extends into the fluid-filled space, the amniotic cavity. The amnion expands as the embryo grows.

Although it is not known exactly how amniotic fluid forms, the volume of fluid increases to between 500 and 1000 mL of clear, slightly yellowish fluid, with a nonfoul characteristic odor, at term. During the first half of pregnancy, the fluid is similar in composition to maternal plasma, except it has a lower protein concentration. Later in pregnancy the fetus contributes to amniotic fluid through urine excretion. The fetus also absorbs amniotic fluid through the gastrointestinal tract by swallowing fluid. As the pregnancy advances, the amniotic fluid is found to contain phospholipids (primarily from the lungs) and albumin, urea, uric acid, creatinine, lecithin, sphingomyelin, bilirubin, fat, fructose, inorganic salts, epithelial cells, some leukocytes, various enzymes, lanugo, scalp hair, and vernix caseosa.

The amniotic cavity in which the embryo/fetus is suspended offers protection in several ways. The fluid acts as a cushion, allows for fetal movement, prevents the embryo/fetus from adhering to surrounding tissues, protects the embryo/fetus from infection, and helps to maintain an even temperature for the embryo/fetus.[6]

Chorion. The chorion develops from hairlike projections along the trophoblast (outer layer of cells) referred to as **chorionic villi.** The villi closest to the uterine wall (chorion frondosum) will form the fetal portion of the placenta. The villi farthest from the uterine wall degenerate into a smooth membrane, the **chorion** (chorion laeve). The inner portion of the chorion adheres to the amnion and surrounds the developing fetus and amniotic fluid. The outer portion of the chorion lies against the decidua vera.

Umbilical Cord. The early embryo is connected to the yolk sac by a connecting or body stalk containing two arteries and one vein. During the rapid development of the embryo, the amniotic cavity enlarges and the amnion begins to envelop the connecting (body) stalk and yolk sac, crowding them together. After the third month, when the amnion has come in contact with the chorion and has obliterated the chorionic cavity, the yolk sac shrinks and is gradually eliminated. The connecting or body stalk then elongates to become the umbilical cord. The vessels in the cord are surrounded by a connective tissue known as **Wharton's jelly.** This tissue is rich in mucopolysaccharides and functions as a protective layer for the blood vessels[3] (Figure 11–4).

Germ Layers. After implantation, the inner cell mass of the blastocyst begins to differentiate in stages into the three primary germ layers: ectoderm, endoderm, and mesoderm.

At the end of the second week of development, the embryonic disc is bilaminar (two germ layers), consisting of the ectoderm and the endoderm. At this time a groove, called the **primitive streak,** appears on the ectoderm. A new cell layer is visible on each side of the streak between the ectoderm and the endoderm. The cells migrate into the bottom of the primitive streak, and form an intermediate germ layer known as the **mesoderm.** From these germ layers—ectoderm, endoderm, and mesoderm—all tissues and organs of the body will develop.

As the embryo develops, the ectoderm gives rise to the entire nervous system, central and peripheral, and the epidermis, with such derivatives as the crystalline lens and hair. The endoderm develops into the lining of the gastrointestinal tract, from pharynx to rectum, and into derivative organs such as the liver, pancreas, and thyroid. In addition, the dorsal portion of the yolk sac, which has developed from the endoderm, in turn develops into the primitive gut. The primitive gut develops into the lining of the trachea, bronchi, lungs, and digestive tract.

The mesoderm gives rise to striated and smooth muscles, connective tissue, blood and lymph cells, the kidneys, the ovaries or testes, the genital ducts, the serous membranes lining the body cavities, the cortex of the adrenal glands, the heart, and the middle ear. The cavity that later divides the somatic and

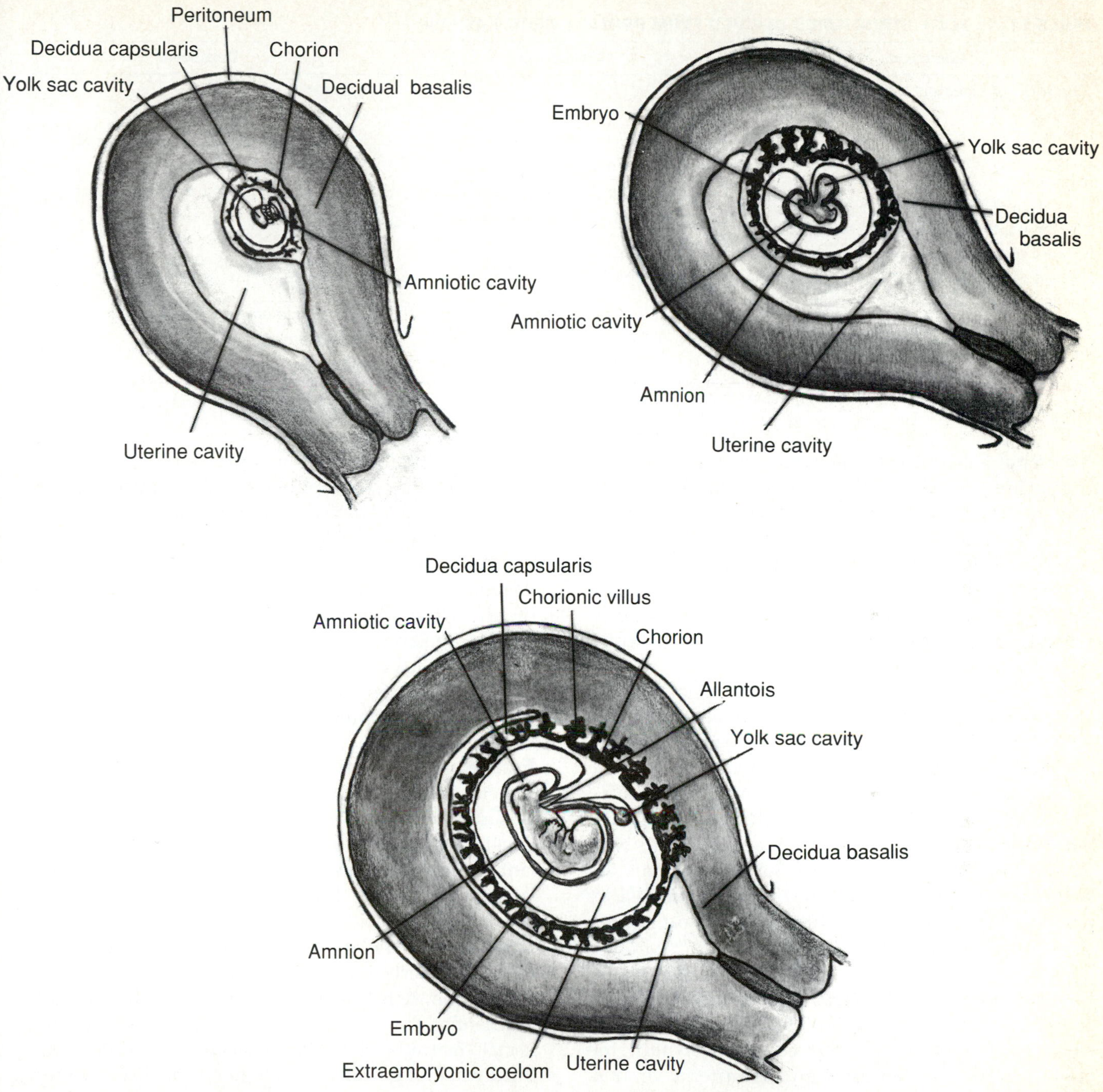

Figure 11–4. Sequence of development of the embryo, fetal membranes, and yolk sac.

visceral sheets of intraembryonic mesoderm is called the coelom[2, 5] (Table 11–1).

Placental Development

The placenta tends to form and to delimit itself in the area of the decidua (decidua basalis), where blood supply is richest. By the fourth month, the placenta has developed two compartments, the fetal portion formed by the chorion frondosum and the maternal portion formed by the decidua basalis. The fetal portion of the placenta is anchored to the maternal portion of the placenta by villi.

As the chorionic villi invade the decidua basalis, a number of wedge-shaped areas are formed; these are known as the placental septa. It is now thought that the placental septa are made up of fetal and maternal tissue.[1] The septa divide the fetal part of the placenta into a number of irregular compartments called cotyledons, consisting of main-stem villi and many branches.[3, 4, 7]

TABLE 11–1. BODY STRUCTURES DERIVED FROM PRIMARY GERM LAYERS

Endoderm	Mesoderm	Ectoderm
Epithelium of digestive tract and its glands	Dermis	Epidermis
Epithelium of respiratory tract	Skeleton	All nervous tissue
Epithelium of urinary bladder, gallbladder, and liver	Smooth and cardiac muscles	Hair follicles, nails, and sweat glands
Epithelium of pharynx, auditory tube, tonsils, larynx, trachea, bronchi, and lungs	Connective tissue (cartilage, bone)	Sebaceous glands
Primary tissue of liver and pancreas	Blood, bone marrow, and lymphoid tissue	Lens, cornea, optic nerve, and internal eye muscles
Epithelium of urethra and associated glands, vagina and associated parts	Endothelium of blood vessels and lymphatics	Internal and external ear
	Fibrous tunic and vascular tunic of eye	Neuroepithelium of sense organs
	Middle ear	Nasal cavity
	Epithelium of kidneys, ureters, adrenal cortex, gonads, and genital ducts	Oral glands and tooth enamel
		Pituitary gland
		Mammary glands

Maternal Placental Structure. During erosion of the decidua basalis by the chorionic villi, blood-filled spaces form and enlarge. These spaces, originally called lacunae, form a large blood sinus, which is bordered by the chorionic plate on one side and the decidua basalis on the other. The placental septa subdivide the blood sinus into many separate but connecting compartments. Each compartment, in turn, has an intervillous space.

Maternal blood enters the intervillous space through 80 to 100 spiral arteries (endometrial arteries) and is temporarily outside of the maternal circulatory system. The oxygenated blood is propelled toward the chorionic plate (fetal side of the intervillous space). The blood slowly circulates around the surface of the villi, allowing exchange of oxygen and nutrients with the fetal blood. The welfare of the embryo/fetus depends on adequate bathing of the chorionic villi by maternal blood; this is considered the most significant factor for embryo/fetal well-being.[3,4,6,8]

Fetal Placental Structure. The chorionic villi are anchored to the chorionic plate of the trophoblast (fetal portion of placental circulation). Within the chorionic villi of the embryo/fetus are arterial-venous-capillary networks. The arteries, which are the terminal end of the umbilical arteries, allow deoxygenated blood from the fetus to diffuse into the maternal blood in the intervillous spaces. In addition, oxygen and nutrients from the maternal blood diffuse into the thin-walled fetal veins that eventually converge to form the umbilical vein. The umbilical vein carries oxygenated blood to the fetus[3,6,8] (Figure 11–5).

Placental Membrane. Normally, fetal and maternal blood do not mingle because of the **placental membrane.** This membrane arises solely from fetal tissues composing the chorionic villi. Up to the 20th week of pregnancy, the placental membrane consists of four layers: (1) syncytiotrophoblast, (2) cytotrophoblast, (3) connective tissue core of the villus, (4) endothelium of the fetal capillary.

As pregnancy progresses, some of these layers degenerate, leaving a thin membrane referred to as the **syncytial membrane.** The fetal circulatory network (capillaries, arteries, and veins) lies in close proximity to the syncytial membrane. This thin, intact membrane separates fetal and maternal blood in the latter part of pregnancy (Figure 11–6).

Embryonic Period

Development of the embryo and fetus follows a cephalocaudal pattern. In other words, the embryo/fetus develops and matures from the head toward the distant extremities. This principle applies to both physical and neurologic development.

Third Week. The **embryonic period** begins the third week after fertilization and continues until approximately the eighth week. During this stage, tissues differentiate into essential organs and the main external features develop. Specifically, during the third week of gestation, the embryonic disc becomes elongated with a broad cephalic and a narrow caudal end.

Fourth Week. By the end of the fourth week, the primitive gut forms and a tubular heart, which develops just outside the body cavity, begins beating, pushing its primitive blood cells through the main blood vessels (Figure 11–7A). By the 19th to 20th days, the chorionic cavity, which has already begun to form, enlarges; the embryo now is attached to its trophoblastic shell by a narrow connecting stalk, which later develops into the umbilical cord.

Somite formation occurs during the fourth week.

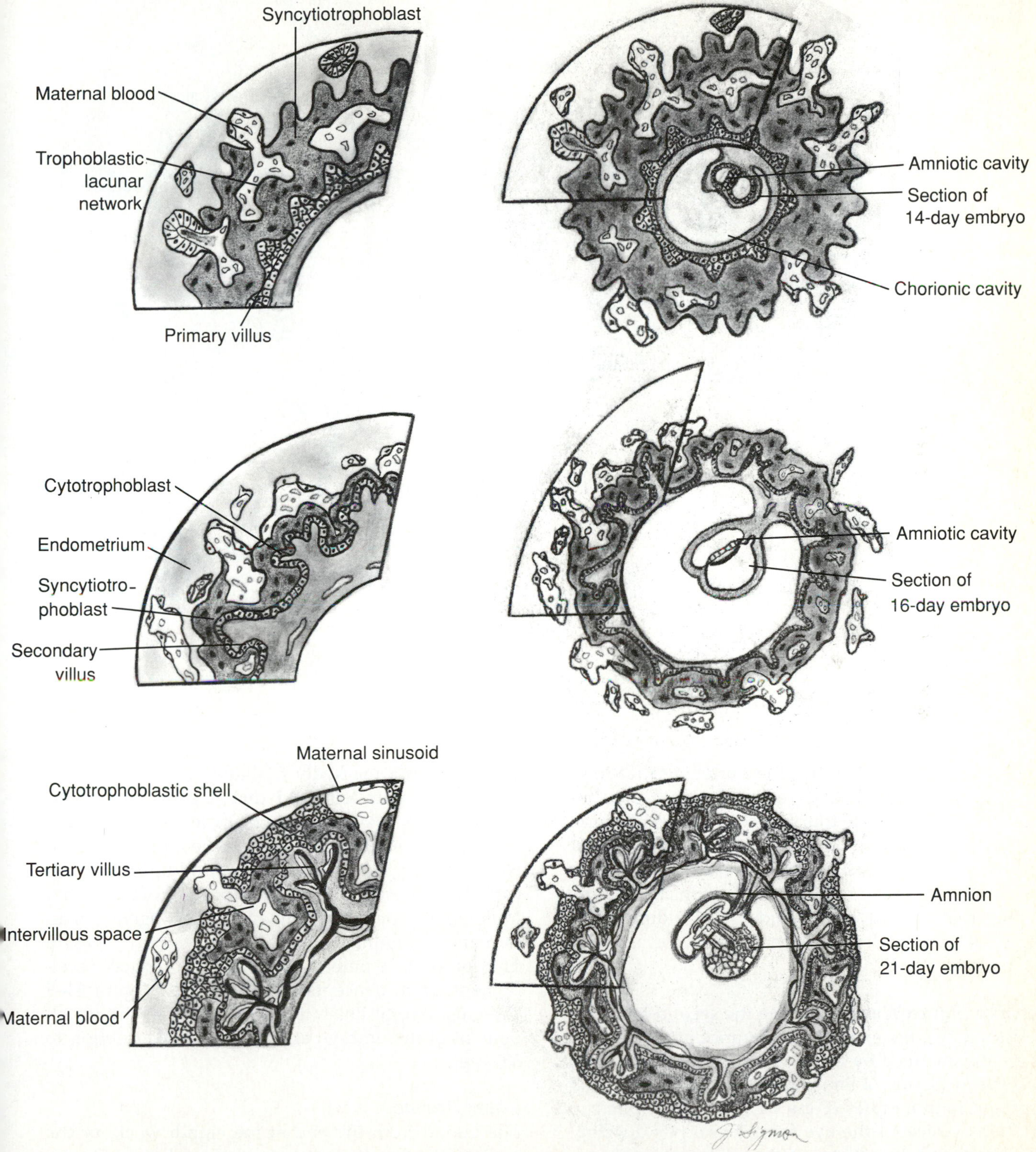

Figure 11–5. Longitudinal section of placental villus, showing three-part development of the amnion and chorion.

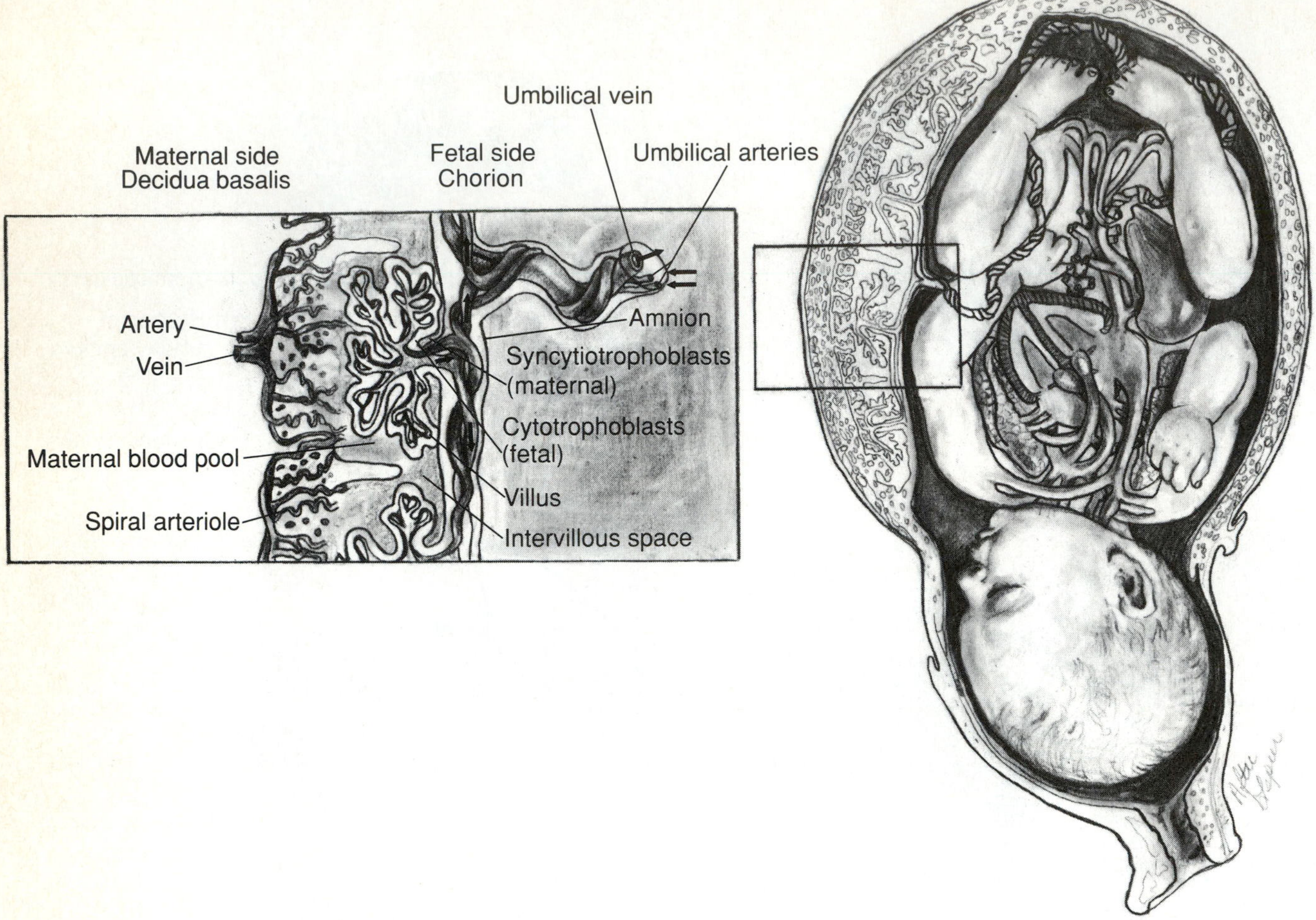

Figure 11–6. Vascular arrangement of the placenta.

These somites develop into the vertebrae that form the spinal column. Pharyngeal arches and pouches also appear during the fourth week. The arches form the lower jaw, the hyoid bone, and the cartilage for the larynx. The pouches form the eustachian tube and the cavity of the middle ear, the tonsils, and the parathyroid and thymus glands. The rudiments of the eyes, ears, and nose appear, as do the arm and leg buds.

Fifth to Eighth Weeks. During the second month of development, the external appearance of the embryo is greatly changed by the enormous size of the head and the formation of limbs, face, ear, nose, eyes, and arm and limb paddles (Figure 11–7B). The optic cup and lens vesicle of the eye form, nasal pits develop, the heart and circulatory system become more advanced, and the brain differentiates into five areas with ten pairs of cranial nerves. The embryo progresses from a markedly C-shaped body to a structure with a rounded head that is nearly erect and measures approximately 3 cm in length. All major organ systems are formed during the fourth to eighth weeks, hence this is called the period of **organogenesis.** The embryo is most susceptible to factors that interfere with development, and most congenital malformations originate, during this period.[3,6] Figure 11–8 presents a timetable of human prenatal development, from conception to 10 weeks. Figure 11–9 presents several illustrations of stages in the development of the embryo and fetus from conception to 38 weeks..

Fetal Period

The period from the end of the eighth week, or the start of the third month, to birth is known as the **fetal period.** This period is characterized by maturation of the tissues and organs and rapid growth of

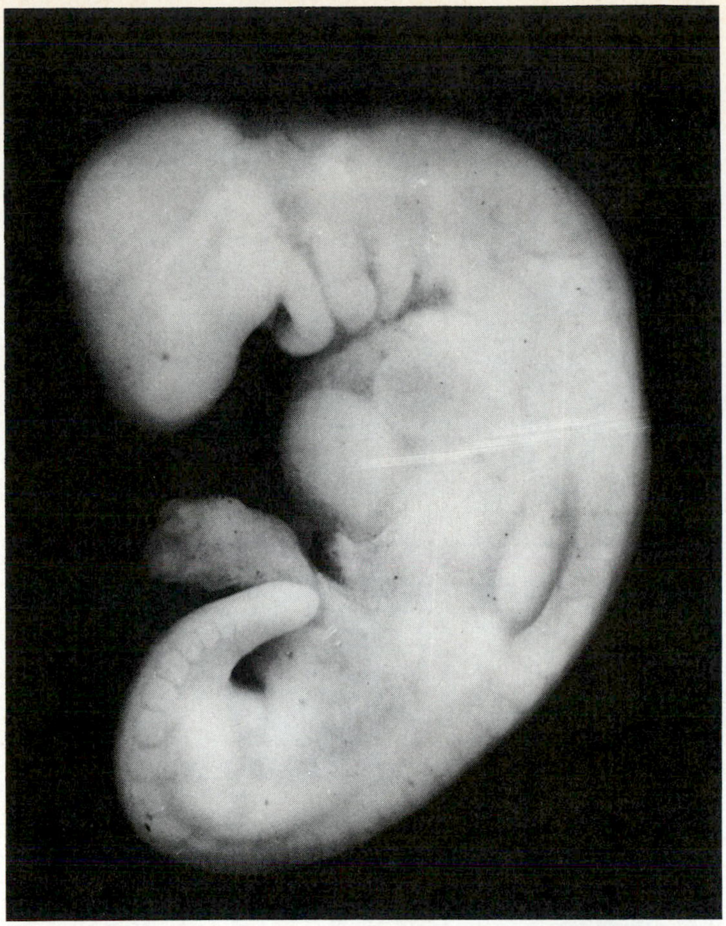

A

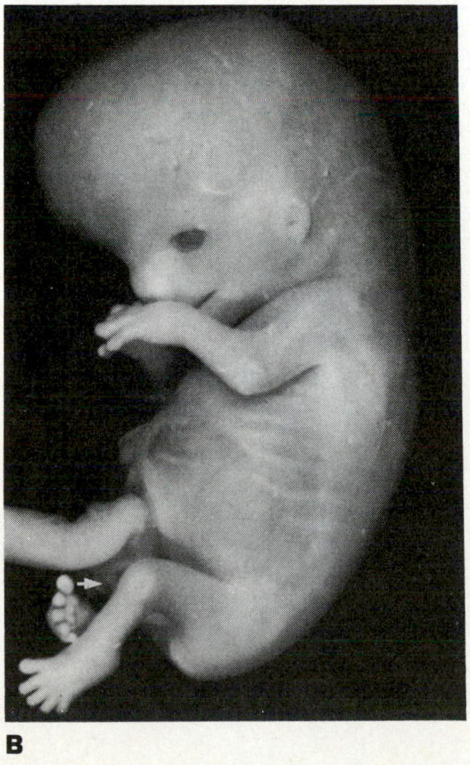

B

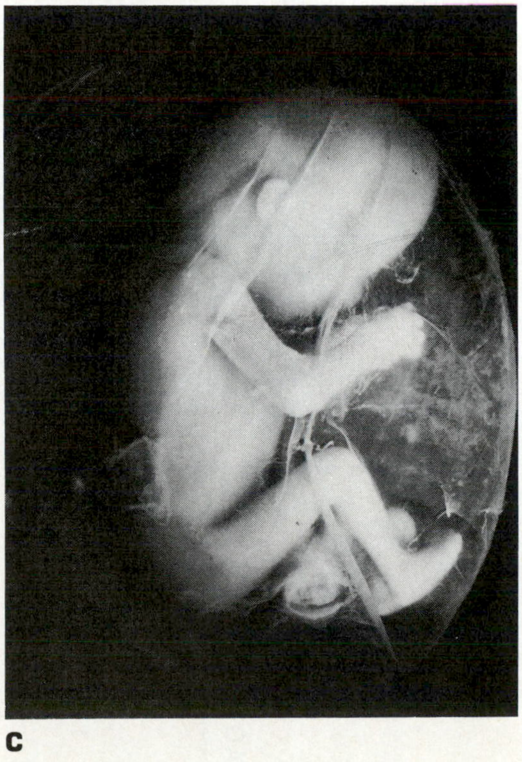

C

Figure 11–7. Development of the human fetus. **A.** 28 days. **B.** 8 weeks. **C.** 12 weeks. (*Reproduced, with permission, from Moore KL.* Before We Are Born. *3rd ed. Philadelphia: WB Saunders; 1989:65,69,100.*)

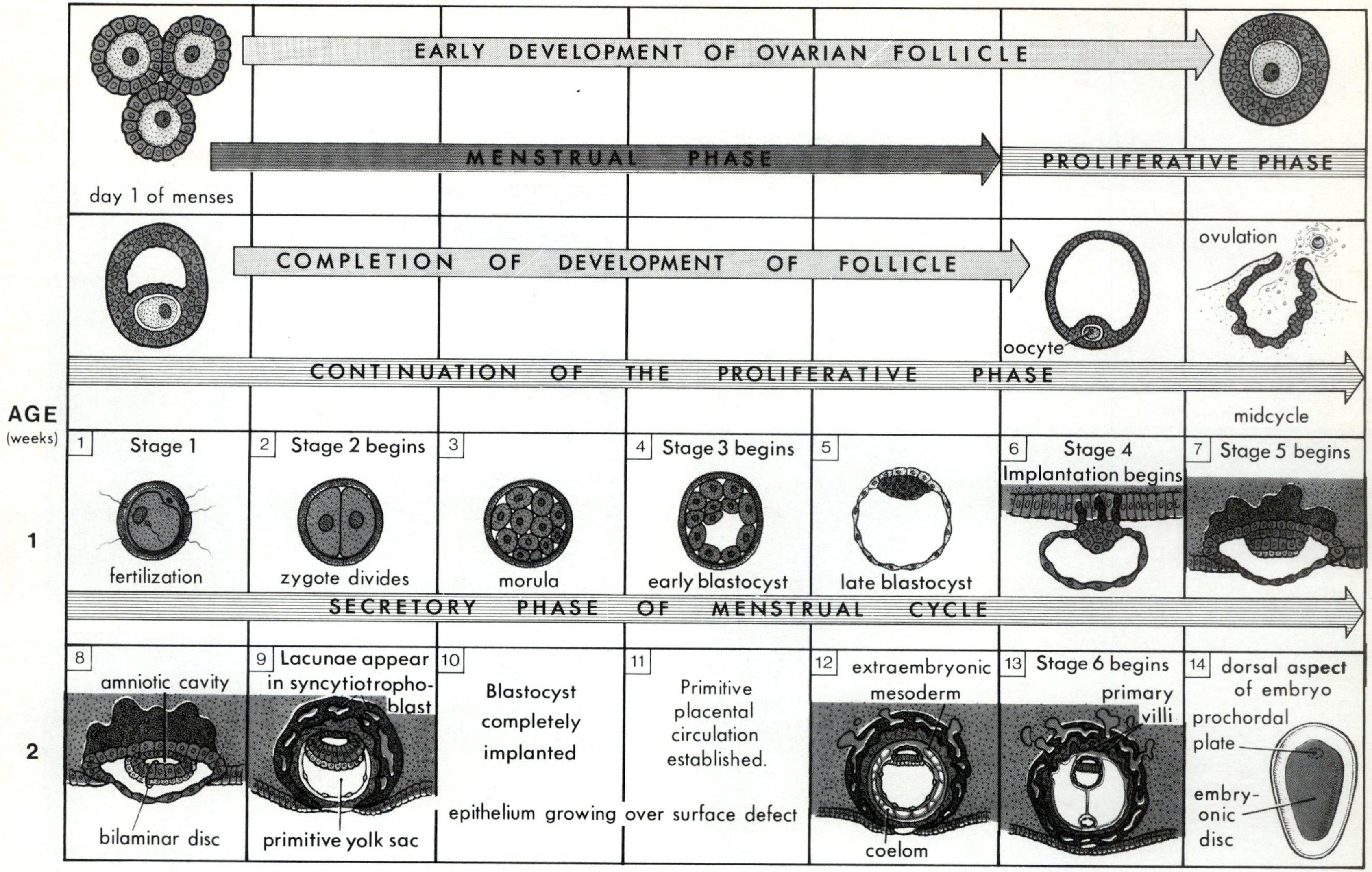

Figure 11–8. Human prenatal development, from conception to 10 weeks. (*Figure continues.*) (*Reproduced, with permission, from Moore KL.* The Developing Human. *3rd ed. Philadelphia: WB Saunders; 1989:2–4.*)

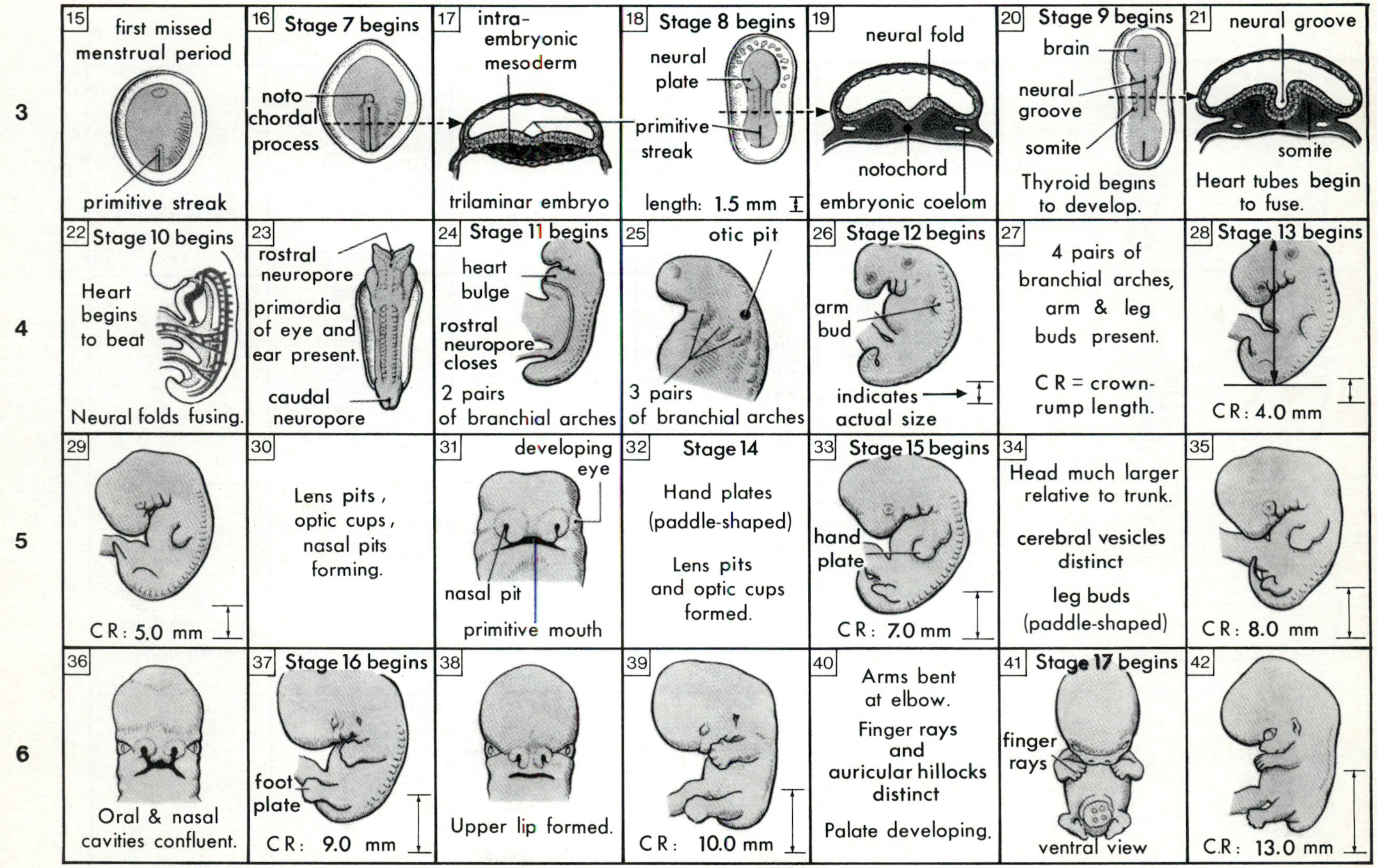

Figure 11–8. (*Continued.*)

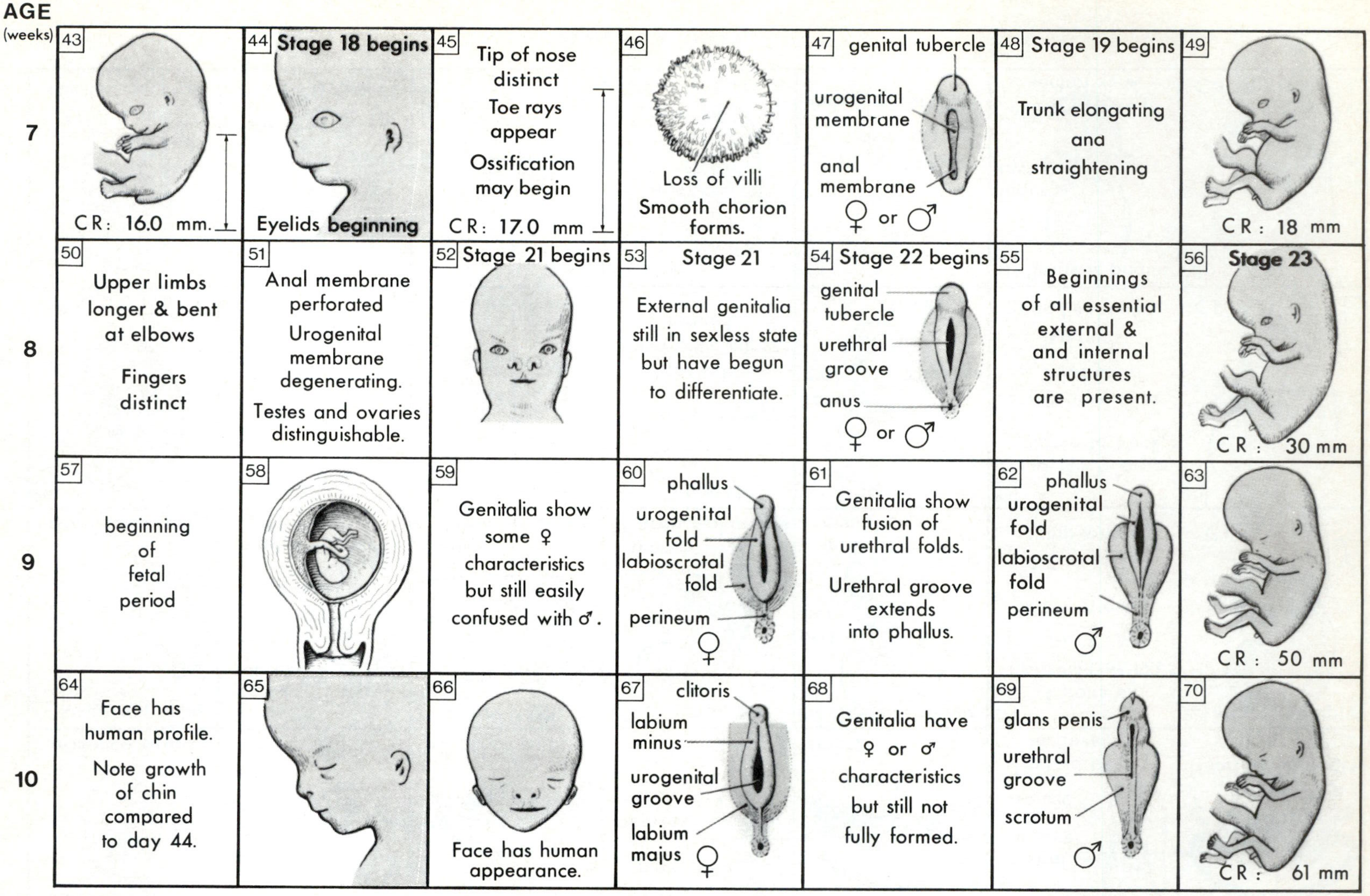

AGE
(weeks)
7
8
9
10
43
CR: 16.0 mm.
44
Stage 18 begins
Eyelids beginning
45
Tip of nose distinct
Toe rays appear
Ossification may begin
CR: 17.0 mm
46
Loss of villi
Smooth chorion forms.
47
genital tubercle
urogenital membrane
anal membrane
♀ or ♂
48
Stage 19 begins
Trunk elongating and straightening
49
CR: 18 mm
50
Upper limbs longer & bent at elbows
Fingers distinct
51
Anal membrane perforated
Urogenital membrane degenerating.
Testes and ovaries distinguishable.
52
Stage 21 begins
53
Stage 21
External genitalia still in sexless state but have begun to differentiate.
54
Stage 22 begins
genital tubercle
urethral groove
anus
♀ or ♂
55
Beginnings of all essential external & and internal structures are present.
56
Stage 23
CR: 30 mm
57
beginning of fetal period
58
59
Genitalia show some ♀ characteristics but still easily confused with ♂.
60
phallus
urogenital fold
labioscrotal fold
perineum
♀
61
Genitalia show fusion of urethral folds.
Urethral groove extends into phallus.
62
phallus
urogenital fold
labioscrotal fold
perineum
♂
63
CR: 50 mm
64
Face has human profile.
Note growth of chin compared to day 44.
65
66
Face has human appearance.
67
clitoris
labium minus
urogenital groove
labium majus
♀
68
Genitalia have ♀ or ♂ characteristics but still not fully formed.
69
glans penis
urethral groove
scrotum
♂
70
CR: 61 mm

Figure 11–8. *(Continued.)*

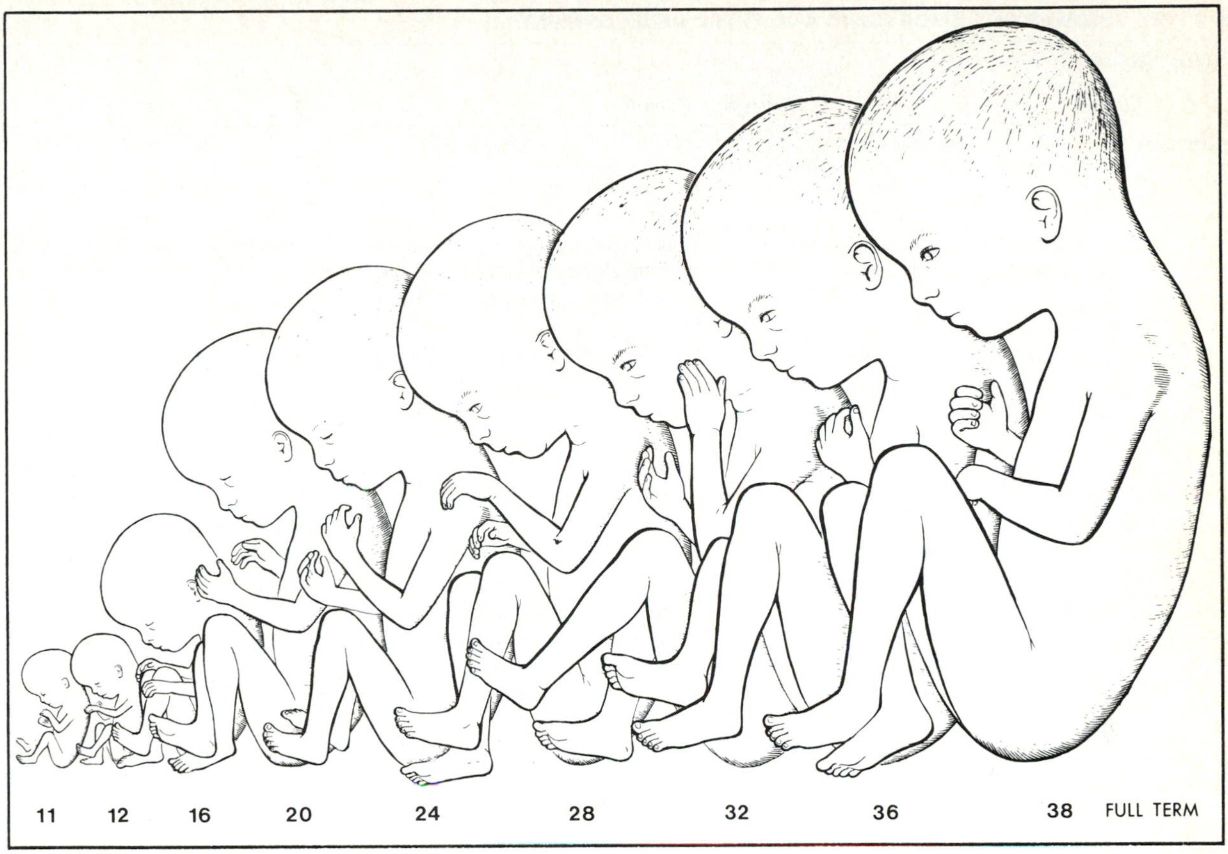

Figure 11–9. Human fetal development, from 11 to 38 weeks. (*Reproduced, with permission, from Moore KL.* The Developing Human. *Philadelphia: WB Saunders; 1989:5.*)

the body. All structures that will be present in the full-term infant are in existence; no new structures will form. Few, if any, malformations arise during this period, although cell death in the central nervous system may be caused by factors toxic to cells and may result in postnatal behavioral disturbances. Growth in length is striking during the third, fourth, and fifth lunar months, whereas increase in weight is most striking during the ninth and tenth lunar months.

In calculating gestational age, most women consider a pregnancy to be 9 months long, starting from their first missed menstrual period. In fact, the average pregnancy is 38 weeks or 266 days in length from the time of conception, or 40 weeks in length or 280 days from the first day of the last menstrual period. When a woman states that she is three months pregnant, she is in fact 12 weeks past her last menstrual period. Thus, most health care providers speak of a pregnancy in terms of lunar or 4-week months. The following discussion uses lunar months and the number of weeks past the last menstrual period to describe the sequence of fetal development.

Third Month (9–12 Weeks). By the end of the 12th week, or third month, the face of the fetus appears more human; the ears come to lie close to their definitive position at the sides of the head; centers of ossification have appeared in most bones; the fingers and toes have differentiated and nail beds form; scattered rudiments of hair appear; and the external genitalia have developed to such a degree that the sex of the fetus can be visually determined. At the end of the third month, reflex activity can be evoked and the fetus is able to make spontaneous movements (Figure 11–7C). By the end of 12 weeks fetal weight is approximately 45 g and crown-rump length is 87 mm.

Fourth Month (13–16 weeks). During the fourth month the fetus achieves a crown-rump length of approximately 120 mm and, at the end of 16 weeks, weighs about 110 g. Fine downy hair called **lanugo** begins to develop, particularly on the head. The muscles and skeleton are able to hold the fetus more erect. Rudimentary kidneys secrete urine, and the liver and pancreas begin to produce their secretions. The fetus is now quite active.

TABLE 11–2. SUMMARY OF EMBRYONIC AND FETAL DEVELOPMENT

FIRST TRIMESTER

Body System	Embryonic Period: Lunar Month 1	Embryonic Period: Lunar Month 2	Fetal Period: Lunar Month 3
Integument	Three germ layers are differentiated	Rapid cell differentiation	Nail beds formed, eyelids fused; teeth begin to appear
Cardiovascular	Begins to function; tubular beating; hemopoiesis in yolk sac	Heart and all structures functionally complete; hemopoiesis in liver as yolk sac is incorporated into embryo	Hemopoiesis by liver and spleen
Respiratory	Differentiation of respiratory system and structure; nasal pits, lung buds, trachea, and larynx formed	Formation of three lobes of right lung and two lobes of left lung; bronchi formed with bronchioles dividing	Some respiratory-like movements exhibited
Gastrointestinal	Differentiation of gastrointestinal tract with accessory structure; liver function begins	Urorectal septum formed; oral, nasal cavities, and upper lip formed	Begins to swallow amniotic fluid; bile begins to be secreted by liver; palate and nasal septum fused
Urinary	Urogenital membrane develops into urethral opening; differentiation of kidney		Kidneys begin to function—urine excreted
Reproductive	Sex determined	Urogenital membrane degenerates; testes and ovaries distinguishable; external genitalia begin to differentiate	Gender distinguishable
Musculoskeletal	Rudimentary body parts formed; limb buds present	Muscles developing; extremities, fingers, and toes differentiate; ossification begins; some movement of limbs	Ossification centers present in bones; fetus moves easily
Neurologic	Neural groove formed; brain formed by closure of anterior neural tube; optic cup of eyes formed	Rapid differention and cellular growth of central nervous system; cranial nerves developing; lens vesicles appear; ear beginning to form final structure	Grasp and sucking reflexes present; brain and spinal cord developed
Immunologic			Rudimentary immunologic system appears; β-lymphocytes appear in liver by 9 weeks

SECOND TRIMESTER

Body System	Fetal Period: Lunar Month 4	Fetal Period: Lunar Month 5	Fetal Period: Lunar Month 6
Integument	Downy hair (lanugo) appears on body	Begins to exchange new cells for old in skin; vernix caseosa appears; permanent teeth buds appear	Fingernails present; skin appears red and wrinkled
Cardiovascular	Hemopoiesis by liver, spleen, and bone marrow	Heart sounds heard with stethoscope	
Respiratory		Alveoli forming	Surfactant formation begins in alveoli; nares open; fetus displays hiccoughs
Gastrointestinal	Meconium present; gastric and intestinal glands developing		
Urinary	Kidneys assume mature structure		
Reproductive	Uterine development in female; external genitalia well developed		
Musculoskeletal	Rapid skeletal development; joint cavities form; greater spontaneous movement	Quickening (movement felt by mother); skeleton begins to harden	Body straightens; may respond to external sound with movement

TABLE 11–2. SUMMARY OF EMBRYONIC AND FETAL DEVELOPMENT *(continued)*

SECOND TRIMESTER (continued)

Body System	**Fetal Period**		
	Lunar Month 4	**Lunar Month 5**	**Lunar Month 6**
Neurologic		Beginning of myelination of spinal cord; sucking reflex present; strong grasp reflex	Alternate periods of sleep and activity; may respond to external sounds; eyes structurally complete
Immunologic	β-lymphocytes are present in the blood and spleen	Detectable level of fetal antibodies	

THIRD TRIMESTER

Body System	**Fetal Period**			
	Lunar Month 7	**Lunar Month 8**	**Lunar Month 9**	**Lunar Month 10**
Integument	Eyelids reopen	Begins to store fat; lanugo begins to disappear from face; skin appears less red	Fat deposition continues; lanugo begins to disappear from body; head hair lengthens; earlobes are soft with little cartilage	Lanugo and vernix caseosa both begin to disappear; skin becomes smooth and plump; earlobes are stiff with thick cartilage
Cardiovascular			Increased iron storage by liver	
Respiratory	Respiratory system sufficiently developed so that babies may survive with intensive care; respiratory-like movements apparent		Increased maturity of lungs and surfactant; excellent chance of survival if born; L : S ratio 2 : 1	
Gastrointestinal		Begins to store fat and minerals		Continues to store fat and minerals
Urinary	Active urine formation			
Reproductive	Testes descend into inguinal canal	One or both testes may descend into scrotal sac		Testes in scrotal sac
Musculoskeletal		Mother may note jerky crying-like movements; minerals stored in bone	Femoral ossification centers formed	Firming of skull and bones; circumference of skull larger than circumference of chest
Neurologic	Central nervous system sufficiently developed so that there is a possibility of survival with intensive care; regulatory activities begin	Fetus can be conditioned to environmental sounds and exhibits good reflex development		All reflexes present
Immunologic				Most IgG is acquired from mother; by term the fetus receives some passive immunity by placental transfer of maternal antibodies

L : S ratio = lecithin : sphingomyelin ratio.

Fifth Month (17–20 Weeks). During the fifth month the fetus increases to a crown-rump length of approximately 200 mm (8 in.) and fetal weight increases to between 435 and 460 g. The lower limbs reach their final relative proportions and the mother begins to feel fetal movements. This sensation is known as **quickening.**

The skin of the fetus becomes coated with sebum, a fatty secretion from the fetal sebaceous glands, and sheds epithelial cells, a mixture known as **vernix caseosa.** This greasy cheeselike material protects the fetus' skin from abrasions, chapping, and hardening that would otherwise result from floating in amniotic fluid. **Brown fat** forms during this period. This brown-pigmented tissue is the first adipose tissue deposited in the developing fetus. Eyebrows, head hair, and nails on both the fingers and toes are visible. By the end of the fifth month, fetal heart tones can be heard with a stethoscope.

Sixth Month (21–24 Weeks). The crown-rump length is now approximately 230 mm (9.6 in.). Weight gain during this period is substantial, with the fetus reaching a weight of 780 g (1 pound 11 oz). The skin is translucent, pink to red, and wrinkled. The organs are rather well developed and a grasp reflex is present. The alveoli in the lungs are beginning to develop.

Seventh Month (25–28 Weeks). The fetus' lungs and pulmonary vasculature develop sufficiently during this period to allow gas exchange to take place. Survival is therefore possible if the infant is born prematurely, although the mortality rate is high. The central nervous system matures dramatically to the stage where it can direct rhythmic breathing movements and control body temperature. The fetus' eyes open and close under neural control. Subcutaneous fat begins to increase.

An infant born at 28 weeks is considered viable (able to live outside the uterus), although morbidity and mortality are greatly increased compared with full-term infants.

Eighth Month (29–32 Weeks). Subcutaneous fat continues to increase during the eighth month, as does body muscle, bringing the weight of the fetus to approximately 2000 g (4 pounds 6.5 oz) and the crown-rump length to 300 mm (12.5 in.). The lungs are not yet fully developed. The bones, although developed, are still soft and flexible. An infant born during this period has a 60 percent chance of survival with special care.

Ninth Month (33–36 Weeks). The skin of the fetus appears pink and less wrinkled by the ninth month. The fetus is beginning to appear plump and the arms and legs may seem chubby. Lanugo is beginning to disappear, and the nails have grown to reach the fingertips.

The surfactant system of the lungs matures at approximately 36 weeks. Surfactant, a surface-active phosopholipid that maintains alveolar patency, is evident in increasing quantities. An infant delivered at this time has a 90 percent chance of survival if he or she receives some special care.

Tenth Month (37–40 Weeks). The fetus is considered full term at 38 weeks. Very little lanugo remains and the amount of vernix caseosa varies, with the largest deposits in the creases and folds of the skin. The skull has the largest circumference of all parts of the body and is generally positioned downward, which is an important factor in preparing for passage of the infant through the birth canal. The sexual characteristics are pronounced; the testes should be in the scrotum.

At term the fetus weighs about 3000 to 3600 g (6 pounds 10 oz to 7 pounds 15 oz), boys being larger than girls. Boys are also longer than girls, with crown-to-heel length, the commonly used measurement for the newborn, ranging from 48 to 52 cm (19 to 21 in.).

The expected delivery date is roughly calculated as 266 days (38 weeks) after fertilization, or 280 days (40 weeks) from the onset of the last menstrual period.[3,6,9,10] Table 11–2 provides a synopsis of embryonic and fetal development, summarizing the major changes and the development of body and organ systems during various stages of gestation.

Fetal Lung Development

Fetal lung development is a very complex process affected by the interrelationship of several hormones. Agents that accelerate lung maturation are corticosteroids, thyroid hormones, growth factors, and cyclic adenosine monophosphate (AMP). The role of estrogen and prolactin in lung maturation is not as clear. On the other hand, insulin and hyperglycemia appear to delay lung maturation.[11]

For the infant to breathe adequately at birth and not to experience respiratory distress syndrome, sufficient quantities of **surfactant,** a phospholipid, must be present to allow expansion of the lungs and free exchange of air. Surfactant reduces the surface tension of the alveoli and prevents collapse of the lung. This reduction in surface tension is necessary for full lung expansion despite the presence of what appears to be adequate respiratory movement.[9]

Movements of the fetal chest have been detected very early in pregnancy. The fetus is capable of respiratory movement from the beginning of the fourth month. By the end of the second trimester, development of air ducts and alveoli, pulmonary vasculature, and muscles of respiration, as well as the coordination of their activities by the respiratory system, reaches a level that allows survival for a short period; however, surfactant sufficient to support adequate respiration is not produced until the third trimester, increasing in quantity as the pregnancy progresses.[1,9,12]

Multiple Gestation

Twins. Twins may be either dizygotic (fraternal) or monozygotic (identical). In the United States, the prevalence of twins is 1.08 percent among the white population and 1.36 percent among the black population. Approximately 70 percent of twin births are dizygotic and 30 percent monozygotic.[3]

Dizygotic twins are delivered more frequently than monozygotic twins. Dizygotic or fraternal twins originate from two separate zygotes; monozygotic or identical twins originate from one zygote. Because they occur as the result of fertilization of two ova, dizygotic twins are genetically different and may be of the same or different sexes. Dizygotic twins are actually no more alike than other brothers and sisters. **Monozygotic twins** result from the fertilization of one ovum. They are therefore genetically identical and of the same sex.[6]

Dizygotic and monozygotic twins also differ with respect to implantation site, placenta, chorion, and amnion. Dizygotic twins have separate implantation sites, placentas, chorions, and amnions, although their placentas have been known to fuse (Figure 11–10).

In monozygotic twins, the zygote splits at various states to form two separate zygotes. Depending on when division occurs, the twins will share different structures. If division occurs within the first 72 hours of fertilization, the two embryos will be diamniotic and dichorionic, developing two amnions and two chorions. If division occurs between the fourth and eighth days, the embryos will be monochorionic, having separate amniotic sacs covered by a common chorion. If division occurs on about the eighth day, the two embryos will share an amniotic sac (Figure 11–11).

Other Multiple Births. Other multiple births—triplets, quadruplets, quintuplets, sextuplets, septuplets, and so forth—may be the result of one zygote (identical), several zygotes (fraternal), or any combination (identical and fraternal).[6] Drugs used to treat infertility may induce multiple births (*see* Chapter 7).

CIRCULATION

Fetal

Fetal circulation differs from the circulation that exists in extrauterine life primarily because the fetus secures oxygen and food from maternal blood through the placenta rather than through its own lungs and digestive organs. Special structures make possible fetal circulation, including the umbilical cord, which contains two umbilical arteries and one umbilical vein; the ductus venosus; and the placenta. In addition, the foramen ovale and ductus arteriosus provide detours by which blood bypasses the lungs.

The umbilical vein carries oxygenated, nutrient-bearing blood from the placenta to the fetus. The umbilical vein enters the fetal body through the umbilicus, or umbilical ring, and ascends along the anterior abdominal wall to the liver, where the vein divides into the portal sinus and the ductus venosus. The portal sinus carries blood to the hepatic veins, located primarily on the left side of the liver. The ductus venosus, or major branch of the umbilical vein, traverses the liver and empties directly into the inferior vena cava.

Highly oxygenated blood from the inferior vena cava mixes with less well oxygenated blood from the veins below the level of the diaphragm and flows into the right atrium of the fetal heart. From the right atrium, the blood passes through the foramen ovale, an opening in the septum between the right and left atria, into the left atrium. Blood then flows into the left ventricle and, finally, is pumped into the aorta. Little or no blood from the superior vena cava, which is less oxygenated, passes through the foramen ovale. The right ventricle and pulmonary circulation are bypassed; thus, the highly oxygenated blood is pumped directly from the left ventricle and perfuses only two vital organs, the heart and the brain. Blood returning through the superior vena cava empties into the right atrium and passes through the tricuspid valve into the right ventricle. For the most part, this blood is shunted into the descending aorta through the ductus arteriosus. The blood nourishes the trunk and lower extremities. A small amount of blood passes through the lungs, and this provides nourishment only.

The ventricles of the fetal heart work in tandem rather than in series, as a result of the action of the foramen ovale and ductus arteriosus shunts. Cardiac output of the fetal heart is about three times that of an adult at rest and is due partly to the rapid heart rate of the fetus and partly to low peripheral resistance.[1,9]

Blood finally returns to the placenta through the two hypogastric arteries, which become the umbilical arteries distally. Carbon dioxide and other waste products are then removed in the placenta, allowing the entire process to be repeated[1,9] (Figure 11–12).

At birth the hemodynamics of fetal circulation undergo profound changes. The umbilical vessels, the ductus arteriosus, the foramen ovale, and the ductus venosus normally constrict or collapse with spontaneous or artificial respiration of the infant, or

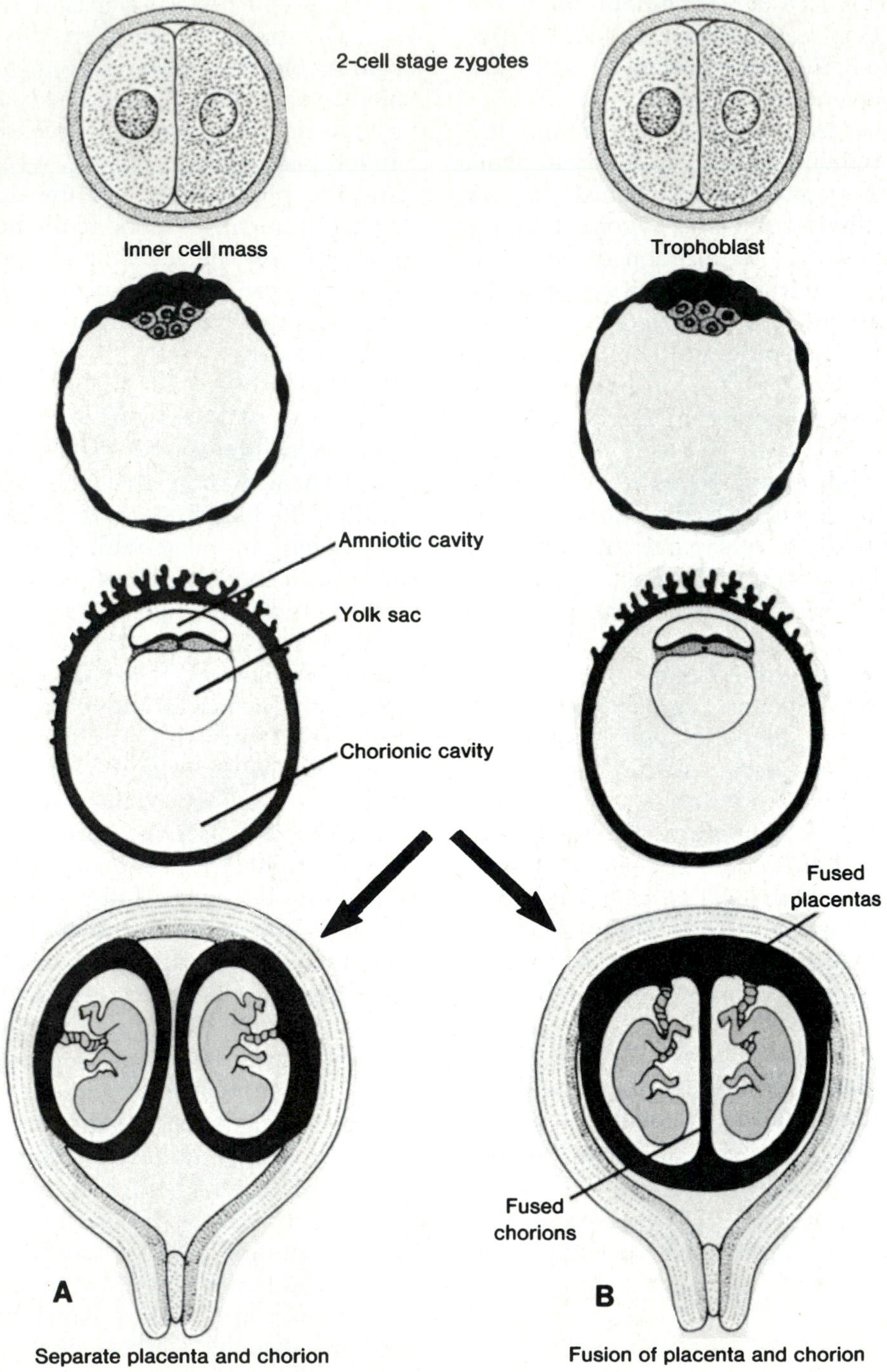

Figure 11–10. Development of dizygotic twins. (*Reproduced, with permission, from Sadler TW.* Langman's Medical Embryology. *5th ed. Baltimore: Williams & Wilkins; 1985:104.*)

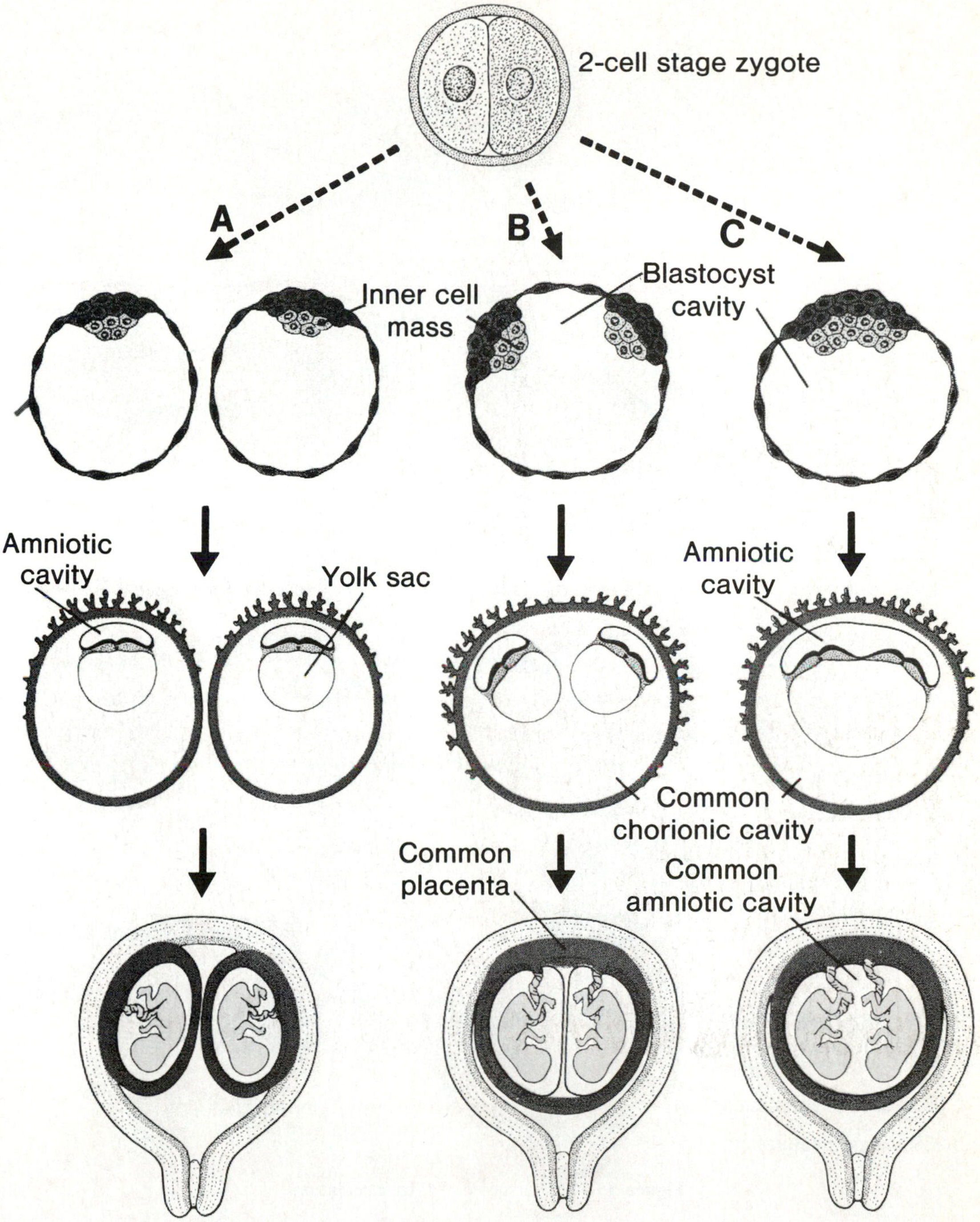

Figure 11–11. Possible relationships among fetal membranes in monozygotic twins. (*Reproduced, with permission, from Sadler TW.* Langman's Medical Embryology. *5th ed. Baltimore: Williams & Wilkins; 1985:105.*)

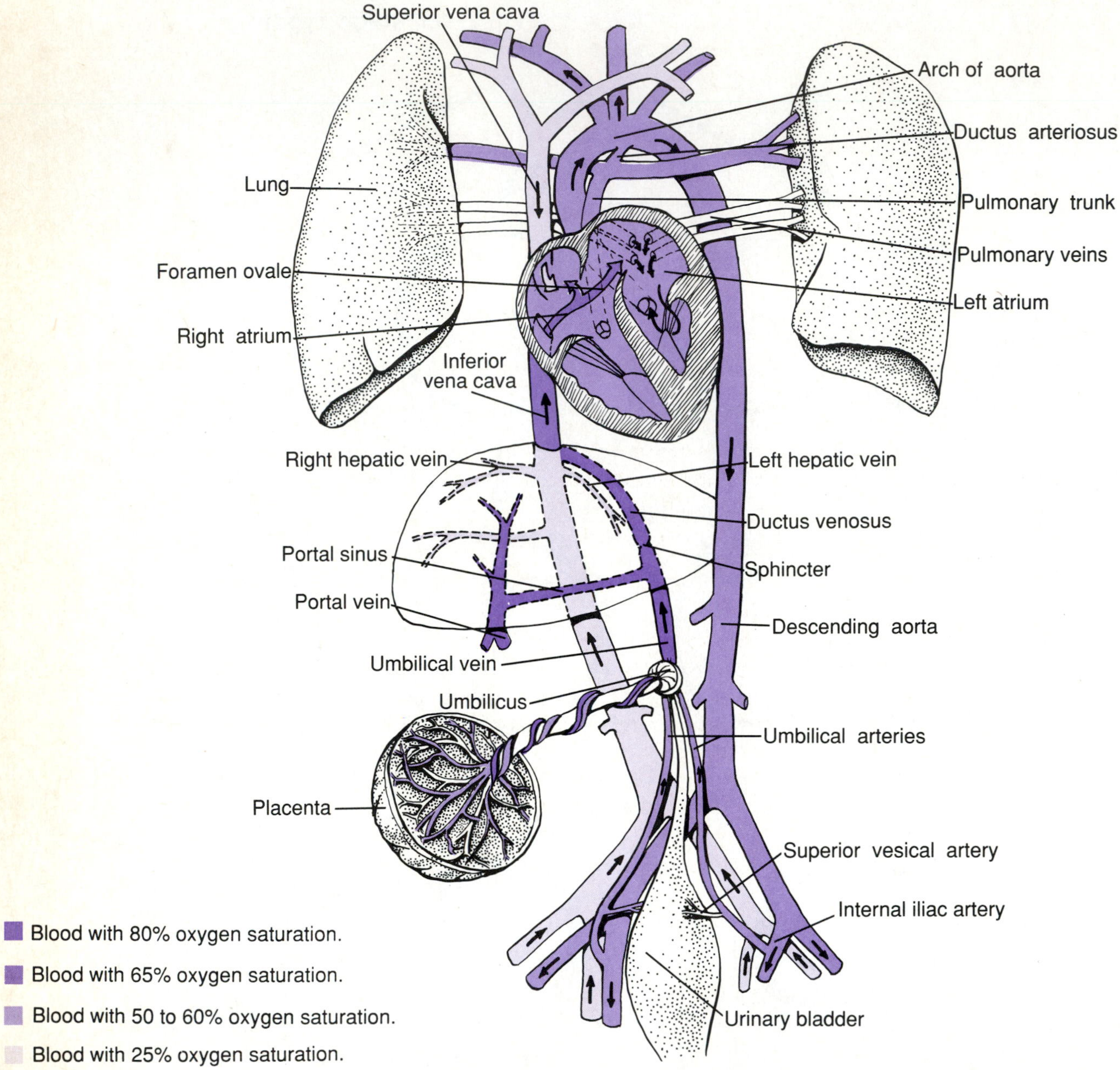
Superior vena cava
Arch of aorta
Ductus arteriosus
Lung
Pulmonary trunk
Pulmonary veins
Foramen ovale
Left atrium
Right atrium
Inferior vena cava
Right hepatic vein
Left hepatic vein
Ductus venosus
Portal sinus
Sphincter
Portal vein
Descending aorta
Umbilical vein
Umbilicus
Umbilical arteries
Placenta
Superior vesical artery
Internal iliac artery
Urinary bladder
Blood with 80% oxygen saturation.
Blood with 65% oxygen saturation.
Blood with 50 to 60% oxygen saturation.
Blood with 25% oxygen saturation.

Figure 11–12. Diagram of fetal circulation.

TABLE 11–3. CHANGES IN FETAL CIRCULATION AFTER BIRTH

Structure	Fetal Circulation	Postnatal Change
Umbilical vein	Transports arterial blood to liver and heart	Becomes round ligament of liver
Umbilical arteries	Transport blood to placenta	Become umbilical ligaments
Ductus venosus	Shunts blood to inferior vena cava	Becomes ligamentum venosum
Ductus arteriosus	Shunts blood from pulmonary artery to aorta	Becomes ligamentum arteriosum
Foramen ovale	Connects right and left atria	Closes
Lungs	Contain no air and little blood; are filled with fluid	Fill with air; begin to oxygenate blood
Pulmonary arteries	Transport small amounts of blood to lungs	Transport blood to lungs for oxygenation
Aorta	Receives blood from both ventricles	Receives blood from left ventricle
Inferior vena cava	Transports atrial blood from placenta and venous blood from body	Transports venous blood to right atrium

shortly thereafter. As the lungs expand, pulmonary vascular resistance decreases considerably, causing the pressures in the right ventricle and pulmonary arteries to fall. This results in equal pressure in both atria, causing the foramen ovale to close. The distal portions of the hypogastric arteries, the umbilical arteries, atrophy to become the umbilical ligaments; intra-abdominal remnants of the umbilical vein become the round ligament of the liver; and the ductus venosus constricts to form the ligamentum venosum.[1,6] These changes are outlined in Table 11–3. (*See* Chapter 32 for an in-depth discussion.)

Maternal Placental

Fetal circulation is dependent on efficient maternal placental circulation. Maternal blood transports nutrients to the fetus and waste materials from the fetus through the process of diffusion. Maternal arterial blood pressure, intrauterine pressure, the pattern of uterine contractions, and factors affecting arteriolar walls are the primary influences on the flow of blood in the placenta. (*See* earlier section on "Maternal Placental Structure" for a discussion of this process.)

PLACENTAL FUNCTIONS

Hormone Production

The corpus luteum, which is maintained throughout the entire pregnancy, continues to secrete estrogens and progesterone for about 8 to 10 weeks after fertilization. The placenta also produces four essential hormones: two protein hormones, human chorionic gonadotropin and human placental lactogen, and two steroid hormones, estrogen and progesterone. (*See* Table 12–2 for a summary of placental hormone functions during pregnancy.)

Estrogen. Throughout pregnancy, the woman is in a hyperestrogenic state. It has been noted that the amount of estrogen produced daily by one woman during pregnancy is equal to that produced by more than 1000 premenopausal women daily.[1] The site of origin of estrogens during most of the pregnancy is the placenta.

Three main forms of estrogen are secreted during pregnancy: estriol, estradiol, and estrone. Estrogen production during pregnancy is dependent on precursors from the mother and the fetus. Estriol is the predominant estrogen secreted during pregnancy. The biosynthetic process of estriol formation in the placenta is dependent on steroid secretions from the fetal and maternal adrenals and further processing by the fetal liver. Estrone and estradiol are also formed in the placenta from steroid precursors secreted by the mother and the fetus.

Estrogen is produced as a result of the interplay of the fetus, placenta, and mother. The so-called fetal-placental unit is an important regulator of the maternal-fetal environment. The fetus is therefore viewed as an active participant in the healthy progress of the pregnancy.

Functionally, estrogens (in particular estriol) are believed to produce an increase in uterine blood flow through vasodilation. In addition, they have a role in increasing the size of the uterus and the ductal system of the breasts.[1,13]

Progesterone. Progesterone is also produced in large amounts during pregnancy. After the first few weeks of gestation, little progesterone is produced in the ovary. The placenta becomes the primary producer of progesterone for the remainder of the pregnancy. At the time of fertilization and during development of the zygote, progesterone functions to increase the secretions of the fallopian tubes and uterus and thereby provide appropriate nutrition. Progesterone must be present in high levels for implantation to occur. Progesterone induces development of the decidual cells in the uterine endometrium

TABLE 11–4. PLACENTAL MECHANISMS OF TRANSPORT

Transport Mechanism	Description
Simple diffusion	The movement of substances from an area of higher concentration to an area of lower concentration. Through this mechanism, gases and other simple molecules cross the placenta. Depends on the differences in concentration of substances in fetal and maternal plasma, nature of substances, and area of the placenta available for transfer. Some substances transported in this manner are sodium, oxygen, carbon dioxide, and exogenous compounds such as drugs.[14]
Facilitated diffusion	Mechanism whereby the molecule to be transported combines with a protein molecule embedded in the membrane of the placenta. When this molecule is released by the protein molecule into the fetus, the protein molecule is again available to facilitate the diffusion of another molecule across the membrane. This mechanism, which is the primary means of transport of glucose and other sugar molecules, is vital because glucose is the primary energy source of the fetus.[15,16]
Active transport	Mechanism which operates against a pressure gradient to move a substance from an area of lower pressure to an area of higher pressure. Essential amino acids and water-soluble vitamins are found in higher concentrations in the fetus than in the mother. Through this mechanism, selective amino acids and vitamins are transferred from maternal to fetal blood.[14]
Pinocytosis	Mechanism by which pseudopodial projections from the syncytiotrophoblastic layer engulf small amounts of maternal plasma substances and carry them intact to the fetal circulation. Through this mechanism, complex proteins, some fats, immune bodies, and even some viruses may be transported across the placenta. The mechanism is, however, highly selective; not all maternal antibodies, viruses, and so on will cross the placental barrier.[14]
Leakage	Defects or breaks in the placental membrane allow for transfer of very large materials, such as red blood cells, between mother and fetus. This occurs most often at delivery and is responsible for maternal Rh sensitization to fetal red blood cells.

and decreases the contractility of the uterus, thereby preventing spontaneous abortions. During pregnancy, progesterone maintains the endometrium and its blood supply, enhances uterine growth, decreases uterine contractility, and aids in alveolar development of the breasts.

Human Chorionic Gonadotropin. Human chorionic gonadotropin (hCG) is believed to be produced primarily by the syncytiotrophoblast. It is a glycoprotein similar in structure to pituitary luteinizing hormone (LH). Human chorionic gonadotropin appears in the maternal blood by the eighth day after ovulation. Levels of hCG increase steadily, reaching a maximum in 60 to 90 days if fertilization occurs. The most apparent and important function of hCG is maintenance of the corpus luteum during the early pregnancy. In the male fetus, hCG acts on the fetal testes as an LH surrogate, to promote testosterone synthesis and secretion and male sexual differentiation.[1]

Human Placental Lactogen. Human placental lactogen (hPL) is detectable in the trophoblast as early as the third week after ovulation, and may be detected in the serum of pregnant women as early as 4 weeks after fertilization. This hormone has an action similar to that of human growth hormone. It facilitates transport of glucose across the placenta by the process of facilitated diffusion, and regulates maternal metabolism to maintain a supply of nutrients for the fetus.[12,13]

Transport and Exchange

The main functions of the placenta are (1) exchange of metabolic and gaseous products between maternal and fetal blood systems, (2) production of hormones, (3) exchange of nutrients and electrolytes, (4) transmission of maternal antibodies, and (5) detoxification of some drugs and chemicals.

During the first few days after implantation, the fertilized ovum receives its nutrition directly from the interstitial fluid of the endometrium and from the surrounding maternal tissue. Once the placenta has developed, there are several mechanisms through which nutrients and other substances are transported from the mother to the fetus.[14] These are described in Table 11–4.

Those substances essential to fetal growth and development, such as oxygen, water, sodium, and glucose, are transported by diffusion. Substances that are required by the fetus for synthesis of tissues, such as amino acids and vitamins, are transported by active processes. Complex proteins such as immunoglobulins are transported to the fetus by pinocytosis.[14]

In addition, several factors affect the efficiency of placental transport mechanisms. Some of these factors are leakage at the placental barrier site, health of the placental surface, the size of the molecules to be transported, adequacy of uteroplacental blood flow, metabolic integrity of the mother and fetus, and the extent to which maternal blood contains oxygen and nutrients.[7,16]

NEW DEVELOPMENTS IN EMBRYOLOGY/FETOLOGY

Research in the field of human embryology and fetology is constrained by the ethical, moral, and legal considerations involved in studying and experimenting on humans; however, if advances are to be made in the field of prenatal development, research is necessary. The physiologic risks to the mother and embryo/fetus require that most experimentation and study in this field be performed in the laboratory on animals. Because this type of study can never fully duplicate the actual effects on humans, broad generalizations to humans cannot be made. Some investigators are attempting to perform some experimental research on the fetuses of women who have elective abortions, but the opposition to this type of research is considerable. Many people regard this as human experimentation, which raises the issue of the rights of the fetus.

Research in embryology and fetology is proceeding in many areas in an effort to advance medical science and to improve pregnancy outcomes. Among these areas are fetal and maternal nutrition; placental and fetal physiology; physiologic effects of drugs and teratogens on the fetus and placenta; physiologic effects of hormones and enzymes of pregnancy on the fetus and mother; fetal and maternal metabolism; fetal, placental, and maternal circulation; fetal, placental, and maternal pathology; fetal and maternal diseases; fetal immunology; and placental transmission of human immunodeficiency virus.

Some of the most exciting work is taking place in the area of infertility. In vitro fertilization (IVF), artificial insemination, gamete intrafallopian transfer (GIFT), cryopreservation of pre-embryos, and IVF with donated oocytes and donated embryos are all being studied and improved daily. (*See* Chapter 7.) These procedures, however, are still generally considered experimental, are very expensive, and are associated with a relatively low success rate. More effective techniques are being developed, but with these improvements come new questions regarding the legal, moral, and ethical issues. Complex issues are raised for which no definitive answers are forthcoming.

Continual improvements in the area of prenatal diagnosis through ultrasonography, amniocentesis, and chorionic villus biopsy are making these techniques relatively safe, acceptable, and reliable. As a result, intrauterine fetal surgery is now an option in the treatment of fetuses with such abnormalities as hydrocephalus, and hydronephrosis associated with posterior urethral valves. In the future, fetuses with a diaphragmatic hernia and meningomyelocele may be subjects for in utero fetal therapy. The goal of fetal surgery is to provide time for fetal maturity and delivery at or near term by reversing or slowing a destructive process. This type of surgery is highly experimental and risky and may result in fetal death. Nevertheless, fetal surgery is being pioneered in at least 13 centers in five countries throughout the world. Many ethical, legal, and moral implications will need to be considered as these highly controversial procedures advance.[17,18]

Research in embryology and fetology is an exciting area that has considerable potential for improving pregnancy outcomes.

ENVIRONMENTAL EFFECTS ON THE EMBRYO/FETUS

Several factors contribute to the risks for the mother and fetus throughout pregnancy. Environmental agents may cross the placenta and affect the developing embryo/fetus. Genetic errors may result in functional defects. Approximately 10 percent of all human malformations are caused by environmental factors, 10 percent are caused by genetic factors, and the remaining 80 percent are presumably the result of an intricate interplay of several environmental and genetic factors.[3]

There are five major risk factors with respect to infant mortality: smoking during pregnancy, alcohol abuse, drug use and abuse, occupational hazards, and injuries.[19] These risk factors may also be referred to as teratogens, agents that can cause congenital anomalies in the fetus. Other teratogens are viruses and nutritional deficiencies. It has been determined that any substance given in large enough doses at critical periods of development can be classified as teratogenic.[20]

The embryo is susceptible to a variety of environmental teratogenic influences that are capable of disrupting the developmental process. The fetus is also susceptible to teratogens that may result in prematurity, abortion, organ or tissue injury, and possibly malformation.[4,21]

Three critical periods of development exist: (1) fertilization and implantation, or the first 17 days of gestation; (2) the embryonic period, from day 18 to day 55; and (3) the fetal stage, from day 56 of gestation to delivery. Exposure to teratogens in the first critical period may lead to improper implantation and spontaneous abortion. The embryonic period is the period when the most extensive organ differentiation occurs, the heart in the first 38 days, the arms and legs in the first 49 days, and the teeth in the first 56 days of gestation. Further, there is differentiation of the palate, external genitalia, and ear in the fetal period.[4] Exposure to teratogens during the embryonic period can cause structural and functional birth defects. During the fetal period, when there is still some organ differentiation, structural defects as well as fetal growth retardation can occur (Figures 11–13 and 11–14).

Infectious agents known to cause malformations are rubella, toxoplasmosis, cytomegalovirus, herpes simplex virus, and group B streptococcus. Environmental and lifestyle hazards causing malformation include exposure to radiation and chemicals, and use of tobacco and drugs.

Infectious Agents

Congenital Rubella Syndrome. Rubella infection is preventable through active immunization, yet it continues to be a major cause of birth defects. Several types of malformation may occur, depending on the stage of embryonic development at which the infection occurs. Cataracts and microphthalmia occur if the infection develops during the sixth week of development. Congenital deafness resulting from destruction of the organ of Corti occurs when the infection is present during the ninth week. Cardiac and dental problems result from infection during the fifth to tenth weeks, and central nervous system defects occur from infection during the second trimester.

Toxoplasmosis. Toxoplasmosis results from exposure to infected excretions of household pets such as cats, rabbits, and birds or from handling of infected animals. The risk of infection may be reduced through the use of suitable preventive measures; for example, pregnant women can refrain from changing cat litter boxes or bird cages and from handling rabbits either as pets or as food. The parasite, *Toxoplasma gondii,* is transmitted during fetal life, not during the birth process. The most frequent sequela is a subclinical infection that is predominantly ocular. In one third of cases, many years may pass before symptoms are observed. If infection occurs during pregnancy, the mother should be treated to reduce the frequency of transmission to the fetus. The infant of an infected mother should be treated after birth.

Cytomegalovirus. Cytomegalovirus infection is the most common cause of congenital infections throughout the world. Severe forms of the disease occur in 0.5 to 1 per 1000 deliveries, subclinical infections in 1 in 100 deliveries. Ten percent of these latter infants will develop significant sequelae later in life.[22] The malformations most frequently seen occur in asymptomatically infected mothers and include microcephaly, cerebral calcifications, blindness and chorioretinitis, and hepatosplenomegaly. Some infants have kernicterus and multiple petechiae of the skin.

Herpes Simplex Virus. Herpes virus is usually transmitted to the infant during the birth process as a result of the virus shedding from the cervix of lower genital tract.[22] About half of the infants exposed to herpes during delivery will become infected. If left untreated it is fatal in 50 percent of these cases, and half of the survivors will have untoward neurologic sequelae. Symptoms of the disease develop during the first 3 weeks of life.[22] The infection may manifest itself as localized inflammatory reactions or as disseminated reactions. The neonate may also be asymptomatic.

Human Immunodeficiency Virus. The agent that was of greatest concern with respect to pregnancy outcome in the late 1980s, and will most likely continue to be of concern in the 1990s, is human immunodeficiency virus (HIV), the virus that can lead to acquired immunodeficiency syndrome (AIDS). It is now known that transplacental transmission of HIV occurs as early as the first trimester.[23] Human immunodeficiency virus has been detected in the amniotic fluid of women known to be HIV positive; it has also been found in the thymus of fetuses at 22 to 23 weeks and in the central nervous system of aborted fetuses of affected mothers. HIV infection may occur in approximately 50 percent of deliveries to affected mothers, according to conversations with Dr. S. Landesman and Dr. H. Mikoff (New York Health Science Center, 1989).

The diagnosis of HIV in the newborn cannot always be made at birth because all newborns receive an antibody from the mother that may not disappear until the infant is at least 15 months old, at which time a positive diagnosis can be made. Controversy exists as to whether HIV has pathologic effects on the embryo. Dr. A. Rubinstein at Albert Einstein College of Medicine, Yeshiva University, New York, has reported that definite congenital defects do occur, yet evidence reported by Drs. H. Minkoff, H. Mendez, and S. Landesman, College of Medicine, State University of New York Health Science Center, Brook-

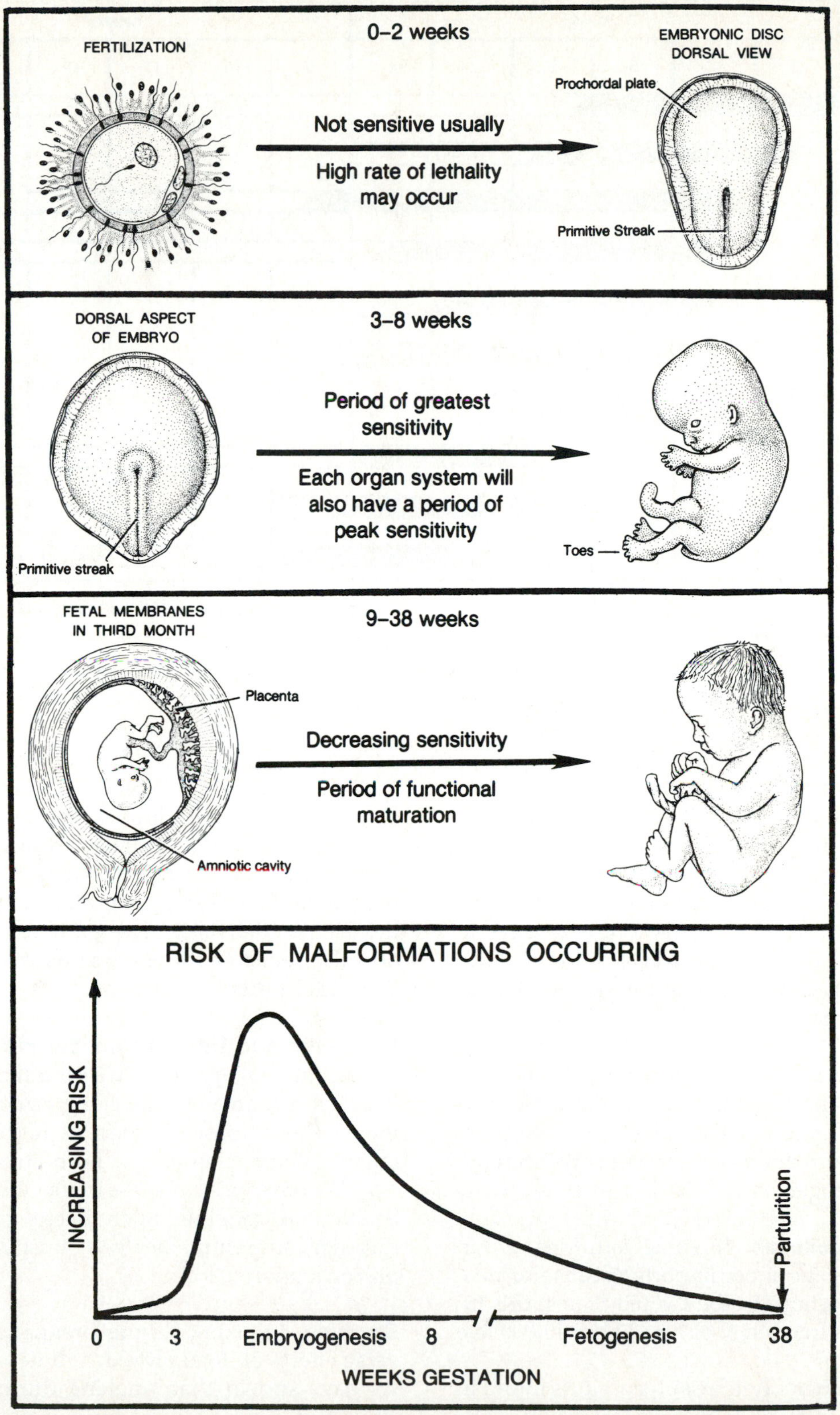

Figure 11–13. Periods of susceptibility to teratogens. (*Reproduced, with permission, from Sadler TW.* Langman's Medical Embryology. *5th ed. Baltimore: Williams & Wilkins; 1985.*)

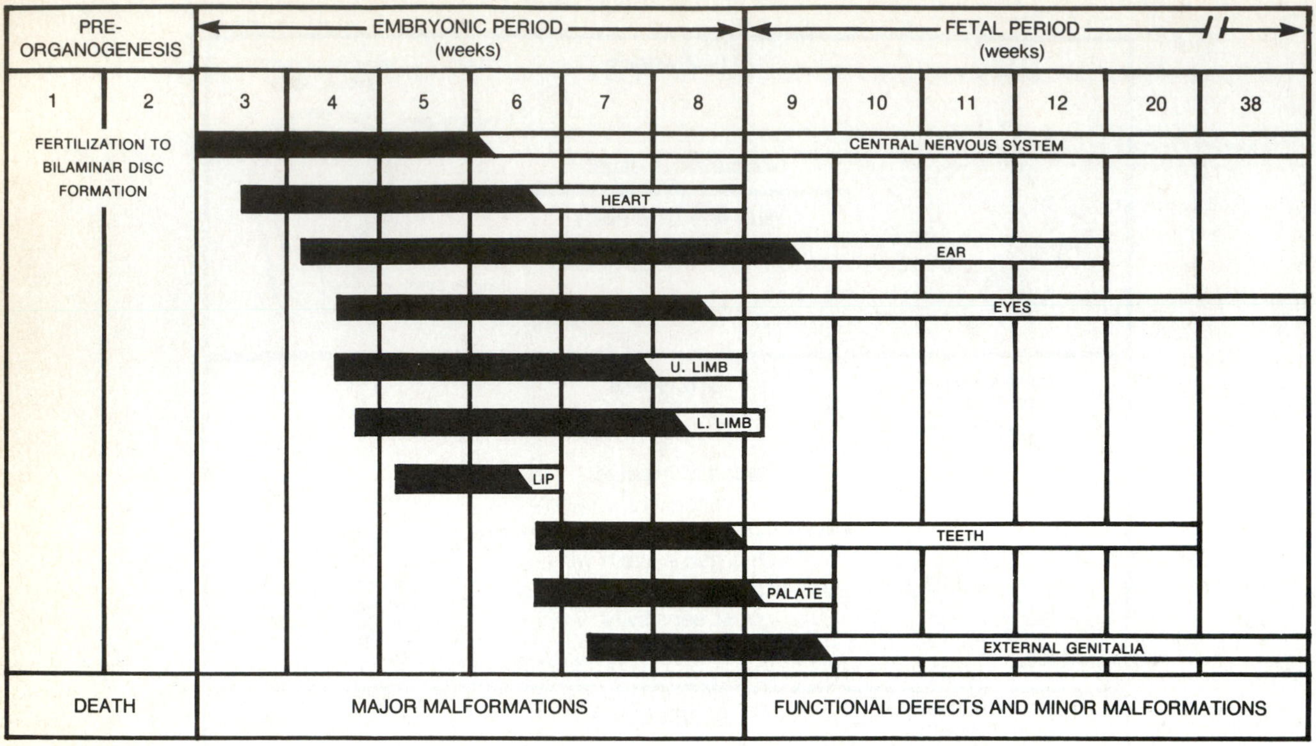

Figure 11–14. Susceptibility of organ systems to teratogens. Solid bars denote highly sensitive periods. (*Reproduced, with permission, from Sadler TW.* Langman's Medical Embryology. *5th ed. Baltimore: Williams & Wilkins; 1985.*)

lyn, indicates that no known congenital defects occur (personal conversation with H. Minkoff, New York Health Science Center, 1989).

All individuals, regardless of age, and especially those who engage in high risk behaviors, need to be educated about HIV, its transmission, and ways to reduce the risk of acquiring or transmitting it. Educational programs are an essential component of family planning and prenatal care.

Other Viral Agents. Malformations rarely, if ever, follow other maternal infections. The hyperthermia (high fever) resulting from viral infections has, however, caused malformations and has recently been implicated as a teratogen.

Group B Streptococcus. In some countries, group B streptococcus is the most important cause of neonatal bacterial infection. In the United States, this infection occurs at a frequency of 1 to 30 per 10,000 live births.

Group B beta-hemolytic streptococcus is found in low-birth-weight infants, especially those born after prolonged rupture of the membranes. When the placental membranes are broken, streptococcus can penetrate the protective barrier, grow in the birth canal, and infect the fetus. Women who are susceptible to early rupture of membranes also tend to harbor colonies of streptococcus B. They are also often asymptomatic.[24] Infants infected by streptococcus B often exhibit a rapid onset of symptoms, with sepsis and death after delivery. Frequently, streptococcus B is also the cause of the meningitis that occurs several days after birth.

Lifestyle and Environmental Hazards

Environmental agents to which a mother is exposed during pregnancy can be categorized into those that the mother chooses as part of her lifestyle, drugs, environmental chemicals, and occupational hazards.

A woman may choose to use tobacco, drugs, alcohol, and caffeine. Such habits can be changed through counseling; ideally, counseling should occur preconception.

Smoking. Smoking during pregnancy can have adverse effects on fetal growth and development. Studies have shown that smoking during pregnancy is associated with reduced birth weight, reduction in uteroplacental oxygen, and delayed neurologic and intellectual development of children.[25–27] The adverse effects of smoking are due to the following factors:

(1) carbon dioxide, which inactivates fetal and maternal hemoglobin, reducing the amount of oxygen delivered to the fetus; (2) nicotine, the vasoconstrictive action of which reduces placental perfusion; and (3) reduction in maternal appetite, leading to a reduction in caloric intake.[1] In addition to the known risks to the mother, smoking increases the risk of spontaneous abortion, bacterial infection, and infant mortality. Although the substances in cigarette smoke place the fetus at risk in the first trimester of pregnancy, smoking can have harmful effects throughout pregnancy, especially on the developing central nervous system of the fetus. If the mother stops smoking by the 12th week of gestation, the effects on the fetus can be minimized.

TABLE 11–5. SELECTED ABUSIVE DRUGS AND THEIR POSSIBLE EFFECTS ON THE EMBRYO/FETUS AND NEONATE

Drug	Effect
Heroin	Intrauterine growth retardation, withdrawal symptoms, respiratory depression, neonatal death
Methadone	Fetal distress, neonatal drug withdrawal
Valium	Possible cleft lip and palate, respiratory depression, hypotonia, hypothermia, low Apgar score
Amphetamines	Possible cleft lip and cleft palate, transposition of the great vessels, learning disabilities
Marijuana	Fetal growth retardation

Recreational Drugs. The use of "recreational" or illicit drugs by the pregnant woman has caused great concern among investigators and clinicians, because of the documented or potential effects of these drugs on the fetus. Chronic use by the expectant mother of such substances as opium derivatives, barbiturates, and amphetamines can result in intrauterine distress, low birth weight, and drug withdrawal in the newborn.[1] The effects of marijuana on the embryo and fetus are not well documented; however, animal studies have shown that maternal marijuana smoking affects both the male and female reproductive systems. Specifically, delta-9-tetrahydocannabinol (THC), found in marijuana, may decrease levels of follicle-stimulating hormone, luteinizing hormone, prolactin, and testosterone, and may inhibit ovulation and spermatogenesis. Further, THC has been implicated in fetal growth retardation.[28] Chronic use of cocaine during pregnancy has also been related to such untoward effects as spontaneous abortion, low birth weight, and possible learning disabilities in the offspring. Table 11–5 lists drugs that may be abused and their effects.

The problem of drug use among pregnant women is complex. The majority of these women receive little or no prenatal care and are at greater risk for malnutrition and infections.[1] Further, women who transmit HIV to their fetuses are frequently intravenous drug users or partners of men who are intravenous drug users. The infection is contracted by the mother through contaminated drug paraphernalia or sexual intercourse with an intravenous drug user. The HIV-infected mother may then transmit HIV to her fetus congenitally. These factors, added to the social and psychologic problems of the mother and the apparent risks to the fetus, require careful health planning by the nurse. The situation becomes quite acute if the expectant mother seeks prenatal care late in the pregnancy. The short-term goal may be to reduce the physiologic problems associated with drug use, for the mother and the fetus. Long-term goals include assessment of the medical, social, and psychologic factors that contribute to drug use and management of the addiction through appropriate resources. Nurses should also become involved in planning educational programs for children and adolescents in an effort to prevent drug use at any stage in a person's life, especially pregnancy.

Medically Prescribed Drugs. Drugs other than those considered "recreational" or illicit also have harmful effects on the developing fetus. Before the thalidomide disaster in the 1960s, it was believed that the placental barrier protected the fetus from drugs taken by the mother. Since that time, the placental barrier theory has been discounted and a number of drugs taken by the mother have been associated with birth defects in the offspring.[29]

Thalidomide, a drug once used as an antiemetic during pregnancy, has been proven to cause deformities of the arms, legs, and face in the fetus. The experience with this drug alerted investigators to the need to exercise caution in applying data obtained from animal studies to the human being. No evidence of the teratogenic effects was found when thalidomide was tested on certain animals before its release, yet thalidomide was found to cause malformations in the human fetus. As the effects of thalidomide have been identified only at the expense of thousands of malformed children, it is imperative that malformations related to drug exposure be carefully documented.[29] *It is also important that the expectant mother exercise caution in relation to any drug she considers using during pregnancy.*

Other drugs that have been proven teratogenic

in human populations are steroid hormones, antineoplastic drugs, and tetracyclines. Early exposure to high doses of androgenic steroid hormones leads to masculinization of female fetuses. It has also been shown that females exposed in utero to stilbestrol may be at increased risk of developing vaginal cancer ten or more years after the exposure. Exposure to antineoplastic drugs during pregnancy results in abortion or malformations in 20 to 30 percent of those fetuses who survive to term. Tetracyclines have been proven to cause dental staining in offspring because of their strong affinity for osseous and dental tissue. Table 11–6 lists known drug teratogens.

In addition to the previously mentioned drugs, which have provided strong evidence of teratogenic effects in human populations, many drugs are suspected to be teratogens on the basis of epidemiologic studies, laboratory reports, and case studies.[29] Drugs taken in the first trimester of pregnancy can cause malformations in the embryo/fetus because organogenesis occurs in this period. Appendix A lists medications and their effects on the embryo/fetus in the first trimester of pregnancy.

Medications can also have an effect on the fetus in the second and third trimesters. Some may even have a delayed effect on the offspring. For example, androgenic agents, such as progestins in general and diethylstillbestrol (DES) in particular, have had a delayed effect on both female and male offspring. Administration of DES to pregnant women to prevent abortion has been related to adenocarcinoma of the genital tract in female offspring and has been associated with genital tract abnormalities, as well as abnormal sperm production and motility, in male offspring.[30]

Another class of teratogens that can affect the fetus is the anticoagulants. All anticoagulants, with the exception of heparin, cross the placental membrane, and may cause hemorrhage in the fetus. Further, maternal intake of anticoagulants, like warfarin, in the second and third trimesters may result in mental retardation, microcephaly, and optic atrophy in the offspring.[31] Appendix B provides a more complete list of medications and their effects on the fetus/neonate in the second and third trimester of pregnancy.

The expectant mother should be aware of the known or possible effects of any medications taken during pregnancy. The old adage "better safe than sorry" applies to the use of any substance during pregnancy. Unless the drug is essential to the mother's health (e.g., insulin for diabetic mothers), it should be avoided; if the drug is deemed essential, careful monitoring of the mother and fetus throughout pregnancy is necessary.

TABLE 11–6. KNOWN DRUG TERATOGENS THAT CAUSE MALFORMATIONS IN THE FETUS

Androgens (e.g., testosterone, methyltestosterone, fluoxymesterone, oxandrolone, oxymetholone, ethylestrenol, methandrostenolone, nandrolone, stanozolol)
Coumarin derivatives (warfarin, dicumarol)
Diethylstilbestrol (DES)
Ethanol (high, chronic doses)
Isotretinoin (Accutane)
Lithium
Methotrexate (and possibly other anticancer drugs)
Paramethadione (Paradione), trimethadione (Tridione)
Phenytoin (Dilantin)
Tetracyclines (demeclocycline, doxycycline, methacycline, minocycline, oxytetracycline, tetracycline)
Thalidomide (no longer available)
Valproic acid (Depakene, Depakote)

Alcohol. Use of alcohol by the expectant mother has been associated with a group of congenital malformations referred to as **fetal alcohol syndrome** (FAS). This syndrome is characterized by such anomalies as intrauterine growth retardation, facial abnormalities, cardiac defects, abnormalities of the limbs and joints, mental retardation, and developmental delays. At birth, the infant is usually small for gestational age, feeds poorly, is irritable, and has a high-pitched cry. The severity of the syndrome varies with the amount of alcohol consumed, so that the heavier the drinker, the greater the probability of severe congenital abnormalities.[32] More recent studies, however, have shown that women who drink alcohol in small amounts have a higher incidence of spontaneous abortion.[33] It is now recommended that women consume no alcohol during pregnancy because of the risks to the fetus.

Caffeine. The effect of caffeine in pregnancy is not well documented; there is no scientific evidence to conclude that caffeine is teratogenic.[34] Heavy maternal caffeine consumption may be related to intrauterine growth retardation as a result of reduction of blood flow to the uterus. Nurses should weigh evidence when counseling pregnant women about caffeine consumption (*see* Chapter 10).

Radiation. Exposure to radiation can have teratogenic effects; the nature of the malformation depends on the dose of radiation and the stage of development at which exposure occurred. Organogenesis is the period of development that is most sensitive to radiation. Gross skeletal and central nervous system anomalies are the most common manifestations. Other malformations include ophthalmic defects, impaired motor performance, spina bifida, cleft palate, and defects to the extremities.

Epidemiologic studies have so far indicated that diagnostic ultrasound does not have any measurable or significant biologic effects on the fetus. Additional studies related to microwaves indicate that this form of electromagnetic energy does not have the capacity to produce mutations. It appears from these studies that microwaves and ultrasound do not have sufficient energy to ionize molecules and disrupt DNA. The data on the effects of microwaves and ultrasound are controversial, however, and continued in-depth investigation of these energy sources is needed.

Properly constructed microwave ovens and video display terminals operated under normal conditions appear to emit no or minimal ionizing radiation; they are thus not currently considered a hazard to pregnant women.[35, 36]

Environmental Chemicals. Exposure to environmental chemicals is often beyond the expectant mother's control. One of the most well-documented teratogens in humans is methyl mercury, which has been found in contaminated coastal waters. Pregnant women who ate fish contaminated with this chemical gave birth to children with severe congenital anomalies. Lead, passive smoke, selenium, and a variety of pesticides are also suspected of causing birth defects.[29]

Occupational Hazards. Several occupational hazards have also been identified that may affect male and female reproduction and cause birth defects in the fetus (Table 11–7). Men and women should be made aware of these possible hazards, especially in the reproductive years, to prevent some of their effects on the parents and their offspring.

Guiding Principles for Client Education. When one considers the number of teratogens or possible teratogens that may affect parents and their offspring, it is essential to incorporate the possibility of exposure to these agents into the health history and nursing care plan. In teaching expectant parents about known and possible teratogens, certain principles guide the nurse:

1. In the broadest sense, a teratogen is any agent that can adversely affect the growth and development of the fetus.
2. The first trimester is a critical period in the development of the fetus. Exposure to teratogens at this time may cause severe congenital malformations.
3. Exposure to teratogens in the second and third trimesters can cause problems related to brain growth, intrauterine growth retardation, and developmental delays in children.
4. Neonatal complications such as drug withdrawal have been attributed to maternal drug intake.
5. Factors that are not associated with birth defects in animals may be teratogenic in humans.
6. Many of the defects caused by teratogens occur before the mother is even aware that she is pregnant; therefore, counseling should be provided prior to pregnancy.
7. Informed decision making concerning avoidance of known or suspected teratogens is the responsibility of the client and her family.

TABLE 11–7. OCCUPATIONAL HAZARDS THAT MAY CAUSE REPRODUCTIVE PROBLEMS OR FETAL CONGENITAL ANOMALIES

Occupation	Hazardous Substance
Textile and garment workers	Cotton and fiber dusts, noise, formaldehyde, dyes, heat, asbestos, solvents, flame retardants
Health personnel	Anesthetic gases, x-rays, alcohol, noise, laboratory chemicals
Electronic assemblers	Lead, tin, antimony, trichloroethylene, methylene chloride, resins
Hair dressers/cosmetologists	Hairspray resins, aerosol propellants, solvents, dyes
Cleaning personnel	Soaps, detergents, heat, enzymes, solvents
Launderers of industrially contaminated clothing	Various industrial chemicals
Photographic processors	Caustics, bromides, iodines, silver nitrate
Plastic workers	Acrylonitrile, formaldehyde, vinyl chloride
Transportation workers	Carbon monoxide, polynuclear aromatics, lead, vibration, microwaves
Painters	Lead, titanium, toluene
Clerks/Clerical workers	Trichloroethylene, carbon tetrachloride, formaldehyde, asbestos, cigarette smoke
Printing personnel	Ink mists, methanol, carbon tetrachloride, lead, noise, solvents, trichloroethylene

Reprinted, with permission, from Samuels M, Bennett HZ. Well Body Well Earth. *San Francisco: Sierra Club Books; 1983.*

With these principles in mind, the nurse should plan health education programs for couples prior to and during pregnancy so that exposure to teratogens can be prevented.

SUMMARY

Human development begins with the fertilization of an ovum by a sperm. The resulting microscopic one-celled organism eventually develops into a 7½-pound newborn. The periods of embryologic and fetal development are the most rapid periods of growth in life. The placenta and membranes protect and provide the essentials of life for the growing embryo/fetus.

Fertilization occurs in the ampulla of the fallopian tube. Both the sperm and the ovum undergo maturation processes prior to fertilization. The mature ovum is surrounded by two membranes, the zona pellucida and the corona radiata. These are the layers the sperm must penetrate to achieve fertilization. Once the sperm penetrates the ovum, the ovum responds by cortical and zona reactions, resumption of the second meiotic division, and metabolic activation.

The first 14 days of development, known as the pre-embryonic period, are characterized by rapid growth and development of the fertilized ovum. During the third to the eighth week of development, termed the embryonic period, all major organ systems are formed. It is during this period that the embryo is most susceptible to infectious or environmental agents. Maturation of the tissues and organs of the fetus occurs during the fetal period, which extends from the third lunar month through the tenth lunar month.

The placenta carries out two important functions during pregnancy, hormone production, and transport and exchange of products between the mother and fetus. Hormone production is essential to maintaining the pregnancy; transport and exchange functions nourish and protect the developing embryo and fetus.

During the period of embryologic and fetal growth and development, a variety of viruses, drugs, and environmental hazards may place the developing human at risk. It is important that the expectant couple understand embryologic and fetal growth and development and the possible risks to development so that they can protect and nurture their infant before he or she is born. The nurse acts as health educator and consultant to the family and provides them with information that will encourage positive health care behaviors during the period of embryologic and fetal development.

REVIEW QUESTIONS

1. Identify the changes in the ovum and the sperm at conception.
2. Describe the fertilization process.
3. Discuss the response of the ovum after penetration by the sperm.
4. Describe the development of the fertilized ovum in the pre-embryonic period.
5. Compare and contrast the decidua basalis, decidua capsularis, and decidua vera.
6. Relate the body structures derived from the ectoderm, endoderm, and mesoderm.
7. Describe the development of the fetus during the fetal period.
8. Describe three environmental agents and their known or possible effects on the embryo/fetus.

REFERENCES

1. Cunningham FG, et al. *Williams Obstetrics.* 18th ed. Norwalk, Conn: Appleton & Lange; 1989.
2. Rugh R, Shettles LB. *From Conception to Birth: The Drama of Life's Beginnings.* New York: Harper & Row; 1971.
3. Sadler TW. *Langman's Medical Embryology.* Baltimore: Williams & Wilkins; 1985.
4. Moore KL. *Before We Are Born: Basic Embryology and Birth Defects.* 3rd ed. Philadelphia: WB Saunders; 1989.
5. Tortora GJ, Anagnostakos NP. *Principles of Anatomy and Physiology.* New York: Harper & Row; 1984.
6. Moore KL. *The Developing Human: Clinically Oriented Embryology.* Philadelphia: WB Saunders; 1982.
7. Danforth DN, Scott JR, eds. *Obstetrics and Gynecology.* Philadelphia: JB Lippincott; 1986.
8. Ramsey EM. What we have learned about placental circulation. *J Reprod Med.* 1985;30:312–317.
9. Koffler H. Fetal and neonatal physiology. *Clin Obstet Gynecol.* 1981;24:545–556.
10. Vorherr H. Factors influencing fetal growth. *Am J Obstet Gynecol.* 1982;142:577–587.
11. Kresch MJ, Gross I. The biochemistry of fetal lung development. *Clin Perinatol.* 1987;14:481–504.
12. Behrman RE, Vaughan VC. *Nelson Textbook of Pediatrics.* 12th ed. Philadelphia: WB Saunders; 1983.
13. Pernoll ML, Benson RC, eds. *Current Obstetric & Gynecologic Diagnosis & Treatment 1987.* Norwalk, Conn: Appleton & Lange; 1987.
14. Knuppel RA, Goodlin RC. Maternal-placental-fetal unit: fetal

& early neonatal physiology. In: Pernoll ML, Benson RC, eds. *Current Obstetric & GynecologicDiagnosis & Treatment 1987.* Norwalk, Conn: Appleton & Lange; 1987:135–160.

15. Creager J. *Human Anatomy and Physiology.* Belmont, Calif: Wadsworth; 1983.
16. Dilts PV. Placental transfer. *Clin Obstet Gynecol.* 1981;24: 555–559.
17. Reedy NJ, et al. Intrauterine fetal surgery: a nursing challenge. *J Obstet Gynecol Neonat Nurs.* 1984;13:291–295.
18. Blakeslee S. Fetus returned to womb following surgery. *The New York Times.* Oct 7, 1986;136:C1, C3.
19. Shepard TH. Human teratogenicity. *Adv Pediatr.* 1986;33: 225–268.
20. Shepard TH. Detection of human teratogenic agents. *J Pediatr Med.* 1982;101:810.
21. Goldman AS. Critical periods of prenatal insults. In: Schwartz, R, Sumner J, eds. *Drug and Chemical Risks to the Fetus and Newborn.* New York: Alan R. Liss, Inc.; 1980:9–31.
22. Desmonts G. General conclusions on the workshop on infectious diseases. In: Marios M, ed. *Prevention of Physical and Mental Congenital Defects, Part B: Epidemiology, Early Detection and Therapy, and Environmental Factors.* New York: Alan R. Liss, Inc.; 1985.
23. Foster SD. Education, the best defense against AIDS. *Am J Matern Child Nurs.* 1987;12:311.
24. Knuppel RA, Drukker JE. *High-Risk Pregnancy: A Team Approach.* Philadelphia: WB Saunders; 1986.
25. Cushner IM. Maternal behavior and perinatal risks: alcohol, smoking and drugs. *Ann Rev Pub Health.* 1981;2:201.
26. Picone T, et al. Pregnancy outcome in North American women: effects of diet, cigarette smoking, and psychological stress on maternal weight gain. *Am J Clin Nutr.* 1982;36: 1205.
27. Stein Z, Kline J. Smoking, alcohol, and reproduction. *Am J Pub Health.* 1983;73:1154.
28. Asch RH, Smith CG. Effects of marijuana on reproduction. *Contemp Obstet Gynecol.* Oct 1982:217.
29. Henomer O, et al. *Birth Defects and Drugs in Pregnancy.* Boston, Mass: Publishing Science Group, Inc; 1980.
30. Offspring of women given DES during pregnancy remain under study. *JAMA* 1977;238:932.
31. Ians JD, Rayburn EF. *Drug Use During Pregnancy.* Portland, Oregon: Perinatal Press. 1980;4:134.
32. Shinono PH, et al. Smoking and drinking during pregnancy. *JAMA* 1986:225.
33. Kuse J, et al. Changes in smoking and alcohol consumption during pregnancy: a population-based study in a rural area. *Obstet Gynecol.* 1986;67:627–631.
34. Dews P, et al. Report of the 4th International Caffeine Workshop, Athens, 1982. *Food and Chemical Toxicol.* 1982; 22:163.
35. Jankowski CB. Radiation and pregnancy: putting the risks in proportion. *Am J Nurs.* 1986;86:260–265.
36. Brent RL. The effects of embryonic and fetal exposure to x-ray, microwaves, and ultrasound. *Clin Perinatol.* 1986;13: 615–648.

The First Trimester of Pregnancy

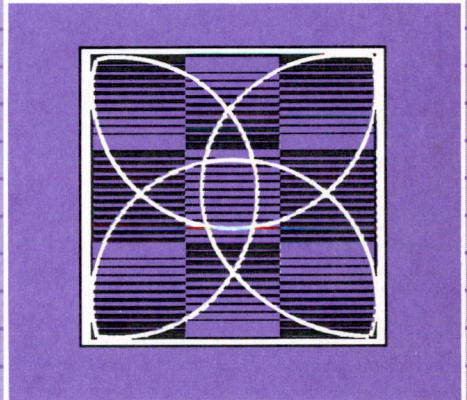

unit 3

Physiologic Changes During the First Trimester

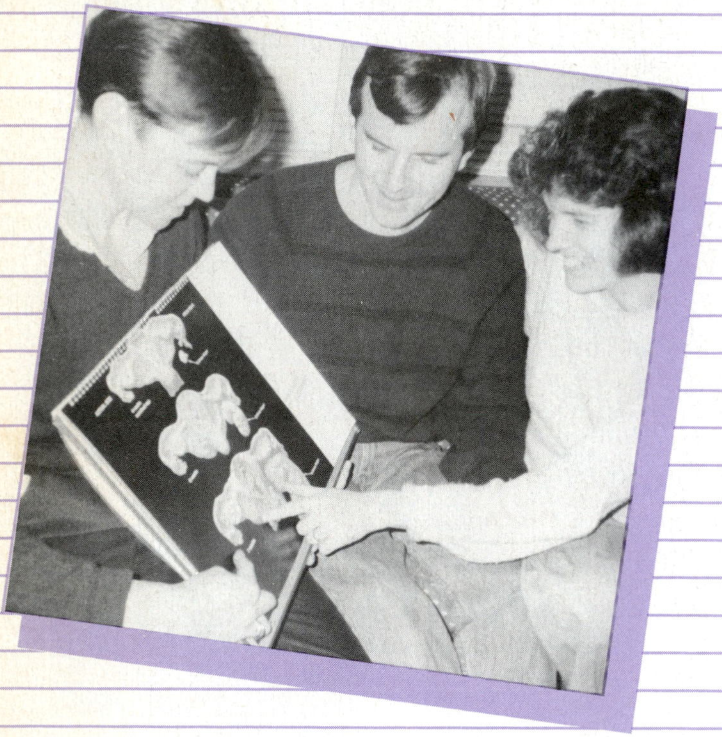

Chapter 12

Key Terms

Braxton Hicks contractions
Braun von Fernwald's sign
Chadwick's sign
Goodell's sign
Hegar's sign
Ladin's sign
leukorrhea
linea nigra
McDonald's sign
mucus plug
Piskacek's sign
ptyalism
telangiectasis
vascular spiders

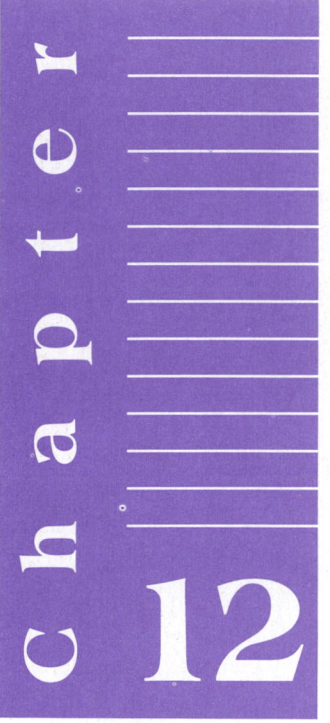

The first 12 weeks of pregnancy are generally referred to as the first trimester. From the moment of conception, changes begin to take place throughout the woman's body. Physiologic adaptation to pregnancy is necessary to sustain the growing products of conception for a total period of about 40 weeks and to maintain a state of wellness as the woman's body prepares for labor, delivery, and lactation. Nursing care during the first trimester is built on an understanding of normal physiologic changes of early pregnancy.

The division of pregnancy into trimesters is artificial and therefore not exact. Profound changes take place among early, middle, and late stages of pregnancy, however, and a trimester approach fosters understanding of these changes. The physiology of pregnancy is extremely complex and in many cases not completely understood. In studying basic changes in pregnancy, the learner must remember that the overall level of wellness reflects the interaction of physiologic and psychosocial factors.

Nutrition is essential to pregnancy and to good health. Nutrition during pregnancy is discussed in Chapter 10, and certain high-risk nutritional concerns are described in Chapters 38 and 39.

GROWTH AND DEVELOPMENT OF THE EMBRYO/FETUS

Prenatal care always encompasses the changes occurring in the embryo/fetus, as well as the changes taking place in the mother. Growth and development of the embryo/fetus have already been discussed in Chapter 11. The first 8 weeks of gestation are called the embryonic period, and week 9 to delivery is known as the fetal period. During the first trimester, rapid cell division occurs in the embryo. By the end of the first lunar month, the foundation for all major organ systems has been laid, the heart begins to beat, and many other changes are taking place. Environmental insults, such as the use of drugs by the

ISSUES AND CONTROVERSIES

Should all women of childbearing age be considered potentially pregnant? This will have major implications for vendors who sell women cigarettes or alcohol, pharmacists who sell women over-the-counter medications, or pediatricians who immunize adolescents of childbearing age for rubella. Should women have to document their nonpregnant status before buying certain potentially toxic products or engaging in activities potentially detrimental to an embryo/fetus? How will current state legislative decisions concerning reproductive health affect women's freedom and health?

mother, can affect the formation of the organ systems in the developing embryo/fetus. By the end of the first trimester, developmental "milestones" include maturation of the fetal gallbladder, spleen, and pancreas. Fingernails and toenails are present, and the external genitalia may often be identified as male or female.[1] To support the developing pregnancy, the placenta is also forming during the first trimester.

MATERNAL PHYSIOLOGIC ADAPTATION

From the time of conception, physiologic changes take place in the woman's body. These changes support and nourish the products of conception; prepare the expectant mother's body for labor, delivery, and lactation; and help to maintain a state of maternal and fetal wellness. The nurse can help the family prepare for and cope with these changes to promote a healthy outcome for mother and fetus. Maternal physiologic responses to the first trimester are discussed in this section and summarized in Table 12–1.

Reproductive System

Uterus. In the nonpregnant woman, the uterus has a capacity of 10 mL or less. During pregnancy, however, this muscular organ has the ability to expand 500 to 1000 times its nonpregnant capacity. After pregnancy the uterus is able to shrink almost to its original size. No other healthy organ in the human body undergoes such enormous change within such a short period.[2,3]

Several days after ovulation, the uterine endometrium is in the secretory phase (*see* Chapter 6). The endometrium responds to progesterone secretion by the ovary to prepare for implantation of the fertilized ovum. After conception, the endometrium of pregnancy is referred to as the decidua. The decidua remains throughout pregnancy; most of it is shed when the pregnancy is completed. Decidual cells hypertrophy, become very vascular, and extend over the entire endometrial surface.

The decidua is divided into three portions. The part of the decidua that lies over the developing embryo is referred to as the decidua capsularis. The portion of the decidua directly beneath the implantation site is called the decidua basalis. The remainder of the decidua, not in contact with the embryo, is referred to as the decidua vera (Figure 12–1).

Estrogen, secreted by the ovarian follicle, and progesterone, secreted by the corpus luteum in the first few months of pregnancy, stimulate hyperplasia and hypertrophy of the uterine myometrial cells. For example, muscle fibers become seven to ten times longer and two to seven times wider during pregnancy. Unlike uterine hypertrophy in later pregnancy, uterine hypertrophy during the first trimester is not thought to result primarily from pressure from the growing products of conception. Indeed, uterine changes occur during ectopic pregnancies when the embryo implants in a fallopian tube or ovary and not in the uterus.[2]

During the first few weeks of pregnancy, the uterus retains its usual pear shape. By the third month, however, the fundus and corpus have become almost spherical. The growth of the uterus is greater in the fundus than in the rest of the organ.

The position of the uterus also changes in the first trimester, to reflect its expanding size. By the end of the first trimester, the uterus is too large to be contained within the pelvis and may be palpated above the symphysis pubis (Figure 12–2).

Beginning in the first trimester and continuing throughout pregnancy, the uterus contracts irregularly. These contractions, known as **Braxton Hicks contractions,** are usually painless, although some women may experience cramping-type sensations. In normal circumstances, these contractions are not associated with bleeding of any kind or with dilation of the cervix. During the first trimester, the Braxton Hicks contractions are mild, occur infrequently, and usually cannot be felt on examination.

Cervix. During pregnancy, the cervix serves the essential function of keeping the fetus within the uterus and avoiding premature delivery.[4] In a classic study, Danforth demonstrated that the human cervix is composed largely of fibrous connective tissue, or collagen.[5] Smooth muscle constitutes about 15 percent of the cervix. As pregnancy progresses, synthesis and breakdown of collagen are thought to increase.

TABLE 12–1. SUMMARY OF PHYSIOLOGIC CHANGES DURING THE FIRST TRIMESTER

Organ	Change
Reproductive System	

Uterus	Uterus increases in size (size doubles by 10 weeks)
	Uterus enlarges asymmetrically until 10 weeks, softens
	  Ladin's sign
	  Piskacek's sign
	  McDonald's sign
	  Braun von Fernwald's sign
	Uterus changes position; rises out of pelvis by end of first trimester
	Number of muscle fibers increases
	Muscle fibers elongate and widen
	Braxton Hicks contractions begin, but are usually not felt
	Endometrium changes to decidua

Cervix	Cervix softens
	  Goodell's sign
	  Hegar's sign
	Vascularity increases
	Vasocongestion causes bluish color (Chadwick's sign)
	Cervical glands increase activity; leukorrhea occurs
	Mucous plug forms
	Lengthens

Vagina	Vascularity increases Vasocongestion causes bluish color (Chadwick's sign) Vagina softens Glycogen content of epithelium increases pH becomes acidic (3.5–6.0) Changes predispose to yeast infections
Fallopian tubes	Few structural changes occur Epithelium flattens Site of fertilization (distal one third) produces ductal fluid to nourish fertilized ovum and help cleavage
Ovary	Ovulation stops after conception Corpus luteum enlarges to about one-third the size of ovary Corpus luteum secretes hormones to support beginning pregnancy (including estrogens, progesterone, relaxin)
Breasts	Mammary ducts and alveoli hypertrophy Breasts swell, become tender Blood flow increases Montgomery tubercles start to become more pronounced Pigment of nipple and areola begins to darken Little or no breast secretion occurs
Cardiovascular System	Cardiac output increases Blood volume begins to increase Resting pulse increases (about 8 beats per minute over nonpregnant rate) Blood pressure remains unchanged Heart murmurs may develop White blood cell count increases Red blood cells show little or no change Certain clotting factors increase
Respiratory System	
Lungs	Tidal volume increases Total oxygen-carrying capacity of red blood cells increases Inspiratory capacity begins to increase Woman breathes more deeply Lungs perform more efficiently Respiratory rate shows little or no change Oxygen consumption by other organ systems increases
Respiratory passages	Hormonally induced vasocongestion and edema of mucous membranes cause nasal stuffiness, nosebleeds, discharge, and general feelings of congestion

(continued)

TABLE 12–1. SUMMARY OF PHYSIOLOGIC CHANGES DURING THE FIRST TRIMESTER *(continued)*

Organ	Change
Urinary System	Kidneys increase in size and weight Glomerular filtration rate and renal plasma flow increase Ureters, renal pelves, and renal calcyes dilate Woman is prone to urinary tract infections Excretion of such substances as glucose and water-soluble vitamins increases Blood urea nitrogen and creatinine levels in urine decrease, blood levels remain unaffected
Musculoskeletal System	Clinical changes are minimal
Integument	
Skin	Pigmentation begins to increase Linea nigra appears Areola and nipples darken Increased blood flow to skin gives feelings of warmth Vascular spiders may develop Some skin conditions improve; some worsen Allergic sensitivity increases Activity of sebaceous and sweat glands increases
Hair	New hair continues to grow at usual pace Hair does not fall out as fast, and thus seems thicker Growth of fine, downy hair begins to increase
Nails	Nails begin to grow faster Nails soften
Gastrointestinal System	Hyperemia of tissues in mouth begins in response to elevated hormones Gums become extra-sensitive to irritants Changes are mostly hormonally induced; uterus as yet too small to cause changes related to its expanding size Motility and tone of gastrointestinal tract decrease Pepsin and HCl decrease Time for absorption of nutrients increases Iron absorption from small intestine increases Water absorption from large intestine increases Nausea and vomiting are experienced Appetite changes Ptyalism occurs Altered taste and smell Nutritional requirements change
Endocrine System	*See* Table 12–2
Pituitary	Anterior pituitary enlarges slightly Hypothalamus inhibits luteinizing and follicle-stimulating hormones Hormones are secreted to foster development of pregnancy and development of breasts
Thyroid	Thyroid enlarges BMR increases Free T_3 and T_4 do not rise significantly; total T_3 and T_4 begin to rise
Parathyroids	Parathyroids enlarge Parathyroid hormone level may decrease
Adrenals	Adrenal cortex begins to hypertrophy Adrenocorticotropic hormone and cortisol decrease Aldosterone increases
Pancreas	Insulin production decreases in response to fetal demands for glucose
Placenta	Placenta develops and becomes fully functioning

T_3 = triiodothyronine, T_4 = 3, 5,3′,5′ = tetraiodothyronine = thyroxine, BMR = basal metabolic rate.

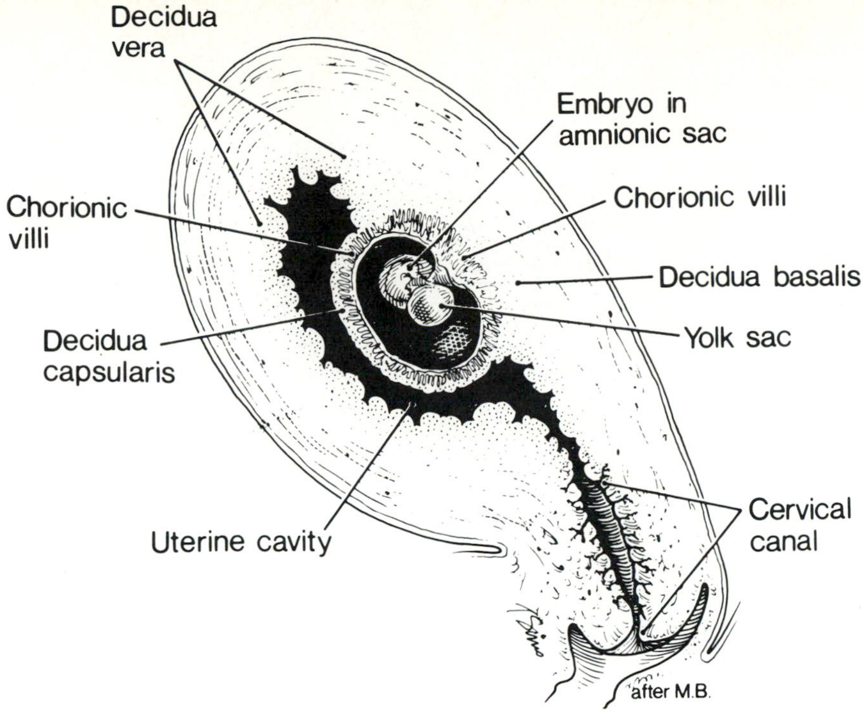

Figure 12–1. The decidua of pregnancy. (*Reproduced, with permission, from Cunningham FG, et al.* Williams Obstetrics. *18th ed. Norwalk, Conn: Appleton & Lange; 1989:53.*)

Through complex processes, the concentration and stability of the collagen content in the cervix decrease. This may contribute to the softening of the cervix.[6] By 10 weeks, connective tissue changes, such as a small decrease in cervical collagen and a moderate increase in collagen breakdown activity, are noted.[7,8]

Hormones such as estrogen may affect cervical softening as early as the first month after conception. The nonpregnant cervix is firm, like the tip of the nose; in pregnancy, it softens to the consistency of the lips. This softening is called **Goodell's sign.**[9] Goodell's sign is thought to be the result of increased blood flow to the cervix and hypertrophy of the cervical glands. Increased vascularity also causes the cervix, as well as the vagina and vulva, to appear dark blue—**Chadwick's sign.**

Hypertrophy of the cervical glands during the first trimester causes a thick mucus to form. The woman may experience a fairly heavy, whitish vaginal discharge, referred to as **leukorrhea.** Mucus also blocks the cervical canal. This **mucous plug** acts as a barrier to protect the fetus from some infections. The mucous plug normally remains in place until the onset of labor, when it is expelled (*see* Figure 16–2). The cervix also begins to increase in length. By 13 weeks the cervix measures about 43.0 mm.[4]

Vagina. The vagina, like the uterus and cervix, demonstrates increased vascularity and softening as a result of increased estrogen secretion. During the first trimester of pregnancy, the vaginal epithelium resembles the epithelium found during the luteal phase of the menstrual cycle. Hyperemia and the proliferation of vaginal cells cause the vagina, like the cervix, to appear dark blue (Chadwick's sign).

As estrogen levels rise, the glycogen content of the vaginal epithelium increases. A thick, white vaginal discharge results. As discussed earlier, active cervical cells also produce thick white secretions at this time. This discharge should never be bloody or have a foul odor. Lactic acid is produced by lactobacillus, an organism normally found in the vagina. This results in an acidic vaginal pH, ranging from 3.5 to 6.0. The acidic vaginal environment helps to control the growth of harmful bacteria and therefore protects the mother and fetus. The glycogen-rich environment also fosters the development of yeast (*Candida albicans*) infections. Although a normal occurrence during pregnancy, yeast infections can be unpleasant and uncomfortable for the woman.

Fallopian Tubes. The fallopian tubes undergo few structural changes during pregnancy. The ovum is fertilized by the sperm in the distal third of the fallopian tube and is transported to the uterus by muscular contractions and ciliary movements within the tube. The fallopian tube produces ductal fluid, which provides nutrition to the fertilized ovum and assists in the cleavage of the gametes. During the first tri-

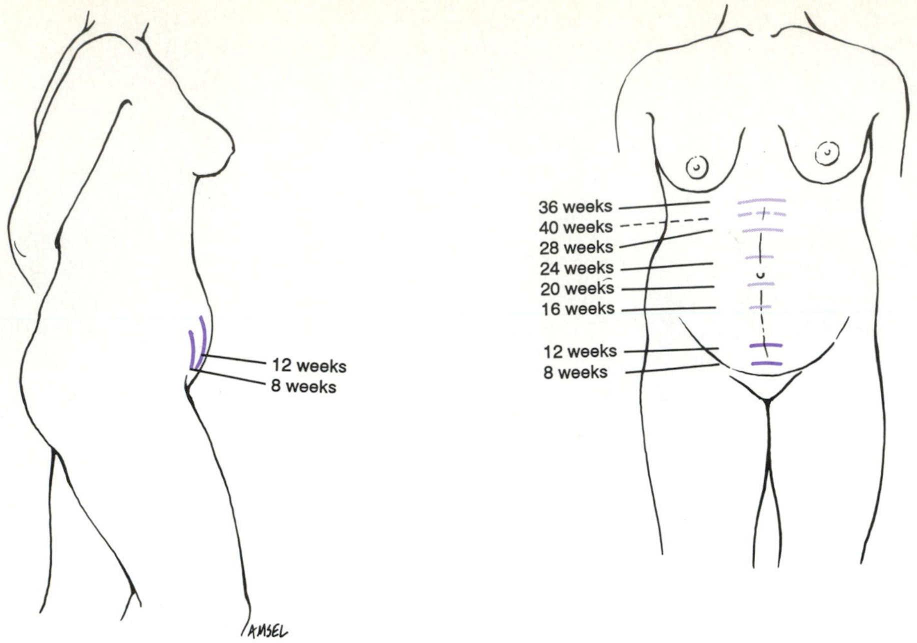

Figure 12–2. Height of the fundus at 8 and 12 weeks.

mester of pregnancy, the epithelium of the mucosa in the tube flattens; it remains flattened throughout gestation.

Ovary. Ovulation does not take place during pregnancy; however, normal ovarian function during the first trimester is necessary for pregnancy to progress. When conception occurs, the corpus luteum of the menstrual cycle becomes the corpus luteum of pregnancy. The corpus luteum is most active during the first 6 to 7 weeks of gestation while the placenta is developing. The corpus luteum of pregnancy secretes progesterone, which (1) prepares the uterine endometrium for implantation, (2) helps to maintain the pregnancy, and (3) assists in the development of the placenta. (*See* Table 12–2, which summarizes the effects of progesterone.)

High levels of estrogens and progesterone help maintain the corpus luteum of pregnancy. Circulating estrogens and progesterone inhibit the secretion of follicle-stimulating hormone and luteinizing hormone by the anterior pituitary. Suppression of new follicles, along with the secretion of human chorionic gonadotropin hormone by the trophoblast, sustains the corpus luteum until the placenta matures.

A functioning corpus luteum is necessary for implantation to take place. Beyond the early part of pregnancy, however, the developing placenta is thought to produce enough progesterone to maintain pregnancy; the corpus luteum is therefore not necessary for a pregnancy to continue.[2]

In addition to progesterone secretion, the corpus luteum of pregnancy also secretes the hormone relaxin. The role of relaxin, which is also produced by the placenta, is unclear and controversial. Some researchers believe that during pregnancy relaxin has a role in "relaxing" the symphysis pubis and other pelvic joints and in "ripening" or softening the cervix in preparation for labor.[10–12] Others believe that relaxin has no significant role in human pregnancy.[2]

The corpus luteum of pregnancy enlarges to about one-third the size of the ovary at its peak during the first trimester. As expected, the ovary containing the corpus luteum remains larger than the other ovary. Once the placenta develops, the corpus luteum degenerates.

Breasts. Changes in the breasts may be one of the woman's first signs of pregnancy. Early in the first trimester, the woman experiences tingling, fullness, and tenderness in the breasts. Some women report that early-pregnancy breast sensations are similar to those experienced immediately prior to the onset of menses. By the second month of pregnancy, the breasts increase in size as a result of hypertrophy of the mammary ducts and alveoli. The Montgomery tubercles, hypertrophic sebaceous glands scattered in the areolae, also become more prominent. Blood flow to the breasts increases. These changes reflect the influence of progesterone and estrogens, which also cause the nipples and areolae of the breasts to become darker and the nipples to become more erectile. Breast secretion does not usually begin until the second trimester, about the 16th week (*see* Chapters 16 and 20).

Cardiovascular System

During pregnancy, the cardiovascular system undergoes profound changes; however, the low-risk, healthy woman should be able to tolerate these changes well. Although changes in the cardiovascular system begin during the first trimester, the major changes occur during the second and third trimesters (*see* Chapters 16 and 20). Factors such as the woman's emotional state, her body position, and the temperature of the environment (e.g., very hot weather) can affect the cardiovascular system.

During the first trimester, cardiac output begins to increase. During the second trimester, cardiac output reaches a peak of 30 to 50 percent above the nonpregnant output. In the later stages of pregnancy, particularly the last 9 weeks, cardiac output actually falls. Cardiac output reflects stroke volume and heart rate. The increase in cardiac output early in pregnancy is due largely to an increase in stroke volume. Later in pregnancy, stroke volume falls but heart rate increases, becoming the major determinant of cardiac output.[13] Cardiac output can be greatly influenced by the mother's position; however, the effects are seen predominantly in the second and third trimesters (*see* Chapters 16 and 20).

During pregnancy there is a change in the resting pulse rate. In the first trimester, the pulse rate may increase about 8 to 10 beats per minute over nonpregnant levels.

Increase in cardiac output and pulse rate might be expected to raise blood pressure, as in the nonpregnant state; however, blood pressure usually remains unchanged during the first trimester and declines in the second trimester. A decrease in peripheral resistance, perhaps associated with factors such as the development of new vascular beds and hormone-related relaxation of smooth muscles within the walls of arterioles, might account for the decline in blood pressure in the second trimester.[14]

As many as 90 percent of pregnant women may develop a physiologic heart murmur during pregnancy.[12] This pulmonic systolic flow murmur reflects increased plasma volume. Any woman with a cardiac murmur should be evaluated carefully to rule out the presence of true cardiac pathology.

Total blood volume increases about 40 percent during pregnancy, and this increase begins during the first trimester (*see* Figure 16–3).[15] The increase in blood volume is probably related to the formation of uterine arteriovenous shunts. Because plasma volume increases faster than red cell mass, the hematocrit decreases in the second trimester. The increase in plasma volume determines maternal cardiac output and the degree of physiologic anemia. The greater the plasma volume expansion, the greater the decline in hematocrit.

Leukocyte count increases during pregnancy, beginning in the first trimester. The leukocyte count ranges from 5000/mm^3 to 12,000/mm^3, with an average of 10,000/mm^3 to 11,000/mm^3. Neutrophils normally peak at the time of ovulation; if conception takes places, the neutrophil count continues to rise. Neutrophils reach a peak during the third trimester and return to prepregnancy levels around the sixth day postpartum.[16] Other white blood cell components, such as lymphocytes and monocytes, remain unchanged during the first trimester.

Several blood clotting factors are also increased throughout pregnancy. These include factors VII, IX, and X, as well as plasma fibrinogen (factor I). Changes in blood clotting factors are detectable from about the third month of pregnancy.[16]

Respiratory System

Changes in the maternal respiratory system take place along with changes in the maternal cardiovascular system.[13,17] The tidal volume, or amount of air breathed in one cycle of ordinary inspiration and expiration, increases, beginning in the first trimester. The total increase during pregnancy is about 35 to 50 percent. Inspiratory capacity, which includes the tidal volume and the greatest volume of air that can be breathed in from the end of the last resting expiration, begins to increase during the first trimester; its peak increase of 5 to 10 percent occurs during the second trimester. Vital capacity remains unchanged.

Beginning in the first trimester, oxygen consumption by various organ systems, as well as by the fetus and placenta, increases (*see* Figure 20–3). To compensate for the increased oxygen demands of the fetus and maternal organs, the woman breathes more deeply. Higher levels of estrogen and progesterone may reduce pulmonary resistance. The respiratory rate changes little throughout pregnancy. Many of the other respiratory changes become more pronounced during the second and third trimesters.

During the first trimester, capillary dilation takes place throughout the respiratory tract. This results in engorgement of the nasopharynx, larynx, trachea, and bronchi. Voice changes and such unpleasant conditions as nasal stuffiness and nosebleeds (epistaxis) may be experienced.[17] Women should not assume they have "colds," and should be advised never to take any medication without first consulting their prenatal care provider.

Urinary System

The pregnant woman's urinary system undergoes structural and functional changes during pregnancy. These compensate for the heavier workload demanded by the increase in maternal metabolic products and the excretion of fetal waste products.

The kidneys increase in size and weight throughout pregnancy. In the first trimester, the ureters, renal pelves, and renal calyces dilate. This may be due to the influence of progesterone, which decreases the tone of smooth muscle. The dilation of these structures contributes to stasis of urine. Therefore, the pregnant woman becomes prone to urinary tract infections.

The bladder is a pressure-sensitive organ. The pressure generated by the collection of urine is responsible for the sensation of having to void.[9] During the first trimester, the growing uterus also puts pressure on the bladder. This may decrease bladder capacity and may mimic the sensation of bladder fullness. The woman may experience urinary frequency and complain of needing to void often. The urine, however, should remain clear; burning sensations are not normal and may indicate the presence of urinary tract infections.

Changes in kidney function during pregnancy are thought to be the result of increased levels of maternal and placental hormones, such as adrenocorticotropic hormone, antidiuretic hormone (ADH), aldosterone, cortisol, and thyroid hormone.[2,18] The glomerular filtration rate (GFR), the rate of movement of substances from the blood to the lumen of the kidney, and renal plasma flow (RPF), the return of substances to the plasma, also increase. The GFR increases by as much as 50 percent and RPF by 25 to 50 percent during the first trimester. With the rise in filtration rate, increased excretion of such substances as glucose, water-soluble vitamins, and amino acids is common during pregnancy. This highlights the importance of adequate nutritional intake during pregnancy (*see* Chapter 10).

Blood urea nitrogen (BUN) and serum creatinine levels decrease during pregnancy. There is more fluid and less solute, because of the higher GFR; therefore, their concentration in urine decreases. During pregnancy, BUN decreases from nonpregnant levels of 13 ± 3mg/100 mL to the pregnant levels of 8.17 ± 1.5 mg/100 mL, and serum creatinine decreases from the nonpregnant levels of 0.67 ± 0.14 mg/100 mL to the pregnant levels of 0.46 ± 0.13 mg/100 mL.[13] Values that would be considered normal in a nonpregnant woman, BUN of 12.0 and creatinine of 0.7, can actually indicate kidney pathology during pregnancy.

In the normal, nonpregnant woman, glucose is usually reabsorbed well in the renal tubules. Glucose appears in the nonpregnant woman's urine at blood levels exceeding 160 to 180 mg/dL. For some reason, this process is not as effective during pregnancy, and 1+ to 4+ glucose levels may be identified in the urine, although blood levels are actually less than 160 mg/dL. Some women do develop diabetes during pregnancy. Women with glucosuria therefore need to be evaluated further (*see* Chapter 39).

A daily total up to 150 mg of protein may normally be excreted in the urine. This can rise during pregnancy to 250 mg of protein per 24 hours.[19] Under healthy conditions, proteinuria should not exceed 10 to 20 mg/100 mL or "trace" by dipstick. Larger concentrations (1+ or greater by dipstick) can signal high-risk conditions, such as renal disease or pregnancy-induced hypertension (*see* Chapter 39). At times, however, readings of proteinuria may be the result of poor urine collection technique.

During pregnancy, fluid and electrolyte regulation alters, progressively, so that by term the pregnant woman is in a state of physiologic hypervolemia.

Several factors influence fluid volume and electrolyte balance during pregnancy. These include[20]:

- complex interactions among hormones such as estrogen, progesterone, prolactin, human placental lactogen, and substances such as aldosterone. Certain actions promote sodium and water excretion, while others oppose these processes.
- increase in glomerular filtration rate (promotes sodium excretion)
- decrease in renal vascular resistance (promotes sodium excretion)
- decrease in plasma albumin concentration (promotes sodium excretion)
- decrease in mean arterial pressure (opposes sodium excretion)
- increase in uterine blood vessels

- increase in renal excretion of bicarbonate, which prevents respiratory alkalosis as the Pco_2 blood levels decrease

Musculoskeletal System

Changes in the musculoskeletal system are thought to evolve from hormonal influences and from expansion of the uterus. Changes are usually clinically unremarkable during the first trimester; however, changes that occur during the second and third trimesters are important (*see* Chapters 16 and 20).

Integument

Integumentary changes occur throughout pregnancy. The most pronounced changes occur during the second and third trimester (*see* Chapters 16 and 20). Integumentary changes involve the skin, hair, nails, and sebaceous glands.

During the first trimester, skin pigmentation begins to darken. For example, the **linea nigra,** a dark line that reaches from the symphysis pubis to the top of the fundus, appears during the first trimester. Estrogen, progesterone, and melanocyte-stimulating hormone have been theorized to have effects on skin pigmentation during pregnancy; however, the exact cause of color changes in the skin is unclear.[2,21]

Telangiectases, often called **vascular spiders,** may occur as early as the second month and continue to appear through the ninth month.[21] Telangiectases are small, dilated end-arterioles that are thought to be related to increased estrogen production. Appearing "spiderlike," telangiectases have a raised red center and may be identified on the face, neck, chest, arms, and legs. Although upsetting to some women, they are not pathologic and disappear shortly after delivery.

Capillary hemangiomas reflect the increase in skin vascularity that occurs during pregnancy.[21] Appearing mostly on the head and neck and on the gums, these hemangiomas do not fade completely after childbirth.

As early as the first trimester, some women report that their skin becomes "oilier." In many women the skin assumes a "pregnancy glow." For the normal woman, the skin mirrors an overall healthy radiance. Certain skin conditions, such as psoriasis, may actually improve during pregnancy. Other dermatologic problems, such as acne vulgaris, may become worse during the first trimester. Some women experience increased sensitivity to skin care products and certain materials. Women may also sweat more, as a result of an increase in hormonally affected sweat production.

Throughout pregnancy, women may experience changes in their hair, possibly related to estrogens. The rate of hair growth does not change; however, hair follicles tend to last longer. The combination of new hair growth and longer life of "old" hair leads some women to report thicker hair throughout pregnancy.[14] An increase in fine, downy hair on the face and other body parts may be noted. This disappears after the birth of the baby, although any new growth of small, coarse dark hairs may remain.

As early as the seventh week, women may observe that their nails have become softer and break more easily; however, fingernail growth tends to increase, possibly in relation to increased blood flow to the hands.[14]

Gastrointestinal System

The gastrointestinal system undergoes several changes in the first trimester of pregnancy. Although pregnancy-related changes produce gastrointestinal discomforts, the function of the gastrointestinal tract is not greatly altered in the healthy woman.[22] Most first-trimester changes are hormonal, as the uterus is as yet too small to exert pressure on abdominal organs.

During the first trimester, under the influence of estrogen and progesterone, the tissues in the mouth become hyperemic. Higher hormonal levels may be related to greater gingival reactions to irritants in dental plaque.[23] Inadequate dental hygiene and poor diet will result in bleeding gums. Clients with bleeding gums should be referred for further dental evaluation.

Under the influence of progesterone, there is relaxation of smooth muscle, associated with decreased motility and tone of the gastrointestinal tract. The stomach takes longer to empty. Beginning during the first trimester, in response to higher levels of estrogens, the stomach produces less hydrochloric acid and pepsin and becomes less sensitive to histamines. A lower incidence of peptic ulcer problems during pregnancy is a beneficial side effect of this physiologic change.

The decrease in motility assists in the absorption of nutrients needed by the fetus at this time. Decreased motility within the small intestine allows more time for nutrients such as iron to be reabsorbed. In the large intestine, an increased amount of water is absorbed. Constipation is an unpleasant related effect (*see* later).

About 50 percent of pregnant women experience nausea and vomiting during the first trimester.[24,25] These symptoms may be related to several factors, including alteration in carbohydrate metabolism, causing the mother to experience hypoglycemia; decreased motility and tone of the gastrointestinal tract; increased levels of human chorionic gonadotropin; emotional reaction to pregnancy; and maternal hypotension.

During the first trimester, women may experience **ptyalism,** defined as "excessive secretion of saliva."[21] This condition almost always is associated with nausea. It is estimated that a normal volume of 1 to 2 L of saliva is secreted each day. The sensation of having too much saliva may occur because of the nauseated woman's difficulty in swallowing her saliva, rather than any real change in secretion. Changes in taste, including a "bitter" or "metallic" taste, may occur in addition to changes in smell.

During the first month of pregnancy, a woman may experience an increase in appetite. During the second month, however, nausea and vomiting, along with alterations in taste and smell, may affect the amount and type of foods and beverages ingested.

The physiologic changes that occur in the mother and the fetus during the first trimester of pregnancy are accompanied by specific nutritional requirements. These are discussed in Chapter 10.

Changes affecting the gallbladder, liver, and pancreas usually are not clinically significant during the first trimester.

Endocrine System

Health and physiologic adaptation to pregnancy evolves, in part, from complex interactions of many hormones secreted by various organs within the body. During the first trimester of pregnancy, hormones are secreted by the maternal endocrine glands, the trophoblast, the corpus luteum, and the developing placenta. Table 12–2 summarizes the major endocrine/hormonal activity throughout pregnancy.

Pituitary. The majority of the changes in the pituitary gland take place in the anterior lobe, which enlarges during pregnancy, mostly in response to increasing secretion of prolactin. For the first 7 to 10 weeks of gestation, the anterior pituitary secretes luteinizing hormone (LH), which helps to maintain the corpus luteum of pregnancy. After this time, elevated progesterone and estrogen levels induce the hypothalamus, for the rest of the pregnancy, to inhibit the release of LH and follicle-stimulating hormone (FSH) by the anterior pituitary.

Other hormones are secreted by the anterior pituitary during pregnancy. These include thyrotropin, or thyroid-stimulating hormone (TSH), and adrenocorticotropic hormone (ACTH). These hormones affect the mother's metabolic processes so that nutrients can be provided to the growing fetus. Thyroid-stimulating hormone is produced throughout pregnancy. Adrenocorticotropic hormone is initially low in the first trimester, but is produced throughout pregnancy. Levels of melanocyte-stimulating hormone rise by the end of the second month of gestation. The exact function of this hormone is unclear, although it possibly has some effect on skin pigmentation.

Prolactin, another hormone secreted by the anterior pituitary, increases steadily during pregnancy. During the first trimester, prolactin levels rise from a nonpregnant level of 25 ng/mL to about 30 to 34 ng/mL.[26] This hormone is also secreted by the anterior pituitary of the fetus and by the myometrium and endometrium of the uterus in response to the elevated progesterone levels found in pregnancy. Prolactin secretion is needed for the process of lactaton.

Thyroid. The thyroid gland enlarges somewhat during pregnancy as a result of increased vascularity and hyperplasia of the glandular tissue.[2] Normal thyroid function is dependent on an adequate intake of iodine, which tends to be excreted in greater quantities through the kidneys, as of the first trimester of pregnancy. The thyroid compensates for this loss by enlarging and trapping additional iodine for synthesis to one of the two circulating thyroid hormones, triiodothyronine (T_3) or thyroxine (T_4). Dietary practices in North Americans, such as the use of iodized salt or iodine-containing prenatal vitamins, tend to keep the plasma iodine concentration above 0.08 ng/ml. Below this level, iodine-deficiency goiter may develop.[27]

Basal metabolic rate, which is a monitor of thyroid function, increases during pregnancy by as much as 25 percent. Most of this increase is related to the metabolic activity of the products of conception. Prenatal changes that take place in aspects of thyroid function are largely related to increased levels of thyroxine-binding globulin. Thyroxine-binding globulin rises to twice normal values during pregnancy, because estrogen stimulates the liver to produce greater amounts of it.

Most of the thyroid hormones T_3 and T_4 are bound to the thyroxine-binding globulin protein; therefore, only a small amount (less than 1 percent) of these hormones is biologically "free."[26] As would be expected, total T_3 and T_4 levels begin to rise during the first trimester and remain elevated until pregnancy is completed. This may produce laboratory values that would indicate hyperthyroidism in a nonpregnant woman; however, the free T_3 and T_4 that actually determine thyroid status do not change substantially.

TABLE 12–2. EXAMPLES OF HORMONAL EFFECTS DURING PREGNANCY

Gland	Hormone	Target Organ	Major Effects
Anterior pituitary (adenohypophysis)	Follicle-stimulating hormone (FSH)	Ovary	Maturation of ovarian follicle Estrogen secretion from follicular fluid Suppressed during pregnancy
	Luteinizing hormone (LH)	Ovary, uterus, breasts	Stimulates ovulation Maintains the corpus luteum of pregnancy for about 7 weeks Stimulates progesterone secretion Prepares uterus for fertilized ovum Prepares breasts for lactation
	Adrenocorticotropic hormone (ATCH)	Adrenal cortex, placenta (role of placental ACTH unclear)	Stimulates adrenal cortex to produce cortisol
	Thyrotropin (thyroid-stimulating hormone, TSH)	Thyroid	Stimulates the thyroid to release thyroxine
Anterior pituitary (of mother and fetus) myometrium and endomentrium	Prolactin	Breasts	Maternal prolactin fosters development of breast in preparation for lactation
Posterior pituitary (neurohypophysis)	Oxytocin	Smooth muscle of uterus and breasts	Stimulates contractions of the uterus during labor, delivery, and involution Stimulates contractions of the breast during lactation
Thyroid	Thyroxine (T_4,T_3)	Body cells	Serum protein-bound iodine increases Increases basal metabolic rate Increases use of nutrients
Adrenal cortex	Cortisol	Body cells	Assists in regulation of glucose in maternal blood by stimulating the liver to synthesize carbohydrates from noncarbohydrates such as amino acids Increases concentration of amino acids in the blood by stimulating degradation of proteins within maternal cells Amino acids and glucose are needed by the mother and fetus for growth and development
	Aldosterone	Kidneys, blood	Regulates sodium content of blood Causes retention of sodium and water when blood sodium levels are low May counteract some effects of progesterone, because progesterone stimulates sodium and water loss by the kidney Helps to increase blood volume
Ovaries, placenta (after 7 weeks of gestation)	Estrogen (estriol is predominant, but many forms of estrogen exist)	Multi-organ effects (especially ova, uterus, skin, stomach, breasts)	Stimulates development of uterine lining Stimulates hypertrophy of uterine muscles and development of additional blood supply; increases uteroplacental blood flow Suppresses secretion of FSH and LH by anterior pituitary Promotes metabolism of nutrients Decreases secretion of hydrochloric acid and pepsin by the stomach Promotes sodium and water retention by kidney Produces increased pliability of connective tissue with relaxation of joints and ligaments Stimulates growth of breasts and development of duct system Stimulates production of melanocyte-stimulating hormone Contributes to integumentary changes, such as darkening of skin pigment Implicated in development of vascular spiders and palmar erythema

(continued)

TABLE 12–2. EXAMPLES OF HORMONAL EFFECTS DURING PREGNANCY *(continued)*

Gland	Hormone	Target Organ	Major Effects
Ovaries, placenta *(continued)*	Progesterone (placental synthesis depends on maternal precursor, lipoprotein cholesterol)	Multi-organ effects (especially uterus, breasts, smooth muscle)	Suppresses FSH and LH by the anterior pituitary gland Maintains corpus luteum of pregnancy until placenta is functional Develops decidual cells of uterus; maintains uterine lining for implantation and early pregnancy Stimulates uterine enlargement in early pregnancy Aids in formation of placenta Increases vascularity of cervix Increases absorption of nutrients Stimulates storage of fat Relaxes smooth muscle; decreases uterine contractility; promotes vasodilatation; decreases tone of bladder and ureters; reduces motility and tone of gastrointestinal tract, including gallbladder Stimulates sodium excretion (naturesis) Promotes lobular-alveolar system of breasts and mammary growth Resets 3 maternal hypothalamic centers, resulting in increase in basal body temperature until mid-pregnancy; an increase in fat storage; stimulation of respiratory center to facilitate pulmonary transfer of carbon dioxide May also prevent rejection of fetus by mother's body
Placenta	Human chorionic gonadotropin (hCG)	Ovary	Synthesized in syncytiotrophoblasts Found in maternal urine and blood; basis for many pregnancy tests Highest levels occur by about 10 weeks of pregnancy and decrease to lowest level by 20 weeks Maintains corpus luteum during early pregnancy Promotes testosterone synthesis, secretion, and sexual differentation in males Used in diagnosis of pregnancy or high-risk conditions such as hydatidiform mole May directly stimulate thyroid activity
	Human placental lactogen (hPL)	Body cells	Secreted by chorionic villi Influences growth and development of fetus and placenta Stimulates growth of breasts Influences metabolic processes Promotes lipolysis and increases free fatty acids, thus offering an energy source for maternal metabolism and fetal nutrition Spares glucose and protein by inhibiting uptake of glucose and also gluconeogenesis Effects raise levels of maternal insulin, which promotes protein synthesis, thus creating a source of amino acids for transport to fetus Possibly serves as a "backup" mechanism; may not be needed for successful pregnancy outcome

T_3 = triiodothyronine, T_4 = 3,5,3,'5' = tetraiodothyronine = thyroxine.

Actual secretion of T_3 and T_4 is related to the mother's expansion in surface area. Through negative feedback, the amount of free thyroid hormones regulates and is regulated by the amount of thyroid-releasing factor from the hypothalamus and of TSH from the anterior pituitary. The thyroid gland may also be stimulated in normal early pregnancy by serum human chorionic gonadotropin.[28]

Parathyroids. Enlargement of the parathyroid glands begins during the first trimester. Parathyroid hormone, which decreases during the first trimester but increases thereafter, has an important role in regulating calcium in the blood by mobilizing calcium from the bones, facilitating absorption of calcium from the small intestine (with the help of Vitamin D), and facilitating reabsorption of calcium from the renal tubule. Actual regulation of calcium metabolism is complex, however, and depends on interactions of magnesium, phosphate, parathyroid hormone, calcitonin, and vitamin D.

Adrenals. The adrenal glands of the healthy pregnant woman show little change morphologically during pregnancy[2]; however, there are changes in hormone secretion. In the first trimester, levels of ACTH, secreted by the anterior pituitary, are reduced. As a result, levels of the glucocorticoid cortisol, produced by the adrenal cortex, are also reduced as compared with later trimesters. Beginning in the first trimester, elevated estrogen levels also influence increases in the secretion of aldosterone, a mineralocorticoid, by the adrenal cortex. Aldosterone secretion is markedly increased during pregnancy, especially if sodium is restricted.

Pancreas. The developing fetus draws glucose from the maternal supply. In addition, use of maternal amino acids by the fetus inhibits glucose formation. The combination of increasing glucose demand by the fetus and decreased supply of glucose results in a reduction in maternal blood glucose. During the first trimester the islets of Langerhans in the pancreas therefore produce less insulin for glucose metabolism.

Placenta. As discussed in Chapter 11, the placenta forms and begins to function during the first trimester of pregnancy. The placenta is a complex organ that is fetal in origin but depends almost completely on maternal blood for its existence. Development of the human placenta is summarized in Table 12–3.

TABLE 12–3. OUTLINE OF PLACENTAL DEVELOPMENT

Days After Ovulation	Placental Development
6–8	Implantation of blastocyst.
7–8	Blastocyst differentiates into inner cell mass (from which embryo develops) and trophoblast, a larger surrounding mass (from which placenta develops). Cells proliferate; trophoblast divides into 2 layers, an inner cytotrophoblast and an outer syncytium.
9–11	Trophoblastic cells invade and break down maternal cells and blood vessels in decidual layer of endometrium. This allows for contact by trophoblastic blood vessels, which soon emerge, and also for production of hormones (such as human chorionic gonadotropin) necessary for the developing pregnancy.
11–13	Trophoblast sends out projections into endometrium; spaces (or lacunae) develop and fill with maternal blood. Fingerlike outgrowths, now called villi, continue to develop.
16–18	Villi continue to branch, becoming treelike. Meanwhile, body stalk of embryo and amnion form. Trophoblastic covering separates fetal vessels from intervillous blood lakes, so that fetal blood does not mix with maternal blood.
by 22	Fetal circulation functional, but sluggish. As growth continues, villi in contact with decidua basalis form the chorion frondosum, whereas those in contact with decidua capsularis atrophy and form chorion laeve. Basal chorion frondosum becomes the fetal part of the placenta and decidua basalis the maternal part.
90–225	Placenta has reached its definitive form. For remainder of pregnancy, placental changes involve degree of branching of villi and increase in intervillous space.

Based on Reference 26.

Placental Hormones. The placenta acts as an endocrine gland during pregnancy, and produces estrogens, progesterone, human chorionic gonadotropin and human placental lactogen (hPL). Major effects of these hormones were summarized in Table 12–2. Placental hormones promote maternal and fetal development during pregnancy. Some of the hormonally induced changes also account for maternal discomforts during pregnancy. Placental hormones and their interactions are extremely complex and not completely understood.

Estrogens. Estrogens are steroid hormones secreted largely by the ovary in early pregnancy. The estrogen secretion by the corpus luteum is dependent on the maternal precursors of cholesterol and acetates.

By the seventh week of gestation, more than half of the estrogen is being secreted by the placenta; as pregnancy advances, the placenta secretes most of the body's estrogens. Placental production of estrogen is dependent on fetal androgens, secreted by the fetal liver and adrenals, as well as by androgens found in the maternal circulation. The fetal-placental unit is thus important in controlling both the secretion of estrogen and the environment of pregnancy. During pregnancy, estrogen secretion increases about one thousand times above nonpregnant levels of the premenopausal woman.[2]

There are many types of estrogen. Indeed, more than 25 have been found in maternal urine. The most common estrogens of pregnancy are estrone, estradiol, and estriol. Estriol, the predominant estrogen produced by the placenta in pregnancy, has many functions, including increasing uteroplacental blood flow and stimulating development of the ductal system in the maternal breasts. Large amounts of estriol are secreted during normal pregnancy. Estriol produced by the placenta is found in maternal blood and urine, as well as in amniotic fluid. For this reason, estriol levels, especially maternal urinary and serum estriol levels, were used as indicators of placental and fetal well-being. For example, decreasing serial urinary estriol levels suggested fetal jeopardy. Today, more direct and accurate measures, such as the nonstress test, are available for fetal assessment in high-risk situations (*see* Chapter 22).

Progesterone. Progesterone is a steroid hormone secreted by the corpus luteum for about the first 7 weeks of pregnancy. During this time, progesterone helps develop the maternal decidual cells and maintain the corpus luteum itself. After the seventh week of gestation, the placenta is the major source of progesterone. Unlike estrogen, no fetal precursors are needed for the production and secretion of progesterone. Instead, maternal cholesterol, which enters the trophoblast as a low-density lipoprotein, is needed for progesterone synthesis. Ten times more progesterone is secreted by the placenta than by the ovary in the nonpregnant state. Progesterone is also produced in greater quantities than estrogens in the course of pregnancy. Progesterone levels rise during pregnancy and peak at term.

Reduction of myometrial contractility during pregnancy is one effect of progesterone. Because of this, progesterone withdrawal was thought to be necessary for the onset of labor. Currently there is no evidence to support this theory. Progesterone withdrawal may only be one step in the complex events leading to labor.

Human Chorionic Gonadotropin. Human chorionic gonadotropin (hCG) is a protein hormone secreted by the syncytiotrophoblast early in pregnancy. It helps sustain the corpus luteum, which in turn secretes progesterone and estrogen necessary for early pregnancy. This protein hormone can be found in maternal blood and urine as early as 8 days after conception and reaches its highest level toward the end of the first trimester, at about 8 to 10 weeks. Thereafter, hCG levels sharply decline. Human chorionic gonadotropin levels are used in the diagnosis of pregnancy and such high-risk conditions as hydatidiform mole (*see* Chapters 14 and 39). Human chorionic gonadotropin has also been reported to stimulate the thyroid gland.[27,28]

Human Placental Lactogen. Human placental lactogen (hPL), a protein hormone, is detectable in the syncytiotrophoblast as early as 2 to 3 weeks after conception.[2] This hormone has been referred to as human chorionic somatomammotropin and chorionic growth hormone because it promotes the growth of the fetus, breasts, and uterus during pregnancy. Human placental lactogen promotes lipolysis, the breakdown of fats. This process increases the level of maternal circulating free fatty acids, which then can serve as an energy source for the expectant mother and the fetus. Human placental lactogen "spares" glucose and protein by suppressing the uptake of glucose and gluconeogenesis in the expectant woman. Protein synthesis is fostered, because more glucose can be mobilized for the rapidly growing energy needs of the fetus. The "anti-insulin" role of hPL is thought to contribute to higher levels of maternal insulin because the pancreas then tries to adapt by producing more insulin. Because of its influence on maternal insulin levels, hPL is thought to contribute to the diabetogenic effect of pregnancy, especially during the second and third trimesters when the demand for maternal insulin production is greatest.

Human placental lactogen is thought to affect growth of the fetus and the placenta, because the level of hPL found in the maternal circulation is directly related to fetal and placental weight. The levels of hPL increase as pregnancy progresses and peak about 35 weeks of gestation. The placenta is the chief source of hPL in the normal pregnant woman.

Women with low or undetectable levels of hPL may have normal pregnancies. For this reason, it is thought that hPL may serve as a physiologic "backup" system able to provide nutrition for the fetus, for example during stresses such as maternal starvation.[2] Human placental lactogen is believed to have no role in human lactation, because lactation occurs during the postpartum period when production of hPL has stopped.

Other Hormones: Prostaglandins. Prostaglandins are substances derived from the precursor unsaturated fatty acid, arachidonic acid. They are found in most body tissues and in high concentrations in the amnion, chorion, and decidua during pregnancy. Prostaglandin synthesis is greatest in the amnion. Their exact function is unknown. Prostaglandin E (PGE) and prostaglandin F (PGF) are believed to have an important role during labor; however, there seems to be an antagonistic relationship between prostaglandin E and prostaglandin F. When concentrations of PGE are elevated, blood vessels dilate. When PGF is elevated, blood vessels constrict. Both prostaglandins contract smooth muscle and are metabolized in the lungs. Tissue levels of prostaglandins remain constant throughout pregnancy.

SIGNS AND SYMPTOMS OF PREGNANCY

The first trimester of pregnancy is an important period for growth and development of the fetus and beginning prenatal adaptation in the mother. Symptoms and signs of pregnancy become apparent and the woman may experience certain related discomforts. For conceptual ease, symptoms and signs of pregnancy have traditionally been divided into three groups: presumptive, probable, and positive. The student should learn to identify and describe these signs and symptoms of pregnancy, because these terms are widely used. Table 12–4 provides a summary of the symptoms and signs of pregnancy.

Presumptive Indications

Presumptive indicators of pregnancy are so called because they can be caused by factors other than pregnancy. Many of the presumptive indicators are subjective, that is, feelings or sensations experienced by the woman. Most presumptive indicators appear during the first trimester.[29]

Presumptive Symptoms. Amenorrhea is often the earliest presumptive symptom. Menses cease after conception in response to the increasing progesterone levels produced by the corpus luteum. In a woman who has regular menstrual cycles, this is a dependable symptom. Amenorrhea cannot be considered a positive symptom of pregnancy, because other factors, such as endocrine problems, emotional stress, chronic disease, certain drugs, and tumors, can be responsible. In exceedingly rare instances, women may have unexplained cyclic bleeding during pregnancy and therefore cannot depend on the absence of vaginal bleeding as a sign of pregnancy.

Nausea and vomiting are experienced by about 50 percent of women. These symptoms are most severe during the first trimester, between 2 and 12 weeks; however, nausea and vomiting can be symptoms of such conditions as gastrointestinal viruses and emotional stress.

Breast changes are early presumptive symptoms of pregnancy, and include breast tenderness (mastodynia). Factors that contribute to breast tenderness include hormonal influences on the mammary ducts and alveolar system of the breasts and increases in blood circulation to the breasts. These changes may also occur with other conditions, such as premenstrual syndrome or chronic cystic mastitis.

Urinary frequency, caused by pressure of the enlarging uterus on the bladder, is also a symptom of urinary tract infections.

Fatigue is a presumptive symptom reported by many women throughout the first trimester. Stress, illness, and lifestyle changes affecting sleep habits are examples of conditions that can also produce fatigue.

Quickening, the first sensation of fetal movement, is a presumptive symptom that usually is experienced during the second trimester. Primigravidas tend to experience quickening around 18 to 20 weeks; multigravidas feel quickening earlier, about 14 to 16 weeks. As peristalsis and "gas" may produce similar sensations, quickening is not a dependable sign of pregnancy; nevertheless, it is helpful in identifying how far the pregnancy has progressed.

Presumptive Signs. Increased basal body temperature that continues longer than 3 weeks may be considered a presumptive sign if the temperatures are conscientiously charted. A low-grade, elevated temperature could also be a sign of infection.

Several changes are also noted in the skin. Linea nigra may be observed. This sign manifests as a dark line on the midline of the abdomen from the umbilicus to the pubis.

Melasma, also called chloasma (*see* Chapter 16), darkening of the skin on the face (forehead, nose, cheekbones), usually appears during the second trimester, after 16 weeks. Melasma is especially pronounced in women with dark complexions and increases in response to sun exposure. Certain illnesses or medications, however, can also be reflected by changes in skin pigmentation.

Stretch marks, called *striae,* on the breasts, abdomen, and legs are presumptive signs that usually appear during the second or third trimester; however, stretch marks may also be the result of such conditions as marked obesity or swelling.

The breasts are also the site of several changes. In response to hormonal stimulation during early pregnancy, the Montgomery tubercles (sebaceous glands) in the areola enlarge at about 6 to 8 weeks of gestation.

Colostrum is secreted (*see* Chapter 16) from the breasts usually beginning during the second trimester, about 16 weeks. Secretion of fluid from both breasts does, however, occur in other conditions, for example, prolactin-secreting pituitary tumors.

Enlargement of and increased pigmentation of

TABLE 12–4. SYMPTOMS AND SIGNS OF PREGNANCY

Symptom/Sign	Physiologic Base	Cause Other Than Pregnancy
Presumptive Symptoms		
Amenorrhea	Increased progesterone; inhibition of FSH and LH	Endocrine disorders, malnutrition, emotional factors, systemic disease, early menopause
Nausea/vomiting	Unknown cause; may be related to altered carbohydrate metabolism increased levels of hCG, decreased gastrointestinal motility, and other factors	Gastrointestinal disorders, acute infections, emotional factors
Breast tenderness	Development of duct system influenced by increased hormone levels	Premenstrual symptoms, chronic cystic mastitis
Urinary frequency	Pressure of enlarging uterus on bladder	Urinary tract infections, stress, tumors
Fatigue	Unknown cause	Stress, anemia, infections, other illnesses
Quickening	Fetal movements felt by mother	Gastrointestinal activity
Presumptive Signs		
Increased basal body temperature	Increased metabolic activity	Infections
Linea nigra	Increase in melanocyte-stimulating hormone	
Melasma-chloasma	Cause unclear, possibly increased estrogen, progesterone, melanocyte-stimulating hormone	Certain contraceptives
Striae	Separation of collagen tissues beneath skin; may be hormonally related; cause unknown	Obesity
Enlargement of secondary breast tissue	Hormonal stimulation	Breast cysts, tumors
Colostrum secretion	Hormonal stimulation (increased prolactin levels)	Pituitary tumors
Probable Indications		
Chadwick's sign	Increased vascularity of vagina, cervix, and vulva	Hyperemia of pelvic organs as a result of non–pregnancy-related hormonal influences
Goodell's sign	Pelvic vasocongestion	Oral contraceptives
Ladin's sign	Anterior uterine softening at midline	
McDonald's sign	Flexibility of uterus where uterus and cervix join	Myomas, tumors
Hegar's sign	Hyperemia of pelvic organs	Anatomically soft walls of nonpregnant uterus
Braun von Fernwald's sign	Hormonal influences, implantation	Myomas, tumors
Piskacek's sign	Softening over implantation site in cornua of uterus	Myomas, tumors
Uterine enlargement	Growing products of conception	Tumors
Braxton Hicks contractions	Irregular contractions of uterus	Hematomas, soft myomas
Ballottement of uterus	Movement of fetus during examination	Ascites, ovarian cysts, tumors
Uterine souffle	Whooshing sound caused by maternal blood moving into placental vessels and sinuses	
Positive pregnancy tests	hCG in urine and blood	Disease states, such as choriocarcinoma, hydatidiform mole
Positive Indications		
Fetal heartbeat heard	Fetus	
Fetal movements felt by examiner	Fetus	
Fetal outline seen	Fetus	

secondary breast tissue can be identified along the nipple line. Hypertrophied axillary breast tissue may be identified as a lump in the armpit. Although normal presumptive signs of pregnancy, these can be confused with true breast pathology; therefore, any breast or axillary lump needs careful and expert evaluation.

Probable Indications

Probable symptoms and signs of pregnancy are the result of physiologic changes in the pelvic organs and hormonal influences. Although they can aid in the diagnosis of pregnancy, probable signs do not definitively identify pregnancy. Probable signs of pregnancy are objective and are identified by the examiner.

Probable Symptoms. Probable symptoms and presumptive symptoms are the same.

Probable Signs. Several, but not all, probable signs of pregnancy appear during the first trimester. Many of these signs are identified on pelvic examination by the physician or by a nurse specialist, such as a certified nurse-midwife. The probable signs include changes in the pelvic organs and positive pregnancy tests.

Several changes occur in the pelvic organs. Chadwick's sign, a bluish coloration of the mucous membranes of the vulva, vagina, and cervix, is related to increased vascularity of the pelvic organs; Goodell's sign, softening of the cervix, is related to vasocongestion (Figure 12–3); and **Ladin's sign,** softening of the anterior part of the uterus at the midline, where the uterus and cervix join (Figure 12–4), occurs at about 6 weeks and is probably related to hormonal changes.

The ability of the uterus to be easily flexed at the site where the uterus and cervix join is referred to as **McDonald's sign. Hegar's sign** is the widening of the isthmus of the uterus to the point where the isthmus can be compressed on bimanual examination (Figure 12–5). Asymmetric softening and enlargement of the uterus at the site of the implantation are known as **Braun von Fernwald's sign** (Figure 12–6). If the irregular softening occurs in the cornual area, the enlarge-

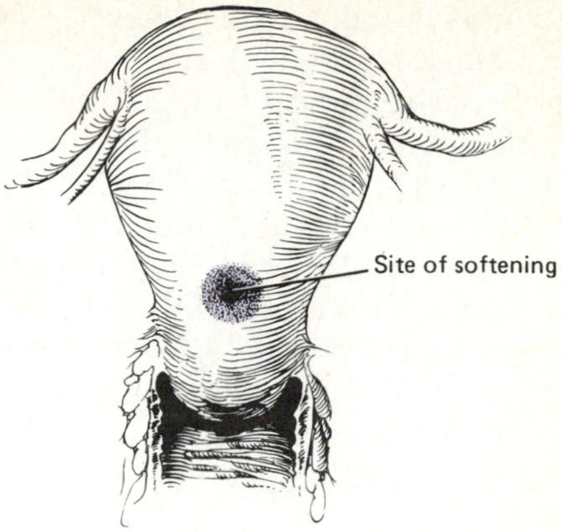

Figure 12–4. Ladin's sign. (*Reproduced, with permission, from Pernoll ML, Benson RC, eds.* Current Obstetric & Gynecologic Diagnosis & Treatment. *Norwalk, Conn: Appleton & Lange; 1987: 164.*

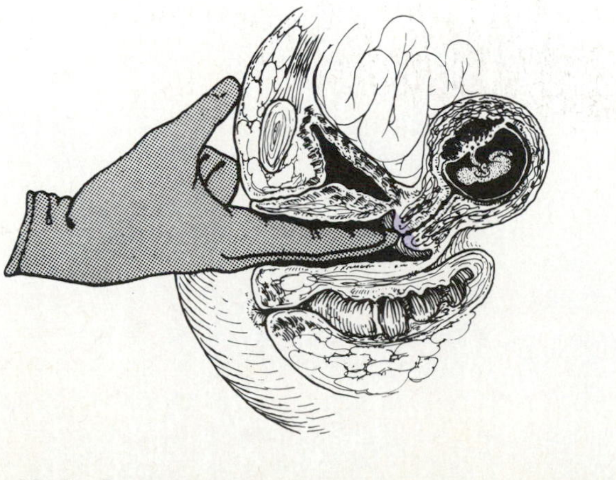

Figure 12–3. Goodell's sign. (*Reproduced, with permission, from Pernoll ML, Benson RC, eds.* Current Obstetric & Gynecologic Diagnosis & Treatment. *Norwalk, Conn: Appleton & Lange; 1987:164.*

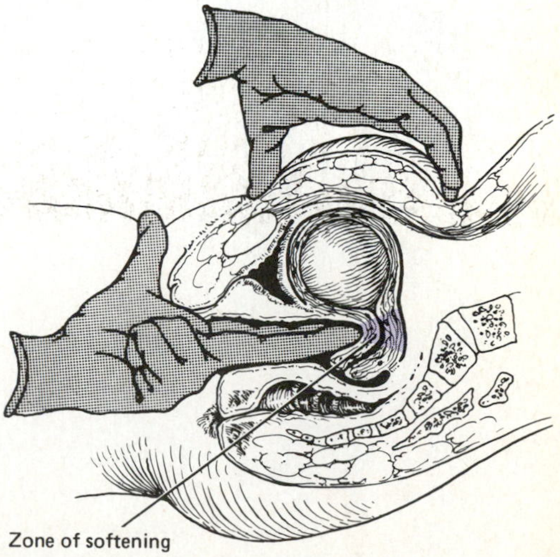

Figure 12–5. Hegar's sign. (*Reproduced, with permission, from Pernoll ML, Benson RC, eds.* Current Obstetric & Gynecologic Diagnosis & Treatment. *Norwalk, Conn: Appleton & Lange; 1987: 164.*

ment is called **Piskacek's sign;** however, by 10 weeks, the uterus enlarges symmetrically.

Other probable signs of pregnancy include: abdominal enlargement, Braxton Hicks contractions, uterine souffle, and ballottement. Abdominal enlargement first becomes noticeable after 7 weeks. Painless uterine contractions (Braxton Hicks contractions) may be felt during the second and third trimesters.

Uterine souffle, the "whooshing" sound made as maternal blood fills the blood vessels and sinuses in the placenta, can be heard through the abdomen after 16 weeks. The rate of uterine souffle is the same as the mother's pulse.

Ballottement is a maneuver used to detect pregnancy. The examiner places two fingers in the vagina and pushes the fetal body upward; the fetus is felt to rise and then fall like a heavy body in water. Later in pregnancy, ballottement may be done abdominally.

A positive pregnancy test is another probable sign of pregnancy. Currently used laboratory tests for pregnancy show positive results because of the presence of hCG in the maternal blood and urine during the first trimester (*see* Chapter 14). These tests are considered *probable* indicators of pregnancy because false negatives and positives can occur.

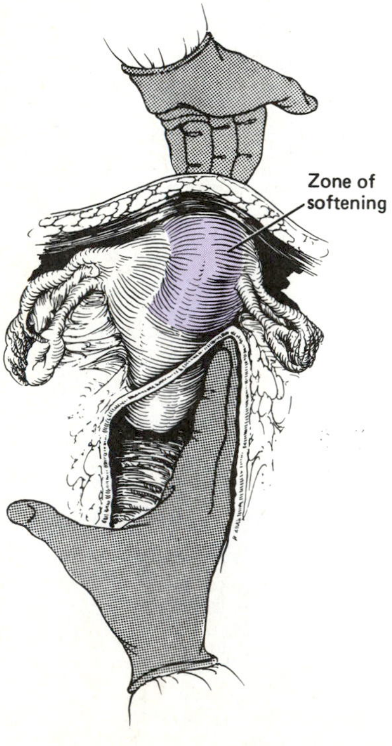

Figure 12–6. Braun von Fernwald's sign. (*Reproduced, with permission, from Pernoll ML, Benson RC, eds.* Current Obstetric & Gynecologic Diagnosis & Treatment. *Norwalk, Conn: Appleton & Lange; 1987: 165.*

Positive Indications

Positive indications of pregnancy clearly demonstrate the presence of a fetus and cannot be due to other conditions. Positive confirmation of pregnancy is made solely on objective signs. In the past, positive diagnosis of pregnancy was not made early in the first trimester. Currently, new methods of assessment (*see* Chapter 14) are making early first-trimester diagnosis possible. Although many symptoms suggest pregnancy, only a few definite positive signs exist.[29] Positive signs of pregnancy include assessment of fetal heart tones, palpation of fetal movements, and visualization of the fetus.

With the use of a fetoscope, fetal heart tones can be auscultated at about 18 weeks, or later if the woman is obese or if implantation was anterior. Blood flow through the fetal heart can be identified with a doppler as early as 10 weeks.

Fetal movements can be palpated by the examiner after 18 weeks. The gestational sac may be visualized on ultrasound as early as 6 weeks from the last missed period.

Clear demonstration of the presence of the fetus, for example, on ultrasound, ends any controversy over whether a pregnancy exists. Sources, however, differ with regard to whether other signs are presumptive, probable, or positive. For example, sometimes, all subjective signs are called "presumptive," and objective signs are referred to as "probable." At other times, signs may be classified as "presumptive" or "probable" according to their reliability in diagnosing pregnancy. An important consideration is that the woman who demonstrates only presumptive signs of pregnancy should begin prenatal care. This will help to ensure early and consistent health care for the mother and fetus.

SUMMARY

The first trimester of pregnancy is a critical period of development for the embryo/fetus. At the same time, physiologic changes occur in many of the mother's organ systems, so that pregnancy can progress. For example, during the first trimester, the uterine walls thicken; the uterus begins to enlarge; and the blood supply to the uterus, breasts, cervix, and vagina increases. The motility and tone of the digestive tract is decreased, as is the emptying time of the stomach. Production of pepsin and gastric acid increases. About 50 percent of pregnant women experience nausea and vomiting during this period. In the first trimester of pregnancy, there are also changes in the urinary system. The ureters begin to dilate, and the glomerular filtration rate begins to rise. Thus, excretion of such substances as glucose, water-soluble vitamins, and amino acids is common during pregnancy. Changes also take place in the integumentary, musculoskeletal and endocrine systems, and levels of circulating hormones change during early pregnancy. To provide comprehensive care to the client during the first trimester, the nurse must understand maternal physiologic changes, as well as fetal growth and development. An understanding of physiologic changes provides the basis for management strategies, such as assessment and client teaching.

Presumptive, probable, and positive symptoms and signs are used to identify pregnancy, especially during the first and second trimesters. Presumptive symptoms of pregnancy include amenorrhea; nausea and vomiting; breast changes, such as tenderness; urinary frequency; fatigue; and perception of fetal movement. Presumptive signs of pregnancy include increased basal body temperature; skin changes; stretch marks on abdomen, breasts, and thighs; breast changes, such as enlargement of Montgomery tubercles and secretion of colostrum; and enlargement and increased pigmentation of secondary breast tissue. Probable signs include Chadwick's sign, Goodell's sign, McDonald's sign, Hegar's sign, Braun von Fernwald's sign, Piskacek's sign, abdominal enlargement, Braxton Hicks contractions, uterine ballottement and souffle, and positive pregnancy tests. Positive signs of pregnancy include identification of fetal heart tones, detection of fetal movements by the examiner, and visualization of the gestational sac on ultrasound. Sources frequently vary according to the classification of signs, particularly as presumptive or probable. Techniques that clearly demonstrate the presence of the embryo or fetus, however, confirm pregnancy.

REVIEW QUESTIONS

1. List changes that take place in the uterus, cervix, ovary, and breasts during the first trimester.
2. Explain why urinary frequency normally occurs during the first trimester.
3. Describe cardiovascular changes in the first trimester.
4. Describe integumentary changes that may be experienced during the first trimester.
5. Define and give examples of presumptive, probable, and positive symptoms and signs of pregnancy.

REFERENCES

1. Knuppel RA, Goodlin, RC. Maternal-placental-fetal unit: Fetal & early neonatal physiology. In: Pernoll ML, Benson RC eds. *Current Obstetric & Gynecologic Diagnosis & Treatment, 1987.* East Norwalk, Conn: Appleton & Lange;1987: 135–160.
2. Cunningham FG, et al. *Williams Obstetrics.* 18th ed. Norwalk, Conn: Appleton & Lange; 1989.
3. Andersen A; Hytten F, Chamberlain G, eds. *Clinical Physiology in Obstetrics.* Oxford: Blackwell Scientific; 1980:328.
4. Kushnir O, et al. Vaginal ultrasonographic assessment of cervical length changes during normal pregnancy. *Am J Obstet & Gynecol.* 1990;162:991–993.
5. Danforth DN. The fibrous nature of the human cervix and its relation to the isthmic segment in gravid and nongravid uteri. *Am J Obstet Gynecol.* 1947;53:541.
6. Ekman G, et al. Cervical collagen: an important regulator of cervical function in term labor. *Obstet Gynecol.* 1986;67: 633–636.
7. Uldbjerg N, et al. The ripening of the human cervix related to changes in collagen, glycosaminoglycans and collagenolytic activity. *Am J Obstet Gynecol.* 1983;147:622.
8. Rechberger R, et al. Connective tissue changes in the cervix during normal pregnancy and pregnancy complicated by cervical incompetence. *Obstet Gynecol.* 1988;71:563–567.
9. Varney H. *Nurse Midwifery.* Boston: Blackwell Scientific; 1987.
10. Porter DG. Relaxin and cervical softening. In: Anderson AM, Ellwood DA; eds. *The Cervix in Pregnancy and Labour.* Edinburgh: Churchill Livingstone; 1980.
11. Steinetx BG, et al. The role of relaxin in cervical softening during pregnancy in mammals. In: Innaftolin R, Stubblefield PG, eds. *Dilatation of the Uterine Cervix, Connective Tissue Biology and Clinical Management.* New York: Raven Press; 1980.
12. Ganong WF. Physiology of reproduction. In: Pernoll ML, Benson RC, eds. *Current Obstetric & Gynecologic Diagnosis & Treatment, 1987.* Norwalk, Conn: Appleton & Lange; 1987: 109–126.
13. Moore P. Maternal physiology during pregnancy. In: Pernoll ML, Benson RC, eds. *Current Obstetic & Gynecologic Diagnosis & Treatment, 1987.* Norwalk, Conn: Appleton & Lange; 1987:127–134.
14. de Swiet M. The cardiovascular system. In: Hytten F, Chamzberlain G, eds. *Clinical Physiology in Obstetrics.* London: Blackwell Scientific; 1980:3–42.
15. McAnulty JH, et al. Cardiovascular disease. In: Burrow GN, Ferris TF, eds. *Complications During Pregnancy.* 3rd ed. Philadelphia: WB Saunders; 1988:180–203.
16. Letsky E. The haematological system. In: Hytten F, Chamberlain G, eds. *Clinical Physiology in Obstetrics.* London: Blackwell Scientific; 1980:43–78.

17. de Swiet M. The respiratory system. In: Hytten F, Chamberlain G, eds. *Clinical Physiology in Obstetrics.* London: Blackwell Scientific; 1980:79–100.
18. Guyton AC. Pregnancy and lactation. In: Guyton AC, ed. *Textbook of Medical Physiology.* 7th ed., Philadelphia: WB Saunders; 1986:983–996.
19. Ferris TF. Renal diseases. In: Burrow GW, Ferris TF, eds. *Complications During Pregnancy.* 3rd ed. Philadelphia: WB Saunders; 1988:277–302.
20. Bruce N. Gestational adaptation: major systems. In: Iffy L, Kaminetzky H, eds. *Principles and Practice of Obstetrics and Perinatology.* New York: Wiley; 1981.
21. Braverman I. The skin in pregnancy. In: Burrow GN, Ferris TF, eds. *Medical Complications During Pregnancy.* 3rd ed. Philadelphia: WB Saunders; 1988:526–539.
22. Connon J. Gastrointestinal complications. In: Burrow GN, Ferris TF, eds. *Medical Complications During Pregnancy.* Philadelphia: WB Saunders; 1988:303–317.
23. Chengar P, Kovacik A. Dental hygiene during pregnancy: A review. *Am J Matern Child Nurs.* 1987;12:342–343.
24. Alley NM. Morning sickness: the client's perspective. *J Obstet Gynecol Neonat Nurs.* 1984;13:185–189.
25. Klebanoff MA, et al. Epidemiology of vomiting in early pregnancy. *Obstet Gynecol.* 1985;66:612–616.
26. Beischer NA, MacKay EV. *Obstetrics and the Newborn: An Illustrated Textbook.* 2nd ed. Philadelphia: WB Saunders; 1988.
27. Burrow GN. Thyroid disease. In Burrow GN, Ferris TF, eds. *Medical Complications During Pregnancy.* 3rd ed. Philadelphia: WB Saunders; 1988;224–253.
28. Kimura M, et al. Physiologic thyroid activation in normal early pregnancy is induced by circulating hCG. *Obstetrics & Gynecology.* 1990;75:775–778.
29. Bennett EC. The first trimester. *J Obstet Gynecol Neonat Nurs.* 1982;13(suppl):93S–96S.
30. Poole CJ. Fatigue during the first trimester of pregnancy. *J Obstet Gynecol Neonat Nurs.* 1986;15:375–379.

Psychologic and Sociocultural Dimensions During the First Trimester

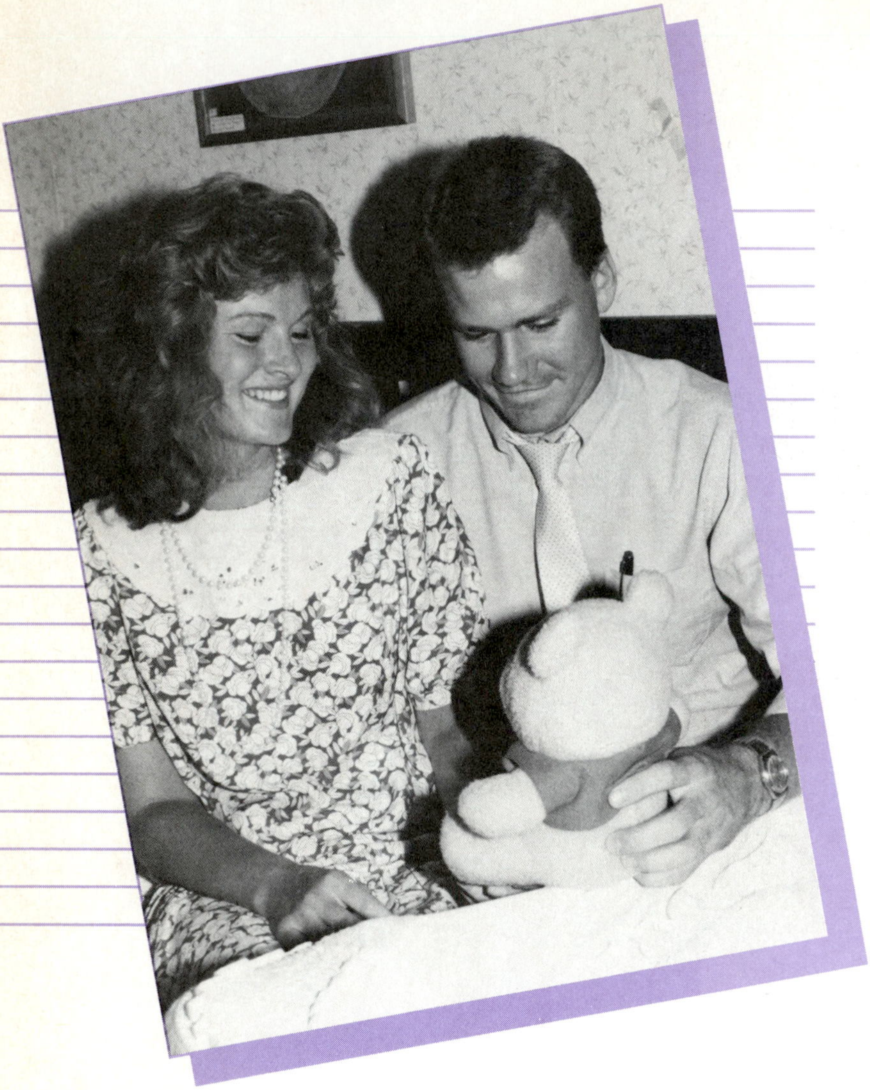

Chapter 13

Psychologic, sociologic, and cultural factors are integral to family adaptation as pregnancy develops. Physiologic changes of pregnancy are restricted to the mother and the developing fetus; however, psychologic changes affect the mother and her significant others, such as the baby's father, siblings, and grandparents.

Psychologic, sociologic, and cultural factors have enormous impact on the expectant mother's physical well-being, affect the couple's transition to parenthood, and influence their ability to parent their child. Chapter 4 presents a theoretical overview of these factors during pregnancy, so that evolution of changes across trimesters can be better understood. This chapter focuses on psychologic, sociologic, and cultural dimensions of pregnancy during the first trimester.

Nurses must understand the implications of culture and heritage for diverse groups of clients, although each client and family must be considered unique. The chapter concludes with a discussion of the impact of cultural background on clients during the first trimester.

PSYCHOLOGIC CHANGES IN THE MOTHER

Psychologic Considerations Prior to Diagnosis of Pregnancy

Pregnancy begins with conception; however, a certain amount of time passes before pregnancy testing indicates that pregnancy is probable. Although some women claim to have no idea they are pregnant during the earliest stages, others "know" they are pregnant within days of conceiving. They are able to detect subtle changes, such as breast enlargement, during the beginning of their pregnancies.

At some point during their reproductive years, sexually active women may experience a "false alarm," or an occasion when their menstrual period is delayed and they suspect they could be pregnant. Some women frequently have irregular menses. The woman who has not had pregnancy diagnosed may therefore doubt whether she is pregnant. During this time of "uncertain-certainty," women may experience various reactions. Whether a woman responds with hopeful excitement, a sense of fatigue, or a feeling of dread depends on many factors:

1. Whether the pregnancy was planned. Women who plan a pregnancy may look for even the smallest changes in their bodies.
2. Whether the pregnancy is wanted. It is important to realize that "unplanned" does *not* necessarily mean "unwanted." For example, some couples who are unable to make a decision may "take a chance." A resulting pregnancy may be greeted with a sense of relief that the decision was made for them.
3. Economic status of the family. Women experiencing financial hardship or potential loss of employment as a result of pregnancy may fear and delay news confirming pregnancy.
4. Number and ages of other children. Mothers who have other young children close in age may respond with a sense of exhaustion. Women with nearly grown children may think they are ill rather than pregnant.
5. Support that the mother perceives from her significant others, especially her husband and own mother. Women who have turbulent or uncertain family relationships, such as impending divorce, may view pregnancy negatively.
6. Woman's cultural and religious background. For example, because of poverty and large populations, certain East Asian countries, have encouraged cultural beliefs in one child per family. This imposes great stress on women with subsequent pregnancies. In other countries, however, such as many within the Middle East, large families are culturally desirable. Religious groups such as Roman Catholics, Orthodox Jews, and Mormons believe that children are a blessing, and large families are encouraged.
7. Whether the couple has had difficulty conceiving or a history of infertility. Women hoping to conceive may be concerned they are not pregnant. They may experience this waiting period with fear of disappointment; however, they may also seek early pregnancy testing.

There is a lack of research on psychologic aspects of the postconception, early-first-trimester period, possibly because women are not readily accessible to researchers within the health care system at this time. Therefore, information about women's earliest reactions often is based on clinical reports, rather than research findings.

Most women seek confirmation of pregnancy at some point during the first trimester. Some may first use home pregnancy tests; others may come to clinic or private office settings for diagnosis of pregnancy. Occasionally, women may deny the symptoms of pregnancy until the second or even third trimester. Indeed, nearly every experienced labor and delivery nurse has worked with clients who arrive at term in the delivery suite with the claim they never knew they were pregnant. Denial that extends into the mid-second or third trimester should not be considered normal. These clients need to be carefully evaluated to identify high-risk psychologic or social conditions. It is important to distinguish between clients who knew they were pregnant and who did not come for prenatal assessment and clients who maintain they never knew they were pregnant.

Concerns

Many of the psychologic processes of pregnancy begin during the first trimester; however, it is often difficult for the woman and her family to believe that she is really pregnant. The woman is not yet able to feel fetal movement, and the pregnancy does not yet "show." As discussed in Chapter 4, pregnancy itself can have many meanings for a woman and her family, including a creative act, a time for rebirth and new beginnings in the family, a rite of passage into adulthood, proof of womanhood, a symbol of sexuality, an expression of the relationship with the woman's own mother or with the baby's father, and a trap.[1] In addition, pregnancy may be viewed as a natural manifestation of the life process.

Although some couples are eager to tell family and friends about the pregnancy, others may hesitate to announce a pregnancy during the first trimester for several reasons:

- Uncertainty over whether or not the pregnancy will be maintained. A couple may worry about miscarriage, especially if previous pregnancies were lost. Women planning diagnostic studies such as chorionic villus sampling or amniocentesis may delay confirming the pregnancy to others until a "normal" result is known. In such situations, women may be concerned about the reactions of and pressures exerted by others.[2] They may also not want to "burden" other family members and friends with responsibility for decision making related to pregnancy termination or continuation.

- Concern related to employment. Many employers still are not supportive of pregnant working women. A woman may fear loss of a potential promotion, salary increase, or job benefit if her pregnancy is known too soon.
- Uncertainty over the reaction of significant others, especially if the woman perceives that news of her pregnancy would not be received with enthusiasm by her significant others.
- Desire to become accustomed to the idea of being pregnant before telling others.

Specific maternal concerns change and differ across the three trimesters. During the first trimester, the woman's concerns are focused mainly on herself, on early physical changes she experiences with the pregnancy and on her feelings about the pregnancy.[3] There is less concern for the infant-to-be at this stage, unless the woman perceives herself to be at some degree of risk. For example, Glazer found that during the first trimester, women's most frequently mentioned concerns related to the self, childbirth, and medical care (safety of medications, diet, and care given by physicians, nurses and others).[4]

Occupational environment and personal habits can place a developing embryo and fetus at risk (*see* Chapter 11). Indeed, pregnant women are advised to avoid exposure to chemicals and other agents that may damage a fetus or harm pregnancy. Some women inaccurately believe they will make changes once they become pregnant. These women may equate the diagnosis of pregnancy with the time for change. By the time their pregnancies are diagnosed, however, the foundation for the fetal organ systems has often been laid. The sense of unreality about the first trimester therefore can contribute to teratogenic problems.

Ideally, women contemplating childbearing should avoid substances and circumstances that could jeopardize pregnancy. In reality, this often does not happen. The nurse needs to be prepared to address client concerns related to lifestyle, occupation, and environment during the first trimester. Nurses working with nonpregnant, sexually active clients of childbearing age need to counsel clients on the importance of this topic.

Currently, most adult women in the United States have some type of employment. One survey found a 60 percent employment rate during pregnancy among American women.[5] During the first trimester, women who are employed experience little change in their general feelings of well-being.[6] One study that compared employed pregnant women with employed men and nonpregnant women found that well-being differed little among the three groups.[7] If the nature of the job and work environment present no problems related to pregnancy, employment during the first trimester is no problem either.

As early as the first trimester, women who plan to continue employment after childbirth may be concerned about their jobs and careers. Many pregnant women have had to contend with the stress of negative societal attitudes toward maternal employment. In the past health care workers have placed little focus on the impact of maternal employment concerns.[8] In providing counseling to expectant mothers, nurses need to assess their own values and attitudes about maternal employment during pregnancy and after childbirth.[9] In addition, employment status must be part of the prenatal history taken at the first visit. Employment options can be discussed if problems are identified. With delivery many months away, the first-trimester expectant mother has time to think about and plan for any employment changes.

Acceptance of the Pregnancy

During the first trimester, women normally experience ambivalence about being pregnant. In an early writing, Caplan estimated that around 80 percent of women initially reject the idea of pregnancy.[10] Even women who planned pregnancy may respond at first with surprise and shock; complete, instant acceptance does not occur often.[11] Some reasons for initial ambivalence during the first trimester include uncertainty over getting what was desired, shock at the major changes in life that will take place, potential economic hardships related to the cost of childbearing and childrearing, potential impact on career goals, potential housing problems, feelings of not being ready on the part of the woman and/or the baby's father, degree of discomfort experienced, and feelings of being "fat."

By the end of the first trimester, most women accept pregnancy.[10] Ambivalence may also normally appear at times throughout the course of pregnancy, and is usually expressed as a desire not to be pregnant.[11] For example, women who experience physical discomfort such as hemorrhoids and women who face potential difficulties in finding child care may ask themselves why they ever wanted to be pregnant. Ambivalence that is normal during the first trimester may, however, signal unresolved conflicts and family problems during the second and third trimesters.

According to Lederman, ambivalence may be assessed according to the following criteria[11]: (1) how honestly ambivalence is expressed, (2) the reason for the ambivalence, (3) the intensity of the ambivalence,

TABLE 13–1. MATERNAL INDICATORS OF ACCEPTANCE OF PREGNANCY

Acceptance
Overall feelings of happiness and enjoyment of pregnancy
Good tolerance of physical discomforts or few discomforts
Minor degree of ambivalence during the first trimester
Minor to moderate mood swings
Feelings that she and her family can handle pregnancy and childbearing; feelings of self-confidence and hope
Lack of Acceptance
Overall feelings of despair or hopelessness
Feelings of being overwhelmed by changes related to pregnancy (physical, lifestyle, and so forth)
Feelings that her world will change for the worse because of the pregnancy (marriage dissolve, career end, and so forth)
Persistent regret at becoming pregnant
Persistent feelings of being ill; excessive subjective physical discomforts

Source: Reference II.

(4) how long the ambivalence is sustained throughout the pregnancy.

Women who are not able to share their doubts about being pregnant, women whose lives or lifestyle may be negatively affected by childbirth, and women who are in vigorous and continuing personal conflict over having a child may be at psychologic risk for acceptance of pregnancy and for childbearing. Lack of acceptance of pregnancy, expressed in various ways during prenatal visits, may alert the nurse to high-risk psychologic and social conditions (Table 13–1). Lack of acceptance of pregnancy may be stated directly or discussed in an indirect or general manner. At times, discussion of feelings during prenatal visits and identification of community resources such as prenatal support groups (usually advertised as early-pregnancy classes) or infant care services can help allay client concerns. Persistent ambivalence indicates the client's need for counseling, social service interventions, or both, and referral for follow-up assessment and intervention is appropriate.

Caplan emphasizes the difference between rejection or ambivalence toward the pregnancy and rejection of the fetus.[10] Ambivalence about pregnancy usually evolves into acceptance and preparation for the coming baby; however, rejection of the fetus presents a potential threat to the mother-infant relationship.

Maternal Role Attainment

During the first trimester, the woman begins to move into the role of mother. According to Rubin, most of the woman's activities at this stage involve replication (*see* Chapter 4).[12] At the very beginning of pregnancy, this may include direct, actual copying of practices and behaviors of other pregnant women or of women who have successfully borne children. Opinions and recommendations of professionals, such as the nurse, also may be modeled by the woman during the first trimester. The newly pregnant woman searches around her for models and tries on the behaviors in an "external" sort of way. This process has also been called "mimicry." The woman may be eager to wear maternity clothes "like" a pregnant woman, although her nonpregnant clothing still fits (Figure 13–1). Mimicking models in the environment around her gives the woman some stable guidelines during a time of uncertainty.

Role models also give the first-trimester pregnant woman guidelines for the experiences of pregnancy.[13] Although they may not yet coincide with her real experiences, the models at least give the mother-to-be some feeling of control over the unexpected. In general, the most important model is the pregnant woman's own mother.

Role playing, another replicative behavior, also begins during the first trimester and continues into the second trimester. Instead of a model, the preg-

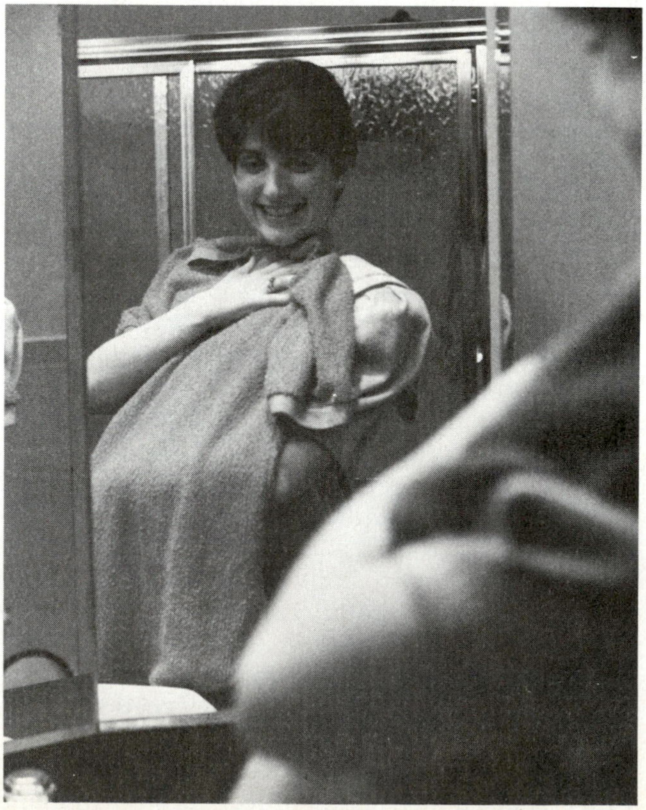

Figure 13–1. Pregnant woman mimics her new role and looks forward to wearing maternity clothes.

MATERNAL PSYCHOLOGIC CHANGES AND CONCERNS DURING THE FIRST TRIMESTER

Psychologic considerations prior to diagnosis of pregnancy

Women's reactions range from hope to despair

Factors influencing reactions include planned pregnancy, wanted pregnancy, economic status, number and ages of other children, support from significant others, cultural and religious background, history of infertility

Psychologic reactions and concerns

Disbelief in reality of pregnancy

Concerns focus on self, feelings about pregnancy, early physiologic changes

Desire to tell everyone or desire to keep pregnancy secret depends on personal, family, or other social factors such as work

Acceptance of pregnancy

Ambivalence common; assessed by honesty of expression, reason for and intensity of ambivalence, duration of ambivalence

Maternal role attainment

Begins during first trimester

Activities include replication, mimicry, search for role models, role playing

Fantasies

Unreal children

Triggered by symbolic objects

Relationship with mother

Own mother is primary role model

Tries to strengthen relationship

Relationship with fetus

Fetus seems unreal

Body image

Does not change much

Time and space

Delivery seems far away

Continues usual activities, unless physical discomforts interfere

nant woman finds a partner with whom to practice role behavior. For example, the pregnant woman may offer to babysit to interact with a baby or child, or she may "mother" a pet. The responses of the partner signal acceptance or rejection of the mothering behaviors, and the mother-to-be can try on new behaviors of the maternal role. Role playing occurs in both primiparas and multiparas. Multiparas tend to explore role behaviors related to having two or more children of different sexes.

Fantasies

During the first trimester, fantasies, both daydreams and nightdreams, are vague.[13,14] They are usually about unreal children and are triggered by symbolic objects in the environment, like an egg. Expectant mothers also report dreams and fantasies about water, for example, oceans, rivers, and lakes.[15] During the second and third trimesters, fantasies become increasingly vivid and provide important clues to the progress of the pregnancy and the woman's feelings about it.

Relationship With Mother

For the expectant mother, the process of rethinking her relationships with her parents begins during the first trimester. Indeed, the woman's own mother is her primary role model.[11] If conflicts exist in the relationship between the newly pregnant woman and her mother, attempts at reconciliation may be made as early as the first trimester.

Relationship With Fetus

Before the use of ultrasound in fetal diagnosis, a woman tended to have a vague relationship with her fetus during the first trimester. Generally, the sensation of fetal movement during the second trimester made the fetus "real" for the mother and ushered in the phase of maternal-fetal interactions. The employment of ultrasound in first-trimester fetal diagnosis, used in the United States for specific indications, makes visualization of the fetus possible before fetal movements are felt. Fetal visualization by ultrasound techniques may affect the mother's (and the father's) relationship with the fetus.[16] Being able to validate the presence of a real fetus as early as the first trimester may alter previous beliefs regarding early perceptions and concerns of the expectant mother, such as the belief that first-trimester mothers have no tactile, visual, or kinesthetic way to identify their embryo or fetus.[11, 17, 18] As yet, the effects of ultrasound visualization on maternal-fetal interaction and attachment have not been extensively documented; the practice of using ultrasound solely to foster attachment to the fetus is controversial.

Body Image

Growth in size of the woman's body during pregnancy represents growth of the child within her. In the pregnant woman's perceptions of the body, these changes in size and weight pertain to the baby, while she herself remains "unchanged."

During the first trimester when there is no obvious growth, there is no real physical evidence of a

PATERNAL PSYCHOLOGIC CHANGES AND CONCERNS DURING THE FIRST TRIMESTER

Psychologic process
Stages include getting ready, stage of conception, end of first trimester

Fantasies
Themes include sex, nurturing, birds nesting, eggs hatching, fear of being left out, images of water

Couvade syndrome
May begin

Any symptoms possible, especially weight gain and gas pains

Concerns
Include income, effect of woman's employment on pregnancy

baby. Although women tend to experience breast fullness, this sensation is similar to that experienced during the premenstrual period. The developing baby still remains vague and unreal. Even a positive pregnancy test does not mean "baby." To the woman, the test results may represent her physiologic situation, not the baby's. Often the woman experiences a slight loss of weight or appetite during the first trimester. As weight gain, rather than loss, is associated with pregnancy in the minds of most people, loss of weight may increase the woman's uncertainty about the reality of a baby.[11]

Changes in body boundary occur with growth in the size of the woman's body.[11] Because there is no change in size during the first trimester, body boundaries also tend to remain unchanged.

Time and Space

According to Rubin, a woman's subjective perceptions of time and space change greatly during the first trimester.[12] During this period, the expected date of confinement (EDC) seems ages away. As the low-risk woman has little sense in the present of really being pregnant, or having a real baby growing in her uterus, her due date seems unreal. The time from the beginning of amenorrhea to the EDC seems empty—nothing is happening that the woman can detect. For some women, this is a time of pride in their ability to become pregnant. During the first trimester, however, a woman tends to use her time in the way she always has, that is, in meeting her adult social commitments and maintaining her normal activities.[11]

THE FATHER'S EXPERIENCE

Psychologic Processes

Expectant fathers undergo unique psychologic processes during pregnancy, although much still remains unknown. During the first trimester, the expectant father is thought to progress through three stages[20]:

1. During the getting ready period, the father and his partner know that they will try to make a child soon. Emotionally, fathers have the feeling of starting something new and foreign. There is a sense of urgency to "get on with it."
2. The stage of conception occurs when pregnancy is medically confirmed. The man who desired pregnancy may experience feelings of joy, manliness, and an increased sexual interest in his partner. The man who did not want pregnancy may react negatively and respond with anger, the feeling of being "trapped," and resentment.
3. The end of the first trimester is a stage in which fathers perceive a great change in their lives. Feelings of "having to give" and nurturing the mother and fetus emerge.

Fantasies

Expectant fathers experience fantasies about pregnancy and the infant-to-be. Fantasy may perform a similar function for the expectant man as for the expectant woman.[21] In American culture, men do not tend to admit day and night fantasies, although both frequently occur. Therefore, men seem to be more reluctant to admit to having fantasies during pregnancy than are their partners.

Toward the end of the first trimester, expectant fathers begin to have new and different fantasies. Sexual fantasies are prevalent, and the father may have images of himself nurturing the pregnancy and fetus. Images and symbols in fantasy during the first trimester include themes of birds nesting and eggs hatching. Night dreams reflect a fear of being "left out" by the pregnancy.[22] Interestingly, dream reports during the first trimester begin to include the imagery of water, for example, lakes, oceans and rivers, which reappears throughout the pregnancy.

Couvade Syndrome

The incidence of the couvade syndrome,[23] that is, almost any physical symptom a man develops during pregnancy but that disappears after childbirth, increases as pregnancy progresses. The couvade syndrome may become evident in some fathers during the first trimester, especially after diagnosis of pregnancy is probable or confirmed.

Mild to severe symptoms may occur at any time during pregnancy. Unintentional weight gain and gas pains are symptoms often reported during the first trimester.

Concerns

Little is known about specific paternal concerns during the first trimester, and this is an area in need of research; however, the woman's career or employment status is one important area of concern. The father, who may feel his role of provider is vital, will be affected by his partner's concerns about her career and employment. If the couple decide that the woman will stay home during her pregnancy or after the baby is born, or both, the father will usually become the primary breadwinner for the family. In the United States today, there is no mandatory employment policy guaranteeing a long-term paid or unpaid parental leave from employment for either mother or father. Therefore, economic worry over absorbing the high costs of a new family member and maintaining the family's lifestyle may affect the father-to-be. In addition, the expectant father may be concerned over the nature of his partner's work or work environment. As the husband of a nurse remarked, "I was always supportive of my wife's love of working with the babies in the intensive care unit. Now that she's pregnant, I find myself worrying about all those in-

RESEARCH ABSTRACT

Clinton JF. Expectant fathers at risk for couvade. Nurs Res. *1986; 35:290–295.*

The couvade syndrome is marked by an expectant father's experience of numerous health complaints and symptoms. The couvade syndrome is viewed in various research reports as a normal response to a developmental crisis, an expression of the father's subjective involvement in pregnancy, and an expression of caring for the partner and unborn child.

The purpose of this study, part of a larger comparative survey, was to determine the risk factors associated with incidence, duration, and perceived seriousness of couvade symptoms as experienced by expectant fathers during each trimester of pregnancy and the early postpartum period. The design used was a repeated-measures survey that monitored physical and emotional health of expectant fathers over pregnancy and the early postpartum. Data were collected at lunar months and at the sixth week postdelivery.

Volunteer subjects were 81 expectant fathers who varied in age (18–48), income ($5,000 to $100,000), years of education, and religion. Most (88 percent) were white; all were currently healthy with no prior history of chronic physical or mental health problems.

Three dependent variables were chosen for the study: total number of couvade symptoms, total duration of symptoms, and total perceived seriousness of symptoms. Three instruments were used to identify potential risk factors (identified from the literature) affecting these three variables: (1) the expectant father's preliminary health interview (PHI), designed to elicit information concerning cultural background, social history, and health events prior to pregnancy; (2) the expectant father's monthly health diary (MHD), designed to elicit monthly information concerning self-perceptions of physical and emotional status, incidence, duration, and perceived seriousness of 39 couvade symptoms, self-initiated actions to alleviate symptoms, perceived effectiveness of self-care, professional health utilization, physical and social role disabilities, work hour loss and salary dollar loss, effective and behavioral involvement in the pregnancy, and perceptions of partner's pregnancy difficulty and ability to help her; (3) Ireton personal inventory (IPI), used to measure stress, including the individual's concern due to health, employment, marriage, sexual life, personal habits, friends, and family.

A regression analysis procedure was used. Six factors were found to significantly account for variance in couvade discomforts: effective involvement in pregnancy, number of previous children, income, ethnic identity, perceived stress, and recent health prior to expectant fatherhood. Interestingly, other variables thought to be associated with the couvade syndrome were discounted in the analysis because of a lack of statistical significance (age, level of education, pregnancy planning/convenience, partner's pregnancy complications, and behavioral involvement in pregnancy, including participation in prenatal classes and attendance at delivery). Additional findings included a descriptive overview of pregnancy couvade events according to trimester and postpartum status. The investigator concluded that the study confirms some theoretical explanations of couvade but not others.

Comment:

This well-designed and controlled study lends factual documentation to speculations about the expectant father's experiences during pregnancy. It further justifies involvement of the father in pregnancy through the practice of family-centered maternity care. Clinically, the study may identify potential risk factors linked to couvade symptoms and serve as a basis for anticipatory health counseling for the expectant father.

fections she is working around and the effects of her many changes in working hours. She keeps going from days to evenings to nights, and is even more tired because of her pregnancy. My greatest fear is that one day, because of her job, we're going to end up as part of the ICU parents' group."

THE FAMILY

During the first trimester, the family is usually eager to determine whether or not the woman is really pregnant. Aside from curiosity, the possibility of a child raises such issues as inheritance and continuation of the family name. First-trimester physiologic changes have an impact on the family. For example, if the mother is nauseated or fatigued, her daily activities may be interrupted. Her husband or other family members may have to assume additional responsibilities. In the "traditional" American family, responsibilities for marketing and household maintenance may need to be divided among other family members, who may not accept their new chores graciously. In addition, the couple's sexual relationship may be affected if the mother simply does not feel well.

Family members may have difficulty in feeling any attachment to the embryo/fetus during the first trimester. The developing baby is not a reality to the expectant father or other family members until fetal movements and the growth of the mother's abdomen makes the baby evident during the second trimester.

Both mother and father begin to evolve new self-concepts, roles, and identities during the first trimester. These intrapsychic processes are also linked to the growth of the fetus, and therefore develop to a much greater degree during the next two trimesters. The first trimester is important, however, as psychologic conflicts can emerge at this time.

Even if they desire the pregnancy and infant, many couples experience ambivalence during the first trimester. Fear and uncertainty about changes they must undergo to become parents and conflicts about the lives they as a couple are leaving behind become apparent.

Role changes in significant others begin during the first trimester. Yet, the reality of a baby is still tentative and uncertain, especially for members of the extended family. The couple may not even tell extended family members about the pregnancy in its early stages. Young children may not be made aware of the pregnancy or may not understand what pregnancy means at this time. In families where children are greatly wanted and valued, news of pregnancy may make the expectant couple the focus of enthusiastic family attention.

Ideally, the pregnant couple begins a new relationship with the broader community during the first trimester. For example, they may come to health care providers for pregnancy diagnosis and early prenatal care. Prenatal health care may be sought from nurse-midwives, physicians, or other culturally prescribed forms of health care delivery. Optimally the couple establishes a collaborative relationship with prenatal care providers in planning for a healthy pregnancy and birth.

FAMILY'S EXPERIENCE DURING THE FIRST TRIMESTER

- Eager to confirm pregnancy
- Issues include continuing family line, inheritance, redistribution of family tasks
- Fetus not a reality
- Psychologic conflicts may emerge
- Couple begins new relationship with broader community (eg, health care system)
- Pregnant couple may become focus of family attention

THE SIBLINGS' EXPERIENCE

Little is known about how children in a family adapt to pregnancy and a new baby.[24] Some 80 percent of children in the United States grow up with siblings,[19] despite a recent trend toward smaller family size. The patterns of sibling interaction seem to be established during infancy of the later-born child and continue throughout childhood. These interactions may influence the nature of future relationships between the siblings and may affect the personality development of each child.[19] Thus, the sibling's experience as early as the first trimester of pregnancy is an area of concern for the nurse delivering family-centered care.

Studies show that the relationships between parents and children in a family begin to change as early as the first trimester. Generally, there seems to be an increase in confrontation between mothers and firstborn children and a decrease in the mother's availability to her firstborn.[25–27] First-trimester physical discomforts, such as nausea and fatigue, affect the amount of energy the expectant mother has to devote to care of other children. Although young children may not understand the normal physical changes of pregnancy, they are certainly aware of changes in their mothers, especially when those changes affect

SIBLINGS' EXPERIENCE DURING THE FIRST TRIMESTER

Relationship with parents begins to change

May or may not be told about pregnancy

Aware of changes, especially if mother is not feeling well

activities of daily living (Figure 13–2). The child may instigate attention-getting behaviors, such as tantrums, that also serve to release frustration at changes he or she cannot understand or control.

Programs dealing with preparation of the child for the birth of a sibling have been reported in the literature. These articles generally do not deal with preparation during specific trimesters. Most programs, however, do not begin during the first trimester. To be effective, sibling education must be based on such factors as the child's age and stage of cognitive development (*see* Chapters 17 and 24). For example, preparation of a 2-year-old is very different from preparation of a 10-year-old.

During the first trimester, children older than 5 can usually comprehend the event of pregnancy, although the concept of "months ahead" is still vague for many 5- to 7-year-olds. Parents need to tailor explanations so that the child can understand the event, based on his or her level of cognitive development.

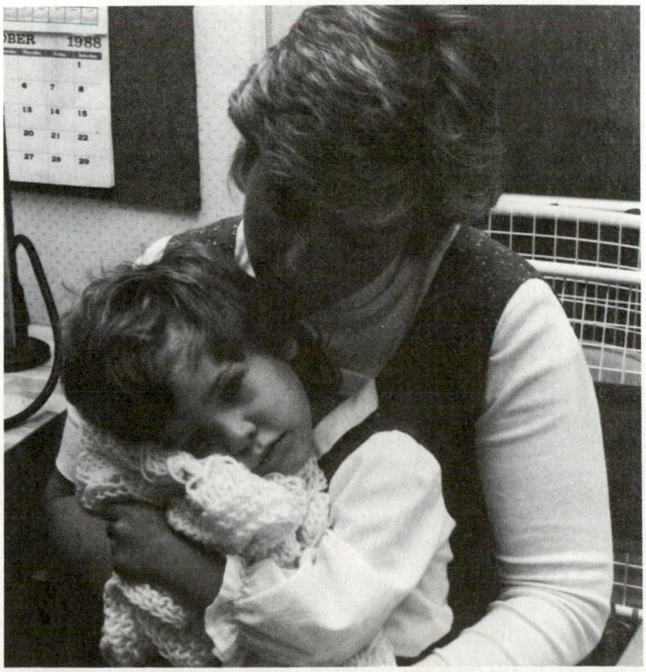

Figure 13–2. Children are aware of changes in their mother's behavior during the first trimester.

Many parents do not tell toddlers or preschool children about pregnancy during the first trimester. Based on his or her state of cognitive development, the child may not understand the concept of a nonvisible baby growing inside the mother. Ultrasound photos also have little meaning to the young child. More extensive preparation for the very young child may best occur after the pregnancy is visible.

Secrets about early pregnancy are not necessary. After discussion of sibling growth and development, parents should be encouraged to present information about the baby at a time they feel is best for themselves and their children.

Parents need to understand how changes in their behavior may be perceived, especially by young children. For example, quiet activities can be suggested for times when first-trimester fatigue alters a usually vigorous schedule. First-trimester prenatal education that provides anticipatory guidance and explanation of physical and psychologic changes can enhance parental well-being and confidence. This in turn may be perceived by the child.

THE GRANDPARENTS' EXPERIENCE

Pregnancy confers the status of grandparent on the parents of the expectant couple. Little research has focused on the special needs of grandparents during the first trimester or at any time during pregnancy. As discussed earlier, both the expectant mother and the expectant father look to their own parents, especially the parent of the same sex, for support and for role modeling. Often grandparents are informed about the pregnancy during the first trimester. The nature of the expectant grandparents' reaction to news of the pregnancy depends on several factors:

- How ready the grandparent perceives the expectant couple to be for parenthood. "Readiness" can include financial independence, completion of education, age, number and spacing of other children, marital status, and acceptance of the spouse.

GRANDPARENTS' EXPERIENCE DURING THE FIRST TRIMESTER

Reactions to pregnancy depend on such factors as couple's readiness for childbearing; relationship with couple; personal feelings about grandparenting (eg, moving up a generation)

Serve as important support and role models for couple

- The expectant grandparent's ability to deal with personal transitions, such as a change in status from parent to grandparent.[28] Indeed, as early as the first trimester, expectant grandparents must realize that they are moving up a generation. Some expectant grandparents equate their new role with cultural stereotypes of grandparents as old, whereas others view impending grandparenthood as a chance to enjoy and indulge grandchildren in ways they were not able to with their own children.
- Whether the expectant grandparents have other grandchildren.
- Nature of the relationship between the expectant couple and grandparents.

SOCIOCULTURAL FACTORS

Within the scope of any textbook, it is impossible to discuss all cultural groups. Indeed, religious and ethnic beliefs are part of cultural considerations. Thus, an individual may belong to several groups at one time. For example, a client may be a Catholic, Protestant, or Jewish Lebanese-American. Actual practices may evolve from a combination of Middle Eastern, American, and religious influences.

A family's culture greatly affects perceptions and behaviors related to childbearing. Cultural ideas and practices may or may not be congruent with those valued by nurses. Indeed, North American nurses themselves may be considered a cultural group. For example, early prenatal care, delivered by a physician or nurse-midwife, is a cultural value that nurses support. Nurses base this belief on scientific research and clinical experience in working with healthy and high-risk clients. Other cultural groups may or may not value early prenatal care for reasons as valid in their cultural belief system as scientific research is in nursing's belief system. In addition, many religious and ethnic groups are represented within the nursing culture. Therefore, although early prenatal care may be valued by nurses in general, Chinese and Irish nurses, for example, may view first-trimester prenatal options differently.

The nurse must strive to understand the cultural backgrounds of clients and to identify specific beliefs and practices related to childbearing. The nurse must determine how cultural groups that are different from the "typical" (eg, dominant) North American culture perceive pregnancy and prenatal care.

Culturally sensitive care evolves from basic respect for clients and curiosity to learn about their cultural background, as well as their personal history. Such differences as language, manner of dress, religious beliefs, attitudes toward personal hygiene, support systems, and attitudes toward health care are among the cultural factors that challenge nursing skills.

Although some clients may come for preconceptional reproductive care prior to pregnancy, the first trimester is often the time of the initial contact between the client and the prenatal health care system. The type and nature of the care presented may determine whether or not the client continues to seek prenatal care. In providing culturally sensitive care beginning prior to pregnancy, during the first trimester, or even after, the nurse must understand certain factors:

- All cultures have specific attitudes and practices related to childbearing. These affect daily activities, dietary intake, and relationships with others.
- Each culture has its own relationship system: who is related to whom and the nature of that relationship vary with the culture.
- Cultures vary as to what constitutes "marriage." For example, the Koran, the Islamic holy book, allows a man to have more than one wife, provided he can treat each the same.
- Cultures tend to prescribe particular male and female roles for childbearing, as well as daily living. These roles, such as the father's lack of participation in birth, may be expected and accepted by members of that culture.
- Cultures tend to have their own ceremonies and rituals related to childbearing.
- Cultural views tend to affect whether or not women seek early or any prenatal care from physicians and nurses.
- The role of nurses varies widely around the world. In the United States, nursing is a profession with increasing status, and members' credentials may include doctorates and postdoctoral study. In certain other countries, nursing is not considered a profession but a menial type of work done by the least advantaged of that society. Nurses need to understand cultural views of nursing to plan effective care.
- Cultures may have a rich heritage, yet may not have extensive technology, financial resources, or educational systems as in the United States.
- Differences in language between health care workers and clients can be a barrier to culturally sensitive care. Use of interpreters, a kind tone of voice, and real interest in the client can be helpful. Teaching sheets can be written with the translation skills of individuals, such as health care workers employed in other departments, faculty and students from local universities, and specific cultural civic groups.

Often, health care workers tend to speak louder when addressing clients who do not understand their language. These clients profit more from the skills of an interpreter.

This chapter will focus on the black American family's experience of pregnancy as an example of how pregnancy is perceived from a cultural perspective. Later chapters of the text will explore how families from other cultural groups perceive pregnancy and the postpartum/newborn period. Stereotyping should, however, be avoided; prenatal care needs to be based on each client's unique perceptions and needs.

Socioeconomic Factors

Socioeconomic level has a distinct impact in addition to culture. Each culture prescribes behaviors women should and should not perform during pregnancy; however, socioeconomic status can place a woman at risk for cultural conflict if the need for financial survival is at odds with her culture's ideal of a pregnant woman's behavior.

Poverty seems to form its own culture, deeply affected by factors such as limited resources, poor housing, and access to services such as health care. Childbearing is a very expensive process. Families who perceive themselves financially stressed may respond to the prospect of pregnancy, childbirth, and childrearing with despair or panic, especially if the mother's income is needed and jeopardized by the pregnancy. Public assistance, the Food Stamp Program, and the Special Supplemental Food Program for Women, Infants, and Children (WIC), and other programs do not cover the increasingly high costs associated with having children. Lack of insurance and ability to pay for private care greatly limits where and when pregnant women seek prenatal health care. Even in urban areas where some sort of prenatal care may be available to women regardless of their ability to pay, transportation and other obstacles may make access difficult. First-trimester prenatal care can become an inaccessible luxury rather than a priority for financially stressed women. In addition, perception of financial hardship can interfere with the psychologic tasks of pregnancy.

Throughout the first trimester, most women can continue to wear their nonpregnant clothes and are thus spared the cost of maternity fashions. Considerable amounts of money can be saved if a woman is able to sew her own clothes; the first trimester can then be a time to prepare a maternity wardrobe. In addition, maternity clothing may be obtained from other sources such as extended family, church, communities, or "second hand" stores. Some women, however, are superstitious about preparing too early during pregnancy, either for themselves or for their infants. Other women cannot sew or cannot afford the sewing equipment and fabric, or reject other options for a variety of reasons.

Most working women can continue with their jobs throughout the first trimester, although work performance may be affected by normal physical discomforts such as nausea and fatigue. Women whose work poses risks at any time during pregnancy may be faced with loss or transfer of employment during the first trimester. In many cases, transfer is difficult to do.

In the United States, the physically healthy pregnant woman usually comes to an outpatient clinic or private office setting for prenatal care. Health care providers thus see her outside her usual living and working environment. A high-risk environment, such as a residence without basic utilities like water or heat, cannot be readily identified. Women who come from middle-class backgrounds may also perceive themselves at financial risk. Mortgages, credit balances, loans, the cost of raising other children, cultural expectations, and other financial responsibilities can contribute to perceptions of financial hardship complicated by pregnancy.

Manner of dress at times can be an unreliable indication of socioeconomic status. For example, a neatly and tastefully dressed client may be struggling to provide the family's next month's rent. In assessing the pregnant client, nurses and other health care providers must include questions focusing on the financial aspect of pregnancy. Health care providers must consider the cost of any recommendations to clients.

When a pregnant family is economically comfortable or well off, the first trimester can be a time of exciting plans. In cases of perceived financial difficulty, however, pregnancy can be a source of additional conflict and psychologic pressure.

Cultural Focus: The Black Family

No single entity can truly be called "the black family" in the United States. Although many are descendants of Africans brought as slaves, blacks in the United States today have originated from a variety of countries.[29] In addition, factors such as geographic location in the United States (eg, urban north, rural south), age, level of acculturation, religious background, and socioeconomic status produce many variations in each family.[30] Socioeconomic status is especially important to consider. Indeed, upper-middle-class blacks are closer in lifestyle and value systems to upper-middle-class whites than to blacks who live in poverty. Likewise, blacks living in poverty share similar social problems with other disadvantaged groups. Nurses should never attempt to stereotype any group, but should base care on the unique needs and patterns of each client and her family.

Although every black American family must be assessed during pregnancy to discover unique characteristics, certain cultural traditions and patterns may help the nurse understand the black family's responses to pregnancy and childbirth. Black families possess many adaptive strengths that help bring about a positive pregnancy outcome. These strengths include strong kinship bonds, flexibility in family roles, and a high value on religion, education, and work.

Kinship Bonds. Strong kinship bonds have helped blacks survive extremely difficult conditions since the days of slavery.[30] Reliance on the kinship network is an important source of support for black families. This kinship is not always drawn along "blood lines," that is, who is directly related to whom. Black families may evolve complex patterns of co-residence and kinship-based exchange networks that link various domestic units together. In addition, black family units often have broad household boundaries and strong bonds to three generations of households. People in this network are involved in many cooperative domestic exchanges among units.[31] A large number of people inside and outside the "nuclear family" may operate within the boundaries of this complex family network. Thus, not only do the pregnant woman's partner, parents, and children affect the course of the childbearing cycle; uncles, aunts, preachers, male and female friends, brothers, sisters, and cousins, may also have influence. Far from being disorganized, as nursing students who make home visits into such flexible families fear, these networks are often organized. They can provide lifelong relationships that offer great stability for the family members.[31]

Family Roles. The role of the black male is difficult. He demands and receives recognition as head of the household; yet, this recognition is often tied to his ability to provide for his family, which may be difficult in the prevailing social structure. In response to this situation, some black men are said to become peripheral to (i.e., exist outside) their family. Current investigators believe this peripheral relationship has been overstated, because the great investment black males have in the family is often overlooked.[30] Black males and females may have great role flexibility in childrearing and household responsibility. Men and women may comfortably reverse roles, especially concerning care of children. Such a pattern has important implications for the nurse providing prenatal care to the couple.

In addition to the parental roles of the black mother and father, other members of the extensive kinship network may assume roles usually reserved for nuclear family members. For example, during childbearing and childrearing, a maternal or paternal aunt or grandmother may share or assume responsibility for child care. A child or infant may be adopted informally and reared by extended family members who have resources not available to the child's parents or who live in a better environment.[30] Thus, the term *significant others* sometimes takes on a different meaning for the black family, and genograms often do not conform to blood lines.

The nurse who explores role responsibilities with the pregnant black family must recognize that the family system may function well, despite its flexible boundaries and role patterns that differ from the "norm" for Caucasian, middle-class groups. For example, that a teenage black mother does not learn to care for her newborn infant may not be a major problem if, in her family system, this will not be her role responsibility. Her own mother, aunt, or sister may actually "mother" the newborn, and the biologic mother's role may be to resume her life as a student. The nurse should determine who will fulfill what roles in care of the newborn and work within the structure of the unique family system of her pregnant client. Role flexibility can be a strength that is mobilized during childbearing and childrearing.

Religion. Religion and the church tend to be strong influences and to serve numerous functions for members of the black community.[30] The religious system provides support in ministers, deacons, deaconesses, and other church members. Spiritual comfort and support are gained from religious beliefs. In addition, numerous church activities may provide a social life for members of the entire black family.

A strong church influence is important during pregnancy, as it is throughout the life process. The church and its members may promote physical health by encouraging young pregnant women to enter early prenatal care and to maintain a lifestyle that can foster a healthy pregnancy outcome. For example, church members have helped provide transportation to prenatal facilities; working collaboratively with health care providers, church members have at times provided space within church properties for mobile prenatal clinics and educational programs related to childbearing.

The Black Family's Experience of Pregnancy. Numerous factors may influence how black women and their families accept pregnancy. Many factors relate to the social and economic circumstances that surround the woman and her family. Satisfaction with her own education and career, along with satisfaction with her partner's education and job, generally fosters a woman's acceptance of pregnancy. A woman married to a man with less education and no stable employment may accept or resent pregnancy, depending on such factors as the number of previous pregnancies, timing of the pregnancy, and the family's economic status. Black women also may reject a pregnancy that is unplanned or occurs out of wedlock.[32] These attitudes are similar for women who are not black.

Although menstruation is a time when some black women view themselves as "sick," pregnancy is seen as a state of wellness. This may be one reason why many black women do not seek early prenatal care; they simply do not see early care as important, because they are healthy. Prenatal care is preventive care, and preventive care may be an unfamiliar concept to some blacks, who enter the health care system only in a health crisis situation.[32] As low-income black women have a high incidence of maternal, fetal, and infant morbidity and mortality, reaching this population is a major responsibility of nurses. Early prenatal care must become meaningful for the low-income black woman. In addition, health care services need to be made accessible so that this minority group seeks early prenatal care.

SUMMARY

The first trimester is a complex time of changes and concerns for the childbearing family. As the embryo develops into a fetus and physiologic changes occur in the mother's body, psychologic adaptation takes place. Pregnancy brings change throughout the family system, and involves not only the mother-to-be, but the expectant father, siblings, and other family members. Psychologic factors have an enormous impact on transition to parenthood and on physiologic well-being during the first trimester.

Factors that affect the way a woman responds to pregnancy include whether the pregnancy was planned, whether the pregnancy was wanted, whether the family feels the baby is affordable, the family's cultural and religious background, and the degree of difficulty the couple had in conceiving. During the first trimester, women normally experience a mixture of such feelings as disbelief, ambivalence, and excitement. The woman's concerns tend to focus on herself and the early physical changes of pregnancy.

During the first trimester, the woman begins to move into the role of mother and tries to model herself after other motherhood role models, especially her own mother; she may also seek to rehearse the motherhood role through role-playing activities. Maternal fantasies tend to be indistinct and focus on unreal, dreamlike children. The maternal relationship with the fetus is vague during the first trimester. The woman's perception of her body image and body boundaries tends to remain unchanged.

Expectant fathers progress through a getting ready period prior to pregnancy; the stage of conception, in which positive feelings may be experienced for a wanted pregnancy and negative feelings may be expressed for an unwanted pregnancy; and the end of the first trimester stage, in which feelings of giving and nurturing ideally emerge. Paternal fantasies include sexual or nurturing themes, but may also include feelings of being left out. Couvade symptoms, such as weight gain and gas pains, may begin during the first trimester.

Relationships between expectant parents and siblings begin to change during the first trimester, especially if first-trimester discomforts affect normal activities. Sibling education about the baby is based on such factors as the child's age and stage of cognitive development. Young children have difficulty conceptualizing early pregnancy.

Expectant parents look to their own parents as role models and as sources of support during pregnancy. Grandparents' reactions are based on complex factors, such as their perception of the couple's readiness for parenthood, their own personal ability to deal with transitions, and the existence and number of other grandchildren.

During the first trimester, the expectant couple begins to establish new roles within the broader community. For instance, contact with health care providers may be established for prenatal care.

A family's cultural and socioeconomic background greatly affects perceptions and behaviors related to childbearing. Nurses need to understand which cultural beliefs and practices are or are not congruent with the health care system. Culturally sensitive care evolves from basic respect for clients and willingness to learn about their cultural background. Nurses also need to identify the impact of socioeconomic factors on a client's perception of pregnancy and on a client's ability to obtain prenatal care. Nurses can do much to overcome barriers to early prenatal care by being aware of culturally prescribed practices so that these practices can be incorporated into the care of the family.

REVIEW QUESTIONS

1. Identify factors that may influence a woman's acceptance of pregnancy.
2. A woman in her first trimester of pregnancy says to you: "I know I planned to become pregnant now, but I feel like I'm giving up everything I've worked for. Sometimes I resent the baby, and he's not even born. Is there something wrong with me?" Your response should be based on what principles?
3. Identify the types of psychologic feelings that fathers might describe during the first trimester.
4. Describe the couvade syndrome.
5. Discuss how the kinship system often found in black families might prove to be a strength during pregnancy.

REFERENCES

1. Colman LL. Psychology of pregnancy. In: Sonstegard L, Kowalski K, Jennings B, eds. *Women's Health, Volume II: Childbearing.* New York: Grune & Stratton; 1983:3–16.
2. Hodge SE. Waiting for the amniocentesis. *N Engl J Med.* 1989;320:63–64. Correspondence.
3. Roberts J. Priorities in prenatal education. *J Obstet Gynecol Neonat Nurs.* 1976;5:18–19.
4. Glazer G. Anxiety levels and concerns among pregnant women. *Res Nurs Health.* 1980;3:110.
5. Marbury MC, et al. Work and pregnancy. *Occup Med.* 1984; 26:415–421.
6. Council on Scientific Affairs. Effects of pregnancy on work performance, *JAMA.* 1984;251:1995–1997.
7. Lips HM. Somatic and emotional aspects of the normal pregnancy experiences: the first five months. *Am J Obstet Gynecol.* 1982;142:524–529.
8. Collins C, Tiedje LB. A program for women returning to work after childbirth. *J Obstet Gynecol Neonat Nurs.* 1988;17: 246–253.
9. Tiedje LB, Collins C. Combining employment and motherhood. *Am J Matern Child Nurs.* 1989;14:9–14.
10. Caplan G. *Concepts of Mental Health and Consultation.* Washington, DC: U.S. Department of Health, Education, Welfare; 1969.
11. Lederman RP. *Psychosocial Adaptation in Pregnancy.* Englewood Cliffs, NJ: Prentice-Hall; 1984.
12. Rubin R. *Maternal Identity and the Maternal Experience.* New York: Springer Publishing Co; 1984.
13. Singer J, Antrobus J. A factor analytic study of daydreaming and conceptually related cognitive and personality variables. *Percept Motor Skills.* 1963; 17 (monograph suppl): whole issue.
14. Sherwen LN, ed. *Psychosocial Dimensions of the Pregnant Family.* New York: Springer Publishing Co: 1987.
15. Rubin R. Fantasy and object consistency in maternal relations. *Matern Child Nurs. J.* 1972;2:101–111.
16. Furlong R, Berkowitz R. Intrauterine treatment: Meeting the psychosocial needs of the family. *Health Soc Work.* 1985: 55–62.
17. Rubin R. Maternal tasks in pregnancy. *Matern Child Nurs J.* 1977;6:67–75.
18. Gay JT, et al. Reva Rubin revisited. *J Obstet Gynecol Neonat Nurs.* 1988;17:394–399.
19. Dunn J. *Sisters and Brothers.* Cambridge, MA: Harvard University Press; 1985.
20. Herzog JM. Patterns of expectant fatherhood: a study of the fathers of a group of premature infants. In: Cath S, Gurwitt AR, Ross JM, eds. *Father and Child.* Boston: Little, Brown; 1982.
21. Sherwen LN. Third trimester fantasies of first time expectant fathers. *Matern Child Nurs. J.* 1986;15:153–170.
22. Gurwitt AR. Aspects of prospective fatherhood. In: Cath S, Gurwitt AR, Ross JM, eds. *Father and Child.* Boston: Little, Brown; 1982.
23. Clinton J. Expectant fathers at risk for couvade. *Nurs Res.* 1986;35:290–295.
24. Kutzner SK. Responses of siblings to pregnancy. In: Sherwen LN: *Psychosocial Dimensions of the Pregnant Family.* New York: Springer Publishing Co; 1987.
25. Dunn J. Kendrick C. The arrival of a sibling: changes in patterns of interaction between mother and firstborn child. *J Child Psychol Psychiatry.* 1980;21:119–132.
26. Dunn J, Kendrick C. Interaction between young siblings in the context of family relationships. In: Lewis M, Rosenblum LA, eds. *The Child and Its Family.* New York: Plenum Press; 1979.
27. Nedelman L, Begun A. The effect of the newborn on the older sibling: mother's questionnaires. In: Lamb ME, Sutton-Smith B, eds. *Sibling Relationships: Their Nature and Significance Across the Lifespan.* Hillsdale, NJ: Lawrence Erlbaum Associates; 1982.
28. Maloni JA, McIndoe JE, Rubenstein G. Expectant grandpar-

ents class. *J Obstet Gynecol Neonat Nurs.* 1987;16:26–29.

29. Spector RE. *Cultural Diversity in Health and Illness.* 2nd ed. Norwalk, Conn: Appleton & Lange, 1985.
30. Hines PM, Boyd-Franklin N. Black families. In: McGoldrick M, Pearch JK, Giordano J, eds. *Ethnicity and Family Therapy.* New York: Guilford Press; 1982.
31. Stack C. *All Our Kin: Strategies for Survival in a Black Community.* New York: Harper & Row; 1975.
32. Carrington BW. The Afro-American. In: Clark A, ed. *Culture, Childbearing, Health Professionals.* Philadelphia: FA Davis Co; 1978.

Assessment During the First Trimester

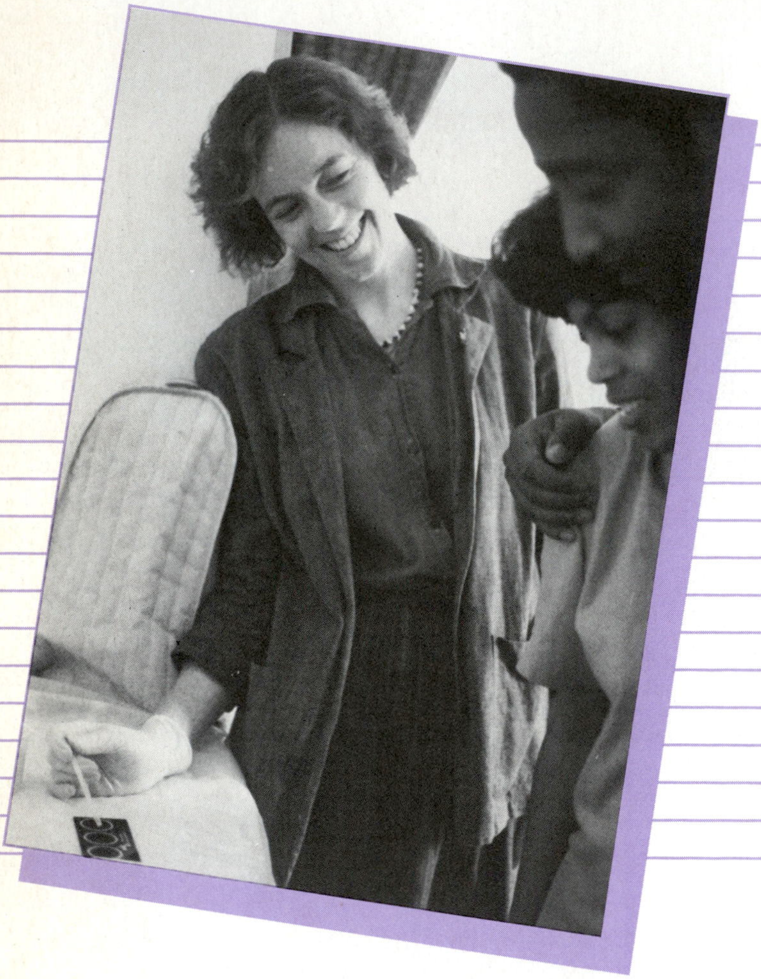

Chapter 14

Key Terms

chorionic villus sampling
diagonal conjugate
false pelvis
gravida
linea terminalis
midpelvis
multigravida
multipara
Nagele's rule
nulligravida
nullipara
obstetric conjugate
parity
pelvic cavity
pelvic outlet
pelvic inlet
pelvimetry
primigravida
primipara
secundagravida
superior strait
true conjugate
true pelvis
ultrasound
x-ray pelvimetry

Prenatal care is defined as a series of interventions received by a woman during her pregnancy, with the goal of promoting her chances for a favorable outcome.[1] Prenatal care has been described as an essential determinant of birth outcome, second only to socioeconomic status.[2] Without prenatal care a woman is at greater risk for harm related to conditions that affect her or the developing fetus. Prior to pregnancy, women may come for regular well woman examinations or for preconceptional assessment; however, actual prenatal assessment and care begin with the first prenatal visit. The earlier in pregnancy that prenatal care is begun, the greater the possibility of healthy outcomes for the mother, fetus and family. First-trimester assessment allows for early identification of the client's and family's risk factors, existing problems, strengths, resources, and educational needs.

Components of prenatal care include obtaining information from the client through history, physical examination, and laboratory testing; setting goals, based on that information; working collaboratively with other health care providers to prescribe appropriate treatments (for example, in relation to diet or activity); and providing client education that will foster health promoting behaviors.[2]

Assessment is the first step in the nursing process. Diagnoses, goals, and interventions evolve from assessment. Because of its importance as a component of prenatal management, assessment is highlighted in separate chapters for each trimester and for the intrapartum and postpartum units of this text.

PRENATAL ASSESSMENT

During the first prenatal visit, the nurse assesses the health of the expectant mother and her family by compiling a comprehensive data base, which includes a health history, physical examination, and laboratory studies. The assessment process is guided by several principles, which are summarized in the box on page 334. Initial assessment of the healthy pregnant client is similar to assessment of the well woman, as described in Chapter 5, but special attention is given to factors related to childbearing and early parenting. This type of detailed assessment is done during the first visit, regardless of the trimester in which the client comes for her initial visit. In some cases women move or change care providers during their pregnancies. Certain laboratory tests may not need to be repeated if clinical documentation can be provided; however, a comprehensive history and a physical examination are performed for any "new" client. Results are recorded in the client's chart and may also be communicated during discussion with other health professionals working with the client.

During return prenatal visits, the health history is updated to reflect the client's and family's current status, and a physical examination is done. Various laboratory tests, such as hemoglobin or glucose assessment, may be part of routine assessment as pregnancy progresses. From thorough assessment at the first and subsequent visits, diagnoses can be determined and strategies for the client's nursing, medical, and self-care management can be developed or modified. Table 14–1 summarizes the assessment focus of the initial prenatal visit and return visits.

Collaborating with other health care providers, the nurse has an important role in initial and ongoing assessment of the pregnant client. During the first visit, the nurse establishes a trusting relationship with the client and family and anticipates their needs at various stages of the pregnancy.

Pregnant women are often very receptive to health teaching. Prenatal visits provide an opportunity to begin or improve positive self-care patterns that may benefit the woman during and after her pregnancy (Table 14–2). The nurse also acts as a teacher and advocate for the family in explaining what the family can expect and in providing information so that the family can make informed decisions regarding their health care.

TABLE 14–1. ASSESSMENT FOCUS AT THE FIRST PRENATAL VISIT AND RETURN VISITS

Focus During First Prenatal Visit
Existence of pregnancy
Past and present maternal health status through a health history, physical examination, and laboratory data
Risk factors for childbearing and early parenting, (including physical, psychologic, and sociologic factors)
Signs and symptoms of pregnancy
Well-being of the embryo/fetus
Psychosocial adaptation to pregnancy
Cultural, socioeconomic, or other factors that influence health care practices
Client/family strengths and resources
Client/family educational needs
Focus During Return Visits
Maternal health status through an updated health history, physical examination, and laboratory testing as indicated
Risk factors (new or ongoing)
Progress of pregnancy
Fetal well-being
Progression of psychosocial adaptation to pregnancy
Cultural, socioeconomic, or other factors that influence health care practices as pregnancy progresses
Client/family strengths and resources
Client/family educational needs

PRINCIPLES TO GUIDE ASSESSMENT DURING NORMAL PREGNANCY

- Childbearing is a normal, although not always comfortable, developmental stage for the family.
- Assessment should focus on the whole client and her significant others and include psychologic and cultural, as well as physiologic aspects.
- Childbearing couples need comprehensive information, so that they can make informed decisions regarding their care. In providing information, nurses should avoid technical jargon and use terms that families can readily understand.
- Risks and benefits of interventions should be explained and informed consent should be obtained before any procedure.
- The childbearing family's self-care practices should be fostered. Participation in self-care necessitates family participation in planning of care.
- Many of the assessment techniques available to assess the expectant client or fetus may carry some type of risk to physical or emotional well-being; the costs of some tests outweigh benefits. Tests should be performed only when indicated; healthy, normal women should not be treated as if they were high risk.
- Childbearing families need advocates who will support them in a nonjudgmental way. Nurses can serve as advocates for the family with other care providers.

Timing of First-Trimester Assessment

In an uncomplicated pregnancy, first trimester prenatal visits are usually scheduled about 4 weeks apart. Ideally, the client and her family are assessed about three times during the first trimester.

PRENATAL HEALTH HISTORY

During the first prenatal visit, health care providers obtain and record a health history that elicits information about the current and past health status of the expectant mother and her family. By collaborating on a health history outline, nurses, physicians, and other prenatal health care providers can avoid asking the

TABLE 14–2. PRENATAL ASSESSMENT OF MATERNAL HEALTH PATTERNS

Self-Care Practice	Nursing Considerations
Breast examination	Assess client's knowledge of breast self-examination, appropriate timing for examination, and technique. Teach breast self-examination by demonstration. Have client return the demonstration. Answer questions related to the procedure.
Frequency of health maintenance examination/Pap smear, self-vulvar examination	Assess client's beliefs and practices with regard to health maintenance examinations/Pap smear, self-vulvar examination. Discuss with client the purpose and recommended practice. Teach procedures and answer questions in a nonjudgmental manner.
Nutrition	Assess client's beliefs and practices regarding nutrient intake. Assess cultural food practices. Teach nutrient requirements during pregnancy. Plan with client a diet, taking into consideration beliefs, practices, and the ability to purchase foods.
Exercise	Assess client's exercise regimen prior to pregnancy. Assess the value the family attributes to exercise and health. Plan with client an exercise program considering tolerance, stage of pregnancy, and desires of the mother.
Substance use/exposure	Assess client's use of or exposure to substances that may be teratogenic. Discuss potential problems related to substance use or exposure. Plan self-care practices with client in an effort to eliminate potentially harmful substances from lifestyle. Refer client to community resources.
Stress reduction	Assess expectant family members' methods of coping with previous stresses. Counsel client regarding psychologic changes during pregnancy. Act as a support person for the family.
Oral care	Assess client's oral health practices; identify any incidence of oral problems, such as bleeding gums. Refer client to dentist and dental hygienist. In collaboration with dentist, reinforce proper techniques for brushing, flossing, and gum stimulation.

TABLE 14–3. SAMPLE OUTLINE FOR A REPRODUCTIVE HISTORY DURING THE FIRST PRENATAL VISIT

Suspicion of pregnancy	Sexual activity, missed menses, home pregnancy test, and so forth
Planned/unplanned pregnancy	Reaction of self and significant others to possibility of pregnancy
Menstrual history	Date when last menstrual period began; history of regular/irregular menses; atypical bleeding or other vaginal discharge; treatments
Family planning history	Birth control practices (attitude toward birth control, type of methods used, length of time used, complications related to the methods); any infertility treatments used to facilitate conception; length of time trying to achieve pregnancy
Obstetric history	Previous pregnancies (planned, unplanned); outcome of previous pregnancies (live, stillborn, aborted, premature); dates and types of deliveries, including length and course of labor; infant's birth weight, sex, and status; obstetric or neonatal complications and treatments Reaction of self and significant others to obstetric events
Gynecologic history	
Breasts	Changes related to early pregnancy, such as increase in size, tenderness; history of breast disease of any kind, including types and dates of treatment; continued practice of breast self-examination; recent screening for breast disease; family history of breast cancer (maternal relatives or sister)
Genitalia	Vaginal discharge (nature, amount, duration, foul odor); itching, burning, lesions; gynecologic problems of infectious (sexually transmitted diseases) or noninfectious (eg, endometriosis, fibroids) origin, including dates and treatments; date of last Pap test; understanding and practice of genital self-examination
Sexual history	Recent change in sexual patterns (especially in relation to suspicion of pregnancy); pain or vaginal bleeding after intercourse; sexual orientation (heterosexual, bisexual); history of multiple sexual partners or sexual partners with other high-risk behaviors, such as intravenous drug use; concerns related to sexuality and pregnancy
Sources and dates of current or previous reproductive care	Private physician, certified nurse-midwife, clinic staff, others

client the same questions. A team approach toward assessment can focus on obtaining new and more complete information about the client and her family.

Information from the health history helps the physician or nurse to individualize the prenatal physical examination, to document the normal progress of pregnancy, to identify any risk factors, and to develop a plan of care. Assessment should be done in a private setting and begin with identification of the client's reason for her visit.

A thorough health history for a first prenatal visit is similar to the health history taken during a well woman visit. Figure 5–1 presents a sample outline for a comprehensive health history. A variety of health history formats may be used to meet the goal of comprehensive assessment. At the first prenatal visit, however, particular attention is paid to the reproductive history (Table 14–3), physical or psychosocial changes characteristic of pregnancy, and the existence of physical, psychologic, socioeconomic, medical, lifestyle, environmental, or occupational factors that could affect pregnancy in a positive or negative way. Adequate nutrition is critical to the well-being of the expectant mother and fetus and is one of the most important aspects of prenatal assessment. (Prenatal nutrition is discussed in detail in Chapter 10.) Terms related to gravidity and parity are employed to interpret the reproductive history. In addition, numeric scoring systems are frequently used in clinical practice to summarize current and past pregnancies (*see* box).

ASSESSMENT OF PHYSIOLOGIC STATE

During the initial prenatal visit, a complete physical examination including a pelvic examination is done for the mother. The physical examination provides

GRAVIDITY AND PARITY

Gravidity

- A **gravida** is a pregnant woman. The word gravida refers to a pregnancy regardless of its duration. A woman's gravidity relates to the total number of her pregnancies, regardless of their duration.
- A **primigravida** is a woman pregnant for the first time.
- A **secundagravida** is a woman pregnant for the second time.
- A **multigravida** is a woman who has been pregnant several times.

Parity

- The prefix *para* refers to past pregnancies that have reached viability.
- **Parity** refers to the number of past pregnancies that have gone to viability and have been delivered, regardless of the number of children involved. (For example, the birth of triplets increase the parity by only one.)
- A **nullipara** is a woman who has never delivered a child that reached viability.
- A **primipara** is a woman who has delivered one pregnancy in which the child has reached viability, without regard to the child's being alive or dead at the time of birth.
- A **multipara** is a woman who has had two or more pregnancies that terminated at the stage when the children were viable.

Gravida and Para

- A woman pregnant for the first time is a primigravida and is described as gravida 1, para 0.
- If she aborts before viability she remains gravida 1, para 0.
- If she delivers a fetus that has reached viability she becomes a primipara, regardless of whether the child is alive or dead. She is now gravida 1, para 1.
- During a second pregnancy she is gravida 2, para 1.
- After she delivers the second child she is gravida 2, para 2.
- A woman with two abortions and no viable children is gravida 2, para 0. When she becomes pregnant again she is gravida 3, para 0. When she delivers a viable child she is gravida 3, para 1.
- Multiple births do not affect the parity by more than one. A woman who has viable triplets in her first pregnancy is gravida 1, para 1.

GTPAL is an acronym for a five-digit numeric scoring system used to summarize a client's obstetric situation. It differs from the two-digit scoring system (above) because it provides more detailed information about parity.

G: Gravidity (total number of pregnancies)
T: Term births
P: Premature births
A: Abortions
L: Living children

Variations on the above system include a four-digit system that omits gravidity and uses only TPAL and a system that adds a final category for the number of pregnancies that resulted in multiple births.

(Adapted, with permission, from Oxorn H. Human Labor and Birth. *5th ed. Norwalk, Conn: Appleton-Century-Crofts, 1986:62–63.)*

TABLE 14–4. SELECTED CLINICAL FINDINGS DURING THE FIRST TRIMESTER

Body System	Clinical Findings
Integumentary	Darkening of pigment of nipples, breast areolae, vulva, and thighs; linea nigra starts to develop (pigmented area extending vertically over midline of abdomen); most noticeable in dark-skinned women
Cardiovascular	Increase in resting pulse rate of, on average, 8–10 beats per minute Slight decrease in base line systolic and diastolic blood pressure Short low-grade, systolic ejection murmur; exaggerated splitting of first heart sound
Respiratory	Increased tidal volume (amount of air breathed in one cycle of ordinary inspiration and expiration) Respiratory rate 16–24 per minute Nasal stuffiness and/or epistaxis
Hematologic	Mean white blood cell count 10,000–11,000 mm^3 Hgb 11–14 g/dL; Hct 33% or greater
Gastrointestinal	Nausea and vomiting Ptyalism and changes in taste
Urinary	Frequency of urination Trace glycosuria
Reproductive	Amenorrhea Uterine enlargement Hegar's sign Braun von Fernwald's sign Piskacek's sign Ladin's sign Goodell's sign Chadwick's sign Increased vaginal secretions (leukorrhea) Breast tenderness

objective data. The nurse prepares the mother for the physical assessment and supports her throughout the procedure.

Physiologic changes that suggest pregnancy may be identified during the initial physical examination during the first trimester (*see* Chapter 12). Table 14–4 summarizes some of these first-trimester clinical findings. Although all systems are not presented, it should be emphasized that a complete physical examination is done on the initial prenatal visit. The outline for an initial prenatal physical examination is similar to that for the well-woman physical examination. (*See* discussion of well-woman assessment in Chapter 5 and Figure 5–2.)

Pelvic Examination

During the first prenatal visit, the pelvis is assessed for abnormalities. Changes related to pregnancy are also assessed through inspection and bimanual examination. As discussed in Chapter 15, the staff nurse participates in this part of the assessment by preparing the couple and assisting the examiner, who may be a physician, a certified nurse-midwife, or a nurse with specialized education in prenatal physical assessment.

Uterine Changes. The uterus undergoes many changes, for example, an increase in size and alteration in shape, to maintain pregnancy and accommodate the developing fetus (*see* Chapter 12). Physical uterine changes are important to assess; they contribute to detection of pregnancy and determination of the gestational age of the fetus.

Softening of the uterine isthmus (Hegar's sign) is apparent at 4 to 6 weeks of gestation. Braun von Fernwald's sign, detectable at 4 to 5 weeks, is the unilateral softening of the uterus, with development of a palpable groove lengthwise between the soft and firm parts. This sign is related to softening of the uterus at the site of implantation of the fertilized ovum (*see* Figures 12–5 and 12–6). The asymmetry of the uterus at the cornual area, an implantation site, is apparent at 6 weeks of gestation and is referred to as Piskacek's sign. The ability to flex the uterine body and cervix against one another during bimanual examination occurs at approximately 7 weeks and is known as McDonald's sign.[3] Nurses should be prepared to explain these signs to any client who asks. Actual physical assessment of these signs is done by the examiner.

During the first trimester, uterine enlargement is noted on bimanual pelvic examination, as the uterus has not yet grown beyond the pelvis. About 12 weeks of gestation, however, the uterus can be palpated 1 to 2 cm above the symphysis (*see* Figure 12–2). The uterus in early pregnancy is pyriform or pear-shaped, but, by the end of the first trimester, becomes ovoid or globular. Initial changes in uterine size result from an increase in the number and size of uterine cells; later in pregnancy, this increase is due to the increased size of the fetus.

Cervical Changes. Under the influence of estrogen and progesterone, the cervix increases in anteroposterior diameter by about 2 to 4 weeks of gestation. The cervical appearance is altered in pregnancy by an outward extension of columnar epithelial tissue where normally squamous epithelium is present[4] (*see* Figure 16–2).

Early in pregnancy the cervix undergoes a noticeable color change to a bluish violet, because of the increased vascularity (Chadwick's sign). This is similar to changes occurring in the vaginal tissue. Hypertrophy of the cervical glands produces an increase in odorless, nonirritating leukorrhea, or discharge. Softening of the cervix (Goodell's sign) may be apparent as early as 4 weeks of gestation. A noticeable softening, midline between the corpus and the cervix (Ladin's sign), is detectable by about 6 weeks[4] (*see* Figures 12–2 and 12–4).

Vaginal Changes. The vaginal tissue undergoes increased vascular congestion in pregnancy, and becomes bluish violet (Chadwick's sign) at 6 to 8 weeks of gestation. The rugae or folds of the vagina become more prominent in nulliparous women. In comparison, the vaginal rugae of multiparous women are smoother or flatter, and the entire vaginal canal may be widened. Estrogenic influences cause vaginal smooth muscle hypertrophy, loosening of connective tissue, and increased thickening, acidity, and production of vaginal mucous discharge.

Pelvic Measurements. Measurement of diameters (or distances) between bony structures of the pelvis is called **pelvimetry.**[4,5] The purpose of pelvimetry is to assess whether the expectant mother's pelvic canal is adequate for passage of the fetus during labor and delivery. A maternal pelvis that is too small or abnormally shaped can alert health care providers to a woman's potential difficulties in labor. Pelvimetry during the first trimester is done through clinical examination.

X-ray pelvimetry has been used late in the third trimester and during labor to provide a fairly accurate assessment of pelvic structures and the distances between them. This procedure also gives precise measurements of the transverse diameter of the inlet and the transverse diameter of the midpelvis, which would not be noted on clinical examination. However, conventional x-ray pelvimetry delivers a radiation dose that approaches 1 rad, the maximum fetal radiation dosage cautioned by the International Commission on Radiologic Protection.[6] No absolutely safe level of radiation has been established for pregnancy. Further, diagnostic radiation has been associated with a small risk of childhood malignancies. Therefore, this procedure is not often done because of concern for effects of prenatal exposure to radiation.[4]

Clinical pelvimetry, done through use of the examining hand as a measurement tool or with an instrument called a pelvimeter, can provide estimates of the size of the true pelvis (Figure 14–1). Prior to clinical pelvimetry, the examiner measures the tip of the middle or longest finger and the fist across the knuckles, as these will be used as the measurement instruments.[7] The experienced examiner will come to know his or her own measurements and therefore not need to take personal hand measurements prior to each clinical pelvimetry evaluation. Measurements of how large a distance exists between bones of the pelvis in anteroposterior (front to back), transverse (sideways), and oblique (diagonal) directions indicate the interior width of the maternal bony passage through which the fetus will pass (Figures 14–2 and 14–8).

Bimanual pelvic examination is part of routine assessment during the first trimester, whereas exter-

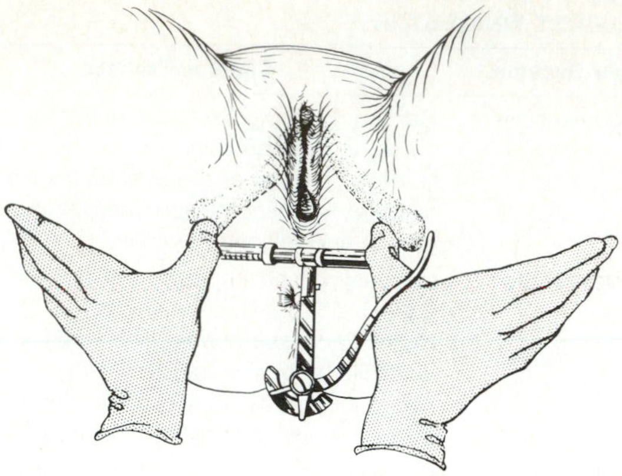

Figure 14–1. Measurement of the bi-ischial or intertuberous diameter with a pelvimeter. (*Reproduced, with permission, from Benson RC.* Handbook of Obstetrics & Gynecology. *8th ed. Los Altos, Calif: Lange Medical Books; 1983.*)

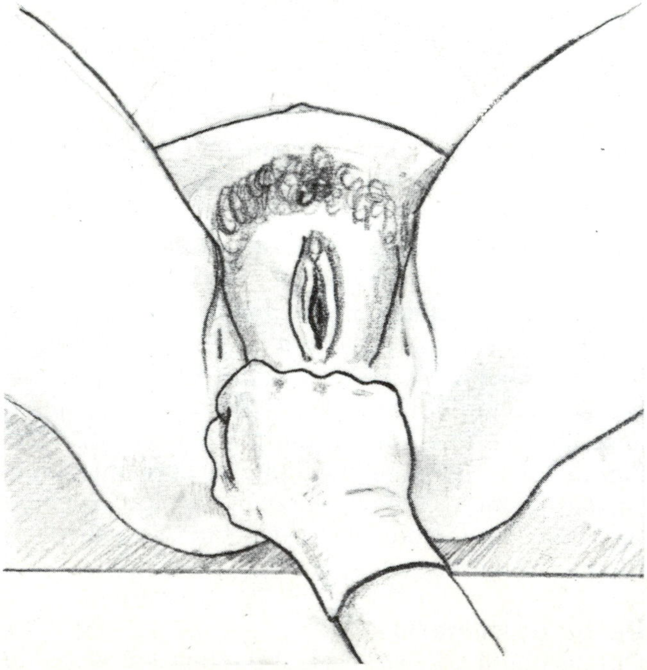

Figure 14–2. Measurement of the pelvic outlet prior to clinical pelvimetry.

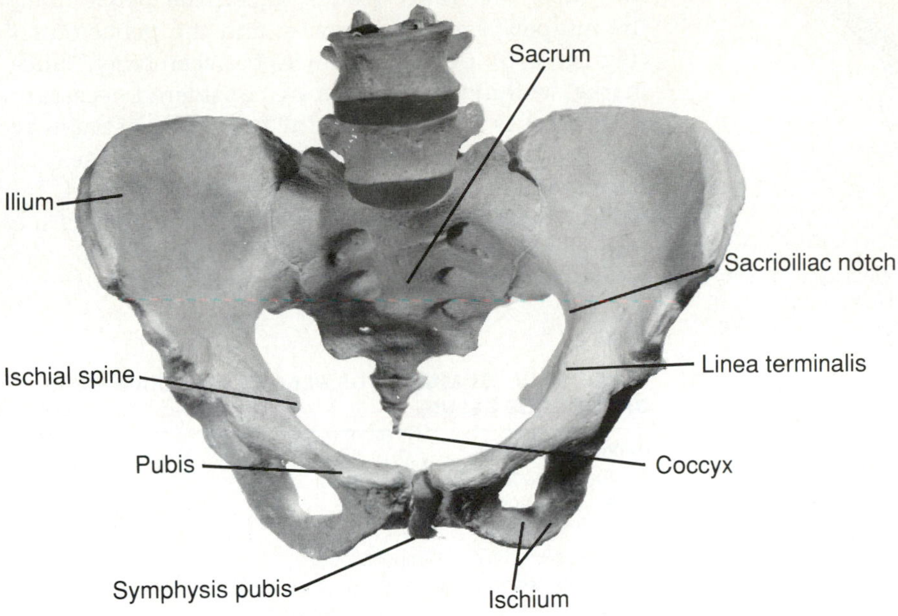

Figure 14–3. Normal pelvis. (*Reproduced, with permission, from Cunningham FG, et al.* Williams Obstetrics. *18th ed. Norwalk, Conn: Appleton & Lange, 1989: 222.*)

nal abdominal assessment is done during the second and third trimesters. Therefore, clinical pelvimetry is performed by the physician or nurse speicalist (often a nurse-medwife) as part of the pelvic examination during the first trimester and usually on the first prenatal visit. Staff nurses need to be able to explain the procedure and provide support to the client during examination.

Prenatal pelvic assessment is based on an understanding of normal female pelvic anatomy, especially in relation to childbearing. The female pelvis contains a bony ring through which the fetus must descend for successful vaginal delivery to take place. The sacrum, coccyx, and two innominate bones form the normal adult pelvis. The ilium, ischium, and pubic bones join to form the innominate bones. At the back, the two innominate bones connect to the sacrum at the place where the sacrum and ilium are joined. In the front, the innominate bones join with each other at the symphysis pubis (Figure 14–3). Men and women have the same number of pelvic bones; however, female pelves are shaped somewhat differently and have special importance for childbearing.[4,5] (*See* Figure 6–20.)

The pelvis is divided into two sections, commonly called the false pelvis and the true pelvis. The **linea terminalis** is a bony line that divides the false pelvis from the true pelvis. As shown in Figure 14–4 the **false pelvis** lies above the linea terminalis. The flared portion of the top of the iliac bones is commonly referred to by clients as the "hip bones." A client mistakenly may think that she will have an easy

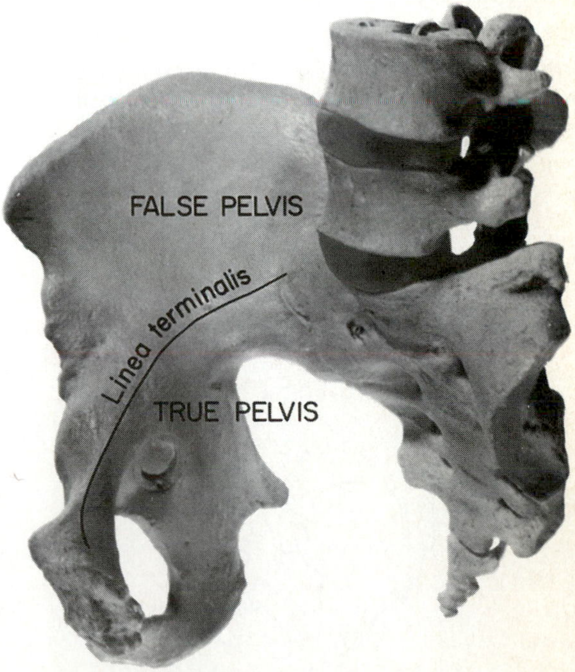

Figure 14–4. Division of false pelvis from true pelvis by linea terminalis. (*Reproduced, with permission, from Cunningham FG, et al,* Williams Obstetrics. *18th ed. Norwalk, Conn: Appleton & Lange; 1989:222.*)

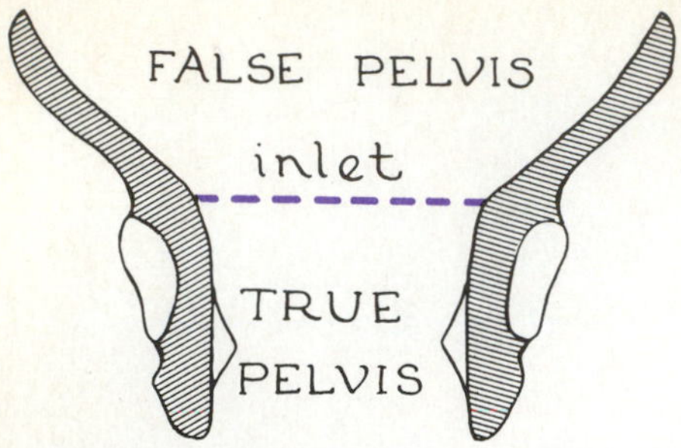

Figure 14–5. False pelvis and true pelvis. (*Reproduced, with permission, from Oxorn H, ed.* Oxorn-Foote Human Labor and Birth. *5th ed. Norwalk, Conn: Appleton-Century-Crofts; 1986: 25.*)

delivery if she has wide hip bones. In reality, the false pelvis has little obstetric importance. The fetus passes through the bony canal of the true pelvis; the shape and size of bones of the true pelvis are therefore of great significance for labor and delivery.

The **true pelvis** is located below the linea terminalis (Figure 14–5). The upper portion of the true pelvis is bounded by the sacral promontory, linea terminalis, and upper margins of the pubic bones. The lower part of the true pelvis is bounded by the lower margins of the ischial tuberosities and the end of the coccyx. The anterior parts of the sacrum and coccyx form its borders in the back. In front, the true pelvis is bordered by the pubic bones, the ascending upper rami of the ischial bones, and the obturator foramina. On the sides, the true pelvis is bordered by the sacroiliac notches and ligaments, as well as by the inner surface of the ischial bones.[4,5]

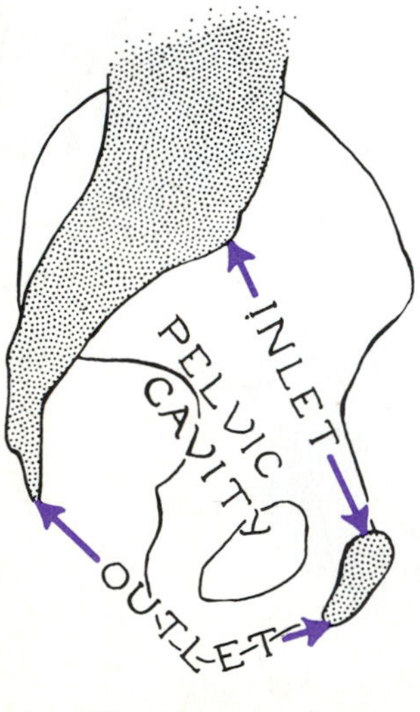

Figure 14–6. True pelvis. (*Reproduced, with permission, from Oxorn H, ed.* Oxorn-Foote Human Labor and Birth. *5th ed. Norwalk, Conn: Appleton-Century-Crofts; 1986:25*)

For conceptual ease, the true pelvis is divided into three imaginary planes, called the pelvic inlet, the midpelvis or pelvic cavity, and the pelvic outlet (Figure 14–6). Certain distances between bony "landmarks" within these planes are considered necessary if the fetus is to fit through the maternal passageway during labor and delivery. Pelvimetry focuses on measurements of distances within the true pelvis. Table 14–5 summarizes the planes and diameters of the true pelvis.

TABLE 14–5. SUMMARY OF PLANES AND DIAMETERS OF THE TRUE PELVIS

Pelvic Inlet

1. Anteroposterior diameters
   a. True conjugate
      11.5 cm
      No obstetric importance
   b. Obstetric conjugate[a] (shortest inlet anteroposterior diameter fetal head passes through)
      11 cm
      Very important; fetus passes through during labor
   c. Diagonal conjugate
      12.5 cm
      Can be measured on clinical examination
      Subtracting 1.5 cm gives an estimate of obstetric conjugate
      Variations in length depend on height and angle of symphysis
2. Transverse diameter[a]
   Widest distance in inlet
   About 13.5 cm
3. Oblique diameters (left and right), about 12.5 cm
4. Posterior sagittal diameter, about 4.5 cm

Pelvic Cavity (Midplane/Midpelvis)

1. Plane of greatest dimension
   Most spacious part of pelvis
   Little obstetric importance
   a. Anteriorposterior diameter, 12.75 cm
   b. Transverse diameter, 12.5 cm
2. Plane of least dimensions
   Important pelvic plane in terms of childbirth
   Has least room
   Most arrested labors occur here
   a. Anteriorposterior diameter,[a] 12.0 cm
   b. Transverse diameter,[a] 10.5 cm
   c. Posterior sagittal diameter,[a] 4.5–5.0 cm

Pelvic Outlet

1. Obstetric anteroposterior diameter[a]
   11.5 cm
   Coccyx can be pushed back by the presenting part of the fetus during labor; this can widen the space
2. Transverse diameter,[a] 11.0 cm
3. Posterior sagittal diameter,[a] 9.0 cm
4. Anterior sagittal diameter, 6.0 cm

[a] Diameters that are important in assessing pelvic adequacy for childbearing.

Pelvic Inlet. The **pelvic inlet** is the upper entrance to the true pelvis. **Superior strait** is another name for this imaginary plane. It is bordered in the back by the sacral promontory, on the sides by the linea terminalis, and in the front by the upper part of the symphysis pubis and horizontal rami of the pubic bones.[5]

There are three anteroposterior diameters of the pelvic inlet (Figure 14–7.)

The **true conjugate** (conjugate vera), which in the typical woman is at least 11.5 cm, is measured from the upper margin of the symphysis pubis to the sacral promontory. The **diagonal conjugate,** is measured from the lower margin of the symphysis to the sacral promontory and is at least 12.5 cm. The diagonal conjugate is the only pelvic inlet distance that can be measured with clinical pelvimetry.

To estimate the diagonal conjugate, the middle finger of the examining hand reaches for the sacral promontory, and the tissue between the index finger and thumb pushes against the pubic symphysis (Figure 14–8). The diagonal conjugate is estimated by measuring the distance between the tip of the examining finger and the point of pressure against the symphysis pubis. The symphysis pubis is thicker in the middle than at the top or bottom. Subtracting 1.5 to 2 cm from the diagonal conjugate (to account for a shorter front-to-back diameter and the angle of the bone) gives an indirect estimation of the actual anteroposterior diameter of the pelvic inlet; this diameter is called the **obstetric conjugate** and is about 11 cm. The obstetric conjugate is important, because it is the smallest front-to-back distance through which the fetal head must pass in moving through the pelvic inlet.[4]

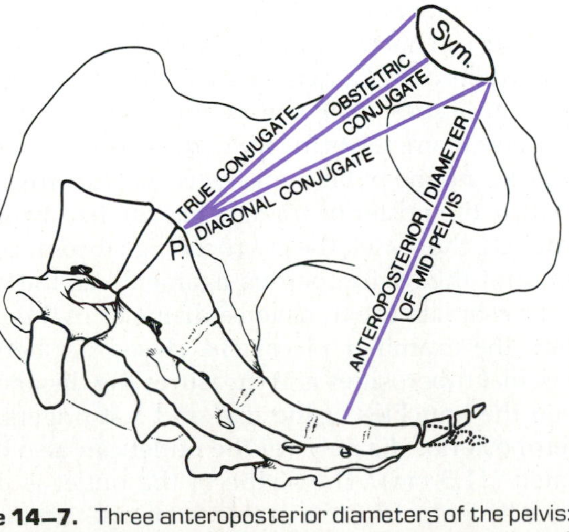

Figure 14–7. Three anteroposterior diameters of the pelvis: the true conjugate, the more important obstetric conjugate, and the clinically measurable diagonal conjugate. The anteroposterior diameter of the midpelvis is also shown. P = sacral promontory, Sym = symphysis pubis. (*Reproduced, with permission, from Cunningham FG, et al.* Williams Obstetrics. *18th ed. Norwalk, Conn: Appleton & Lange; 1989:165.*)

Other measurements of the pelvic inlet are the transverse diameter, the diagonal diameters, and the posterior sagittal diameter. The transverse diameter (about 13.5 cm) is the largest diameter of the pelvic inlet and is located at right angles to the true conjugate. The transverse diameter is the distance measured between the linea terminalis on each side of the pelvis. The diagonal (oblique) diameters of the pelvic inlet are about 12.5 cm and cannot be measured clinically. The posterior sagittal diameter of the pelvic inlet reaches from the point where the anteroposterior and transverse diameters cross each other to the middle of the sacral promontory (about 4.5 cm).

Pelvic Cavity. The area between the pelvic inlet and the pelvic outlet is called the **pelvic cavity,** pelvic canal, **midpelvis,** or midplane of the pelvis. The diameters of greatest dimensions (largest distance) and diameters of least dimensions (shortest distance) are located in this portion of the pelvis.

As expected, the plane of greatest dimensions is the roomiest part of the pelvic canal. It is bounded in the front by the midpoint of the posterior surface of the pubis, on the sides by the upper and middle thirds of the obturator foramina, and in the back by the junction of the second and third sacral vertebrae. The plane of greatest dimensions has little obstetric management importance; because of the large size, it can readily accommodate an average sized, normal fetus. From front to back (from the midpoint of the posterior surface of the pubis to the junction of the second and third vertebrae), the plane of greatest dimension measures about 12.75 cm. The widest distance between the lateral parts of the plane, the transverse diameter, is about 12.5 cm.[8]

The plane of least dimensions is important in obstetrics because it has the smallest amount of room. As the narrowest part of the bony maternal passageway, the plane of least dimensions can be a place where labor fails to progress. The plane of least dimensions extends from the top of the subpubic arch, through the ischial spines, to the sacrum, at or near the point where the fourth and fifth sacral vertebrae join. From front to back, this plane is bordered by the lower boundary of the symphysis pubis, the white line on the fascia over the obturator foramina, the ischial spines, the sacrospinous ligaments, and the sacrum.

Important diameters within the plane of least dimensions include the anteroposterior, transverse, and posterior sagittal diameters. The anteroposterior diameter, about 12.0 cm, extends from the lower boundary of the symphysis pubis to the junction of

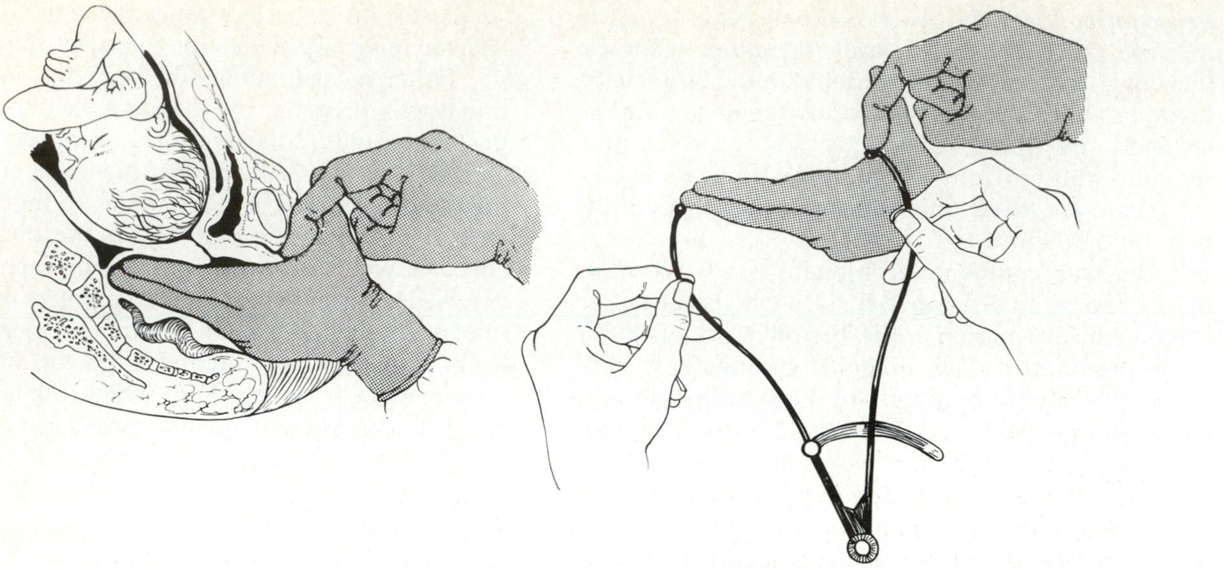

Figure 14–8. Measurement of the diagonal conjugate. (*Reproduced, with permission, from Benson RC.* Handbook of Obstetrics & Gynecology. *8th ed. Los Altos, Calif: Lange Medical Books; 1983.*)

the fourth and fifth sacral vertebrae. The transverse diameter, also called the interspinous diameter, stretches between the ischial spines and measures about 10.0 or 10.5 cm. This is the smallest pelvic distance through which the fetus must pass. The distance can be decreased if a woman has ischial spines that are especially sharp or large or that protrude into the pelvic cavity; this situation could place her at risk for labor problems related to adequacy of pelvic size. The posterior sagittal diameter of the pelvic cavity is generally at least 4.5 cm, and extends from the bispinous diameter to the junction of the fourth and fifth sacral vertebrae.[5,8]

Pelvic cavity measurements cannot easily be determined clinically; however, adequacy of pelvic cavity size may be estimated by noting the prominence of the ischial spines. During vaginal examination, the ischial spines are palpated for prominence and distance. Spines that are flat or blunt are optimal for birth, whereas prominent or encroaching spines can decrease the size of the pelvic cavity. The distance between the two ischial spines is estimated by placing one examining finger on one spine and spreading the other to the opposite spine. The length of the sacrospinous ligament is also determined by following the ligament to the point of insertion on the sacrum. This measurement is the same as the width of the sacrosciatic notch. A length of two to three fingerbreadths indicates a good anteroposterior diameter of the midpelvis. If the sacrosciatic notches are narrow, the midpelvis may be inadequate for a vaginal delivery. The shape of the sacrum is determined by moving the examining fingers down the sacrum to the coccyx. Optimally the sacrum should feel hollow, rather than flat or curved, and the coccyx should feel movable, rather than fixed.[5,7,8]

Pelvic Outlet. The **pelvic outlet** is described as two triangles (Figure 14–9). The transverse diameter of the outlet forms the common base of the triangles. The transverse diameter of the outlet is the distance between the inner parts of the lowest aspect of the ischial tuberosities. This distance is also called the bi-ischial or intertuberous diameter and is about 10 cm.[5] As shown in Figure 14–9, the anterior triangle has the transverse diameter as the base, the subpubic angle as the apex, and the pubic rami and ischial tuberosities as the sides; the posterior triangle has the transverse diameter as the base, the sacrococcygeal joint as the apex, and the sacrotuberous ligaments as the sides.

To estimate the transverse diameter of the pelvic outlet, the examiner places the closed fist between the ischial tuberosities and measures the distance between the knuckles of the first and last fingers. The anteroposterior diameter of the outlet can also be estimated (11.5 cm). The shape of the outlet is determined by palpating the pubic rami and noting the angle of the rami. Pubic rami are short and concave; a subpubic angle of more than 90° suggests inadequacy of the outlet.[3] The examiner also determines if the coccyx is movable by placing firm but gentle pressure on the coccyx with the examining fingers. A coc-

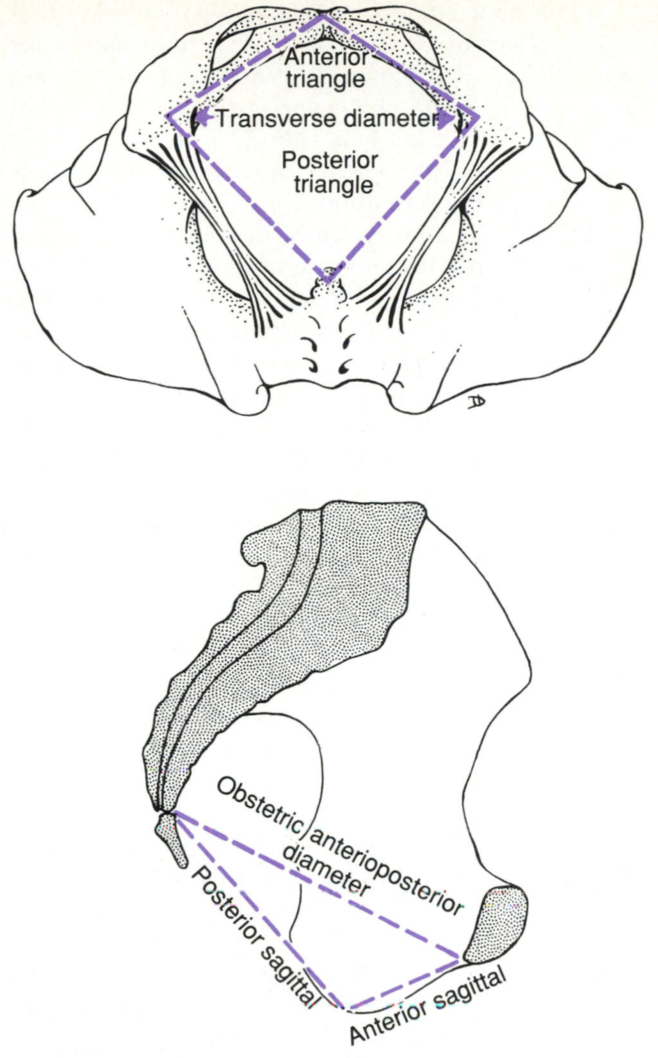

Figure 14–9. Pelvic outlet. (*Reproduced, with permission, from Oxorn H, ed.* Oxorn-Foote Human Labor and Birth. *5th ed. Norwalk, Conn: Appleton-Century-Crofts; 1986:33.*)

cyx that is not movable can reduce the diameter of the outlet.

Advantages and Limitations of Pelvimetry. The goal of first-trimester pelvic measurement theoretically is to determine whether the passage provided by the bony pelvis will be able to accommodate the descending fetus at term. Internal examination of bony pelvic structures provides a way to identify women whose pelves are normally shaped or abnormally narrowed, or contracted. If a woman's pelvis does not have certain measurements, then she is thought to be at potential risk of not being able to deliver vaginally. Prenatal health forms often have space for inclusion of clinical pelvimetry measurements; however, assessment of pelvic measurements early in the first trimester does not allow for firm confirmation of pelvic disproportion. As described in Chapter 25, whether or not a healthy woman delivers vaginally depends on factors at term, such as size and position of the fetus in relation to the maternal pelvis. Indeed, women who have smaller-than-average pelvic measurements may uneventfully delivery a healthy baby, especially if the baby is in the 5- to 6-pound range. In most cases, first-trimester pelvic measurements would not alone be sufficient to prevent a trial of labor, although they could alert staff to potential difficulties.

Discomforts Related to Clinical Pelvimetry. When performed by an experienced health care provider, clinical pelvimetry takes only a few moments during a bimanual pelvic examination. The woman may experience a sense of pressure as the examiner presses against bones and soft tissues. The healthy woman will not have any acute physical pain. The client should, however, receive an explanation of the purpose and process of pelvimetry, as well as the results of the assessment. An educational approach, as described in Chapter 5, helps to allay anxiety and to include the client in her own care.

Assessment of Pregnancy

Pregnancy Tests. Pregnancy tests are used together with thorough history and physical examination to confirm pregnancy. Early diagnosis of pregnancy, along with early prenatal care, can promote maternal and fetal well-being. Pregnancy testing has been done by detection of human chorionic gonadotropin (hCG) in a woman's blood or urine, by biologic animal assays, and by ultrasound. As described in this chapter and in Chapter 18, ultrasound can provide a positive diagnosis by visualizing the developing pregnancy. Ultrasound is expensive, however, and is used to confirm pregnancy only for high-risk indications, such as diagnosis of ectopic pregnancy.

Detection of Human Chorionic Gonadotropin in Blood or Urine. Testing for the presence of hCG in a woman's blood or urine can be readily, reliably, and relatively inexpensively conducted. For these reasons, tests for hCG in blood or urine are currently the most frequently performed pregnancy tests. Pregnancy tests for urinary hCG may be performed as a single service at minimal or no charge by women's health centers; as part of comprehensive assessment for a first prenatal visit; as part of assessment of the woman with amenorrhea; and at home using over-the-counter test kits. Blood (serum) tests for hCG are performed in laboratory, clinic, or office settings as part of comprehensive client evaluation.

In the healthy woman, the hormone hCG is produced only during pregnancy. Low levels of hCG are present after fertilization, but increase rapidly after implantation when trophoblastic cells profilerate and produce greater amounts. Under healthy conditions, hCG levels follow a predictable pattern. As shown in Figure 14–10, hCG levels rise rapidly during early pregnancy, peak about 60 to 70 days after conception, and then drop to a lower level for the rest of pregnancy. Abnormally high levels of hCG can indicate pathologic conditions such as hydatidiform mole (*see* Chapter 39); abnormally low levels of hCG can occur with disturbances of pregnancy, such as a threatened or incomplete abortion or fetal death.[10–13] (*See* Chapter 38.)

Tests for hCG in blood or serum are based on the principle that hCG, or a subunit of hCG, is recognized by an antibody to the hCG molecule. The hCG molecule has an alpha subunit and a beta subunit. The alpha subunit of hCG is similar in molecular structure to such hormones as luteinizing hormone (LH). For this reason, false-positive results can occur in pregnancy tests that simply detect the whole hCG molecule, including the alpha subunit. Tests that detect the beta subunit have less incidence of false-positive results, because the beta subunit is specific for pregnancy and does not cross-react with other hormones in the body. Table 14–6 summarizes pregnancy tests based on the detection of hCG in blood or urine samples.[4, 9–12]

In normal circumstances, pregnancy tests that simply detect hCG provide enough information for confirmation of pregnancy. When high-risk conditions are suspected, however, pregnancy tests that specifically detect the beta subunit or hCG tests that identify the quantity of hCG, or both, provide important diagnostic information.

Blood or urine tests for hCG are not 100 percent accurate, although many are quite reliable. For this reason, these pregnancy tests are considered probable, rather than positive, indicators of pregnancy. Table 14–7 lists conditions in which false-negative or false-positive pregnancy tests can occur.[10] Therefore, pregnancy tests should be used as adjuncts, rather than substitutes, for the history and physical examination in the diagnosis of pregnancy.

Home pregnancy test kits are currently available without prescription to consumers and can be purchased in pharmacies and supermarkets. These are urine tests for hCG that can be performed by the client in the privacy of her home. Some home tests involve simple color changes as the result of monoclonal antibody reactions. Others are hemagglutination inhibition tests that use sheep erythrocytes, antibodies to hCG, and a sample of the woman's urine.

Pharmaceutical research has focused on the development of consumer tests that are increasingly easy to use. One currently available test simply requires a woman to place the absorbent tip of the testing device in her urine stream and to cap the device immediately afterward. The appearance of a blue line in a "window" on the test stick indicates a positive

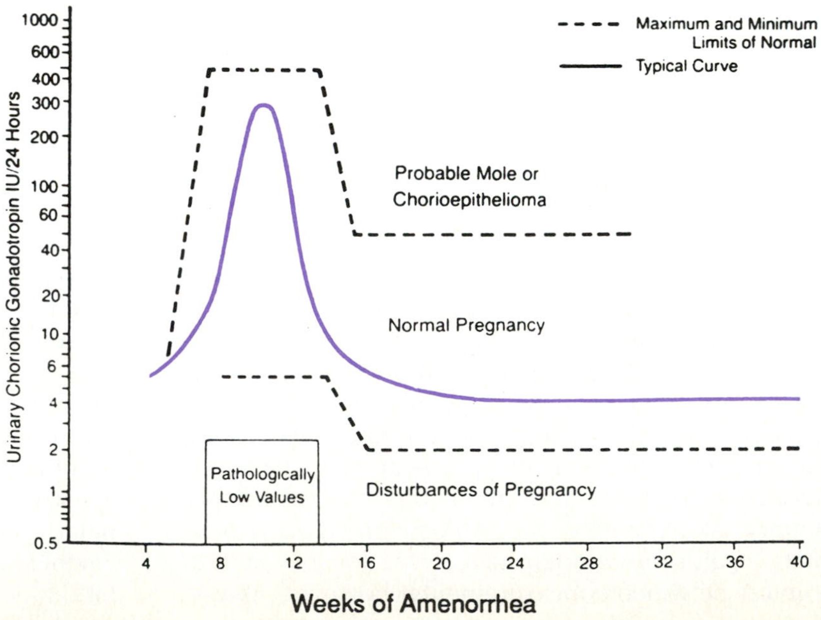

Figure 14–10. Human chorionic gonadotropin levels during pregnancy. (*Reproduced, with permission, from Hatcher RA, et al.* Contraceptive Technology, 1988–1989. *14th ed. New York: Irvington; 1988:381*)

TABLE 14–6. MAJOR TYPES OF PREGNANCY TESTS BASED ON DETECTION OF HUMAN CHORIONIC GONADOTROPIN IN BLOOD OR URINE

TESTS FOR hCG

Immunoassay (IA; test "tube" or slide; serum or urine)

- Accurate within 7 to 28 days of conception
- Tests for the hCG molecule; does not specifically identify the beta subunit, so cross-reaction with LH can occur
- Readily accessible; widely used as a pregnancy test in routine situations
- Does not require radioisotopes and sophisticated laboratory analysis
- Based on antigen-antibody reaction. Most tests are positive if the solution stays homogeneous and no agglutination occurs; most are negative if agglutination is noted; directions *must* be read carefully, as not all tests are conducted or read in the same way.
- Examples
  - Latex agglutination inhibition test (LAI), which uses a specimen from the client, a reagent containing hCG, antibody, and latex particles bound to hCG as the antigen (slide test)
  - Hemagglutination inhibition test (HAI), which uses a specimen from the client, a reagent containing hCG antibody, and reagent containing animal erythrocytes, coated with hCG, as the antigen (tube test)

Radioreceptor Assay (RRA; serum)

- Accurate within 14 days of conception
- Tests for the hCG molecule; does not specifically identify the beta subunit, so cross reaction with LH can occur
- Used for early confirmation of normal pregnancy (A small amount of radioactive isotope is used to "tag" hCG; this method allows for early detection because the test can be positive with the smaller amounts of hCG present in early pregnancy or with high-risk conditions involving low levels of hCG.)
- Requires laboratory analysis with specialized equipment
- Uses hCG receptors from the corpora lutea of animal tissue and radiolabeled hCG (The amount of radio labeled hCG that remains unbound to the specific receptor sites increases in relation to the amount of hCG in the client's serum.)

TESTS FOR BETA SUBUNIT OF hCG

Enzyme-Linked Immunoassay (EI)/Enzyme-linked Immunosorbent Assay (ELISA) (Urine or Serum)

- Accurate within 12 days of conception
- Specific for the beta unit of hCG; no cross-reactions with LH, FSH, or other hormones occur
- Particularly helpful for testing perimenopausal women who normally have higher levels of LH and might otherwise have a positive result based on cross-reaction with this hormone
- Urine tests usually positive when maternal serum levels are at least 25 mIU/mL, but do not quantitate level of beta-hCG
- Results have less interference from urinary blood or protein if present
- Uses a monoclonal antibody specific for the beta subunit of hCG and an antigen-enzyme conjugate (A simple color change takes place when the beta subunit is present.)
- Method used in newer home pregnancy kits

Radioimmunoassay (RIA)

- Highly accurate within 7 days of conception during normal pregnancy
- Specifically tests for beta unit of hCG; no cross-reactions with LH, FSH, or other hormones occur
- Used for evaluating abnormal pregnancy, for example, threatened abortion, hydatidiform mole
- Sensitive in detection and quantification of beta-hCG and, therefore, a sensitive indicator of trophoblastic activity (Information about the exact level of beta-hCG provides more accurate interpretation of any findings from ultrasound, often also done for high-risk evaluation.)
- Uses a radiolabeled hCG in a fixed amount (The amount of radiolabeled hCG that can bind to the anti-hCG in a solution decreases in relation to the amount of hCG in the woman's serum, permitting quantitative measurement of hCG.)

Source: References 4, 10, 11, and 13.

result. Test results are available in 3 minutes and are not affected by such factors as movement; however, false-positive results can occur if the woman is receiving hCG injections or if the readings are not taken within the recommended time frame. False-negative results can occur if the test is performed too early in pregnancy, that is, less than 14 days after conception (Clearblue Easy, Whitehall Laboratories, New York, 1989).

Although consumer tests have advantages such as privacy and early detection, many of the tests can occasionally produce inaccurate results, especially if they are not done correctly. False-negative results tend to occur more frequently than false-positive results, often because the test is not sensitive enough to identify hCG early in pregnancy when urinary levels are low. A client may falsely believe she is not pregnant and participate in lifestyle behaviors that could harm pregnancy. Some women may use positive results to seek prenatal care early; other women may delay prenatal care if the test does not indicate that pregnancy actually exists or if they do not recognize

TABLE 14–7. CONDITIONS CONTRIBUTING TO FALSE-NEGATIVE OR FALSE-POSITIVE PREGNANCY TEST RESULTS[a]

False-Negative Results (test fails to detect pregnancy)
Test misread by examiner
Test done too early or too late in pregnancy
Urine too dilute (possibly because a random sample, rather than a first morning urine used)
Urine stored too long or improperly
Missed or impending spontaneous abortion
Ectopic pregnancy
Drug interference
False-Positive Results (test inaccurately read as pregnant)
Test misread by examiner
LH cross-reaction
Protein in urine
Blood in urine
Lipemia or turbidity (in serum specimen)
Continuing cyst of the corpus luteum
Recent pregnancy (less than 10 days after pregnancy terminated)
Residue on glassware used for test (especially detergent)
Premature menopause
Certain drugs, for example, aldomet, marijuana, phenothiazines, antidepressants
hCG treatment, eg, fertility treatment injections
Thyrotoxicosis
Malignant tumors that secrete hCG (eg, ovary, breast, melanoma)

[a]Directions for performing each pregnancy test must be read and followed carefully, as false results can often be attributed to improper testing procedures. Certain tests may also require use of a stopwatch for precision in timing. Tests indicating surprising results should be repeated. *Adapted from Hatcher RA, et al.,* Contraceptive Technology: 1988–89. *14th ed. New York: Irvington; 1988: 383–384.*

the importance of comprehensive early prenatal evaluation. Through information provided in product package inserts and at well-woman visits, women should be advised of the importance of following product directions carefully, repeating negative tests within a week if amenorrhea persists, and scheduling an appointment for clinical examination as appropriate.

Biologic Animal Assays. Biologic animal assays were the first tests developed to aid in pregnancy diagnosis. Positive results occurred as a result of the presence of hCG. Biologic animal assays depended on examination of the reproductive tracts of animals such as frogs, rabbits, or mice after the animals were injected with a pregnant woman's urine. Biologic animal assays tended to be clumsy, time consuming, and expensive and required the support and then destruction of numerous laboratory animals. They have been replaced in clinical practice by the simpler, chemical tests for hCG, discussed earlier.

Ultrasound. Ultrasound (sonography) is a technique that involves the use of high-frequency sound waves. Ultrasound is defined as "any sound with a frequency of greater than 20,000 Hz (undetectable by the human ear)."[14] The sound waves are bounced off tissues of differing acoustic density. Ultrasound frequencies are usually in the range 1 to 10 MHz (1 to 10 million cycles per second).[14, 15] A frequency range of 3.5 to 5 MHz is usually used in obstetrics, although it may be higher. Currently, the piezoelectric crystal is the material used to generate the high-frequency sound waves.

Ultrasound was first applied medically in the United States in the late 1940s; Donald and associates in Glasgow, Scotland, pioneered the use of ultrasound in gynecology in the mid 1950s. Donald applied industrial ultrasound equipment used in the engineering city of Glasgow to identify flaws in metals, to the detection of human tumors. With further development of ultrasound and application to obstetrics, by 1965 measurement of the fetal skull was possible as early as 7 weeks.[16] Ultrasound equipment and techniques have continued to develop. Today, ultrasound is one of the most valuable and widely used means of fetal and maternal assessment.[4, 17]

Pulse echo imaging and Doppler systems (described later) are two classifications of ultrasound used often in obstetrics. Pulse echo systems transmit high-frequency sound pulses and receive back echoes that are then displayed as a two-dimensional image on a television type monitor. Static scanners and real-time scanners are two types of pulse echo ultrasound equipment. Static scanners emit a pulse of sound waves from the transducer. These waves move through soft body tissues. Some of the energy is reflected back (echoed) to the transducer when an interface between different tissue densities is reached. The transducer then emits a small electrical voltage that is magnified and shown on a screen. Static scanners give a "still" image in the same way that a photograph freezes a moment in time. Static scanners are able to present still views from several different points, because the transducer, which is responsible for the imaging, is moved across the woman's abdomen. Real-time scanners show movement as it happens, because the transducers send out many pulse echo systems.[4] In clinical practice with prenatal clients, real-time scanners are often used because they allow fetal movements, as well as heart and breathing activity, to be observed.

Pulse echo scanning may be done by an ultrasound technician, nurse, or physician. The American College of Obstetricians and Gynecologists recommends that this test be done by "a trained professional."[14] Final interpretation of ultrasound tests is done by a physician. Pulse echo ultrasound scanners may be located in hospital outpatient clinics or in physicians' offices. Ultrasonography is also considered a subspecialty of radiology, and diagnostic ultrasound may be performed in radiology departments.

Uses During Pregnancy. Ultrasound may be used alone for the assessment of the pregnant client, developing fetus, or both. Ultrasound may also be used to visualize internal maternal and fetal structures to guide other diagnostic procedures, such as chorionic villus sampling and amniocentesis.

Basic and Targeted Ultrasound. Basic (level I) and targeted (level II) ultrasound studies provide different types of information. The basic ultrasound, used most frequently, is done to assess the presence of intrauterine pregnancy, the number of fetuses, the position of the fetus (second and third trimesters), and whether or not the fetus is alive.[14] The yolk sac can be identified during the first 12 weeks. A yolk sac without an embryo indicates a missed abortion. Fetal death at any time throughout pregnancy may also be confirmed. Basic ultrasound is also used to determine location of the placenta, size and maturity of the placenta, abnormalities of the placenta, amount of amniotic fluid, and gestational age of the fetus.[14] The gestational sac, embryonic poles, yolk sac, fetal heart, and crown-rump length (when visualized up to 12 weeks) can quite accurately predict gestational age within 4 days. Repeat (serial) ultrasounds, performed when indicated, can help identify a growth-retarded fetus. In addition, maternal pelvic pathology, such as pelvic masses (most useful when done in the first trimester), and gross abnormalities in fetal anatomy are assessed by basic ultrasound.

Targeted (level II) ultrasound is done for a client who is thought to be carrying an anatomically or physiologically abnormal fetus. Indications for this examination include a history of previous offspring with anomalies that could be viewed by sonogram, abnormal findings on clinical examination (especially with polyhydramnios [excessive amniotic fluid] or oligohydramnios [little amniotic fluid]), and elevated alpha-fetoprotein levels[14] (*see* Chapter 18). The targeted ultrasound is performed by someone who specializes in high-risk sonography. During this procedure, attention is directed toward specific evaluation of fetal anatomy and physiology.

Safety. Over the years many questions have been raised about the safety of ultrasound. Pregnancy is a physically vulnerable period for the developing fetus. The experience with adverse effects of other technologic advances applied during pregnancy has shown that caution is required with any type of technology. To date, specific harmful effects directly related to ultrasound have not been documented in any human fetus or mother.[14, 17, 18, 19] Ultrasound, performed for a specific indication, is thought to be beneficial to the mother and infant, because the information provided can be important to diagnosis and treatment.[20]

Controversy exists over whether ultrasound should be routinely used for all pregnant clients. Well-designed, controlled large-scale studies would be needed to establish benefits of routine screening; however, concern for potential damage that has not yet been identified continues to make ultrasound in the United States a procedure that should be done only when specifically indicated.

Transabdominal and Transvaginal Approaches. Transabdominal and transvaginal approaches are currently used for first-trimester ultrasound. Transabdominal approaches are used during the second and third trimesters. Until the mid-1980s, a transabdominal approach was most frequently used whenever ultrasound was indicated during pregnancy. With a transabdominal approach, a transducer is passed over the woman's abdomen and images of internal structures are produced on a television-type monitor. With a transvaginal approach, a transducer is placed in the vagina.

During the first trimester, the uterus has not yet grown out of the pelvis. With a transabdominal approach, the first-trimester embryo, as well as maternal pelvic structures such as the ovaries and fallopian tubes, is difficult to visualize. To obtain clearer images during the first trimester, women are required to drink one to two quarts of clear fluid. Within an hour the urinary bladder fills and pushes the uterus higher in the abdomen where it can be more accurately scanned. The test is performed with the woman lying on her back. Side-lying positions may be requested to provide better visualization of certain structures. Unfortunately, a highly distended bladder can be very uncomfortable or embarrassing for the woman. Waiting for the bladder to fill enough or for the ultrasonographers to be ready to perform the scan prolongs the discomfort. Although the transabdominal approach may still be used during the first trimester, transabdominal ultrasonography is frequently an approach used during the second and third trimesters, when the uterus is an abdominal organ.

Transvaginal ultrasonography allows small, deep pelvic organs, such as the ovaries, to be visualized more clearly, because these structures are closer to the transducer probe. Factors such as greater distance or other body tissues can affect the quality of sonographic pictures; accurate diagnosis depends on clear pictures.[21, 22]

Transvaginal ultrasound during the first trimester has advantages over a transbdominal approach. A transvaginal approach is especially useful with obese clients, whose thick abdominal layers cannot be adequately penetrated by the ultrasound when a transabdominal approach is used. Transvaginal ultrasonography can provide for earlier detection of ectopic pregnancies.[21] Serious complications, such as tubal rupture resulting from ectopic tubal pregnancy, may then be prevented. In addition, transvaginal ultrasonography can be used to monitor the developing embryo and can help both in identification of abnormalities and in establishment of gestational age.

Transvaginal ultrasound is performed with the client in the lithotomy position.[18] A small reversed Trendelenburg tilt to the examining table allows the slight amount of peritoneal fluid that normally occurs to pool in the pelvis and create tissue/fluid interfaces. These interfaces help to identify the normal or pathologic structures in the pelvis and fetus by enhancing visualization[18, 22] (Figure 14–11).

After being coated with a special coupling gel, the transvaginal probe is covered with a protective sheath. A condom, a clean rubber surgical glove, or a probe cover provided by the manufacturer may be used. Gel is also used to lubricate the covered probe to promote conductivity and client comfort. The probe is placed in the vagina by the person performing the sonogram; however, the client may insert the probe herself if she feels embarrassed by the sonographer's placing the probe. During the examination the angle or position of the probe may be changed and the electrical control panel adjusted to provide nearly complete access to the whole pelvis.[18]

Transvaginal ultrasound takes about 10 minutes. The length of the procedure can vary, depending on whether pathology is identified. The procedure should not be physically painful. Discomfort relates mostly to being in the lithotomy position or to the existence of a pathologic condition. The covered probe may feel cool and like a speculum; the client may experience a sense of pressure as the probe is moved.

Doppler Ultrasound. Unlike ultrasound techniques, which provide actual images of body structures, Doppler ultrasound provides information about blood moving within living blood vessels and body organs. Sound waves of known frequency are directed at blood vessels containing moving red blood cells. The waves "bounce off" the moving red blood cells and return at a different frequency. The change in frequency depends on how fast the red blood cell is moving. The difference between the ultrasound wave frequency "sent out" and the frequency "re-

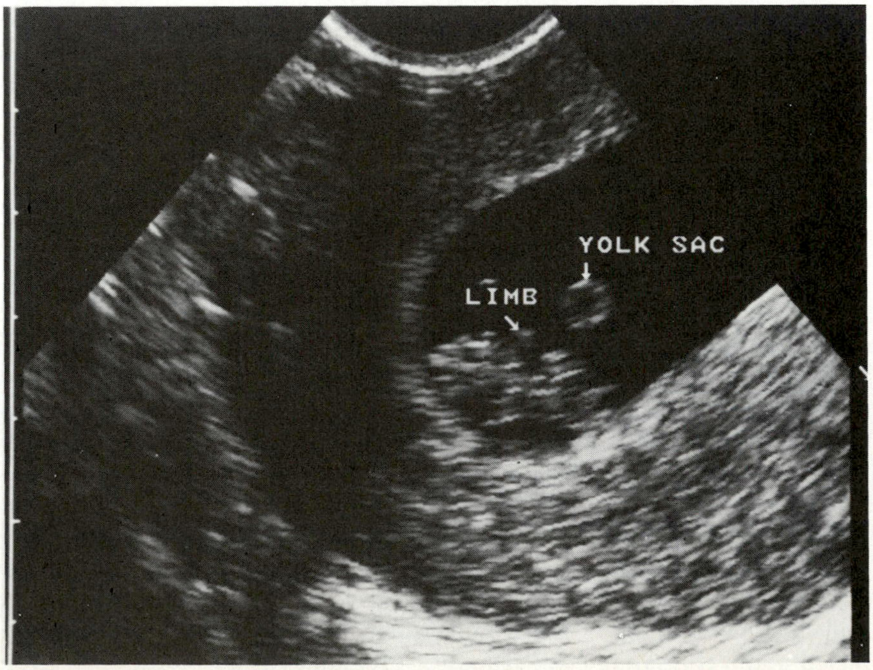

Figure 14–11. Transvaginal ultrasound image at 7 to 8 weeks demonstrating yolk sack and embryo. (*Reproduced, with permission, from Fleischer AC, et al.* The Principles and Practice of Ultrasonography in Obstetrics and Gynecology. *4th ed. Norwalk, Conn: Appleton & Lange; 1991:48.*)

ceived back" is called the Doppler shift (named for the Austrian physicist who made this discovery during his study of light waves).[23]

Blood cells in a vessel's center travel faster than blood cells near the sides of the vessel. At any time within a blood vessel, red blood cells are moving at different speeds. Therefore, at any one time during the cardiac cycle, a range of shifted frequencies exists in each blood vessel. Special Doppler imaging equipment can sample blood flow in the entire vessel or specific areas within the vessel. In obstetrics, circulation is assessed using transducers with frequencies of 2 to 8 MHz.[23]

Several types of Doppler instruments may be used.[24] Continuous-wave (CW) Doppler instruments send a continuous beam of ultrasonic waves. The velocity of red blood cells in the path of the beam is then recorded. This easily performed type of Doppler evaluation is commonly used in prenatal clinics or private offices for electronically monitoring fetal heart rate and for detecting blood flow through the fetal heart. Physicians, nurses, or technicians may perform this type of testing. Continuous-wave Doppler instruments facilitate identification of blood flow through the fetal heart and are used for this reason during the first trimester. With use of a Doppler instrument, flow of blood through the fetal heart may be detected around 8 weeks, whereas auscultation of fetal heart sounds is possible at 17 to 20 weeks. Doppler readings may be affected by such factors as the mother's breathing, position of the fetus, and fetal movements.

To take a CW Doppler reading, the transducer head is coated with gel and then positioned against the woman's abdomen. With simple, hand-held Doppler instruments, fetal heart rate activity may be heard and counted. More sophisticated fetal heart rate monitors provide recorded tracings of fetal heart rate activity and can also amplify the sound of fetal heart tones. As described in Chapter 27, fetal heart tones may be monitored externally with a belt holding the transducer against the mother's abdomen or internally with the probe fastened to the presenting part of the fetus.

Pulsed-wave Doppler instruments differ from continuous-wave instruments by sending out pulses of waves each second rather than a continuous beam of ultrasound waves. These pulses of sound waves bounce off different areas within the blood vessel, depending on how far they have traveled. If the returning waves are sampled at different time intervals as they return to the transducer head, velocity of flow in specific areas of the blood vessel can be measured.

The combination of the pulsed Doppler with real time ultrasound is known as duplex scanning. Modern transducer heads have both modalities within a single unit. Using real time ultrasound, specific blood vessels can be located. The velocity of blood flow within the vessels then can be determined using the pulsed Doppler instrument. Structures such as the uterine placental vessels, umbilical vein, fetal aorta, carotid arteries, and the fetal heart can be precisely imaged, and blood velocity can be quantified. For example, measurement of increasing resistance to blood flow in these vessels has been done with duplex scanners and is associated with problems such as fetal intrauterine growth retardation. Duplex scanning is therefore a diagnostic tool that can be used for second and third trimester high-risk vascular conditions.

Color flow imaging is an extension of duplex scanning. A specific area of a blood vessel, for example, is first imaged with real time ultrasound. Using the pulsed Doppler instrument, multiple samples of velocity of blood flow are taken within the visualized area of the blood vessel. A mean velocity of each sample is calculated and assigned a color by the machine. The result is the blood vessel's image, portrayed in color on a monitor screen. Direction and mean velocity of blood flow are represented by color changes during the cardiac cycle. Color coding facilitates identification of the blood vessels and the actual direction of flow.

Although Doppler ultrasound signals are easy to record from the expectant woman and fetus during pregnancy, interpreting and understanding the significance of the findings are more difficult. Results can be affected by such factors as problems in obtaining measurements of the same place in the same blood vessel or measurements taken by different operators.[24]

Client Reactions. A wide variety of client and family reactions may be expected in relation to ultrasound. Some clients may fear any study; however, client reactions may also relate to the reason for the ultrasound study. For example, the first-trimester client who will have a Doppler ultrasound done during her prenatal visit may excitedly bring the expectant father or significant others to hear the heartbeat. Some clients may feel that first-trimester visualization helps them feel close to their developing fetus.

Clients referred for ultrasound to assess for a blighted ovum or a missed abortion may respond with fear. During ultrasound procedures, clients may intensely search the faces of the sonographer and other health care providers for clues as to what the ultrasound shows. Positioning for the ultrasound or the need for a full bladder during a first-trimester transabdominal ultrasound may present actual physical discomfort. When maternal or fetal abnormalities are detected or when fetal death is confirmed, clients react with grief.

Role of the Nurse. Providing education and support to the client and her family before, during, and after ultrasound studies are important roles of the nurse. Table 14–8 outlines the topics to be addressed. Clients may worry about the reason for the study, the safety of ultrasound, and discomforts related to the procedure. Advance staff planning can clarify ways in which collaboration can provide information and deal with client anxiety or grief. Ways to support clients who receive bad news need to be planned. For example, the nurse and the physician may talk with the client together, or they may enlist the help of a chaplain or other grief specialist. Interdisciplinary staff conferences may also help health care providers to deal with their own feelings about diagnosis of fetal abnormalities.

Staff nurses in prenatal and labor and delivery settings may frequently use Doppler ultrasound in assessing and monitoring fetal heart rate patterns. Familiarity with the equipment and procedure, as well as with principles of basic Doppler ultrasound, is necessary.

TABLE 14–8. TOPICS FOR EDUCATIONAL PREPARATION OF THE CLIENT UNDERGOING DIAGNOSTIC ULTRASOUND

Why is the procedure being done?
Is the procedure safe?
Who will perform the ultrasound?
Who will be with the client during the test?
Where will the ultrasound be done?
What will the ultrasound be able to show?
Is any preparation necessary?
What does the procedure entail?
What will the client feel during the ultrasound?
How may the client deal with any discomfort (eg, breathing, imagery)?
How long with the ultrasound study take?
How much time can the client expect to commit to the ultrasound (includes waiting and follow-up testing)?
Who will interpret the ultrasound findings?
When will the client be informed of the results?
Should a relative or friend accompany the client? (Especially in high-risk conditions, presence of a significant other is helpful in ensuring that the client returns home safely.)
What specifically does the client question and fear in relation to the ultrasound?
Will photos of the fetus be given to the client? (Photos are often desired by clients having ultrasound for gestational dating or other nonthreatening conditions, but may also be desired by clients with abnormal fetuses.)

Determination of Delivery Date

The average pregnancy has a gestation of 266 days or 38 weeks postconception. The delivery date or the expected date of confinement (EDC) can be estimated by a variety of methods. **Nagele's rule** is the most common method of delivery date determination: subtract 3 months from the first day of the last normal menstrual period (LMP) and then add 1 year and 7 days to this date. For example, if the woman's LMP began on December 20, subtracting 3 months provides a date of September 20, to which 7 days are added to derive the due date of September 27 of the following year:

$$\underset{(12/20/90)}{\text{First day of LMP}} - \underset{(9/20/90)}{\text{3 months}} + \underset{(9/27/91)}{\text{1 year, 7 days}} = \text{EDC}$$

The fundal height is considered a gestational estimation but may be inaccurate if there is a multiple gestation, intrauterine growth retardation, or maternal obesity. Estimation of the delivery date may be guided by fundal height if the LMP is unknown; however, other clinical data should be obtained for confirmation. McDonald's method of fundal height determination corresponds to the gestational week within a 2- to 4-week range after 22 to 24 weeks. With McDonald's method, the fundal height is measured in centimeters, with a tape measure, from the superior border of the symphysis pubis to the fundus. If the woman is at 24 weeks of gestation, the measurement should be 24 cm ± 2 to 4 cm. At 12 weeks of gestation, the fundus is level with the symphysis. Before the fundus reaches the umbilicus (at 22 to 24 weeks), 4 cm is added to the measurement to determine gestation. To ensure accuracy, consistency of measurement should be used (for example, a tape measure instead of finger breadths) and the same practitioner should perform the initial and subsequent assessments if possible.

Sonographic determination of gestation can be accomplished by comparisons of measurements of gestational sac, crown-rump length, crown-heel length, and biparietal diameter to expected development. The dimensions of the gestational sac can be assessed at 8 weeks of gestation. The crown-rump length progressively increases each week as the C-shaped embryo develops into a fetus (Table 14–9). Femur length, crown-heel length, and biparietal diameter can be obtained after 12 weeks for gestational age assessment. When repeat ultrasounds are indicated, serial ultrasounds may be performed approximately 3 to 4 weeks apart to determine gestational age accurately.

TABLE 14–9. SONOGRAPHIC DETERMINATION OF CROWN-RUMP FETAL LENGTH AS AN ESTIMATION OF AGE

Weeks of Gestation	Length (cm)
4	3.5
5	8.0
6	14.0
7	20.0
8	30.0
9–12	Doubles in size

DETERMINATION OF RISK STATUS

Pregnancy may carry some risk of perinatal morbidity or mortality. Thus, the expectant mother and her family should be screened for potential risk factors during the initial prenatal visit and at each subsequent visit, because risk factors may emerge during the course of pregnancy. Research has indicated that perinatal morbidity and mortality are affected by such factors as maternal socioeconomic status, quality of prenatal care, age, nutrition, past obstetric history, current pregnancy problems, and associated illness.[1,2,25] Risk assessment during pregnancy is therefore based on the evaluation of physiologic, psychosocial, socioeconomic, lifestyle, and environmental factors that may affect perinatal outcome. Examples of risk factors in pregnancy are presented in Table 14–10. As indicated in Table 14–11, risk factors are also related to specific pregnancy problems. Once risk status is determined, appropriate nursing and collaborative management can be initiated to promote maternal, fetal, and family well-being. It is important to remember that risk factors vary in the degree to which they can negatively affect the childbearing process (*see* Chapter 35 for further discussion of risk status).

Screening Tools

Various screening tools, such as risk rating scales or questionnaires, are available for determining risk status during pregnancy. The usefulness of any risk screening tool in a particular situation depends on the ability of the tool to predict outcome criteria (maternal complications, fetal problems, or neonatal status).

Unfortunately, no screening tool identifies all possible problems with complete certainty. Scoring systems predict approximately half the problems experienced during pregnancy.[26] Screening tools do, however, have several advantages. For example, many high-risk conditions are actually identified through use of the tools. In addition, uniform data can be obtained for populations of pregnant clients. Uniform data can then assist in diagnosis and management of high-risk conditions and in better definition of high-risk indicators among differing socioeconomic groups.[3,25]

Management Guidelines

Once high-risk status has been determined, a plan of care, based on the unique needs and condition of each family, is developed. The primary objective of management is to provide appropriate and timely preventive or restorative care with a minimum of technologic intervention and financial or emotional cost.[22,23] Management strategies may include health education, continued observation, further assessment procedures, specific interventions, or referrals to regional antenatal centers that specialize in management of pregnant clients with specific high-risk conditions. Management guidelines for the client identified as high risk are discussed in later chapters of this text.

Many clients who are screened for high-risk conditions turn out to be normal and deliver healthy infants at term; however, the screening process can be extremely stressful for clients who worry they may be, as one client stated, "part of that small percentage of women who do have a real problem." By using a calm, supportive and knowledgeable approach, nurses can do much to help clients through emotionally difficult screening processes. The nurse should encourage the woman, her partner, and other family members to verbalize their concerns, fears, and needs, without fear of ridicule or judgment. Continuous communication throughout pregnancy is necessary, as pregnancy is an evolving process and even careful screening cannot always predict complications.

BIOCHEMICAL SCREENING TECHNIQUES

The initial biochemical screening during the first trimester of pregnancy provides baseline data and allows for early intervention to ensure optimal maternal-fetal well-being. After the initial confirmation of pregnancy, the following tests may be routinely ordered: urinalysis, complete blood count (CBC), blood typing and Rh determination, rubella titer, serology for syphilis, gonorrhea culture, and Papanicolaou (Pap) smear. The prenatal assessment is an ongoing process and some screening tests warrant repetition at specific times as the pregnancy pro-

TABLE 14–10. RISK FACTORS AFFECTING PREGNANCY

Physiologic Factors

Maternal age
Parity
Late or no prenatal care
Maternal health status (conditions occurring before or during pregnancy)
- Neuromuscular disorders
- Seizures or other neurologic disorders
- Mental illness
- Cardiovascular disease, history of rheumatic heart disease
- Respiratory disease (chronic conditions, severe infections)
- Gastrointestinal disorders, liver or gallbladder disease
- Urinary tract disorders (renal disease, repeated urinary tract infections, anomalies)
- Metabolic disorders (eg, diabetes mellitus and thyroid, pituitary and adrenal disorders)
- Blood disorders (eg, anemias, hemoglobinopathies)
- Major anomalies of the reproductive tract
- Poor nutritional status (obesity, underweight, eating disorders, poor-quality nutrition, weight losses between visits)
- Severe skin diseases
- Malignancy
- Infections (sexually transmitted diseases and other infections)

Pregnancy-related risk factors
- Grand multiparity
- Previous pregnancy loss
- History of previous prenatal risks
- Risk of inherited disorders
- Risk of neural tube defects
- Multiple fetuses
- Vaginal bleeding
- Isoimmunization
- Lack of immunization to diseases such as rubella and hepatitis B (at-risk groups)
- Premature labor
  - Risk of spontaneous abortion (first and second trimesters)
  - Risk of premature delivery (second and third trimesters)
- Premature rupture of membranes
- Ectopic pregnancy (first trimester)
- Hydatidiform mole (first and second trimesters)
- Pre-eclampsia/eclampsia (second and third trimesters, first trimester with hydatidiform mole)
- Gestational diabetes
- Disproportionate uterine growth, oligohydramnios, polyhydramnios)
- Abnormal fetal growth
- Abnormal results of tests for fetal well-being
- Abnormalities of placenta formation or function, infarction, previa, abruptio, infections)

Psychosocial Factors

Unwanted pregnancy
Previous obstetric loss
Real or potential high-risk condition
No previous contact with young children
Severe career-parenting conflict
Client raised with no maternal role model or with poor maternal role model
Resentment/rejection of fetus
Inability to attach to fetus
Lack of support from significant others, persistent feelings of isolation
Severe social problems affecting self and others
- Turbulent marriage
- Pending divorce
- Problems with children already in family
- Crises/catastrophe in family system
- Client, expectant father, or family member incarcerated

Abuse (current or past, physical or emotional)
Pregnancy resulting from rape (by husband or other)
Other

Socioeconomic Factors

Inability to provide basic needs for self and family
Perceived financial stress, complicated by pregnancy
Poor housing/lack of housing (homelessness)
Unemployment, threatened loss of income from usual source of support

Lifestyle Factors

Smoking
Alcohol use
Use of drugs that could affect fetus or pregnancy
Hazardous, stressful, or strenuous occupation
Number of sexual partners; sexual partners with high risk behavior (eg,IV users)

Environmental Factors

Potentially hazardous home environment (eg, lack of plumbing; no potable water source; lack of heat, electricity, or other utilities; exposure to chemicals such as lead; unsafe housing structure, infestations of rodents and vermin)
Potentially hazardous work environment (eg, exposure to teratogens or carcinogens in the workplace; occupation that requires strenuous physical activity, balance, or other)
Potentially hazardous recreational environment (eg, swimming in polluted waters, exposure to teratogens during recreational activities)

gresses. Subsequent prenatal visits include urinalysis for albumin and glucose and periodic determinations of hemoglobin and hematocrit. More extensive screening may also be warranted on the basis of maternal history and clinical indications; for example, if glucose is found in the urine, serum glucose testing may be ordered.

Urinalysis

A freshly voided urine sample is tested for glucose, protein, and ketones at each prenatal visit in order to identify complications of pregnancy. A clean catch technique may be used if microscopic examination and culture are to be done to screen for asymptomatic bacteriuria. A single specimen with a colony count of

TABLE 14–11. RISK FACTORS RELATED TO SPECIFIC PREGNANCY PROBLEMS

Preterm Labor
Age below 16 or over 35
Low socioeconomic status
Maternal weight below 50 kg (110 lb)
Poor nutrition
Previous preterm birth
Incompetent cervix
Uterine anomalies
Smoking
Drug addiction and alcohol abuse
Pyelonephritis, pneumonia
Multiple gestation
Anemia
Abnormal fetal presentation
Preterm rupture of membranes
Placental abnormalities
Infection
Polyhydramnios
Diabetes mellitus
Multiple gestation
Fetal congenital anomalies
Isoimmunization (Rh or ABO)
Nonimmune hydrops
Abnormal fetal presentation
Intrauterine Growth Retardation (IUGR)
Multiple gestation
Poor nutrition
Maternal cyanotic heart disease
Chronic hypertension
Pregnancy-induced hypertension
Recurrent antepartum hemorrhage
Smoking
Maternal diabetes with vascular problems
Fetal infections
Fetal cardiovascular anomalies
Drug addition and alcohol abuse
Fetal congenital anomalies
Hemoglobinopathies
Oligohydramnios
Renal agenesis (Potter's syndrome)
Prolonged rupture of membranes
Intrauterine growth retardation
Intrauterine fetal demise
Post-term Pregnancy
Anencephaly
Placental sulfatase deficiency
Perinatal hypoxia, acidosis
Placental insufficiency
Chromosomal Abnormalities
Maternal age 35 years or more at delivery
Balanced translocation (maternal and paternal)

From Pernoll ML, Benson RC. Current Obstetric and Gynecologic Diagnosis and Treatment. *Norwalk, Conn: Appleton & Lange; 1987.*

100,000 (10 mL) or more per milliliter is considered asymptomatic bacteriuria.[9] Recently, the rapid detection of gram-negative bacteriuria by chromogenic limulus amoebocyte lysate assay has been recommended as a reliable and simple screening test for asymptomatic bacteriuria of pregnancy.[12,27] A freshly voided urine specimen for the detection of glucose and protein should be obtained form the woman at each prenatal visit.

Blood Studies

A variety of blood studies are performed at the initial prenatal visit. Additional studies may be ordered if there are specific indications. In many settings, a complete blood count and differential analysis is performed in the first prenatal visit to screen for blood disorders and infections. (*See* Appendix C for normal laboratory values during pregnancy.) Elevation of the white blood cell count may indicate infection. Hemoglobin and hematocrit indices detect anemia, which may have serious implications during pregnancy. Levels below 11 to 12 g/100 mL for hemoglobin or 33 to 36 percent for hematocrit suggest anemia in the first trimester.[12] Hemoglobin or hematocrit levels are again determined early in the third trimester, unless there is indication for testing to be done sooner.[17] Pathologic causes of anemia during pregnancy should be excluded and dietary counseling with iron supplementation prescribed as needed.

A sample of the expectant woman's blood is analyzed to identify the specific type (A, B, O, or AB) and presence of the Rh factor or antibodies. Eighty-five percent of the population has a positive Rh factor (Rh+) and the remaining 15 percent has a negative Rh factor (Rh−).[13] If the mother is Rh negative and the fetus is Rh positive, isoimmunization can occur during future pregnancies. If the father is Rh negative, isoimmunization will not occur. Therefore, paternal blood may be tested for Rh factor if the mother is Rh negative. Rh incompatibility is the most common cause of fetal hemolytic disease; however, other antibodies can be implicated (*see* Chapters 39 and 42). An irregular antibody screen may also be done.[17]

Rubella susceptibility during pregnancy is significant, as rubella (German measles) can be teratogenic to the fetus, especially if the disease occurs during the first trimester. Rubella screening is routinely performed to determine past maternal rubella infection or adequate immunization. A serum antibody titer is performed to determine the level of immunity to rubella. A titer less than 1:8 is considered indicative of maternal susceptibility to rubella or lack of immunity; a titer of 1:8 to 1:32 indicates past rubella exposure;

and a titer over 1:32 indicates that immunity exists.[27]

Susceptible women should be counseled to avoid contact with individuals who have been exposed to rubella or who are thought to have rubella. Women should *not* be immunized for rubella when pregnancy is suspected or being attempted. Postpartum vaccination is recommended, with counseling to use a means of contraception for a minimum of 3 months. It is generally considered safe to administer the rubella vaccine during lactation.[4, 28]

Screening for syphilis is part of the blood studies done at the first prenatal visit. Syphilis, a sexually transmitted disease caused by the spirochete *Treponema pallidum,* not only harms the mother, but also can transplacentally infect the fetus. A variety of serologic tests may be used to detect syphilis. The Venereal Disease Research Laboratories (VDRL) test and the reactive plasma reagin (RPR) test are widely used nontreponemal antibody screening tests. Fluorescent treponemal antibody absorption (FTA-ABS) and *T. pallidum* immobilization (TPI) are treponemal antibody tests that are more specific and sensitive to spirochete infections. Certain chronic diseases can produce biologic false-positive results for the VDRL; however, tests can then be performed on a blood sample to identify the organism specifically. Additionally, the VDRL may be negative in the early infectious phase of syphilis.

The human immunodeficiency virus (HIV) presents a life-threatening condition that can potentially be transmitted to the fetus. Currently, universal screening of all prenatal clients is controversial; however, HIV screening may be offered to clients at risk.

Cytology

At the first prenatal visit, a Pap smear is taken to detect cytologic abnormalities (*see* Chapter 5).

Cultures

In some settings, cervical cultures for *Neisseria gonorrhoeae* (gonorrhea) and chlamydia may be routinely performed. In other settings, the tests are done only for clients at risk or with a history of the diseases. On the basis of the client's history or observations made by the examiner during the vaginal examination, cultures for other organisms, such as gardnerella, trichomonas or herpes, may be done.

PSYCHOSOCIAL AND CULTURAL ASSESSMENT

Psychosocial Assessment

The nurse can help the family cope with various psychosocial tasks of pregnancy through counseling and support of family members. Thorough prenatal assessment during the first trimester allows the nurse to identify normal and abnormal patterns of adaptation.

Patterns of Self-Perception/Concept. Pregnancy can bring changes in a woman's self-image (*see* Chapter 13). The expectant woman experiences changes in body image as her pregnancy progresses. She may feel as though the pregnancy is a manifestation of femininity and react positively to the beginning changes in her body during the first trimester. Conversely, she may be uncomfortable with the changes and may feel unattractive or undesirable. The father, too, may have an altered self-perception related to the pregnancy and the role he envisions for himself.

A thorough prenatal assessment can reveal the expectant mother's and father's self-concepts or perceptions of the pregnancy. The nurse should assess whether the expectant couple views the pregnancy as reinforcing or as threatening to their self-image. The nurse may then intervene to validate the positive aspects or offer guidance to alter threats to self-image.

Cognitive/Perceptual Aspects. Cognitive ability is variable and needs to be assessed individually to establish a realistic plan of prenatal care. The nurse should discuss the instructional plan in terms that the woman and her partner will understand. The educational needs of the couple should be assessed throughout pregnancy; a variety of culturally appropriate instructional means should be available because learning ability is unique for each person.[29] Visual aids, demonstrations, and seminar presentations may be used by the nurse as methods to meet the educational needs of the couple.

Pregnancy may temporarily alter sensory perceptions, causing distress for some women. The woman may develop an aversion to certain smells or tastes. She may experience transient alterations in vision or hearing related to congestion or edema. Some women find they are unable to wear contact lenses comfortably or that their sense of smell is diminished.

Behavioral Aspects. The first trimester is typified by uncertainty, ambivalence, and the need for attention and reassurance. Disbelief and questioning as to timing may dominate the first trimester as the woman begins to accept the reality of pregnancy (*see* Chapter 13). Assessment of the woman's behaviors specific to pregnancy guides the nurse in comprehensive pregnancy management.

Coping/Stress Tolerance. Pregnancy can be a stressful event, because of the many changes that take

ISSUES AND CONTROVERSIES

Issues and controversies in first-trimester prenatal assessment focus on such topics as the use of invasive assessment techniques, the use of new technology, and the role of various health care providers in the assessment process. Questions such as how much technology should be used routinely and should all clients be assessed as potentially high risk or low risk remain unanswered.

Concern continues to be raised about potential long-term effects of such tests as diagnostic ultrasound. Methodologic problems with existing research studies leave questions about widespread use. Chorionic villi sampling is a fairly new procedure that offers an earlier alternative to amniocentesis in the diagnosis of chromosomal abnormalities; however, the nature of complications, the lack of long-term experience with the procedure, and the lack of experienced staff to perform the procedure except in relatively few perinatal centers are sources of controversy. As new technology for prenatal and fetal assessment emerges, so do concerns about the effect of the technology on the physical development of the fetus and the psychologic state of the expectant family. When assessment techniques reveal information of severe fetal anomalies, clients are faced with decisions about continuing the pregnancy. The choice between continuing and terminating the pregnancy is enormously controversial.

Controversy continues to exist over which health care providers should direct and implement prenatal assessment. Such issues as the choice of a certified nurse-midwife or physician persist.

place within the woman and within the family. Pregnancy may tax the financial and physical resources of the family. The nurse must evaluate the stress perceived by family members during pregnancy, as well as the effectiveness of coping patterns. High life stress occurring with pregnancy may present problems for the client and her family.

The couple may need assistance in identifying stresses related to pregnancy, support for beneficial coping patterns, and, at times, referral to community resources that can provide help in dealing with stress. Interaction with health care providers at prenatal visits offers enough professional support to help some clients cope with normal prenatal stress. Others benefit greatly from group support provided by early pregnancy classes. Still others, who have few resources for dealing with stress or who are experiencing severe stress, benefit from referral to counseling services, which may be available through private or clinic mental health services, social services, or pastoral care.

Roles/Relationships. The transition to motherhood and fatherhood is accompanied by changes in roles and relationships within the family, within employment situations, and within the societal structure.[30] The pregnant woman, expectant father, and other family members are influenced by their own perceptions of appropriate roles. In interviews with the client during the first trimester, the nurse assesses the ways in which the expectant family is adapting to pregnancy and identifies potential conflicts in roles and relationships.

Cultural Assessment

The cultural and spiritual needs of the expectant family should be assessed, because various beliefs and practices influence the couple's interpretation of and receptiveness to health care. The expectant family may have religious beliefs that prohibit care by males at certain times, use of transfusions, or consumption of certain foods. Some women may have had female circumcision, which may affect childbirth because of the resulting anatomic changes.[31] Cultural practices may influence the family to seek health care and may affect adherence to instructions. In addition, language difficulties may influence whether and to what extent services are received. Prenatal assessment must encompass the spiritual and cultural differences of each expectant family. Spiritual and cultural influences can then be incorporated into a care plan tailored to the unique needs of the client and family.

PRENATAL DIAGNOSTIC ASSESSMENT

Fetal assessment during the first trimester may be done through a variety of means. Fundal height can be used to estimate growth (*see* Figure 12–2). As early prenatal enlargement of the uterus takes place even with ectopic pregnancies, however, it can be a misleading sign. As described earlier, fetal heart blood flow may be identified with Doppler ultrasound as early as 8 weeks. Ultrasound imaging, especially with a transvaginal approach, may provide information about the fetus, such as gestational age. Chorionic villus sampling is yet another first-trimester procedure for fetal assessment.

Chorionic Villus Sampling

Chorionic villus sampling (CVS) is a first-trimester procedure, performed to obtain fetal cells for diagnosis of chromosomal abnormalities.[32] It is indicated for women of advanced maternal age; women with a previous history of a fetus or child with a genetic disorder; couples who express or carry a genetic abnormality; and any other women for whom there is reason to suspect a genetically abnormal fetus.

In the United States, desire to know sex of the fetus is not considered reason enough to justify this invasive procedure; however, sex of the fetus is reported as part of the results of CVS.

Chorionic villi, which are fetal in origin, reflect the chromosomes, enzymology, and DNA content of the fetus. CVS is able to detect a variety of cytogenic, biochemical, and DNA-linked abnormalities. Identification of chromosomal disorders, such as trisomy 21, trisomy 18, translocations and X-linked disorders; enzyme deficiencies or biochemical disorders such as Tay-Sachs disease; and hematologic diseases such as sickle cell anemia, thalassemia, and hemophilia is possible. Unlike amniocentesis, CVS cannot detect such disorders as neural tube defects, because alphafetoprotein levels currently can be tested only on serum or amniotic fluid. The procedure is relatively simple, takes about 20 minutes, and can be performed on an outpatient basis.[32, 33]

During the 1970s, CVS was performed in China for sex determination.[34] Later, CVS was tested in women prior to elective termination of pregnancy to determine the feasibility, safety, and accuracy of its use as an alternative method to amniocentesis for prenatal diagnosis of genetic disorders. (For discussion of amniocentesis, *see* Chapter 18.)

Chorionic villi are microscopic hairlike projections of the outer membrane surrounding the embryo. Chorionic villi burrow into the maternal decidua basalis. The villi, which are genetically similar to the fetus, develop around 2 weeks after implantation and proliferate until the tenth week, when placental formation is taking place. After that time, the thinning chorion interfaces with the amnion. Although villi on the implanting side of the chorion develop into the placenta, by about 14 weeks, the villi that were not on the implanting side disappear. Chorionic villus sampling is optimally performed between 8 and 12 weeks after the first day of the last menstrual period, when the chorionic tissue is thickest and the amnion and chorion are still separated by a fissurelike excoelomic fluid-filled cavity, but before the villi begin to disappear.[33–35]

Advantages. CVS has several advantages[33] that stem from its availability as a first-trimester assessment technique. Test results from CVS are available within a few days (*see* later), as compared with the 3 to 4 weeks usually needed for results from amniocentesis. Normal results may help allay clients' anxieties about certain genetic disorders. Abnormal results may allow clients who choose to continue the pregnancy to receive special support and to have a considerable amount of time to prepare for the baby. Some clients will elect to terminate the pregnancy. First-trimester terminations are medically safer, quicker, and easier than second-trimester terminations. Because first-trimester pregnancy is less visible, the client may have greater privacy in decision making than during the second trimester.

Disadvantages/Risks. Chorionic villus sampling can be associated with complications or inaccurate results.[33] A 1.7 percent discrepancy rate between the apparent villus karyotype and the fetus has been reported.[36] The possibility of maternal cell contamination requires meticulous cell separation and skilled interpretation of samples. Additionally, true mosaicism within the placenta can lead to false results. Follow-up amniocentesis or percutaneous umbilical blood sampling may then be suggested.

Possible risks of CVS include ruptured amniotic sac, chorioamnionitis, altered fetomaternal fluid dynamics (severe oligohydramnios), pregnancy loss, intrauterine growth retardation, placental dysfunction or accidents, rh isoimmunization, and fetal anomalies.[34] Chorionic villus sampling does not ensure that the fetus will be completely healthy, as other conditions can develop during gestation or delivery, and certain abnormalities, such as neural tube defects, cannot be detected by CVS.

Pregnancy loss has been estimated to range from 3.8 to 6 percent. Spontaneous abortion rates by gestational week are often compared with use of CVS; however, the time of actual fetal demise is unknown, as spontaneous abortion rates are derived from the time of actual passage of tissue. Procedure-related losses need further study, as do natural loss rates, which have been estimated to range from 2 to 20 percent during the first trimester.[35, 37]

An inadequate specimen may prevent accurate analysis. The localization of cord insertion as a marker for catheter placement and accurate gestational assessment, based on crown-rump length (9 to 41 mm) is suggested for optimal specimen collection.[38] If adequate specimens cannot be obtained after three attempts, the procedure is repeated a week later.[38] Although CVS seems to be fairly safe, it is a relatively new procedure. Further CVS experience and study are needed to determine whether long-term adverse effects exist.

Procedure. Prior to CVS, a negative cervical culture for gonorrhea may be requested to avoid the possibility of spreading the organism into the blood of an infected client.[32] A client diagnosed with gonorrhea would therefore need to be treated successfully prior to the procedure.

The client who elects CVS receives genetic counseling. The procedure, its risks, and its benefits are explained, and the client signs a consent form.[32] At the time the test is scheduled, the client should be made aware of the time commitment necessary. For example, preparation, procedure, and recovery may entail about 2 hours, although the procedure takes only about 20 minutes. Delays in the testing center may prolong this time. The client should be informed of the need for rest at home after the procedure, so that she can make appropriate adjustments in her own usual schedule and responsibilities.

Various approaches have been used for CVS and include direct vision biopsy with a hysteroscope, transabdominal aspiration with ultrasound guidance, and transcervical aspiration with ultrasound visualization. Currently, the transcervical approach is most often employed (Figure 14–12). A physician performs CVS.

In preparation for transcervical CVS, the client must have a full bladder. She is then placed in the lithotomy position, a pelvic examination is done, and a speculum is inserted so that the cervix can be seen. A slender catheter is passed through the cervix. Under direct visualization with real-time ultrasound, a small sample of chorionic villi is aspirated through the catheter into a syringe. The catheter never penetrates the amniotic sac. The aspirated chorionic villi are put into a sterile medium and sent for cytogenic analysis. As first-trimester cells divide rapidly, time is not needed for them to grow in a laboratory. Theoretically, preliminary reports can be available within a few hours, as karyotyping is done during metaphase of mitosis through use of direct microscopic preparation. Unless there is some pressing reason to attend at once to a specimen, laboratory personnel realistically have preliminary reports within 24 to 48 hours and confirmed reports within 5 to 10 days of CVS.[32]

Discomforts. The client undergoing CVS may experience discomforts related to a full bladder, the lithotomy position, or the presence of the speculum. Mild cramping related to cervical manipulation may be felt. In the healthy woman the procedure does not require anesthesia[32]; however, CVS may be psychologically distressing to a client, and unrelieved anxiety may amplify discomforts.

Role of the Nurse. Working collaboratively with the physician in an antenatal testing unit, the nurse has several important roles, including client education, assessment, and support. The nurse's role involves teaching the client and her partner about CVS, its risks and benefits; acting as a client advocate for the couple when they make an informed decision regarding the procedure; and caring for the client before, during, and after CVS.[32] In addition, the nurse's role may involve teaching about choices the woman may face if an abnormality is detected.[39]

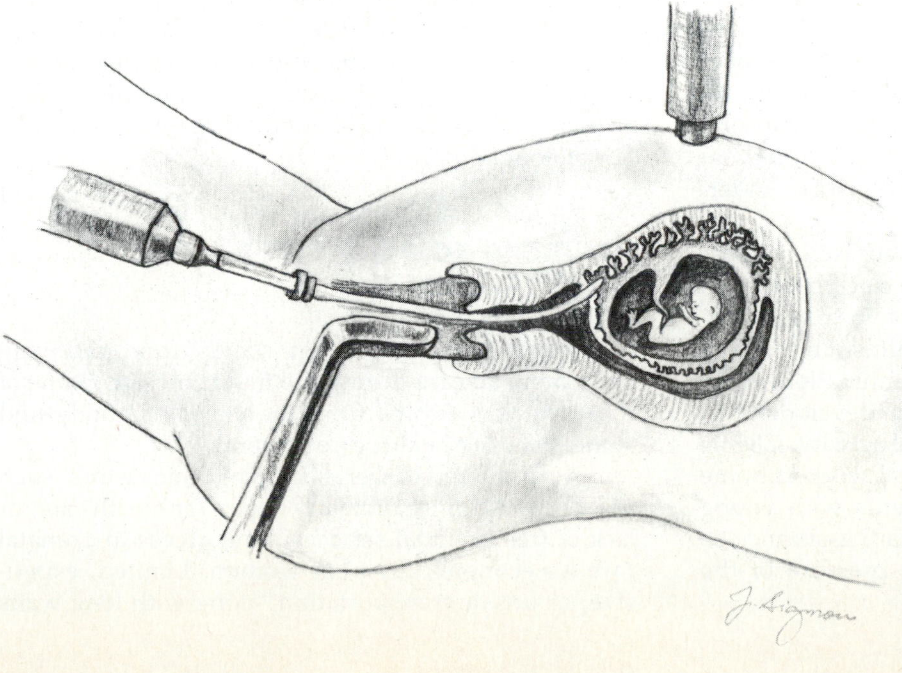

Figure 14–12. Chorionic villus sampling.

Prior to the procedure, the nurse may provide anticipatory guidance and help with the timing of the test so that the client's discomfort related to a full bladder is minimized. Most clients are frightened at the thought of CVS. Fear may be verbalized or expressed by tears or even by silence during the procedure. Chorionic villus sampling is a secondary screening procedure, done because some degree of risk is suspected. The nurse needs to anticipate fears, and to offer support throughout the procedure. Including the woman's partner (or significant other), showing the ultrasound images on the monitor during the procedure, reassuring the client that the catheter does not enter the amniotic sac, and using relaxation techniques such as touch and deep breathing can help comfort the client through CVS.[32] Unfortunately, some clients will have a fetus with a genetic disorder; therefore, support during CVS needs to be provided without assuring the client that the fetus is genetically normal.

After the procedure, the client is assisted out of the lithotomy position. Blood pressure and pulse are taken. If vital signs are normal, the client may void in a collection container in the bathroom. Although a small amount of spotting may appear, heavy bleeding or the passage of amniotic fluid, clots, or tissue is not normal and should be reported to the physician at once. A clear or pink-tinged specimen may be discarded, whereas tissue passed may be sent for laboratory analysis.

Chorionic villus sampling is an outpatient procedure, and the client leaves for home if her vital signs are stable, she is not experiencing cramping, and she is having no vaginal discharge other than spotting. The nurse remains accessible to the client and provides an opportunity for the client to express her feelings, which may include relief that the test is over and fear related to possible results. A client with associated complications is kept in the antenatal testing unit until stable or, if necessary, admitted. Interventions based on the type of complications are undertaken.

After the procedure the client is advised to avoid sexual activity for 48 hours, contact her physician if bleeding, cramping, or flulike symptoms are experienced, return for examination and ultrasound 1 week later, return for an ultrasound examination at 16 weeks (to evaluate fetal and placental development), and avoid heavy or vigorous physical activity. Clients should plan to rest that day. Physical work at home or at a job should be avoided. Clients with young children should plan to have child care assistance so that they may recover without the pressure of the usual daily childcare activities.

SUPPORT OF THE CLIENT UNDERGOING DIAGNOSTIC ASSESSMENT

The purpose of diagnostic assessment during the first trimester is secondary prevention, that is, the early identification of abnormalities. Many clients do not have uncomfortable symptoms during the early stages of disease processes. Prompt treatment may help cure or control pathologic conditions. For example, infections such as gonorrhea can be successfully treated during pregnancy, and diabetes can be controlled. Early identification of conditions that cannot be changed, such as genetic abnormalities or human immunodeficiency virus, may help the client make decisions about whether to continue the pregnancy.

By concluding that a client is normal and at low risk, health care providers rule out a broad range of potential pathologic conditions. Clients need to be informed about the type and purpose of any diagnostic test performed. Care needs to be taken to present information accurately, yet in a manner that does not needlessly alarm the client and her family. For example, a client may be told that a blood specimen is being obtained to confirm that her blood count is normal and that blood analysis is a routine part of early prenatal care. Such an approach is preferable to informing a client she needs a blood test to identify evidence of anemia.

All diagnostic tests can be a source of misinterpretation and worry for the client and her family. Unfortunately, no one test can answer all questions about the well-being of the developing fetus. In addition to providing teaching about the test and support during procedures, health care providers need to make sure that clients receive test results as soon as possible. At times, clients with abnormal findings are notified promptly, while equally worried healthy clients are left wondering about their normal test results for prolonged periods.

BARRIERS TO CARE DURING THE FIRST TRIMESTER

Numerous barriers prevent clients from receiving early prenatal care during the first trimester. Some of these barriers evolve from the client or family and some from the health care system.

As discussed earlier, socioeconomic factors, such as lack of insurance, inability to pay for health care, or lack of free prenatal services, limit access to prenatal care for economically poor women. Limited, expensive, or unsafe transportation, along with long waits in prenatal clinics, makes regular trips for prenatal care unfeasible. For example, the woman who has to travel for 2 hours to receive care and who has other responsibilities, such as preschool or school-aged children, may simply not be able to attend a prenatal visit that will keep her away from home after the school bus comes. Certain cultural groups may not value or accept the need for prenatal care during the first trimester.

Nurses can do much to help surmount barriers to early prenatal care, as shown in these examples:

1. Prenatal sessions can be scheduled to include evening or weekend hours. In this way, working women do not have to choose between their jobs and their health care.
2. Through professional nursing organizations, direct contact with legislators, and networking with private corporations, nurses can seek support to provide funds to make prenatal care accessible to all women.
3. Through roles as authors, speakers, producers, and consultants to the media, nurses can raise public awareness about the importance of early prenatal care.
4. By providing a welcoming and supportive attitude at all prenatal contacts, nurses can encourage clients to keep their first and subsequent prenatal visits.
5. By assessing barriers to prenatal care that individual clients may face, nurses can provide appropriate referrals to resources, for example, to social services or to prenatal clinics closer to the client's home. Nurses may also initiate change to reduce carriers in their own settings.

NURSING DIAGNOSES

The first-trimester assessment process provides extensive information about the client and her family. Diagnoses are then developed from the subjective and objective data collected and reflect conclusions about the client and her family. Planning, intervention, and evaluation evolve from assessment data and nursing diagnosis. Many professions use this process; however, the nursing process presents a unique perspective. Nursing diagnoses provide summary statements of information that reflect the client's healthy and unhealthy responses or potential responses to differing levels of wellness.[40]

Despite changes and discomforts related to early pregnancy, the first trimester is part of a healthy life process. Nursing diagnoses therefore focus on well-

NURSING DIAGNOSES RELATED TO THE FIRST TRIMESTER

Physiologic

Problem-Oriented

Fatigue, related to demands of pregnancy during first-trimester

Nutrition, altered: potential for nutritional deprivation related to first-trimester nausea and vomiting

Strength-Oriented

Asset in health of mother related to normal physical changes in the first trimester

Progressive normal embryo/fetal growth and development, related to maternal health and nutritional status during the first trimester

Psychosocial

Problem-Oriented

Anxiety, related to
- Initial encounter with the health care system
- Financial pressures related to economic impact of childbearing

Knowledge deficit, related to
- Lack of understanding about first-trimester changes
- Lack of information about first-trimester discomforts
- Lack of understanding about early prenatal assessment techniques
- Lack of information about the nature and extent of services available in the prenatal health care system

Strength-Oriented

Potential asset in self-care practices, related to early initiation of prenatal care

Cultural

Problem-Oriented

Social isolation, related to cultural differences in perception of roles during early pregnancy

Impaired social interaction, related to differences in language between client and care providers

Strength-Oriented

Positive self-concept, related to congruence between cultural beliefs and
- Achievement of pregnancy
- Expectations of prenatal care

ness and on the need to identify potential risk factors. (*See* the box on page 359 for nursing diagnoses related to the first-trimester of normal pregnancy.)

SUMMARY

The first trimester of pregnancy is an important time for the childbearing family. Early and thorough assessment allows health care providers to get to know the client, to identify her overall health status, real or potential risk factors, strengths, and resources. Comprehensive assessment includes physical, psychosocial, socioeconomic, and cultural dimensions and focuses on the client's family, significant others, home, and work environment. Diagnoses of wellness and illness evolve from assessment.

Ideally, the client comes for her first visit during the first trimester and returns at 4-week intervals during the first trimester. Initial assessment includes a thorough health history, physical examination, and appropriate laboratory studies. Assessment during return visits updates the history, identifies any new problems, confirms that pregnancy and prenatal adaptation are progressing normally, and identifies educational needs. Several diagnostic tests, such as ultrasound and chorionic villus sampling, may be performed if certain risk factors are identified.

Collaboration between nurses and other health care providers is necessary to provide complete care in an effective, efficient manner. First-trimester assessment provides an opportunity to establish a trusting relationship with the client and to develop a plan of care that will maximize well-being throughout the childbearing process.

REVIEW QUESTIONS

1. Discuss the importance of history, physical examination, and laboratory data in prenatal assessment.
2. Describe maternal assessment techniques that are used during the first trimester.
3. Identify at least two techniques available to confirm pregnancy.
4. Identify psychosocial and cultural dimensions of the childbearing family that should be assessed during the first trimester.
5. How would the nurse explain the following techniques to a pregnant couple: transvaginal ultrasonography, chorionic villus sampling?
6. Discuss several psychologic implications for the pregnant family related to first-trimester assessment techniques.
7. Discuss the role of the nurse in initiating and participating in interdisciplinary, collaborative approaches to care of the pregnant family.

REFERENCES

1. Nagey, DA. The content of prenatal care. *Obstet Gynecol* 1989;74:516–528.
2. Feeg VD. *Pediatric Nursing: Forum on the Future: Looking Toward the 21st Century.* Pitman, NJ: Anthony J. Jannetti, Inc, 1989.
3. Pernoll M. Benson, R, eds. *Current Obstetric & Gynecologic Diagnosis & Treatment.* 6th ed. Norwalk, Conn: Appleton & Lange; 1987.
4. Cunningham FG, et al. *Williams Obstetrics.* 18th ed. Norwalk, Conn: Appleton & Lange, 1989.
5. Varney H. *Nurse-Midwifery.* 2nd ed. Boston: Blackwell Scientific; 1987.
6. Varner MW, et al. X-ray pelvimetry in clinical obstetrics. *Obstet Gynecol* 1980;56:296.
7. Block G, Nolan J. *Health Assessment for Professional Nursing: A Developmental Approach.* Norwalk, Conn: Appleton-Century-Crofts; 1986.
8. Oxorn H, ed. *Oxorn-Foote Human Labor and Birth.* 5th ed. Norwalk, Conn: Appleton-Century-Crofts; 1986.
9. Kee JL. *Laboratory and Diagnostic Tests with Nursing Implications.* 2nd ed. Norwalk, Conn: Appleton & Lange; 1987.
10. Hatcher RA, et al. *Contraceptive Technology, 1988–1989.* 14th ed. New York: Irvington; 1988.
11. Lichtman R, Papera S. *Gynecology: Well Woman Care.* Norwalk, Conn: Appleton & Lange; 1990.
12. Corbett JV. *Laboratory Tests and Diagnostic Procedures with Nursing Diagnoses.* 2nd ed. Norwalk, Conn: Appleton & Lange; 1987.
13. Jones HW, et al. *Novak's Textbook of Gynecology.* 11th ed. Baltimore: Williams & Wilkins; 1988.
14. American College of Obstetricians and Gynecologists. *Ultrasound in pregnancy.* Technical Bulletin, 116. Washington, D.C.: The College; 1988.
15. O'Brien W. Ultrasound bioeffects: a view of experimental studies. *Birth.* ll;1984:149–157.
16. Oakley A. The history of ultrasonography in obstetrics. *Birth.* 1986;13:5–10. (Special Supplement: Royal Society of Medicine: Forum on Maternity and the Newborn: Ultrasonography in Obstetrics.)
17. American Academy of Pediatrics, American College of Obstetricians and Gynecologists. In: Frigoletto FD, Little GA, eds. *Guidelines for Perinatal Care.* 2nd ed. March of Dimes Birth Defects Foundation; 1988.
18. Modica MM, Timor-Tritsch IE. Transvaginal sonography provides a sharper view into the pelvis. *J Obstet Gynecol Neonat Nurs.* 1988;17:89–95.
19. Grant A. Controlled trials of routine ultrasound in pregnancy. *Birth.* 1986;13 (special suppl):16–22.
20. Mole R. Possible hazards of imaging and Doppler ultrasound in obstetrics. *Birth.* 1986;13 (special suppl):23–33.
21. Cacciatore B, et al. Comparison of abdominal and vaginal

sonogrpahy in suspected ectopic pregnancy. *Obstet Gynecol.* 1989:770–774.
22. Steinkampf MP. Transvaginal sonography. *J Reprod Med.* 1988;33:931–938.
23. Spencer JAD, et al. Latest Obstetric uses of Doppler ultrasound. *Contemp Obstet Gynecol.* 1989;33:154–165.
24. Platt LD, et al. Assessing the fetus with Doppler ultrasound. *Contemp Obstet Gynecol.* 1989;33:168–199.
25. Klaus M, Fanaroll A. *Care of the High Risk Neonate.* 3rd ed. Philadelphia: WB Saunders; 1986.
26. Warshaw J, Hobbins J. *Principles and Practice of Perinatal Medicine.* Menlo Park, Calif: Addison-Wesley; 1983.
27. Nachum R, et al. Gram negative bacteruria of pregnancy: rapid detection by a chromogenic limulus amoebocyte lysate assay. *Obstet Gynecol.* 1986;62:215–219.
28. Guyton A. *Textbook of Medical Physiology.* 7th ed. Philadelphia: WB Saunders; 1986.
29. Nichols FH, Humenick SS. *Childbirth Education: Practice, Research, and Theory.* Philadelphia: WB Saunders; 1988.
30. Sherwen LN, ed. *Psychosocial Dimensions of the Pregnant Family.* New York: Springer Publishing Co; 1987.
31. Shaw E. Female circumcision. *Am J Nurs.* 1985;85:684–687.
32. Stringer MR. Chorionic villi sampling: nursing perspective. *J Obstet Gynecol Neonat Nurs.* 1988;17:19–24.
33. Hogge JS, et al. Chorionic villus sampling. *J Obstet Gynecol Neonat Nurs.* 1986;15:24–30.
34. Jeavons G. Detecting fetal abnormalities. *Nurs Mirror.* 1985;161:22–24.
35. Hammer R, Tufts M. Chorionic villi sampling for detecting fetal disorders. *Am J Matern Child Nurs.* 1986;11:29–31.
36. Hogge W, et al. Chorionic villus sampling: experience of the first 1000 cases. *Am J Obstet Gynecol.* 1986;154:1249–1252.
37. Elias S, et al. Chorionic villus sampling for first trimester prenatal diagnosis: Northwestern University Program. *Am J Obstet Gynecol.* 1985;152:204–213.
38. Perry T, et al. Chorionic villi sampling: clinical experience, immediate complications and patient attitudes. *Am J Obstet Gynecol.* 1985;151:161–166.
39. Diekemper MA. Chorionic villi sampling. *J Obstet Gynecol Neonat Nurs.* 1988;17:233. Correspondence.
40. Pinnell NN, de Meneses M. *The Nursing Process: Theory, Application and Related Processes.* Norwalk, Conn: Appleton-Century-Crofts; 1986.

Nursing Care of the Family During the First Trimester

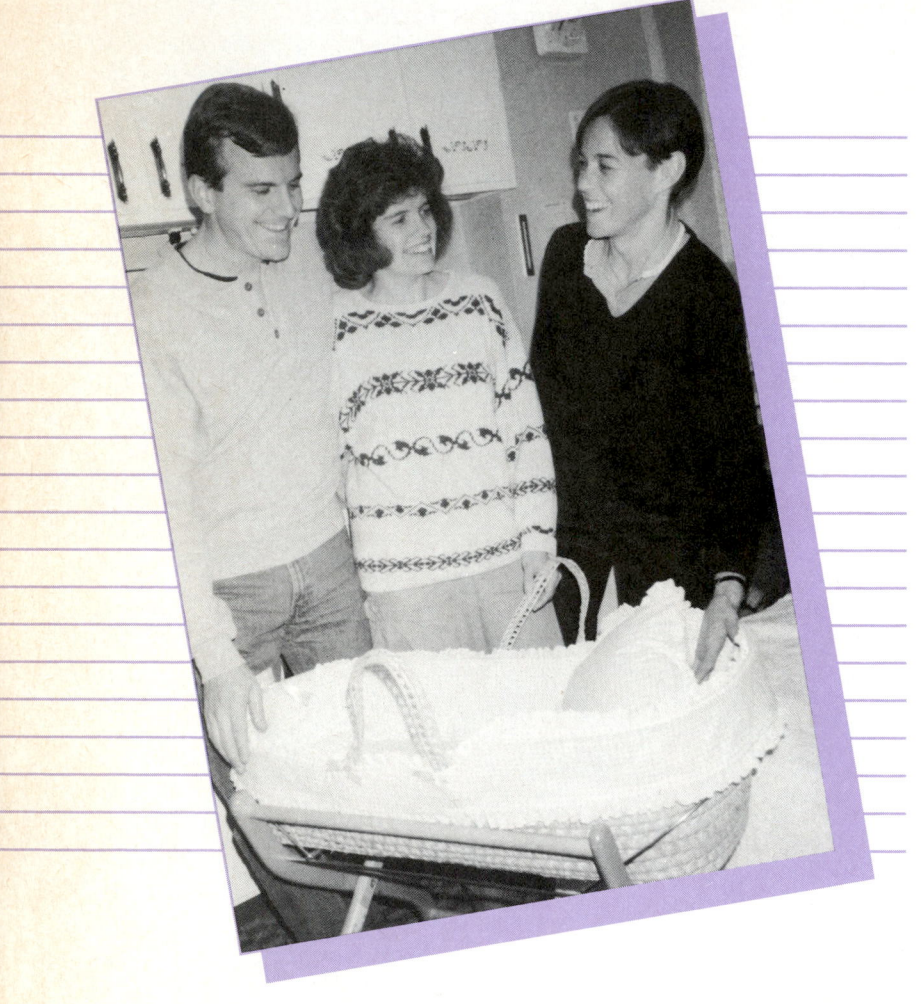

Chapter 15

Key Terms

"morning sickness"
ptyalism

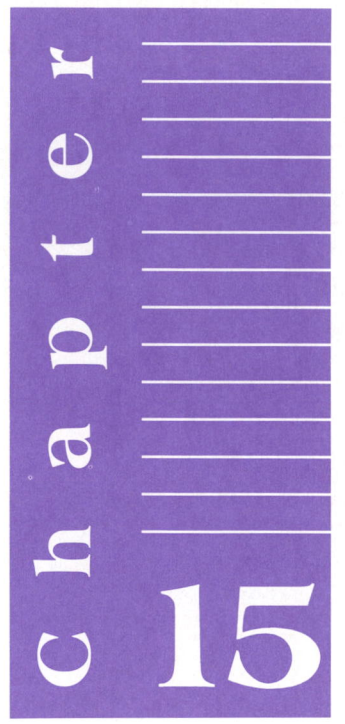

Nursing management involves the delivery of care to the client and family. Nursing care depends on a thorough knowledge of normal and abnormal physiologic, psychosocial, and cultural parameters. Through the management process, a large body of information is gathered, organized, and then individualized so that effective care, based on the unique needs of each client and family, may be delivered. The nursing process of assessment, diagnosis, planning, intervention, and evaluation supplies the ideal tool.

An understanding of what is normal is crucial to interpretation of data from assessment, to formulation of diagnoses, to planning, and to implementation of care. Most clients have a low-risk pregnancy that results in the birth of a healthy newborn. Differentiating between healthy, normal pregnant clients and clients at risk presents a nursing care challenge. High-risk diagnostic techniques and interventions can be costly and threatening to the client's physical and emotional well-being.

The preceding chapters provide information about fetal development; prenatal physiologic, psychosocial, and cultural adaptations; and methods of assessment of the pregnant family. This chapter discusses nursing care according to specific nursing goals that help to organize care (Table 15–1).

The role of health care providers during the first trimester is to support and to guide pregnant families in their self-care practices and to identify and to treat alterations in health. A collaborative approach is necessary to ensure that pregnant families receive optimal care. The nurse is in an excellent position to assist the family, because of nursing's focus on the total health status of the client and her family.[1]

Nursing interventions extend beyond the individual client to families of childbearing age in general. For this reason, a nursing care goal, focused on community education strategies, is included.

ESTABLISH A PHILOSOPHY OF CARE WITH WELL-DEFINED GOALS

Antenatal health care providers should collaborate to develop a philosophy of care with well-defined goals and objectives. The philosophy should be communicated in writing and in discussion with the family[2] (Figure 15–1). Ways in which the philosophy is incorporated into routine client care should

TABLE 15–1. GOALS OF NURSING CARE DURING THE FIRST TRIMESTER

Establish a philosophy of care with well-defined goals
Incorporate recent literature into nursing care
Prepare the client and family for antenatal health care
Evolve a data base from which diagnoses are developed
Develop a care plan
Provide support to the client
Incorporate the client's cultural background into care
Begin the process of informed decision making
Promote psychologic adaptation to early pregnancy
Foster beginning family attachment
Meet early-pregnancy educational needs of the client and her family
Promote nutritional well-being
Assist the client in coping with first-trimester discomforts
Promote client safety
Evaluate antenatal care
Ensure appropriate referrals for the client
Contribute to general antenatal public health

be outlined. For example, staff can show their commitment to childbearing as a normal, family-centered process by encouraging family members to attend all prenatal visits, to participate in prepared childbirth activities, and to be present for labor and delivery.

INCORPORATE RECENT LITERATURE INTO NURSING CARE

Numerous publications related to principles, practice, ethical issues, and research in antenatal care are increasingly available. Optimal prenatal care requires that nurses, as well as other health care providers, keep up with current advances that affect practice. Attendance at professional meetings, in-service programs that focus on different childbearing topics, "journal club" meetings at which staff take turns presenting relevant articles from the professional literature, and regular reading of childbearing literature (personal subscription or borrowed from a library with a nursing collection) help nurses provide state-of-the-art care. Nurses without research backgrounds can be aided in interpretation of research studies by attending basic research continuing education programs, by requesting unit in-service programs on how to read research, and by consulting with nurses who do have research backgrounds.

PREPARE THE CLIENT AND FAMILY FOR ANTENATAL HEALTH CARE

Preparation of the client and her family for antenatal health care includes orientation to health care providers and the antenatal health care system. Indeed, the initial contact may influence a client's willingness to come for early prenatal care; the first visit begins a pattern for client-health provider relationships. The nurse who welcomes clients and encourages their active participation in their own care may foster attendance. An approach to clients is suggested in Chapter 5. Table 15–2 presents a sample outline for an antenatal visit. It is important to realize that variations exist among antenatal care facilities.

During the initial visit, the first-trimester client should be oriented to the antenatal facilities, personnel who will provide care, what to expect during each visit, and the scheduling of prenatal visits.

Antenatal Facilities

Careful directions to the clinic or office, including transportation or parking arrangements, minimize stress related to arrival in a new setting. Many obstetric centers routinely offer tours of the obstetric facilities at the first visit.

Personnel

Primary prenatal care is delivered by certified nurse-midwives, physicians, or house staff physicians (under supervision of attending physicians in clinic settings). Nurse practitioners, antenatal staff nurses, dietitians, nutritionists, social workers, and chaplains are also part of the prenatal care team. Student participation, under instructor and staff supervision, is often welcomed. Student activities in antenatal settings are based on such factors as the student's level, course objectives, nature of the courses, and length of time the student will be able to work with the client. Students who follow childbearing families through pregnancy, childbearing, and the postpartum period have unique opportunities to facilitate the meeting of client care goals and to ensure continuity of care. Antenatal settings vary widely with respect to the type and number of health care personnel interacting with the client. The client needs to be informed of the identity of all personnel directly involved in her care.

Obstetric personnel, such as midwives and/or obstetricians, often join together in group practices. These arrangements relieve grueling obstetric schedules and also offer clients the advantage of access to health care providers with different backgrounds. In

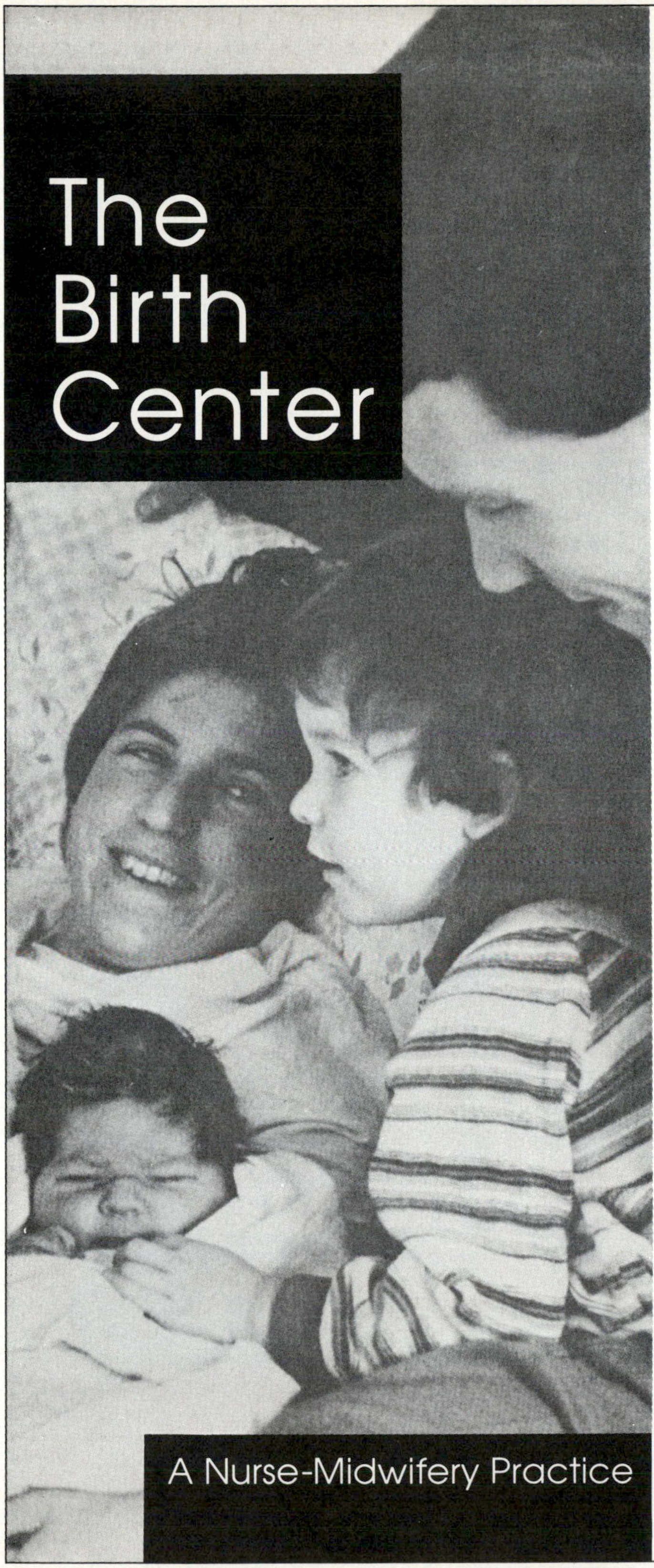

Our Expert Prenatal Care

Throughout your pregnancy, labor and birth, most of your care will be provided by Certified Nurse-Midwives (CNMs). CNM's are highly trained registered nurses who have completed post-graduate study in nurse-midwifery, are certified by The American College of Nurse-Midwives and licensed to practice in The Commonwealth of Pennsylvania. Our nurse-midwives work in a team relationship with you, your spouse or support person and an RN birth attendant. An obstetrician and other health care professionals are available if necessary.

Your initial prenatal visit at The Birth Center will be one hour long, with most successive visits being 30 minutes. This gives you plenty of time to talk with the CNM and ask questions about the physical and emotional changes of pregnancy, development of the baby and the natural process of labor and birth. You will be involved in every decision regarding your care.

During your third trimester of pregnancy, we offer an eight-week Childbirth Education Series for first time parents. The course content covers a variety of topics including: becoming parents, support and pain coping strategies during labor, styles of birthing, breastfeeding, needs of the newborn and postpartum adjustment. We also offer a Birth Rehearsal class which is a one-time refresher class for parents who have already been through at least one birth; and, a Sibling Preparation class to enable parents to help prepare their child for the coming of a new baby.

The Birth of Your Child

Your birth will be a very personal experience. Some of our clients want their birth to be an intimate experience to be shared by two–others welcome siblings, grandparents and other family members and friends to participate in the celebration of birth. The choices are yours, and we invite you to write a birth plan before your due date specifying how you would like your birth to proceed.

Figure 15–1. Pamphlets describe the childbearing facility and program for the childbearing family. (*Courtesy of The Birth Center, Bryn Mawr, PA.*)

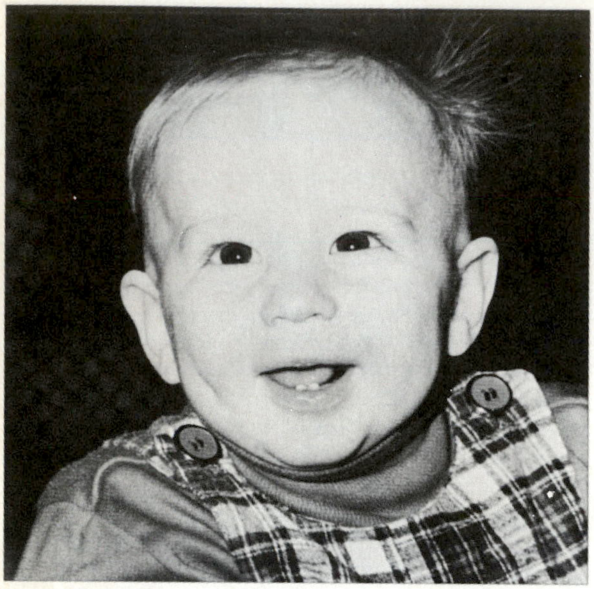

Birth Center parents assume maximum responsibility within the security of professional guidance. The well-being of mother and child are paramount, but of course, we'll do all we can to follow your birth plan.

Should a complication arise that necessitates transfer to Bryn Mawr Hospital, a Birth Center CNM will be with you to smooth the transition to hospital care, and one of our consulting physicians will attend your birth.

Our Unique Postpartum Care

After your baby is born he or she will stay with you, and you will have uninterrupted time with your family to bond with your new baby. One of our RN birth attendants is always available to assist you as needed. A pediatrician will examine the baby, and within 6 to 12 hours after the birth you can go home with your newborn. Your care continues in a number of ways:

- Two days of phone contact—We'll monitor you and the baby each day.
- Third day home visit—One of our RNs will come to your home for a physical exam and routine blood tests on you and the baby. The RN will answer any questions you have regarding infant care, your recovery, and breast feeding.
- Newborn Housecall—At two weeks, a special home visit by a Maternal-Infant Nurse helps the family understand the newborn as a competent, communicating person. The visit includes an assessment of the baby's needs, signals, language and behavior, massage for both the mother and baby, parenting strategies, and safe play with baby for siblings.
- Six-week postpartum check-up—You'll return to The Birth Center at six weeks for a one hour visit with the midwife who attended your birth. Newborns are more than welcome.
- Listening Moms Program—Another woman who has had Birth Center care is available to be a telephone buddy for as long as you wish.

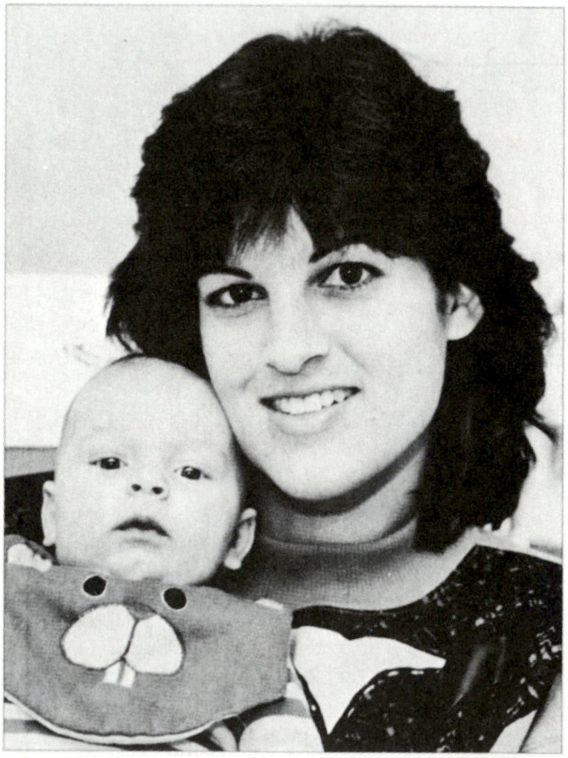

Figure 15–1. *(continued)*

TABLE 15–2. SAMPLE OUTLINE OF AN ANTENATAL VISIT

Appointment made
- Directions to facilities
- Information about length of visit
- Expectations for reimbursement

Waiting area
- Assessment begun (self-report forms, eg, demographic information, health history)
- Health promotion: teaching materials available, eg, posters, audiovisual programs, pamphlets, other literature

Before client undresses for examination
- Nurse and physician or certified nurse-midwife meet with client (separately or together)
  - Assessment continued; review of client's self-report form, history taken; blood pressure, pulse, respiration, temperature, weight; in some settings, fingerstick for hemoglobin/hematocrit analysis; assessment data recorded
  - Diagnoses made: information shared between nurse and physician or nurse-midwife prior to further examination

Preparation of client for examination
- Gown given; location for clothing shown (locker, closet, or hooks in examining room; anticipatory guidance; client instructed in collection of urine specimen; urine sample tested in unit or sent to laboratory

Physician or nurse-midwife meets with client
- Assessment continued: physical examination performed with female staff member in room
- Diagnoses made
- Teaching performed (in some settings, client may dress before meeting for postexamination interview)

Client may meet again with nurse for continued teaching on topics such as nutrition

Next antenatal appointment scheduled

Client referred to laboratory for further testing (eg, blood sampling; blood samples may be drawn by staff in some antenatal settings)

private group practice settings, clients may see several physicians or midwives throughout their pregnancy; the primary care provider who is on call on the client's delivery day attends the delivery. Clients need to be aware of this arrangement and to schedule appointments with all staff members. The client then has the opportunity to get to know and feel comfortable with each physician or midwife prior to delivery.

In clinics where physicians or certified nurse-midwives rotate through the antenatal setting, a client may not have the opportunity to become acquainted with the staff who will attend her delivery. The nurse has a particularly important role in group practice and clinic settings, as she or he may be the only health care provider the client sees consistently at each antenatal visit throughout pregnancy. The nurse therefore can do much to ensure continuity of care.

Expectations of Visit

Table 15–3 lists topics to be included in preparation of the client for antenatal care. The client coming for an initial visit may be advised of what to expect over the phone or sent information describing the antenatal visits. Preparation includes the amount of time, including estimated waiting time, for the visit. Nurses should be aware of client responsibilities such as work or children's coming home from school. Antenatal sessions that are constantly overbooked and require extended waiting periods make prenatal visits unpleasant and discourage attendance. Every effort should be made to fulfill all health care needs in one visit, especially for clients who must take time off from work or who live at a distance.

Unfortunately, financial considerations make some antenatal settings inaccessible to some clients. Prior to the first visit, the client should be informed of the cost of care for childbearing and the type of payment plans that are or are not accepted. Personnel working in settings that do not provide care to all clients regardless of their type of insurance or ability to pay should be prepared to offer referrals to health care providers who will care for these clients. Ideally, grants could be sought to supply start-up funding for prenatal care without restriction.

Schedule of Prenatal Visits

The client needs to be informed of the need for prenatal visits at least every 4 weeks during the first trimester. More frequent visits can be scheduled to meet client needs. Clients should also be given phone

TABLE 15–3. TOPICS THAT CAN BE USED TO PREPARE CLIENTS FOR ANTENATAL CARE

- Name and location of facility
- Directions from major travel routes
- Description of antenatal facility, range of services offered
- Specific focus of antenatal facility (eg, a birth center specializing in low-risk healthy clients or a tertiary care center focusing on high-risk care)
- Philosophy of staff
- Personnel who work with childbearing client
- Usual pattern of visits, adaptation of frequency of visits based on client's individual needs
- Length of visits
- What client may expect at visits
- Who is encouraged to attend with the client, any policy related to attendance of children
- Cost of care, method of payment accepted, any provisions for clients unable to pay
- Whom to contact for information about care (name, phone number, address)

numbers to call for advice and for answers to any questions they may have between visits.

EVOLVE A DATA BASE FROM WHICH DIAGNOSES ARE DEVELOPED

A comprehensive data base is established at the first visit through the assessment process, which first identifies the reason for the client's visit (eg, confirmation of pregnancy or continuing prenatal care) and includes a complete history and physical examination with appropriate laboratory tests (*see* Chapter 14). The history is updated at subsequent visits throughout pregnancy. Assessment forms for the history portion of assessment may be filled out by clients who are able to read and write. These self-report forms are reviewed and additional information is included during the interview that precedes the physical examination at each visit. Collaboration in history taking among health care providers ensures that clients are not repeatedly asked the same questions and that time can be efficiently used to cover all topics related to assessment.

Staff nurses participate in antenatal physical assessment and testing. Prior to the examination, the nurse ensures that equipment is prepared for the client. Table 15–4 lists suggested facilities and equipment used for antenatal examination.[3] The client is requested to void, as an empty bladder facilitates accurate pelvic assessment and minimizes discomfort, and is instructed in the collection of urine samples. The nurse may perform urine tests for pregnancy confirmation (when appropriate) and may test urine for protein, glucose, and ketones. The nurse may also label and send specimens for laboratory urinalysis, culture, and sensitivity. As discussed in Chapter 5, the nurse provides the client with support and anticipatory guidance for pelvic examination.

TABLE 15–4. FACILITIES AND EQUIPMENT FOR ANTENATAL EXAMINATION

Facilities
- Private examining area (ideally, private room)
- Adequate ventilation, temperature control
- Handwashing facilities in the room
- Toilet facilities
- Writing surface for charting
- Examination table with stirrups for pelvic examination
- Movable light in working order

Equipment
- Clean barrier (paper or cloth) for examining table
- Examination gloves
- Specula in a variety of sizes
- Water-soluble lubricant for vaginal/rectal examinations
- Culture tubes, slides, and fixative for cultures and smears
- Stethoscope (considered a personal item and not shared among personnel)
- Sphygmomanometer
- Fetoscope (however, does not detect fetal heart rate during first trimester)
- Doppler device (may detect fetal blood flow through fetal heart during first trimester)
- Hand mirror for educational examination
- Emergency equipment (including oxygen and suction)

Prior to the client's examination by the nurse-midwife or physician, the nurse takes and records the client's weight, blood pressure, pulse, respirations, and temperature. The nurse makes certain to bring any abnormalities in history or physical assessment to the attention of the nurse-midwife or physician before his or her assessment begins. In some settings, nurses may draw blood samples from fingersticks (for hemoglobin or hematocrit) or from the cephalic or brachial veins near the antecubital fossa. Nurses may perform hemoglobin or hematocrit testing in the antenatal setting or prepare and send blood tubes to specified laboratories for further analysis. As indicated by the nurse-midwife or physician at the initial visit, staff nurses may perform tuberculosis screening, for example with tine testing, for clients who are not known to be positive.[4]

The nurse assists the client in getting onto the examining table, positioning properly for examination, and getting up from the table, as described in Chapter 5. For the protection of both the client and the examiner, a female staff member remains in the examining room throughout physical assessment as witness to proper conduct of the examination.

During the pelvic examination, the nurse helps the examiner as needed. For example, the nurse makes sure that equipment, such as the speculum, is accessible to the examiner.

DEVELOP A CARE PLAN

After examination during the first visit, while the client dresses, the nurse and examiner collaborate on development of a care plan. On the basis of assessment, specific diagnoses are identified, behavioral outcomes are projected, health care interventions are planned, and evaluation criteria are noted. After the client is dressed, the examiner and, in some settings, the nurse may meet with the client to discuss these. The nurse may also meet separately with the client to address identified educational needs on such topics as nutrition, weight management, or signs and symptoms of pregnancy. At times, information from laboratory data, such as results of blood studies or urinalysis, will not be available until after the visit. Results are communicated to the client and incorporated into the plan of care.

Client participation in development of the care plan is important. In this way a plan of care that is realistic, feasible, and acceptable for each client is devised. For example, on the basis of thorough assessment, health care providers may identify a client's fatigue as a normal symptom during the first trimester. The client may collaborate on identification of coping strategies that will help her deal with her fatigue and lifestyle.

The care plan is recorded in the client's chart, reviewed before each antenatal visit, and updated as necessary. At times generic care plans may be used. These provide general approaches to care of healthy clients or particular high-risk conditions and save time related to rewriting information on similar topics when many clients are seen. Childbearing families are never identical, although care plans may seem to be similar. Generic care plans must always be individualized to meet each family's needs.

PROVIDE SUPPORT TO THE CLIENT

Nursing strategies to provide support to the client during antenatal visits include remaining accessible and using therapeutic communication skills. The nurse stays with the client during her examination and is available to answer any questions. The nurse needs to avoid chatting about unrelated subjects with other staff members who are present in the room. Attention should be directed to the client and her partner or toward collaboration with other staff in working with the client. As one client recalled, "All through my examination the nurse and physician were talking about the recent elections. I was afraid to interrupt." A client in another setting observed, "The nurse and the doctor always explained everything to me. I felt as if all three of us were working together." Communication skills such as attentive listening and interest in client well-being promote the nurse-client relationship and are essential to the assessment process.

Some clients are frightened and uncomfortable during pelvic examinations. Identifying reasons for the fear, providing anticipatory guidance, using an educational approach to the examination (*see* Chapter 5), and, when needed, providing the comfort of a hand to hold during the examination can be helpful in reducing anxiety.

INCORPORATE THE CLIENT'S CULTURAL BACKGROUND INTO CARE

Success of any antenatal care strategy depends on the nurse's ability to recognize and incorporate the client's cultural background into care (*see* Chapter 13). Stereotyping, however, should be avoided. The nurse needs to identify individual prenatal cultural influences on each pregnant family. An open-minded, flexible approach and willingness to learn about very different childbearing practices are essential to provision of culturally sensitive care. In general, support may be given to any practices that do not jeopardize the health and safety of the client, the fetus, or the family.

Nurses need to be aware of ways in which antenatal care and scheduling may conflict with the client's cultural background. For example, some expectant fathers, such as men from Orthodox Jewish or Moslem groups, may not wish to be present while their wives are immodestly garbed and positioned during pelvic examination. Nurses may invite the client to bring a support person with her; however, the decision of the client not to have the expectant father present should be respected. In addition, clients should not be pressured to attend antenatal visits at times that conflict with religious or cultural practices. For example, Orthodox Jewish women must be home to observe the Sabbath, which begins with sundown on Friday, and therefore should not be scheduled for the last late Friday afternoon antenatal visit. Asking the client if a particular times poses a hardship for her can help identify cultural needs.

Several strategies may be used to communicate with clients who do not speak English. Clients should be encouraged to bring adult family members or friends who can serve as interpreters at their prenatal visits. In certain ethnic areas, staff who speak the language of the surrounding community are hired. Clinics may draw on resources of larger hospital settings where staff who speak different languages volunteer as interpreters and then meet with antenatal clients and staff during clinic visits. Interpreters should be individuals who would be considered culturally appropriate to discuss intimate topics related to pregnancy with the client. Antenatal literature may be translated into a variety of languages; however, translations should be done only by individuals who have a strong command of the language and an understanding of antenatal care. Languages do not translate word for word. Poor translations can present material in an offensive or inaccurate manner.

BEGIN INFORMED DECISION MAKING

The client and her family have the right and responsibility to make informed decisions about pregnancy and prenatal care. Many clients who come for prenatal care are not aware of their rights as clients. A copy of the Pregnant Patient's Bill of Rights and the Pregnant Patient's Responsibilities can be provided and discussed (*see* Appendix D). Risks and benefits of all pregnancy and birth options should be explained.

During the initial visit, the family's plans for birth are discussed. As described in Chapter 23, specific aspects of the birth plan are finalized during the third trimester. In the first trimester, the client selects caregivers and a setting that will make desired aspects of childbirth possible. Some families already have particular wishes for a childbirth experience and want to develop the birth plan early; others need much assistance in making this decision.

The nurse orients the client and her family to the childbearing setting and provides referrals for the client whose birth plan would be better implemented elsewhere. For example, clients who desire a complete birthing room experience would not be able to fulfill their birth plan in a hospital setting that did not have a birthing room and routinely transferred all clients to separate labor, delivery, recovery, and postpartum areas. Their plan would, however, be feasible in a hospital where a single labor, delivery, and recovery room was routinely used.

The client must understand that no birth plan can be guaranteed. The need for alternative plans in case of complications must also be considered, as must the setting in which those alternative plans will take place.

Clients may have to make decisions about altering their lifestyle. For example, if the woman's daily activities at home or at work involve potential teratogens, the woman needs to make an informed choice about the activity. Nurses therefore need to be able to identify real risks and to provide reassurance to clients whose activities do not place them at risk during pregnancy.

RESEARCH ABSTRACT

Jordan PL. Laboring for relevance: expectant and new fatherhood. Nurs Res. *1990;39:11–20.*

This qualitative study described the experience of expectant and new fatherhood. The Grounded Theory Method, a rigorous qualitative technique for analyzing subjective data to produce a theory, guided the study.

The sample consisted of 56 expectant and recent first-time fathers. Twenty-eight expectant fathers were followed. They were interviewed six to seven times, beginning close to conception and ending 1 year after birth. In addition, the 28 fathers of the second group were interviewed once, at one of the same time periods. "What can you tell me about your experience of being an expectant/new father?" and "When was your baby real to you?" were two questions asked in the interview. Similarities and differences in fathers' responses during the interviews were noted and grouped into clusters. The core concepts were then developed into a theory concerning expectant and new fatherhood. Results described the father as "laboring" to perceive the paternal role as relevant. Jordan found that relevance is a process comprising three developmental subprocesses: (1) grappling with the reality of the pregnancy and the child; (2) struggling for recognition as a parent from partner, coworkers, friends, family, baby, and society; (3) persevering at the role-making aspects of involved fatherhood.

Jordan concludes that this theory provides an understanding of the male experience of expectant and new parenthood, and serves as a beginning point for the development of interventions to promote positive paternal behavior.

Comment:

This qualitative study provides the nurse with a theory related to expectant and new fatherhood. From this theoretical perspective, fatherhood can be seen as a developmental process beginning as early as conception. Nursing interventions can be tailored to support and promote fatherhood, beginning in the first trimester and continuing throughout pregnancy. Concepts from this theory can now be tested by quantitative research methods.

PROMOTE PSYCHOLOGIC ADAPTATION TO EARLY PREGNANCY

As discussed in Chapter 13, early pregnancy is normally accompanied by a mixture of feelings on the part of the expectant mother and father. Even those who desire pregnancy may feel overwhelmed during this time. Clients' concerns may also include uncertainty about ways to inform others about the pregnancy, their own physical well-being, early pregnancy changes, and discomforts such as nausea and fatigue.[4,5]

Among the nursing strategies that promote psychologic adaptation and parental role attainment are the following:

- Providing opportunities for the couple to discuss concerns during prenatal visits.
- Encouraging clients to telephone if they have questions or concerns between visits.
- Reassuring the couple about normal feelings and uncertainties.
- Reassuring the couple that the first trimester still allows much time to prepare emotionally for the baby.
- Encouraging the client to talk with her own mother, sister, or other female relatives and friends, as evolving her own concept of the maternal role is an important part of maternal role attainment and prenatal adaptation.
- Encouraging similar behaviors for the expectant father. Unlike men in previous generations, expectant fathers in the United States today are encouraged to be nurturing and expressive. Therefore, some expectant fathers may encounter surprise or reluctance about discussing paternal feelings on the part of their own fathers or men of older generations.
- Informing the couple about early pregnancy classes, which can provide an environment of group support and information.
- Assisting the couple to identify whom they are concerned about informing of the pregnancy.
- Discussing ways that news of the pregnancy can be shared.
- Providing referrals for couples who need counseling.

FOSTER BEGINNING FAMILY ATTACHMENT

As early as the first trimester, the nurse encourages behaviors that allow family members to support each other throughout pregnancy and develop feelings of closeness, although at this time the expectant parents may still be ambivalent about the pregnancy and siblings may not yet have been told (Figure 15–2). Scheduling prenatal visits at convenient times and encouraging family members to attend the visits together help to foster family attachment.[1] The nurse can also assist the couple in planning how and when to inform siblings about the pregnancy.

The initial contact a family has with the antenatal care team, the manner in which family members are oriented to antenatal care, and the manner in which the first health visit is conducted can also foster attachment among expectant family members.

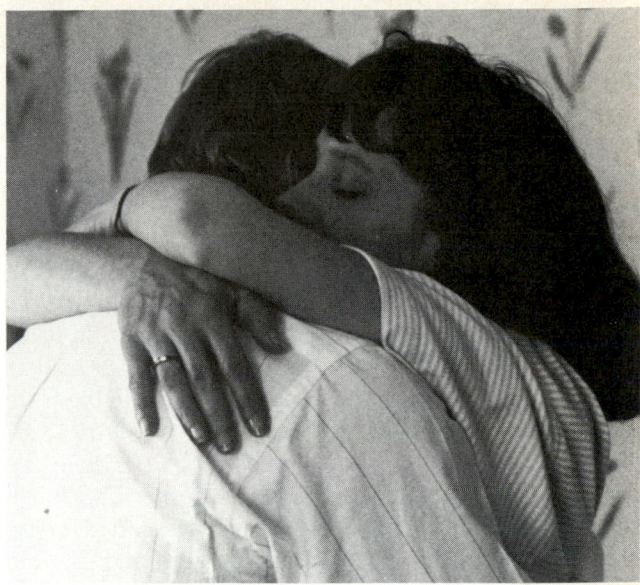

Figure 15–2. An expectant father provides support to the mother.

MEET THE EARLY-PREGNANCY EDUCATIONAL NEEDS OF THE CLIENT AND HER FAMILY

Client and family education constitutes one of the most important nursing roles during antenatal care. Education focuses on health promotion, for example, teaching the client how to maximize feelings of wellness during the first trimester, on primary prevention, for example, teaching the client to avoid hazardous substances and situations; and on secondary prevention, for example, teaching the client to identify warning signs of pregnancy.

As discussed in Chapter 24, teaching involves cognitive, affective, and psychomotor skills. Effectiveness of teaching depends on many factors, such as the way in which information is provided, the readiness of the learner, the involvement of the learner, and the amount of time available for teaching. All clients, including pregnant nurses, physicians, and others with backgrounds in obstetrics, should receive basic teaching.

Teaching should never be done in a haphazard manner. Working together, health care providers need to assess what subjects are essential for all clients to learn about, to develop client learning objectives, to specify methods and interventions, to devise ways to ensure teaching is done, and to identify means for evaluation. The assessment process identifies specific diagnoses focusing on client education, such as lack of knowledge related to normal physiologic changes of the first trimester.

Client education takes place throughout the antenatal visit. Antenatal waiting areas can be used for visual and audiovisual displays and can include pamphlets and other printed literature for clients to take home. Literature for client education is available from such sources as the Organization for Obstetric, Gynecologic and Neonatal Nurses (NAACOG), the March of Dimes, and the International Childbirth Education Association (ICEA). Nurses can develop learning aids, such as pamphlets, videotapes, and sound-slide learning packages, specific to the antenatal setting. Health care providers can also collaborate with nursing faculty and with nursing students performing graduate or undergraduate student projects. Teaching strategies, based on behavioral objectives, can be implemented on a one-to-one basis during physical assessment and during an educational session afterward.

Table 15–5 summarizes topics for educational preparation during the first trimester and lists chapters in this book in which the topics are discussed further. Client education focuses on explanations of current and future changes related to pregnancy.

All pregnant clients and family members have questions. Although some clients bring specific questions to antenatal visits, others are too shy to ask or "forget" their questions in the presence of the nurse, nurse-midwife, or physician. Time and encouragement are needed for clients to ask their questions. Clients can be encouraged to write down questions as they occur at home and bring them to antenatal visits. An approach such as "What questions do you have?" or "What is concerning you about your pregnancy?" tends to elicit more of a response than questions that imply a one-word answer, eg, "Do you have any questions?"

Many pregnant women share concerns about certain topics. Questions commonly asked are presented in Table 15–6. The nurse may anticipate these concerns and initiate discussion of these subjects.

As discussed earlier, clients should be provided with literature about the antenatal care facilities and personnel, as well as about aspects of prenatal health. Clients should leave any prenatal visit with a clear idea of whom to call for questions and concerns they may have between visits.

TABLE 15–5. SAMPLE TOPICS FOR EDUCATIONAL PREPARATION DURING THE FIRST TRIMESTER

Normal physiologic changes in the first trimester	*See* Chapter 12
Normal fetal growth and development	*See* Chapter 11
Client safety Hazards during pregnancy; Use of drugs and alcohol, smoking Threats to safety and security (seat belts, environmental hazards related to lifestyle, and high-risk behaviors)	*See* Chapter 11
Pets	*See* Chapter 24
Warning danger signs of pregnancy	*See* Chapter 15
Nutrition and weight management	*See* Chapter 10
Dental health	*See* Chapters 12, 14, 15
Discomforts of pregnancy during the first trimester	*See* Chapter 15
Sexuality	*See* Chapters 8 and 24
Normal psychologic reactions to first trimester—client, expectant father and family; informing others of pregnancy; worries and concerns; adaptation	*See* Chapter 13
Self-care practices to promote wellness Breast care Relaxation and stress reduction Posture and movement Exercise Clothing Food preparation Gardening activities Bathing and swimming Personal hygiene Travel	*See* Chapter 24

PROMOTE NUTRITIONAL WELL-BEING

As discussed in Chapter 10, nutritional counseling is one of the most important aspects of prenatal management. The type of foods selected and the time of day when foods and beverages are ingested may vary in response to pregnancy-related discomforts. For example, a first-trimester client experiencing nausea (described later) may tolerate only simply prepared foods without heavy spices, sauces, or odors. Small portions, spaced between periods of nausea, may ensure adequate intake.

Nutritional assessment begins at the initial visit and continues at each visit throughout pregnancy for *every client*. In establishing nursing diagnoses related to positive nutritional practices and well-being, the nurse assesses such parameters as the client's weight

TABLE 15–6. ANSWERS TO QUESTIONS COMMONLY ASKED DURING THE FIRST TRIMESTER

Why am I so tired all the time, especially when I'm not doing anything differently?

Fatigue is normal during the first trimester and occurs regardless of the woman's activity level. The cause of fatigue has never been clearly identified. Fatigue is thought to occur in response to hormonal levels, physical changes, psychologic changes, and other factors.

Does "morning sickness" occur only in the morning?

No. Nausea and vomiting, "morning sickness," can occur at any time. Although most women experience episodes of nausea and vomiting during the first trimester, some women report that periods of nausea continue into the second and third trimesters.

Will cutting back on fluids help having to urinate frequently?

Frequency of urination occurs as the uterus enlarges and presses on the bladder. Urinary frequency will occur regardless of fluid restriction. Greater amounts of fluid do produce more urine and more frequent urination. Because of the risks of dehydration, and the importance of fluids, for normal pregnancy development, however, a daily fluid intake of 6 to 8 glasses of noncaffeinated bev rages is recommended.

Are bleeding gums anything to be concerned about?

Gum changes during pregnancy are thought to occur because of increased hormone levels. During pregnancy, gums may be more sensitive to irritants in the mouth; however, bleeding need not occur and may be a sign of poor dental hygiene or peridontal (gum) disease. Any pregnant woman with bleeding gums needs to be evaluated by a dentist. It is also important to remember to inform the dentist of pregnancy, as pregnancy usually does not "show" during the first trimester. Dentists need to be aware that the client may be pregnant, because some dental medications and procedures may be contraindicated during pregnancy.

If I want to be in good physical condition should I start exercising vigorously now?

No. Pregnancy is no time to begin vigorous exercise programs, especially for the woman unaccustomed to heavy exercise; however, mild exercise such as walking is encouraged.

Will my working harm my pregnancy?

Employment alone is no reason to quit work during the first trimester. Daily activities at home and at work should, however, be evaluated. Any activity that poses a risk to safety and health, such as exposure to potentially teratogenic chemicals, should be avoided. This may involve a change in employment status or a transfer to another type of employment.

Before I was pregnant, my husband and I thought we wanted a baby so very much. Now that I am pregnant, we are both uncertain. Are these feelings normal?

Yes. Most women and men have mixed feelings about having a baby, especially during the first trimester of pregnancy. These feelings are normal and expected.

Is it too early to start thinking about plans for childbirth?

No. It is a good idea to begin thinking about the type of delivery you would like and to make certain that the health care providers and childbirth setting you select will support your decisions, such as for a birthing room delivery. Your actual birth plan, ie, your written plan for the birth experience, can be finalized during the third trimester.

Is it all right to have wine with dinner during the first trimester?

Wine, beer, or other alcoholic beverages are never recommended at any time during pregnancy, because of the potential for harm to the developing embryo and fetus. No safe level of alcohol has been established during pregnancy.

in relation to her height; history of current and past weight management practices; pattern of prenatal weight gain; hemoglobin and hematocrit; condition of skin for eruptions possibly related to poor diet; usual dietary intake; pattern of intake; and consumption of nonfood items (*see* pica, described later). It is important to remember that clients whose weight is within normal limits or clients from both wealthy and financially disadvantaged backgrounds may not eat a nutritionally adequate diet for pregnancy.

Prior to attempting any nutritional counseling, the nurse who works in an antenatal setting should visit local food stores and shops. The nurse should become knowledgeable about the availability and price of foods and beverages recommended for pregnancy and be prepared to counsel clients from a variety of cultural and financial backgrounds. In general, recommendations of foods that are expensive or out of season should be avoided, as clients may be embarrassed about admitting their inability to afford these foods. Sample diets, based on a variety of religious and cultural preferences, can be developed with consultation from nutritionists and should be part of advance staff planning. Nutrition management counseling may then tailor the diets to the individual needs of the client and family.

Nutrition management encompasses identification of the client at nutritional risk, either for physical, educational, psychologic, or financial reasons. The physician or certified nurse-midwife may order nutritional supplements, such as vitamins and iron, for the woman at physical or psychologic risk; dietary counseling for any client may be provided by nurses and by nutritionists. Some women maintain their prepregnancy weight by constant dieting and may be extremely anxious about "losing" their figures and "getting fat." Nutritional counseling related to healthy prenatal patterns and weight management is necessary. Clients who gain more than the recommended weight between visits should be advised against vigorous dieting or exercising to "make up" for this. Referral to social services may make nutritional supplements available to financially disadvantaged women through such programs as the Special Supplemental Food Program for Women, Infants, and Children.

ASSIST THE CLIENT IN COPING WITH FIRST-TRIMESTER DISCOMFORTS

Although pregnancy is a time of health, it also can be a time of discomfort. Discomforts evolve from such factors as hormonal changes and the growing uterus. In addition, a client's fear and anxiety may magnify perceptions. Careful assessment assists the nurse in differentiating between normal discomforts related to healthy first-trimester changes and high-risk conditions. Through anticipatory guidance and counseling, the nurse can help the client cope with discomforts as temporary, although unpleasant, manifestations of pregnancy. Discomforts related to the first trimester are described below.

Nausea and Vomiting—"Morning Sickness"

Symptoms of nausea and vomiting, also referred to as "**morning sickness,**" occur in about 50 percent of pregnant women. As discussed in Chapter 12, these symptoms usually appear shortly after the first missed menses and end by the 12th week of gestation. Nausea with or without vomiting can occur at any time of the day. Indeed, some women report feeling "constantly morning sick." Severe, prolonged episodes of nausea and vomiting (hyperemesis gravidarum) are not normal and present threats of electrolyte imbalance and nutritional deprivation (*see* Chapter 38).

No known treatment provides relief of nausea and vomiting for all women during the first trimester. The nurse must therefore thoughtfully assess the client to identify the client's unique reaction to this discomfort and to suggest individual interventions.[6] The following strategies may help relieve nausea and vomiting:

- Teach the mother to increase her intake of dry carbohydrate foods, such as plain crackers, which are easily digested. If the nausea occurs in the morning, the nurse may advise the mother to keep soda crackers at her bedside and to eat one or two before arising.
- Teach the mother to eat smaller but more frequent meals.
- Teach the mother to avoid greasy, fatty foods.
- Teach the mother to avoid fluids during meals; however, fluid intake should be encouraged at other times so that fluid needs can be met.
- Teach the mother to avoid odors that precipitate nausea and vomiting. The nurse can assist the client who cooks for her family in selecting family menus that she can tolerate preparing. When possible, improving ventilation by opening windows or turning on stove fans can help to decrease odors. The use of artificial room deodorants is not recommended, as their smell can add to, rather than relieve, nausea. When possible, enlisting the aid of other family members in meal preparation can help remove one potential source of nausea.
- Teach the mother to change positions slowly, especially when getting up in the morning.

Many women benefit from knowing that nausea and vomiting are normal during pregnancy.[6] Indeed, the literature indicates that nausea and vomiting are associated with favorable pregnancy outcome, possibly because nonviable pregnancies have lower estrogen and human chorionic gonadotropin (hCG) levels.[7] It is, however, necessary for the nurse to realize that nausea and vomiting are real discomforts that occur at a time when many other changes take place.

Ptyalism

Ptyalism, an uncommon discomfort that includes the client's perception of excess saliva in the mouth, can occur during the first trimester of pregnancy. Ptyalism usually occurs in women who also experience nausea, possibly because of the difficulty in swallowing anything while feeling upset. Avoidance of swallowing increases the amount of saliva, which in turn may increase nausea.[3] Although higher estrogen levels are suspected, the cause of this symptom is not well understood. Treatment methods vary and include encouraging women to swallow consciously, use good oral hygiene, use mouthwash, suck on hard candy, and chew gum. Ingestion of starch, which may stimulate salivary glands, should be discouraged.

Altered Taste

During the first trimester the woman may experience a bitter or sour taste in her mouth. The nurse can advise her to brush her teeth well, use mouthwash, chew gum, or suck on hard candies (particularly mint or "tart" candies) in an effort to relieve the symptoms.

Gingivitis

Beginning in the first trimester, hyperemia of the gums, perhaps related to increased estrogen secretion, may cause these tissues to be more friable. Because of the condition of the gums, periodontal disease may be accelerated during pregnancy and may contribute to tooth loss. Bleeding of the gums during pregnancy is common. With a well-balanced diet, regular dental examinations, prophylactic professional cleanings as indicated, and conscientious home care (regular brushing, flossing, gum stimulation, and so forth), the incidence of sore, inflamed, bleeding gums can be reduced or eliminated.[9] Nurses should never ignore this condition, but should refer clients who report bleeding gums for dental evaluation.

Breast Tenderness

Breast tenderness, caused by elevated estrogen and progesterone levels, is particularly noticeable in the first trimester of pregnancy. Although tenderness usually resolves within the first trimester, the breasts often continue to enlarge throughout pregnancy.[10] The mother should be encouraged by the nurse to wear a well-fitting support brassiere (*see* Chapter 24). Warm showers may also provide the mother with some relief.

Urinary Frequency

Urinary frequency is a common discomfort during the first trimester of pregnancy. The symptom begins around the 6th week and usually subsides as the uterus rises out of the pelvic cavity, around the 12th week.[10] Urinary frequency may again be normally experienced during the third trimester, when the baby "drops" or "lightens" (*see* Chapter 20). Urinary frequency is sometimes accompanied by leakage of urine, especially when the mother coughs or sneezes late in the pregnancy. The expectant mother can be reassured that these symptoms will subside when the pregnancy is completed. She can also be taught to perform Kegel exercises, contracting the muscles of the pelvic floor for 5 seconds frequently during the day (may be as many as 100 times per day).[11] Kegel exercises tighten the pubococcygeal muscle, maintain good perineal muscle tone, and strengthen the urinary sphincter. Fluid intake should not be decreased in an effort to relieve urinary frequency. The nurse should advise the client to have a clear path between her bed and the toilet and to leave a nightlight burning, as getting to the bathroom during the night poses a potential safety risk.

Urinary frequency can be a sign of urinary tract infection. Any reports of frequency therefore need to be evaluated carefully. Women need to be taught about signs of urinary tract infection and advised to call their health care provider should the signs appear.

Nasal Stuffiness and Epistaxis

The increased estrogen levels during pregnancy can cause edema of the mucous membranes of the nasal cavity. Nasal stuffiness, nasal discharge, and epistaxis (nosebleeds) may occur. The expectant mother should be advised by the nurse to avoid the use of nasal decongestants and sprays, as well as other medications. Humidifiers, cool mist vaporizers (without medications added), or normal saline drops may relieve some of these symptoms.

Increased Vaginal Secretions (Leukorrhea)

Increased vaginal secretions (leukorrhea) begin during the first trimester. As discussed previously, these thick white secretions result from hyperplasia and increased activity of cervical and vaginal cells. Some clients become distressed about this condition, which many women regard as one of the less "glamorous" aspects of pregnancy. Some clients may also worry they have an infection. Before providing advice, the nurse needs to identify why the client feels she may be infected and to assess the client for signs of infection, for example, burning, itching, change in color of vaginal discharge, foul odor of the discharge and temperature elevation. The client needs to be advised to call her health care provider should any of these signs occur.

Douching for the pregnant woman is not recommended. The pregnant client may experience sensitive allergic reactions to the douching solution. In addition, during pregnancy women are more susceptible to air and fluid embolisms resulting from vaginal instillation of air or fluid under pressure. Pregnant women should be advised not to wear tampons as a means of absorbing secretions, because of the risk of infection. Good personal hygiene, including daily washing of the perineal area with water and a mild soap, is usually sufficient. Cotton underpants or absorbent external minipads may promote comfort.

Fatigue

Early in the first trimester, the woman may begin to experience fatigue, which is possibly related to increased levels of hormones such as progesterone and to the physiologic and psychologic changes taking place.[12] This symptom decreases in the second trimester. Fatigue is felt again in the third trimester because of such factors as insomnia and cumbersome size.

Fatigue can be an upsetting symptom, especially when women become tired out of proportion to their activities.[10] Many women continue to work outside the home through the first trimester; nearly all women have active responsibilities within the home. Indeed, some women do not even announce their pregnancies at this time. The woman must fulfill all her usual activities and responsibilities without her usual level of energy.

Before a woman's fatigue can be identified as a normal manifestation of pregnancy, anemia needs to be ruled out. Women then may need to be treated for this condition.

The goals of nursing management for first-trimester fatigue help the woman to deal with fatigue-related concerns and to relieve or minimize the fatigue.[12] The best treatment for fatigue in the healthy woman is more frequent rest periods during the day; however, nurses need to be realistic and creative in their counseling. Evaluation of daily activities at work and at home can aid in planning rest periods or relaxation exercises that are acceptable to the client. Indeed, even during a work day, brief relaxation exercises, such as closing the eyes and visualizing oneself in a restful environment, can promote feelings of well-being. Although rest means inactivity, relaxation involves knowledge of the muscular system and the ability to learn ways to release tension.[12] Encouraging family members to assist with specific tasks, such as laundry or shopping, not only promotes a woman's rest, but also fosters family communication.

Other Discomforts

The preceding conditions occur regularly during the first trimester of pregnancy. Although other discomforts, such as varicose veins, hemorrhoids, and heartburn, can occur at this time, they frequently emerge after the first trimester. These discomforts are therefore discussed in Chapters 19 and 23.

PROMOTE CLIENT SAFETY

Management includes a focus on client safety throughout pregnancy. Meeting the goal of promotion of safety during the first trimester involves strategies to prevent client injuries during the prenatal visit and client teaching related to safety.

As described in Chapter 5, the nurse assists the client during physical examination and thus prevents falls from the examining table. Examination gowns and, in some places, slippers may be worn; however, hospital "slippers" should not be used if they will not remain securely on the client's feet while she walks or if the soles are made of slippery materials, such as paper. Instead, the client may wear her own shoes and remove them before or after getting onto the examining table. Most first-trimester clients can put their own shoes on again without difficulty. Nevertheless, the nurse assists the client as needed. The nurse also advises the client to select slippers and shoes that provide good support and that will not add to the risk of injury as advancing pregnancy changes balance and center of gravity. This information is important to clients who make first-trimester purchases.

As noted in Chapter 24, topics related to safety are important aspects of educational preparation. The nurse counsels the client about the importance of using seatbelts in automobiles, even though first-trimester discomforts, such as nausea and fatigue, may make even the smallest tasks seem burdensome. A pregnant woman normally has urinary frequency related to the pressure of the expanding uterus against the bladder during the first trimester. The nurse advises the client about the importance of maintaining a clear pathway between her bed and the bathroom and leaving a nightlight on. In this way, falls related to walking sleepily in the dark may be prevented.

Through the assessment process, the nurse helps the client to identify threats to safety posed by the client's lifestyle or environment and to design ways in which these can be avoided or minimized. Counseling related to safety includes daily activities, such as preparation of foods, caring for pets, especially cats, and gardening (*see* Chapter 24). Care strategies include referrals, for example, to smoking cessation groups. At times, a client may need to change responsibilities at work to avoid contact with teratogenic materials or high-risk situations. Nursing care then includes providing the client with verification of the need to transfer or take leave for pregnancy-related reasons.

Promotion of client safety includes education

about warning and danger signs related to pregnancy (Table 15–7). Clients who experience any of these signs are advised to contact their health care provider without delay. Some clients become anxious when talking about warning and danger signs. The nurse needs to reassure the low-risk client of her current normal status.

EVALUATE ANTENATAL CARE

Evaluation is part of the nursing process and allows the nurse to identify effective care strategies as well as strategies that need to be changed. Evaluation evolves from client care objectives and depends on factors, such as accurate identification of behaviors, that will indicate client care objectives have been met. Strategies that result in a healthy outcome for mother, infant, and family are regarded as effective. Despite the best strategies, the outcome at times may be poor. Unfortunately, there is no perfect "recipe" for care.

TABLE 15–7. WARNING/DANGER SIGNS IN PREGNANCY

Headache
Persistent
Severe
Otherwise unusual
Altered vision
Blurring
Seeing double
Seeing spots
Nausea
Persistent
Intense
Interfering with food or fluid intake
Vomiting
Intense
Frequent
Interfering with food or fluid intake
Epigastric pain
Abdominal pain
Intense
Persistent
Unusual
Muscular irritability/seizures
Signs of infection
Fever of 101°F or above
Burning with urination
Flank pain
Diarrhea
Other
Vaginal bleeding
Other vaginal discharge (excluding leukorrhea)
Gush of fluid
Leakage of fluid
Decrease or cessation of fetal movement

Evaluation as part of the nursing process is discussed in greater detail in Chapter 2. During the first trimester, effectiveness of interventions may be reflected by such factors as regular attendance at prenatal visits, behaviors that indicate prescribed strategies have been carried out, and the client's meeting with sources of referral.

Evaluation of the effectiveness of teaching is at times difficult. Written tests are usually not appropriate for use in antenatal settings. Learning objectives therefore, need to focus on other behaviors. For example, a weight gain of a pound and a half between monthly visits during the first trimester and client reports of a diet that is assessed as well balanced indicate the client's ability to meet nutritional needs of pregnancy.

ENSURE APPROPRIATE REFERRALS FOR THE CLIENT

Through the assessment process the nurse frequently identifies client needs that require specialized referrals. For example, the nurse may refer clients for early prenatal education and exercise classes, social services, or nutritional counseling. Working with the physician or nurse-midwife, the nurse can ensure that appropriate referrals are made for such services as ultrasound and chorionic villus sampling.

Priests, ministers, rabbis, and other spiritual leaders are often considered members of the health care team. Although their services are indispensable during periods of crisis and grief, they can be excellent sources of spiritual support during times of wellness. The nurse needs to recognize the importance of spiritual needs of low-risk as well as high-risk clients and to be able to make appropriate referrals; however, nurses should never pressure clients or try to convert clients to the nurse's belief system.

Nurses need to be knowledgeable about any referral, including the nature and scope of services offered, the quality of the services, how clients can receive the services, and the costs involved.

CONTRIBUTE TO GENERAL ANTENATAL PUBLIC HEALTH

Preconceptional health and lifestyle have great impact on pregnancy; however, many well women and men do not come for health care unless they are ill or required to do so for reasons such as employment. Public education campaigns are effective in teaching people of childbearing age about preconceptional and early prenatal health. Nurses can participate in public education by serving as expert consultants to the media, schools, and community groups, as speakers on topics related to preconceptional and antenatal health, and as authors and producers of articles and programs. Through professional organizations, lobbyists, and direct contact with legislators, nurses can have further meaningful impact on prenatal health care.

CASE STUDY/CARE PLAN: CARE OF THE FAMILY DURING THE FIRST TRIMESTER

Rosa and Anthony Martucci, ages 30 and 31, respectively, have come to the obstetrician's office because they suspect that Rosa is pregnant. They have been married for 2 years and this is their first pregnancy. Rosa was born in the Dominican Republic and came to the United States with her mother and older sister when she was 8 years old. She has a master's degree in business administration and is presently employed as a computer analyst. She expects to return to work after the baby is born. Anthony, an engineer, was born in the United States and is of Italian descent. The couple's religious affiliation is Roman Catholic.

Present Health Status

Rosa states that she has been in excellent health. She has regular health examinations, the last being 6 months ago when she was found to be in good health. She is presently "2 weeks late with my period." A home pregnancy test performed 4 days ago was positive for pregnancy. Rosa admits that she is "compulsive" about not gaining weight. She tries to eat a well-balanced diet, avoiding red meat and caffeine. She also walks about 3 miles a day. Rosa states that she has recently been bothered by a "sour taste in her mouth from some foods" and tingling and fullness of her breasts. She also does not feel as energetic as she had prior to missing her period.

Anthony states that he has no health problems. He also tries to eat a balanced diet and exercise regularly.

Past Health Status

Childhood Illnesses

Rosa reports that her mother told her that she had the childhood diseases: measles, mumps, chicken pox, and rubella before the age of 12. She has no history of scarlet fever or strep infections.

Immunizations

She was immunized for diphtheria, pertussis, and tetanus (DPT), polio, and smallpox. Her last tetanus booster was 6 months ago.

Allergies

She has no known allergies to foods or medications. She occasionally complains of sinus congestion after cutting the lawn.

Hospitalizations and Other Illnesses

None.

Accidents and Injuries

None.

Medications

Acetaminophen approximately once a month for premenstrual headache. Ocassionally takes decongestant for sinus congestion.

Habits
Client is in bed by 10 PM and arises at 6 AM during the work week. On weekends, she goes to bed "later and gets up later." She eats three meals a day, with no snacking between meals. She does not smoke cigarettes, has never experimented with drugs, and has not ingested caffeinated beverages or álcohol since hoping to become pregnant. She admits that her mother believes in certain cultural folklore with respect to pregnancy. "Certain foods should be avoided so that the baby will not be born with marks." Rosa, herself, does not ascribe to these beliefs, but tries to keep her mother happy when she is in her company.

Review of Systems

General
Height 5 ft. 6 in. Usual minimum-maximum weight 118 to 120 pounds. She states that she watches her weight carefully. Since missing her menses, she has been feeling somewhat fatigued.

Integument
Denies rashes, bruising, color changes. States that sometimes her skin feels dry, especially in the winter. Skin lotions help the dryness.

Nails
No peeling, cracking, splitting, or biting of nails.

Hair
Does not use dyes, hairsprays, or gels. No loss of hair. Washes hair daily with baby shampoo.

Head
Complains of headache about once a month, over the eyes. Headache occurs 1 week prior to menstruation and is relieved by Tylenol Extra-Strength, 1 tablet.

Eyes
States that visual acuity is 20/20 for both eyes. Denies blurred vision, infection, double vision, cataracts, or problems with night vision.

Ears
No discharge, pain, tinnitus, or history of hearing loss.

Nose and Sinuses
States that she occasionally has sinus congestion after cutting grass, which is relieved by a decongestant. Denies sinus pain, nasal discharge, problems with olfaction.

Mouth
Sees dentist every 6 months; has not had a cavity in 6 years. No history of gingivitis or bleeding gums. No swelling of mouth, lips, or tongue. Flosses teeth every day; brushes teeth three times a day.

Throat
No history of hoarseness or frequent sore throats.

Neck
Denies stiffnes, pain, limitation of motion.

CASE STUDY/CARE PLAN: Care of the Family During the First Trimester (continued)

Lymph Nodes
Denies node enlargement or tenderness.

Respiratory
No history of bronchitis, pneumonia, tuberculosis, asthma, emphysema. No history of difficulty breathing, cough, hemoptysis, orthopnea, or night sweats. Mantoux test done last summer—negative.

Cardiovascular
No palpitations, cyanosis, precordial pain, edema, or varicose veins. No history of heart disease, rheumatic fever, high blood pressure.

Gastrointestinal
No diarrhea, constipation, hemorrhoids, jaundice, or food intolerances. Lately she has experienced a sour taste in her mouth with some nausea in the morning.

Urinary
No history of kidney or bladder infection, hematuria, urgency, frequency, nocturia, incontinence, polyuria, or veneral disease.

Musculoskeletal
Reports occasional lower back pain when sitting at her desk, relieved by getting up and walking for a few minutes. No problems with range of motion.

Extremities
No history of arthritis, deformities, varicosities, phlebitis, discoloration, limited range of motion, coldness. No joint pain, swelling, or redness.

Neurologic
No episodes of fainting, weakness, difficulty with balance, disorientation, hallucinations, depression, tremors, numbness, speech disorders, tingling. No history of seizures, aphasia, loss of memory, paralysis, pain, or paresthesias. States she rarely has mood swings.

Hematopoietic
Denies any history of blood diseases, bleeding tendencies, transfusions. Blood type O+.

Endocrine
No polyuria, polydypsia, polyphasia. No problems with thyroid, heat or cold intolerances, hirutism.

Reproductive Data

Menstrual History
Menarche 13 years. Since onset, menstrual cycle is 26 to 28 days, duration 5 to 7 days. No cramping; complains of headache 1 week before menses and breast tenderness. No dysmenorrhea, menorrhagia, infection, pruritis. Has had Pap smear within last year. Denies use of tampons. Last menstrual period October 9 (6 weeks ago).

Obstetric History
Has never been pregnant.

Presumptive Signs
Tingling and fullness of breasts, nausea, fatigue, amenorrhea.

Breasts

No masses or discharge. Self-examines breasts every month 1 week after menses. Experiences fullness in breasts prior to menses. Now feels fullness and tingling of breasts.

Nutritional History

Tries to eat a nutritionally sound diet, but admits to being very weight conscious. For breakfast, she eats a bowl of oatmeal with one cup milk and a glass of water, fruit; for lunch, cottage cheese, decaffeinated tea with skimmed milk; and for dinner, two portions of vegetables, one small slice of fish or chicken, salad with dressing, one glass of skimmed milk. Drinks water between meals; tries not to snack.

Family History

Significant family health histories include: hypertension (both Rosa's mother and Anthony's father are being treated for chronic hypertension).

Social Data

Support Systems

Rosa feels that her husband is her greatest support. She would like them to experience the pregnancy, labor, and delivery together. She is close to her sister and her mother, and states she never knew her father. Her husband's family is close knit and he counts on them for emotional support during periods of crisis. Rosa and Anthony have a few close friends at their places of employment and some others maintained since school.

Home Environment

The couple recently purchased a one-family home, which has eight rooms, including three bedrooms and a spacious kitchen. Rosa states that she worries about the mortgage payments and feels she needs to return to work shortly after the baby is born. Her mother has agreed to come to live with them so that she can care for the baby, allowing Rosa to return to work.

Economic Status

The couple is in the middle-income socioeconomic group with potential for advancement in their careers. They both believe that the two incomes are necessary to maintain their household.

Occupational History

Rosa is a computer analyst and Anthony is an engineer. She experiences backache when sitting for prolonged periods. Both admit to stress in their employment, but also like their jobs.

Cultural Affiliations

The couple denies any customs that might affect their response to pregnancy. Rosa does admit that her mother has certain health beliefs regarding pregnancy. These include that pregnancy is a "hot" condition so that vitamins or iron tablets, which are considered "hot" medications, should be avoided. Rosa's mother also believes that antacids should be taken in the first 6 months of pregnancy so that the baby will not be "marked," and that the postpartum woman should not leave the house for 40 days after the birth of the baby. Rosa states that she herself does not hold to these beliefs, but that there may be some conflicts with her mother because she will come to live with them.

Sexual History

Rosa states that they both feel good about themselves and their sexual relationship. They feel they have a loving relationship. Both deny any problems with sexuality. Rosa used a diaphragm for 1 year. She stopped using the diaphragm 2 months ago. Both admit that the pregnancy was planned. Rosa states that she has some ambivalent feelings because of her career and wonders how she is going to handle motherhood and employment. She also has fears and anxieties regarding the pregnancy.

CASE STUDY/CARE PLAN: Care of the Family During the First Trimester (continued)

Exercise and Activity
The couple enjoys movies, music, and going out to dinner for relaxation. Both exercise daily; Rosa walks 3 miles a day.

Stress
Rosa states that when she experiences stress, she walks or reads a book. At work, she will close her eyes for a minute in an attempt to relax. Anthony states that if he feels stressed at work, he "takes a walk" during lunch break.

Supporting Assessment Data	Expected Client/Family Outcome	Nursing Action/Intervention	Rationale	Criteria for Evaluation
PHYSIOLOGIC STATE				
Nursing Diagnosis: Alteration in physiologic responses, related to pregnancy				
Presumptive signs of pregnancy: tingling and fullness of breasts, nausea, fatigue, amenorrhea	The client and her support person will: Be prepared for physical assessment prior to the first examination	Teach couple about the physical examination including the pelvic examination.	Preparing the couple will alleviate anxiety associated with a new process.	If asked, client is able to report that she has received teaching in preparation for the examination. Client behaviors may include familiarity with the procedure.
	Describe the health care setting and program by end of first visit	Introduce couple to personnel and setting; provide literature about the prenatal program.	Orientation of couple to health care personnel and setting helps establish a trusting relationship and alleviate fear of unknown.	Client completes tour and orientation program provided by staff. Client discusses the program with the nurse or other health care provider.
	Identify physical changes that occur during the first trimester by end of first visit	Teach couple the basic physiologic changes during the first trimester and the reasons for these changes.	Education regarding physiologic changes will help couple cope with changes and alleviate fear of the unknown.	When asked, client is able to discuss physiologic changes that occur during the first trimester by the end of the first visit.
	Identify warning signs of pregnancy complications by end of first visit	Teach couple warning signs of pregnancy.	Knowledge of warning signs will allow couple to seek prompt treatment.	When asked, client is able to describe warning signs of pregnancy by the end of the first visit.
		Provide couple with outline of warning signs, including instructions of what to do and whom to call if they occur.		Client leaves first visit with a written outline of warning signs of pregnancy and instructions about what to do and whom to call if they occur.
	Identify physical changes of second trimester by end of first trimester	Teach couple regarding the basic physiologic changes that occur in the second trimester, including growth and development of the fetus.	Anticipatory guidance will help couple cope with changes in the second trimester.	By the end of the first trimester, client is able to discuss changes that occur during the second trimester.
	Identify resources for information about pregnancy by end of first visit	Explore with couple community resources related to pregnancy; provide a list of resources.	Couple often require information and support beyond the scope of antenatal services.	By the end of the first visit, client is able to identify resources appropriate for her.

Supporting Assessment Data	Expected Client/Family Outcome	Nursing Action/Intervention	Rationale	Criteria for Evaluation
				Client leaves first visit with a written list of resource agencies and programs. The list includes descriptive information, addresses, and phone numbers.
	State purpose, procedures, and time required for first-trimester screening and assessment by end of first visit	Inform couple of screening procedure; give relevant information concerning purpose, procedure, time required, and so on.	Anticipatory guidance relieves anxiety.	Couple is able to make informed decisions. Couple describes and schedules screening procedures for the first trimester; they realistically plan to fit the procedure into their schedule.
	Couple determines the husband's participation in procedures during first trimester	Give husband the option of remaining with his wife throughout the prenatal examination.	Clients have the right to make informed decisions about degree of participation of support persons.	Couple makes decision about husband's level of involvement.
Nursing Diagnosis: Potential asset in health care during pregnancy, related to positive health practices				
Early prenatal care Regular health examination Regular exercise: walks 3 miles No use of drugs, eg cigarettes, caffeine, alcohol.	By the end of the first trimester, the client will: Continue prenatal self-care practices, such as pregnancy exercise	Encourage client to continue to exercise, but allow for fatigue. Encourage couple to continue prenatal care; teach that their continued positive health-care practices are an asset to pregnancy.	Effective coping with changes occurring during pregnancy is helped by positive health care practices prior to pregnancy. Positive health care practices during pregnancy are helped by positive health care practices prior to pregnancy. Couples should be given positive feedback as motivation to continue health care practices.	For a typical 24-hour period, client is able to describe healthy self-care practices, such as exercise, rest, and nutrition.
		Teach couple self-care practices specific to pregnancy.	Self-care allows people to participate in their health care. Participation helps people feel in control of their lives.	
Nursing Diagnosis: Potential asset for healthy newborn, related to normal development of fetoplacental unit				
Normal growth and development of the embryo/fetus and placenta Physical examination reveals uterine enlargement and changes consistent with early pregnancy	Throughout the first trimester, the client will: Avoid potentially hazardous behaviors and substances related to intake or environment. Identify deviations from healthy prenatal development Identify health-promoting behaviors	Encourage client to continue activities that foster fetal development: to obtain adequate rest and nutrition and avoid harmful substances and exposure to infections and teratogens. Teach couple about fetal growth and development during the first trimester.	Teratogens have the greatest impact during the first trimester; safe practices are the responsibility of the client, but health care providers need to offer the client the necessary information.	Client is able to identify any hazards in the home or workplace. Client is able to identify positive health care practices: nutrition, rest, exercise. Couple describes their fetus during the first trimester.

(continued)

CASE STUDY/CARE PLAN: Care of the Family During the First Trimester (continued)

Supporting Assessment Data	Expected Client/Family Outcome	Nursing Action/Intervention	Rationale	Criteria for Evaluation
Nursing Diagnosis: Potential asset for healthy mother, related to normal pregnancy development				
Normal maternal assessment data Low risk history Vital signs: T 98°F, P 72, R 18, BF 110/70 Height = 5 ft 6 in. Weight = 118 pounds Urinalysis (protein, blood, glucose, acetone) = negative Blood studies: Hematocrit = 39, hemoglobin = 13%, serology = negative, glucose = 80 Physical examination: all systems within normal limits	Throughout the first trimester, the client will: Be screened for normal prenatal development Identify warning signs of pregnancy Identify health-promoting behaviors	Discuss with client the Pregnant Patient's Bill of Rights. Participate in screening hemoglobin, hematocrit, glucose, vital signs, urinalysis, height, weight, pelvic exam for size of uterus, clinical pelvic measurements. Teach couple about normal pregnancy changes during the first trimester. Teach couple warning signs of pregnancy.	Preparing a couple will minimize anxiety related to uncertainty; an understanding of the warning signs of pregnancy will help clients promote their own health by early identification and follow-up of problems. Ongoing screening ensures early identification of risks.	Couple discuss Pregnant Patient's Bill of Rights with understanding. Client regularly attends prenatal visits. Couple reports normal changes to nurse as they occur. Couple will verbally identify warning signs of pregnancy.
Nursing Diagnosis: Alteration in comfort, related to normal physiologic pregnancy changes				
Discomforts related to pregnancy Nausea in morning Fatigue Breast tenderness, tingling Sour taste in mouth	Client will describe comfort measures for nausea, fatigue, breast tenderness, and sour taste by end of visit	Teach client to eat dried soda crackers before arising in the morning; to decrease fluids during mealtimes. Reassure her that symptoms usually abate by the end of the first trimester.	Eating dried carbohydrates and decreasing fluids during meals may help alleviate nausea. Nausea and vomiting abate by the second trimester.	When asked, client is able to identify normal discomforts of pregnancy.
		Counsel client to elevate her feet and close her eyes for a few minutes every hour during work, and to get 8 hours sleep.		Client relates discomforts she is experiencing and comfort measures that were successful.
		Counsel client to wear a support bra, and take warm showers in an effort to provide comfort for breast tenderness	Warm showers and supportive bra provide comfort for breast tenderness. Client uses method of closing her eyes to alleviate stress. Increasing rest periods may help with fatigue.	Client leaves visit with a written outline of normal discomforts related to pregnancy.

Supporting Assessment Data	Expected Client/Family Outcome	Nursing Action/Intervention	Rationale	Criteria for Evaluation
		Teach client to brush teeth as desired, use mouth wash, chew gum, or suck on hard candy.	Use of interventions will improve taste in mouth.	Client is able to identify specific relief measures she may use for discomforts related to the first trimester. Client leaves visit with a written outline of home relief measures to use for discomforts related to the first trimester. On subsequent visits, client reports effectiveness of any relief measures tried. By end of visit, client is able to demonstrate her ability to select resources should discomforts require professional attention before the next prenatal visit.
NUTRITIONAL STATE				
Nursing Diagnosis: Potential for altered fetal and maternal nutrition, related to rigid control of weight gain				
24-hour dietary recall indicates avoidance of carbohydrates and fats and low protein intake. Height and weight appropriate Hgb and Hct within normal range Physical parameters indicate good current nutrition: hair, nails, skin, eyes, hydration, color, muscle tone. Height = 5 ft 6 in. Weight = 118 pounds States "I am compulsive about not gaining weight"	Client will increase intake of nutrients by end of first trimester By next prenatal visit, client will prepare diet so that nutrient requirements are met. The diet will be one with which client can cope	Teach couple about nutrient requirements during pregnancy. Teach client elements of a nutritionally sound diet.	A couple who is motivated toward good health practices will be helped through education regarding nutrients needed during pregnancy.	Client is informed of the results of all screening assessments. Client is able to state the importance of nutrition for a healthy pregnancy outcome. Client will leave first visit with a list of nutrients important for pregnancy and sample menus based on her cultural background.
		Examine with couple current nutritional practices.	Education should begin by first exploring current practices and incorporating these practices into the care plan.	
		Teach client to keep diary of foods eaten and patterns of eating.	A 24-hour recall is not sufficient to ascertain nutritional practices. Keeping a diary makes the person aware of patterns of eating as well as food eaten over a longer period.	
	Client will explore feelings regarding weight by next prenatal visit	Explore with client her feelings related to weight and body image.	Exploration of feelings will help to guide health practices for the couple and the nurse.	By the end of second visit, client will develop a personal menu, based upon nutrient requirements for pregnancy. Client's 24-hour dietary recall or dietary diary demonstrates appropriate nutrition for pregnancy. Client identifies specific nutritional practices based on her culture.

(continued)

CASE STUDY/CARE PLAN: Care of the Family During the First Trimester (continued)

Supporting Assessment Data	Expected Client/Family Outcome	Nursing Action/Intervention	Rationale	Criteria for Evaluation
			Satisfaction with weight promotes adaptation to pregnancy. Normal weight gain is needed for fetal and maternal health during pregnancy.	Client is able to insert culturally prescribed foods in her prenatal menu and maintain proper nutrition. Client demonstrates a normal pattern of weight gain during pregnancy.

PSYCHOSOCIAL STATE

Nursing Diagnosis: Potential asset in coping, associated with healthy family dynamics

Supporting Assessment Data	Expected Client/Family Outcome	Nursing Action/Intervention	Rationale	Criteria for Evaluation
Planned/wanted pregnancy Couple's relationship mutually supportive Support from significant others Beginning acceptance of future changes in family dynamics Awareness of fetus Acceptance of pregnancy Acceptance of need for health care	By the end of the first trimester, the client will: Develop new problem-solving strategies to deal with challenges occurring in first trimester of pregnancy Identify and use available support systems Continue supportive relationship with nurses and other health care providers	Explore with couple successful and unsuccessful ways they have dealt with stress in the past.	Previously successful coping strategies may or may not be adequate to deal with pregnancy changes.	Couple discusses with the nurse strategies to meet real or potential psychosocial challenges of the first trimester.
		Explore with couple potential conflicts and stressors that will emerge during the first and subsequent trimesters.	Stressors related to news of being pregnant may be especially pronounced during the first trimester.	
		Have couple identify support systems.	Support systems (grandparents, friends) may have a beneficial effect on the manner in which the pregnant couple deal with stress.	Through health history, couple identifies their significant others on whom they rely for support, eg, mother, sister, friend.
		Encourage couple to discuss fantasies about the infant-to-be.	Fantasies assist parents to bond to the infant-to-be.	Client involves significant others in her plans for childbearing and childrearing. Client names specific health care providers on whom she can rely for support. Couple maintains open communication about feelings toward pregnancy. Client consults health care providers when appropriate. Client discusses with the nurse strategies to meet real or potential psychosocial challenges of the second trimester.

Supporting Assessment Data	Expected Client/Family Outcome	Nursing Action/Intervention	Rationale	Criteria for Evaluation
Nursing Diagnosi: Potential asset in maternal role development associated with positive mother-daughter relationship				
Regular contact with grandmother Grandmother informed early about pregnancy Grandmother shared information about her own pregnancy Grandmother accepts daughter as an adult	By end of first trimester, client will begin to use her own mother and other pregnant women as role models for motherhood	Encourage sharing of pregnancy experiences between mother and daughter.	A daughter's relationship with her own mother influences her ability to mother. (Other pregnant women may also serve as role models.)	Client demonstrates stage-appropriate role behaviors, and relates a positive relationship with her mother.
Nursing Diagnosis: Potential alteration in coping associated with conflicting beliefs between client and her mother				
Client's mother adheres to folklore regarding pregnancy related to cultural beliefs. Client tries "to keep mother happy." Client's mother will live with couple after baby is born.	Couple will begin to verbalize their feelings regarding cultural beliefs by the end of the visit. Client's mother attends next prenatal visit and expresses her beliefs Couple will identify beliefs regarding child care by end of first trimester	Allow couple to describe their feelings regarding cultural beliefs. Have client describe how she has dealt with cultural beliefs in the past. Include client's mother in planning care. Assess the strength of these beliefs and the degree of conflict they may create. Elicit information from client and her mother regarding child care beliefs. Allow couple and mother to express these beliefs in a nonjudgmental atmosphere.	Allowing the couple to verbalize their feelings in a nonjudgmental way helps them identify their feelings and begin the problem-solving process. Coping strategies that have been successful in the past can be successful in other stressful situations. Support for beneficial cultural practices reduces conflict between client and health care system. Including family members in planning care fosters positive communication. Conflict resolution begins with identification of conflict situations. The degree of change that occurs results from identification of the strength of the beliefs. Anticipatory guidance helps in the resolution of potential conflicts. Nutritional recommendations based on cultural practices decrease cultural conflict.	Client's mother attends a prenatal visit. Couple and mother communicate with each other concerning pregnancy practices. All family members have input into planning care. Client maintains cultural practices not harmful to pregnancy.

SUMMARY

The first trimester of pregnancy is a critical period of development for the childbearing family. During this time, the basis for meeting future tasks of pregnancy is set, and self-care practices related to pregnancy are begun. Ideally, at this time, a therapeutic relationship is begun between the expectant family and their health care providers. Most expectant couples are healthy, and seek health care personnel to confirm their normal status and for guidance and consultation. Nursing care of the healthy first-trimester family is therefore based on assessment and focuses on teaching. Referrals or further interventions are then developed for clients who are at risk or who have other specialized needs.

This chapter presented nursing care according to specific goals for the childbearing family during the first trimester. It is important to realize that other goals are possible. At all times, nursing care should be tailored to the unique needs of each client and should encompass physiologic, psychosocial, and cultural aspects of the childbearing family. The care plan included in this chapter demonstrated ways in which nursing care strategies can be applied to a pregnant family during the first trimester.

REVIEW QUESTIONS

1. Describe information that should be imparted to the client to prepare her for antenatal health care.
2. Discuss the importance of an interdisciplinary approach to care of the first trimester pregnant family.
3. Identify topics that would be important for client education during the first trimester.
4. Describe nursing care strategies that may be used to promote psychologic adaptation of the first trimester client.
5. Identify discomforts related to the first trimester of pregnancy and describe strategies to help clients cope with the discomforts.

REFERENCES

1. McKay S, Phillips C. *Family Centered Maternity Care.* Rockville, Md: Aspen; 1984.
2. American Academy of Pediatrics, American College of Obstetricians and Gynecologists. In: Frigoletto FD, Little GA, eds. *Guidelines for Perinatal Care.* 2nd ed. White Plains, NY: March of Dimes Birth Defects Foundation; 1988.
3. Varney H. *Nurse Midwifery.* 2nd ed. Boston: Blackwell Scientific; 1987.
4. Roberts J. Priorities in prenatal education. *J Obstet Gynecol Neonat Nurs.* 1976;5:18–19.
5. Cox B. Time perception during pregnancy. Poster presentation at Seventh National Meeting, Organization for Obstetric, Gynecologic, and Neonatal Nurses (NAACOG); April 1989; St. Louis, Mo.
6. Alley NM. Morning sickness: the client's perspective. *J Obstet Gynecol Neonat Nurs.* 1984;13:185–189.
7. Klebanoff MA, Koslowe PA, Kaslow R, Rhoads GC. Epidemiology of vomiting in early pregnancy. *Obstet Gynecol.* 1985;66:612–616.
8. Cunningham FG, et al. *Williams Obstetrics.* 18th ed. Norwalk, Conn: Appleton Lange; 1989.
9. Chenger P, Kovacik A. Dental hygiene during pregnancy: a review. *Am J Matern Child Nurs.* 1987;12:342–343.
10. Bennett EC. The first trimester. *J Obstet Gynecol Neonat Nurs.* 1982;13 (suppl): 935–965.
11. Aukamp V. *Nursing Care Plans for the Childbearing Family.* Norwalk, Conn: Appleton-Century-Crofts; 1984.
12. Poole CJ. Fatigue during the first trimester of pregnancy. *J Obstet Gynecol Neonat Nurs.* 1986;15:375–379.

The Second Trimester of Pregnancy

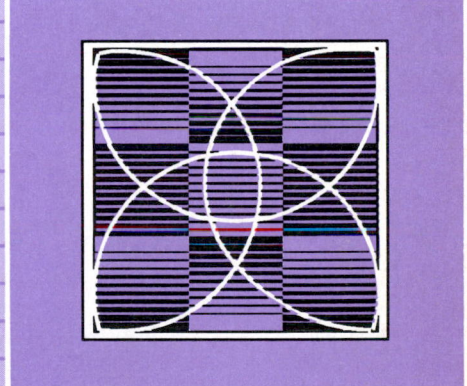

unit

4

Physiologic Changes During the Second Trimester

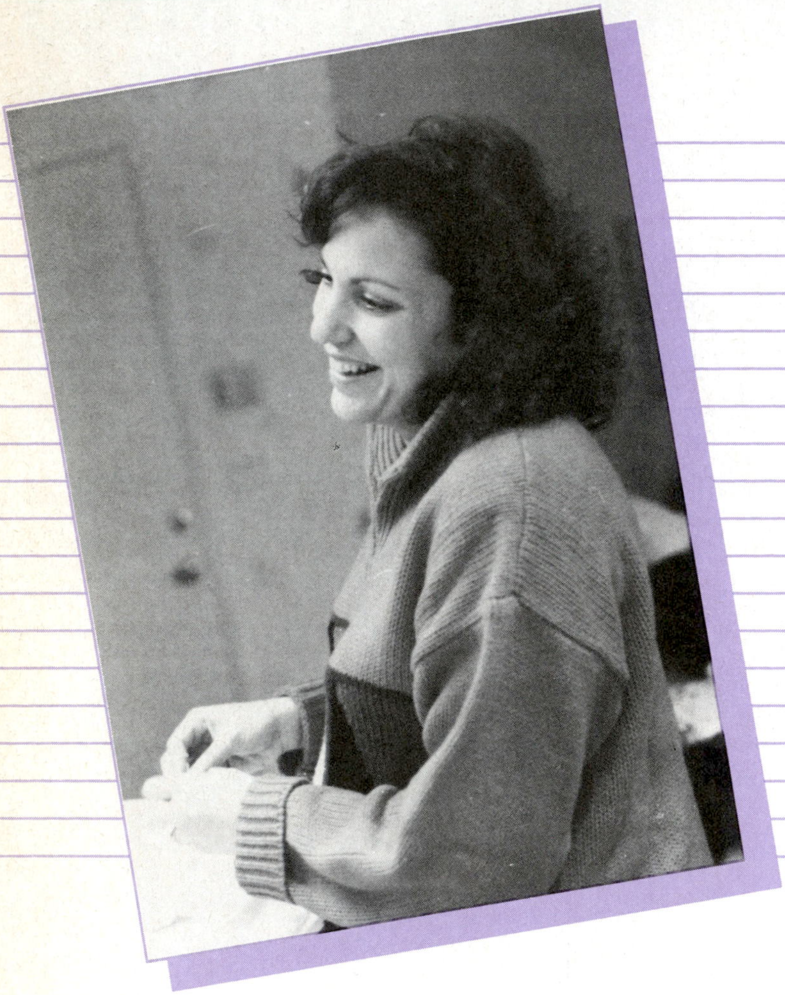

Chapter 16

Key Terms

colostrum
"mask of pregnancy"
melasma/chloasma
palmar erythema
physiologic anemia of pregnancy

The second trimester begins with the 13th week of gestation and extends through the end of the 24th week. During this period, maternal changes take place as the fetus continues to grow and develop. The expectant mother's body changes to provide for the increasing growth and needs of the still immature fetus, to continue pregnancy for an additional trimester, and to maintain the mother's own state of wellness. As such first trimester discomforts as nausea, vomiting, and extreme fatigue fade during the second trimester, the healthy expectant mother develops a sense of physical well being that is unequaled in either early or late pregnancy.

GROWTH AND DEVELOPMENT OF THE FETUS

During the second trimester of pregnancy, major body systems of the fetus become functional (*see* Chapter 11). By the end of the 16th week of gestation, the fetus looks like a very thin baby; at this time the head accounts for one third of the total length of the fetus. The musculoskeletal system continues to develop with advancing ossification of bone and movement of the arms and legs. The fetus begins holding the head in a more erect position, as the back and neck muscles develop. Fetal movements (quickening) may be first felt by the mother during the fourth month. Fine, downy hair (lanugo) begins to develop over the body of the fetus. Blood vessels can be seen through the transparent skin, and pads develop on the fingers and toes. The digestive system begins functioning during the fourth month. The fetus swallows amniotic fluid and produces meconium in the intestinal tract.

By the 20th week of gestation, subcutaneous deposits of brown fat develop in the neck, chest, and inguinal areas. Glands in the skin begin to produce a cheesy, fatty substance (vernix caseosa) to help protect the skin from the amniotic fluid. Lanugo increases. The mother feels many fetal movements, as the activity level and strength of the fetus continue to increase. Maximum brain growth begins with the fifth month. By the sixth month of gestation, the alveoli of the lungs begin to develop, and mature hemoglobin can be identified in fetal blood. Grasp, startle, and blink reflexes are present, and the fetus makes muscular breathing movements. By the second trimester, organ systems are formed. The fetus remains vulnerable, especially to environmental insults that could impair function of the brain or other organ systems. The pregnant woman must therefore continue to pay attention to potential effects of environmental and lifestyle factors such as drug use and alcohol consumption.

MATERNAL PHYSIOLOGIC ADAPTATION

In the second trimester of pregnancy, physiologic changes in the mother occur along with and in response to the increasing needs of the fetus. Table 16–1 summarizes physiologic changes that take place during the second trimester.

Reproductive System

Uterus. The uterus continues to enlarge during the second trimester. During the first trimester, uterine growth took place primarily through hyperplasia and hypertrophy of muscle cells. These changes were stimulated by such hormones as estrogen and progesterone. After the first trimester, growth of the myometrium can be attributed mainly to hypertrophy of muscle cells. This hypertrophy is stimulated both by distension from the growing products of conception and by hormonal activity.

By the end of the first trimester, the uterine wall, which had previously thickened, thins and softens. As the second trimester progresses, the fetus can be palpated through the abdominal wall. The uterus becomes ovoid, as it increases more in length than width. The uterus enlarges beyond the pelvic cavity, rotates to the right, and displaces the intestines to the side and above. By the end of the second trimester, the uterus can be felt above the umbilicus (Figure 16–1).

As pregnancy progresses, the uterus becomes a soft muscular sac, which exerts increasing pressure on the broad and round ligaments.[1] The uterus is a movable organ. When the woman stands, the uterus is supported by the abdominal muscles in a longitudinal position along the pelvic axis. When the pregnant woman lies on her back, the uterus rests on the vertebral column, the inferior vena cava, and the aorta.

During the second trimester, Braxton Hicks contractions may be experienced by the woman. These may become more frequent as the pregnancy progresses. Women have described second-trimester Braxton Hicks contractions as "tightening," "mild pressing," or "light cramping" sensations. Vaginal bleeding, cervical dilation, sharp continuing pain, and pain that increases in intensity are not normal manifestations of Braxton Hicks contractions. Women who experience these problems should contact their health care provider without delay.

Cervix. Through a combination of complex factors, the collagen framework of the cervix continues to change and cervical softening progresses during the second trimester.[1,2] The precise mechanisms responsible for these changes are unknown, although prostaglandins and hormones such as estrogen may be involved.

Glands of the cervical mucosa continue to proliferate. The thin walls (septa) that separate the spaces between the glands get thinner. The cervix takes on a "honeycomb" appearance with the honeycomb spaces filled with mucus (Figure 16–2).

Eversion or extension of glands and epithelium from the inner cervix takes place frequently. The cervix then appears to have lesionlike red velvety patches. Although called "cervical erosions," these patches represent a normal occurrence during pregnancy, rather than an inflammatory or ulcerating process.[1]

The cervix continues to lengthen. Between 20 and 25 weeks, the cervix reaches a maximum length of about 48 mm, as assessed by vaginal ultrasound.[3]

Vagina. The smooth muscle cells of the vagina hypertrophy during the second trimester. The vaginal mucosa thickens. The vaginal wall elongates and becomes looser as a result of the loosening of the connective tissue. Vaginal, as well as cervical, secretions

TABLE 16–1. SUMMARY OF PHYSIOLOGIC CHANGES IN THE SECOND TRIMESTER

Organ	Changes
Reproductive System	
Uterus	Continues to enlarge, mainly by hypertrophy of muscle cells Uterine wall thins, softens Fetus is palpable abdominally Uterus becomes ovoid Braxton Hicks contractions are felt
Cervix	Continues to lengthen, reaching greatest length between 20 and 25 weeks Mucous plug forms and is in place Muscle cells hypertrophy Cervical glands are active
Vagina	Smooth muscle cells hypertrophy Mucosa thickens Walls elongate and loosen Leukorrhea continues pH is acidic, 3.5–6.0
Fallopian tubes	No new changes occur
Ovary	Corpus luteum degenerates
Breasts	Mammary ducts and alveoli continue to hypertrophy Areolae and nipples enlarge and pigment deepens Colostrum secretion begins
Cardiovascular System	Blood volume expands (red blood cells and plasma) Hemoglobin may decrease as a result of greater expansion of plasma than red blood cells Position of heart changes Cardiac output increases Stroke volume increases Heart rate increases Blood pressure remains the same or decreases slightly Supine hypotension may occur, especially in late second trimester
Respiratory System	Oxygenation of blood increases Woman breathes more deeply Tidal volume increases Oxygen consumption increases Expanding uterus displaces diaphragm and causes rib cage to expand and to flare Thoracic, rather than abdominal, breathing takes place by 24 weeks Nasal congestion continues Shortness of breath develops
Urinary System	Size and vessel tortuosity of bladder increase Physiologic edema occurs in bladder tissue Urinary frequency decreases Kidneys increase in size Kidneys and ureters, especially on right side, dilate Mother is susceptible to urinary tract infections Glomerular filtration rate rises about 50% Renal plasma flow remains elevated at first trimester's level Excretion of glucose, amino acids, polypeptides, electrolytes, and water-soluble vitamins increases
Muscoloskeletal System	Sacroiliac, sacrococcygeal, and pubic joints relax Woman's center of gravity shifts as a result of expanding uterus Gait widens Physiologic lordosis develops Pressure and strain on round ligament causes abdominal and inguinal pain
Integument	
Skin	Pigment deepens, especially on areolae, nipples, vulva, perineal area Melasma is observed Linea nigra is apparent

(continued)

TABLE 16–1. SUMMARY OF PHYSIOLOGIC CHANGES IN THE SECOND TRIMESTER *(continued)*

Organ	Changes
Integument *(continued)*	
Skin *(continued)*	Vascular spiders may develop Palmar erythema may appear
Hair	Hair does not shed as quickly as when nonpregnant; along with new hair growth, gives impression of hair thickening
Nails	Are softer than prior to pregnancy Rate of growth increases
Gastrointestinal System	
Mouth and gums	Hyperemia continues Sensitivity to irritants continues Epulis may form
Esophagus and stomach	Esophagus shifts to side Angle at which esophagus enters stomach changes Stomach capacity perceived to be decreased Cardiac valve works less efficiently with resulting gastric reflux Secretion of hydrochloric acid and pepsin in stomach decreases
Liver	Size, structure, and form remain unchanged Changes occur in function, eg, increased serum alkaline phosphatase, decreased plasma albumin and plasma globulins
Gallbladder	Capacity increases Empties more slowly Woman becomes predisposed to gallstones
Pancreas	Hypertrophy, hyperplasia, and hypersecretion occur in beta cells Physiologic demands of pregnancy can precipitate gestational diabetes or aggravate existing diabetes mellitus
Intestines	Emptying time increases Absorption of nutrients and water increases
Endocrine System	
Pituitary	Enlarges Suppression of luteinizing and follicle-stimulating hormones continues Prolactin levels increase
Thyroid	Vascularity increases Increased T_3 and T_4 levels reflect increase in thyroxine binding globulin Hyperplasia continues Basal metabolic rate increases, dietary iodine continues to be important
Parathyroids	Enlarge Parathyroid hormone increases
Adrenals	Adrenocorticotropic hormone level increases Cortisol level rises Aldosterone level increases
Placenta	Fully functioning

increase during this trimester and continue to have a thick, white appearance. Vaginal pH remains acidic (3.5 to 6.0). The woman continues to be susceptible to yeast infections, which may cause considerable discomfort during the second trimester. Yeast infections are also fostered by conditions that raise serum glucose levels, such as a high sugar intake or diabetes.

Fallopian Tubes. Few significant changes occur in the fallopian tubes during the second trimester of pregnancy.

Ovary. During the first trimester, substantial enlargement took place in the ovary that produced the ovum and then sustained the corpus luteum. By the second trimester, the placenta is developed and the corpus luteum is not needed to maintain pregnancy. The degenerative process that began late in the first trimester continues; therefore, during the second trimester, the ovary regresses in size.

Breasts. Breast changes, which began in the first trimester, continue through the second trimester.[1,4]

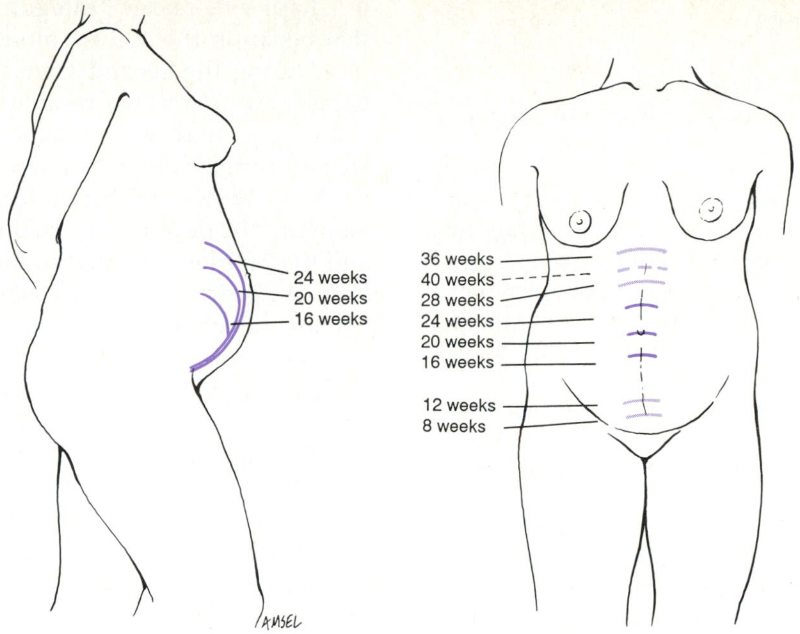

Figure 16–1. Height of the fundus at 16, 20, and 24 weeks.

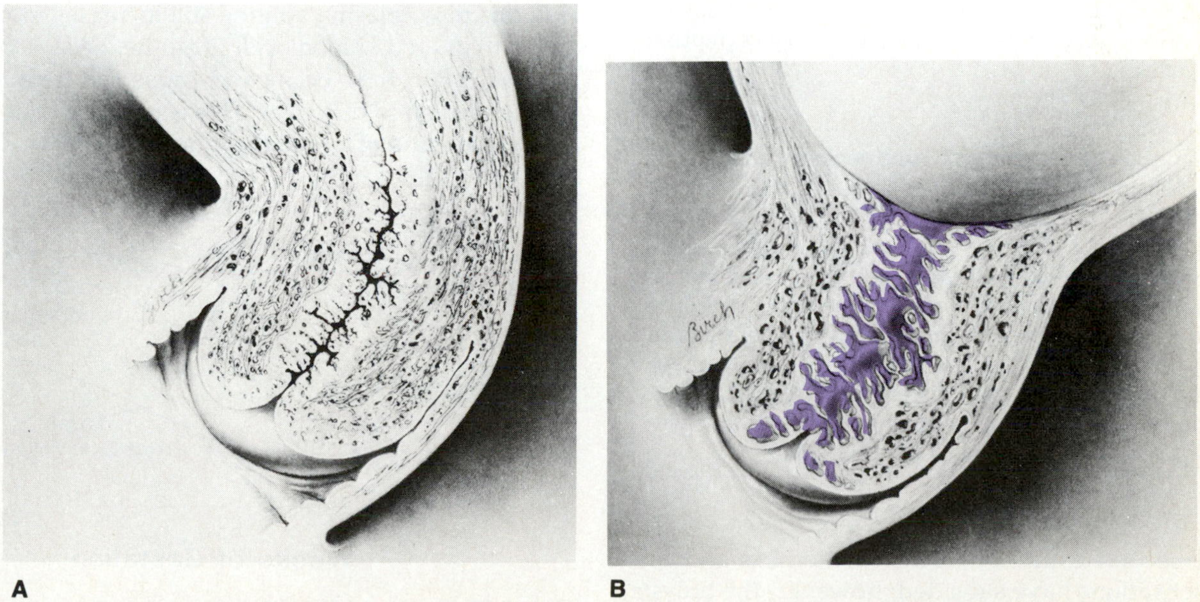

Figure 16–2. A. Cervix in the nonpregnant woman. **B.** Cervix in the pregnant woman. Note the elaboration of the mucosa into a honeycomb-like structure, filled with a tenacious mucus—the so-called mucous plug. (*Reproduced, with permission, from Cunningham FG, et al.* Williams Obstetrics. *18th ed. Norwalk, Conn: Appleton & Lange; 1989:134.*)

RESEARCH ABSTRACT

Fawcett J, York R. Spouses' physical and psychological symptoms during pregnancy and the postpartum. Nurs Res. *1986;35:144–148.*

This study used a descriptive design to investigate the types and frequency of physical and psychologic symptoms experienced by women and their spouses at various stages of pregnancy and the postpartum period. The sample consisted of 70 married couples in three groups: 23 couples in the third to fourth month of pregnancy, 24 in the ninth month of pregnancy, and 23 in the sixth postpartum week. A symptom checklist was developed by the investigators to measure the types and frequency of physical and psychologic symptoms experienced by the participants.

The physical symptoms most frequently reported by the women in the early-pregnancy group were fatigue, increased urination, reduction in activity, bloating, increase in appetite, sensitivity to odors, and nausea and vomiting. Physical symptoms most frequently reported by women in the late pregnancy group included increased urination, fatigue, indigestion, backache, reduction in activity, clumsiness, nausea and vomiting, increase in appetite, sensitivity to odors, and difficulty in breathing. This group of women reported the most physical symptoms. Two physical symptoms were most frequently reported by women in the postpartum group: fatigue and constipation.

Men experienced physical symptoms in early and late pregnancy and in the postpartum period. The physical symptom reported by men in the early pregnancy group was increased appetite, and in the late pregnancy group, craving for certain foods. All groups of women and men experienced the psychologic symptom of anxiety.

Comment:
Identification of discomforts experienced by clients at various stages of pregnancy assists nurses in providing anticipatory guidance and teaching. Clients in this study reported symptoms that are not usually associated with late pregnancy, such as nausea and vomiting, as well as symptoms well documented during the periods examined. Results of the study indicate a wide range of physical symptoms that can normally occur for both women and men in relation to childbearing. Findings also support the existence of the couvade syndrome in an American middle-class population.

By the second trimester, breast tenderness and tingling sensations have subsided; however, the breasts continue to enlarge. Delicate blue veins may be seen beneath the skin of the breasts. Striae, or "stretch marks," may appear (these are described more fully in Chapter 9, under "Integument"). The nodularity that began in the second month continues.

During the second trimester, the areolae of the breasts are noticeably broader. The nipples also become larger and more erectile. The color of the areolae and nipples deepens to a dark red in fair-skinned women, brown in brunettes, and black in black women. The depth of the pigmentation in the areolae and the nipples is related to the color of the woman's skin. As pregnancy progresses, the Montgomery tubercles, which are subaceous glands on the areolae, become more prominent. Although they appear nodular or "lumplike," they are not pathologic and should not be confused with true breast masses.[5,6]

During the second trimester, the lobule-alveolar formation of the breasts dominates. **Colostrum,** a fluid precursor of milk that is composed mainly of serum and white blood cells, is usually secreted from the breasts after the 16th week[7]; however, colostrum may be expressed earlier.

Cardiovascular System

Responses of the maternal cardiovascular system are pronounced during the second trimester of pregnancy. The blood volume of the pregnant woman expands more rapidly in the second trimester than at any other time during the pregnancy (Figure 16–3). Mean red blood cell volume is increased because the rate of red cell production is greater than that of red cell destruction. The diameter of the red blood cells decreases, and the cells become more spherical. Although the red blood cells increase by one third during this time, plasma volume still increases more rapidly than red blood cell volume. As a result, hemodilution may occur and cause the hemoglobin concentration to decrease. This is referred to as **physiologic anemia of pregnancy;** however, at sea level a

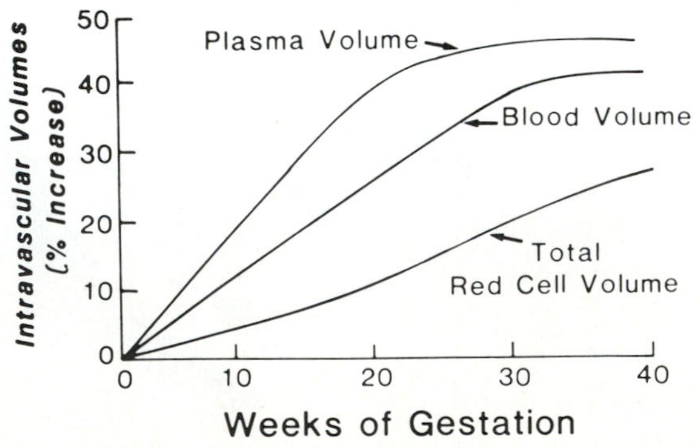

Figure 16–3. Increase in blood volume during pregnancy. (*Reproduced, with permission, from Burrow GN, Ferris TF, eds.* Medical Complications During Pregnancy. *3rd ed. Philadelphia: WB Saunders; 1988:181.*)

hemoglobin level below 11.0 g/dL is considered low and not a result of physiologic hemodilution of pregnancy.[1] During the second trimester the iron needs of the fetus and mother increase as a result of the increased maternal blood volume and the fetal and maternal storage of iron.

As pregnancy progresses, the heart is displaced upward and to the left. The apex of the heart is moved to the side. Cardiac output, which rose markedly by the end of the first trimester, rises to about 40 percent beyond nonpregnant levels during the second trimester. As shown in Figure 16–4, this increase peaks around 20 weeks and is sustained for the remainder of the pregnancy. The rise in cardiac output is necessary to meet increased blood flow needs to the uterus and to the kidneys for maternal-placental circulation, and to adapt to the increase in plasma volume during the second trimester.

During the second trimester, the amount of blood ejected by the heart per minute (stroke volume) may increase by as much as 30 percent over the prepregnant level. The heart rate, which rose about 8 beats per minute during the first trimester, increases an additional 2 to 7 beats per minute during the second trimester and is, therefore, about 10 to 15 beats higher than it was before pregnancy.

Despite the greater cardiac workload during the second trimester, blood pressure tends to decrease, because the total peripheral resistance continues to decline.[4,7,8] The relaxation of the small blood vessels counterbalances the increased volume load on the heart until late in the second trimester. This reflects the influence of hormones such as progesterone.[8] Blood pressure is affected by the position of the pregnant woman, with the highest reading in the sitting position (Figure 16–5), and the lowest reading in the left side-lying position.

Blood flow to the skin increases partly as a result of the decrease in peripheral resistance. This may serve an excretory function by dissipating heat released by increased metabolic processes during pregnancy. Erythema of the hands (**palmar erythema**) may occur around the fifth to sixth month and may be related to peripheral vascular changes.

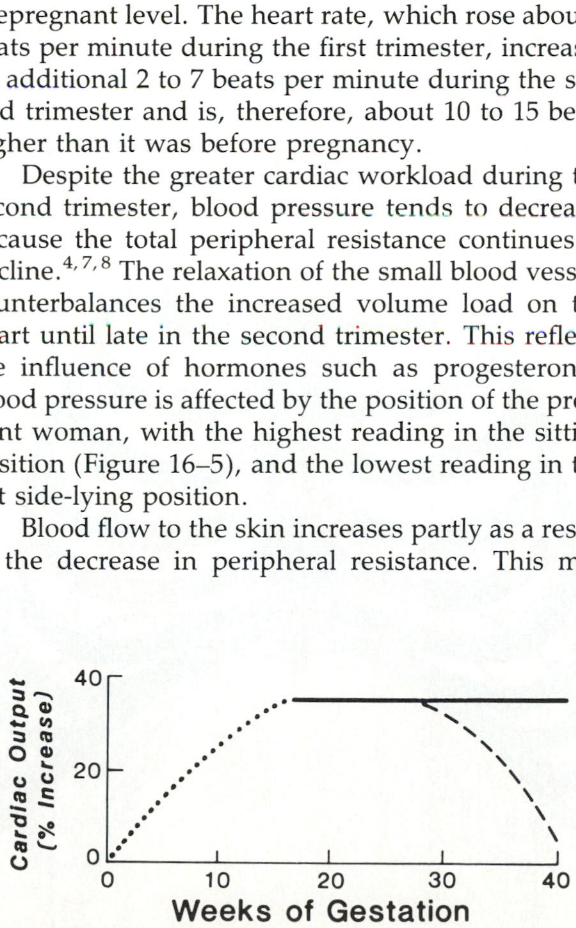

Figure 16–4. Cardiac output during pregnancy. (*Reproduced, with permission, from Burrow GN, Ferris TF, eds.* Medical Complications During Pregnancy. *3rd ed. Philadelphia: WB Saunders; 1988:181.*)

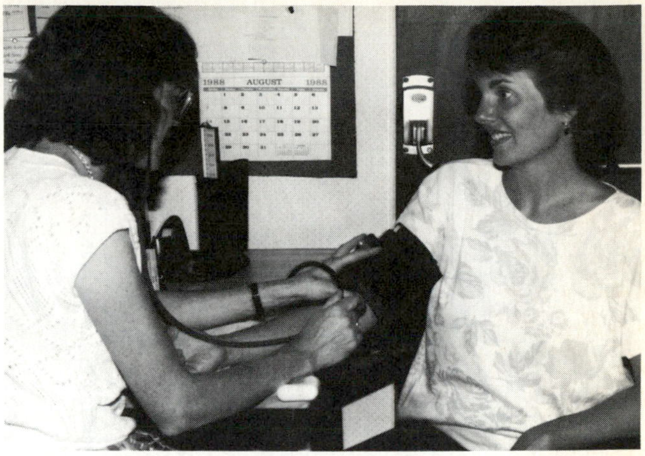

Figure 16–5. Nurse taking mother's blood pressure.

As the uterus increases in size, pressure may be placed on large blood vessels, especially when the mother is supine (*see* Chapter 20). The large uterus causes partial compression of the inferior vena cava and abdominal aorta, resulting in return of less blood to the heart. A decrease in stroke volume may then occur. During late pregnancy, increased pressure in the legs may also contribute to the development of varicose veins and edema in the lower extremities.

Respiratory System

As the blood volume increases, the maternal respiratory system responds, so that the lungs can oxygenate the additional blood required during pregnancy. The increase in oxygenation of blood is accomplished without structural changes in the lungs.

Estrogen and progesterone decrease the pulmonary resistance, and progesterone helps to reset the respiratory center in the brain. Decreases in the blood P_{CO_2} and in the bicarbonate concentrations take place. No respiratory alkalosis occurs during pregnancy, because of the resetting of the respiratory center in the hypothalamus. Under the influence of progesterone, there is a reduction in the P_{CO_2} from 40 mm Hg in the nonpregnant state to 32 mm Hg during pregnancy. The decrease in P_{CO_2} facilitates the increase in oxygen consumption and oxygen tension. Maternal respiratory rate does not vary much during pregnancy from its usual frequency of 14 to 15 per minute.[9] The expectant mother does, however, breathe more deeply, so that tidal volume (volume of air inspired and ex-

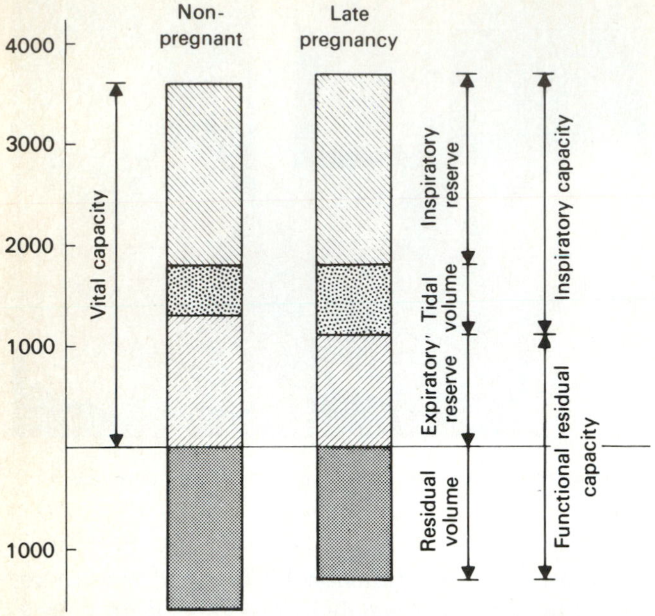

Figure 16–6. Comparison of components of lung volume in late pregnancy and in nonpregnant women. (*Reproduced, with permission, from Hytten F, Chamberlain G, eds.* Clinical Physiology in Obstetrics. *London: Blackwell Scientific; 1980:81.*)

pired with each respiration) and minute volume (amount of air exhaled per minute) increase. Tidal volume progressively increases 35 to 50 percent (about 200 mL over the nonpregnant volume of 500 mL) as pregnancy develops, and minute ventilation rises about 50 percent.[10] Residual volume (amount of air remaining in the lungs after maximal expiration), functional residual capacity (a combination of the expiratory reserve and residual volume), and expiratory reserve volume (the greatest amount of air that can be exhaled from the resting end-expiratory position) decrease about 20 percent. The greater tidal volume and smaller residual volume result in about a 65 percent more efficient gas exchange in the alveoli during pregnancy.[8] By 22 to 24 weeks, the greatest increase (5 to 10 percent) in inspiratory capacity (the greatest amount of gas that can be breathed in from the resting and end-expiratory position) is reached. Figure 16–6 illustrates and compares components of lung volume before pregnancy and during advanced pregnancy.

Around the 16th week of pregnancy, oxygen consumption increases by about 15 percent. Although oxygen consumption needs of the fetus, placenta, and various organs begin to increase substantially during the second trimester, the greatest oxygen consumption needs occur during the third trimester (*see* Chapter 20, especially Figure 20–4). Vital capacity, the total amount of air that can be moved in and out of the lungs with maximum effort in one breath, also increases during the second trimester for some women. The increase may be around 100 to 200 mL. Such factors as body build and weight may affect whether and to what extent vital capacity changes; obese women may have a decrease in vital capacity.[9]

During the second trimester, the expanding uterus presses against the diaphragm. The diaphragm elevates and the substernal angle is increased, causing the rib cage to expand and to flare (Figure 16–7). The increase in the circumference of the chest compensates for the elevated diaphragm, so that diaphragmatic excursions (elevation and lowering of the diaphragm during breathing) are greater, and tidal volume increases. By 24 weeks of gestation, the pregnant woman breathes thoracically, rather than abdominally. As pregnancy progresses, the mother may experience shortness of breath.

Congestion of the respiratory passages and nosebleeds, presumably effects of estrogen, continue into the second trimester.

Urinary System

During the second trimester the changes in renal function may be attributed to such factors as expanded plasma volume and increased maternal and placental hormones, such as adrenocorticotropic hor-

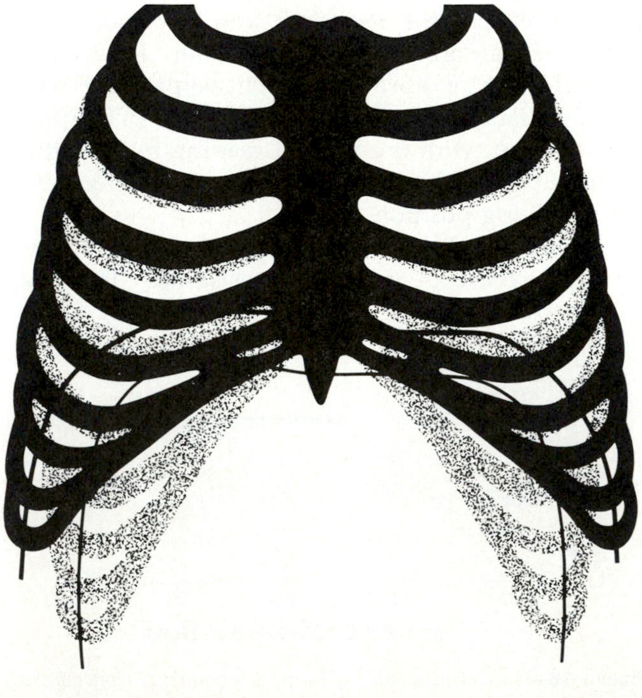

Figure 16–7. Comparison of rib cage in pregnant and nonpregnant women. (*Reproduced, with permission, from Hytten F, Chamberlain G, eds.* Clinical Physiology in Obstetrics. *London: Blackwell Scientific; 1980:86.*)

mone (ACTH), antidiuretic hormone (ADH), aldosterone, and thyroid hormone.[10] The kidneys continue to increase in size. Dilation of the kidneys and ureters, particularly on the right side, takes place. Ureteral dilation may be caused by the expanding uterus, pregnancy-enlarged pelvic blood vessels through which the ureters pass en route to the bladder, and the influence of progesterone and prostaglandins in decreasing the smooth muscle tone of the ureter. These conditions contribute to urinary stasis and make the expectant mother vulnerable to such problems as urinary tract infections and pain caused by overdistension in the ureters.[11]

During the second trimester, the glomerular filtration rate (GFR) rises by as much as 50 percent above the nonpregnant level to process waste materials from the mother and fetus. About 20 percent of cardiac output flows to the kidneys during rest. By midpregnancy, renal plasma flow (RPF) has increased as much as 50 percent over the nonpregnant level; maximum RPF is reached by the end of the second trimester and stabilizes thereafter.[10]

In the nonpregnant healthy woman, nutrients are returned to the plasma from the proximal tubule of the kidney. These substances include glucose, amino acids, and polypeptides, as well as sodium, electrolytes, and water-soluble vitamins. For unknown reasons, during pregnancy, these solutes are excreted in increased quantities.

About 80 percent of the glomerular filtrate is reabsorbed by the proximal tubules. Despite the large increase in the GFR, the volume of urine excreted daily does not rise much; therefore, during normal pregnancy, the urinary system seems to work harder.[10]

As discussed in Chapter 12, the renal threshold for glucose may normally be lower during pregnancy. During the second trimester, glucose may at times appear in the urine because of the increased GFR. Women with glucosuria need to be evaluated carefully. Although occasional episodes may be normal, they may also be a sign of diabetes, which may become apparent in the second trimester of pregnancy.

As discussed in Chapter 12, renal clearance of urea and creatinine from the blood rises during pregnancy; however, the production of urea nitrogen and creatinine does not change significantly. Therefore, during the second trimester, as the GFR increases, the levels of blood urea nitrogen and creatinine decrease.[10]

After the fourth month of gestation, the trigone of the bladder (the smooth triangular area on the inner surface of the bladder between the openings of the two ureters and the internal urethral opening) is elevated, and the posterior margins thicken. This process continues through the rest of pregnancy and results in deepening and widening of the trigone. The only changes in the mucosa of the bladder involve increases in size and in tortuosity of the blood vessels.[10] These changes may be caused by the hyperemia of pregnancy and the hyperplasia of muscle and connective tissue associated with pregnancy.

During the second trimester, there is less pressure on the bladder because the uterus rises out of the pelvis. Urinary frequency thus subsides during this trimester, and the woman feels more comfortable.

Musculoskeletal System

Under the influence of hormones, possibly including relaxin and progesterone, the sacroiliac, sacrococcygeal, and pubic joints relax. As the uterus increases in size, the expectant mother's center of gravity begins shifting, and compensatory changes in posture occur (*see* Figure 20–5). During the second trimester, the gait widens. Accentuation of the lumbodorsal spinal curve results in lordosis and may contribute to lower back pain. The weight of the uterus can also pull on the round ligament and cause lower abdominal and inguinal pain (*see* later discussion).

Increased size and weight of the breasts place a strain on the muscles of the upper back and chest. Some women may experience upper back pain during the second trimester. Upper back pain is accentuated by activities such as sitting for prolonged periods at a desk and by slouching.

Integument

Pigmentation changes that began in the first trimester continue through the second trimester of pregnancy. These changes are more noticeable in dark-skinned women. During the second trimester skin around the nipples and areolae of the breasts, the vulva, and the perianal area darkens considerably.

Melasma, also called **chloasma** and the **"mask of pregnancy,"** is a blotchy, irregular area of deeper pigmentation that may develop on the forehead, cheeks, temples, and upper lip during pregnancy. As with other skin pigment changes in pregnancy, the cause of melasma is unclear. Estrogen, progesterone, and melanocyte-stimulating hormone, however, have been theorized to have some effect.[1,12] Melasma tends to appear during the second trimester, although it may be seen earlier and later. This condition lightens after delivery, but may not fade completely.

During pregnancy, the number and size of capillaries increase.[13] Telangiectases, or vascular spiders, are manifestations of dilated capillaries and may become prominent during the second trimester (*see* Chapter 12). These occur more commonly in white women than in black women.[1] **Palmar erythema**, or redness of the palms of the hands, tends to occur at the same time. These conditions are of cosmetic concern to clients, but are otherwise of no clinical significance. Both tend to disappear after pregnancy. It is thought that these changes take place because of the high levels of estrogen.

During the second trimester, hemangiomas may develop or pre-existing hemangiomas may enlarge. After delivery, they shrink but do not disappear completely.[12] Pre-existing moles (nevi) may darken or enlarge and new moles may develop. Although most will regress after pregnancy, any suspicious lesion should be evaluated carefully, because melanomas do occur in women of reproductive age.

Gastrointestinal System

Mouth and Gums. Hyperemia of the gums, as discussed in Chapter 12, continues, in response to the high circulating levels of hormones. In addition, higher hormonal levels may be related to greater reactions to irritants in dental plaque.[14] Inadequate dental hygiene and poor diet will result in bleeding gums, especially as pregnancy progresses. Clients with bleeding gums should be referred for further dental evaluation.

During the second trimester, epulis of pregnancy, small very vascular swellings on the gum, may become apparent. Epulis subsides after pregnancy.[1]

Esophagus and Stomach. As the uterus enlarges during the second trimester, the stomach shifts to the side and the intestines are pushed upward. Because of these postional differences, the angle at which the esophagus enters the stomach changes. Pressure on the stomach decreases capacity and requires the consumption of smaller meals, especially late in the second trimester.

As discussed in Chapter 12, hormones such as progesterone may exert a relaxing effect on smooth muscles. This also takes place in the gastrointestinal tract. For example, pregnancy's changes cause the cardiac valve to work less efficiently as pregnancy progresses. Acidic stomach secretions may reflux into the esophagus. The resulting pyrosis, or "heartburn," is experienced by about 80 percent of women during pregnancy and usually becomes noticeable in the second trimester. Occasionally, reflux and pyrosis can be so severe that stomach contents may extend as far as the pharynx. This can put the woman at risk for aspiration or wheezing and may induce asthma attacks in women with asthmatic histories.[15]

During the second trimester, there continues to be decreased secretion of hydrochloric acid and pepsin in the stomach. Conditions such as peptic ulcer continue to be uncommon.

Liver. The liver does not change much in size, structure, and form during pregnancy, although functional changes do take place. Changes in liver function considered normal in pregnancy would indicate liver disease in the nonpregnant woman. For example, serum alkaline phosphatase and serum lipids increase, but plasma albumin and plasma globulins decrease as pregnancy progresses.

Gallbladder. The emptying time of the gallbladder is prolonged during pregnancy, possibly as an effect of progesterone. After the first trimester, gallbladder volume also increases. Therefore, the gallbladder holds more and empties more slowly. Conditions promoting increased cholesterol saturation and cholesterol crystal formation predispose the pregnant woman to the formation of gallstones, although the precise mechanism is unclear.[1,15]

Decrease in bile flow and increased retention of bile salts in the gallbladder may be implicated in the development of generalized itching (pruritis gravidarum). This subsides after pregnancy.

Pancreas. Hypertrophy, hyperplasia, and hypersecretion take place in the beta cells of the islets of Langerhans as pregnancy progresses, although the precise mechanism explaining these changes remains unknown.[1] The increasing physiologic demands of pregnancy can precipitate gestational diabetes or can complicate existing diabetes mellitus. Therefore, carbohydrate metabolism and insulin metabolism become important concerns as pregnancy progresses (*see* Chapters 18 and 39). Pregnant women are often screened routinely for diabetes between the 24th and the 28th weeks.

Intestines. Decreased tone and motility of smooth muscle in the gastrointestinal tract mean that food and its breakdown products remain longer in the stomach and intestines. During the second trimester, there continues to be the benefit of increased time for maximum absorption of nutrients and water from the small and large intestines. Increased water absorption in the large intestine tends to make the stool hard. The hard stool and decreased intestinal motility contribute to constipation. The pregnant woman may strain during bowel movements. This causes additional venous pressure on the rectal vessels and fosters the development of hemorrhoids during the second trimester.

Endocrine System

Pituitary. During the second trimester, elevated progesterone and estrogen levels suppress production of luteinizing hormone (LH) and follicle-stimulating hormone (FSH) by the anterior pituitary gland. This suppression continues for the remainder of pregnancy. Maternal plasma levels of prolactin continue to increase, however. The hypothalamus regulates secretion of prolactin by the pituitary. Thyrotropin-releasing hormone stimulates this release and dopamine serves as an inhibitor to maintain physiologic balance. Estrogens stimulate prolactin production by the pituitary, as early as the first trimester. Because of the high circulating levels of estrogens, prolactin becomes the major hormone secreted by the pituitary as pregnancy progresses.[16]

As discussed in Chapter 12, FSH and LH are necessary for pregnancy to occur; however, a functioning pituitary gland is not necessary for pregnancy to continue. This is evidenced by pregnant women who have undergone removal of the pituitary gland (hypophysectomy) and then successfully completed pregnancies with supplementation of glucocorticosteroids, thyroid hormone, and vasopressin.[1]

Thyroid. During the second trimester of pregnancy, vascularity and hyperplasia of the glandular tissue of the thyroid continue to increase. The basal metabolic rate continues to rise in this trimester, although most of the activity is related to the metabolic requirements of the fetus and uterus and to the work of the mother's heart and lungs.[1,17] Dietary iodine continues to be needed to synthesize both triiodothyronine (T_3) and thyroxine (T_4).

Thyroid-binding plasma proteins rise to their highest level during the second trimester (Table 16–2); however, although the overall concentrations of T_3 and T_4 increase, the concentrations of free, unbound hormones remain within normal nonpregnant limits.[1] Thyroid stimulating hormone levels remain elevated during the second trimester.

Parathyroids. The parathyroids continue to have important roles in metabolism, particularly of calcium, during the second trimester. Serum parathyroid hormone levels steadily increase in the second trimester and produce a so-called "physiologic hyperparathyroidism" of pregnancy, although the reason why this occurs is unclear. Approximately 47 percent of serum calcium is bound to proteins, especially albumin. About 47 percent is found in serum as ionized calcium. The remaining 6 percent is bound to organic anions such as the phosphates. During the second trimester, when hemodilution occurs, serum albumin levels fall and total serum calcium also decreases. The expanding extracellular volume, increasing urinary calcium loss, and increased placental transfer of calcium to the fetus may contribute to overall lower total serum calcium levels and stimulation of parathyroid hormone secretion. Ionized or unbound calcium is believed to be the major regulator of parathyroid hormone production; however, this does not change significantly during pregnancy. High levels of estrogens may contribute to a blocking effect of parathyroid hormone on bone resorption and may therefore foster increased secretion of parathyroid hormone. The relationship between ionized calcium and parathyroid hormone secretion may differ between the pregnant and nonpregnant state and this may also account for higher levels of parathyroid hormone.[1,7]

TABLE 16–2. AVERAGE LEVELS OF THYROID-BINDING GLOBULIN IN PLASMA

Nonpregnant	3.6 mg/dL
First trimester	7.1 mg/dL
Second trimester	9.0 mg/dL
Third trimester	8.9 mg/dL

Source: Reference 1.

Adrenals. The morphology of the adrenal glands does not change much during pregnancy.[1] Adrenocorticotropic hormone levels progressively rise after a decrease during the first trimester of pregnancy. The concentration of circulating cortisol increases, and much of this hormone is bound by transcortin, a cortisol-binding globulin. Unlike thyroid hormones, concentrations of both free and bound cortisol rise. The rate of secretion of cortisol by the maternal adrenal cortex does not rise. Instead, the metabolic clearance of cortisol is lower in pregnancy and this accounts for the greater amount of this hormone in the blood. Higher cortisol levels are thought to be maintained because a physiologic "resetting" of the woman's feedback mechanisms causes the mother's body to adjust to higher levels.[1,18]

The secretion of aldosterone by the adrenal cortex also increases during the second and third trimesters. Aldosterone may counteract some of the effects of progesterone during pregnancy. For example, progesterone stimulates increased excretion of sodium and water by the kidney, whereas aldosterone fosters their retention. Sodium and water balance is therefore maintained, despite the changes of pregnancy. Major effects of cortisol and aldosterone are summarized in Table 12–2.

Placenta. By the 14th to 16th week of gestation, the placenta is fully formed and functioning. During the rest of pregnancy, changes relate to the degree of branching of the villi and enlargement in the intervillous spaces.[8] The size and weight of both the fetus and the placenta increase, although fetal increases are larger than placental increases. Placental hormones continue to have complex, important, and not thoroughly understood roles during the second trimester of pregnancy. Examples of placental hormones and their effects are summarized in Table 12–2.

SUMMARY

In the second trimester of pregnancy, the fetus continues to develop and the major body systems become functional. Physiologic changes in the mother occur rapidly during this trimester. The uterus enlarges beyond the pelvis, breasts continue to develop, cardiac output increases, blood volume makes its greatest increase, glomerular filtration rate increases, and most other organ systems are affected in some way. Changes take place in response to complex interactions of circulating hormones and to displacement of organs by the enlarging uterus.

REVIEW QUESTIONS

1. Identify changes that occur in the uterus, cervix and vagina during the second trimester of pregnancy.
2. Explain why the blood pressure is thought to remain the same or decrease during the second trimester despite a rise in cardiac workload.
3. Explain why a blood urea nitrogen level of 12 mg/100 mL and a serum creatinine level of 7.0 mg/100 mL might be cause for concern during the second trimester.
4. Discuss normal skin changes during the second trimester.
5. Identify normal physiologic changes in the stomach that can lead to discomforts such as heartburn during the second trimester of pregnancy.

REFERENCES

1. Cunningham FG, et al. *Williams Obstetrics.* 18th ed. Norwalk, Conn: Appleton & Lange; 1989.
2. Rechberger T, et al. Connective tissue changes in the cervix during normal pregnancy and pregnancy complicated by cervical incompetence. *Obstet Gynecol.* 1988;71:563–567.
3. Kushnir O, et al. Vaginal ultrasound assessment of cervical length changes during normal pregnancy. *Am J Obstet Gynecol.* 1990;162:991–993.
4. Varney H. *Nurse Midwifery.* 2nd ed. Boston: Blackwell Scientific; 1987.
5. Mitchell MS, Capizzi RL. Neoplastic diseases. In: Burrow GN, Ferris TF, eds. *Medical Complications During Pregnancy.* 3rd ed. Philadelphia: WB Saunders; 1988:540–569.
6. Haagensen CD. Anatomy of the mammary gland. In: Haagensen CD, ed. *Diseases of the Breast.* 3rd ed. Philadelphia: WB Saunders; 1986:1–46.
7. Taylor CM, Pernoll ML. Normal pregnancy and prenatal care. In: Pernoll ML, Benson, RC, eds. *Current Obstetric & Gynecologic Diagnosis & Treatment.* Norwalk, Conn: Appleton & Lange; 1987:161–177.
8. Beischer NA, Mackay EV. *Obstetrics and the Newborn: An Illustrated Textbook.* 2nd ed. Philadelphia: WB Saunders; 1988.
9. de Swiet M. The respiratory system. In: Hytten F, Chamberlain G, eds. *Clinical Physiology in Obstetrics.* London: Blackwell Scientific; 1980:79–100.
10. Moore PJ. Maternal physiology during pregnancy. In: Pernoll ML, Benson RC, eds. *Current Obstetric & Gynecologic Diagnosis & Treatment.* Norwalk, Conn: Appleton & Lange; 1987:127–134.
11. Meyers SJ, et al. Dilatation and nontraumatic rupture of the urinary tract during pregnancy: a review. *Obstet Gynecol.* 1985;66:809–815.
12. Braverman IM. The skin in pregnancy. In: Burrow GN, Ferris TF, eds. *Medical Complications During Pregnancy.* 3rd ed. Philadelphia: WB Saunders; 1988:528–539.
13. de Swiet M. The cardiovascular system. In: Hytten F, Chamberlain G, eds. *Clinical Physiology in Obstectrics.* London: Blackwell Scientific; 1980:3–42.
14. Chenger P, Kovacik A. Dental hygiene during pregnancy: a review. *Maternal Child Nurs.* 1987;12:342–343.
15. Connon J. Gastrointestinal complications. In: Burrow GN, Ferris TF, eds. *Medical Complications During Pregnancy.* 3rd ed. Philadelphia: WB Saunders; 1988:303–317.
16. Jouppila P, Ulikorkala O. The role of maternal prolactin in early pregnancy failure. *Obstet Gynecol.* 1984;64:373–375.
17. Ramsay ID. The thyroid gland. In: Hytten F, Chamberlain G, eds. *Clinical Physiology in Obstetrics.* London: Blackwell Scientific; 1980:400–410.
18. Ramsay ID. The adrenal gland. In: Hytten F, Chamberlain G, eds. *Clinical Physiology in Obstetrics.* London: Blackwell Scientific; 1980:411–423.

Psychologic and Sociocultural Dimensions During the Second Trimester

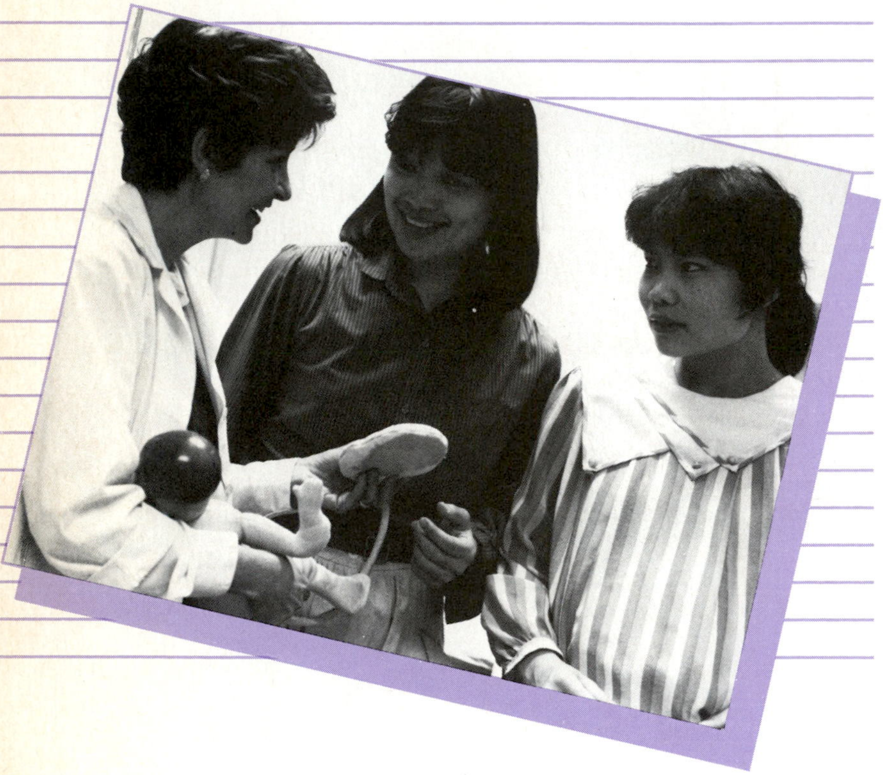

Chapter 17

Key Terms

internalization **prenatal attachment**

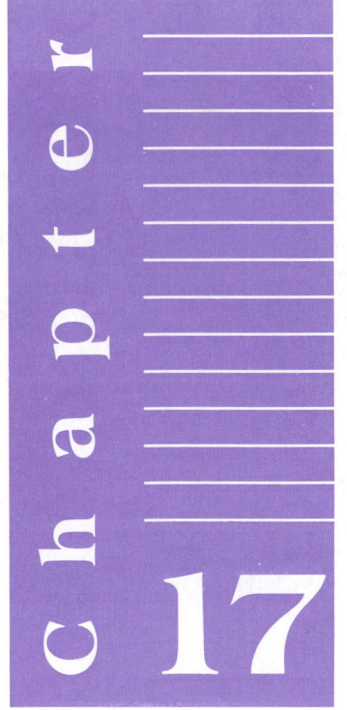

The expectant mother, father, and family undergo distinct psychologic changes during the second trimester of pregnancy. Many of these changes began during the first trimester. For the expectant parents and family members, pregnancy and the baby no longer seem unreal. The expectant mother, father, and siblings can "see" the baby because of changes within the mother's body. After quickening occurs around 16 to 18 weeks, family members also may perceive the baby's movements. Family members who attend prenatal visits with the expectant mother may hear the baby's heartbeat. As pregnancy becomes readily identifiable to others, societal and cultural expectations of family behaviors during pregnancy are activated, and family members attain a different status.

Realization of the pregnancy and the infant-to-be means that decisions and plans concerning life with an infant will have to be made and specific family goals set. Accomplishment of certain psychologic, social, and cultural tasks will allow the family to move into their new lifestyle and prepare for the newest member, the infant.

PSYCHOLOGIC CHANGES IN THE MOTHER

Psychologic Reactions and Concerns

For most low-risk expectant mothers, the second trimester is characterized as a "happy, content" period, marked by confirmation of the pregnancy, presence of a live fetus, and developing affection for the fetus. The uncertainty and ambivalence of the first trimester are generally resolved, and the expectant mother moves toward achieving the changed lifestyle of "woman and child." Discomforts of the first trimester, such as nausea and fatigue, subside, and the mother feels physically well.

RESEARCH ABSTRACT

Aaronson LS. Perceived and received support: effects on health behavior during pregnancy. Nurs Res. *1989;38:4–8.*

This study was undertaken to examine the effects of perceived and received social support on three health practices during pregnancy—abstinence from alcohol, cigarettes, and caffeine.

The sample consisted of 529 pregnant women who were less than 36 weeks pregnant and who were not appearing for their first prenatal visit.

Several measures of social support were used in this study. A modified version of the Personal Resources Questionnaire (PRQ) was used as a measure of five aspects of perceived support: worth, intimacy, social integration, nurturance, and assistance. Four-item scales were used for specific measures of the women's perceived social support in avoiding alcohol, cigarettes, and caffeine. For a measure of specific received support the women were asked if any person in their home drank alcoholic or caffeinated beverages or smoked. Data on the pregnant woman's abstinence from alcohol, cigarettes, and caffeine were obtained from telephone interviews.

T tests were used to analyze the impact of various measures of perceived and received support on the pregnant women's health behaviors. Regression analysis was also done to determine if perceived support and received support could predict the women's health behavior.

The findings of this study demonstrated that specific perceived and received support were significant for all three health behaviors. General social support, however, did not significantly predict any of the behaviors. The findings suggest that the effects of social support and social networks on an individual's health behavior are complex. Although others have found perceived support rather than received support to be the critical component of social support in its effects on health, this study has provided evidence that received support is also important. Both forms of social support are therefore important in planning care for pregnant women.

Comment:
This study suggests that social support influences positive health care practices. Nurses should give attention to this information in caring for pregnant women and their families. Abstinence from negative health behaviors such as smoking and alcohol consumption during pregnancy will positively influence the health of the fetus, as well as that of the mother.

Many women continue to work during the second trimester. Indeed, for the healthy woman, work by itself is no problem at any time during pregnancy.[1] Physiologic changes related to advancing pregnancy may, however, require changes for women who hold jobs that involve vigorous physical activity and balance (eg, police, firefighter, professional athlete). Extreme fatigue or job-related stress may also be reasons for changes.

Working women without the luxury of housekeepers often have household responsibilities that continue after their employment day is finished. Even when a couple shares tasks, activities such as cooking, shopping, and cleaning can be especially tiring during pregnancy. These responsibilities can be particularly stressful if the woman has other children.

The pregnant woman who works part-time may receive reduced benefits or no benefits.[1] She may therefore be reluctant to stop work during the second trimester and lose wages needed to maintain family lifestyle or meet basic expenses. During the second trimester, employed women are concerned with whether and when maternity leave should be taken, how to find child care, how significant others feel toward their working before and after the baby is born, and what effects working will have on the baby and family. Although they will not deliver for several months, women who intend to return to work may want to discuss and begin planning their future employment. In working with these mothers, nurses need to clarify their own values regarding employment and motherhood and to provide guidance in a nonjudgmental manner.[2]

Acceptance of the Pregnancy

In a classic study, Caplan noted that by the middle of the second trimester, the pregnant woman's feelings of ambivalence usually give way to joy over being pregnant.[3] He felt that "quickening," the first sensation of fetal movements, was the event that ushered in this change. For the pregnant woman, quickening meant that a real baby, not just a "pregnancy," existed. In fact, Caplan felt that any rejection experienced by the emotionally healthy pregnant woman was rejection of the physical state of pregnancy, not of the baby.

Lederman did not find complete joy and acceptance during the second trimester in her sample of healthy pregnant women.[4] She found that the expectant woman's ambivalence could be repeated occasionally throughout the pregnancy as a wish not to be pregnant. This wish may reflect the woman's uncertainties about the immensity of her step into motherhood. All of the women in Lederman's sample were primiparas; however, adding another child to a family is also a great step in the family life cycle. According to Lederman, ambivalence about pregnancy can range from low to high.[4] Although occasional, low levels of ambivalence are common, persistent, high levels of ambivalence may signal emotional difficulties. Each expectant client and her family needs to be assessed with care.

Though some feelings of ambivalence toward the physical pregnancy may surface throughout the second trimester, the expectant mother has essentially accepted the pregnancy and the fetus, who has become a real "baby" to her with the advent of fetal movement.

Maternal Role Attainment

During the first trimester of pregnancy, processes related to attaining the maternal role included replication, that is, mimicking pregnant "models" in the woman's environment, and role playing, that is, playing at being a mother[5] (*see* Chapter 13). During the second trimester, replication continues. Rubin believes that each stage of the pregnancy cycle involves new models for replication.[5] Once a stage is completed, former models are no longer relevant and, psychologically, the woman moves on. For example, the woman who has completed the prenatal role must progress into the role of woman in labor.

During the second trimester, activities begin to be internalized into the woman's personality system; they begin to become part of the woman. Like Caplan, Rubin sees the presence of a "real" fetus/baby and fetal movement as the catalyst for **internalization**.[5] This leads to fantasy, which is another operation of role attainment during the second trimester.

Fantasies

Fantasies, both daydreams and nightdreams, become an important part of the expectant mother's prenatal experience during the second trimester of pregnancy. The presence of a "real" fetus/baby who provides stimuli through fetal movement initiates maternal fantasies about a variety of topics. In addition to helping the woman to attain the maternal role, fantasy during pregnancy may serve other important functions for the expectant parents. A woman's life history and attitudes toward the pregnancy can influence both her dreams and the course of her labor.[6] Investigators have noted relationships between the content of certain dreams and length of labor, maternal anxiety, and mother's attitude toward the infant.[7,8] One function of fantasy may be to work through unresolved problems from everyday life.[6,8] This "day residue" becomes the material for dreams during sleep. The pregnant woman's concerns thus may be revealed openly in her daydreams and nightdreams. This information can provide the nurse with many insights into the pregnant woman's current concerns.

Few investigators have researched maternal fantasies during the second trimester. Most focus on third-trimester fantasies, which seem to be the most vivid, anxiety-filled, and troublesome to the pregnant woman. Rubin's descriptions of second-trimester fantasies tend to confirm the second trimester as a relatively happy, content phase of childbearing.[5,9] In Rubin's study, the infant-to-be is first imagined to be like a 6-month-old baby floating peacefully in space. The woman's wished-for child is literally an "angel."

MATERNAL PSYCHOLOGIC CHANGES AND CONCERNS DURING THE SECOND TRIMESTER

Psychologic Reactions and Concerns
Sense of well-being; aware that pregnancy can be easily recognized by others; concerns over employment

Acceptance of Pregnancy
Ambivalence mostly resolves; pregnancy accepted

Maternal Role Attainment
Replication continues; new role models are sought; fetal movement fosters internalization and fantasy

Fantasies
Continue; help woman to attain maternal role, "bind-in" to infant; provide clues to concerns about pregnancy, significant others, and life events

Relationship With Mother
Relationship with own mother becomes increasingly important; needs to perceive own mother as supportive; desires to share experiences and to feel mother's acceptance of her as an adult and a mother

Relationship With Fetus
Enhanced with fetal movement; beginning attachment behaviors evident; fetal movement experienced as an intimate form of communication

Body Image
Begins to view fetus as separate from own body; signs of pregnancy readily observable; changes represent "baby"; increased perception of body boundary as protective barrier for fetus

Time and Space
Pregnancy no longer feels endless; woman focuses inward on fetus; woman may seem to withdraw from significant others

The expectant woman may fantasize about a baby of a specific sex, as indicated by dreams of dressing the baby, and later the child, in gender-specific clothing. By the middle of the second trimester the age of the baby in the mother's fantasies begins to vary. The expectant woman may fantasize about her child (either sex) as an adolescent, as a school-aged child, or as an infant usually no smaller or younger than 6 months. The expectant mother's fantasies tend to be based on events from her own childhood. The infants and children portrayed on television, in magazines, and through other media may also have an impact on maternal fantasies.

Fantasies during the second trimester are therefore important for several reasons: (1) they help the pregnant woman to attain the maternal role; (2) they help the pregnant woman to "bind-in" to her future child; (3) they provide clues to the woman's concerns about her pregnancy, significant others, and life events.

Relationship With Mother

In the second trimester, the expectant woman's adaptation is influenced by her relationship with her own mother (Figure 17–1). Five components of this relationship develop as pregnancy progresses[4]: availability of the grandmother; grandmother's reaction to the pregnancy; grandmother's respect for her daughter's autonomy; willingness of the grandmother to reminisce; and empathy with the grandmother.

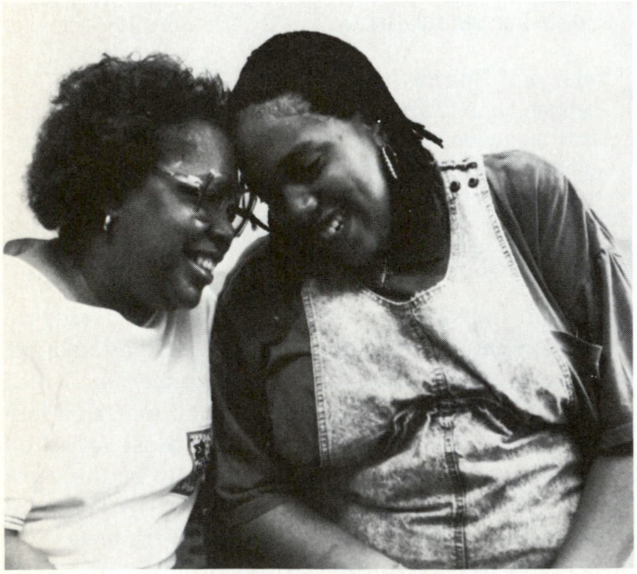

Figure 17–1. The quality of her relationship to her own mother is important to the expectant woman preparing to assume a maternal role.

Availability of the Grandmother. In ideal situations, pregnancy and childbirth provide the expectant mother and grandmother with an opportunity to move their relationship to a higher level. In healthy relationships the expectant woman's own mother is interested in her daughter and able to provide emotional support. The original mother-child relationship has evolved into a relationship between two adults. The expectant grandmother recognizes her daughter's development in becoming a mother. She offers not just assistance, but closeness and support. Availability is fostered when the grandmother lives near her daughter; however, adult women can perceive close relationships despite distance.[10] The quality of the relationship with mother, rather than the amount of time spent together, has been noted to be critical for the health of members of this dyad.[11]

Grandmother's Reaction to the Pregnancy. Ideally, the grandmother reacts to the pregnancy by accepting her daughter as a mother. Lederman found that most mothers of the women in her sample were happy and excited over their daughter's pregnancy[4]; however, the grandmother can be enthusiastic about the grandchild and still offer limited emotional support to her daughter. Attitude toward the grandchild therefore does not automatically mean acceptance of the daughter as a mother.

The woman has a great desire to receive her mother's support during pregnancy. If the grandmother is not available to her, the expectant woman may react with resentment or hostility.

The pregnancy of an adult daughter confirms that the grandmother-to-be has moved up a generation. This may be personally difficult to accept at first, especially if the expectant grandmother has prided herself on being youthful. The later and middle years of adulthood have provided new lifestyles and opportunities for older women. Grandmothers who in previous generations might have lived near or with their daughters and cared extensively for grandchildren are now actively pursuing independent lifestyles. Adult children, especially middle-and upper-middle-class groups, frequently move great distances to further careers, and grandparents may retire to "sunbelt" locations such as Florida and Arizona. The roles and role conflicts between these "new" grandmothers and their adult children are in need of research and study.

Grandmother's Respect for Her Daughter's Autonomy. In a healthy, autonomous relationship, the expectant mother and grandmother relate to each other as two independent adults. The grandmother's belief in her daughter's independence and maturity fosters decision making by the pregnant woman and promotes her confidence in herself as a mother.[4] The grandmother who is critical of, interferes with, or attempts to control the expectant woman may still see her daughter as a dependent child. She literally cannot "let her go."

Willingness of the Grandmother to Reminisce. The expectant mother's early childhood experiences and the grandmother's childbearing experiences are topics shared between expectant mothers and their own mothers. When done in a positive manner, this form of close communication tends to increase the ego strength and self-confidence of the mother-to-be.

Empathy With the Grandmother. In a relationship that includes mutual sharing, the expectant woman may also be supportive of her own mother. She can empathize with her mother's experiences in parenting and with the tasks she must accomplish to become a grandmother. As one client observed, "Not until I was having my own child did I really come to understand my mother. I felt us become closer as *women* and not just as mother and daughter. For me it was a new and beautiful feeling."

Not every mother and daughter enjoy a strong, positive relationship. During pregnancy, however, the expectant woman may attempt efforts at reconciliation. As Lederman indicates, reconciliation is most readily achieved when both women become aware of and accept each other's differences.[4]

Relationship With Fetus

The mother's relationship to her infant-to-be is greatly enhanced during the second trimester, when the presence of a "real" fetus/baby is evident. Quickening naturally encourages the development of this relationship. Ultrasound may begin this relationship as early as the first trimester, although promoting maternal-fetal acquaintance is not a reason for ultrasound.

Prenatal attachment can be seen in such maternal behaviors as identifying the fetus as a separate individual; imagining the attributes of the fetus (eg, hair, eye color, personality); imagining the role of mother; selecting names for the baby; talking to the fetus; touching and stroking fetal parts as they are outlined against the abdomen; considering feeding methods; or calling the fetus by a pet name.

According to Rubin, the infant-to-be becomes prominent in the expectant mother's thoughts when the uterus rises out of the pelvis during the second trimester.[5] Quickening reorients the mother's attention and awareness to the growing baby in her uterus. Maternal perception of fetal movement is seen by Rubin as a form of "intimate communication" that no one but the pregnant woman can experience.[5] This private, pleasurable feeling may enhance the mother's love for the developing fetus.

There is growing speculation that the fetus, in some manner, also establishes a relationship with the mother before birth.[12] The fetus responds to such stimuli as music. Most studies, however, have focused on maternal responses during the third trimester (*see* Chapter 21).

Body Image

The woman's body image changes during the second trimester, as the signs of pregnancy become increasingly obvious.[13] During the first trimester, the fetus is viewed as part of the woman's body. After quickening the woman may begin to view the fetus as separate from her body.[14] During the second trimester, the mother wears maternity clothes from necessity, not for validation of pregnancy, as in the first trimester.

Body image during the second trimester is more gratifying and stable than in the first trimester.[5] The growth of the uterus is obvious to others; however, the woman's abdomen does not enlarge enough to cause discomfort, as in the third trimester. Abdominal prominence and weight gain represent "baby" to the woman (Figure 17–2).

During the second trimester the woman searches her body for additional physical signs of pregnancy. She may enjoy noting breast changes and is interested in deepening of pigmentation of the areolae. Striae, or stretch marks, are seldom viewed negatively during the second trimester as they too signify the growth of the baby.

ISSUES AND CONTROVERSIES

During the second trimester, much attention is directed toward facilitation of parental-fetal attachment. One issue is the proposed benefits of ultrasound in enhancing parent-fetal attachments. Is ultrasound visualization of the fetus an acceptable method for promoting attachment? Are better results achieved by teaching parents to note fetal movement and identify fetal body parts? (Identification of fetal movement and body parts does not expose the mother and fetus to unknown potential hazards.) On the other hand, is paternal-fetal attachment at a disadvantage because the father cannot "feel" his fetus move within him?

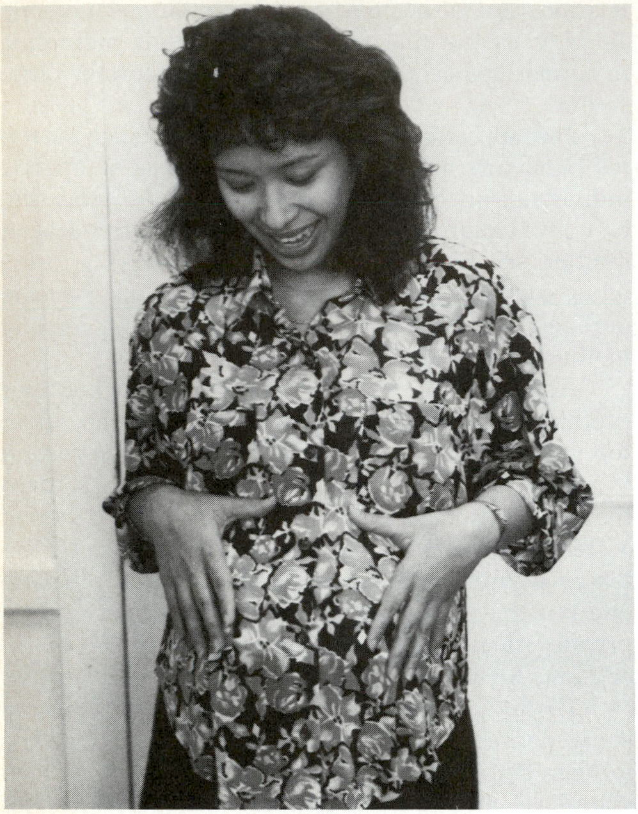

Figure 17–2. Abdominal prominence represents "baby" to the second-trimester woman.

The concept of body boundary can be studied in at least two ways: (1) the degree to which the body is perceived by the woman to be an effective barrier, and (2) the amount of space the body is perceived to occupy. The expectant woman's perception of her body boundary as a protective barrier or container for the fetus increases during the second trimester.[15] The woman also begins to see her body as potentially vulnerable to the environment. Crowded rooms may make the pregnant woman feel especially uncomfortable. Indeed, in busy, crowded clinics, second-trimester pregnant women may be observed to sit in defensive positions with their arms clasped around their sides.

Perception of body space, or how far the pregnant woman's body boundary seems to extend into her environment, is another way to assess body boundary and body image. The pregnant woman's perception of the large amount of space her body occupies does not necessarily coincide with her actual body size.[16,17]

Toward the end of the second trimester, the woman's body size is actually quite large. Her movements therefore may be impeded and she may feel increasingly vulnerable. Some women may try to curtail their social activities because of this, although there is no physiologic reason for doing so.

Time and Space

Perception of time and space during the second trimester is influenced primarily by quickening. This provides the companionship of a "real" fetus/baby and replaces the endless feeling of the first trimester.[5] Time has an identifiable present and an endpoint (delivery) in the future. According to Rubin, the growing fetus and changing hormones encourage feelings of serenity and composure in the woman's relation to time.[5] As the woman begins to focus on her fetus during the second trimester, she becomes more introspective and may be perceived as withdrawing from significant others as her attention shifts to her inner space.

THE FATHER'S EXPERIENCE

Psychologic Processes

As discussed in Chapter 4, the psychologic processes of expectant fathers can be divided into six stages based on specific time periods[18]: (1) the getting ready period, (2) conception, (3) the end of the first trimester, (4) midpregnancy, (5) the stage of turning toward father and fathering, and (6) the end of pregnancy. The first three stages were discussed in Chapter 13. The fourth and fifth stages occur during the second trimester of pregnancy.

PATERNAL PSYCHOLOGIC CHANGES AND CONCERNS DURING THE SECOND TRIMESTER

Psychologic Process
Stages include midpregnancy and turning toward own father and fathering role; father tries to clarify relationship with members of family of origin, especially own father; looks to own father as role model and for support

Fantasies
May parallel psychologic stages

Couvade Syndrome
High incidence; may include such symptoms as stomach ache and weight gain; pathology needs to be ruled out before couvade syndrome diagnosis is made

Body Boundaries
Perception of body boundaries blurs and may expand

During the midpregnancy stage, fathers who are "tuned in" to their feelings about pregnancy may report gastrointestinal symptoms.[18] (These may also be viewed as couvade symptoms, as discussed later.) Herzog found that some fathers report wishing they could both fertilize and bear a child; some may feel "emptiness" inside, experience greater appetite, increase their food consumption, and gain weight.[18]

During the second trimester, the father-to-be enters the stage of turning toward his own father and the fathering role. Between 15 and 25 weeks of pregnancy, "tuned in" fathers studied by Herzog reported increased pressure to sort out things with their families of origin.[18] There was special focus on the fathers' relationships with their own fathers (Figure 17–3). Expectant fathers seemed to want to reestablish ties with past generations of family. Without this sorting out phase, the men seemed to be less able to participate in expectant fatherhood.

Some similarities exist between the psychologic experiences of expectant mothers and fathers. For example, both mother and father seem to perform similar tasks of resolving issues with their families of origin and reestablishing relationships with the parent of the same sex. The manner of expression, degree, and type of parental need may differ between males and females; however, the expectant father needs the support of his father, as the expectant mother needs the support of her mother.

Fantasies

Very little information exists on paternal fantasies during the second trimester. Paternal fantasies during the second trimester are thought to parallel closely the psychologic stages and can provide insight into the expectant father's psychologic state. The expectant father during the second trimester is aware of the presence of the fetus. In addition to seeing the woman's enlarged abdomen, he may feel fetal movements and may hear the fetal heartbeat by pressing his ear against the woman's abdomen or by listening through a fetoscope or with a Doppler device, usually at prenatal visits. Ambivalent feelings about the woman may surface, possibly in relation to the way she looks or his feelings about becoming a father.

In one case during the midpregnancy stage, a father's dreams concerned symbolic representations of a "full uterus" that had no room for the father. His feelings also included increased emotional mood swings.

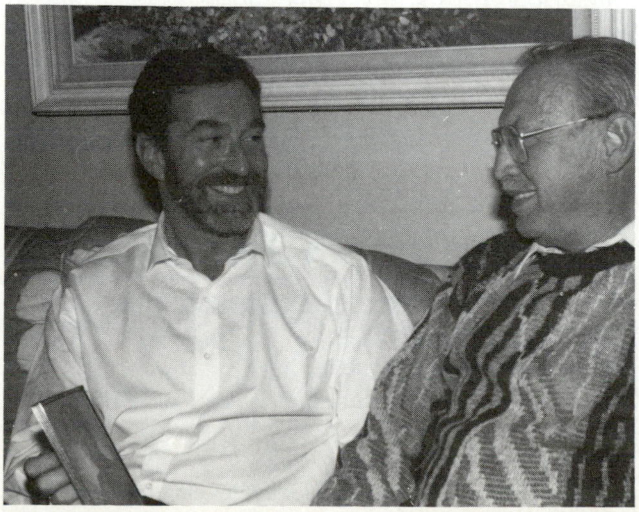

Figure 17–3. An expectant father reminisces with his own father.

Couvade Syndrome

Couvade symptoms are a dramatic expression of the father's involvement in pregnancy, as described in Chapter 13. Clinton was one of the few researchers to focus on couvade experiences by trimester.[19] During the second trimester, men in her study reported an average of 12.4 couvade symptoms per month. This is a higher number of symptoms than was reported during the first or third trimester or postpartum. Symptoms included stomachache and weight gain.

Although the couvade syndrome occurs widely in the United States, some men may worry that they are silly or abnormal. Nurses should assess for the presence of the couvade syndrome and provide reassurance that mild symptoms are real and normal. Any severe or persistent symptom, or any symptom accompanied by physical signs, for example, abdominal pain with fever, change in bowel patterns, or rectal bleeding, should be evaluated carefully.

Body Boundaries

The father's perceptions of his own body boundaries may begin to blur as his partner's pregnancy becomes increasingly evident[20,21]; however, the significance of this change is unclear.

THE FAMILY

The second trimester is often considered a "happy" time for the healthy pregnant client and her family. The now visible pregnancy does, however, produce concerns such as anxiety about medical care, childbirth, and future pregnancies.[22] Stress can be the result of biologic, psychologic, interpersonal, and sociocultural factors.[23] For example, the biologic stress of the growing pregnancy, the psychologic stress of

FAMILY'S EXPERIENCE DURING THE SECOND TRIMESTER

Generally a happy time

Visible pregnancy may evoke concerns such as health status, health care, or delivery

Sources of family stress include emotions related to life changes, altered body image, economic fears, career concerns, and quality of family relationships

accomplishing maternal tasks, interpersonal stress of moving into new roles, or conflict arising from cultural expectations or financial concerns may become apparent during the second trimester. Although stress may be present in some form throughout pregnancy, the nature of stress changes in each trimester.

The following are among the psychosocial and biologic factors that may produce stress during the second trimester.[24]

Emotions. The emotions that may accompany life change may produce stress in the family. Once the pregnancy and infant-to-be are a reality to them, the woman and her family acknowledge that life with an infant will be different and that they must undergo life changes. Indeed, pregnancy is a developmental crisis or challenge (*see* Chapter 13).

Body Image. The idealized woman in Western culture is young, thin, glamorous, sexy, and exciting.[24,25] Pursuit of the perfect body is stressful to many women. The growing abdomen and weight gain during the second trimester may contribute to the development of a negative body image,[13,15] if either or both the expectant mother and the expectant father view the pregnant body poorly. Conflict between the expectant parents therefore can be stressful for the entire family. (It is important to note that many men and women view prenatal changes as beautiful and enjoy a positive body image throughout pregnancy.)

Economic Concerns. During the second trimester, financial stresses may increase as the childbearing family anticipates expenditures related to the prenatal, delivery, and infant periods. For further discussion of socioeconomic factors, *see* discussion later in this chapter.

Career Concerns. During the second trimester, when pregnancy is readily apparent, the expectant mother may experience various types of discrimination at work. For example, she may be "passed over" for a promotion, because of perceived factors like the need for maternity leave, traditional prejudices about women with young children working, or "concerns" that a new mother might be too distracted to fulfill employment obligations. Although direct discrimination is not lawful in the United States, many other excuses, for example, "someone else was better for the job" and "the woman needs more experience," can be used. Although in certain cases these situations may be true, in others they can reflect employment prejudice toward pregnant women and women who intend to work after childbirth. Some companies assure women of continued employment; however, they may not be guaranteed their former jobs, but may face being shifted to other departments, according to company need.

During the second trimester, as the woman focuses more on the fetus, she may question how long she will work before delivery and when and whether she will return. Long-term career goals, employment policies, current career opportunities, and financial need influence these choices.

Perception of Quality of Relationship With Baby's Father and Significant Others. Perceived support from significant others, especially from the husband or baby's father, has been identified as a critical factor in prenatal adaptation.[3,26–29] A strong relationship with the baby's father has been theorized to help protect against the effects of high life stress and to promote better feelings about pregnancy and parenting.[27]

THE SIBLINGS' EXPERIENCE

Changes occurring physically and psychologically in the mother during the second trimester make pregnancy obvious to even the young child. Although the mother feels physically well during the second trimester, the child may feel deprived of the mother's attention as she psychologically focuses on aspects of her pregnancy and fetus.

SIBLINGS' EXPERIENCE DURING THE SECOND TRIMESTER

Become aware of pregnancy

Activities with mother may change as mother focuses inward

Responses depend on such factors as age and developmental patterns (psychosocial development, cognitive development, separation-individuation)

How the child experiences the mother's pregnancy depends largely on his or her stage of development. Three major developmental patterns may affect the sibling's experience of pregnancy:

- *Stage of psychosocial development.* According to Erikson, the growing child evolves behaviors that allow him or her to interact in social situations with others.[30] This process begins in infancy with parents and family and expands to others outside the family as the child grows to adolescence and adulthood. For conceptual ease, psychosocial development is subdivided into six stages.
- *Stage of cognitive development.* According to Piaget, cognitive development relates to ways in which a child develops thinking processes and the ability to solve problems.[31] Cognitive ability begins in infancy and continues to develop through adulthood.
- *Separation-individuation.* As described by Mahler, separation-individuation is the process by which the child becomes an independent and interdependent individual.[32] Not only is the person able successfully to function alone, but she or he can live and work with others.

All three developmental patterns begin in infancy and develop through childhood, adolescence, and adulthood. All involve mental and interactional processes; however, each pattern focuses on different, yet essential aspects of development. Along with physiologic maturation, they describe how children grow and develop.

Table 17–1 summarizes developmental patterns during childhood. Nurses need to understand developmental patterns to provide appropriate guidance to parents who are preparing a sibling for the new baby. An outline of developmental patterns is included in this chapter, because the second trimester is the time when children become aware of the mother's changing shape.

Guidelines for Preparation of Siblings

There is no "best" time for telling siblings about a pregnancy and birth. Pregnancy is readily apparent during the second trimester, and this may be the time couples choose to discuss a coming baby with a sibling. Sibling preparation is a topic of great concern to the healthy pregnant couple. Although negative sibling reactions to the prospect of a new baby have been discussed in the popular press and professional literature, many siblings respond to the news of the coming baby with interest and curiosity[33,34] (Figure 17–4). Through anticipatory guidance and counseling the nurse can provide some guidelines:

- Realize that there are normal psychologic changes related to childbearing. By understanding the inward focus of women during the second trimester, couples can take steps, such as providing extra attention, to ensure that the child does not feel rejected or left out.
- Identify ways in which psychologic changes related to pregnancy can conflict or coincide with the child's developmental patterns.
- Consider the child's age. As noted in Table 17–1, a child less than 3 years old may not understand the meaning of pregnancy or the abstract concept of future. Chronologic age, however, does not always coincide with developmental patterns. Discussion therefore needs to be based on assessment of each sibling.
- Realize the need of the sibling to continue to feel loved, wanted, and valued. This is important regardless of the age of the child, although the manner of expression varies with the child's developmental pattern.
- Realize that children should not be expected to shoulder adult responsibilities. Expectant parents need to understand that what may appear to be a small contribution to them, such as bringing a tired mother a glass of juice, may actually be seen as a large contribution by the child.
- Understand that news of a new baby may not be greeted with joy by the sibling. School-aged children may wonder what their own role will be, especially if they have no other siblings. Adolescents may be uncomfortable at the confirmation of their parents' sexuality or may worry about changes in their family. Strategies that include attention, loving support, and developmentally appropriate discussion can help the child to receive a sibling positively.
- Appreciate the value of sibling preparation aids, such as books and sibling preparation classes.

GRANDPARENTS' EXPERIENCE

During the second trimester, the couple's parents must also accept the reality of the pregnancy and the

GRANDPARENTS' EXPERIENCE DURING THE SECOND TRIMESTER

Accept reality of coming infant

Provide necessary support to couple

Deal with own feelings about infant and moving up a generation

TABLE 17–1. SUMMARY OF CHILDHOOD DEVELOPMENTAL PATTERNS AFFECTING THE SIBLING'S EXPERIENCE OF PREGNANCY

PSYCHOSOCIAL DEVELOPMENT (Erikson)[30]	
Basic Trust Versus Mistrust (Birth to 1 Year)	Infant gains basic sense of security in self and in surroundings. Infant needs to "receive and accept" attention, love, food, and so on. Infant has difficulty coping with decreased attention from primary caregiver (usually mother). Development of trust is the successful completion of this stage and is highly dependent on the caregiver. Mother's attention to another pregnancy creates a need for additional attention from others (such as father or grandparent).
Autonomy Versus Shame and Doubt (1 Year to 3 Years)	Child learns to control own body. Child develops a sense of "self." Child starts to balance autonomy with parents' wishes. Child needs much attention from caretakers to develop autonomy and avoid feelings of shame and doubt.
Initiative Versus Guilt (3 Years to 6 Years)	Child is becoming the type of person he or she will be later in life. Child wants to be like parents. Sexual curiosity develops; notes differences between parents. Child needs to maintain a sense of worth and initiative, while recognizing she or he is not a grownup. Child starts to develop a conscience. Child without adequate support can develop feelings of guilt. Child notices mother's pregnancy as a manifestation of being a woman. Child may ask sexually oriented questions, although she or he will not understand detailed answers. Child may make contact with others outside family if in a preschool program.
Industry Versus Inferiority (6 Years to 12 Years)	Child wants to learn all he or she can about the world. Child makes contact with people outside the family, especially through school, and develops friendships. Child is interested in making and collecting things; participation in team efforts becomes important. Child may worry about whether her or his efforts are valued; may have worries about being not good enough. Child is likely to be interested and pleased about mother's pregnancy and birth of baby, and may understand changes in mother. Child especially between ages 8 and 12, usually relates well to friends. Peer groups lessen the need for mother's attention. Child with a sense of "industry" may want to help prepare for the baby; can do simple chores, help select baby's name, and so on.
Identity Versus Identity Diffusion (12 Years to 18 Years)	Adolescent solidifies continuing personal sense of self. Adolescent may be threatened by "identity diffusion," that is, he or she feels unable to keep an independent sense of self, but gains identity only through cliques, organizations, or identification with "heroes." Adolescent with healthy sense of self may be excited about mother's pregnancy. Adolescent with fragile sense of self may be angry, ashamed, or jealous of mother's pregnancy. Adolescents will have stated or unstated questions about pregnancy and relationships. Parents may initiate discussion of sexuality, love, and marital bond with adolescents. Mother's pregnancy presents opportunity to help adolescent incorporate a model of mature sexual love, childbearing, and birth into his or her own identity.
COGNITIVE DEVELOPMENT (Piaget)[31]	
Sensorimotor Period (Birth to 2 Years)	Child progresses through action sequences in which the result of a behavior stimulates repetition of that behavior (especially when behavior is pleasing). Child learns to gain desired results by various willed activities. Action sequences are carried out in actual behavior alone; child does not think about them in complex manner. Child cannot really grasp cognitively the meaning of pregnancy. Child's experience of pregnancy is at a feeling level.

TABLE 17–1. SUMMARY OF CHILDHOOD DEVELOPMENTAL PATTERNS AFFECTING THE SIBLING'S EXPERIENCE OF PREGNANCY *(continued)*

Preoperational Stage (2 Years to 7 Years)	More complex thinking can take place, especially for the preschool and school-age child. Thinking is very concrete. Child tends to believe that everyone sees the world the same as he or she does (egocentrism). Child tends to think that real events have intentional causes, eg, the child causes rain by putting on a raincoat (called animism). Child views pregnancy in a simplistic, concrete way. Child is usually unable to understand abstract explanations of pregnancy. The 2- to 3-year old can perceive the growth of the mother's abdomen; however, understanding that there is a growing baby inside may be difficult. This becomes easier for children of 6 or 7. Time (past and future) is still a difficult concept, especially for children 2 to 5 years of age. Patience and repetition ("talks" with parents, age-appropriate sibling preparation books, and so on) needed to help child understand about future baby. Child may repeatedly ask the same questions. Questions need to be answered simply and concretely; explanations should be based on what a child can see.
Concrete Operations (7 Years to 11 Years)	Child develops reasoning ability. Child can conceive of events that would be impossible in the real world. Child has a better perception of time; he or she can go back in time or reverse the directions of a thought sequence. Child is less egocentric. Thought still depends on concrete experiences. Parents can discuss pregnancy and birth with child; explanations should be concrete and direct. Child will have specific questions about childbirth. Child may participate in preparation for baby.
Formal Operations (11 Years Onward)	Child can reason abstractly about things and events that cannot be represented in reality. Child is able to understand relationships beyond events and things represented in reality. Child can appreciate alternatives in any situation. Child can understand adult-type explanations about pregnancy and birth. Child can understand abstract notions, such as parental motivations for having another child. Child can participate in preparation for the baby; can assume greater responsibilities.
SEPARATION-INDIVIDUATION (Mahler)[32]	
Symbiosis (Pregnancy to after birth)	Closeness, "bondedness." Not applicable to sibling, as child must be at least 10 or 11 months old before sibling is born. Mother who remains in close symbiosis with baby as he or she develops may have difficulty attaching to the fetus in a future pregnancy.
Rapprochement (18 months to 2 years)	Child is aware of her or his growing separation and autonomy from parents. Child desires autonomy but may fear loss of mother; may cry when well liked babysitter arrives and mother leaves. Child has little tolerance for frustration. Child wants mother to participate in all activities even though he or she no longer requires this participation. Child may have "arguments" or tantrums if mother does not provide enough attention. Child may become more demanding as mother becomes more emotionally unavailable in relation to pregnancy; developmental phases of child and mother may thus be in conflict. Parents need to ensure that child receives adequate attention; parents need support to deal with demanding child behaviors.
Separation-Individuation (2 Years to 3 Years)	Continues; the child perceives self as a separate individual. The more separate and individuated the child is from the mother, the better is the child's ability to cope with pregnancy and a new sibling.

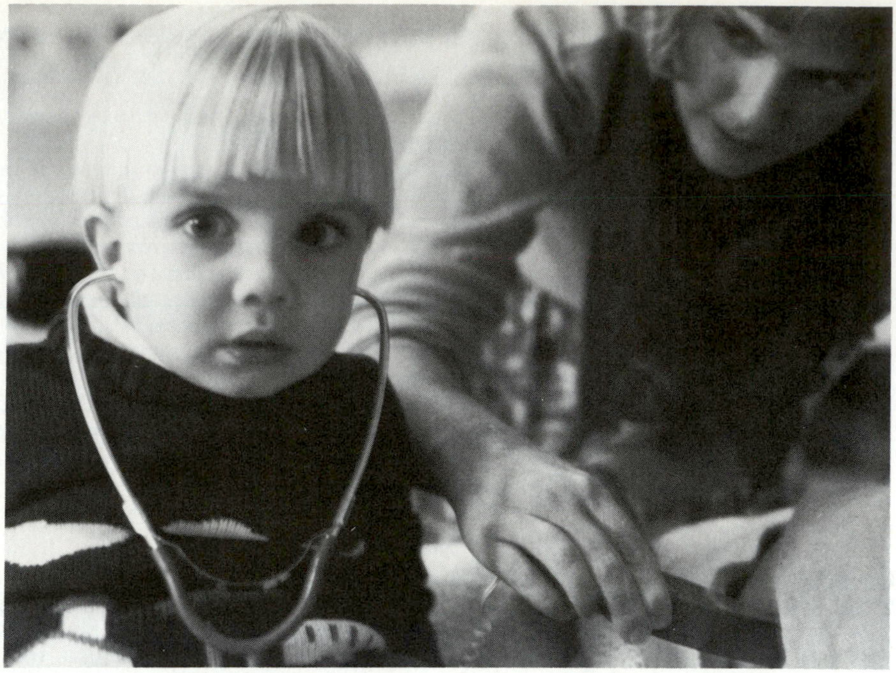

Figure 17–4. A 2½-year-old sibling responds to hearing the fetal heartbeat.

coming grandchild. Some grandparents-to-be express disappointment about not being informed sooner; others react with excitement about the prospect of a baby. Chapter 13 identified potential reactions of grandparents to news of pregnancy.

When feasible, the nurse can encourage the pregnant couple to bring the expectant grandparents to prenatal visits during the second trimester. A class for expectant grandparents may be devised, focusing on such topics as changes in obstetric care, the importance of the grandparenting role, and the bridging of generation gaps.[35] Literature can be made available at the classes or in waiting room areas. Grandparent support groups may provide an enjoyable setting for the sharing of thoughts and feelings about this developmental step. Current trends in American culture encourage more open sharing of information about childbirth than was widely available during the 1950s, 1960s, and early 1970s, when many of today's childbearing clients were born. Indeed, expectant grandparents may have need for information about developing pregnancy. In addition, expectant grandparents may need information about the psychologic changes of pregnancy and their own importance to their expectant daughter or son. In working with grandparents-to-be, the nurse must remain sensitive to cultural patterns of communication between the expectant parents and grandparents, especially with respect to presence during physical examination.

SOCIOCULTURAL FACTORS

Cultural patterns exist in nearly every family and affect internal family dynamics and interactions with others in the environment. Health care providers working with the pregnant family during the second trimester must therefore understand cultural proscriptions surrounding family members during childbearing. In addition, nurses should be aware of the influence of socioeconomic factors on the childbearing family.

In Chapter 13, the black family was used to illustrate how membership in a specific cultural group may affect perceptions and practices during pregnancy and childbirth. In this chapter, the Japanese-American family is considered as one example of East Asian cultural groups.

Socioeconomic Factors

Financial stresses may increase during the second trimester. For example, a maternity wardrobe is needed. Maternity clothes are costly, especially if the woman requires winter coats or "business" type clothing. Many women who dress professionally do not enjoy economic freedom. In addition, the cost of prenatal care, delivery, and infant care present economic stresses. Not every family has full and unrestricted maternity and pediatric care insurance coverage. Family lifestyle may depend on income from the expectant mother's job. The prospect of maternity leave, often at reduced pay or no pay, may become an economic concern during the second trimester. Women who work in areas considered unsafe during advanced pregnancy, such as construction jobs or jobs that require physical balance, may face transfer to other areas or layoffs. Lack of benefits for part-time work makes potential loss of employment especially stressful.[1]

East Asian Cultural Groups

Japanese, Chinese, Korean, and Vietnamese are a few of the many cultural groups that originated in East and Southeast Asia; there are numerous sub-groups within each of these groups, as well. In addition to readily apparent differences in physical characteristics and language, East Asians differ greatly from other cultural groups in the United States, especially in philosophic approaches to life. These approaches are generally influenced by traditional belief systems, for example, Confucianism and Buddhism.[36]

East Asian philosophic systems do not tend to stress the individual's independence and autonomy, but rather emphasize that the wishes of the individual are superceded by those of the family.[36] The East Asian family adheres to the tradition of specific hierarchic roles with formal rules of behavior for all members. Each person's response and loyalty to this code are more a reflection of the family than of the individual. The extended family then is responsible for maintaining the status of the family. All relationships, such as those among husband and wife and parents and children, have particular definitions. Males are valued more than females, and there are different expectations for men and for women.[36]

In addition to the broad distinction between East Asian and Western cultures, each of the many East Asian groups is unique. East Asian groups differ in vital developmental aspects of life, such as language, history, and social and economic backgrounds.[36,37] People from the different groups are unique and need to be assessed individually; however, an understanding of common features of family structure gives the nurse a starting point for a plan of care. Nursing care planning can then be tailored to the specific needs of each family and client. Further assessment is based on key factors, including the family's social class, geographical origin, birthplace, and generation of family members living in the United States. Broad cultural concepts are most applicable when considering recent immigrants and others with strong traditional ties. Although East Asians born in the United States may be considered to be more assimilated into the "American" culture, they may yet retain deep cultural ties to their East Asian heritage and practices.

Time. In the United States, the primary family unit is the nuclear family, which has a time-limited life span. In other words, the nuclear family dissolves when children grow to adulthood and have their own families and when their parents die. Unlike the American family, the East Asian family is not time limited. For the East Asian person, the family extends both backward and forward in time. The individual is seen as the product of all the generations of his or her family since the beginning of time. Because of the extended sense of family existence, a person's behavior has a different meaning than does the behavior of a person from a nuclear family. For the Asian, personal actions reflect not only on the individual, the immediate family, and the extended family, but also on all preceding generations and all future generations of the family. East Asians thus may perceive responsibility that goes far beyond personal concerns.[36]

Marriage. Marriage and choice of a partner are also different for the Asian person. The family of both partners may greatly influence the choice of partners. This is true even among East Asians living in the United States. Marriage does not necessarily mark the beginning of a new nuclear family unit. Marriage may instead be viewed as a continuation of the man's family line. The woman is considered to have left her family of origin on her marriage and to have been absorbed into her husband's family. In this arrangement her status as a young wife may be low. From this perspective, cultural emphasis on male children as preferable to females can be better understood. Indeed, a male expands the family even after his marriage, whereas a daughter represents a reduction of the family.

Family Roles. Within the traditional East Asian family, roles are clearly defined. The father is the leader. He makes decisions, has responsibility for the "success or failure" of the family's well-being and status, and enforces family rules. His authority was traditionally unquestioned by other family members. To his children, he may be a stern disciplinarian.

The mother, on the other hand, nurtures husband and children. East Asian women have not been free to engage in the same kinds of work and activities as men. Care of the family and childrearing are the mother's traditional roles. Children establish the strongest emotional tie to their mother. This emotional tie has importance later in the mother's life, in case the father dies and the oldest son becomes the family leader. The oldest son's great emotional attachment to his mother influences his behavior to fulfill her wishes. Thus, East Asian women often have much power, albeit covertly, through their influence on men. Indeed, they have much power over their daughters-in-law.

Children in East Asian families also have defined roles. The most important role is that of eldest son, who is groomed to become the family leader. He may be treated better than other children, has authority over them, and commands their respect. He also has much responsibility and is expected to be a role model. His siblings are expected to follow his guidance, even as adults. In traditional Asian families, daughters are not valued as highly as sons, possibly because they join their husbands' families at the time of marriage. The daughter's role is primarily caretaker of the home. There has, however, been some change and loosening of tradition as attitudes toward women change. Daughters now do have some freedom in choice of a partner and career. In some families, a daughter may fill the role of eldest, if the oldest son vacates his role as leader or if there are no male heirs.

One consideration for maternity nursing is the East Asian husband's lack of involvement during pregnancy and birth. This separation of men's and women's roles is mutually agreeable in traditional families. Although traditional patterns of interaction are being influenced by increased contact with the West, they nevertheless remain. Westernized Asian women may desire greater involvement of their husbands when their husbands are reluctant to participate and this may be a potential source of conflict. Shared childbirth is a cultural value; nurses must not try to impose their own value systems on any cultural group.

Family Dimensions. Among other important dimensions of traditional East Asian family life are the concepts of obligation, shame, and communication.[36] These concepts may affect the nurse's interactions with East Asian families during pregnancy.

Obligation. Traditionally, East Asians do not tend to see themselves as self-reliant, self-sufficient individuals in the same way individuals from a Western culture might see themselves. Instead, East Asians may view themselves as products of their relationships to nature and to other people. To maintain harmony in relationships with others, the concept of obligation is vital. Obligation arises through ascribed roles or status and through helpful or kind actions toward another person. This person then incurs obligation. The greatest obligation of the East Asian is to parents.

Shame. Shame and shaming reinforce societal expectations and proper behavior in traditional East Asian society. The desire to avoid "loss of face" is a powerful motivating force.

Communication Process. Western society values the ability to express ideas and feelings openly. The process of communication is very different for people of the East Asian cultures. What may be communicated between people is determined by specific characteristics of those individuals. Some characteristics that determine individuals' relationships to each other and their manner of communication are age, sex, education, occupation, social status, family background, marital status, and parenthood. These specific characteristics influence both verbal and nonverbal communication patterns between people, for example, who can begin a conversation or who must be most accommodating and tolerant. Ambiguous situations in which the East Asian may not know the attributes of the person to whom he or she is speaking may cause anxiety. Often, this anxiety is due to the fear of making a social error in speech and thus losing face. In such situations, the East Asian may withdraw, be silent, and watch for cues from the unknown individual.[36] Certain health care providers, especially physicians, may be regarded with respect because of their knowledge. The East Asian client may feel that questions present challenges and therefore should be avoided. American health care providers working with the childbearing client usually expect questions. Differences in communication expectations may unfortunately result in the health care provider's assumption that the client has no questions and the client's fear that the health care provider will be insulted if questions are asked. The health care provider with an understanding of cultural communication patterns might offer information in a manner culturally acceptable to the client. The nurse working with East Asian clients must appreciate the importance of harmony in relationships for East Asian people. Directness may lead to disagreement, disharmony, and loss of face for both client and health care provider. Direct confrontation is therefore avoided whenever possible. East Asian people often rely on the sensitivity of the conversation, as they are able to do. Such sensitivity requires that both people be familiar with the culture.[36]

Family Transition. Transition to the culture of the United States can be difficult for East Asians, because of the very different life philosophies of East Asian and North American families. Family members may experience conflict and grief-type reactions. These reactions may comprise six stages[36]:

1. Cultural shock, resulting from differences between what was expected in the United States and what really exists, especially if expectations were for a better economic life
2. Disappointment about what exists
3. Grief at separation and loss of what was left behind
4. Depression because of the current family situation
5. Acceptance of the current situation
6. Mobilization of family resources and energy to cope with the new environment

The last stage may be difficult, as the family may try to use familiar traditional problem-solving methods that worked in their former culture, but may not be effective in the United States. The nurse must keep this in mind when attempting to use crisis intervention techniques with East Asian families.

Not all families or all family members pass through the six stages. In ideal circumstances, the acculturated family comes to value both the old and the new culture.

The Nurse's Role. The East Asian family can be very different structurally from the typical family in the United States. The nurse must assess the unique nature of any pregnant East Asian family to avoid stereotyping. The extent of the East Asian family's acculturation in the United States affects nursing actions.

Nurses in prenatal clinics may attempt to counsel a traditionally oriented pregnant East Asian woman on prenatal diet and medications. If this woman follows traditional family practices, she may not be the correct person for the nurse to address concerning family or individual dietary changes. The husband's role as leader of the family may require him to "approve" dietary changes. The husband may decide whether it is necessary to consult his mother, as she has a major influence on the manner in which the husband may make family decisions. It may be unwise to try to convince the pregnant East Asian client to go against her mother-in-law's wishes; this may end in the pregnant woman's avoiding American prenatal care altogether.

The nurse who works with an ethnic or cultural population must learn about specific cultural family patterns. If not, the nurse's culturally ignorant behaviors might have undesired results.

Cultural Focus: The Japanese-American Family

Japanese-American families comprise a cultural group which came originally from the East Asian cultural tradition. These families challenge the nurse's sociocultural assessment skills. Adherence to traditional cultural beliefs and practices may vary depending on how many generations of the family has lived in the United States. The majority of third-, fourth-, and fifth-generation Japanese Americans are well assimilated into the dominant North American culture; however, extent of assimilation may vary with socioeconomic status, geographic location, and where the person has been educated (Japan or the United States). Okamoto describes the generations of Japanese Americans.[38] The first generation, or the original Japanese immigrants, called the *Issei,* migrated to the United States in the early 1900s. The *Nisei,* or the second generation, are all descendants born to Japanese immigrants in the United States. Specifically, the term designates the offspring of the pioneer Issei of the 1900s. The third generation of Japanese-Americans born in the United States is the *Sansei,* the fourth is the *Yonsi,* and the fifth is the *Gosei.* The term *Kibei* designates Japanese Americans born in the United States who were sent back to Japan to be educated. This practice was fairly common between 1920 and 1940.

Okamoto interviewed women from various generations about their attitudes and beliefs about pregnancy, birth, and childbearing.[38] She concluded that Japanese Americans have managed pregnancy and birth in a variety of ways. Certain aspects of traditional Japanese beliefs, affiliations, and practices are retained; others are replaced by those of their sociocultural environment. Each woman interviewed, regardless of her generation, kept some ethnic affiliation and identity. Ethnicity was demonstrated in food preparation, use of the Japanese language in the home, and participation in traditional rituals or practices related to pregnancy and birth. Although this sample represented three generations with diverse levels of acculturation, all women retained a strong affiliation to the Japanese identity.

In general, Japanese-American women sought and received prenatal care similar to that obtained by members of the dominant culture. All generations saw pregnancy and birth as natural events. Further, Japanese-American women in this sample seemed to take a more active, pragmatic interest in health education concerning the pregnancy cycle than many members of the dominant culture.

Belief in the Western health care model was quite evident in this sample, especially among the Sansei. Younger women stated that they would have liked an Asian birth attendant. Okamoto concluded that the cultural assimilation process was quite complete in this sample. There was nearly total acceptance of majority culture practices concerning pregnancy or a blending with traditional ethnic values. Okamoto warns, however, that "care must be taken not to assume that assimilation to Western culture entails the rejection of ethnic identity and values.[38] Indeed, the highly assimilated Sansei often desire to recover elements of the culture of Japan. Although Japanese Americans have shown altered values and behaviors over time, much still remains unclear concerning ethnically based aspects of the Japanese American.

In many ways, Japanese-American families see pregnancy in the same manner as do North American families of the dominant culture; however, as pregnancy involves the extended family, being of Japanese background may produce some changes in the psychologic processes involved in becoming parents. For example, although many childbearing Japanese-American women may be highly assimilated, there is no guarantee that their mothers are also assimilated into the dominant culture. Traditional attitudes and values may still prevail in the grandmother's life. This traditional orientation may greatly affect the pregnant woman's relationship with her mother and her mother's availability to her, especially if the expectant grandmother sees her daughter as "belonging" to her husband's family. A mother-in-law may expect to control the expectant mother's decisions concerning pregnancy and childbearing. This may cause conflict between generations. The nurse should assess the cultural orientation and level of assimilation not only of the expectant mother, but also of her partner and both maternal and paternal families of origin.

Specific cultural practices place emphasis on rest and warmth during pregnancy. For example, pregnant Japanese women may wear knee socks for warmth. Beginning around the fifth month, traditional women may use a white abdominal binder (*obi*) as an undergarment to promote warmth.

During the second trimester, when the pregnancy becomes apparent, culturally related conflicts may arise between generations. Other potential problems in the Japanese-American family during pregnancy may be geographic separation of the nuclear family from families of origin. If unable to be united with their families, Japanese Americans may experience a sense of isolation at this time.

SUMMARY

For the low-risk, healthy family, the second trimester of pregnancy tends to be a period marked by contentment and acceptance of the pregnancy. In moving toward attainment of the maternal role, the woman continues processes of replication, internalization, and fantasy. Fantasies help the pregnant woman to bind-in to her baby and also illustrate her special concerns. The woman's relationship with her own mother assumes increasing importance to her. The woman's relationship with her fetus is enhanced by such factors as quickening, continued fetal activity, and the enlarging uterus. As pregnancy progresses, the woman becomes increasingly aware of her expanding size, although body image can be more gratifying than in the first trimester. Pregnancy seems to have a definite end point; the woman begins to focus inward.

Expectant fathers pass through the psychologic stages of midpregnancy and turning toward father and fathering. Couvade symptoms may be experienced. Like expectant mothers, expectant fathers begin to place increasing attention on their relationship with the parent of the same sex, although factors such as the manner of expression and type of parental need differ. The expectant father also experiences fantasies and changes in body boundaries during the second trimester.

Stresses on the expectant family come from sources such as emotional reactions to life changes or body image, and economic or career concerns. Quality of relationship with the expectant father and significant others affect maternal prenatal adaptation at this time.

During the second trimester, pregnancy becomes obvious to even the young child. A child's reactions to pregnancy depend on such factors as the age of the child and the stages of psychosocial and cognitive development, and the degree of separation-individuation. Anticipatory guidance and counseling can help the couple prepare the sibling for the coming infant. Sibling preparation classes and literature can be especially helpful.

Whenever appropriate, the participation of expectant grandparents is encouraged. Attendance at prenatal visits, literature for grandparents, and expectant grandparent programs are some ways to foster their involvement.

Socioeconomic factors, especially financial stress, have a profound effect on an expectant family's adaptation to the second trimester of pregnancy. Cultural background continues to influence beliefs and behaviors as pregnancy progresses. The importance of understanding each family's unique cultural background is emphasized.

REVIEW QUESTIONS

1. Discuss four tasks the expectant woman must accomplish to attain the maternal role.
2. Describe the maternal-fetal relationship during the second trimester of pregnancy.
3. Cite two examples of the expectant father's psychologic experiences during the second trimester of pregnancy.
4. Identify the types of reactions children may have to pregnancy.
5. Describe psychologic responses of grandparents during the second trimester.

REFERENCES

1. Bryant H. Antenatal counseling for women working outside the home. *Birth.* 1985;12:227–232.
2. Tiedje LB, Collins C. Combining employment and motherhood. *Matern-Child Nurs.* 1989;14:9–14.
3. Caplan G. *Concepts of Mental Health and Consultation.* Washington, DC: US Department of Health, Education, Welfare; 1969.
4. Lederman RP. *Psychosocial Adaptation in Pregnancy.* Englewood Cliffs, NJ: Prentice-Hall; 1984.
5. Rubin R. *Maternal Identity and the Maternal Experience.* New York: Springer Publishing Co; 1984.
6. Krippner S, et al. An investigation of dream content during pregnancy. *J the Am Soc Psychosomat Dent Med.* 1974; 21:111–123.
7. Winget C, Kapp F. Manifest dream content and length of labor. Paper presented at the First International Congress of Sleep and Dreams; 1971; Bruges, Belgium.
8. Sherwen LN. Fantasies during the third trimester of pregnancy. *Am J Matern Child Nurs.* 1981;6:398–401.
9. Rubin R. Fantasy and object constancy in maternal relations. *Matern Child Nurs J.* 1972;2:101–111.
10. Martell LK: The mother-daughter relationship during daughter's first pregnancy: the transition experience. *Holistic Nursing Practice.* 1990;4:47–55.
11. Patsdaughter CA, Killien M. Developmental transitions in adulthood: mother-daughter relationships. *Holistic Nursing Practice.* 1990;4:37–46.
12. Verny T. The psycho-technology of pregnancy and labor. *Neonat Network.* April 1985:12–22.
13. Schuzman E. Body image in pregnancy. In: Sherwen LN, ed. *Psychosocial Dimensions of the Pregnant Family.* New York: Springer Publishing Co; 1987.
14. Tanner L. Developmental tasks of pregnancy. In: Bergersen B, et al, eds. *Current Concepts in Clinical Nursing.* St. Louis, Mo: CV Mosby; 1969.
15. Gray L. *A Study of Pregnancy: Body Image and Anxiety.* Los Angeles: California School of Professional Psychology; 1977. Doctoral dissertation.
16. Fawcett J. The relationship between identification and patterns of change in spouse's body images during and after pregnancy. *Int J Nurs Stud.* 1977;14:199–213.
17. Shuzman E. *Body Image with Respect to Completion of Psychological Tasks of Pregnancy.* Cleveland, Ohio: Case Western Reserve University; 1980. Master's thesis.
18. Herzog JM. Patterns of expectant fatherhood: A study of the fathers of a group of premature infants. In: Cath S, et al, eds. *Father and Child.* Boston: Little, Brown; 1982.
19. Clinton J. Expectant fathers at risk of couvade. *Nurs Res.* 1986;35:290–295.
20. Colman LL. Psychology of pregnancy. In: Sonstegard L, et al, eds. *Women's Health: Childbearing.* New York: Grune & Stratton, 1983.
21. Fawcett J. Body image and the pregnant couple. *Am J Matern Child Nurs.* 1978;3:227–233.
22. Glazer G. Anxiety levels and concerns among pregnant women. *Res Nurs Health.* 1980;3:107–113.
23. Jenkins C. Psychosocial modifiers of response to stress. *J Hum Stress.* 1979;5:3–15.
24. Callison T. Understanding and managing stress. In: Littlefield V, ed. *Health Education for Women.* Norwalk, Conn: Appleton-Century-Crofts; 1986.
25. Sherwen LN. An investigation into the effects of psychoprophylactic method training and locus of control on fantasy production and body cathexis in the primiparous woman. In: Sherwen L, Toussie-Weingarten C, eds. *Analysis and Application of Nursing Research: Parent-Neonate Studies.* Monterey, Calif: Wadsworth Health Sciences; 1983.
26. Weingarten CT, et al. Married mothers' perceptions of their premature or term infants and the quality of their relationships with their husbands. *J Obstet Gynecol Neonat Nurs.* 1990;19:64–73.
27. Mac-Elveen-Hoehn P, Eyres SJ. Social support and vulnerability: State of the art in relation to families and children. In: Barnard K et al, eds. *Social Support and Families of Vulnerable Infants.* Birth Defects Series 20:11–29. White Plains, NY:March of Dimes, 1984.
28. Tilden V. The relation of life stress and social support to emotional disequilibrium during pregnancy. *Res Nurs Health.* 1983;6:167–74.
29. Brown MA. Support, health and stress in expectant mothers and fathers. *West J Nurs Res.* 1984;6:28.
30. Erikson E. *Childhood & Society.* New York: Norton; 1963.
31. Piaget J. *Genetic Epistemology.* New York: Columbia University Press; 1970.
32. Mahler M, et al. *The Psychological Birth of the Human Infant.* New York: Basic Books; 1975.
33. Kutzner SK. Responses of siblings to pregnancy. In: Sherwen LN, ed. *Psychosocial Dimensions of the Pregnant Family.* New York: Springer Publishing Co; 1987:177–192.
34. Dunn J. *Sisters and Brothers.* Cambridge, Mass: Harvard University Press; 1985.
35. Maloni JA, et al. Expectant grandparent class. *J Obstet Gynecol Neonat Nurs.* 1987;16:26–35.
36. Shon S, Ja D. Asian families. In: McGoldrick M, Pearce J, Giordano J, eds. *Ethnicity and Family Therapy.* New York: Guilford Press; 1982.
37. Choi E. Unique aspects of Korean American mothers. *J Obstet Gynecol Neonat Nurs.* 1986;15:394–400.
38. Okamoto N. The Japanese American. In: Clark A, ed. *Culture, Childbearing, Health Professionals.* Philadelphia: FA Davis; 1978.

Assessment During the Second Trimester

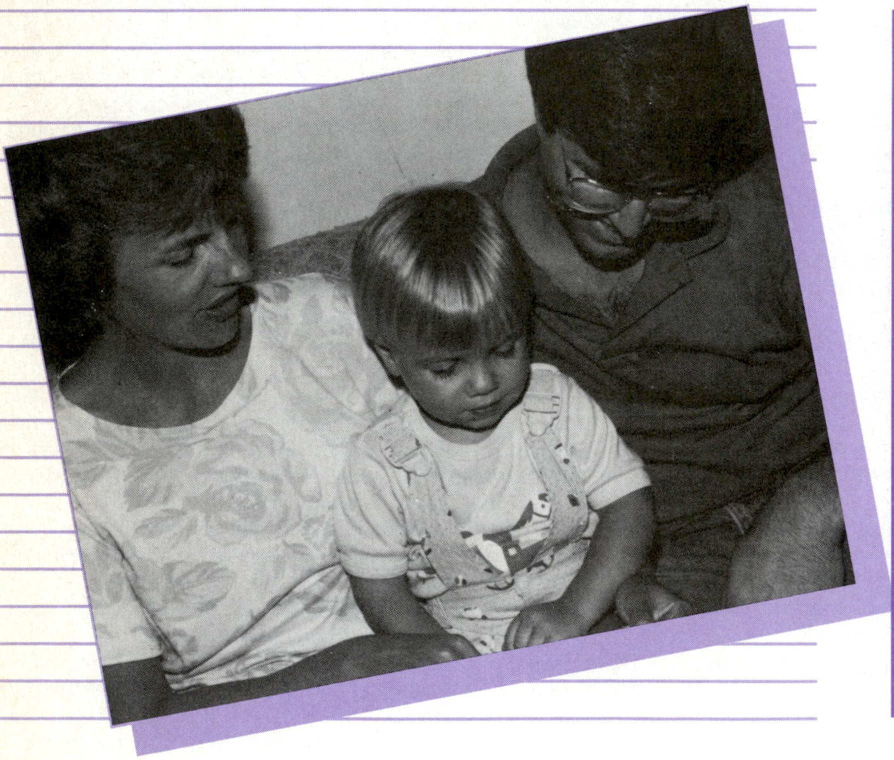

Chapter 18

Key Terms

alpha-fetoprotein
amniocentesis
fetoscopy
neural tube defects
percutaneous umbilical blood sampling
quickening

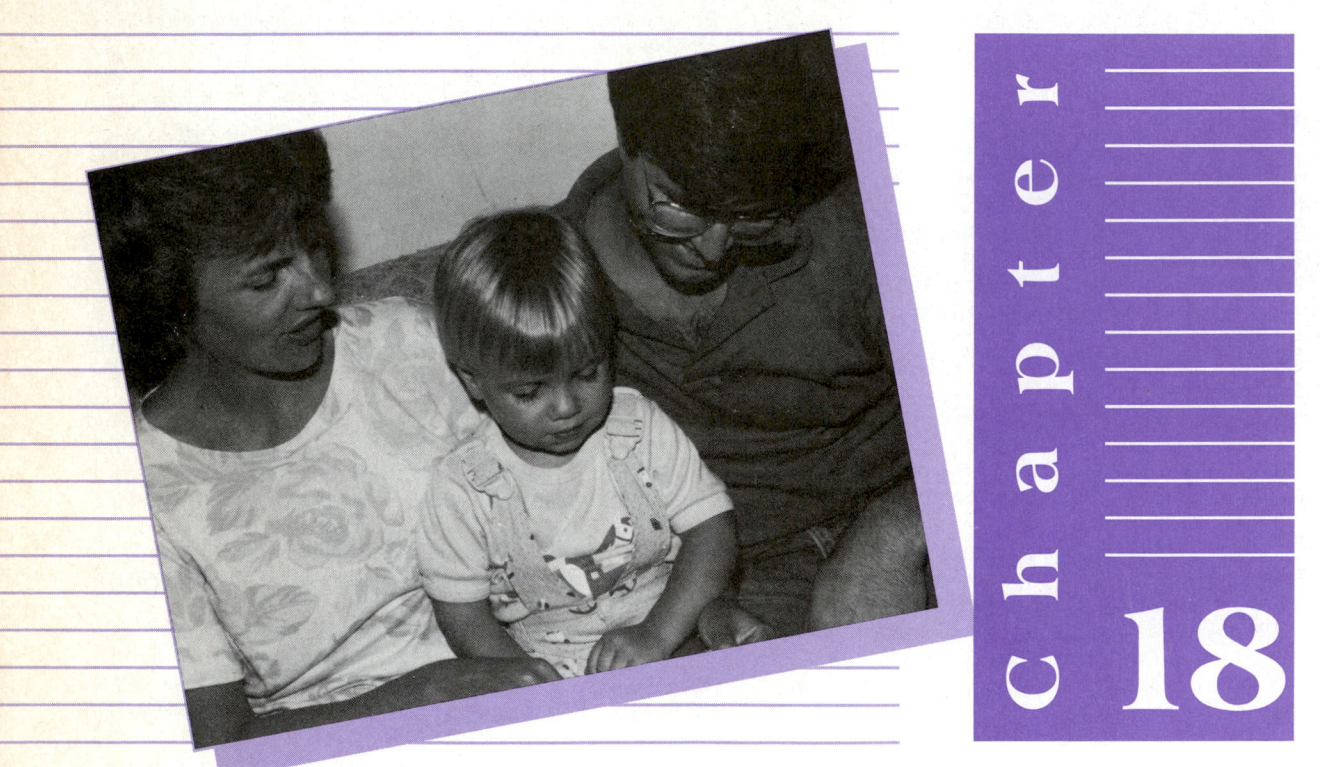

By the beginning of the second trimester, the woman with an uncomplicated pregnancy optimally will have seen her health care provider two or three times. During the second trimester the healthy woman will be assessed every 4 weeks. The pregnant family may have additional contact with health care providers through attendance at prenatal education classes during this period. Prenatal care during the second trimester is designed to monitor fetal and maternal adaptations to pregnancy and to identify and to intervene with clients at risk. Several goals for assessment are therefore developed to guide this process. Table 18–1 lists some targets of assessment during the second trimester.

In providing care to the pregnant client during the second trimester, the nurse may obtain information to update the health history, participate in physical assessment by evaluating physiologic parameters such as blood pressure and fetal heart rate, provide information related to current and future prenatal needs, and offer referrals to a variety of health and community resources such as childbirth education programs.

THE WOMAN WHO BEGINS PRENATAL CARE DURING THE SECOND TRIMESTER

Women may begin care during the second trimester for a variety of reasons, including lack of awareness of being pregnant, travel or residence during early pregnancy in areas where prenatal care was not accessible, financial concerns, fear of health care systems, and fear of confirmation of pregnancy. The assessment approach used for the initial visit during the first trimester is employed for the client at whatever point in pregnancy she first seeks care. In addition, reasons for delay in seeking care are assessed. Nurs-

TABLE 18–1. TARGETS OF ASSESSMENT DURING THE SECOND TRIMESTER

Maternal adaptations to pregnancy
Development of new risk factors
Effects of existing risk factors on the pregnant family
Fetal well-being
Psychosocial status and adaptations to pregnancy
Educational needs
Resources available to the pregnant client and her family

Source: Reference 1.

ing diagnoses and interventions are based on the unique needs of the client during the second trimester.

ASSESSMENT OF MATERNAL ADAPTATIONS TO PREGNANCY

Updating the Health History

During the first trimester, the client history was thoroughly assessed by health care providers. Ideally, a collaborative approach continues to be used. Current records that document physiologic and psychosocial findings and related interventions must be maintained. Accurate records chronicle progress during pregnancy, identify management strategies, and provide for early identification and treatment of risk factors throughout pregnancy.

The care plan was based in part on information obtained from the client's initial history, taken by the nurse-midwife, physician, or staff nurse. As the woman returns for subsequent visits in the second trimester, her history and care plan (for example, with respect to nutrition and exercise/activity) are revised in response to changes.

Physiologic Assessment

Prenatal visits are recommended every 4 weeks during the second trimester for the healthy, low-risk client. Assessment of the healthy client is performed in a prenatal clinic, private office, or birth center setting. Clients with high-risk conditions are seen more frequently. Care for high-risk clients is given in settings and by staff prepared to meet high-risk needs.

During each prenatal visit, a standard set of parameters is assessed to obtain information about maternal physiologic adaptations to pregnancy and fetal well-being. Table 18–2 lists parameters assessed at each visit during the second trimester. In addition, certain screening tests may be performed during the second trimester. Serum alpha-fetoprotein levels, described later in this chapter, may be drawn around 16 weeks to detect conditions such as neural tube defects in the fetus.[2] As diabetes in pregnancy is believed to be related to maternal age, the American College of Obstetricians and Gynecologists recommends diabetic screening for all pregnant women over age 30 and any pregnant woman with risk factors such as family history of diabetes, obesity, glycosuria, hypertension, previous delivery of a stillborn, and malformed or macrosomic infant.[1,3] A recent trend, however, is for diabetic screening of all pregnant women. For example, Coustan and associates found that 70 (56 percent) of 125 cases of gestational diabetes identified were less than 30 years of age.[4] Forty-four (35 percent) of the gestational diabetics would not have been diagnosed if screening criteria had been followed.

TABLE 18–2. PHYSIOLOGIC PARAMETERS ASSESSED DURING THE SECOND TRIMESTER

Assessment Parameter	Frequency of Assessment	Purpose
Vital signs, including blood pressure, pulse, respiration	Monthly	Detect any changes from normal/baseline that may indicate development of complications (eg, pre-eclampsia)
Uterine growth, measured by fundal height; fetal well-being, measured by fetal heart tones and, after quickening, fetal movement	Monthly	Assess for disproportionate enlargement, which may indicate multiple gestation, inadequate fetal nutrition, and so on; assess location and quality of fetal heart tones (fetal heart tones and activity indicate fetal well-being)
Maternal weight and nutritional status	Monthly	Assess pattern of weight gain and nutritional adequacy and detect fluid retention
Urinalysis for protein and glucose	Monthly	Detect development of complications (eg, pre-eclampsia and need for diabetic screening)
Suggested blood studies		
Alpha-fetoprotein	16 weeks	Screen for neural tube defects
Glucose	24–28 weeks	Screen for diabetes

During second-trimester visits, the nurse may obtain the client's blood pressure, pulse, respirations, and weight and may test urine for protein and glucose. In some settings, staff nurses, nurse practitioners, nurse-midwives, or physicians may draw blood samples in the clinic or office. In other settings, blood samples are drawn by technicians in the clinic, office, or laboratory. Fundal height and fetal heart rate are usually measured by the nurse practitioner or physician.

Knowledge about normal and abnormal findings and their relation to physiologic adaptations is necessary so that effective interventions can be planned and implemented. Table 18–3 presents an overview of nursing assessment of maternal physiology during the second trimester.

TABLE 18–3. SELECTED CLINICAL FINDINGS DURING THE SECOND TRIMESTER

Body System	Clinical Findings
Integumentary	Darkened breasts and areolae, chloasma (mask of pregnancy); linea nigra; increased perspiration; stretch marks; hot flashes (cutaneous flushing of skin); hair seems to thicken and nails grow faster; flushing
Cardiovascular	Increase in heart rate of an average of 10–15 beats per minute over nonpregnant rate
	Decrease in blood pressure from baseline during first 24 weeks of an average of 5 mm Hg systolic and 10 mm Hg diastolic
	Supine hypotension may occur and be accompanied by nausea, lightheadedness, tachycardia, sweating
	Increased splitting of heart sound with loudness of S_1, S_2; systolic murmur may be heard
	Dependent edema of the legs; edema that disappears after elevating legs; hemorrhoids; varicose veins in legs, vulva
Respiratory	Dyspnea on exertion; respiratory rate 16–24 per minute
Hematologic	Hgb 11 g/dL or greater; Hct 32 g/dL or greater
Gastrointestinal	Constipation
	Pyrosis (heartburn)
	Hemorrhoids
	Hypercholesterolemia; lipid intolerance
Musculoskeletal	Backache, especially in lower sacral area
	Pregnancy "waddle"; loosening of pelvic joints
Urinary	Nocturnal voiding
	Trace glycosuria
	Trace proteinuria
Reproductive	Progressive enlargement of uterus
	Round ligament pain
	Braxton Hicks contractions
	Vaginal leukorrhea
	Breasts—fullness, tingling, and heaviness; colostrum may appear; everted nipples
Neurologic	Alert, appropriate
	Normal (+1 to +2) deep tendon reflexes in all four extremities

Risk Assessment

Assessment of risk factors continues at each prenatal visit, because high-risk conditions can appear at any time during pregnancy. Early identification of the woman with a complication is necessary to minimize poor maternal-fetal or neonatal outcome.[5,6] Second-trimester risk assessment focuses on current pregnancy risk factors, and any changes in physiologic, psychosocial, demographic, lifestyle, or socioeconomic factors. Table 18–4[1,7] lists risk factors that may be identified during the second trimester. These factors are identified from interviews, physical examinations, laboratory studies, and prenatal diagnostic tests. The plan of care should be designed to reduce risk factors or the effects of risk factors. For example, if the mother smokes during the second trimester, the nurse may discuss possible strategies for smoking cessation and provide referral to smoking cessation programs.

Biochemical Screening Techniques

Urinalysis. At each prenatal visit, a freshly voided urine specimen is assessed for the presence of protein, glucose, and ketones. The nurse may perform this analysis with a laboratory kit (usually a dipstick) that detects the presence of such substances. If a urinary tract infection is suspected through the report of symptoms, such as painful and frequent urination, fever, or lower back pain, a clean catch urine specimen should be obtained for microscopic study and culture.

The healthy woman does not have significant proteinuria during pregnancy. Normal protein loss through the kidneys is 200 to 300 mg per 24 hours. Proteinuria of more than 500 mg per 24 hours may indicate a disease process.[8] Trace to 1+ proteinuria on a urine sample may be considered negligible. Readings of 2+ and above require further assessment. Pre-existing signs, such as elevated blood pressure, excessive weight gain, and generalized edema, are likely to be present if pregnancy-induced hypertension exists, because proteinuria occurs late in the course of the disorder[9] (*see* Chapter 39). A 24-hour urine collection test to measure the total amount of protein being lost may be performed for the client who has 2+ proteinuria.

TABLE 18–4. RISK FACTORS OF THE SECOND TRIMESTER

Socioeconomic Factors
Inadequate finances
Poor housing
Severe social problems
Nutritional deprivation
Hazardous, strenuous, or stressful occupation
Maternal Health Status
Maternal diseases, such as cardiac, pulmonary, or metabolic disease
Chronic hypertension
Maternal hemoglobinopathies
Seizure disorder
Venereal and other infectious diseases
Weight loss greater than 5 pounds
Malignancy
Surgery during pregnancy
Major congenital anomalies of the reproductive tract
Maternal mental retardation, major emotional disorders
Urinary tract infections
Febrile illness
Pregnancy-induced hypertension/albuminuria
Current Obstetric Status
Late or no prenatal care
Disproportionate uterine growth
Exposure to environmental hazards and teratogens
Need for antenatal diagnosis of inherited disorders
Multiple gestation
Vaginal bleeding
Rh isoimmunization
Preterm labor
Premature rupture of membranes
Disproportionate weight gain
Cervical dilation/effacement
Lifestyle
Smoking
Alcohol/drug use
Psychosocial Factors
Problems in acceptance of pregnancy
Lack of support from partner, own parents, and significant others
Difficulty adapting to changes of pregnancy
Hospitalization or illness of other family members
Resentment of, or failure to follow, therapeutic regimen; resentment of fetus for the demands of pregnancy

Adapted, with permission, from Auman G, Baird M. Screening for high risk pregnancy. In: Knuppel RA, Drucker JF, eds. High Risk Pregnancy. *Philadelphia: WB Saunders; 1986: 12–13; and Frigolelte FD, Little GA, eds.* Guidelines for Perinatal Care. *2nd ed. Washington, DC: American Academy of Pediatrics, American College of Obstetricians and Gynecologists; 1988 56–57.*

Slight glycosuria may be present because of the physiologic decrease in the renal threshold for glucose. About 50 percent of women excrete glucose in their urine at some point during pregnancy.[8] As discussed in Chapter 12, this may be normal in pregnancy[10,11]; however, serum glucose analysis would be done for any client with persistent glycosuria.

Blood Studies. Blood glucose screening may be performed between 24 and 28 weeks of gestation to detect the development of gestational diabetes. Urine testing alone is not an adequate screen for glucose intolerance during pregnancy. A random blood glucose sample or a 1-hour abbreviated glucose tolerance test are two approaches used in screening for gestational diabetes.[10,11] A random blood glucose level greater than 120 mg/dL indicates the need for a full glucose tolerance test. The 1-hour abbreviated glucose tolerance test assesses blood glucose 1 hour after a 50 g standard oral glucose solution is ingested. A value or 140 mg/dL or greater is considered a positive result and an indication for full glucose tolerance testing.

Psychosocial and Cultural Assessment

Psychosocial Assessment. The first trimester is often marked by a woman's ambivalence and then gradual acceptance of the reality of pregnancy. By the second trimester, the pregnant woman has accepted the fact that she is going to have a baby and begins to focus more on the fetus. This response is heightened as the pregnancy becomes more physically evident and the woman begins to feel fetal movement.[12] Completion of these tasks is important for the pregnant woman to perceive the fetus as becoming differentiated from the self and finally, at birth, separated.[13]

During the second trimester, a woman with no past history of psychologic disturbances may feel vulnerable and uncertain. In addition, the pregnant woman may normally experience a certain amount of anxiety. Anxiety may focus on fears concerning her own health, the health of the fetus, or a perceived loss of physical attractiveness, especially to her partner.[14,15,16]

Thorough psychosocial assessment, with follow-up at each prenatal visit, is an essential aspect of prenatal care during the second trimester and throughout pregnancy (Table 18–5). Information about the woman's psychologic well-being prior to pregnancy is important. For example, a woman with a previous history of emotional disorders may be at higher risk of developing emotional problems as pregnancy progresses and may not deal well with the psycho-

TABLE 18–5. COMPONENTS OF SECOND-TRIMESTER PSYCHOSOCIAL ASSESSMENT

Psychologic Factors
General emotional status
Previous history of emotional problems
Level of stress

Socioeconomic, Cultural, and Environmental Factors
Family integrity, structure, and level of functioning
Cultural, community, and family support systems
Economic status of family
Availability of adequate housing and food
Access to appropriate prenatal care
Knowledge about and accessibility of community resources
Employment outside of the home, nature of job
Cultural beliefs and practices affecting reproduction
Lifestyle
Health beliefs and practices
Work and home environment

Adaptation to Pregnancy
Feelings at this time about pregnancy
Anxiety in relation to concern about fetus, maternal well-being, and physical testing
Sexual functioning: changes in, feelings about, and problems with
Perception of pregnancy affecting present activities and responsibilities
Perception of physiologic changes and body image
Accomplishing "tasks of pregnancy"

Coping Patterns
Ability of client and her partner to cope with stressful situations
Effectiveness of coping methods (Do they result in positive outcomes? If not, what follows?)

Network of Support
Father's present attitude toward pregnancy
Amount of emotional support from parents, siblings, other family members, and friends
Accessibility of family, distance client lives from family
Amount and types of support client expects from family and friends during pregnancy, childbirth, and early parenting

logic transitions of pregnancy.[16] Social support networks should be identified and encouraged. Studies suggest an association between social support and factors such as adaptation to pregnancy or actual health practices.[16,17]

Attentive listening is another important aspect of nursing assessment. The nurse ideally builds on a trusting relationship begun at previous visits (Figure 18–1). By listening to the woman's concerns about herself and her pregnancy, the nurse can complete assessment, individualize nursing interventions, facilitate the woman's psychologic adjustment to the second trimester of pregnancy, support coping mechanisms, and become an active member of the woman's support system.[18]

Cultural Assessment

Assessment of cultural beliefs and responses to pregnancy and prenatal care continues throughout pregnancy. Returning for wellness evaluation and adhering to health care prescriptions may reflect religious and cultural backgrounds. The low-risk client usually feels well during the second trimester. Groups that equate health care with illness and pregnancy with wellness may not perceive the need for second-trimester assessment and may not make or keep appointments. Clients from poor socioeconomic backgrounds may view loss of work for second-trimester prenatal visits, costs of transportation to visits, or cost of prenatal care beyond confirmation of pregnancy and delivery as inaccessible luxuries. Conversely, certain groups may highly value prenatal care and pay close attention to any advice given. For example, education and health are valued among most upper-middle-class persons. Learning about second-trimester changes, questioning various aspects of prenatal care, and planning for the future are culturally expected. Through interviews with and observations of the client, such as the way in which she responds to health care, the nurse can identify cultural influences on the family during the second trimester of pregnancy.

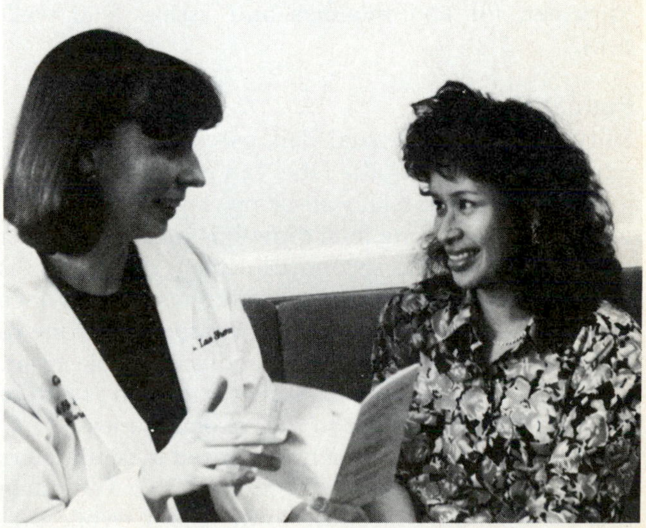

Figure 18–1. A trusting relationship is the basis for effective nursing assessment.

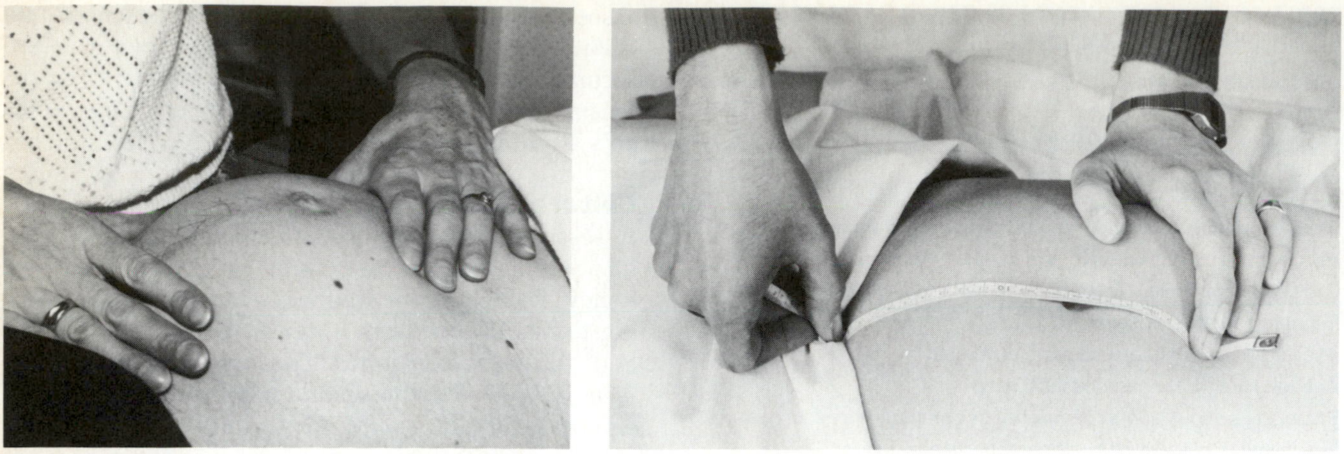

A B

Figure 18–2. **A.** Palpation of the uterus during the second trimester. **B.** Measurement of uterine size during the second trimester. (**B** *is reproduced, with permission, from Block GJ, Nolan JW.* Health Assessment for Professional Nursing: A Developmental Approach. *2nd ed. Norwalk, Conn: Appleton-Century-Crofts; 1986:462.*)

ASSESSMENT OF FETAL WELL-BEING

Assessment of fetal well-being during the second trimester has two aspects, low-risk and high-risk assessment. Low-risk assessment involves physical examination techniques such as measurement of fundal height and fetal heart rate. Maternal reports of lifestyle behaviors and reports of fetal activity after quickening are also useful indicators of fetal health. High-risk assessment involves screening for abnormalities (for example, genetic disorders). Techniques such as diagnostic ultrasound, maternal serum screening for alpha-fetoprotein levels, amniocentesis, fetoscopy, and percutaneous umbilical blood sampling are used to screen for abnormalities and assess fetal well-being.

Fundal Height

During a routine prenatal visit, assessment of uterine size and palpation of the fetus can provide important information about fetal well-being (Figure 18–2). One method of evaluating fetal growth is measurement of uterine size. By the second trimester, the fundus is palpable above the maternal symphysis pubis (see Figure 16–1). By 20 weeks, the fundus is felt one to two fingerbreadths below the umbilicus (Table 18–6). Pelvic examination is not usually performed as part of the ongoing assessment in the second trimester.

Fundal height is usually measured in centimeters by use of a tape measure (Figure 18–2B). The nurse first explains the procedure to the client. While preparing the client, the nurse can obtain information about the tone, irritability, and consistency of the uterus. The examiner measures the distance between the upper border of the maternal symphysis pubis, over the midline of the abdomen, to the top of the uterine fundus. This measurement is then inserted into McDonald's formula:

$$\frac{\text{Distance in centimeters} \times 8}{7} = \text{Total weeks of gestation}$$

This finding should correlate with gestation after 22 to 24 weeks. If a difference exists between actual find-

TABLE 18–6. PREGNANCY MILESTONES IN THE SECOND TRIMESTER

Quickening
Placenta in anterior part of uterus
19 weeks—primigravidas
17.5 weeks—multiparas
Placenta in posterior part of uterus
18 weeks—primigravidas
16.1 weeks—multiparas
Fetal heart tones
17–20 weeks with unamplified auscultation
8–10 weeks with Doppler ultrasound
Fundal heights and estimated gestation[a]
12 weeks—at level of symphysis pubis
16 weeks—halfway between symphysis pubis and umbilicus
20 weeks—one to two fingerbreadths below umbilicus
24 weeks—one to two fingerbreadths above umbilicus

[a] See *also Figure 16–1.*

ings (in centimeters) and gestational age, further assessment is necessary to rule out conditions that could alter fundal height. Fundal height may be altered by increased uterine size as a result of polyhydramnios, hydatidiform mole, and multiple gestation or by decreased size as a result of oligohydramnios or intrauterine growth retardation.

Uterine Activity

Uterine activity also is assessed during each second-trimester visit. During the second trimester, uterine activity normally consists of mild, low-intensity contractions. These Braxton Hicks contractions are characterized by irregular, painless tightening of the uterus. As pregnancy progresses, Braxton Hicks contractions increase in frequency and intensity. Some women may experience pain related to Braxton Hicks contractions, although many women do not.

Women should be taught the distinction between false and true contractions so that the onset of labor can be recognized. This is particularly important during the second trimester because of problems related to preterm birth. Educating low-risk women at 22 to 26 weeks and high-risk women at 13 to 15 weeks about symptoms of preterm labor and the importance of notifying their health care provider without delay if symptoms occur may help prevent preterm birth.[19] (*See* Chapter 39 for symptoms of preterm labor).

Fetal Heart Tones

Fetal heart tones can be detected as early as 8 weeks with Doppler ultrasound amplification.[1,9] Without amplification, fetal heart tones can be auscultated at 17 to 20 weeks' gestation.[20,21] Fetal heart sounds during the second trimester are usually found at the midline of the maternal abdomen or slightly to the left or right of the midline, depending on fetal position (Figure 18–3). The average fetal heart range is 120 to 160 beats per minute; a fetal heart range of 150 to 160 may be common during the second trimester. The baseline fetal heart rate generally decreases as pregnancy advances and the fetus matures.

Quickening

Quickening may be used to determine gestational age in conjunction with other assessments. As discussed in Chapter 16, quickening may be perceived by the mother between the 14th and 20th weeks of pregnancy as a gentle fluttering feeling in the abdomen.[20] Quickening alone, however, cannot be used as a positive identification of gestational age.

RESEARCH ABSTRACT

Heidrich SM, Cranley MS. Effect of fetal movement, ultrasound scans, and amniocentesis on maternal-fetal attachment. Nurs Res. *1989;38:81–84.*

This study examined the effects of fetal movement, ultrasound scans, and amniocentesis on maternal-fetal attachment and perception of fetal development in normal pregnancy during the second trimester. There were four specific research questions: (1) What is the effect of fetal movement on maternal-fetal attachment during the second trimester? (2) What is the effect of ultrasound performed to determine fetal age on maternal-fetal attachment during the second trimester? (3) What is the effect of amniocentesis performed for genetic diagnosis in advanced maternal age on maternal-fetal attachment during the second trimester? (4) What is the relationship between women's perceptions of fetal growth and development and maternal-fetal attachment during the second trimester?

Ninety-one women in the second trimester participated in the study. The majority of the women were married. Thirty-five percent of the women were primiparas; 65 percent were multiparas.

The findings of this study indicate that women who report feeling fetal movement early in pregnancy have higher maternal-fetal attachment scores and higher perception of fetal development than women who do not report early fetal movement. Ultrasound scans had no effect on maternal-fetal attachment or fetal development scores. Women who underwent genetic amniocentesis had lower attachment scores before the procedure was done and before the results were known. The investigators suggest the sensation of fetal movement may be more important to maternal-fetal attachment than ultrasound visualization of the fetus.

Comment:

This study supports the importance of noninvasive techniques, such as teaching parents to feel fetal movement, in the development of maternal-fetal attachment. The study findings do not support a relationship between screening techniques, such as ultrasound visualization, and attachment. The study should be replicated to confirm these findings.

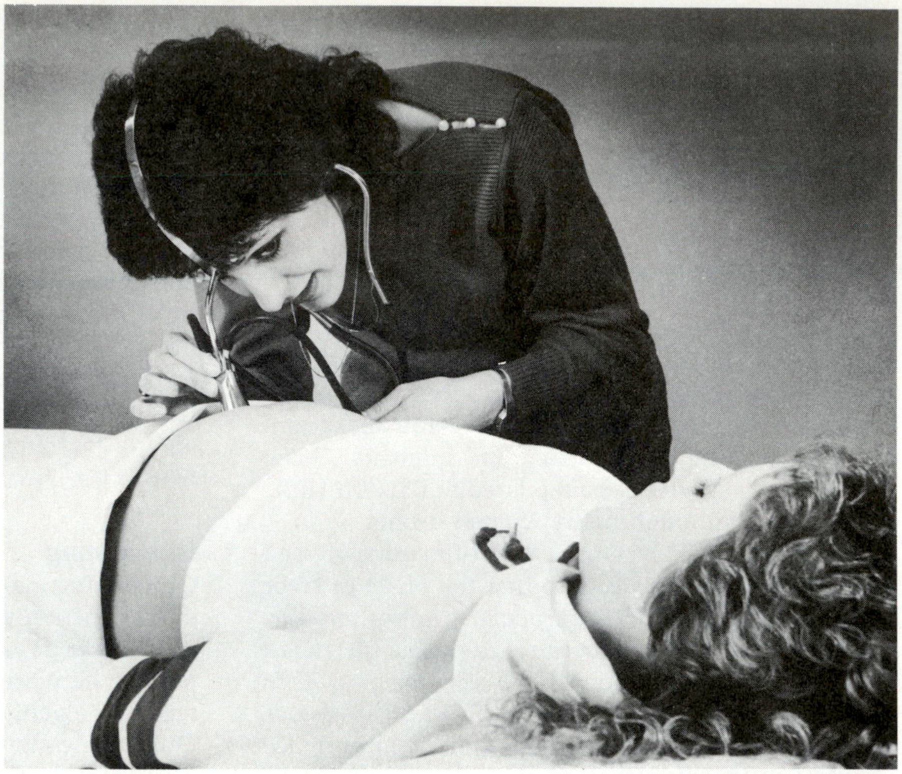

A

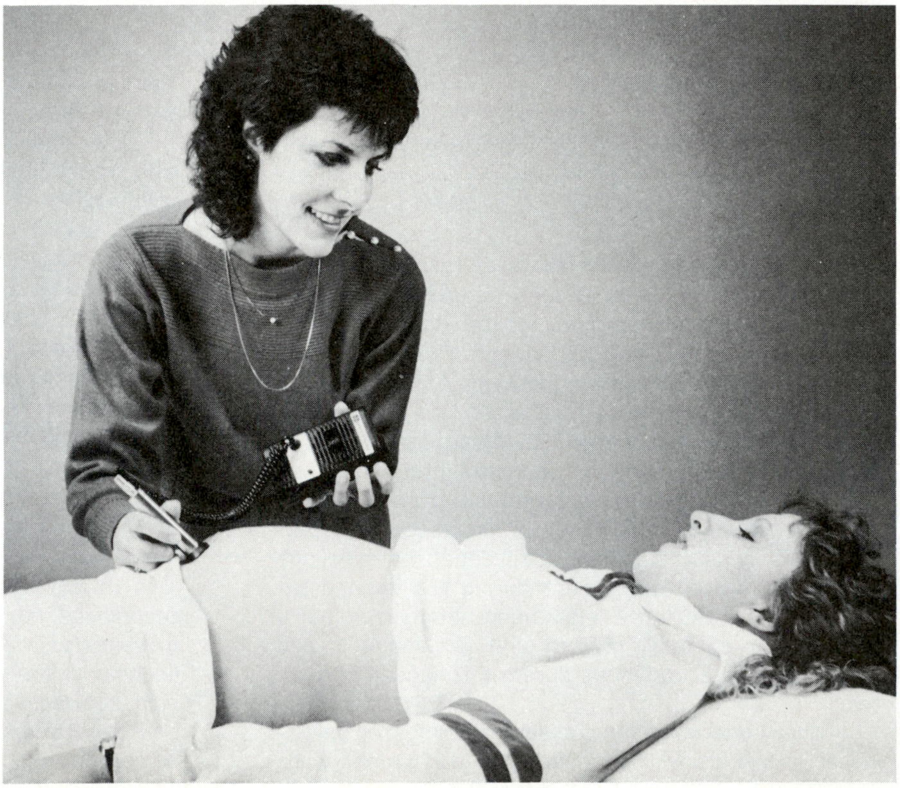

B

Figure 18–3. Listening for fetal heart activity with (**A**) the fetoscope and (**B**) the Doppler. (*Reproduced, with permission, from Block GJ, Nolan JW.* Health Assessment for Professional Nursing: A Developmental Approach. *2nd ed. Norwalk, Conn: Appleton-Century-Crofts; 1986: 462–463.*)

PRENATAL DIAGNOSTIC ASSESSMENT

Diagnostic Ultrasound

As described in Chapter 14, ultrasound has become an important diagnostic technology throughout pregnancy. During the second trimester, ultrasound's major uses are fetal assessment, visualization of internal structures during invasive diagnostic procedures and treatments, and identification of maternal abnormalities. For example, gestational age may be calculated based on biparietal diameters of the fetal head. Fetal growth can be followed by serially estimating fetal weight and plotting the values against gestational age. This is done in cases of suspected intrauterine fetal growth retardation.[22]

Fetal evaluation for structural malformations, estimation of fetal head size, and identification of the symmetry and proportional growth of the fetal brain and liver are among factors that provide information about fetal well-being. Ultrasonic visualization of internal structures promotes client safety and facilitates invasive procedures such as amniocentesis, fetoscopy, or percutaneous umbilical blood sampling (*see* later). Ultrasonic measurement of length of the femur and thickness of the nuchal skin fold has been noted to be helpful in identifying second-trimester fetuses with Down's syndrome.[23] The location, thickness, and condition of the placenta may be evaluated, especially in cases of second-trimester bleeding.[22] Table 18–7 presents some indications for ultrasound diagnosis in midpregnancy.[22]

TABLE 18–7. INDICATIONS FOR ULTRASOUND DIAGNOSIS IN MIDPREGNANCY

Estimation of gestational age for women with uncertain clinical dates
Evaluation of fetal growth
Vaginal bleeding of undetermined etiology
Suspected multiple gestation
Adjunct to amniocentesis or percutaneous umbilical blood cord sampling
Significant uterine size/clinical dates discrepancy
Suspected hydatidiform mole
Adjunct to cervical cerclage placement
Suspected uterine abnormality
Suspected polyhydramnios or oligohydramnios
Estimation of fetal weight
Presentation with premature ruptured membranes
Premature labor
Abnormal serum alpha-fetoprotein value
Serial evaluation of fetal growth in multiple gestation

Adapted, with permission, from Hohler C. Ultrasound and high-risk obstetrics. In: Kuppel R, Drukker J, eds. High Risk Pregnancy, A Team Approach. *Philadelphia: WB Saunders; 1986:59.*

Some clinicians recommend diagnostic ultrasound examination for every fetus at 16 to 20 weeks of gestation. The rationale for this approach is the benefit and potential cost savings related to early diagnosis and treatment of high-risk fetal conditions such as multiple gestation, intrauterine growth retardation, and congenital anomalies.[24] Opponents to this approach urge caution with this technology, as the safety of ultrasound's use in pregnancy has not been conclusively tested.[25,26] In addition, ultrasound is a very costly procedure that is not needed by lower-risk clients. In the United States, ultrasound is currently recommended only when there is a specific indication.[1,27,28]

The decision to schedule an ultrasound is made by an obstetrician or nurse-midwife in consultation with the client and, when indicated, the perinatologist. The test itself may be performed during the second trimester in settings such as a physician's office or special antenatal testing unit of a hospital or clinic. The procedure may be done by a physician, by a nurse with specialized training, or by a technician.

Procedure. The procedure for ultrasound was described in Chapter 14. A transabdominal approach is used for ultrasound during the second trimester when the uterus has enlarged beyond the pelvis. If a full bladder is requested to promote visualization early in the second trimester, the client is instructed to drink 32 to 40 oz of fluid 1 hour before the test and not to empty her bladder until after the test is completed.

During the procedure the woman is placed in a semirecumbent position. When appropriate, she and her support person are positioned so that both can see the monitor screen. One concern of positioning of the client during ultrasound relates to the enlarging uterus. Supine hypotension, related to the compression of the inferior vena cava by the uterus, may occur during the second and third trimesters (*see* Chapter 20 for discussion of supine hypotension). The potential for supine hypotension increases as the uterus becomes heavier with advancing pregnancy. The client is therefore assessed for signs and symptoms of hypotension during the procedure. These include tachycardia, hypotension, diaphoresis, pallor, and reports of lightheadedness or nausea. If this condition occurs, the client is assisted in turning onto her left side to displace the uterus from the inferior vena cava.

The ultrasound procedure takes about one-half hour to an hour, depending on the type of test. Ul-

ISSUES AND CONTROVERSIES

Many issues and controversies surround second-trimester assessment. For example, what constitutes adequate screening for healthy women? Should routine ultrasounds be done for all clients? Do potential but unknown risks justify benefits of information gained from routine ultrasound? Should women undergo procedures that are as yet considered experimental, such as percutaneous umbilical blood sampling? If these procedures are not tested, how can future clients benefit?

Controversy continues over whether clients should undergo fetal screening procedures if they would not consider abortion as an option. Cost of the procedure and the physical risks involved are arguments used against testing; however, information about the fetus and decisions about the pregnancy are also viewed as separate issues. Prenatal diagnosis may allow the couple to receive help and support throughout pregnancy.

As technology continues to develop and to allow for increasingly sophisticated fetal assessment, issues and controversies will continue to emerge. Nurses need to be well informed about current procedures and about the nature of debate surrounding each one.

trasound itself is painless. Discomforts relate to a full bladder and emotional concern related to the need for the test. The person performing the test should explain the image on the screen for the couple. Positive aspects, such as fetal thumbsucking and the heart beating, may be pointed out. Photographs of the fetal image may be taken and given to the client as a keepsake.

The results of the ultrasound should be interpreted by a physician skilled in ultrasound. In certain antenatal testing units, staff physicians are available to meet with the client immediately after the scan to discuss results and thereby decrease fear and anxiety related to waiting. If the client has been referred, reports of the ultrasound are sent to the referring physician or nurse-midwife. Clients who are referred by nurse-midwives for conditions such as gestational age assessment or identification of a single fetus may continue to be cared for by the nurse-midwives; however, identification of a high-risk condition, such as intrauterine growth retardation, may necessitate transfer to a high-risk specialist.

Ultrasound and Attachment. Does ultrasound promote attachment? Visualization of the fetus confirms the reality of pregnancy. It is logical to assume that a mother's ability to observe the fetus and fetal movements would foster feelings of attachment; however, research findings have had conflicting results. For example, results of some descriptive studies have indicated that ultrasound increases maternal feelings of attachment to the fetus[29,30]; however, findings of one study did not support a relationship between ultrasound and attachment during the second trimester, although a relationship between the mother's feeling fetal movement and attachment was identified.[31] Depending on the results of the scan and the woman's treatment during the procedure, some women may feel more worried or vulnerable after the scan.[29,32] In light of the various research findings, attention must be given to assessing the individual responses of each client. Further research on this topic is also warranted.

Role of the Nurse. The need for diagnostic ultrasound, as well as the test itself, can cause anxiety for the woman and her partner. The nurse's role includes providing anticipatory guidance and support to the couple before, during, and after the procedure and encouraging them to express their feelings regarding the procedure. Clients who have been referred to an antenatal testing unit must deal with assessment procedures performed by strangers in an unfamiliar environment and therefore need a warm, supportive approach. Strong communication between referring staff and staff in the antenatal testing unit is necessary. It is important to emphasize that the information obtained from diagnostic ultrasound is integrated with other diagnostic information and clinical observations before an accurate diagnosis can be reached. (*See* Chapter 14, for a discussion of the nurse's role during diagnostic ultrasound.)

Assessment for Neural Tube Defects

Neural tube defects are potentially major, central nervous system malformations that occur when the embryonic neural tube does not develop normally.[33] This embryonic structure may not close properly, or it may close normally, but then overdistend and rupture. The brain, spinal cord, and overlying tissues may be affected. Disabilities ranging from mild to severe neurologic impairment may result; some neural tube defects are incompatible with life. (*See* Chapter 42 for additional discussion of neural tube defects.)

The incidence of neural tube defects in the United States is 1 to 2 per 1000 live births.[1,2] Certain countries, particularly the Great Britian (Ireland, Scotland, Northern Ireland, Wales), parts of northern India,

Pakistan, Egypt, and the Arab countries, have a higher incidence.[33] The etiology of neural tube defects is multifactorial. Both environmental and genetic factors are thought to influence the development of these defects; however, 90 to 95 percent of women who have a fetus or child with a neural tube defect have no identifiable risk factors.

Neural tube defects may be closed, that is, covered by skin or a thick membrane, or "open," as in cases when neural tissue is totally exposed or covered only by a thin, transparent membrane. The three most common neural tube defects are anencephaly, spina bifida, and encephalocele.[33]

1. *Anencephaly*. In this condition, the cranial vault is absent and the brain is poorly developed. It is almost always incompatible with life for a prolonged period after birth. Most cases of anencephaly are open defects.
2. *Spina bifida*. This condition ranges in severity from a mild, barely noticeable defect with minimal if any nerve tissue affected (spina bifida occulta) to extensive nerve tissue involvement as a result of protrusion of the meninges from the spinal canal (meningocele) or protrusion of the meninges and spinal cord through the defect (meningomyelocele). About 80 to 90 percent of spina bifida cases are open defects.
3. *Encephalocele*. This defect occurs in the head and refers to the protrusion of meninges and brain tissue through a cranial defect. Most encephaloceles are closed defects.

"Open" neural tube defects leak **alpha-fetoprotein (AFP).** Alpha-fetoprotein is a glycoprotein that is synthesized in the embryonic yolk sac, developing gastrointestinal tract, and fetal liver.[2,33] Alpha-fetoprotein is present in healthy pregnancies and enters amniotic fluid as a result of fetal urination, gatrointestinal secretions, and transudation from exposed blood vessels. Alpha-fetoprotein normally may gain access to maternal serum by crossing the placenta or through the amniotic fluid membranes. Levels of AFP change during pregnancy (Figure 18–4). For this reason, correct gestational age is important for interpretation of findings. Abnormal AFP results often reflect inaccurate estimates of gestational age, rather than true pathology. The highest level of AFP normally occurs in fetal serum about 15 weeks of gestation; AFP concentrations slowly decrease after that. The amniotic fluid level of AFP shows a similar pattern, although there is a lower concentration of AFP in amniotic fluid than in fetal serum. As shown in Figure 18–4, the concentrations of AFP in the mother's serum follows a different pattern. During the second trimester, the level of AFP in amniotic fluid is about 100 times the level of AFP found in the mother's serum.[1,2] Elevated AFP levels in maternal serum and in amniotic fluid may indicate open neural tube defects. Closed defects cannot be identified in this way.

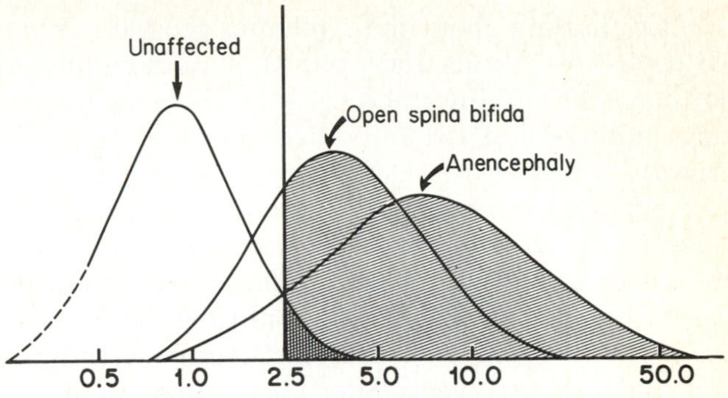

Figure 18–4. Levels of alpha-fetoprotein in maternal serum during pregnancy. (*Redrawn from American College of Obstetricians and Gynecologists.* Prenatal Detection of Neural Tube Defects. *Technical Bulletin 99. Washington D. C.: ACOG;* 1986:2. Reproduced, with permission, from Cunningham FG, et al. Williams Obstetrics. *18th ed. Norwalk, Conn: Appleton & Lange; 1989: 585.*)

Multiple gestation, contamination of an amniotic fluid specimen with fetal blood, different fetal abnormalities (eg, hydrocele, esophageal atresia, certain chromosomal disorders), and laboratory error may account for an abnormal AFP level in amniotic fluid.[1,2,33] Several factors may also produce an abnormal AFP level in maternal serum (Table 18–8).[9]

Because of methodologic differences among laboratories, normal levels for AFP are set by each laboratory; results are thus evaluated in reference to the standards of each laboratory.[2] False-negative and false-positive results can, however, occur, regardless of the normal value range set by a laboratory.

Neural tube defects may be identified by assessment that includes serum testing of pregnant women at 16 to 18 weeks of gestation, diagnostic ultrasound, and amniocentesis. Blood sampling is the least expensive, least invasive, and most economical approach. Although the results are not as precise, serum evaluation for AFP is therefore a useful, initial screening approach. If AFP levels are normal, results are shared promptly with the client, and routine prenatal care proceeds. Diagnostic ultrasound and amniocentesis are recommendations reserved for clients at risk.

Counseling about the screening program, along with possible results and options, should be offered to the client and informed consent obtained. Expectant mothers and fathers with a personal or family history of neural tube defects are considered at risk and offered screening. As these defects occur frequently in women without risk factors, nurse-midwives or physicians may routinely perform or order blood sample screening for all pregnant women at 16 to 18 weeks of gestation. Serum screening is done again 1 to 2 weeks later for clients with abnormal AFP results. The repeat serum AFP level is at times omitted if advancing pregnancy makes time considerations a factor, if no significant new information is expected, or if the client feels strongly about proceeding without delay for further diagnostic assessment. Diagnostic ultrasound for fetal assessment is then done. Neural tube defects may be seen on ultrasound. In addition, conditions that may affect AFP levels, such as gestational age, other congenital anomalies, and multiple gestation, may be identified.

TABLE 18–8. SOME CONDITIONS ASSOCIATED WITH ABNORMAL MATERNAL SERUM ALPHA-FETOPROTEIN CONCENTRATIONS

Elevated Levels
Neural tube defects
Pilonidal cysts
Esophageal obstructions
Liver necrosis
Cystic hygroma
Sacrococcygeal teratoma
Abdominal wall defects (omphalocoele, gastroschisis)
Urinary obstruction
Renal anomalies (polycystic or absent kidneys)
Congenital nephrosis
Osteogenesis imperfecta
Congenital skin defects
Cloacal exstrophy
Low birth weight
Oligohydramnios
Multiple gestation
Decreased maternal weight
Underestimated gestational age
Low Level
Chromosomal trisomies
Gestational trophoblastic disease
Fetal death
Increased maternal weight
Overestimated gestational age

Reproduced, with permission, from Cunningham FG, et al. Williams Obstetrics. *18th ed. Norwalk, Conn: Appleton & Lange; 1989:584.*

Amniocentesis to test AFP levels would be recommended for clients with positive serum AFP tests whose ultrasound evaluation revealed no condition that could affect AFP levels.[2] Results of the tests need to be communicated promptly to clients at all phases of screening, options regarding the pregnancy presented, and strategies for follow-up implemented.

Role of the Nurse. Alpha-fetoprotein testing programs are collaborative endeavors in which nurses work closely with clients, obstetricians, genetic counselors, ultrasonographers, and perinatologists. The nurse's role differs among settings and depends on such factors as his or her own specialized educational background and whether the client will be cared for in a high-risk testing unit or a low-risk environment. Nurse specialists may provide genetic counseling or may assist in the coordination of antenatal testing.

Staff nurses must be knowledgeable about the screening programs, about the advantages and limitations of AFP screening, about procedures that will be recommended for clients with positive results, about options available to clients, about the staff who will work with the client, and about support resources. Blood samples may be drawn by a physician, by a nurse, or by a laboratory technician. Nurses may also have key roles in coordination of services, as second-trimester assessment does not allow a great deal of time for further testing and decision making.

Low-risk healthy women may not be screened in the setting where primary care is delivered, for example, in a birth center. Clients need to be well prepared for their experience in a testing laboratory or center. Nurses who work in an antenatal testing setting must be sensitive to clients' unique concerns related to AFP screening and to receiving care in an unfamiliar setting. Nurses also need to provide support to clients during the difficult period of waiting for test results.

All staff need to be prepared to deliver emotional support for the client with prenatal diagnosis of a fetus with a neural tube defect. Procedures and protocols must be ready for implementation in advance of any client care. Options available to the client are discussed, and the client makes her own decision. Support groups for clients who decide to terminate pregnancy and also for clients who decide to continue the pregnancy can be important sources of assistance.

Amniocentesis

Amniocentesis involves the transabdominal withdrawal of fluid from the amniotic sac (Figure 18–5). The development of the amniocentesis procedure and the successful cultivation of amniotic cells for genetic

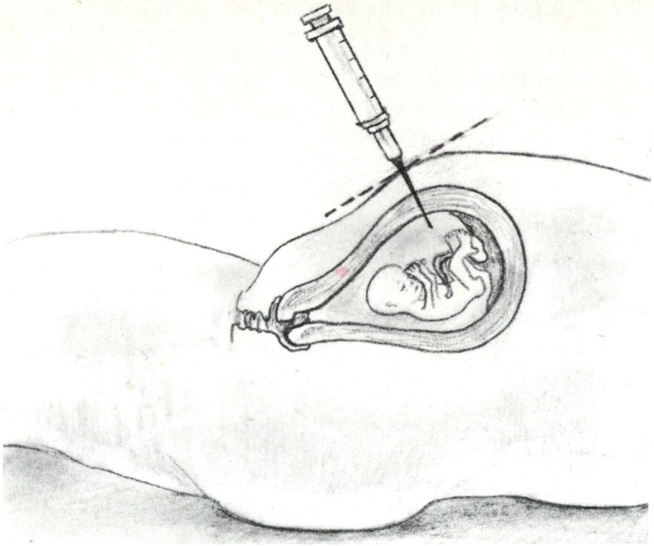

Figure 18–5. Amniocentesis: cross-sectional view.

determination have made it possible for clients to find out whether their fetus has abnormal conditions, for example, a genetic abnormality or a neural tube defect. News of a genetically normal fetus may allay anxiety. Information about an abnormal fetus may be used by the client to make an informed choice to terminate the pregnancy or to prepare for the birth of an infant with special needs. Amniocentesis is an invasive procedure that is performed only for specific reasons. Table 18–9 lists indications for amniocentesis.[9]

Amniocentesis for prenatal diagnosis of genetic abnormalities or neural tube defects is usually performed between 15 and 18 weeks of gestation, when there is enough amniotic fluid present for aspiration. Using continuous ultrasound, some centers are able to perform this before 15 weeks.[34] Results of cell cultures usually take about 2 to 4 weeks.[1] Scheduling of the procedure is therefore important so that adequate time is left for the couple to consider reproductive options.

TABLE 18–9. INDICATIONS FOR AMNIOCENTESIS

Maternal age 35 years or greater
Previous chromosomally abnormal offspring
Chromosomal abnormality in either parent, including balanced translocation carrier state, aneuploidy, and mosaicism
Down's syndrome or other chromosomal abnormality in a close family member
Pregnancy after three or more spontaneous abortions
Previous fetus/infant with multiple major malformations
Risk of a serious X-linked hereditary disorder
Risk of a serious autosomal or X-linked recessive disorder
Risk of a neural tube defect (eg, personal or family history, exposure to drugs such as valproic acid and aminopterin, maternal conditions such as diabetes mellitus)[31]
Elevated maternal serum alpha-fetopretein level, obtained by routine screen

Analysis of amniotic fluid and cultured cells, drawn during one amniocentesis, can provide a diagnosis of chromosomal abnormalities and biochemical disorders. Table 18–10 lists certain biochemical and genetic disorders detectable in the second trimester.[35] In addition, amniotic fluid analysis can give information about general fetal well-being, as in the case of a fetus compromised by Rh isoimmunization, uteroplacental insufficiency, or impending preterm delivery. The latter two conditions are usually third-trimester indications for amniocentesis. Analysis of amniotic fluid does not screen for all possible abnormalities; a "clean" report is *not* a guarantee that the baby will be normal in every way. In addition, results of an amniocentesis may be inconclusive. For example, in a laboratory setting, fetal cells obtained during amniocentesis may not divide properly. Occasionally, a falsely abnormal result, such as pseudomosaicism related to laboratory artifact, may emerge. Although the overall pattern of chromosomes may be normal, the report reflects the possibility of chromosomal defect. More precise analysis of fetal blood cells, obtained through percutaneous umbilical blood sampling, described later, would then be indicated.

The presence of fetal cells in amniotic fluid allows for chromosomal analysis. In this way genetic disorders can be directly identified. Women are referred for amniocentesis to detect neural tube defects if they or a family member have had a previous fetus or child with the defect, if they have elevated serum AFP levels, or if either partner has a neural tube defect.[3,9]

Amniotic fluid analysis can be performed to assess fetal well-being in the presence of Rh isoimmunization (*see* Chapter 39). Rh-immune globulin has greatly reduced the incidence of Rh isoimmunization from approximately 14 to 2 percent. Antenatal prophylaxis, administered to the Rh-negative mother at 28 weeks, has further reduced the incidence to 0.07 percent.[36] Despite this reduction in the incidence, Rho(D) isoimmunization remains an important problem. In cases in which a known Rh-negative mother has a high antibody titer (1:8 to 1:16), amniotic fluid analysis is done. Approximately 50 to 100 mL of amniotic fluid is withdrawn and placed in collection tubes. The tubes must be covered with opaque material to prevent the breakdown of bilirubin by light rays. The fluid is analyzed for optical density, which measures the quantity of bilirubin in the fluid. Elevated levels indicate hemolysis. The levels are plotted

TABLE 18–10. DISORDERS THAT ARE DETECTABLE IN THE SECOND TRIMESTER OF PREGNANCY

Chromosomal abnormalities: essentially all significant cytogenetic disorders

Sex-linked recessive disorders, by fetal sex determination

Neural tube defects (especially open defects that leak alphafetoproteins)
- Anencephaly
- Myelomeningocele
- Encephalocele

Inborn errors of metabolism
- Disorders of lipid metabolism
  - Cholesterol ester storage disease
  - Fabry's disease
  - Familial hypercholesterolemia
  - Farber's disease
  - Gaucher's disease, infantile and adult types
  - GM1 gangliosidosis, types I and II
  - GM2 gangliosidosis, type I (Tay-Sachs disease)
  - GM2 gangliosidosis, type II (Sandhoff's disease)
  - GM2 gangliosidosis, type III
  - GM3 gangliosidosis
  - Krabbe's disease
  - Metachromatic leukodystrophy
  - Niemann-Pick disease, types A, B, and C
  - Refsum's disease
  - Wolman's disease
- Disorders of carbohydrate metabolism
  - Fucosidosis
  - Galactokinase deficiency
  - Galactosemia
  - Glucose-6-phosphate dehydrogenase deficiency
  - Glycogen storage disease, types II, III, IV, VI, and IX
  - Mannosidosis
  - Pyruvate decarboxylase deficiency
  - Pyruvate dehydrogenase deficiency
- Disorders of mucopolysaccharide metabolism
  - Hurler's syndrome (MPS I)
  - Scheie's syndrome (MPS I)
  - Hunter's syndrome (MPS II, A and B)
  - Sanfilippo's syndrome (MPS III, A and B)
  - Morquio's syndrome (MPS IV)
  - Maroteaux-Lamy syndrome (MPS VI, A and B)
  - Beta-glucuronidase deficiency (MPS VII)
- Disorders of amino acid and organic acid metabolism
  - Arginase deficiency
  - Argininosuccinic aciduria
  - Aspartylglucosaminuria
  - Citrullinemia
  - Cystathioninuria
  - Dihydropteridine reductase deficiency (phenylketonuria variant)
  - Histidinemia
  - Homocystinuria (cystathionine synthetase deficiency)
  - Hypervalinemia
  - Isovaleric acidemia
  - Maple syrup urine disease, severe and intermittent types
  - Methylmalonic acidemia
  - Propionic acidemia (ketotic hyperglycinemia)
- Miscellaneous disorders
  - Adenosine deaminase deficiency
  - Congenital erythropoietic porphyria
  - Congenital nephrotic syndrome
  - Cystinosis
  - Hypophosphatasia
  - I-cell disease
  - Lesch-Nyhan syndrome
  - Lysosomal acid phosphatase deficiency
  - Lysyl-protocollagen hydroxylase deficiency
  - Menke's kinky hair syndrome
  - Oriotic aciduria
  - Xeroderma pigmentosum

Hemoglobinopathies
- Sickle cell anemia
- Thalassemia

MPS = mucopolysaccharidosis.
Reproduced, with permission, from Quilligan E, Kretchmer N. Fetal and Maternal Medicine. *New York: John Wiley & Sons; 1980:102–103, 190.*

on optical density graphs according to gestational age. The placement on the graph gives an indication of the extent of hemolysis and fetal compromise. Intrauterine exchange transfusions may then be done to correct fetal anemia, if needed.

Procedure. Amniocentesis is an outpatient procedure that is performed by a physician (obstetrician). Amniocentesis may be done in a physician's private office or in a special antenatal testing unit.

The pregnant woman is placed in the supine position, and ultrasound is used to identify the location of the placenta and fetus. The gestational age of the fetus is assessed, and the presence of multiple gestation is ruled out. The uterine cavity is then searched through ultrasonography for a pool of fluid that can be reached with a needle without being obstructed by the placenta or fetus. The safety of the procedure and the success of obtaining a specimen of blood are enhanced by the use of sonography.[37] A specimen contaminated with blood may alter results, especially if maternal and fetal blood mix.

Once a pool of amniotic fluid is located, the insertion site is marked on the abdomen. The abdomen is then washed with an iodine solution and draped, to create a sterile field. This reduces the risk of introducing infection into the uterine cavity. The physician may inject a local anesthetic subcutaneously around the intended puncture site. A 20- or 22-gauge needle, 3 to 6 in. long (depending on the thickness of the abdominal wall and location of the pool) is then inserted into the uterine cavity; up to 30 mL of amniotic fluid may then be withdrawn.[9] The woman may feel pressure and slight cramping at the puncture site. The character of the amniotic fluid is assessed for the presence of blood, discoloration, or foul odor. The fluid is transferred from the syringe to specimen tubes and sent to the clinical laboratory for culture and analysis.

The client is discharged approximately 30 minutes after the procedure if no complications occur. She is instructed to keep the puncture site clean and to report any complications such as vaginal discharge, severe, persistent cramping, or the onset of fever. Normally, the client may experience some mild cramping for several hours. After the procedure she is instructed to rest, but may resume normal light activity after the cramping subsides.[38]

Risks. Three major risks associated with amniocentesis (1) trauma to the fetus, placenta, umbilical cord, or maternal structures, (2) infection, and (3) premature labor and spontaneous abortion. Hemorrhage can result from perforation of the placenta. A hematoma may develop at the perforation site, and the transfer of nutrients between the placenta and uterus may be decreased. Uteroplacental insufficiency and intrauterine growth retardation may result. Additionally, placental hemorrhage and transfer of fetal blood to the mother may cause maternal isoimmunization for the Rho(D)-negative mother carrying an Rh-positive fetus. Thus, hemolytic disease of the fetus may occur.[39] In such instances, anti-Rho globulin is administered to nonsensitized Rh-negative women to prevent isoimmunization from taking place.[9]

The risk of injury to the fetus and umbilical cord is minimal with an experienced physician, using a well-guided needle insertion. At times, even the most skillful clinician cannot obtain enough fluid, and another puncture is necessary. Repeated punctures may increase the risk of fetal injury. Most reported cases of injury occur late in pregnancy, although no figures are available for the exact incidence of this complication; however, when amniocentesis is performed during the third trimester close to the time of delivery, the newborn is examined immediately for any puncture wounds.[9]

Infection can result when pathogens are inadvertently introduced into the uterine cavity, as may occur when surgical aseptic technique is broken. Amnioitis, with complications such as preterm labor and delivery, may occur. Signs and symptoms of infection include fever, chills, uterine cramping, and possibly prurulent discharge at the puncture site.

Fetoscopy

Fetoscopy was developed in the early 1970s and has expanded prenatal diagnostic potential. Some disorders are not detectable by amniocentesis because the gene or substance of interest may not be expressed in amniotic fluid or chorionic villus cells. Therefore, morphologic or biochemical evaluation of such cells cannot provide information concerning the presence or absence of the disorder. If the gene is expressed in the skin, blood, or liver, however, the disorder can be diagnosed through analysis of samples of fetal tissue obtained through fetoscopy.[40,41]

Fetoscopy provides direct visualization of the fetus through insertion of a fiberoptic telescope transabdominally into the uterine cavity (Figure 18–6). This invasive procedure enables fetal blood sampling and skin and liver biopsies to be done. Fetoscopy is done by a physician after careful ultrasound examination of the uterus. A puncture site is located and marked on the mother's abdomen, so that the placenta and fetal parts will not be injured. The skin is cleansed; a local anesthetic may be used at the puncture site. Intravenous sedation may be administered to reduce maternal anxiety and fetal activity. Using surgical aseptic technique, the physician inserts the fetoscope. Under direct visualization through the fetoscope, samples of fetal blood or tissue are obtained.

Complications of the procedure include spontaneous abortion, infection, rupture of membranes, bleeding from the placenta or fetal puncture site, and fetal death.[40] Fetoscopy is as yet considered an experimental procedure, although continued research and physician training may change this situation. For

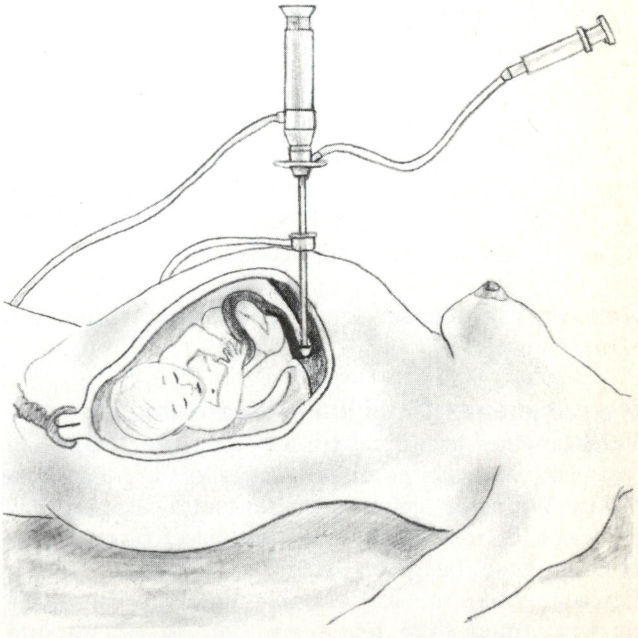

Figure 18–6. Fetoscopy: cross-sectional view.

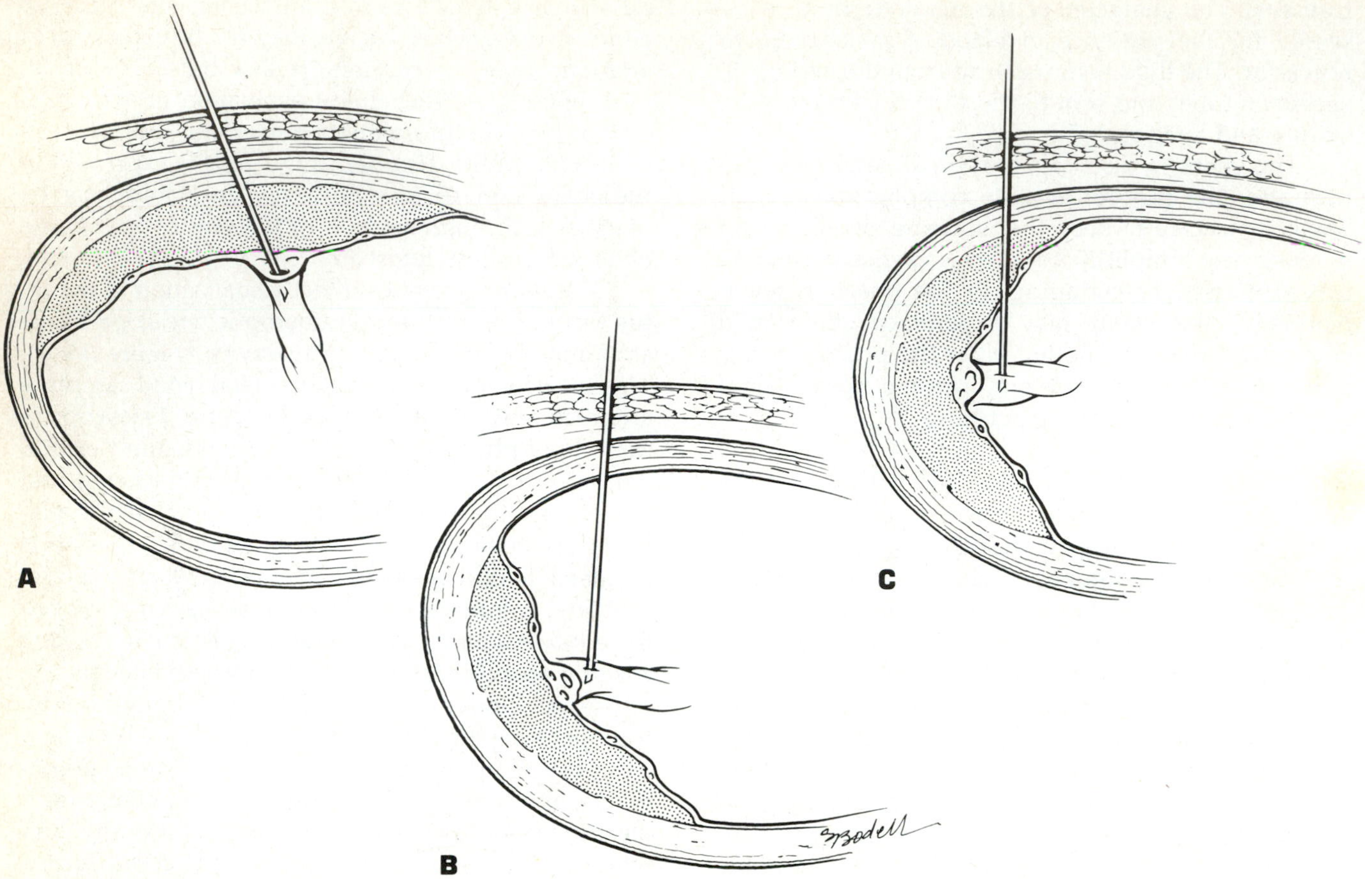

Figure 18–7. Percutaneous umbilical blood sampling. Access to the umbilical artery or vein varies, depending on both the placental location and the position of cord insertion into the placenta. **A.** With an anterior placenta, the needle may traverse the placenta. **B.** With a posterior implantation, the needle usually passes through the amnionic fluid before penetrating an umbilical vessel. **C.** With a lateral or fundal placenta, the needle may pass through the placenta and amnionic cavity to enter the umbilical vessel. (*Redrawn after Queenan and King.* Contemp Ob/Gyn. *1987:30:51. Reproduced, with permission, from Cunningham FG, et al.* Williams Obstetrics. *18th ed. Norwalk, Conn: Appleton & Lange; 1989:283.*)

this reason the nature, extent, and rates of some complications have not yet been confirmed. Clients who may benefit from this procedure are counseled extensively about the risks and benefits, as well as the experimental nature of the procedure.

Role of the Nurse. *See* "Percutaneous Umbilical Blood Sampling."

Percutaneous Umbilical Blood Sampling

Percutaneous umbilical blood sampling (PUBS) or *funipuncture* provides direct access to the fetal circulation. With this technique, fetal blood samples may be taken or treatments, such as direct blood transfusions, may be given to the fetus (Figure 18–7). Percutaneous umbilical blood sampling is more easily performed than fetoscopy, can be on an outpatient basis, and has been replacing fetoscopy as a method of fetal blood sampling.[1] Table 18–11 lists some indications and contraindications for PUBS.[42–45] The table is not all-inclusive, as the indications for PUBS are continual developing. Although PUBS has expanded possibilities for fetal assessment and treatment, it has not been widely evaluated. It is an invasive and costly technique, done after 16 weeks of gestation and only for clients who require this type of testing. PUBS should not be done when a procedure that is less invasive or more easily used could provide similar information. Percutaneous umbilical blood sampling should be performed only by an experienced team in an antenatal testing center. Table 18–12 summarizes some risks and special considerations associated with PUBS.

TABLE 18–11. SOME INDICATIONS AND CONTRAINDICATIONS FOR PERCUTANEOUS UMBILICAL BLOOD SAMPLING

Indications, Assessment/Diagnosis
Coagulation abnormalities
Hemophilias, such as hemophilia A and hemophilia B
Hemoglobinopathies
Congenital infections, such as toxoplasmosis and rubella
Metabolic or cytogenetic abnormalities that cannot be identified by amniocentesis or other types of screening
Karyotyping, for example, when results of amniocentesis are inconclusive, when fetal anomalies or severe growth retardation exist, or when rapid results are necessary
Rh disease
Blood gas concentration
Immune deficiency
Administration of blood products for treatment of fetal anemias and Rh disease
Administration of medications to the fetus
Contraindications
Fetal distress
Infection
Cases in which less invasive, safer, or easier methods (eg, ultrasound, amniocentesis) could give similar information
Cases in which delivery and neonatal care could be more effective or could be given with lower chance of risk than the procedure
Lack of client acceptance of the procedure or willingness to come for follow-up care

Source: *References 42–45.*

Procedure. Informed consent is needed prior to the procedure. The client must understand the reason for PUBS and the risks, benefits, and nature of follow-up care. Preprocedure counseling usually involves the client's meeting with a genetic counselor. Nurses with specialized educational backgrounds in genetic counseling may serve in this role.

Percutaneous umbilical blood sampling is an outpatient procedure that is performed with sterile technique in an operating room environment.[42] To prevent supine hypotension, the client with a greatly enlarged uterus is positioned on her left side. A support person of the client's choice may be encouraged to stay with the client.

A physician performs PUBS and is assisted by a nurse and an ultrasonographer. All team members must be skilled in their unique roles. Ultrasound is used for visualization during PUBS. The mother may need a full bladder, depending on the size of the uterus. The client's abdomen is cleansed with an iodine solution and draped, as with any surgical procedure. A sterile sleeve is placed over the ultrasound transducer, and the ultrasound is used to identify the area for puncture. A local anesthetic is injected by the physician into the client's abdominal wall, to minimize physical discomfort. A spinal needle may be used for obtaining access to the fetal circulation by way of the umbilical cord vessels. The stylet of the spinal needle is withdrawn, appropriate fetal blood samples are taken and sent for laboratory analysis, and any treatments are administered. Obtaining fetal blood samples takes about 10 minutes. Physical discomfort is minimal and is similar to the sense of pressure with possible cramping experienced with amniocentesis. After the procedure, the client is monitored until the fetus is noted to be normally reactive.

Care after PUBS is similar to care after amniocentesis (*see* earlier in chapter); however, the risk of infection is greater for PUBS than for amniocentesis. The physician may prescribe antibiotics prophylactically for the client. In addition, the client is advised to check her temperature twice daily and to contact her health care provider promptly if her temperature exceeds 100°F. She is advised to return at specified intervals for evaluation, which may include ultrasound. Further assessment and treatment are prescribed according to individual needs and conditions.

Role of the Nurse. As with each of the techniques for second-trimester assessment, the nurse caring for

TABLE 18–12. RISKS AND SPECIAL CONSIDERATIONS ASSOCIATED WITH PERCUTANEOUS UMBILICAL BLOOD SAMPLING

Risks
Injury to fetal structures
Placental or fetal hemorrhage, placenta abruptio[46]
Thrombus of umbilical vessel
Fetal arrhythmias
Chorioamnionitis
Preterm labor
Rupture of amniotic membranes
Fetal death
Special Considerations
High-risk specialized personnel and setting required
May need to be repeated at another time if cord vessels are too difficult to reach
May not be covered by insurance
Expensive
Nature of and reason for the procedure may frighten clients
Accessibility to follow-up care essential, but may be difficult for clients who live far from testing center

a client undergoing PUBS has important roles in educating and supporting the client before, during, and after the procedure. Working with the physician and the genetic counselor, the nurse makes certain that the client understands the reason for the procedure, the procedure itself, its risks and benefits, and any interventions that will be offered based on the results of PUBS. The nurse also makes sure that the client understands postprocedure instructions and is able to perform self-care practices, such as recognizing and reporting complications and returning for follow-up care.

Prior to and after the procedure, nurses monitor the client's vital signs. During the procedure the nurse assists the physician performing PUBS and provides support to the client and her support person. The nurse assesses fetal monitor tracings done after the procedure, promptly reports signs of fetal distress, and undertakes emergency measures, such as position changes and administration of oxygen, according to the unit's protocols. The nurse is responsible for ensuring that emergency equipment is accessible and in working order. The nurse's role may also involve telephone outreach to clients after their discharge home.

Nurses have important roles in coordinating care for the client undergoing PUBS. Nurses who work in high-risk antenatal settings may network with nurses in the referral site. Staff education, including invitations to visit the test center, can ensure continuity of care and understanding of the testing process. Nurses in low-risk settings can remain in touch with clients. Clients undergoing PUBS need support that may involve crisis counseling. Being responsive to the client's unique emotional needs and collaborating with physicians, social workers, and representatives from pastoral care, as appropriate, help nurses deliver optimal care to high-risk clients undergoing PUBS.

PSYCHOLOGIC CONCERNS RELATED TO ASSESSMENT

Second-trimester assessment can be an exciting and pleasant process for the low-risk, healthy client and her family. The expectant parents may look forward to hearing the fetal heartbeat, to confirming that pregnancy is progressing normally, and to discussing concerns and plans with their health care providers. Some clients, however, may fear physical examination for a variety of reasons or may worry about their own health or the health of their fetus. Nurses should evaluate each client's unique responses to the assessment process and make certain that clear explanations are given to allay anxiety. Normal test findings should be promptly communicated, and healthy clients need to be assured that they are progressing normally. Efforts should be made to ensure that a welcoming, educative approach is used with any assessment procedure.

As described earlier, a variety of techniques are available for the evaluation of fetal abnormalities and well-being in the second trimester. Some clients may be terrified of high-risk screening procedures. Feelings of crisis may be expected whether or not results of the screening procedures are positive. Loss of appetite, tears, inability to sleep, as well as silence, may be observed. Couples who would not consider abortion may seek prenatal diagnosis to allay anxiety and to allow them time to prepare for an infant with special needs.[47] Nurses need to be sensitive to their concerns, to ensure that they also receive test results without delay, and to provide referrals to support groups as appropriate.

Waiting days or weeks for the results of procedures may be especially stressful for clients. For example, Hodge described how much pregnancy seemed to slow while she awaited results of amniocentesis, performed because of advanced maternal age.[48] In addition she noted that her attitude toward the pregnancy was affected and that she tried to deny being actually pregnant and to "hold back" on bonding with the fetus until the results were known. Hodge felt this attempt at emotional restraint did not spare her or her husband from pain, but did deprive them of the love and support they subsequently received when faced with making decisions about a fetus with trisomy.[48] She urged clinicians to assess and to appreciate the negative effects of a long wait before the woman can accept that she is "really pregnant." In their research with second-trimester women, Heidrich and Cranley found that women who underwent genetic amniocentesis had lower attachment scores before the procedure than other second-trimester women studied[31]; however, a month after normal results, these women had attachment scores that did not differ significantly from the scores of the other women in the study. Such findings support clinical reports that suggest women withhold personal investment in the fetus and in the pregnancy until a normal result has been received.

Nurses, physicians, and other health care providers who participate in high-risk assessment need to be prepared to intervene with clients who do have abnormal results. Several strategies can be employed with these clients:

- Remain accessible to the client
- Support the client through further evaluation procedures when indicated
- Encourage verbalization
- Be able to answer questions
- Discuss options regarding the pregnancy and future treatment
- Coordinate care to minimize delays in testing, especially when advancing pregnancy makes time a concern
- Help clients meet their spiritual needs during this time
- Obtain support for clients from other sources.

Health care personnel should avoid imposing their own values and beliefs on clients; however, health care providers may pray with clients at their request and if they are comfortable doing so. Representatives from pastoral care may also be helpful, and clients may welcome the special support they can provide.

Many communities have support groups for people who have experienced prenatal or neonatal loss or for those who have children with special needs. Representatives of these groups can provide a strong and supportive community network for clients.

BARRIERS TO CARE DURING THE SECOND TRIMESTER

Not all clients have equal access to high-quality prenatal care during the second trimester. Barriers to care evolve from a variety of sources:

- Socioeconomic level
- Cultural backgrounds that do not promote understanding or acceptance of the health care system
- Lack of money or insurance to pay for services; lack of access to affordable prenatal care
- Lack of transportation or ability to afford transportation for prenatal care
- Lack of education about the importance of prenatal care during the second trimester
- Bureaucratic systems that make access to care difficult
- Geographic location far away from or inaccessible to prenatal care centers
- Scheduling of prenatal care at times that are incompatible with a client's work or personal activities
- Client's fear about the assessment process or potential results
- Beliefs of clients and health care providers about various screening procedures

NURSING DIAGNOSES

Nursing diagnoses for the healthy client during the second trimester are based on adaptation to the normal changes of pregnancy and responses to screening procedures. (*See* the box for nursing diagnoses related to the second-trimester client and her family.) Diagnoses related to the high-risk client are presented in later chapters of this text.

NURSING DIAGNOSES RELATED TO THE SECOND TRIMESTER

Physiologic

Problem-Oriented

Potential for constipation, related to second-trimester changes in gastrointestinal system

Potential for altered tissue perfusion, related to decreased iron absorption during the second trimester

Strength-Oriented

Asset in health of mother and fetus, related to physiologic adaptation in the second trimester

Progressive normal fetal growth and development, related to maternal health-promoting behaviors during the second trimester

Psychosocial

Problem-Oriented

Potential altered maternal role performance, related to lack of maternal role model (grandmother)

Potential for decisional role conflict, related to
- Career conflicts
- Need for income from work

Strength-Oriented

Positive family coping during the second trimester, related to adequate support from significant others and few role conflicts

Beginning maternal-fetal attachment, related to statements about perception of fetal movement (quickening)

Cultural

Problem-Oriented

Alteration in family process, related to cultural differences in perception of roles during pregnancy and parenting

Strength-Oriented

Positive partner self-concept, related to congruence between perceptions of appropriate maternal and paternal role behavior

SUMMARY

Assessment of the client and her family continues into the second trimester with prenatal visits every 4 weeks. The health history is updated. Physical examination, including maternal weight, blood pressure, pulse, fundal measurement, and fetal heart rate assessment, reveals normal physical changes in pregnancy. Appropriate laboratory tests, for example, urinalysis, are done. Assessment also includes psychosocial, socioeconomic, and cultural dimensions. Second-trimester assessment confirms that prenatal adaptation and fetal development are progressing normally, identifies emergence of risk factors, evaluates ways in which the client has been responding to health care recommendations, and identifies educational needs. An initial visit approach is used for the client who begins care during the second trimester; attention is given to reasons why the client delayed seeking care.

The second trimester is usually the period of greatest feelings of well-being. First-trimester discomforts such as fatigue and nausea subside and third-trimester discomforts related to the large uterus and advanced pregnancy changes are not prominent. Delivery is still far off and psychologically the woman continues to prepare for motherhood. During the second trimester the mother-to-be experiences quickening and becomes aware of fetal movements.

Risk assessment is important during the second trimester. Diagnostic tests and procedures such as ultrasound, alpha-fetoprotein screening, amniocentesis, fetoscopy, and percutaneous umbilical blood sampling may be used in diagnosis and treatment of many high-risk conditions. The emotional impact of these procedures and their implications must be considered in providing supportive care. Clients who would not elect termination of pregnancy may seek assessment such as alpha-fetoprotein screening or amniocentesis to allay anxiety, as even most high-risk individuals have normal results, or to have time to prepare for an infant with special needs.

As in the first trimester, assessment focuses on the client, her significant others, and her home and work environment. Nursing diagnoses identified in the first trimester are updated to reflect client strengths and the meeting of previous goals. Continuing diagnoses or the emergence of new diagnoses of wellness and illness emerge from ongoing assessment. A collaborative approach between nurses and other health care providers fosters client trust and promotes efficient, effective care during second-trimester visits.

REVIEW QUESTIONS

1. Identify the importance of comprehensive prenatal assessment, including physical, psychologic, socioeconomic, and other factors that reflect the level of wellness of the prenatal client and her family during the second trimester.
2. Describe routine maternal assessment techniques used during the second trimester.
3. Discuss indications for and implications of techniques used for fetal assessment during the second trimester, such as ultrasound, alpha-fetoprotein levels, amniocentesis, fetoscopy, and percutaneous umbilical blood sampling.
4. Discuss psychologic implications of assessment techniques for clients during the second trimester.
5. Summarize barriers to care during the second trimester.

REFERENCES

1. American Academy of Pediatrics, American College of Obstetricians and Gynecologists. *Guidelines for Perinatal Care.* 2nd ed. Frigoletto FD, Little GA, eds. White Plains, NY: March of Dimes Birth Defects Foundation; 1988.
2. American College of Obstetricians and Gynecologists. *Prenatal Detection of Neural Tube Defects.* Technical Bulletin *99*. Washington, DC: The College; 1986.
3. American College of Obstetricians and Gynecologists. *Management of Diabetes Mellitus in Pregnancy.* Technical Bulletin 92. Washington, DC: The College; 1986.
4. Coustan DR, et al. Maternal age and screening for gestational diabetes: a population based study. *Obstet Gynecol.* 1989;73:557–561.
5. Bouden ES. *Health Practices to Improve Pregnancy Outcomes.* Harrisburg: Commonwealth of Pennsylvania; 1984: 14.
6. Ryan GM Jr, ed. *High Risk Pregnancy Outcome: Ambulatory Care in Obstetrics and Gynecology.* New York: Grune & Stratton; 1980.

7. Auman G, Baird M. Screening for high risk pregnancy. In: Knuppel RA, Drucker JF, eds. *High Risk Pregnancy.* Philadelphia: WB Saunders; 1986.
8. Moore PJ. Maternal physiology during pregnancy. In: Pernoll ML, Benson RC, eds. *Current Obstetric & Gynecologic Diagnosis & Treatment.* Norwalk, Conn: Appleton & Lange; 1987:127–134.
9. Cunningham FG, et al, eds. *Williams' Obstetrics.* 18th ed. Norwalk, Conn: Appleton & Lange; 1989.
10. Coustan DR, Felig P. Diabetes mellitus. In: Burrow GN, Ferris TF, eds. *Medical Complications During Pregnancy.* 3rd ed. Philadelphia: WB Saunders; 1988;34–64.
11. Winick M. *Nutrition, Pregnancy and Early Infancy.* Baltimore: Williams & Wilkins; 1989.
12. Rubin R. Maternal tasks in pregnancy. *Matern Child Nurs. J* 1975;4:143–153.
13. Lederman RP. *Psychosocial Dimensions of the Pregnant Family.* Englewood Cliffs, NJ: Prentice-Hall; 1984.
14. Sherwen LN, ed. *Psychosocial Dimensions of the Pregnant Family.* New York: Springer Publishing Co; 1987.
15. Zajicek E, Wolkind S. Emotional difficulties in married women during and after the first pregnancy. *Br J Med Psychol.* 1978;51:379–385.
16. Brown MA. Social support, stress and health: A comparison of expectant mothers and fathers. *Nurs Res.* 1986;35:72–78.
17. Aaronson LS. Perceived and received support: effects on health behavior during pregnancy. *Nurs Res.* 1989;38:4–8.
18. Nichols FH, Humenick SS. *Childbirth Education: Practice, Research and Theory.* Philadelphia: WB Saunders, 1988.
19. Johnson F. Assessment and education to prevent preterm labor. *MCN* 1989;14:157–160.
20. Jiminez JM, et al. Clinical measures of gestational age in normal pregnancies. *Obstet Gynecol.* 1983;61:438–443.
21. Varney H. *Nurse Midwifery.* 2nd ed. Boston: Blackwell Scientific; 1987.
22. Graham D, Jacques S, Degeorges V. The role of ultrasound in the diagnosis and management of the obstetrical patient. *J Obstet Gynecol Neonat Nurs.* 1983;12:307.
23. Benacerraf RB, et al. Sonographic identification of second trimester fetuses with Down's syndrome. *N Eng J Med.* 1987;317:1371–1375.
24. Hohler C. Ultrasound and high-risk obstetrics. In: Knuppel R, Drukker J, eds. *High Risk Pregnancy: A Team Approach.* Philadelphia: WB Saunders; 1986.
25. Grant A. Controlled trials of routine ultrasound in pregnancy. *Birth.* 1986;13:16–22.
26. Mole R. Possible hazards of imaging and Doppler ultrasound in obstetrics. *Birth.* 1986;13:23–33.
27. Diagnostic ultrasound imaging in pregnancy. National Institute of Health Consensus Statement; 1984: Vol 5, No. 1.
28. American College of Obstetricians and Gynecologists. *Ultrasound in Pregnancy.* Technical Bulletin 116. Washington, D.C.: The College; 1988.
29. Kohn C, et al. Gravidas responses to real time ultrasound fetal image. *J Obstet Gynecol Neonat Nurs.* 1980;9:77.
30. Fletcher JC, Evans MI, Maternal bonding in early fetal ultrasound examination. *N Engl J Med.* 1983;308:392–393.
31. Heidrich SN, Cranley MS. Effect of fetal movement, ultrasound scans, and amniocentesis on maternal-fetal attachment. *Nurs Res.* 1989;38:81–84.
32. Stewart N. Women's view of ultrasonography in obstetrics. *Birth.* 1986;13 (special suppl):34–38.
33. Cohen FL: Neural tube defects: epidemiology, detection and prevention. *J Obstet Gynecol Neonat Nurs.* 1987;16:105–115.
34. Hanson FW, et al. Ultrasonography-guided early amniocentesis in singleton pregnancy. *Am J Obstet Gynecol.* 1990; 162:1376–1381.
35. Quilligan E, Kretchmer N. *Fetal and Maternal Medicine.* New York, John Wiley & Sons: 1980;102–103, 190.
36. Chibber G, et al. Rh isoimmunization following abdominal trauma: A case report. *Am J Obstet Gynecol.* 1984;151: 692.
37. Harrison R, et al. Risks of fetomaternal hemorrhage, resulting from amniocentesis with and without placental localization. *Obstet Gynecol.* 1976;48:557.
38. Simpson J. Genetic counseling and prenatal diagnosis. In: Gabbe S, et al, eds. *Obstetrics in Normal & Problem Pregnancies.* New York: Churchill-Livingstone; 1986.
39. Mennute M, et al. Fetal-maternal bleeding associated with genetic amniocentesis. *Obstet Gynecol.* 1980;55:48.
40. Golbus M. The current scope of antenatal diagnosis. *Hosp Pract.* 1982:179.
41. Simpson J. Genetic counseling and prenatal diagnosis. In: Gabbe S, et al, eds. *Obstetrics in Normal & Problem Pregnancies.* New York: Churchill-Livingstone; 1986:235.
42. Dunn PA, et al. Percutaneous umbilical blood sampling. *J Obstet Gynecol Neonat Nurs.* 1988;17:308–313.
43. Daffos F, et al. Fetal blood sampling during pregnancy with use of a needle guided by ultrasound: a study of 606 consecutive cases. *Am J Obstet Gynecol.* 1985;153:655–659.
44. Benacerraf BR, et al. Fetal abnormalities: diagnosis or treatment with percutaneous umbilical blood sampling under continuous ultrasound guidance. *Radiology.* 1988;166:105.
45. McColgin SW, et al. Group B streptococcal sepsis and death in utero following funipuncture. *Obstet Gynecol.* 1989;74: 464–465.
46. Feinkind L, et al. Abruptio placentae after percutaneous umbilical cord sampling. *Am J Obstet Gynecol.* 1990;162: 1203–1204.
47. Clark SL, Devore GR. Prenatal diagnosis for couples who would not consider abortion. *Obstet Gynecol.* 1989;73: 1035–1037.
48. Hodge SE. Waiting for the amniocentesis. *N Engl Jour Med.* 1989;320:63–64.

Nursing Care of the Family During the Second Trimester

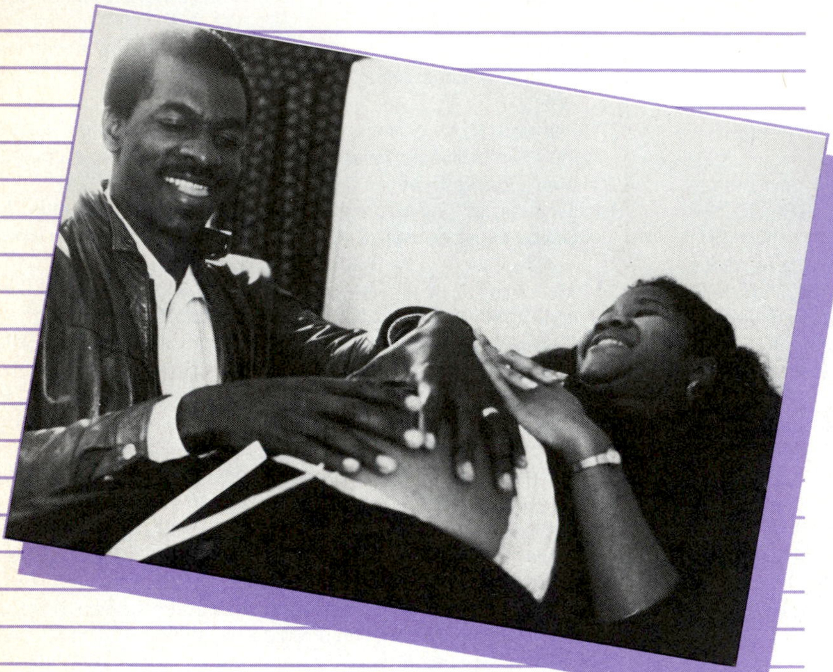

Chapter 19

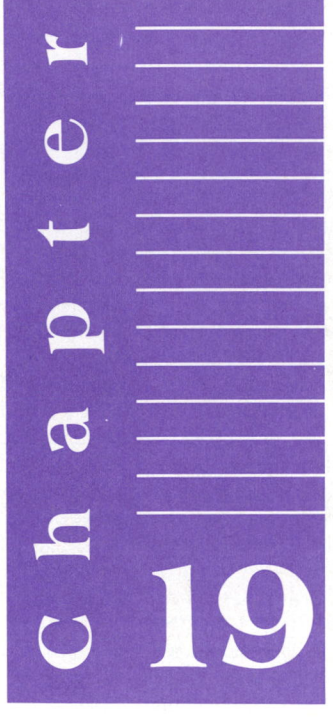

Continue a Philosophy of Care With Well-Defined Goals
Continue to Incorporate Recent Literature into Nursing Care
Prepare the Client and Family for Continued Care
Continue Assessment and Update Data Base from Which Diagnoses Are Developed
Update and Continue Strategies Identified in the Care Plan
Continue Support to the Client
Continue to Incorporate the Client's Cultural Background into Care
Continue to Encourage Informed Decision Making
Promote Psychologic Adaptation to Midpregnancy
Foster Family Attachment During Midpregnancy
Meet the Midpregnancy Educational Needs of the Client and Family
Promote Nutritional Well-Being
Assist the Client in Coping With Second-Trimester Discomforts
- Heartburn
- Constipation
- Hemorrhoids
- Faintness or Dizziness
- Round Ligament Pain
- Cosmetic Concerns

Promote Client Safety
Evaluate Antenatal Care
Ensure Appropriate Referrals for the Client
Summary

By the second trimester, a trusting relationship among the childbearing family, the nurse, and other health care providers ideally has been established. This relationship is critical to effective nursing care, which requires a partnership between the client and her health care providers.

The nursing process continues to provide an ideal means for organizing information and implementing nursing strategies. Health promotion, primary prevention, and secondary prevention remain essential to nursing care during the second trimester. Goals of nursing care identified in Chapter 15 for the first trimester continue; however, changes in management related to nursing care goals reflect the unique adaptations of the second trimester.

This chapter continues the format used in Chapter 15 and addresses nursing care according to specific goals. These goals are outlined in Table 19–1.

CONTINUE A PHILOSOPHY OF CARE WITH WELL-DEFINED GOALS

As discussed in Chapter 15, the philosophy, goals, and objectives for antenatal care should be discussed with clients and communicated in writing by the end of the first visit. During interviews at subsequent visits, the nurse assesses the client's understanding of these important components and makes certain that care provided is individualized, yet congruent with philosophy, goals, and objectives.

Through periodic assessment of the antenatal unit, done internally by staff or by external reviewers, antenatal staff can evaluate the degree of congruence between philosophy of care and actual care delivered

TABLE 19–1. GOALS OF NURSING CARE DURING THE SECOND TRIMESTER

Continue a philosophy of care with well-defined goals
Continue to incorporate recent literature into nursing care
Prepare the client and family for continued care
Continue assessment and update data base from which diagnoses are developed
Update and continue strategies identified in the care plan
Continue support to the client
Continue to incorporate the client's cultural background into care
Continue to encourage informed decision making
Promote psychologic adaptation to midpregnancy
Foster family attachment during midpregnancy
Meet the midpregnancy educational needs of the client and family
Promote nutritional well-being
Assist the client in coping with second-trimester discomforts
Promote client safety
Evaluate antenatal care
Ensure appropriate referrals for the client
Contribute to general antenatal public health

throughout pregnancy. Problems such as staff who rotate on a monthly basis, lack of time during busy clinic days, or inexperience with teaching can be addressed and possible solutions identified. For example, orientation programs for all new staff could inculde philosophy of care, goals, objectives, approach to clients, and ways in which these may be implemented. Periodic in-service programs can do much to ensure that all staff evolve care strategies congruent with the unit's philosophy.

CONTINUE TO INCORPORATE RECENT LITERATURE INTO NURSING CARE

As discussed in Chapter 15, recent clinical and research literature contributes to the design of optimal nursing care strategies. Nurses' own observations made in clinical practice may also stimulate research on care of the childbearing family. For example, nursing observations of clients' reactions to screening may stimulate research on ways to reduce anxiety during these procedures.

PREPARE THE CLIENT AND FAMILY FOR CONTINUED CARE

Chapter 15 discussed client and family preparation for prenatal health care. Before the end of each visit, a subsequent prenatal visit should be scheduled and the client should be informed about what to expect at the next visit. During the second trimester, visits continue to take place every 4 weeks, unless there is some reason for more frequent evaluations.[1] The client should be introduced to any new staff members involved in her care and should be informed about any changes in policies or protocols that affect her.

CONTINUE ASSESSMENT AND UPDATE DATA BASE FROM WHICH DIAGNOSES ARE DEVELOPED

As discussed in Chapter 18, continued assessment is an essential part of care during the second trimester. Through assessment, existing or potential high-risk conditions can be diagnosed; interventions may then be developed to minimize, eliminate, or rule out negative outcomes. Assessment also leads to diagnoses of strengths and assets, such as independence in self-care practices and healthy progress of pregnancy. Teaching and support provided by the nurse can help the client to maintain or to develop these strengths and assets further.

At each visit during the second trimester, the client's history is updated. The process of physical examination during the second trimester is similar to the process described in Chapter 15. Complete physical examination is performed on the first visit. During the low-risk woman's subsequent visits, physical assessment focuses on assessment parameters outlined in Table 18–2. Other health aspects are evaluated further if indicated. Pelvic examination is not routinely performed during the second trimester, as the uterus can be measured above the symphysis through use of a tape measure (*see* Chapter 18). By 16 weeks of gestation the fetal heart can usually be heard with a fetoscope. Doppler ultrasound makes it possible to defect fetal heart activity throughout the second trimester.

Components of each second-trimester visit include continued interdisciplinary assessment, anticipatory guidance and education based on the unique needs of each family during the second trimester, supervision in self-care procedures, and referrals to appropriate resources. All relevant information gathered during the assessment process, interventions, responses to interventions, and evaluation of client responses continue to be recorded clearly in the client's chart. Health care providers review the chart prior to seeing the client at each visit and update the records during the visit or shortly after seeing the client.

RESEARCH ABSTRACT

Brown MA. How fathers and mothers perceive prenatal support. Am J Matern Child Nurs. *1987; 12:414–418.*

The purpose of this descriptive study was to compare the perceptions of first-time mothers and fathers regarding the importance of their partner's support during pregnancy. The sample consisted of 313 couples ranging in age from 16 to 42 years. The mother was in the second half of pregnancy and both partners planned to assume joint parental responsibility for the child.

The instrument used in the study was developed specifically to evaluate participants' perceptions of supportive behaviors. The Support Importance Scale (SIS) consisted of questions based on a conceptualization of social support. The investigator requested that the partner respond to the questionnaire independently, without consulting the other.

The mean scores of each of the 45 items of the SIS were ordered to identify which behaviors were most and least important to the subjects. The highest-ranked behaviors were similarly valued by both men and women. The behaviors focused on two themes: (1) involvement in the pregnancy and (2) physical affection. In general, women tended to value supportive behaviors more than did men. The greatest differences between the ranking of men's and women's perceptions were the men's need for acceptance of their work schedule and the women's need for assurance about being attractive.

Comment:

This study developed an instrument, the SIS, that may provide valuable information to nurses planning care for expectant clients. Additional studies are needed for further validation of this instrument. Findings from this study highlight the importance of support for the well-being of expectant parents.

UPDATE AND CONTINUE STRATEGIES IDENTIFIED IN THE CARE PLAN

Throughout pregnancy, the care plan, based on the nursing process, provides an important tool for implementing management strategies. As discussed in Chapter 15, during the initial visit, the nurse and other health care providers collaborate on identification of relevant diagnoses and the development of a comprehensive care plan. Certain diagnoses, such as knowledge deficit related to discomforts of pregnancy, will remain. Although the need for teaching and anticipatory guidance continues, the topics change as pregnancy progresses. Careful and complete recording of information, including the client's participation in self-care practices and responses to previously prescribed interventions, ensures continuity of care. The case study and care plan presented later in this chapter illustrate nursing care of a family during the second trimester.

CONTINUE SUPPORT TO THE CLIENT

The nurse's supportive role remains unchanged throughout the second trimester. Continued contact at numerous prenatal visits provides the opportunity for development of a strong and trusting nurse-client relationship. By getting to know the client, the nurse is able to anticipate times when the client will need special support. Nursing strategies to support the client include remaining accessible, encouraging verbalization, providing anticipatory guidance, and acting as the client's advocate in the health care system (Figure 19–1).

For reasons such as family history or maternal age, clients may undergo diagnostic testing during the second trimester. As discussed in Chapter 18, ultrasound, genetic amniocentesis, and alpha-fetoprotein screening require nursing strategies that help clients make their own informed decisions. Nursing interventions also help clients cope with stress related to the tests. Most women who undergo screening tests do deliver healthy, normal infants; however, a small percentage do not. As one client recalled, "We had a small but definite risk of Down's syndrome. I was terrified of the test but felt I had to have it . . . [the nurse]

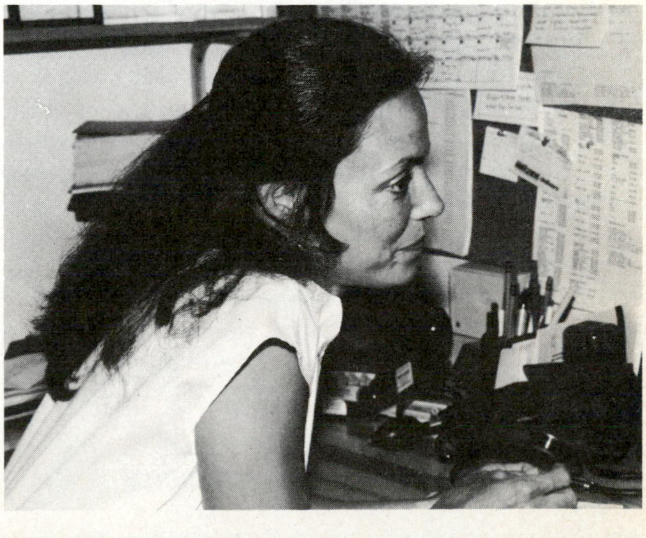

Figure 19–1. A nurse-midwife listens attentively to her client's concerns.

. . . stood by me. Never once did she ignore my concerns. She was there to listen, to explain, to help us pull through."

CONTINUE TO INCORPORATE THE CLIENT'S CULTURAL BACKGROUND INTO CARE

Throughout the second trimester the nurse continues to incorporate the client's cultural background into antepartal care, as discussed in Chapter 15. For example, the nurse may continue to provide nutritional teaching based on culturally prescribed dietary patterns identified at the first antenatal visit.

With an understanding of the cultural backgrounds of clients, the nurse can identify potential areas of conflict. For example, in Japan, a woman's commitment to a child's well-being is highly valued, begins before conception, and extends throughout the child's life.[2] Therefore, women in Japan may quit work when they marry and may alter their dietary patterns, style of dress, and lifestyle (eg, give up caffeinated beverages, stop smoking) to promote fetal health during pregnancy. Depending on the type of work, women in the United States may remain at their jobs through much of the third trimester. A potential source of conflict therefore arises between traditional Japanese cultural values and the actual practices of the Japanese-American woman who needs or wants to work as pregnancy progresses.

CONTINUE TO ENCOURAGE INFORMED DECISION MAKING

By the second trimester, the client ideally has decided on the birthing facility and selected caregivers. The childbearing family is encouraged to think about as the birth plan, although this is not finalized until the third trimester. The need for the client to make informed decisions related to aspects of antenatal care continues, especially in regard to antenatal tests such as ultrasound, genetic amniocentesis, and alphafetoprotein screening. The nurse ensures that the client is fully informed about the risks and benefits of any second-trimester screening procedure. The client can then make an informed decision about the test.

PROMOTE PSYCHOLOGIC ADAPTATION TO MIDPREGNANCY

Psychologic adaptation normally takes place throughout pregnancy. During the second trimester, nurses can do much to assist families in meeting psychologic tasks of pregnancy. Experiencing pregnancy together and preparing for a new family member require new family patterns of interpersonal interaction and adaptation. A basic, yet essential, care strategy is to encourage couples to share their feelings and concerns with each other. Through anticipatory guidance and teaching about physiologic and psychologic changes, nurses can also do the following:

- Identify and discuss clients' concerns about topics such as sexuality.
- Identify clients' concerns about body image, which is affected by the rapidly changing shape during the second trimester.[3]
- Explain normal psychologic processes of the second trimester. For example, family members may be upset as the woman seems to withdraw during the second trimester and to focus inward on the fetus.
- Prepare or help the couple cope with tensions in other family members, related to "moving up" a generation. These tensions may manifest during the second trimester when the pregnancy is visible.
- Discuss changing interpersonal family relationships and clients' reactions to them.
- Discuss the importance of thinking about characteristics they would like to have as a mother and changes motherhood may bring.
- Reassure clients about normal fantasy processes.
- Explore paternal reactions to pregnancy during the second trimester and explain the couvade symptoms that may normally occur.
- Encourage sharing of feelings between the expectant father and his own father.

Ambivalence about pregnancy usually resolves by the end of the first trimester, although some ambivalence may occur any time thereafter.[4] Through assessment of second-trimester psychologic adaptation, the nurse can identify high-risk situations that require futher counseling and referral. Examples of these are listed in Table 19–2.[4]

FOSTER FAMILY ATTACHMENT DURING MIDPREGNANCY

During the second trimester, pregnancy becomes visible and more "real" to family members. Attachment can be fostered by encouraging the client to bring significant others to prenatal visits, by welcoming them and including them in teaching about pregnancy, and by helping them to hear the fetal heart-

TABLE 19–2. BEHAVIORS INDICATING HIGH-RISK PSYCHOLOGIC ADAPTATION DURING THE SECOND TRIMESTER

Maternal Ambivalence Toward the Pregnancy, the Fetus, or Both
No questions asked about pregnancy, labor and delivery, and infant care; plans about these topics remain fuzzy and vague
No interest in the fetus; not interested in listening to the fetal heartbeat, feeling fetal parts, or discussing fetal growth
Unrealistic expectations of labor, delivery, and postpartum
Past negative experiences with pregnancy or labor and delivery
Denial of pregnancy and of fetal movement actually felt by caregiver
Pregnancy and parenthood seen as interfering greatly and negatively with lifestyle and self-image
Continuation of activities that could damage self or fetus, eg, heavy drinking and drug use
Reporting persistent and many physical complaints
High Stress Experienced by the Pregnant Family or Members
Reports of high-stress life events
Ineffective means of coping with stress
Lack of Nuclear and Extended Family Support Systems
Lack of support from expectant father
Lack of support from own parents, siblings, and family members
Feelings of isolation

Source: *Reference 4.*

beat and to feel fetal body parts or movements.[5] Understanding the importance of a woman's relationship with her own mother during pregnancy, the nurse may encourage the client to share her thoughts about pregnancy with her own mother if possible.

The client undergoing diagnostic testing may be encouraged to bring a significant other with her. During ultrasound procedures, the client and her companion may be positioned so that they can see the fetus on the monitor screen, if they so desire.

Expectant parents are frequently concerned about encouraging siblings to accept the pregnancy and new baby. The nurse can encourage the couple to express their thoughts; provide anticipatory guidance about normal sibling reactions, based on the age and developmental level of the child; suggest ways in which siblings can be made to feel included in decisions about the baby (for example, helping to select items for the baby); encourage the couple to bring siblings to prenatal visits; and include siblings in teaching about the developing baby.[6]

The second trimester is an appropriate time to establish support groups for expectant parents, who are then able to share thoughts and concerns and to network with others who are also experiencing the same phase of pregnancy. Expectant fathers' meetings and expectant mothers' meetings may provide special opportunities for sharing.

MEET THE MIDPREGNANCY EDUCATIONAL NEEDS OF THE CLIENT AND FAMILY

Throughout pregnancy, education continues to be a major focus of nursing care (*see* Chapter 24). The nurse explains current physiologic and psychosocial adaptations of the second trimester and provides anticipatory guidance so that the client is reassured about her normal progress and knows what to expect about the next phase of pregnancy. Table 19–3 lists topics for educational preparation during the second trimester and identifies chapters in this book in which the topics are discussed further. Table 19–4 summarizes answers to questions commonly asked during the second trimester. Education is based on each family's individual needs, rather than on a set schedule of content; family participation in determining educational needs is encouraged.[5]

As the second trimester progresses, the client may enroll in prepared childbearing classes. Childbirth preparation programs vary greatly according to method, approach, number, and length. Clients should be advised to select classes that will end within a month of their due date, so they benefit from all information presented in advance of their own labor and delivery. As discussed in Chapter 24, the nurse needs to be able to describe available programs and to make client referrals, based on an understanding of the client's unique needs.

PROMOTE NUTRITIONAL WELL-BEING

Nutrition is a major focus of nursing care throughout pregnancy because of its importance to fetal growth and development and to maternal health status. Strategies related to nutritional management were described in Chapter 10. Throughout pregnancy, nutritional status is reflected by parameters such as general appearance, the client's weight in relation to her height, history of current and past weight management practices, pattern of prenatal weight gain, hemoglobin and hematocrit (which may be assessed in the second trimester if indicated), usual dietary intake, pattern of intake, and consumption of nonfood items.

TABLE 19–3. TOPICS FOR EDUCATIONAL PREPARATION DURING THE SECOND TRIMESTER

Normal physiologic changes	*See* Chapter 16
Normal fetal growth and development	*See* Chapter 11
Client safety Hazards during pregnancy; use of drugs and alcohol; smoking; threats to safety and security (seat belts, environmental hazards, related to lifestyle and high-risk behaviors)	*See* Chapters 11 and 19
Warning signs of pregnancy and what to do	*See* Chapter 15
Nutrition and weight management	*See* Chapter 10
Dental health	*See* Chapters 16 and 19
Discomforts	*See* Chapter 19
Sexuality	*See* Chapters 8, 19, and 24
Normal psychologic reactions—client, expectant father, and family; reaction of others to pregnancy; concerns; adaptation	*See* Chapters 17 and 19
Self-care practices that promote wellness Relaxation and stress reduction Posture and movement Exercise Clothing Food preparation Gardening activities Bathing and swimming Personal hygiene Travel	*See* Chapter 24
Employment	*See* Chapters 19 and 24
Breast self-examination	*See* Chapter 5
Preparation for childbirth/early parenting	*See* Chapter 24

Weight management may be a problem during the second trimester, because women tend to feel well. Excess intake causes many women at this time to gain weight rapidly. Dietary changes may also be necessary to minimize second-trimester discomforts such as heartburn, described later in this chapter.

ASSIST THE CLIENT IN COPING WITH SECOND-TRIMESTER DISCOMFORTS

A sense of well-being usually characterizes the second trimester of pregnancy. By this time some distressing first-trimester symptoms, for example, nausea, fatigue, and urinary frequency, have subsided. Although the uterus rises out of the pelvis and the woman begins to look pregnant, uterine enlargement has not yet produced the uncomfortable changes of the third trimester.

The discomforts experienced by the expectant mother during the second trimester are not necessarily restricted to this stage of pregnancy. Some women may develop these discomforts earlier or later in their pregnancies. Nursing assessments must therefore be individualized.

A great deal of advertising money is spent yearly to entice consumers to purchase remedies to deal with physical discomforts. Many of these discomforts, such as heartburn and constipation, frequently occur in nonpregnant adults. Widespread advertising campaigns on television, on radio, and in the print media are also seen by pregnant women who may inaccurately assume that "safe and effective" slogans apply during pregnancy. The pregnant client should be advised that many over-the-counter medications should not be used during pregnancy. The pregnant client should be advised to check with her health care provider before using any relief remedy in topical, tablet, liquid, inhalant, or any other form.

Heartburn

Gastric reflux affects up to 80% of women during pregnancy.[8] During the second and third trimesters, the altered position of the stomach, the relaxation of the cardiac valve, and the progesterone-induced decrease in muscle tone and motility of the gastrointestinal tract combine to make pyrosis (heartburn) a common discomfort. If reflux becomes so severe that the client is at risk of aspiration or mucosal damage or is unable to perform daily activities, further evaluation is necessary; however, the healthy client who experiences occasional reflux can be assured that this condition is normal during pregnancy and will subside after delivery.

The client can make use of several strategies to relieve pregnancy-related heartburn[7,8]:

- Eat smaller, more frequent meals
- Avoid fatty or spicy foods or any foods that increase heartburn
- Eat the last meal at least 3 hours before bedtime
- Avoid lying down immediately after a meal
- Keep the head elevated when lying down, especially if heartburn episodes are frequent or severe (this may help counteract the effects of gravity on gastric reflux)
- Maintain good posture to provide more room for the stomach to function

TABLE 19–4. ANSWERS TO QUESTIONS COMMONLY ASKED DURING THE SECOND TRIMESTER

When will I first feel the baby move?

Women having their first baby usually feel first fetal movements around 18 to 20 weeks of gestation. Women who have already borne a child may experience these movements around 16 weeks or, in some cases, earlier. These movements often feel like a "fluttering" sensation. Experiencing fetal movements for the first time is called quickening.

How often should I feel the baby move?

After quickening occurs, fetal movements are felt about once or twice daily. By 22 to 24 weeks, fetal movements are frequently felt. During the second trimester, fetal movements most often feel like "kicks" and "punches." A pregnant woman who has already experienced quickening should call her health provider without delay if fetal movement decreases or stops or if marked increases in fetal movement are noted.

If fetal organ systems are formed during the first trimester, are there any restrictions on medications during the second trimester?

Yes. Fetal organ systems, for example, the lungs and central nervous system, continue to develop throughout pregnancy. Many medications cross the placenta and affect the maturing fetus; therefore, no medication should ever be taken during pregnancy unless it is prescribed by the obstetric health care provider or unless the health care provider in another specialty (eg, dentist, ophthalmologist) is informed that the client is pregnant.

If I eat a lot over the weekend, is it harmful to "fast" to make up for excess weight gain?

Possibly. Binging and fasting are never healthy dietary patterns and should be avoided throughout pregnancy. Such conditions as electrolyte imbalance and ketosis can result from fasting and adversely affect the fetus. Any day of heavy eating should be followed by a return to a normally prescribed dietary pattern. Pregnant women should seek nutritional counseling if they are unable to maintain healthy eating patterns during pregnancy.

What can I do about heartburn? I'm so uncomfortable and never had this before I was pregnant.

Heartburn, related to gastric reflux, is a normal yet uncomfortable occurrence that often begins during the second trimester. Attention to dietary habits may minimize this unpleasant condition. For example, avoiding heavy spices, fried foods, acid-forming foods (such as tomatoes); drinking milk, and eliminating beverages with meals (but maintaining fluid intake between meals) may provide some relief. Antacids such as Tums (which also provides calcium), Maalox, or Mylanta may be taken if prescribed by the certified nurse-midwife or physician. Sodium bicarbonate (baking soda) is a base; it should be avoided because of its potential for causing acid-base imbalance and also because of its sodium content.

Is it safe to have vaginal intercourse during the second trimester?

Yes. In general, there is no reason for the healthy pregnant woman not to continue sexual activity during the second trimester. Indeed, many women experience increased libido in this stage of pregnancy.

Is it safe to take a bath during the second trimester?

Yes. Tub bathing can be relaxing during pregnancy and may be recommended as long as membranes are intact and bath water does not fill the vagina. Bath water should not, however, exceed 102° F to avoid raising the core body temperature.

Can I use a sauna during the second trimester?

Use of saunas is not recommended. Intense heat can produce increased body temperature and generalized vasodilation. The shunting of blood to the skin can lower blood pressure. Increased sweating can contribute to dehydration and electrolyte imbalance.

Is swimming hazardous during the second trimester?

Swimming, like tub bathing, may be encouraged as long as membranes are intact; however, concern about the water quality itself should be raised and areas at high risk for pollution avoided. Diving is not recommended, because of the possibility of trauma.

May I travel during the second trimester?

There is no reason why the healthy, low-risk woman cannot travel by plane, car, or train during this stage of pregnancy and enjoy vacation or business trips. Changing the position while in transit, stopping or getting up to walk every hour and a half, maintaining adequate fluid intake, and wearing clothing that does not constrict or inhibit circulation from the lower extremities promote well-being. Before undertaking any long trip, it is wise to investigate the nature and availability of prenatal health care. Trips to areas of the world where there are poor facilities, high incidence of disease, and lack of available health care are not encouraged during pregnancy. Vacations that involve unusually strenuous or stressful activities, as well as activities that require balance for safety, should be avoided.

Should I quit my job?

A healthy pregnant woman who does not work in an emotionally or physically hazardous environment may continue to work throughout the second trimester. Women who do work in high-risk areas may need to use special precautions, transfer from the area, or stop working in that environment.

- Try sips of water during heartburn episodes to "clear" the esophagus

Some women have also been helped by drinking milk and eating ice cream, or by drinking cultured milk rather than sweet milk.[8]

Antacids should be used as prescribed. Low-salt antacids such as magnesium trisilicate (Gelusil) and magnesium hydroxide (Maalox) may be used by the healthy pregnant woman with normal renal function. Calcium carbonate (Tums) can also provide calcium supplementation; however, sodium bicarbonate, a popular "home remedy," should be avoided. Excessive intake of sodium bicarbonate can affect acid-base balance and contribute to the development of such conditions as metabolic alkalosis. The expectant mother should be reminded that antacids are medications, whether in tablet or liquid form. Women should check with their health care providers as to type and dosage of any medication, including antacids.

Constipation

Constipation is a change in the client's normal bowel patterns and includes decreased frequency of bowel movements, increased stool consistency, and increased difficulty with defecation.[7] Normal bowel patterns vary considerably among people. Indeed, daily bowel movements are not normal for everyone. Normal bowel patterns can range from three stools per week for some clients to three per day for other healthy individuals. Certain clients, however, think they should have a daily bowel movement. This belief may result from the client's social upbringing or from media advertising.

Constipation clinically becomes problematic during the second and third trimesters of pregnancy. For some women, however, constipation becomes a problem during the first trimester. As discussed in Chapter 16, pressure and displacement of the intestines by the enlarging uterus, decreased gastrointestinal tone and motility, and increased absorption of water from the stool contribute to this condition. Constipation is also a side effect of iron supplementation, which may be recommended during the second trimester (*see* Chapter 10). Prior to counseling the expectant mother, the nurse should discuss previous bowel patterns with the client to identify whether constipation exists. The expectant mother experiencing constipation should be counseled to maintain a noncaffeinated fluid intake of at least 6 to 8 glasses per day. If heartburn is a problem, fluids should be taken between meals. She should eat foods that contain roughage, bulk, and natural fiber, for example, prunes, figs, bran, lettuce, and fresh apples. Good posture and daily light exercise such as walking (up to one mile at a moderate pace) can foster venous circulation in the large intestine and facilitate intestinal motility. Exercises such as contraction of the lower abdominal muscles may also be helpful.[8]

The use of laxatives or suppositories should be avoided unless prescribed by the health care provider. Stool softeners may be safely taken during pregnancy; however, the client should check first with her health care provider. She should establish regular bowel patterns and not postpone bowel movements. This is difficult advice for some women who do not perceive that their work allows them adequate time to attend to personal bodily functions.

Hemorrhoids

A combination of factors, such as increased pressure of the expanding uterus on the hemorrhoidal veins, the influence of progesterone on the walls of blood vessels and on the large intestine, conditions predisposing to constipation, and straining during bowel movements, contribute to the development of hemorrhoids during the second and third trimesters. Although hemorrhoids subside and may disappear after pregnancy, they can be a source of considerable discomfort as pregnancy progresses. The expectant mother may experience itching and throbbing rectal pain that increases after a bowel movement or after long periods of sitting or standing. Irritation of swollen hemorrhoids may produce bleeding; however, any client with rectal bleeding requires further evaluation (physical examination, hematocrit, possible sigmoidoscopy, and so forth).

Pregnancy-related hemorrhoids are rarely "cured" during pregnancy, although relief may be obtained with the following measures[9]: strategies to decrease constipation (*see* earlier text); avoidance of straining during bowel movements; warm baths to increase circulation and provide topical relief (eg, full baths or partial sitz baths); ice packs or astringent solutions (witch hazel) to reduce the hemorrhoids; certain positions to relieve pressure and facilitate circulation, including resting in bed with hips and legs elevated and lying on the left side with a pillow between the legs; gentle replacement of the hemorrhoids into the rectum; stool softeners as prescribed; and nonsteroidal ointments or sprays to reduce swelling and provide analgesia (eg, Preparation H) as prescribed.

Faintness or Dizziness

Faintness or dizziness is caused by sudden changes in position, being in warm, crowded areas, or standing for prolonged periods. Faintness or dizziness is attributed to postural hypotension, which causes pooling of blood in the dependent veins in the legs when the pregnant woman stands too long or stands suddenly. The gravid uterus also may place pressure on the vena cava when the expectant mother lies in a supine position. The result is supine hypotensive syndrome (*see* Chapter 20).

The nurse should encourage the expectant mother to move slowly, avoid sudden changes in position, avoid warm crowded areas if possible, lie on her side rather than supine, and lower her head or lie down on her side if she feels faint.[8]

Round Ligament Pain

Early in the second trimester, the expectant mother may experience round ligament pain. As the uterus enlarges, the round ligaments stretch and lengthen. This results in a throbbing or sharp pain from the fundus to the pubic bone. The pain may extend or localize in the inguinal area. Pathologic conditions, such as appendicitis, may present with similar types of pain. Therefore, the client needs to be examined before the normal diagnosis of pregnancy-related round ligament pain can be confirmed.

Unfortunately, round ligament pain cannot be prevented or "cured." Reassurance that this is a normal discomfort related to healthy pregnancy may, however, help many women. In addition, to obtain some relief the woman should be advised to take warm baths (not to exceed 102°F), apply a heating pad, support the uterus with pillows while lying on the left side, wear a nonconstricting yet supportive maternity girdle, and avoid further stretching of the ligaments when getting out of bed by first rolling on the side and then pushing upward with the hands.

Cosmetic Concerns

Vascular spiders (telangiectases), melasma, and palmar erythema are painless changes associated with the second trimester of pregnancy. Nevertheless, they may be cosmetically distressing to women. No treatment is effective, although the client can be reassured that they will subside after pregnancy.

Client concerns, especially for facial changes, are real and should never be dismissed. The darkening of areas on the face and neck, although perfectly normal, is not always viewed as beautiful. Although direct sunlight may deepen melasma, it occurs even if the woman stays indoors.

Corrective cosmetics can "normalize" the skin's appearance and help the woman not to be self-conscious about changes in skin pigment or the development of vascular spiders. Many department stores carry these moderately priced cosmetics and have cosmetic consultants who can assist clients in learning about their application. In addition, corrective cosmetology is an emerging specialty in nursing. Clients who have pronounced skin changes related to pregnancy and who are self-conscious about them may be referred to these specialists for consultation, although such services may be costly.

PROMOTE CLIENT SAFETY

Nursing goals to promote safety continue to focus on prevention of client injuries during the prenatal visit and teaching related to safety. During the second trimester, safety and safe passage for self and fetus become emotionally important to the pregnant woman. Teaching about pregnancy and childbirth-related topics becomes of special interest. The mother may be very receptive to alteration of potentially harmful activities, such as smoking or ingestion of alcohol.

During the second trimester, the woman's center of gravity and balance change as the uterus enlarges in size and weight. This physiologic alteration can place the woman at risk of injury during activities that require balance or quick movements, such as skating and skiing. The nurse helps the client to identify which of her activities can be safely continued and which hold risk of injury.

Some second-trimester clients avoid using seatbelts for fear of harming the fetus; however, clients may be more severely injured if they are in an accident while not wearing seat restraints. The nurse advises the client about the importance of seatbelts throughout pregnancy and demonstrates ways the seat harness should be worn in the second and third trimesters (Figure 19–2).

At each visit, the nurse helps the client recognize potential safety hazards related to lifestyle or environment and to develop ways to minimize or avoid these. Warning or danger signs of pregnancy are reviewed at each visit (*see* Table 15–7). Signs and symptoms of preterm labor are also presented. In addition, the nurse reinforces the importance of continuing self-care screening practices, such as

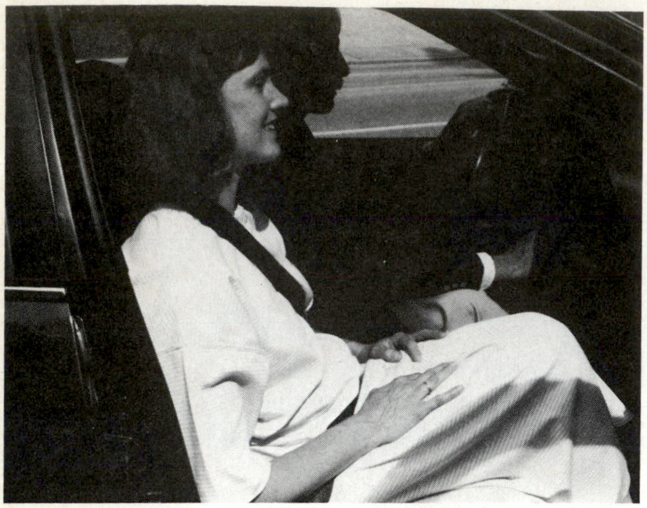

Figure 19–2. Seat harnesses should always be worn properly when traveling in an automobile.

breast self-examination. The client is advised to contact the health care provider if any abnormal signs occur.

Some low-risk clients may become anxious about safety during pregnancy. Throughout pregnancy, the nurse needs to reassure the low-risk client about her healthy, normal status.

EVALUATE ANTENATAL CARE

During the planning phase of care, desired maternal and fetal outcomes are stated in measurable, behavioral terms. Throughout pregnancy, evaluation continues to reflect the degree to which these behavioral objectives are met. For example, meeting objectives related to maintenance of adequate nutritional status may be observed by the client's reports of feeling well, a normal weight gain between monthly visits, and the client's report of a well-balanced diet. Evaluation, related to outcome behaviors identified in the care plan, is recorded in the client's chart.

ENSURE APPROPRIATE REFERRALS FOR THE CLIENT

In addition to the types of referrals described in Chapter 15, nurses frequently refer second-trimester clients to childbirth education classes. In some areas, clients may need to explore and select a prepared childbirth series early in the second, or even in the first, trimester to hold their places in the program.

Advancing pregnancy at times precipitates emotional upheaval within the family system. Through assessment, the nurse identifies clients at social or emotional risk and refers them appropriately to social service or counseling resources.

CASE STUDY/CARE PLAN: NURSING CARE DURING THE SECOND TRIMESTER

Yuri Yamaguchi is a 28-year-old Japanese-American woman who teaches home economics in the local high school. Her husband, Hideo, is a 29-year-old math teacher in the same school. They are in the second trimester of pregnancy with their second child. Their first child, Kenji, is a healthy 4-year-old boy.

The Yamaguchis live with Hideo's mother and father in a two-family house in the town where they teach. Hideo's mother emigrated to the United States as a young child, prior to the Second World War. Hideo's father was born in the United States. As a mother-in-law, Mrs. Yamaguchi has tried to adhere to the Japanese culture in her lifestyle, and she takes great pride in teaching her grandson about Japanese ways.

Yuri has had prenatal care since early in the first trimester. The pregnancy was planned, and although Hideo's parents would like another grandson, Yuri and Hideo express no sex preference for their second child.

The pregnancy is progressing normally. During her prenatal visit, Yuri tells the nurse, "I'm starting to look so fat; my clothes look terrible on me." Also, she states "I seem to get a lot of heartburn after I eat."

Supporting Assessment Data	Expected Client/Family Outcome	Nursing Actions/ Interventions	Rationale	Criteria for Evaluation
PHYSIOLOGIC STATE				
Nursing Diagnosis: Potential asset for healthy mother, related to normal physiologic indices				
Normal maternal assessment data for second trimester Vital signs: temperature 98.6, pulse 72, respirations 15, blood pressure 106/68 Uterine size appropriate for gestation Fundus felt slightly above umbilicus Urinalysis negative for glucose, protein, acetone Physical examination appropriate for stage of gestation (*see* Chapter 18)	The client will: Continue positive health care practices throughout the second trimester	Provide positive reinforcement regarding positive health care practices.	Positive feedback is a teaching technique that supports people's efforts and encourages learning.	If asked, client reports that she is engaging in positive health-related behaviors, such as moderate exercise.
	Identify physiologic changes occurring during this stage of pregnancy by the end of the initial second-trimester visit	Teach family members expected physiologic changes throughout second trimester, focus on pregnant woman and fetus.	Enlargement of the uterus and onset of quickening make the fetus a reality to family members so that teaching can be focused on the fetus as well as the mother.	Indices such as blood pressure and uterine growth remain within normal limits throughout the second trimester. Client describes how fetus will look during the second trimester. Client relates subjective experiences of second-trimester pregnancy to physiologic changes.
		Give anticipatory guidance on physiologic changes expected during third trimester. Prepare couple and family members for second-trimester visits and testing.	Anticipatory guidance by the nurse and other health care providers alleviates uncertainty and helps family members cope with ongoing changes of pregnancy.	
	Identify behaviors that do not promote optimum childbearing health by the end of the initial second-trimester visit			Client can discuss her own behaviors and differentiate between health-promoting behaviors and behaviors that will negatively affect her and her fetus.
	Identify health-promoting behaviors for the third trimester of pregnancy by the end of the second trimester			Client discusses intentions to continue positive self-care practices during the third trimester and acknowledges need to alter practices that negatively alter own or fetus' health. Client makes a resource list after discussion with the nurse, evaluates those resources that have been helpful, and indicates which resources she and her family will continue to use during this phase of pregnancy.
	Continue to use childbearing resources throughout the second trimester of pregnancy			Client questions nurse about new or additional resources as needed.

(*continued*)

CASE STUDY/CARE PLAN: Nursing Care During the Second Trimester (*continued*)

Supporting Assessment Data	Expected Client/Family Outcome	Nursing Actions/ Interventions	Rationale	Criteria for Evaluation
Nursing Diagnosis: Potential asset for healthy newborn, related to normal fetal growth parameters				
Continued normal growth and development of fetus	Throughout the second trimester, the client will:	Support health-promoting behaviors: nutrition, exercise, stress reduction, rest, and avoidance of drugs, alcohol, and cigarettes	Holistic nursing views pregnancy as a normal state; low-risk clients should not receive high-risk care.	When asked, the client describes quickening and health care practices such as nutrition, exercise, rest, and avoidance of alcohol and drugs.
Uterine size appropriate for gestation	Identify behaviors that will continue to foster healthy fetal development	Evaluate quickening felt by the mother.		When asked, client can identify the warning signs of pregnancy.
Fetal heart tone: 160 regular	Identify deviations from healthy fetal prenatal development (eg, cessation of fetal movement)	Advise client to contact health care providers without delay if fetal movement decreases or ceases.	All clients must be able to identify warning signs, as prompt treatment often improves outcome.	Client identifies stress-reduction strategies that promote health.
Quickening felt by mother at 20 weeks	Continue to avoid situations and substances that are potentially hazardous to the health of the fetus	Measure fundal height with a tape measure and explain procedure to client and other family members.		
		Assess fetal heart rate.	Assessment of fetal heart activity confirms presence of a live fetus.	
		Teach health-promoting behaviors and effects on fetal development during the second trimester.	Anticipatory guidance reduces anxiety, and social support given by the nurse relates to positive health care practices.	When asked, client can identify hazardous situations and substances in her own environment. Client identifies methods and strategies for avoiding hazardous situations and substances.
		Teach about assessment techniques during the second trimester.	Explanations of risks and benefits of various procedures allow the couple to make informed decisions and cope with uncertainty about the unknown.	

Supporting Assessment Data	Expected Client/Family Outcome	Nursing Actions/ Interventions	Rationale	Criteria for Evaluation
Nursing Diagnosis: Alteration in comfort, related to physiologic changes in the gastrointestinal tract during the second trimester and growth of the gravid uterus				
Client reports burning sensation in epigastric area after meals: "I seem to get a lot of heartburn after I eat."	The client will: Identify, by the end of the prenatal visit, changes that can be made in eating habits to decrease discomfort	Identify how client has coped with the discomfort of heartburn, what measures she has used in relieving the discomfort, and how her discomforts may be affecting family functioning.	Anticipatory guidance helps the expectant couple cope with discomforts of pregnancy. Identification of successful health-related coping measures motivates the client to continue these practices.	When asked, client can identify foods that produce heartburn or other gastric distress. Client can produce a menu plan and dietary pattern that will help to alleviate discomfort.
	Describe the physiologic basis for the discomfort by the end of the visit	Discuss with client and other family members relief measures and the physiologic basis for the discomfort.	Knowledge of physiologic causes of discomfort helps alleviate anxiety.	Client discusses with the nurse normal discomforts of pregnancy and their physiologic bases.
	Identify strategies to promote relief of heartburn	Advise client to eat smaller more frequent meals, and to avoid spicy or fatty foods.	Smaller meals produce less gastric distention. Fatty, spicy foods contribute to heartburn.	Client makes a plan to alter behaviors that increase discomfort. Client's dietary diary reflects changed eating habits. Client reports decrease in heartburn and other gastric discomforts.
		Advise client to avoid lying down right after eating.	Lying down after eating promotes reflux.	
		Advise client to keep her head elevated when lying down.	Elevation helps counteract reflux.	
		Encourage good posture.	Proper body mechanics provide more room for stomach to function normally.	
		Suggest sips of water during heartburn episodes.	Sips of water help "clear" esophagus.	
		Teach about antacids, as prescribed by nurse-midwife or physician.	Antacids neutralize stomach acid.	
		Advise against use of sodium bicarbonate.	Sodium bicarbonate can contribute to acid-base imbalance.	

(continued)

CASE STUDY/CARE PLAN: Nursing Care During the Second Trimester (*continued*)

Supporting Assessment Data	Expected Client/Family Outcome	Nursing Actions/ Interventions	Rationale	Criteria for Evaluation
NUTRITIONAL STATE				
Nursing Diagnosis: Potential asset in maternal and fetal health, related to adequate nutrient intake				
Gained 2 pounds in 1 month Twenty-four-hour recall of diet reveals adequate nutrient intake when iron and folacin supplements are used Additional laboratory values reveal deficiency in iron and folic acid	The client will: State the need for additional nutrients during pregnancy by the end of the visit	Explore with client and family dietary intake practices.	Nutrition during pregnancy is an important component in optimal maternal-fetal health status.	Client lists nutrients needed during pregnancy.
		Reassess nutritional intake through 24-hour recall and dietary diary.	24-hour recall and dietary diary provide comprehensive assessment. Planning with clients instead of for clients helps ensure motivation toward positive health care practices. Knowledge and anticipatory guidance help to motivate client toward continued positive health practices.	Client identifies from a 24-hour diet recall assets and deficiencies in her diet. Client plans a nutritious diet. Client's 24-hour recall and diary reflect adequate folic acid and iron intake through food and supplementation. Client relates necessary nutrients to the four food groups, taking into account her cultural preferences.
	Continue to eat a nutritionally sound diet and continue iron and folacin supplements as prescribed	Explain and support client's prescribed supplementation of folacin and iron.	Iron and folacin supplement dietary intake to meet prenatal nutrition requirements.	When asked client identifies foods containing iron and folacin. Client also reflects knowledge in cooking practices, such as those designed to maximize folic acid retention in food. Client can identify reasons for laboratory studies such as those for hemoglobin and hematocrit values.

Supporting Assessment Data	Expected Client/Family Outcome	Nursing Actions/ Interventions	Rationale	Criteria for Evaluation
PSYCHOSOCIAL STATE				
Nursing Diagnosis: Potential alteration in maternal dietary practices, related to possible negative perceptions of pregnant body				
Client expresses reluctance to gain weight Client states that she has always "worried about my weight"	The client will: Discuss feelings about weight gain and body image by the end of the visit	Explore with client her feelings with regard to nutrient intake and perceptions of body image. Explore with client factors that influenced her body image prior to and during pregnancy.	Body image and body boundary are important parameters for assessment when providing nursing care for the pregnant family. Perception of body image is developmental and occurs prior to pregnancy. During the second trimester, the woman's body image changes as a result of changes in the gravid uterus and normal weight gain. Strengthening of the expectant family's support networks facilitates psychologic adjustment during pregnancy.	Client discusses feelings about body image prior to pregnancy as well as during pregnancy.
	Describe normal weight gain parameters	Encourage client to continue to eat a well-balanced diet.	Good nutrition promotes maternal-fetal well-being	Client continues to gain weight normally and maintains adequate intake.
	Participate in discussion of weight related issues in prenatal classes	Encourage discussion of weight-related issues during prenatal classes.	Group discussion helps client to deal with feelings also shared by others.	Client and husband attend prenatal classes. Client participates in group discussion about weight related issues.
Nursing Diagnosis: Potential asset in mother-child attachment, related to positive binding-in of mother to fetus				
Client expresses delight at fetal movement Client refers to fetus alternately as "she" or "he" Client gives fetus a pet name Client describes a dream about having a baby	The client and her family will continue attachment behaviors to the fetus throughout the second trimester	Discuss with client and husband the psychosocial processes that occur during this and later stages of pregnancy. Explore with husband paternal attachment behaviors and his feelings regarding the pregnancy and his role as father. Explore with the couple maternal and paternal fantasies.	Binding-in of the mother to the fetus helps the mother to identify a maternal role and attain a maternal identity. Fathers also begin attachment and role assumption during pregnancy. Fantasies foster parental attachment and role assumption.	Family members jointly assess fetal movements. Family members palpate fetal movements, talk about coming baby. Family members begin to seek resources connected to child care (eg, books, groups, and other resources).

(continued)

CASE STUDY/CARE PLAN: Nursing Care During the Second Trimester (*continued*)

Supporting Assessment Data	Expected Client/Family Outcome	Nursing Actions/ Interventions	Rationale	Criteria for Evaluation
Nursing Diagnosis: Potential alteration in family relationships, related to knowledge deficit of 4-year-old son				
Client describes inability to thoroughly discuss pregnancy with 4-year-old son Family members state that child believes that baby will be a boy and will quickly grow up to be "as big as him"	The client and family will: Identify ways to teach a 4-year-old child about pregnancy and newborn by the next prenatal visit.	Explore with parents problems that they have in explaining the pregnancy to their child. Explain the psychosocial and cognitive development of a 4-year-old. Encourage client and husband to bring their child with them to prenatal visits.	Children differ in their ability to understand and cope with pregnancy based on their developmental level. Teaching of children should be age appropriate.	When asked, client and family identify strategies to teach child that are appropriate to developmental level. Parents enroll their child in a sibling preparation class.
	Identify informational resources available to help parents teach children about pregnancy by the end of the visit	Give parents a list of books and videos that can be used to assist them in teaching their child about pregnancy.	Helping parents prepare their children for the new child will facilitate sibling relationships after the baby is born and facilitate coping by the sibling.	Parents buy books appropriate to the child's developmental level.
Nursing Diagnosis: Potential conflict in family relationships, related to cultural beliefs of paternal grandmother				
Nuclear family is a "Westernized" Japanese family Traditional mother-in-law lives with family Couple states that paternal grandmother wants them to adhere to traditional Japanese birth and childrearing practices	The client and her family will: Discuss their feelings about cultural beliefs by the end of the second trimester	Reassess family function and family dynamics.	Acculturation affects how family members cope with pregnancy.	Parents and grandmother discuss cultural rituals and beliefs regarding family and pregnancy.
	Discuss potential conflicts that may arise related to beliefs by the next prenatal visit	Reassess potential family conflict based on cultural differences.	Cultural prescriptions influence family members' roles and attitudes.	When asked, family members identify differences in beliefs between culture of origin and Western cultural norms. Family members acknowledge conflicts between cultures.
	Identify strategies for resolving culturally based conflicts by the end of the second trimester	Help family members identify potential conflicts and strategies to deal with conflicts, such as compromise.	The family controls relationships of its members so that conflict resolution is dependent on strategies they can use to foster positive relationships.	Family members plan strategies for conflict resolution.
		Encourage communication among family members.		Family members communicate with each other.

SUMMARY

By the second trimester of pregnancy, the client and family have ideally developed a trusting relationship with health care providers and have become well acquainted with the antenatal facility and the services provided. Nursing care strategies, identified during the first trimester, are continued or modified to meet the unique changes of the second-trimester client and her family. For the low-risk, healthy family, second-trimester management continues to focus on assessment, guidance, and teaching. Self-care practices that promote wellness or identify high-risk conditions are encouraged.

As in Chapter 15, management for the second trimester was discussed according to nursing care goals. Management topics, such as strategies to relieve discomforts related to the second trimester and answers to questions commonly asked during the second trimester, were addressed. Application of the nursing process to a low-risk, second-trimester pregnant family was illustrated by a case study and care plan.

REVIEW QUESTIONS

1. Discuss nursing care related to psychosocial/cultural influences on the second trimester childbearing family.
2. Identify topics that would be considered important for client education during the second trimester.
3. Describe advice about work or travel that could be given to a pregnant client during the second trimester.
4. Identify discomforts related to the second trimester of pregnancy and discuss strategies to help clients cope with the discomforts.
5. Discuss advice that should be given to promote safety during the second trimester.

REFERENCES

1. American Academy of Pediatrics, American College of Obstetricians and Gynecologists. In: Frigoletto FD, Little GA, eds. *Guidelines for Perinatal Care.* 2nd ed. White Plains, NY: March of Dimes Birth Defects Foundation; 1988.
2. Engel N. An American's experience of pregnancy and childbirth in Japan. *Birth.* 1989;16:81–86.
3. Shuzman E. Body image in pregnancy. In: Sherwen LN, ed. *Psychosocial Dimensions of the Pregnant Family.* New York: Springer Publishing Co; 1987:129–156.
4. Allen E, Mantz M. Are normal patients at risk during pregnancy? *J Obstet Gynecol Neonat Nurs.* 1981;*10*:348–353.
5. McKay S, Phillips C. *Family Centered Maternity Care.* Rockville, Md: Aspen; 1984.
6. Kutzner S. Responses of siblings to pregnancy. In: Sherwen LN, ed. *Psychosocial Dimensions of the Pregnant Family.* New York: Springer Publishing Co; 1987:177–192.
7. Connor J. Gastrointestinal complications. In: Burrow GN, Ferris TF, eds. *Medical Complications During Pregnancy.* 3rd ed. Philadelphia: WB Saunders; 1988:303–317.
8. Varney H. *Nurse Midwifery.* 2nd ed. Boston: Blackwell Scientific; 1987.

The Third Trimester of Pregnancy

unit

5

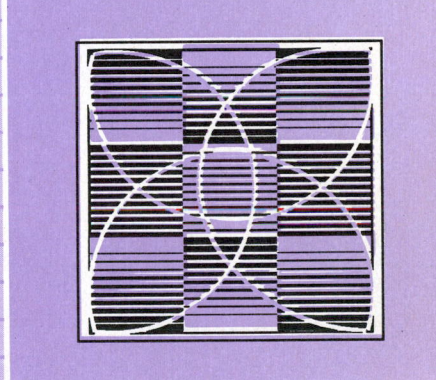

Physiologic Changes During the Third Trimester

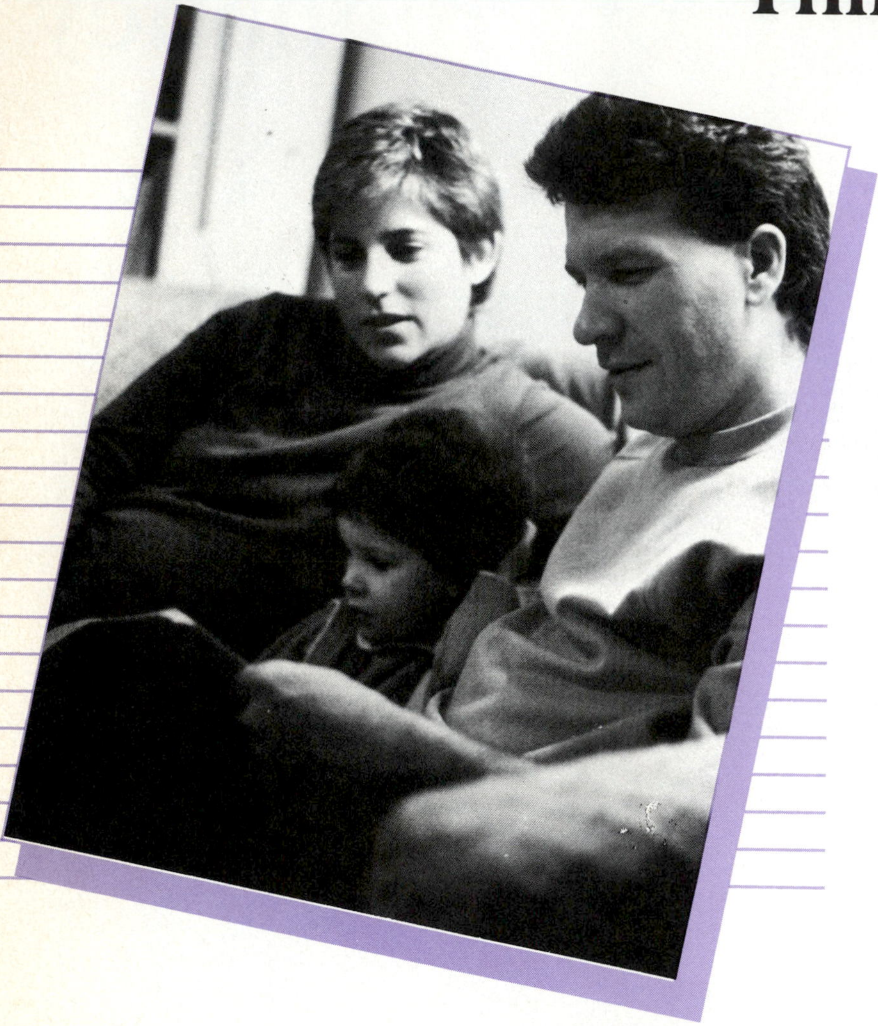

chapter 20

Key Terms

bloody show
carpal tunnel syndrome
cervical ripening
diastasis recti
effacement
striae gravidarum
supine hypotensive syndrome
vena caval syndrome

The third trimester of pregnancy extends from the beginning of the 25th week until the end of pregnancy. Full-term delivery takes place anytime from the beginning of the 38th week of gestation through the end of the 42nd week.[1] Maternal physiologic adaptation during the third trimester of pregnancy supports the final phases of intrauterine fetal development and prepares the expectant mother for labor, delivery, and lactation.

Although each trimester includes specific physiologic changes, pregnancy is a continuous process. Many changes discussed in Chapters 12 and 16 begin during the first trimester, but become most noticeable at later dates. The nurse must realize that body changes are complex and that body systems, as well as psychosocial and environmental factors, are interrelated.

GROWTH AND DEVELOPMENT OF THE FETUS

The third trimester of pregnancy is highlighted by rapid growth and maturity of the organ systems of the fetus (*see* Chapter 11). During the seventh lunar month, the fetal lungs are capable of gas exchange and the alveoli continue to manufacture surfactant, the surface-active lipid that maintains alveolar patency. As the third trimester progresses, increasing amounts of surfactant are produced, preparing the fetus for respiration after birth. The central nervous system also matures during this time, with the maturation process continuing after birth. The cerebral cortex proliferates, and myelin, the fatty sheath that

RESEARCH ABSTRACT

Cahill C. Beta-endorphin levels during pregnancy and labor: a role in pain modulation? Nurs Res. *1989; 38:200–203.*

The endogenous opiate system (endorphin system) is anatomically located in central nervous system structures known to participate in transmission and interpretation of pain impulses. An understanding of the endorphin system has served as a basis for development and testing of new approaches to pain management by nurses and other professionals.

This study explored the association between plasma beta-endorphin–like peptides, known as neuroendocrine modulators, implicated in pain perception, and reports of pain perception. A convenience sample of 10 healthy pregnant women, 16 nonpregnant women, and 18 men (both nonpregnant women and men served as controls) were studied to determine if changes in plasma beta-endorphin–like immunoreactivity affected pain perception during labor. The three groups were reported to be similar in age and health status.

Two types of measurement were used: a measurement of pain (a visual scale of pain perception) and a measurement of beta-endorphin–like peptides in blood plasma. Blood samples were collected from female controls at the midpoint of their menstrual cycle. Collections were made one time only for both nonpregnant women and men. The 10 pregnant women were studied weekly during the last month of pregnancy, during labor, and 24 hours postpartum. During labor (which was arbitrarily divided into three stages based on degree of cervical dilation to better examine findings), women reported pain levels between and during contractions and had blood drawn for later analysis.

Findings indicated that pregnant women had plasma levels of beta-endorphins significantly higher than those of nonpregnant women at the midpoint of their menstrual cycle. There were no differences in hormone level between pregnant women and men. During labor, there was no statistical association between reported pain levels and plasma beta-endorphins. In all cases, the amount of pain reported between contractions rose steadily throughout labor as did the amount of pain reported during contractions; however, the amount of pain reported between contractions rose much more rapidly. This pattern suggested that opiate-active beta-endorphin may increase the ability of women to tolerate acute pain. The complexity of the function of such hormones in the body needs to be further considered.

Comment:

This study presents preliminary physiologic data concerning mechanisms of pain perception during pregnancy and labor. This research points to many areas for future investigation, such as the complex nature of the pain experience. Future studies could examine possible interactions between plasma beta-endorphins and use of childbirth preparation techniques, which also may affect perception of pain.

transmits nerve impulses, is laid down around the neurons. By the 28th week of gestation, there is a growth spurt with regard to brain size, surface area, and cells.[2] At this time the senses of the fetus begin maturing. The fetus can taste, hear, smell, and perceive light.

Beginning in the seventh lunar month, subcutaneous fat (white fat) forms under the skin of the fetus. By 30 weeks of gestation, the quantity of white fat constitutes about 8 percent of the fetal weight, so that the skin becomes smooth and the legs and the arms fill out. The lanugo begins to disappear in the eighth lunar month. By the 28th week of gestation, the bone marrow is producing red blood cells.

The ninth and tenth lunar months are times of slower fetal growth. Although the rate of growth slows, weight increases are greater. In the last few weeks of gestation, about 14 g of white fat is laid down each day. The body of the fetus, as well as the extremities, appears plump. The fingernails are well developed. The tenth lunar month is considered the "finishing" period, as the fetus prepares for adaptation to the extrauterine environment.

During the tenth lunar month, the fetus is usually positioned head down in the pelvis in preparation for labor and delivery. The fetus has developed biorhythms, such as sleep-wake cycles, so that a distinct pattern of behavior has been established by birth. At term the average newborn weighs 3400 g (7½ pounds).

MATERNAL PHYSIOLOGIC ADAPTATION

A great deal of physiologic adaptation is required as the end of pregnancy approaches because the expectant mother's body must simultaneously nourish a rapidly enlarging, active fetus and prepare for childbirth and lactation in the near future. Table 20–1 summarizes physiologic changes of the third trimester.

TABLE 20–1. SUMMARY OF PHYSIOLOGIC CHANGES IN THE THIRD TRIMESTER

Organ	Change
Reproductive System	
Uterus	Enlarges to its greatest size Myometrium distends Uterine walls thin and soften Braxton Hicks contractions increase in strength and frequency
Cervix	Ripens in preparation for labor Effacement may take place Mucous plug may be expelled
Vagina	Continues to relax and distend as a result of physiologic changes Epithelial cells continue to change Growth of *Lactobacillus*, which maintains acidic environment, increases Leukorrhea increases Hyperemia of connective tissue continues
Fallopian tubes	No new changes
Ovary	No new changes
Breasts	Enlarge Colostrum is present
Cardiovascular System	Cardiac output remains elevated up to 40% over prepregnant levels Maternal blood volume increases 30% to 50% over nonpregnant levels Circulation to decidua, myometrium, placenta, kidneys, and skin increases Heart is pushed upward and to left Heart rate continues to be increased about 15 beats over nonpregnant levels Stroke volume continues to be elevated over nonpregnant levels until term, when decrease begins Cardiovascular workload peaks at beginning of third trimester, presenting a risk to women with pre-existing cardiac disease
Respiratory System	Changes are due to displacement by uterus and to hormonal factors Diaphragm rises Anterior-posterior and transverse chest diameters increase Ribs flare; rib cage expands Oxygen consumption increases.
Urinary System	Some dilation of renal calyces, pelves, and ureters occurs, especially on right side Urinary frequency results from pressure of presenting part settling into pelvis Physiologic hypervolemia occurs Fluid and electrolyte balance continues to be affected by complex hormonal interactions, increased glomerular filtration rate, decreased renal vascular resistance, decreased plasma albumin concentration, and other factors
Musculoskeletal System	Joints continue to relax and become mobile Center of gravity continues to shift forward Lordosis progresses Balance is altered Walking and changing positions become more difficult Women waddle, develop wide gait Numbness and tingling in upper extremity, carpal tunnel syndrome, and diastasis recti may develop
Integument	
Skin	Striae increase and become more pronounced Sweat and sebaceous gland activity increases Vascular spiders and palmar erythema may be present or develop Skin pigmentation darkens
Hair	Continues to seem thicker Some women may have hair loss
Nails	Continue to grow faster than in nonpregnant state Continue to be softer and break more easily than in nonpregnant state

(*continued*)

TABLE 20–1. SUMMARY OF PHYSIOLOGIC CHANGES IN THE THIRD TRIMESTER *(continued)*

Organ	Change
Gastrointestinal System	
Mouth and gums	Hyperemia continues Gums continue to be sensitive to irritants
Esophagus and stomach	Second trimester changes continue Gastric reflux continues or increases Stomach capacity decreases because of enlarging uterus Hydrochloric acid and pepsin remain lower than in prepregnant state
Liver	Is pushed upward and to right by uterus No change occurs in liver size or morphology Alterations in liver function continue
Gallbladder	Capacity continues to be greater Continues to empty more slowly than in nonpregnant state Predisposition to gallstones continues
Pancreas	Responds to greater demands for glucose metabolism Production of insulin increases Gestational diabetes may develop
Intestines	Pushed upward and to side Decreased motility and tone continue and foster increased absorption of nutrients and water Changes predispose to constipation
Endocrine System	
Pituitary	Continues to be enlarged Prolactin increases until about 36 weeks, then decreases Levels of follicle-stimulating and luteinizing hormones remain suppressed Growth hormone decreases Oxytocin production increases Melanotropic hormone increases
Thyroid	May be palpable Vascularity and hyperplasia increase Basal metabolic rate increases Free T_3 and T_4 remain within normal nonpregnant limits; thyroid-binding globulins remain elevated
Parathyroids	Parathyroid hormone remains elevated Calcium and phosphorus metabolism increases
Adrenals	Adrenocorticotropin level continues to be elevated Concentration of cortisol rises, although rate of cortisol secretion does not Aldosterone continues to be elevated
Placenta	Remains fully functional to term Grows in size and weight

T_3 = triiodothyronine, T_4 = 3,5,1^{2x}, 5^{2x} – tetraiodothyronine = thyroxine.

Reproductive System

Uterus. The uterus grows substantially during the last trimester of pregnancy. The average weight of the uterus increases 20-fold, from a prepregnant weight of 50 g (1.7 oz) to 1100 g (2.4 pounds) at term. The volume of the uterus increases from 10 mL prior to pregnancy to about 4 to 8 L at term. This includes the fetus, amniotic fluid, and placenta. The myometrium distends, mainly as a result of stimulation from the growing fetus during the third trimester. This distension helps maintain the contractile proteins of the myometrium and promote their synthesis.[3]

The uterine walls continue to thin and soften; at term the walls of the uterus measure 0.5 cm or less. During the third trimester, the uterus continues to be saclike and freely movable. Because of the growth of the fetus and the thinning of the uterine wall, the fetus can easily be palpated and fetal movement observed.[1]

The position of the uterus also changes during the third trimester (Figure 20–1). By 8 months of ges-

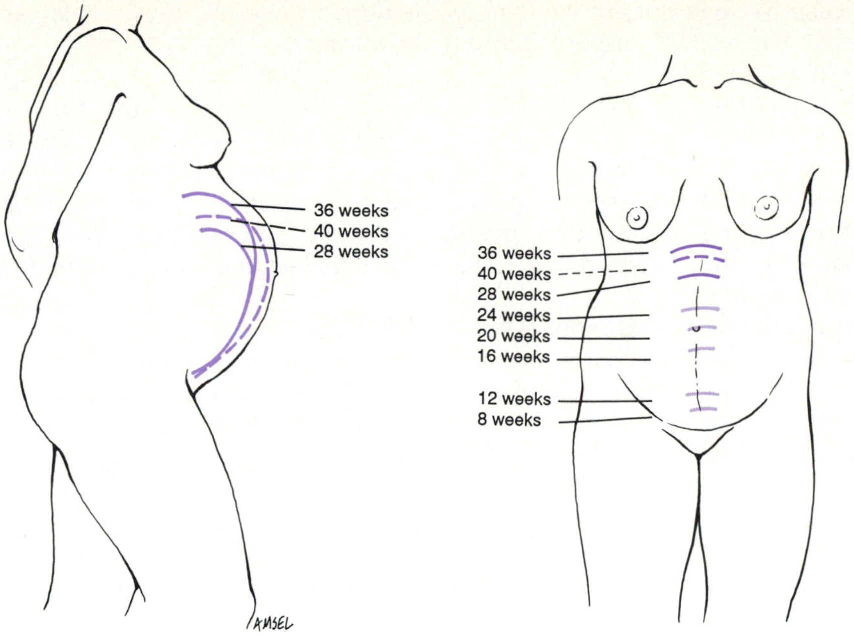

Figure 20–1. Height of the fundus at 28, 36, and 40 weeks of gestation.

tation, the height of the fundus can be felt three quarters of the way between the umbilicus and ensiform cartilage. Toward the end of the ninth month, the fundus can be felt at the ensiform cartilage and has reached its highest point of upward growth.

Approximately 1 to 2 weeks before term, especially in primigravidas, the presenting part of the fetus, that is, the fetal part closest to the cervical os, descends into the pelvis. This process occurs suddenly and is called lightening. The expectant mother may report that "the baby has dropped." With the lowering of the fetus into the pelvis, the uterus also lowers to about its level at 8 months of gestation (*see* Figure 20–1).[4] The expectant mother may have less shortness of breath; however, she may experience discomforts related to pressure of the presenting part of the fetus within the pelvis. For example, she may have urinary frequency, pelvic pressure, increased leg cramps, or dependent edema. In multiparas, lightening may occur at the time of labor.

During the third trimester, Braxton Hicks contractions may become stronger, more frequent, and rhythmic. Indeed, they sometimes mimic labor; however, Braxton Hicks contractions are not accompanied by cervical dilation, bleeding, or vaginal discharge.

Cervix. During pregnancy, there is marked proliferation of the cervical mucosa. By the end of the third trimester, the endocervical glands take up approximately half of the total mass of the cervix[1] (*see* Figure 16–2).

As discussed in Chapters 12 and 16, there is a progressive change in the collagen framework of the cervix. For example, the collagen fibers that at one time had been fairly rigid are rearranged. A flexible pattern develops, and fibers are able to slide over each other more freely. This gradual process may start as early as 24 to 28 weeks.[5] The process accelerates during the third trimester and contributes to the softening of the cervix in preparation for labor and delivery. Cervical softening during late pregnancy occurs spontaneously. No exact mechanism accounting for this process has been identified, although it is thought that prostaglandins may have an important role.[6,7] After 25 weeks, the cervix begins to shorten to an average of 40.0 mm by 37 weeks, as assessed by vaginal ultrasound.[8] Late in the third trimester or during labor, the process of cervical thinning, as well as shortening, is called **effacement** (*see* Chapter 25).

The process by which the cervix softens to a puddinglike consistency and begins to efface is called **cervical ripening.** This process prepares the cervix to open during labor. Late in the third trimester, the internal cervical os may open slightly as the cervix ripens, and the lower uterine segment tends to expand.[9] Assessment of cervical ripeness is unique for each woman. For example, the cervix of a woman having her first baby may change and soften, yet remain closed; however, the cervix of a woman having her fifth baby may normally be dilated 2 cm.[4] A cervix may be said to be ripe when it becomes soft, less than 1.3 cm in length, admits an examining finger easily, and is dilatable.[5]

Up to several days before the onset of labor, or during labor, the mucous plug may be expelled. As the plug separates, small capillaries rupture, staining the mucus with blood. This is referred to as the **bloody show,** and is a sign of labor (*see* Chapter 25). Bloody show is a small amount of blood-streaked mucus, usually not exceeding a quantity of two to three tablespoons. Gushes of bright red or deep red blood should not be mistaken for the bloody show. Heavy bleeding is never normal during pregnancy or labor and may be a sign of a high-risk condition, such as abruptio placentae and placenta previa (*see* Chapter 39).

Vagina. The vaginal epithelial cells continue to change as pregnancy progresses.[1] During the third trimester, proliferation of cells, hyperemia of the vaginal connective tissue, and increased vaginal secretions cause the vaginal wall to become relaxed and distensible to permit passage of the fetus during labor and delivery. Vaginal pH remains acidic (3.5 to 6.0), and the woman continues to be susceptible to yeast infections.

Fallopian Tubes. Few clinically significant changes occur in the fallopian tubes during the third trimester of pregnancy. (*See* Chapter 12 for discussion.)

Ovary. Changes to the ovary during early pregnancy and midpregnancy were discussed in Chapters 12 and 16. During the third trimester, ovarian changes are not clinically significant.

Breasts. During the third trimester, the breasts grow larger as the lobule-alveolar cells mature. These mature cells are secretory during this phase of pregnancy in preparation for lactation. Colostrum can be readily expressed from both breasts throughout the third trimester. Striae may become more prominent.

Cardiovascular System

Cardiac output, which reaches a maximum about 20 to 24 weeks of gestation, remains elevated about 40 percent above nonpregnant levels (Figure 20–2).[10] The increase in cardiac output during pregnancy is associated with redistribution of blood to the kidneys, uterus, breast, and skin. Cardiac output and stroke volume are greatest when the mother is lying on her left side.[11] For any given level of exercise, the cardiac output is increased during pregnancy as compared to the nonpregnant state. Maximum cardiac output is reached at lower levels of exercise in pregnant clients, suggesting a lowered cardiac reserve during pregnancy.

By the end of the third trimester, the maternal blood volume is 30 to 50 percent greater than the nonpregnant level, or about an additional 1500 mL[10,12] (*see* Figure 16–3). The increase in blood volume is the result of an increase in both plasma and red blood cells. Although plasma volume increases more than the red blood cell volume, the volume of circulating red blood cells still increases by as much as 33 percent at term. This increase is due to accelerated production of red blood cells, rather than extension of the life span of the red blood cells.[1] Despite the rise in

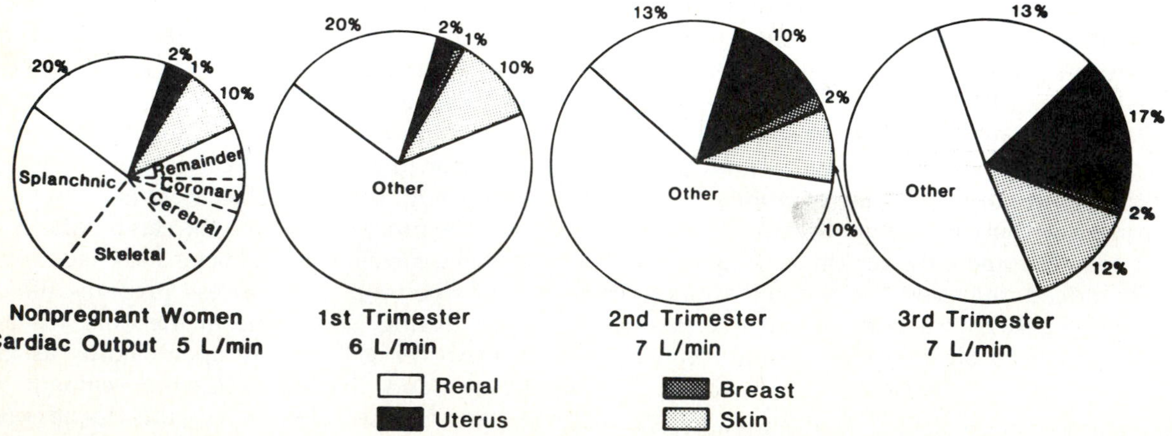

Figure 20–2. Distribution of increased cardiac output during pregnancy. (*Reproduced, with permission, from Burrow GN, Ferris TF, eds.* Medical Complications During Pregnancy. *3rd ed. Philadelphia: WB Saunders;1988:183.*)

circulating red blood cells, the expansion of plasma volume is still greater than the red cell mass. Therefore, as in the second trimester, hematocrit and hemoglobin may decrease and result in physiologic anemia. As discussed in Chapter 10, iron is necessary for hemoglobin formation. Dietary iron may not meet the increased demand for iron during the third trimester. Iron supplementation, begun by the second trimester, is continued through the third trimester.

Blood flow increases during pregnancy in response to the greater workload of the maternal organ systems. To meet the needs of the expanding uterus and products of conception, there is increased circulation to the myometrium, decidua, and placenta. Estimates of uterine blood flow range from 50 mL/min at 8 weeks of gestation to 500 mL/min at term.[3] The kidneys and skin also receive increased circulation during pregnancy. Both the kidneys and the skin help in the removal of waste products. The kidneys "filter" the expanded blood volume of pregnancy. The skin helps dissipate the large amount of heat that is generated by the increase in basal metabolic rate (BMR) during pregnancy.[1] The total increase in cardiac output is distributed largely to the uterus, kidneys, and skin as a result of needed blood flow to these areas (*see* Figure 20–2).[9]

During the third trimester, the enlarging uterus further pushes the heart upward and to the left. The heart rate continues to be elevated about 15 beats per minute over the nonpregnant level. A woman whose heart rate was normally 70 beats per minute before pregnancy might be expected to have a heart rate of about 85 beats per minute during the third trimester of pregnancy. The stroke volume, which increased about 30 percent over the nonpregnant level in the second trimester, remains elevated. At term, however, the stroke volume begins to decrease toward the nonpregnant level.

When the expectant mother lies on her back late in pregnancy, the large, heavy uterus compresses the inferior vena cava and other vessels that return blood from the lower portion of the body (Figure 20–3). Less venous return results in less blood filling the heart and decreased cardiac output. Arterial hypotension ensues and causes the woman to feel agitated and lightheaded or even to lose consciousness. These symptoms are referred to as the **supine hypotensive syndrome.** Supine hypotensive syndrome was initially called **vena caval syndrome;** however, as the uterus also compresses the abdominal aorta, the term *supine hypotensive syndrome* describes the condition with greater accuracy. The blood flow to the uterus and therefore to the fetus also is decreased and may produce fetal hypoxia and distress. This syndrome is especially problematic in high-risk conditions where additional stress on the fetus must be avoided.

Anticipatory guidance and planning to prevent supine hypotensive syndrome are the best interventions. In situations in which a supine position is necessary, such as during examinations, placing a pillow or wedge beneath the woman's right hip can shift the weight of the uterus off the vena cava and the abdominal aorta. Supine hypotensive syndrome can be remedied by turning the woman to her left side. Women who feel lightheaded should not be raised to a sitting or standing position, as fainting may occur and injury result.

Standing for prolonged periods can cause an increase in the femoral venous pressure and a decrease in blood flow to the upper extremities, because of pressure from the uterus and the effects of gravity. Swelling in the legs and feet (dependent edema), as well as varicose veins in the rectum, vulva, and legs, may develop.

Healthy women do not have difficulty sustaining the cardiac and hemodynamic changes of pregnancy; however, women with pre-existing heart disease are at greater risk of morbidity and mortality because of

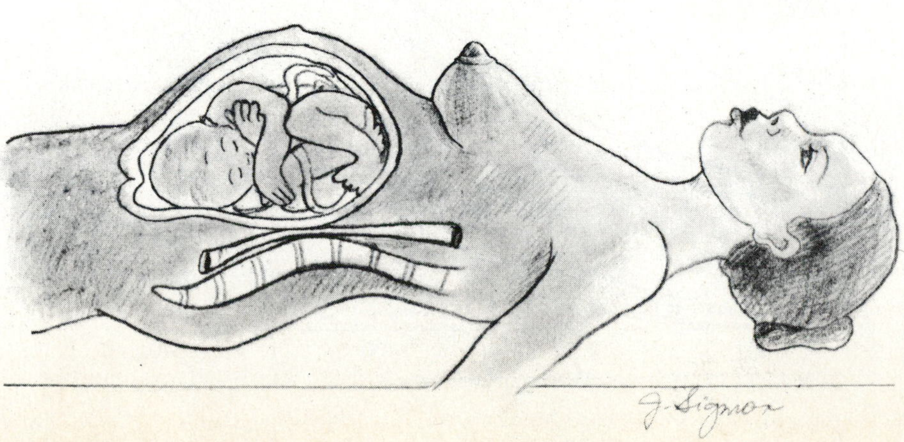

Figure 20–3. Supine hypotensive syndrome. When the woman lies on her back, the large uterus compresses the vena cava and abdominal aorta.

these changes, especially at the beginning of the third trimester when the cardiovascular workload peaks and is no longer counterbalanced by decreased peripheral resistance related to the effects of progesterone on vasodilation.[12] In addition, certain pathologic conditions of pregnancy, such as pregnancy-induced hypertension syndrome, may manifest after 20 weeks of gestation. As described in Chapter 39, these conditions have major cardiovascular effects. Careful evaluation of cardiovascular indicators such as blood pressure is necessary at each prenatal visit to identify promptly any high-risk cardiovascular condition.

Respiratory System

Anatomic and physiologic changes in the respiratory system continue to take place through a combination of mechanical displacement by the expanding uterus and the influence of hormones such as estrogen and progesterone. Most of the respiratory changes have been discussed in Chapters 12 and 16.

During the third trimester, the diaphragm is elevated about 4 cm, and the anterior-posterior and transverse diameters of the chest increase. This results in an overall increase in thoracic circumference of about 6 cm. The substernal angle continues to increase so that the ribs flare and expand the rib cage. The mother's chest and back therefore appear wider than at any previous time during pregnancy (*see* Figure 16–7).

During the third trimester, oxygen consumption increases substantially (Figure 20–4). This increase reflects the higher oxygen demands of the fetus, placenta, uterus, and breasts as well as the workloads of the heart, lungs, and kidneys.[13]

Urinary System

By the third trimester, nearly all pregnant women have some dilation of the calyces, renal pelves, and ureters, especially on the right side.[14, 15] In the last 2 weeks of pregnancy, particularly in women having their first babies, lightening occurs, and the presenting part settles into the pelvis. This causes the bladder to be pushed forward and upward. The normally convex-shaped bladder becomes concave, and its retention capacity is reduced. With pressure from the uterus against the bladder, the expectant mother once again experiences frequency of urination. Frequency does not, however, mean additional, large quantities of urine, burning, or bleeding. These can indicate abnormal conditions such as diabetes, urinary tract infection, and damage.

The fluid and electrolyte regulation of the body adapts to the changing needs of pregnancy and particularly the third trimester. There is a cumulative retention of about 950 mEq of sodium during pregnancy. This is distributed among the products of conception, the increased plasma volume, and the ma-

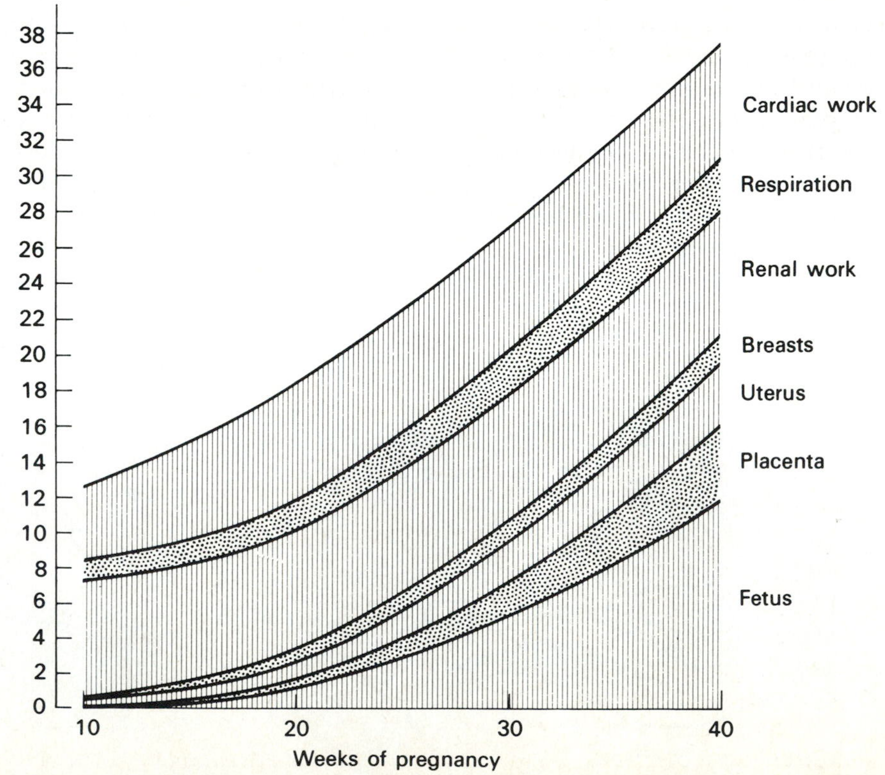

Figure 20–4. Increase in oxygen consumption among body organs during pregnancy. (*Reproduced, with permission, from Hytten F, Chamberlain G, eds.* Clinical Physiology in Obstetrics. *London: Blackwell Scientific; 1980:91.*)

ternal extracellular volume. At term, approximately 6 L of fluid is retained by the expectant mother, resulting in a physiologic hypervolemia[14]; however, the woman's daily fluid requirements remain and the healthy woman should not have fluids restricted.

Because of the increase in waste products during pregnancy, there is greater clearance of creatinine, uric acid, and urea. As discussed in Chapters 12 and 16, the blood levels of these substances are normally lower in pregnant women than in nonpregnant women. Glucosuria may be common during the third trimester of pregnancy as a result of a change in the renal threshold for glucose, although the precise mechanism of this change remains unclear.

During the third trimester, the expectant mother may experience edema of the lower legs, ankles, and feet (dependent edema). Although this may be related to sodium and water retention, swelling in the lower extremities also reflects pressure of the expanding uterus and increased plasma volume. The degree of dependent edema can also be related to the size of the fetus.

Musculoskeletal System

During the third trimester, there is further relaxation and increased mobility of the joints, especially the sacroiliac, sacrococcygeal, and pubic joints. The mobility of the joints, accentuated by the anterior position of the uterus at this stage, shifts the woman's center of gravity forward. To compensate for this change, the woman develops a progressive lordosis. This tends to strain the lower back muscles, and many women experience lower back pain. Weight gain and its distribution around the pelvis and abdomen contribute to the stress and pain.[16] Any situation that increases the lordosis, such as wearing high-heeled shoes, can intensify the back pain.[17] In addition, the mother's center of gravity changes greatly. This presents a threat to safety, as the woman's ability to balance herself is impeded. Activities such as climbing on chairs or ladders and sports that require balance (such as skiing) should therefore be discouraged. Figure 20–5 illustrates changes in maternal posture during pregnancy.

Walking and changing positions in general become difficult during the third trimester, especially in multigravidas, because of the cumbersome size of the woman and the changes in joints. The woman may develop a wide, waddling gait. Small women tend to have greater difficulties than tall women. They simply are not large enough to accommodate a full-sized uterus and maintain normal activities without some extra creativity in movement.

Numbness, tingling, and weakness in the upper extremities may be attributed to musculoskeletal changes during the third trimester (*see* Chapter 23). Changes in posture may cause the mother to slump her shoulders and bend her neck forward; this contributes to the development of upper back pain. In relation to increased fluid retention during pregnancy, **carpal tunnel syndrome** may develop[17] (*see* Chapter 23).

The tension of the pregnant uterus on the abdominal muscles may result in separation of the rectus abdominis during the third trimester of pregnancy. This separation, called the **diastasis recti,** is very common and usually causes no discomfort to the mother (*see* Figure 31–6). In rare and extreme cases, the uterus may herniate through the opening in the abdominal wall. The rectis abdominis muscle usually returns to normal after delivery; this process may be facilitated by exercise.

Integument

Skin. **Striae gravidarum,** often called "stretch marks," are reddish or purplish streaks that develop in the skin over the maternal abdomen, breasts, thighs, and hips, possibly as a result of such factors as hormonal influences and the loosening and stretching of connective tissue. Striae may appear or become more pronounced during the third trimester. About half of pregnant women develop striae; women also vary greatly with regard to the amount of striae they develop during pregnancy. Although striae fade to a silvery white color after pregnancy, they do not completely disappear. Expectant mothers may attempt to treat the striae with creams and lotions, such as cocoa butter. There is no evidence, however, that any of these remedies are successful in controlling striae, although some women enjoy using the products.

During the third trimester, the sebaceous and sweat glands may become hyperactive, causing the mother discomfort, especially in the summertime. Melasma, vascular spiders, and palmar erythema may also develop during the third trimester, if they have not already become evident (*see* Chapter 16).

Hair. The hair continues to appear thickened; however some women report that their hair tends to fall out more during pregnancy.

Nails. Nail growth continues at a faster rate throughout pregnancy, although the nails remain softer and more easily broken.

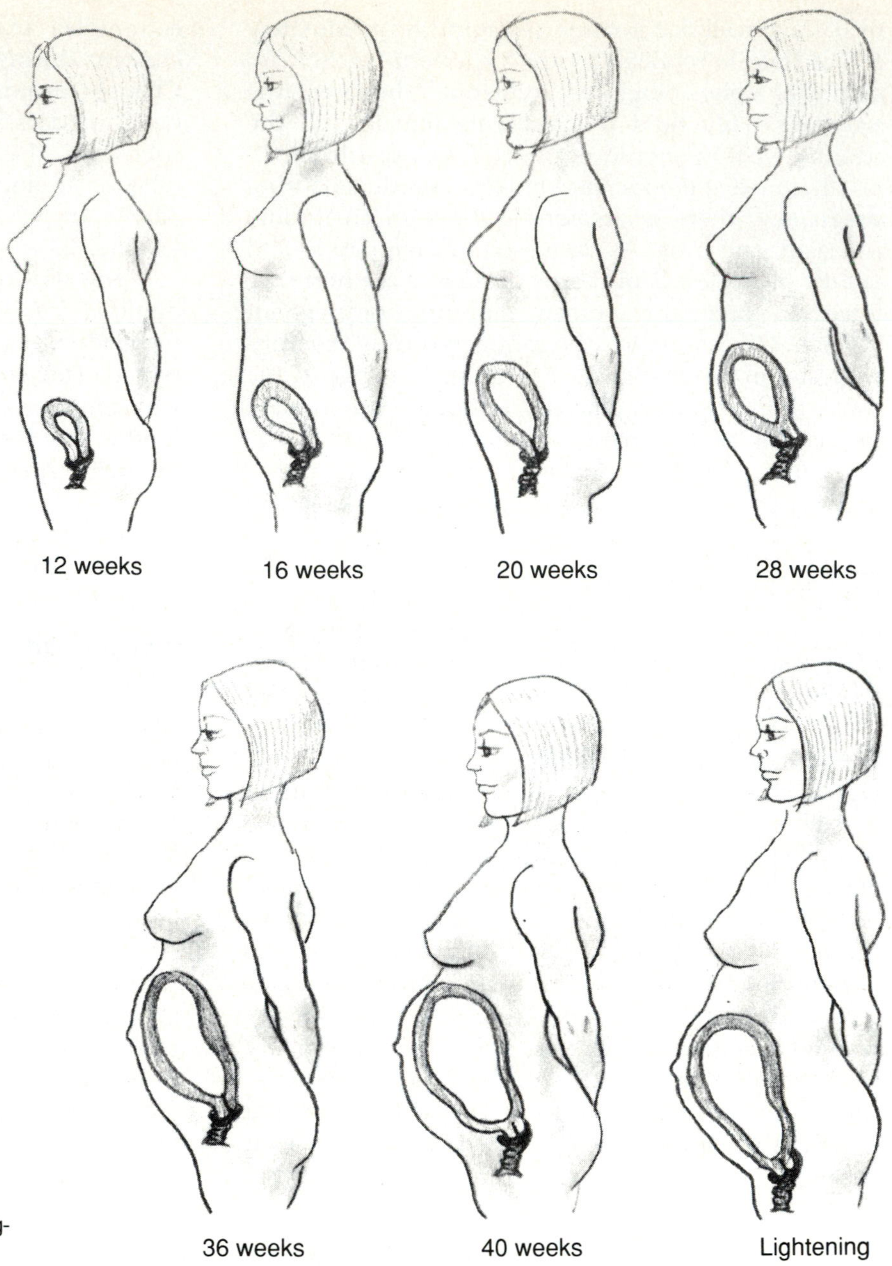

Figure 20–5. Postural changes during pregnancy.

Gastrointestinal System

The third trimester continues and accentuates changes that became noticeable during the second trimester. Most of these changes affect the stomach, gallbladder, and intestines, and have been discussed in Chapter 16.

Mouth and Gums. "For every child a tooth," was a saying used to describe dental problems related to pregnancy. Actually, the fetus does not draw calcium and phosphorus from the mother's teeth, and tooth loss does not take place for these reasons. As discussed in Chapters 12 and 16, changes in gum tissue (hyperemia) take place in response to higher circulating maternal hormones during pregnancy.[18] Without scrupulous, thorough attention to brushing, flossing, and, as prescribed, gum stimulation, gums bleed. By the third trimester women who have not consciously attended to dental hygiene may have considerable amounts of bleeding. Changes in gum tissue may contribute to loosening and loss of teeth at this time; therefore, even small amounts of bleeding should be investigated further.

Esophagus and Stomach. The pregnant woman's stomach is displaced upward during the third trimester because of the large gravid uterus. Esophageal reflux, discussed in Chapter 16, may continue or increase. Stomach capacity is decreased. Despite an appetite for food, the woman may need to eat smaller meals to feel comfortable. The woman continues to produce less hydrochloric acid and pepsin than she did before pregnancy.

Liver. During the third trimester the gravid uterus pushes the liver upward and backward to the right. As discussed in Chapter 16, in normal pregnancy, the expectant mother manifests symptoms and signs that may be seen in nonpregnant women with abnormal liver function.

Gallbladder. During the third trimester, changes to the gallbladder described for the second trimester continue (*see* Chapter 16).

Pancreas. The demand for glucose metabolism increases during the third trimester (*see* Chapter 10). This requires increased production of insulin by the maternal islets of Langerhans. Maternal insulin does not cross the placenta. If the maternal pancreas is unable to meet the needs for greater insulin production, diabetes may develop (*see* Chapter 39).

Intestines. During the third trimester, the intestines are further pushed upward and to the side. Under the influence of hormones such as progesterone, motility and tone continue to be decreased. Slower emptying of the gastrointestinal tract continues to foster absorption of nutrients; however, increased time for the absorption of greater quantities of water contributes to continued problems of constipation.

Endocrine System

Pituitary. By late pregnancy, the anterior pituitary may double or triple in size, mostly in relation to increases in prolactin secretion.[19] In rare cases, the pituitary may become so large as to result in problems, such as decreases in the visual fields. Plasma prolactin concentration increases steadily throughout pregnancy but begins to decrease after 36 weeks of gestation. During the third trimester, prolactin is synthesized by the decidua, as well as by the maternal and fetal pituitary glands. A major role of prolactin is the stimulation of lactation; however, it is thought that one of the effects of estrogen is the prevention of milk production by the mammary gland. After delivery, when hormonal levels fall, the effects of prolactin on lactation emerge. The maternal pituitary gland is not necessary during pregnancy to stimulate estrogen and progesterone secretion, because these hormones are manufactured by the placenta.

High levels of estrogen and progesterone continue to inhibit production of follicle-stimulating hormone and luteinizing hormone.[19] Growth hormone levels also decrease. The mechanism for this is unclear, although hormones such as human placental lactogen and progesterone may have roles.

The posterior pituitary produces increasing amounts of oxytocin, a hormone that promotes uterine contractions.

Production of melanotropic hormone continues to rise during the third trimester.

Thyroid. By the third trimester the thyroid has undergone moderate enlargement and may be palpated. The basal metabolic rate (BMR) continues at its highest level in the third trimester, i.e. about 25 percent over non-pregnant levels. Thyroid-binding globulins remain elevated to levels of 8.9 mg/dL as compared to nonpregnant levels of 3.6 mg/dL.[1] As during the second trimester, total triiodothyronine (T_3) and thyroxine (T_4) levels continue to be higher than nonpregnant levels;[20] however, free or unbound T_3 and T_4 levels remain within normal nonpregnant limits, because of the binding capacity of thyroid-binding globulins. Although elevated during the first and second trimesters, serum levels of thyroid-stimulating hormone decrease to about nonpregnant levels by term, because secretion of this hormone is thought to be related to secretion of human chorionic gonadotropin which has also decreased substantially by this time. Dietary intake of iodine continues to be important for normal thyroid function.

The fetal thyroid functions separately from the maternal thyroid. Thyroid hormone supplements therefore may be taken during pregnancy, if indicated, because of an effective placental barrier.

Parathyroids. Parathyroid function was discussed in Chapters 12 and 16. During the third trimester, secretion of parathyroid hormone continues to rise, peaks around 37 weeks, and then begins to decrease. Through mechanisms such as increased maternal absorption and placental transfer, calcium is available to meet the larger fetal needs posed by greater skeletal development during the third trimester. Nevertheless, maternal calcium balance is maintained and demineralization of the expectant woman's skeleton is avoided.[21]

Adrenals. The size and structure of the adrenal glands do not change much during the third trimester. As discussed in Chapter 16, cortisol concentrations and secretion of adrenocorticotropin and aldosterone increase. Major effects of these hormones are summarized in Table 12–2.

Placenta. Throughout the third trimester until term, the placenta continues to be fully functioning. The placenta and fetus continue to increase in size and weight, although fetal increases continue to be greater than placental increases. By 40 weeks of gestation, the average fetal weight is about 6 times the placental weight. At term the placenta is about 1 cm thick at the edges and 4 cm thick in the center and measures about 18 to 20 cm. Estrogens, progesterone, and human placental lactogen continue to be supplied in large quantities during the third trimester, although human chorionic gonadotropin levels decrease. Examples of hormones produced by the placenta and their major effects are summarized in Table 12–2.

SUMMARY

The physiologic responses of the mother during the third trimester support the final phase of fetal development and maintain the maternal body systems in a state of balance. In addition, physiologic changes prepare the mother's body, as well as the fetus, for labor and delivery. Changes in the mother's body during the third trimester take place by the influence of hormones and by the greatly expanding uterus, which mechanically displaces or strains body structures. The healthy, low-risk woman is well able to sustain the many changes and increased physiologic workload of pregnancy.

REVIEW QUESTIONS

1. Identify changes that occur in the uterus, cervix, and vagina during the third trimester of pregnancy.
2. Describe the process of "lightening."
3. Discuss cardiovascular changes during the third trimester.
4. Define supine hypotensive syndrome and identify ways in which this condition can be avoided and treated.
5. Discuss the old saying "for every child a tooth" in light of physiologic changes in the mouth during the third trimester.

REFERENCES

1. Cunningham FG, et al. *Williams Obstetrics.* 18th ed. Norwalk, Conn: Appleton & Lange; 1989.
2. Dobbling J. Human brain development and its vulnerability. In: *Biological and Clinical Aspects of Brain Development.* Mead Johnson Symposium on Perinatal and Developmental Medicine, Evansville, In: Mead Johnson; 1975:vol 6, pp 3–5.
3. deSwiet M: The cardiovascular system. In: Hytten F, Chamberlain G, eds. *Clinical Physiology in Obstetrics.* London: Blackwell Scientific; 1980:3–42.
4. Varney H. *Nurse Midwifery.* 2nd ed. Boston: Blackwell Scientific; 1987.
5. Oxorn H, ed. *Oxorn-Foote Human Labor & Birth.* 5th ed. Norwalk, CT: Appleton-Century-Crofts; 1986.
6. Ekman G. et al. Cervical collagen: An important regulator of cervical function in term labor. *Obstet Gynecol.* 1986;67: 633–636.
7. Rechberger T, et al. Connective tissue changes in the cervix during normal pregnancy and pregnancy complicated by cervical incompetence. *Obstet Gynecol.* 1988;71:563–567.
8. Kushnin O, et al. Vaginal ultrasound assessment of cervical length changes during normal pregnancy. *Am J Obstet Gynecol.* 1990;162:991–993.
9. Papiernik E, et al. Precocious cervical ripening and preterm labor. *Obstet Gynecol.* 1986;67:238–242.
10. McNulty JH, et al. Cardiovascular disease. In: Burrow GN, Ferris TF, eds. *Medical Complications During Pregnancy.* Philadelphia: WB Saunders; 1988:180–203.
11. Milsom I, Forssman L. Factors influencing aortacaval compression in late pregnancy. *Am J Obstet Gynecol.* 1984; 148:764.
12. Beischer NA, MacKay EV. *Obstetrics and the Newborn: An Illustrated Textbook.* 2nd ed. Philadelphia: WB Saunders; 1986.
13. deSwiet M. The respiratory system. In: Hytten F, Chamberlain G, eds. *Clinical Physiology in Obstetrics.* London, Blackwell Scientific; 1980:79–100.
14. Davison JW. The urinary system. In: Hytten F, Chamberlain G, eds. *Clinical Physiology in Obstetrics.* London, Blackwell Scientific; 1980:289–327.
15. Meyers SJ, et al. Dilatation and nontraumatic rupture of the urinary tract during pregnancy: A review. *Obstet Gynecol.* 1985;66:809–815.
16. Urowitz MB, Gladman DD. Rheumatic diseases in pregnancy. In: Burrow GN, Ferris TF, eds. *Medical Complications During Pregnancy.* 3rd ed. Philadelphia: WB Saunders; 1988:499–525.
17. Donaldson J. Neurologic complications. In: Burrow GN, Ferris RF, eds. *Medical Complications During Pregnancy.* 3rd ed. Philadelphia: WB Saunders; 1988:485–498.
18. Chenger P, Kovacik, A. Dental hygiene during pregnancy: A review. *Am J Matern Child Nurs.* 1987;12:342–343.
19. Burrow GN. Pituitary and adrenal disorders. In: Burrow GN, Ferris RF, eds. *Medical Complications During Pregnancy.* 3rd ed. Philadelphia: WB Saunders; 1988:254–276.
20. Burrow GN. Thyroid diseases. In: Burrow GN, Ferris RF, eds. *Medical Complications During Pregnancy.* 3rd ed. Philadelphia: WB Saunders; 1988:224–253.
21. Pitkin RM. Calcium and the parathyroid glands. In: Burrow GN, Ferris RF, eds. *Medical Complications During Pregnancy.* 3rd ed. Philadelphia: WB Saunders; 1988:271–276.

Psychologic and Sociocultural Dimensions During the Third Trimester

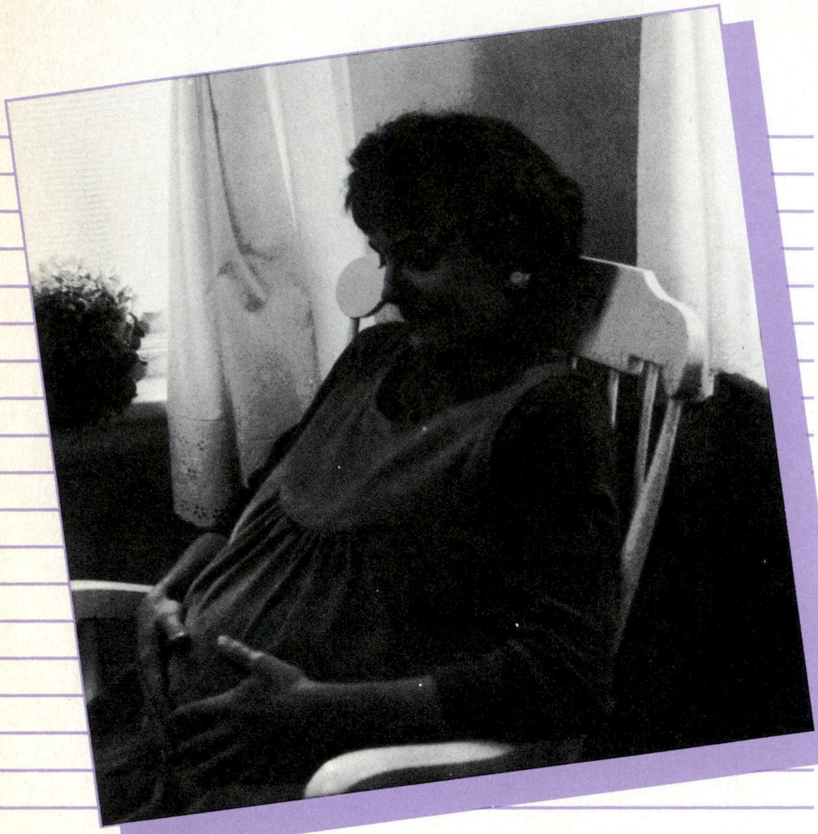

Chapter 21

The third trimester differs in many ways from the preceding two trimesters. The pregnancy is obvious to everyone because of the woman's size. Labor and delivery are no longer far off. The family must actively prepare for the new baby.

This chapter discusses psychosocial and cultural aspects of the expectant family during the third trimester. As in Chapters 13 and 17, the experiences of the expectant mother, father, siblings, and grandparents are described. The chapter concludes by examining the prenatal experiences of another cultural group, the Chicano family.

PSYCHOLOGIC CHANGES IN THE MOTHER

The second trimester is generally a calm period for the pregnant woman. The third trimester, however, marks the return to emotional turbulence. The woman is now faced with the impending birth and a new baby. Her lifestyle will soon be changed. She is not as physically comfortable as she was during the second trimester. Time needs to be scheduled for prenatal visits at 2-week and then weekly intervals. As she approaches her due date, the woman must complete many psychologic preparatory activities to move into the changed lifestyle of mother and child.[1]

MATERNAL PSYCHOLOGIC CHANGES AND CONCERNS DURING THE THIRD TRIMESTER

Acceptance of pregnancy
Negative feelings about being pregnant; acceptance of fetus

Maternal role attainment
Moving into maternal role; able to give birth and nurture infant; fantasy and differentiation occur

Fantasies
Increase in fearful and anxiety-related images; toward end of pregnancy, a focus on labor and delivery experience; greater focus on real experiences than imaginary events; reflection of life history, current concerns, attitudes toward pregnancy

Relationship with fetus
Continues to develop; eager to have and to hold infant

Relationship with mother
Strives to improve relationship with own mother; depends on own mother for support

Body image
Size of body and physical discomforts contribute to negative image for many women

Body boundaries
Body expands; perceived as more fragile

Body size and position
Increase in perceived body space; increased awareness of body size, change in balance, and decreased mobility

Time and space
Time slows; pregnancy seems endless; plans for delivery; continues inward focus

Preparation for labor
Rehearses for labor; attends prenatal classes; nesting behaviors (eg, preparation of infant clothes, schedule arrangements for labor)

Acceptance of the Pregnancy

By the third trimester, the pregnant woman normally may again have negative feelings about "being pregnant." She is anxious for the pregnancy to end and often becomes tired of her pregnant body and the restrictions it places on her; however, the mother-to-be should demonstrate general acceptance of the fetus. Rejection of the fetus during the third trimester is an ominous sign for the future mother-child relationship. Women who consistently express negative feelings about the coming baby may be considered at emotional risk; further assessment of the woman and her family situation is warranted.

A woman who rejects her fetus often depersonalizes him or her. She may think of the fetus as a foreign body or a tumorlike growth. She may be annoyed by fetal movement.[2] When speaking of the fetus, the woman may refer to him or her as "it."

A mother's intense ambivalence about being pregnant and becoming a parent may indicate unresolved conflicts in the third trimester.[3] Severe conflicts that are not resolved may interfere with the woman's acceptance of the newborn.

Maternal Role Attainment

By the third trimester, the expectant mother has taken on enough of the maternal role that she may give birth and be able to nurture her newborn; however, maternal role assumption is not completed until many months after the birth of the infant.[4] Fantasy and dedifferentiation are among activities of maternal role assumption that occur during the third trimester.[5] (*See* Chapter 4 for a discussion of the stages of role assumption.)

The stage of fantasy in role taking, which began during the second trimester, changes dramatically in the third trimester. Second-trimester fantasies are idyllic and pleasurable and concern an idealized life with a new baby. In the third trimester, the mother's increasing sense of vulnerability and desire to have the pregnancy end produce an increase in fantasies filled with fearful and anxiety-producing images. The image of the infant-to-be shifts from the desired angelic infant to the "feared" infant. Fantasies of the child change toward the end of pregnancy to fantasies about the experience of labor and delivery.[5] The nature of these third-trimester fantasies is described in more detail later in this chapter. Some negative fantasies about pregnancy and the infant-to-be are necessary parts of role assumption for the woman.[6–8] If her fantasies are only positive, the woman may not have the benefit of problem solving in fantasy about ways to cope with potential negative events (such as a cesarean delivery) that may actually occur during childbirth.

The final stage of maternal role assumption, which Rubin terms dedifferentiation, occurs during the third trimester.[5] This final stage is both similar to and different from Rubin's first stage of replication (these stages are described in Chapter 4). The woman still tries to "match" or "replicate" her role with role models in the environment. She still searches for her concept of the "ideal" mother. At this point, however, the expectant mother no longer simply mimics maternal behaviors of women she observes. Instead, she builds on the core of a maternal identity that she has already developed. During the third trimester, the expectant mother critically examines and evaluates maternal behaviors of other women as they relate to her concept of the ideal. She rejects behaviors and attitudes that do not "fit" her vision of the maternal role. In Rubin's terms, these behaviors reflect a trying on (or introjection) of a new modeled element (ie, behavior or attitude), a fantasy of the mental image of herself with the new element in action or in appearance, and a decision to accept or reject the new element as a congruent part of herself in her maternal role. This process is much more complex and critical than mimicry and involves choice as to which modeled elements (attitudes or behaviors) are taken as part of a woman's maternal role.

Fantasies

During the third trimester, fantasies (daydreams and nightdreams) are felt more as real experiences than as unreal imaginary events. Fantasies may have greater meaning for the woman during the third trimester.[5] Third-trimester fantasies may be accompanied by worry, anxiety, and fear, despite the woman's attempts to orient herself to the "real world" and to keep her mind off unpleasant thoughts. The pregnant woman may fear for herself and for her infant during the coming labor and delivery; she may also hope and wish for her child to be born and the tiresome burden of pregnancy to end.[5] Fantasies about the child during the third trimester may be frightening. They may center on images of a hairy, animal-like child or a dismembered or incomplete child. As she approaches labor, the woman may increasingly fantasize about herself in dangerous and destructive situations.[8] Fears for the baby's safety, as shown in third-trimester fantasies, may also indicate that the woman has established bonds with her infant-to-be.[5]

Not all women are able to fantasize through daydreams.[3] Indeed, some women may find this type of effort too abstract. From reports of primiparous women who did fantasize during the third trimester, Lederman theorized that at least three different types of fantasies help prepare the woman to identify with the maternal role. First, the woman envisions herself as a mother in a positive manner. Second, she imagines the characteristics desired in a mother; all women in Lederman's research expressed some desire to be available, warm, loving, and close to their children and fantasized about interacting in this manner. Third, the woman anticipates future life changes as a mother, that is, the changes the baby will make in her life.

During the third trimester, nightdreams may tend to parallel real-life concerns.[3] Lederman identified five categories of nightdreams:

1. *Dreams of reliving childhood.* Women had an opportunity to resolve their own childhood conflicts, as preparation for helping their own children through conflicts. This was congruent with Caplan's classic work in which pregnancy was identified as a time when the woman has a second chance to try to resolve old conflicts that surface from her subconscious.[2]
2. *Dreams about being in school.* Women interpreted these dreams as a wish to return to the prepregnant state. Motherhood also may represent a developmental step equivalent to the separation from family that occurs with going to school.
3. *Dreams about the motherhood-career conflict.* Women in Lederman's study often expressed preoccupation with the problem of combining motherhood with a career. These dreams were associated with anxiety.
4. *Dreams reflecting confidence (or lack of confidence) in maternal skills.* Many women dreamed about their babies and about their ability to take care of them. Fear of failure in mothering and lack of confidence in the child's ability to thrive were often mirrored. Themes involving infant anomalies or other misfortunes occurred.
5. *Dreams of food and infant intactness.* Many women in Lederman's sample reported dreams about food of various types. Food was seen as the equivalent of a "baby" (eg, "The fruit of the womb") or as nourishment for the baby in terms of milk or love.

Sherwen reported on a survey of fantasies experienced by pregnant women in their third trimester.[7,9] Women recorded their nightdreams and daydreams during a 6-week interval. Fantasies fell into certain thematic categories or groupings. A frequent symbol was water, for example (oceans, lakes, swimming pools, and rivers). In addition, the fantasies in the various categories seemed to be divided further into those associated with positive emotions, such as pleasure, joy, peace, and those associated with negative emotions, such as fear, guilt, and panic. Sherwen classifies these third-trimester maternal fantasies into eight categories:

1. *Fantasies about having an abnormal infant.* The woman dreams that she will have a deformed infant, an infant of abnormal size or with extraordi-

nary ability such as flying, multiple infants, or delivery complications that will affect the infant: "About a week ago, I dreamed that we had a newborn baby girl who could already talk, and she never wet her diapers; she had a funny nose that had to be filled out, kind of like a balloon." "I dreamed that I gave birth to a large girl in a very few minutes of labor. She was the size of a 10-year-old child! I was upset because I had no baby to hold." Many of these fantasies are accompanied by fear, anxiety, or other unpleasant emotions and are often viewed as premonitions by the pregnant woman; however, fantasies about multiple births, usually twins, are often associated with positive, happy feelings.

2. *Fantasies about being attacked.* The mother, or a symbol, is attacked in some manner. Some women dream that pets are attacked by larger animals or that intruders or burglars violate their dwellings. Sometimes, unknown people are the targets of attacks. As one mother noted, "I was in the labor room with about five other women. We all had our babies with us. I saw tiny, tiny red bugs crawling in bunches all over the women and babies. I woke up frightened and itching all over." Slipping or being pushed down stairs is a frequent event in these fantasies. The spiral staircase was a symbol repeated in many dreams.
3. *Fantasies about being enclosed or drowning.* In these fantasies, mostly nightdreams, the woman is inside a tunnel, a car, a small room, or another type of enclosure. Sometimes she tries or is unable to get out. As one woman reported, "I dreamed that my husband and I were in his car about to go through a car wash. For some reason, my husband got out of the car, and I went through the car wash alone. At the end of the car wash, the car, with me inside, dropped off into a deep lake of snowy slush. I spent the rest of the dream trying to figure out how to get out of the car without drowning, freezing to death, or suffocating. I awoke before I was killed or saved."
4. *Fantasies about losing things.* During the third trimester, women frequently report unpleasant fantasies about losing objects or people who are important to them, especially the infant-to-be. These fantasies are often accompanied by guilt: "I was doing routine things and forgetting about the baby. Or I'd go out and then remember the baby."
5. *Fantasies about being unprepared.* In this recurring fantasy, the woman dreams she is unprepared for labor, either in direct terms or symbolically: "I had recurring dreams of not being prepared for final exams at college and high school. I felt panic because I had done no work all semester."
6. *Fantasies about sexual encounters.* Sexual fantasies can evoke positive or negative emotions, depending on such factors as who the fantasized partner is. Fantasies about sexual encounters with the husband seem to be a great source of pleasure for the pregnant woman: "I dreamed my husband and I made love very, very slowly on a waterbed that moved back and forth, side to side." On the other hand, fantasies about sexual encounters with someone perceived as taboo for the pregnant woman, such as old boyfriends, or relatives, can produce great guilt.
7. *Fantasies about restoration.* These fantasies are unusual because they deal primarily with death; however, they are accompanied by positive feelings. As noted earlier, during pregnancy women may have an opportunity to rework and resolve old crises through fantasy. The pregnant woman who reports having this type of fantasy seems to be resolving the loss of someone close to her. In addition, these dreams seem to provide a link among generations and a means to connect the infant-to-be with ancestors. Women restore the family chain that has been broken by death, and add another link to the chain with a new baby, as in the following example: "I had one dream in which I was pushing my newborn boy in a baby carriage. I passed large groups of people sitting on long benches. One of these people was an uncle of mine who had died two years ago. He winked and smiled at me. The overall feeling was happy, but also rather anxious and tense."
8. *Everyday fantasies.* These fantasies deal with the concerns, plans, and problems faced by any family having a new baby. Some common themes are life changes and restructuring of living space for the new baby; characteristics of the new baby-to-be, for example, sex, health, hair and eye color, beauty, and family resemblances; strategies for coping with labor; checklists of chores for preparation; living with and caring for the baby-to-be, for example, loving, playing with, or feeding the baby; reactions of the father or significant others to the baby; the expectant mother's own childhood experiences; and the baby in different stages of growth and development.

Sherwen regards the presence of such everyday fantasies as "bonding clues."[7] As these fantasies seem to be instrumental to "binding-in" to the child, their absence or suppression may indicate a block in maternal attachment to the fetus.

Through exploration of maternal fantasies during the third trimester, the nurse may gain much insight into the pregnant woman's current concerns.

These fantasies may be unsettling to the expectant mother. The nurse should be aware of the often disturbing nature of these fantasies and should be prepared to discuss them with the client, when asked.

Relationship with Mother

As labor approaches, the expectant mother strives for a positive balance in her relationship with her own mother and, in many cases, the mother-daughter relationship improves.[3, 10, 11] The expectant woman's perception of her mother as reassuring, tolerant, and supportive of her contributes to her self-esteem and modifies her anxiety in the days before delivery. Indeed, as Lederman observed, a poor relationship with mother and unresolved conflicts by the end of the third trimester can be manifested by such childbirth problems as prolonged labor.[3]

The expectant mother often depends on her own mother to provide support to her and to her family, although the nature and extent of desired support depends on the mother-daughter relationship. She may also experience conflict between her partner's and her parent's involvement surrounding birth and early parenting, particularly if she is having her first baby and her mother is becoming a grandparent for the first time.[10] Open discussion with significant others, clarification of roles and responsibilities, and avoidance of using mother or husband as scapegoat in dealings with the other person can foster harmony in the third trimester.

Relationship with Fetus

During the third trimester, the woman's desire for pregnancy to end and her perception of pregnancy as a burden conflict with her attachment to her fetus. The woman's love for her infant-to-be and her desire to help him or her be a full-term healthy infant allow her to "get through" these trying last months of pregnancy.[5] As pregnancy goes to term, the expectant mother becomes increasingly aware of the fetus and fetal activity patterns. A woman may talk to the fetus, call the fetus by a pet name, or stroke her abdomen in response to fetal movements.

Toward the end of the third trimester, the mother becomes eager and ready to have and hold the infant.[3] Both high-risk and low-risk pregnant women demonstrate attachment to their fetuses.[12] Such prenatal attachment allows for the evolution of maternal-infant bonding after birth of the infant.

Body Image

During the third trimester of pregnancy, the woman perceives many differences in the size of her body, her body boundaries, and the space her body occupies. The size of the body in the third trimester begins to be a nuisance to many women.[5] The pregnant woman becomes progressively less tolerant of abdominal growth, increasingly anxious about how much more childbearing will demand of her body, and generally feels irritable. Many women view third-trimester body changes, such as stretch marks, as unpleasant. The woman may wish to be rid of the pregnancy, but not the child. Examples of negative third-trimester body images have been presented in the literature. For example, Shuzman discussed the woman's disenchantment with the pregnant body during the third trimester.[13] None of the subjects in Lederman's sample of primiparas expressed pride in body size during the third-trimester interviews.[3] Imle theorized that concerns about lack of body predictability in the third trimester might have an impact on adjustment to parenthood.[14]

Some women may delight in the body changes and maintain a positive body image during the third trimester, viewing all of pregnancy as a time of beauty (Figure 21–1). Women's perceptions of their bodies may reflect complex factors such as their overall self-image, whether they feel their partners consider them beautiful, and what the cultural standards of beauty are. American cultural standards of beauty, reinforced by media images of slender, nonpregnant,

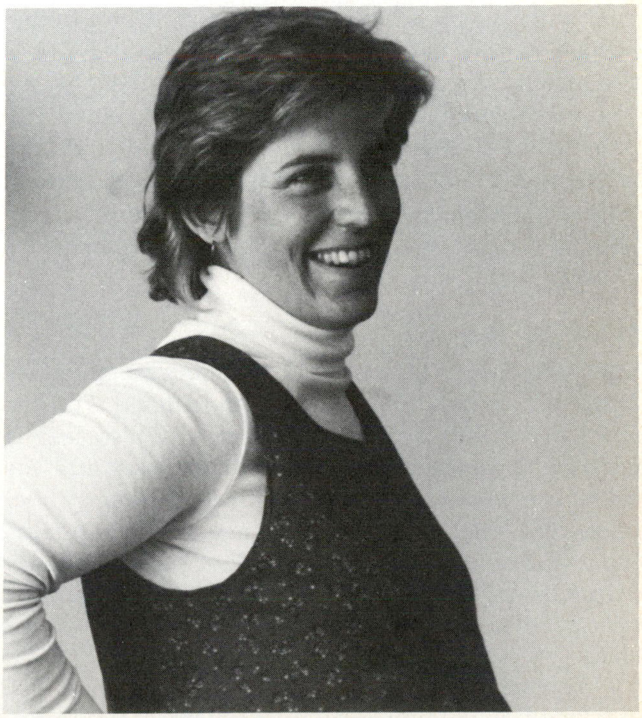

Figure 21–1. Some women have a positive body image in the third trimester.

ISSUES AND CONTROVERSIES

During the third trimester, women tend to "tie up loose ends" and essentially prepare themselves to give birth. Some people refer to these actions as "nesting" behaviors.

1. Nesting behaviors are instinctive in animals. Are they instinctive or learned in humans?
2. Certain cultural groups have prohibitions against preparations for an infant prior to birth (eg, baby showers, preparing a room). Does lack of prenatal ceremony interfere with integration of the infant into the family? Should nurses encourage nesting behaviors in families from these cultural groups?

young women, can also lead to feelings of conflict over the pregnant body.

Body Boundaries. During the third trimester, the woman's thinning abdominal walls and increased size make her feel that her fetus is more vulnerable to external influences.[5] The woman feels that her body, as a barrier, is more fragile and may express this feeling in fantasies.

Body Size and Position. The woman's experience of her body in space changes radically after the second trimester of pregnancy.[5] As the woman approaches the end of pregnancy, she becomes more preoccupied with her body's position in space. Contributing factors include the change in balance resulting from the increased size and the shift of body weight, decreased mobility, and perceptions of the body as vulnerable. In a classic study Fawcett found that both women and their husbands may have an increase in their perceived body space, compared with perceptions of body space in the first and second postpartal month.[15]

Time and Space

During the third trimester, time again creeps for the pregnant woman, and she may be irritated with the slowness of her actions; however, she also feels a growing urgency to get ready for delivery and the baby. The woman makes plans for the running of her home and her family while she is gone (if not delivering at home) and if she does not return. Shortly before labor, the woman often experiences a burst of energy and takes care of personal and household tasks.

Toward the end of pregnancy, the woman also may emotionally pull away from others. Time, space, and her body are all burdensome to her. She increasingly focuses on her "inner time and space" as opposed to her external work[5] (Figure 21–2).

Preparation for Labor

The pregnant woman must take specific steps, including concrete actions and imaginary rehearsals, in preparation for labor and parenting. Maternal preparation includes nesting behaviors (practical activities such as taking childbirth classes and preparing infant clothes) as well as gearing up psychologically for labor.[3] From her research, Lederman identified three ways that women may plan for labor:

1. Practical activity, for example, gathering information about labor and delivery, taking prenatal classes, talking to other women, reading books and viewing films, preparing a layette for the baby, arranging for additional help in the home after the birth, and arranging transportation to the place for birthing
2. Imaginary rehearsals
3. Dreaming about labor

Imaginary rehearsals and dreams about labor have already been discussed (*see* "Maternal Fantasies"). Third-trimester activities have the overall goal of helping the expectant mother prepare psychologi-

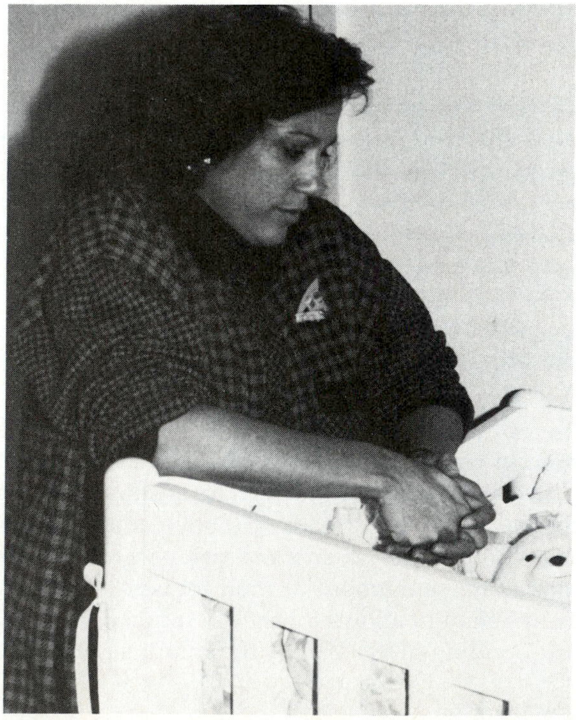

Figure 21–2. The third-trimester mother turns inward, becoming introspective.

cally for pregnancy to end and for the birth of the infant. By 38 weeks of gestation, the low-risk healthy pregnant woman is psychologically as well as physiologically ready for her baby.

Nurses have important roles in helping the expectant mother prepare for childbirth and beginning parenthood. Chapter 24 discusses educational preparation for parenthood.

THE FATHER'S EXPERIENCE

Psychologic Processes

The nature of paternal feelings and psychologic experiences during the third trimester has not been documented consistently in research. As discussed in Chapter 4, Herzog divided the emotional course of pregnancy for a man into six stages.[16] The last of these Stage 6, the end of pregnancy, covers the period from 26 weeks to delivery. Fathers in Herzog's study reported that something powerful, magical, and "big"—beyond their ability to control—was happening. These fathers turned their interests toward getting things ready in the real world for the coming baby. Observations of children in the father's environment and concern with possible methods of childrearing and preparing for the infant's arrival (for example, fixing up a room) replaced the father's focus on his inner thoughts.

The expectant father may have his most negative feelings during the third trimester of his partner's pregnancy.[17] The last half of the third trimester can be a stressful time for expectant fathers. One study found that third-trimester expectant fathers had higher overall anxiety than nonexpectant men.[18] Many expectant fathers experience a loss both of personal freedom and of the partner's time and attention. Some fathers report feeling a sense of being in the background, outside the maternal-fetal dyad. Expectant fathers also may report a need for increased attention, which they generally do not feel they receive.

> **PATERNAL PSYCHOLOGIC CHANGES AND CONCERNS DURING THE THIRD TRIMESTER**
>
> **Psychologic processes**
> End of pregnancy stage; various reactions, including increased need for attention, increased anxiety, perceived loss of personal freedom, excitement; preparation for coming infant
>
> **Fantasies**
> Infant's coming, water, anxiety regarding birth; nature of themes reflects paternal involvement in pregnancy and relationship with expectant mother; themes provide clues to current concerns
>
> **Couvade syndrome**
> May be severe; symptoms include gastrointestinal discomforts and weight gain
>
> **Attachment to fetus**
> Associated with relationship with partner; many popular beliefs based on media images, rather than scientific sources
>
> **Preparation for parenthood**
> Reading, planning, classes, fantasizing, talking to other fathers, exposure to media; fostered by strong relationship with partner

Fantasies

Like the expectant mother, the expectant father has specific fantasies during the third trimester. Symbols of water and diving may appear in nightdreams, and dreams begin to include the baby's coming and the birth process. Magic and mysticism may be prevalent in paternal fantasies.[19]

Sherwen found that, in comparison to nonexpectant men, expectant third trimester fathers had more fantasies oriented in the present.[20] Expectant fathers' fantasy patterns were similar to those of their partners, except that the expectant women had more nightdreams than the men. The extent of the father's involvement in his partner's pregnancy also affected the nature of his fantasies. The more involved the father was in the pregnancy, the more positive were his fantasies and the more the fantasies contained visual images. Conversely, the less involved the father was in the pregnancy, the less he fantasized about the future.

Like maternal fantasies, paternal fantasies during the third trimester can be grouped into major themes, which Sherwen identified as:[7]

1. *Anxiety about upcoming events* (eg, being a good father, the condition of his wife, cesarean delivery, lack of money). As one father reported: ". . . they (nightdreams) seem to have originated from fear. In one . . . my wife gave birth to a boy that seemed to be deformed or disfigured."
2. *The father's happiness about coming events.* One father stated: "I always have this picture in my mind of coming home from work and being greeted on the front porch by children, wife and the dog barking happily in the background."

RESEARCH ABSTRACT

Norbeck J, Anderson J. Psychosocial predictors of pregnancy outcomes in low-income black, Hispanic, and white women. Nurs Res. *1989;38:204–209.*

Incidence of infant mortality and low birth weight is much higher in nonwhite ethnic groups. Regardless of ethnicity, low-birth-weight rates increase as family income decreases. This study was designed to extend the findings of an earlier study by Norbeck and Tilden in 1988 of middle-income white women. The purpose was to determine if the variables of high stress, low social support, and high anxiety predict pregnancy outcomes with this population, and to learn whether ethnic differences exist in these relationships.

Life stress and social support were thought to have major effects on short-term responses to stress. These responses were expected to be related to pregnancy outcomes. Social support and life stress were expected to neutralize each other and to predict short-term responses and pregnancy outcomes.

The short-term responses to stress used in this study were anxiety and substance abuse. Pregnancy outcomes were gestation, labor and delivery, infant condition, gestational age, birth weight, and Apgar score (which ultimately was not used as most infants had high Apgar scores).

Subjects were 208 low-income, healthy women. The ethnic composition of the sample was 28 percent black, 37 percent Hispanic, and 35 percent white. Study instruments included the Revised Life Events Questionnaire (LEQ) developed by Norbeck in 1984, the Norbeck Social Support Questionnaire (NNSQ), the Spielberger State-Trait Anxiety Inventory, a demographic data sheet, and a one-page self-report substance use questionnaire. Data were collected during midpregnancy and late pregnancy (the midpregnancy data are reported here).

Stress and social support were usually not significant for the full sample. For black women, social support from the woman's partner or mother accounted for 33 percent of the variance in gestation complications and 14 percent of the variance in prolonged labor or cesarean section complications. For white women, high rather than low social support was significant in accounting for pregnancy outcome and substance abuse, indicating that the social network might reinforce negative health practices for this group. None of the variables were found to be statistically significant for the group of Hispanic women. The investigators concluded that the lack of significance for life stress and anxiety in predicting pregnancy outcomes, as well as the lack of significant stress-support interactions, suggests that the theoretical model used in this study may not be valid for use with lower-socioeconomic-class pregnant women.

Comment:

The researchers attempted to replicate findings of their previous study with a different population. This study focuses on the prenatal experience of women from minority and lower-socioeconomic-class groups. Replication of such studies and development of appropriate models have the potential to improve care delivery to these populations who demonstrate consistently high infant morbidity and mortality rates despite current attempts at correction. The investigators note that this group actually had unexpectedly good pregnancy outcomes, inconsistent with typical statistics on similar populations. Future research might focus on testing less healthy women, who demonstrate the poorest pregnancy outcomes.

3. *Fear of injury or trauma to the self, spouse, or significant other* (eg, the wife being mugged or attacked).
4. *Fantasies about the father's winning or coming into large sums of money.*
5. *Concerns about being prepared.* As one father reported: "I keep imagining that the baby will arrive and I won't be prepared—no film, not packed for the hospital, the Lamaze bag not ready."
6. *Concerns about loss and/or death:* ". . . I imagine where my deceased friends have gone to."
7. *Fantasies about the father's own "creative" acts or dependents that he must care for* (as acquiring and caring for a dog).
8. *Concerns about the reactions of others, especially the father's father, to the child.*

Fantasy themes can give the nurse clues to a father's current concerns and provide a basis for anticipatory guidance.

Couvade Syndrome

Many expectant fathers experience couvade symptoms during the third trimester.[21,22] Although the incidence of symptoms was reported in one study to be highest during the second trimester, the severity of symptoms was noted to be greatest during the third trimester and the first trimester.[23] Examples of couvade symptoms during the third trimester include unintentional weight gain, gastrointestinal discomforts, and difficulty in concentrating.

Couvade symptoms may add to or be a manifestation of stress during the third trimester. Nurses need to discuss the existence of this syndrome with expectant parents and to treat this topic as a genuine client concern.

Attachment to Fetus

The process of paternal attachment to the coming baby is likely to be somewhat different from maternal attachment, as the expectant father does not carry the fetus in his body and experience prenatal physical changes. There is, however, little doubt that fathers do attach to their fetuses prenatally. The nature of the father's relationship with his partner is one factor that influences his attachment to the fetus. One study found that during the third trimester, a strong association exists between the stability of a couple's marriage and the father's prenatal attachment to the infant.[24] Thus, a father with a strong marriage during pregnancy is likely to be highly bonded in the third trimester to his unborn infant. As one client recalled: "Marrying my wife was one of the best decisions I ever made. Having a baby seemed to be a special expression of our love and we both wanted to be parents together. I loved feeling the baby move inside my wife. I felt the baby was real long before I actually held her."

The concept of paternal-infant bonding is not new; however, the popular press and mass media, rather than scientific studies or information from health care professionals, may be the primary source of information for the general public.[25] Expectant fathers may approach delivery with preconceived ideas about the "scientific" importance of attending delivery to foster their attachment to their infant. They may worry about not being good fathers if they do not attend every prenatal class or labor and delivery. Through individual client teaching and prepared childbirth classes, nurses can discuss attachment with expectant fathers. As authors of articles in the popular press, producers, and consultants to media sources, nurses can have a considerable impact on information received by expectant parents.

Preparation for Parenthood

In general, expectant fathers come to terms with the reality of a baby in a process similar to the way in which the expectant mother identifies with the maternal role. Expectant men prepare for fatherhood by reading and planning, fantasizing and thinking about the baby and the changes in their lifestyle, attending classes, talking to other fathers, and being exposed to television, radio, magazines, and other types of media.[3,25] Men who relate poorly to their wives may have difficulty accepting the responsibilities of fatherhood.

Although the modern American father is currently expected to be involved in childbearing and childrearing, specific roles are as yet unclear. Men are also greatly affected by their families' cultural background and expectations for the role of the father. Through thoughtful discussion of paternal concerns, the nurse can assist the couple in evolving their new roles as parents.

THE FAMILY

During the third trimester, concerns of the family and the expectant mother in particular may place stress on the pregnancy and fetus and affect pregnancy outcome. This may happen during a first or subsequent pregnancy.

Many studies document the effects of psychosocial and physical stress on pregnancy. In a comprehensive review of the literature, Carlson and Labara found that maternal stress, called "emotionality," was related to habitual abortions, hyperemesis gravidarum, toxemia, deviant infant behavior, and a variety of other pregnancy and birth complications.[26]

Other studies verify that prenatal stress can produce obstetric complications. Stress during pregnancy has also been found to relate to prematurity and delivery of low-birth-weight infants,[23] prenatal anxiety,[27] failure to progress in labor,[28] and postpartum depression.[29] One study identified the pregnant woman's ability to cope with stress as a factor in how

FAMILY'S EXPERIENCE DURING THE THIRD TRIMESTER

Changes/concerns
Coping with stresses of late pregnancy; coping with biologic changes; expectant parents attach to fetus and see fetus as separate being; family roles and relationships shift; adjusting to moving up a generation; establishing new relationships within the community and society; preparing for birth

Multiparas
Experience stress, as do primiparas; nature and source of stress may vary

damaging stress may be to the pregnancy and fetus. The less able a woman was to cope with stressors, the higher the level of negative pregnancy outcomes.[30]

Stress or negative emotional states can be higher during the end of pregnancy than at other times during the childbearing cycle. Most pregnancy-related concerns seem to be voiced during the third trimester.[31]

Many studies on stress and pregnancy outcome have been done during the third trimester of pregnancy. Among the stress-producing factors identified by these studies are[31] fear of damage to the self, childbirth, effects of birth on the baby, finances, family, future pregnancies, negative self-concept,[29] previous loss of a fetus,[29] terminating work,[29] major life changes,[26, 27] and concern about pain in labor and delivery.[27]

Denial of stressful concerns may also be damaging to the pregnancy.[32] The stressful problems do not simply disappear and may result in increased obstetric complications. Family-centered nursing care focuses on encouraging the family and the pregnant woman to deal with stressful pregnancy-related concerns.

Family Changes and Concerns

The third trimester marks the end of the first phase of the childbearing cycle—pregnancy. The family must now accept the reality of the coming child and anticipate the changes this new member will make in their patterns of life. To do this, the family members complete several tasks.[1] (These tasks were outlined earlier in Chapter 3.)

1. *Coping with biologic changes.* In the final months of pregnancy, the expectant mother must begin to prepare herself for delivery. Birth is the only major life passage that directly involves two individuals. Both must complete the birthing safely and in a manner that fosters family integrity.
2. *Attaching to the infant-to-be.* By the third trimester, both expectant mother and father should have a beginning attachment to the fetus and consider him or her as a real and separate person. Additional attachment (bonding) occurs after birth, as do additional separation and eventual individuation of the infant.
3. *Coping with intrapsychic changes.* Both expectant mother and father, and often children in the family, experience intense intrapsychic or emotional changes as pregnancy draws to an end. The family is a system, and psychologic changes in one member affect all family members as they interact.
4. *Coping with shifts in roles and relationships.* Many role changes may occur toward the end of pregnancy. For example, the expectant mother may leave work several weeks before her due date. This may result in a loss of income, depending on the type of maternity leave. The woman then becomes a dependent, especially if she does not receive paid maternity leave. The expectant father may now become the sole breadwinner. These new roles and relationships may require much adaptation, especially on the part of couples used to two incomes.
5. *Adjusting to moving up a generation.* The reality of "moving up" continues to be important in the third trimester. Not only must the expectant mother and father accept the status of being new parents, or the parents of another child, so must grandparents accept a new role. Other children in the family must make a transition to being a "big" brother or sister. Many preparatory activities are undertaken during the third trimester to allow family members to make this transition (*see* Chapter 24).
6. *Establishing new relationships within the community and society.* Giving birth to a child ushers in new social responsibilities for and cultural expectations of the couple. Certain activities and rituals during the third trimester help prepare the couple. For example, the expectant parents may plan and decorate a nursery and select baby clothing and equipment. Relatives and friends may host baby "showers" for the expectant couple. Attendance at third-trimester prenatal classes has become an American cultural trend, especially among middle-class and upper-middle-class couples.

The Multipara and Stress

Multiparas must deal with challenges different from, but no less challenging than, those of a primigravida. Table 21–1 summarizes sources of stress and concern for multiparas. Specific maternal tasks have been identified for the multipara.[36] Based on Rubin's concept of maternal tasks, these include securing approval of the firstborn child(ren) for the new baby; resolving the loss of an exclusive parent-child relationship with the first child; managing time, space, and resources for child care; redefining a relationship with the first child(ren); claiming the second child by comparing him or her with the first; and evaluating her own emotional ability to meet the needs of all family members.

Multiparous women are vulnerable to the specific demands and stressors of their situations. It should never be assumed that multiparas know everything about pregnancy and childbirth simply be-

TABLE 21–1. SOURCES OF STRESS FOR MULTIPARAS

Increased fears for the unborn baby and the self with each successive pregnancy
Distress related to lack of nursing support with each successive pregnancy (multiparas should not be assumed to know everything)
Stress from too much company
Stress from interfering relatives
Concern about weight reduction during the postpartum period, especially if she failed to return to prepregnancy weight after first pregnancy
Concern with housework and family routines with increased family size
More fatigue in the postpartum period
Increased depressive episodes
Increasingly complex family interaction patterns
Fear of not having enough love for everyone
Fear of not having enough time for self and others; lack of time and poor time management
Disillusionment with parenting and child care
Increased physical discomforts
Focus of less attention than with the first child, because baby is no longer a family novelty

Source: *References 33–35.*

cause they have previously borne a child. Certain topics discussed with multiparas and primiparas differ (*see* Chapter 9) because of the need to prepare for a first or additional infant.

THE SIBLINGS' EXPERIENCE

Third-trimester pregnancy can have a major impact on siblings. The mother has become large and noticeably pregnant. Third-trimester discomforts, as well as the mother's size, may restrict her usual schedule. The mother may wish to engage in quiet rather than physically demanding activities. Her attention may be directed more toward preparation for the baby and less toward entertaining the older sibling(s). Working mothers may begin maternity leave during the third trimester. This may actually afford them additional time with the sibling.

Most children are aware of their mothers' pregnancies. All children have questions, although the level of questions and the child's ability to comprehend and to verbalize vary with the child's age and developmental level. Table 21–2 outlines some topics of concern to children during the third trimester. Sibling responses to pregnancy were also discussed in Chapter 17. Negative sibling responses to late pregnancy and birth include sleep disturbances, frequent crying, and regressive behaviors, especially in relation to toilet training.[37] In addition to being a potential source of disturbance, however, advancing pregnancy and the prospect of a new baby can be a source of great interest, particularly to firstborn children[37] (Figure 21–3).

As the pregnancy becomes increasingly visible, the older child or children need reassurance of their parents' love. Baking cookies, reading aloud, and undertaking a quiet project special to the child are activities that can promote parent-child relationships. Indeed, a strong and loving parent-child relationship can help the sibling, as well as the parent, get ready for the baby. Expectant parents also need to feel that they are adequately preparing siblings for the arrival of the baby.[38]

When planned, pregnancy is a decision made between parents and is based on what the parents believe will be "best" for themselves and their existing family. Although some children may ask their parents for a brother or sister, the final decision belongs to the couple. Nevertheless, the siblings' lives are greatly affected by a new baby and family member.

SIBLINGS' EXPERIENCES DURING THE THIRD TRIMESTER

- Very aware of pregnancy
- Activities may be affected by mother's decreased mobility and inward focus
- May have increased time with mother if she begins maternity leave from work
- Need to be gently prepared, especially if sibling's former possessions are to be used for infant
- Need attention to reinforce feelings of being loved and valued
- May participate in sibling preparation programs

TABLE 21–2. TOPICS THAT MAY CONCERN SIBLINGS DURING THE THIRD TRIMESTER

What does the baby look like?
What does the baby do?
What will become of me when Mommy goes to have the baby?
What will happen when Mommy is having the baby?
Will Mommy be all right? Will she come back to me?
Will I still be loved as much?
Will the baby use my things?
Can I choose the baby's name (blanket, toys, and so on)?
Will I get to help?
Will I know who is going to take care of me?
Can I stay home and "help" Mommy?

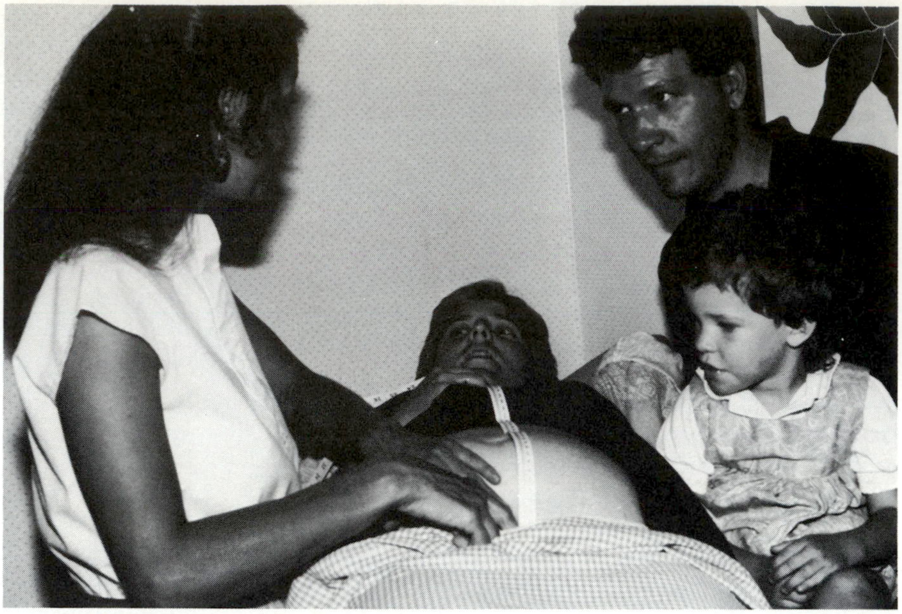

Figure 21–3. Advancing pregnancy can be a source of great interest, particularly to firstborn children.

The activities for most families change because of infant care concerns. Many families cannot afford the luxury of separate bedrooms for each child. The sibling(s) may therefore be expected to share bedrooms, time, and often toys with the new family member. Although frequently not considered at the time, the arrival of a sibling divides family inheritance, a situation that has provoked conflict throughout history.

Infant furniture, clothing, and accessories are very expensive. Parents may want to reuse items, especially if the new baby is the same sex as a sibling. The siblings' crib is one major item that may be used by the new baby. During the third trimester, the sibling may make the transition from crib to bed, and the bedroom furniture may be rearranged. Although most young children want to feel "grown up," they may still miss the crib or feel upset that their possessions are being passed along. Gentle parental strategies that allow the sibling to feel she or he is "giving" items to the baby or no longer "wants" them are necessary to smooth transition and to maintain the sibling's feelings of love and belonging.

In families with two or more siblings, parents may require help in daily activities from the older siblings. School-aged and adolescent expectant siblings may need to help care for younger children in the family or help in meal preparation or other household chores. Children often want to help out and view their contributions as important in preparation for the baby; however, their contributions should be age appropriate. The nurse can help parents to base their expectations on what a child, and not an adult, can emotionally and physically contribute. In addition, siblings of any age need to continue to feel loved and valued.

With the addition of a new baby to the family, the status and roles of siblings change. As plans are made for the baby during the third trimester, the siblings in families where there are already two or more children may vie with each other over who will do what for the baby. Sibling rivalry may provide temporary quarrels, with siblings taking sides for and against the baby. Through such squabbles, siblings may try to assert themselves as important, yet independent of each other. By providing anticipatory guidance, nurses can help parents prepare each child in the family for the new baby.

THE GRANDPARENTS' EXPERIENCE

With the birth of the first grandchild, grandparents assume a new role and status in life.[39] During the third trimester, as the time for birth of the infant draws closer, expectant grandparents may participate actively in making plans for the new baby. They may assist the expectant parents with care of older siblings, may make arrangements to stay with the children while the mother delivers and recovers, and may contribute to overall preparations. During the third trimester, expectant grandmothers, especially the woman's mother, may share experiences and demonstrate support by participating in prenatal rituals, for example, a baby shower for the parents-to-be.

GRANDPARENTS' EXPERIENCE DURING THE THIRD TRIMESTER

May assist in plans for infant

May provide caretaking and support role for expectant parents and siblings

Concerns focus on health of mother and infant, safe delivery; may serve as labor coach (especially grandmother)

Shopping together is an American ritual; expectant grandmothers and mothers may want to be with each other to select baby and other household items.

During the third trimester, expectant grandparents may have concerns, such as the health of the expectant mother and baby and the safety of labor and delivery. As one grandmother expressed, "I know my daughter has had a normal pregnancy and that she is healthy. But she is still my daughter, and I'll worry about her until I know that she and her baby are safe." For the expectant grandparents, the third trimester, and especially the last month of pregnancy, may seem long.

Becoming a grandparent and moving up a generation can be important to older adults. One researcher suggests that becoming a grandparent can add to the overall quality of life and thereby increase physical and mental health and adjustment to old age.[40] Another researcher describes the most valued aspects of grandparenting as an increased sense of identity and feelings of personal meaning; recognition as a valued elder who is a resource person for children and who identifies with grandchildren; assurance of immortality through continuation of the family line and through contact with the grandchild; reinvolvement with a personal past as grandchildren evoke memories of early life and experiences with the grandparent's own grandparents; and the opportunity to indulge grandchildren and, especially for the grandfather, to be lenient without worrying about "spoiling" the grandchildren.[41]

Expectant grandparenting can generate a renewed sense of excitement about life as the process ensures continuation of the family. The prospect of grandchildren can be an especially pleasing way to fill the "activities gap" that older men and women may face at retirement.[42]

Unlike their own parents, however, who may have been able to help when the now-expectant parents were born, contemporary grandparents may not be accessible or have regular childcare within their life goals. These grandparents may thus have to deal with adult children who wish they would be around to help them, not only with child care, but also in their preparations for delivery during the third trimester. As one pregnant woman expressed: "I'm due in 4 weeks . . . my parents went off to Florida and my in-laws are on a winter cruise. They said they love me, they were glad I would be well cared for, and that they would be back when the baby came. But I need them now. How could they do this to me?"

Moving up a generation evokes fears of getting older and dying for some expectant grandparents. For others, there may be role conflicts. For example, in the past they were responsible for teaching their child; now their child assumes that responsibility.[39] As a result of changes in social structure and the increase in technology in the United States, health care workers, rather than grandparents, may be seen as the experts on pregnancy and parenthood. Indeed, the information shared by grandparents about pregnancy and childbirth may be regarded by their children as outdated, rather than valuable. Increasing emphasis on paternal involvement in pregnancy and birth may strengthen the marital bond during advancing pregnancy, yet make the expectant grandparents feel distanced. Although expectant parents may welcome contact with their own parents, grandparents' suggestions may be regarded as interference. Expectant and new parents may be caught in conflicts between suggestions of their parents, those of health providers, and their own wishes. Such conflicts may be minimized if expectant grandparents are prepared through clarification of changes in childbearing and childrearing.[43]

Childbirth education programs for expectant grandparents can facilitate the transition to grandparenthood by discussing changes in birthing and parenting practices between generations, providing tips for being a welcome grandparent, discussing labor support, and providing a forum for grandparents to share ideas and concerns with each other.[39] Most expectant grandparent programs are offered during the third trimester. Considering the important role of the parent's parents in maternal and paternal role development, grandparent preparation might be encouraged earlier in the pregnancy. Grandparent education is discussed further in Chapter 24.

At times an expectant grandmother, rather than an expectant father, will plan to be the woman's support person during labor. Among certain ethnic groups, an expectant grandmother or another female relative may be the primary support person. Women who do not have support from the expectant father and wives of men who cannot be present for births, such as military servicemen or men whose work takes them overseas, may look to their own mother for support. In accepting this responsibility, the expectant grandparent may also need support, education, and guidance. The grandparent may be encouraged to attend prenatal visits and also to accompany the expectant mother to prepared childbirth classes.

Role of the Grandfather

Grandparenting can hold a special meaning for the older man. Being a grandfather may provide an outlet for long suppressed nurturing instincts. Often, the grandfather assumes a more maternal role toward his grandchild than he did with his own children.[42] Current societal emphasis on male involvement with childbearing has done much to legitimize the involvement of grandfathers, as well as fathers, in the nurturing process.

SOCIOCULTURAL FACTORS

Preparation for birth in the third trimester of pregnancy will reflect the cultural orientation of the expectant family. The way birth is viewed and the rituals and customs that surround birth differ among cultural groups. The nurse might expect a third-generation white middle-class American family and a first-generation Filipino-American family to have different expectations of childbearing. Cultural sensitivity and appreciation of differing beliefs and traditions are essential components of holistic care.[44] In addition, nurses must be aware of the influence of socioeconomic factors on the childbearing family during the third trimester.

Socioeconomic Factors

Socioeconomic concerns can have great importance during the third trimester. For clients with stable and sufficient family incomes, the realization in the third trimester that birth is near is accompanied by shopping for maternity and infant clothing and accessories. Most women have financial concerns precipitated by the coming infant; these can become sources of conflict. Clients who live in poverty have difficulty meeting basic needs; other clients may perceive themselves to be in financial jeopardy. High mortgages and other financial responsibilities may stress families who have comfortable addresses. Several sources of conflict are cited here.

The need for maternal clothing increases during the third trimester. In geographic areas where seasons change, second and third trimesters require warm or cold weather clothing. Maternity clothing can strain an already fragile family budget, and conflict about expenses can arise.

Infant equipment, such as crib, clothing, diapers, and accessories, is very expensive. Even though multiparas may have infant items and clothing from a previous child or children, the coming baby adds financial stress to the family budget.

Health care and delivery are also expensive. Although many women have some form of health insurance, many have no insurance. Not all plans provide maternity benefits. Women may depend on public assistance to help them gain financial access to prenatal care, which takes place on a weekly basis during the third trimester. These women may have to travel long distances to reach health care providers who will provide services without charge. Some clients who are unable to buy insurance or qualify for public assistance are forced to forego prenatal care, even in late pregnancy.

To help meet family expenses, women may choose to work until delivery; however, the woman's cumbersome size and other physiologic changes during the third trimester may make certain jobs difficult, especially if long periods of standing, lifting, or heavy physical activity are required. The prospect of decreased family income can be stressful, especially if maintaining the family's lifestyle depends on income contributed by the expectant mother.

Hispanic Cultural Groups

Hispanic-Americans originated in such Spanish-speaking areas as Mexico, Puerto Rico, Spain, Cuba, and countries in Central and South America.[45] Hispanic-Americans are predominantly Roman Catholic and share the Spanish language as a common heritage, but each country has its own cultural beliefs and practices. Care must be taken to identify the unique characteristics of each Hispanic cultural group and to avoid the erroneous assumption that all Hispanic groups are alike. Indeed, even the Spanish language varies according to such factors as geographic area. This chapter focuses on the Chicano family as one example of a Hispanic group. The Puerto Rican family is considered in Chapter 26.

Cultural Focus: The Chicano Family

Chicano refers to all Americans of Mexican descent. Mexican-American, Spanish American, Latin American, Latin, or Mexican are terms also used to identify this group.[45] Chicano families constitute one of the largest ethnic groups of childbearing families in the United States.

Many Chicanos were born either in Mexico or to parents born in Mexico; however, many Chicanos are also descendants of early settlers in California and the Southwestern part of the United States.[45] Many Hispanic cultural traditions may be practiced by this group, because they have met barriers to full assimilation into the dominant culture in the United States. Although Chicanos hold all types of employment, many have found themselves relegated to low paying jobs. Unemployment remains high. Depending on the amount of time lived in the United States and the opportunity to learn English, Chicanos may be bilingual, speak English to some degree, or speak no English.

Many Chicanos are *mestizos*—of mixed Mexican and Native American descent. Both these heritages are fused in their cultural practices. Although the predominant religion is Roman Catholic, the Native American belief system is often evident.[46]

Family Patterns. Broad cultural generalizations cannot explain all the unique behaviors in any Chicano family. Cultural norms tend to refer to "public" realities—how things ought to be in a cultural group—whereas each family within a culture has its own "private" reality—how things really are for that particular family. The nurse must remember to assess and treat each family as unique, regardless of the cultural heritage. Cultural norms and patterns merely provide a framework to organize thoughts about a family and its members.

Many Chicano immigrants to the United States in the past 30 to 40 years were poor or working class families from rural or semi-rural areas of northern and central Mexico.[46] The following descriptions relate to these families. Like many other groups, Chicano nuclear families are embedded in an extended family which includes many relatives, such as grandparents, uncles, aunts, cousins, and even compadres (childrens' godparents). Cousins, even up to the third or fourth cousins, are very close to each other. Boundaries among these individuals are very flexible, and there is often a sharing of many family functions such as the care and discipline of children, financial or emotional support, and problem solving. The extension of kinship ties has been called *familism*.[47] To help the kinship network function, affiliation and cooperation among individuals are stressed, and confrontation and competition are discouraged. Chicanos generally perceive membership in some kind of family, so that all life-cycle events and rituals, such as birth, are *family* events that affirm family unity.

The family protects the individual but expects loyalty. Autonomy and individuality in members are not emphasized, but honesty and dignity are very important. Although the extended family is cohesive, nuclear families do live in separate dwellings, thus preserving their own boundaries and identity. Family size is a final factor that greatly affects family function. The Chicano nuclear family is typically large and may include parents and four or five children.[46]

Marital Relationships. The roles of husband and wife in Chicano culture are set by tradition. The husband is the provider and protector; the wife is the homemaker and caretaker. The cultural ideal male and female sex roles of male dominance (*machismo*) and female submission support these marital role patterns. Within individual families, couples often arrange their own balance of power and control. In fact, the wife is often very powerful, as she exerts much psychologic control as the "self-sacrificing" mother.[46]

Because many newly married couples live with the husband's family, another important relationship is that between the mother-in-law and daughter-in-law. The success of the marriage may be affected by how well these two women work out their respective role relationships.

Parent-Child Relationship. The romantic ties of marriage traditionally are not viewed as important as the parent-child relationship in the Chicano family. Preservation of the marriage is important, and children validate the marriage. This perhaps reflects the strong Roman Catholic religious tradition. Motherly love is seen as stronger than marital love, and the father is also involved with his children. As the parent-child relationship is primary, the couple has little freedom from parental functions throughout the childbearing and childrearing phases of the family life cycle.

Chicano children tend to leave the family at an older age. Thus, the Chicano couple has a long parenthood period. A primary focus throughout life is parenting and then grandparenting.

Traditional parental roles are seen as complementary: the father disciplines and controls, and the mother nurtures and supports. Both parents receive the respect of the children. Parent-child interaction occurs in a hierarchic fashion with children having low status and parents high status. Chicano parents are very nurturing to children and generally relaxed in their childrearing as compared with Anglo-American parents.

Extended family members may perform many parental functions for children. Chicano children thus receive nurturance and support from many different sources.[46]

Sibling Roles. Ties among brothers and sisters in Chicano families are very strong. Siblings and cousins are often constant companions during childhood. Competition and fighting among siblings are discouraged; cooperation, sharing, and sacrifice for each other are stressed. As siblings become adolescents, roles become more sex segregated, and girls and boys develop complementary functions. For example, a sister may do chores for her brother, and he will protect her.[46] As they grow to adulthood, Chicano siblings maintain close ties and become part of the extended family network. Life-cycle events of one sibling, such as birth, will affect the other siblings and their nuclear families as well.

Chicano families are in a state of cultural transition, as are other ethnic groups who have immigrated to the United States; however, close proximity and interaction with Mexico and kin still living in Mexico tend to reinforce cultural identity in many of these families.

Spiritual Dimensions. Health care providers must appreciate the importance that spiritual dimensions and religion often hold for Chicano families. Families frequently have shrines in their homes and participate in religious rituals, for example, in relation to health and illness.

The Chicano Family During Pregnancy. The traditional Chicano family may have a variety of cultural beliefs related to pregnancy. For example, while pregnant, Chicano women may follow a series of "pregnancy rules," described by Kay.[48] Pregnancy rules are a series of prescriptions and taboos to which the pregnant woman adheres, especially during the first pregnancy. These rules, which are believed to protect the fetus and provide for easy delivery, evolved from practices of traditional midwives and folk healers. Some of the more noteworthy activities used to prepare the woman for labor, delivery, and birth of her baby are described here.[48]

1. *Control of the environment.* The pregnant woman should avoid cool, moving air and especially night air. Moonlight is thought to be particularly hazardous. The sun's rays, coming through glass, are seen as dangerous as well, and pregnant women should not sit in drafts or by closed windows. Bathing in water, however, is encouraged during pregnancy.
2. *Food taboos and prescriptions.* Consuming or avoiding certain foods calls attention to the status of pregnancy for Chicano women. Cravings must be satisfied, or the infant may be marked by the food that was craved. Pica is not a common practice, but takes the form of eating ashes or dirt when it does occur. Women may avoid drinking to prevent the baby from growing too large and being hard to deliver.
3. *Control of the gastrointestinal tract.* Chicano women treat nausea and vomiting by drinking flour and water, flour and lemon juice, or chamomile tea. Heartburn is believed by some to predict a long-haired baby and is treated by baking soda and commercial antacids. (This practice is at odds with the current recommendation to avoid baking soda, which may cause acid-base imbalances.) Constipation is treated by over-the-counter medications and herbal teas (which are said to cause "violent purges" and must be used with care). During pregnancy, Chicano women may readily take vitamin and iron preparations, which they believe will enrich their blood.
4. *Sleep and exercise.* According to Kay, Chicano women believe that sleeping on their back will protect the fetus.[48] It is believed that activity helps the mother to keep the fetus from becoming too big and aids delivery. Chicano women remain very active and mobile and avoid only the heaviest chores during pregnancy. Massage is an important activity and is thought to help put the fetus in a good position for delivery. Reaching up high, crossing legs, or sitting in tailor positions are believed to cause knots in the umbilical cord and are therefore to be avoided.
5. *Affective states.* The pregnant woman tries to avoid feelings of rage or anger, as these may have harmful consequences for the pregnancy. The pelvic examination is frightening and may cause the woman shame. It is also not acceptable to her partner and should be performed in complete privacy and only when necessary. Sexual relationships are maintained throughout pregnancy to keep the birth canal well lubricated.
6. *Rituals.* Baby showers are not held until delivery time is very near. To have one earlier is perceived as bad luck. Chicano women also undertake the prediction of their baby's sex.
7. *Preparation for delivery.* According to Kay, Chicano women in Arizona and New Mexico favored midwife and home deliveries. Women were attended primarily by a *partera,* or lay midwife. Although many Chicano women in the United States cur-

rently deliver in hospitals, this may still be the custom in Mexico.

Maintaining the balance between "hot" and "cold" or "wet" and "dry" elements is believed to foster good health in general.[45] Treatments may be based on restoring the body's "balance." For example, delivery, considered a "hot" experience, would be balanced by the eating of "cold" foods. Hot and cold refer to specific substances and not their temperature or amount of spices used. Because rules related to hot and cold differ from person to person, an understanding of the nature of the concept of hot-cold imbalance is important to health care providers working with Chicano clients.

SUMMARY

Preparations for childbirth and the coming baby are finalized during the third trimester. For the expectant family, this period alternately seems to drag or go too quickly. By the final weeks of pregnancy, however, the expectant woman and her family seem to count the days until pregnancy ends. Concerns of the expectant parents focus on a safe delivery and ways in which the family will cope with a new baby. Although educational preparation is important throughout pregnancy, the third trimester is the time during which most clients attend classes in preparation for birth. Preparatory activities also focus on getting siblings ready for the new baby. Contact with health care providers increases, as prenatal visits are scheduled biweekly and then weekly.

Expectant parents may look to their own parents for support and role modeling during the third trimester. Expectant grandparents may also be relied on for assistance, such as in providing child care for siblings. Although many expectant grandparents relish this role, others have lifestyles that do not make them readily accessible to their adult children. In situations where expectant fathers cannot attend birth, grandparents may attend prenatal visits and preparatory classes.

Socioeconomic factors affect the way families prepare for childbirth during the third trimester. Financial hardship can affect many aspects of life, including the ability to receive prenatal care. Cultural beliefs and practices also influence the family's preparation for birth and must be considered in providing care to the childbearing family.

REVIEW QUESTIONS

1. Discuss maternal and paternal fantasy patterns during the third trimester.
2. Describe psychosocial tasks of the pregnant family during the third trimester.
3. Compare the stresses experienced during pregnancy by multiparous and primiparous women.
4. Describe activities designed to prepare children for the birth of a sibling.
5. Describe psychologic aspects of becoming a grandparent.

REFERENCES

1. Oklan E. Psychological midwifery during the birth of a family. *Mobius.* 1985;5:6–20.
2. Caplan G. *Concepts of Mental Health and Consultation.* Washington, DC: US Department of Health, Education, Welfare; 1969.
3. Lederman RP. *Psychosocial Adaptation in Pregnancy.* Englewood Cliffs, NJ: Prentice-Hall; 1984.
4. Mercer RT. *First-Time Motherhood.* New York: Springer Publishing Co; 1986.
5. Rubin R. *Maternal Identity and the Maternal Experience.* New York: Springer Publishing Co; 1984.
6. Levy J, McGee R. Childbirth as a crisis: a test of Janis theory of communication and stress resolution. *J Pers Soc Psychol.* 1975;31:171–179.
7. Sherwen LN, ed. *Psychosocial Dimensions of the Pregnant Family.* New York: Springer Publishing Co; 1987.
8. Rubin R. Fantasy and object consistency in maternal relations. *Matern Nurs J.* 1972;2:101–111.
9. Sherwen LN. Fantasies during the third trimester of pregnancy. *Am J Matern Child Nurs.* 1981;6:398–401.
10. Martell LK. The mother-daughter relationship during daughter's first pregnancy: the transition experience. *Holistic Nursing Practice.* 1990;4:47–55.
11. Patsdaughter CA, Killien M. Developmental transitions in adulthood: mother-daughter relationships. *Holistic Nursing Practice.* 1990;4:37–46.
12. Kemp V, Page C. Maternal prenatal attachment in normal and high risk pregnancy. *J Obstet Gynecol Neonat Nurs.* 1987;16:179–184.
13. Shuzman E. Body image in pregnancy. In: Sherwen LN, ed. *Psychosocial Dimensions of the Pregnant Family.* New York: Springer Publishing Co; 1987:129–156.
14. Imle MA. Third trimester concerns of expectant parents in transition to parenthood. *Holistic Nursing Practice.* 1990; 4:25–36.
15. Fawcett J. The relationship between identification and patterns of change in spouse's body images during and after pregnancy. *Int J Nurs Stud.* 1977;14:199–211.
16. Herzog JM. Patterns of expectant fatherhood: a study of the fathers of a group of premature infants. In: Cath S, et al, eds. *Father and Child.* Boston: Little, Brown; 1982.
17. Robinson B, Barret R. *The Developing Father.* New York: Guilford Press; 1986.
18. Gerzi S, Berman E. Emotional reactions of expectant fa-

thers to their wive's first pregnancy. *Br J Med Psychol.* 1981;54:259–265.
19. Gurwitt AR. Aspects of prospective fatherhood. In: Cath S, et al, eds. *Father and Child.* Boston: Little, Brown; 1982.
20. Sherwen LN. Third trimester fantasies of first time expectant fathers. *Matern Child Nurs J.* 1986;15:153–170.
21. Clinton J. Expectant fathers at risk of couvade. *Nurs Res.* 1986;35:290–295.
22. Fawcett J, York R. Spouses' physical and psychological symptoms during pregnancy and the postpartum. *Nurs Res.* 1986;35:144–148.
23. Newton R, Hunt L. Psychosocial stress in pregnancy and its relation to low birth weight. *Br Med J.* 1984;288:1191–1194.
24. Robson B, Mandel D. Marital adjustment and fatherhood. *Can J Psychiatry.* 1985;30:169–172.
25. Palkowitz R. Sources of father-infant bonding beliefs: implications for childbirth educators. *Matern Child Nurs J.* 1988; 17:101–113.
26. Carlson D, Labarba R. Maternal emotionality during pregnancy and reproductive outcome: a review of the literature. *Int J Behav Dev.* 1979;2:343–376.
27. Perez R. Effects of stress, social support and coping style on adjustment to pregnancy among Hispanic women. *Hispan J Behav Sci.* 1983;5:141–161.
28. Lederman R, et al. The relationship of maternal anxiety, plasma catecholamines, and plasma cortisol to progress in labor. *Am J Obstet Gynecol.* 1978;132:495–500.
29. Fink R, Windt A. Depression during the prepartum and postpartum period. *Birth Psychol Bull.* 1984;5:1–22.
30. Obaywana A, et al. Psychosocial distress and pregnancy outcome: a three year prospective study. *J Psychosomat Obstet Gynecol.* 1984;3:173–183.
31. Glazer G. Anxiety levels and concerns among pregnant women. *Res Nurs Health.* 1980;3:107–113.
32. Rosenberg S, et al. Mothers' emotional responses to pregnancy and delivery. *Birth Psychol Bull.* 1984;5:1–8.
33. Mercer R. She's a multip . . . She knows the ropes. *Am J Matern Child Nurs.* 1979;4:301.
34. Grubb C. Perceptions of time of multiparous women in relation to themselves and others during the first postpartal month. *Matern Child Nurs J.* 1980;9:226
35. Westbook M. The effect of the order of birth on women's experience of childbearing. *J Marriage Fam.* 1978;40:165.
36. Walz B, Rich O. Maternal tasks of taking on a second child in the postpartum period. *Matern Child Nurs J.* 1983;12:185.
37. Kutzner SK. Responses of siblings to pregnancy. In: Sherwen LN, ed. *Psychosocial Dimensions of the Pregnant Family.* New York: Springer Publishing Co; 1987:177–192.
38. Dunn J. *Sisters and Brothers.* Cambridge, Mass: Harvard University Press; 1985.
39. Maloni JA, et al. Expectant grandparents class. *J Obstet Gynecol Neotat Nurs.* 1987;16:26–29.
40. Quinn W. Personal and family adjustment in later life. *J Marriage Fam.* 1983;45:57–73.
41. Kivnick H. Grandparenthood: an overview of meaning and mental health. *Gerontologist.* 1982;22:59–66.
42. Cath S. Vicissitudes of grandfatherhood: a miracle of revitalization? In: Cath S, et al, eds. *Father and Child.* Boston: Little, Brown; 1982.
43. Horn M, Manion J. Creative grandparenting: bonding the generations. *J Obstet Gynecol Neonat Nurs.* 1985;14: 233–236.
44. Fong C. Ethnicity and nursing practice. *Top Clin Nurs.* 1985; 7:1–10.
45. Spector RE. *Cultural Diversity in Health and Illness.* 2nd ed. Norwalk, Conn: Appleton-Century-Crofts; 1985.
46. Falicov C. Mexican families. In: McGolrick M, et al, eds. *Ethnicity and Family Therapy.* New York: Guilford Press; 1982.
47. Mindel C. Extended families among urban Mexican Americans, Anglos and Blacks. *Hispan J Behav Sci.* 1980;2:21–34.
48. Kay M. The Mexican American. In: Clark A, ed. *Culture, Childbearing, Health Professionals.* Philadelphia: FA Davis; 1978.

Assessment During the Third Trimester

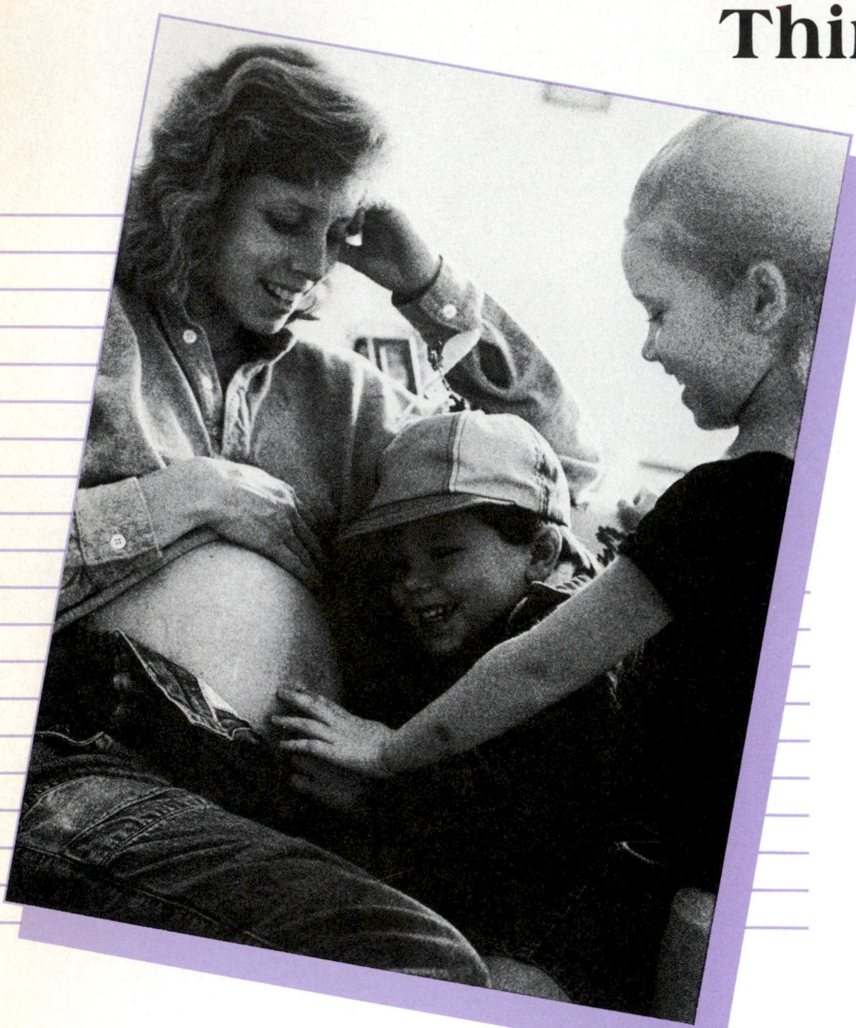

chapter 22

Key Terms

ballottement
biparietal diameter
cephalic index
contraction stress test
fetal biophysical profile
lecithin:sphingomyelin (L:S) ratio
Leopold's maneuvers
nonstress test

By the beginning of the third trimester of pregnancy, the low-risk, healthy expectant mother and her partner will have seen the health care provider five to six times. During the third trimester, client visits increase in frequency. Prenatal education classes also supply other opportunities for contact with health care providers. Around 36 weeks, clients and health care providers meet on a weekly basis. In addition to monitoring changes related to pregnancy, health care providers assess the expectant family's preparation for labor, delivery, and early parenting. Table 22–1 lists targets of assessment during the third trimester.

By collaborating with other health care providers, such as physicians, certified nurse-midwives, and nutritionists, the nurse ensures that comprehensive third-trimester assessment is performed. The nurse's role includes client interviews for the purpose of updating the health history and providing client education about the third trimester of pregnancy, labor, delivery, and the postpartum period. The nurse also participates in aspects of physical assessment of the expectant mother and the fetus, such as measuring the client's blood pressure and taking the fetal heart rate. In addition, the nurse serves as a client advocate in the health care system and may provide referrals to health and community resources, for example, prepared childbirth classes.

THE WOMAN WHO BEGINS PRENATAL CARE DURING THE THIRD TRIMESTER

As discussed in Chapter 18, women may delay prenatal care because they lack the finances, lack access to prenatal care (lack of transportation, timing of prenatal care sessions, geographic distance, and so on), fear the health care system, do not value wellness-oriented prenatal services, or have other reasons.

The comprehensive assessment approach used for the initial visit during the first trimester is employed for the client who seeks care for the first time during the third trimester. Reasons for the delay in

TABLE 22–1. TARGETS OF ASSESSMENT DURING THE THIRD TRIMESTER

Maternal adaptations to the third trimester of pregnancy
Development of new risk factors, including those associated with preterm birth, gestational diabetes, and pregnancy-induced hypertension
Effects of existing risk factors on the pregnant family during the third trimester
Fetal well-being
Psychosocial status and adaptations to the third trimester
Educational preparation and readiness for labor, delivery, and early parenting
Development of a birth plan
Resources available to the pregnant client and her family during the last trimester of pregnancy

seeking care are identified. Clients who do not obtain prenatal care until the third trimester frequently come from lower-socioeconomic-class backgrounds, although clients without care may come from any group. Socioeconomic status and the prenatal care a woman receives rank first and second as the most important determinants of birth outcome.[1] Women who seek initial prenatal care during the third trimester may therefore be considered at risk on the basis of either or both of these important factors; however, the nature of any alternate sources of prenatal care, such as self-care or reliance on culturally acceptable "wise" women or men, needs to be recognized. As with the client who first presents for care during the second trimester, nursing diagnoses, interventions, and assessment methods are based on the special needs of the client during the third trimester.

ASSESSMENT OF MATERNAL ADAPTATIONS TO PREGNANCY

Updating the Health History

Using a collaborative approach, as described in Chapters 14 and 18, health care providers update the health history at each prenatal visit throughout the third trimester. Assessment identifies client and family strengths as well as potential or actual risk factors during the third trimester.

Assessment of Physiologic State

For the low-risk client, assessment during the third trimester usually takes place according to the following schedule:[2] every 4 weeks for the first 28 weeks, every 2 to 3 weeks until 36 weeks of gestation, and every week from 36 weeks to labor. Women who are considered at risk are seen more often.

The parameters for assessment of maternal physiologic state are similar to those presented in Chapter 18. The nurse bases her assessment of the mother's physiologic state on knowledge of changes that normally occur during the third trimester and high-risk conditions that may be present at this time. Table 22–2 outlines physiologic parameters assessed during the third trimester, and Table 22–3 summarizes selected clinical findings.

During the third trimester the fetus assumes position for delivery; by term, full growth and development are attained. Around 32 weeks of gestation, fetal presentation and position and engagement of the fetus are assessed at each visit through the use of Leopold's maneuvers, described later in this chapter. The uterus continues to enlarge steadily (*see* Figure 20–1), and fundal growth and fetal size are assessed at each visit (Figure 22–1). Ultrasound evaluation of the fetus and amniotic fluid may be recommended if marked differences exist between uterine or fetal size and dates of the pregnancy. In this way conditions such as fetal intrauterine growth retardation may be identified.

Near term some clinicians perform pelvic examinations at each prenatal visit to assess the readiness of the cervix for delivery and engagement of the presenting part in the pelvis. Others see little need for third-trimester pelvic examination unless there is specific indication, for example, contractions that might be related to preterm labor. Appropriate laboratory analysis of body fluids or secretions may be obtained if symptoms of infection are present or the client is in a high-risk group. Examples include cervical and vaginal smears for gonorrhea, chlamydia, and monilia; blood tests for syphilis; and urine for culture and sensitivity.

Risk Assessment

Risk assessment is continued at each prenatal visit, because high-risk conditions, such as preeclampsia may develop during the third trimester. Approximately 20 percent of women have high-risk conditions recognizable during pregnancy; this constitutes about 55 percent of poor pregnancy results.[2] Prompt identification and intervention can often minimize complications and foster delivery of a healthy infant.

Table 18–4 lists risk factors that can be identified during the second trimester. The nurse continues to assess for these risk factors during the third trimester by updating the data base through history, physical

TABLE 22–2. PHYSIOLOGIC PARAMETERS ASSESSED DURING THE THIRD TRIMESTER

Assessment Parameter	Frequency of Assessment	Purpose
Vital signs, including blood pressure, pulse, respirations	Each visit	Detect any changes from normal/baseline that may indicate development of complications (eg, pre-eclampsia); determine maternal adaptation to third trimester
Uterine growth, measured by fundal height	Each visit	Assess for disproportionate uterine enlargement, which may indicate multiple gestation, polyhydramnios, inadequate fetal nutrition, and other conditions
Uterine characteristics such as present contractility, soreness, irritability	Each visit	Assess for signs of infection, preterm labor, and so on
Abdominal muscle tone	Each visit	Assess for poor muscle tone, contributing to discomforts such as low back pain
Fetal presentation, engagement, lie, and position, measured by Leopold's maneuvers	Each visit	Identify potential labor and delivery problems related to fetal presentation, position, or lie (especially when engagement has occurred)
Fetal heart rate auscultated with fetoscope or assessed with Doppler; fetal movements felt by examiner, reported by mother	Each visit	Fetal heart tones, fetal movement, and activity indicate fetal well-being
Maternal weight and nutritional status	Each visit	Assess nutritional patterns and detect fluid retention
Urinalysis for protein, glucose, ketones	Each visit	Detect development of complications, such as pre-eclampsia and diabetes
Suggested blood study for:		
Hemoglobin or hematocrit	Early in third trimester (some facilities routinely screen more often)	Detect anemia of pregnancy
Glucose	28 weeks, if not done during second trimester	Screen for diabetes
Rh antibody titer (in unsensitized Rh-negative clients)	28 weeks	Identify clients at risk for Rh hemolytic disease

Source: *Reference 2.*

examination, biochemical screening, fetal assessment, and other prenatal diagnostic tests.

As prematurity remains the most significant perinatal problem, risk assessment for preterm delivery is essential. The nurse assesses socioeconomic status, past history, daily habits, and current prenatal events; however, signs and symptoms of preterm labor are reviewed with all third-trimester women, because many women who deliver prematurely have no identifiable risk factors.

The third-trimester expectant woman and her partner are also assessed for risk factors that may indicate a potential problem with accepting or caring for the newborn. Attainment of maternal and paternal roles, as well as accomplishment of psychologic tasks, is assessed by the nurse throughout pregnancy.

Socioeconomic status and related living conditions can present great risks to family health during pregnancy and after childbirth. Financially impoverished clients may not be able to provide adequate nutrition, shelter, or clothing for themselves or an infant. Through antenatal assessment, nurses identify clients in such high-risk situations. Nurses' collaboration with other health care personnel, such as social workers, and, when appropriate, representatives from charitable organizations, may result in a client's receiving emergency shelter, food, and clothing.

Biochemical Screening Techniques

Urinalysis. During third-trimester visits, urine is assessed for protein, glucose, and ketones, as during the second trimester. Proteinuria of 2+ or more on a standard dipstick testing may indicate the onset or progression of high-risk conditions, such as pre-eclampsia. The presence of glucose in the urine may or may not be considered abnormal, as about 50 percent of pregnant women have glucosuria at some point.[3] When glucosuria occurs, blood glucose screening is recommended to assess for carbohydrate intolerance as found, for example, in diabetes mellitus.

TABLE 22–3. SELECTED CLINICAL FINDINGS DURING THE THIRD TRIMESTER

Body System	Clinical Findings
Integument	Stretch marks over abdomen, breasts, and thighs (striae gravidarum)
	Pruritis of the skin and vulva
	Melasma, vascular spiders, or hemangiomas may develop or increase
Cardiovascular	Continued increase in heart rate of an average 10–15 beats per minute above baseline
	Return of blood pressure to baseline from decrease during the first 24 weeks of gestation
	Supine hypotensive syndrome—drop in systolic and diastolic blood pressure from baseline if client is in supine position
	Leg cramps
	Varicosities of the legs and vulva
Respiratory	Shortness of breath, difficulty breathing (dyspnea)
Hematologic	White blood cell count 5000–12,000/μL (Counts as high as 16,000/μL have been seen in the third trimester.)
	Hgb 11 g/dl or greater; Hct 32 g/dl or greater[6]
	Rh-negative mother, Rh-positive father, antibody screening negative
Gastrointestinal	Pyrosis (heartburn)
	Increased flatulence
Musculoskeletal	Low backache
	Diastasis recti (separation of abdominal rectus muscles)
Urinary	Frequency of urination similar to that of first trimester
	Edema of the legs and ankles
Reproductive	Braxton Hicks contractions
	Round ligament pain
	Effacement of the cervix
	Vaginal leukorrhea
	Fullness and heaviness of the breasts; presence of colostrum
Neurologic	Alert, appropriate
	Continued normal reflexes in all four extremities
	Possible numbness and tingling of fingers and toes (paresthesias); carpal tunnel syndrome

Blood Studies

Hemoglobin or Hematocrit. Around 32 weeks, hemoglobin or hematocrit levels are drawn to assess for anemia. A hemoglobin value below 11 g/dL or a hematocrit below 32 percent is considered anemic.

Antibody Screening. Screening for antibodies is done to identify hemolytic disease in the fetus and newborn (*see* Chapter 42). The Rh (rhesus) system is no longer limited to Rh-positive and Rh-negative blood group factors, as many other red blood cell antigens have been recognized. Exposure to any antigen, for example as a result of a blood transfusion, may trigger an antibody reaction if that antigen does not already exist on the client's red blood cells. Most red blood cell antigens occur rarely or do not severely affect the fetus, that is, cause hemolytic disease. Absence of the D antigen on the mother's red blood cells, a condition referred to as Rh(D) negativity, can be a major cause of hemolytic disease in the fetus and newborn if the mother has in the past built antibodies, that is, become isoimmunized. If the mother-to-be is Rh(D) negative, a sample of the expectant father's blood is examined for Rh(D) status. In usual circumstances, if the father is Rh(D) negative, the fetus will not be affected by this type of incompatibility (*see* Chapter 42 for further discussion of blood incompatibilities). Nevertheless, there is a chance that even Rh(D)-positive women may have acquired antibodies as a result of exposure to antigens at some point in their lives. All pregnant women should therefore be screened at their initial visit for D(Rho) antigen on their erythrocytes, as well as for the presence or absence of other antibodies in their serum. Ideally, this visit would take place in the first trimester.[4]

Antibody screening is done again around 28 weeks of gestation if the expectant father is Rh positive and the unsensitized expectant mother is Rh negative or if the expectant father is unavailable for testing.[2] Antibody screening may be done earlier and more frequently if additional risk is suspected.

Initial assessment of Rh immunization may be done through antibody titration. Two methods that have been used for assessment of antibody titers are the albumin titration method and the indirect antiglobulin Rh antibody titration (IDAT).

With the albumin titration method, a titer greater than 1:16 indicates a significant risk of fetal morbidity and mortality from Rh disease. When there is no history of a previously affected fetus, a steady titer of 1:16 at any time during pregnancy is an indication for supplementary testing, such as ultrasound and amniocentesis, or for delivery if the fetus is mature.[4] Antibody titers less than 1:8 have not been associated with stillbirths prior to term.[5]

The IDAT screening is believed by some to be a more accurate measure of fetal risk because of its increased sensitivity. With this method, titers of 1:32 or

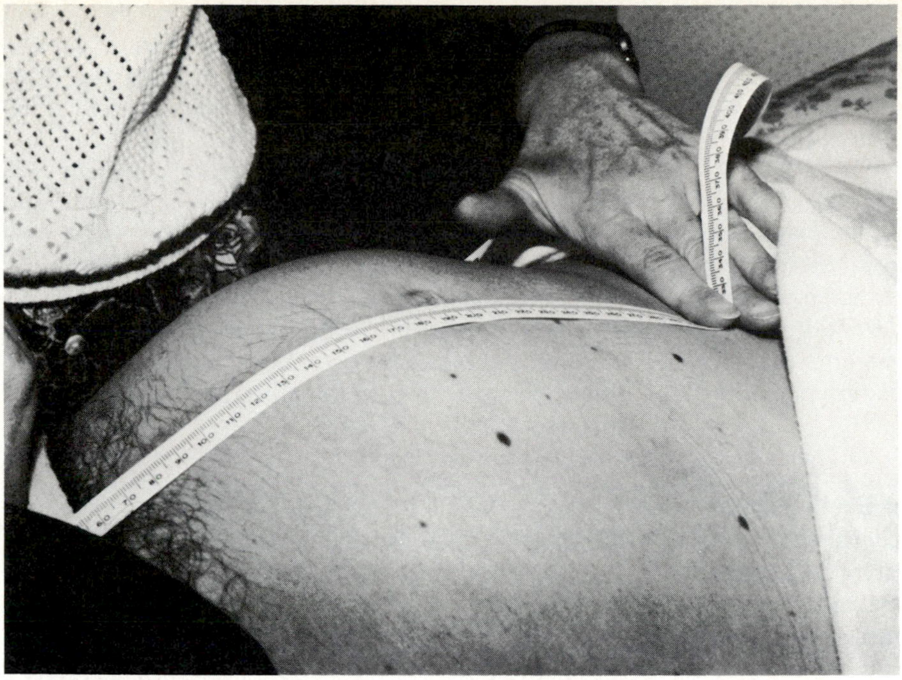

Figure 22–1. The height of the fundus is measured at prenatal visits during the third trimester.

higher may indicate fetal risk. It is more costly than the albumin method and is therefore used less frequently.[6]

Amniotic fluid and fetal blood analysis provide direct means to evaluate hemolytic disease in the fetus, although both procedures are more invasive than drawing a sample of the expectant mother's blood. When fetal hemolytic disease is suspected, assessment of bilirubin may be done using amniotic fluid, obtained by amniocentesis. Fetal blood samples, taken during percutaneous umbilical blood sampling (PUBS), may be used for fetal blood typing and antibody screening, direct Coombs testing, and complete blood count.[7] As discussed in Chapter 18, by providing a direct route to fetal circulation, PUBS may also be used for treatments, for example, fetal blood transfusions for anemia resulting from hemolytic disease.

Glucose Screening. Glucose screening is usually performed between the 24th and 28th week.

Psychosocial and Cultural Assessment

Psychosocial Assessment. During the third trimester the client and her family actively prepare for the birth of the baby and their changing roles within the family structure. Fears and worries regarding the labor and delivery process surface during this trimester. Family members also accomplish certain psychosocial developmental tasks. These tasks include coping with the biologic changes of the third trimester, preparing for labor and delivery, attaching to the infant-to-be, coping with changes in family roles and relationships, adjusting to moving up a generation (becoming parents or grandparents), and establishing new relationships within the community and society.[8]

The nurse provides support to the family as third-trimester feelings toward the pregnancy and the fetus are discussed. The expectant mother's negative feelings, such as desire to have the pregnancy completed or dissatisfaction with her large size, are distinguished from negative feelings about the fetus, which may indicate problems with attachment to the newborn. Intense parental ambivalence about becoming a parent at this stage may indicate unresolved conflicts that may interfere with acceptance of the newborn.[9] The nurse also assesses maternal and paternal fantasies, which may indicate concerns and fears.[10, 11] The nurse can help allay these fears and provide support to the couple as they move into their new roles.

The preparation of siblings for the baby's arrival is important during the third trimester. The nurse assesses such factors as the age, developmental level, and number of siblings, as well as the family's cultural background and the parents' involvement in sibling preparation.[12] Family members may decide to have siblings attend the prenatal visits. The children may be encouraged to listen to fetal heart tones, palpate the uterus, and ask questions. The client may or may not want the sibling to be present if pelvic examination is to be done.

The nurse and parents can use a variety of teaching aids such as books, dolls, and role playing to prepare children for the new baby and for their role in the family. Parents may also decide to have children share in the birth experience. This decision is based on such factors as the desire of the parents and siblings and the availability of such an experience in the health care system.[12]

Assessment of Plans for Birth and Early Parenting. The goal of assessment of the client's plans for birth and early parenting is to identify client preparation for childbirth, the puerperium, and care of a neonate. Through assessment the nurse can ensure the following:

- The client's birth plan remains feasible within the selected birthing environment.
- The client has a basic understanding of the labor and delivery process and what to expect in the selected birthing environment.
- The client receives educational preparation regarding labor and delivery techniques (eg, prepared childbirth classes).
- The client is prepared for alternatives in the event of emergency.
- The client is prepared for postpartum changes and care.
- The client is able to care safely for a newborn with existing resources.
- The client who requires supplementary services is able to receive them.
- The client has identified options in infant feeding methods.
- The client can identify health care and community resources related to childbearing.

Cultural Assessment. During the third trimester, the nurse assesses cultural values and beliefs related to late pregnancy, to the labor and delivery experience, and to early childrearing practices. For example, some Orthodox Jewish sects follow a traditional and strict interpretation of Jewish law.[13] Tsniut is one category and refers to laws of modesty. A Jewish man who observes Tsniut will not directly view his wife while she is immodestly exposed, for example, during pelvic examinations. For this reason, the couple may not want the expectant father to be present throughout prenatal physical assessment. Nevertheless, they may share a loving relationship. This type of religious belief contrasts with current antenatal philosophy and practice that encourage and expect that both partners in a strong marriage will want to share all aspects of prenatal care, labor and delivery. As illustrated by this example, what may appear as new and family centered to American nurses may actually be regarded as odd and unacceptable to clients from different backgrounds. Nursing interventions are most therapeutic when factors related to cultural patterns and values are considered.[13,14]

ASSESSMENT OF FETAL WELL-BEING

Fundal Height

Measurement of fundal height with a tape measure is one method used to assess fetal growth during the third trimester (*see* Chapter 18). Between 22 and 34 weeks, the measurement of the fundal height in centimeters should correlate with the gestational age in weeks. After 36 weeks, the presenting part may descend into the pelvis, and the fundal height may decrease (*see* Figure 20–1). Figure 22–1 shows a nurse-midwife measuring the height of the fundus during the third trimester.

Johnson's Calculation of Fetal Weight

Fundal height measurement can also be used to estimate fetal weight in the third trimester. Johnson's formula for estimation of fetal weight has been found to be accurate within 375 g in 75 percent of newborns. Johnson's formula has been used late in the third trimester when decisions must be made about labor and delivery. In high-risk situations, however, other studies such as ultrasound provide more accurate information about fetal size and weight; decisions regarding delivery would not rely on clinical weight estimation alone.

The formula for estimation of fetal weight in vertex (head first) presentations is[15]

$$\text{fetal weight (g)} = \text{fundal height (cm)} - n \times 155$$

where

n = 12 if vertex is above the ischial spines or
n = 11 if vertex is below ischial spines.

Using Johnson's formula (with fundal height measured from the symphysis pubis), if fh = 33 cm, station = −2 (present part is 2 cm above ischial spines)

then

$$(33 - 12) \times 155 = 3255 \text{ g}$$

Leopold's Maneuvers

Fetal lie, presentation, position, and engagement (*see* Chapter 25) can be determined by abdominal palpation of the mother through use of **Leopold's maneuvers.** Abdominal palpation also provides other information, such as uterine irritability, tone, tenderness, current contractility, fetal movement, and estimation of fetal weight.[16] To prevent discomfort related to a full bladder during abdominal examination, the client is asked to void. The expectant mother then lies on her back on the examining table with the shoulders raised by a pillow and the knees drawn up slightly[17] (Figure 22–2).

After explaining the procedure, the examiner performs Leopold's maneuvers (Figure 22–3), by assessing the part of the fetus located in the fundus, the location of the back of the fetus, the presenting part, and whether the part is engaged in the pelvis. During abdominal palpation, the examiner also makes observations noted earlier.

During third-trimester visits, Leopold's maneuvers are routinely performed by the primary health care provider, that is, a certified nurse-midwife or physician; however, the staff nurse who works in prenatal testing units or in labor and delivery settings needs to be able to perform this technique to aid, for example, in positioning fetal monitoring equipment.

First Maneuver. The examiner stands at the mother's side and palpates the fundus with the fingertips of both hands to assess which fetal part is in the fundus. The fetal head feels firm and round and is gently movable. When pressing down on the head, the examiner will feel the head move against the fingertips. This is referred to as **ballottement.** If the fetal breech (sacrum) is found in the fundus, the fetal part will feel large and nodular with less movement; there will be no ballottement.

Second Maneuver. After identifying which part of the fetus lies in the fundus, the examiner places the palms of the hands on either side of the maternal abdomen and exerts gentle pressure. Through this maneuver, the examiner determines where the back and small parts (feet and hands) of the fetus are located. The back feels like a hard, consistent structure, whereas the small parts feel like nodules. If the expectant mother is obese or there is a large amount of amniotic fluid, the back may be felt by putting pressure on the side of the abdomen with one hand, while palpating with the other.

Third Maneuver. The third maneuver is done to determine the presenting part of the fetus. The lower uterine segment, just above the symphysis pubis, is held between the thumb and fingers of one hand. This maneuver is similar to the first maneuver in that the fetal head feels hard and globular, while the breech feels large and nodular. An attempt is also made to move the presenting part (usually the head) from side to side to determine whether it is free (floating) or in the pelvis and fixed (engaged).[17] After completion of the third maneuver, the examiner has located the fetal head, breech, back, and extremities. The fourth maneuver then provides information regarding the attitude of the head.

Fourth Maneuver. During the fourth maneuver, the examiner stands at the mother's shoulder and faces toward her feet. The fingertips of each hand gently move down the uterus toward the symphysis pubis. When the head is the presenting part, one hand is stopped sooner than the other hand by a rounded body, the cephalic prominence. When the fetal head is flexed, the forehead is the cephalic prominence and is found on the same side as the fetal small parts. If the fetal head is extended, the occiput is the cephalic prominence and can be felt on the same side as the fetal back. A fetal attitude of flexion is the most desirable for the labor and delivery process.

Palpation of the maternal abdomen provides a good opportunity for the nurse to teach the client and her support person about fetal growth, lie, position, and presentation. The expectant father and siblings

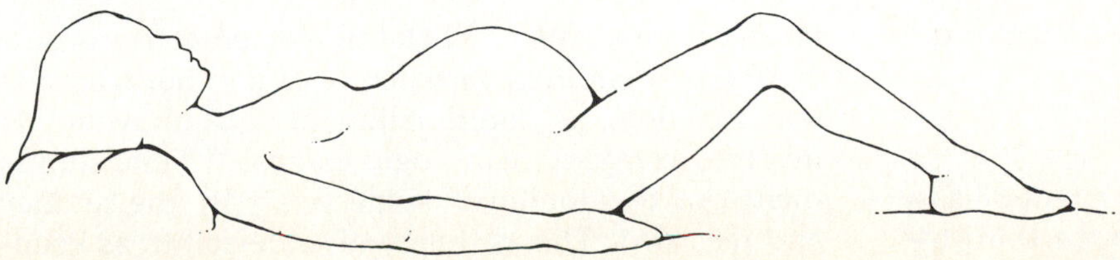

Figure 22–2. Position of mother for abdominal palpation. (*Reproduced, with permission, from Oxorn H, ed.* Oxorn-Foote Human Labor and Birth. *5th ed. Norwalk, Conn: Appleton & Lange; 1986:75.*)

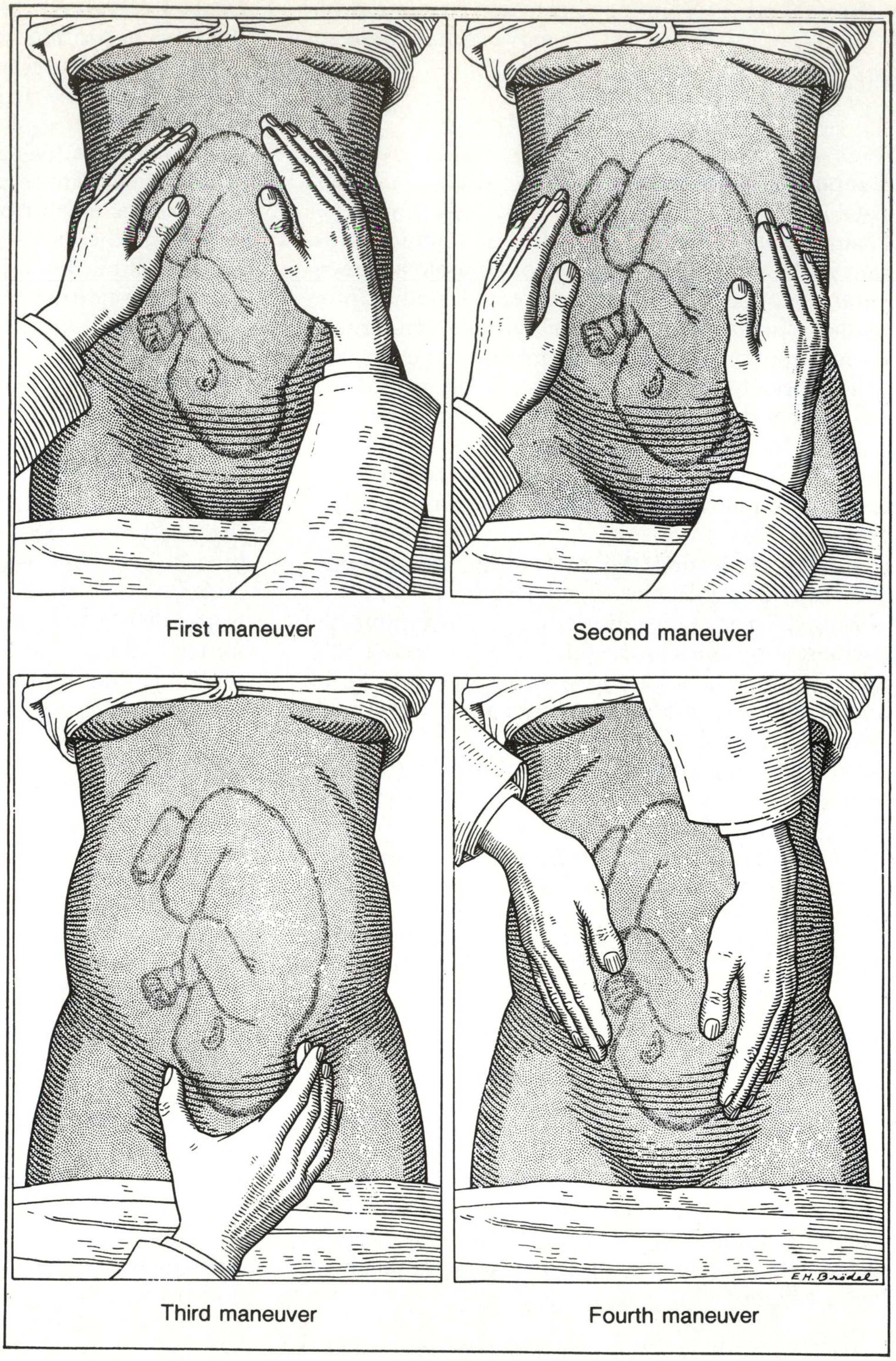

Figure 22–3. Leopold's maneuvers. (*Reproduced, with permission, from Cunningham FG, et al.* Williams Obstetrics. *18th ed. Norwalk, Conn: Appleton & Lange; 1985:183.*)

can also participate in this assessment as part of the plan of care.

Assessment of Fetal Movement

Fetal movement has received increased attention as a method of assessing fetal well-being in the third trimester of pregnancy.[18] Fetal movements are considered to be an indirect measure of central nervous system function, as coordination of fetal movements involves complex neurologic control.[19] Fetal movement can be monitored subjectively by the mother and recorded. This is frequently referred to as keeping a fetal "kick count." One approach has the mother note the time required for ten movements to occur daily. The expectant mother begins to count movements at 8 AM (or some other specified time) and notes the time when the tenth movement is felt. If ten movements are not felt by 8 PM (or 12 hours later), or if it takes twice as long to feel ten movements as in prior days, the mother reports these findings to the health care provider. Figure 22–4 depicts a fetal movement record; the expectant mother's name, the date, and the estimated gestational age (EGA) of the fetus are included.[15] Another way of measuring fetal activity is to have the expectant mother set aside time each day or evening to count fetal movements. Fetal activity, with this method, is defined as three or more movements in 1 hour. If fewer than three movements occur, the expectant mother should report these findings.[18]

Monitoring fetal movements provides information about fetal well-being. For example, it has been estimated that 46 to 81 percent of inactive fetuses will have a negative perinatal outcome, such as stillbirth, fetal distress during labor, asphyxia, or delays in neurobehavioral development after birth.[20] Although evidence of an active fetus is reassuring, an inactive fetus is not necessarily an ominous sign. Reduction in activity may instead reflect a normal fetal state such as sleep.[18] Some clinicians feel that the absolute number of fetal movements per day is less important than the degree of change in fetal movements.[4] Using this criterion, the mother would report findings if the number of fetal movements decreases. Monitoring of fetal movements is a highly subjective measure of assessment that depends on client perceptions, understanding, and actual use of the procedure. Errors in interpretation can result from lack of client perception of all types of movement and lack of attention to recordkeeping as a result, for example, of distractions from everyday activity.

The opportunity for the expectant mother and her partner to participate in the assessment of the fetus is one positive aspect of monitoring fetal movements. They are also able to become more aware of the fetus; this may foster attachment behaviors. Persistent focusing on the presence or absence of fetal movement may also cause anxiety about fetal well-being. Although counting fetal movements may be used as one means of fetal surveillance, other tests are used to identify the compromised fetus.[4] These tests should not be done routinely with all pregnancies, but are helpful in estimating fetal well-being in pregnancies considered at risk. Additional tests, described later, include the nonstress test, the contraction stress test, and the fetal biophysical profile.

Electronic Fetal Monitoring

Electronic fetal monitoring records fetal heart activity through use of Doppler ultrasound. At the same time, uterine activity is assessed with a tocotransducer. This apparatus is held painlessly in place by a belt or adhesive pad placed on the expectant mother's abdomen (Figure 22–5). The tocotransducer records the duration and frequency of uterine contractions at the same time that the ultrasound transducer records the fetal heart rate. In this way the response of the fetus to any contractions, including the rhythmic, usually painless contractions experienced during pregnancy, can be assessed; in addition, information about fetal activity during contraction-free periods can be provided. Electronic fetal monitoring can be used for fetal surveillance during pregnancy, as well as during labor (*see* Chapter 27).

In the nonstress test, the contraction stress test, and the fetal biophysical profile, a fetal heart tracing must be obtained with an electronic fetal monitor. The nurse needs to know certain parameters of the fetal heart rate tracing when interpreting test results:

1. The fetal heart rate (FHR) has a baseline usually in the range of 120 to 160 beats per minute (BPM). By

Fetal Movement Record

	M	Tu	W	Th	F	Sat.	Sun.
8 AM							
10 AM							
12 PM							
2 PM							
4 PM							
6 PM							
8 PM							

Name:

Date:

EGA:

Figure 22–4. Fetal movement record. (*Reproduced, with permission, from Pernoll ML, Benson RC, eds.* Current Obstetric and Gynecologic Diagnosis and Treatment. *6th ed. Norwalk, Conn: Appleton & Lange; 1987:286.*)

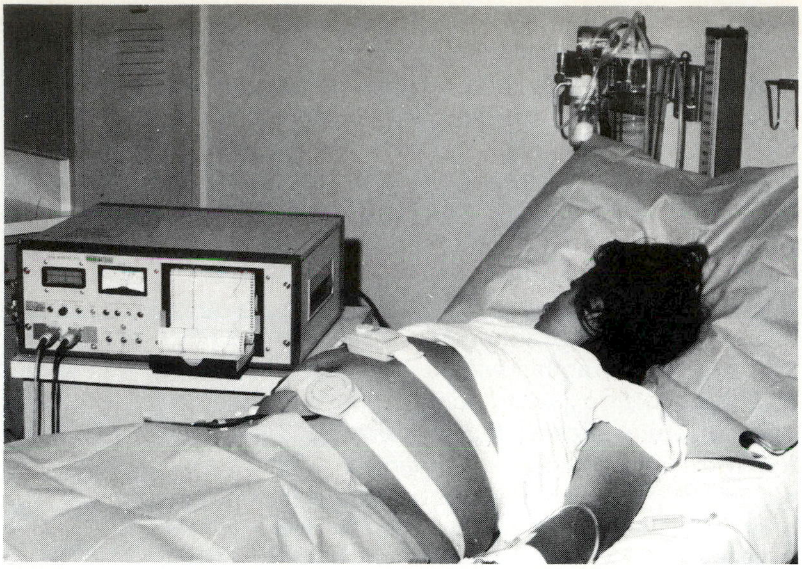

Figure 22–5. Antepartum electronic fetal monitoring (Doppler and transducer). (*Reproduced, with permission, from Cunningham FG, et al.* Williams Obstetrics. *18th ed. Norwalk, Conn: Appleton & Lange; 1989:290.*)

evaluating the FHR for a 10-minute period, the nurse can determine the FHR baseline of the individual fetus.

2. The FHR has variability, or fluctuations, if the fetus has normal neurologic functioning. The beat-to-beat variability of the FHR can be 6 to 25 BPM. Lack of variability or decreased variability may indicate fetal sleep state or fetal distress. When an external fetal heart monitor is used, fetal heart rate variability may be artificially increased.[15] This parameter is therefore less reliable as an indicator of fetal distress in the antepartum period when noninvasive external electronic fetal monitoring must be used.
3. The fetal heart rate will accelerate above the baseline in response to fetal movement. This is referred to as a *reactive pattern* of the FHR and is an indication of fetal well-being.
4. The fetal heart rate may fall below the baseline in response to uterine contractions. This is referred to as *fetal heart rate deceleration* and may be classified as follows:
   a. *Early decelerations* occur early in the contraction, usually in the latter stages of labor, in response to pressure on the fetal skull. Transient decelerations occur at the beginning of the contraction and do not indicate fetal distress.
   b. *Variable decelerations* occur any time during the contraction and are associated with cord compression. These can sometimes be relieved by turning the mother from back to side (especially onto her left side) or from side to side.[15] If they are not relieved, they may indicate fetal distress.
   c. *Late decelerations* occur late in the contraction (after the acme), and indicate uteroplacental insufficiency. These can be an ominous sign.

The Nonstress Test. The **nonstress test** (NST) has become a widely used method for assessment of fetal condition.[21] The NST uses Doppler ultrasound to monitor baseline fetal heart activity, accelerations of fetal heart rate with fetal movement, and absence of fetal heart rate decelerations.[22] Fetal movement typically is accompanied by fetal heart rate acceleration above the baseline. When this occurs, the NST is considered reactive (normal); when fetal heart rate accelerations do not occur with fetal movement, the test is considered nonreactive (abnormal). A fetus that does not have heart rate accelerations as a reflex response to movements may potentially be asphyxiated.[23] The NST is often done as a primary method of third-trimester fetal surveillance. Other tests, such as the contraction stress test or the biophysical profile may be performed if NST results indicate a need for further testing.[24] The greatest advantage of the NST is that it is easy to administer.[23]

Procedure. The expectant mother is placed in the left lateral or semi-Fowler position to prevent maternal supine hypotension. A reclining chair may also be used as a comfortable alternative. The examiner monitors maternal blood pressure initially and at 10- to 15-minute intervals throughout the testing procedure. If hypotension occurs, interventions such as changing the expectant mother's position are initiated.

External fetal monitoring equipment is applied to the maternal abdomen and a fetal heart rate tracing is obtained (*see* Chapter 27 for further discussion of electronic fetal monitoring). The externally placed detector most often used is an ultrasound transducer, because both phonocardiography and fetal electrocardiography can be unsatisfactory in tracing the fetal heart rate through maternal tissue.[4] Fetal movements are noted with an external tocotransducer, which is secured to the maternal abdomen.

Fetal movements can be recorded by the mother using a remote event marker that she presses each time she senses movement.[26] The event marker records the movement on the same moving paper strip on which the fetal heart rate is recorded.[4] The nurse also monitors fetal activity and writes "FM" (fetal movement) on the strip when movement is noted.[27]

Interpretations

Reactive Pattern: Normal Nonstress Test. Several different protocols have been used to define a reactive test; each prescribes a certain number of fetal heart rate accelerations in a defined time period; each identifies particular values of the amplitude and duration of fetal heart rate accelerations.[28] According to two widely used definitions, the NST is considered reactive (normal) when there are two or more fetal heart rate accelerations, coinciding with fetal movement, during a 10- or 20-minute observation period. Each acceleration must have an amplitude greater than 15 beats per minute and a duration of more than 15 seconds. Additionally, the baseline fetal heart rate should be within the normal range of 120 to 160 with no periodic decelerations[17] (Figure 22–6). Fetal heart rate accelerations do not need to occur during the first part of the NST, but may normally take place during any 10- to 20-minute portion of the test.

Because the normal fetus has sleep-wake cycles, the fetus may be asleep when the NST is performed. The test then may be interpreted as nonreactive, thereby necessitating further assessment of an otherwise normal fetus. Waiting for the fetus to become reactive can prolong the time for the test substantially. If the fetus does not move perceptibly during the first five or ten minutes of the test, stimulation may be used to produce fetal movement and thereby shorten the NST.[28] A reactive test produced by stimulation is thought to be similar to a reactive test produced by spontaneous fetal movement.

At present no clear guidelines about fetal stimulation techniques exist, and further research is needed. Several fetal stimulation techniques have been used with varying success and include having the mother drink juice to raise her blood sugar, manipulation of the fetus by the mother or nurse in order to arouse the fetus, and fetal auditory stimulation (acoustic stimulation), such as ringing a bell next to the mother's abdomen and using loudspeakers to deliver varying levels of sound.[23,28,29] Vibroacoustic stimulation is a technique that has been reported to be effective in converting nonreactive tracings to reactive tracings in healthy fetuses and in shortening the time of the NST.[30] In one approach to vibroacoustic stimulation, an artificial larynx is held against the maternal abdomen over the area of the fetal head, after the baseline fetal heart rate has been documented.[30,31] The vibrating buzzing sound (100 to 110 decibels at 1,000 hertz in open air) that is delivered provides both an auditory and vibratory stimulus which causes the healthy fetus to react. Fetal reactions can be so pronounced that fetal heart rates may remain elevated for up to an hour or longer, possibly reflecting a change in the fetal state of arousal.[31] No long-term negative effects of vibroacoustic stimulation have been substantiated.

Nonreactive Pattern: Abnormal Nonstress Test. The NST is considered nonreactive when fewer than two accelerations occur during a 20- to 40-minute period.

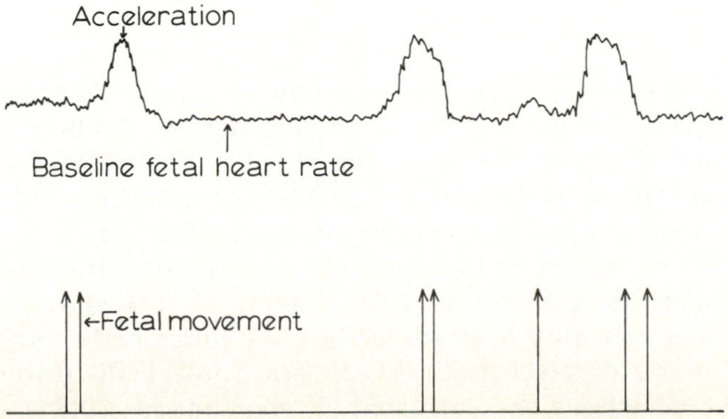

Figure 22–6. Reactive NST—normal finding. (*Reproduced, with permission, from Oxorn H, ed.* Oxorn-Foote Human Labor and Birth. *5th ed. Norwalk, Conn: Appleton & Lange; 1986:599.*)

If accelerations do occur, the test is considered nonreactive when their amplitude is less than 15 beats per minute and their duration is less than 15 seconds[17] (Figure 22–7).

Errors in Interpretation: False Negatives and False Positives. Problems can occur in interpretation of the NST. With a true false-negative test, a reactive pattern is identified but the fetus dies before the next testing date or delivery.[23] This situation occurs in only about 1 percent of cases, as a reactive test is usually indicative of fetal well-being;[32] however, the future is always uncertain, and many unrelated events (such as trauma, drug use, placental abruption, complications during labor) may cause fetal death after the test date. Certain high-risk conditions such as diabetes, postmaturity, and intrauterine growth retardation require at least twice weekly testing to assess fetal status.

In as many as 50 to 80 percent of cases, the NST can be falsely positive, that is, a fetus with a nonreactive NST has a normal outcome.[29] Lack of agreement about what actually represents normal fetal reactivity is one reason for the high false-positive rate. Studies have demonstrated that nonreactivity of the test may be a function of gestational age rather than of fetal jeopardy. They conclude that such tests should not be performed prior to 30 weeks of gestation. Further, they suggest that extending test duration when accelerations are absent initially, accepting lower thresholds for reactivity, or both may reduce errors in the interpretation of test results.[21,23] Using fetal stimulation techniques, such as vibroacoustic stimulation, may also elicit fetal reactivity. In addition, variation among individuals who interpret tests can account for some differences.

Risks. The NST is considered a noninvasive test. Unknown effects of ultrasound might be mentioned as a possible risk related to the NST; however, as yet no harmful effects on humans as a result of ultrasound have been documented.[2] Attention to maternal position should avoid or promptly correct supine hypotensive syndrome, which could be a risk related to the procedure. Like any fetal surveillance test, the NST carries a potential emotional risk, as clients may be anxious about fetal well-being, especially if the test is read as nonreactive. Anticipatory guidance, emotional support, and strategies to foster fetal reactivity and minimize false positive results can address these possible problems.

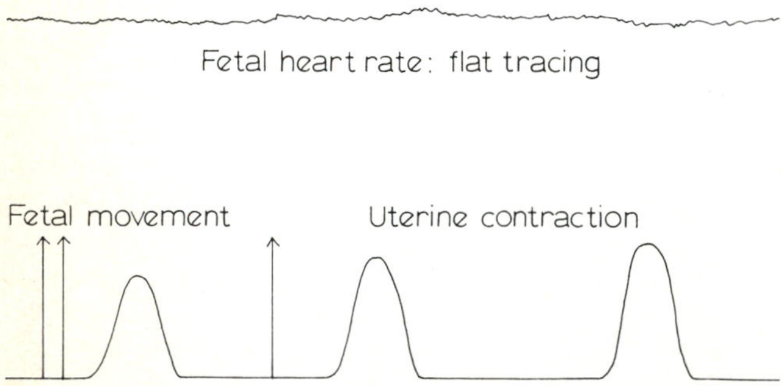

Figure 22–7. Nonreactive NST—abnormal finding. (*Reproduced, with permission, from Oxorn H, ed.* Oxorn-Foote Human Labor and Birth. *5th ed. Norwalk, Conn: Appleton & Lange; 1986:605.*)

The Contraction Stress Test. A **contraction stress test** (CST) is a third trimester assessment method that is performed when the NST is nonreactive and when the expectant mother is at risk because of such conditions as hypertension, insulin-dependent diabetes, and renal disease. Scheduling of the CST is based on clinical evaluation of the client late in the third trimester. The test may be performed weekly or more frequently if the client has a change in status or a high-risk condition such as diabetes. The CST subjects the fetus to uterine contractions that compress the arteries supplying the placenta, thus reducing placental blood flow and the flow of oxygen to the fetus. The fetus with adequate oxygen reserve will tolerate transient reductions in the flow of oxygen; the heart rate will remain relatively unchanged. When the fetus has minimal metabolic reserve, contractions will cause late decelerations of the fetal heart rate. With late decelerations, the FHR does not return to the baseline until after the contraction ends. Late decelerations are associated with factors that reduce uteroplacental gas exchange. The presence of late decelerations may therefore suggest fetal compromise; their absence suggests, but does not ensure, fetal well-being.[33]

The CST can be performed by observing the FHR tracing with spontaneous or stimulated uterine contractions. Uterine contractions can be stimulated through nipple stimulation/breast massage or with an intravenous infusion of oxytocin.

Procedure. The positioning of the mother and the frequency of blood pressure monitoring are similar for the CST and the NST. The client is placed on the electronic fetal monitor. An NST is performed first. Baseline spontaneous uterine contractions and fetal heart rate are recorded for 15 to 30 minutes. If spontaneous uterine contractions lasting 40 to 60 seconds and recurring approximately three times in 10 minutes are detected, the responses of the FHR to the contractions are evaluated. If spontaneous contractions meeting the preceding criteria do not occur, uterine contractions are induced by breast stimulation (nipple stimulation/breast massage) or with an oxytocin intravenous infusion pump.[4]

Nipple/Breast Stimulation Test. Nipple stimulation is a noninvasive technique that has been used to stimulate contractions needed for the CST. This test is based on the premise that tactile stimulation of the nipple also stimulates the release of exogenous oxytocin from the maternal posterior pituitary gland.[4] Studies have indicated that the nipple stimulation test is comparable to the oxytocin challenge test in obtaining contractions needed for the CST.[33,34]

Protocols for the nipple stimulation test may vary. For example, some investigators and clinicians suggest that warm moist towels be placed on each breast, and then the nipple on one breast be rolled and massaged for 10 minutes.[33] Some suggest massaging the breasts with mineral oil, concentrating the tactile stimulation on the nipple and alternating sides every 10 minutes for a maximum of 40 to 60 minutes.[34] Others recommend that the client roll one nipple between her thumb and forefinger for 1 minute[35]; if a contraction occurs the technique is repeated on the other side 60 seconds after its end. If no contraction takes place within 3 minutes of nipple stimulation, the procedure is then performed on the other nipple. According to this protocol, the procedure is usually not repeated more than three times. If some uterine activity has been identified, nipple stimulation may be attempted twice more.

Whatever protocol is used, the principle to be followed is that, once the contractions begin, the nipples, breasts, or both are massaged intermittently, so that the desired contractions are stimulated. If no contractions result, oxytocin infusion may be used.[17] The CST takes about 1 to 2 hours.

Nipple stimulation and breast massage make use of the body's own natural resources; however, hyperstimulation of the uterus (contractions lasting 90 seconds or more) has been reported in some studies in which nipple stimulation was used.[34]

Oxytocin Challenge Test. In the absence of spontaneous uterine contractions for the CST, oxytocin may be administered intravenously. A dose of 0.5 mU per minute may be used to begin the test. A controlled-rate infusion pump is used to regulate the infusion of oxytocin in normal saline or Ringer's lactate solution. The oxytocin infusion should be "piggybacked" to a main intravenous line. In case of complications related to oxytocin infusion, the medication can be easily discontinued while the vein is kept open and accessible.[36] The oxytocin infusion should be connected close to the mainline needle site.[28] There is greater risk of inadvertently giving the client a bolus of oxytocin when the infusion is piggybacked higher in the tubing. The dose, administered in milliunits, is increased every 15 to 30 minutes until at least three uterine contractions, lasting 60 seconds, occur per 10 minutes. The typical rate of oxytocin infusion used to elicit uterine contractions is 4 to 5 mU per minute. The expectant mother will rarely require more than 8 mU per minute to stimulate uterine contractions. The oxytocin infusion is stopped once satisfactory contractions occur. The procedure is discontinued if no contractions occur by the end of 30 minutes and the infusion has been working properly, if contractions occur more often than every 2 minutes or last longer than 60 seconds, if uterine tetany takes place, or if continued fetal heart rate decelerations are noted.[27] After the test, the client is not discharged until contractions are at least 10 minutes apart.

Interpretation. Interpretations of the CST are summarized in Table 22–4. Categories such as positive (abnormal), negative (normal), suspicious, hyperstimulated, and unsatisfactory have been used and are based on frequency of contractions and FHR decelerations; however, concern related to accuracy of results, especially false-positive readings, have prompted additional categorization of the CST into reactive negative, nonreactive negative, reactive positive, and nonreactive positive. These categories, also included in Table 22–4, are based on the presence or absence of FHR accelerations as well as decelerations.[21]

Errors in Interpretations: False Negatives and False Positives. The CST is a valuable technique for assessing fetal well-being; however, results that do not accurately reflect fetal status, that is, false results, can occur.

A negative test generally indicates that the uteroplacental unit will continue to support fetal life for at least a week longer. There is, however, no absolute assurance that the fetus will be well. A test is said to have a false-negative result when fetal death occurs within the next 7 days.[28] Fetal death within that time could occur as the result of many factors. New complications or unrelated conditions, such as trauma, abruptio placentae, and drug abuse, could arise after the test. Problems in test administration or interpretation or lack of sensitivity of the test to actual fetal status could also contribute to a false-negative result.

Unfortunately, the CST can have a high rate of false-positive results, as high as 50 to 70 per-

TABLE 22–4. INTERPRETATIONS OF THE CONTRACTION STRESS TEST

The CST may be interpreted according to frequency of contractions and FHR decelerations:

Positive CST: Abnormal	Consistent and persistent late decelerations of the FHR occur with 50% or more of the contractions.[12,37] A true positive CST indicates fetal compromise related to uteroplacental insufficiency.
Negative CST: Normal	No late decelerations of the FHR take place, and at least three contractions, each lasting at least 40 seconds, occur within 10 minutes. Usually fetal heart rate reactivity (accelerations of the FHR with fetal movement) are also seen on the tracing. About 80% to 85% of CSTs are negative. A negative CST usually indicates that fetal well-being related to uteroplacental function will continue for at least another week. The negative CST may therefore be repeated weekly unless complications emerge and either require testing at a shorter interval or necessitate other types of interventions.
Suspicious	Inconsistent late decelerations of the FHR take place but do not continue with subsequent contractions.[4] About one fifth of suspicious tests become positive on repeated testing. The test is usually repeated within 24 hours after the suspicious test results are noted.[37] Timing of the repeated test is based on clinical assessment; the test may be repeated the same day. For example, when variable decelerations occur, ultrasound may be indicated to assess whether cord compromise, related to oligohydramnios or fetal presentation, is present.[28]
Hyperstimulated	Contractions occur more often than every 2 minutes or last longer than 90 seconds. Late decelerations of the FHR with this excessive uterine activity do not necessarily indicate uteroplacental insufficiency.[4] Caution should be used when administering oxytocin by intravenous infusion or when exogenous oxytocin is obtained through nipple stimulation. Excessive uterine activity may cause fetal compromise because of decreased oxygen. In this situation, the test itself may cause the compromise. The hyperstimulation test may be repeated within 24 hours and with careful observation.
Unsatisfactory	This term refers to a test that cannot be read adequately. For example, inability to stimulate at least three contractions within 10 minutes or unsatisfactory tracings, related to such factors as positioning or fetal movement, may account for unsatisfactory test results. Attentive, one-to-one nursing care with appropriate positioning and adjustment of the transducer may avoid an unsatisfactory test result. The unsatisfactory test may be repeated within 24 hours.[28]

CST results may be interpreted according to presence or absence of FHR accelerations as well as decelerations[17]:

Reactive Negative CST	Normal accelerations of the FHR (more than 15 BPM, lasting 15 seconds) occur with fetal movement and no FHR decelerations. Results indicate a normal, healthy fetus with good oxygen reserve (Figure 22–8).
Nonreactive Negative CST	There is an absence of accelerations of the FHR following fetal movement and no late decelerations occur with contractions. This pattern is observed in only 0.4% of CSTs and could be related to subtle late decelerations that are being missed, a congenital anomaly of the fetus, or maternal therapy with a central nervous system depressant[17] (Figure 22–9).
Reactive Positive CST	Normal accelerations of the FHR following fetal movement occur with the presence of late decelerations with some uterine contractions[17] (Figure 22–10). These reactive-positive tests are often false-positive tests and thus require careful assessment. The test may be repeated or an alternative method of fetal assessment, such as the fetal biophysical profile, may be considered.
Nonreactive Positive CST	Fetal heart rate accelerations following fetal movement are absent and persistent late decelerations occur with uterine contractions[17] (Figure 22–11). The nonreactive positive CST is more accurately indicative of fetal compromise.[4] The false-positive rate is less than 5%.[17] If this interpretation is made on the CST, delivery is usually needed for the near-term fetus. If the fetus is very immature, a biophysical profile may be done to document fetal status.[17]

cent.[15,17,32,39] A false-positive test occurs when an abnormal test result is then followed by normal fetal heart rate patterns in labor and normal fetal outcome. False-positive results can reflect several conditions, such as problems in interpretation of test results or technical difficulties in obtaining tracings. Improvement in fetal status after the test may be related to treatment of maternal conditions like hypoglycemia or dehydration.[28] Categorization of CSTs based on the presence or absence of FHR accelerations, as well as decelerations, has promoted better specificity and reliability of the test, but problems remain. Positive test results pose difficult management questions: Should delivery take place without delay? What happens if a normal fetus is delivered too early? Other tests, for example, a fetal biophysical profile or ultrasound, may be used for assessment of fetal well-being.

Risks/Contraindications. Certain risks and contraindications are associated with the CST, because oxytocin can cause powerful uterine contractions. (Chapter 27

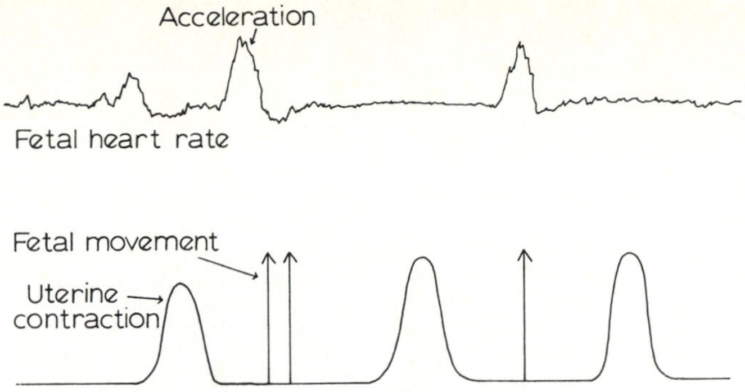

Figure 22–8. Reactive-negative CST shows normal acceleration of the fetal heart with movement; no decelerations are present. (*Reproduced, with permission, from Oxorn H, ed.* Oxorn-Foote Human Labor and Birth. *5th ed. Norwalk, Conn: Appleton & Lange; 1986:605.*)

identifies risks associated with oxytocin administration.) Contraindications to the CST include[35] predisposition to uterine rupture, predisposition to premature labor (especially in women with a history of preterm birth or who are carrying more than one fetus), and bleeding, for example, in placenta previa.

Fetal Biophysical Profile. The **fetal biophysical profile,** first developed by Manning and associates to assess fetal well-being, consists of five parameters: fetal heart rate reactivity, fetal breathing movements, gross fetal body movements, fetal tone, and volume of amniotic fluid.[32] Fetal heart rate reactivity is measured with the nonstress test, and the other four parameters are measured with real-time ultrasound scanning.[42]

The basic premise behind the biophysical profile is that multiple variable assessment of fetal biophysical activities is a more reliable test of fetal well-being than the examination of a single fetal parameter, such as fetal heart rate.[17] The purpose of the biophysical profile includes the identification of fetuses with chronic asphyxia, or congenital anomalies. Table 22–5 summarizes advantages and limitations of this method of fetal assessment. Indications for biophysical profile testing include postdate pregnancy, maternal hypertension (chronic or pregnancy induced), diabetes mellitus, premature rupture of membranes, vaginal bleeding, maternal reports of decreased fetal movement, maternal Rh sensitization, and maternal history of previous stillbirth. Life's complexities make absolute prediction of good health impossible. Therefore, the biophysical profile may be most useful in identifying a fetus that is in jeopardy, rather than in predicting future fetal well-being.[4]

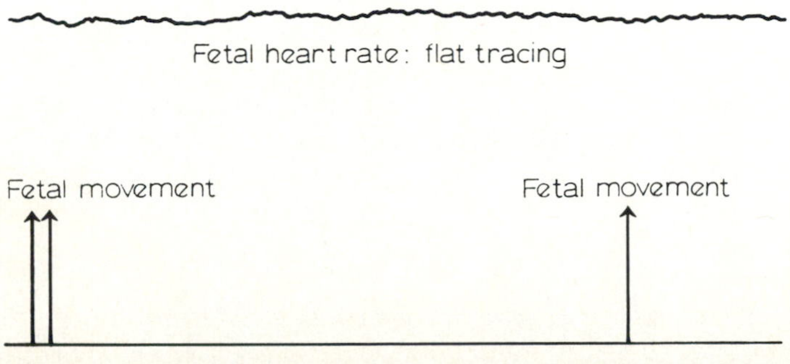

Figure 22–9. Nonreactive-negative CST.

Fetal Heart Rate Reactivity. Fetal heart rate reactivity is measured and interpreted in the same manner as the nonstress test. The fetal heart rate is considered reactive when there are movement-associated FHR accelerations of at least 15 beats per minute above baseline and 15 seconds in duration over a 20-minute period.[23] A score of 2 is given on the fetal biophysical profile if fetal heart rate reactivity is noted; a score of 0 means that the FHR is nonreactive.

Fetal Breathing Movements. In utero, the fetus makes chest wall and diaphragmatic movements that mimic respiratory movements.[40] Assessment of this parameter is based on the assumption that fetal breathing movements indicate fetal well-being and their absence may indicate hypoxemia. Fetal breathing tends to occur periodically after 28 weeks and becomes increasingly regular in frequency and uniformity after the 36th week of gestation.[41] To earn a score of 2, the fetus must have at least one episode of fetal breathing of at least 60 seconds' duration within a 30-minute observation period. The absence of fetal breathing movements of at least 60 seconds' duration within a 30-minute observation period is scored 0 on the fetal biophysical profile.[42] Several factors can alter fetal breathing movements. For example, fetal breathing movements have been shown to increase during the second and third hours after maternal meals and at night (1 AM to 7 AM) during maternal sleep; increased blood glucose levels after eating and stable blood glucose levels during sleep were thought to account for this.[43] Fetal breathing movements may not be regarded as a sign of well-being in diabetic mothers, because hyperglycemia can increase them.[44] Fetal breathing movements may be decreased as a result of such conditions as hypoxemia, hypoglycemia, nicotine use (cigarette smoking), or ingestion of even small amounts of alcohol. For some as yet unexplained reason, fetal breathing movements normally decrease several days before spontaneous labor.[24] This observation is

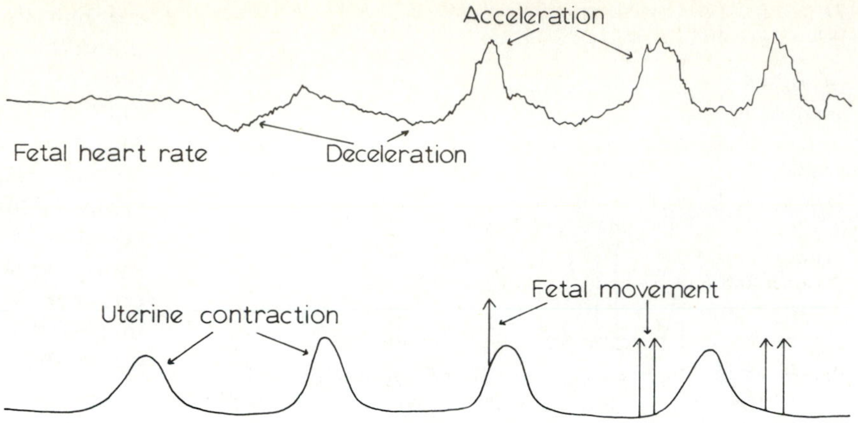

Figure 22–10. Reactive-positive CST. (*Reproduced, with permission, from Oxorn H, ed.* Oxorn-Foote Human Labor and Birth. *5th ed. Norwalk, Conn: Appleton & Lange; 1986:607.*)

useful in the treatment of premature labor. If fetal breathing movements are noted, it is unlikely that premature delivery will take place, whereas the absence of fetal breathing movements suggests that preterm delivery may occur soon.[41] The episodic nature of fetal breathing movements, the multiple factors that can affect the movements, and the long period that may be necessary for documentation of a normal pattern detract from the usefulness of this parameter in identifying the fetus in jeopardy.

Fetal Body Movements. Fetal activity reflects neurologic integrity and function. Fetal movements have been noted to differ in certain abnormal conditions, such as intrauterine growth retardation and diabetes.[41] The presence of at least three discrete episodes of fetal movements within a 30-minute observation period is given a score of 2. Simultaneous limb and trunk movements are counted as a single movement. In the event of decreased fetal movements, two or fewer discrete fetal movements in a 30-minute observation period, a score of 0 is given.[42]

The fetus does rest; therefore, fetal rest periods must be distinguished from those related to a compromised uterine environment.[40] Fetal activity, as well as fetal breathing movements, is greatest 1 to 3 hours after the mother has consumed a meal. Some therefore suggest that testing should be arranged in relation to meals or by offering the mother caloric liquids prior to testing.[15]

Fetal Tone. In utero, the fetus is normally in flexion; however, the fetus also stretches, rolls, and moves in the uterus, and the arms, legs, trunk, and head may be flexed and extended.[40] The fetus earns a score of 2 when there is at least one episode of active extension with return to flexion of fetal limb(s) or trunk, for example, the opening and closing of the hand. A score of 0 is given for slow extension with return to partial flexion, fetal movement not followed by return to flexion, limbs or spine in extension, and an open fetal hand.[23,39]

Amniotic Fluid Volume. By midpregnancy, the amniotic sac contains about 324 mL of fluid; by 36 weeks the volume is about 1000 mL, but decreases afterward. Amniotic fluid volume is believed to indicate the chronic state of the intrauterine environment, as opposed to the acute condition of the fetal central nervous system.[19] Fluid should be evident throughout the uterine cavity. Oligohydramnios (too little amniotic fluid) has been associated with fetal anomalies, especially of the genitourinary tract, with intrauterine growth retardation, and with post-term

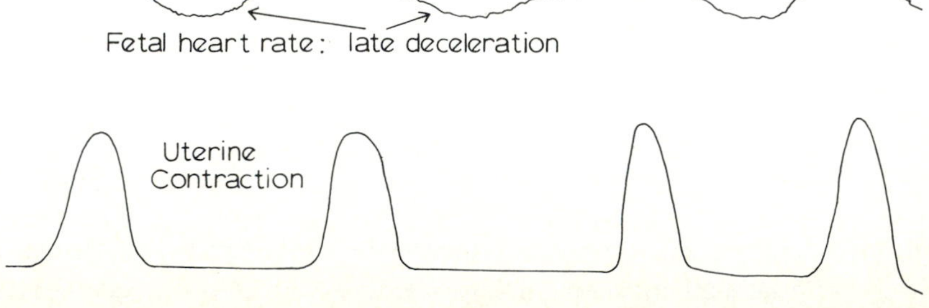

Figure 22–11. Nonreactive-positive CST. (*Reproduced, with permission, from Oxorn H, ed.* Oxorn-Foote Human Labor and Birth. *5th ed. Norwalk, Conn: Appleton & Lange; 1986:607.*)

TABLE 22–5. ADVANTAGES AND LIMITATIONS OF THE FETAL BIOPHYSICAL PROFILE

Advantages
Noninvasive
Results are available as soon as test is completed and interpreted
Testing can be done on outpatient basis, thereby reducing hospital admissions and associated financial and emotional costs
Provides other types of useful information, eg, fetal number, placental location, risk of intrauterine growth retardation, congenital anomalies
May help in monitoring clients with premature rupture of membranes for impending infection, thereby preventing neonatal or maternal sepsis
May decrease false-positive or false-negative results associated with NST
Indicates current fetal well-being, especially in high-risk groups, thereby allowing for conservative treatment and avoidance of certain intervention, eg, early delivery, iatrogenic prematurity, and cesarean delivery
Limitations:
Duration and frequency of hypoxemia and effects on the fetus are unknown
Exogenous factors can affect the central nervous system and change fetal activities and test results
Each variable is given equal weight; it is possible that certain variables are indeed more important than others
Testing intervals are arbitrary
Long-term development outcomes of fetuses with low scores is unknown
Research related to use of this technique and meaning of scores is lacking
May not accurately predict continued fetal well-being

Compiled courtesy of N. Hoffman, MSN, RN.

pregnancy.[45] Immediate delivery is recommended for a post-term client with oligohydramnios, even if other tests are normal, because of the high risk of associated problems such as umbilical cord compromise.[32] A score of 2 for this parameter on the fetal biophysical profile indicates that at least one pocket of amniotic fluid that measures 1 cm in two perpendicular planes has been identified. A score of 0 indicates that either fluid is absent in most areas of the uterine cavity or that the largest pocket of fluid measures 1 cm or less in the vertical axis.[39, 42]

Interpretations. Table 22–6 describes the interpretations of scores for the five parameters of the fetal biophysical profile. Each of the five parameters of the fetal biophysical profile contributes either 2 or 0 points to the total score. A score of 10 is a perfect score; a score of 0 is the worst score. A score of 8 or 10, with a normal amount of amniotic fluid, indicates a healthy fetus. No interventions would be indicated other than repeat testing at weekly intervals. Testing at twice weekly intervals would be appropriate for high-risk conditions. A score of 8 with oligohydramnios or a score of 4 or 6 is equivocal. An equivocal test score is interpreted as possibly abnormal. The false-positive rate in the equivocal group has been estimated to be 44 percent.[17] Some clinicians recommend repeating the test within 24 hours; however; others advocate extending testing after any equivocal or abnormal test result.[39, 44] In this way a sleeping fetus may be distinguished from the asphyxiated fetus; impending fetal death between the time of the nonreassuring result and the repeat test done on the following day can be avoided. A score of 0 or 2 is abnormal and indicates the need for assessment for immediate delivery. The abnormal rating (0 or 2) has a low false-positive rate and is considered a reliable measure of severe fetal compromise. It is important to remember that fetal biophysical activities can be suppressed by any factor that causes fetal central nervous system depression. For example, hypoxemia, drugs (sedatives, analgesics, anesthetics, and so on), and trauma decrease fetal biophysical activities, whereas central nervous system stimulants such as certain seizure-inducing malformations, catecholamines, and hyperglycemia can increase activities.[23]

Investigators have also related each abnormal parameter of the fetal biophysical profile with consequences to the fetus during labor and delivery and the perinatal period.[44] For example, the absence of fetal movements was noted to predict abnormal fetal heart rate patterns in labor, the nonreactive nonstress test was noted to be associated with meconium-stained amniotic fluid, and decreased fetal tone was associated with perinatal death. The biophysical profile was also described as being superior to the contraction stress test in predicting the oxygen-deprived fetus. Oligohydramnios has been discussed in relation to congenital anomalies, fetal growth retardation, and post-term pregnancy.[39]

Despite the useful information provided by the biophysical profile, management decisions for client care cannot be based solely on the composite scores of this test.[44] Any diagnosis or treatment strategy needs to evolve from assessment of the individual components of the biophysical profile and, most of all, of the total client and her unique situation.

Variations. Several variations of the biophysical profile have been developed; their use varies among antenatal testing units.[46] In one variation, ultrasound is used to assess fetal breathing movements, gross body

TABLE 22–6. FETAL BIOPHYSICAL PROFILE[a]

Nonstress test	Reactive pattern: at least 2 FHR accelerations of ≥ 15 BPM and ≥ 15 seconds' duration, associated with fetal movement in a 20-minute period	Nonreactive pattern: fewer than 2 FHR accelerations of ≥ 15 BPM and 15 seconds' duration associated with fetal movement in 40 minutes
Fetal breathing movements	Present: presence of at least one episode of fetal breathing of ≥ 60 seconds' duration within a 30-minute period of observation	Absent: absence of fetal breathing movements or the absence of an episode of fetal breathing movements of ≥ 60 seconds' duration during a 30-minute period of observation
Gross fetal body movement	Present: presence of at least three discrete episodes of fetal movement within a 30-minute period; simultaneous limb and trunk movements are counted as a single movement	Decreased: two or fewer discrete fetal movements in a 30-minute period of observation
Fetal tone	Upper and lower extremities in full flexion; trunk in position of flexion and head flexed on chest; at least one episode of extension of limbs with return to position of flexion, extension of spine with return to flexion, or both	Decreased: limbs in position of extension or partial flexion; spine in extension; fetal movement not followed by return to flexion; fetal hand open
Volume of amniotic fluid	Fluid evident throughout the uterine cavity; largest pocket of fluid greater than 1 cm in vertical diameter	Decreased: fluid absent in most areas of uterine cavity; largest pocket of fluid 1 cm or less in vertical axis; crowding of fetal small parts

[a] Normal: score = 2; abnormal: score = 0. The intermediate score of 1 is not used with this scoring system.
Reproduced, with permission, from Oxorn H. Oxorn-Foote Human Labor & Birth. *5th ed. Norwalk, Conn: Appleton & Lange; 1986:609.*

movements, fetal tone, and volume of amniotic fluid. The nonstress test is not done if these four parameters of the biophysical profile are normal.[47] A perfect score on this variation is "8," as four parameters are scored. Another variation uses a score of 0, 1, or 2 and includes assessment of placental maturity (placental grading), as discussed later.[48]

Nursing Role in Antenatal Fetal Assessment Using the Nonstress Test, Contract Stress Test, and Fetal Biophysical Profile. In many antenatal testing settings, nurses may perform NSTs and CSTs, do initial assessment of the tracings, and initiate appropriate strategies for nonreassuring findings. By remaining with the client during the tests, the nurse is in a unique position to document maternal and fetal events during each procedure and to make certain that the tests are administered correctly. The tests are also evaluated by a physician, ideally on the same day. A collaborative approach that incorporates test interpretation by the nurse and physician can offer the client a better assessment than one individual reading.[28, 49] Interpretation of antenatal tests requires education and skill on the part of nurses and physicians. False-positive or false-negative readings, related to inaccurate interpretation, may result in failure to diagnose fetal compromise or in unnecessary interventions. As in any area of practice, nurses are accountable for their interpretation of tests. In addition, nurses involved in antenatal testing need to make certain that procedures for test administration and interpretation are developed and followed, that all personnel performing the tests are qualified to do so, and that the antenatal settings allow for adequate staffing for the tests.

The nursing role in antepartal fetal assessment using the NST, CST, and fetal biophysical profiles involves technical aspects, reassessment of the physical condition of the mother, client teaching, and psychosocial support for the client and her family.

Technical Aspects. Proper test procedure is necessary for accurate findings.[35] The mother must be positioned correctly. A semi-Fowler's position with a wedge under the right hip to prevent supine hypotension is desirable. Supporting the abdomen with a pillow, rolled blanket, or towel may increase comfort. This may also minimize client movements and increase the chance of obtaining satisfactory tracings. A reclining chair can also be used as a comfortable alternative during NST or CST.

The transducers or leads must be properly placed. Leopold's maneuvers are used to identify fetal position (*see* Figure 22–3), so that the ultrasound transducer can be located over the fetus' back, ideally at shoulder level. When properly positioned, a clear pattern of uniform shapes will be seen if the monitoring device has an oscilloscope. The tocotransducer, used to record uterine activity, is placed to the right or left at the level of the fundus. Because the pregnant uterus is not perfectly symmetrical, the center of the abdomen is not the best location. During the test the abdomen should be observed and palpated to make certain that all contractions are being recorded.

RESEARCH ABSTRACT

Chez BF, et al. Interpretations of nonstress tests by obstetric nurses. J Obstet Gynecol Neonatal Nurs. *1990;19:227–232.*

This is one of the first studies that assessed the reliability of obstetric nurses' interpretations of nonstress tests. Four hundred and twelve of 1000 surveyed members of the Organization for Obstetric, Gynecologic, and Neonatal Nurses (NAACOG) interpreted and returned five 20-minute nonstress-test strips that had been mailed to them. Subjects were nurses who identified labor and delivery or antepartum as their primary clinical focus, according to NAACOG's records. The same five strips had been interpreted by obstetricians in a previous study.

Subjects interpreted the strips in three ways. They first identified the strips as reactive or nonreactive, then interpreted them as reactive, equivocal, or nonreactive, and finally rated them on a 5-point scale, ranging from most healthy to most ill. Noteworthy observations included the finding that between 84 and 98 percent of the nurses' answers were in agreement on each of the five steps when a reactive or nonreactive interpretation was elicited. As a group, nurses performed in a manner similar to the way physicians as a group performed in correctly identifying and interpreting nonreassuring fetal heart rate patterns. Nurses' responses differed significantly from physicians' interpretations of strips as reactive or nonreactive on only one strip on which 92 percent of nurses concurred as compared to 98 percent of the obstetricians. Nurses' interpretations were not related to experience, education, formal courses in electronic fetal monitoring, or other demographic variables.

Comment:

Nurses are highly involved in many areas of nonstress testing. Nursing roles often extend beyond client education and administration of nonstress tests, to initiation of appropriate actions based on interpretation of test results. Questions at times arise as to the breadth of nursing roles in relation to nonstress testing. The findings of this study highlight nursing expertise and nurses' ability to screen and interpret nonstress tests effectively. The findings also suggest that nurses' interpretations can be similar to physicians' interpretations. In clinical practice it is sometimes difficult to identify whether or not a pattern is reassuring. As the authors noted, errors in interpretation by physicians as well as nurses indicate a need for more than one interpretation of nonstress tests.

Electrodes must be properly positioned on the expectant mother's abdomen if an abdominal wall electrocardiogram is to be done. In this way the fetal heart rate can be monitored and the beat-to-beat variability can be measured to assess fetal well-being. First, Leopold's maneuvers are used to identify fetal position. The skin over the three areas where electrodes will be placed to record the fetal electrocardiogram is then cleansed with alcohol. This facilitates conduction of the fetal electrocardiogram by removing any oils, creams, or lotions that may be on the skin. An electrode is placed over the fetal head, over the fetal buttocks, and just beneath the expectant woman's umbilicus. The monitor senses the electrocardiograms from the expectant mother and the fetus, displays both on the screen, and may also record the tracings.[35]

The NST and CST must be conducted according to unit protocols.[35] Several important aspects of client care during NST or CST must be considered whatever the protocol. For example, NSTs or CSTs should be performed only by nursing and medical staff educated in this technique. If a technician performs the NST, then a physician needs to interpret the test. The CST should be done only by nursing and medical staff skilled in the use of oxytocin and capable of responding effectively to oxytocin-induced emergencies.

A client should never be left unattended during the CST and should be monitored carefully throughout the test, because of the risks associated with oxytocin.[35] The nurse should observe the client for signs of uterine hyperstimulation. The mother's abdomen must be checked by observation and palpation to make certain that all contractions are recorded and that hyperstimulation is not occurring.

The physician must be promptly notified if nonreassuring patterns are noted on the NST or CST or if any complications occur during the CST. Although the physician needs to be accessible to clients undergoing CSTs, nurses are often responsible for administering the CST according to unit protocol.[35]

Accurate records of the NST or CST must be prepared for inclusion in the client's chart.[35] Records for the NST include the client's identifying data; blood pressure before the NST, every 15 minutes during the test, and after the test; fetal heart rate, especially in relation to fetal movement (recorded on the test strip with an event marker); the time the test started and ended; and any techniques used to stimulate fetal activity. For the CST, records include the client's identifying data; blood pressure before the CST, every 15 minutes during the test, and after the test; the manner in which contractions were stimulated; the nature, frequency, and duration of contractions; fetal heart rate, especially in response to contractions; the time the test started and ended; and any complications or treatments. Client responses to the antenatal test and any teaching done are also recorded.

Reassessment Aspects. The client's history is updated at the time of the test. Any factors that could have impact on test results, for example, use of drugs or alcohol, are identified. The expectant mother's overall physical health at time of the test and changes in physical status since the last prenatal evaluation are documented.[35]

Teaching Aspects. The nurse assesses the client's understanding about the test, provides teaching about the test (Table 22–7), and notes the client's response to teaching.[35]

Psychosocial Support. The client's response to potential or actual high-risk status is assessed. Clients referred for antepartal testing may be terrified about the health of the fetus; they may also worry about the possibility of fetal death during pregnancy, fetal compromise during labor, or premature birth. Some clients may have experienced fetal loss during previous pregnancies. The need for bedrest may interfere with the usual schedule or perception of self as healthy and may add to the stress of antenatal testing.

Tests should be conducted with respect for the client's reaction to the nature of the test and her need for privacy. For example, many clients may feel shy about nipple stimulation for CST. Calm explanation of the physiologic rationale for the test and provision of privacy can do much to promote emotional comfort. A private room or room dividers such as curtains or screens, as well as restriction of personnel coming to see the client during the test, may be used. A sheet may be used to cover the client during the NST or CST.

Clients undergoing antepartal tests may have blocks of free time, especially during NSTs. This provides a special opportunity for the nurse to undertake assessment of client and family responses to pregnancy and testing and to provide appropriate teaching.

Antepartal testing may be done in specialized units. When appropriate, clients coming for testing may be encouraged to support each other.[35]

TABLE 22–7. TOPICS FOR TEACHING RELATED TO ANTENATAL TESTING

Type of test (NST, CST, fetal biophysical profile)
Reason for test/implications of the test for fetal well-being
Nature of the test
Length of the test; total time commitment needed for test
Site of the test
Personnel who will conduct the test
Significant other who may accompany client during test
Discomforts related to the test
Possible complications related to the test/reassurance related to lack of risks of NST
Interpretation of test results/need for any further testing (what the test can and cannot indicate)
Cost of test
Posttest teaching
Signs and symptoms of labor (especially for CST)
Advice *not* to try nipple stimulation at home to induce contractions or labor

Settings for Antenatal Testing. The NST, CST, and fetal biophysical profile may be performed on an outpatient basis in an antenatal testing area. The CST requires backup for delivery, if complications related to oxytocin administration occur, and therefore may be performed in an antenatal testing unit accessible to the delivery area. The labor and delivery unit is not an ideal setting for antenatal testing because of staffing patterns that can result in conflicting nursing priorities.[24,28] The need to care for a laboring or delivering client takes the nurse away from the client undergoing antenatal testing. Interruption of observations can affect the interpretation of the tests and can deprive clients of teaching and support. Antenatal testing units may be equipped with ultrasound and personnel for biophysical profile testing. The NST may be performed in any setting equipped for fetal monitoring.

Recently, mobile outpatient monitoring services have made it possible to perform NSTs in the client's home.[50] The nurse makes a home visit for the purpose of the NST. Use of a telephone strip transmitter and a cellular telephone allows for instant transmission of any questionable strip to the test center, where a perinatologist is available for immediate consultation.

In other situations, clients are taught to apply monitoring equipment at home. Contraction patterns are sent through telephone strip transmitters to antenatal testing centers. Specially educated nurses or physicians interpret the patterns and provide telephone counseling to the clients.

Home monitoring is especially helpful for clients who must remain at home on bedrest and who may be at risk for complications, such as preterm labor, that may be increased by activity related to travel for periodic antenatal surveillance.

PRENATAL DIAGNOSTIC ASSESSMENT

Delivery may be recommended when prenatal testing indicates the fetus is seriously compromised. The fetus therefore needs to be assessed for maturity and ability to survive outside the uterus. Amniocentesis and ultrasound are examples of tests for fetal maturity that can be used during the third trimester of pregnancy.

Amniocentesis

Amniocentesis may be used in the third trimester to estimate the maturity of the fetal lungs. As discussed in Chapter 18, amniocentesis is also used earlier in pregnancy, most commonly for diagnosis of chromosomal and neural tube disorders.

Type II pneumonocyte cells of the fetal lung alveoli produce surfactant. This is a mixture of surface-active phospholipids[4] needed to prevent collapse of the alveoli during neonatal respirations, thus preventing respiratory distress or death of the newborn.

Surfactant appears in the amniotic fluid by 24 to 26 weeks of gestation. As the fetus approaches maturity, the amounts of surfactant phospholipids in the amniotic fluid increase.[15] Lecithin (phosphatidylcholine) is a major component of the pulmonary surfactant and constitutes about 80 percent of the phospholipids. Other phospholipids include phosphatidylglycerol, the phospholipid that has the second largest concentration in surfactant; phosphatidylinositol; and sphingomyelin. Measurements of the ratio of amniotic fluid lecithin to sphingomyelin and of phosphatidylglycerol concentration have been used to assess the maturity of the fetal lungs.[15]

Lecithin:Sphingomyelin Ratio. Mean proportions of lecithin and sphingomyelin do not differ markedly until about the 30th week of gestation. The level of sphingomyelin stops rising at week 32, whereas the level of lecithin rises gradually above that of sphingomyelin. In assessing fetal maturity, a **lecithin:sphingomyelin (L:S) ratio,** equal to or greater than 2:1 indicates a positive result, eg, fetal lung maturity with little likelihood of immaturity-related respiratory distress syndrome in the newborn. A ratio of 1.5:1 to 1.9:1 indicates the possibility of mild to moderate respiratory distress in the newborn. A ratio of 1.0:1 to 1.49:1 usually reflects immaturity of the fetal lungs and a possibility of moderate to severe respiratory distress in the newborn. A ratio less than 1.0:1 indicates immaturity of the lungs and predicts severe respiratory distress in the newborn.[15]

About 5 mL of amniotic fluid is needed for measurement of the L:S ratio. Phospholipid is extracted from the amniotic fluid and evaluated by thin-layer chromatography. This method assesses the size and density of the lecithin and sphingomyelin "spots," which then indicate the stage of fetal lung maturity.[15]

The reliability of the L:S ratio may at times be questioned. Contamination of amniotic fluid by blood or meconium may alter the L:S ratio and produce inaccurate results. The false-positive rate, whereby the infant develops respiratory distress syndrome despite a prenatal L:S ratio of 2:1 or more, is around 2 percent. With a false-negative test, the infant does not develop respiratory distress syndrome, even though the L:S ratio indicates immaturity. False-negative rates of 25 percent have been estimated for infants when the L:S ratio is less than 1.5; false-negative rates as high as 60 percent have been estimated when the L:S ratios are between 1.5:1 and 2.0:1.[17] The occurrence of false-negative and false-positive results highlights the difficulty of accurately predicting a future neonatal course.

Certain high-risk conditions alter fetal lung maturation; therefore the L:S ratio must be interpreted with caution. For example, misleading results may be obtained from expectant mothers with diabetes. In this situation, fetal lungs may be immature despite an L:S ratio of 2:1. Some physiologically stressful conditions, such as chronic heavy smoking or membranes that have been ruptured longer than 24 hours, may actually promote fetal lung maturation. (This should never be used to justify smoking, because smoking has many harmful effects on the mother and fetus.)

Foam Stability (Shake) Test. In an effort to reduce the time needed for the precise measurement of the L:S ratio, the foam stability (shake) test was introduced. This test is based on the idea that surfactant will foam when mixed with ethanol. In theory, if enough surfactant is present, that is, the fetal lungs are mature enough to avoid respiratory distress, a ring of bubbles (foam) will form on the top of the liquid mixture. The procedure takes about one-half hour and requires 1.5 mL of amniotic fluid. Recently collected amniotic fluid (1 mL) and 1 mL of 95 percent ethanol are placed into a test tube. In another tube, 0.5 mL of amniotic fluid, 0.5 mL of .09 percent saline, and 1 mL of 95 percent ethanol are combined. Each tube is then vigorously shaken for 15 seconds and placed in an upright position in a rack for 15 minutes.

Persistence of an intact ring of bubbles at the air-liquid surface after 15 minutes is considered a positive test for surfactant; the risk of respiratory distress syndrome, related to lung immaturity, is then considered low.[52] Commercially manufactured kits, such as the Lumadex-FSI test, are based on foam stability and may be used to test amniotic fluid surfactant.[4]

Although the foam stability test provides a rapid and inexpensive way to estimate pulmonary surfactant, problems also have been noted with the reliability of the test. Contamination of the amniotic fluid, test containers, or errors in conducting or interpreting the test may alter the results. Additionally, false-negative results can occur. In this situation, the infant would be at low risk for immaturity-related respiratory distress syndrome; however, the ring of foam does not stay intact.[4]

Phosphatidylglycerol Test. Phosphatidylglycerol (PG) has become a useful indicator of fetal lung maturity. In the healthy woman, PG is found in amniotic fluid late in gestation, after 35 weeks; its concentration in amniotic fluid then gradually increases to term. Phosphatidylglycerol is found solely in amniotic fluid, in lungs, and in semen. Therefore, contamination of the amniotic fluid by blood or meconium does not influence the test results because these substances contain no PG. Further, the presence of PG in the amniotic fluid in the vagina when membranes are ruptured usually indicates low risk for respiratory distress syndrome of the newborn.[17]

The test for PG indicates a more mature surfactant complex than that found in the L:S ratio, because PG appears late in gestation. It has been noted that PG was absent in cases where the L:S ratio indicated pulmonary maturity and respiratory distress occurred (false-positive result). Conversely, when PG was present, respiratory distress syndrome did not develop.[17] The absence of PG is not necessarily an indication that respiratory distress *will* develop; its absence indicates that respiratory distress syndrome *may* develop.[4] Elective delivery in the absence of at least 0.5 percent PG in amniotic fluid is discouraged.[15]

A commercial test (Amniostat-FLM) is available to detect PG in the amniotic fluid. The test takes about 15 minutes to perform. If the test is positive for PG, the fetus is unlikely to develop respiratory distress syndrome at birth.[52]

Other Amniotic Fluid Parameters of Fetal Maturity. Other parameters of fetal maturity have been analyzed using amniocentesis; however, they do not predict fetal maturity well and are rarely used today. These tests include analyses of amniotic fluid bilirubin, creatinine, and lipids (fat cells).

Amniotic Fluid Bilirubin. The concentration of bilirubin in amniotic fluid falls progressively in the later stages of pregnancy, and usually is about zero at 36 weeks of gestation. A bilirubin reading greater than 0.01 in the amniotic fluid was thought to indicate a gestational age of less than 35 weeks. Today, this test is rarely used as a predictor of fetal maturity. Amniotic fluid bilirubin analysis *is,* however, considered a reliable indicator of fetal hemolytic disease from maternal isoimmunization[4, 17] (*see* Chapter 42).

Amniotic Fluid Creatinine. The level of creatinine in amniotic fluid rises progressively throughout pregnancy; at term, the increase is more rapid. A level of 2.0 mg/dL in amniotic fluid may indicate fetal maturity; however, fetal pulmonary function may prove to be mature even when creatinine concentrations are less than 2.0 mg/dL. Additionally, an increase in maternal plasma creatinine may cause an increase in the amniotic fluid creatinine even when the fetus is immature.[4]

Lipids (Fat Cells) in the Amniotic Fluid. Staining of a drop of amniotic fluid with Nile blue sulfate reveals two types of cell particles. Blue-stained cells represent fetal epithelial cells; orange-stained cells represent sebaceous glands. When more than 20 percent of the cells are orange stained, the gestational age is estimated at 36 weeks or more, because the sebaceous cells mature late in gestation. Problems with this analysis include difficulty in quantifying the cells and the finding that lower percentages of orange-stained cells do not always indicate prematurity.[4, 17]

Problems With Amniotic Fluid Analysis for Fetal Maturity. Several problems are associated with assessment of fetal maturity through substances in amniotic fluid. Early methods used to measure fetal maturity included analysis of bilirubin, creatinine, and fetal fat cells in the amniotic fluid. These provided some indication of fetal size and gestational age, but were inadequate predictors of pulmonary maturity. Interpretations of the L:S ratio and the foam stability tests may be hampered by false-negative or false-positive results, which can be related to such maternal conditions as hypertensive disease, diabetes, and sickle cell disease.[15] The use of analyses such as the L:S ratio has declined in certain high-risk situations. For example, intervention may be necessary regardless of the risk of respiratory distress syndrome in cases where severe hemorrhage or fulminating pre-eclampsia threaten the mother's life. The development of ultrasound has also made more precise dating of gestation and fetal maturity possible, so that amniotic fluid analysis need not be the sole method of assessment for fetal maturity.[53]

Risks. As discussed in Chapter 18, risks associated with amniocentesis include bleeding, infection, and premature labor. Maternal supine hypotension may be avoided through proper positioning, as for any examination. The large size of the fetus and fetal movements during the third trimester contribute to a greater risk of trauma to the fetus; however, the use of ultrasound to guide amniocentesis promotes safety of the procedure. Nevertheless, when amniocentesis is performed during the third trimester, the newborn is assessed carefully for any evidence of trauma.

Percutaneous Umbilical Blood Sampling

Percutaneous umbilical blood sampling (PUBS) is discussed in Chapter 18. This technique can be used for fetal assessment and treatment during the third trimester in situations where direct access to the fetal circulation is needed. For example, third-trimester PUBS may be done for assessment and management of fetal hemolytic disease.

Diagnostic Ultrasound

During the third trimester, ultrasound is used to provide information about maternal and fetal structures and fetal activity and to guide invasive procedures such as amniocentesis or PUBS. Indications for third trimester ultrasound are summarized in Table 22–8. Chapters 14 and 18 provide further discussion of ultrasound.

Procedure. The procedure for ultrasound in the third trimester is similar to that used in the second trimester (*see* Chapter 18); however, special consideration is given to testing in light of physiologic changes of late pregnancy and of the reason for the test. After 20 weeks of gestation, a full bladder is not necessary for examination and may cause unnecessary discomfort to the client. A full bladder may be requested, however, if the examination is done for evaluation of placenta previa.[54]

The client lies on her back with a wedge or firm pillow under her right buttock to elevate the presenting part and to avoid supine hypotension, which can be a problem in the third trimester. Signs and symptoms of maternal supine hypotensive syndrome should be promptly identified: decrease in blood pressure, increase in pulse, irritability, lightheadedness, diaphoresis, and pallor. The client's position should be changed without delay if supine hypotension develops.

During the third trimester, the fetus is readily identifiable on the monitor screen during ultrasound. Clients often appreciate the opportunity to see the fetus depicted on the monitor screen and to receive a photograph of the fetus taken during the examination.

TABLE 22–8. INDICATIONS FOR ULTRASOUND IMAGING DURING THE THIRD TRIMESTER

Estimation of gestational age for uncertain clinical dates; verification of dates for women who are to have scheduled elective cesarean delivery or induction of labor
Assessment of fetal growth
Vaginal bleeding of undetermined etiology
Determination of fetal presentation
Adjunct to amniocentesis
Significant difference between uterine size and clinical dates of gestation
Suspected fetal death
Biophysical assessment for fetal well-being (fetal breathing movements, gross body movements, fetal tone, heart rate, amniotic fluid volume)
Suspected polyhydramnios or oligohydramnios
Suspected abruptio placentae
Follow-up evaluation of placental location for identified placenta previa
Serial evaluation of fetal growth in multiple gestation

Fetal Measurements Obtained During Ultrasound. Certain fetal parameters are used to assess fetal growth and gestational age through ultrasonic evaluation. Among these are fetal biparietal diameter, circumference of the head, abdominal circumference, head circumference:abdominal circumference ratio, and femoral length.

Biparietal Diameter. The **biparietal diameter** (BPD) is the widest diameter of the fetal skull; it is the most widely used determinant of fetal growth and gestational age. Between 14 and 28 weeks of gestation, the BPD is accurate to within plus or minus 7 to 10 days. After 28 weeks of gestation, the accuracy is only within 3 weeks. The BPD may be difficult to measure late in pregnancy because of fetal position or engagement of the fetal head in the maternal pelvis. It has been estimated that if serial BPD alone were used to determine fetal growth, some 20 to 50 percent of growth-retarded fetuses would not be detected.[55] This is especially true when fetuses have unusual head shapes (flattened or elongated).

Cephalic Index. The **cephalic index** (CI) is the ratio of the BPD to the occipitofrontal diameter (OFD) of the fetal skull. This parameter provides a means of quantifying fetal head shape. The CI remains constant throughout fetal development, and the normal shape index is 79 ± 8 percent. A CI less than 71 percent indicates a flattened BPD; a CI greater than 87 percent indicates an elongated shape. In the first case, the BPD would underestimate, rather than properly reflect, gestational age. In the second case, the BPD would overestimate gestational age. In cases where the CI is out of the normal range, the BPD should not be used for gestational age or estimates of fetal weight.[54]

Tables relating BPD with period of gestation may vary in the actual values presented; however, these tables are used frequently with different populations of expectant mothers. Table 22–9 lists biparietal diameters in centimeters by week of gestation.[56] By using a table such as this, the examiner can observe a serial picture of fetal growth.

Circumference of Head. The OFD also may be used to estimate the head circumference (HC) in an effort to calculate gestational age:

$$\text{BPD} + \text{OFD} \times 3.14/2 = \text{HC (cm)}$$

Table 22–10 lists mean head circumferences by week of gestation during the third trimester.

Abdominal Circumference. To estimate abdominal circumference (AC), the anteroposterior abdominal diameter (APAD) and the transverse abdominal diameter (TAD) are measured at the level of the umbilical vein or fetal liver. The formula used to calculate abdominal circumference is

$$\text{APAD} + \text{TAD} \times 3.14/2 = \text{AC (cm)}$$

Abdominal circumference is used mainly as an estimate of intrauterine growth retardation rather than as an estimate of gestational age.[57]

Head Circumference : Abdominal Circumference Ratio. The head circumference : abdominal circumference (HC:AC) ratio is used as an indicator of fetal growth and nutrition, rather than of gestational age.[57] The adequacy of liver stores of glycogen primarily determines liver size and, therefore, abdominal circumference. The HC:AC measurement directly compares brain size with liver size.

Before 36 weeks of gestation, the HC:AC ratio is greater than 1.0; that is, the HC is greater than the AC. After 36 weeks of gestation, the ratio is less than 1.0; the HC is less than the AC. Disproportionate HC:AC ratios may indicate problems with fetal growth. A low HC:AC may indicate a large baby, for example, a fetus of a diabetic mother. A high ratio may indicate intrauterine growth retardation. The HC:AC may be calculated by the following formula[57]:

$$\text{HC:AC} = (\text{BPD} + \text{OFD} \times 3.14/2):(\text{APAD} + \text{TAD} \times 3.14/2)$$

Femoral Length. Femoral length (FL) is used as an estimate of gestational age. It is less affected by changes in growth than the head or abdomen; thus, FL is considered a useful aid in determining gestational age and in identifying the fetus with abnormal

TABLE 22–9. BIPARIETAL DIAMETER BY WEEKS OF GESTATION (THIRD TRIMESTER)

Weeks of Gestation	Biparietal Diameter (cm)
28	7.0
29	7.2
30	7.5
31	7.7
32	7.9
33	8.2
34	8.4
35	8.6
36	8.8
37	9.0
38	9.1
39	9.3
40	9.5

Reproduced, with permission, from Hadlock FP. Computer assisted analysis of fetal age in the third trimester, using multiple growth parameters. J Clin Ultrasound. *1983;11:313.*

TABLE 22–10. MEAN HEAD CIRCUMFERENCE BY WEEKS OF GESTATION (THIRD TRIMESTER)

Weeks of Gestation	Head Circumference (cm)
28	26.2
29	27.1
30	28.0
31	28.9
32	29.7
33	30.4
34	31.2
35	31.8
36	32.5
37	33.1
38	33.6
39	34.1
40	34.5

Reproduced, with permission, from Hadlock FP. Computer assisted analysis of fetal age in the third trimester, using multiple growth parameters. J Clin Ultrasound. *1983;11:313.*

growth.[15] Femoral length is the length of the shaft of the femur (excluding the femoral head). Femoral length increases in a linear fashion with gestational age; FL should be measured after 13 weeks of gestation, because before that time the FL measurements are unreliable.[57]

Placental Maturation/Placental Grading. Assessment of placental maturation has been used together with fetal parameters to estimate fetal maturity. Ultrasonographic examination has identified changes in the chorionic plate, placental substance, and basal layer of the placenta with maturation. Four distinct phases of placental maturation have been identified and "graded" from 0 (immature) to III (most mature).[17] Grade 0 placentas are noted during the first and second trimesters. Grade I placentas appear between 30 and 32 weeks and, in as many as 40 percent of cases, may persist until term. Grade II placentas usually can be observed on ultrasound at around 36 weeks, and have been estimated to continue until term in 45 percent of cases. Grade III reflects the phase of greatest placental maturity and is seen at 38 weeks in about 15 percent of gestations. Clinical evidence supports a relationship between a fully mature placenta and maturity of fetal lungs; therefore, in most cases a grade III placenta might be used to predict that the fetal lungs were developed enough to support breathing after birth.[59]

Early studies on placental grading found a 100 percent correlation between grade III placentas and L:S ratios of 2:1 or greater. It was concluded that placental grading could therefore be used as an assessment technique to predict fetal lung maturity[60]; however, further studies did not document this strong relationship between placental grading and L:S ratio. False-positive correlations of placental grading and L:S ratio were noted.[61] It also has been estimated that grade III placentas are found in only 15 percent of pregnancies at term.[17] These limiting features suggest that placental grading should not be used alone in predicting fetal maturity or fetal lung maturity.

Risks. Ultrasound scanning in the third trimester, as during the first and second trimesters, is recommended only for specific indications, as more information is needed on possible short-term and long-term effects on mother and fetus.[2] Ultrasound has been widely used, however, and to date no harmful effects on humans have been substantiated.

Role of the Nurse. The role of the nurse during ultrasound assessment has been discussed in Chapters 14 and 18. All clients having third-trimester ultrasound are at risk for some real or potential problem. The nurse needs to recognize that anxiety and emotional pain may be experienced by the client and her partner. The nurse provides anticipatory guidance and teaching about the procedure (*see* Table 14–8); encourages the client and her partner to remain together during the test; promotes the client's physical comfort during the procedure through such techniques as proper positioning; identifies maternal and fetal structures seen on the monitor (may be done by the person performing the ultrasound); remains accessible and supportive to the client regardless of the outcome of the test; and makes certain that clients are appropriately referred for additional counseling when needed.

Placental/Fetal Function Tests

The placenta produces various substances that are either quantitatively or qualitatively specific to pregnancy. Placental function tests are based on the assumption that the level of a given substance in the mother is directly related to the overall functioning of the fetal-placental unit. The concentration of a substance measured in an expectant mother is compared with a normal range. The result is either within this range (a negative test) or outside the normal range (a positive test). This basic interpretation does, however, pose problems[62]: the exact nature of the substance being tested and related to fetal-placental function is not clearly understood, and the overlap between normal and abnormal populations creates false-positive and false-negative results.

Placental function tests at times were used with other prenatal assessment parameters to identify the fetus at risk for such conditions as intrauterine growth retardation, neonatal asphyxia, neurologic impairment, and perinatal mortality; however, tests for placental function are currently not considered very accurate and are therefore not used widely or used alone to determine fetal outcome. A decrease in amniotic fluid tends to be a better indicator of poor placental function, as the placenta is a source of amniotic fluid. Decreased amniotic fluid, however, tends to be an indicator of an existing problem, rather than an accurate predictor of a problem that does not yet exist.

In the past, maternal urine and plasma estriol determination was considered the principal assessment technique in determining fetal condition late in pregnancy; for this reason, estriol determination is described here.

Estriol, one of the forms of estrogen, is synthesized by a series of maternal-fetal-placental biochemical reactions, most of which are dependent on the fetus and the placenta. The fetal adrenal gland secretes a precursor that is converted in the fetal liver.

Finally, free estriol is produced in the placenta. Ninety percent of estriol production can be accounted for by the fetal-placental biosynthesis of estrogen. The other 10 percent can be accounted for by a metabolic process in the mother. In theory, the biosynthesis of estriol depends on an intact maternal-fetal-placental unit.

Normally, estriol levels increase in an almost linear fashion as pregnancy progresses. They can be measured by assessment of the maternal plasma or the maternal urine. Serial (over time) determinations were used because of the variations in levels day by day and problems associated with inaccurate or incomplete urine collection. Low or decreasing levels in late pregnancy were believed to indicate fetal compromise or future neonatal problems such as apnea, cyanosis, and neurologic abnormalities.[63]

For assessment of urinary estriol, the client collects all urine voided within a 24-hour period in a special container. The excretion of estriol in the maternal urine after 30 weeks of gestation should be 10 to 14 mg per 24 hours; values of 4 mg per 24 hours or less were thought to indicate severe fetal compromise or death. At 30 to 40 weeks of gestation, plasma estriols should be 5 to 40 ng/mL; to avoid circadian variations, serial samples needed to be done at the same time of the day.[15]

Estriol determinations are used far less frequently today because of the advent of more reliable and useful tests, such as the nonstress test and fetal biophysical profile. In addition, estriol determinations were estimated to relate to actual fetal outcome in only about 60 percent of cases. This fact, along with inconvenient collection techniques, cost of testing, a wide range of normal values seen (5 to 40 ng/ml for plasma, 5 to 40 mg/24 hours for urine) and the false negative results have made estriol tests unpopular.[15]

Current Imaging Techniques: Nuclear Magnetic Resonance Imaging

Nuclear magnetic resonance imaging (MRI or NMR), is an assessment technique which provides computer-derived images based on the detection of energy in the nuclei of atoms within the body. Magnetic resonance imaging depends on the physical property of magnetism, which is possessed by some of the nuclei of the body's atoms, and MRI is based on the principle that protons within the nucleus of the atom have magnetic spins with different energy levels. In a normal state all energy seeks the lowest level. Magnetic resonance imaging creates an intense magnetic field that raises the energy of the protons within the nucleus of the atoms. The magnetic field is then turned off. As the protons revert to their original state, energy is released; the magnetic moments are detected and translated into images by the computer. Not all nuclei within the body have magnetic moments; therefore, such structures as bone are not seen on MRI, although soft tissues in the reproductive system are well visualized. In this way, MRI differs from x-ray studies that provide information about bony structures and their relationships. Nuclear magnetic resonance imaging studies are interpreted by a physician specially educated in MRI. Table 22–11 lists uses for MRI during pregnancy.[4, 64–66]

Procedure. The expectant mother lies in a supine position on a sliding couch which moves into a cylindrical unit containing a magnet with coils and a transmitter.[64] During the procedure the woman's body is encased in the MRI unit. She may not be able to see staff members, although they remain in voice contact with her.

Risks/Limitations. At present there are no documented adverse reactions or harm to a human mother or fetus as a result of the use of MRI; however, ample study of the safety of MRI has not yet been done, and caution in using this technique should be taken. MRI is used only when other more traditional methods cannot provide the same information and maternal or fetal condition provides strong indication for the test. Limitations of the test include higher cost than other diagnostic tests such as ultrasound and problems with obtaining images because of fetal movement.[65]

TABLE 22–11. EXAMPLES OF USES FOR MRI DURING PREGNANCY

Replacement for x-ray diagnostic imaging
Adjunct to ultrasound; MRI offers additional information on fetal development, growth or structures (such as the central nervous system and subcutaneous tissues) which are not seen well on ultrasound.
Identification of soft tissue relationships between the fetus and the birth canal; thus helpful in identifying whether a client carrying a fetus in a breech position would be at risk during a vaginal delivery
Confirmation of fetal anomalies, such as anomalies associated with oligohydramnios (Unlike ultrasound, MRI does not need amniotic fluid to visualize the fetus)
Diagnosis of ectopic pregnancy in complicated situations
Definition of the size of the pregnant uterus and the position of the placenta; assessment of areas of poor placental perfusion or infarction.

Sources: *References 4, 64–66.*

NURSING DIAGNOSES RELATED TO THE THIRD TRIMESTER

Physiologic

Strength-Oriented
Asset in health of mother and fetus, related to normal physical changes in the third trimester

Problem-Oriented
Potential sleep pattern disturbance, related to fetal activity, shortness of breath, pressure on bladder

Impaired physical mobility, related to relaxation of joints and muscles and altered balance

Psychosocial

Strength-Oriented
Positive parental self-image, related to support from extended family and friends

Potential for positive sibling interaction, related to sibling preparation during the third trimester

Problem-Oriented
Anxiety, related to:
- Third-trimester discomforts
- Financial pressures associated with costs of childbearing and potential loss of income

Anxiety, related to:
- Impending labor and delivery
- Caring for a first or additional child
- Third-trimester diagnostic techniques
- Diagnostic tests for fetal well-being
- Having a normal fetus and infant

Knowledge, deficit, related to:
- Lack of understanding about third-trimester changes
- Lack of preparation for labor and delivery
- Lack of understanding about fetal assessment techniques

Altered sexuality patterns, related to
- Physical changes in third trimester
- Fear of hurting fetus
- Lack of comfort during third trimester

Cultural

Strength-Oriented
Positive self-care practices, related to incorporation of cultural beliefs and practices into plan of care

Problem-Oriented
Altered family process, related to cultural differences in perception of roles during third trimester of pregnancy, labor, delivery, and early parenting

Because MRI is a fairly new technique, there is a lack of well-documented imaging parameters. This situation at times complicates diagnosis.

Role of the Nurse. High-risk clients undergoing MRI during pregnancy require support and teaching. Although MRI is not physically painful, the client's positioning in the unit, along with the reason for the test, may be stressful and upsetting to her. Nurses can do much to ensure that staff members conducting the test provide reassurance to the client during this potentially frightening procedure, that results of the test are communicated promptly, and that the client receives adequate and appropriate support if pathology is diagnosed.[66, 67]

BARRIERS TO CARE DURING THE THIRD TRIMESTER

Barriers to care were previously discussed in Chapters 14 and 18. Obstacles may come from the health care system, from the client herself, from her home or work environment, or from significant others. Assessment includes client attendance at prenatal visits and identification of any factors that interfere with the client's receiving antenatal care.

NURSING DIAGNOSES

Third-trimester assessment continues to enrich the data base from which nursing diagnoses are developed. Nursing diagnoses for the low-risk client during the third trimester evolve from the client's adaptation to the changes of advanced pregnancy, responses to screening procedures, and preparations for childbirth and early parenting. In the box are listed nursing diagnoses related to the third-trimester client and her family.

SUMMARY

Assessment during the third trimester of pregnancy focuses on physiologic, psychosocial, cultural, and nutritional parameters that have an impact on the childbearing family. Nursing diagnoses and interventions are guided by a comprehensive data base, which is obtained through thorough, individualized assessment of the childbearing family.

The goals of third-trimester assessment include identification of normal third-trimester adaptation, recognition and management of any high-risk conditions, and determination of readiness for labor and delivery. The assessment techniques of choice for a normal pregnancy are those that provide adequate information with the least degree of associated risk, that is, history and physical examination. At each visit the history is updated. Normal physical assessment includes weight, blood pressure, transabdominal measurement of uterine size, fetal position, fetal heart rate, and fetal activity. Pelvic assessment may be done near term to assess cervical readiness for labor. Laboratory testing for the healthy woman may include urine screening at each visit and blood sampling for hematocrit early in the third trimester. The woman with no prenatal care prior to the third trimester is considered at risk and attention is given to reasons why care was delayed. Interviews with the expectant family will provide the nurse with valuable information regarding the health status of the expectant mother, her fetus, and family members.

Several prenatal diagnostic techniques are available for assessing the maternal and fetal condition for clients at risk. These include the nonstress test; the contraction stress test; the fetal biophysical profile; amniotic fluid analysis; percutaneous umbilical blood sampling; ultrasonic assessment of maternal structures, the fetus, and placenta; and nuclear magnetic resonance imaging. Advancing technology continues to evolve techniques for increasingly comprehensive assessment; however, no single technique provides all possible information safely, reliably, and effectively in all situations. Diagnostic techniques are therefore ordered for specific indications and with an understanding of their risks, benefits, and limitations. Results are interpreted in the light of total client assessment.

Nurses collaborate with physicians and other health care providers to ensure that comprehensive assessment takes place. Nursing responsibilities in third-trimester assessment include technical aspects, psychosocial support, teaching, and advocacy. The nurse also encourages the family's participation in planning care to enhance the self-care practices of the expectant client and her family.

REVIEW QUESTIONS

1. Describe normal findings and alterations commonly seen in the cardiovascular, reproductive, integumentary, gastrointestinal, and renal systems during the third trimester.
2. Identify third trimester risk factors that may have an impact on labor and delivery and the nenonatal period.
3. Describe criteria of the psychosocial assessment of the family during the third trimester.
4. Develop a nursing assessment worksheet to be used for expectant families during the third trimester.
5. Describe three diagnostic assessment techniques that would be appropriate for assessment of fetal well-being and fetal maturation during the third trimester. What information would be obtained from these techniques?

REFERENCES

1. Feeg VD. *Pediatric Nursing: Forum on the Future: Looking Toward the 21st Century.* Pitman, NJ: Anthony J. Jannetti, Inc; 1989.
2. American Academy of Pediatrics, American College of Obstetricians and Gynecologists. In: Frigoletto FD, Little GA, eds. *Guidelines for Perinatal Care.* 2nd ed. White Plains, NY: March of Dimes Birth Defects Foundation; 1988.
3. Moore PJ. Maternal physiology during pregnancy. In: Pernoll ML, Benson RC, eds. *Current Obstetric & Gynecologic Diagnosis & Treatment.* 6th ed. Norwalk, Conn: Appleton & Lange; 1987:127–134.
4. Cunningham FG, et al. *Williams Obstetrics.* 18th ed. Norwalk, Conn: Appleton & Lange; 1989.
5. Kelton JG, Cruickshank M. Hematologic disorders of pregnancy. In: Burrow GN, Ferris TF, eds. *Medical Complications During Pregnancy.* 3rd ed. Philadelphia: WB Saunders; 1988:65–94.
6. Wald NJ, ed. *Antenatal and Neonatal Screening.* New York: Oxford University Press; 1984.
7. Dunn PA, et al. Percutaneous umbilical blood sampling. *J Obstet Gynecol Neonat Nurs.* 1988;17:308–313.
8. Oklan E. Psychological midwifery during the birth of a family. *Mobius.* 1985;5:6–20.
9. Lederman RP. *Psychosocial Adaptation in Pregnancy.* Englewood Cliffs, NJ: Prentice-Hall; 1984.
10. Sherwen LN, ed. *Psychosocial Dimensions of the Pregnant Family.* New York: Springer Publishing Co; 1987.
11. Sherwen LN. Third trimester fantasies of first-time expectant fathers. *Matern Child Nurs J.* 1986;15:153–170.
12. Kutzner SK. Responses of siblings to pregnancy. In: Sherwen LN, ed. *Psychosocial Dimensions of the Pregnant Family.* New York: Springer Publishing Co; 1987:177–192.
13. Lutwak RA, et al. Maternity nursing and Jewish law. *Am J Matern Child Nurs.* 1988;13:44–46.
14. Leininger M. Transcultural nursing care diversity and

universality: a thoery of nursing. *Nurs Health Care.* 1985; 10:209–212.
15. Certanzarite VA, et al. Assessment of fetal well-being. In: Pernoll ML, Benson RC, eds. *Current Obstetrics and Gynecology: Diagnosis and Treatment.* 6th ed. Norwalk, Conn: Appleton-Lange; 1987:279–302.
16. Varney H. *Nurse Midwifery.* 2nd ed. Boston: Blackwell Scientific; 1987.
17. Oxorn H, ed. *Human Labor and Birth.* 5th ed. Norwalk, Conn: Appleton-Century-Crofts; 1986.
18. Klaus MH, Fanaroff AA. *Care of the High Risk Neonate.* Philadelphia: WB Saunders; 1986.
19. Buerle J, Behamroun B. The fetal biophysical profile: interpretation and nursing implications. *Crit Care Nurse.* 1988; 8:52–55.
20. Rayburn WF. Monitoring fetal body movements. *Clin Obstet Gynecol.* 1987;3:899–911.
21. Bishop E. Fetal acceleration test. *Am J Obstet Gynecol.* 1981;141:905–909.
22. Knuppel RA, et al. A review of the nonstress test. *J Reprod Med* 1982;27:120–126.
23. Keegan KA. The nonstress test. *Clin Obstet Gynecol.* 1987; 30:921–935.
24. Porto M. Comparing and contrasting methods of fetal surveillance. *Clin Obstet Gynecol.* 1987;30:956–967.
25. Brar HS, et al. The biophysical profile. *Clin Obstet Gynecol.* 1987;30:936–947.
26. Devoe LD, et al. Nonstress test: dimensions of normal reactivity. *Obstet Gynecol.* 1985;66:616.
27. Knuppel RA, Drucker JE. *High Risk Pregnancy: A Team Approach.* Philadelphia: WB Saunders; 1986.
28. Dauphinee JD. Antepartum testing: A challenge for nurses, *J Perinat Neonat Nurs.* 1987;1:29–48.
29. Kisilevsky BS, et al. Human fetal responses to sound as a function of stimulus intensity. *Obstet Gynecol.* 1989;73: 971–976.
30. Sleutel MR. An overview of vibroacoustic stimulation. *J Obstet Gynecol Neonatal Nurs.* 1989;18:447–452.
31. Sleutel MR. Vibroacoustic stimulation and fetal heart rate in nonstress tests. *J Obstet Gynecol Neonatal Nurs.* 1990; 19:199–204.
32. Platt LD. Predicting fetal health with the biophysical profile. *Contemp Obstet Gynecol.* 1989;33:105–119.
33. Freeman RK. Contraction stress testing for primary fetal surveillance in patients at high risk for uteroplacental insufficiency. *Clin Perinatol* 1982;9:265–270.
34. Gantes M, et al. Breast massage to obtain contraction stress test. *Nurs Res.* 1985;34:338–341.
35. Kogut EA. The nurse's role in antepartum fetal assessment. *J Perinatol.* 1986;6:108–113.
36. Govoni LE, Hayes JE. *Drugs and Nursing Implications.* 6th ed. Norwalk, Conn: Appleton & Lange; 1988.
37. Huddleston JF, Freeman RK. Assessment of fetal well being by antepartum fetal heart rate testing. In: Bolongnese RJ, et al, eds. *Perinatal Medicine: Management of High Risk Fetus and Newborn.* 2nd ed. Baltimore; Williams and Wilkins; 1982:129.
38. Resnik R, et al. NST or CST? What's best for spotting the high risk fetus? *Contemp Obstet Gynecol.* 1982;19:92–94.
39. Manning R, et al. Antepartum determination of fetal health: composite biophysical profile scoring. *Clin Perinatol.* 1982; 19:285–296.
40. Ferguson H. Biophysical profile scoring: The fetal Apgar. *Am J Nurs.* 1988;88:662–663.
41. Johnson TRB, et al. New clues to fetal behavior and well being. *Contemp Obstet Gynecol.* 1988;32:108–123.
42. Manning RA, et al. Antepartum fetal evaluation: development of a fetal biophysical profile. *Am J Obstet Gynecol.* 1980;136:785–787.
43. Patrick J. Fetal breathing movements. *Clin Obstet Gynecol.* 1982;25:787–800.
44. Vintzileos AM, et al. The use and misuse of the fetal biophysical profile. *Am J Obstet Gynecol.* 1987;156:527–533.
45. Manning FA, et al. Fetal assessment based on fetal biophysical profile scoring: experience in 19,221 referred high-risk pregnancies: II. An analysis of false-negative fetal deaths. *Am J Obstet Gynecol.* 1987;157:880.
46. Vintzileos AM, et al. The fetal biophysical profile and its predictive value. *Obstet Gynecol.* 1983;62:271–278.
47. Manning FA, et al. Fetal biophysical profile scoring: selective use of the nonstress test. *Am J Obstet Gynecol.* 1987; 156:709.
48. Brar HS, et al. The use and misuse of the fetal biophysical profile. *Am J Obstet Gynecol.* 1987;156:527–532.
49. Chez BF, et al. Interpretations of nonstress tests by obstetric nurses. *J Obstet Gynecol Neonatal Nurs.* 1990;19: 227–232.
50. Harmon JS, Barry M. Antenatal testing, mobile outpatient monitoring service. *J Obstet Gynecol Neonatal Nurs.* 1989; 18:21–24.
51. Clements J, et al. Assessment of the risk of the respiratory distress syndrome of a rapid test for surfactant in amniotic fluid. *N Eng Med.* 1972;286:1077–1081.
52. Garite TJ, et al. A new rapid slide agglutination test for amniotic fluid phosphatidylglycerol. *Am J Obstet Gynecol.* 1983;147:681–684.
53. Turbull AC. The lecithin/sphingomyelin ratio in decline. *Br J Obstet Gynecol.* 1983;90:993.
54. Hohler C. Ultrasound and high risk obstetrics. In: Knuppel R, Drukker J, eds. *High Risk Pregnancy: A Team Approach.* Philadelphia: WB Saunders; 1986.
55. Gough DJ. Ultrasound. In: Wald NJ, ed. *Antenatal and Neonatal Screening.* New York: Oxford University Press; 1984: 423–434.
56. Hadlock FP, et al. Computer assisted analysis of fetal age in the third trimester using multiple fetal growth parameters. *J Clin Ultrasound,* 1983;11:313–316.
57. Shepard MJ, et al. An evaluation of two equations for predicting fetal weight by ultrasound. *Am J Obstet Gynecol.* 1982;142:47.
58. Hohler CW, Queter RA. Femur length: equations for computer calculation of gestational age from ultrasound measurements. *Am J Obstet Gynecol.* 1982;143:479.
59. Key TC, Moore TR. Evaluation of high risk pregnancy using ultrasonography. *J Perinatol.* 1984;5:49–53.
60. Grannum P, et al. The ultrasonic changes in the maturing placenta and their relation to fetal pulmonic maturity. *Am J Obstet Gynecol.* 1979;133:15–18.
61. Quinlan RW, et al. Changes in placental ultrasonic appearance: I. Incidence of grade III changes in the placenta in correlation to fetal pulmonary maturity. *Am J Obstet Gynecol.* 1982;144:468–470.
62. Chard T. Placental function tests. In: Walk NJ, ed. *Antenatal and Neonatal Screening.* New York: Oxford University Press; 1984:510–522.
63. Kochenour NE. Estrogen assay during pregnancy. *Clin Obstet Gynecol.* 1982;25:659–572.

64. Johnson IR, Kean DM, et al. Imaging the pregnant uterus with nuclear magnetic resonance. *Am J Obstet Gynecol.* 1984;148:1136–1139.
65. Williamson RA, et al. Magnetic resonance imaging of anomalous fetuses. *Obstet Gynecol.* 1989;73:952–956.
66. Mattison DR, et al. Magnetic resonance imaging in maternal and fetal medicine. *J Perinatology.* 1989;9:411–419.
67. Philips CR. Rehumanizing maternal-child nursing. *Am J Matern Child Nurs.* 1988;13:313–318.

Nursing Care of the Family During the Third Trimester

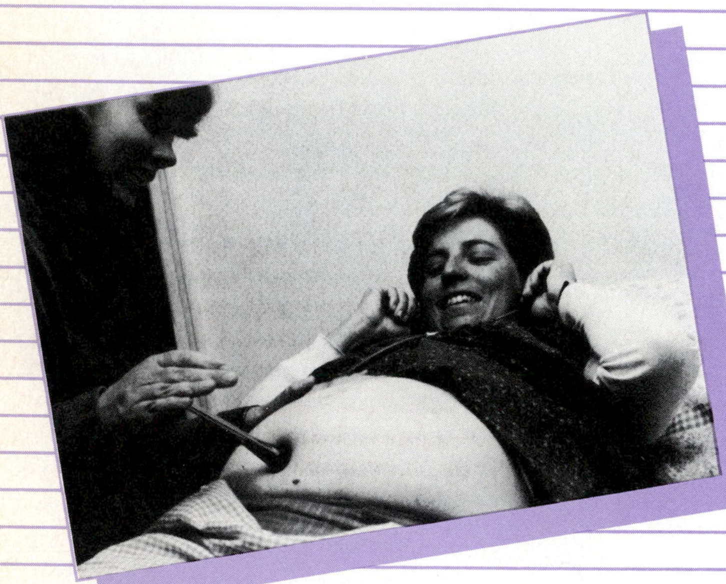

chapter 23

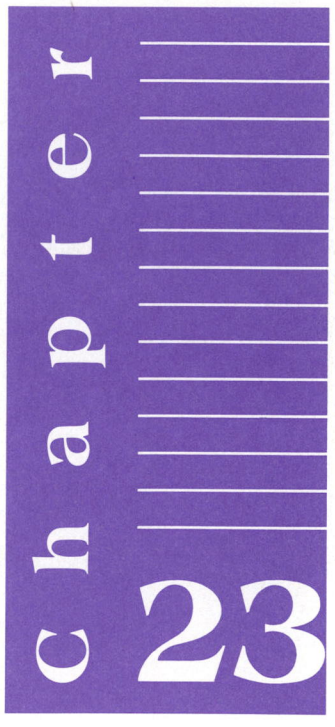

Nursing care during the third trimester focuses on goals that foster healthy fetal, maternal, and family development and that prepare the family for labor, delivery, and early parenting. Advanced pregnancy is accompanied by changes in many aspects of the expectant mother's body and life. For the low-risk, healthy family, the third trimester is a time of expectation and increasing readiness for childbirth. The large abdomen makes pregnancy highly visible. Fetal movements are no longer perceived only by the expectant mother, but may be easily felt by others. By term, the family has completed many psychologic tasks and is ready for the new family member.

Nursing care during the third trimester continues to focus on assessment; anticipatory guidance and teaching become especially important so that clients can participate actively in labor and delivery and prepare for the newborn. Antenatal visits increase in frequency from every other week to every week, providing an excellent opportunity for a strong, ongoing relationship to continue to develop between the third-trimester family and their health care providers. Indeed, at no other time during the life cycle are healthy, low-risk clients in such frequent touch with the health care system. Third-trimester care continues to require a collaborative approach between nurses and other health care providers so that comprehensive care is ensured. Nursing care continues to focus on specific care goals (see Table 23–1).

CONTINUE A PHILOSOPHY OF CARE WITH WELL-DEFINED GOALS

As discussed in Chapters 15 and 19, every antenatal care facility should have a philosophy of care with clearly defined goals and objectives related to care of the childbearing family. All staff members need to be well informed about the philosophy, goals, and objectives and to be able to translate them into practice. For example, in a unit committed to provision of wellness care to low-risk childbearing families, screening tests such as fetal biophysical profiles would not be routinely ordered for the third-trimester client, but would be reserved for specific indications.

Ideally, the philosophy of wellness care for low-

TABLE 23–1. GOALS OF NURSING CARE DURING THE THIRD TRIMESTER

Continue a philosophy of care with well-defined goals
Continue to incorporate recent literature into nursing care
Prepare the client and family for continued care
Prepare the client for intrapartum care and early postpartum care
Continue assessment and update the data base from which diagnoses are developed
Update and continue strategies identified in the care plan
Continue support to the client
Continue to incorporate the client's cultural background into care
Continue informed decision making and assist the client in finalizing birth plans
Discuss alternatives in the event of high-risk intrapartum, postpartum, or neonatal conditions
Promote psychologic adaptation to late pregnancy
Foster family attachment during late pregnancy
Meet the late-pregnancy educational needs of the client and family and promote preparation for labor, delivery, and early parenting
Promote nutritional well-being
Assist the client in coping with third-trimester discomforts
Promote client safety
Evaluate antenatal care
Ensure appropriate referrals for the client
Contribute to general antenatal public health

risk clients extends throughout the childbearing experience. Through networking with staff in labor, delivery, postpartum, and newborn nursery settings, antenatal staff can identify and ensure practices that support low-risk, wellness care. For example, staff from prenatal and intrapartum settings can jointly consider whether electronic fetal monitoring, important in high-risk cases, is appropriate for all low-risk clients.

A philosophy of wellness and interventions only when necessary for the low-risk childbearing family can be implemented in any setting, regardless of the availability of sophisticated diagnostic equipment. Indeed, staff who do have ready access to high-risk equipment and screening procedures are challenged not to use them except when necessary.

CONTINUE TO INCORPORATE RECENT LITERATURE INTO NURSING CARE

As discussed in Chapters 15 and 19, nursing care cannot be current unless based on the most recent clinical and research literature. Published findings must also be assessed carefully and not simply applied to practice. Nurses will find a substantial and ever-expanding literature on physiologic and psychologic adaptations to late pregnancy. For reasons such as pronounced physical changes and more frequent antenatal visits, more studies have been done during the third trimester than at other times during pregnancy. The current literature provides background for all aspects of client care and may stimulate research questions on the part of the nurse working with third-trimester clients. With appropriate consultation from others with research backgrounds, the nurse may replicate certain studies in his or her own prenatal practice setting or may use previous findings to stimulate research on related topics. For example, a nurse may wish to replicate findings of a study on third-trimester maternal attachment or may wish to study attachment in expectant fathers or grandparents.

PREPARE THE CLIENT AND FAMILY FOR CONTINUED CARE

Around 28 weeks of gestation, the client's prenatal visits increase to every other week; around 36 weeks of gestation, the client begins weekly visits.[1] The client may be seen more often, if needed. Before the end of each visit, the client continues to make future appointments. Third-trimester clients often schedule several advance appointments, to be better able to make their own plans, such as transportation and child care, and to ensure they will not have difficulty finding an available appointment at a convenient time. (First- or second-trimester clients who need to make plans 2 months ahead may also do this.) Frequent prenatal visits can be difficult to manage, especially for clients who are employed, live at a distance, or have other regularly scheduled responsibilities. Attention therefore needs to be paid to making certain that appointments progress on time. Flexible scheduling of prenatal sessions, including evening hours, does not force the working client to choose between prenatal care and a paycheck.

PREPARE THE CLIENT FOR INTRAPARTUM CARE AND EARLY POSTPARTUM CARE

During the third trimester, the nurse ensures that the client and her family are prepared for intrapartum care and for early postpartum care. Clients who attend childbirth preparation classes at the same facility where they will deliver may receive information about intrapartum and postpartum care through their prepared childbirth classes. In some settings members of the nursing staff may also be certified childbirth educators and teach the childbirth preparation classes. Many clients, however, attend childbirth education programs elsewhere in the community; therefore, as part of third-trimester care, the nurse makes certain that the client is informed about what to expect in the particular setting during labor and delivery and what she, her family, and her newborn will experience after birth there.

As part of a birth center experience, clients become well educated about all aspects of the center by delivery. Birthing areas are usually adjacent to antenatal assessment areas, and clients have ample prenatal opportunity to become familiar with them and to select the room they wish to use for labor and delivery, if available. Clients who come for prenatal care in private office or clinic settings usually have little contact with the intrapartum facilities, although many have toured the facilities in selecting their birthing environment. During the third trimester, clients should therefore be encouraged to tour the facility again, as new questions may arise with advanced pregnancy. Antenatal nurses should make certain that clients do not see the intrapartum facility for the first time when they arrive in labor.

During the third trimester, the client should be prepared for changes that will take place in her body after delivery and in the early postpartum period, although postpartum teaching will also be given in the postpartum setting. For example, such topics as postpartum lochial discharge (which can be a source of surprise and anxiety to the unprepared woman), what postpartum assessment will involve, care of the newborn, and contact between mother, family members, and the newborn should be discussed.

CONTINUE ASSESSMENT AND UPDATE THE DATA BASE FROM WHICH DIAGNOSES ARE DEVELOPED

Chapter 22 explained assessment strategies for the third-trimester client. Screening for high-risk conditions continues to be a major focus of third-trimester assessment, because high-risk conditions, such as pregnancy-induced hypertension, can emerge suddenly and jeopardize maternal and fetal well-being. Assessment continues to identify client and family strengths and assets, so that successful self-care practices can be reinforced, independence fostered, and the family included in care decisions. Through assessment the nurse collaborates with other health care providers in updating or formulating new nursing diagnoses and evaluating client responses to previous strategies. As the third trimester progresses, new diagnoses also include readiness of the client for labor, delivery, and early parenthood.

The format for repeat prenatal visits remains similar throughout pregnancy, although certain screening tests, such as hemoglobin/hematocrit, repeat testing for syphilis or other infections (in women at risk), irregular antibody screen, and Rh antibody testing for Rh-negative women may be done during the third trimester.[1] In some settings, pelvic examinations are again begun around 36 weeks of gestation to assess cervical ripening and dilation and fetal station. The third-trimester client should not lie flat on her back on an examining table, to avoid supine hypotensive syndrome.[2] In other settings, pelvic examinations are not routinely done for the low-risk client until labor begins.

UPDATE AND CONTINUE STRATEGIES IDENTIFIED IN THE CARE PLAN

Throughout pregnancy, the care plan serves as a vehicle to express management strategies.[3] The client's chart and care plan are always reviewed by the nurse and the examiner prior to meeting with the client at each antenatal visit.

Some management strategies, such as preparation of the client for childbirth and early parenting, assume special importance during the third trimester as delivery approaches. Many management strategies change as pregnancy progresses, although particular goals continue. For example, knowledge deficits related to pregnancy may continue as a diagnosis throughout pregnancy. Nursing care related to knowledge deficits in the third trimester will focus on: assessment of client responses to teaching during the first and second trimesters, client mastery of topics covered at prior visits, and client initiatives in addressing knowledge deficits; identification of specific subjects for third-trimester teaching and educational preparation for labor, delivery, and early parenthood; development or continuation of intervention strategies that will best meet the unique educational needs of the client; and, identification of ways in which the client's mastery of the subjects taught may be evaluated (return demonstrations of proper body mechanics when bending, breathing exercises for labor and delivery, and so on).

Sample management strategies for a low-risk client during the third trimester are illustrated later in this chapter. Assessment and diagnoses related to the third trimester are presented in Chapter 22.

CONTINUE SUPPORT TO THE CLIENT

Support of the pregnant family remains essential throughout pregnancy. The nurse should continue to remain accessible and to anticipate client concerns, such as late-pregnancy discomforts, altered physical appearance, weight gain, increased feelings of vulnerability, and lack of confidence in ability to cope with labor, delivery, or a new family member. During the third trimester, many couples need to be reassured that their fetus is developing normally and that their concerns are also normal. By 40 weeks of gestation, the low-risk client will ideally have made around 15 visits. Thus, during pregnancy, and especially the third trimester, the nurse frequently has more contact with the client than do some members of the client's own family.

Third-trimester diagnostic testing focuses on assessment and fetal well-being, and maintenance of the pregnancy to term. Such assessment measures as the nonstress test, the contraction stress test, and the fetal biophysical profile may be particular sources of anxiety to couples who are fearful about the health of their developing fetus. Lack of conclusive results or the need for repeat tests contributes to stress. Nurses have an important role in providing emotional support to expectant families throughout the diagnostic process.

CONTINUE TO INCORPORATE THE CLIENT'S CULTURAL BACKGROUND INTO CARE

The client's cultural background must be integrated into any management strategy. This is especially important during the third trimester, as the nurse provides anticipatory guidance and counseling for intrapartum, postpartum and neonatal care.

The health care system and lifestyle of women in the United States at times are in conflict with beliefs and practices of other cultures. For example, Chicano women may avoid milk because of a cultural belief that milk may make the fetus too large and hard to deliver.[4] Alternate sources of protein and calcium may therefore be suggested. Control of the environment is also culturally valued by pregnant Chicano women, who may then view cool moving air or even the sun's rays, coming through glass, as dangerous during pregnancy. Nursing care might thus involve positioning clients during visits so they are not in direct sunlight. Nursing strategies related to care of Chicano women would include specific caution about the use of laxatives and purgative teas, which culturally are often believed to be remedies for constipation during the third trimester. Certain cultural beliefs, such as the Chicano woman's emphasis on activity, exercise, and massage can be encouraged as health-promoting strategies.

Clients should be encouraged to discuss ways in which their own cultural expectations differ from health care practices in the United States. Interpreters for non–English-speaking clients should be present for each visit and should accompany clients on tours of the birthing facility.

Physical examination, particularly pelvic examination during early and late pregnancy, is stressful for women from all cultural groups; however, certain groups, such as some Chicano women or Arab-American women, may find examination particularly difficult. Management strategies must therefore always be explained carefully and implemented in a professional manner that ensures the client's privacy.

Special arrangements may need to be made antenatally to accommodate cultural variations within the intrapartum and postpartum settings. For example, some facilities do not have arrangements for kosher diets. Jewish clients who follow kosher dietary practices need to be prepared to bring their own foods and beverages. During the third trimester, the nurse, working with an interpreter whenever necessary, can assist the couple to develop a birth plan that reflects their cultural beliefs. In this way staff can work with the client toward realizing a satisfying birthing experience within the health care delivery system.

Cultural conflict during the third trimester is not restricted to religious or ethnic groups, but may affect women whose lifestyles or responsibilities are incongruent with past beliefs regarding late-trimester behavior. Identification of conflict is part of the assessment. For example, in the United States women traditionally were expected to leave their jobs well in advance of delivery. A woman who works because of necessity, work responsibilities, or need to maximize maternity leave after birth of the infant may experience personal or interpersonal conflict related to her continued working. In this type of situation, nursing strategies include providing support for the client's decision to continue working. As one client reported, "Friends, family, even coworkers keep asking me why I'm still working at my secretarial job. I get 6 weeks' paid maternity leave and I want to save it for being with the baby. We need my income too much for me to take unpaid leave. I felt so relieved when the nurse and doctor reassured me there was no medical reason why I had to stop working."

CONTINUE INFORMED DECISION MAKING AND ASSIST THE CLIENT IN FINALIZING BIRTH PLANS

During the third trimester, the nurse serves as a consultant to the client in finalizing birth plans. The expectant couple is encouraged to discuss a draft of their birth plan with health care providers around 34 weeks of gestation, although some couples may choose to do this sooner. After discussion, the birth plan is modified as necessary, and then signed by the client and the health care provider.[5]

The nurse advises the couple in developing a plan that is congruent with available facilities. For example, certain birthing facilities may have jetted tubs for use by clients in labor; clients may then realistically include use of the tub in their birth plan.

Around 34 weeks, you will be asked to formulate a birth plan with your partner/support person(s). This birth plan is a very simple document written to let the nurse-midwives and nurses know how you visualize your labor and delivery. It is a way to communicate what is *specifically* important to *you*. Some people find it helpful to describe the environment they would like. For example:

- Would you like something special with the lighting, music?
- What roles do you wish your partner/support person(s) to take during labor and at the actual delivery?
- Do you have children who will be present at this birth, and how will they be supported?
- Do you have special fears or desires you would like us to know about?
- What room do you prefer for the birth?
- Do you wish to have pictures taken of the birth?

Please feel free to list anything that will assist us in making your birth experience everything you would like for it to be.

Figure 23–1. Example of guidelines for a birth plan. (*Courtesy of The Birth Center, Bryn Mawr, Pennsylvania. Reproduced with permission.*)

During labor and delivery I would like my husband and sister to be present with me. My sister will bring her camera and take photos. I want to stay out of bed as long as I am able and would prefer to be able to walk, to use the jetted tub for relaxation, or to be up in the chair in the birthing suite. I would like to be able to listen to the tapes that we will bring and do not want the television to be on at any time. My husband and I have attended the prepared childbirth classes, but I know we will need "on the job" teaching which I would like from the staff. If all goes well, my husband would like to cut the cord. Please delay the baby's antibiotic eyedrops long enough for me to be able to look into the baby's eyes. After delivery I would like to introduce the baby to his or her grandparents and three-year-old brother and to spend time with my family in the birthing suite.

In the event that I require transfer I would like my husband and the nurse-midwife to remain with me through delivery. If I need a cesarean delivery, I would like to remain awake, if feasible, to have a low transverse skin incision if circumstances allow, and, if the baby's conditions permits, to see and touch the baby as soon as possible.

Figure 23–2. Example of a birth plan.

Siblings may be welcomed to attend birth in a birth center; however, "special" permission may be needed in advance in hospital settings. A birth plan including a sibling that is "approved" in advance may prevent client disappointment or conflict with staff at the time of labor.

A copy of the client's written birth plan is placed in the client's chart, and one copy is kept by the parents. When feasible, clients may request that staff who may substitute for their antenatal caregivers review the birth plan and discuss any areas of disagreement. The birth plan ideally then becomes standing orders for the midwife or physician who will attend the birth.[6] The couple is therefore "spared" the necessity of re-explaining their birth plans or negotiating with intrapartum staff during labor, especially if attended by staff who did not work with them prenatally. Figure 23–1 presents an example of guidelines for a birth plan, and Figure 23–2 presents an example of an actual birth plan.

Currently, childbirth education supports shared decision making between clients and health care providers, as evidenced by the implementation of birth plans. Unfortunately, health care providers in traditional hospital settings have not always welcomed the use of birth plans. Birth plans, as well as other attempts by clients to participate actively in their own care, have been viewed suspiciously by some health care providers, for example, as demonstrations of lack of client trust.[6] A goal of birth plans is to meet the unique needs of each family for a personally satisfying childbirth, while fostering mutual participation and sharing of information between expectant families and their health care providers.

DISCUSS ALTERNATIVES IN THE EVENT OF HIGH-RISK INTRAPARTUM, POSTPARTUM, OR NEONATAL CONDITIONS

During the third trimester, health care providers and the client should discuss alternatives in the event high-risk intrapartum, postpartum, or neonatal conditions emerge. The client should also be encouraged to develop an alternative birth plan to be included in the chart with the original birth plan. If feasible at the time, the alternative birth plan would be used in the event of unexpected outcomes. For instance, if an unplanned cesarean delivery becomes necessary, the client may request that her partner remain with her; she may also ask to receive regional, and not general, anesthesia if possible to be awake for the delivery.

Clients who expect to deliver in a free-standing birth center or in a low-risk obstetric facility may also visit the hospital units to which they or their infants would be transferred if complications arise. Although the possibility of transfer is never a pleasant topic, familiarity with these units may allay anxiety if transfer becomes necessary. Some clients become upset at the discussion of high-risk topics. Health care providers therefore need to reassure clients about their current healthy, normal status.

ISSUES AND CONTROVERSIES

One issue related to nursing management concerns the determination of risk status. Should a well, pregnant woman with a history of high-risk delivery be cared for in a high-risk center, or can she be managed in a low-risk environment, if her problem is unlikely to recur? If the woman is managed as "high-risk," will she have unneeded diagnostic tests and procedures? Such issues need to be addressed, especially in light of the current emphasis on use of technology in obstetrics.

PROMOTE PSYCHOLOGIC ADAPTATION TO LATE PREGNANCY

During the third trimester, nurses continue to have an important role in helping families to meet emotional tasks of late pregnancy and to complete their preparations for childbirth and early parenting. Continuing to encourage couples to share their feelings with each other remains a basic management strategy. Other components of psychosocial care are important during the third trimester:

- Meeting with the client (and family members, if present) prior to physical examination by the midwife or physician at each visit.[7] The nurse assesses the progression of the client and the family's preparation for childbirth and parenting, provides anticipatory guidance and counseling, formulates or revises nursing diagnoses, and communicates any client care problems to the physician or certified nurse-midwife for collaborative follow-up.
- Reassessing family functioning in late pregnancy.[7] Psychosocial factors, such as acceptance of the pregnancy and the coming infant, are crucial during the third trimester, when birth of the baby is imminent. At this time some ambivalence about being pregnant may occur, although this should be neither prolonged nor intense. The pregnant woman may be uncomfortable and desire to no longer be pregnant; however, these feelings should not involve rejection of the fetus, as the third trimester woman and family should look forward to the newborn. As indicated later, rejection of the fetus is a psychologically high-risk situation requiring further evaluation. Through observation, interview, or the use of screening tools (*see* Chapter 14) the nurse may identify whether the third trimester family is continuing to adapt normally or whether high-risk psychosocial conditions have emerged.
- Explaining normal psychologic processes of the third trimester. For instance, as the woman continues to focus inward, family members may feel increasingly isolated from her. Other topics include altered time perception (time seeming to "creep") and changes in body space and body image in late pregnancy.
- Providing anticipatory guidance and teaching. Topics include rearrangement of time and space for a new infant or additional child, the mother's employment plans, the family's plans for care of the new mother and infant at home, paternal feelings of being "left out" of the mother-infant dyad, feel-

ings of paternal attachment to the fetus and infant, and sexuality during the third trimester.

- Discussing changing interpersonal family relationships and the client's own reactions as delivery approaches.
- Fostering the expectant grandmother's involvement in the pregnancy by continuing to encourage the client to bring her to antenatal visits and by encouraging the client to share her feelings with her own mother. Indeed, the expectant woman's relationship with her own mother is one of the most important psychosocial dimensions of pregnancy.[8,9]
- Reassuring the client about normal fantasy processes. As discussed in Chapter 21, dreams and concerns about an abnormal infant are normal for women during the third trimester. They can, however, be extremely upsetting to clients who worry that these fantasies are prophetic. During the third trimester, healthy expectant women may feel they and their fetuses are increasingly vulnerable, as reflected by fears or dreams of being attacked.[10] (It is important to identify that these are part of normal fantasy patterns and not reflections of actual abuse.) Clients and families may greatly benefit from the nurse's anticipating these concerns, identifying the nature of maternal and paternal fantasies, and providing appropriate reassurance.
- Exploring paternal reactions to pregnancy during the third trimester. Expectant fathers should be encouraged to discuss concerns related to pregnancy, feelings about the pregnant partner, sexuality during late pregnancy, the paternal role during labor and delivery and early parenting, and couvade symptoms that normally may occur during the third trimester.[11] In addition, discussion should include the expectant father's concerns in the event that alternative birth plans need to be used.
- Assisting the expectant couple to cope with stress in themselves and other family members, related to the birth of the baby in the near future.
- Encouraging sharing of feelings between the expectant father and his own father, as this relationship assumes special importance as childbirth approaches.
- Encouraging the expectant couple to discuss plans for integrating the newborn into the family and providing anticipatory guidance as appropriate.

Through assessment of third-trimester psychologic adaptation, the nurse can identify high-risk situations that require additional counseling and referral. Examples of these are presented in Table 19–2.

FOSTER FAMILY ATTACHMENT DURING LATE PREGNANCY

During the third trimester, attachment to the fetus normally progresses, not only for the expectant mother, but for the expectant father, grandparents, and siblings (Figure 23–3). Nurses can assess attachment behaviors by encouraging clients to talk about their fetuses. Such questions as "Can you describe your developing baby's personality?" and "What does your developing baby seem to like and dislike?" encourage clients to focus on the fetus as a separate being. Facial expression, tone of voice, and nature of description provide clues to maternal and paternal attachment as well as to psychologic adaptation in the third trimester.

Including significant others in prenatal visits, identifying fetal parts, encouraging family members to listen to the fetal heartbeat, and providing learning materials, such as charts, to illustrate fetal growth and development are activities that reinforce the reality of the developing baby and promote attachment on the part of family members. Nurses can encourage the expectant parents to share their thoughts and feelings with each other and with their own parents, as both the marital relationship

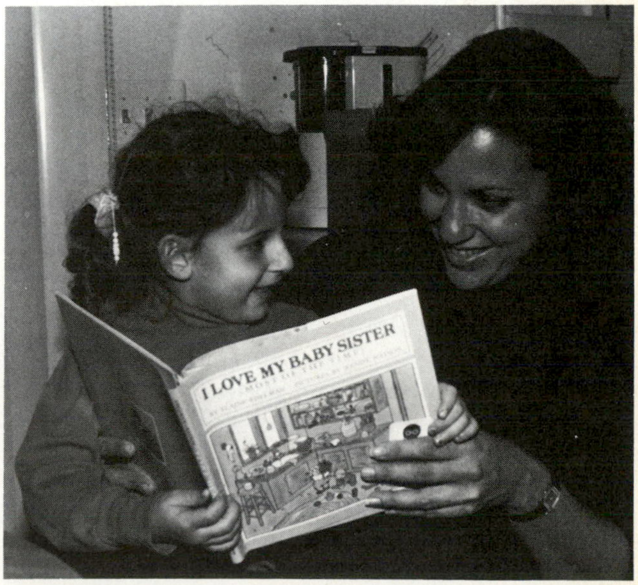

Figure 23–3. As birth approaches, attachment to the fetus progresses for family members, including siblings.

and the expectant parents' relationships with their own parents become especially important as pregnancy progresses. Failure to attach to the fetus by the third trimester indicates an emotionally high-risk situation in need of further assessment.

Many pregnant clients in the United States attend childbirth preparation classes during the third trimester. Through their content and process, the classes also foster attachment to the fetus. Expectant grandparents classes and sibling classes focus on the special needs of these groups in preparation for and attachment to the infant (*see* Chapter 24).

MEET THE LATE-PREGNANCY EDUCATIONAL NEEDS OF THE CLIENT AND FAMILY AND PROMOTE PREPARATION FOR LABOR, DELIVERY, AND EARLY PARENTING

Throughout the third trimester, educational preparation remains an essential component of nursing care. Education during the third trimester assumes special importance, as the expectant couple must learn not only about third trimester adaptations, but also about labor, delivery, the early postpartum period, and the newborn. Before the end of pregnancy, the family should have resources mobilized for independent self-care practices in late pregnancy and after returning home with the newborn. Table 23–2 lists some questions commonly asked during the third trimester. (*See* also Chapter 24, particularly Table 24–3, which presents an outline for prenatal education.)

Third-trimester education includes advice and teaching about items that will be needed for care of the newborn. To avoid confusion and additional stress in the busy days after childbirth, expectant families may be encouraged to prepare items that will be used for the new baby (Figure 23–4). Some families may be reluctant to bring major baby items into the home before the baby is born because of fears that "all will not be well." Such beliefs may be culturally supported. The families may, however, plan, select, and order items such as a crib that can be delivered after the baby is born.

Table 23–3 lists items related to care of the newborn in the United States. Items used for infants vary among cultures and among different socioeconomic groups within the same culture. Creativity, resourcefulness, and access to community groups or programs that assist the disadvantaged are important for nurses working with clients who are experiencing economic hardship. Currently, a huge number of beautiful infant items are creatively marketed and widely available; however, these are often costly and may only be used for a short time by the healthy, rapidly growing baby. Nurses therefore need to be aware of the cost and alternative sources of infant items, for example, borrowing or buying used items and attending yard sales.

Some families feel guilty if they are not able to provide new, "top-of-the-line" equipment and clothing for their baby, and therefore benefit from the nurse's emphasis on aspects of parenting that are not financially related, such as the quality of parent-infant interactions. By touring the community and visiting various stores to note the cost of infant items, the nurse can provide the third-trimester couple with helpful advice. For example, the same brand of disposable diapers or infant formula may be much more expensive in a local supermarket than in a large "discount" chain store where larger-size packages can also be purchased. (This is not always true, and therefore comparison shopping in each neighborhood is advised.)

Specialized prepared childbirth programs enhance teaching that takes place during prenatal visits in the third trimester. Although prenatal education classes may be available throughout pregnancy, many couples attend series that begin late in the second trimester or early in the third trimester. Nurses are often consulted by clients and other health care providers for referrals to prepared childbirth programs. Childbirth education programs vary greatly; nursing referrals are therefore based on the individual needs and preferences of each family. Nurses working with third-trimester clients may also be asked to discuss or explain topics presented in these classes.

During third-trimester antenatal visits, the nurse explains current physiologic and psychosocial adaptations related to the third trimester. The nurse continues to provide anticipatory guidance to allay potential client anxiety about her normal, low-risk status and to inform her of what she may expect at future visits or in the intrapartum unit. The healthy client needs to understand that the need for increasing the frequency of prenatal visits during the third trimester reflects standard protocols of care rather than problems with her pregnancy.

In the United States, obstetric care for the healthy childbearing family is completed with the final postpartum checkup, usually scheduled around 6 to 8 weeks after delivery. The antenatal nurse advises the

TABLE 23–2. ANSWERS TO QUESTIONS COMMONLY ASKED DURING THE THIRD TRIMESTER

How often should I feel the baby move?

About ten fetal movements are usually felt in a 6-hour period; However, a fetus normally has different activity periods during a 24-hour period. The health care provider should be consulted promptly if a change in the usual patterns of fetal movements, for example, a marked decrease, increase, or absence of fetal movements, is noted.

What can I do to get to sleep at night? I can't seem to get comfortable and I'm tired all day. Is a glass of wine or a beer advisable?

Sleeplessness is a common problem during the third trimester. Helpful strategies include preparing a restful environment before sleep (comfortable room temperature, smoothed bed, soft lights or no light, restful music, tapes of waves, rain, or other relaxing sounds); engaging in relaxation techniques (back rub from partner, relaxation exercises such as imagery); reading nonstressful material; trying to put stressful topics aside at least half an hour before sleep; avoiding stressful confrontations with others before bedtime if possible; drinking a glass of warm milk; avoiding caffeinated foods and beverages, such as chocolate and caffeinated coffee or tea; trying not to focus on insomnia. **Alcoholic beverages of any kind are never recommended during pregnancy because of potential hazards to the fetus.**

Should I abstain from intercourse during the third-trimester? Does sexual intercourse hurt the baby?

There is no reason why the healthy woman with intact membranes should not have intercourse during pregnancy. Sexual intercourse does not hurt the baby.

Is swelling in my feet normal during the third trimester?

Many women normally experience swelling in their feet during the third trimester, especially if they sit or stand for long periods. The large uterus tends to slow circulation from the legs and contributes to the swelling. Sudden swelling in the legs should be reported promptly to the health care provider, particularly if accompanied by swelling of the hands, face, or lower back, headache, altered vision, abdominal pain, or nerve or muscular irritability.

Can I take a bath or go swimming during the third trimester?

Yes, as long as membranes have not ruptured. During late pregnancy, women need to be especially careful not to fall, as increased size and altered center of gravity and balance make trauma a real risk. Skid protectors should be used in bathtubs and showers; women who have difficulty getting in or out of the bathtub may find showering safer.

Is there any problem with traveling for business or vacation until my due date?

Possibly. A due date is calculated for the 40th week of gestation; however, many women deliver at term up to 2 weeks earlier. Planning vacation trips at the end of pregnancy is therefore not advised. Women who must travel should bring a copy of their prenatal health records with them. Strenuous, stressful trips are not recommended during the third trimester, nor is travel to areas of the world where obstetric health care is inaccessible, where there is poor sanitation, and where there is a high incidence of infectious disease.

My dreams are so vivid. Sometimes the baby I dream about doesn't look normal. Is this a cause for worry?

These types of dreams are upsetting, but common occurrences in the third trimester. They do not normally mean that a couple will have a handicapped infant. Talking about the dreams with the health care provider or a supportive significant other may help to decrease anxiety.

At times I feel like my husband is withdrawing from me. He seems so interested in his new hobby. Is this normal?

Yes. During the third trimester, expectant fathers may focus on their own concerns, and may worry about providing for the enlarged family and coping with additional responsibilities. In addition, expectant fathers may fulfill their own desires to create by undertaking a hobby or acquiring a pet at this time. Sharing your feelings about this with your husband may be helpful.

Why is a birth plan important?

A birth plan gives the expectant family a chance to think in advance about what would make their childbirth experience especially meaningful and what they would like to avoid. Finalizing plans in consultation with health care providers during the third trimester and having those plans incorporated into your chart minimize confusion or negotiations at the time of labor and delivery.

What can I do to prevent stretch marks?

Unfortunately, there is currently no known treatment that prevents stretch marks. Moisturizers may prevent dry skin and associated itching.

My hips seem to feel "loose"; sometimes I also have a feeling of pelvic pressure. What can I do for relief?

These are normal symptoms during the third trimester and are related to relaxation of joints and additional, increasing weight of the uterus. Many women experience these symptoms at night in relation to sleeplessness when they cannot seem to get comfortable in bed. Strategies that provide some relief include wearing a support garment, such as a maternity girdle, using good body mechanics, and assuming a side-lying position, with pillows between the legs and supporting the abdomen, when in bed.

During this trimester I have been having a heavy clear to whitish vaginal discharge like I did during my first trimester. Is this normal?

Leukorrhea, which can manifest as a heavy, clear to whitish vaginal discharge, is a normal but common discomfort, especially during the first and third trimesters of pregnancy. Examination is important, however, to confirm that the discharge is indeed normal leukorrhea.

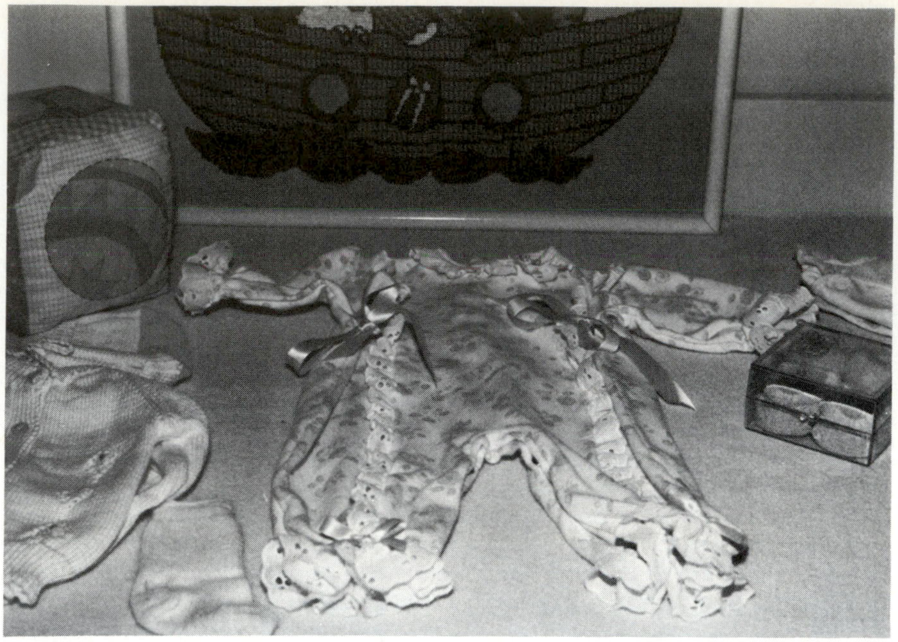

Figure 23–4. Baby layette.

client about the importance of this visit, and encourages the family to call with any questions that may arise.

PROMOTE NUTRITIONAL WELL-BEING

Throughout pregnancy, nutrition remains an essential component of management because of its impact on fetal development and maternal adaptation.

During the third trimester, nutritional status continues to be reflected by such factors as general appearance, the client's pattern of weight gain, fetal growth, previous weight management history and patterns, hemoglobin/hematocrit, usual dietary intake, and consumption of nonfood items.

Weight gain may be perceived by the client as problematic during the third trimester. Careful assessment is needed to diagnose that weight gain is not due to fluid retention related to pathologic conditions, for example, pregnancy-induced hypertension. Dietary counseling can also help the client cope with third-trimester discomforts, such as constipation.

ASSIST THE CLIENT IN COPING WITH THIRD-TRIMESTER DISCOMFORTS

The third trimester is an uncomfortable time for most women. Many discomforts are related to the large size of the uterus and to continuing hormonal changes. Discomforts experienced during the second trimester may continue through the third trimester. In addition, the woman may experience edema of the lower extremeties, varicose veins, lower backache, shortness of breath, and tingling or numbness in the fingers.

The discomforts that the expectant mother experiences during this stage of pregnancy may cause anxiety. Simple explanations of the basis of the discomforts and measures of relief can help relieve the worries experienced by the woman.

Edema of the Feet, Ankles, and Lower Legs

Edema of the feet, ankles, and lower legs is a common discomfort during the third trimester. Women may experience a sense of tightness or pulling in the swollen areas. Shoes worn prenatally may become tight and no longer fit. Some women report an increase in shoe size at this time. Edema of the feet, ankles, and lower legs results from sodium and water retention, which is influenced by such factors as estrogen, cortisol, prolactin, and human placental lactogen. In addition, the pregnant uterus presses on the veins in the legs and impairs return of blood flow from the legs. Posture also influences ankle edema. Sitting or standing for prolonged periods results in increased edema.

The expectant mother should be advised that edema of the ankles, feet, and lower legs is a normal finding in the third trimester. She should be counseled to avoid prolonged sitting or standing and to

TABLE 23–3. ITEMS FOR CARE OF THE NEWBORN

Crib or cradle with well-fitting sturdy mattress.

To promote infant safety, the source and composition of the mattress need to be considered, especially if the mattress is not new. If a crib or cradle cannot be obtained, a large dresser drawer or heavy-duty plasticized laundry basket may be padded and placed on the floor for the infant. A heavy, folded blanket placed inside a pillow case can serve as a mattress. Pillows should not be used as "crib" mattresses, because their softness does not provide adequate support for the infant.

Carriage or stroller that will support the infant when lying flat

An "umbrella"-type stroller is easy and lightweight. The infant and young child will use this for a longer period of time than a heavy carriage; however, not all umbrella-type strollers provide adequate support for the newborn.

Strap-on infant carrier

Car seat

If the infant will travel in an automobile, a car seat is necessary. A car seat can be used as an infant feeding seat and can foster an infant's interest in the environment by providing a wide viewing area. Any infant seat support should have shoulder restraints to prevent injury related to falls.

Clothing

6 undershirts, 2 with cuffs (The 6- to 12-month size allows room for growth and saves the additional cost of infant wear.)

6 receiving blankets

6 "stretchies" or other types of seasonal infant outfits

1 or 2 infant sweaters or sweatshirts

2 infant hats (in hot weather, for sun protection; in cool weather, for protection and warmth)

1 infant snowsuit or heavy outerwear (in cold climates)

Bedding items

1 heavy blanket

2 or 3 infant crib sheets

2 crib pads (cotton on one side, plastic or rubber on the other side)

Diaper bag

This does not have to be a special "diaper" bag, but could be any spacious bag made of canvas or other sturdy material.

Diapers

1 large (48 count) box or package of disposable diapers, if these are to be used

36 diapers, if cloth are to be used and laundered at home (more may be obtained, depending on how often laundry will be washed.)

12 thin "birdseye" diapers (These are versatile for folding and dry more quickly than heavier diapers.)

36 diaper liners

1 deep diaper bucket for soiled diapers and neutralizing solution such as baking soda (one-half cup dissolved in warm water)

Diaper service (If this service will be used, initial delivery will be scheduled before infant is born or comes home.)

4 diaper pins (2 for use, one extra set) (Avoid plastic heads, as they tend to break with frequent use. Pins may be stored open in a bar of soap. The soap allows pins to slide easily into diaper fabric. **Pins must be kept out of reach of other children and of the infant**.)

6 or 12 (one package) cloth diapers for clients who use disposable diapers (These make excellent shoulder or crib sheet protectors.)

3 to 6 pairs of plastic pants

1 container of diaper wipes to be used to clean infant when away from home. (For a less expensive alternative, cut a disposable cloth in two, soap one piece, wet the other piece, and place in separate plastic bags or containers to use when traveling.)

Items related to infant feeding

6 baby bibs (plastic lined, remove after feeding)

6 baby bottles with nipples, 8-oz size (Bottles may also be obtained by breastfeeding mothers who will be expressing milk for infant feeding.)

1 manual breast pump for breastfeeding mothers (cylinder type, eg, Kanason) For bottle feeding mothers, 1 week's supply of infant formula, as prescribed by the pediatrician (When finances are a major concern, formula may be purchased in advance at intervals and in accordance with the family's budget. Many retailers will accept returned formula if in unused condition with seals intact, should this become necessary.) Powdered formula is the most economical, because the client needs to mix only what will be consumed.

1 small nipple brush for cleaning bottle nipples

1 bottle brush

3 pacifiers

Mild soap for laundering infant clothing

White vinegar (one-half cup in rinse water) may be used to soften baby clothes.

(continued)

TABLE 23–3. ITEMS FOR CARE OF THE NEWBORN *(continued)*

Infant bath items
Special infant bathing tubs are an unnecessary expense for the family with financial concerns. Once the umbilical cord stump has dried and healed, a large plastic dishpan, used exclusively for the infant, or a clean bathroom tub may be used.
Mild soap for use on infant's skin
2 bath towels, 3 thin washcloths (easier to use with an infant), and 1 hand towel (to be placed under the infant in the bath to prevent sliding)
Infant skin care items
Emollient (avoid baby oils, make certain to remove before reapplying)
1 box of corn starch
White petroleum jelly without additives (especially for use with circumcised male infants)
Paper nail file for fingernails (Avoid scissors or metal files to prevent injury.)
Storage items, eg, dresser and cabinet
If lack of furniture is a problem, heavy-duty cartons, available free from supermarkets or other stores, can be obtained, covered with contact paper for a bright look and stacked sideways to form open shelves.

Courtesy of Kathleen Y. Donnelly, RN.

avoid restrictive clothing around the legs.[12] "Knee high" stockings should be discouraged, because the elastic bands prevent adequate venous drainage and contribute to edema. She should continue to meet fluid requirements of 6 to 8 full glasses of noncaffeinated beverages each day. Normal edema in the lower extremities or fingers does not require fluid restrictions. Resting with the legs elevated or lying down on the left side should help reduce swelling by facilitating venous drainage from the lower extremeties. The supine position should be discouraged because of the risk of supine hypotensive syndrome.

Edema of the face may be a sign of pregnancy-induced hypertension; the woman with this type of edema requires further evaluation.

Urinary Frequency

As discussed previously, the presenting part of the fetus may settle into the pelvis during the last month of pregnancy, placing pressure on the bladder. The woman again experiences urinary frequency. Nursing interventions focus on evaluation of the woman to make certain that the urinary frequency is a normal manifestation of third-trimester pregnancy and not a sign of urinary tract infection or other pathology. Fluids should not be restricted. Other than reassuring the woman of the normalcy of this condition and its indication that pregnancy will soon be completed, there are no measures that can provide adequate relief.

Nocturia

In addition to the nuisance of urinary frequency during the third trimester, the woman may experience increased production of urine at night or during prolonged rest periods, especially when in a side-lying position. When the weight of the uterus is removed from the vena cava and other venous blood vessels, venous drainage and renal blood flow are facilitated. More urine is produced, and the woman may be awakened during the night.[2,12] This condition complicates insomnia for some women and may lead to sleep deprivation. Explanations of this normal condition may help relieve anxiety. Although reducing fluid intake after dinner may provide a small amount of relief, women should be careful to space a fluid intake of six to eight full glasses of noncaffeinated beverages throughout the day. In addition, care should be taken to avoid falls when getting up during the night. There should be a clear path to the bathroom; a nightlight is also helpful.

Insomnia

Insomnia during the third trimester may be attributed to several factors, such as difficulty in finding a comfortable position as a result of the enlarged uterus, fetal activity, heartburn, nocturia, and emotional concerns. For a woman accustomed to falling asleep on her abdomen, the third trimester requires changes in a lifelong practice. Suggested relief measures may work for many women.[12]

- Have a warm drink before bedtime. Alcoholic beverages, including wine and beer, should not be recommended, because of potential effects on the fetus.
- Avoid stimulation found in caffeinated foods such as chocolate and coffee.
- Seek quiet activities before bedtime. (For some women, reading a textbook has an excellent sedative effect!)
- Never take sleeping pills or other medications without first consulting the health care provider.

- Attempt relaxation techniques such as deep breathing or visualizing herself in a quiet and peaceful environment.
- Have her partner provide a backrub to promote relaxation.

Varicose Veins

Varicose veins in the legs, vulva, and rectum may be especially problematic during the third trimester, although they also cause discomfort earlier in pregnancy (Figure 23–5). Discomfort from varicosities may be experienced as a dull, throbbing-type pain. Varicose veins are aggravated by venous congestion, which worsens because of pressure from the expanding uterus. Progesterone, which relaxes smooth muscles and the walls and valves of veins, may also contribute to the development of varicosities. Unfortunately varicose vein formation may also be familial. The expectant mother should be advised to avoid restrictive clothing around the legs; to avoid prolonged sitting and standing; to wear supportive pantyhose, which should be put on before getting up in the morning; to keep the legs uncrossed when sitting; to rest with legs elevated or in a left side-lying position (placing a pillow between the legs may also provide relief for varicosities of the vulva and rectum); to provide support for vulvar varicosities (this may be done by using a sanitary belt to hold a foam rubber pad in place); and to call her health care provider if signs of phlebitis (areas of hardness, redness, swelling, increased pain) should occur.[12]

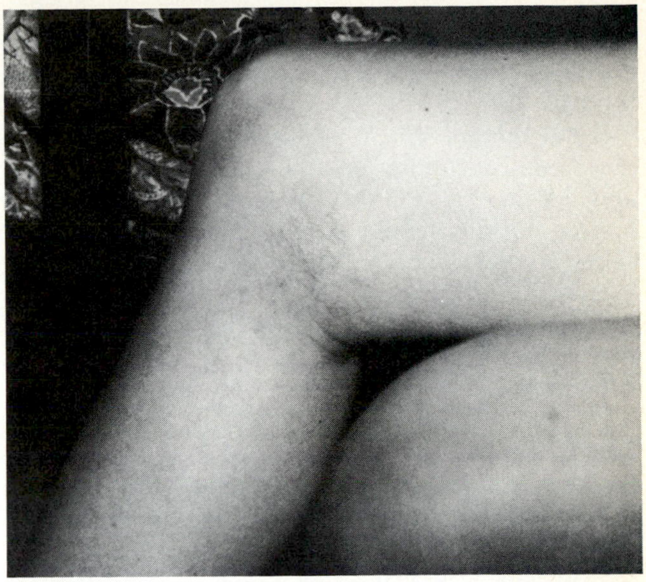

Figure 23–5. Varicose veins.

Lower Backache

Lower backache is very common as pregnancy progresses because of the compensatory changes in

RESEARCH ABSTRACT

Jacobs MK, et al. Leg-volume changes with EPIC and posturing in dependent pregnancy edema. Nurs Res. *1986;35:86–89.*

The purpose of this study was to explore the differential effects of external pneumatic intermittent compression (EPIC) and posturing on leg-volume changes in healthy pregnant women with dependent leg edema. The sample consisted of 35 healthy pregnant women who had 3+ to 4+ pretibial and pedal edema. All women were in the third trimester of pregnancy. The women were randomly assigned to one of two groups. The treatment (experimental) group (17 women) received EPIC and posturing; the control group (18 women) received only posturing.

The EPIC treatment was administered by use of a pump with leg boots that had varying pressure controls. This device allowed the investigators to apply a set amount of pressure in a set amount of time. Leg circumference measurements were taken prior to and after treatments. After the second set of measurements, both groups walked for 10 minutes; a third set of measurements was then taken.

Analysis of covariance indicated that volume losses were greater for the experimental group than for the control group immediately after the EPIC procedure. Although some of this effect was lost after the experimental group subjects walked, volume loss was still greater than for the control group subjects; however, volume decreases were also significant for the control group subjects after posturing in the left lateral position. The researchers concluded that EPIC may be a useful treatment for relieving dependent edema.

Comment:

A large amount (3+ and 4+) of edema in the lower extremities can be an uncomfortable and unsightly condition in late pregnancy. This study suggsts that the EPIC treatment may provide one source of relief. The study also highlights the value of the left lateral position in reducing lower extreity edema. The study offers additional empirical support for teaching about positioning, a strategy that may relieve edema comfortably and without cost.

posture resulting from the enlarging uterus (*see* Figure 20–4). As discussed previously, musculoskeletal changes in the third trimester result in a progressive lordosis.

The mother should be taught to use correct body mechanics, including positions for sitting, standing, and lifting (Figure 23–6); to avoid back strain from improper or excessive lifting; to wear low-heeled shoes to reduce back strain; to practice pelvic tilt exercises (*see* Chapter 24) to help strengthen the muscles supporting the uterus; and to use a well-fitting, nonconstricting maternity girdle to provide support.[12]

Leg Cramps

Sudden, painful leg cramps may occur during the third trimester. The physiologic reason is unclear. Explanations attributing leg cramps to calcium-phosphorus metabolism or pressure from the enlarging uterus on pelvic blood vessels have never been supported.[12] Several measures may provide relief. Dorsiflexing the foot ("toes pointed toward the nose") may relieve cramping. Pressing the bottom of the foot against a firm flat surface, such as the footboard of the bed or the floor, is also helpful. Good body mechanics should be employed to facilitate circulation. An adequate diet is always advised. If prescribed by a certified nurse-midwife or physician, milk intake can be stopped and strategies such as supplemental calcium and vitamin E implemented.[12]

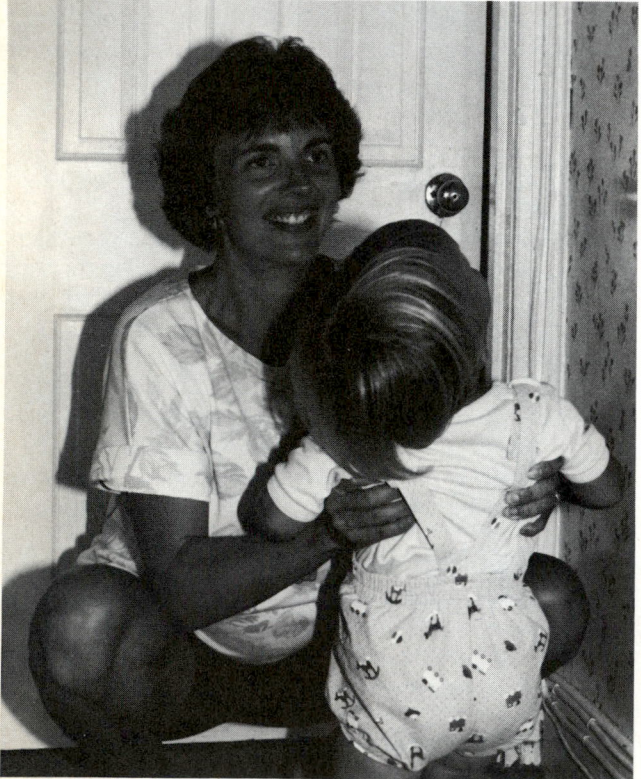

Figure 23–6. A woman should use correct body mechanics when picking up a child.

Shortness of Breath

During the third trimester the expectant mother may experience shortness of breath as the uterus pushes the diaphragm upward. The nurse may advise the woman to avoid hyperventilation and consciously try to regulate her breathing when she realizes she is hyperventilating; to practice correct body mechanics to allow for maximum expansion of the lungs; to use two or more pillows at night to identify a comfortable position; and periodically to stand and take a deep breath while stretching the arms overhead.[12]

Carpal Tunnel Syndrome

Carpal tunnel syndrome is a condition in which feelings of tingling, numbness, and burning are felt in the fingers and hands. It is thought to result from edema, which compresses the median nerve within the carpal tunnel at the wrist. The woman's posture, such as holding the shoulders too far back and flexing the head forward to counterbalance the heavy uterus and curved back of late pregnancy, contributes to this condition. Discomfort may be present on awakening. Relief measures include raising the affected hand above the head and flexing and slowly extending the fingers upward to relieve symptoms, paying attention to good posture, and, if necessary, using a splint, applied to the slightly flexed wrist and worn during sleep.[2,12,13]

PROMOTE CLIENT SAFETY

Safety continues to be an important aspect of nursing care during the third trimester. As delivery approaches, the woman continues to be concerned about safety for herself and her fetus.

The woman's large size, altered center of gravity, and balance make trauma related to falls a concern during the third trimester. Often, normal physiologic changes will provide women with clues regarding activities they can no longer undertake; however, women should be advised to avoid activities that require balance, such as climbing ladders or using a chair as a ladder at work or at home. Recreational sports that require balance and speed, such as skiing, are not recommended during late pregnancy. Health care providers may need to provide the expectant mother's employer with written verification of the need for her to refrain from certain work-related activities that jeopardize the safety of the woman or her fetus during late pregnancy.

Showering and bathing are permitted as long as membranes remain intact; however, the third-trimester pregnant woman's large size makes getting out of a tub difficult. Special care must be taken to avoid falls. Early in pregnancy, skid protectors, available inexpensively in hardware stores, bath shops, and other retail settings, can be applied to the bottom of tubs and showers to make these surfaces less slippery when wet. (Skid protectors also promote safety for nonpregnant family members.) The temperature of hot water can be lowered to prevent scalding. This also promotes safety for the newborn and young child, lowers the water heating bill, and still provides water hot enough for comfortable bathing.

Seat harnesses should continue to be used, although during the third-trimester women may need to shift position frequently to remain comfortable. Figure 19–3 illustrates the proper way to wear a seat harness during late pregnancy.

At each visit, the nurse continues to assist the client in identification of safety concerns and of potential safety hazards related to lifestyle or environment. The nurse also assists the client in developing ways to minimize or avoid these. Warning or danger signs of pregnancy continue to be reviewed (*see* Table 15–7).

As discussed in Chapter 39, high-risk conditions such as pregnancy-induced hypertension and premature labor can appear during the third trimester and present severe complications. Signs and symptoms of preterm and term labor are discussed with the client (*see* Table 18–7). As term approaches, signs and symptoms of normal labor are presented, along with appropriate strategies.

The nurse continues to provide positive reinforcement and support for self-care practices that promote wellness, such as breast self-examination and good nutritional patterns.

Discussion of safety issues includes plans for care of the newborn. During the third trimester, the nurse discusses the importance of always using an infant car seat when traveling in an automobile, as the family may wish to obtain a seat prior to the baby's birth. Many hospitals or charitable groups will provide infant seats at minimal or no charge. The nurse can identify and appropriately refer clients in need of these services.

Expectant parents may "babyproof" their home during late pregnancy. Many people enjoy all preparations for the newborn, and the postpartum period is often too hectic for some parents to make this aspect of safety a priority. (Ideally, parents who have young children will have done this already.) The infant develops so rapidly within the first year that potential hazards can become actual hazards suddenly. Table 23–4 lists ways to "baby proof" a home.

Concerns for safe passage for self and fetus are especially important during the third trimester as delivery approaches. By encouraging the client to express her concerns and by listening intently, the nurse encourages the client to express her fears related to safety, provides relevant teaching, and offers appropriate reassurance.

TABLE 23–4. WAYS TO "BABYPROOF" A HOME

Walk through each room in your home. Look carefully from the floor to the ceiling in each room. Are there any potential or real hazards to the safety of an infant? Assume that babies are curious, will pull, chew, or swallow anything, and have no "judgment."
Place protectors on each electric outlet.
Examine the area around the baby's crib or cradle. Remove wires, extension cords, and other items that could be pulled or could fall into the baby's crib.
Examine all baby toys carefully. Do not use any toys with sharp or removable pieces that could cut the baby or be swallowed by the baby. Do not use any large toys or objects that could possibly smother an infant. For example, large stuffed animals or crib bumpers are not appropriate for use with the newborn.
Reduce the temperature of the hot water so that it is not able to scald directly from the tap.
Use cribs with slats that are less than 2⅜ in. apart to avoid head injuries. Check cribs that are more than 2 years old for dangers that might result in injuries (Figure 23–7).
Remove all medications, matches, household cleaners, and other chemicals from areas accessible to young children (this becomes important as the child develops).
Place guard rails on any windows that can be opened.
Discuss plans for supervision of pets around the newborn. Make certain that the infant can rest in a crib or cradle inaccessible to pets.
Repair peeling paint or plaster on ceiling or walls near the infant's personal areas.
Use only products that are nontoxic to infants and young children. Follow the manufacturers' directions carefully; contact manufacturers for additional product information related to use around children.

DANGER!

Protect Your Baby

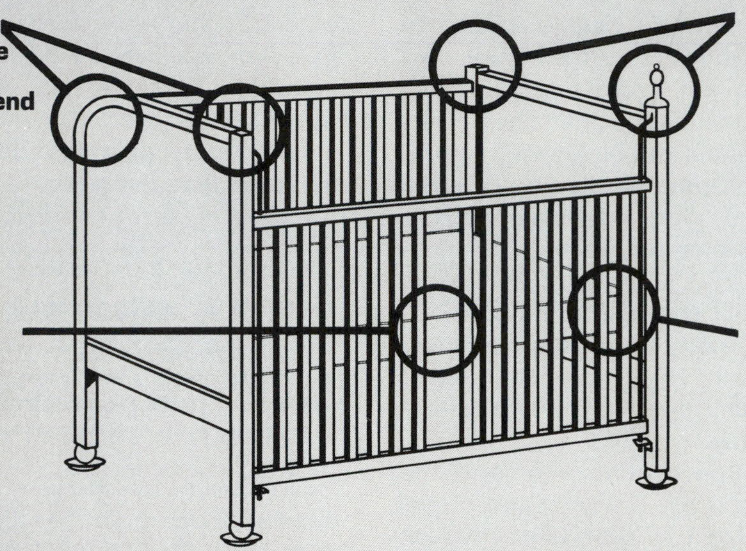
YES! Corner posts should be same height as the end panels, and NOT extend above end panels.
NO! Decorative corner posts present entanglement hazard to child climbing out of crib.
BEWARE! Space between slats must be less than 2⅜" wide, and no slats should be missing.
BEWARE! Mattress must fit snugly next to the crib so that there is NO gap.

CHECK YOUR CRIB FOR THE FOLLOWING DANGERS:

- ☐ **Corner Posts:** Should be the same height as the end panels, and NOT extend above end panels. Remove extended corner posts by unscrewing or sawing off and sanding smooth. Children's clothing catches on extended corner posts.
- ☐ **Slats:** Space between slats should be less than 2⅜" and no slats missing. Children attempt to squeeze feet first through wider slats, but their heads get caught.
- ☐ **Mattress Fit:** Mattress must fit snugly next to the crib so that there is no gap. If two adult fingers can fit between mattress and crib, mattress should be replaced. Sleeping or active child may become trapped in wider gaps and suffocate.
- ☐ **Placement of Crib:** Do not place a crib near a window where cords from blinds or drapes may strangle a child. Once an infant is able to crawl or kneel, remove mobiles and all other hanging cords and strings from the crib.
- ☐ **End Panels:** Be sure end panels extend below mattress at its lowest position. Child can strangle by becoming trapped in space between mattress and end panel.
- ☐ **Crib Hardware:** All screws, bolts, and hardware must be in place and tight to prevent crib's collapse. Mattress support hangers and brackets should be securely attached to end panels and no wooden parts should be cracked. Child's activity can cause crib to collapse, trapping and suffocating child.
- ☐ **Side Latches:** The drop side latches must not be easily releasable by a child, and must hold securely in a raised position to prevent fall.
- ☐ **Cutouts:** Cribs with cutout designs in end panels must not be used. Child can strangle by becoming entrapped in cutout.
- ☐ **Teething Rail:** Remove or replace if damaged or loose.
- ☐ **Child's Height:** When a child first climbs out of the crib or is 32"–35" tall, it has outgrown the crib and should sleep in a bed. A crib is not a playpen. Top rails of drop-sides, when raised, should be at least 26" above the top of the mattress support. The top rail of a lowered side should be at least 9" above the mattress support to prevent falls.
- ☐ **Paint:** Any paint used on a crib must be high-quality non-toxic household enamel. Be very careful of the paint on a hand-me-down. If the crib was made prior to February 1978, the paint may have a higher lead content than current safety standards allow. All wood surfaces should be free of splinters and cracks.
- ☐ **Plastic Bags:** Do not use plastic bags or plastic material for mattress covers. Children suffocate when plastic material clings to face.

35 BABIES TREATED FOR CRIB INJURIES EVERY DAY

IF YOUR CRIB IS MORE THAN TWO YEARS OLD, EXAMINE IT CAREFULLY FOR DANGERS LISTED ON THIS POSTER

Please report crib injuries, deaths and crib hazards to the Consumer Product Safety Commission at 1-800-638-CPSC. For more information or a crib safety pamphlet, write: The Danny Foundation, Post Office Box 680, Alamo, CA 94507, or call toll free 1-800-83-DANNY.

Figure 23–7. Cribs should be checked for safety features and potential dangers. (*Courtesy of the Danny Foundation, Alamo, California.*)

EVALUATE ANTENATAL CARE

Third-trimester evaluation continues to address the extent to which behavioral objectives are achieved. For example, meeting self-care objectives related to third-trimester edema of the legs and feet would be noted by a decrease in swelling after implementation of such strategies as resting on the left side, elevating the legs, and no longer wearing knee-high stockings with constricting bands. The value the client places on prenatal care is evidenced by verbal reports, regular attendance at prenatal visits, and willingness to implement prescribed care strategies. Evaluation, related to outcome behaviors identified in the care plan, continues to be carefully documented in the client's chart.

Prenatal written records, kept in the client's chart, allow for continuity of care by intrapartum and postpartum staff who may not have known the client personally before her delivery, as frequently happens in hospital settings.

ENSURE APPROPRIATE REFERRALS FOR THE CLIENT

Except for routine well-woman examinations or in situations where family practitioners provide care across the life span, the healthy family will have the most contact with pediatric health care providers after the postpartum period. In many situations, this relationship extends until the child reaches young adulthood. Antenatal nurses and physicians should encourage clients to select and to meet with their pediatric health care provider prior to the birth of the infant. Health care providers should also be prepared to provide referrals for pediatric care.

As discussed earlier, nurses frequently provide referrals to educational programs for childbirth preparation and early parenting and to other care providers such as social service workers.

CASE STUDY/CARE PLAN: CARE OF THE FAMILY DURING THE THIRD TRIMESTER

Belinda and Luis Mendez are a Chicano couple who are expecting their second child in 10 weeks. They have an 8-year-old daughter, Yolanda, who was born after a difficult labor at 38 weeks' gestation. She is currently at the appropriate developmental level and attends public school.

Belinda (34 years old) is a loan officer at a local bank and plans to return to work 6 weeks after delivery. Luis (40 years old) is a partner in a law firm. Luis' father, who has a small apartment in the Barrio, keeps in constant touch with the family.

Since early in her first trimester, Belinda has received care from a certified nurse-midwife at a birth center. Luis, who did not attend the first delivery, would like to be present at the birth. Yolanda is attending the sibling preparation program at the birth center and would also like to be with her parents when the baby is born.

Although Belinda has had a normal pregnancy, she has been experiencing backache and inability to "fit into her shoes." At the current visit she is upset because she has had dreams of her baby being malformed.

(continued)

CASE STUDY/CARE PLAN: Care of the Family During the Third Trimester *(continued)*

Supporting Assessment Data	Expected Client/Family Outcome	Nursing Action/ Intervention	Rationale	Criteria for Evaluation
PHYSIOLOGIC STATE				
Nursing Diagnosis: Alteration in comfort, related to physiologic changes during the third trimester				
Client reports lower backache especially when sitting and standing too long; ankle edema, "can't even get my shoes on anymore"	By end of visit, the client will: Identify changes in body mechanics that will decrease discomfort	Reinforce pelvic tilt exercises and use of proper body mechanics when standing, bending, and lifting.	Physiologic changes that occur as pregnancy progresses produce predictable discomforts. Knowledge of physiologic changes allows the client to remedy the discomforts.	Client describes changes in body mechanics that will decrease discomfort (eg, postural changes, demonstration of pelvic tilt exercises, and proper body mechanics).
	Describe the physiologic basis for discomforts in late pregnancy	Teach couple possible factors that cause back pain during late pregnancy: gravid uterus, stretching of abdominal muscles, increased curvature of spine.	Discussion of discomforts and their physiologic bases can reduce stress. Reinforcement facilitates learning.	Client discusses with the nurse the basis for backache, and ankle edema.
	Implement self-care practices to increase comfort	Encourage client to wear comfortable clothing and shoes; take frequent rest periods with legs elevated; avoid prolonged standing and sitting; use techniques of leg extension and foot dorsiflexion for leg cramps; check for physiologic alterations that might produce the same symptoms (eg, pregnancy-induced hypertension, phlebitis).	Comprehensive assessment includes ruling out pathophysiology.	The client relates changing self-care practices to increased comfort (eg, resting with legs elevated, stooping instead of bending, and so forth.
NUTRITIONAL STATE				
Nursing Diagnosis: Potential asset for lactation, related to nutritional status of the mother				
Weight gain appropriate for gestation. Hgb 12.5 g/dL Hct 36% Client reports that diet includes nutrients from four food groups	By end of seventh month, the family will: Describe the physiology of lactation	Assess the family's knowledge of lactation. Assess the family's knowledge about nutrition for breastfeeding.	Good maternal nutritional status promotes lactation and infant nutrition.	Family members point to diagram of the breast, identify the anatomy and discuss basic physiology of lactation. Family members can identify techniques to promote lactation.
Clients states that she and her husband have chosen to breastfeed their baby	Describe a culturally acceptable, nutritious diet that will facilitate lactation	Teach maternal nutrient needs during lactation: Increase protein by 20 g per day; Increase vitamins and minerals; Increase calories by 500 per day. Plan with family a sample daily diet that will facilitate lactation, taking into consideration cultural food preferences	Prenatal nutritional counseling will influence the adequacy of the diet during lactation.	Client and family members describe the type and amount of nutrients necessary to maintain lactation. Family members plan a diet that fits their cultural background and meets the requirements of lactation.

Supporting Assessment Data	Expected Client/Family Outcome	Nursing Action/ Intervention	Rationale	Criteria for Evaluation
	Identify community resources that will foster nutrition and lactation	Provide a list of community resources such as LaLeche League or lactation consultants that will assist in the breastfeeding experience.	Support systems in the community and family are often instrumental in the success of breastfeeding.	Client and family leave visit with listing of appropriate community resources, such and LaLeche League. Family members identify resources that are accessible in the neighborhood.
PSYCHOSOCIAL STATE				
Nursing Diagnosis: Potential alteration in family coping, related to maternal fantasies of the third trimester				
Client reports being upset by having several dreams of her baby being born malformed: "I dream about having a little boy with no ears and a strange nose." Father states "I hate to hear that she has dreams like that. I've been very worried about this baby being normal throughout the pregnancy."	By eighth month of pregnancy, the family will: Identify maternal fantasies as normal aspect of pregnancy	Inform the couple that it is normal to have such fantasies, especially during the third trimester.	Women's nightdreams and other fantasies increase during the third trimester and are often about frightening situations.	When asked, family members discuss fantasies.
	Discuss feelings about fantasies together and with nurse and other members of health care team and family	Encourage couple to relate any daydreams or nightdreams about pregnancy, childbirth, or infant.	It is common for both men and women to fantasize during pregnancy.	Family members discuss positive and negative reactions to fantasies.
	Identify underlying concerns that might be connected with maternal fantasies	Explore with couple their feelings concerning their fantasies.	Fantasies may be connected to some underlying concern.	Family members link fantasies with concerns such as childcare.
	Identify coping strategies to manage concerns that might be connected with maternal fantasies	Assist the couple in identifying strategies to cope with any concerns that might be connected with specific fantasies, eg, "talking it out."	Discussion of fantasies and coping strategies can reduce anxiety.	Family members devise a plan for managing identified concerns such as childcare preparation classes, parenting support groups, and so on.
Nursing Diagnosis: Potential alteration in self-esteem, related to fear of labor and delivery				
Couple expresses fear regarding labor and delivery Couple attends preparation for childbirth classes	By eighth month of pregnancy, the family will: Express their fears concerning labor and delivery	Encourage couple to express their fears regarding labor and delivery.	Fear of the unknown or previous negative experiences causes anxiety.	Family members identify and discuss labor and delivery fears with nurse.
Client practices relaxation exercises several times each day Couple reads and rereads literature concerning labor and delivery	Discuss specific fears concerning labor and delivery	Encourage the couple to identify specific fears such as pain and loss of control	Allowing the family to communicate their fears in a nonthreatening atmosphere will foster identification of fears and problem-solving processes.	
Client describes own previous negative labor experiences and the negative experiences of family members and friends	Discuss previous labor and delivery experience	Explore with couple previous labor and delivery experiences and methods they used to cope with them, eg, breathing, support systems.		Family members discuss positive and negative aspects of previous birth experience.

(continued)

CASE STUDY/CARE PLAN: Care of the Family During the Third Trimester *(continued)*

Supporting Assessment Data	Expected Client/Family Outcome	Nursing Action/ Intervention	Rationale	Criteria for Evaluation
		Review with couple knowledge gained in childbirth education classes.	In the teaching-learning process, it is important to identify what the learner knows and any apprehensions he or she may have about labor and delivery.	
	Identify several strategies to cope with fear of labor and delivery experience	Review family's birth plan.		Couple identifies coping strategies from content learned in childbirth education. Couple describes birth plans
Nursing Diagnosis: Potential asset in sibling bonding, related to total family participation in the childbearing experience				
Couple states that they would like their daughter to attend the birth 8-year-old daughter also expresses excitement about seeing the baby born Daughter has begun to attend sibling classes, but has several questions	By end of eighth month, the family will: Identify their respective roles in the childbearing experience Discuss their daughter's role in the birthing process	Explore with family their perceptions of their roles during the childbirth experience.	The third trimester is seen as the most appropriate time to begin preparation of siblings for childbirth.	Family decides that daughter will witness birth
	Evaluate their daughter's preparedness concerning the birthing experience	Explore with daughter what was learned in sibling preparation class. Use a model and a doll to reinforce learning at daughter's developmental level. Explore with daughter her feelings and wishes with regard to participation in the birth experience.	Strategies used for teaching children about birth should be age appropriate, eg, books, dolls, movies.	Through play, the daughter will demonstrate knowledge of the birth and readiness to participate.
	Identify resources that will facilitate a positive experience for the sibling	Refer family to other community resources that prepare siblings for the birth experience.	Referring the family to appropriate community resources assists in sibling and family coping.	
		Explore possibility of having a separate support person for daughter present at the birth.	Children need support persons during new and different procedures or experiences. Parents involved in delivery cannot also attend to child care.	Family members identify specific support person for the child during the birth process.
Nursing Diagnosis: Potential alteration in paternal self-esteem, related to cultural conflict				
Client's husband states that his father, who was born in Mexico, keeps telling him that "it is not manly to be around women in labor"	By end of eighth month, the husband will identify cultural conflicts concerning paternal participation in the childbirth experience	Explore with husband his cultural beliefs and practices. Encourage open communication between husband and his own father.	Acculturation is an important factor to be considered when caring for the childbearing family. Men from the expectant grandfather's culture did not traditionally attend births. Families may be influenced by the attitudes of significant others.	Client's husband describes his relationship with his own father, his cultural background, and family expectation of roles.

SUMMARY

By the end of the third trimester, the low-risk, healthy client is physiologically ready for labor, and the pregnant family is psychologically prepared for the birth of the infant. Management during the third trimester continues, modifies, or adds to first- and second-trimester strategies to meet the unique needs of the expectant family during late pregnancy. An interdisciplinary approach is needed to provide comprehensive care to the expectant family.

Third-trimester management for the healthy client includes assessment every other week and then weekly until delivery, anticipatory guidance, and teaching. During late pregnancy, clients normally feel negative about being pregnant. Nurses must differentiate between normal wishes to have pregnancy finally end and high-risk emotional conditions, including rejection of the fetus.

During the third trimester, nurses assist clients in finalizing their birth plans and alternative birth plans. Educational preparation focuses not only on adaptations during late pregnancy, but on topics related to labor and delivery, postpartum, and newborn care. Safety during late pregnancy and in care of the newborn is an important subject. Teaching includes topics that will be important in the care of the newborn, such as "babyproofing" the home.

As in Chapters 15 and 19, management for the third trimester was organized according to nursing care goals. Management subjects, such as strategies to relieve discomforts related to the third trimester and answers to questions commonly asked during the third trimester, were presented. Application of the nursing process to a healthy, third-trimester pregnant family was demonstrated by a case study and care plan.

REVIEW QUESTIONS

1. Discuss advice regarding development of a birth plan that should be given to the client and describe the rationale for the development of alternative birth plans.
2. Describe strategies that may be used to promote psychologic adaptation of the client and family during the third trimester.
3. Identify topics that would be included in client education during the third trimester.
4. Discuss advice related to infant safety that would be given to expectant parents making preparations during the third trimester.
5. Identify discomforts related to the third trimester of pregnancy and describe strategies to help clients cope with the discomforts.

REFERENCES

1. American Academy of Pediatrics, American College of Obstetricians and Gynecologists. In: Frigoletto FD, Little GA, eds. *Guidelines for Perinatal Care*. 2nd ed. White Plains, NY: March of Dimes Birth Defects Foundation; 1988.
2. Cunningham FG, et al. *Williams Obstetrics*. 18th ed. Norwalk, Conn: Appleton & Lange; 1989.
3. Aukamp V. *Nursing Care Plans for the Childbearing Family*. Norwalk, Conn: Appleton-Century-Crofts; 1984.
4. Kay M. The Mexican American. In: Clark A, ed. *Culture, Childbearing, Health Professionals*. Philadelphia: FA Davis; 1978.
5. Simkin P, Reinke C. *Planning Your Baby's Birth*. Seattle: Pennypress; 1980.
6. McKay S. Consumer-provider relationships. In: Nichols FH, Humenick SS, eds. *Childbirth Education: Practice, Research, and Theory*. Philadelphia: WB Saunders; 1988: 485–503.
7. McKay S, Phillips C. *Family Centered Maternity Care*. Rockville, Md: Aspen; 1984.
8. Sherwen LN. Maternal role attainment. In: Sherwen LN, ed. *Psychosocial Dimensions of the Childbearing Family*. New York: Springer Publishing Co; 1987:85–108.
9. Lederman RP. *Psychosocial Adaptation in Pregnancy*. Englewood Cliffs, NJ: Prentice-Hall; 1984.
10. Sherwen LN. Fantasy patterns of the pregnant woman. In: Sherwen LN, ed. *Psychosocial Dimensions of the Pregnant Family*. New York: Springer Publishing Co; 1987:109–127.
11. Sherwen LN. The pregnant man. In Sherwen LN, ed. *Psychosocial Dimensions of the Pregnant Family*. New York: Springer Publishing Co; 1987:157–176.
12. Varney H. *Nurse-Midwifery*. 2nd ed. Boston: Blackwell Scientific; 1987.
13. Kitzinger S. *The Complete Book of Pregnancy and Childbirth*. Revised ed. New York: Knopf; 1989.

Educational Needs of the Healthy Childbearing Family

unit 6

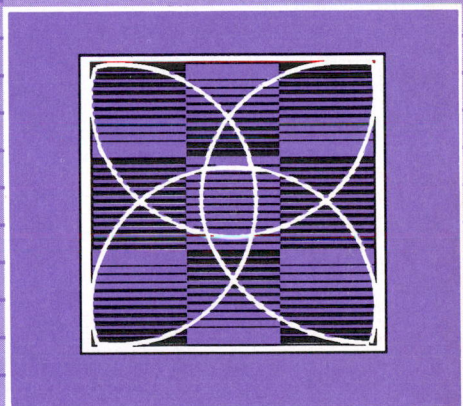

Educational Preparation for Childbirth

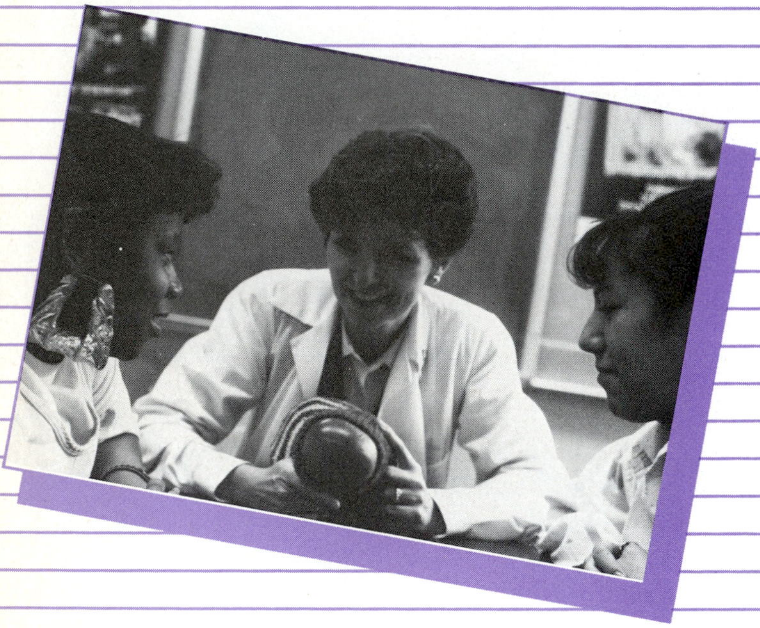

chapter 24

Key Terms

- birth center
- birth plans
- certified nurse-midwife
- hospital birthing room
- Lamaze technique
- lay midwife
- "natural childbirth"
- psychoprophylaxis

Client education is a major component of the nursing care of the childbearing family as the opportunity for client teaching arises in nearly every setting in which nurses interact with pregnant families. The teaching roles of the nurse include one-to-one explanation and discussion, client education classes, and nurse-authored pamphlets, articles, books, and audiovisual packages directed toward education of the childbearing family. These roles are equally important; however, the scope and focus of the roles are not the same and, therefore, different objectives and strategies are required.

All clients require and benefit from educational preparation for childbearing and early parenting. Differences in cultural and educational background among clients challenge the nurse to present material that is acceptable and understandable to the client. Educational preparation includes teaching related to physical and psychosocial changes of childbearing, childbirth alternatives, and ways in which the client and her family can best be prepared for advancing pregnancy, labor, delivery, and the newborn.

TEACHING-LEARNING CONSIDERATIONS DURING CHILDBEARING

Much has been written about how people learn. Mastery of a subject involves not only information (cognitive domain), but an individual's attitude and readiness to learn (affective domain) and ability to perform whatever skills are necessary (psychomotor domain).[1] For example, if a couple want a birth using **psychoprophylaxis,** they need to acquire basic information about childbirth and the breathing techniques necessary for this method, be motivated to seek and attend teaching sessions about this method, and master their ability to perform the appropriate breathing patterns. If their knowledge base is incomplete, if they do not care to learn about the method, or if they are unable to do the breathing patterns, they cannot be expected to have a successful birth experience using psychoprophylaxis. If the nurse presents information on a level the couple cannot understand, if classes are held at times incompatible with the couple's work schedules, or if opportunity for supervised practice is not provided during the classes, the nurse, rather than the clients, establishes an ineffective teaching-learning situation.

The nurse must consider several factors before attempting to provide client education. This is as important for nurses expecting to give "on the spot" teaching in a clinic or labor room setting as for nurses conducting a series of prepared childbirth classes.

Who are the learners? What are their demographic characteristics, especially with regard to their cultural background and socioeconomic and educational levels? Although it may be assumed that almost all individuals are capable of learning, teaching strategies differ greatly for different learners. For example, diet counseling for women from financially poor backgrounds needs to focus on low-cost nutritious foods, whereas price might not even be a consideration for women from wealthy backgrounds. A frightened adolescent who has had no prenatal care and arrives ready to deliver does not have the same learning needs as the prepared, mature couple who comes to the labor suite with a list documenting the frequency and duration of each contraction. The client's cultural background must also be considered when devising appropriate teaching strategies. The box presents teaching strategies appropriate for clients from various cultural backgrounds.

What is the purpose and length of the teaching-learning situation? Is the nurse providing anticipatory guidance for one clinic visit? Is the nurse assuming a major ongoing responsibility for assisting couples to prepare for childbirth through a series of classes? Definition of the purpose and length of the teaching-learning situation is essential to the planning of any content.

In what setting will the teaching-learning situation take place? Will the nurse be interacting with the client in an examination room, a labor and delivery suite, a postpartum room, a birth center, or a classroom? Will more than one client or client-family be present, as in a prepared childbirth class? Assessment of the setting is crucial to the development of effective strategies.

What does the nurse expect the learners to be able to do after attending the teaching sessions? Will they be able to state in their own words reasons to avoid over-the-counter medications? Will they be able to demonstrate Lamaze breathing patterns as taught in the prepared childbirth classes? Will the adolescent in the labor room be able to follow simple directions and mimic breathing patterns as directed by her nurse-coach? Whether teaching takes place in a clinic or classroom, the nurse needs to specify in advance behavioral objectives for each client. These objectives need to be stated in terms of readily observable or measurable client behaviors. Such expressions as "clients will *know*, will *feel*, will *understand*," need to be avoided, as these are not possible to evaluate as stated. Clients could, however, demonstrate knowledge by defining "false labor" or by performing a certain breathing technique appropriately.

In a classic project, Bloom and colleagues developed a taxonomy of educational objectives.[1,2] This taxonomy provided a means for classifying educational goals from the simplest to the most complex learning behaviors. It dealt with three major domains of learning. The cognitive domain focused on the recall or identification of knowledge and on the development of intellectual abilities and skills. The affective domain dealt with objectives describing interest, attitudes, and values and the evolution of appreciations and adequate adjustment. The psychomotor domain focused on the development of manipulative or motor skills.[1] Developed as a means to facilitate communication, the taxonomy allowed an individual in a teaching role not only to identify what behaviors or goals were expected of the learners but also to state those goals in an appropriate fashion. (Nursing students sometimes find first attempts at objective writing to be difficult; however, as with any skill practiced repeatedly, objective writing can become "second nature," and can then readily be incorporated as the teaching component of the nursing care plan.)

What is to be taught? How much content can realistically be presented? What content *must* be presented by the nurse? What material can be presented through teaching aids, such as written literature or audiovisual presentations in a clinic or class? What content will be presented by other health professionals? The nurse must realize that "everything" cannot be taught at once or by one person. For example, it is more important for a woman contemplating pregnancy to be taught about the potential hazards of drugs and alcohol than it is for her to be taught about infant care. From the current literature dealing with the childbearing family, from discussions with colleagues, and from clinical

TEACHING STRATEGIES FOR CLIENTS FROM DIVERSE CULTURES

Respect the client's traditions and ideas. Know your limits. Be kind. Share your knowledge.

Understand belief systems surrounding pregnancy, labor and birth, and postpartum/infant care for the client population (anthropologic approach). Listen to the client's questions. Let them direct the client education. Clients will tell you their values, customs, and priorities through their questions.

Plan a teaching strategy:

- Teach the smallest amount needed to do the job. List only a few words at a time.
- Make your points as vivid as you can. Use simple language. Illustrate. Use active voice. Use headings.
- Have clients restate and demonstrate the information. Have clients share in group and translate information into real-life situations.
- Review repeatedly. Skip records and calendars; different cultures have different time orientations.

The plan must be "by the people, for the people."

Use the teaching methods available:

Environment

- Make your environment acceptable to your population.
- Make the location a place in which clients can find *sameness* with themselves.
- Provide clients with positive role models: posters, artwork from community members or organizations, enlargements of 35-mm photographs of members of the community.

One-on-One Counseling

- A file of commonly asked questions; many illustrations, not many words.
- Flip chart with illustrations of common cultural beliefs and expected health care practices.
- Flash cards with common procedures in clients' language, including illustrations.
- Language bank: bilingual staff, client education materials in clients' language, list of common phrases for clinical area, on-site community college language course.

Group Education

- Encourage group discussion.
- Avoid questions that require "yes" or "no" answers.
- Encourage discussion of cultural approaches.
- Role-play what to do in various situations, and have the learners provide the cues.
- Grandmother connection: instruct one member from each neighborhood to act as a resource for health-related questions; set up link on community level for referral for health care.

Videos

- Interact with your audiovisual.
- The more you interact, the more your audience will interact.
- Turn off video, show certain sections, talk over parts.
- In previewing films, choose those not longer than 10 minutes. Look for people from the culture in the film. Note use of street or professional language. Determine accuracy of information and target audience.

Written Materials

- Present written materials in a culturally acceptable manner.
- Use advance organizers. Put first things first. Summarize and review.
- Use active voice and conversational style. Use short words and sentences. Keep concept density low. Use words consistently.
- Avoid stylized pictures. Cartoons can confuse. Use simple pictures, drawings, or diagrams. Include all anatomic parts; this makes it easier for clients to locate body parts and also provokes less fear.
- Develop written materials in languages used by clients. To avoid inaccurate or insulting translations, have translations done only by individuals who know the language and subject well.
- Some people cannot read; however, clients can learn effectively despite their inability to read or write. Alternative strategies should be used in this situation. Any printed material should rely on a pictorial presentation.

Courtesy of Christina Ippolito Moore, RN, MS.

experience, the nurse needs to decide what information must be presented to all clients. Client assessment then helps the nurse to tailor an educational program to meet the unique learning needs of the pregnant family. The nurse must prioritize this information so that the most important concepts are adequately presented. This type of decision making evolves from consideration of where the client is in the childbearing cycle, the extent of the teaching role of the nurse, the setting in which the teaching will take place, and the amount of time available for teaching. One *ineffective* strategy is to present large amounts of detailed information in a short period.

What other health professionals are involved in client teaching and what content will they present? Although teaching is a major nursing role, it is not solely the domain of nursing. Indeed, nurses often refer clients to childbirth education programs that are taught in part by other health professionals. Nurses caring for the childbearing family should identify topics that they will present and topics that will be presented by other health professionals. Other health professionals include fellow nurses, nurse-midwives, physicians, and nutritionists. Through a collaborative approach, duplication of teaching is avoided, and the expertise of each professional can be employed. In collaborating with others, the nurse has the responsibility to find out what is being taught and to make certain that other health professionals working with the childbearing family are aware of topics that have been covered by the nurse. One way to implement a collaborative teaching plan is through discussions at interdisciplinary planning meetings. Another way is through development of instruction guides, identifying teaching content and including individuals covering the content, dates, and special remarks.[3]

Nurses, and especially nursing students, may at first be uncomfortable in the teaching role. To deal with this discomfort, they may rely on learned patterns of social interactions and spend teaching time discussing such topics as the weather or babies' names. They may later wish they had more time to meet objectives. It is essential that nurses assess their own feelings regarding teaching and identify behaviors they use to deal with their own feelings of discomfort in teaching-learning settings. It is helpful to note the amount of time available for nurse-client interaction, and to make an effort to adhere to a presentation schedule. In such situations, teaching plans become especially important, because they give the nurse an agenda to ensure that a standard of information is provided to all clients. The practice of "just going to do some prenatal teaching" without any advance idea of what will be taught, the amount of time to be spent on each topic, and what will be expected in terms of client behaviors should be avoided.

What strategies will be most effective in helping clients achieve objectives? Which methods will present the material most clearly? These are topics in which nursing creativity is necessary. People learn in different ways, and strategies that work effectively with one client or group of clients may not be as helpful with others. The nurse therefore needs to assess potential learners and to devise strategies that will best convey the information that needs to be taught. For example, if a woman cannot read, the nurse should consider using visual presentations along with discussions. Although teaching aids such as films, models, and games can facilitate learning, they should not eliminate opportunities for nurse-client discussion.

Which methods of evaluation are appropriate for the clients and for the teaching-learning situation? Although paper-and-pencil tests are a common evaluate method in academic programs, they may not be the best choice in clinical settings. Return demonstrations or a client's ability to present information in her own words may be more suitable. The nurse should remember that methods of evaluation in teaching should always directly relate to the objectives. For example, if the objectives for a class on infant bathing specify that mothers will independently bathe their infants according to the procedure shown in the class, the evaluative component should assess whether mothers who attended the class can bathe their infants in the prescribed manner.

What questions will aid in evaluation or provide additional information needed by the nurse for client assessment? The ability to ask effective questions is an art that can be developed by the nurse with careful thought, consultation, and practice. The nurse should not rely on questions that require culturally conditioned "yes" or "no" answers or that assume that the client already has a great deal of obstetric expertise. Table 24–1 presents examples of questions that do and do not assist the nurse in obtaining information.

Providing effective teaching does not mean that the nurse needs to discuss each piece of content. Alternative strategies, for example, filmstrips shown in clinic waiting rooms or at the bedside on the postpartum units, can provide information and allow more nurse-client time for teaching on other important topics. A wide assortment of client education materials has been developed by a variety of private and nonprofit groups for the childbearing family. After identification of recurrent teaching needs, nurses might consider including the cost of appropriate audiovi-

TABLE 24–1. EXAMPLES OF EFFECTIVE AND INEFFECTIVE QUESTIONS FOR USE WITH THE CHILDBEARING FAMILY

Ineffective Questions

How are you?

Do you have any questions?

Are you following the diet instructions you received at your last visit?

Is everything okay?

Do you know how to do the breathing exercises for labor and delivery?

Do you like the prepared childbirth classes?

Alternative Questions

What brings you to the clinic today?

What has been making you feel uncomfortable since your last visit?

What worries or concerns do you have about this pregnancy, labor and delivery, your new baby, and so forth?

What have you liked about the prepared childbirth series? What did you find not to your liking about the prepared childbirth series? What things would make the classes more helpful to future expectant parents?

Can you describe the diet you have been following since your last visit? In what ways have you found the prescribed prenatal diet to be easy to follow (or difficult to follow)?

Show me how you do the psychoprophylactic breathing exercises.

sual packages into unit and program budgets. Nurses can also serve as authors of these types of packages and seek grants for the financial support in their development. A less expensive method is to collaborate on the production of health promotion programs with faculty and students from nursing programs at a local university. Frequently, students can receive course credit for working on such projects. In addition, nursing faculty who desire to remain clinically involved may find that collaborative projects, dealing with production of educational materials for the childbearing family, are a way to meet this personal objective. Such collaborative projects between nursing faculty and nurses in clinical practice can do much to foster relationships between nursing education and nursing service.

What factors related to physical and other such needs of childbearing clients need to be considered in teaching-learning situations? For example, classes planned for third-trimester clients need to incorporate opportunities for breaks, movement, and change of position, as pregnant women have difficulty sitting for extended periods. Classes should be scheduled so that couples can easily attend.

An extensive literature exists on the topics of teaching and learning. Table 24–2 lists categories of learning objectives with examples of their application to childbearing clients. Broad consideration of teaching-learning theory and its application to nursing is, however, beyond the scope of this textbook. Students are referred to other sources for in-depth discussion.[4,5]

PREPARATION OF THE EXPECTANT PARENTS

Preparation During Different Phases of Childbearing

The childbearing process represents the time of most rapid physical and emotional change during the reproductive years. Although procreation is a normal cultural expectation, it is not easy. The physical and emotional changes of childbearing, frequently accompanied by alterations in lifestyle, can produce situational and developmental crises in the childbearing family (*see* Chapter 4). Educational preparation can do much to allay fears and to involve clients in the selection and practice of lifestyle behaviors that promote optimal obstetric health. Ideally, prenatal edu-

TABLE 24–2. SELECTED CATEGORIES OF LEARNING OBJECTIVES

Category	Example of Objective ("The pregnant couple will . . .")
Cognitive[1]	
Knowledge	
Define	Define terms specific to pregnancy.
Identify	Identify the components of a healthy pregnancy diet.
Comprehension	
Interpret	Interpret experienced physiologic changes during pregnancy.
Translate	Translate health practices to self-care during pregnancy.
Application	
Apply	Apply exercises learned during childbirth classes to a 15-minute practice session.
Affective[2]	
Valuing	
Accept	Accept responsibility for developing a birth plan.
Commit	Commit to health care practices during pregnancy.
Psychomotor	
Skill Acquisition	
Acquire	Acquire skills in caring for a newborn.
Physical Ability	
Endure	Endure labor and delivery with the help of learned breathing techniques.

cation should begin prior to pregnancy; formalized classes should start early in pregnancy and extend across the childbearing year, that is, from conception to 3 months after delivery.[6] This gives the childbearing family time to assimilate information, to understand the processes of childbearing and beginning parenthood, and to make informed choices about their childbearing experience.[7]

Preconception. Educational preparation for parenting evolves from the complex interaction of many factors. These include the individual's own experiences with parents or parenting figures, cultural heritage, religious background, personal attitude, school educational programs, and exposure to media programs and publications portraying families and parents. Such factors extend from earliest childhood and have impact on parenting perceptions and practices throughout the adult years.

During the 18th century, the French philosopher-writer Voltaire wrote a political and social satire of contemporary society. In his book *Candide,* Voltaire describe how wonderful life was and how everything always worked out well in the best of all possible worlds inhabited by his fictional characters. In the best of all current childbearing worlds, a woman contemplating childbearing would be emotionally and developmentally mature and would have a loving spouse and a stable marriage. She would have grown up in a household in which there was adequate food and clothing and where she had loving parental role models. Parenting would be a developmental commitment that she and her husband looked forward to and felt ready for. The couple anticipating parenthood could also expect to offer their infant a clean, furnished home that included a crib and perhaps a special room for the newborn. They would be in complete agreement about their beginning roles as parents and would not be experiencing conflicts about career or finances. In addition, they would have ready access to high-quality child care whenever needed.

Contemporary American society is as different from the preceding scenario as Voltaire's best of all worlds was from 18th-century France. For example, it has been noted that about 40 percent of American adolescent females will become pregnant, and that 80 percent of these pregnancies will be unintentional.[8] About 3.3 million (55 percent) of the 6 million pregnancies that occur each year in the United States are unplanned. About half of American marriages are expected to end in divorce. Single-parent families and blended families incorporating children from previous partners are commonplace. Changing social attitudes toward working mothers, expanding career opportunities for women, and economic necessity are making working mothers the norm rather than the exception. Indeed, it has been estimated that in the 1990s, 75 percent of American mothers will be in the work force.[9,10] The trend toward smaller American families and the greater mobility of families is also important, as women contemplating pregnancy may have fewer family members and fewer accessible family members on whom to depend for support during childbearing and childbearing experiences. All of these hold the potential for role conflict and family crisis.

In his classic book *Awake and Aware,* Chabon noted the lack of contact with childbearing for 20th-century children whose mothers' pregnancies were cared for and delivered outside the home.[11] He also observed that American children spent years in school where their preparation for adulthood rarely included information about pregnancy and childbirth; it was not until their own pregnancies that women were educated specifically about childbearing. Although Chabon's comments were published more than 20 years ago, they unfortunately remain true.

The diversity of American family patterns and the complexity of factors dealing with preconceptional preparation for childbearing offer a major nursing challenge. As noted by Sutterley and Donnelly, "Nurses need to liberate themselves from some of the myths of motherhood and parenting if they are to assist others in making rational choices about parenting issues."[12] A primary nursing goal is nonjudgmental assessment of the client, including her informal and formal preparation for parenthood. It is important for the nurse to realize that not all of life's preparatory experiences are desirable or positive. For example, an adult who had been physically or emotionally abused as a child may approach parenting from a negative parenting perspective. A woman whose family depends heavily on her income may realistically be worried about the amount of time she can manage to be away from work or the kind of child care that she can afford.

During the preconceptional phase, clients expecting to get pregnant may become interested in learning about or selecting obstetric caregivers and care settings. Education dealing with obstetric choices is therefore important.

Nurses can participate in preconceptional education in several ways. They can serve as consultants, speakers, and teachers in schools, community, or religious organizations; they can author, produce and consult on media projects dealing with parenting; and they can counsel clients in clinical settings. Topics related to preconceptional preparation for childbearing might include physical health, safety (including environmental safety), use of drugs and alcohol, family planning, and strategies for selecting obstetric caregivers and obstetric facilities.

First Trimester. Early-pregnancy education involves teaching efforts directed toward the pregnant family during the first trimester. Early-pregnancy education programs have been sponsored by individuals and groups such as childbirth education associations, clinics, private physicians, certified nurse-midwives, and obstetric nurses. The media are also important sources of early pregnancy education and reach large viewing, listening, and reading audiences. Unfortunately, formalized early-pregnancy education has been a neglected area. Most prenatal teaching has been done during the third trimester to prepare clients for the "big event" of childbirth. Until recently, teaching during this critical, early period of pregnancy was relegated to on-the-spot instruction or responses to clients' questions.

The first trimester is the period during which most women seeking early obstetric care begin a relationship with health care providers that will continue at least through the postpartum period. Although some women will have had prior contact through gynecologic care visits or previous obstetric experiences, others will be making contact for the first time. For many women, this is when choice of caregiver (physician, certified nurse-midwife, or lay midwife) and setting (hospital, birth center, or home) is specified. At a time when there is fierce competition for obstetric clients, it may be difficult for clients to obtain information about alternative obstetric settings from individuals working within those settings. Client education presented through the media or by groups that do not have a vested interest in a particular agency therefore assumes great importance in representing the range of obstetric choices available to the pregnant family. The source of the information should, however, be carefully evaluated, as an individual's not being associated with a childbirth agency does not ensure objectivity. Nurses need to evaluate the extent to which their teaching presents obstetric options in an objective or biased manner.

In developing a prenatal education program, the nurse must first understand the psychologic phases that women experience while pregnant (*see* Chapters 13, 17, and 21). During the first trimester of pregnancy, women normally tend to focus on themselves. Pregnancy as yet may have a feeling of unreality, and women may be dealing with ambivalence about the prospect of being pregnant. The major purposes of first-trimester prenatal education are to explain the changes currently taking place within the women's body, to identify changes within the family system, to assist clients in identifying normal reactions to being newly pregnant, to furnish anticipatory guidance, and to offer information that may help pregnant clients make lifestyle changes that can promote good health for themselves and their unborn babies.

From experience in the development of first-trimester counseling classes within a private practice setting, Carey observed that early prenatal education tended to reduce confusion and anxiety preceding late pregnancy (when classes were most often offered), as well as to foster interest among women to learn more about pregnancy, childbirth, and parenting.[13] Early prenatal classes helped establish a foundation to assist women in building their own knowledge according to their unique needs. Carey further noted that the potential for first-trimester prenatal counseling was as great as nurses in these settings chose to make it.

A variety of formats for pregnancy education classes have been suggested. Although discussed here in relation to early pregnancy, they are relevant to each trimester. The formats range from single-class sessions for pregnant women only[13] to a series of classes open to each woman and her support person.[14] There is probably no "best" format that can be recommended for use in all first-trimester teaching settings.

Success of first-trimester programs depends largely on the commitment of the nurse and the sponsoring agency. Commitment extends beyond philosophic support to the provision of adequate funds, space, time, and personnel to implement such a program. In designing first-trimester classes, the nurse needs to assess such factors as the current literature, client population, factors that will motivate attendance by the client population, and resources available in his or her own setting. Networking with nurse colleagues who have been involved in first-trimester prenatal education elsewhere is also suggested. Table 24–3 presents a suggested content outline for prenatal education.

Teaching Plan Versus Birth Plan. **Birth plans** and teaching plans are sometimes confused by those new to childbirth preparation. Indeed, both focus on clients' needs. Every client should have a birth plan as well as a teaching plan, begun as early as the first prenatal visit, updated whenever appropriate, and included within the client's records.

With a birth plan, a couple identifies a list of

TABLE 24–3. OUTLINE FOR PRENATAL EDUCATION

At the earliest contact between client and nurse, a teaching plan is developed. This reflects the unique learning needs of each client and incorporates information that health care providers identify as essential for all pregnant women to know and information that clients identify as learning priorities. The outline is reviewed with the client and updated whenever necessary. Client referral to individuals or organizations sponsoring childbirth education can also be appropriate for meeting overall learning objectives.

Preconception

How pregnancy occurs (menstrual cycle)

Lifestyle factors with potential impact on becoming pregnant and on early pregnancy: drugs, such as alcohol, nutritional status, general health, occupational and environmental considerations

Alternatives in childbirth settings and in obstetric caregivers

Pregnancy tests

Myths about conception and pregnancy

First Trimester

Feelings about pregnancy, ambivalence, developmental tasks of early pregnancy, age-related issues

Family reactions to pregnancy, first-trimester emotional responses of expectant fathers

Early-pregnancy physical changes

Sexuality during the first trimester[15, 16]

Lifestyle factors with potential impact on early pregnancy: drugs, alcohol, nutrition (including prescribed vitamin and iron supplements), general health, exercise, rest, occupational and environmental considerations

Warning signs of early pregnancy

Fear of miscarriage (suggested presentation as a topic in a group setting)

First-trimester diagnostic tests for maternal/fetal well-being (as appropriate)

Client expectations for pregnancy and childbirth

Options available to client within the selected prenatal and delivery setting, tour of birthing facility

Anticipatory guidance regarding what to expect at prenatal visits

Sibling concerns, telling other children about pregnancy

Resources within the caregiving agency or private practice and within the community (including relevant literature)

Second Trimester

Feelings about pregnancy, acceptance of pregnancy, developmental tasks of midpregnancy, age-related issues

Family responses to progressing pregnancy, second-trimester responses of expectant fathers

Fetal growth and development

Midtrimester physical changes, relief of discomforts associated with enlarging fetus and physical changes

Sexuality during the second trimester

Lifestyle factors with potential impact on midpregnancy: drugs, such as alcohol, smoking, nutrition (including prescribed vitamin and iron supplements), general health, exercise, body mechanics, rest, occupational and environmental considerations, stress

Changes in activities of daily living related to midtrimester

Warning signs of midpregnancy

Diagnostic tests for assessment of maternal/fetal well-being (as necessary)

Client's expectations for pregnancy and birth

Client's fears and anxieties related to second trimester

Sibling concerns

Client expectations for pregnancy and childbirth, confirmation of registration for third-trimester prenatal classes

Third Trimester

Feelings about pregnancy, developmental tasks of third trimester

Preparation for labor, delivery, and parenting (Content may be given by health care providers during prenatal visits, or can be offered in greater depth during a series of prepared childbirth classes.)

Client expectations for labor and birth, progress of prepared childbirth classes

Family reactions to advanced pregnancy; third-trimester emotional responses of expectant fathers; sibling preparation

Late-pregnancy physical changes, management of discomforts related to late pregnancy

Sexuality during the third trimester

TABLE 24–3. OUTLINE FOR PRENATAL EDUCATION (*continued*)

Third Trimester (*continued*)
Lifestyle factors with potential impact on late pregnancy: drugs such as alcohol, nutrition (including prescribed vitamin and iron supplements), smoking, general health, exercise, body mechanics, rest, occupational and environmental considerations
Signs of labor, "true" labor versus "false" labor, physiology of labor and delivery, passenger, passage, powers, and psyche in labor
Techniques useful during labor and delivery (eg, psychoprophylactic method, Bradley method)
Analgesia and anesthesia during labor and delivery, medications used during labor and delivery
Technology and childbirth, assessment of fetal maturity, potential for induction or augmentation of labor, potential use of electronic fetal monitoring, intravenous infusions, and so on
Variations in labor
The high-risk experience: potential for operative obstetrics (eg, forceps, episiotomy, cesarean childbirth), potential for transfer from birthing center, home, or birthing room because of obstetric complications; potential for family-centered birth despite operative obstetrics
Warning signs of late pregnancy, signs and symptoms of premature labor
Review of birth plan, anticipatory guidance regarding what can be expected within the selected labor and delivery setting
Discussion of fears and concerns related to late pregnancy, labor and delivery, or postpartum
Tour of labor and delivery setting
Preparations for client's stay in hospital or birth center, preparations for a home birth
Preparations for other family members during client's birthing experience and immediate recovery (eg, child care for siblings)
Preparations for the newborn, selection of a pediatric caregiver (may include a prenatal introductory meeting)
Infant nutrition, preparation for breastfeeding or bottle feeding
Early parenting
What to expect from caregivers and the health care system during labor, delivery, and postpartum
Anticipatory guidance for postpartum (includes physical and emotional changes, family changes, and strategies for coping)
Resources available during third trimester and postpartum

options preferred for their birth, whether the birth is normal or high risk (see Figure 23–2). Developed as a flexible, cooperative effort between caregivers and the pregnant couple, the birth plan can be incorporated into the client's chart to serve as a vehicle for communication between the pregnant couple and the staff.[17] To foster a satisfying birth experience, high-risk as well as low-risk couples should have the opportunity to develop a birth plan with their caregivers. The birth plan can be reviewed periodically with the client during the course of the pregnancy. As the outcome of the birth plan will depend on the actual labor and delivery situation, a birth plan can be evaluated only during the postpartum period. It is important to realize that the birth plan is *not* a list of demands or a binding contract restricting maternity nursing or medical practice.

A teaching plan is based on assessment of the pregnant family's learning needs. It identifies learning objectives in terms of client behaviors, specifies content that needs to be presented to help the woman and her family during childbearing and early parenthood, suggests strategies to assist clients in meeting the learning goals, and designates criteria to be used to evaluate client achievement of learning goals. It can readily be seen that the teaching plan follows the steps of the nursing process. The teaching plan is reviewed for each prenatal visit and attainment of learning objectives is marked accordingly as pregnancy progresses. It is not appropriate to wait until the postpartum period to evaluate all objectives for the teaching plan.

Second Trimester. Discussion of midpregnancy educational programs is rare in the literature. As noted earlier, most nursing attention is given first to late-pregnancy classes and next to early-pregnancy classes. Formal mid-pregnancy classes are not widely available. Indeed, those in existence tend to be focused on exercise during pregnancy and tend to be taught not by nurses, but by individuals with interest in physical fitness. For couples seeking prenatal care through hospital or private physician-based practices, educational preparation evolves mainly from office and clinic visit encounters with individual health care providers. A more comprehensive, educationally oriented approach is often provided by nurse-midwives. A strong philosophic emphasis on collaboration between client and caregiver is a highlight of midwifery services, and client teaching is a major midwifery priority throughout the childbearing year.

Early-pregnancy classes may actually include couples in midpregnancy. As discussed earlier, these classes may be designed as a series offered to clients new to a service. Clients may not come for prenatal care until they are nearly at the end of the first trimester or may not be able to attend the series early in their pregnancies. "Early"-pregnancy classes may therefore begin with couples who are in the first or second trimester of pregnancy. Careful assessment of class members allows the nurse to identify the particular learning needs of the group and to direct course content accordingly. Table 24–3 presents a suggested outline of content relevant to midpregnancy.

Third Trimester. Traditionally, most formalized prenatal education programs have been directed toward development of a series of classes for couples during the third trimester of pregnancy. At a time when delivery is truly within the forseeable future, attempts have been made by health care providers to bring clients closer in preparation for the impending "big event." These classes tend to focus on physical, emotional, and lifestyle factors associated with the third trimester and on preparation for a couple's performance during labor and delivery. In response to criticisms that third-trimester classes did not provide adequate preparation for beginning parenthood, many now include content relevant to concerns of the early postpartum and newborn period. Some series include a class that takes place after all participants have delivered. Table 24–3 presents a suggested outline of content for late-pregnancy classes.

Originally, many third-trimester pregnancy classes focused on a particular method of childbirth; most educational preparation was therefore devoted to mastery of a particular technique, such as psychoprophylaxis. Drawbacks of this type of approach included a sense of failure on the part of couples who were unable to follow the method exactly or who were unable to experience a low-risk vaginal delivery and anger at delivery in a setting where medical or nursing staff were unsupportive of the selected method. Other criticisms of the classes dealt with the limitation of content to pregnancy, labor, and delivery. Today, as third-trimester childbirth educational programs have spread across the United States and as some type of third-trimester education has become available to most pregnant couples, the approaches used tend to be more eclectic. Indeed, at the start of the 1990s, third-trimester education tends to focus less on adherence to a particular method than on approaches that incorporate aspects of various methods.

Childbirth Educators. Currently, anyone with an interest in childbirth preparation can call herself or himself a childbirth educator. No local, state, or national board regulates who teaches or what is taught. Certain major organizations, such as the American Society for Psychoprophylaxis in Obstetrics (ASPO) and the International Childbirth Education Association (ICEA), offer programs that can lead to certification in this specialty. They also specify standards for childbirth preparation classes, and sponsor educational programs on childbirth-related topics; however, simple membership in the organization does not signify that an individual has advanced training in childbirth education.

Nurses need to become knowledgeable about the nature of childbirth education programs offered in their geographic areas and about the backgrounds of the people offering those programs. In addition, evaluation of couples' satisfaction with the classes, and their level of preparation for labor and delivery and the postpartum can provide additional clues to the quality of the educational programs. Nurses who provide childbirth education need to accept their own responsibility to remain current in this specialty through attendance at appropriate conferences, membership in childbirth education groups, completion of continuing education courses, and continual review of relevant literature. Nurses should not assume that their own personal or clinical experiences, although necessary and important, provide them with all they need to know about childbirth education.

Information for Prenatal Clients

Education throughout pregnancy focuses on the physiologic and psychosocial needs of the pregnant family. Information for clients that is specific to a particular trimester of pregnancy is usually introduced prior to that stage. In addition, much content has relevance for more than one trimester of the pregnancy.

Relaxation/Stress Reduction. Pregnant couples can learn to reduce stress by active relaxation (Figure 24–1). Relaxation can be taught as a coping strategy to deal with the changes encountered during pregnancy. Clark[18] identifies several stress management interventions that can be taught to clients:

- *Breathing awareness.* The client is taught to concentrate on inhalation and exhalation while lying on a blanket on the floor with legs straight and slightly

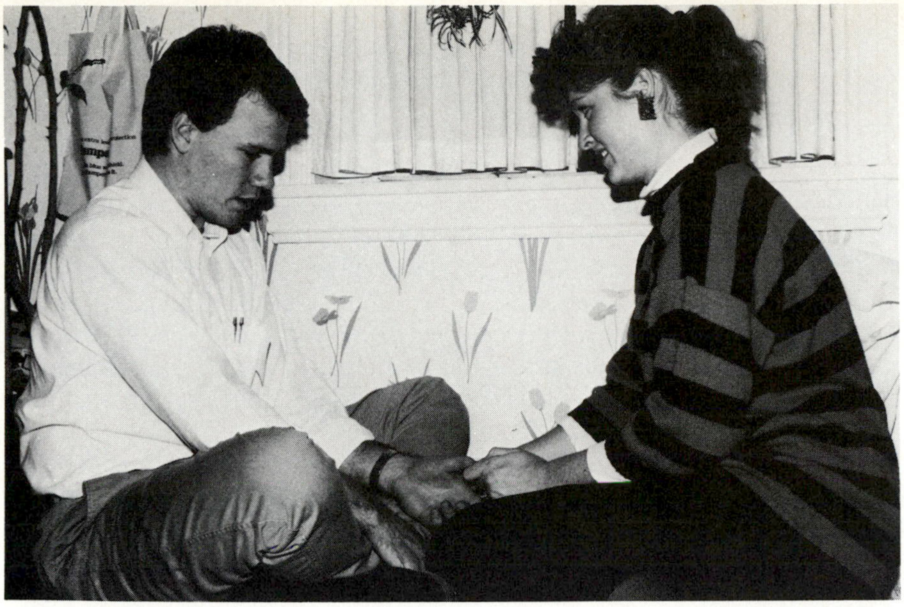

Figure 24–1. Pregnant couple practicing relaxation technique.

apart, arms at sides away from the body, palms up, and eyes closed.

- *Relaxation sigh.* The client is taught to sigh deeply on exhalation while standing or sitting.
- *Breathing and imagery.* The client is taught to breathe using imagery while in a comfortable position. On inhalation, the client is told to picture energy rushing into the lungs. On exhalation, energy is pictured flowing to all parts of the body.
- *Biofeedback.* When taught biofeedback, the client develops the ability to identify tensions in various parts of the body, and then is taught to "let go" of the tension.
- *Progressive relaxation.* The client is taught to tighten and relax muscle groups of the body, beginning with the hand and moving down to the foot. The client checks for relaxation in each muscle group before moving on to the next muscle group. This exercise is sometimes accompanied by *imagery,* whereby the client lets her mind drift to a pleasant image.
- *Self-hypnosis.* This technique is a wakeful state of deep relaxation. Positive suggestions are used to reduce stress-related discomforts. Someone knowledgeable in hypnosis must train the client in this technique.
- *Thought stopping.* The client is taught to interrupt unwanted thoughts with the command "stop." It is an assertive response and can be followed by reassuring and accepting self-statements.
- *Coping skills training.* Progressive relaxation is combined with stress/coping self-statements. Some stress/coping self-statements are listed in Table 24–4.

Self-Care Practices. Education about self-care practices focuses on information the pregnant couple may need to cope with activities of daily living.

Posture and Movement. The pregnant woman is taught proper body mechanics as early in the pregnancy as possible. Thus, as her center of gravity shifts because of the enlarging uterus, she will be able to move safely and easily. When standing, the woman should keep her shoulders, back, hips, knees, and feet in a straight line. She is taught to use her legs rather than her back muscles when stooping or lifting. (Refer to Figure 23–6 for body mechanics when lifting a child.) The pregnant woman is also encouraged to sit with her legs crossed (tailor sitting). This strengthens the inner thigh muscles (Figure 24–2). The position of choice when resting is lying on the

TABLE 24–4. EXAMPLES OF STRESS/COPING SELF-STATEMENTS

There's nothing to worry about.
I'm going to be all right.
I can get help if I need it.
Take it step by step.
I did well!
Situations don't have to overwhelm me anymore.
Deep breathing really works.

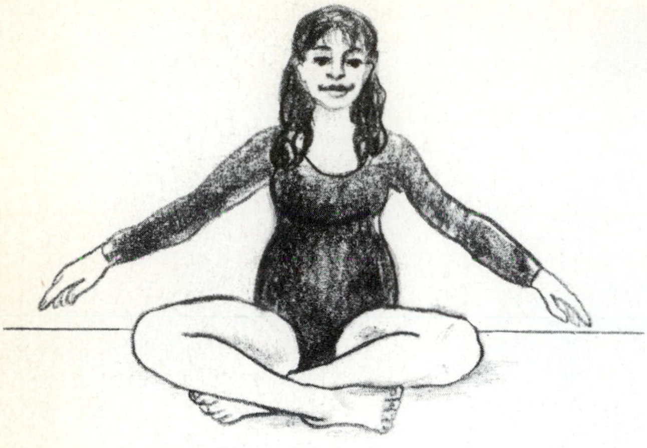

Figure 24–2. Tailor sitting. (*Redrawn, courtesy of Coalition for the Medical Rights of Women, San Francisco. From* Natural Remedies for Pregnancy Discomforts, *p. 8.*)

left side in a lateral Sims position, with pillows supporting the upper legs.

Clothing. In general, loose-fitting skirts and pants that stretch are most appropriate for pregnancy. Maternity clothing can be fashionable as well as comfortable for the mother and need not be costly or new. In fact, many women share maternity clothing.

Maternity girdles are usually not necessary unless the abdomen is large and pendulous. Constricting items such as garters and tight waist bands may interfere with venous return and should be avoided.

The pregnant woman should also avoid high-heeled shoes, as they may cause back discomfort and affect balance. Maternity bras may be used to support the breasts (see additional discussion later). Cotton–crotch underpants should also be worn, as they absorb moisture, which may give rise to vaginitis.

Lifestyle/Habits. The pregnant couple is taught positive health care practices. Rationales for changing behaviors such as smoking and intake of alcohol are explained. The couple is also taught about environmental factors that may cause potential harm to the mother and fetus. For example, expectant mothers may acquire toxoplasmosis (an infection caused by the protozoan *Toxoplasma gondii*) through contact with infected cat feces or by eating raw or undercooked infected meat. The expectant mother who owns a cat is advised that the cat's litter box should be placed in an area where she will not come in direct contact with it. Someone who is not pregnant should change the litter box daily, as *T. gondii* mature within 24 hours of leaving the cat's body. In addition, the woman should wash her hands well after contact with the cat and should wear gloves when gardening (neighborhood cats often have access to home garden areas and organisms such as *T. gondii* can survive actively in soil long after feces decompose). She should also prepare and eat only well-cooked meat. Women may be screened for toxoplasmosis antibodies before pregnancy or at the initial prenatal visit and are advised to report any flu-like symptoms to the health care provider without delay. (For additional information concerning nursing management of lifestyle factors that may influence pregnancy, *see* Chapter 11.)

Employment/Daily Activities. Working per se is not contraindicated during pregnancy. Pregnant women should be able to work as long as they feel comfortable and can be taught various exercises and relaxation techniques that can be used on the job; however, attention needs to be paid to daily acts that may put the client at physical or psychologic risk during pregnancy. These include exposure to teratogenic chemicals or medications or working in a high-stress occupation. (*See* Chapter 11 for additional discussion of this topic.)

Sexuality. Sexual desires and behaviors may change during pregnancy. The nurse needs to be aware of clients' individual responses to sexuality throughout the childbearing cycle. Women and their partners may worry about having sexual desires while pregnant. A variety of responses may be normally experienced by either partner and include fear of hurting the fetus, conflict over the "presence" of the fetus during lovemaking, conflict related to sexual desire during a culturally "taboo" period, lack of interest, and embarrassment regarding the pregnant shape.

During the first trimester, clients who experience discomforts such as nausea and vomiting may have decreased sexual desires. In the second trimester, with quickening, the woman becomes aware of fetal movements; these may also be perceived by her partner later in the second trimester. Yet, many women enjoy sexual expression more during the second trimester than at any time during pregnancy. In the third trimester, the woman's large abdomen, discomforts, and fatigue may be expected to have considerable impact on sexual adaptation[15]; however, clients may also continue to enjoy sexual activity, may identify more comfortable positions, and may view third-trimester changes with loving humor.

Desire for physical closeness and expression of sexuality are normal and may be encouraged for the low-risk, healthy couple. To provide client teaching, the nurse needs to assess the couple's attitude toward sexuality, the influences of their cultural backgrounds, and their fears and concerns. It is important to remember that sexuality encompasses more than intercourse. Kissing, touching, and cuddling are also examples of sexual expression.

Bathing/Swimming. Bathing, swimming, and showering are allowed throughout pregnancy. Tub baths and swimming should be avoided after rupture of the membranes because of the possibility of infection. Women should use caution in taking tub baths late in pregnancy because their center of gravity has shifted, making them vulnerable to falls. Exposure to very high temperatures, as found in saunas or hot tubs, should be avoided because of the possible harmful effects on the fetus related to increase in the mother's own body temperature.

Personal Hygiene. Daily bathing controls odors related to sweating and normal vaginal secretions. Douching is not recommended for the pregnant woman.

Travel. Long-distance travel by train or plane is not contraindicated during pregnancy. Travel to regions of the world where health care is not available or where incidence of disease is very high is not recommended during pregnancy. Parents should be aware of the health and medical care available at their destination. It is important that pregnant women protect themselves and their fetuses from physical trauma during travel. Seat belts, including lap and shoulder straps, should be worn when traveling in a car. Fetal loss in automobile accidents is most frequently caused by maternal injury or death. Another frequent sequela of maternal involvement in automobile accidents is placental separation.[19, 20]

Exercise. Currently much attention in the professional and public media has been directed toward regular exercise as a means of promoting health. Benefits of physical exercise during pregnancy include toning and strengthening of maternal muscles, toning and strengthening of the cardiovascular system, promotion of physical stamina, release of tension, improved body image, and an overall sense of well-being.[21] Various prenatal exercises are recommended to strengthen muscle tone in preparation for delivery and for the postpartum period.

Kegel Exercises. Kegel exercises are done to strengthen the pubococcygeal muscle (the perineal area). Kegel exercises help increase the tone and elasticity of the vagina in preparation for labor and delivery. Increased tone may also influence sexual pleasure during pregnancy and after the birth of the baby. Many different techniques are used to teach Kegel exercises. In one, the mother is taught to tighten the pubococcygeal muscle while her finger is in the opening of the vagina. If the exercise is done correctly, she will feel the muscle tighten around her finger. Kegel exercises can be broken down into four steps[22]: (1) The client squeezes the pubococcygeal muscle for 3 seconds, relaxes for 3 seconds, then squeezes again. (2) She then squeezes and releases the pubococcygeal muscle as quickly as she can (flutter exercises). (3) She imagines she has a tampon in her vagina that she is pulling in with her pubococcygeal muscle. (4) The client bears down as she would during a bowel movement but tries to concentrate more on the vagina than on the anal area. The client can perform Kegel exercises anywhere. The increased tone of the pubococcygeal muscle can have beneficial effects during and after pregnancy.

Pelvic Tilt. Pelvic tilt exercises help alleviate backache and also help strengthen the abdominal muscles. The client tucks the buttocks under the back; this flattens the lower back. She then relaxes the back muscles, which allow the hips to return to the natural position. It is basically a rocking movement. Pelvic tilt exercises can be done in three different positions[22]: (1) The client stands against a wall and presses her lower back against the wall. (2) The client positions herself on her hands and knees, arching her lower back and then relaxing to a flat back (Figure 24–3). (3) The client lies on the floor on her back and bends her knees; she presses her lower back flat against the floor and then relaxes.

Knee-Chest Twist. The knee-chest twist is an exercise the mother may do during pregnancy to alleviate backstrain. The client is taught to lie on her back on a firm surface while pulling her knees to her chest. She places her arms straight out to the sides and rolls her knees to one side while turning her head to the opposite side. She then switches sides and repeats the exercise[22] (Figure 24–4).

Concerns About Sports and Exercise. Moderate exercise during pregnancy has many benefits, but exer-

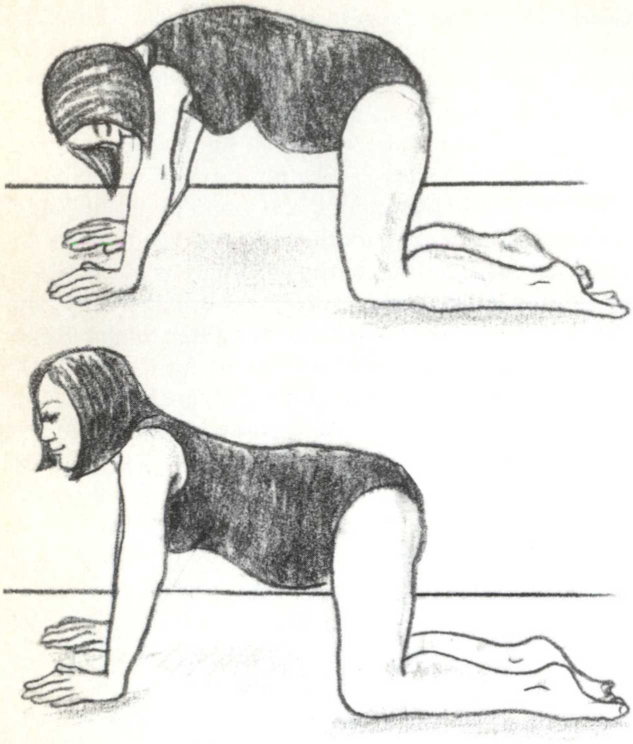

Figure 24–3. Pelvic tilt exercises: hands and knees. (*Redrawn, courtesy of Coalition for the Medical Rights of Women, San Francisco. From* Natural Remedies of Pregnancy Discomforts, *p. 13.*)

cise during pregnancy has also provoked concerns.[21,23] Fetal hyperthermia results from increased production of heat during exercise; however, in a temperate climate without extremely hot or humid weather, the body is usually able to dissipate heat efficiently. Vigorous exercise may cause fetal hypoxia; the increased oxygen demands of peripheral muscles may draw blood away from the uterus, thereby providing less blood to the fetus. Maternal safety is also threatened by exercise. Throughout the first trimester there is little effect on the mother's ability to perform sports or exercises. As the uterus expands during the second and third trimesters and hormonal influences cause changes in the musculoskeletal system, the mother's center of gravity, balance, and gait change, and joints and ligaments weaken. She then becomes at risk for injury, especially in sports that require speed, precision, and balance. Changes brought about by softening of ligaments and joints predispose women to tearing of these structures.

The literature varies with regard to how much exercise and what type of exercise is safe during various stages of pregnancy. The healthy pregnant woman should be encouraged to exercise; however,

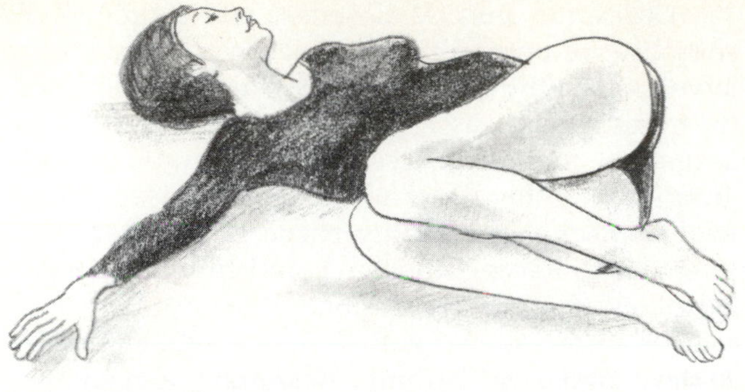

Figure 24–4. Knee–chest twist. (*Redrawn, courtesy of Coalition for the Medical Rights of Women, San Francisco. From* Natural Remedies for Pregnancy Discomforts, *p. 12.*)

advice about exercise and sports should be provided with caution. The nurse needs to identify the client's plans for participation in exercises or sports and to assess the client's interpretation of mild, moderate, and heavy exercise. Good sense and evaluation of the client's unique physical condition and responses are necessary when providing advice about exercise and sports. In addition, the pregnant woman should be advised about warning signs and told to call her health care provider if they occur during or after exercise (Table 24–5).

Currently there exist many types of prenatal exercise classes. Nurses need to familiarize themselves with the differing programs before referring clients.

Preparation of the Breast for Breastfeeding. A well-fitting bra is essential for maintaining good posture and minimizing discomfort such as upper backache related to increasing weight of the breasts. Char-

TABLE 24–5. WARNING SIGNS RELATED TO PRENATAL EXERCISE

Persistent pain or tenderness, especially chest, back, pubic, or hip pain; ripping sensation followed by pain
Onset of uterine contractions
Headache, "lightheadness"
Vaginal bleeding
Leakage of fluid from the vagina
Nausea and vomiting (not the usual morning sickness)
Difficulty in breathing
Palpitations
Increase, decrease, or cessation of fetal movements
Heart rate above 130 beats per minute
Dyspnea

Source: Reference 21.

acteristics of a well-fitting bra include nonelastic shoulder straps that minimize movement of the breast; a cup that completely covers the breast and allows for a small amount of breast growth; and proper size that does not constrict in any area. Plastic-lined bras should be avoided. Plastic tends to hold moisture against the skin, which can foster irritation and skin breakdown, especially later in pregnancy when colostrum is produced. Colostrum secretion can easily be washed from the breasts with warm water.

Preparation of the breasts during the antepartum period has long been advocated for mothers who intend to breastfeed. It has been thought to toughen the nipple and thus prevent soreness during actual breastfeeding. An interesting early study on preparation of the breast for breastfeeding indicated that there were no significant differences in either objective or subjective measures of nipple sensitivity or trauma in the postpartum period among three groups of women, each using one of the common breast preparation methods.[24] Little has been done since to replicate these findings, although nipple preparation is still advocated by some health care providers. Although this text discusses common nipple preparation methods, the reader should remember that the efficacy of these methods is open to question. Additional empiric evidence is necessary to support the usefulness of nipple preparation methods.

Common breast preparation methods include rolling of nipples, application of a lanolin-based cream, and correction techniques for inverted nipples. Breast preparation is usually done in the third trimester.

- *Rolling of the nipples.* The mother is taught to place her thumb and forefinger around the nipple and gently roll the nipple several times a day. Women who have histories of preterm birth are discouraged from nipple rolling because of the possibility of stimulation of uterine contractions.
- *Application of lanolin-based cream.* The mother is taught to cleanse her nipples with warm water and then to apply a lanolin-based cream such as Masse.
- *Correction techniques for inverted nipples.* For those women who have inverted nipples, preparation of the breast includes having the mother press on the alveoli with the thumb and forefinger and move toward the nipple. Nipple rolling also helps for some mothers. If the nipple remains inverted, special breast shields can be worn to increase the protractility of the inverted nipples (*see* Figure 31–5).

CHOICES IN CHILDBIRTH

Currently, the pregnant family has a variety of childbearing options that were not available prior to the latter part of the 20th century. To appreciate the childbirth alternatives that now exist, it is important to understand historic and social trends in childbirth. These hold major implications for the nurse providing educational preparation to the pregnant family. No single person or social factor quickly alters childbearing practices and beliefs. As always, current practice is the result of a complex and ever-changing process. The choices possible for pregnant families today have evolved from years of professional and lay groups' working with each other and against each other. Nurses need to realize that no educational program or delivery alternative is unconditionally accepted for the childbearing family. Nevertheless, the heterogeneous nature of the American population requires availability of safe choices in childbearing and educational preparation to enable clients to make informed choices.[25–27]

Trends in Childbearing: Development of Current Delivery Alternatives

Before the 20th century, nearly all births in the United States occurred out of the hospital. Women planned to deliver at home, where they would be assisted by a woman who was experienced in childbirth, a midwife, or by a local physician. Limited transportation, fewer hospitals, and the low level of hospital technology did not make hospital birth a desirable choice for many families. Throughout this period, hospitals were regarded as places for the sick, the feeble, and the dying, certainly inappropriate for women undergoing a normal event. This trend persisted into the early 20th century.[25]

Changes in patterns of obstetric care and location of childbirth accompanied social and technologic changes in the early 20th century. One difference was in the delivery attendant. For instance, it is estimated that midwives performed 38 percent of all deliveries in New York City in 1913.[28] In the following years, however, there was a decrease in midwife-attended births. By 1935, midwifery came to be centered mainly among the poor and among blacks in the rural South. This change may have occurred for several reasons, including a lack of programs for the education of midwives and the decrease in the number of women aspiring to be midwives. Over time, the United States came to have no well-educated group of people skilled in home births; in contrast, continental European countries had well-trained and accepted childbirth attendants.[29] Through the beginning of the 20th century, immigrant women from these countries continued to deliver at home where they were attended by midwives. As they began to move upward, however, many started to identify the physician and the hospital as symbols of their new status and of their integration into the American way of life. As medical technology became more advanced, this type of midwifery began to be opposed; physicians also started to resent midwives as treading on their medical practice.[30,31]

Midwifery did not completely disappear. For instance, a physician-supported nurse-midwifery program was started at the Maternity Center Association in New York City during the 1930s. This program was begun to educate nurse-midwives who could care for the poor.

Location of delivery also started to change at the beginning of the 20th century. National statistics on place of birth are not available before 1935; however, the rate of hospital births increased from 39.6 percent in 1935 to 96 percent in 1960.[29] Also, pregnancy and birth began to be viewed as pathologic phenomena that required technologic treatment during this period. Some of these interventions, such as the use of forceps, were thought to be a greater hazard to client health if used in a home rather than in a hospital setting; this fostered physicians' support of in-hospital deliveries. In addition, obstetrics had developed into a separate, major specialty of medical practice by 1930.[32] The professional movement to organize obstetrics as a specialty reinforced the abnormal aspects of birth. With the development of obstetric analgesia and anesthesia, women received the message that childbirth in the hospital would mean a safer, less painful delivery experience.

Handling obstetric cases at a central location such as a hospital helped deal with the problem of availability of physicians. During the first half of the 20th century, a lack of physicians was compounded by the occurrence of two world wars, which claimed physicians through draft or enlistment. At a time when the national birth rate was increasing, centralizing obstetric cases in hospitals allowed for more efficient use of a physician's time and services.[28] The Hill-Burton Act of 1946 made funds available to build hospitals in rural parts of the United States. Rural women, whose only accessible birth option had been the home, were now able to deliver in a hospital.

Changed in the location of delivery and the shift from midwife to physician were accompanied by changes in hospital practices. During the early 20th century restrictive isolation policies developed over concern for the high rate of morbidity and mortality of hospitalized children with infectious diseases. Visiting was cut back, because it was thought that visitors were responsible for bringing the diseases. Thus evolved the practice of separating parents from their hospitalized child, whether the child was ill or in a well-baby nursery.[33] Eventually, physicians and hospital systems, rather than the childbearing family, provided the leadership and control over the childbearing process.

Just as there were few birthing choices for the childbearing family at the beginning of the 20th century, there were few childbearing choices at the middle of the century, although the country had moved from the totally home-centered birth to the hospital birth, directed by health care providers. Women were treated as surgical patients who received the maximum in technological advances and who experienced labor and delivery accompanied only by hospital staff. The father was regarded as a helpless intruder when it came to childbirth and relegated to a separate waiting room. This scenario became widely accepted as part of the "unpleasant" process of childbirth. Women were frequently given amnesic drugs to help them forget what having a baby was actually like.

During the 1950s, opposition to this type of childbirth began to take root; however, it was not until the late 1960s that major changes in American obstetric practices began to take place. The women's movement had a great impact. Women's groups joined together to foster women's rights. Emphasis also centered on women's understanding and accepting control over their own bodies. Opposition to obstetric practices was directed toward a woman's lack of control over her body, rigidity of hospital policies, separation of women from their support people during childbirth, and the definition of childbirth as high-risk pathology even for healthy women. By the 1970s, extensive media coverage, focusing on women's issues and childbearing, was reaching all segments of society. As feminists strongly presented the case for pregnancy as a normal life event, attention was directed toward educational preparation for childbirth, settings for childbirth, delivery attendants, and the right of women to make choices regarding their own birthing experiences. Organizations consisting of concerned professionals and lay people began to form; their goals dealt with returning childbearing to a more normal, less risk-oriented process. Two such organizations, ASPO and ICEA, remain in existence today and continue to exert influence on current obstetric practice. (*See* Appendix G for addresses of these organizations.)

By the late 1960s and early 1970s, in response to consumer demand, nurse-midwifery programs in the

United States began to grow and nurse-midwives became more widely available. With their focus on childbirth as a normal, natural process, nurse-midwives strove to ensure a satisfying, family-centered birth experience for their clients. Their background in nursing, advanced training in obstetrics, and success on a national certifying examination for the American College of Nurse Midwives established a professionally educated group of birth attendants whose philosophy evolved from commitment to childbirth as a manifestation of health. The availability of nurse-midwives offered a choice of childbirth attendant to healthy, low-risk women.

Today, childbearing in the United States is a topic that appears in the popular literature on a daily basis. Parents can find any type of childbirth management, although not within each geographic area.[34] Professional and moral commitment toward family-centered childbirth, as well as fierce competition for obstetric clients among health care providers, has fostered the establishment of these options. The pregnant family, more than at any time in history, is confronted with many choices. Knowledgeable explanation of these choices is within the teaching role of nurses.

Prepared Childbirth

The prepared childbirth movement in the United States developed from the belief that there were psychologic and physiologic advantages in a woman's being prepared for and being able to participate in her own labor and delivery. As of the 1920s, several behavioral approaches to reduce perception of pain in childbirth had emerged. It was not until the late 1940s, however, that these approaches were put into practice. After World War II, few technologic resources were available in the Soviet Union; the shortage of analgesics and anesthetics for healthy women during labor and delivery encouraged, through necessity, a greater dependence on more "natural" methods of dealing with pain in childbirth. These methods were more widely accepted in Europe than in the highly technologically oriented United States. In comparison with other countries that had experienced firsthand the hardships, destruction, and shortages brought about by the world wars, the postwar United States enjoyed plentiful resources, including analgesics and anesthesics for use during labor. Several major prepared childbirth methods eventually emerged, a few of which are described here.

Grantly Dick-Read: Psychophysical Preparation. Grantly Dick-Read, a British physician, was a pioneer in the development of the childbirth preparation methods available to families today. Dick-Read evolved his belief in the emotional beauty of childbirth by designing a process of prenatal and intrapartum education and exercise. He questioned why young people were not routinely educated for childbearing in the way they were prepared in school for other aspects of adulthood. He also discussed the lack of opportunity afforded to children of the 1940s for understanding what pregnancy and delivery entailed. He attributed this to the control of health care providers over childbearing. Dick-Read felt this lack of education and experience contributed to high levels of anxiety for pregnant women. He believed that, with a prescribed educational program, women could be assisted in decreasing their fears and, therefore, muscular tension in childbirth.[35] Through studied relaxation methods, women could learn to control specific muscle groups and prevent or inhibit a spiral of fear, tension, and pain. According to Dick-Read, many of the body's physiologic reactions were related in their intensity to the body's muscle tone. For Dick-Read, muscular relaxation was "a condition in which the muscle tone throughout the body is reduced to a minimum."[35] The primary goal of his work was childbirth without fear.

Dick-Read refused to specify a time when educational preparation was to begin; however, he believed that lessons in relaxation could be given during the earliest stages of pregnancy, "if there is the slightest tendency to nervous symptoms."[35] Dick-Read included among these symptoms such presumptive signs of pregnancy as morning sickness and frequency of urination. During the late 1940s, when Dick-Read's book became available in the United States, obstetric practices were technologically and pathologically oriented (see early discussion). What today seems to be a gentle, commonsense approach was at the time thought to be radical and revolutionary.

Dick-Read's techniques were never completely developed as a method. His version of "natural childbirth" depended on each woman's taking cues from her own body to respond in a manner that would ensure relaxation.[36] Thus, it was difficult to offer a specific mass-market type of prepared childbirth prescription.

A modified Dick-Read approach, psychophysical preparation, focused on a woman's ability to work along with the forces of labor. A woman could do this by relaxing and breathing more rapidly and more deeply with the increasing intensity of contractions. This in turn would help her to be in harmony with her body's demands. Prenatal preparation was to evolve from unstructured class discussions. During these classes, group members could raise topics to meet their own learning needs; breathing and relaxation techniques could be presented as aids for breaking the fear-tension-pain spiral[36] (*see* box).

Dick-Read was the first to use the term **natural childbirth.** This readily caught on and eventually was applied to any method of preparation and education for labor that prevents or decreases the need for pain-relieving medications. Chabon felt that the term *natural childbirth* was unfortunate, because childbirth was a natural, normal life event.[11] Although writing in reference to psychoprophylaxis (described below), Chabon noted that childbirth preparation was an "artificial, completely contrived and manmade way of dealing with contractions in labor."[11] Far from "natural!"

BREATHING TECHNIQUES FOR THE DICK-READ METHOD

The breathing technique is primarily abdominal, with the depth and rapidity of the breathing increasing as the uterine contractions increase during the first stage. Toward the end of the labor, if the abdominal breathing is not sufficient, rapid chest breathing is done by the mother. During the second stage of labor, the mother uses panting and breath holding: panting to prevent pushing, and breath holding to aid in pushing.

Psychoprophylaxis: Lamaze Technique. Psychoprophylaxis is the training of mind and body to select an appropriate reaction to stressful stimuli.[11] The psychoprophylactic method is based on principles first developed in the Soviet Union and used widely there and in China. It was introduced in France in 1951 by the French physician Ferdinand Lamaze. Originally it was called the Pavlov method, because it was based on the stimulus-response, conditioned reflex theory of the Russian physiologist Pavlov. Psychoprophylaxis was popularized in the United States by Marjorie Karmel, whose book *Thank You, Dr. Lamaze* joyously describes the satisfaction the author experienced using this technique during her delivery in Paris.[37] Karmel's book was published in 1959, a time when American women had a very passive, medically managed role in childbirth; it was widely read. Her work made a landmark contribution to the changing of obstetric practice and was instrumental in raising support for establishment of the ASPO, a childbirth education organization that remains active today.

The main focus of the psychoprophylactic technique (commonly referred to as the **Lamaze technique**) was the alteration of the perception of pain in childbirth through the use of the mind. As noted earlier, this method evolved from the stimulus-response theory. According to this method, women would attend prenatal classes where they would learn activities and breathing patterns that would allow them to control their experience of pain during uterine contractions. By maintaining a high level of alertness and conscious activity during labor and delivery and by using conditioned responses, a woman could keep control over her muscles and alter her perception of pain.[34] The techniques were best used with the active support of the woman's husband and members of the attending health team. According to Chabon, "the greater this support, the more successful the exercise techniques."[11] Prenatal classes, especially those beginning prior to the third trimester, could facilitate communication between parents-to-be. They could then work more effectively together during labor.

The psychoprophylactic technique is a very structured method that evolves from conditioning, concentration, and discipline to produce an expected response.[36] These are developed and practiced through a series of prenatal classes, ideally beginning prior to the third trimester. The exercises and relaxation and breathing patterns of psychoprophylaxis are simply tools that the couple can enlist to deal with the stress of childbirth, rather than goals in themselves. As coping measures, the pain reduction techniques may diminish distress associated with labor by helping the woman to remain in control of the painful experience; in doing so, they might also lessen the laboring woman's perception of pain.[38] Figure 24–5 presents a model depicting responses to the pain of labor contractions in women who have had psychoprophylactic preparation and in women who have not had psychoprophylactic preparation.[36] The box outlines specific breathing techniques used in the psychoprophylactic technique.

Some proponents interpreted psychoprophylaxis as a problem-solving technique that could be used by couples throughout the childbearing year.[38] They felt that the prenatal classroom could provide an environment in which parents could discuss and learn effective responses. These responses could be applied not only to the stress of labor, but also to crises in other areas of their lives. These advocates believed that with proper guidance from the childbirth educator, it was "just a simple step from choosing appropriate responses in labor to reacting effectively to the stresses of postpartum and parenting."[38] Clearly, this is an optimistic viewpoint.

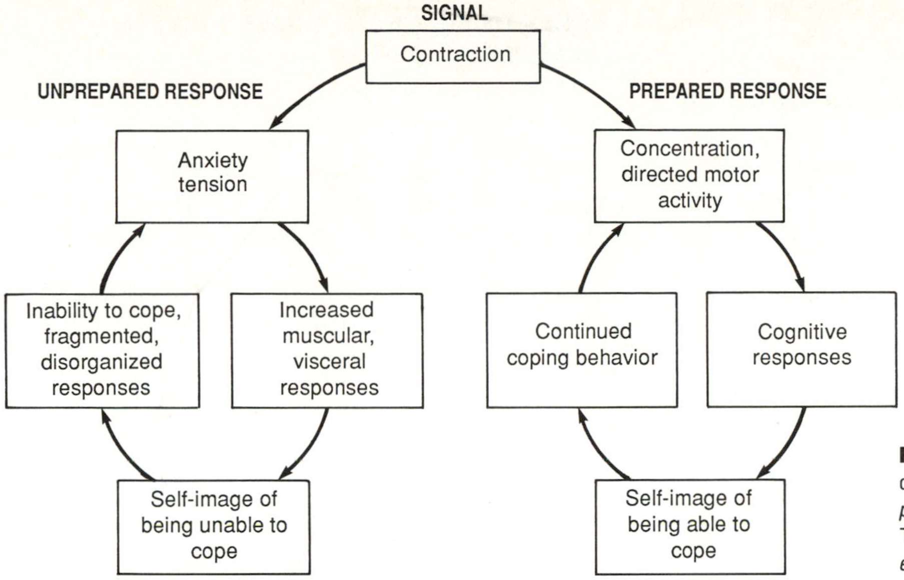

Figure 24–5. Model depicting pain of contractions in labor. (*Redrawn and reproduced, with permission, from Hassid P.* Textbook for Childbirth Educators. *2nd ed. Philadelphia: JB Lippincott; 1984:33.*)

Childbirth Without Violence (the LeBoyer Method). In 1975, Frederick LeBoyer introduced a delivery technique that was intended to improve the birth experience from the perspective of the newborn. In this method, basic steps are taken to ensure a gentle birth experience for the baby. LeBoyer's method included dimming the lights in the delivery room, placing the baby on the mother's warm abdomen, waiting up to 6 minutes before cutting the umbilical cord while the mother gently massages the baby, and submerging the baby in warm water after the cord is cut. This proposed delivery technique would alleviate the so-called "birth trauma" of concern to psychotherapists. Therapists have described negative effects of the traumatic births of clients with psychiatric problems. Currently, there is no scientific evidence that the LeBoyer method of birth actually helps an individual in future psychosocial development. Many

BREATHING TECHNIQUES FOR THE PSYCHOPROPHYLACTIC METHOD OR LAMAZE

The psychoprophylactic or Lamaze method is a conditioned pain response that results from a combination of techniques. The first breathing pattern is called slow paced breathing. This pattern begins with a deep cleansing breath, and involves a focal point or focus of attention, effleurage (light touch massage of the abdomen), and slow paced breathing (about 6 to 10 breaths per minute), ending with a deep cleansing breath. The support person or practitioner may breathe with the woman to help her focus her attention, massage her, and check for relaxation.

For stronger contractions, modified paced breathing is used. The woman begins to breathe slowly in and out either through her nose or mouth, increasing speed as the contraction reaches its peak, slowing as the contraction goes away, and ending with a cleansing breath.

For very strong contractions, modified paced breathing with increased concentration is used. The modified paced breathing is, at its maximum, twice the normal breathing rate or about one breath every 2 seconds (about 30 breaths per minute maximum). The woman is taught that the faster the breathing the more shallow it must be, the slower the deeper, to ensure the proper amount of oxygen-carbon dioxide exchange and to prevent hyperventilation.

Other techniques are used with these breathing patterns. The woman may use a one-two-three-four count or four-four musical beat while mentally (or with her coach) singing a song like Yankee Doodle. If the woman also has a premature urge to push this can be used with a blowing out exhalation or puff, at regular intervals; for example, four breaths and one puff. The blowing out helps to counteract any voluntary urge to push as the diaphragm cannot push both up and down at the same time. The coach is also taught numerous other techniques to help with labor and variations (like back labor) that might occur.

Courtesy of Diane Moore, CNM, PhD.

parents, however, report a positive birthing experience with the LeBoyer method.

Other Methods. A number of other prepared childbirth methods have been developed. The Kitzinger psychosexual method (1950s), the Wright method (1960s), and the Bradley method (1960s) all have loyal supporters. The hallmark of the Bradley method is that the husband or partner of the mother serves as the primary labor coach (*see* box). In fact, the role of the father is so central to this method that it is referred to as "husband-coached childbirth." The American Academy of Husband-Coached Childbirth (AAHCC) was founded to certify teachers of this method.

Hypnosis has also been claimed to be an effective approach to pain control in labor; this technique has gained less support, mostly because of the great deal of time, training, and intensity it requires. Childbirth educators may offer eclectic approaches that incorporate aspects of different methods. The many different childbirth education programs currently available may make the choice of an approach difficult.[39]

Childbirth preparation methods differ in their explanations of why they work and the specific activities that are taught, for example, breathing patterns. Despite these variations, however, all involve a combination of physical and psychologic techniques. All methods require that a process of prenatal education take place, that the educational program include discussions of what labor and delivery are like, that the laboring woman be attended by a support person (ideally the baby's father), and that the woman learn to relax specific muscles, breathe in a controlled manner, and use her muscles effectively in delivery (Figure 24–6).[7,36]

Acceptance. Today, some type of childbirth education is available to nearly every family in the United States who has access to prenatal care. Prenatal education classes are now considered to be part of standard obstetric practice. In some geographic areas, pregnant clients must decide among many educational options; however, nurses should never take this for granted. None of the methods currently avail-

BREATHING TECHNIQUES FOR THE BRADLEY METHOD

The physiologic components of the Bradley method involves breath control, abdominal breathing, and general body relaxation in harmony with the body, labor, and contractions. The major breathing technique used is slow abdominal relaxed breathing, which may become more rapid as the contractions intensify. The Bradley method focuses on breath control while the mother is in a comfortable position; this can be individualized to each woman. Deep mental relaxation is used along with controlled abdominal breathing.

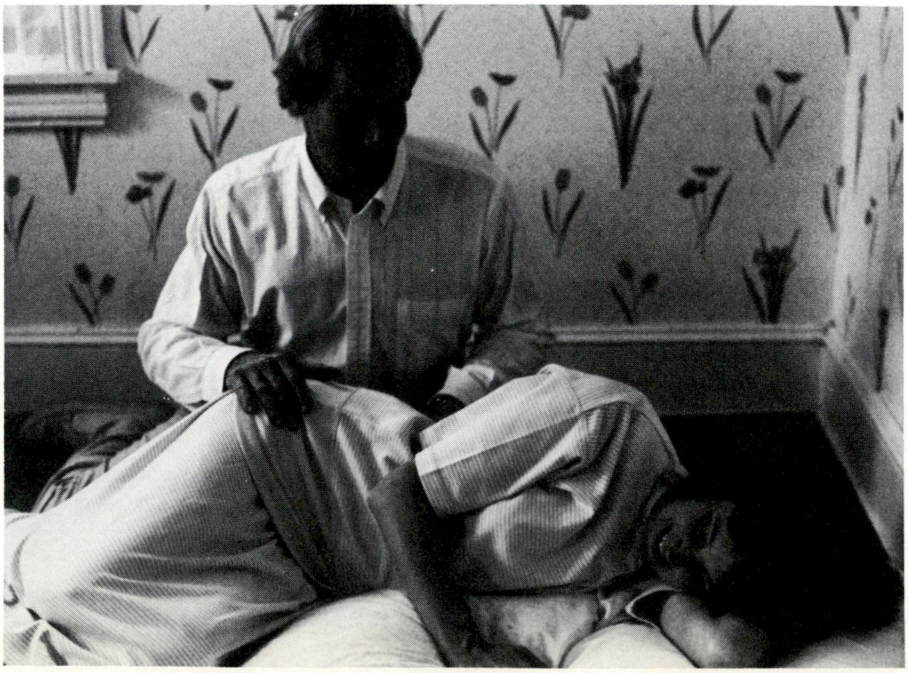

Figure 24–6. Couple practicing childbirth education technique.

able was enthusiastically welcomed in the United States. Indeed, initially Grantly Dick-Read was considered a radical.[28] During the 1950s and early 1960s, women who wanted to use the prepared childbirth methods often had problems in locating physicians who were willing to work with them during their hospital births. These women frequently were opposed by hospital staff members and by other women who tended to view them as upstarts willing to sacrifice the health of their infants for the politics of obstetrics.

During the 1970s, social forces such as the women's movement, the proliferation of self-help groups, and extensive media coverage contributed to a broader acceptance of prepared childbirth in the United States. As the public began to view prepared childbirth more positively, pregnant couples started to look for settings and health care providers who would assist them in obtaining prepared childbirth instruction and in fostering deliveries using these techniques. Economic concerns and the desire to continue to attract clients forced changes in policy and procedures used by some agencies and health care providers. If clients kept bringing business, anything safe, reasonable, and acceptable to the professional staff would be allowed.[25] This is one example of how consumers can have an impact on health care practices.

Effectiveness. How effective is prepared childbirth? The answer to this often-asked question must be given with caution and depends on how the term *effective* is being used. For instance, educational preparation that affords a pregnant couple the opportunity to learn about and discuss pregnancy, labor, and delivery can be effective in establishing a care partnership between clients and health care providers. Educational preparation that focuses on a shared delivery experience between the client and her support person can also foster communication between family members.

Support for prepared childbirth has ranged from passionate endorsement to more pragmatic views that knowledge is better than ignorance in almost all of life's situations. Likewise, claims of benefits have also covered the spectrum from near-religious experiences to more modest reports of research studies. Genest conducted a substantial review of studies dealing with pain and psychoprophylaxis in relation to preparation for childbirth.[40] He observed that childbirth education classes had the benefit of lowering anxiety levels and altering clients' assessments of their coming labors. The classes helped clients to develop feelings of resourcefulness, excitement over sharing a major life effort, acceptance of birth as a rewarding problem they were capable of solving, and greater control during childbirth. When clients (not the childbirth instructors) had positive self-appraisals, they tended to perceive less pain during birth and to have better feelings about the birth and their babies. Indeed, positive feelings were among the strongest benefits Genest reported; he also suggested that such good feelings might be the most important single factor contributing to the popularity of prepared childbirth classes among both clients and health care providers.[40] Research evidence does not, however, clearly support claims that prepared childbirth techniques alone ensure healthier babies for everyone or that there will be fewer labor and delivery complications. In addition, no single method has been shown to be the best.

Disadvantages. A possible, unintentional disadvantage of prepared childbirth classes is the sense of failure that may be experienced by women who are unable to follow through with the program as taught. In American society, where schooling is required of all children, many tend to view prepared childbirth as classes helping them to get ready for the big test of childbirth. Women and their partners may feel they have "failed" a major course in parenthood if they cannot perform a particular technique well. Indeed, in some situations even receiving anesthesia or analgesia could be a source of disappointment. For example, advocates of the Bradley method are so strongly opposed to analgesia and anesthesia that teachers must keep a high rate of medication-free deliveries to remain certified by the AAHCC.[36] This could be a subtle (or not so subtle) burden on the pregnant couple.

At times, couples undertake prepared childbirth education with unrealistic expectations of easy, pain-free deliveries. Such hopes can foster a sense of failure and negative feelings if the delivery experience is very different.

A major problem exists for women who develop complications requiring cesarean delivery. After receiving prepared childbirth education, expecting to have a low-risk delivery experience, and hoping to have a birth shared in all aspects with a partner, these women instead undergo a high-risk, surgical birth (*see* Chapter 28). Such women are at risk for a situational crisis related to the operative birth and may grieve the loss of the expected birth experience. Today, the availability of cesarean birth classes and attempts by nurses and other health care providers to ensure a satisfying birth experience for cesarean couples have done much to address this problem; however, such classes are not yet universal.

Currently, many childbirth educators attempt to present labor and delivery in a realistic manner and strive to help clients feel good about themselves whatever the delivery outcome. In their roles as childbirth educators, nurses need to be sensitive to the potential untoward effects of these classes. In addition, nurses need to identify client expectations at the beginning of the educational program and to deal with these as appropriate. As discussed earlier, development of alternative birth plans may also help reduce disappointment should a high-risk condition arise. Support partners should be specifically included, as women may

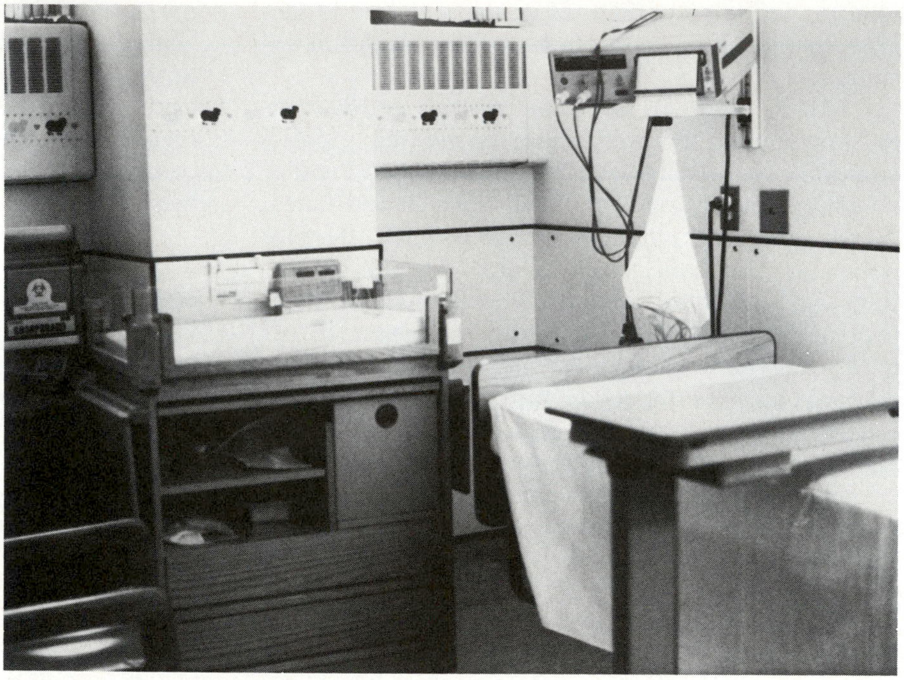

A

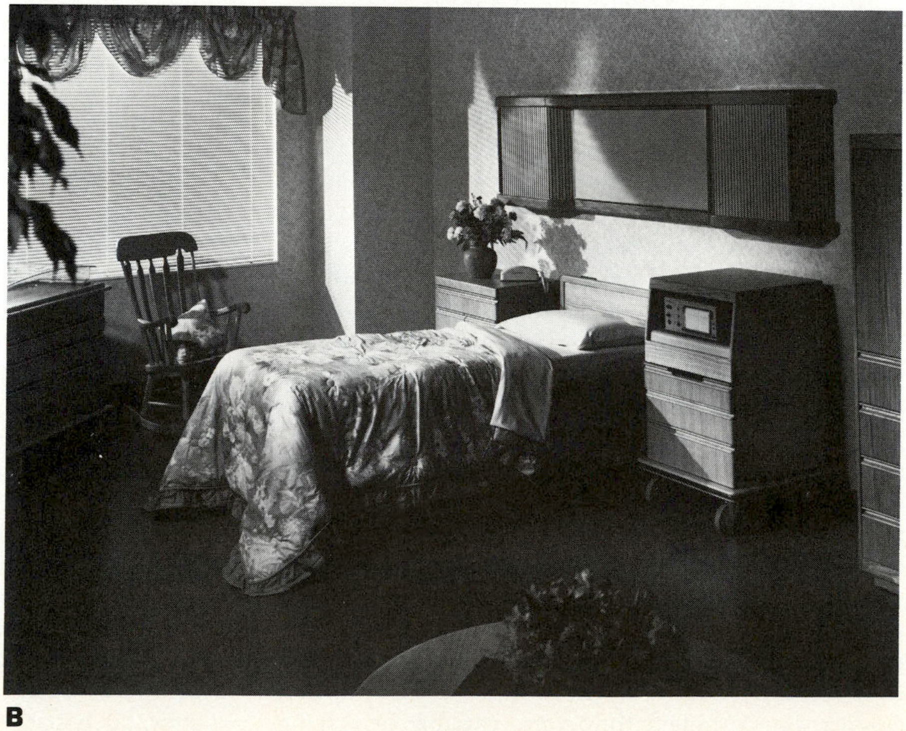

B

Figure 24–7. Childbirth alternatives. **A.** hospital labor and delivery room. **B.** Hospital birth suite (courtesy of Hill-Rom). (*Figure continues.*)

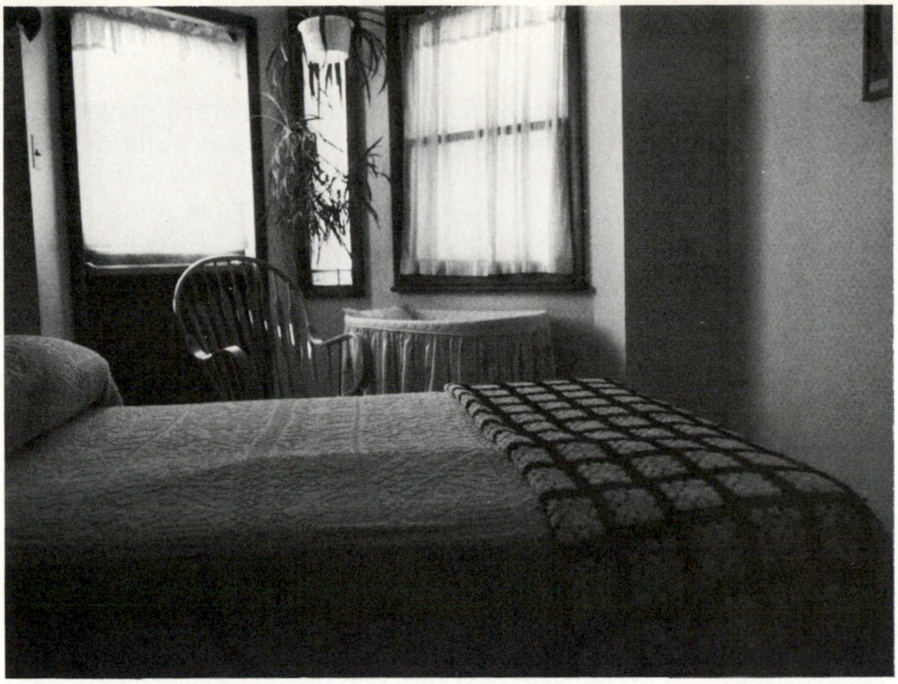

C

Figure 24–7. *(Continued.)* Childbirth alternatives. **C.** Birth center.

have a difficult time if they feel that their family members think they have failed. Nurses in labor and delivery and postpartum settings need to be aware of clients' birth plans and to provide for additional support if the plans do not work out.

Prepared Childbirth and Technology. Technologic developments have a goal of improving physical outcomes for women and infants. Technologic advances range in complexity from simple fetoscopes used to auscultate fetal heart tones to electronic fetal monitors and include such entities as intravenous infusions, forceps, scalpels, and sutures. These are all obstetric tools devised to assist childbirth. In several instances, technologic advances have made a family-centered birth possible. For example, regional anesthesia now allows a woman to be awake during a cesarean delivery and to share the birth event with her support person. Prenatal genetic testing allows a couple at risk for genetic defects to anticipate the birth of a genetically normal child or to have time to prepare for an infant with special needs.

Problems have arisen, however, when technology has controlled childbirth and has been used as an excuse to prevent a family-centered birth experience. For example, focusing only on fetal monitor tracings can lead to restriction of movement of laboring women and selection of an unphysiologic, supine position. In addition, the tendency to read monitors away from the bedside can decrease the nature of nurse-client communication; by auscultating fetal heart tones and feeling contractions, the nurse had to physically touch the laboring client at regular intervals. Implications of barring a support person from the cesarean delivery room will be discussed in Chapter 28. In some settings, there is such a high-risk, high-tech focus that the humanizing aspects of birth and the importance of integrating childbirth preparation techniques are only given lip service.

It would be as silly to suggest that technology be abolished from obstetrics as it would be to suggest that people again should rely on horses for their transportation. Nurses working with childbearing clients need to assess carefully the ways in which technology is used to augment or detract from the childbearing experience. Nurses need to include appropriate information about the existence of technical equipment and procedures and to provide clients with the opportunity to discuss them. In addition, nurses need to employ strategies that allow clients to use their prepared childbirth methods along with any necessary technology.

Choice of Setting and Childbirth Attendant

In contemporary society, delivery alternatives are available to pregnant families. These alternatives include the hospital birth experience, free-standing birth centers, and home births (Figure 24–7). In addition, several types of birth attendants are available to the family: the physician (most often an obstetrician), **certified nurse-midwife** (CNM), or **lay midwife** (Table 24–6).

Decisions about where and with whom to deliver involve the interaction of family members, availability of choices in the geographic area, and the goals for the birth experience.[25,41] A family's past experiences and attitudes, level of risk, and socioeconomic background are important factors. In addition, ability to pay for services influences selection of delivery alternatives. For example, a family that does not have obstetric insurance may simply seek obstetric care from the cheapest source or opt for no prenatal care.

TABLE 24–6. WHO DOES THE DELIVERIES?

Physicians

Physicians constitute the largest group of professionals performing deliveries in the United States. Educational preparation includes graduation from medical or osteopathic school, successful completion of at least one year of post–medical school clinical training, passage of a national board licensing examination, and ability to meet physicians' requirements for licensure in each state. Although deliveries can legally be performed by any physician, most are done by obstetricians. These are physicians who have completed several years of postgraduate specialty training in obstetrics; many have also successfully passed national certification boards sponsored by the American College of Obstetricians and Gynecologists.

Certified Nurse-Midwives

Certified nurse-midwives (CNMs) are registered nurses who have successfully completed postgraduate training in nurse-midwifery. This is a specialized program focusing on maternal and newborn health and normal deliveries. Certified nurse-midwives have passed a certification examination sponsored by the American College of Nurse-Midwives and are licensed by the states in which they practice. Restrictions on the scope and location of practice of CNMs are decided by individual states. Locations for CNM practice include hospitals, birth centers, and occasionally home settings.

Lay Midwives

Lay midwife is the general term used for an individual who attends births, but who is not a nurse-midwife or physician. The educational preparation varies greatly. It is not possible to identify a lay midwife as a person who has met certain educational standards. Some lay midwives may have had much training and may have served apprenticeships; they may be able to attend childbearing families with great skill. Others may simply have an interest in birth and may have very little educational preparation or experience. Some states do have licensing requirements for lay midwives; however, currently, lay midwives remain mostly beyond the scope of professional regulation. Lay midwives rarely have hospital or licensed birth center privileges; they attend clients most often in home settings. The term *midwife* frequently causes confusion between CNMs and lay groups. As noted, these birth attendants are different from each other, although they share a philosophy of birth as a normal life event.

In other instances, couples may be reimbursed by their insurance companies only if they deliver in a hospital.

Despite the availability of birth options, most pregnant families in the United States still choose to deliver in hospitals. To determine the best place for the delivery, the woman and family must be well informed about each choice, what is available in the community, and the implications of the choice for family and baby. The benefits to the woman and family of choosing the place of birth stem mainly from the psychologic and physiologic stress reduction that occurs when the woman feels that she is in a safe place and in good care.

Table 24–7 summarizes the advantages and disadvantages of each type of birth experience. The hospital setting and obstetrician-attended birth are the primary recommendations for the high-risk client. Alternatives in delivery settings and attendants are therefore restricted to obstetrically low-risk clients.

Hospital. Hospitals differ tremendously in the types of obstetric services offered and in the ability to provide care to high-risk clients. Facilities may range from low-risk services, focusing only on healthy mothers and infants, to second-level units able to care for certain types of high-risk conditions, to third level care settings that can provide technology and staff expertise for those at highest risk. For financial and staffing reasons, high-risk care has tended to be concentrated in regional centers (for further discussion, *see* Chapter 35).

Transport of a sick neonate to a high-risk neonatal unit at another hospital may result in the separation of mother and infant. Desire to avoid anguish caused by potential separation and quick access to staff skilled in high-risk care are reasons why some families may elect such a setting for all of their care.

If a hospital birth is necessary either because of maternal choice or complications, an appropriate location should be chosen as follows:

- Women who have no or minimal problems are usually referred to a low risk community hospital or to a community hospital with a neonatal special care unit that can handle many but not all neonatal problems.
- Women who have moderate to high complications (eg, severe diabetes, cardiac or thyroid disorders, premature labor) or who have a fetus with a diagnosis of abnormalities (eg, Rh disease, hydrocephaly, certain genetic disorders) should deliver in a medical center with the availability of a perinatologist and neonatologist, high-risk maternal-fetal unit, and neonatal intensive care unit.

TABLE 24–7. ADVANTAGES AND DISADVANTAGES OF DIFFERENT BIRTH SETTINGS

Type	Advantages	Disadvantages
Hospital	Security, availability of emergency equipment Potential use of birthing room Availability of professional staff Availability of latest technology For multiparas, some quiet time alone Contact with other new mothers Insurance coverage of birth expenses Availability of analgesia and anesthesia, if necessary	Impersonal and routine care Potential rigid rules Restrictive visiting policies Increased risk of unnecessary interventions Use of unnecessary medications Hospital limitation of options (eg, ambulation) Separation from other children at home Separation from other family members
Birth center	Continuity of care Homelike setting Opportunity for couple to participate actively in care Wellness oriented Less expensive Extensive information on childbirth readily available Discharge within 24 hours Early and extended contact with newborn Ability to have any significant others present	Possibility of transfer to another facility Appropriate only for low-risk women (may be "risked out" at any time) Limited accessibility Possibility of needing emergency care Insurance may not cover birth center deliveries Regional anesthetics may not be available Sense of failure if client needs to be transferred to acute care facility
Home	Emotionally satisfying for all family members Familiar environment Opportunity for family members to participate actively in birth Wellness orientation Least expensive birth option Early and extended contact with newborn	Possibility that emergency interventions may be needed Difficulty in finding qualified birth attendants Difficulty in accessing transportation to acute care setting if needed Insurance may not cover home birth Analgesia and anesthesia not available Appropriate only for low-risk women

It is important to note that family-centered care and CNM-attended deliveries can also exist in hospitals offering high-risk care.

Hospitals, in response to consumer demand for family-centered birth, now offer a variety of options. The expectant family may labor and deliver in traditional, separate labor and delivery rooms (which require that the woman be transferred from one room to another to deliver), in a combined labor and delivery room (Figure 24–7A), or in a birthing room (Figure 24–7B).

With the exception of women requiring operative obstetrics or in situations in which the health status of mother or fetus requires specialized equipment and a high-risk team, there is little reason to transfer a woman from a labor room to a delivery room. This time-consuming practice is uncomfortable for the client, difficult for the staff, and a financial waste of space and of housekeeping services. In a study of women who had used a hospital birthing room, Maloney noted that elimination of the transfer was identified as a major strength of the birthing room experience.[42]

The woman delivering in a hospital may choose from a variety of equipment, such as a birthing bed (Figure 24–8), a birth chair, or a delivery table. All equipment is designed to allow the mother to assume a variety of positions (sitting, knee-chest, supine, and so on). Other equipment that may be available for the birth includes forceps, stirrups, anesthesia sets, infant warmer, intubation and resuscitation supplies, infant identification sets, clamps and bulb syringes, fetal monitoring equipment, delivery room garb, infant eye prophylaxis, infant wrappers, and other items.

Hospital Birthing Room. Many women today labor, deliver, and recover in a **hospital birthing room** (*see* Figure 24–7B). There is no transfer to a delivery room, unless the mother or fetus is in distress. In many hospitals that offer birthing rooms, women are moved to the postpartum unit after a recovery and bonding period; however, in a few places, women remain in the same room until discharge. A support person, and at times other relatives or friends, may remain with the client. Sibling attendance at birth is generally uncommon in hospital settings. By establishing birthing rooms, hospitals have attempted to create a family-centered, homelike birth experience. This represents attempts to make institutional goals more congruent with a family's emotional needs as well as with consumer and professional desires.

A great deal of thought usually goes into the design of birthing rooms. Indeed, this is a subject in which nursing involvement is important. Nursing expertise can help create an environment that blends homelike decor with professional practice. Birthing rooms may contain a specially designed birthing bed that can adjust to different positions and can be separated in two, if necessary; skillfully concealed medical equipment; home-type furnishings such as a rocking chair, television, cradle, wallpaper, and soft lighting; and a private bathroom with shower.

Studies of clients who have used birthing rooms have demonstrated consumer satisfaction.[42–45] In Kieffer's study of 109 women, 33 percent reported they would have delivered at home if their hospital had not had a birthing room.[45] This indicates that the presence of birthing rooms may attract clients who otherwise would opt to deliver elsewhere.

The implementation of homelike, family-centered care in birthing rooms has had a subtle impact on procedures and policies used elsewhere in hospital obstetric units. One effect is to build into the organizational structure of the hospital a vehicle for family-centered care, regardless of the high-risk care capability of the units.

Unfortunately, the existence of a birthing room in a hospital does not ensure that it will be supported as a delivery alternative. Hospitals may advertise lovely rooms as a way of enticing clients to deliver there. Through their lack of commitment to providing birthing room experiences, however, nurses and physicians can prevent this option from becoming a reality for clients. For instance, by assuming each client is a possible high-risk client, hospital staff can convince women they should not use a birthing room.[42] Nurses must remember that it is the philosophy, attitudes, and interventions of hospital staff, rather than the room decor, that foster satisfying birth experiences.[42]

Which clients are able to use a birthing room? Criteria differ among hospitals. For example, some units have very strict criteria[47]; only women at lowest risk are considered candidates. Other units are more lenient in their criteria and routinely allow women expecting to deliver vaginally to use the birthing room, even if they are not at lowest risk. As part of prenatal education, pregnant couples who hope for a birthing room experience need to identify whether or not their hospital has a birthing room and whether they would be able to use it.

The hospital birthing room offers couples the chance to have an emotionally supportive, homelike birth within ready access of the backup facilities of a hospital. In addition, the creation of birthing rooms illustrates a shift in obstetric practice toward a greater client role in childbirth. Conversely, inability to meet criteria for a birthing room, arriving in labor at a time when the birthing rooms are being used by other clients, or being transferred as a result of labor complications can foster a sense of failure and frustration for some clients.

Free-Standing Birth Centers. **Birth centers** provide homelike birthing experiences outside a hospital setting. This is why they are often called "free-standing." Birth centers are usually licensed by their states. They are able to give some emergency care on the premises and are able to provide transportation to a backup hospital, should the need arise.

Birth centers are based on the belief that childbirth for most women is a normal life event; thus, safe, satisfying, health-oriented, family-focused births can take place away from an acute care hospital setting. Birth centers provide homelike decor (Figure 24–7C). Staff usually encourage the client to include any family and friends she desires to participate in the birth. Prenatal care is given at the center, and the family has much opportunity to get to know the birth center and its staff. The birth center may be owned by a physician, by CNMs, by lay groups, or any combination of these. Licensed birth centers have physicians available for consultation whenever appropriate.[48]

It has been estimated that 1 to 2 percent of births outside hospitals take place in birth centers, although Lubic reported that as many as 11 percent of women might select this alternative.[49] Personal feelings of alienation, lack of control, lack of participation in decision making, and frustration with inflexible hospital policies are among reasons clients seek an alternate birth experience. These are also reasons why clients choose birthing rooms within hospitals. According to Lubic, families who felt alienated from hospital practices engaged in home births without professional attendants.[49] The availability of a birth center offered a compromise between hospital and home birth.

In 1975, the Maternity Center Association in New York City became the first free-standing birth center in the United States. It served as a model for other American birth centers.[50] In 1981, the Cooperative Birth Center Network was created to provide information on a national level and to foster the growth of birth centers.[49] As of 1985, it was estimated that there were more than 150 birth centers located in 32 states. Professional motivation, as well as client demand, has promoted the establishment of birth centers, because birth centers provide settings in which CNMs can practice full-scope midwifery.

Only women who have no history or foreseeable possibility of medical, obstetric, or psychiatric problems qualify for care in a birth center. No client can be assured that the birth will take place there, because development of a high-risk condition during preg-

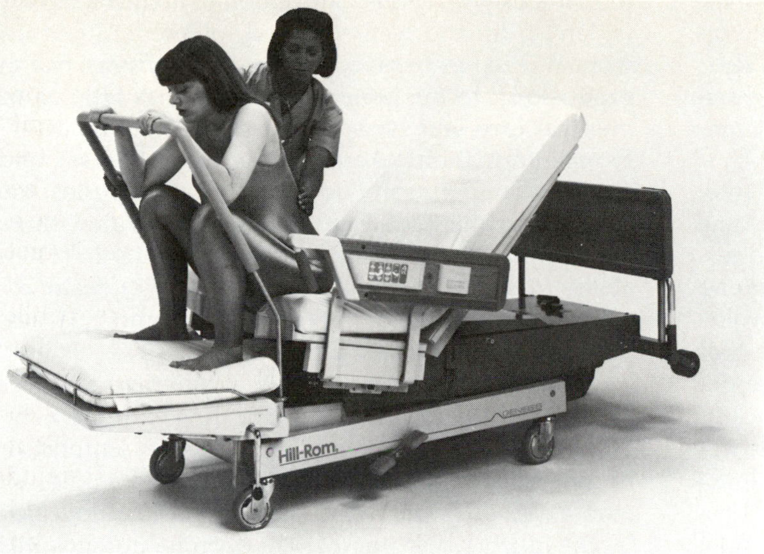

A

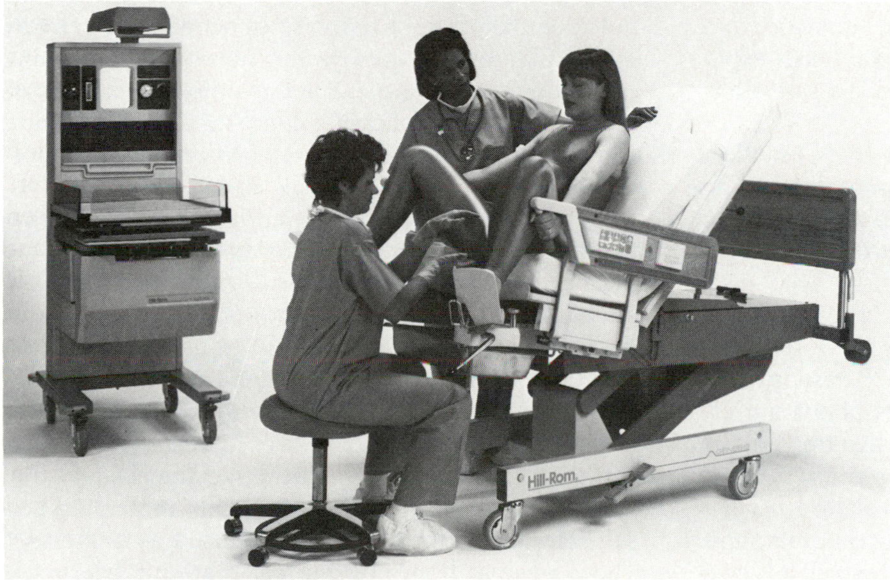

B

Figure 24–8. Birthing bed. **A.** Labor. **B.** Delivery. (*Courtesy of Hill-Rom.*)

nancy or labor will necessitate transfer to an acute care hospital. Inability to realize a birth plan and having to deliver in an unfamiliar and unwanted setting can contribute to frustration, anger, and a sense of failure for some clients. To deal with this potential problem, the CNM may remain with the couple as a support person during transport and throughout the hospital delivery.

Information is not available on rates of transfer for all birth centers. Indeed, actual transfer rates may reflect subjective practitioner interpretation of who is and who is not at risk, despite the existence of qualifying criteria. Transfer rates in some cases have been reported to approach 20 percent.[51]

Delivery at a birth center necessitates a client's active involvement and willingness to accept personal responsibility during pregnancy and childbirth. Not every pregnant woman desires to do this. From a study of 11 birth centers, Bennets and Lubic drew a profile of birth center clients.[50] The women tended to have a mean age of 25; 64 percent were urban residents, 63 percent were Caucasian, and 88 percent were married. The women tended to be highly motivated toward learning; 95 percent had attended prepared childbirth courses and 82 percent had come for at least nine prenatal visits. It is important to remember that this profile does not describe every client. Note how different this profile is from the poor, rural women attended by midwives in the early 20th century.

As with any childbearing alternative, a freestanding birth center is the best choice for some women and a poor selection for others. Indeed, questions are often asked about the safety of birth centers, especially when transfers for complications involve time delays. Advocates of birth centers believe that attentive screening, client cooperation, and care delivered by CNMs with appropriate physician backup made this a safe option. From a retrospective study of two matched low-risk groups of women, Feldman and Hurst found that women who delivered in hospitals had more medical interventions than women who delivered in a birth center; however, the obstetric outcome was the same for both groups. Their results, consistent with other studies, indicate that place of birth did have an impact on childbirth experience and that birth centers did provide a safe alternative to hospital delivery.[52]

Whatever the setting in which they practice, nurses caring for the childbearing family need to be familiar with birth centers in their geographic area and to be knowledgeable about birth centers in general.

A great nursing challenge is presented to hospital-based maternity nurses who work with clients transferred from birth centers. These nurses must first evaluate their own feelings about out-of-hospital births. They must welcome the transferred client, her support person, and her midwife and strive to work together with them to ensure a satisfying birth experience. Nurses working on units serving as backup for birth centers would be well advised to plan meetings with birth center staff and to devise collaborative strategies in the event of transfer. It is possible to work toward the goal of client well-being, even if professionals do not share identical views on settings for childbirth. Unfortunately, in some instances, an "us" versus "them" attitude exists, and the client is caught in the middle; on transfer to the hospital setting, she and her support person are treated as if they are undesirable revolutionaries.

Home. Although once the choice of nearly every woman, home birth today is an option that is not often intentionally practiced throughout the United States. It is difficult to identify how many women actually deliver at home, because those undertaking home delivery or providing care for home delivery do not have extensive statistical recordkeeping priorities. Individuals who choose the option of home birth vary widely, from the well-educated, older, multiparous woman who has received thorough care from a health professional to the poor woman who has little or no prenatal care and no specialized birth attendants.[55] From information taken from birth certificates and records of midwife and out-of-hospital deliveries, the U.S. Department of Vital Statistics identified three main reasons why women choose home birth: (1) inability to reach a hospital (geography), (2) desire for a family-centered birth experience, and (3) unplanned delivery at home.

A major controversy in obstetrics revolves around the safety of home birth. It is extremely difficult to use any statistical argument to support or oppose home birth, because of the lack of ample, accurate data on home birth. This is further complicated by the much larger numbers of documented hospital births and the more complete records available on hospital births. In addition, birth certificates often do not identify place of delivery or whether a delivery was a planned or unexpected home birth. Birthing centers may also be classified in state records as hospitals, further complicating comparisons of birth outcomes among births at home, birth centers, and hospitals.

Home birth has been defended as a safe alternative to hospital birth in certain medically and obstetrically low-risk populations using skilled birth attendants.[54] Women delivering at home have been described as having low rates of transfer to hospitals and thus lower rates of interventions, such as cesarean deliveries or use of forceps, than women delivering in hospitals. Opponents of home birth maintain that such comparisons are deceptive; they believe that home birth couples tend to be highly motivated and self-selected when home birth is used as a choice.[55] Those against home births feel that childbearing is unpredictable and that birth at home presents an unneeded risk to mother and infant. Opponents also claim that decreases in perinatal morbidity and mortality may be the result of the shift to hospital deliveries and the use of technologies that have developed over the last 50 years. Supporters of home birth counter with the argument that most complications can be predicted and that major obstetric difficulties are rare.

As may be seen, the option of planned home birth is the most controversial of birth alternatives. The nature of obstetric problems and the dearth of credible research demonstrating the safety of home birth indicate that this controversy is likely to continue. Nevertheless, some clients do elect home birth, and nurses working with pregnant couples need to be aware of this.

RESEARCH ABSTRACT

Morse JM, Park C. Home birth and hospital deliveries: a comparison of the perceived painfulness of parturition. Res Nurs Health. *1988;11:175–181.*

The purpose of this study was to obtain information about the amount of pain associated with childbirth by parents electing home birth or hospital deliveries. The study was conducted in a western Canadian city. Two hundred and eighty-two subjects including 149 women and 133 male partners made up the home birth group. The hospital group included 102 women and 89 male partners. All of the participants in the study had attended prenatal classes, which taught Lamaze labor relaxation exercises.

The investigators constructed the Morse Pain Stimulus Scale, a questionnaire containing 36 items reflective of common pain conditions. Questionnaires were sent to the participants. Sixty-nine percent of the home birth group and fifty-nine percent of the hospital birth group returned questionnaires.

Childbirth was perceived to be more painful in the hospital birth group than in the home birth group. The hospital birth group ranked childbirth as the third most painful stimulus, whereas the home birth group ranked it the eighth most painful stimulus. Analysis also showed a discrepancy in the rating of childbirth pain between men and women. In the hospital birth group, the women rated the pain of childbirth higher than the men; the reverse was true for the home birth group.

Comment:
This study alerts the nurse to differing perceptions of labor pain in different birthing environments; however, the labor pain that women experienced was ranked against other forms of pain, such as that associated with a heart attack or kidney stone, which these women had not experienced and with which they were not familiar. Although investigators reported similar demographic characteristics for the home and hospital birth groups, there may have been initial differences in perceptions about birth pain between the groups. Individuals who choose a home birth may hold very different attitudes from individuals who choose a hospital birth. Reports of pain may therefore reflect what the home birth group believes should be their responses. These issues aside, this study contributes to a needed literature explaining perceptions of pain in alternative childbirth settings.

In many states, lay midwives, rather than physicians or CNMs attend home births. In general, lay midwives do not have delivery privileges at hospitals or licensed birth centers. Physicians and CNMs may hesitate to attend scheduled home births in places where hospitals or licensed birth centers are readily accessible. Beyond the issue of the safety of home birth itself is the issue of defense in a malpractice suit. There currently continues to be a perceived crisis in the number and size of obstetric malpractice suits against physicians and nurses. Fear of litigation and difficulty in defending one's actions in an unlicensed and unsupported setting are deterrents to the most well-intentioned obstetric professional.

PREPARATION OF SIBLINGS

It has been estimated that around 80 percent of American and European children have siblings.[56] Siblings can be less than one year apart in age or more than 20 years apart. Children raised together as siblings can have the same mother and father. Children from blended families can share one common biologic parent; in cases where pregnancy occurs after another child has been adopted, the older child or children may not share biologic parents with the new baby. Despite the variation in family relationships, sibling education should be provided for any child who resides with the pregnant client.

Any time a family adds—or loses—a member, changes in the emotional patterns of the family may be expected. Although there may be very positive outcomes associated with the addition of a new baby, these do not always evolve easily or without thoughtful preparation.

For the most part, the decision to have another child is made by the parents, although there may be strong influencing factors such as desire for a child to have future sibling companionship. The sibling-to-be is told at some point that a new baby is coming; if events proceed normally, the infant arrives, grows, and ends up staying until late adolescence or early adulthood. Especially in the case of a first child, time alone with Mommy or Daddy may become a scheduled "date" rather than an everyday occurrence. Much has been written about sibling rivalry. Negative sibling behaviors manifested in relation to childbearing have included regressive behaviors, sleep disturbances, frequent crying, and demanding behaviors. Conversely, the arrival of a new baby has been described as a source of great interest to siblings.[57–60]

Changes associated with advancing pregnancy may be identified by even young children who may be aware not only of their mother's new silhouette but also of changes in her energy levels. When labor and delivery take place in hospital settings, children are suddenly separated from their mothers, usually for several days. In cases of high-risk pregnancies, the mother may be gone from the home for months. These situations can be distressing to the young child.

The impact of the media, especially television, has been noted frequently in this text. Sibling reactions to a new baby may also be influenced by television programs. Although some programs, especially those designed for educational enrichment, portray the arrival of new babies in a responsible, informative, and interesting manner, others do not. In planning educational preparation for siblings, nurses therefore need to be aware of the kinds of positive and negative programs that siblings may be viewing. (As writers, producers, and consultants to program companies, nurses could potentially have a major impact on the presentation of this topic.)

When to tell a sibling about the pregnancy and coming baby depends on the age and maturity level of the child (*see* discussions in Chapter 17). Because very young children have difficulty with abstract concepts of time, parents may wait until the pregnancy becomes visible. Parents should take care that news of the pregnancy comes from them, rather than from some well-meaning relative or friend. Parents of young children frequently need to be reminded that these children do understand their verbal and nonverbal actions. Unless they have told the child about the coming baby, parents should not converse with others as if the child were unable to decipher what they were saying.

It is difficult to prescribe prenatal classes for siblings in the same way it is possible to plan prenatal classes for adults. The nature and extent of prenatal teaching depend on such factors as the number of siblings already present at home, the age of the siblings, the nature of family dynamics preceding and during pregnancy, and possibly the extent to which the sibling perceives the new baby is taking his or her place in the affections of family members. Prenatal classes, delivered at a level the child can comprehend, might cover how a baby develops, what happens when the baby is born, where the child's mother (and father) will go when it is time for the baby to be born, who will remain with the child at home or at the birth center, what the new baby will be like, what it will be like for the child to be a "big" brother or "big" sister, and what it will be like to have another sibling.

Nursing Strategies

Nursing strategies focusing on sibling preparation can be devised to be implemented from both informal and formal approaches, depending on such factors as parental support of sibling education (provided by the parents with or without assistance from health care providers), characteristics of the siblings (eg, age, developmental level, number of siblings in the family, siblings' prior experiences with new babies), the setting where prenatal care and childbirth will take place, the philosophy of the health care providers and of the setting where prenatal care and childbirth will take place, and whether or not the sibling will be present at birth.

Nursing strategies can be designed to advise parents in their preparation with direct sibling teaching. Parents may be uncomfortable about speaking to their children about pregnancy and may seek information and guidance from nurses. Direct sibling teaching could be done on an individual basis during prenatal visits and through scheduled sibling tours and classes.

The topic of siblings should be included in all teaching plans for multiparas and should be dealt with during each trimester and at visits prior to delivery. Siblings who are brought to prenatal visits can be included by assisting them to hear the fetal heartbeat and to feel the baby's movements. If possible, mothers can be encouraged to bring the sibling to at least one prenatal visit. Visual aids such as child-oriented books, pamphlets, and charts can help explain how a baby develops and what childbirth entails.

Presence at Delivery

The presence of older children at delivery has been common in many cultures and has occurred frequently in the United States prior to the shift of birth location from home to hospital. Currently, siblings do not routinely attend deliveries. Most sibling preparation has therefore focused on what takes place during pregnancy and after the baby arrives.

A child's presence at delivery may not be desired by all families. Nevertheless, it is important for nurses to realize that there is no scientific reason to deny this as a viable positive option for some families. A family's wish to have a child view a delivery is not to be considered weird or strange. Indeed, nurses need to be able to provide information about settings that will support this option.

Of all alternatives for delivery settings, the hospital has been traditionally the most restrictive about siblings at births. In response to consumer pressures for more family-centered bonding experiences, many hospitals permit postpartum sibling visits (Figure 24–9); however, siblings tend to be invited only during certain periods after delivery. They usually view the new baby through a nursery window, and may be allowed to visit within the mother's hospital room. In

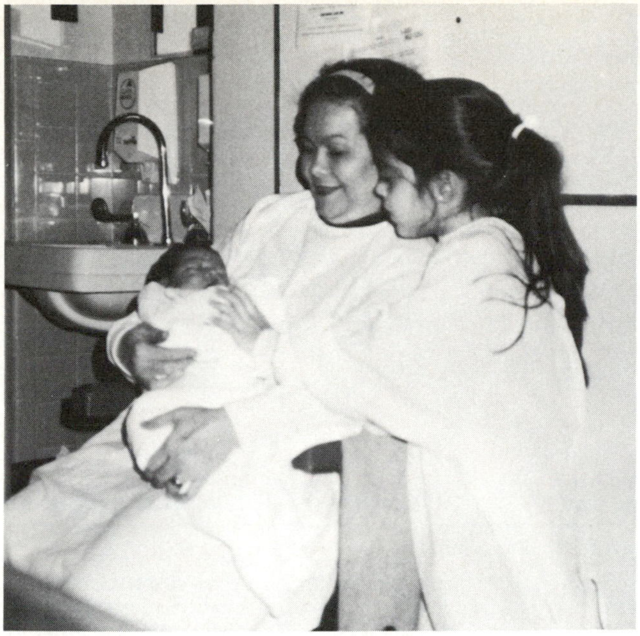

Figure 24–9. Sibling and grandmother visiting with newborn after hospital delivery.

addition, hospitals may have "bonding rooms" for siblings so that they can touch and hold the new baby. Sibling attendance at deliveries within a hospital setting is still the exception. DelGiudice observed that many of the reasons given by staff for preventing children from attending deliveries in hospitals are similar to reasons used in the past by those opposing fathers in the delivery room, that is, effects of seeing the birth on the child, potential for increased infections, staff inconvenience, and distraction of laboring mothers by their children.[61]

The wellness and family orientation of birth centers, as well as home environments, supports the option for a client to have anyone she desires, including siblings, to be with her during labor, witness the birth, and join her during the immediate recovery period. Indeed, such a family-based philosophy is part of the educational background of CNMs and nurses.

To ensure that the client and her support person can focus on labor and that the special needs of the sibling can be met, an adult of the family's choosing should be present with each child in a birth center. Ideally, these should be individuals who are well known to the child, who have received some education for childbirth, and who have been prepared for their role in supporting the sibling at birth. Although there are no policies available in a home setting, this tends to be helpful advice for sibling-attended births.

It is not possible to set absolute age limits for sibling attendance at births. Such decisions are based on assessment of each child and family and are made by clients in collaboration with health care providers.

PREPARATION OF GRANDPARENTS

Changes in styles of childbirth and infant care practices have contributed to a communications gap between today's parents and their own parents. Indeed, as noted earlier in this chapter, obstetric and neonatal care were very different at the time many grandparents gave birth. Disparities in beliefs and options can be a source of conflict between parents-to-be and grandparents-to-be. In addition, the literature has highlighted the importance of perceived parental support in a new mother's own adaptation to motherhood.[62–65]

Maloni and coworkers described a grandparent education class, established to acquaint grandparents with current maternity and pediatric care, abilities of the newborn, current and past approaches to infant care and feeding methods, and infant safety.[66] The purpose of the class was to foster communication by sharing information being learned by new parents Figure 24–10). The class did not focus on ways to be a grandparent. Of 200 grandmothers and grandfathers attending during the first year, 83 percent registered at the request of the expectant parent; the authors felt this indicated expectant parents' desires to have the support of their parents and the grandparents' desires to respond.[66]

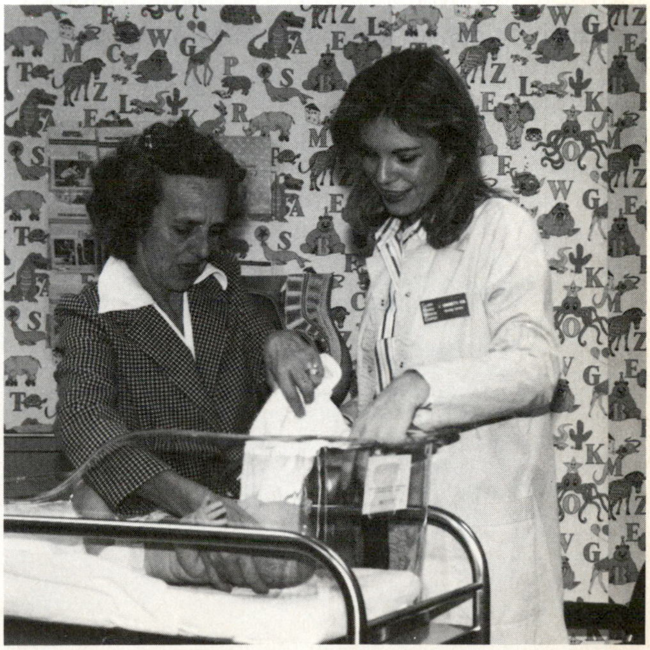

Figure 24–10. Grandparents class. (*Courtesy of Clara Maas Memorial Hospital, Belleville, New Jersey.*)

CASE STUDY/CARE PLAN: FAMILY PREPARATION FOR CHILDBIRTH

Kathleen and George Mulligan are expecting their third child. Kathleen, 34 years old, is 28 weeks pregnant. Since her first child was born 10 years ago, Kathleen has been a homemaker. George is a lineman for the telephone company. Their children, Coleen (10) and George Jr (6) are in good health and attend public school. The couple relates that the whole family is looking forward to the new baby.

At her routine appointment at the birth center, Kathleen says to the nurse: "I would really like to try the Lamaze method and have George in the labor and delivery room with me. We didn't take classes with the other two kids, because George never wanted to. He now would like to see the baby born." Kathleen delivered her previous babies with an epidural block. They were normal spontaneous deliveries.

Supporting Assessment Data	Expected Client/Family Outcome	Nursing Action/Intervention	Rationale	Criteria for Evaluation
Nursing Diagnosis: Coping, family: potential for growth, related to childbirth preparation				
28-week pregnant multipara; no childbirth preparation classes with previous births; delivered previous pregnancies with epidural block; two previous normal spontaneous deliveries; states "I would really like to try the Lamaze method and have George [husband] in the labor and delivery room with me." Two siblings, a girl aged 10 and a boy aged 6.	By the end of the visit, the client will be able to identify childbirth preparation classes (Lamaze) and sibling preparation classes available in the area.	Discuss differences in types of childbirth preparation (eg, Lamaze, Bradley). Provide client with a list of dates, places, instructors, and goals of Lamaze classes and sibling classes.	Childbirth preparation should fit the family's needs and lifestyle.	When asked, client identifies potential childbirth preparation classes she and her husband might attend.
	During the third trimester, the couple will attend a series of childbirth preparation classes (Lamaze).	Assess client's understanding of Lamaze childbirth preparation and knowledge of labor and delivery.	Learning begins with the individual's level of knowledge regarding the subject matter.	When questioned, couple relates that they are attending a childbirth preparation class.
	During the third trimester, the siblings will attend a sibling preparation class.	Give client supplemental reading materials related to Lamaze preparation and sibling preparation.	Supplemental reading materials help to reinforce concepts and clear up misunderstandings.	When questioned, client relates that her children are attending a sibling preparation class.
		Discuss client's perceptions of previous deliveries. Discuss how couple previously prepared their daughter for their son's birth.	Previous experiences identify knowledge deficits, misconceptions, and also strengths.	Client discusses perceptions of previous deliveries.
Nursing Diagnosis: Knowledge defict (husband), related to participation in childbirth preparation and labor and delivery				
Client wants to try Lamaze method; couple did not attend preparation classes with previous two pregnancies; husband has not been exposed to labor and delivery experience, although he now states he would like to see this baby born.	By the end of this visit, couple will identify goals and contents of Lamaze preparation	See earlier interventions.	See earlier rationale.	See earlier evaluation.
	The next prenatal visit will be scheduled during the birth center's evening hours so that husband can attend.	Encourage client to bring husband to prenatal visits.	Including the supporting other in health care encourages active participation and informed decision making.	Husband attends next prenatal visit with client and asks questions. Husband discusses pros and cons of attending classes and birthing; couple makes decision.
		Schedule visits at a time convenient to husband.	Prenatal care should be accessible and available at times congruent with family members' needs.	

Supporting Assessment Data	Expected Client/Family Outcome	Nursing Action/Intervention	Rationale	Criteria for Evaluation
		Discuss husband's feelings about attending classes and birthing, perceptions of wife's previous labors and deliveries.	Considering the clients' feelings and perceptions helps formulate a trusting relationship.	Couple decides whether husband will coach or if an alternative is more desirable.
	By the end of the third trimester, if husband agrees to participate, he will be prepared in the role of support person, or agree to attend labor and delivery, with an alternative person being coach	Provide husband with information and supplemental reading materials regarding childbirth preparation.	Supplemental material reinforces learning.	
		Discuss the role of support person with husband and alternatives available.	Information regarding role and alternate strategies for participation allows for informed decision making.	

SUMMARY

Educational preparation during childbearing is an integral part of prenatal care. Today nearly all pregnant clients who receive prenatal care have access to some type of educational program. This emphasis on education during pregnancy has evolved from the vocal and persistent efforts of professional and lay groups.

Contemporary educational efforts focus on preconceptional parenting education as well as early-pregnancy, midpregnancy, and late-pregnancy education for the family. Topics for preconceptional preparation for childbearing include physical health, safety, use of drugs and alcohol, family planning, and strategies for selecting obstetric caregivers and facilities. Early-pregnancy educational programs explore such topics as feelings about pregnancy, family reactions to pregnancy, physical changes, sexuality, warning signs of pregnancy, sibling concerns, and resources within the community. Among the topics discussed in midpregnancy preparation classes are fetal growth and development, mid-trimester physical changes, changes in activities of daily living, and client's expectations for pregnancy and birth. Late-pregnancy classes focus on preparation for labor and delivery and parenting. The couple may choose to attend a class that teaches them a specific method of prepared childbirth that they will be able to use during labor and delivery.

Educational prenatal preparation involves family members in addition to the pregnant couple. Current teaching strategies have been broadened to include siblings and grandparents.

The nursing role in educational preparation of clients during childbearing cannot be overstated. Nurses serve as childbirth educators, as expert sources of referral of pregnant clients to educational programs, as practitioners who work with clients who have had (or not had) various types of childbirth education, and as authors, producers, and evaluators of childbirth education materials. Nurses serve as teachers in formal and informal settings. The wide assortment of childbirth education programs and the complexity and diversity of each client's needs necessitate that nurses be knowledgeable about educational programs and options.

REVIEW QUESTIONS

1. Discuss factors that should be considered in planning client prenatal education.
2. Identify content to be included in educational programs during early, middle, and late pregnancy.
3. Distinguish between teaching plans and birth plans.
4. Discuss trends in childbearing practices in the United States during the 20th century.
5. Describe common features of prepared childbirth methods.

Some content in this chapter was adapted with permission from Weingarten CT, Jacobwitz JT. Alternatives in childbearing: choices and challenges. In:

Sherwen LN, ed. *Psychosocial Dimensions of the Pregnant Family.* New York: Springer Publishing Co; 1987: 193–218.

REFERENCES

1. Bloom B, ed. Taxonomy of Educational Objectives: Cognitive Domain. 25th ed. New York/London: Longman; 1982.
2. Krathwohl DR, et al, *Taxonomy of Educational Objectives: Affective Domain.* 13th ed. New York/London: Longman; 1982.
3. Walls JL. An instruction guide for educating expectant mothers. *Am J Matern Child Nurs.* 1983;8:274–276.
4. Reilly DE. *Behavioral Objectives: Evaluation in Nursing.* 2nd ed. Norwalk, Conn: Appleton & Lange; 1980.
5. Van Hoozer HL, et al. *The Teaching Process: Theory and Practice in Nursing.* Norwalk, Conn: Appleton & Lange; 1987.
6. Cameron J. Year-long classes for couples becoming parents. *Am J Matern Child Nurs.* 1979;4:358–362.
7. Bean CA. *Methods of Childbirth.* New York: Quill William Morrow, 1990.
8. Klein L. Our willy-nilly childbearing: Unintended and teenage pregnancy in the United States. *Pharos, Alpha Omega Alpha Honor Medical Society.* 1986;49:27–32.
9. Kutzner SK, Toussie-Weingarten CG. Working parents: The dilemma of child rearing and career. *Top Clin Nurs.* 1984;6: 30–37.
10. Siegel-Gorelick B. *The Working Parent's Guide to Child Care.* Boston: Little, Brown; 1983.
11. Chabon I. *Awake and Aware.* New York: Delacorte Press; 1966.
12. Sutterley DC, Donnelly GF. From the editors. *Top Clin Nurs* 1984;6:vi.
13. Carey J. First-trimester prenatal counseling in private practice. *J Obstet Gynecol Neonatal Nurs.* 1981;10:336–339.
14. Bretschneider JU, Minetola AC. Another look at early-pregnancy classes. *Am J Matern Child Nurs.* 1983;8:268–273.
15. Bing E, Colman L. *Making Love During Pregnancy.* New York: Noonday Press; 1989.
16. May K. Men's sexuality during the childbearing year: implications of research findings. *Holis Nurs Practice.* 1987;1: 60–66.
17. Simkin P. The birth plan: vehicle for trust and communication. *Birth.* 1983;10:184–185.
18. Clark CC. *Wellness Nursing: Concepts, Theory, Research and Practice.* New York: Springer Publishing Co; 1986.
19. Daddario JB. Trauma in pregnancy. *J Perinat Neonatal Nurs.* 1989;3:14–22.
20. Krozy RE, McColgan JJ. Auto safety, pregnancy and the newborn. *J Obstet Gynecol Neonatal Nurs.* 1985;14:11.
21. DeGrez SA. Bend and stretch. *Am J Matern Child Nurs.* 1988;13:357–359.
22. Department of Health Services. *Natural Remedies for Pregnancy Discomforts.* Sacramento, Calif: Coalition for the Medical Rights of Women and Educational Programs Associates, Inc; 1987.
23. Ketter DE, Shelton BJ. Pregnant and physically fit, too. *Am J Matern Child Nurs.* 1984;9:120–122.
24. Brown MS, Hurlock JT. Preparation of the breast for breastfeeding. In: Sherwen LN, Weingarten CT, eds. *Analysis and Application of Nursing Research: Parent-Neonate Studies.* Monterey, Calif: Wadsworth Health Sciences; 1983.
25. Weingarten CT, Jacobwitz JT. Alternatives in childbearing: choices and challenges. In: Sherwen LN, ed. *Psychosocial Dimensions of the Pregnant Family.* New York: Springer Publishing Co; 1987:193–218.
26. Maloney, R. Childbirth education classes: expectant parents expectations. *J Obstet Gynecol Neonatal Nurs.* 1985;14: 245–248.
27. Taubenheim AM, Sibernagel T. Meeting the needs of expectant fathers. *Am J Mat Child Nurs.* 1988;13:110–113.
28. Yankauer A. The valley of the shadow of birth. *Am J Public Health.* 1983;73:635–638.
29. Devitt N. The transition from home to hospital birth in the United States. *Birth Fam* 1977;4:47–58.
30. Donahue MP. *Nursing, the Finest Art: An Illustrated History.* St. Louis, Mo.: CV Mosby; 1985.
31. Gordon IT. The birth controllers: limitations on out-of-hospital births. *Nurse Midwifery.* 1982;27:34–39.
32. Varney H. *Nurse Midwifery.* Boston: Blackwell Scientific; 1987.
33. Klaus MK, Kennel J. *Parent-Infant Bonding.* 2nd ed. St. Louis, Mo: CV Mosby; 1982.
34. Beernink HE. Choice in childbirth. *Birth.* 1983;10:182–183.
35. Read GD. *Childbirth Without Fear.* New York/London: Harper & Brothers; 1944.
36. Hassid P. *Textbook for Childbirth Educators.* 2nd ed. Philadelphia: JB Lippincott; 1984.
37. Karmel M. *Thank You, Dr. Lamaze.* New York: Dolphin Books; 1959.
38. Roberts J. Factors influencing distress from pain during labor. *Am J Matern Child Nurs.* 1983;8:62–66.
39. Ellis J. What to choose in childbirth? *Birth.* 1983;10:183–184.
40. Genest M. Preparation for childbirth: evidence for efficacy. *J Obstet Gynecol Neonatal Nurs.* 1981;10:82–85.
41. Hurzeler C. Finding a qualified home-birth attendant. *Genesis.* 1985;7:14–26.
42. Maloney J. The birthing room: Some insights into parents' experiences. In: Sherwen LN, Toussie-Weingarten C, eds. *Analysis and Application of Nursing Research: Parent-Neonate Studies.* Monterey, Calif: Wadsworth Health Sciences; 1983.
43. Dobbs KB, Shy KK. Alternative birth rooms and birth options. *Obstet Gynecol.* 1981;58:626–631.
44. Faxel AM. The birthing room concept at Phoenix Memorial Hospital, Part I: development and eighteen months' statistics. *J Obstet Gynecol Neonatal Nurs.* 1980;9:151–154.
45. Kieffer MJ. The birthing room concept at Phoenix Memorial Hospital, Part II: consumer satisfaction during one year. *J Obstet Gynecol Neonatal Nurs.* 1980;9:155–164.
46. Rothman BK. Anatomy of a compromise: nurse-midwifery and the rise of the birth center. *J Nurse Midwifery.* 1983; 28:3–7.
47. Averitt SS. Adapting the birthing center concept to a traditional hospital setting. *J Obstet Gynecol Neonatal Nurs.* 1980;9:103–108.
48. DeJong RN, et al. An out of hospital birth center using university referral. *Obstet Gynecol.* 1981;58:703–706.

49. Lubic R. Free standing birth centers: Where are we now? *Genesis.* 1985;7:11–13.
50. Bennetts AB, Lubic R. The free standing birth center. *Lancet.* 1982;1:378–380.
51. Eakins PS, et al. Obstetric outcomes at the Birth Place in Menlo Park: the first 7 years. *Birth.* 1989;16:123–129.
52. Feldman E, Hurst M. Outcomes and procedures in low risk birth: a comparison of hospital and birth center settings. *Birth.* 1987;14:18–24.
53. DeClerq E. Out of hospital births, U.S., 1978: birth weight and Apgar scores as measures of outcome. *Public Health Rep.* 1984;99:63–72.
54. Mehl L, Peterson GH, Whitt M, Hawes W. Outcomes of elective home births: a series of 1146 cases. *J Reprod Med.* 1977;19:281–190.
55. Adamson GD, Gare D. Home or hospital births? *JAMA.* 1980;243:1732–1736.
56. Dunn J. *Sisters and Brothers.* Cambridge, Mass: Harvard University Press; 1985.
57. Kutzner SK. Responses of siblings to pregnancy. In: Sherwen LN, ed. *Psychosocial Dimensions of the Pregnant Family.* New York: Springer Publishing Co; 1987:176–192.
58. Johnsen NM, Gaspard ME. Theoretical foundations for a prepared sibling class. *J Obstet Gynecol Neonatal Nurs.* 1985;14:237–242.
59. Amderberg GJ. Initial acquaintance and attachment behavior of siblings with the newborn. *J Obstet Gynecol Neonatal Nurs.* 1988;17:49–52.
60. Krutsky C. Siblings at birth: impact on parents. *J Nurs Midwifery.* 1985;30:269–276.
61. DelGiudice GT. The relationship between sibling jealousy and presence at a sibling's birth. *Birth.* 1986;13:250–254.
62. Kutzner SK. *Adaptation to Motherhood from Postpartum to Early Childhood.* Ann Arbor: University of Michigan; 1984. Doctoral dissertation.
63. Lederman R, et al. The relationship of maternal development to progress in labor and fetal-newborn health. In: Lederman R, Raff B, eds. *Perinatal Parental Behavior: Nursing Research and Implications for Newborn Health.* March of Dimes, OAS, XII. New York: Alan R. Liss; 1981.
64. Lederman R, et al. The postpartum self-evaluation questionnaire: Measures of maternal adaptation. In: Lederman R, Raff B, eds. *Perinatal Parental Behavior: Nursing Research and Implications for Newborn Health.* March of Dimes, OAS, XII. New York: Alan R. Liss; 1981.
65. Horn M, Manion J. Creative grandparenting: bonding the generations. *J Obstet Gynecol Neonatal Nurs.* 1985;14:233–236.
66. Maloni JA, et al. Expectant grandparents' class. *J Obstet Gynecol Neonatal Nurs.* 1987;16:26–29.

The Intrapartum Period

unit

7

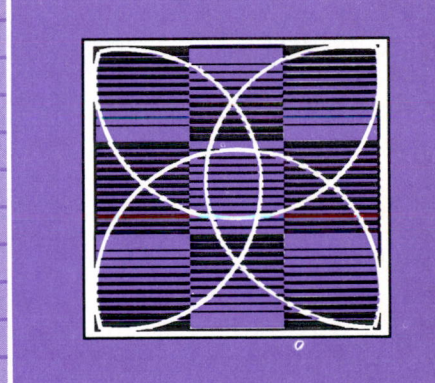

Physiologic Aspects of Labor and Delivery

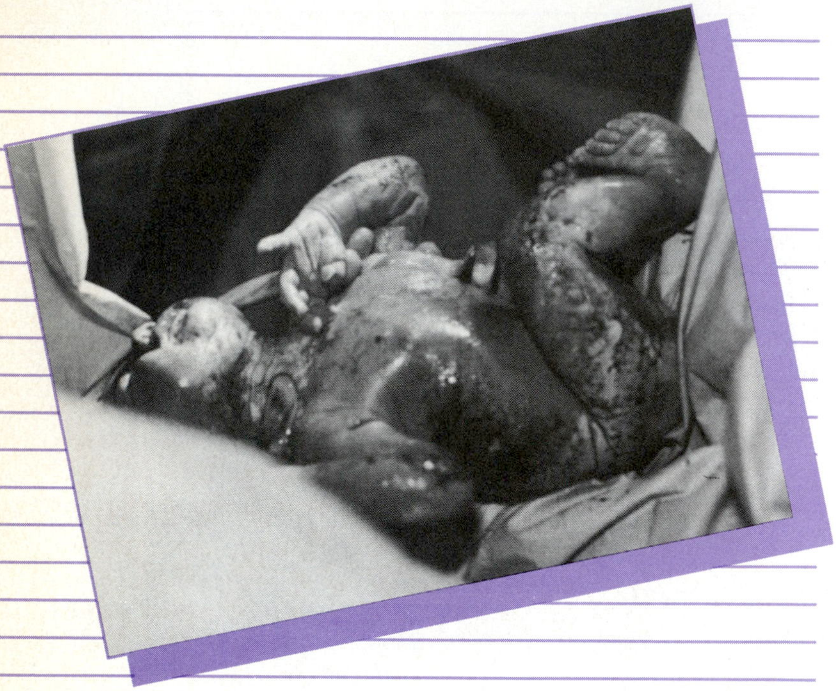

chapter 25

Key Terms

acceleration
anterior fontanelle
asynclitism
attitude
brachystasis
cardinal movements of labor
contraction
coronal sutures
denominators
dilation
engagement
external rotation
fetal station
flexion
Friedman curve
frontal suture
internal obstetric conjugate
internal rotation
labor
lambdoidal sutures
lie
mentum
molding
occiput
phase of maximum slope
position
posterior fontanelle
presentation
restitution
sagittal suture
sinciput
stations of descent
synclitism
transverse diameter
vertex

The processes of labor and delivery require complex physiologic responses by the mother and fetus; among them, the initiation of uterine contractions, effacement and dilation of the cervix, and fetal accommodation and passage through the maternal pelvis and birth canal. These responses are important factors in a healthy pregnancy outcome. This chapter examines physiologic responses during the labor and delivery processes, beginning with theories of labor onset and ending with the initial postpartum recovery of the mother.

MATERNAL PHYSIOLOGIC ADAPTATION AT TERM AND DURING LABOR

The complex adaptations of maternal anatomy and physiology required to promote and support successful pregnancy have been explored in Chapters 12, 16, and 20. The following description of the pregnant woman at term and during labor highlights those anatomic and physiologic changes from the nonpregnant state that influence the planning and delivery of care during birthing.

Reproductive System

Uterus. The uterus attains its greatest weight by midpregnancy (at 20 weeks). At term, the uterus is 30 to 35 cm long and 20 to 25 cm wide, with walls 0.5 cm or less in thickness. The uterine walls are quite elastic, permitting palpation of the fetal outline in the absence of excess maternal adipose tissue. Uterine blood supply and return have increased approximately 50 percent, reaching 700 mL per minute at term.

Over the course of pregnancy, the uterine isthmus elongates and is incorporated, along with the internal os, into the lower segment of the uterus. At term, the upper cervix is also incorporated into this lower segment. The lower segment thus comprises 70 percent isthmus and 30 percent cervix. This lower segment tissue differentiation is responsible for the functional differences between upper (fundal) and lower uterine segments during labor; the upper segment contracts and shortens while the lower segment effaces and dilates.

At term, the Braxton Hicks contractions that have been felt in the uterus throughout pregnancy strengthen and become more rhythmic.

Cervix. In addition to the changes in the upper cervix, several other changes characterize the cervix at term. The mucous plug, which filled the cervical canal, is expelled prior to or during the labor process. During expulsion of the plug, some bleeding of the walls of the os occurs, producing the "bloody show." The process of effacement, which is the thinning and shortening of the cervix, takes place prior to or during the onset of labor.

Vagina. During pregnancy there is a proliferation of cells in the vagina, along with hyperemia of the vaginal connective tissue. By the end of the pregnancy, the vaginal walls have become relaxed and distensible to permit passage of the fetus during labor and delivery.

Breasts. Under the influence of estrogen and progesterone an average of 1½ pounds is gained in each breast during pregnancy. At term, colostrum fills the alveoli, ducts, and ampullae. Breasts, particularly the nipples, are sensitive and nipple stimulation causes a sensory response that can elicit a uterine contraction.

Cardiovascular System

Cardiac volume increases by 70 to 80 mL, or about 12 percent, during pregnancy. Cardiac output rises by 1.5 L at 10 weeks and then stabilizes. There is a moderate increase in cardiac output during the first stage of labor, and a significant increase in the second stage because of the expulsive efforts of the mother.

In labor, approximately 300 mL of blood is expelled from the uterine muscle with each contraction. This blood suddenly enters the maternal circulation and is as rapidly withdrawn, re-entering the uterine musculature again with the relaxation between contractions. Perfusion of uterine tissue progressively lessens as the interlacing fibers of the upper segment constrict blood vessels. Diminished perfusion exerts a protective function by decreasing the probability of excessive bleeding, but is also responsible for some degree of maternal discomfort.

Systolic blood pressure remains at the prepregnancy level throughout pregnancy. Diastolic pressure decreases in the first two trimesters and returns to normal in the third. In young women, systolic blood pressure may range from 100 to 120 mm Hg and diastolic blood pressure, from 60 to 80 mm Hg. As pregnancy progresses, an increase in lower-extremity venous pressure (caused by the weight of the gravid uterus on pelvic vessels) predisposes the woman to edema of the legs, which disappears with bedrest, particularly when a side-lying position is maintained.

From a prepregnancy volume of 2600 mL, blood volume increases 1250 mL in the primigravida and 1500 mL in the multigravida; red blood cell mass increases from 240 to 400 mL. Without supplementation, serum iron proportionately decreases by 35 percent in pregnancy. A general increase in blood coagulability also occurs.

Blood levels of total globulin, plasma lipids, carotenoids (precursors of vitamin A), and vitamin E (tocopherol) rise, whereas levels of most amino acids, retinol, vitamin C, and B-complex vitamins fall. At term, maternal levels of calcium, magnesium, and inorganic phosphate have decreased from early pregnancy, reflecting fetal absorption of elements required for growth.

A positional shift of the heart occurs as it is pushed upward, moved to the left, and rotated forward by the enlarging uterus during pregnancy. This may explain the systolic murmur or split sounds that are often auscultated at the base of the heart. The cardiac status of the mother at term is of primary importance in assessing projected labor and delivery capability.

Respiratory System

During pregnancy, a sharp increase in progesterone levels stimulates an increase in inspiratory capacity and tidal volume. Although the diaphragm rises approximately 4 cm, this is offset by an increase in the transverse diameter of the rib cage (*see* Chapter 20); hence inspiratory capacity remains increased. These physiologic changes cause the mother to breathe deeply with no increase in respiratory rate. Maternal oxygen consumption increases during pregnancy by 16 percent, with alveolar and arterial Pco_2 reduced, leading to a reduction in plasma bicarbonate and sodium. Consequently, osmolarity decreases. Increases in arterial Pco_2 vary slightly. At term, functional residual capacity is greatly reduced, leading to more efficient gas exchange in the alveoli. Thus, prolonged deep breathing, as in the controlled breathing of labor, can lower Pco_2 and raise pH very quickly.

Urinary System

Changes in the urinary system occur throughout pregnancy. In the last 2 weeks of pregnancy, lightening occurs and the presenting part of the fetus engages in the pelvis, causing the bladder to be pushed forward and upward. The bladder, which is normally convex, becomes concave and its retention capacity is reduced.

At term, blood flow to the kidneys increases 400 mL per minute over the prepregnancy flow rate of 1000 to 1200 mL per minute. The kidneys enlarge by up to 1 cm during pregnancy.

Body fluids increase gradually until term and may reach 7.5 L over the prepregnancy measurement. Increase in maternal volume, coupled with an estimated 2.5 L of interstitial fluid and a rise in sodium levels, accounts for the fluid increase. Fluid excretion is related to maternal posture, with greatest output efficiency in the lateral recumbent position.

During pregnancy, there is also greater clearance of creatinine, uric acid, and urea in response to the increase in waste products. The glomerular filtration rate (GFR) is increased, so that some women have glycosuria during the latter part of pregnancy.

Musculoskeletal System

By the end of the pregnancy, the combined weight of the fetus, amniotic fluid, and enlarged uterus often strains the musculature of the lumbar spine, resulting in lower back pain.

Integument

Blood flow to the skin of the hands and feet increases at term. Swollen mucous membranes of the nasal passages may cause difficulty in nose breathing and episodes of epistaxis during labor.

Gastrointestinal System

The mother is generally unable to consume a full meal at term unless lightening has occurred. There is reduced motility of the esophagus, stomach, and large and small intestines. Gallbladder motility and emptying rate are also reduced. A meal ingested immediately preceding labor may be followed by emesis during labor.

Endocrine System

Thyroid. During pregnancy, there is an increase in vascularity and hyperplasia of the glandular tissue of the thyroid gland. The basal metabolic rate may increase more than 20 percent in late pregnancy as thyroid hormones, which regulate cell metabolism, respond to the increasing metabolic requirements of pregnancy. At the end of the pregnancy, the thyroid gland may be palpable.

Adrenals. The adrenals are also important in regulating metabolism. Adrenocorticotropic hormone (ACTH) levels rise progressively during pregnancy. There is also an increase in the concentration of circulating cortisol, which helps break down fats to fatty acids. By the end of the pregnancy, 1 mg of aldosterone is secreted per day to regulate the sodium content of maternal blood.

Pituitary. During pregnancy, the anterior pituitary enlarges, sometimes to double or triple its prepregnancy size, mostly in response to increases in prolactin secretion. Plasma prolactin concentrations are 10 to 20 times higher in the pregnant woman at term than in the nonpregnant woman.

The posterior pituitary produces the hormones oxytocin and vasopressin. Some oxytocin is secreted throughout pregnancy, but does not cause the contractions that stimulate cervical effacement and dilation until term.

Placental Hormones

Estrogen. Throughout most of the pregnancy, the placenta synthesizes estrogens. Late in pregnancy, estrogens are thought to contribute to the softening of the collagen tissues of the cervix. Moreover, they make the uterus sensitive to prostaglandins, hormones that may contribute to the onset of labor (*see* later discussion). Toward the end of the third trimester, estrogens are influential in increasing the concentration of fibrinogen, which facilitates maternal blood clotting during and after the delivery process.

Progesterone. Progesterone levels rise sharply during pregnancy. This hormone has important roles in maternal metabolism, facilitating the breakdown of nutrients for needed energy. During pregnancy, progesterone also reduces myometrial contractility. Although this once led to the belief that progesterone withdrawal was necessary for the onset of labor, the current view is that it may be only one step in the complex events leading to labor (*see* later discussion).

Human Placental Lactogen. During pregnancy, human placental lactogen stimulates formation of glycogen from noncarbohydrate sources such as proteins and fats. In this role, it is considered glucose sparing, inhibiting the use of maternal glucose while providing glucose for the fetus. Both mother and fetus will require glucose for energy production during the demanding processes of labor and delivery.

Other Hormones

Prostaglandins. Prostaglandins are hormones that are synthesized from arachidonic acid, which is found in large quantities in the amnion and chorion. During labor, the stores of arachidonic acid, which become available to the decidua, contribute to uterine contractions and cervical effacement and dilation (*see* later). A role for prostaglandins in the initiation of labor has not, however, been confirmed.

Relaxin. Relaxin is a polypeptide hormone that is thought to relax the symphysis pubis and other pelvic joints and to soften the cervix, although its role is unclear. Preliminary evidence from animal and human research suggests that synthesis of relaxin occurs principally in the corpus luteum, although the placenta and decidua have also been cited as sources of relaxin.[1]

Neurologic System

The neurologic system should remain stable during pregnancy, labor, and delivery; however, expectant mothers who experience pregnancy-induced hypertension (PIH) may demonstrate hyperactive deep tendon reflexes during pregnancy, labor, and delivery.

ONSET OF LABOR

Hypotheses

Several mechanisms have been hypothesized to influence the initiation of labor, among them the uterine stretch mechanism and both maternal and fetal hormonal stimulation. To date, biomedical research has been unable to document a single cause-and-effect correlation between any of these mechanisms and the onset of labor. It seems most likely that a combination of factors is responsible for labor onset. Research in this area concentrates almost exclusively on possible physiologic mechanisms, with a notable absence of investigation into any psychologic components. As hormonal response to emotion and emotional response to hormonal shifts have been documented in other contexts, it appears that there may be causes of onset that are as yet unexplained.

Uterine Stretch Mechanism. One of the earliest hypotheses about labor onset proposed that distension of the uterus eventually results in increased irritability and contractility. The increased irritability of the uterus may be heightened by an increase in oxytocin levels or may cause an increase in production of the hormone. Support for this hypothesis came from the observation that mothers with multiple gestations or polyhydramnios may experience preterm labor and delivery. The physiologic secretion of oxytocin during labor may, however, vary; in fact, oxytocin may be secreted more in the expulsive phases of labor than in the early phases. This would seem to contradict the uterine stretch-oxytocin relationship.

Hormonal Stimulation. Hormonal stimulation hypotheses focus on the interplay among the mother, fetus, and placenta. Maternal, fetal, and placental hormones, possibly controlled by fetal adrenal cortisol activity, are believed to contribute to the onset of labor. Specific hypotheses involve (1) oxytocin, (2) prostaglandins, (3) fetal cortisol, and (4) estrogen and progesterone.

Oxytocin. It is supposed that the greatly distended uterus contains cells especially sensitive to oxytocin. It is further supposed that the fetus plays an active role in the production of oxytocin. From this perspective, fetal oxytocin and maternal oxytocin combine to exert a contractile influence on the uterus.[2]

Support for this hypothesis initially came from research that appeared to demonstrate a consistent pattern of delayed onset of labor for anencephalic fetuses, who lack oxytocin. This seemed to support the need for fetal oxytocin as a stimulant to labor onset.[3,4] Later research, however, indicated no significant difference between mean gestational ages of anencephalic fetuses and normal fetuses.[3]

In general, physiologic evidence for the role of both fetal oxytocin and maternal oxytocin in the initiation of labor is inconclusive. Animal and human research has demonstrated increased levels of oxytocin in amniotic fluid during labor; however, researchers have been unable to document conclusively a rise in oxytocin immediately prior to onset of labor.[5] Some would conclude from these data that oxytocin has little importance in the initiation of labor and that its major role occurs during labor and after delivery.

Prostaglandins. The sites of prostaglandin production during pregnancy appear to be primarily fetal membranes (amnion and chorion) and the decidua.[6] Estrogen appears to stimulate prostaglandin production. Prostaglandins are reported to initiate a wide variety of biologic activities including vasodilation, inhibition of gastric acid secretion, and hormone-induced lysolysis. Prostaglandins stimulate the uterus and can induce effective uterine contractions at any stage during the pregnancy.[7,8] Infusion of one of the prostaglandin compounds, prostaglandin $F_{2\alpha}(PGF_2)$ can result in cervical effacement throughout pregnancy.

Researchers attempting to document prostaglandins as initiators of labor have measured a minor increase in maternal blood levels at term and a 10- to 30-fold increase during labor.[6] As significant increases have not been demonstrated prior to the onset of labor, there is no conclusive evidence as to the role of prostaglandins as an initiator of labor.

Cortisol. Animal studies have demonstrated that a sharp increase in the rate of production of cortisol by the fetal adrenal acts on the placenta, reducing progesterone formation and increasing production of prostaglandins. The same findings, however, are not conclusive in humans. Specifically, no significant increase in cortisol concentrations in fetal blood has been found before the onset of labor. Further, there is no evidence of a decline in human maternal plasma progesterone levels before or during labor.[1] Thus, the role of cortisol as an initiator of labor is inconclusive.

Estrogen and Progesterone. In animals, estrogen increases the number of uterine receptor sites for oxytocin. Progesterone (also in animal studies) acts to quiet the uterine response.[9] In humans, the balance between estrogen and progesterone serves to stabilize and maintain the pregnancy. In the past it was believed that a decrease in progesterone levels at term allowed estrogen to excite the contractile response of the uterus. However, newer studies have failed to consistently document decreased progesterone in maternal blood, leaving this hypothesis of labor onset in question.[10]

Interplay Among Factors Affecting Labor Onset

As the preceding discussion indicates, research has been unable to document any single hypothesis regarding the onset of labor. Each of the hormones discussed can influence uterine contractions; however, each taken separately fails to explain the initiation of labor. A variety of factors, both maternal and fetal, act in concert to initiate labor in the normal parturient.[11] Further research will likely focus on the interactions among various factors that may combine to trigger the onset of labor. Examples of these factors are summarized in Table 25–1.

FACTORS INFLUENCING ONSET, DURATION, AND OUTCOME

Traditionally, the "three P's"—passage (pelvis), passenger (fetus), and powers (contractions)—were considered to be the major factors determining the outcome of labor and delivery. The maternal psyche is an important factor affecting labor and delivery; therefore psychologic influences on labor and delivery are also discussed briefly in this section. For additional discussion, the reader is referred to Chapter 26.

TABLE 25–1. FACTORS BELIEVED TO INFLUENCE LABOR ONSET

Factors that may constitute a primary stimulus
Fetal oxytocin
ACTH and related peptides
Factors fairly specific to parturition but dependent on a primary stimulus
Estrogen
Progesterone
Cortisol
Maternal oxytocin
Oxytocin receptors
Relaxin
Nonspecific factors involved in the activation of smooth muscle at any site
Prostaglandins
Autonomic mediators
Calcium
Cyclic nucleotides

Adapted, with permission, from Chard T, Lilford R. Basic Sciences for Obstetrics and Gynecology. *3rd ed. Heidelberg; Germany: Springer-Verlag; 1990.*

Passage

Bony Pelvis. The bony pelvis of the pregnant woman is assessed in relation to the size, lie, and presentation of the fetus. As the pelvic structure is relatively unyielding (except for the coccyx, which may be somewhat movable) and is the passage through which the fetus must descend for a successful vaginal delivery, internal and external pelvic diameters are measured.

Ideally, skeletal assessments are made at least twice during pregnancy, after a detailed history is taken to identify factors that may have impact on the development of the pelvis. Conditions such as ricketts, polio, and trauma resulting in pelvic fracture or a history of previous cephalopelvic disproportion aid in the estimation of delivery outcome. An initial assessment is performed in the first trimester to identify any gross abnormalities or obvious barriers to vaginal delivery (*see* Chapter 14). Assessment of the pelvis is essential for estimating successful passage of the fetus during labor and delivery (*see* section on "passenger"). Usually, the smallest diameter of the fetal skull will descend in the largest diameters of the true pelvis.

Anatomy of the Pelvis. The anatomy, diameters, and planes of the pelvis were described in Chapter 14. This section highlights several key anatomic landmarks; the reader is referred to the earlier chapter for a more complete discussion.

The bony pelvis consists of the following bones and joints: two innominate bones (front and sides), sacrum and lumbar vertebrae (posterior), coccyx (posterior, may be somewhat movable), sacroiliac joint (links sacrum to iliac portion of the innominate bones), symphysis (links the anterior pubic bones at midline), and sacrococcygeal joint (links sacrum and coccyx). Additionally, the pelvis is differentiated into two sections: the false pelvis and the true pelvis.

False Pelvis. The basin-shaped superior portion of the bony pelvis lying above the true pelvis is termed the false pelvis. It is bounded inferiorly by the linea terminalis, posteriorly by the lumbar vertebrae, laterally by the iliac fossae, and anteriorly by the wall of the abdomen. This latter boundary gives some latitude to false pelvis dimensions. The function of the false pelvis is support of the uterus and its contents.

True Pelvis. The portion of the pelvis below the linea terminalis is termed the true pelvis. It is composed of the pelvic inlet, cavity, and outlet.

Pelvic Inlet. The pelvic inlet is bounded anteriorly by the pubic bones, laterally by the linea terminalis, and posteriorly by the sacral promontory (*see* Figures 14–6, 14–8, and 14–9). The obstetric conjugate of the inlet (middle of the sacral promontory to posterior superior margin of the symphysis pubis) normally measures about 11 cm. This critical inlet measurement determines whether the largest fetal diameter can successfully negotiate entry.

Additional anteroposterior inlet measurements include the anatomic or true conjugate (middle of sacrum to middle of pubic crest, normally about 11.5 cm) and the diagonal conjugate (suprapubic angle to promontory of sacrum, normally about 12.5 cm). The diagonal conjugate, which is measured manually, is used in turn to estimate the **internal obstetric conjugate,** obtained by subtracting 1.5 to 2 cm (the width of the pubis) from the diagonal conjugate.

The **transverse diameter** (normally about 13.5 cm) is the largest diameter of the pelvic inlet and is the greatest distance between the linea terminalis on each side of the pelvis. Two other dimensions of the pelvic inlet are the right and left oblique diameters (about 12.5 cm), which cannot be measured clinically.

Pelvic Cavity. The pelvic cavity consists of a curved cavity between the inlet and outlet with a straight anterior wall bounded by the pubis; a curved posterior wall bounded by the sacrum, which is roughly twice the length of the anterior wall; and side walls bounded laterally by the ischium and part of the ilium (Figure 25–1). Pelvic planes are imaginary surfaces used to describe points of critical dimension. The anteroposterior diameter, measured from the midpoint of the interior surface of the pubis to the juncture between the second and third sacral vertebrae (12.75 cm), and the transverse diameter (12.5 cm) are the important diameters of the plane of greatest dimension. The plane of least dimension is the most critical pelvic dimension because it is the narrowest plane through which the fetus must pass. The anteroposterior diameter (lower border of the pubis to the juncture of the fourth and fifth sacral vertebrae, about 12 cm), the transverse diameter (between the ischial spines, about 10 to 10.5 cm), and the posterior sagittal diameter (bispinous diameter to the juncture of the fourth and fifth sacral vertebrae, about 4.5 to 5 cm) are the important diameters of the plane of least dimension.

Pelvic Outlet. The pelvic outlet is made up of an anterior and posterior triangular plane, sharing a common base. The anterior triangle has the following components: the transverse diameter or the inner

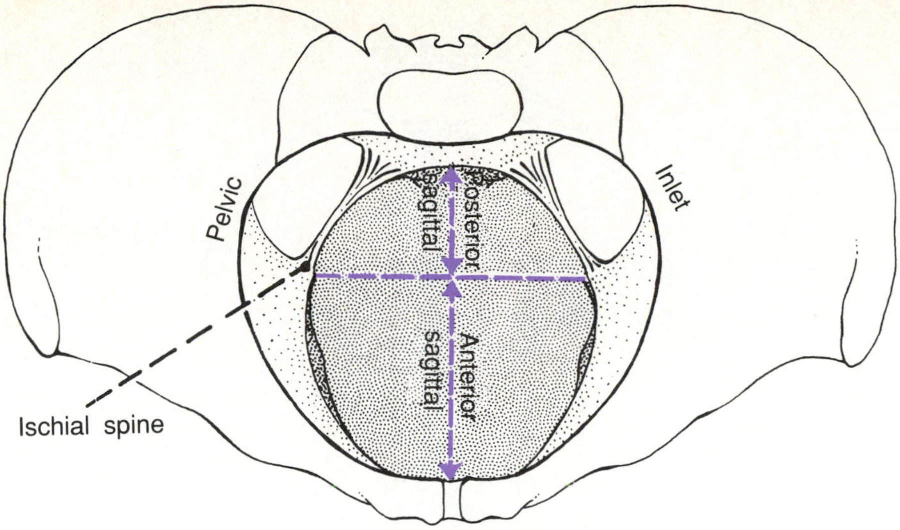

Figure 25–1. Pelvic cavity: plane of least dimensions. The anterior-posterior view showing anterior-posterior and transverse diameters. (*Reproduced, with permission, from Oxorn H, ed.* Oxorn-Foote Human Labor and Birth. *5th ed. Norwalk, Conn: Appleton-Century-Crofts; 1986: 31.*)

edges of the ischial tuberosities as the base, the subpubic angle as the apex, and the pubic rami and ischial tuberosities as the sides.

The posterior triangle is bounded by the transverse diameter as the base, the sacrococcygeal joint as the apex, and the sacrotuberous ligaments as the sides.

The diameters of the pelvic outlet are the obstetric anteroposterior diameter, from the inferior margin of the symphysis pubis to the sacrococcygeal joint (11.5 cm); the transverse diameter, the distance between the inner surfaces of the ischial tuberosities (11.0 cm); the posterior sagittal diameter, from the middle of the transverse diameter to the sacrococcygeal junction (9.0 cm); and the anterior sagittal diameter, from the middle of the transverse diameter to the subpubic angle (6.0 cm) (*see* Figure 12–12).

The box below summarizes pelvic measurements that determine whether the pelvis is adequate to allow passage of the fetus.[12]

Vagina. Bounded by the vulva, the uterus, the bladder, and the rectum, the vagina is composed of muscular tissue with a mucosal overlay. This tube, 6 to 8 cm in length, with the cervix at one end and the introitus or vaginal opening in the perineum at the other, is vastly elastic and readily distends to accommodate passage of the fetus.

CRITICAL PELVIC MEASUREMENTS

Obstetric conjugate of the inlet
Distance between the ischial spines
Subpubic angle and transverse diameter
Posterior and sagittal diameters of the three planes
Curve and length of the sacrum

Passenger

Fetus. The fetal head is the most important parameter of the fetal body because it is the largest and least yielding fetal part. It is also most frequently the part that presents first in the maternal pelvis.

Fetal Skull. The fetal skull is made up of three parts: the face, the vault, and the base. The bones of the face are heavier than those of the vault and are fused. The vault is composed of two frontal bones anteriorly, two parietal bones on the sides, and one occipital bone posteriorly. The bones of the vault are not fused. Instead, they are separated from each other by membranes that allow the head to change shape, or **mold**, as it descends through the maternal pelvis.

Fetal Skull Sutures. The skull sutures are membrane-occupied spaces between the bones of the vault. The sutures in the cranial vault allow for molding of the fetal skull during labor and delivery. The **sagittal suture** is located between parietal bones and follows the anteroposterior direction of the skull. The **frontal suture** is an anterior continuation of the sagittal suture, and is found between the two frontal bones. The **coronal sutures** are found between the parietal and frontal bones, extending transversely on both sides of the anterior fontanelle. The **lambdoidal sutures** are located between the occipital bone and the two parietals, extending transversely on either side of the posterior fontanelle (Figure 25–2).

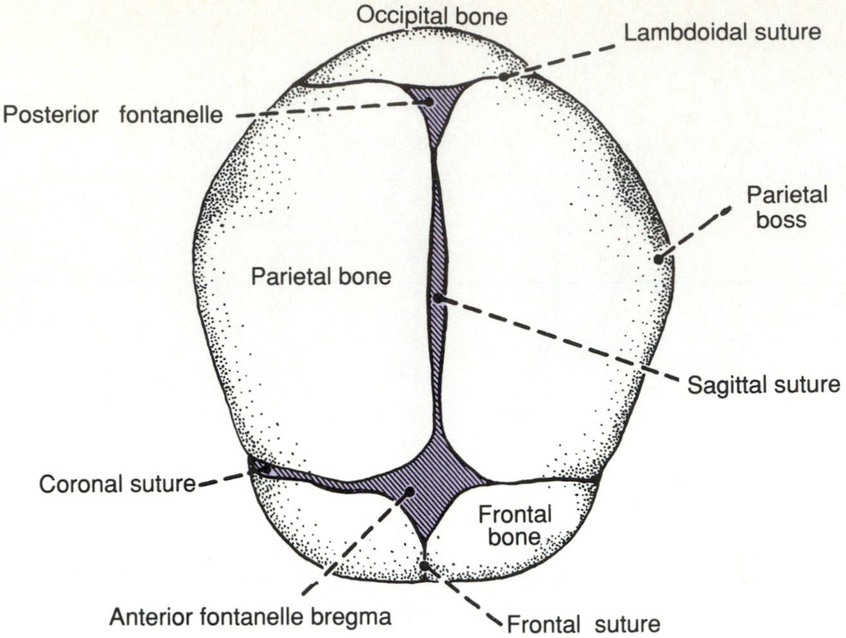

Figure 25–2. Superior view of the fetal skull. (*Reproduced with permission, from Oxorn H, ed.* Oxorn-Foote Human Labor and Birth. *5th ed. Norwalk, Conn: Appleton-Century-Crofts; 1986:43.*)

Fontanelles. The fontanelles are membrane-covered spaces found where the sutures intersect. The **anterior fontanelle** or bregma is located at the anterior junction of the sagittal and coronal sutures. It is diamond-shaped and measures on average 3 × 2 cm. The anterior fontanelle remains open for 12 to 18 months after birth to allow for growth of the brain. The **posterior fontanelle** or lambda is located at the posterior junction of the lambdoidal and sagittal sutures. It is triangular in shape, measures on average between 0.5 cm and 1 cm at its widest diameter, and closes 6 to 10 weeks after birth (*see* Figure 25–2).

Landmarks of the Fetal Skull. Certain landmarks of the fetal skull are important in describing the relationship of the fetal presenting part to the maternal pelvis during delivery. These landmarks are referred to as **denominators**:

1. The **occiput** is the region in the back of the head, behind and inferior to the posterior fontanelle.
2. The **sinciput** or brow is the region bounded by the anterior fontanelle and the coronal sutures superiorly and by the orbital ridges inferiorily.
3. The **vertex** is located between the anterior and posterior fontanelles and is bounded laterally by the parietal bones.
4. The **mentum** or chin is the guiding point for face presentations (*see* later), which occur when the head is in complete extension.

There are additional denominators that are not landmarks of the fetal skull. These denominators are discussed later in this chapter.

Diameters of the Fetal Skull. The diameters of the fetal skull are important in judging the ability of the fetus to fit through the maternal pelvis. The most important dimensions are the anteroposterior and transverse diameters.

Anterior-Posterior Diameters. The actual size in centimeters of the anteroposterior diameter of the fetal skull that presents to the maternal pelvis depends on the extent of extension or flexion of the fetal head.

The suboccipitobregmatic diameter extends from the undersurface of the occipital bone to the center of the anterior fontanelle. It is the shortest anteroposterior diameter of the head, measuring 9.5 cm. This diameter presents to the maternal pelvis when the fetal head is well flexed. (Figure 25–3A).

The occipitofrontal diameter extends from a point just above the top of the nose to the most prominent portion of the occipital bone. It measures 11.5 cm (Figure 25–3B).

The occipitomental diameter extends from the chin to the most prominent portion of the occiput. It is found when the head is extended and normally measures about 12.5 cm (Figure 25–3C).

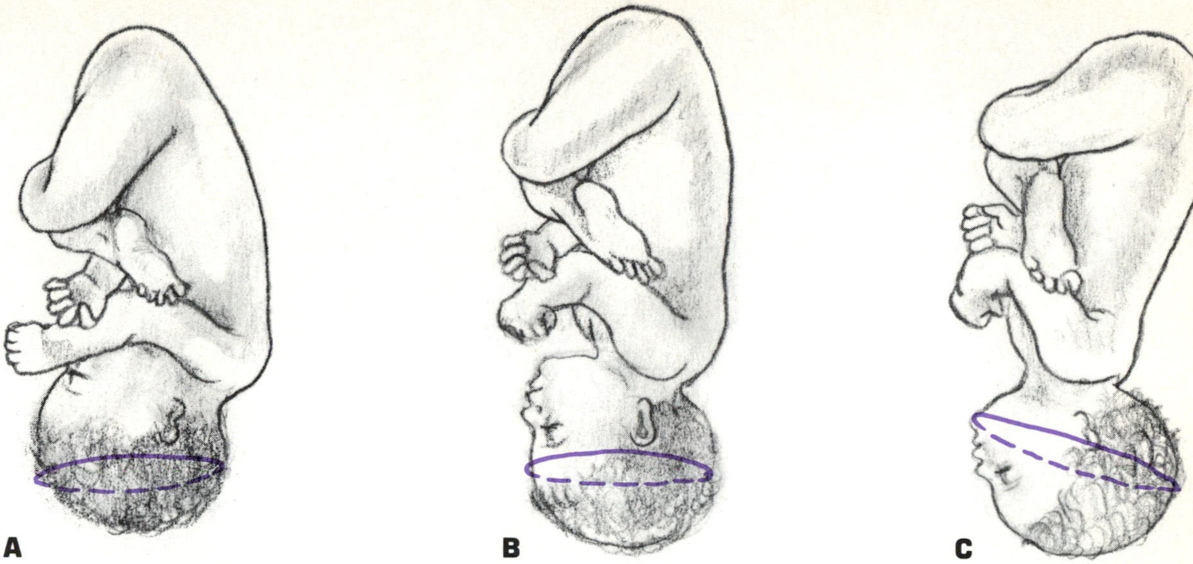

Figure 25–3. **A.** Suboccipitobregmatic diameter. **B.** Occipitofrontal diameter. **C.** Occipitomental diameter.

Transverse Diameters. The biparietal diameter is the largest transverse diameter of the head, measuring 9.5 cm. It extends from one parietal prominence to the other (Figure 25–4).

The bitemporal diameter extends between the lateral sides of the temporal bones. It is the shortest transverse diameter of the fetal skull, measuring 8 cm (Figure 25–4).

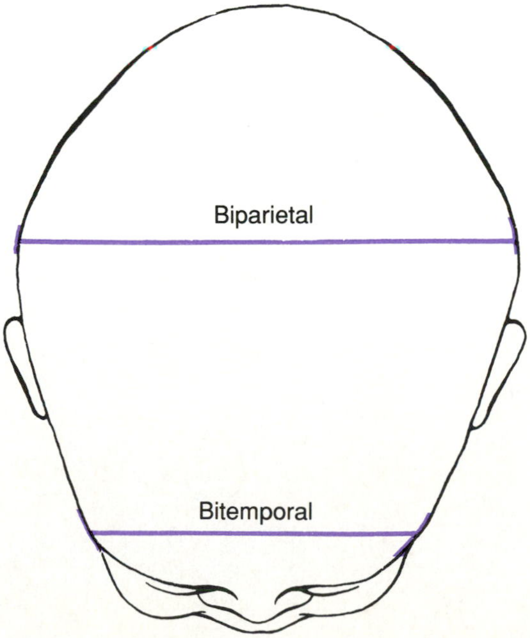

Figure 25–4. Transverse diameters of the fetal skull. (*Reproduced, with permission, from Oxorn H, ed.* Oxorn-Foote Human Labor and Birth. *5th ed. Norwalk, Conn: Appleton-Century-Crofts; 1986:43.*)

Fetopelvic Relationships

Attitude. Fetal **attitude** is the relationship of the fetal parts to each other. The typical fetal attitude is one of **flexion**, whereby the arms and legs are folded in front of the body, the back is curved forward, and the head is bent on the chest. This attitude occurs as a result of growth of the fetus and the process of fetal accommodation to the uterine cavity. The extent of flexion of fetal parts, especially the head, determines which diameter will enter the maternal pelvis.

In certain circumstances, fetal parts may also be in a state of extension in relation to each other, as occurs in a frank breech presentation (*see* Chapter 40).

Lie. **Lie** is the relationship of the long axis of the fetus to the long axis of the mother, and can be longitudinal, transverse, or oblique. Longitudinal lies are present in more than 99 percent of term pregnancies. In a longitudinal lie, the head or buttocks may enter the maternal pelvis first. A transverse lie finds the long axis of the fetus at right angles to the long axis of the mother. In this lie, the shoulder of the fetus enters the maternal pelvis first. A transverse lie is rare, and the fetus cannot be delivered vaginally in this position. Occasionally, the long axis of the mother and fetus cross at a 45° angle, forming

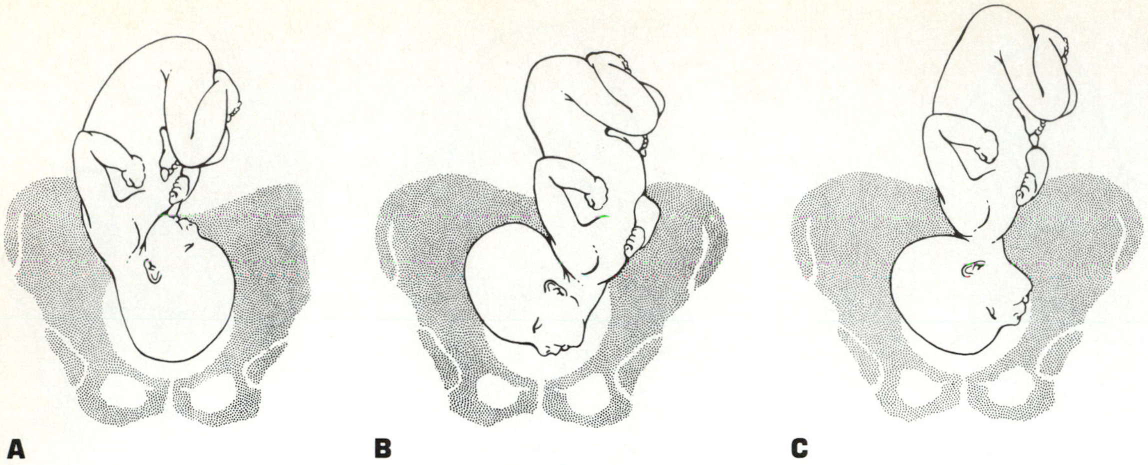

Figure 25–5. Cephalic presentations. **A.** Vertex/occiput presentation. **B.** Face presentation. **C.** Brow presentation. (*Reproduced, with permission, from Oxorn H, ed.* Oxorn-Foote Human Labor and Birth. *5th ed. Norwalk, Conn: Appleton-Century-Crofts; 1986:55.*)

an oblique lie. This lie will become either longitudinal or transverse during the course of labor.

Presentation. **Presentation** denotes the part of the fetus that is closest to the pelvic inlet of the mother. This part of the fetus is termed the **presenting part.** In longitudinal lies, the presenting part is either the head or the fetal pelvic parts; these are termed cephalic and breech presentations, respectively. In a transverse lie, the presenting part is the shoulder, arm, or trunk; this is termed a shoulder presentation.

Cephalic Presentation. Cephalic presentations are classified according to the attitude of the fetal head (Figure 25–5). If the head is flexed, the occiput is the presenting part. This is referred to as a **vertex** (or **occiput) presentation** (Figure 25–5A). The vertex presentation is the most efficient presentation for delivery, and also the most common, occurring in 95 percent of all term pregnancies.

A **face presentation** occurs when the fetal head is completely extended, with the widest part of the face presenting for delivery (Figure 25–5B). When the fetal head is partially extended, the presenting part is the brow; this is referred to as a **brow presentation** (Figure 25–5C).

Breech Presentations. Breech presentations are classified according to the attitude of the fetal hips and

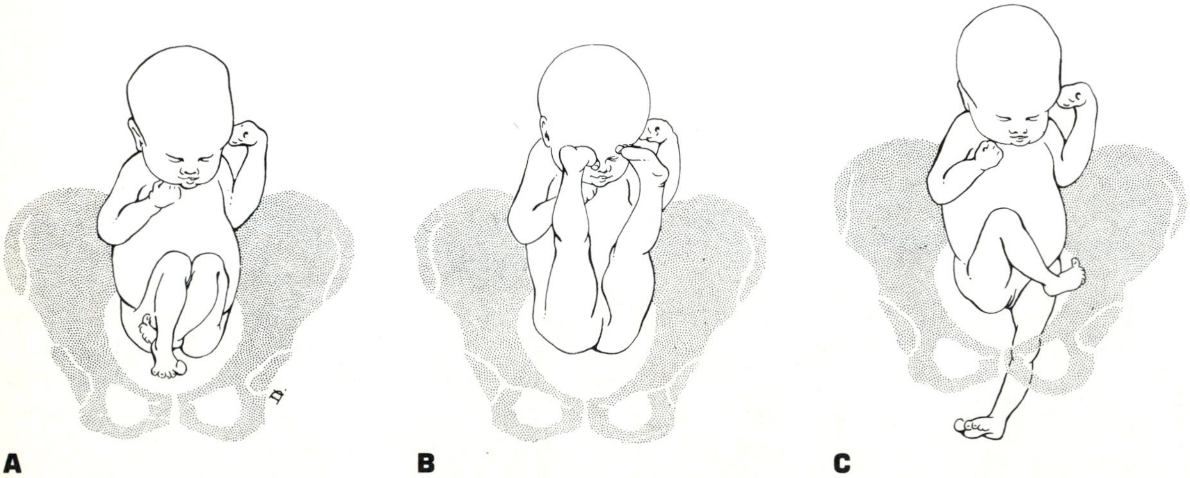

Figure 25–6. Breech presentations. **A.** Complete breech. **B.** Frank breech. **C.** Footling breech. (*Reproduced, with permission, from Oxorn H, ed.* Oxorn-Foote Human Labor and Birth. *5th ed. Norwalk, Conn: Appleton-Century-Crofts; 1986: 57.*)

knees (Figure 25–6). In a **complete breech presentation,** the fetus presents buttocks first with flexion at both the hips and the knees (Figure 25–6A). In a **frank breech presentation,** the thighs are flexed and the legs extend over the anterior surfaces of the fetal body (Figure 25–6B); the presenting part is still the buttocks. An **incomplete** or **footling breech presentation** occurs when the presenting part is one or both feet, with extension at both the hips and knees (Figure 25–6C).

Shoulder Presentation. A shoulder presentation (also called a transverse lie) occurs when the long axis of the fetus is perpendicular to the long axis of the mother (Figure 25–7). The most frequent presenting part is the shoulder; however, the fetus may also present the trunk or arm. Although shoulder presentations occur in less than 1 percent of deliveries,[12] they are considered a serious malpresentation. Unless the fetus converts to a longitudinal lie, vaginal delivery cannot occur. (*See* Chapter 40 for discussion of complications of childbirth.)

Position. Fetal **position** refers to the relationship of landmarks (denominators) of the fetal presenting part to the sides, front, or back of the maternal pelvis.[13] Each presentation has its own denominator. Table 25–2 lists the fetal denominators for each presenting part.

When describing the fetal position in the mother's pelvis, three sets of terms are used: (1) denominator, (2) right or left, depending on which side of the mother's pelvis the denominator is in; and (3) anterior, posterior, or transverse, according to whether the denominator is located in the front, back, or side of the mother's pelvis. There are eight possible positions (Figure 25–8) for each fetal presentation:

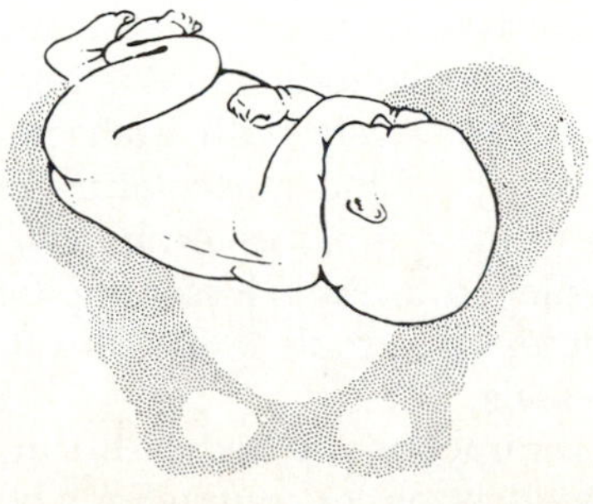

Figure 25–7. Shoulder presentation (transverse lie). (*Reproduced, with permission, from Oxorn H, ed.* Oxorn-Foote Human Labor and Birth. *5th ed. Norwalk, Conn: Appleton-Century-Crofts; 1986:57.*)

Vertex Presentations

- Left occiput anterior (LOA)
- Left occiput posterior (LOP)
- Right occiput anterior (ROA)
- Right occiput posterior (ROP)
- Right occiput transverse (ROT)
- Left occiput transverse (LOT)
- Occiput anterior (OA)
- Occiput posterior (OP)

Face Presentations

- Left mentum anterior (LMA)
- Left mentum posterior (LMP)
- Right mentum anterior (RMA)
- Right mentum posterior (RMP)
- Right mentum transverse (RMT)
- Left mentum transverse (LMT)
- Mentum anterior (MA)
- Mentum posterior (MP)

Breech Presentations

- Left sacrum anterior (LSA)
- Left sacrum posterior (LSP)
- Right sacrum anterior (RSA)
- Right sacrum posterior (RSP)
- Right sacrum transverse (RST)
- Left sacrum transverse (LST)
- Sacrum anterior (SA)
- Sacrum posterior (SP)

Brow presentations are rarely described in this manner, because they usually convert to a vertex or face presentation during labor.

Powers

Three variables—the uterine contraction, intraabdominal pressure, and the passive counterpressure of the pelvic floor—constitute the powers or energy

TABLE 25–2. DENOMINATORS FOR FETAL PRESENTING PARTS

Presenting Part	Denominator
Vertex (occiput)	Occiput (O)
Face	Mentum (chin) (M)
Brow	Frontum (forehead) (Fr)
Buttocks	Sacrum (S)
Feet	Sacrum (S)
Shoulder, arm	Scapula (Sc)

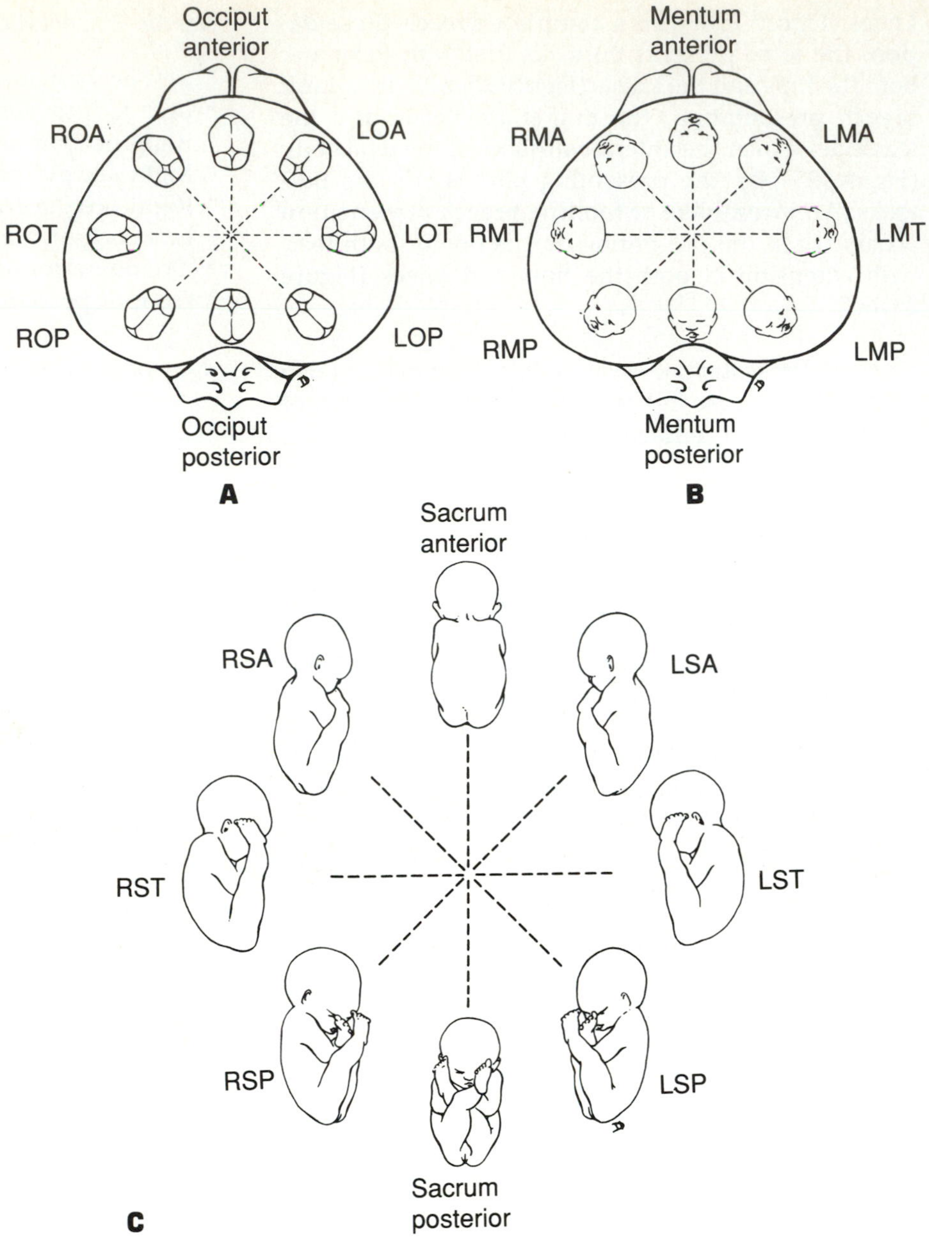

Figure 25–8. Fetal positions. **A.** Vertex presentations. **B.** Face presentations. **C.** Breech presentations. (*Reproduced, with permission, from Oxorn H, ed.* Oxorn-Foote Human Labor and Birth. *5th ed. Norwalk, Conn: Appleton-Century-Crofts; 1986:59.*)

component of birth. These powers may be further described as primary (involuntary) or secondary (voluntary).

The uterus is a muscular organ composed of three layers: the outer (maternal side) layer or perimetrium; the middle, thickest layer or myometrium; and the internal (fetal side) layer composed of glandular tissue and termed the endometrium. The myometrium is itself structured in three interlacing layers that encircle the uterus. Each muscle cell in the myometrium has a double curve so that the interlacing of the cells forms a figure-eight configuration. The muscle fibers of the myometrium are permeated in all directions by blood vessels (*see* Figure 6–16).

The musculature of the myometrium has a unique characteristic termed **brachystasis,** the ability to contract in response to a stimulus and to shorten and thicken progressively with each stimulus. The meshlike structure of the musculature of the myometrium acts to exert pressure on uterine blood vessels, and is believed to aid in lessening the blood loss that would otherwise result from disruption of multiple small vessels.

Uterine contractions, whether Braxton Hicks or the progressively stronger contractions of true labor, are primary or involuntary. Several mechanisms seem to enhance involuntary labor contractions. The first of these mechanisms is oxytocin, which is thought to enhance rhythmic labor contractions. At term, when the cervix is ripe (softened and in the earliest stage of dilation and effacement), the uterus is sensitive to oxytocin,[1] although the degree of sensitivity varies with the individual.

The second mechanism involves pacemakers in the uterus. Very early research into this phenomenon indicated that cells acting as pacemakers (analogous to sinoatrial node cells in the heart) existed in the myometrium and were in part responsible for the initiation of the rhythmic labor contractions.[14] Later investigation discovered that although any cluster of myometrial cells is capable of acting as a pacemaker, significant clusters are located in the fundus, near the sites where the fallopian tubes open into the uterus.[1,15,16]

The third mechanism is the mechanical stretching of the cervix. This appears to cause an increase in prostaglandin levels in women at term, and prostaglandins are capable of causing contractions of the uterus. It is not known whether the natural softening of the cervix elicits a similar response.

All three mechanisms—hormonal stimulation, pacemaker cell activity, and cervical change and consequent prostaglandin response—may act together to establish rhythmic contractions. The uterine contractions provide the power that shortens, thickens, and straightens the body of the uterus and further dilates and effaces the cervix.

Dilation is the widening of the cervical os from an opening that will not admit a finger to an opening that is 10 cm when fully dilated. Effacement is the thinning and shortening of the cervical os from a 2.5-cm structure to a part of the lower uterine segment. Ideally, the cervix is ripe when labor begins. A ripe cervix is soft, less than 1.3 cm in length, and admits a finger easily.

Fibers of the lower uterine segment behave contrarily to those of the body (brachystasis). Once stretched and thinned by pressure from the uterine corpus on the fetus, they do not return to prepressure status. This phenomenon explains the ability of cervical tissue to change progressively from firm, rubbery, and thick to thin, elastic, and capable of allowing passage of the fetus (Figure 25–9).

Once the first stage of labor (from 0 to 10 cm dilation with full effacement) is completed, the second stage of expulsion occurs, and is characterized by the overwhelming urge of the laboring client to exert abdominal muscle pressure with each contraction, or to "push." This is considered the secondary power of labor. The pelvic floor exerts a passive counterpressure as the fetal presenting part encounters resistance and is guided to the vaginal opening.

Psyche

The physical process of labor and delivery is affected by the level of excitement, tension, and fear experienced by the client and her family and by the degree to which the client's self-esteem is threatened or supported. Somatic manifestations of fear—elevated blood pressure, increased heart and respiratory rate—should not be confused with normal excitement. Caregivers must be alert to body language indicating extreme stress. Careful interviews will foster accurate assessment of the client's and family's emotional status. The nurse should be aware that baseline vital signs, taken when the client first enters the birthing area, may be affected by anxiety and therefore less reliable than those read when the client has calmed. Fear and panic are extreme responses to real or perceived threats to bodily or psychic integrity. Labor can be experienced as a loss of control, particularly to the primiparous client or the client without childbirth preparation. The nurse should explore with the frightened client and family the reasons for their fear, whether they be loss of control, pain, the unfamiliar environment, or the strange sensations experienced. Once the source of fear is identified, the nurse is able to explain, support, and comfort and, in so doing, promote the stability essential for an optimal outcome while preventing the unnecessary expenditure of energy that is the result of unrecognized and unresolved terror. Psychologic aspects of labor and delivery are discussed in Chapter 26.

PREMONITORY PHASE

Occasionally, it is difficult for the woman to determine if labor has truly begun. It is important for the nurse to distinguish between false and true labor. True labor includes a premonitory phase and results in dilation and effacement of the cervix. False labor, on the other hand, does not dilate or efface the cervix. (*See* Chapter 27 for a discussion of nursing management of false labor.)

Signs that the onset of labor is imminent may be noted subjectively by the mother or may go unnoticed. Primigravidas may experience lightening, or the descent of the presenting part of the fetus into the pelvis, more frequently than multigravidas. Lightening is more common when the fetus presents in a vertex position, the mother has good abdominal muscle tone, and there is no cephalopelvic inlet disproportion. The expectant mother reports relief from pressure on the upper abdomen and diaphragm and quite possibly an easing of the problem of heartburn.

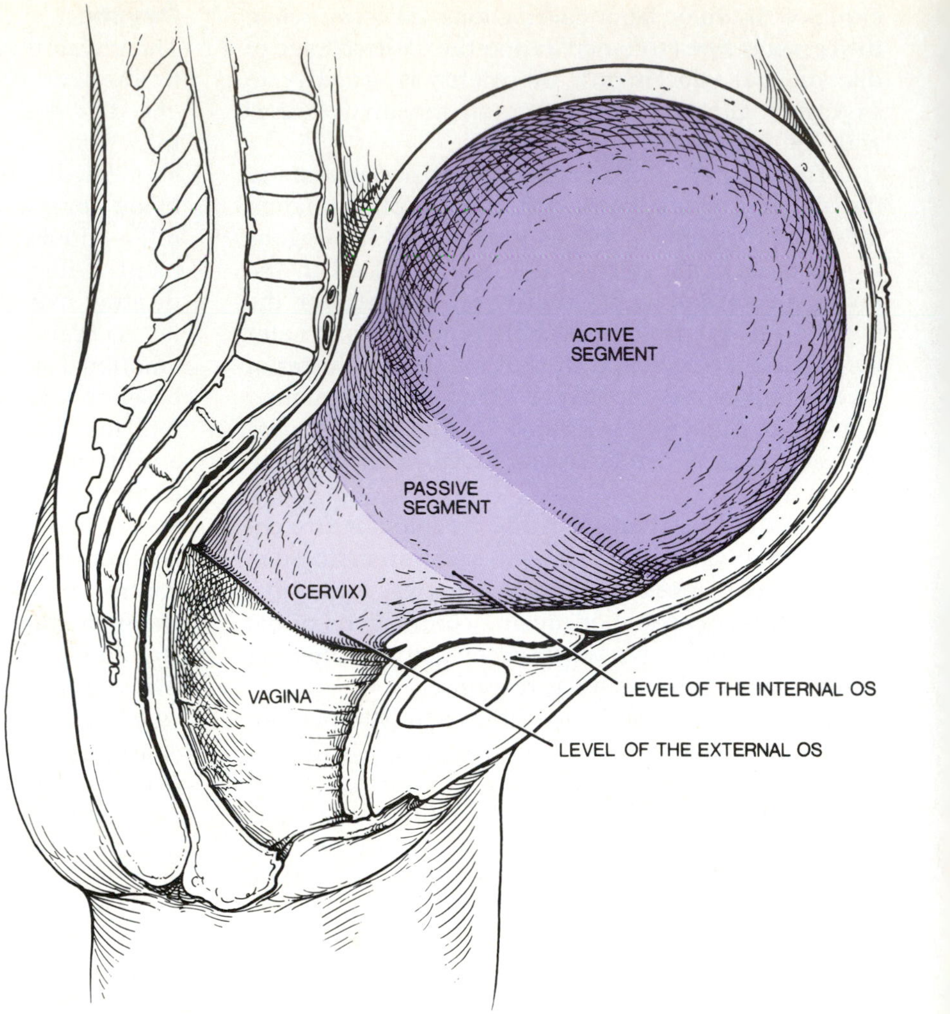

Figure 25–9. The uterus at the time of vaginal delivery. The active upper segment retracts about the fetus as the fetus descends through the birth canal. In the passive lower segment there is considerably less myometrial tone. (*Reproduced, with permission, from Cunningham FG, et al.* Williams Obstetrics. *18th ed. Norwalk, Conn: Appleton & Lange; 1989:215.*)

Pelvic pressure, frequent urination as a result of bladder compression, increase in leg cramps and the characteristic waddling gait are other symptoms that accompany lightening. This initial uterine/fetal descent may occur several weeks before the onset of labor; the indeterminate time frame makes lightening a weak predictor of labor.

The Braxton Hicks contractions that have "exercised" the uterine musculature throughout pregnancy become more perceptible to the mother near term. As anxiety heightens awareness and impatience magnifies each somatic change, the pregnant woman may experience the Braxton Hicks contractions as painful. Multiparous women report that these preparatory contractions become more uncomfortable with each succeeding pregnancy, probably as a result of loss of uterine tone. Braxton Hicks contractions are irregular and experienced primarily in the abdomen.

Many women experience a rush of energy several days before the onset of true labor. In the 72-hour period before onset the woman at term often can be found cleaning, washing windows, waxing floors, or rearranging the nursery. Such "nesting behavior" is also exhibited in species other than humans and appears to be a deep-seated, biologically patterned response to impending birth. Because sleep is often difficult as the woman nears term (as a result of the need to void frequently, difficulty in breathing, fetal activity, and the general discomfort of a cumbersome body), this short period of intense physical activity further depletes energy stores. Antepartum teaching must include caution against overdoing. Walking or short periods of light activity might be suggested as a substitute. The mother who is made aware of the significance of the energy burst can use this time to review preparations for the trip to the hospital and to practice prepared childbirth techniques.

A slight weight loss of 1 to 4 pounds may directly

precede labor as the hormonal balance between progesterone and estrogen causes a shift in electrolytes.

An increase in vaginal mucous secretions may be confused with amniotic leakage. The increase is caused by congestion of tissues. A "bloody show" of pink-stained mucous may be present for several days preceding labor onset. Women often report that walking results in a feeling of instability, which may result from the pelvic pressure of lightening and the more relaxed pelvic joints. Safety is important throughout pregnancy, but at this time it is important to take special precautions against falling.

In summary, there are several signs of the premonitory stage of labor. The nurse should make the pregnant couple aware of these signs, but should explain that the signs may not be experienced by all women.

STAGES AND PHASES OF LABOR

For purposes of assessment, labor is divided into stages and phases using the variables of time, effacement/dilation of the cervix, and changes in maternal behavioral responses. Each stage and phase has characteristic landmarks and parameters that are useful in determining progress or lack of progress. Patterns of labor are highly individual. The nurse should listen carefully to the woman who reports that her labors in the past have "gone from 3 cm to 10 cm in 90 minutes." What appears to be a history of abnormally long or startlingly short labors may reflect inherited pelvic anatomy and, for that individual woman, present a normal pattern.

Definitions

The following terms and definitions are used throughout this chapter.

- **Labor.** Involuntary physiologic process by which the fetus and placenta are propelled from the uterus of the mother into the external environment.
- **Contraction.** Wavelike tightening and shortening of the muscles of the uterine fundus that also exert pressure on the lower uterine segment through the fetal presenting part.
- **Acme.** Point of maximum intensity in a uterine contraction.
- **Increment.** Curve that builds to the acme of a contraction, starting with the onset.
- **Decrement.** Curve descending from the acme of a uterine contraction to a resting plateau.
- **Effacement.** Softening and thinning of the cervix. On palpation the prelabor cervix feels soft and rubbery, with a discernible raised ridge. When completely effaced, the cervix is paper thin with no palpable ridge.
- **Dilation.** Progressive widening of the external cervical os, which cannot occur without effacement. Effacement may precede dilation or occur simultaneously with it.
- **Fetal station.** Relationship of the presenting part of the fetus to the ischial spines of the mother.
- **First stage of labor.** Process of dilation whereby the cervix opens from 0 to 10 cm, or to a diameter wide enough to accommodate passage of the fetus. The first stage begins with the onset of true labor and is complete when dilation is accomplished.
- **Second stage of labor.** Process that begins with the complete dilation and effacement of the cervix and ends with the birth of the baby.
- **Third stage of labor (placental stage).** Process that begins with the birth of the baby and ends with the expulsion of the placenta and membranes.
- **Fourth stage of labor.** Process that begins with the delivery of the placenta and membranes and ends with the initial physiologic adjustment and stabilization of the mother's body systems. The fourth stage may last approximately 1 to 4 hours postpartum.

First Stage

The first stage of labor is made up of two phases: the latent phase and the active phase.

The **Friedman curve** is a graphic representation of these phases in the normal progress of labor. It is used by health care professionals to monitor the progress of labor. On this graph, cervical dilation, in centimeters, is the vertical axis and time, in hours, is the horizontal axis (Figure 25–10). The Friedman curve has been particularly useful for more than 20 years. The nurse who is caring for more than one woman during labor will find the graphic method an aid to early identification of a trend toward deviation from normal.

Latent Phase. The **latent phase** begins with the onset of true labor and ends when the cervix dilates approximately 3 cm (*see* Figure 27–5). The latent phase has traditionally been considered to be longer for primigravidas (8.6 hours) than for multigravidas (5.3 hours, with outer limits of normal of 20 hours for primigravidas and 14 hours for multigravidas). In their study of women with uncomplicated labors, Peisner and Rosen noted that women expectant for

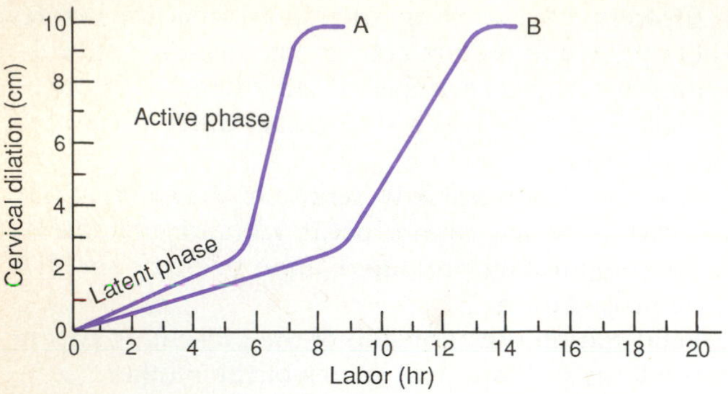

Figure 25–10. Friedman's curve, showing first stage of labor for (A) a multipara and (B) a primigravida. (*Reproduced, with permission, from Oxorn H, ed.* Oxorn-Foote Human Labor and Birth. 5th ed. Norwalk, Conn: Appleton-Century-Crofts; 1986: 120.)

the first time sought hospital admission earlier in labor than multiparous women.[17]

Contractions during the latent phase are widely spaced (15 to 30 minutes) and of mild to moderate intensity. The graph of the Friedman curve is nearly flat during the latent phase. Nulliparous women frequently assume that because of the relative comfort of the latent phase, the remaining labor will not be difficult. "This isn't bad . . . certainly not what my sister told me it was like." "If this is as bad as it gets, I won't have any problems." The nurse caring for the nulliparous client supports the client in building confidence in her ability to accomplish the tasks of labor, for example, "You have certainly managed the contractions very well so far. I'm sure that as labor becomes more intense you will do equally well." Such responses imply that the client retains the control essential to her self-image and self confidence (the word *manage* is chosen deliberately).

Active Phase. Once the cervix is dilated to 3 cm, the woman enters the **active phase** of labor. The active phase lasts from the end of the latent phase until full dilation of the cervix. Contractions grow stronger and longer (30 to 60 seconds). They are more frequent, occurring every 2 to 3 minutes. The graph of the Friedman curve during the active phase becomes a nearly vertical incline until the second stage of labor is almost reached, when the curve flattens again. The active phase is further subdivided into the acceleration phase, phase of maximum slope, and deceleration phase.

Acceleration Phase. A prelude to the intense activity that follows, the **acceleration phase** is characterized by an intense increase in the rate of dilation from approximately 3 cm to 4 to 5 cm.

Phase of Maximum Slope. The greatest increase in the rate of cervical dilation is referred to as the **phase of maximum slope.** Rapid cervical dilation during this phase averages 3 cm per hour. An increase of less than 1.2 cm in a primigravida or 1.7 cm in a multipara is considered abnormal. The use of such fractional measurements may give the impression that complete precision in measuring cervical dilation is possible; however, normal variations occur among laboring women.

Deceleration Phase. Also termed the transition phase, the deceleration phase is characterized by cervical dilation to 8 to 10 cm. Effacement of the cervix is either complete or almost complete, with only a rim remaining (analogous to the mouth of a balloon) on vaginal examination. The rim may completely encircle the os, or may be partial if a portion of the cervix is trapped between the presenting part (particularly in a vertex presentation) and the pubic arch. Contractions are moderate to strong and occur at 1- to 2-minute intervals.

Behavior of the laboring woman often changes markedly in transition. Although earlier in labor she may have welcomed the soothing touch of her support person or the nurse as backrubs and a cool washcloth on the forehead provided comfort, the woman now tends to be irritable and dislikes being touched. (*See* Chapter 26 for discussion.) Nausea and vomiting may add to her discomfort. She concentrates totally on the labor process and may experience a loss of control with subsequent panic as contractions increase in intensity. The so-called "bloody show" becomes more profuse during this phase; however, *bright red, steady, or clotted flow is not normal* and should be reported and further assessed.

If relaxation techniques have been learned, the laboring woman may sleep in the brief intervals between contractions to conserve strength. The first stage of labor ends with complete effacement and dilation of the cervix. The longest period of labor is over, and preparation of the birth passage has been completed. The nurse should be aware that sedation may prolong the latent phase. According to Friedman,[18] it is possible to analyze the active phase of the first stage by drawing inferences *about* the relationship (fit) of fetus to maternal pelvis during the deceleration phase, *about* the outcome of labor from the acceleration phase, and *about* the competent interrelationship of power, passage, and passenger from maximum slope.

Rupture of Membranes. The membranes that constitute the sac containing the fetus and amniotic fluid are subject to extreme pressure in the lower uterine segment as the presenting part of the fetus descends into the pelvis. A pocket of fluid, is trapped and applies pressure against the cervix. Membranes may rupture at any time during labor, or may rupture in the prelabor period before admission. Characteristically, however, rupture occurs at the height of a moderate to strong contraction, with the fetal presenting part well engaged and descended. (*See* Chapter 27 for nursing actions during the rupture of membranes.) The membranes can also be ruptured artificially through the procedure of amniotomy. (*See* Chapter 27 for discussion.)

Second Stage

The second stage of labor begins at full dilation, that is, 10 cm, and ends with delivery of the neonate.

Mechanisms of Labor. The terms mechanisms of labor and **cardinal movements of labor** are used to describe the simultaneous accommodation of the fetal anatomy to the maternal pelvis and birth canal and passage of the fetus from the abdominal site to the outside world. Although the mechanisms are traditionally described in a "list" fashion, such a presentation may be misleading as several of the mechanisms occur either at the same time or in an overlapping time frame (Figure 25–11).

The relatively unyielding planes of the maternal pelvis require that the fetus accommodate to the pelvic contours. In 95 percent of deliveries, presentation involves the fetal head; therefore, in the description of the mechanisms that follows, fetal skull designations, particularly the occiput, will be used to indicate the fetal presenting part during descent.

Descent. The fetus descends throughout labor. Descent, therefore, is a variable of normal labor that is continuous, is measurable, and provides one item of data by which progress can be measured against a known standard.

The ease with which the fetus is born is a result of the interaction between fetal accommodation and maternal internal structures. The progress of fetal movement through the maternal pelvis is monitored by the stations of descent.

The **stations of descent** is a measurement, in centimeters, of the progress of the descending fetal presenting part to the maternal ischial spines. On this scale, the point where the presenting part reaches the ischial spines is identified as zero. Measurements above the ischial spines are denoted in negative numbers (-1 through -5) and those below, in positive numbers ($+1$ through $+5$), depending on how many centimeters above or below the ischial spines the presenting part is located.

The degree of advancement of the fetal presenting part is assessed using this scale as pictured in Figure 25–12. When the presenting part is at a -5 station, it is at the level of the pelvic inlet. When the presenting part is at zero station, it is at the level of the ischial spines. Below the spines, the presenting part is considered at $+1$, $+2$, $+3$, and so on. At $+5$, crowning occurs and birth is imminent.

Protocols for recording assessment of station may vary according to established custom; for example, some institutions use a -4 to $+4$ notation[1] rather than the -5 to $+5$ scale noted here. Station is assessed by vaginal examination and the use of Leopold's maneuvers. The station is assessed at the same point in the contraction cycle each time an examination is done because the fetus may advance and recede with each contraction.

Flexion. Flexion of the fetal head is necessary to bring the smaller suboccipital diameter into and out of the midpelvis of the mother. Flexion occurs when the fetal head meets resistance from the bony pelvis and soft tissue. Two additional factors make the extreme flexion of the fetal head possible: (1) The fetus has the typical receding chin that characterizes the neonate. The mandible recedes even further in response to pressure and permits hyperflexion of the head. (2) The hormone relaxin may contribute to the process described, permitting a degree of hyperflexion that will never again be possible after birth.

Flexion of the fetal head should occur as the fetus in vertex presentation enters the pelvic inlet. Flexion allows the largest transverse diameter (biparietal) to pass through the pelvic inlet after the fetus has entered with the sagittal suture in a transverse or oblique relationship to the pelvic inlet. Refer to Figure 25–11, which illustrates the mechanism or cardinal movements of labor.

The dimensions of the fetal presenting part and of the pelvis of the mother must always be studied in relation to each other and not separately. The pelvis of the mother is relatively fixed in dimension, with the only pelvic accommodation occurring when the coccyx is movable. The fetal skull changes in dimensions throughout labor as compression against

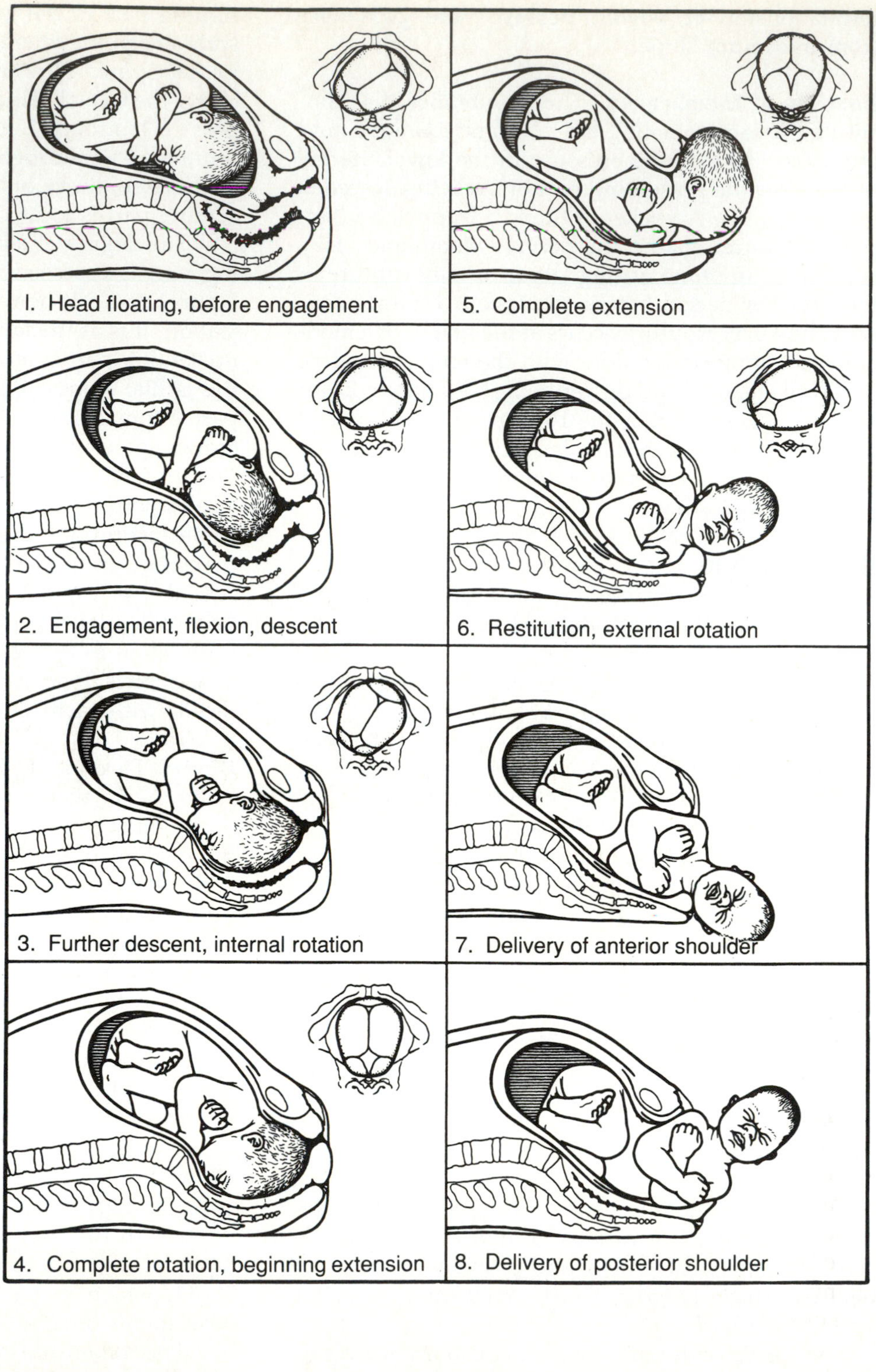

Figure 25–11. Mechanism of labor: left anterior occiput position. (*Reproduced, with permission, from Cunningham FG, et al.* Williams Obstetrics. *18th ed. Norwalk, Conn: Appleton & Lange; 1989:228.*)

the maternal pelvis causes narrowing in one dimension with a consequent widening in another. The joints of the fetal skull (sutures) allow for this accommodation both through compression and through override, but total skull volume does not change.[1] This process of skull change is termed *molding*. The degree of molding is related to such factors as the length of labor and the size of the fetal head in relation to maternal structures.

When the fetal head is in flexion (truly, hyperflexion) the chin of the fetus is tucked down so that in a vertex presentation when descent and degree of dilation permit, both the anterior and posterior fontanelles can be palpated on vaginal examination.

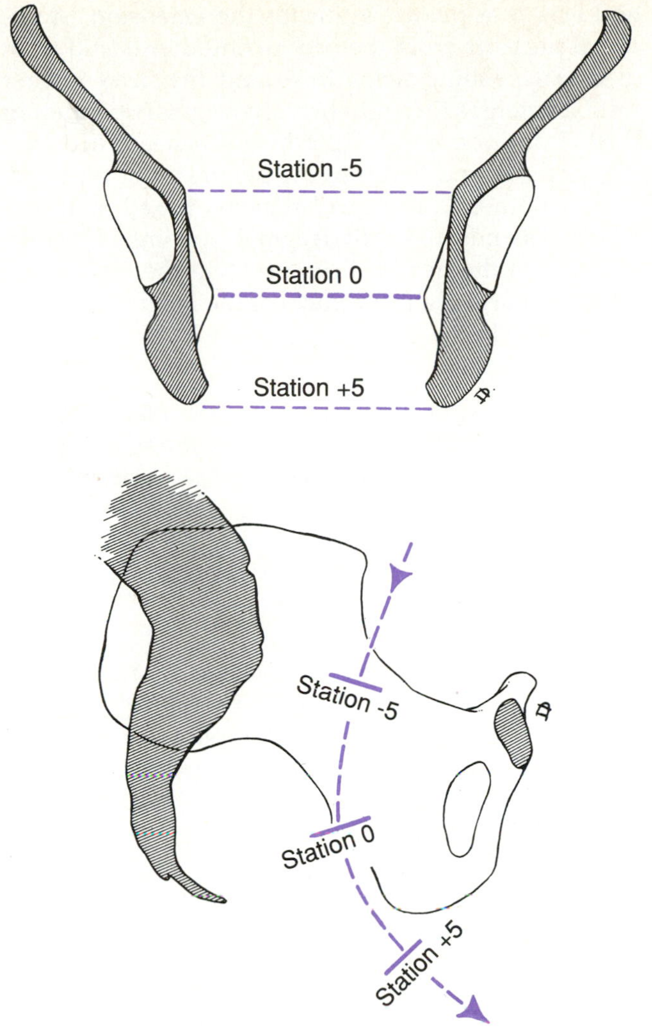

Figure 25–12. Stations of descent. (*Reproduced, with permission, from Oxorn H, ed.* Oxorn-Foote Human Labor and Birth. *5th ed. Norwalk, Conn: Appleton-Century-Crofts; 1986:69.*)

Engagement. When the presenting part of the fetus has entered the true pelvis, **engagement** has occurred. Specifically, in a vertex presentation, engagement occurs when the largest transverse diameter (biparietal) of the fetal head has passed through the maternal pelvic inlet. The pelvic inlet is described as an imaginary plane extending from the superior surface of the symphysis pubis through to the promontory of the sacrum.

The fetal head engages most often with its anteroposterior diameters in the transverse diameter of the pelvis. Thus, the most common position of the fetal head during engagement is the left occiput transverse position, with the biparietal diameter parallel to the planes of the pelvis. This position of the fetal head in the pelvic inlet is termed **synclitism.** In this position, the smallest diameter of the head (suboccipitobregmatic) enters the widest diameter of the pelvic inlet (transverse). It is thus the best position for an effective descent. **Asynclitism,** on the other hand, is the term used when the fetal head is not parallel to the planes of the pelvis on engagement, and thus is in a less optimal position for descent (Figures 25–13 and 25–14).

The head may enter the pelvic inlet in positions other than vertex, for example, brow, mentum, or face presentations. Brow presentations often convert spontaneously to vertex and can initially be considered as on the normal continuum. If conversion does not occur, a cephalopelvic disproportion may result in dystocia, or an abnormality in the labor process (*see* Chapter 40). Face presentations rarely convert and lie outside the normal continuum.

Internal Rotation. **Internal rotation** of the fetal head results in the anteroposterior diameter of the fetal head being in alignment with the anteroposterior diameter of the maternal pelvis. Usually this rotation brings the fetal head from a LOA or ROA position into a direct anterior position, resulting in an OA position; that is, the fetus is looking down to the floor if the mother is on her back. In about 4 percent of cases, the fetus enters the pelvis in a LOP or ROP

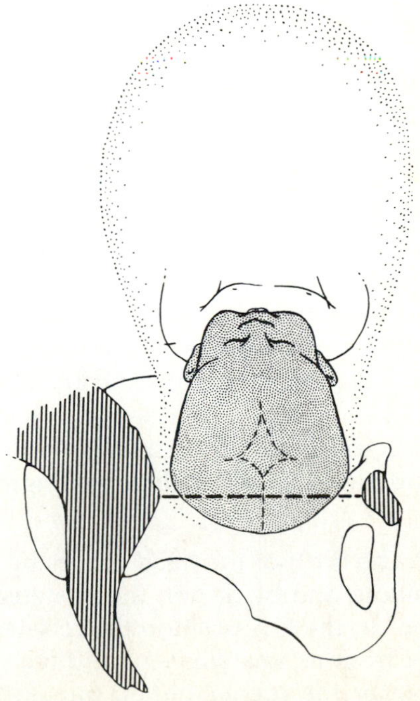

Figure 25–13. Synclitisms at the inlet. (*Reproduced with permissin, from Oxorn H, ed.* Oxorn-Foote Human Labor and Birth. *5th ed. Norwalk, Conn: Appleton-Century-Crofts; 1986:71.*)

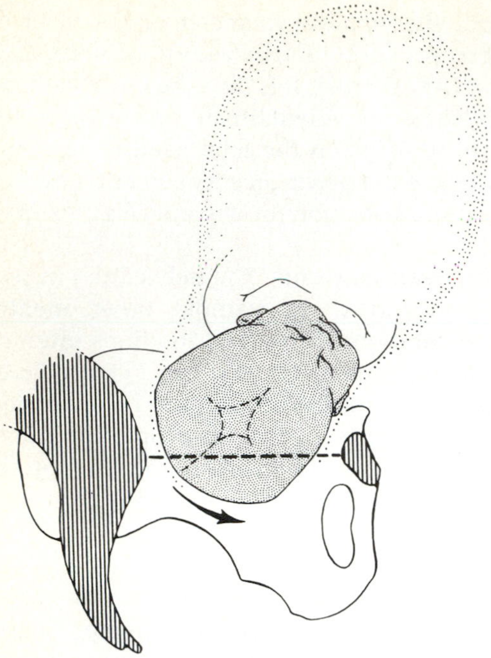

Figure 25–14. Anterior asynclitism. (*Reproduced, with permission, from Oxorn H, ed.* Oxorn-Foote Human Labor and Birth. *5th ed. Norwalk, Conn: Appleton-Century-Crofts; 1986:73.)*

position and rotates into a direct OP position; that is, the fetus is looking up to the ceiling if the mother is lying on her back.

Internal rotation is caused by a combination of factors: (1) the powerful pressure exerted by uterine contractions on the fetus, (2) the curved shape of the pelvic floor, and (3) the relationship of the vertex to the projection of the ischial spines in the midpelvic cavity.

The ischial spines act as guides or tracks, aiding the fetal skull to assume the position that will facilitate birth. Because the fetal skull and fetal shoulders are at right angles to each other, the ischial spines aid the body of the fetus in passage through the pelvis. As internal rotation takes place (a 45° turn) the pelvis of the mother compels the limbs and body of the fetus to assume the most compact shape possible. Once complete internal rotation occurs the fetus has usually descended to the pelvic floor (*see* Figure 25–11).

Extension. The birth of the head occurs by extension in OA position, and by flexion then extension in the OP position. In the OA position the resistance of the pelvic floor from its anatomic curve directs the head upward toward the vaginal outlet, causing extension of the fetal head. The back of the fetal head in the suboccipital region moves under the symphysis pubis and acts as a pivotal point for the extension. Additional pressure from the contracting uterus and from maternal pushing helps to extend the head further until it emerges through the vulvovaginal opening. In the OP position the sinciput moves beneath the symphysis pubis and becomes the pivotal point for delivery of the head. The head remains flexed as it (occiput) distends the vulvovaginal opening. In effect the back of the head is born first and then extension takes over and the front (face) of the head is born (*see* Figure 25–11).

Restitution. After the birth of the infant's head (with the sagittal suture parallel to the mother's long axis) the head rotates 45°, returning to the position it assumed when it first entered the pelvis. This maneuver, known as **restitution,** restores the normal anatomic alignment of the infant's neck and shoulders (*see* Figure 25–11).

External Rotation. **External rotation** occurs as the shoulders (which are still in the pelvis) rotate 45° to bring them in line with the anteroposterior diameter of the pelvis. When the shoulders rotate, the head rotates another 45° into the LOT or ROT position (*see* Figure 25–11).

Expulsion. The birth of the shoulders is by lateral flexion. The anterior shoulder is usually born first and is seen at the anterior portion of the vulvovaginal opening. Like the head in the OA position, the anterior shoulder moves under the symphysis pubis. With the continued forces of maternal pushing and contractions, the posterior shoulder distends the perineum and is born by lateral flexion following the pelvic curve. The remainder of the body follows the same curve and is readily born, as it is much smaller and more flexible than either the head or shoulders.

ISSUES AND CONTROVERSIES

In the United States controversy continues to surround several practices related to labor and delivery. For example, a variety of researchers have demonstrated that positions other than the lithotomy delivery position aid the physiologic process of delivery. The question becomes, whose well-being is served when the woman is placed in a lithotomy position to deliver: the practitioner's or the mother's?

Another question concerns the practice of encouraging the mother to bear down vigorously during the second stage of labor.

RESEARCH ABSTRACT

Liu YC. The effects of the upright position during childbirth. Image. *1989;21:14–18.*

This research replicated an earlier study done by the investigator. Its focus was to identify the effects of the angle of the mother's position during the second stage of labor on the duration of labor.

The sample consisted of 68 primigravid married women between the ages of 18 and 25 years. All women met the criteria of (1) appropriate age, (2) no pregnancy complications, (3) active participation of their husband, and (4) between 38 and 42 weeks of gestation. Additionally, no women who had cephalopelvic disproportion or psychiatric disorders and only those with fetuses in left or right vertex presentation were admitted to the study.

The women were assigned to one of three groups. Women in group A (n = 24) used a 30° upright position and were not given instructions to bear down during the second stage of labor. The women in group B (n = 22) used a 30° upright position and were given instructions to bear down. Group C, the control group (n = 22), used a 0° recumbent position and were given instructions to bear down.

The subjects were instructed to call the investigator or her research assistant when signs of labor began. Second-stage management was monitored by the labor and delivery nurses.

Descent of the fetal head was measured by vaginal examination. Duration of labor was measured for both the first and second stages in hours and minutes. Instructions to bear down, if applicable, were given by the labor and delivery nurses.

Results indicated that mothers in the 30° upright position enhanced the descent of the fetal head and had a shorter duration of labor in both first and second stages than mothers in the recumbent position. For mothers in the upright position but not given instructions to bear down, the second stage of labor was even shorter. This study confirms the results of previous research that indicated position during labor and delivery has significant influence on duration of labor.

Comment:
This replication study further documents the possibility that position during labor and delivery affects such variables as descent of the fetus and duration of labor. In providing care during labor, nurses can encourage and assist clients to assume upright rather than supine positions. The study further stimulates consideration of factors within birthing environments that do or do not foster the use of upright positioning during childbirth.

Delivery of the Newborn. At full dilation and effacement with the fetal presenting part (vertex) at +5 station, caput (fetal scalp) will be visible with each contraction. The mother feels an uncontrollable involuntary urge to push out the contents of the uterus. The perineum distends further with each contraction, bulging as the presenting part applies pressure. Labia minora and labia majora disappear with distension and rectal mucosa often protrudes with the effort of expulsion. The fetal head advances with each contraction, then slips back in the resting plateau. Each advance moves the fetus farther until the widest diameter of the fetal skull (biparietal) is rimmed by the introitus, and with the next contraction or two, the head emerges.

Duration of Second Stage. The Friedman graphic analysis of normal labor indicates that on average the second stage of labor lasts about 1 hour in primigravidas and about 20 minutes in multigravidas. Both time designations represent means, not absolutes. In primigravidas, second-stage labor can last up to 2 hours and still be considered "normal" if there is a measurable rate of descent and no indication of fetal distress.

Third Stage

The third stage of labor encompasses the time between delivery of the neonate and expulsion of the placenta. With the birth of the neonate the formerly distended uterus contracts, beginning the process of placental disengagement. The sight of the newborn and the first sounds may also form a powerful primary stimulus to the production of maternal oxytocin, which in turn promotes further contraction of the uterus. Blood specimens for the Coombs test (antibody test), hematocrit/hemoglobin, and type with Rh analysis may be taken from the remnant of the umbilical cord that protrudes from the vagina.

Separation of the Placenta. The placenta may safely remain attached to the uterine wall for as long as 30 minutes before being termed "retained."[19] In most births, placental separation occurs from 5 to 10 minutes after delivery of the neonate.

Failure of the placenta to fully separate or reten-

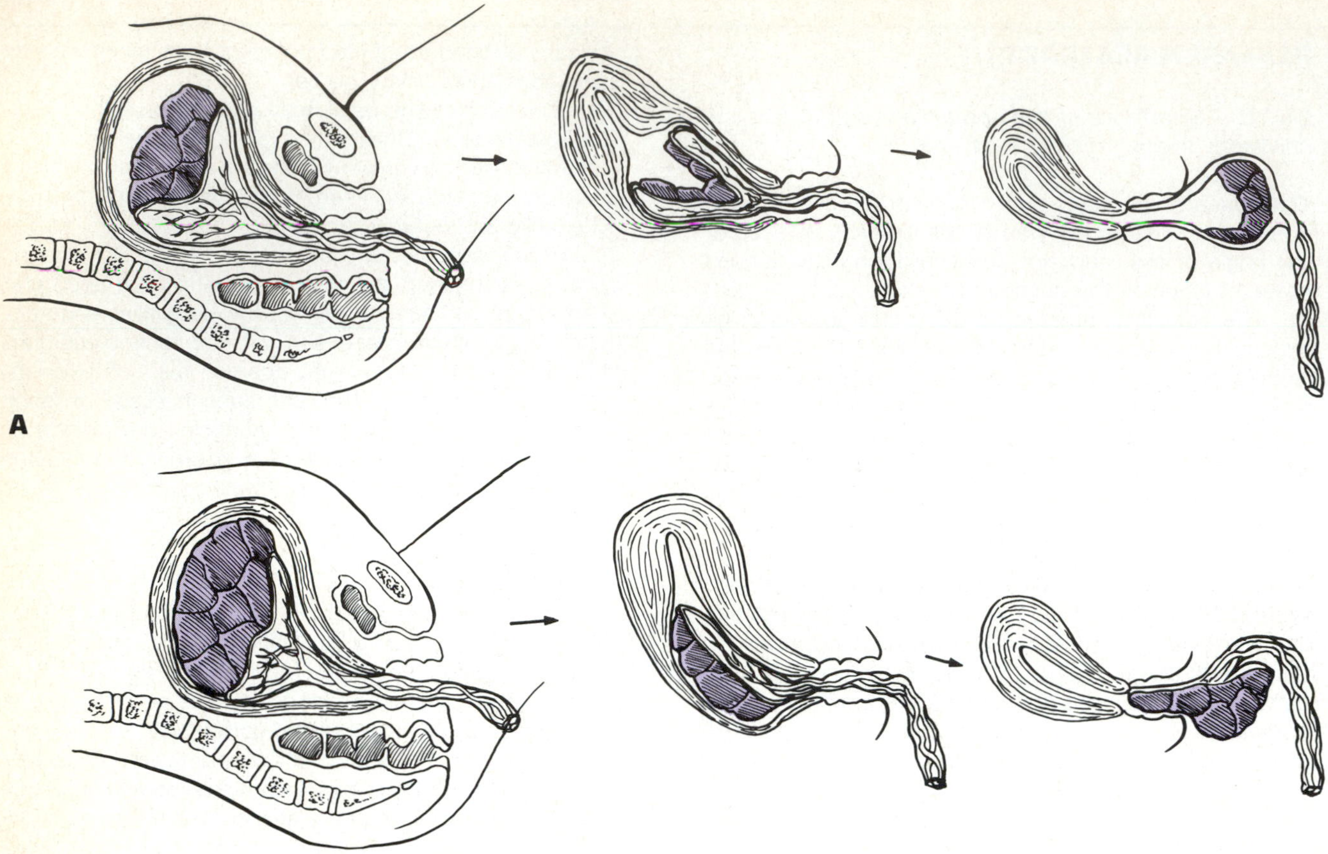
A
B

Figure 25–15. Placental separation. **A.** Schultze mechanism. **B.** Duncan mechanism.

tion of placental fragments may require manual removal under anesthesia. The totally retained placenta is a rare complication. Retention of placental fragments, although not common, occurs more frequently than total retention and may cause immediate or delayed hemorrhage (*see* Chapter 41).

The separated placenta presents in one of two ways. In the Schultze mechanism, dubbed "Shiny Schultze," the placenta first separates from the uterine wall at its center with the edges releasing last so that the shiny membranous fetal side is seen first, trailing the membranes. In the Duncan mechanism, dubbed "Dirty Duncan," the maternal side presents first, indicating that separation has occurred first at an edge and progressed. The maternal surface which has adhered to the uterine wall is rough and bumpy in appearance (Figure 25–15).

Fourth Stage

The fourth stage of labor has traditionally been identified as the period after or within 4 hours of delivery of the placenta. In practice it is viewed as the period required for stabilization of the mother's physical and emotional state after the stresses of labor and delivery. In the hospital setting, this postdelivery period may therefore be very short and encompass only the time required for hygienic care and assessment of the mother's status before transport to a postpartum unit, or it may include a stay of several hours in a delivery recovery area.

With the fourth stage of labor the mother's body systems begin a phase of physiologic restoration. The final outcome of the adjustments will be return of the woman's body to a physiologic state similar to the prepregnancy state. Chapter 26 discusses psychologic aspects of the restorative process; physiologic adaptations are presented in Chapter 29.

SUMMARY

Labor and delivery represent the culmination of the physiologic process of pregnancy. By the end of pregnancy, significant physiologic changes will have occurred in the mother's body to facilitate delivery of the fetus. At term, the cervix begins the process of effacement—softening, thinning, and shortening in preparation for onset of labor. In addition, the vaginal walls relax to allow passage of the fetus.

Researchers have proposed several hypotheses for labor onset. Although no one hypothesis can be used to explain onset of labor, contributing factors include the uterine stretch mechanism and maternal and fetal hormones. Progress of labor is influenced by the four P's: passage or true pelvis, consisting of the inlet, the pelvic cavity, and the outlet; passenger or fetus; powers, the uterine contractions; and psyche, the maternal cognitive emotional responses.

The terms *fetal attitude, lie, presentation,* and *position,* collectively referred to as fetopelvic relationships, describe characteristics of the fetus in relation to himself, herself, or the maternal pelvis. The most frequent fetal presentation is the vertex (or occiput) presentation, with the head flexed and the occiput presenting.

Onset of labor is often mild and difficult to distinguish from false labor. Patterns of early labor may be irregular, and a progressive pattern may not develop until the woman is well into active labor. Common signs of labor onset include lightening (descent of the fetus into the pelvis), primarily in primigravidas, and more pronounced Braxton Hicks contractions. Many women also experience "nesting behavior," a heightened level of energy in the 2 to 3 days before onset of true labor.

Labor may be divided into four stages. The first stage begins with the first true labor contraction and ends with complete dilation of the cervix and is further divided, using Friedman's curve, into the latent phase and the active phase. The second stage begins with complete dilation and effacement of the cervix and ends with birth of the baby. The third stage begins with birth of the baby and ends with delivery of the placenta. The fourth stage is the immediate postpartum period.

Mechanisms of labor or cardinal movements of labor are terms used to describe the accommodation of the fetal anatomy to the maternal birth canal and the passage of the fetus into the outside world during second-stage labor. The mechanisms or movements are descent, flexion, engagement, internal rotation, restitution, external rotation, and expulsion. Progress of fetal descent is measured in centimeters using a scale termed the *stations of descent.*

Placental separation during third-stage labor occurs in one of two ways: the Schultze mechanism, in which the membranous fetal (shiny) side is seen first, or the Duncan mechanism, in which the maternal (bumpy) side appears first. Placental separation usually occurs from 5 to 10 minutes after delivery of the neonate, but may be delayed as long as 30 minutes before being termed *retained.*

Nursing care of the woman and family during labor is based on a thorough knowledge of maternal physiology and the stages and phases of labor.

REVIEW QUESTIONS

1. Describe and compare at least two major theories of labor onset.
2. Identify the powers of labor. List three mechanisms that enhance these powers.
3. Identify the passage. Describe at least three important diameters of the passage.
4. Identify the passenger. Describe two aspects of the passenger that influence progress of labor.
5. Identify the factors influencing onset, duration, and outcome of labor.

REFERENCES

1. Cunningham FG, et al. *Williams Obstetrics.* 18th ed. Norwalk, Conn: Appleton & Lange; 1989.
2. Lipshitz J. Initiation of labor. In: Givens JR, Andrews GD, eds. *Endocrinology of Pregnancy Year Book.* Chicago: Yearbook Medical Publishers; 1981.
3. Challis JR, Mitchell BF. Hormonal control of preterm and term parturition. *Semin Perinatol.* 1981;5:192.
4. Chard T. The role of maternal and fetal posterior pituitary gland in parturition. In: MacDonald PC, Porter JC, eds. *Initiation of Parturition: Prevention of Prematurity, Fourth Ross Conference on Obstetric Research.* Columbus, Ohio: Ross Labs; 1983:121.
5. Soloff MS. The role of oxytocin receptors in parturation. In: MacDonald PC, Porter JC, eds. *Initiation of Parturition: Prevention of Prematurity, Fourth Ross Conference on Obstetric Research.* Columbus, Ohio: Ross Labs; 1983:160.
6. Hillier K, et al. Concentrations of prostaglandin F in amniotic fluid in spontaneous and induced labors. In: Givens JR, Andrews GD, eds. *Endocrinology of Pregnancy Year Book.* Chicago: Yearbook Medical Publishers; 1981.
7. McCosten JA, et al. Prostaglandin E_2 release on the fetal

and maternal sides of the amnion and chorin decidua before and after term labor. *Am J Obstet Gynecol.* 1987;156:173.

8. Giannopoulos G, et al. Prostaglandin E and F_2 receptors in human myometrium during the menstrual cycle and in pregnancy and labor. *Am J Obstet Gynecol.* 1985;153:904.
9. Huzar G. *The Physiology and Biochemistry of the Uterus in Pregnancy and Labor.* Boca Raton, Fla: CRC Press; 1986.
10. Thorburn GD. Past and present concepts on the initiation of parturition. In: MacDonald PC, Porter JC, eds. *Initiation of Parturition: Prevention of Prematurity, Fourth Ross Conference on Obstetric Research.* Columbus, Ohio: Ross Labs; 1983:2.
11. Hariharan S, et al. Initiation of Labor. In: Sciarri JJ, ed. *Gynecology and Obstetrics.* Philadelphia: WB Saunders; 1986.
12. Oxorn H, ed. *Oxorn-Foote Human Labor and Birth.* 5th ed. Norwalk, Conn: Appleton-Century-Crofts; 1986.
13. Hughy MJ. Fetal position during pregnancy. *Am J Obstet Gynecol.* 1985;153:885.
14. Ivy AC, et al. The contractions of the monkey uterus at term. *Am J Obstet Gynecol.* 1931;22:388.
15. Huzar G. Biology and biochemistry of myometrial contractility and cervical maturation. *Semin Perinatol.* 5 July, 1981, 216.
16. Berg G, et al. Androgenic receptors in human myometrium during pregnancy. *Am J Obstet Gynecol.* 1986;154:601.
17. Peisner DB, Rosen MG. Latent phase of labor in normal patients: a reassessment. *Obstet Gynecol.* 1985;66:644–647.
18. Friedman E. Assessing labor progression. In: Friedman E, ed. *Obstetric Decision Making.* St. Louis, Mo: CV Mosby, 1982.
19. Oskowitz SP. Retained placenta. In: Friedman E, ed. *Obstetric Decision Making.* St. Louis, Mo: CV Mosby, 1982.

Psychologic and Sociocultural Dimensions of the Intrapartum Family

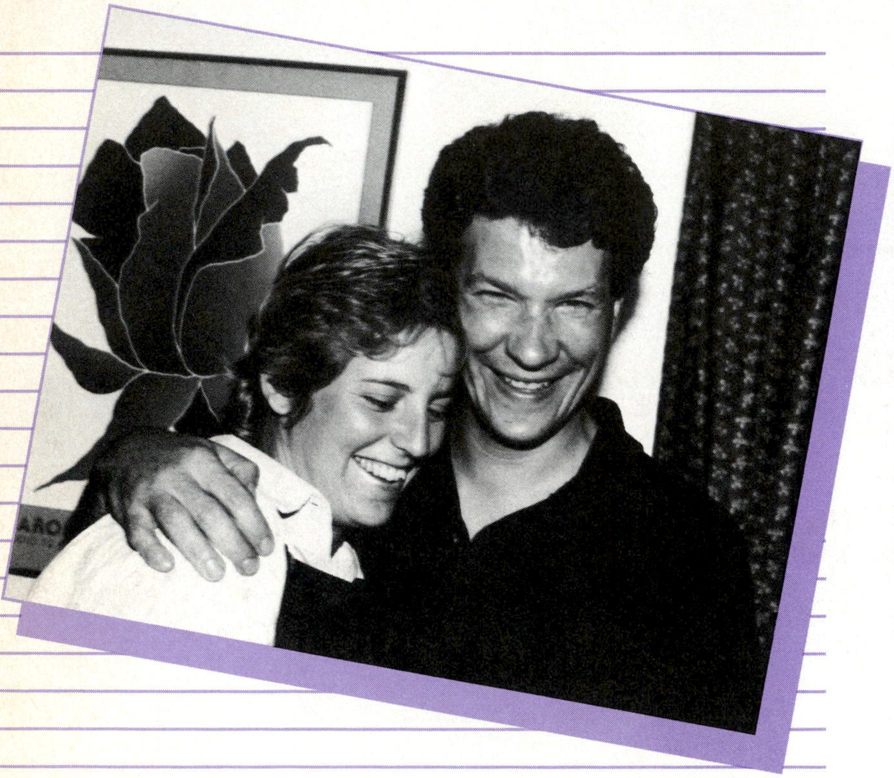

chapter 26

Key Terms

body boundary
body image
claiming
contemporary father
identification
personal space
traditional father

In recent years, many advances have been made that have improved care directed to the physical needs of the woman during labor; however, care directed to the psychologic needs of the woman and family in this period is also vitally important. The psychosocial reactions of the laboring woman and her family influence the physiologic labor process and the amount of discomfort the laboring woman experiences. Cultural factors will also influence the woman's and family's reaction to childbirth. This chapter explores the dynamics of the family during the intrapartum period and concludes with a focus on the birthing experience as viewed by various cultures. An understanding of these psychosocial and cultural dimensions enables the nurse to give care that assists the family to master childbirth and to have a satisfying birth experience.

COUPLE'S REACTIONS TO LABOR AND DELIVERY

Not long ago care during the intrapartum focused solely on the laboring woman. Today, caregivers recognize that childbirth involves a family. Each member reacts individually and as part of a family unit to the birth experience. Each family member experiences psychosocial reactions to the birth process, although only the childbearing woman actually gives birth. The woman's physiologic progress influences both her own and her family's psychosocial reactions. The psychosocial reactions thus in a cyclic manner both influence and are influenced by the woman's physical progress in labor. Understanding how these reactions interact enables the nurse to provide comprehensive, individualized care for the intrapartum family.

First Stage of Labor

Maternal Reactions. Maternal reactions to labor are unique and varied. Past experiences, cultural background, the marital relationship, fatigue, personality, and parity all contribute to the expectant mother's responses. Variations also occur in relation to frequency, intensity, and timing of the mother's psychologic reactions. Common reactions to labor include feelings of excitement and concern, anxiety, recruitment and use of support, use of role models, alterations in body image, expression of pain, maintenance of control, and feelings of hostility and aggression. The nurse needs to understand these reactions to interpret a woman's progress in labor and to provide supportive care for the intrapartum family.

Excitement and Uncertainty. Expectant mothers tend to respond to signs of labor with excitement, an "emotional high." The long wait finally has come to an end and the birth of the baby is imminent. In the initial hours of labor the mother typically is alert. She focuses vigilant attention on the early contractions. If contractions begin during the night, rest or sleep becomes difficult. Each uterine contraction causes the mother to cease activity and to focus on her body. She "listens" intently to orient herself to what is happening within; she questions whether labor has begun. If unable to interpret the inner sensations, she seeks added information by palpating her abdomen to help determine whether a contraction has truly occurred.

Sometimes an uncertain mother misreads her body's cues, thinking labor has begun when it has not. If these inner cues are not verified as "true" labor, the mother often feels embarrassed. Her self esteem may be affected and she may tearfully ask, "If this is not real labor, how will I know when it really begins?" She vows not to repeat the error again to prevent continued loss of self-esteem. This often results in a tendency to delay responding to signs of true labor when it actually occurs. Some women carry this resolve to such an extreme that they wait too long to seek assistance, arriving at the health care facility when delivery of the baby is imminent. The nurse should consider the potential for loss of self-esteem when sending the mother home undelivered, and provide support and reassurance that this is a common experience (*see* Chapter 27).

Anxiety. Not all women respond to the onset of labor with elation and excitement. Some experience feelings of ambivalence over the onset of labor. The desire to deliver the baby conflicts with a reluctance and fear to experience labor and delivery. This "push-pull" conflict may heighten the woman's feelings of anxiety. Women who initially reacted with excitement to labor onset may also begin to experience anxiety as labor progresses.

Anxiety demonstrated at the onset of labor tends to be of mild or moderate degree. Mild anxiety enhances the perceptual field, sharpening perceptions so that the woman sees, hears, and understands more than before. As a result she is more alert and aware of her environment. Moderate anxiety, on the other hand, results in narrowing of the perceptual field so that less is seen, heard, and understood. The focus is on immediate concerns, and peripheral matters are blocked out. An individual experiences selective inattention at this level of anxiety, but she can focus attention if directed to do so.[1] Women experiencing such levels of anxiety mobilize their inner resources in response to the labor process. They react positively, and welcome and learn from explanations about their environment and what to expect during labor.

Anxiety and fears evidenced during labor tend to center around concerns for the self and the baby, frequently existing at an unconscious level. Despite technology, which has greatly reduced the risk of childbirth, the threat of death for mother or baby has not been eliminated. Along with the fear of death is the fear of separation from the baby, who is perceived as a part of the self.

The birthing environment selected by the woman may contribute to her anxiety. If she seeks care in an institutional setting, she encounters unfamiliar persons and a strange environment. In the unfamiliar surroundings she encounters additional stress from unfamiliar sights, sounds, and smells; lack of privacy; and the use of medical terminology and expectations placed on her by health care providers. Institutional routines and procedures, so familiar to the health care providers, are strange and even overwhelming to the expectant mother. On admission to the institution the woman is asked to take off her own familiar clothes and put on a hospital gown. Her possessions are locked away or given to another family member for safekeeping. Stripped of the familiar physical items that contribute to her identity, she takes on a new role, that of a patient or client. Taking on an unfamiliar role often produces anxiety. In this unfamiliar role the mother may also experience many anxiety-producing procedures, depending on institutional policy.

Reactions of anxiety and fears for self occur along with inner physiologic changes over which the woman has no control. Escape of amniotic fluid, bloody show, and intensifying uterine contractions often contribute to feelings of anxiety and fear. These events present a threat to body integrity and self-concept.

Women frequently experience anxiety in response to experienced pain. In the early phase of labor, each contraction provides a pain signal that labor has begun. Rubin suggests that women react cognitively to early labor.[2] They may even experience pleasure in their ability to recognize labor and cope with the pain. The tendency exists, however, to anticipate how painful the next contraction will be, and this heightens anxiety.

Anxiety may escalate to high levels and become panic, as labor progresses to the active phase. Perception of the intensifying inner sensations as pain threatens the woman's integrity. A startled look on the woman's face may reflect her fear and anxiety as the baby suddenly descends within her pelvis. Stretching of muscle tissue and increasing sensations of pressure contribute to the perception that she is being torn and ripped apart. A sudden, quick placement of a hand on the lower abdomen or perineum also reflects the woman's anxiety over her sense of threatened integrity. The woman may use her hand to determine if she has actually come apart and to help hold her body together.[3]

The very anxious client uses all her energy to maintain control. All of her attention focuses on obtaining relief. In this state, her cognitive control is threatened as she fears the next contraction will be even worse. Unless reassured, she may panic and lose her ability to maintain self-control; however, anxiety reactions of such severe intensity during labor can generally be prevented through the use of support systems and supportive nursing interventions.

Failure of labor to progress as quickly as the woman expected or in a sequence as described by childbirth teachers, family, and friends also generates anxiety. A multipara, for example, may anticipate that her membranes will rupture right before the birth of her baby because that is what happened when her other babies were born. If this time the membranes rupture before labor becomes well established, she may perceive this occurrence as abnormal and become very anxious. Women tend to become anxious when labor continues for several hours in the early phase or if no documented change in the cervix occurs after a prolonged period of active labor. Anxiety results, in such instances, from the belief that something is wrong and both self and baby are threatened.

Excessive anxiety often negatively affects the woman in labor. Anxiety alters perceptions and intensifies the pain experience, contributing to fatigue and increased anxiety. The cyclic influence of the woman's anxiety and pain is a primary concern for caregivers during labor. Intensification of anxiety increases tension, which in turn leads to experiencing more intense pain. The woman's anxiety increases in anticipation of even more intense pain, so the cycle repeats itself with greater and greater intensity. Lederman and others[5] demonstrated a relationship between excessive anxiety and the secretion of catecholamine, which inhibits uterine activity. Inhibition of uterine activity by anxiety prolongs labor and increases the risk of intrapartum complications.

Nursing Strategies. Strategies for the woman experiencing anxiety include assessing the level of anxiety of the woman; identifying factors such as fear and pain that contribute to anxiety; educating the woman about institutional routines and procedures; intervening in a nonjudgmental manner (the caregiver should not belittle the woman's fears); providing supportive nursing interventions to the woman and family members; and intervening in a timely fashion before the cycle of fear, pain, and tension becomes established.

Recruitment and Utilization of Support. Once she believes labor has begun, the woman recruits and uses support persons to ensure safe passage for herself and her baby. Whom she recruits and when she recruits them vary. Some women quickly alert significant others, including the father, grandparents, siblings, other family members, and friends that labor has begun. Other women inform only the immediate family. Couples today frequently feel that birth is a private intimate experience that should be shared only with each other. They wish to wait until after the birth to inform others.

Many factors influence who is recruited to provide support during the labor and delivery. In our mobile society, family members may be too far away to attend the birth. Even if available, some families do not interact positively and would not be perceived as supportive. The expectant parents also may decide not to notify family members because of the fear they would become too anxious. Cultural factors also influence whom one recruits for childbirth support (*see* later section). Some cultures believe having men in attendance during childbirth is unacceptable. Other cultures desire, even expect, the baby's father to be present at birth.

Exactly when the woman seeks health care assistance for childbirth also varies. Some women seek assistance early in labor. Others wait until labor is well established before they seek assistance. Children may need to be cared for, and the woman may take time to see that the person she has recruited to care for them is present. Generally these activities delay but do not prevent the woman from seeking care. At times, however, these responsibilities delay seeking health care assistance until delivery is imminent. In such situations, the nurse should quickly prepare the woman for delivery. The nurse should use a nonjudgmental approach and not scold the woman for waiting so long.

Nursing Strategies. Strategies related to the recruitment and use of support include identifying cultural factors that influence selection of support persons during labor; establishing institutional policies that allow for flexibility in attendance of significant others during labor and at the birth; and identifying approaches to support the support person.

Use of Role Models. Women often use role models as a guide for their expectations during childbirth. Childbirth is a new or relatively unfamiliar experience for most women. The role model's childbirth experiences thus provide a standard against which the woman measures her own birthing experiences, both in anticipating what to expect and in guiding her behavior during labor and delivery.

Family, peers, and the woman herself may provide these role models. A primigravida tends to use her own mother as her primary role model although sisters, other female relatives, and peers also serve as role models. A multigravida usually uses herself, that is, her previous childbirth experiences, as her main role model.[2]

Role models are commonly used to anticipate the length of labor, sequence of events, or how painful labor will be. Laboring women also use role models as a guide for their behavior. If they believe that a behavior is a good example, they will try to act in the same way. On the other hand, if they believe that a behavior, such as screaming, is not good, they will try to avoid it.

The woman's reaction may also be an attempt to prevent having a labor experience similar to her role model's. For instance, a role model may have delivered so quickly that she had no time to receive an epidural anesthetic she had requested. In an attempt to prevent this from happening to her a woman may request or demand that she be given an epidural before it is really needed.

Nursing Strategies. Gathering data about the laboring woman's use of role models is part of a nurse's assessment. These data help the nurse to identify actual and potential stressors that affect the mother's psychosocial and physical reactions during the intrapartum experience. Other nursing strategies include assessing the possible influence of role models on the course of the mother's labor; assessing coping methods that the mother used in previous labors; maintaining a nonjudgmental attitude toward the mother's chosen coping strategies (such as screaming); and assisting the mother to substitute more effective coping strategies for less effective ones (for example, controlled breathing for screaming).

Alterations in Body Image. Women commonly experience alterations in their body image during labor. As discussed in Chapter 4, **body image** refers to the mental picture each person has about the structure of his or her own body. Each woman begins labor with a subconscious knowledge of her body image that she uses to orient and differentiate herself as a separate being within the environment. Knowledge of her body image enables her to function actively and to be in control of herself. The borderline between body image and the environment is called the **body boundary.** This boundary consists of an obvious physically visible outer layer of skin, hair, and nails and the immediate area around the body, sometimes called **personal space.**[2] The actual distance this space encompasses varies because it expands and contracts depending on the situation. The body boundary serves to protect the woman physically and in a psychosocial sense. Many threats or actual invasions of the body boundary occur during labor, resulting in alterations of the body image.

Invasion of the body boundary often occurs during the implementation of caregiving procedures, such as performing a vaginal examination, inserting needles or catheters, applying monitoring devices, rubbing a back, and other tactile actions. When a threatened or actual invasion of the body boundary occurs, a woman tends to use defensive actions in an attempt to prevent the invasion. In some instances, she may try to move away from or repel an approaching invasive object. The sight of a needle may result in sudden pulling away of the approached body part. The client may resist the attempt to insert a catheter or to conduct a vaginal examination by bringing the knees tightly together, pushing the body upward toward the head of the bed to elude the approaching invasive object, or using the hands to repel the approaching object. A woman may hold up a hand in front of her abdomen to prevent being touched during a uterine contraction. In some instances a woman will grasp the hand of another when it is placed on her abdomen, and seek to remove it.[3] The client also may cover or constrict a body part to prevent invasion. Usually these reflexive defense reactions cease once the body boundary has been penetrated (for example, once the vaginal examination is performed).[2] Some women, however, are unable to end the defense reaction until the invasive procedure is over, causing the procedure to be uncomfortable or even painful.

A sense of loss of a definite, defined body boundary, called body boundary diffusion, sometimes occurs in response to experienced pain or to altered levels of awareness resulting from medication or falling asleep. Pain seems to spread and radiate so that an aching body part feels several times bigger than usual. Radiation of pain results in the body boundary around the aching part becoming less defined and more diffuse. When this happens during labor, a client may experience a diminished ability to determine her body boundary. Contact of the painful part by her hands, objects, or others helps the laboring woman to localize the pain and restore the body boundary. A woman may hold, press, rub, or massage a painful area to contain the pain, helping to restore the body boundary.[3]

When the nurse understands how alterations in body image affect women during labor, and why a woman reacts as she does, the nurse is better able to assist the woman in regulating nonproductive behavior. For instance, a woman may suddenly put her hand over her perineum when she feels internal stretching and pressure. If asked why, she probably will say she wants to keep the area from tearing apart or to see if it already has torn.

Nursing Strategies. Some strategies to assist the mother in coping with alterations in body image include assessing the mother's response to stimuli, such as pain; teaching the mother about the procedures that may be used during labor and delivery prior to their use; alerting the mother before touching her for a procedure; and performing nursing interventions in such a way that the mother maintains a sense of intactness.

Pain. Women universally tend to experience some degree of pain as a reaction to labor (Figure 26–1). Each woman's experience of pain is subjective and unique, ranging in intensity from mild to severe. As labor progresses, pain and discomfort intensify as the uterine contractions increase in frequency, duration,

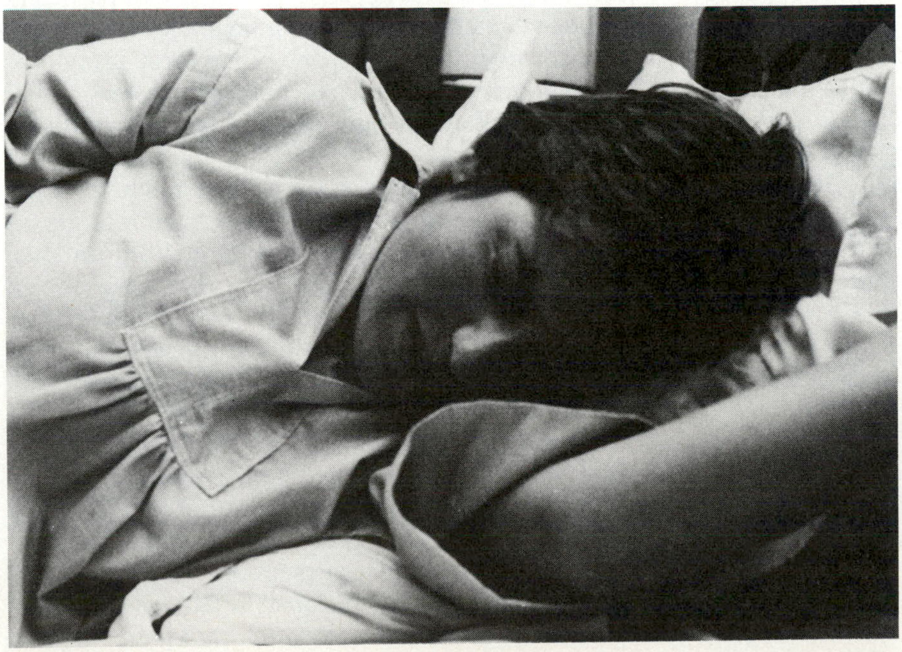

Figure 26–1. A woman reacts to pain in early labor.

and intensity.[6] Women report that the pain of childbirth is very intense despite childbirth education techniques.[7]

Factors Affecting Pain Reactions. Pain experienced during labor results from many interacting physical and social factors. The woman's parity, age, history of menstrual problems, and expectations of pain and discomfort influence her experience pain.[8] Size of the fetus, fetopelvic relationships, and physical characteristics play a role in the perception of pain and discomfort.

Cultural norms also influence the pain experienced during childbirth. Culture particularly affects the expectation and expression of pain. Some cultures emphasize the fact that labor will be extremely painful and allow free expression of pain, whereas other cultures downplay the pain experience and view expression of pain as unacceptable behavior.[9] The nurse should not overgeneralize such findings. Each person's experience of pain should be assessed as unique.

Other factors have a major impact on the pain experience during childbirth. Key factors include the presence of support persons and the relationship the woman establishes with the physician or midwife, nurses, and other health care professionals. The reports of the progression of labor pain may differ between primiparas and multiparas.[10] Another factor that influences the pain a woman experiences is her attitude toward childbirth, that is, whether she views childbirth as a normal process or as an illness during which her role is to act sick.

Childbirth pain results in many reactions that often occur even though the experience of pain varies from woman to woman. The following discussion of the more commonly occurring pain reactions includes only the psychosocial reactions. One should remember that pain responses include many physiologic reactions as well. Together these psychosocial and physiologic pain reactions contribute important information about the labor process. This information provides clues about the progress of normal labor and also serves to alert the health care team when something is not right (*see* Chapter 27).

Labor pain, as many other types of pain, is "whatever the experiencing person says it is, and exists whenever she says it does."[11] This definition does not mean that all women in labor always make clear verbal statements about their pain. It means that both verbal and nonverbal behavior contribute information about pain, whether voluntarily or involuntarily.[11] These behaviors transmit information about the presence, location, characteristics, quality, and tolerance of pain.

Verbal Expression of Pain. Verbal expression of childbirth pain ranges from no verbalization of pain to many pain verbalizations. Some women talk easily and spontaneously about their pain. Others talk about their pain only when they are asked to give information about it. Many times a woman will not or cannot express her pain with words.

Women may verbally tell others about their pain. Their reports describe the pain briefly or in detail. Usually pain reports correlate with descriptions of uterine contractions. Early labor uterine contractions are often described, with a smile, as a little one, not too bad or good. Words such as aching and cramping also are used by both primiparas and multiparas to describe the contractions of early labor.[10] As the uterine contractions intensify, the smile changes to a more serious expression and the contractions are reported as being stronger, worse, really bad, hard to deal with, unbearable, or excruciating. Words such as pressing, troublesome, or tiring are used frequently during the transitional phase of labor.[10] Other common ways of expressing pain verbally include comments about the ability to tolerate pain. Pain may also be expressed as a request for help or medication.

Nonverbal Expression of Pain. Some women only express their pain nonverbally. Nonverbal indications of pain are found in facial expression, vocalizations, body movements, and posture. The face in particular provides a readily observable indication of expressed pain; however, the face is one of the most easily controlled nonverbal means of pain expression. Other nonverbal behaviors may reveal a more accurate expression of pain.

Women frequently respond to pain with vocalizations, including various levels of moaning, groaning, crying, gasping, and screaming. Vocalizations, as well as verbal statements, vary in volume and pitch. Differences in the quality of sounds tend to reveal the intensity of the pain and the woman's ability to tolerate existing pain. Such vocalizations of pain tend to have an impact on other laboring women who can hear the vocalizations. Some women respond by expressing themselves in a similar manner. Others become frightened and worry whether they will find their own experiences to be equally as painful.

Body movements and posture express reactions to pain during childbirth. Early in labor, when most women experience the least amount of pain, they are mobile and position themselves without assistance.

As labor intensifies, overall body movement decreases. Women may cease activity when painful uterine contractions occur and then resume activity once the contraction ends. Posture also tends to change also as pain intensifies. When pain is absent or mild, the body tends to assume an open relaxed posture. As pain becomes more intense, the body is drawn and held rigid, often in a protective fetal position.

As discussed earlier, tension contributes to a cycle of anxiety, tension, and pain that escalates. Women who are able to relax instead of becoming tense when the pain becomes stronger find the pain is not as intense as when the body is rigid. Learned coping strategies as well as the use of music and imagery during labor helps to break the anxiety-tension-pain cycle.[12,13] Use of relaxation techniques, such as those taught in childbirth education classes, also helps to break this cycle. (*See* Chapter 24.)

Purposeless movements are another nonverbal means of reacting to pain. These movements tend to be rhythmic, repetitive motions that express pain and provide an outlet for increased body tension. In some instances, the motions include movement of the whole body, such as rocking or tossing and turning restlessly in bed. At other times less global movements, such as shaking a foot or rolling the head from side to side, serve as more controlled reactions to pain.

Other nonverbal reactions to pain include more purposeful activities such as rubbing, massaging, pressing, or holding a painful area. These actions can have a soothing effect. Women frequently massage, rub, or press their lower back when it hurts during labor. They also respond to discomfort resulting from fetal activity by pressing on the abdomen where the activity occurs.

At times women react reflexively to pain in an effort to protect the painful area. When a painful uterine contraction occurs, a hand or arm may be quickly used to block contact with the abdomen until the contraction ceases. This is the same type of protective reflex reaction used when procedures that are expected to be painful are to be carried out.

Nursing Strategies. The nurse should understand the varied reactions a woman can have to childbirth pain. The nurse then assesses the pain experience and to identify when intervention is needed. Knowledge of childbirth pain and the relationship of pain to the physical changes that occur during labor provides a basis for determining progress or failure to progress in labor. Understanding the many pain variations and

RESEARCH ABSTRACT

Geden E, Lower M, Beattie S, Beck N. Effects of music and imagery on physiologic and self-report of analogued labor pain. Nurs Res. *1989;38:37–40.*

The purpose of the two experimental studies was to examine the effects of music on analogued (simulated) labor pain. The first study hypothesized that subjects listening to "easy listening music" would report lower pain ratings and have less cardiovascular responses than subjects listening to "rock music" and subjects in a no-treatment control group. The sample for the first study consisted of 50 nulliparous women between the ages of 18 and 30. The subjects were randomly assigned to one of five treatment groups: easy listening music, rock music, self-selected music, a placebo group, and no-treatment control. Simulated labor pain was produced by a device that caused continuous and uniform pressure on the subject's left index finger. The subjects also were fitted with earphones according to the group assignment. Subjects reported their own pain experiences on a Likert-type scale, which ranged from 0 (no pain) to 10 (very severe pain). No statistically significant effects of type of music on self-reported pain, heart rate, or blood pressure were found, although the treatment results were in the predicted directions.

In the second study, the dependent measures (self-reported pain, heart rate, and blood pressure) were identical to those in the first study. The subjects included 50 nulliparous women between the ages of 18 and 30. The subjects were randomly assigned to one of five groups. The first group listened to the musical selection while using self-generated imagery, the second group used self-generated imagery without music, the third group listened to the musical selection while using guided imagery, the fourth group used guided imagery without music, and the fifth group was the no-treatment control group. Pain was induced in the same manner and was measured by the same instruments. No statistically significant group effects were obtained from this second study; however, the subjects in the first group reported less subjective pain when using their own imagery with music.

Comment:
This was an interesting study in its attempt to demonstrate that nonpharmacologic methods have efficacy in reducing the laboring woman's pain perception. A limitation, however, is that the simulated pain did not reproduce the pain experienced with labor contractions. Ideally the study should be replicated using women in labor, although it might not be as well controlled and a number of other variables might be introduced.

their causes also helps the nurse to accept each woman's expression of pain in a positive nonjudgmental manner and to give the support each family needs throughout the childbirth experience.

Specific nursing strategies in response to the laboring woman's expressions of pain include manipulating the environment to remove or decrease surrounding stimuli, for example, noise, heat, glare, traffic flow in the room; providing comfort measures such as position changes, backrubs, effleurage, as desired by the woman; giving appropriate medications as requested by the woman; encouraging relaxation between contractions and with contractions; using transcutaneous electrical nerve stimulation (TENS) and acupressure if requested and available (*see* Chapter 27), and teaching imagery techniques; supporting childbirth education methods or teaching breathing techniques if the couple is not prepared; and providing encouragement to the couple with regard to the progress of labor.

Control. During labor, women continually work to maintain control. They try to regulate their behavior, emotions, body functions, interpersonal relations, and ability to manipulate the environment. Frequently many stressors simultaneously affect a woman in labor. Examples of such stressors are pain, sensory overload, sleep loss, a strange environment, new role requirements, and the physiologic changes resulting from the labor process. These stressors place increasing demands on the woman's ability to maintain control.

During early labor, an observer often does not realize when a contraction occurs unless the woman mentions the contraction or the uterus is monitored for activity. When their anxiety level is not too high, women watch television, read, play cards, and interact socially during early labor. They converse in normal tones and in a normal manner. Social conversation focuses on topics related to the self and others.[14] Multigravidas sometimes review what happened during past labors.

Most women in early labor demonstrate an awareness and focus of attention that extend beyond the immediate environment. Often they are hypervigilant and attuned to what is taking place around them. Women search for information as a means to help maintain control. They seek information by asking about themselves, the baby, other people, procedures, and the environment. Information is taken in visually, as women follow all of the activity around them. Women also may share or withhold information about themselves as a means of control.[15]

Regulation of behavior further reflects the woman's attempts to maintain control during early labor. Women hold their bodies in an alert, relaxed posture and move purposefully at a normal pace both during and between contractions. When not restricted to bed, they walk without assistance, often continuing to walk throughout contractions. If in bed they change position without assistance. They also meet their own bodily needs and demonstrate concern for their physical appearance. Frequently, women who have ruptured membranes or a bloody show will request repeatedly that soiled linens be changed. Normally these women keep themselves clean and unsoiled. Their efforts to maintain themselves as they usually would reflects their functioning in a controlled manner. When uncovered for an examination or other procedure, the women may not verbally express concern for modesty, but quietly may pull their gowns or the covers back over their bodies.[3] The ability to void spontaneously reflects normal control of bodily functions. Women who receive enemas in early labor usually have no difficulty with retention of fluid, although they may express concern about this.

In early labor women make decisions readily, and most women want this responsibility. Decision making about themselves, the baby, and the care they are to receive is a vital component of control for most women. Sometimes women delegate this task to another person such as a support person or caregiver. Women tend to prefer to share rather than surrender all decision making and responsibility, and conflict may arise if control is completely taken away from them. As labor progresses, making even minor decisions, such as whether to eat an ice chip, becomes difficult.

As labor progresses to the active phase, women expend increasing amounts of energy to maintain control. Control may become tenuous and some women experience loss of control as labor intensifies. Autonomous behavior gives way to more and more dependent behavior. Awareness and focusing of attention become increasingly restricted as efforts to maintain control become more difficult. Interest in events occurring outside the room ceases and the woman withdraws, focusing attention inward. Once the active phase of labor begins, women respond to questions directed toward them, but they generally do not respond to other activity within their immediate vicinity. They continue to withdraw, turn inward, and shut out extraneous stimuli, and they respond more slowly to activities directed toward them.

As the second stage approaches, a normal tone of voice becomes interspersed with whispers or shouts. Verbalizations become more and more fragmented until only separate words are used as great effort is required to maintain control. The woman's cognitive processes are directed to the work of control and little energy remains for conversation. Topics of conversation narrow, with the laboring woman focusing mainly on the context of giving birth; she includes others only in relationship to herself.[14]

Women may ask for pain medication or anesthetics as well as other measures that will decrease their discomfort and help them maintain self-control. As labor intensifies, requests for pain medication or anesthetics become commands. They want help now! *Right now!* Some women protest that the pain is too much, saying they cannot stand it any longer. Women may even say they want to go home to get out of the hospital. Such comments reflect the woman's desire to flee, to get away from an intolerable situation, and should not be taken literally. Often when help is most needed, women will tell support persons to go away. Such a request, if taken literally, would cause much distress. Some women tell caregivers what comfort measures they want done, saying very specifically "Get me this!" or "Do that!" Words are limited to specific content. The woman does not have the energy to make polite requests at this time. Other women are unable to put their needs into words and actually do not know what will help. In these situations a trial-and-error approach to the use of comfort and support measures helps to identify what will be most helpful. This help should not be thought of as a "hit-or-miss" type of care. Rather, the nurse bases interventions on the woman's coping style and identified needs. In such instances all unnecessary stressors should be eliminated. Eliminating stressors such as wet or soiled bedding, high room temperature, and sensory overload helps to improve the woman's self-control. What was supportive and comforting in an earlier stage may no longer be as helpful as labor intensifies.

The woman's search for information as a means of maintaining control continues into active labor. Requests for information now tend to focus more narrowly on self, baby, and procedures. Less information is taken in with the eyes. Women begin to close their eyes between contractions, opening them at the onset of a contraction to inform others that a contraction has begun, then closing them again. At first women respond to the entrance of someone into the room or activity nearby by opening their eyes to see what is happening, afterward closing their eyes. Later in active labor the woman's eyes frequently are kept closed even when activity occurs within the room. To maintain self-control when the inner sensations and stimuli increase, the laboring woman limits sensory input from the environment.

Once active labor begins, women tend to become tense and relaxation becomes much more difficult as the contractions become stronger. Some women brace themselves, tensing their bodies with each contraction in an effort to maintain self-control.[3] Their control of body movement lessens as the contractions become stronger, often to a point where they require assistance even to turn to the side. As the time of delivery approaches, women often must be urged to move. Movement becomes difficult and they move as if their bodies have become very heavy. Control needed for purposeful movement takes considerable effort once labor intensifies.

The woman's ability to meet bodily needs and her concern about physical appearance also lessen as labor progresses. A woman's mouth tends to become dry and parched; however, oral fluids on a nearby stand often remain untouched until someone picks up the cup and gives it to the woman. Bodily secretions contribute to discomfort and the woman will express appreciation of being cleansed, but will tend not to cleanse herself or ask for changes of linen. The nurse can contribute to the woman's comfort by anticipating these needs. Women who are very much in control, on the other hand, may make frequent requests for cleansing and linen changes.

Late in labor, when control becomes difficult, requests for change of linen or cleansing of the perineum cease. Women have little energy for modesty. They do not attempt to cover their exposed bodies and may in fact cast aside the covers themselves when they feel hot. Comfort takes precedence over modesty, reflecting decreasing control of compulsive actions.

Limitation or loss of control of body function occurs frequently during active labor. Women often experience problems with elimination during advancing labor. They have difficulty determining whether they have an urge to void or whether the sensations they perceive are related to changes resulting from the labor process. Women report increased lower abdominal discomfort, but the discomfort often is not identified as being caused by a full bladder. Others cannot empty their bladders even when they attempt to void in the bathroom.

Nursing Strategies. Strategies for helping the mother maintain control during the labor process include assessing the mother's level of awareness and focus of attention during labor; reducing surrounding stimuli in the environment that may cause sensory overload; keeping the mother and her support person informed of the progress of labor and procedures that may be

TABLE 26–1. BEHAVIORAL CHARACTERISTICS DEMONSTRATED BY WOMEN DURING THE FIRST STAGE OF LABOR

Behavior	Latent	Active: Early	Active: Transition
Nonverbal			
General	Makes decisions readily Anxiety mild to severe Excited labor has begun Hypervigilant Functions independently Tolerates being alone for intervals of time Can be distracted—reads, plays cards, watches TV Sociable Demonstrates awareness of activities beyond immediate environment Responsive to auditory stimuli	Makes decisions slowly, may ask support person to help determine choices Anxiety level either diminishes or escalates Demonstrates dependency Desires presence of others; does not tolerate being alone very well Distraction becomes increasingly less possible Less sociable Withdraws awareness to immediate environment Responds to auditory stimuli directed toward her; may not respond to other auditory stimuli in room	Does not make or has difficulty making decisions Anxiety may be severe Increased dependency Does not want to be left alone Irritable, especially when touched Withdrawn Responds slowly to auditory stimuli directed toward her Hiccups
Response to uterine contractions	Continues previous activity May pause, cease conversation, and feel contraction Easily distracted from focus on contraction Tolerates external stimuli; usual breathing pattern Pain: generally not identified or designated as cramping located more in lower back	Anticipates onset Ceases all other activity Increasing body tension Squeezes support person's hand, siderail, pillow, and so on Implements control of breathing Pain: evidences increasing discomfort located in the pelvic area; may rub lower back, which aches	Disoriented as to onset and completion Self-control tenuous Body very tense Vicelike grasp May refuse to grasp another's hand, preferring an inanimate object May hyperventilate Pain: evidences extreme discomfort located in pelvic area; if back ached previously, now very intense; indicates sensations of internal pressure
Facial cues			
Eyes	Open Follows activities in environment Maintains eye contact when interacting with others	Begins to close eyes between contractions Opens eyes with onset of contraction then closes; looks toward activity in environment then closes May make initial contact while interacting with others, then closes eyes	Closes eyes May open eyes at onset of contraction, then close Does not visually indicate awareness of activity in environment Closed, no contact when interacting with others
Expression	Generally smiles spontaneously Facial muscles relaxed May demonstrate anticipation, excitement, or fear	A forced smile, if any Facial muscles may be tense Takes on a serious demeanor May reflect pain	Grimace Facial muscles fixed and tense May clench teeth Serious May reflect pain Worried or startled expression
Posture	Alert Generally relaxed body	Body tension noticeable Flexes or extends extremities depending on position	Body tension very noticeable, difficulty relaxing Increasing flexion of extremities depending on position May brace body

TABLE 26–1. BEHAVIORAL CHARACTERISTICS DEMONSTRATED DURING FIRST STAGE LABOR *(continued)*

Behavior	Latent	Active: Early	Active: Transition
Movement	Purposeful Normal pace Moves during and between contractions Able to control body movement Alters position without assistance	Purposeful or aimless More slowly paced Moves between contractions Less sense of control of body movement May utilize help to move Reflects a feeling of body heaviness Restlessness may begin	Purposeful motion may occur Very slowly paced Moves between contractions with encouragement Minimal sense of control of body movement When necessary to move, usually needs help and considerable urging Reflects a feeling of extreme body heaviness Movement appears to take much effort Marked restlessness may be noted
Verbal			
Quantity	Very verbal Complete sentences Elaborate	May talk between, not during, contractions Less, more fragmented, partial sentences Less elaboration	Speaks only to impart messages Short fragments of sentences Separate words No elaboration
Quality	Normal tone Distance appropriate Normal pace or very rapid	Quiet, subdued tone Not distance appropriate Normal pace	Some normal tones Whispers, shouts Not distance appropriate
Content	Seeks information about self, baby, others, environment, procedures Discusses previous labors Shares information about self Social talk	Seeks information about self, baby, procedures Asks for help Tells what she wants done Answers questions briefly Cries out in pain, may moan or groan	Cries for help at once Commands Protests pain is too much May scream, moan, or groan May ask to go home or tell others to go away
Subject	Self Self in relation to others Others	Self Self in relation to others	Self Self in relation to others
Orientation to time			
Past	30%	20%	1%
Present	58%	72%	98% right now!
Future	12%	8%	1%

done; allowing the mother to make decisions during labor; allowing the mother to maintain privacy; limiting social interaction when the mother needs to focus attention on a contraction; and supporting the mother and support person in use of childbirth preparation techniques.

Aggression and Hostility. Aggressive and hostile behaviors occasionally occur when women experience frustration resulting from threats to self-control or an actual loss of control.[2] Generally, these threats to self-control or loss of control during labor are associated with the inability to hasten progress in labor or with a feeling that the uterine contractions are overwhelming. If she is unable to control her behavior or body functioning, a woman sometimes begins to feel incompetent, inadequate, and powerless. She may then demonstrate her powerlessness by hostile behavior, criticizing and belittling her support persons or caregivers. Nurses and other caregivers should recognize that this type of behavior is not directed at them personally.

Nursing Strategies. Strategies useful when mothers exhibit feelings of aggression and hostility include accepting the mother's behavior in a nonjudgmental manner; keeping the mother informed about the progress of labor; encouraging the mother and her support person throughout labor; helping the support person understand the mother's behavior; and explaining to the mother and her support person that the phase of transition, which is when feelings of hostility commonly occur, is the shortest phase of labor.

In summary, women demonstrate a variety of behaviors during the first stage of labor. Table 26–1 outlines maternal behavioral characteristics during the latent and active phases of the first stage of labor. These guidelines are generalizations that prove helpful in assessing progress in labor and establishing nursing diagnoses.

Paternal Reactions

Level of Paternal Involvement. Paternal attendance and participation during childbirth have become accepted practice. An expectant father attends labor and delivery to provide support to his partner and to see his baby born. The father should be regarded as a unique human being who is sharing a challenging experience with his partner and not as merely a "coach."[16] Unlike mothers, fathers may choose how involved they will be during this important event. As a result, their levels of participation during birth will differ. May has identified two levels of paternal participation, termed the **contemporary father** and the **traditional father.**[17] Contemporary fathers tend to be totally and actively involved; traditional fathers tend to be less involved and more passive.[17]

Contemporary fathers want to know as much as possible about what the mother experiences. These fathers usually have attended childbirth classes and demonstrate an understanding of the birth process. They usually remain calm and emotionally supportive throughout labor and seem to enjoy coaching, caregiving, and supporting the mother. These fathers want to share as much as possible so that they participate as equal partners in the experience. A few fathers identify completely with the mother, internalizing the experience. These fathers are more anxious about what is happening, and may actually experience the labor with the mother. They also tend to lose control of themselves if their efforts to help the mother fail and she has difficulty coping.[18]

The more traditional father tends to be an onlooker, an observer. These fathers are more detached, distancing themselves emotionally from the experience. They view childbirth in an objective manner. Some men may be delighted with the thought of becoming a father, but be unable to imagine themselves actually involved in the birth process. Others are naturally unemotional and matter-of-fact. They may accompany the mother during childbirth but do not become obviously involved in the event. They talk and interact with the mother while she is comfortable and needs distraction. When the mother withdraws and focuses inward, these fathers also seem to withdraw. They may read, watch television, or even sleep.[17] Other fathers in the traditional group believe childbearing is women's work. These fathers have no desire to take part in the birth experience and may wish to be elsewhere when the birth occurs. They may reluctantly accompany the mother out of a sense of duty or to please her. Very little interaction occurs between the traditional father and the mother during childbirth; however, it is important for the nurse to recognize that these fathers care and are concerned. For them, being actively involved is not a father's role.[17]

Nursing Strategies. Strategies that focus on assisting the father to maintain his desired level of involvement in labor and delivery include assessing his desired level of involvement and respecting his choices in participation; supporting his chosen level of involvement in a nonjudgmental manner; and caring for the father's needs during labor and delivery.

Supportive Actions. Fathers provide various forms of support for the laboring woman. Fathers who choose to attend the birth provide support just by their presence. Fathers frequently use touch to convey support nonverbally.[19] Fathers also provide support verbally, praising the laboring woman's efforts, coaxing and encouraging her to continue to maintain control during contractions.

Fathers do not always use the most helpful coaching techniques. Nor do they always use support measures at the most appropriate times. Although most fathers will sensitively limit conversation to the task of coping with the labor situations, at times an anxious or overly excited father fails to realize the concentration required by the laboring woman to deal with the contractions. As a result, he does not regulate his use of verbal or tactile support actions. At other times, a father may overly empathize, repeatedly saying how sorry he is or that he did not know that childbirth was such a terrible experience. Instead of helping the woman, these comments can contribute to her loss of control.

Involved fathers generally coach the woman during labor. Most often these fathers coach relaxation and breathing techniques. As labor coaches, fathers may use various methods to time contractions. If an electronic monitor is being used, fathers quickly learn to use the monitor to help their coaching.[20] If a monitor is not in use, fathers may write down the time each contraction begins. As labor progresses fathers frequently identify the contraction pattern. They recognize when a contraction is beginning and begin coaching in anticipation of the next contraction.

Nursing Strategies. Strategies designed to foster the role of the father in supporting the laboring woman include avoiding competition with the father in supporting the mother; offering the father respite from his role as support of the laboring woman (encouraging him to take a rest break, letting him know that the nurse will stay with the mother in his absence, assuring him that someone will call him if there is a change); offering the father nourishment; praising the father's role as support person; informing the father of the progress of labor and the procedures to be performed; and making the father feel valuable as a person himself.

Control. Fathers want to be in control during the childbirth situation. Regardless of how well prepared a father is, the childbirth situation is unfamiliar and strange, especially for first-time fathers.[21] As a result fathers do not always know what is expected of them.

In Western society, fathers may act as protectors and providers for their partners. During pregnancy, however, fathers often feel excluded by their partners and by health care workers.[22] In the birth setting, the woman's responses to labor may be overwhelming, and the father may perceive that he has little control over rules and events deemed routine by caregivers. To retain control, fathers seek information through questioning and observation.

Fathers' ability to maintain control varies widely. Some fathers remain calm and relaxed throughout labor. They may be involved actively and effectively in coaching their partners. Less actively involved fathers may consciously give control of their partners' care to others. Involved fathers also may recognize a need for help and give control to others.[21]

There are times when the father loses control. Often his loss of control occurs in response to his partner's loss of control.[23] In such instances the father may persist in use of measures that are not helpful. He may be unable to change his coaching techniques, either because he does not recognize a need to or because he does not know any other technique. This type of behavior often continues until the couple receives help.

Nursing Strategies. Strategies to assist the father in maintaining control during labor and delivery include preparing the father for changes in the mother's behavior; anticipating factors such as fear that might cause the father to feel out of control; modifying surrounding stimuli such as noise, glare, traffic, and so on; informing the father of the progress of labor and explaining the procedures to be performed for the mother; and giving positive reinforcement of his participation in the labor and delivery.

Protective Actions. Fathers try to protect their partners during childbirth.[23] They act protectively to ensure the safety of both mother and baby throughout the birth process (Figure 26–2). As a protector, the father may request care for the woman's bodily needs, pain relief, and assistance with labor. As the demands of labor become all consuming, the woman may be unable to request help. The father may then communicate her wishes to the caregiver or even demand that something be done. These demands often occur in relation to requests for pain relief, perceived failure to make progress toward delivery, or perceived risk.

The father protectively seeks information and asks questions about procedures, equipment, and caregivers.[24] He seeks, through questioning, to assure himself that the best available care is being given and that what is being done will not cause any harm.

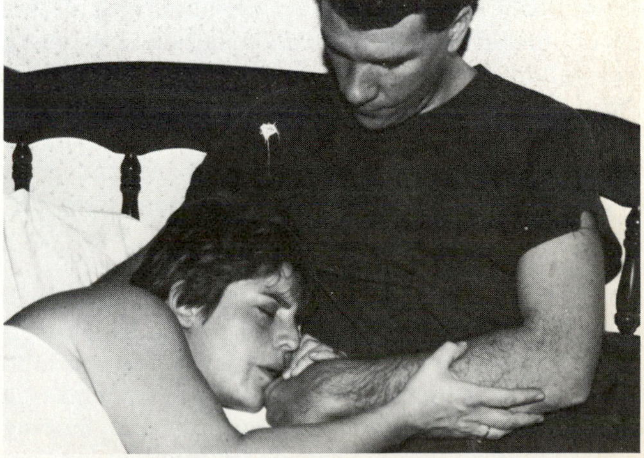

Figure 26–2. An expectant father acts protectively toward the expectant mother during labor.

He will also monitor equipment to be sure it functions as explained.

Protective reactions also include defending goals set for the labor experience prior to its onset. For example, expectant parents sometimes plan not to use analgesics or anesthetics during labor. The mother may be afraid that she may change her mind once labor begins. As a precaution she may ask the father to promise that he will not let her use medication even if she asks for it. Should labor fail to progress as expected, or if she has unbearable pain or fatigue, the woman may change her mind and ask for medication. The father, based on his promise, may then refuse to allow the medication to be given. It is important to remember in such cases that the father is not acting harshly. Caregivers need to consider his promise as well as the woman's distress. In other cases the father evaluates the situation and encourages the use of medication. This type of situation also may occur in relation to other interventions such as use of fetal monitors.

Nursing Strategies. Strategies designed to support the father's protective behaviors include nurturing the father; communicating potential maternal behavioral changes that may occur during the progress of labor; explaining procedures carefully; and respecting the coping style of the father.

Anxiety. Fathers experience a range of feelings and emotions during labor. These feelings and emotions arise as reactions both to the partner's birth experience and to the experience of becoming a father. As discussed earlier, the amount of the father's involvement also influences his emotional reactions to labor.

Fathers concerned for the well-being of their partners and babies frequently experience anxiety during labor (Figure 26–3). Anxiety occurs at all levels of intensity. Mildly anxious fathers frequently seek information as a way to manage their anxiety. Often, they are unsure and hesitant about what to do and what they are allowed to do in the unfamiliar birthing environment. These fathers respond positively to reassurance and encouragement from caregivers. They welcome instruction about what they can do to be of assistance.

As his partner's labor intensifies and she experiences distress, an anxious father may become disorganized. This is particularly true when his efforts to help seem to be ineffective. Such fathers respond well to caregivers' redirecting their activity and helping them to understand that changes in interventions are needed as labor progresses.

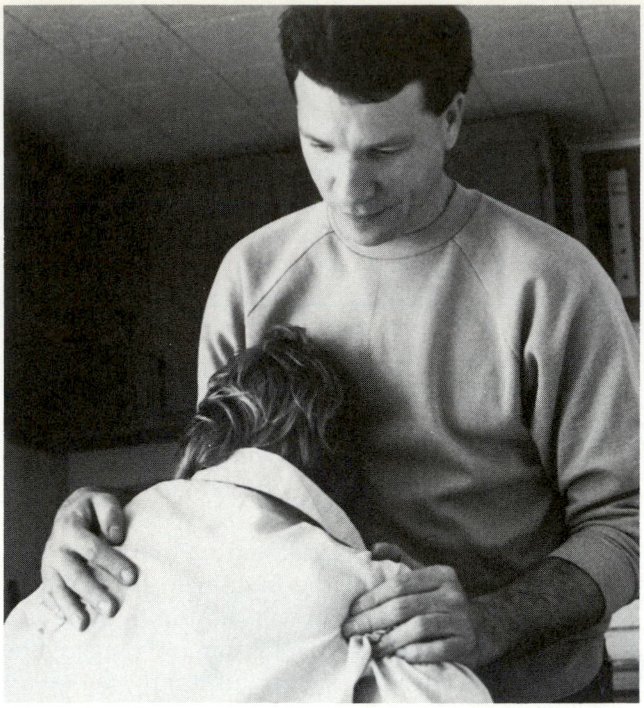

Figure 26–3. Fathers often experience anxiety during labor.

Nursing Strategies. Strategies related to the anxiety of the father during labor include assessing the father's level of anxiety; orienting the father to the labor and delivery areas; explaining procedures and the progress of labor; answering the father's questions; supporting the father in his role as support person; and maintaining a nonjudgmental attitude concerning the father's display of anxiety.

Guilt. Fathers may feel guilty when they observe their partners in acute distress, particularly if the father was the one who suggested having the baby. This feeling of guilt may be verbalized openly or expressed nonverbally, for example, by crying.

Fathers also may feel guilty because of subtle messages received from caregivers. Caregivers may inappropriately convey a value judgment about how involved the "ideal" father should be in childbirth. This judgment fails to consider the capability of each father as an individual, as well as his cultural background. As a result, a father who is not totally involved in active coaching may feel guilty and stressed. A sense of guilt can result in an unsatisfactory birth experience for the father.[17]

Nursing Strategies. Strategies for fathers who may feel guilty include assessing the cultural background of the father; assessing the father's satisfaction or dissatisfaction with any previous birth experience; allowing the father to verbalize his feelings; and being nonjudgmental about the father's chosen level of involvement in the birthing experience.

Anger and Hostility. Fathers may react with anger and hostility during labor. Generally, these strong emotions erupt when the father has done all he can to help his partner and sees few results for his efforts. The father does not know how to help and begins to feel inadequate, helpless, and powerless. If this continues, he may become frustrated and angry, striking out at others. His anger may be directed at his partner, or he may accuse the nurse and other caregivers of not helping enough.

Nursing Strategies. Strategies useful when fathers appear angry or hostile include assessing the father's reasons for anger, including feelings of helplessness; providing the father with comfort and support; maintaining a nonjudgmental attitude toward paternal behaviors; and allowing the father to verbalize his feelings.

Attention to Own Needs. Fathers often pay little attention to their own physical and emotional needs during the childbirth experience.[23] They feel that they should support their partners.[24] Many fathers choose not to take a break for rest or nourishment because they are concerned something will happen while they are away or that their partner will be upset if they go.

All fathers become fatigued without sleep or food over an extended period. Standing near the bedside or sitting in an uncomfortable chair for hours is fatiguing. Fathers may also remain in awkward positions as they give sacral pressure or hold their partners without admitting their own discomfort. Fathers also may be unaware of the effects unaccustomed sights, sounds, or odors have on them until they become nauseated or emotionally upset.

Nursing Strategies. Strategies to foster the father's attending to his own needs include providing a comfortable chair; offering nourishment; showing the father how to use proper body mechanics; minimizing surrounding stimuli in the environment, such as sights, sounds, or odors as much as possible; and reassuring the father that his responses are normal.

Pride and Self-esteem. Fathers experience a sense of pride and self-esteem when they feel they are needed and helpful during labor. A father who coaches his partner while providing her physical comfort and psychologic support has a sense of achievement during labor. He realizes he is able to help when his partner needs him and thus shares a mutually satisfying experience. Other fathers who accompany their partners but do not actively participate also experience a sense of pride. The father who may have questioned his ability to remain throughout labor experiences pride in his ability to overcome his concern and remain nearby. A sense of achievement and self-esteem results from each father giving what he is able to do successfully.[24]

Nursing Strategies. Strategies to foster paternal pride and self-esteem include providing the father with positive reinforcement for his role in supporting the mother; valuing the father as a person; and focusing on his successful supportive interventions.

Second Stage of Labor

Maternal Reactions. A sense of relief often accompanies the onset of the second stage of labor. The woman knows that the baby will be born soon and the pain and discomforts of labor will end. At this time pushing to deliver the baby is encouraged. This active form of participation also contributes to the woman's feelings of relief.

Sometimes women react to the inner sensations that occur at the onset of second stage labor with surprise or panic; especially when the changes happen suddenly. As the cervix reaches full dilation and the baby moves downward in the birth canal, sensations of extreme pressure and stretching occur. Women who are unfamiliar with what is happening may fear that they are "coming apart." If a woman is alone when this happens, she fears the baby is coming and no one will help her. The nurse can prevent this from happening by ensuring that women in active labor are never alone.

Behaviors of women in second-stage labor are uninhibited and feelings are expressed openly. Feelings of helplessness and frustration are most likely to be expressed as anger. Women also may demonstrate an apparent lack of modesty at this time. Most women become very warm when labor is intense and they may remove any covering in an attempt to cool themselves. This happens no matter who is present or where they are. In these situations caregivers should maintain the woman's privacy by making certain curtains or doors are closed.

In the second stage, the woman becomes totally absorbed in the task of giving birth (Figure 26–4). She

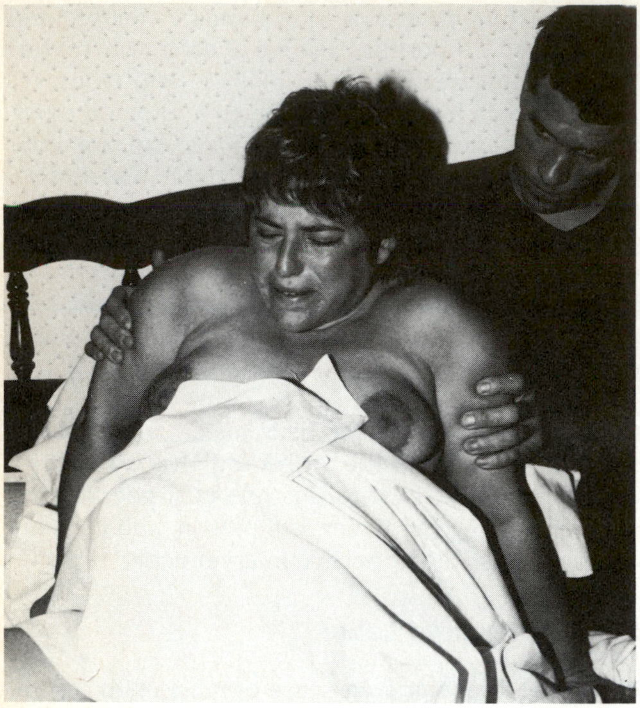

Figure 26–4. A woman becomes absorbed in the task of giving birth.

often withdraws between contractions, closing her eyes and appearing to be asleep[2] (Figure 26–5). Some women talk, responding to questions with single words between contractions. Some women have difficulty following even short specific commands. Therefore, the nurse should break any instructions into simple steps, allowing the woman to focus on and complete each part successfully.

Even women who adapted well early in labor may find second-stage sensations difficult. Self-control is often tenuous and the caregiver's help is needed to prevent loss of control. At this point, women usually respond when "talked through" a contraction. With each contraction constant repetition of what to do helps them to remain in control. Difficulty also is experienced in control of body movement. Assistance is needed for turning or moving; these activities require energy and concentration that overwhelm the woman.

Throughout the second stage most women focus on what is happening to themselves rather than on the baby. Completely absorbed with the expulsive effort, they may close their eyes. Many women who desire to watch the baby's birth need to be reminded and encouraged to open their eyes.

Nursing Strategies. Strategies supportive of the mother in the second stage of labor include "talking" the mother through a contraction; giving the mother simple instructions; removing distractions to the mother's concentration during pushing; assuring the mother that she will not be left alone during the second stage; allaying the mother's fears concerning body intactness; performing desired comfort measures; and informing the mother that labor is nearly over.

Paternal Reactions. Fathers tend to interact with their partners during the second stage of labor much as they did earlier. Those who coached actively continue to do so. They encourage and praise their partner's pushing efforts, doing all they can to encourage her. Less assertive fathers sometimes feel they are in the way once pushing begins and will watch from the sidelines.

In institutions where the mother is transported to a delivery room, fathers will be required to change into special attire for the delivery. The father may be separated from his partner at a point where the woman needs support and coaching. Some fathers find this a very difficult time and become angry if their partner pleads for them to stay. Other fathers may be willing to be present during labor but may wish not to be present during the birth. It is important for caregivers to support the father's choice and not cause him to feel guilty about what he is doing.

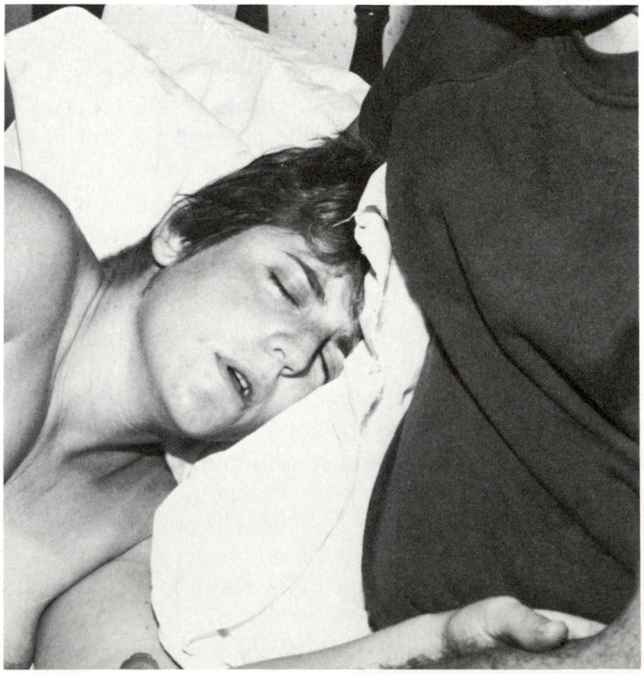

Figure 26–5. Resting between contractions.

Birth is a very emotional time for fathers as well as mothers. For some men, fatherhood becomes a reality only as the birth of the baby takes place.[22] Suddenly they realize the extent of the responsibility that fathering entails. Often tears and laughter accompany the delivery of the baby. Some fathers express their feelings openly, sharing their joy and delight with their partners. They are proud of their partners' efforts and proud to be fathers. Other fathers do not express their feelings openly. Their inner feelings may be expressed in a quick look shared with their partners. Occasionally a father may feel faint at the time of delivery, and the nurse should be alert to this possibility. As a rule, fathers who may be feeling overwhelmed tend to regulate the sights they take in by looking away. They relax visibly once assured that both mother and baby are well.

Nursing Strategies. Strategies designed to support the father during the second stage of labor include allowing the father to change into delivery room attire in ample time (if birth occurs in a hospital setting); allowing the father to choose his level of involvement; encouraging the father and praising his efforts; keeping the father informed on the progress of the birth; and allowing the father to freely express emotion.

Third and Fourth Stages of Labor

Maternal Reactions. Immediately after delivery mothers want to know if the baby is healthy and normal. The first cry, awaited in silence, is greeted with smiles and excitement. This is a very emotional time and new mothers often laugh or cry. They may reach down to touch the baby even before the cord is cut. Some mothers, fatigued after a long labor with little sleep, fall asleep after learning the baby is healthy. Others experience an emotional high; in a state of elation they are very excited and talkative. They may hug and kiss the father telling him they could not have made it through the labor without his help. They also express pride in the baby, ask questions, and exclaim over the baby's sex, size, and appearance.

In the immediate postdelivery period, most mothers want to hold the baby. Those planning to breastfeed usually want to begin at this time while the baby is awake and alert. Mothers try to make eye contact as they hold their baby[2] (Figure 26–6). The baby is wrapped in a blanket to prevent chilling and the mother explores the face and hands with her fingers. She may offer the father an opportunity to hold the baby also. She then will share her observations of the baby with the father as they both observe the baby or as she watches the father and baby interact.

In the postpartum period, women are able to recall the different phases of labor and distinguish between variations of pain.[25,26] They need to talk about the labor and should be encouraged to do so.

Nursing Strategies. Strategies related to maternal reactions in the immediate postdelivery period focus on

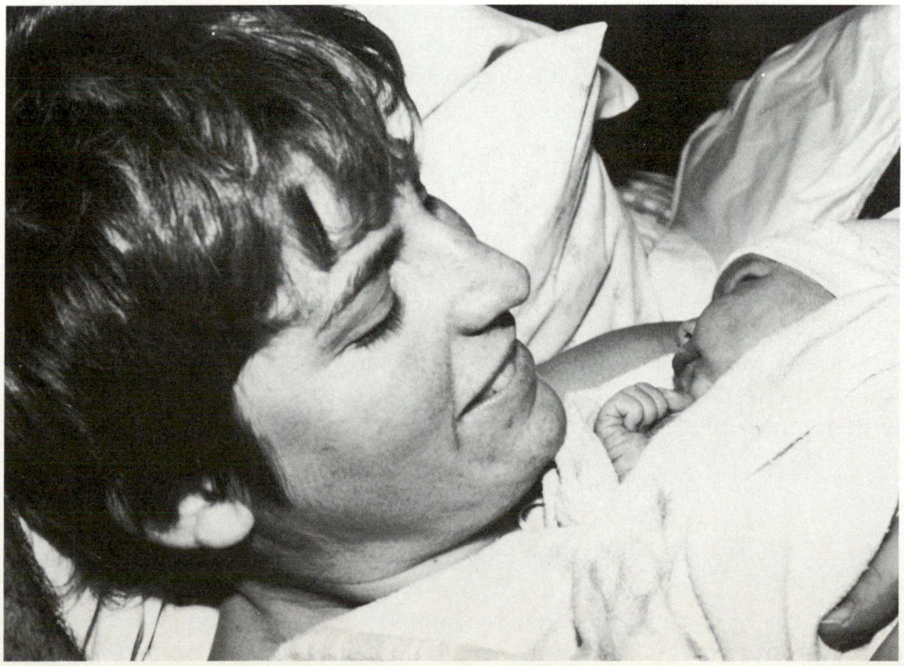

Figure 26–6. A mother makes eye contact with her baby immediately after delivery.

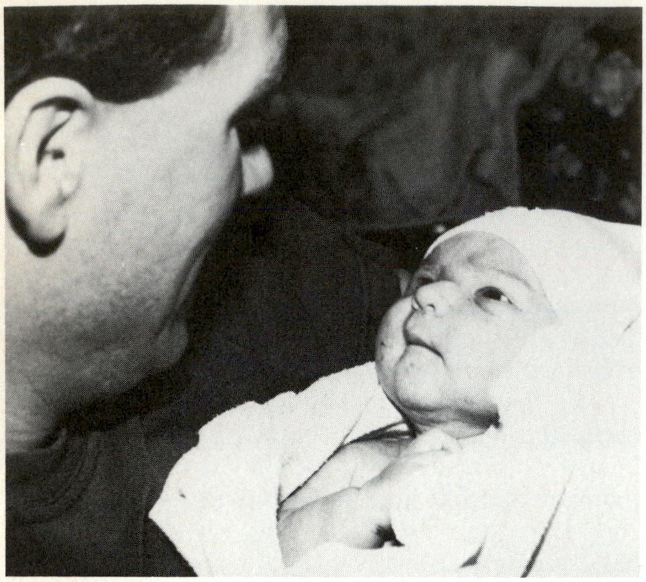

Figure 26–7. Father makes eye contact with baby.

bonding with the infant and include encouraging the mother to hold and inspect the baby; delaying routine newborn care such as eye prophylaxis until the mother and her support person have time with the baby; putting the baby to breast for those mothers who choose breastfeeding; and encouraging the new family to remain together.

Paternal Reactions. When the delivery is over the father watches the newborn and may hold the baby. Fathers will try to make eye contact with the baby while holding and talking to the baby (Figure 26–7). Fathers also share their observations about the baby with the mother. Once they are sure that mother and baby are settled, fathers will attend to their own physical needs.

Nursing Strategies. Strategies related to paternal reactions also focus on beginning bonding behaviors. Specifically, these include allowing the father to hold the baby as soon as possible after delivery; encouraging the father to support and nurture the mother as she makes the acquaintance of the baby; supporting the father as he makes the acquaintance of the baby; and encouraging the father to meet his own needs after the initial interaction period with infant and mother.

OTHER FAMILY MEMBERS' REACTIONS TO LABOR AND DELIVERY

Some expectant couples want significant others to be present for birth. Others want to share childbirth only with each other. Family members and close friends may be present at some time during childbirth. When significant others accompany the childbearing parents, the nurse needs to consider the entire group as she or he provides care.

Institutional visitation policies vary and certain restrictions may be imposed as to when and who is permitted to be present during childbirth. Siblings attend births most often in the home or in an alternative birthing center.[27] Attendance of siblings at birth is infrequent in hospital settings, although the number of hospitals allowing children to be present during birth is increasing. Hospital policies regarding the presence of grandparents during childbirth tend to be more flexible, as the term "adult significant other" is not restricted to the expectant father.

Grandparents' Reactions

A grandparent, particularly the woman's own mother, may attend childbirth. Grandparents may come to the birth experience with little knowledge of what to expect about current birthing practices.[28] Much of what they know about childbirth is based on their own experiences a generation ago. Their experiences may have occurred in a different setting and at a time when mothers were heavily sedated and delivered with a general anesthetic[29] so that they were not awake for the birth of their babies. It is likely that the grandmother experienced her labor apart from significant others, although if she and her spouse had attended childbirth education classes they may have been allowed to remain together. The father and family usually waited in a separate room and wondered what was happening. It is also possible that the grandparents' birth experiences occurred in another culture or country where birth practices differ.

Some grandparents do not understand the changes in birthing practices that now exist as a result of technology nor the choices available during childbirth. Practices that differ from what the grandparents experienced may communicate that something is wrong rather than indicating that all is progressing safely.[28] The use of electronic monitors or oxytocin and the artificial rupture of membranes often arouse distrust and suspicion. The grandparents then convey their feelings to the childbearing parents, increasing the parents' stress.

In some instances a grandparent competes with the father. Each strives to be the primary source of support. This is especially apt to happen in families in which tension already exists among the members. The nurse needs to be alert to such occurrences and help support persons and family members to work together to avoid increasing the laboring woman's stress.

Grandmothers sometimes identify strongly with the laboring woman. They may recall their own birth experiences, and relive their own discomfort and suffering as they watch the laboring woman. They may need to verbalize how they felt and what they went through. A grandmother who had a long, slow, and difficult labor may feel guilty as she watches her daughter having a similar labor. She may believe her daughter is experiencing difficulty because of something she has passed along genetically.[29] The grandmother who either identifies with the labor or feels guilty may herself be in need of support and thus be unable to provide support to the laboring woman.

Some grandparents are very supportive and nurturing toward the childbearing parents. They may provide temporary relief for the father, allowing him to meet his own personal needs. They also encourage and express pride in the childbearing parents. Their presence has a calming and stabilizing effect.

Grandparents display a wide range of emotional reactions to the childbirth experience. They may express anxiety and concern about what the laboring woman is experiencing, and concern for the welfare of the baby and father. Envy of current practices is frequently expressed by grandparents.[28] They may wish that these practices had been available when they were having babies. In contrast, some grandparents distrust the new methods and want to see the "old ways" used. Changes in childbirth practices cause them to feel insecure and uneasy.

Grandmothers, when present for the delivery, usually continue the support and coaching behaviors they used during labor. If they have never actually seen the birth of a baby, they may become caught up in watching the delivery. After the delivery, the grandparents congratulate the new parents and exclaim over the baby. Attention then turns to the newborn. Grandparents proceed to identify with the baby, much as the parents do (Figure 26–8). Knowledge of the baby's sex and weight helps them in this process. They often comment about resemblences between the baby and other family members. When possible, grandparents often want to touch or hold the baby.

Nursing Strategies. Strategies related to grandparents' experiences during childbirth depend on the level of participation that the family has chosen. If grandparents are present during the labor and delivery, specific nursing strategies include educating the grandparents about current birthing care and equipment; encouraging their support of the childbearing couple; allowing grandparents to talk about their own birthing experiences; and allowing the grandparents to be alone with the childbearing couple with and without the baby present.

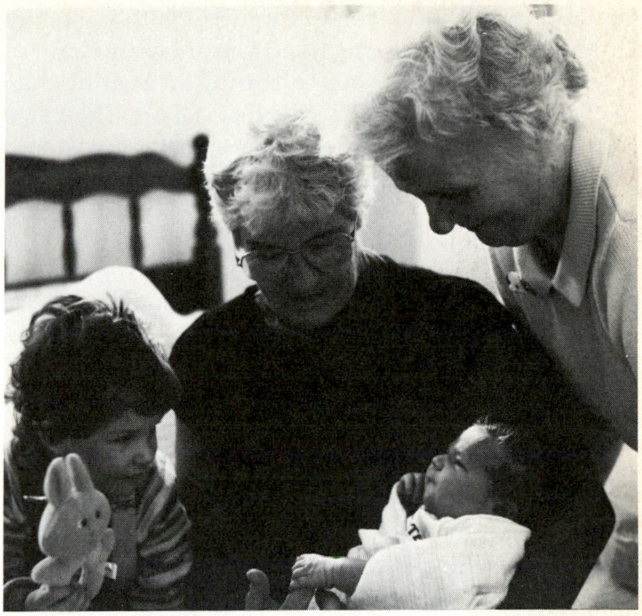

Figure 26–8. Grandmothers and sibling get acquainted with a new baby.

Siblings' Reactions

Parents sometimes wish to include their children in the birth experience. Generally, siblings who attend the birth are free to remain in the immediate birthing area or to leave whenever desired. Young children with a short attention span often come and go frequently. They play in an adjacent room or nearby in the birthing room, even on the mother's bed when allowed. In early labor the mothers sometimes play and interact with the children. As labor intensifies, some mothers continue to make an effort to interact with their children between contractions. Other

> **ISSUES AND CONTROVERSIES**
>
> Sibling presence during birth is a controversial practice in hospital settings. One issue related to sibling participation involves the wishes of the sibling. What if the sibling does not want to be present, despite the parent's desire for a family experience? What is the nurse's responsibility if the sibling becomes upset when the mother cries out or when the child sees vaginal bleeding? What are the advantages and disadvantages of sibling participation in birthing?

mothers are too involved in coping with the labor and need to be free of distraction from their children.

Siblings often act in a nurturing and caring manner toward their mothers during labor. They may wipe their mother's face with a cool cloth, give her ice chips or water, pat her arms or legs, or copy other adult actions.

Young children may become bored or tired during labor.[30] They may continue their usual routine of eating, sleeping, or playing. When delivery is imminent, they are awakened or brought back to observe the birth of the baby.

Siblings, like their parents, have varied emotional reactions. Children's reactions depend on factors such as age and stage of development. To date, however, children's reactions to sharing the birth experience are not fully understood.[31] Most siblings react to the birthing experience with their usual coping techniques. Quiet children tend to become quieter and active children more active.[32]

Frequently, children express fear and concern about their mother's expression of pain and the noises she makes during labor. Sounds related to the mother's pushing efforts are a major source of fear and concern for children.[33] Older children are more likely to ask questions at such times to determine what is happening.[34] Younger children, on the other hand, need assurance that everything is all right. They usually look to their mother for comforting when they experience such feelings. This is usually not possible at this time because she is distracted by the labor process. Children in need of comfort do not understand their mother's inaccessibility in their time of need. Parents are advised to plan to prevent such a problem by asking an adult to care for the child throughout the birth process.[35]

When the birth occurs, children usually watch very intently, positioning themselves so they can see the baby delivered.[30] Siblings may regulate how much they watch by looking away or closing their eyes. In some instances, instead of watching the birth of the baby a child may become preoccupied with the equipment or what is happening elsewhere in the room.

Sibling reactions to the birth vary. Some children watch with awe and excitement. Others become frightened and overwhelmed. Children also may feel left out as they watch from the sidelines when the adults become preoccupied with the mother and the birth.[35]

Once the baby is born the siblings usually focus their attention on the baby[36] (*see* Figure 26–8). In some instances, the sibling may need acknowledgment from the mother before shifting full attention to the baby.[35] In the period following the birth, the siblings reach out to touch the baby.[30] The children also want to hold or carry the baby. They become excited, smile, and laugh, and try to get the baby to relate to them.[35] A toy or other article may be offered as a present. Overall, siblings react positively, watching the baby intently. They will often admonish caregivers to be careful of "my baby."

Nursing Strategies. Strategies with regard to siblings' experiences during childbirth depend on the level of participation that the family has chosen and the age of the siblings. Specific strategies include supporting the sibling according to his or her developmental level; allowing the sibling(s) to come and go from the birthing site as he or she desires; providing the sibling(s) with a toy, such as a doll, so that she or he can model parents' actions with the newborn; advising parents prenatally to arrange for a support person to be available for the sibling(s) throughout labor and delivery; answering the sibling's questions and explaining the sights and sounds that accompany the birth; and allowing the sibling(s) to see and interact with the baby when she or he is ready.

RESTRUCTURING THE FAMILY SYSTEM

Birth of a baby enlarges and alters the family system. Each family member acquires a new role and status in the family at the time of the baby's birth; however, it takes weeks, even months, of effort to integrate the baby into the family system. Each family member must work to know and build a unique relationship with the new baby.[2]

Newborn as Object

At first parents tend to view the newborn as an object or possession rather than as a person, particularly in the case of a firstborn child. Each parent may view the baby as a gift to the other; for example, a mother may comment that she is happy she had a son for her husband. After birth, the baby "belongs" to the parents; thus, parents display the newborn for friends and loved ones to exclaim over and proudly accept praise of their new acquisition. It takes repeated interactions over time before the parents view the baby as a person.[2]

Identification and Claiming

Immediately after the birth family members begin working to integrate the baby into the family. Parental and family tasks include getting to know the baby and finding associations that bind family and baby together. Rubin calls these processes identification and claiming.[2]

Identification is the process of learning about the characteristics, appearance, and behaviors of the baby. It begins with learning whether the baby is healthy. The sex and size of the baby are important factors that help with identification. Once the condition, sex, and size are known, further identification of the baby includes learning about the baby's appearance and behaviors. This information is obtained primarily by looking at and touching the infant.[2]

Claiming involves the development of an awareness of a unique composite of family attributes in the baby. In this manner the baby is linked to the family by association. Claiming often begins simultaneously with identification. As each feature or behavior is identified and examined it is compared with the same attribute of another family member. Each attribute is "like" that of another person within the family system. For example, the baby has big feet "like" father, a dimple "like" mother, red hair "like" grandmother, or a pushed-in nose "like" the brother had at birth. Each association contributes to the integration of the baby into the family.

Identification and claiming usually begin as soon as the baby is born. Each family member—parent, grandparent, sibling, aunt, uncle—goes through this process of identifying and claiming the newborn. When the birth occurs in an institutional setting this process initially may be limited to looking at the baby.

Nursing Strategies. Strategies designed to foster restructuring of the family system focus on identification and claiming of the newborn by family members and include giving the family time to inspect and explore the newborn and encouraging family members to discuss the newborn's attributes and compare these with those of other family members.

CULTURAL ASPECTS OF CHILDBIRTH

Chapters 13, 17, and 21 presented the family structure of several different cultural groups. These cultural groups were chosen as examples of the varied people that a nurse will meet in the course of delivering health care to individuals and families. Although thorough discussion of many cultural groups is not the intent of this text, it is hoped that the nurse will be encouraged to develop cultural sensitivity and motivated to learn about clients' cultural backgrounds.

This chapter focuses on the Puerto Rican family, and discusses some birth practices of several other cultural groups. This section begins, however, by examining the cultural birth experience in the United States today.

Birth Experience in the United States

The birth experience in the United States has been studied in comparison to that of other countries.[37,38] Several features of the birth event are common to all birth situations, regardless of the country or cultural group, and may serve as a basis for describing childbirth in the United States. These features are the group's definition of the event, modes of preparation for the birth, the attendants and support systems present at the birth, the nature of the birth territory, the use of medication in childbirth, the technology of birth, and the nature of the decision-making process during labor and delivery.

Definition of the Event. How a society or cultural group conceptualizes birth is the best indicator of what its birthing system is like. The definition of the birth event provides participants with a shared view about the appropriate "who," "where," and "how" of birth. This societally shared definition allows participants in the birth to have a similar view regarding the course and management of events and provides a "guide" for conducting the process of birthing.[37,38]

The United States today demonstrates at least two opposing views or definitions of the birth event: on the one hand, birth is seen as a "high-tech" medical event; on the other hand, it is also seen as a highly natural event. In either case, there is currently a strong belief that the family, as a whole, should have a positive birth experience.

Preparation for Childbirth. Society prepares a woman and her family for the experience of childbirth in two ways. The first is the manner in which girls and boys are socialized into the roles of parents, and prepared for the event of pregnancy in their lives. The second concerns the knowledge that couples, once pregnant, are expected to acquire and the physical preparation they must undergo in preparation for the birth itself.[37]

Chapter 8 describes the way men and women become socialized to a sexual and reproductive role in the United States. Chapter 24 describes the manner in which families prepare themselves for the birth event. Additionally, each society transmits knowledge about birth to the woman and her family through formal and informal channels. In the United States, much information is transmitted to the family through formal channels connected to the health care delivery system (that is, clinics, physician's offices, birth centers, prepared childbirth classes). Information also comes to the family through informal channels. Often, this information has a "cultural flavor" and contributes to the variability in perceptions of different cultural groups, even when these groups have been acculturated into the dominant culture.

Information coming from these formal or informal channels may or may not help prepare the family members for the "realities" of the birth situation. For example, prepared childbirth philosophy may present an idealized picture of the birth experience. Couples who do not experience their concept of an "ideal" birth may feel guilty and disappointed, believing that they have failed. On the other hand, sometimes information received through informal channels may be so negative about the birth experience that the couple is terrified and is unable to cope with labor and delivery.[9] Information that is either too positive or too negative can be equally detrimental to the expectant couple's experience of childbirth.

Childbirth Territory. Societies also prescribe an appropriate place for giving birth. Two types of birth environments may be identified: (1) specifically designated and specialized, or (2) unspecific, within the family's normal sphere of living.[37] Thus, the woman and her support persons may go to a special-purpose facility to give birth (i.e., a hospital or birth center) or the family may experience the birth in their routine environment (i.e., their own home or other familiar setting). Currently most families in the United States prefer to give birth in specialized facilities; however, couples are electing to give birth in their homes with greater frequency. (*See* Chapter 24 for further discussion of alternative birthing environments.)

Use of Medication in Childbirth. The use of medication in labor provides an indication of how much a society sees fit to intervene in the process of childbirth. In general, medications do two things during labor and delivery: they affect the course of labor (speed it up, slow it down), or provide pain relief for the laboring woman.[37]

Medication use in the United States is fairly common, but may depend on the location of the birth, preparation of the woman and her support persons for the labor, and other techniques used to moderate the surrounding stimuli of labor (*see* Chapter 27 for further discussion). Medication use during the process of birth is still quite controversial in the United States. Many individuals feel that pharmacologic intervention is overused, whereas others believe that the benefits of medication use outweigh the risks. Couples need to understand the advantages and risks of medications and their effects during labor, and take decision-making responsibility for medication use.

Technology of Childbirth. Birth, like other events in a society, is seen as having a variety of "artifacts," equipment, and instruments necessary for managing the process in a culturally appropriate manner.[37] Birth technology in the United States is highly advanced, with new, more sophisticated equipment being constantly developed. Birthing instruments (forceps, electronic monitoring, and so on) represent the American belief in the necessity of medical intervention during the birth process; however, not all individuals in the United States today believe in the appropriateness of use of extensive birth technology. Many believe that the benefits of this technology and equipment in the United States is likely to remain a controversial issue for many years to come.

Cultural Focus: The Puerto Rican Family

The Puerto Rican family living in the United States or Puerto Rico today represents a complex cultural tradition. Although racial and cultural ancestry may be a mixture of African, Taino Indian, Corsican, and Spanish, ethnic identification is Puerto Rican.[39] Thus, families who identify their background as Puerto Rican may differ as much from each other as do members of different cultural subgroups.

Puerto Rican families also differ on the basis of the economic life in which the family participated when in Puerto Rico. Families have different characteristics, structural organizations, and even different communication patterns depending on whether they came from agrarian groups (sugar cane workers or coffee growers), middle-class groups, or upper-class groups.[39] Although Puerto Ricans cannot be viewed as one distinct cultural group, some values present in all classes and groups can be characterized as Puerto Rican.[39] These include the belief in spirituality, dignity of the individual, respect for authority, and control of aggression.

1. *Belief in spirituality.* The Puerto Rican family places an emphasis on spiritual values, and often is willing to sacrifice material goods for spiritual goods. Family members live in the present; the future and past are seen as less important in the scheme of things. Though not resigned, families accept "fate." Many Puerto Ricans are Roman Catholic. Many individuals believe in spiritualism (the belief that the visible world is surrounded by an in-

visible world inhabited by good and evil spirits who influence human behavior).[40]

2. *Dignity of the individual.* Puerto Rican family members define self-worth in terms of inner qualities that give them self-respect and earn them the respect of others.[39] This form of individualism is called "personalism." This focus on inner qualities allows a person to experience self-worth regardless of whether she or he is rich or poor.
3. *Respect for authority.* Respect is vital in the interpersonal relationships of the Puerto Rican family and plays a major role in maintaining social networks. Failure to show proper respect to a Puerto Rican male insults his manliness, his self-esteem and even his family integrity.[39] Respect is learned in the family, and extends to the outside society.
4. *Control of aggression.* The Puerto Rican individual fears losing impulse control and expressing violence. It is important for the individual to preserve an appearance of outward dignity and calm.[39]

Family Structure. The focus in Puerto Rican families is on the extended rather than the nuclear family. Relationships are often intense, and members experience a deep sense of family commitment, obligation, and responsibility.[39,41]

The Nuclear Family. Traditionally, Puerto Rican families have been patriarchal. The father's responsibility is to protect and provide for his family. *Machismo* (maleness, virility) is a desirable trait for the man to possess.

The role of the woman is to care for the home and keep the family together. She is expected to perform household tasks and childrearing (without her husband's help), and is further expected to respect him. Yet, the Puerto Rican woman can often become the "power behind the scenes" in the family system.[39]

Traditionally, Puerto Rican couples marry early and have large families. Children are valued, and parents (especially the mother) often feel obligated to sacrifice for their children. During infancy, children receive much love and attention from all adults in the family. After age 2, children are trained by their mother and grandmother.[42] Children are trained to show gratitude and respect, and are not seen as autonomous individuals by their parents. Discipline may include spanking, and parents may hesitate to reward their children's good behavior for fear that they will lose respect.[39]

The Extended Family. The extended family includes not only those individuals related by blood or marriage, but also *compadres* (godparents) and *hijos de crianza* (informally adopted children). Ritual kinship systems bind individuals together with mutual obligations for economic assistance and support.[43] Transferring children between families in time of crisis is a common practice in extended families, and is not seen as neglecting a child.[39]

The extended family is a source of strength for the nuclear family, and can provide much needed emotional and physical support. For example, female extended family members often help the Puerto Rican woman during childbearing and childrearing, as the Puerto Rican male is not expected to perform domestic tasks. Birth is a major life event for the extended family, and is joyfully celebrated by the family and community.

Emigration and the Puerto Rican Family. Many families from the island of Puerto Rico emigrate to the mainland United States seeking economic opportunity. Emigration may have several negative effects on the family. If the family lived in poverty in Puerto Rico, it is likely that they will be poor in the mainland. Further, in the mainland they are often the targets of racism.

Cultural values and attitudes are not reinforced by the dominant culture of the United States, and families may experience culture shock. For example, sex roles may be reversed, with the woman supporting the family economically. Children may learn English before their parents, thus gaining power over parents and losing respect for them. Finally, emigration to the mainland may separate the nuclear family from the extended family, increasing feelings of loss and isolation. Some Puerto Rican families thus opt to return to Puerto Rico, and movement between the island and the mainland is common.

Birth Experience. Puerto Rican women may have fears about the labor process, their ability to parent a newborn, and their change in body image. They may fear losing their partners' interest as term approaches and their bodies grow larger.[40] Pain during labor is seen as a means of achieving the goal of giving birth as soon as possible. Many Puerto Rican women do not see the necessity of the father's presence at delivery.[40] This may reflect traditional masculine and feminine roles in the Puerto Rican family.

Birthing Experience of Selected Cultural Groups

Studies concerning the reactions of families from differing cultural groups during labor are rare. The following descriptions represent selected observations of the birth experience of various cultural groups. The reader should not generalize from the limited observations presented here to all families in a cultural group. Each family, regardless of culture, should always be assessed as unique individuals.

Several clinicians and investigators[45] have observed that black women tend to remain stoic during labor, refraining from crying out and making a fuss. According to one hypothesis, this behavior stems from the early days of slavery and segregation, when it was inadvisable for blacks to call attention to themselves.[46] Some investigators feel that this factor also may account for the fact that many black women come to the delivery place in well-advanced labor.

Religion may influence the behavior of the black woman during labor, as it does so many other aspects of life.[46] If outcries are made during labor, they may reflect a strong religious foundation.[45] Praying may be one coping mechanism for the black woman in labor. In addition, the laboring black woman may call out for her mother.

Women have traditionally provided the emotional support for black women during labor and birth. A man's role was to "stand by" and do errands.[45,47] It is not unusual for black women to say that they would rather have their mother with them in the labor area than the baby's father.

Several observations concerning the behaviors of Asian-American women during birthing have been made. One author[48] reported that Chinese women are stoic in labor, rarely crying out. These Chinese women reported that they would be embarrassed to cry out and shamed in front of others. Other Asian-American women who were studied also hesitated to cry out, for fear of embarrassment.[49,50]

Although today most Chicano women deliver in hospitals, prior to 1950, many Chicano women living in the southwestern United States delivered at home with a native midwife. During that era, birth was seen as natural and not to be hastened. A birth chair often was used, and the woman was encouraged to walk until the moment of birth.[51] Such practices are very different from current practices and may produce conflicts for Chicano women who received information about birth from their mothers or other women who delivered during this period.

As the preceding descriptions illustrate, a family's cultural orientation will influence their behaviors and reactions during the intrapartum period. Much more needs to be learned, however, concerning specific cultural practices and beliefs of diverse groups so that nurses and others may give culturally sensitive care at this crucial time.

SUMMARY

During the labor and delivery process, the mother experiences many psychologic reactions along with physiologic changes. In the early phases of labor, excitement, uncertainty and anxiety dominate the woman's perceptions. The use of role models and presence of support persons during labor, add to the woman's coping abilities. The ability to cope with pain is a primary aspect of the woman's experience of labor, as is her ability to maintain control of the self and bodily processes. Body image and, in particular, invasions of a woman's body boundary, are factors in the experience of labor and delivery. The laboring woman may respond to the labor and delivery experience with aggressive and hostile behaviors.

The father also undergoes many psychologic reactions during his partner's labor and delivery experience. Unlike his partner, however, he can choose his level of involvement in the birthing. This may range from observation to high levels of involvement. Many fathers assume a supportive and protective role toward the mother and her labor. Maintaining control is important for the father, as it is for the mother. The father may feel anxiety as to the outcome of the labor process; he also may experience feelings of guilt for his part in the pregnancy and labor. He may respond with anger and hostility, often directed toward caregivers. He may become so concerned and involved in the progress of labor that he pays little attention to his own needs. The birth of a baby adds to the father's sense of pride and self esteem.

Other family members also may be involved in the birthing experience. Grandparents, if present, will need preparation, as differences between current and past birthing practices may produce anxiety or conflict. Siblings also may be present at the birth. Much thought must go into plans for preparing siblings for a positive birthing experience. Nursing support is necessary for both siblings and grandparents who participate in the birth experience.

With the birth of the infant, the family system must begin to restructure to incorporate the new family member. All family members engage in the processes of claiming and identifying the infant. The nurse can facilitate these processes by selected nursing interventions designed to support family interactions.

Cultural orientation plays an important role in the family's perception of the birth experience. This chapter concluded with a focus on the Puerto Rican family as one example of a cultural group that the nurse may encounter in practice.

REVIEW QUESTIONS

1. Describe at least five psychologic reactions of the mother during the first stage of labor.
2. Describe four psychologic responses of the father during labor and delivery.
3. Identify two reactions of siblings and grandparents to the labor and delivery process.
4. Discuss conflicts the family experiences between expectations and reality during the intrapartum period.
5. Discuss how a family's cultural orientation may affect their reactions during labor and delivery.

REFERENCES

1. Peplau H. A working definition of anxiety. In: Burd SF, Marshall MA, eds. *Some Clinical Approaches to Psychiatric Nursing.* London: Macmillan; 1963:323–327.
2. Rubin R. *Maternal Identity and the Maternal Experience.* New York: Springer Publishing Co; 1984.
3. vanMuiswinkel J. Hand behaviors of women during childbirth. *Am J Matern Child Nurs J.* 1984; 13(monograph 14):205–288.
4. Lederman R, et al. The relationship of maternal anxiety, plasma catecholamines, and plasma cortisol to progress in labor. *Am J Obstet Gynecol.* 1978;132:495–500.
5. Lederman R, et al. Anxiety and epinephrine in multiparous women in labor: relationship to duration of labor and fetal heart rate pattern. *Obstet Gynecol.* 1985;153:870.
6. Lynn N. ICEA review: pain theory and childbirth. *Int Childbirth Educ.* 1987;2:21.
7. Melzack R, et al. Labour is still painful after prepared childbirth training. *Can Med Assoc.* 1981;125:357–363.
8. Fridh G, et al. Factors associated with more intense labor pain. *Res Nurs Health.* 1988;11:117–124.
9. Morse JM, Park C. Differences in cultural expectations of parturition. In: Michaelson, ed. *Childbirth in America: Anthropological Perspectives.* South Hadley, Mass: Bergin and Garvey; 1988;121–129.
10. Gaston-Johansson F, et al. Progression of labor pain in primiparas and multiparas. *Nurs Res.* 1988;37:86–89.
11. McCaffery M. *Nursing Management of the Patient with Pain.* 2nd ed. Philadelphia: JB Lippincott; 1979.
12. Geden E, et al. Effects of cognitive and pharmacologic strategies on analogued labor pain. *Nurs Res.* 1986;35:301–306.
13. Geden E, et al. Effects of music and imagery on physiologic and self-report of analogued labor pain. *Nurs Res.* 1989;38: 37–40.
14. Rich O. Temporal and spatial experience as reflected in the verbalizations of multiparous women during labor. *Am J Matern Child Nurs.* 1973;2 (monograph 2):239–325.
15. Highley B, Mercer R. Safeguarding the laboring woman's sense of control. *Am J Matern Child Nurs.* 1978;3:39–41.
16. May K. The father's role: is it time to fire the coach? *Childbirth Educ.* 1988; winter:30–35.
17. May K. The father as observer. *Am J Matern Child Nurs.* 1982;2:319–322.
18. Jackson B. *Fatherhood.* London: George Allen & Unwin; 1983.
19. Klein R, et al. A study of father and nurse support during labor. *Birth Fam J.* 1981;8:161–165.
20. Greenberg M. *The Birth of a Father.* New York: Avon; 1985.
21. MacLaughlin S. First-time father's childbirth experience. *Nurse-Midwifery.* 1980;25:17–21.
22. Jordan PL. Laboring for relevance: expectant and new fatherhood. *Nurs Res.* 1990;39:11–16.
23. Leonard L. The father's side. *Can Nurse.* 1977;Feb:6–20.
24. MacLaughlin S, Taubenheim A. A comparison of prepared and unprepared first-time father's needs during the childbirth experience. *J Nurse-Midwifery.* 1983;28:9–16.
25. Lowe NK, Roberts JE. The convergence between in-labor report and postpartum recall of parturition pain. *Res Nurs Health.* 1988;11:11–21.
26. Stolte K. A comparison of women's expectations of labor with the actual event. *Birth.* 1987;14:99–103.
27. Van Dam S. Siblings at birth: A survey and study. *Birth Fam J.* 1979;6:80–87.
28. Horn M, Manion J. Creative grandparenting. *J Obstet Gynecol Neonat Nurs.* 1985;May/June:233–236.
29. Stephany T. Supporting the mother of a patient in labor. *J Obstet Gynecol Neonat Nurs.* 1983;Sept/Oct:345–346.
30. Perez P. Nurturing children who attend the birth of a sibling. *Am J Matern Child Nurs.* 1979;4:215–217.
31. DelGiudice G. The relationship between sibling jealousy and presence at a sibling's birth. *Birth.* 1986;13:250–254.
32. Kuhn J, Kopcinski E. Siblings at birth: professional philosophy and preparation. *Health Care Women Int.* 1984;5:223–232.
33. Leonard C, et al. Preliminary observations on the behavior of children present at the birth of a sibling. *Pediatrics.* 1979; 64:949–951.
34. Mehl L, et al. Children at birth: effects and implications. *J Sex Marital Ther.* 1977;3:274–279.
35. Daniels M. The birth experience for the sibling. *Nurse-Midwifery.* 1983;28:15–22.
36. Amderberg GJ. Initial acquaintance and attachment behavior of siblings with the newborn. *J Obstet Gynecol Neonat Nurs.* 1988;17:49–52.
37. Jordan B. *Birth in Four Cultures.* 3rd ed. Montreal: Eden Press; 1983.
38. Eakin P. *The American Way of Birth.* Philadelphia: Temple Univ. Press; 1986.
39. Garcia-Preto N. Puerto Rican families. In: McGoldrick M, Pearce J, Giordano J, eds. *Ethnicity and Family Therapy.* New York: Guilford Press; 1982.
40. Sanavitis AM, Murillo-Rohde I: The Puerto Rican. In: Clark AL, ed. *Culture, Childbearing, Health Professionals.* Philadelphia: FA Davis; 1978.
41. Delgado M. Folk medicine in Puerto Rican culture. *Int Soc Work.* 1978;21:46–54.
42. Papajohn J, Spiegel J. *Transactions in Families.* San Francisco: Jossey-Bass; 1975.

43. Rodriquez CE, et al. *The Puerto Rican Struggle: Essays on Survival.* New York: Puerto Rican Migration Research Consortium; 1980.
44. Mizio E. *Puerto Rican Task Report—Project on Ethnicity.* New York: Family Service Association, 1979.
45. Carrington BW. The Afro-American. In: Clark AL, ed. *Culture, Childbearing, Health Professionals.* Philadelphia: FA Davis; 1978.
46. Boyd-Franklin N. *Black Families in Therapy.* New York: Guilford Press; 1989.
47. Flaherty MS, et al. Grandmother functions in multigenerational families: an exploratory study of black adolescent mothers and their infants. *Am J Matern Child Nurs.* 1987; 16:61.
48. Rose PA. The Chinese American. In: Clark AL, ed. *Culture, Childbearing, Health Professionals.* Philadelphia: FA Davis; 1978.
49. Stringfellow L. The Vietnamese. In: Clark AL, ed. *Culture, Childbearing, Health Professionals.* Philadelphia: FA Davis; 1978.
50. Ellis J. Southeast Asian refugees and maternity care: the Oakland experience. *Birth.* 1982;9:191.
51. Kay MA. The Mexican American. In: Clark AL, ed. *Culture, Childbearing, Health Professionals.* Philadelphia: FA Davis, 1978.

Assessment and Nursing Care of the Family During Childbirth

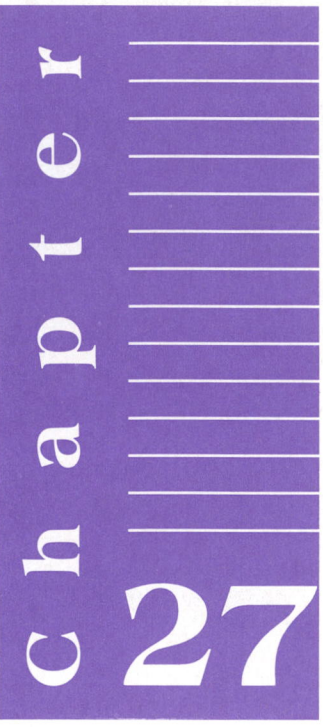

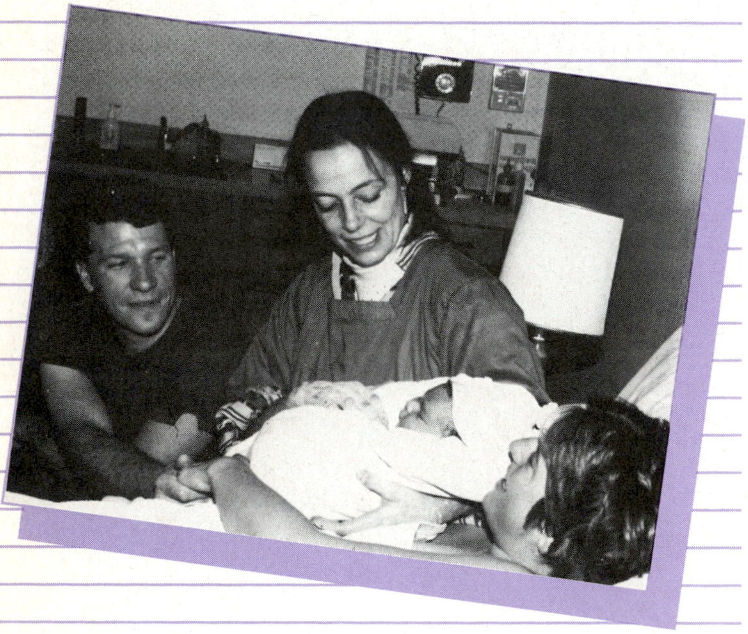

chapter 27

Key Terms

augmentation
continuous external monitoring
continuous internal monitoring
effleurage
epidural anesthesia
epidural block
episiotomy
forceps delivery
general anesthesia
induction
paracervical block
premature rupture of membranes
pudendal block
regional anesthesia
saddle block
spinal anesthesia
spinal block
spontaneous rupture of membranes
surrounding stimuli of labor
vacuum extraction

Birth is a normal physiologic and spiritual process, not a medical event. For families, it can be a joyful period in life, but it may be a positive or negative experience. For the woman, labor is a compelling experience that overtakes her body. For however many hours it takes to give birth to the child within her, the laboring woman has no choice but to give her undivided attention to the events that follow. Perinatal events not only have profound effects on the physical safety of the mother and infant, but also on the psychologic health of the mother, father, and family, and on the developing relationship between parents and the new infant.

The goal of maternity care is the safe delivery of a viable, healthy newborn to a healthy, participating mother and family. Throughout the antepartal period the efforts and concerns of the community, the health care team, the parents, and the family are devoted to this outcome. In providing care, the caregiver must also consider the culture from which the person comes and accommodate those needs as much as possible. "The touch of a caring hand is needed as well as the ultrasonic . . . probe."[1]

When nurse professionals assume the multifaceted role of manager, coordinator, advocate, and facilitator of the pivotal event of labor and delivery they also assume responsibility for the health of the family structure. Maternity nurses base care on those principles that support the adaptive strengths of the client and family and promote healthy role definition and self-concept. The intrapartum presents a unique opportunity to the nurses who nurture and support clients through crises and peak events and who are privileged to share in the miracle of each birth.

Childbearing is a significant life event, and families seek the assistance of the health care team because they believe these care providers can help them have a safe and satisfying birth experience. Health care providers must remember that birth is a natural life event, and as such, the care and services offered the family should facilitate that process. The woman and her family have the right and responsibility to plan for and participate in their birth experience. This includes prenatal education, birth plans, and informed consent regarding management.

The nurse acts as an advocate for the family, providing coordination among members of the delivery team. Nursing care during labor and delivery means one-to-one care for the woman giving birth and her support persons. The nature of the care will vary with the risk factors and strengths the woman brings to the labor, the wishes of the mother and family, the events of the labor, and where the labor and birth takes place.

THE DELIVERY TEAM

The delivery team consists of many different professionals and may vary considerably among various birth sites, institutions, and communities (Table 27–1). The nurse, as part of the team, works with each of the other members to effect the best outcome for mother, baby, and family.

ASSESSMENT OF THE WOMAN AND FETUS IN LABOR

Throughout the prenatal course, the nurse has acted as a facilitator to client care. In doing so, the focus has been on health promotion and prevention of complications, to help clients enter into labor and delivery with a high level of wellness.

Admission to the Birthing Facility

Most couples who arrive at the birthing facility for delivery are excited that the birth of their baby is imminent and anxious that everything will go well. The nurse can allay much of this anxiety by ensuring that the couple understands the events of labor and delivery and the care that will be provided. From the

TABLE 27–1. MEMBERS OF THE DELIVERY TEAM

Team Member	Role
Perinatologist/Maternal-fetal medicine obstetrician	Most medical technically prepared team member; a physician trained in the obstetric care of the high-risk woman and fetus. Usually works in a level III medical center and takes referrals from all other personnel (usually other obstetricians, family practitioners, or nurse-midwives) when the mother or fetus has had or is having considerable problems. Also may care for the low-risk woman.
Neonatologist	Pediatric physician trained in the care of sick neonates who works in a level III center, and usually receives referrals from obstetricians or perinatologists, and sometimes nurse-midwives.
General obstetrician	Physician who in this country cares for most women during their childbearing years. May work in a variety of settings, but most often at a community level I or II hospital. Can handle all normal pregnancies and most complications of pregnancy and birth. In cases of high-risk mothers or babies, will either consult with or directly refer the client to the perinatologist.
Family practitioner	Modern and more educated version of the general practitioner or family doctor. Trained to handle normal births, minor complications, normal newborns, and general family health care. May act in the same capacity as the obstetricians and pediatricians in communities in which these practitioners are not available.
Pediatrician	Physician trained in the care of children; the member of the delivery team who examines the baby after birth and cares for the normal neonate in the birthing institution and community.
Pediatric nurse practitioner (PNP)	Nurse with additional education in the care of children. Many PNPs have masters degrees and also function as nurse specialists. Affiliated with a pediatrician. May perform all the normal newborn examinations and provide care in the birthing institution or community. Like the pediatrician, cares for the normal newborn and also handles minor illnesses of childhood.
Certified nurse-midwife (CNM)	Individual educated in the two disciplines of nursing and midwifery who possesses evidence of certification according to the requirements of the American College of Nurse-Midwives.[2] Education can be at the certificate, master's, or doctoral level. More than 3000 nurse-midwives have been certified in the United States to date. In collaboration with a physician, cares for the woman during her pregnancy, birth, and postpartum and also does family planning and well-woman gynecology. May work in a variety of settings ranging from own midwifery private practice to a physician's private practice, either as a partner or employee of the physician, and in a variety of health care agencies.
Maternity clinical nurse specialist (CNS)	Registered nurse with master's level clinical specialist preparation in the care of women during the childbearing cycle. The title "clinical specialist" designates a nurse who has expertise in a defined area of knowledge and practice.[3] It is mastery of the domain of maternity nursing that allows the clinical specialist to coordinate care for childbearing clients in a variety of settings.
Maternity (OB) nurse	Registered nurse with additional formal or informal education in the care of the mother and fetus during the prenatal, intrapartum, and postpartum periods.[4] May work in a variety of settings although most work in hospitals. Role is to provide nursing care needed to give the woman and her family a safe and satisfying birth experience.

ISSUES AND CONTROVERSIES

In the light of increased malpractice litigation, many physicians use technology and interventions that may not be needed medically but will cover them in the event of a bad outcome. The reasoning is that the bad outcome occurred despite the use of available interventions; the physician, therefore, was not at fault. Although this reasoning may or may not have merit legally, it does not address the issue that each intervention carries risks and that cumulatively these risks may create problems. This, of course, does not address the larger issue that the legal tort system is not the place to resolve problems of bad outcomes and malpractice. Nor does it fairly address the problems of families who have damaged babies to care for, physicians who have to pay more than $100,000 per year in malpractice insurance, nurse-midwives who have had difficulty practicing because they cannot get malpractice insurance despite an excellent outcome record and few suits, and the health care systems' skyrocketing medical costs, which are linked to the insurance problems.

Another area of controversy centers on the place of birth. In several of the developed countries of the world home birth is a norm; these countries also boast a much lower infant mortality rate than the United States. The difference is that the home birth is part of an integrated system of care from the beginning of the pregnancy. The United States has resisted this approach and insisted that all women should give birth in hospitals. It is interesting that in an era when diagnosis-related groups and cost containment are pushing many sick clients out of the hospital and to their homes sooner than optimal and dying clients are being cared for in hospices, maternity clients are being forced into hospitals when many would rather be at home or in a birth center. The reality is that when the woman has no medical or obstetric complications, the birth is planned as an out-of-hospital one, there is a qualified practitioner caring for the woman, and there is a good transport, physician, or hospital backup system in place, the home and birth center outcomes can be as good or better than the hospital outcomes.

outset, the childbearing couple needs to feel that the birthing facility and staff are there for them and not that they are strangers with others in control. This tone is set by the nurse who welcomes the couple into the system. Nursing assessment, which includes obtaining the health history and performing a physical examination, is done in this same empathetic manner throughout labor and delivery.

Health History

When the couple contacts the delivery team, an assessment must be made about whether the expectant mother is in labor, her risk status, and the birthing plans. The information obtained in the history helps determine who on the health team needs to be notified about this client and her progress in labor. Ideally, much information is obtained during the prenatal period. If this is not the case, the labor and delivery nurse obtains the history (*see* Figure 5–1, Chapter 5).

Demographic and Descriptive Data. The labor and delivery nurse asks the mother and her support person their names and how they would like to be addressed while in labor. Other descriptive data that are important include the age of the client (may determine risk status), ethnic and religious group, and the estimated date of confinement (EDC).

The reason for admission is stated in the client's own words and should include at least the following:

- *Contraction pattern.* Time and date of onset, frequency, duration, intensity, change of pattern.
- *Amniotic membranes (Bag of waters).* Intact or ruptured; if ruptured, color and odor of fluid, date and time the membranes ruptured, and anything unusual surrounding the event.
- *Bleeding/Bloody show.* Date, time, color, and amount; bright red bleeding, date, time and amount, circumstances, associated pain, and other associated symptoms or problems, eg, nausea, vomiting, diarrhea, pain (location).

Obstetric History. The client's obstetric history is important because it gives the nurse an idea of the client's risk status and what other personnel (eg, obstetrician, perinatologist, pediatrician, neonatologist, nurse-midwife) should be notified, and it affects the plan of care. A good prenatal record provides this information; if it is not already available, this information should be elicited quickly but completely, if possible (*see* Chapter 14).

The nurse asks the client when she had her first prenatal visit and the place and provider of prenatal care. The course of the present pregnancy is also important information. Any prenatal complications, hospitalizations, and special tests alert the nurse to potential problems during the labor and delivery period.

Information about the client's present and past

pregnancies also adds information about her risk status and helps the nurse determine which members of the delivery team need to be notified (*see* Chapter 14).

Maternal-Fetal Examination

A physical examination of the woman and fetus is performed when the mother is first seen in labor by the nurse or other professional; elements of the examination are repeated during the course of labor. In addition, other factors that affect the progress of the labor, such as the woman's psyche and cultural background, are assessed.

During labor, the changes that the mother and fetus experience are so interconnected that they cannot be considered two distinct entities. Thus, assessment and care are of the maternal-fetal dyad rather than the mother and fetus separately. The following discussion considers assessment of the mother and fetus together, as they interrelate.

The complete examination is performed once the diagnosis of true labor is made and the woman is to be admitted to the hospital or birthing center. Even if a complete physical examination has been performed during the prenatal period, another examination is often done as part of the admission procedure. This examination is usually brief, but it encompasses all of the organ systems and the mother's psychologic state as well. Several areas that are specific to the woman in labor are examined in more detail or differently during the physical examination.

Physical assessment data further includes indicators of fetal well-being, the parameters of fetal heart tones, fetal movement. fetal presentation and position, estimated fetal age, and estimated fetal weight.

Fetal Assessment

Fetal Heart Rate

Manual Assessment. Fetal heart rate (FHR) or heartbeat is an indication of fetal well-being and is taken on evaluation of labor or admission to the care of the nurse or birth setting. FHR can be obtained manually using a fetoscope or electronically using a fetal monitor.

If the nurse listens manually using a fetoscope (Figure 27–1), the timing depends on the stage of labor. In early labor, assessment every 30 minutes is acceptable; in active labor, every 15 to 20 minutes; and in second stage, every 5 minutes or after each contraction. The nurse using a fetoscope should listen to the FHR as soon as the peak of the contraction passes and the sounds are audible. The nurse counts for at least 30 seconds and notes if there are any changes in the rate, quality, or regularity.

With a Doppler device (Figure 27–2), the nurse can usually listen throughout the contraction. In addition to giving the rate, quality, and regularity, the location of the sound is also important and should be recorded in terms of quadrants of the mother's abdo-

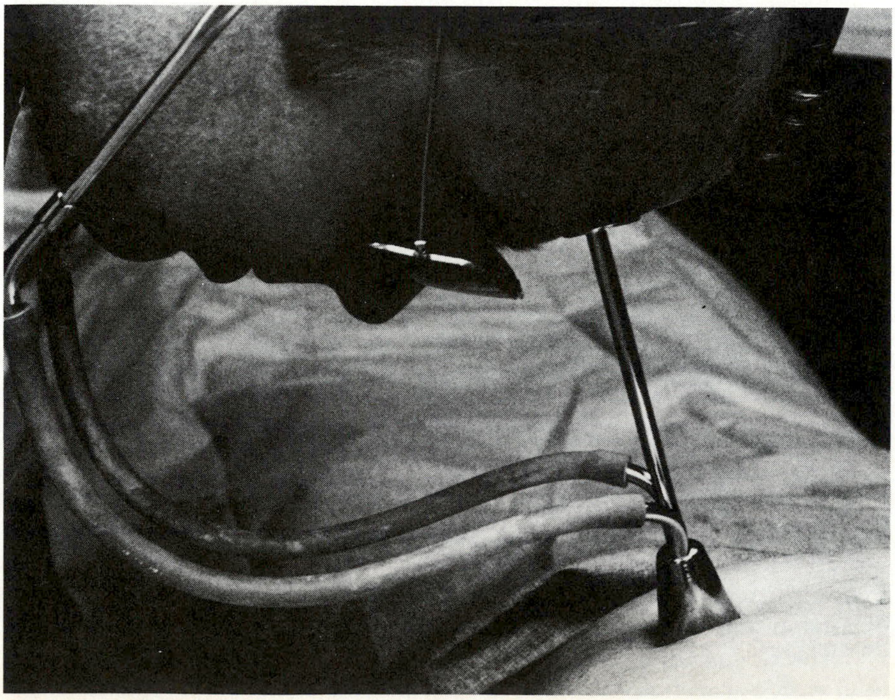

Figure 27–1. Monitoring fetal heart rate with fetoscope. (*Reproduced, with permission, from Cunningham FG, et al.* Williams Obstetrics. *18th ed. Norwalk, Conn: Appleton & Lange; 1989:311.*)

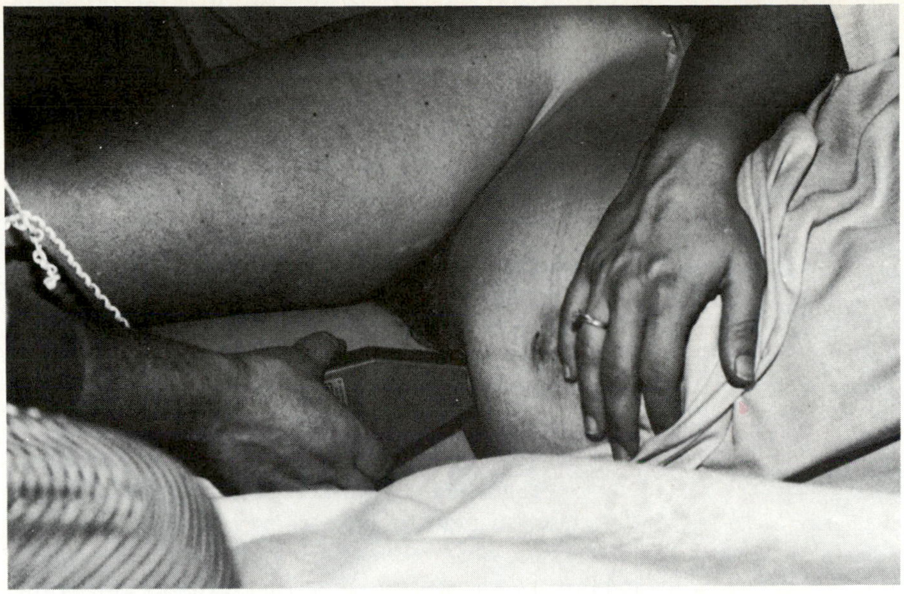

Figure 27–2. Assessing the fetal heart rate with a Doppler device during labor.

men. The nurse often uses a "+" to represent the quadrants of the abdomen and places an "×" on the spot where the fetal heart tones are the loudest. The fetal heart tones are then located under the "×" or in the opposite quadrant.

Electronic Monitoring. FHR can also be measured with the electronic fetal monitor, either externally or internally (Tables 27–2, 27–3).

The reading from the external monitor is obtained using an ultrasound transducer, which is attached to a belt that goes around the mother's abdomen and is placed where the FHR can be heard the loudest (*see* Figure 22–5). This registers a continuous recording of the FHR and any changes that may occur in response to contractions. The external reading provides a relative degree of variability but not an exact reading; only the internal fetal electrode can do that.

TABLE 27–2. PRINCIPLES FOR ASSESSMENT OF FETAL WELL-BEING THROUGH FETAL HEART MONITORING

Principle	Intervention
The FHR is an indicator of fetal well-being. Any deviation from the normal range of 120–160 beats per minute or any precipitous rise or fall within the normal range requires intervention.	Continuous electronic monitoring will be instituted at any stage of labor when the FHR deviates from normal limits or responds acutely (precipitous drop or rise) within normal limits.
The fetus of a mother who has been identified as belonging to a risk category is more likely to be hypoxic during part or all of labor than the fetus of a mother not at risk.	Careful identification of mothers as currently at risk or potentially at risk is sufficient indication for continuous monitoring of the FHR beginning with admission.
Significant shifts in the FHR may occur at any time in the cycle of contractions. Fetal heart sounds are least audible during a contraction when a stethoscope is used for auscultation.	If the decision is made to assess the FHR sporadically in low-risk labor, at least three FHR auscultations, beginning at the increment of a contraction and continuing for one full minute, should be performed sequentially.
Hypoxia resulting from cord compression occurs at the same rate in high-risk and low-risk fetuses.	Continuous FHR assessment is essential in any stage of labor when the fetal presenting part is not firmly engaged, membranes have been ruptured, or amniotomy has taken place. As the danger of cord compression, occlusion, or knotting is greater in second-stage labor, continuous FHR monitoring may be instituted in second-stage labor if first-stage labor has been monitored by other means.
The fetus of a low-risk mother may fall within a higher-risk category if assessment indicates small for gestational age (SGA), a positive oxytocin challenge test, or a nonstress test that indicates an inappropriate fetal response.	Antepartum assessment that reveals a fetus at risk indicates the necessity for continuous fetal monitoring at each stage of labor.

TABLE 27–3. COMPARISON OF VARIOUS METHODS OF FHR ASSESSMENT

Method	Benefits	Risks
Fetoscope	Easily portable, noninvasive	Sporadic auscultation may miss problems
Doppler stethoscope	Magnifies beat	Same as above
Ultrasonic transducer	Continuous record, noninvasive	Equipment may inhibit maternal movement and encourage supine position
Internal fetal scalp electrode	True fetal electrocardiogram, less inhibition of maternal movement	Dilation must be 3–4 cm, membranes ruptured, station −2 or lower, possibility of infection—maternal or fetal (sterile abcesses)

The internal electrode (Figure 27–3) is a tiny corkscrew-shaped wire that is gently screwed into the fetal scalp or presenting part and gives an exact reading of fetal heart rate variability. The fetal monitor is described in more detail under "Procedures and Treatments" under "Nursing Care During the First Stage of Labor," later in this chapter.

Fetal Movement. Fetal movement is another indicator of fetal well-being. The nurse should ask the mother when she last felt fetal movement. If, during the examination, the nurse also feels fetal movement, this should be noted. Decreased fetal movement during labor is normal, but it is not normal for the woman to have decreased fetal movement in the days before labor. One way to test for fetal movement before labor is to have the woman begin recording fetal movements at 40 weeks. One method of doing this is to have her count fetal movement for one hour, one hour after eating breakfast, lunch, or dinner. If the woman feels four or fewer movements, she should count for another hour and, if the pattern persists, should contact the nurse, physician, or nurse-midwife for further evaluation.[5,6]

Fetal Parts, Presentation, and Position. Fetal presentation, position, lie, attitude, and descent are usually determined by means of Leopold's maneuvers, uterine measurements, and vaginal examination, in that order. The nurse or other professional should not rely solely on vaginal examination, as a great deal of information can be overlooked, such as FHR, estimated length of gestation, multiple-fetus gestation, estimated fetal weight, polyhydramnios, and uterine abnormalities. The method for performing Leopold's maneuvers was described in Chapter 22 as part of the prenatal assessment. The same method is used in the intrapartum period except that it is done between contractions; the process itself may bring on contractions.

Assessment of fetal parts, presentation, and position through vaginal examination includes the following components:

- *Presenting part.* Cephalic, shoulder, limb, breech. In cephalic presentations, the following is also necessary: molding of fetal head, overriding of sutures.
- *Station.* The relationship of the lowermost presenting part of the fetus to the maternal ischial spines. It is measured in −5 to +5 cm, with 0 station meaning that the biparietal diameter of the fetal skull has cleared the inlet of the maternal pelvis and is at the level of the ischial spines (*see* Figure 25–12) (unless there is molding or caput succedaneum).[6] An unengaged head in a nullipara may indicate ceph-

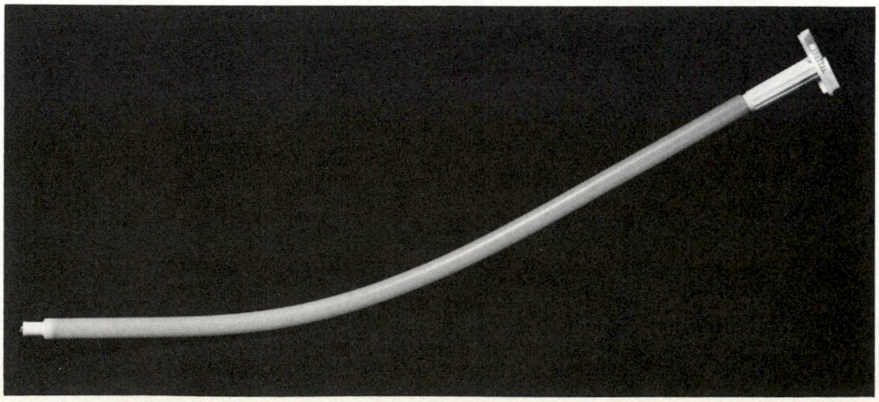

Figure 27–3. Internal probe. (*Photo courtesy of Corometrics Medical Systems, Inc., Wallingford, Conn.*)

alopelvic disproportion (CPD), or malpresentation. The higher the station at the beginning of labor, the longer the labor is likely to be. High station when the amniotic sac ruptures can be associated with prolapse of the umbilical cord.

- *Lie.* The relationship of the long axis of the maternal pelvis to the long axis of the fetus. The lie could be transverse or oblique or there might be no presenting part palpable. For delivery, the lie must be longitudinal.
- *Position.* The relationship of the fetal part (denominator)—occiput (O), frontum or forehead (Fr), mentum or chin (M), sacrum (S)—to the right (R), left (L), anterior or front (A), or posterior or back (P) of the mother's pelvis. The most common vertex positions in labor are left occiput anterior (LOA), left occiput posterior (LOP), left occiput transverse (LOT), right occiput anterior (ROA), right occiput posterior (ROP), and right occiput transverse (ROT). In the second stage of labor, the fetal head turns to the direct occiput anterior (OA, about 90 percent of births) or occiput posterior (OP, 3 percent of births). In breech births (3 percent) the positions are left sacrum anterior (LSA), left sacrum posterior (LSP), left sacrum transverse (LST), right sacrum anterior (RSA), right sacrum posterior (RSP), right sacrum transverse (RST), sacrum anterior (SA), and sacrum posterior (SP). (*See* Chapter 25 for in-depth discussion of fetal position.)

Estimated Fetal Age and Weight. Uterine measurements (*see* Chapters 16 and 20) help to determine length of gestation or fetal age and EDC, to estimate fetal weight, and to uncover twins and abnormalities of the fetus or reproductive tract of the mother. This makes Leopold's maneuvers and uterine measurements a type of maternal and fetal obstetric vital sign.

A less commonly used method of determining duration of gestation is McDonald's rule (*see* Chapter 18). Another infrequently used but useful measurement is Johnson's calculation of fetal weight (*see* Chapter 22). Using this calculation, about 50 percent of infants will be within 240 g and 70 percent within 375 g of the estimated weight.[5] The average infant in the United States weighs 7½ pounds or 3400 g. Estimated fetal age and weight are important in determining possible problems in the labor, delivery, and neonatal period.

Fetal Oxygenation. Although the assessment of fetal cardiac function has become more sophisticated, and additionally more accurate with the advent of electronic internal and external monitors, the instrumentation provides data that may be far from definitive. Variations of rate, baseline, and reactivity may be a fetal response or a characteristic of the equipment. (*See* later discussion of electronic monitoring.) When such a question arises, it is often necessary to obtain a blood sample from the fetal presenting part for pH analysis. There is always a correlation between FHR changes and pH shifts. Fetal blood is collected when membranes are ruptured, dilation is at least 3 to 4 cm, and station is −1, 0, or lower. Under sterile conditions and direct visualization through an endoscope, the clinician uses long, heparinized capillary tubes to collect a blood sample. Normal fetal scalp blood has a pH of 7.25. Fetal hypoxia and acidosis are suspected when fetal blood pH falls below 7.15 and maternal blood pH is within normal limits. Blood loss resulting from fetal sampling may be significant and difficult to control. The sampling site is frequently the site of neonatal infection. The process of sampling is therefore undertaken only to clarify a confusing or unclear FHR pattern.

Signs and Symptoms of Fetal Distress. The nurse, throughout labor, assesses the fetus for signs of distress. Signs and symptoms of fetal distress include deviations in the FHR (transient tachycardia, over 160 beats per minute, if the episode precedes a variable or late deceleration), fetal scalp blood pH below 7.15 when maternal blood pH is normal, and meconium-stained amniotic fluid with a vertex presentation (staining with a breech presentation is not considered to be ominous).

Important maternal assessment data include maternal vital signs; pattern of contractions; vaginal examination including the external genitalia, vagina, cervix (dilation, effacement), and membranes; maternal bowel patterns; maternal bladder; maternal bony pelvis, and pelvic measurements; and maternal psyche.

Maternal Assessment

Maternal Vital Signs

Blood Pressure. The maternal blood pressure (BP) is measured on evaluation of labor or admission and thereafter every hour during the active phase of labor if normal, and between contractions, never with them. The normal blood pressure range is 100 to 120 systolic and 60 to 80 diastolic. A BP above 120/88, an increase of 30 mm Hg systolic and 15 mm Hg diastolic above the prepregnancy or first-trimester blood pressure, or both may be indicative of pregnancy-induced hypertension, or other anxiety or disease states. A BP below 90/60 could be indicative of anemia or supine hypotension syndrome. If the blood pressure is abnormal, the reading should be repeated while the woman is lying on her left side. The nurse should record the pressures as well as the position of the woman when taking the blood pressure. In addition, the nurse should be careful to use the correct size cuff.

Temperature. The temperature is an important vital sign because it is an indicator of hydration and infection. The woman's temperature is taken orally on admission and every 4 hours thereafter unless the membranes are ruptured, in which case is it taken every 2 hours or more frequently. Use of electronic temperature devices are helpful as they register the temperature quickly and accurately. This can be important to the client when she is in active labor with her mouth open doing breathing exercises and contractions are frequent. An elevated temperature in labor could mean that the woman has simply not had enough fluids to compensate for the amount of work she is doing or that some infectious process is occurring. If the woman has ruptured membranes, particularly if more than 12 hours have elapsed since the membranes broke, an elevated temperature could be indicative of chorioamnionitis. This infection can be dangerous to mother and infant during the labor and postpartum period. Intervention in the form of intravenous fluids and antibiotics is often indicated. If the elevation is not alleviated by providing fluids, either orally or intravenously (IV), then the midwife or physician must be notified.

Pulse and Respirations. Pulse and respirations are reflective of anxiety, hydration, infections, temperature, and exertion of the mother during labor. They are measured between contractions, along with the temperature. There is a normal rise in pulse rate during pregnancy, but elevations in pulse above 110 beats per minute may be indicative of stress, pain, infection, hemorrhagic shock, or dehydration and should be investigated. Respirations above or below the normal of 14 to 20 beats per minute may be associated with particular types of breathing techniques or hyperventilation. A change in the oxygen-carbon dioxide exchange caused by breathing too deeply and too rapidly at the same time can lead to hyperventilation. This can be corrected by having the woman put a paper bag over her face and rebreathe the exhaled air in the bag.

Nurses should not be alarmed at more rapid respirations during contractions if the woman is using breathing patterns, like Lamaze, for coping with contractions. These techniques should not lead to hyperventilation if done properly, that is, about 30 breaths per minute or about one breath every 2 seconds at the peak of the contraction. Nurses should be familiar with the different breathing patterns used in childbirth education. These techniques are used to cope with labor, and the nurse may provide the teaching, support, and encouragement needed by the laboring woman and family (*see* Chapter 24).

Maternal Contraction Pattern. Contractions are the power of labor and one of the means used to determine the progress of labor. Measurement is usually done manually but may be done using the fetal monitor as well. In some settings, the monitor is placed on the mother on admission to the labor area and this gives the nurse similar information to a contraction stress test (CST) as well as contraction pattern information (Figure 27–4). The frequency, duration, intensity, and pattern of contractions are recorded.

Frequency of Contractions. Frequency of contractions is recorded in minutes.[7] The easiest method to remember and teach when manually recording frequency is to measure from the beginning of one contraction to the beginning of the next contraction. The nurse places her fingertips over the client's fundus and palpates the duration of the contraction from beginning to end. When using the fetal monitor, the contractions are usually measured from the peak of one contraction to the peak of the next. This peak method cannot, however, be used when recording manually.

Duration of Contractions. Duration is recorded in seconds and is measured from the beginning of the contraction until the end of that same contraction.

Intensity or Quality of Contractions. Intensity is recorded either manually or electronically. Using the manual method, the nurse places the flat of his or her fingers on the fundus of the uterus to determine if the contraction feels mild, moderate, or strong. This requires some experience on the part of the nurse before an accurate assessment can be made but the following correlation offers a good rule of thumb in evaluating the contracted uterus:

- *Mild.* Feels like the tip of the nose.
- *Moderate.* Feels like the chin.
- *Strong.* Feels like the forehead.

Electronically, the only accurate method of determining intensity is by using the internal fetal monitor via the maternal uterine catheter. This produces an exact pressure recording on the monitor strip. Some practitioners use the external monitor to measure inten-

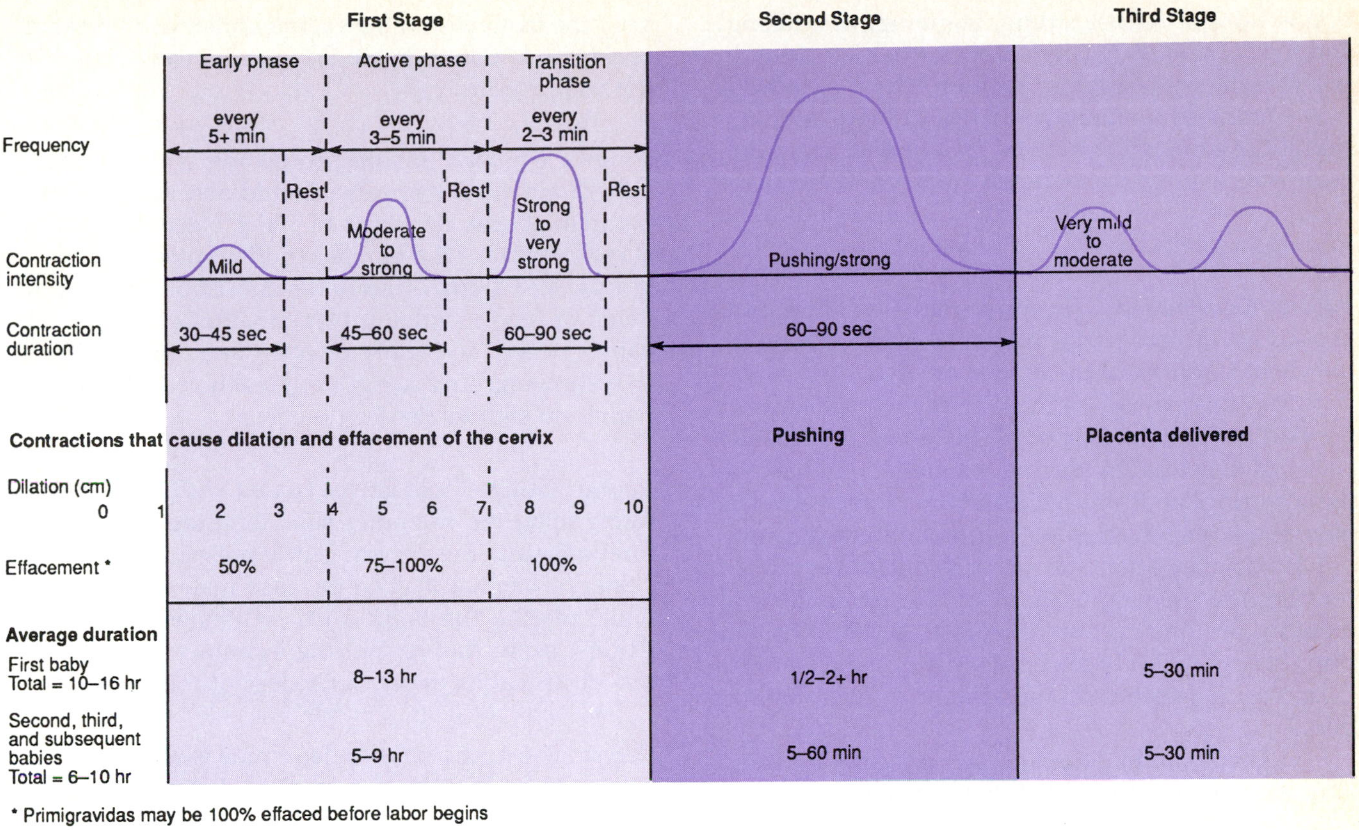

Figure 27–4. Contraction patterns in first, second, and third stages of labor.

sity. If the machine is calibrated correctly, it is possible to obtain a relative picture of intensity; that is, the nurse can determine that one contraction appears more intense than another, provided the woman does not change position or push during this period.

Pattern of Contractions. The pattern of contractions is important because it may indicate the stage of labor, whether the woman or fetus is having difficulty, and possible dysfunctional labor.

On the average, labor starts with contractions of mild intensity, 10 to 20 minutes in frequency, and 30 seconds in duration. Another way of describing the frequency is to say that the interval between contractions is 10 to 20 minutes.

As labor proceeds, the contractions become progressively more frequent, of longer duration, and stronger in intensity. The pattern may show a smooth progressive change or the labor may start off immediately with contractions 3 to 4 minutes in frequency. Another pattern is coupling, in which the woman has two or three very intense contractions, 2 minutes in frequency and about 60 seconds in duration, and then another contraction 5 minutes later, repeating this pattern.

A regular repeating pattern, no matter how irregular it may seem, is one of the factors that determines whether the woman is in true labor as opposed to false labor. The coupling (or early, extremely intense) contractions may be very difficult for the woman. They can also put the fetus under stress, causing fetal heart rate decelerations.

Other Factors Affecting Contraction Patterns. Contraction frequency, duration, and intensity may be affected by a number of other variables. These include rupture of the membranes, enemas, medication, anesthetics, change in position, and the mother's fear or anxiety. Amniotomy, or artificial rupture of the amniotic membranes, has a variable effect on contractions, sometimes arresting and sometimes accelerating labor.[8] Enemas also have no consistent effect on the quality of contractions or the length of labor.[9] Both medication and anesthetics may decrease the frequency and intensity of contractions in the early or latent phase, but regional block anesthetics may improve uncoordinated contractions in the active phase of labor.[10] The position the woman assumes during labor does affect the frequency and quality of the contractions. The most effective position is upright (either sitting, standing, or walking) and next is side lying (preferably on her left side). In the upright or side-lying position, the contractions may occur less frequently but the strength or intensity of the contraction may be greater and, therefore, more effective for the progress of labor. Women are usually more comfortable and require less medication in upright positions.[11]

Vaginal Examination. The nurse-midwife, physician, or staff nurse may perform vaginal examinations for the client throughout the course of labor. This procedure may be stressful for the laboring woman and her support person and should be done judiciously. Some of the reasons vaginal examinations may be done during labor are for determination of cervical effacement and dilation on admission and throughout labor; after spontaneous or artificial rupture of membranes; for application of the internal fetal monitor; for introduction of regional anesthesia; and prior to application of forceps by the obstetrician. (*See* Chapter 5 for further discussion of vaginal examination.)

Vaginal examinations should not be done if there is frank bleeding or when there is rupture of membranes and the woman is not in active labor. A sterile speculum examination to make an initial admission diagnosis of rupture of membranes is, however, done.

When performing or assisting with a vaginal examination, the nurse should: (1) explain to the woman and her companions why the examination is being done; (2) have the woman empty her bladder; (3) give perineal care to the perineal area; (4) help the woman place her arms alongside her body or in a comfortable relaxed position away from the examiner; (5) help her with relaxation and breathing throughout the examination; use a very gentle verbal and physical approach; (6) give explanations of what is being done throughout the procedure; (7) give a description of how it might feel; and (8) communicate the results of the examination and their meaning in terms of labor progress and management.[6]

When doing the initial vaginal examination for labor, it is important to determine if the fetus can be accommodated by the woman's pelvis. Before doing the vaginal examination, an abdominal examination consisting of Leopold's maneuvers, uterine measurements, and estimated fetal weight is done. The following is a guide to consider when doing the vaginal examination in labor. The basic procedure is the same as that outlined in Chapter 5 but in labor, other factors must be considered. When doing the examination, the nurse should follow a consistent pattern, keep the hand within the vagina until the information is obtained, and compare findings between and during contractions.

External Genitalia. Before proceeding with the internal examination, the nurse should observe the external genital area for signs of frank bleeding, bloody show, rupture of membranes (noting color and consistency), and signs of second-stage labor (passing of flatus or stool), bulging of perineum, caput (top of baby's head), and puffy or open anus or rectal mucosa showing. Any scars or other abnormalities of the perineum should also be noted.

Vagina. Using sterile gloves coated with sterile lubricating jelly, the examiner slips the index finger and forefinger into the vagina, gently pressing against the posterior vaginal wall to increase maternal comfort, while placing the hand on the abdomen. Once the fingers are in the vagina, the examiner should note any obstructions or any tenseness of the muscles.

Cervix. The next step is to determine the status of the cervix. The examiner assesses the following parameters:

- Location of the cervix. Posterior, midposition, anterior.
- Consistency of the cervix. Firm, medium, soft.
- Effacement. Thickness or thinness of the endocervical canal. Uneffaced = 2 cm long and thick, 25 percent effaced = 1.5 cm long, 50 percent effaced = 1 cm long, 75 percent effaced = 0.5 cm long, 100 percent or completely effaced = no endocervix remains, feels paper thin.
- Dilation of the cervix, 0 to 10 cm. Maximal measurement is relative, that is, however many centimeters are required to allow birth of the infant's head. *See* inside back cover. A premature infant may require less than 10 cm dilation and a very large baby somewhat more.

The nullipara will usually efface first and then start to dilate as effacement nears completion. The multipara usually dilates and effaces simultaneously. Women often enter labor already dilated about 2 cm or more, particularly if they are multiparas or have had false labor. Figure 27–5 illustrates dilation of the cervix in the primigravida.

Membranes. With the examiner's fingers in the cervix, the membranes are assessed to determine whether they are ruptured or intact. If they are intact, the examiner determines if they are tightly applied to

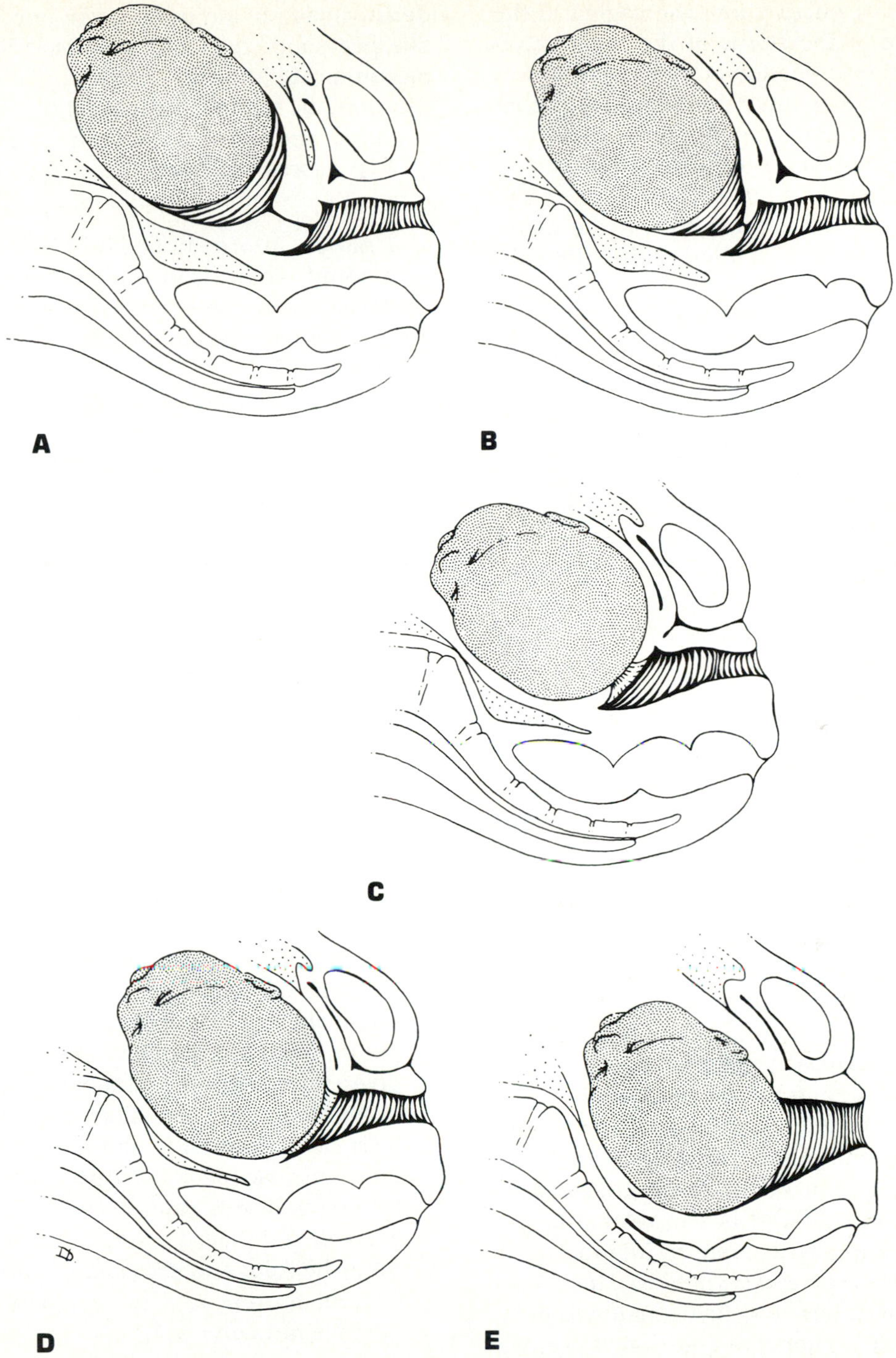

Figure 27–5. Cervical effacement and dilation of the cervix in a primigravida. **A.** Cervix thick and closed. **B.** Cervix effaced. **C.** Cervix effaced and dilated 2 to 3 cm. **D.** Cervix half open. **E.** Cervix fully dilated and retracted. (*Reproduced, with permission, from Oxorn H, ed.* Oxorn-Foote Human Labor and Birth. *5th ed. Norwalk, Conn: Appleton-Century-Crofts; 1986:119.*)

the presenting part or bulging into the vagina. If the examiner is unsure of the status of the membranes when the speculum examination is completed, she or he should observe for leaking or pooling. In addition, pH changes and ferning are noted. Sometimes there can be a leak only from the hindwaters, the part of the membranes higher up in the uterus. Further, the cervix may not be dilated enough to feel the membranes, making assessment of their status difficult. (*See* sterile speculum examination under "Examination of Membranes and Amniotic Fluid.")

The **spontaneous rupture of membranes** (SROM) results in a hole in the membranes, leading to a gush, trickle, or seepage of fluid from the vagina. **Premature rupture of membranes** (PROM) is SROM before the onset of active labor, that is, before contractions begin. Of women who have PROM at term, 80 percent go into labor within 24 hours and 95 percent within 72 hours.[12] In preterm PROM, 35 to 50 percent go into labor within 24 hours and 70 percent within 72 hours. The incidence of spontaneous rupture of membranes before the onset of contractions is 7 to 12 percent. During labor, 5 percent of women experience rupture spontaneously in early labor and 95 percent in later labor, transition, or second stage.[12,13] It is important to distinguish between PROM prior to term and PROM at term but before the onset of contractions, as the former is an ominous sign for mother and fetus.

Assessment of the membranes is important because once the uterine and fetal seal to the outside world is broken, the environment of the fetus and mother is open to the risk of infection and other complications. PROM is also associated with infection, incompetent cervix, increased maternal age and parity, trauma, manipulation of the sac, malpresentation of the fetus, prematurity, respiratory distress syndrome, floating presenting part, prolapse of the cord or limb and increased perinatal mortality and morbidity. On the other hand, PROM is also related to increasing fetal lung maturity in preterm infants.[7]

Examination of Membranes and Amniotic Fluid. The speculum part of the internal vaginal examination is not routine but is done if there is a question of vaginal infection, status of the amniotic fluid (i.e, presence of meconium), or status of the membranes.

The status of the amniotic fluid is assessed by placing a speculum or long cone-shaped device (amnioscope) in the vagina and using a light to view the membranes and fluid behind them for color, density, and particles. The normal fluid looks clear or opaque to whitish in color, with some occasional whitish particles (vernix). The presence of meconium changes the color to yellow, brown, or dark green, and the density may remain transparent or become very thick like pea soup. It is also possible to see particles of meconium floating in the fluid. This description of the amniotic fluid also applies if the membranes have ruptured and the fluid is seen on pads or clothing.

To assess whether the membranes have ruptured, the examiner should complete the following:

1. *History.* Information is obtained as to time, amount, color, and odor of fluid loss, and last sexual intercourse (loss of semen from the vagina can sometimes be mistaken for the rupture of membranes).
2. *Physical examination.* Abdominal palpation is performed to determine amniotic fluid volume.
3. *Sterile speculum examination.* Sterile gloves, nitrazine pH paper, clean glass slide, and microscope are required equipment. Wearing the sterile gloves and using a sterile speculum (using no lubricating jelly), the examiner inserts the speculum into the vagina and locates the cervix. The woman is asked to cough or bear down (while abdominally moving the fetal head up) and the examiner observes the fluid that escapes onto the lower blade of the speculum.
4. *Laboratory tests.* At the conclusion of the speculum examination, the examiner removes the speculum and tests the fluid with the nitrazine paper. A color code is used to determine any pH changes. Presence of amniotic fluid indicates a pH of 7 to 7.5 and turns the paper dark blue. Occasionally, urine will be alkaline and give a false-positive result if it gets on the nitrazine paper. The examiner must take care to avoid touching the nitrazine paper onto the cervix or any other fluids, as this will give a false reading. In a separate step, a few drops of amniotic fluid are allowed to dry undisturbed on a clean glass slide and then are examined under a microscope on low power. The presence of ferning indicates amniotic fluid. Some of the fluid is taken and placed against a white field to determine the color and presence of particles. The presence of ferning is a more reliable result than a positive nitrazine test.[6]

Bowel. Assessment of whether there is stool in the mother's bowel may be important in early labor to determine whether an enema may be helpful. An enema is contraindicated for the woman with a history of diarrhea within the last 24 hours, a presenting part below zero station, frank bleeding, or fetal distress or for the woman in advanced labor. If emptying the bowel is indicated, it can be done with a suppository, warm tap water, or normal saline enema (not a soap

RESEARCH ABSTRACT

Formato L-S. Routine prophylactic episiotomy: is it always necessary? J Nurse-Midwifery. 1985;30: 144–148.

The routine use of episiotomies was first introduced in 1918 by Pomeroy and 1920 by DeLeé. In 1980 Banta and Thacker undertook an extensive review of the literature from 1960 and found that there was no scientific evidence to support the routine use of episiotomies. Nevertheless, episiotomies continue to be performed and major textbooks continue to list their advantages but not their disadvantages.

This retrospective descriptive study involved 100 uncomplicated spontaneous vaginal births that occurred in client homes in the New York City area and were attended by the author. Routine episiotomies were not performed. Rather, delivery was gentle and controlled, with the woman in a semireclining or left lateral position, with knees and feet no more than 14 to 16 in. apart; and the nurse-midwife placed her hands so she could flex the infant's head as it emerged and support the woman's perineum. The woman pushed until just before the parietal bones of the head were born, at which time she was instructed to blow with contractions and not push.

As a result, 64 percent of the primiparous and 70 percent of the multiparous women had intact perineums. Sixteen percent of each group had first-degree lacerations not requiring repair, and 11 percent of primiparous women had first-degree tears that required repair. Nine percent of primiparous women had second-degree lacerations equivalent to small episiotomies, and 14 percent of multiparous women had second-degree tears, 50 percent of which were along previous episiotomy scars. There were no third-degree or fourth-degree lacerations.

Ninety-five infants had Apgar scores of 9 and 10 at 1 and 5 minutes. Two had Apgar scores of 7 and 9, and one infant had 1- and 5-minute Apgar scores of 4 and 9 primarily because of a tight nuchal cord. All infants and mothers were in good condition at 2 and 3 days, 2 weeks, and 6 weeks as determined by the nurse-midwife and pediatrician. The infants ranged from 5 pounds 8 oz to 9 pounds 5 oz in weight, with a median weight of 7 pounds 12 oz. The duration of the second stage of labor ranged from 7 minutes to 3 hours.

Comment:

This study demonstrates that episiotomy need not be a routine procedure at least in the hands of this nurse-midwife, in this setting, with these clients, and in terms of the outcome variables described, that is, infant outcome and maternal lacerations. Such retrospective studies generally suffer from the problem of not entirely convincing the audience and of needing other studies to confirm their results. The author recognizes this problem, however, and states "it is hoped that this study will provide impetus for further studies on infant outcome and perineal integrity." In fact, this study does not address one of the key arguments for use of routine episiotomy, namely, that episiotomy reduces the stretching of the perineal muscles that leads to problems of stress incontinence, cystoceles, and rectoceles later in life.

suds enema). If an enema is given, it should be stopped during the contractions; however, enemas are not routinely given in current practice.[7]

Bladder. On admission and periodically throughout labor, the mother's urine should be evaluated for acetone, sugar, and protein. If the woman is having symptoms of urinary tract infection (UTI), a clean-catch urine specimen for urinalysis, microscopic examination, culture, colony count, and sensitivity should be sent to the laboratory.

The bladder has limited capacity during labor so the woman needs to be encouraged to void every 2 hours. The urine should be measured and tested and results charted at each void. Retention of urine can occur because of hypotonus of the bladder, pressure of the presenting part on the bladder neck or urethra, or analgesia or regional anesthesia. If the woman is having difficulty voiding, she can be helped to void by using the bathroom or bedside commode (unless contraindicated because of sedation, anesthesia, bleeding, unengaged head and ruptured membranes, or other reasons) or other self-help or imagery techniques. Catheterization is reserved until all other measures fail and is used to permit descent of the fetus, relieve discomfort for the woman, or prevent injury to the bladder during delivery, particularly if forceps are to be used. Catheterized urine is sent to the laboratory for urine analysis and culture and sensitivity. (*See* Appendix C for Standard Laboratory Values.)

Bony Pelvis. Assessment of the bony pelvis by manual pelvimetry is important because as pregnancy progresses the musculature of the pelvis relaxes and the nurse or other professional develops a more realistic picture of the adequacy of the pelvis for delivery of the fetus. In addition, once the fetal weight is estimated, the nurse can use that determination to assess whether the pelvis can accommodate the fetus.

A pelvis that may be adequate to accommodate an average 7½-pound baby may not accommodate a 9-pound baby. If the woman has a large baby and a questionable pelvis, by size or shape, she is usually given a trial of labor but then more careful attention is paid to the progress of labor and the fetal tolerance of labor. (*See* Chapter 14 for discussion of pelvic measurement.)

On completion of the assessment, the pelvis is commonly termed either *adequate* (if, in the opinion of the examiner, passage of the fetus is possible) or *inadequate* (if the reverse is true). This terminology, although descriptive, may be misinterpreted as appearing to lay responsibility for this physiologic situation on the client. Substituting other language, for example, saying that the passage is "big enough" or "roomy" rather than "adequate," or alternatively stating that "the baby appears to be too big for the passage" rather than using the term *inadequate,* removes any inadvertent inference of blame or inadequacy from the woman. It is also important to recognize that ultimately the fetus, with inherent elastic capabilities of the movable fetal skull plates, will determine pelvic efficiency.

Psyche. The psyche is an important dimension to assess when planning care for the laboring woman and her support person(s). Research with women in labor or anticipating labor indicates that body image, value of self as indicated by assertiveness, and tolerance of self are indicators that yield important data[14] that may have an effect on labor progress. The ability to trust—both the efficiency of her own body and the abilities of the caregivers—is another indication of the client's psyche. The mind-body continuum is nowhere more evident than during labor and delivery.

Maintenance and support of the psyche require a variety of nursing strategies:

1. *Concrete definition of the role of the woman and her partner.* If the couple has undertaken childbirth education prior to labor, a beginning knowledge has been established and can be developed. Without prior education, the entire sequence must be taught on admission. It is necessary to explain not only current procedures ("This is an instrument to measure and record your contractions. It works like this") but to describe the sequence of events to follow ("Each time a contraction is traced we can count the time elapsed, how far apart they are, and how labor is progressing. They will become stronger and closer together as the baby is closer to being born"). A description of expected behaviors related to the process helps the woman to maintain her image as a competent person: for example, "You can change position in any way that makes you comfortable. We will adjust the monitor to you."
2. *Consistent positive feedback.* Efforts of the mother and family members must be recognized and supported. Positive reinforcement of healthy coping behaviors and gentle redirection of responses that are counterproductive send the message that the client and her support persons are valued and that their efforts are those of competent individuals.
3. *Establishment of a trusting relationship with caregivers.* When needs, both present and anticipated, are answered promptly the client and family members quickly learn to trust that those who care for them are capable and caring. It may not always be possible or desirable to meet a need instantly but it is usually possible to give the client or family members a time frame and a reason for a delay or denial. If a pain medication cannot be administered for another hour, a short explanation of why, coupled with institution of alternate comfort measures, recognizes both the validity of the request and the availability of other measures from a caregiver willing to use them.

Psychosocial dimensions of labor and delivery are discussed in depth in Chapter 26.

Cultural Influences. Culture also influences the process of labor and delivery, and may be considered a component of the mother's "psyche." The folklore of childbirth helps the nurse understand the client and family members' reactions to labor and delivery. (*See* Chapter 26 for fuller discussion of cultural responses during labor.) An important consideration for the nurse is the relationship between the birth site and the culture of the laboring family. The nurse must realize that the very familiarity that allows him or her to function smoothly may be frightening to the client and family, who are not familiar with the "culture" of the health care institution.

SURROUNDING STIMULI OF LABOR

The term **surrounding stimuli of labor** is used rather than pain in the following discussion because many feelings that are associated with the progress of labor are not necessarily painful. In addition, some stimuli during labor may provide support for the woman. Most texts concentrate on only the pain when these other factors are also important and the interventions that help them often decreases the pain as well.[15]

It is important to note that not all women experience labor as painful. The degree of discomfort associated with labor can be represented on a bell-shaped curve. Some women are at the left end of the curve; they experience no pain and do not even recognize that they are in labor until the birth is imminent. Most women are near the top of the curve; but a few women experience labor at the extreme right of the curve, as excruciatingly painful. These women are often in obstructed or dysfunctional labor over many hours. Some women are so fearful of the labor process that all feelings are interpreted as extremely painful. In addition, as the labor progresses and the hours pass, most women find it more difficult to cope, because this is when the stimuli increase and fatigue makes it more difficult to help oneself.

Again, using the concept of the bell-shaped curve, some women have labors of less than an hour whereas others may labor 48 hours or longer. The average length of labor for a primigravida is around 14 to 16 hours; this may be difficult enough but for the woman at the extreme end of the labor curve, the lack of sleep and the attention necessary to cope with the forces of labor make this the most demanding work a woman must do. The only person who might come close to appreciating this work is the coach who stays and works with her through the entire process. Labor is like no other work a woman will ever do in her life. There are no coffee breaks, no "I'm tired and want to stop" breaks; it simply continues until the birth of the infant, however long and difficult or wonderful that may be.

Given this background, surrounding stimuli fall into several categories, namely, the environment; presence or absence of support systems; maternal or fetal position in labor; fatigue; nausea, vomiting, and diarrhea; fear; and pain. Most of these surrounding stimuli tend to interact with one another, influencing aspects of the others.

The specific interventions used to help the woman and her family cope vary with the individual, the situation, the type of stimuli, the progress of labor, and many other factors. The nurse can use the following basic guidelines when trying to control or eliminate the unpleasant feelings associated with the laboring process.

Birth Place Environment

The environment in which the woman labors and gives birth is very important because it may influence the progress and experience of labor. For example, research findings have demonstrated that women who delivered in hospitals rated childbirth pain significantly higher than those who delivered at home.[16] More couples in the United States are having only one or two children, so where they have them and the overall experience become more important to them. At the least, the surroundings should be clean, safe, quiet, free from obnoxious odors, and esthetically pleasant and should permit the woman some privacy to progress physiologically and psychologically in her labor. The place or room may also have other items like music or a TV that the woman can use as additional stimuli if she so chooses. Wherever it is, the health care team should make an effort to keep the birth place as free from other distracting noises as possible. This includes staff conversations in the hall or by the nurses' station and the noise of other women in labor.

Many hospitals today have birthing suites or provide for the women and her family to labor, deliver, and recover in the same room. The philosophy of a birthing suite (whether it is in or out of the hospital) is to allow labor to progress as naturally as possible with as much freedom to the woman and family, close nursing supervision, and as little technologic intervention as possible. Women react differently to different environments but a setting that offers friendly, caring, competent, and understanding practitioners, in a clean cheery atmosphere that encourages the presence of family members, has the best possibility of allowing the woman the freedom to experience her labor in a positive manner.

Support Persons for Labor

The overall environment also includes those persons who are with the woman while she labors. The presence of support persons can make the difference in how the woman feels and copes with labor, and the presence of good nursing care makes an overall difference in the family's emotional and physical health. There is no substitute for the professional nurse who provides the expertise in a caring and thoughtful manner.

The support persons with the woman should provide comfort measures, coach with breathing patterns, act as an interpreter, and generally provide positive support. If the support person is not knowledgeable about how to help the laboring woman, the nurse can teach useful techniques while acting as a role model. The nurse must also observe the interaction between the woman and the support person. Occasionally, a support person or coach may misinterpret the needs of the laboring woman. This misinterpretation may produce conflicts between the woman and her support person. For example, a woman may wish analgesia, while her coach, adhering to earlier intentions against medications, refuses to let her have analgesia. The nurse can assist the support person in a more realistic assessment of his or her partner's current needs.

In addition, it is important for the nurse to remember that there are a wide variety of family structures. It is not always the father of the baby who will supply support to the mother. If it is not possible for more than one support person to be present during labor, it is quite feasible to change the support person for a brief period if the woman desires, for instance, to see and be comforted by a mother or sister. Recognition and respect for the family unit, whatever the structure, increases the probability that birth will be a unifying factor in the evolution of the family. The family unit should be strengthened and enriched by the birth experience. (*See* Chapter 26 for a more complete discussion of the psychological dimensions of labor and delivery.)

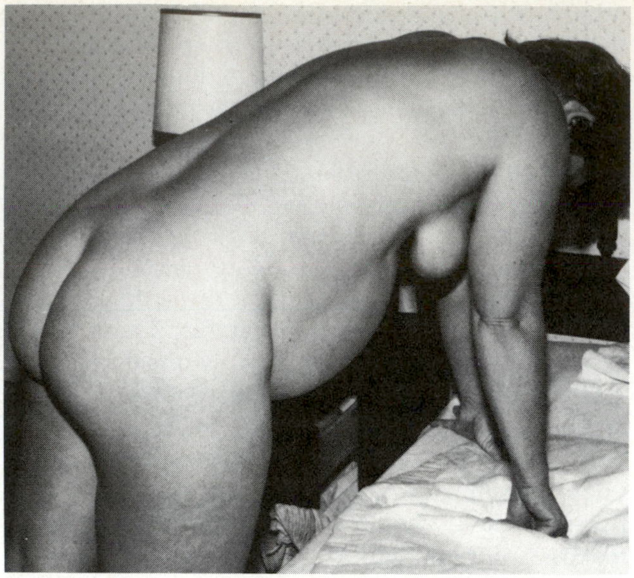

Figure 27–6. Change in position relieves discomfort in labor.

Maternal and Fetal Positions in Labor

The position the woman assumes in labor and the position of the fetus in utero will greatly affect the maternal perception of stimuli. The best maternal positions (in descending order) to assist with the first stage of labor and reduce pain are standing and walking, sitting, lying on left side, and lying on right side. Women should avoid lying on their backs, not only because it is more uncomfortable but also because it may induce the supine hypotension syndrome. This syndrome is caused by the pressure of the uterus and fetus lying on the inferior vena cava and aorta and interfering with the return of blood from the lower extremities to the heart, which also leads to lowering of the maternal blood pressure and decreased oxygen supply to the fetus.

Back pain is usually a result of the pressure of a fetus in the LOP, ROP, or OP position. In these cases, the occiput (back) of the fetal head is pressing against the mother's sacrum, which has a large nerve supply. This type of back pain can be controlled in several ways:

- Changes in position with the mother either standing (Figure 27–6), sitting, lying on the side opposite the baby's back, or kneeling on her hands and knees and being massaged from her back to front on the side of the fetal back (these last two positions encourage the fetus to rotate to the anterior position in addition to helping the immediate feelings of pain).
- Change in temperature, which can be accomplished by application of direct heat to the area with a hot pack, bath, or shower[17] or by application of direct cold to the area with an ice pack.
- Counterpressure by means of acupressure or direct firm massage with the fist or heal of the hand, a rolling pin, tennis balls, or a can filled with frozen fluid (Figure 27–7).

Many of these techniques can be performed by the nurse or other support person. Allowing the couple some privacy to interact in whatever intimate manner that feels good can also be very helpful to the laboring woman.

Fatigue

The methods used to counteract fatigue depend on the stage of labor, the health of the woman and fetus, the desires of the mother, and the need for the mother's cooperation at different stages of labor. Fatigue is caused by a number of factors, principally the number of hours with or without sleep prior to the start of labor, the amount of fluid and calories the mother consumes during the labor period, the amount of calories used for the labor process, how much the woman is able to work with the forces of labor, how much rest she is able to get during the labor process, her general conditioning and previous exercise, and how much she has learned and is able to apply from her childbirth education.

If the woman is having a long latent phase of labor or it is difficult to distinguish true from false labor and the woman has had little or no sleep recently, the obstetrician may prescribe medications,

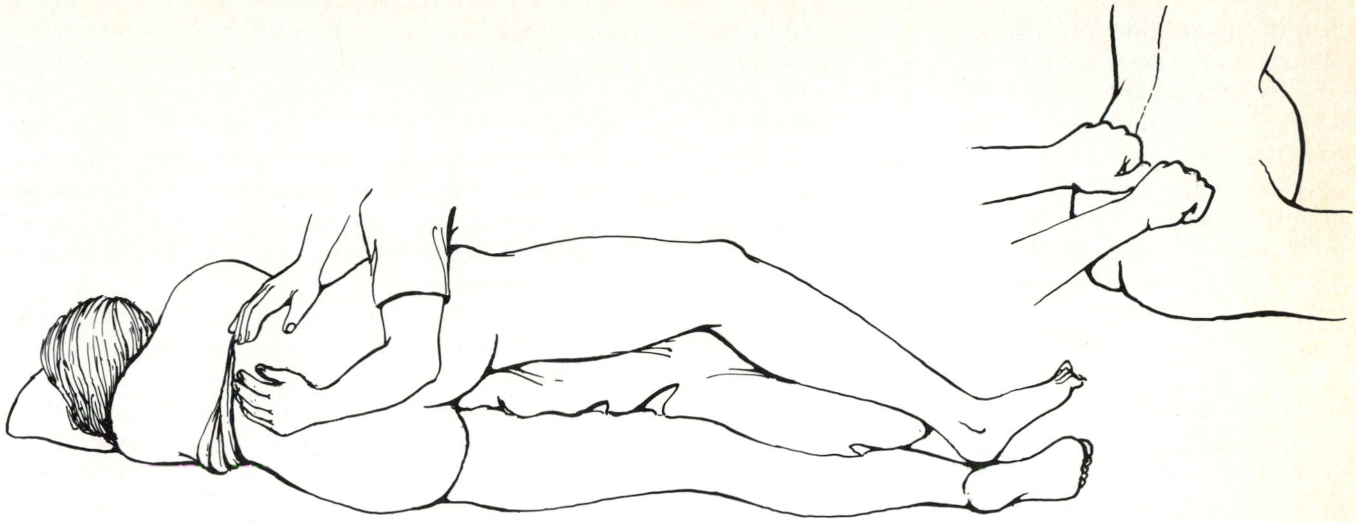

Figure 27–7. Massage techniques for back labor. (Redrawn, with permission, from Whitley N. *Manual of Clinical Obstetrics.* Philadelphia; JB Lippincott; 1985.)

for example, morphine, meperidine (Demerol), or a tranquilizer, to help her sleep for several hours. If she has been in false labor, the medication will arrest it; if she was in early latent phase, it will give her the time to rest while the labor progresses. Medication is sometimes used in this manner with labors that have hypertonic or dysfunctional contractions. In these cases, the goal is to significantly decrease or stop labor temporarily, with the hope that when it starts again it will have a more normal pattern.

Another technique that is sometimes used to promote sleep is hypnosis. If the woman has been prepared beforehand or a suitable practitioner is available, this method may help her to sleep. Some Eastern techniques, such as acupressure, also may be used by knowledgeable practitioners to eliminate or relieve pain and help the woman to sleep.

If the woman does not wish to receive medication, it is very important to provide her with a quiet environment and methods of relaxation so that she can obtain as much rest as possible. Allowing the woman to sleep between contractions is also helpful during any stage of labor. Whether the woman has chosen to labor with doses of medication (that do not eliminate the feelings of the peak of the contractions) or without medication, she may request to be awakened when a new contraction is starting so that she can be prepared to use her coping techniques for the sensations of the contractions. A combination of adequate high-calorie fluids and changes in position can also help the woman avoid the extreme effects of fatigue. It must be emphasized that for the majority of women, labor is a normal physiologic process that requires comprehensive care on the part of the woman's support persons, the health care team, and herself. Labor is like a marathon athletic event with a very tangible outcome, a baby.

Nausea, Vomiting, and Diarrhea

Other stimuli that can occur in labor are nausea, vomiting, and diarrhea. Many women, whether they take analgesics or not (some analgesics, like meperidine, have side effects of nausea and vomiting), have at least one of these symptoms at some point in the labor process, particularly in transition, and a few women experience all of them.

In addition to discomfort, these symptoms deplete the woman of fluids, calories, and electrolytes needed for the labor process. If the woman is taking oral fluids, the nurse should be sure she is sipping high-calorie clear fluids that "agree" with her (like juices that contain calories and fluid). If she is receiving intravenous fluids, they may need to be increased or monitored more carefully in terms of her urine output and fluid requirements for labor. In either case, her fluid output needs to be measured and at least replaced.

In some cases, an antiemetic medication, for example, hydroxyzine (Vistaril) and promethazine (Phenergan), may need to be given either alone or with the analgesic to stop the vomiting. If the woman has had diarrhea, an enema is not indicated because the bowel is already empty and irritated.

Fear

Fear of the unknown is a very powerful negative influence on the actions of the woman and her family. Grantly Dick-Read first discussed women's fear of the labor process and discussed the fear-tension-pain syndrome. Another aspect of this syndrome is having one's feelings or wishes ignored or dismissed as unimportant. Being misunderstood (or not understood in the case of language differences) can be very frustrating and both situations may lead to the fear-tension-pain syndrome.

These problems can be addressed by open communication with the woman and her support persons. The nurse should always introduce himself or herself, explain what is being done, and why it is needed. The nurse should try to anticipate why the woman might be afraid and explain why her cooperation is needed. An example in the second stage of labor may be the woman's fear of pushing because she is afraid of passing a stool. An interpreter should be brought in if necessary. Childbirth education can be extremely helpful to the woman and her support person before labor or, if needed, during labor.

Pain and Pain Management

Pain is a highly subjective and personal experience often described as an unpleasant sensation, emotion, affect, or feeling that may or may not produce suffering in the woman.[7, 18–20] Pain is whatever the woman says it is and exists if she says it does. The nurse therefore should never deny, admonish, or belittle the woman who says she has pain, but simply acknowledge it and help her overcome the negative sensations.

Pain may be viewed as having benefits, drawbacks, causes, and relief measures. Pain often provides the first warning sign that injury is occurring. In the first stage of labor, pain is due primarily to dilation and effacement of the cervix (thoracic nerves 10 to 12), and is usually not indicative of tissue damage. In second-stage labor, pain may cause the woman to forcefully bear down, which might result in lacerations. The causes of pain in this stage are related to stretching and possible tearing of the perineum (sacral nerves 2, 3, and 4 and the pudendal, ilioinguinal, and genital-femoral nerves). In addition, distension of the bladder or lower uterine segment, hypoxia to the uterine muscle, tissue damage as in vaginal tissue lacerations, and emotional tension caused by fear and anxiety may produce pain.

The intensity of the pain felt by the individual woman during labor is determined by her cultural expectations,[21] previous experience with pain or childbirth,[22] her understanding of the causes and consequences of the pain, intensity of the contractions, the speed of cervical dilation, position of the fetus (eg, LOP), complications such as abruptio placentae, duration of labor, type and extent of tissue damage, and type and amount of pain relief used. Pain also affects other body functions and may cause increased cardiac output, tachycardia, cardiac arrhythmias, tachypnea, hyperventilation, sweating, and decreased uterine blood flow.

Interruption of pain impulse transmission can be accomplished in some clients by acupuncture and is also affected, to some degree, by **effleurage,** the rhythmic stroking and massage of the abdomen. Both techniques use the gateway theory of pain control and block or interrupt transmission of the pain message. The use of acupuncture in labor and delivery is experimental in the United States, but is used often in Eastern cultures especially for cesarean deliveries. The application of transcutaneous electrical nerve stimulation (TENS) technology is also experimental at this time, as the effect on the fetus has not yet been determined by animal testing. Effleurage during a contraction has some minor effect on pain transmission, but is hampered by the belts required for external fetal monitoring.

Comfort measures are quite effective in reducing stress and, therefore, in reducing pain. Bed linen must be clean and dry, wrinkle free, and nonrestricting. Massage of the lower back, the thighs, or legs is often welcome until transition. A cool washcloth on the forehead or sponging of the face and neck is refreshing. Rinsing the mouth with either water or mouthwash and expectoration of the fluid help to relieve the discomfort of a dry mouth. Frequent perineal care maintains medical asepsis and provides comfort for the woman. Caregivers should demonstrate respect for the modesty of the client by appropriate draping and curtaining at all times. These comfort measures are basic nursing techniques that carry a message of caring.

Distraction is an effective method of pain control, and finding an appropriate source of distraction for the individual client challenges the creativity of the labor and delivery nurse. Many clients enjoy watching television during the latent phase; others may prefer listening to music. Use of a radio or earphones can be encouraged to promote relaxation and distraction for the laboring woman. The nurse should assess each client by interview and observation to ascertain individual preferences. Would the woman prefer silence? Conversation? Being able to view the monitoring screen? Music? Many women find the sound of the fetal heartbeat, as amplified by the monitor, to be reassuring and hypnotic, whereas others appear to be made more anxious by the variability of the FHR.

Ambulation during labor can influence the woman's perception of pain. Low-risk clients in an acute care facility are usually permitted to walk with assistance and support if the fetal presenting part is well engaged, to diminish the possibility of cord prolapse. If the mother chooses to remain in bed, or if there are indications that require bedrest, changes in position can aid in pain relief. The range of possible positions should include squatting, knee/elbow position, or sitting with a support person or pillows behind her.

Childbirth Education as a Means of Pain Relief. The subject of prenatal or childbirth education is a very broad area for discussion. This chapter focuses briefly on the application of this education to labor and birth. Several different breathing techniques can be taught in the prenatal or intrapartum period. (*See* Chapter 24 for descriptions of these various techniques.)

Role of the Nurse

First Stage of Labor. The nurse should identify the method of prepared childbirth that the couple will be using in labor. During the first stage, the practiced technique should be encouraged. This may include the use of different methods of breathing at different points in the first stage.

For example, when the Dick-Read method is used, deep breathing, both abdominal and chest, as well as shallow breathing may be used. In the Lamaze method, the breathing begins at a slow pace and then changes to a modified pace as the first stage progresses. The Bradley method, on the other hand, involves breath control and abdominal breathing during the first stage.

If the couple has not attended childbirth education classes, controlled relaxation techniques can be taught by an experienced nurse.

Second Stage of Labor. Each of the methods just mentioned uses basically the same pushing technique during the second stage of labor. The woman takes one or two cleansing breaths, pushes at the peak of the contraction, and uses the cleansing breath again at the end.

Recommendations about the force to be used in pushing and the length of time the woman holds her breath have changed over the years. In the past, the woman was told to hold her breath for as long as she could and push down as hard as she could. Today there is more flexibility in instructing the woman to push for the length of time and with the force that feels right for her. Long hard pushing is discouraged as it may lead to fetal bradycardia. Some women naturally push about 10 seconds, take a deep breath, and push again, continuing the pattern until the contraction ends.

Other Nonpharmacologic Methods of Pain Relief. Other nonpharmacologic methods used to relieve pain during labor and delivery depend on an altered stage of consciousness called the alpha state. It is thought that the pain of labor can be decreased by decreasing generalized muscle tension through relaxation measures,[23,24] such as hydrotherapy, acupressure, therapeutic touch, and imagery/visualization.

- *Hydrotherapy.* In hydrotherapy (water therapy), the mother submerges herself in a warm bath, which causes local vasodilation and muscle relaxation (Figure 27–8).
- *Acupressure.* Acupressure is based on the principle that pain is an imbalance of energy within the body. During labor, to help the pain caused by the imbalance, pressure is applied with the fingertips on three major body points. The first is between the first and second metacarpal bones on the dorsum of the hand. The second is below the tibial tuberosity on the side of the tibialis anterior muscle. The third is behind the tibia.[23]
- *Therapeutic touch.* Therapeutic touch operates on the principle that the human body is an energy field. The relief of pain may be mediated through a person, like the nurse, who transmits energy to an area on the pregnant woman's body. This transmits recuperative powers that may alleviate pain.
- *Imagery/Visualization.* Relaxation may be enhanced if the laboring mother pictures the process of birth in a positive light. For example, the mother would imagine her vagina gently and easily opening to allow the passage of the fetus. Imagery is sometimes accompanied by music.

Pharmacologic Management of Pain. Labor and delivery can cause the mother to experience discomfort and pain that may sometimes require pharmacologic as well as nonpharmacologic interventions. Judicious use of medications may be an acceptable alternative coping measure for the laboring woman. The pharmacologic means of pain relief include the use of analgesics, tranquilizers, sedatives, and anesthetics. Some overlap exists in the use of these terms. Fc example, some practitioners consider a continu lumbar epidural a form of analgesia, as it re' pain during labor. For purposes of this disc

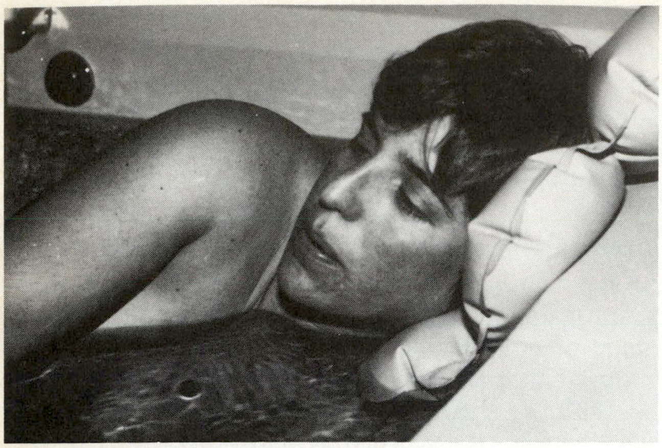

A

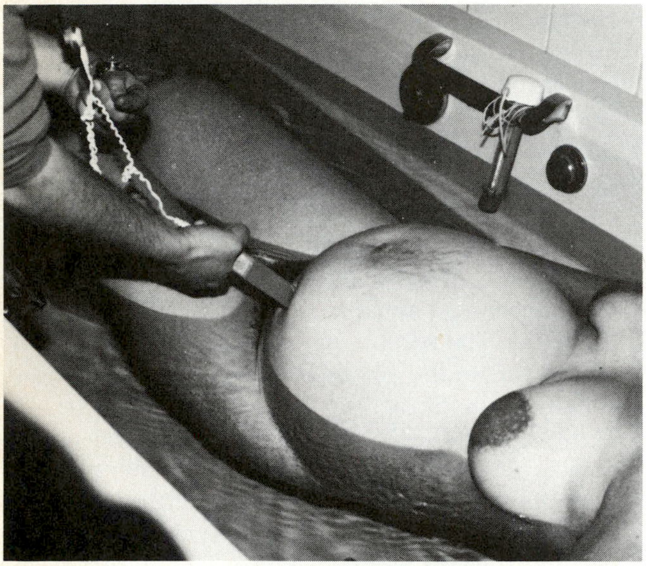

B

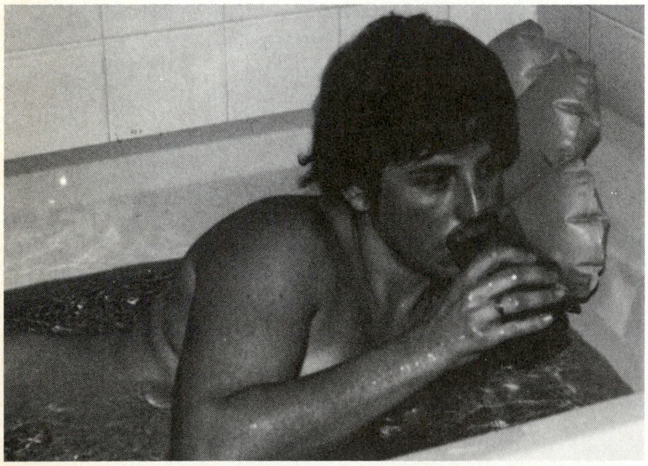

C

Figure 27–8. Hydrotherapy in labor. **A.** Breathing with contraction. **B.** Assessing fetal heart rate between contractions. **C.** Relaxing between contractions.

however, the following classification will be used, although others are possible.

Analgesics, Tranquilizers, and Sedatives. Before the nurse administers systemic medications to the laboring woman, maternal and fetal status must be thoroughly assessed. Any medication given will have an effect on the mother, fetus, and labor. The mother's respirations and blood pressure should be assessed prior to administering the medication and at regular intervals thereafter, including the approximate time that the medication reaches its peak. Any decrease in maternal respirations and blood pressure not only affects the mother, but may also produce fetal hypoxia.

The fetal heart rate should also be assessed prior to administering the medication. Medications cross the placenta by means of diffusion so that timing and route of medication are essential; that is, the fetus needs time to metabolize and excrete the medication before birth to prevent fetal depression.

Medications can have an effect on the progress of labor. The contractions may occur farther apart and their intensity may decrease. In general, medications should be timed so that they are not given too early, which may slow labor and delivery, or too late, which will not give the mother and fetus ample time to metabolize and excrete the medication.

The more common analgesics used for labor are meperidine (Demerol) and morphine (for sleep in early labor). The tranquilizers often given with them are antihistamines such as hydroxyzine (Vistaril), phenothiazines such as promethazine (Phenergan), and benzodiazepines such as diazepam (Valium). Tranquilizers alone do not provide analgesia, but used with narcotics may provide sedation. They may, however, produce additional depression of mother and fetus. Barbiturate sedatives such as secobarbital (Seconal) and pentobarbital (Nembutal) are rarely used today in labor as they may actually antagonize the effects of the analgesics.

The particular drugs used in labor are somewhat a preference of the physician or nurse-midwife. The nurse has the responsibility to monitor the mother and fetus prior to and after medications are given. (*See* Table 27–4 for an overview of common systemic medications given during labor.)

Anesthetics. Common anesthetic methods used for labor and delivery include local, regional (pudendal, paracervical, epidural, and spinal) and general (gas, volatile, intravenous) anesthetics. The same drug, administered by alternative routes and doses, may produce the anesthetic effect in several of these types of anesthetic methods. As with analgesics used during labor, broad, general principles govern the use of an-

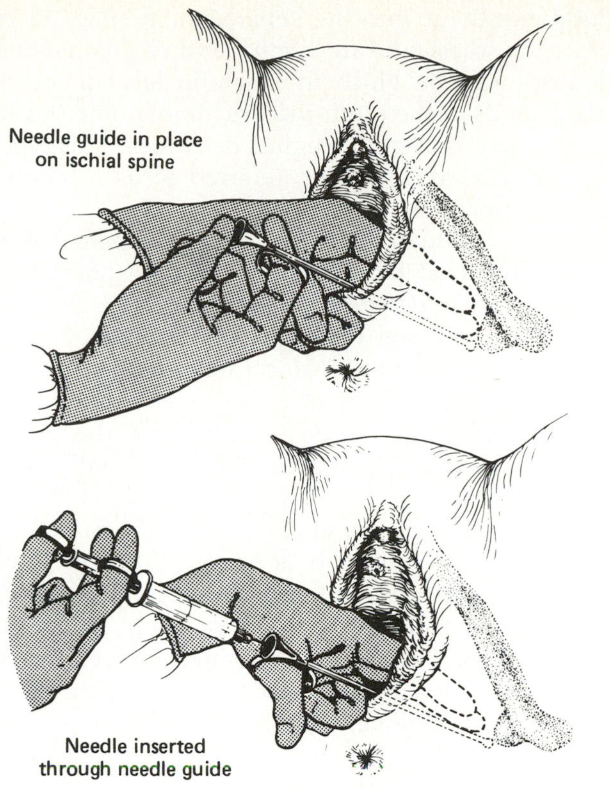

Figure 27–9. Technique of transvaginal pudendal block. (*Reproduced, with permission, from Pernoll ML, Benson RC.* Current Obstetric and Gynecologic Diagnosis and Treatment. *6th ed. Norwalk, Conn: Appleton & Lange, 1987:468.*)

esthetic agents during labor and delivery. The anesthetic should be simple to use, preserve maternal and fetal health, be safe, and be administered by a competent practitioner (eg, an anesthesiologist or nurse anesthetist) with expertise in obstetric anesthesia.

The same concerns relevant to analgesics are important here, namely, the effects of the anesthetic agent on the mother, the fetus, and the progress of labor. Although the maternity nurse does not administer anesthesia, she or he is responsible for closely monitoring the mother and fetus. This is especially the case during labor, when the nurse is the primary care provider.

Local Anesthesia. The simplest anesthetic method for the delivery process is local infiltration of the subcutaneous and intramuscular tissue of the perineum. This is done to numb the area of the site of the episiotomy for incision and repair. Some commonly used local anesthetics include lidocaine (Xylocaine), mepivacaine (Carbocaine), and chloroprocaine (Nesacaine). This method has minimal side effects on the mother and fetus.[25]

Regional Anesthesia. Today, regional anesthesia is in fairly wide use for pain relief. Several methods of nerve blocks may be used to relieve pain during labor or delivery, including pudendal, paracervical, epidural, and spinal blocks. Paracervical block provides pain relief during labor. True saddle block (a form of spinal anesthesia) and pudendal nerve block alleviate the discomfort of the second stage of labor. Epidural block (including both lumbar epidural and caudal epidural) and spinal block may provide relief of pain for both labor and delivery.

A **pudendal block** is so named because it blocks sensations around the vagina, which is innervated by the pudendal nerve. The procedure involves injecting a local anesthetic agent such as lidocaine in the vicinity of each of the two pudendal nerves as they pass between the ischial spines. The approach to the pudendal nerves may be either through the vagina (transvaginal) or through the perineum (transcutaneous). Bilateral pudendal blocks alleviate most of the discomfort from perineal distension at the time of delivery. They also allow the use of low forceps or vacuum extraction and provide pain relief for performing and repairing an episiotomy. In rare cases, an intravascular injection of the anesthetic agent may lead to maternal convulsions. Other side effects include hematoma and infection. Figure 27–9 illustrates a pudendal block.

The **paracervical block** is a technique used to relieve the discomfort of uterine contractions and cervical dilation during labor (Figure 27–10). Lidocaine

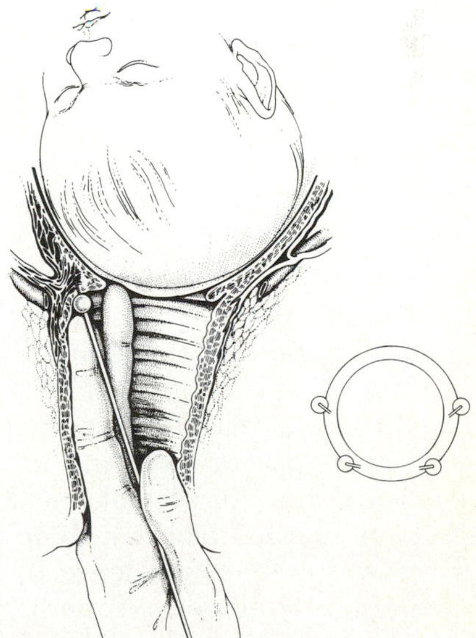

Figure 27–10. Technique of paracervical/uterosacral block. (*Reproduced, with permission, from Zuspan, FP, Quilligan EJ.* Douglas-Stromme Operative Obstetrics. *5th ed. Norwalk, Conn: Appleton & Lange; 1988:134.*)

or another local anesthetic agent is injected directly into the cervix at the positions of 3 and 9 or 4 and 8 o'clock. The block does not relieve perineal pain; therefore additional anesthesia, such as pudendal block, may be needed for delivery.

Although pain relief is achieved during the first stage of labor, paracervical blocks may cause fetal bradycardia associated with fetal asphyxia in 10 to 70 percent of cases.[25] Thus, the technique is rarely used today and if used is limited to women with low-risk pregnancies. The nurse must carefully monitor fetal heart rate pattern when a laboring woman receives a paracervical block.

Relief from the pain of uterine contractions and perineal distension may also be accomplished by **epidural anesthesia,** the injection of a local anesthetic agent into the epidural space. **Epidural block** may be one of two types, lumbar epidural and caudal epidural. A continuous lumbar epidural may be administered through a catheter placed in the lumbar area. For vaginal delivery, this provides complete anesthesia from the tenth thoracic to the fifth sacral dermatomes. For cesarean delivery, the effects of the epidural block begin at the level of the fourth thoracic dermatome.

The spread of the epidurally injected anesthetic agent depends on the location of the catheter, the dose and concentration of the medication, and to some extent the position of the laboring woman (head-down, horizontal, or head-up position).

Caudal epidural anesthesia is accomplished through the injection of an anesthetic agent into the epidural space through the sacral hiatus, which is found at the lower end of the sacrum. Continuous caudal epidural, like continuous lumbar epidural, usually involves the placement of a catheter, in this case through the sacral hiatus. This method of anesthesia decreases the sensation of pain by anesthetizing the nerve roots from the tenth thoracic through the fifth sacral nerves as they pass through the epidural space. Lumbar and caudal epidurals have been used for both labor and delivery, but because of its easier placement, greater reliability, and requirement of less drug, lumbar epidural block has for the most part replaced caudal block in current practice.

Side effects of epidural blocks include puncture of the dura, causing a high incidence of maternal headache; maternal hypotension; and, possibly, slowing of the progress of labor and delivery. The most important side effect is a sudden fall in maternal blood pressure, which can rapidly produce fetal distress and demise.[25] Ephedrine is used as a treatment for side effects of epidural blocks.

Spinal anesthesia, also called subarachnoid or **spinal block,** is produced by the introduction of a local anesthetic into the subarachnoid space to produce anesthesia during vaginal and cesarean deliveries. A low spinal block, in which the level of anesthesia extends to the tenth thoracic dermatome (level of umbilicus), is used for vaginal deliveries. This type of anesthesia has also been referred to as a modified **saddle block.**

For cesarean delivery, the anesthetic should reach the level of the fourth thoracic dermatome. With cesarean deliveries, a larger dose of anesthetic agent is necessary, increasing the frequency of side effects. (*See* Chapter 28 on cesarean delivery.)

Some side effects of spinal anesthetics are hypotension, spinal headaches, bladder dysfunction postdelivery, and total spinal blockade with respiratory paralysis.

A spinal or postpuncture headache may follow the spinal procedure. It is characterized by severe headache often associated with neck stiffness when the woman is in the upright position. Much controversy exists concerning methods to treat or prevent spinal headaches. Keeping the client flat in bed for any number of hours has generally been demonstrated to be without effect. Vigorous hydration with intravenous or oral fluids may be of value, but this procedure still lacks conclusive empirical documentation. Abdominal support with a tight abdominal binder or girdle when the client is upright has been shown to provide some relief. Fortunately, most spinal headaches resolve by themselves within a few days (usually 3 to 5) using conservative therapy. Those that do not can be treated with a procedure called an epidural blood patch. In this procedure, 10 mL of maternal blood is injected into the epidural space through a catheter to seal the leak.

Nonpharmacologic and pharmacologic methods of pain management are used to lessen the perceived pain of labor or to block the pain pathways during labor and delivery. The perceived pain and discomfort differ according to the stage of labor. Figure 27–11 illustrates pain pathways in the first and second stages of labor.

General Anesthesia. **General anesthesia** for routine vaginal delivery is rarely used today for several reasons. General anesthesia depresses the mother's and fetus' central nervous systems. Moreover, there is the danger that the mother may aspirate gastric contents.[25] In addition, general anesthesia denies the mother the experience of birth itself, and of interacting with her baby and the baby's father at birth. When general anesthetics are used, the nurse must closely monitor the woman as she recovers from the agent. The newborn also requires close observation and as-

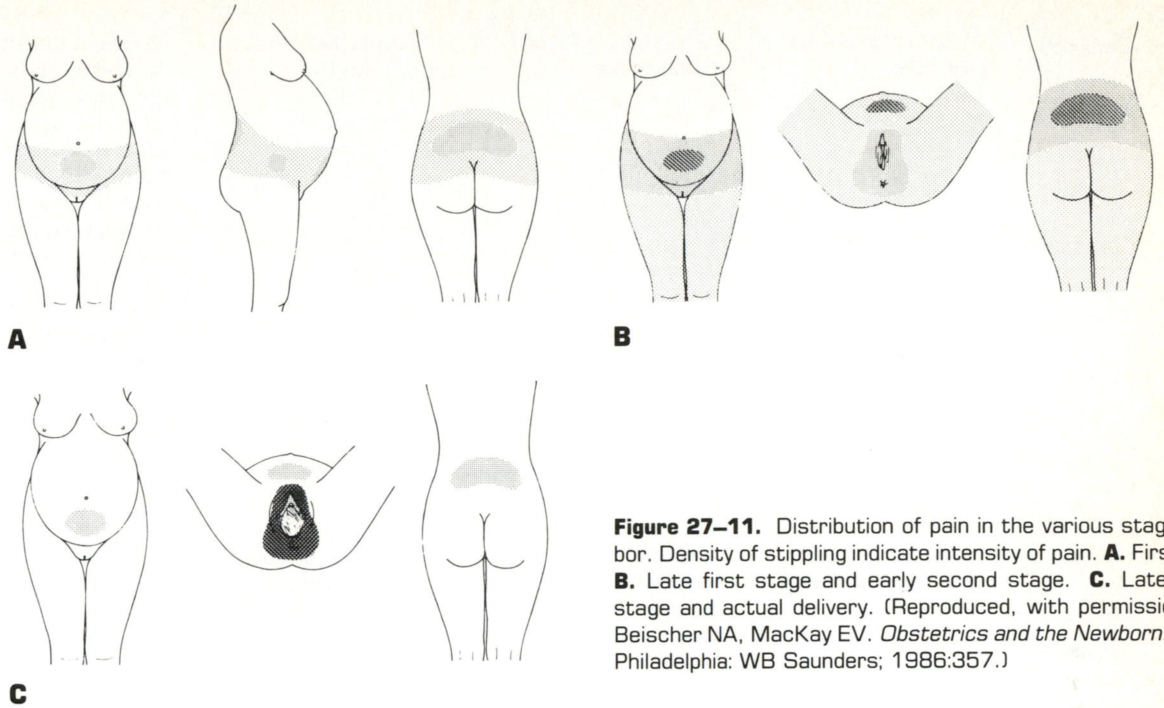

Figure 27–11. Distribution of pain in the various stages of labor. Density of stippling indicate intensity of pain. **A.** First stage. **B.** Late first stage and early second stage. **C.** Late second stage and actual delivery. (Reproduced, with permission, from Beischer NA, MacKay EV. *Obstetrics and the Newborn.* 2nd ed. Philadelphia: WB Saunders; 1986:357.)

sessment. Thus, general anesthesia is usually reserved for emergency cesarean and operative vaginal deliveries.

General anesthetics include gas anesthetics, volatile anesthetics, and intravenous drugs.

Nitrous oxide is the only anesthetic gas currently used for maternity clients in the United States.[25] By itself, nitrous oxide is not a potent or complete anesthetic and must be supplemented to ensure freedom from pain.

Volatile anesthetic agents include halothane (Fluothane) and enflurane (Ethrane). They are used to supplement nitrous oxide during delivery. These agents readily cross the placenta and are capable of producing severe fetal depression.

Intravenous anesthetic agents are also used to produce general anesthesia. They are usually used in combination with inhalation agents, for example, thiopental (Pentothal) and ketamine (Ketalar).

General anesthesia usually involves a combination of several of the above-mentioned agents. After preoxygenation, the woman is rendered unconscious by a rapidly acting drug such as thiopental or ketamine. She then receives a rapid-acting muscle relaxant to allow placement of a cuffed endotracheal tube in the trachea, which assures an open and clear airway and protects against pulmonary aspiration. Anesthesia is then maintained with various inhalation agents. As mentioned, nitrous oxide must be supplemented by other agents to ensure the proper anesthetic effect. Before delivery, 50 percent nitrous oxide in oxygen is usually supplemented with a low concentration of a potent inhalation agent such as 0.5 percent halothane or 1.0 percent enflurane. Higher concentrations of these drugs are avoided as they will be associated with decreased uterine activity predisposing to postpartum uterine bleeding.

Following delivery, anesthesia is deepened by increasing the nitrous oxide concentration to 60 to 70 percent. This is supplemented by narcotics and a low dose of a potent inhalation agent. Although the woman cannot experience pain and does experience amnesia, she is usually in a light plane of anesthesia. Therefore, additional muscle relaxants are needed to ensure lack of movement and adequate relaxation. At the conclusion of the surgical or other birthing procedure, the client is not extubated until she is awake, responsive with upper airway reflexes intact, and with no residual muscle weakness. In general, the time between induction of anesthesia and delivery is kept as short as possible. The woman is only lightly anesthetized to assure minimal neonatal depression at birth.

In addition to Table 27–4, which gives the basic information about the more commonly used analgesics in labor, Table 27–5 gives information about anesthetics used in labor and delivery.

For each medication or anesthetic agent used in labor and birth, the nurse should be knowledgeable about the type of medication; the indications, routes,

TABLE 27–4. COMMON ANALGESICS USED DURING LABOR

Drug Name	Indications	Administration	Onset and Duration of Action	Intended Effects
Analgesics				
Meperidine (Demerol)	Maternal desire for pain relief Early labor, to help sleep	25–100 mg IM or IV in active labor	IV: immediate effect and lasts 2–3 hours. IM: 15–30 minutes to take effect and lasts 2–3 hours	Sedation of mother and good (but not complete) pain relief without loss of consciousness Analgesics rarely relieve all the painful feelings of contractions; they usually relieve the pain associated with the beginning and end but not the peak of the contractions
Alphaprodine (Nisentil)	Same as for *meperidine*, however rarely used today	30–60 mg SC or IV in active labor	IV (30 mg): immediate effect 1–2 minutes; duration 30 –90 minutes SC: 5–10 minutes; duration 2 hours	Same as for *meperidine*
Morphine	Same as for *meperidine*	8–15 mg IM: 4–10 mg IV	IV: immediate: duration 2–4 hours IM: within 15–30 minutes; duration 3–4 hours	Same as for *meperidine*
Tranquilizers				
Hydroxyzine (Vistaril)	Tense anxious mother; administered with meperidine to potentiate analgesia and to counteract nausea and vomiting	IM only 25–100 mg	Onset 15–30 minutes; duration 2–4 hours	Sedation of mother lessens anxiety, raises pain threshold Muscle relaxant Potentiates narcotics and barbiturates Antinauseant
Promethazine (Phenergan)	Same as for *hydroxyzine*	25–50 mg IM or IV	Rapid onset; 6–8 hours duration	Same as for *hydroxyzine*
Diazepam (Valium) (used mostly in England)	Same as for *hydroxyzine*	15–20 mg IM or 5–15 mg IV	Rapid onset; duration 1–1½ hours	Same as for *hydroxyzine*
Sedatives				
Secobarbital (Seconal)	Helps mother who may be in false or prolonged early labor to sleep; also helps anxious mother	Up to 100 mg PO, IM, or IV	PO: 30–60 minutes IM: about 15 minutes IV: 30–60 seconds	Sedation of mother
Pentobarbital (Nembutal)	Same as for *secobarbital*	Same as for *secobarbital*	Same as for *secobarbital*	Same as for *secobarbital*

IV = intravenous(ly), IM = intramuscular(ly), SC = subcutaneous(ly), PO = oral(ly) (by mouth), CNS = central nervous system.

Effects on Labor	Maternal Effects	Placental Transfer	Fetal/Newborn Effects
In early labor, there may be a decrease in intensity and frequency of contractions Excessive doses prolong labor Heavy medication may lead to use of forceps	Respiratory and circulatory depression, dizziness, confusion, nausea, vomiting, cough suppression, gastrointestinal stasis, lowered blood oxygen With any drug that may cause respiratory depression in the mother or fetus there must be resuscitative equipment and personnel available in the event this should happen Naloxone (Narcan) 0.4 mg IM or IV should also be available to counteract effects of drug	Within 30 seconds of IV dose	Effects dependent on dose or administration relative to time of birth, size, health, and maturity of fetus. Side effects (respiratory depression, poor sucking, decreased weight gain, less visual attentiveness, hypothermia, poor consolability, greater irritability), if they occur, are most pronounced in the first few minutes and days, as fetus/newborn cannot easily metabolize the drugs, but can also be seen weeks and months later. Naloxone (Narcan) 0.01 mg/kg may be given IM into infant's thigh to counteract immediate respiratory depression
Same as for *meperidine*	Same as for *meperidine*, except maternal respiratory depression is more pronounced and may lead to rapid respiratory arrest; should not be given with other CNS-depressing drugs: resuscitative equipment should be available	Rapid	Same as for *meperidine*
Same as for *meperidine*	Same as for *meperidine*	Rapid	Same as for *meperidine*
Unknown	Drowsiness, confusion, drop in blood pressure, urinary retention, dry mouth, fat embolism, amnesia, pain at injection site	Rapid	Unclear but possible CNS depression and hyperbilirubinemia
Unknown	Same as for *hydroxyzine*, except no fat embolism	Within 1–2 minutes of injection	Unclear but possible CNS depression and impaired neonatal behavior for several days
Unknown	Same as for *promethazine*	Rapid	Hyperbilirubinemia, hypothermia, hypotonia, hypoactivity, loss of beat-to-beat variability in heart rate, reduced sucking, decreased attentiveness
May stop false labor; may slow early labor	Decreases pulse and blood pressure and general responsiveness, reduces anxiety and allows rest but client may have difficulty dealing with contractions as this is not a pain reliever	Rapid, 30–60 seconds IV and 3–5 minutes IM	Drug accumulates in tissue, may cause CNS depression (especially given with a narcotic), poor sucking, decreased muscle tone, altered waking state, alterations in electroencephalogram No effective antidote; have resuscitative equipment and personnel available
Same as for *secobarbital*	Same as for *secobarbital*	Same as for *secobarbital*	Same as for *secobarbital*

TABLE 27–5. COMMON ANESTHETICS USED IN LABOR AND DELIVERY

Type of Anesthetic	Indications	Administration	Onset and Duration of Action	Intended Effects
Local	Numbs tissue at site of episiotomy for incision and repair of laceration	Interstitially, directly into tissue to be repaired Carbocaine and Xylocaine are amide-type local anesthetics, 1% solution up to 200 mg or 20 ml Ester-type local anesthetics are Nisacaine and Pontocaine	Onset 1–10 minutes; duration 1 hour	Numbs site
Regional: paracervical/ uterosacral block	Maternal request of pain relief from uterine contractions and cervical dilation	2.5 mL of local anesthetic (like those medications used for local anesthesia) per site just below the vaginal mucosa, given into 3 and 9, or 4 and 8 o'clock positions of lateral vaginal fornices when dilation is between 4 and 6 cm, the presenting part is 0 to +2 station, and delivery is not expected within 1 hour	Onset within 5–10 minutes; duration depends on drug used and varies from 45 minutes to 2 or 3 hours	Relief of pain from uterine contractions and dilating cervix
Regional: pudendal block	Given into pudendal nerve through anesthesia of perineal area rather than local anesthetic May be used for forceps or difficult delivery, large or extensive incision, laceration and repair	Same as for *local agent*	Same as for *local agent*	Numbs lower vagina and perineum
Regional: epidural block	In active labor for the relief of pain from contractions and pelvic pressure/pain, at request of mother after 4 cm and establishment of regular pattern of contractions; in second-stage labor for delivery, particularly if manipulation or forceps anticipated Also for cesarean delivery	Given by anesthesiologist into epidural space at L2, L3, L4, or L5, while woman lies on her side with legs drawn up in a fetal position or sitting position	Takes 20–45 minutes to administer and 20–60 minutes to act Can be given in one bolus injection through catheter or by continuous infusion through implanted catheter (via bolus injections as medication wears off or through infusion pumps, which measure dose and provide continuous small amounts to keep anesthetic working)	Complete pain relief in lower part of body
Regional: spinal block	For delivery or if excessive manipulation or forceps anticipated; also for cesarean delivery	Given by anesthesiologist into spinal column at L2, L3, L4, or L5 while the mother lies on her left side in the fetal position	Onset 3–5 minutes; duration 1–3 hours	Numbs body from waist to feet

Effects on Labor	Maternal Effects	Placental Transfer	Fetal/Newborn Effects
None known especially because given at delivery	When used locally, rare maternal side effects, including cardiac depression, CNS depression, and restlessness, dizziness, and, in large doses, convulsions Amide-type anesthetics penetrate tissue better and act more rapidly and longer than ester-type drugs and hence are used more frequently	2–3 minutes	None if given after birth and rare even before birth, but may cause bradycardia, tachycardia, fetal acidosis, and, in high blood levels, convulsions Metabolism of amide drugs requires liver enzymes that are not mature in the fetus
Rarely might slow contractions	Pain relief for first-stage labor; only rarely systemic toxic effects	Rapid, particularly as so close to uterus and to placenta	Bradycardia reported in 2–70% of cases, which varies with drug and dose used Convulsions and death if injected into fetus and vaginal area together Risk to fetus if delivered during episode of bradycardia
If given in second-stage labor, woman may have decreased bearing down reflex	*See* "Effects on Labor"	Same as for *local agent*	Same as for *local agent*
If given too early, improperly, or in too large a dose, may stop or slow labor, necessitating the use of a labor stimulant like oxytocin Eliminates the urge to push and may necessitate use of forceps	Must remain in bed, frequent vital signs needed because of hypotension danger Fetal monitor needed to detect possible labor, fetal effects, IV fluids, and need for oxytocin and forceps Possible postpartum backache or spinal headache, and toxic reaction Epidural block is difficult to administer; puncture of dura leads to spinal anesthesia, possible respiratory arrest (if anesthetic goes too high in the spinal column), and paralysis (rare)	7–15 minutes depending on agent used	May cause poor muscle tone, hypoxia, fetal heart rate decelerations, and drug may concentrate in infant
May stop labor if given by accident when attempting an epidural	Loss of sensation, motor function, and pushing reflex; therefore forceps need Hypotension, possible spinal injury, and headache Possible infection at puncture site and meningitis	Rapid	Same as for *epidural block*

(continued)

TABLE 27–5. COMMON ANESTHETICS USED IN LABOR AND DELIVERY (*continued*)

Type of Anesthetic	Indications	Administration	Onset and Duration of Action	Intended Effects
General: halothane, nitrous oxide, enflurane	Complete loss of sensation and consciousness for cesarean delivery, difficult delivery, uterine relaxation or postpartum uterine manipulation	Volatile anesthetics used to supplement nitrous oxide during maintenance of general anesthesia	Rapid onset; duration varies with length and dose of anesthetic	Complete anesthesia and loss of consciousness with complete muscle relaxation
General: intravenous thiopental (Pentothal), ketamine (Ketalar)	Rapid induction of general anesthesia, usually followed by inhalation agents	IV: Pentothal usually given in a dose less than 4 mg/kg maternal body weight so side effects to mother and fetus are minimized Ketamine given in a dose less than 1 mg/kg maternal body weight with same anesthetic effect; can also be used as alternative to inhalation anesthesia in a dose of 0.25 mg/kg body weight	Immediate	Rapid induction of general anesthesia

and dosages of administration; methods or procedures for administration and monitoring; onset and duration of action; intended effects; effect on labor; maternal side effects; placental transfer; and potential fetal and newborn effects. There is continued debate concerning the safety of these anesthetics for use in the pregnant woman or her fetus. Analgesia or anesthesia should be given judiciously for pain relief. *Do not* continually ask the mother if she wants pain medication regardless of her behavior. Provide supportive touch and other nursing care techniques outlined in this chapter to assist a woman in labor.

NURSING CARE DURING THE FIRST STAGE OF LABOR

Nursing care for the childbearing family during the first stage of labor begins with admission of the woman to the labor and delivery unit or birthing area. During the first stage of labor, the nurse determines whether the mother is in true or false labor, obtains informed consent, and ascertains the maternal and fetal progress in labor. Several procedures may be performed during the first stage of labor. The following discussion highlights some of these treatment modalities that may be used during labor. They are not used in all cases or all settings. As with delivery of care throughout pregnancy, the nurse maintains conscientious adherence to universal precautions against the Human Immunodeficiency Virus (HIV) (*see* Appendix F). The intrapartum period is a time when the nurse may be exposed to maternal body fluids and blood—and potentially, to HIV. Thus, a special reminder to use universal precautions is warranted.

False versus True Labor

Women frequently have difficulty knowing whether or not true labor has begun. Most pregnant women, particularly nulliparas, fear they "will not know whether labor is real or just a false alarm." Because the symptoms of labor onset may be mild and perceptible only to the woman experiencing them, there is a tendency on the part of spouses, family, and friends to regard the mother as the "expert" in determining whether labor has indeed finally begun. Clients therefore should be taught the difference between true and false labor and given a reference such as the information in Table 27–6. They should be advised to contact their health care provider. Most important, the mother and her family must understand that medical and nursing personnel can usually determine onset, and that mistaking false labor for true labor is a common event. For example, if the nurse says, "We're glad to see you, even if we do have to send you home again. It happens to so many peo-

Effects on Labor	Maternal Effects	Placental Transfer	Fetal/Newborn Effects
Would stop labor if given during first stage labor, but is reserved for delivery only	Complete loss of consciousness, no pain felt, extreme uterine relaxation, cardiopressant and hypotensive effects, increased bleeding, aspiration of vomitus, rarely death	Rapid	Depending on drug, dose, and length of anesthesia, there may be respiratory depression, decreased alertness, decreased orientation and responsiveness to visual and auditory stimuli, poor consolability, and greater irritability
If recommended doses are used, effects on labor are minimal	Pentothal: possible hypotension and laryngospasm Ketamine: if recommended doses are used, little effect on maternal CNS; in addition, ketamine stimulates maternal cardiovascular system and may be used in situations of maternal hypotension and hemorrhage	Pentothal: rapidly crosses placenta within 4 minutes of injection into mother's vein; concentrations in fetal and maternal blood will be equal Ketamine: rapidly crosses placenta, but little fetal depression with recommended dose Because of rapidity of placental transfer, IV agents are rarely employed as primary anesthetic agent for delivery	Pentothal: when rapid delivery occurs after injection into vein, severe fetal depression may occur Ketamine: doses greater than 1 mg/kg maternal body weight increase the incidence of respiratory depression in mother and should not be used in any situation involving fetal distress

ple," the mother may feel reassured. A failure in communication occurs between health care professionals and clients when a woman fears the embarrassment of a false labor admission so much that the true labor results in delivery in a car, the parking lot, or a hospital elevator.

Early labor does not always follow the textbook picture. Contractile patterns occasionally vary with a pattern of irregularity in place of the progressive regular series. The client must be aware that it is not wise to wait until a regular progressive pattern develops, as the irregular "sets" of contractions may persist well into the active phase. Because labor does not always follow a textbook picture, other factors that must be considered in the management include distance to the birthing facility (or practitioner to the home), maternal history of rapid labors or problems with the cervix, gravidity, parity, anxiety of the woman, and risk status.

The assessment to determine if the woman is in true labor includes abdominal and pelvic examination, observation of contractions, vital signs (maternal and fetal), and a differential diagnosis of other factors that may mimic labor, for example, UTI, acute abdomen resulting from other conditions (appendicitis), red degeneration of fibroid tumors of the uterus,

TABLE 27–6. CLIENT TEACHING GUIDE: DIFFERENCES BETWEEN FALSE AND TRUE LABOR

False Labor	True Labor
Contractions mainly abdominal	Contractions felt in abdomen and spread to lower back
Irregular contractions that may disappear during sleep or with activity	May be widely spaced and somewhat irregular at onset; usually progress with increasing intensity and progressively shortened resting interval; do not decrease with activity
Vaginal mucus clear or slight threads of pink; may expel mucous plug	May expel mucous plug; show of definite pink-tinged mucus
Fetus more active or unchanged	Fetal activity may lessen; should never disappear
Membranes intact	Membranes may rupture with "gush" of amniotic fluid or slow continuous seepage
Cervix may be ripe and slightly dilated on sterile vaginal examination	Cervical dilation and effacement are palpable on sterile vaginal examination, and continue to progress

and muscular aches or ligament pain resulting from pregnancy.

To assess maternal and fetal status, some practitioners run a 30-minute fetal monitor strip and, at the end of that time, re-evaluate the progress of labor. If there has been no progress and there are no other signs of true labor, and if no other problems are present, the woman may be sent home or kept for further observation.

The end of pregnancy can be a difficult time for the expectant family, particularly if the mother has been having any problems. If she is told she is having false labor, she may be embarrassed or angry. The nurse needs to discuss the reasons for the diagnosis and the woman's and family's feelings. Assessment of the woman's knowledge level, cultural attitudes regarding the signs and progress of labor, and why she is anxious for the pregnancy to be over can be very revealing and allow the nurse to support the family through this stressful period.

Informed Consent

Before any procedures, interventions, or medications are used, informed consent is obtained. Informed consent involves a verbal explanation of what is to be done and includes the risks, benefits, and alternatives to all interventions or medications. Occasionally, audio or video tapes may be used to ensure consistent and accurate information for the consent, with time for the client to ask questions later. The client signs the consent form after her questions have been answered. This conversation is documented in the client's chart. Ideally, obstetric consents for procedures or medications should be given prenatally when the woman is not so anxious or preoccupied with labor and has the time to think and read about issues of particular concern (in some states, the law requires that these consents be given prenatally when possible).

Whatever format is used, certain elements of informed consent must be followed: an explanation of the procedure and its purpose in a manner that the client can understand; a description of how it will feel; benefits and risks to mother and fetus; alternatives to the place, procedure, or medication and their benefits and risks; how complications can be treated; an indication that the client is free to withdraw consent at any time; and an offer to answer any questions. A consent form must be written in the client's primary language with the purpose, benefits, and risks carefully explained. It must have the client's signature, date of consent, and a signature of the witness certifying that the client was given a fair explanation and appeared to understand the explanation. It is helpful to have the client explain the elements of consent in her own words and have a witness sign that the client gave an accurate explanation. The client should also be given a copy of the consent.

Maternal Progress in Labor

The nurse assesses maternal progress in labor by observing the following:

1. *Maternal vital signs.* Blood pressure, temperature, pulse, respirations.
2. *Perineal signs.* Bleeding, bloody show, rupture of membranes, color and odor of amniotic fluid, passing of gas, bulging of perineum, enlargement of anus, rectal mucosa showing.
3. *Maternal behavior.* Facial expressions, positions, what and how mother says things, noises or crying out, restlessness, breathing patterns, grunting or breath holding, response to comfort measures and coaching, need for human presence, reassurance of safe outcome, acceptance of her behavior.[7]
4. *Labor progress.*
   - Vaginal examination. Dilation and effacement of cervix, status of membranes, bony pelvis, fetal progress such as position, descent, station, and molding.
   - Contraction pattern. Frequency, duration, and intensity.
   - Friedman's curve (*See* Figure 25–10). Pictorial analysis used as a guideline for assessing progress of labor over time; useful in spotting disorders of arrest of dilation or failure of fetal descent of the presenting part, which are indicative of dystocia or cephalopelvic disproportion (CPD) of labor. (Keep in mind, however, that the data used to develop this curve represent labors that occurred in hospitals with women undergoing routine medical interventions. It is unknown at this point if this labor curve is a truly normal representation of labor or if the time frame it implies is truly predictive of good perinatal outcome in all settings.)
5. *Maternal hydration.* Need for fluid and calories whether by mouth or intravenously.
6. *Maternal elimination.* Amount and presence of sugar, ketones, or protein in urine; urinary output; presence of stool in lower bowel and need for emptying it.
7. *Presence of surrounding stimuli.* A need for a control of environment or additional coaching, change in position or temperature, medications for nausea or pain relief.
8. *Level of maternal comfort.* Need for ice chips, mouth care, cool wash cloth, back rub, cleansing of body

area soiled from blood, feces, vomitus, and so on, change of bed clothes or underpads, and someone to remain with woman for comfort.

Fetal Progress in Labor

In monitoring the progress of the fetus, the nurse must be aware of a variety of fetal parameters, including fetal heart rate, color and odor of amniotic fluid, scalp pH, descent of presenting part, progress of the fetus in rotation, molding of the head, and synclitism of head (the position in which the biparietal diameter of the fetal head is parallel to the planes of the pelvis and the sagittal suture is midway between the front and back of the pelvis; the fetal head can also be in anterior or posterior asynclitism).[15]

Procedures and Treatments

Shaving of Pubic Hair

Indications. The major indication for shaving of perineal and pubic hair is cesarean delivery, which requires removal of the hair on the abdomen and pubic region. Shaving is done to reduce the possibility of infection, as hair is known to carry bacteria and may interfere with the incision, repair, or healing. For vaginal births, shaving of the hair has been shown to increase the possibility of infection, not decrease it.

In the past, complete preparation involved shaving of the entire mons, perineal, and rectal areas. A lesser procedure, which requires shaving hair from the clitoral area to the rectum, generally replaced complete preparation. In many situations, shaving is not done at all.

An alternative to shaving the client who has a great deal of hair in the perineal region is to clip the hair in this area, making it easier for the practitioner to see when performing an episiotomy or repairing an episiotomy or laceration. The nurse should explain the procedure to the client and wash his or her hands before beginning. Good lighting is required, and it is important that the woman be placed in a position that allows good visibility of the area and is also comfortable to her. It may be necessary to have her turn on her side for part of the procedure.

Procedure/NursingCare For shaving, the nurse uses a sterile shaving kit, sharp blade in the razor, special soap or betadine, sterile gloves, and sponges and towels. While wearing the sterile gloves, the nurse cleanses the skin, leaving it soapy while the skin area is shaved. In areas where the skin is not taut, it is helpful to hold the skin tight in one direction while shaving the hair in the other direction. Care must be taken in the pubic and perineal area in particular as the skin has many folds, is soft, and is often edematous. The nurse should be sure to cleanse and dry the area when done. In addition, shaving should not be done during contractions for the mother's comfort.

Benefits. Complete shaving has not been shown to have any benefits for a vaginal birth; however, clipping the hair or partial shaving makes it easier for the practitioner to see when performing an episiotomy or repairing lacerations.

Risks. Complete shaving may increase the risk of infection, particularly if the skin is nicked or bruised in the process. The woman also experiences considerable itching when the hair begins to grow back. Shaving is also an embarrassing procedure for many women.

Evacuation of the Lower Bowel/Enema

Indications. Today, enemas are no longer used routinely in many places. An enema or rectal suppository may be used to evacuate stool in the rectum in early labor or at midlabor as determined by examination of the vagina. This should *not* be done if the woman has had diarrhea in the last 24 hours; if she is in advanced labor, the presenting part is low in the pelvis, or both; or if there is frank bleeding or fetal distress. Evacuation of the lower bowel may also be done if the woman requests it because of constipation when there are no other contraindications. Some practitioners use it as a means of stimulating labor although the scientific basis of this is not proven.

Procedure/Nursing Care. Evacuation of the lower bowel may be done using a rectal suppository inserted by the woman herself. This eliminates the problem of watery fecal contamination and embarrassment.

If an enema is chosen, a warm tap water or normal saline enema is instilled into the rectum between contractions. The nurse should pinch off the tubing during contractions and be sure the bed has sufficient protective covering in case some enema solution is returned during a contraction.

Benefits. Evacuation of the lower bowel may result in a small reduction of fecal contamination during the second stage and increase the pelvic space available for the fetal head. It may spare the woman the embarrassment from defecation while bearing down in second-stage labor. It may provide the extra room needed in the event a forceps delivery is necessary.

Risks. The evacuation procedure is uncomfortable, painful, and embarrassing. If the amniotic membranes have broken, there is the possibility of introducing bacteria. In some women, evacuation of the bowel may cause extremely rapid labors and the baby may be born with the expulsion of the enema (for this reason, *never* leave a laboring client alone after giving an enema, particularly if she is a multipara). The enema may also result in watery fecal contamination in the second stage of labor.

Hydration and Calories

Oral Nourishment

Indications. Fluids and nutrients are needed in labor to prevent dehydration and to provide calories to the laboring woman.

Nursing Care. If the woman takes solid food in labor, it is usually in the early first stage. A meal that is high in carbohydrates, low in protein and fats, and high in carbohydrate fluids is recommended (like the meal taken by athletes before a sporting event). Oral fluids may be taken throughout labor but the fluids are usually limited to water, ice chips, and high-calorie clear fluids, as tolerated by the particular woman.

Benefits. Providing oral nourishment allows the woman to take fluids and calories as she feels the need. Keeping the stomach full also maintains the gastric acidity closer to neutral, thus reducing the risk of complications from acid-pulmonary-aspiration syndrome.

Risks. The greatest risk from provisions of oral nourishment comes if the woman should vomit and aspirate the acidic gastric contents or solid food particles into her lungs. This situation is potentially life threatening to the woman and fetus. The risk of aspiration occurs when the woman needs general anesthesia for a difficult vaginal delivery or cesarean delivery. Although antacids can be given to neutralize the acid contents, nothing helps eliminate the solid particles in the stomach.

Intravenous Fluids

Indications. Intravenous infusion provides fluids and calories to the laboring woman via a vein, usually in the hand or arm, thereby keeping the stomach free of food. An intravenous line also provides an emergency route for medications or blood.

Procedure/Nursing Care. The nurse or other professional inserts a small catheter (or needle) into the vein of the hand or forearm and connects this to tubing attached to a bottle or bag filled with sterile fluid. This fluid usually contains normal saline or lactated Ringer's solution (an electrolyte solution). The sole use of 5 percent dextrose in water (D_5W) is no longer recommended because it results in an increased incidence of hypoglycemia in the newborn.[26]

The nurse should have the proper solution ready along with betadine or other bacteriocidal cleansing wipes, tubing, tape, blood tubes for the laboratory tests, and protective pads to place under the intravenous site to prevent any blood from spilling on the floor or bedding. Although the intravenous line can be inserted alone, it is helpful to have someone to assist with the procedure.

Benefits. Intravenous infusion provides a steady source of calories and fluid to the mother, and is especially beneficial when she does not want or is unable to drink or is vomiting. It decreases the possibility of aspiration of undigested food from the stomach contents into the lungs, but does not eliminate the possibility of acid aspiration from the stomach contents if the woman vomits. The intravenous line also provides a ready access to the blood for giving medications or additional blood in the event of emergency.

Risks. Insertion of an intravenous line is painful and places the woman at risk for infection at the site or in the vein. It may cause bruising, and restricts movement of the affected limb and of the woman in general.

Bathing

Indications. Bathing in labor, either shower or tub bath, is a noninvasive means of providing comfort and also assists with cleanliness in the first stage of labor. Research is in progress at this time regarding bathing in labor, but there is little in the literature to advise of any harmful effects. Careful consideration should be given regarding tub baths when the membranes are ruptured, as the effects in terms of infection or fetal outcome are only minimally known. Showers do not produce this same concern.

Procedure/Nursing Care. The woman either immerses herself in warm water in a tub, comfortable to her touch, or lets the warm water from the shower cover her body while she stands or sits in the shower. How long she remains is somewhat up to the woman and the comfort she obtains from the hydrotherapeutic effects of the water. In either case, the woman needs direct supervision while she is receiving the shower or bath to ensure her safety, particularly during contractions. The woman needs to remove herself from the bath or shower periodically to assess fetal status and cervical dilation.

Benefits. It has been reported by Odent in Pithivers, France, that contractions become more efficient and less painful and that labor is sometimes shortened dramatically, a point that is underscored, by the birth of babies underwater; in Odent's clinic there were no adverse effects to mother or baby.[27] The heat and water exert a soothing action on the cutaneous nerve endings and all organs with which the skin is in reflex connection.[23] In addition, the thermal effects of the warm bath cause vasodilation, increased urine output, and promote psychologic and physiologic relaxation.[17]

Risks. The risks of bathing in labor are scientifically unknown at this time. There is a possibility that infection may be passed from the tub bath water to the vagina. Although this is no longer a concern during pregnancy, it warrants consideration in labor, particularly if the mucous plug has been discharged or the membranes are ruptured. The research presently underway in the United States and other countries needs to be thoroughly examined before maternal body immersion in a warm bath becomes a standard procedure. The only physical risk to a shower in labor might be if the woman were to slip and fall, an event that could happen at home as well but would be better controlled in a birth setting because she would not be unattended.

Fetal Monitoring. The fetal heart is assessed for tone (FHT) and rate (FHR). In this text, FHT refers to the ausculated sound, and FHR refers to the electronic tracing.

Ausculation of Fetal Heart Tones

Indications. In low-risk women having a normal birth, the FHTs as well as fetal movement and uterine contractions can be determined using the human senses of hearing and touch, coupled with use of equipment such as fetoscope or Doppler device for auscultation of FHTs.

Procedure/Nursing Care. To auscultate FHTs, the nurse places the fetoscope or Doppler device on the mother's abdomen over the shoulder or back area of the fetus (doing Leopold's maneuvers first as needed to determine fetal position and thereby the best place to listen for FHTs). The nurse listens for and counts FHTs at the end of and between contractions to determine fetal well-being. Listening at the end of contractions is also important because the nurse can pick up heart rate decelerations occurring with or at the end of the contractions, both of which are ominous signs.

It is recommended that the heart tones be auscultated every 30 minutes in the first phase of the first stage of labor, every 15 to 20 minutes in the active phases of the first stage, and every 5 minutes or after each contraction in second-stage labor. If abnormalities are noted, electronic monitoring can be used.

To obtain the greatest accuracy when using the fetoscope or Doppler device, the nurse needs to assess to the FHTs between contractions to obtain the fetal baseline and then during contractions to determine if the fetus is stressed during contractions. To obtain the best information on variability of the fetal heart, the nurse should count 5 seconds, wait 5 seconds, count 5 seconds, wait 5 seconds, and so on, until the end of the contraction. Looking at each count provides a better picture of how the fetus is reacting to the contraction, the variability of the fetal heart, and the occurrence of heart rate decelerations.

Benefits. Auscultation of FHTs is a noninvasive method, which is not restricting for the mother and is relatively easy to use for the nurse. It is also inexpensive as the care provider is already present. This method also ensures that the nurse will be close by the woman frequently during labor. The cesarean delivery rates for women who are monitored by auscultation are significantly lower than those for women who are electronically monitored. Women who are auscultated also have lower infection rates with no increase in neonatal problems.[28–30] Use of the fetoscope, specifically, avoids exposure to ultrasound in labor.

Risks. One drawback to auscultation as a method of fetal monitoring is that the mother or support person may not be able to hear the FHTs. Many couples relate that hearing FHTs during labor reassures them of fetal well-being. There is also no permanent record of the FHT other than the nurse's note, and monitoring is intermittent rather than continuous.

Use of auscultation as a method of fetal monitoring may increase the risk of perinatal mortality in some situations. For example, fetal distress might occur in the intervals between the times the heart rate is listened to, but this would not be detected by human auscultation. The nurse using a fetoscope would not be likely to hear the FHT during the contraction and, therefore, could miss late decelerations, the most ominous of the heart rate decelerations. There is also the possibility of human error in hearing and counting FHTs. They might be confused with placental souffle, cord pulse, or maternal heart rate. A large study done in Ireland by MacDonald and colleagues[31] showed no difference in perinatal mortality between the auscultated and electronically monitored groups,[31] but did show an increased incidence in neonatal seizures (suggesting undetected fetal hypoxic episodes in labor).

An additional risk of auscultation may occur if the nurse uses a Doppler device to obtain FHTs rather than a fetoscope, namely, the still unknown risk associated with the ultrasound. Ultrasound is a relatively new diagnostic technique that is now replacing former diagnostic methods, such as x-ray. There is a lack of completed research on latent or long-term effects of ultrasound on humans, although, to date, no adverse effects have been noted. When tested on animals in the laboratory, cell damage and genetic alterations appear to result from ultrasound at levels much higher than that used in clinical obstetric situations. The levels of ultrasound used in a Doppler device or electronic monitor are small, but some practitioners are concerned that these effects, whatever they might be, could be cumulative. Until conclusive evidence is reported, it is wise to use any ultrasonic diagnostic tool with some caution.[32,33]

Electronic Fetal Monitoring

Indications. Electronic fetal monitoring is indicated either if the woman did not have a normal pregnancy or if she is not having a normal labor and the fetus has or is demonstrating abnormalities. Maternal conditions indicating use of electronic monitoring include maternal hypertension, diabetes, renal or cardiac disease, blood abnormalities or bleeding, previous uterine surgery, anesthesia, induced or augmented labor, poor obstetric history, infection, and abnormal labor patterns. Fetal conditions requiring use of electronic monitoring include meconium-stained fluid, abnormal heart rate, abnormal presentation, prematurity, growth retardation, and postmaturity.

Procedure/Nursing Care. The procedure for electronic fetal monitoring varies depending on whether it is external or internal or a combination of both.

Continuous external monitoring involves the use of an electronic monitoring machine attached to two belts that are placed on the woman's abdomen to record the FHR and the uterine contractions. To obtain the FHR, these steps are followed:

1. The nurse explains the procedure and obtains the woman's consent.
2. All of the necessary equipment is gathered, namely, fetal monitor, ultrasound transducer, tocodynamometer, ultrasonic gel, and abdominal belts.
3. The nurse places the belts around the woman while she is in a semilateral position (ie, head of bed raised, with the woman on her left side).
4. The ultrasonic cable plug is inserted into the appropriate connector on the fetal monitor; the same is done for the tocodynamometer plug.
5. The power is turned on to elicit an audible response.
6. The nurse applies the gel to the underside of the transducer and places it on the mother's abdomen in the area where FHTs were previously heard. In a full-term cephalic presentation, this will be below the level of the umbilicus. In a full-term breech, this will be above the level of umbilicus.
7. The nurse moves the transducer to the place where the FHT signal is the loudest and, once found, secures the belt in place.
8. The tocodynamometer is placed on the woman's abdomen over the fundus in an area where the uterus would be closest to the pressure-sensing button. The belt is secured. Beltless tocotransducers are now available. These devices use adhesive base plates to secure the transducer.
9. After the recorder is set to a 3 cm/min paper speed, the nurse observes the FHR on the strip chart. The baseline FHR is obtained between contractions. To interpret FHR patterns, it is necessary to have the monitor simultaneously record the contraction pattern. The pen-set knob should be adjusted between contractions to make the stylet print out at about the 20-mm-Hg line on the strip paper. This establishes a baseline and can be tested by applying some pressure on the woman's abdomen. The stylet should show an increase in pressure just as it should when the woman has a contraction. The tocodynamometer does not measure intensity of contraction; only an internal uterine catheter can measure the intrauterine pressure of contractions.
10. The nurse depresses the test button and makes a notation on the strip chart that this was done.

11. On the paper strip, the nurse charts the woman's name, identification number, date, time the monitor was attached and type of monitoring, any risk conditions, status of fetal membranes, gestational age/EDC, dilation and effacement, maternal temperature, pulse, respirations, blood pressure, maternal position, IV, medications, maternal activity, fetal movements, and any change of equipment. These items should be charted at the start of the monitor strip and as each item is done or noted in the course of providing care. All of this information also should be charted.

Continuous internal monitoring involves an electrode attached to the fetal scalp and a uterine pressure catheter placed inside the uterine cavity, both of which are attached to the electronic monitoring machine providing a continuous paper readout of FHR and intrauterine pressure (Figure 27–12). The mother may also be attached to a telemetry unit (if the hospital has one), which allows more freedom of movement while still recording FHR and maternal uterine contractions. The procedure for inserting the fetal electrode is as follows:

1. The nurse explains the procedure and obtains informed consent from the woman.
2. The nurse gathers the necessary equipment, namely, fetal monitor, disposable spiral electrode, leg plate with cable, leg plate strap, electrode paste, disposable intrauterine catheter kit, strain gauge, injectable sterile distilled water, three-way stopcock, 10-mL syringe, 18-gauge 1½-in. sterile needle, two sterile towels, sterile gloves of appropriate size, and any other items necessary for a sterile vaginal examination.
3. The nurse positions the leg plate strap around the woman's thigh, using a small amount of electrode paste on the leg plate, and secures it.
4. The cable is inserted into the fetal monitor electrocardiograph connection.
5. The physician or nurse-midwife inserts the fetal electrode and intrauterine catheter using the following procedure:

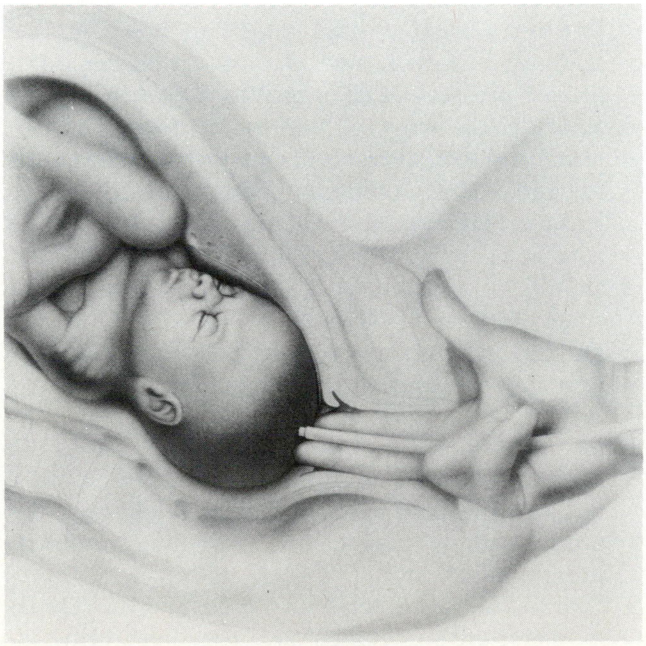

Figure 27–12. Continuous internal fetal monitoring. (Courtesy of Corometrics Medical Systems, Wallingford, Conn.)

- *Uterine catheter.* Prior to insertion, the uterine catheter is filled with sterile water. To insert the uterine catheter, the physician or nurse-midwife puts the catheter into the introducer and then positions his or her fingers at the posterior section of the cervix, gently guiding the introducer to the fingertip but no further. The catheter is then gently advanced through the introducer, past the fingertips into the uterine cavity. It is advanced only to the 18-cm. mark on the catheter. The nurse then removes the needle adaptor from the end of the catheter so that the physician or nurse-midwife can slide the introducer back over the catheter. The stopcock must be positioned to allow filling of the dome and flushing of the catheter. The catheter is flushed with 5 to 10 mL of sterile water to remove any air bubbles. The woman is asked to bear down, which should give a reading above zero and indicate the patency of the catheter. The catheter is then taped to the leg to ensure it is not accidently pulled out.
- *Fetal electrode.* To apply the fetal scalp electrode, the physician or nurse-midwife first performs a sterile vaginal examination using a bactericidal solution as a lubricant and cleansing agent for the fetal scalp. An amniotomy is done if the membranes are intact. The physician or nurse-midwife advances the inserter with the electrode in it to the fingertips. The fingers are positioned over the fetal skull away from the fontanelles. The electrode is then placed against the fetal scalp and the drive tube rotated clockwise to insert the electrode into the scalp. The physician or nurse-midwife next releases the lock on the drive tube and slides the inserter back over the electrode wires and out of the vagina. Finally,

the wires are attached to the leg plate (following the color codes) and the leg plate wires to the monitor, and the recorder is turned on.

6. The nurse turns the power on and observes the oscilloscope for the fetal electrocardiogram. The machine must be allowed to warm up if it has not been in use recently.
7. The recorder paper is set to a 3 cm/min paper speed; the nurse then observes the FHR and uterine contraction pattern on the strip chart.
8. The button is depressed to produce a test pattern. A notation is made indicating that this was done.
9. On the paper strip, the nurse charts the woman's name, identification number, date, time the monitor was attached and type of monitoring, any risk conditions, status of fetal membranes, gestational age/EDC, dilation and effacement, maternal vital signs, maternal position, IV, medications, maternal activity, fetal movements, and any change of equipment. These items should be charted at the start of the monitor strip and as each item is done or noted in the course of providing care. All of this information should also be charted in the nurse's notes.

Benefits. Continuous electronic monitoring provides a constant readout of the FHR and uterine contractions. This allows the nurse to monitor such details as beat-to-beat variability of the FHR and late or variable decelerations of the FHR, both of which are not easily obtainable by any other means. Poor beat-to-beat variability and late or variable decelerations are indicative of possible fetal distress, and early diagnosis allows the practitioner to investigate further or provide treatment. With continuous monitoring, it may also be possible to diagnose false labor, to perform nonstress or stress testing, and to reassure the mother by having a visual and auditory record of the FHR.

With the fetal monitor in place, the mother or her labor support person can see that contractions are starting even before the woman may feel it. This can be very helpful to the coach, as he or she can alert the mother and she can prepare herself for the contraction by relaxation and breathing techniques. Each method of continuous monitoring has specific benefits:

1. *External monitoring.* A non-invasive procedure but the nurse still can obtain a continuous readout of the FHR and uterine contractions.
2. *Internal monitoring.* The nurse can obtain the beat-to-beat variability and more accurate FHR tracing, and can obtain actual readings of the uterine pressure, which are important when labor is induced or augmented.
3. *Combination.* A combination of internal fetal electrode and external tocodynamometer monitoring is often used, particularly if the FHR is difficult to obtain or there is a question about the external fetal tracing. Frequently, it is the FHR that is the more difficult to obtain externally and the fetal electrode is relatively easy to apply. Thus, an accurate FHR can be obtained without invasion of the uterus by the uterine catheter.

Risks. Electronic monitoring is associated with high cesarean delivery rates, without documented maternal or neonatal benefits to justify the increased rate. Increased mechanization also has led to decreased personal care. At times more attention may be paid to the monitor than to the client. In addition, the long-term effects of ultrasound use in fetal monitoring are unknown. The presence of the machine, straps, and cables tends to make the woman and her family feel that birth is an abnormal event. This equipment also keeps the woman in bed and often on her back. The machinery is expensive to buy and maintain and it takes skilled professionals to read the tracings accurately. Some women have negative reactions to being monitored electronically and being confined to a machine for an extended period. The three methods of continuous monitoring are associated with these specific drawbacks or risks:

1. *External monitoring.* The nurse obtains a relative picture of what is happening but not a precise reading; however, one cannot determine intrauterine pressure at all or beat-to-beat variability as accurately as with the internal monitor. The maternal and fetal movements may require the straps to be moved each time the mother or fetus moves and the FHR can often be detected best when the mother is on her back, the precise position that should be avoided by a laboring woman. Even small maternal movements show up on the graphs, and in obese women the contraction pattern may be difficult to obtain, thereby making interpretation more difficult at times.
2. *Internal monitoring.* This procedure is invasive. The membranes must be ruptured and the scalp electrode can lead to infection of the fetal scalp; the uterine catheter may lead to uterine perforation or uterine infection.
3. *Combination.* The fetal electrode and tocodynamometer are sometimes used together during induction or augmentation of labor. They do not, however, provide sufficient information concern-

ing the strength of the contraction. The practitioner must know the strength of the contraction to determine whether more or less oxytocin is needed and thereby ensure that the woman receives enough medication for a good trial of labor, but not so much as to rupture her uterus.

Parameters of Fetal Heart Rate Tracing. Several parameters of the FHR tracing are assessed.

Baseline Fetal Heart Rate. The baseline FHR is the average rate assessed when the mother is not in labor or is between contractions. The baseline FHR is usually between 120 and 160 beats per minute. The baseline FHR is the least sensitive indicator of fetal distress. A compromised fetus could have a normal baseline rate. Conversely, changes in the baseline should be considered a possible sign of fetal distress. The baseline fetal heart rate is assessed using the following criteria.[15, 34]

- *Normal range:* 120 to 160 beats per minute
- *Tachycardia*
  Mild: 161 to 180 beats per minute
  Severe: greater than 180 beats per minute
- *Bradycardia*
  Mild: 90 to 119 beats per minute
  Moderate: 70 to 89 beats per minute
  Severe: less than 70 beats per minute

To be accepted as a baseline change, the change in FHR should be sustained for more than 10 to 15 minutes.

Baseline Beat-to-Beat Variation. The normal FHR has a beat-to-beat variability of 6 to 25 beats per minute. This beat-to-beat variability in labor indicates that the fetus has an intact central nervous system that is capable of controlling the FHR during contractions.

Variability of the baseline FHR is a more significant parameter of fetal well-being than is assessment of the baseline alone. Baseline variability of the FHR may be divided into two types.[15]

Short-term variability (STV) is an indication of the normal variance in intervals between successive cardiac cycles. It is not as useful an assessment parameter as long-term variability because it is difficult to identify.

Long-term variability (LTV) is an indication of the cumulative changes in the FHR occurring over 6 to 30 seconds. It is recognized by the waviness of the FHR tracing. The usual frequency is 3 to 5 cycles per second, with an amplitude of at least 6 beats per minute, lasting at least 5 seconds. Artificial increases in the LTV may occur with external monitoring.

Interpretation of Long-Term Variability. When the amplitude of the cycle exceeds 30 beats per minute, the long-term variability is said to be increased. Possible explanations include mild fetal hypoxia, fetal hemorrhage, and compression of the umbilical cord.

A decrease in the long-term variability may be related to fetal hypoxia, physiologic sleep cycle, central nervous system–depressing drugs, or parasympatholytic or sympatholytic drugs.

Another pattern to evaluate is a baseline FHR that is persistently flat, although within the normal range. This pattern may be caused by congenital anomalies of the cardiac or central nervous systems, prematurity, or previous hypoxia, or it may be idiopathic.[15] Figure 27–13 illustrates FHR baselines and variability.

Fetal Heart Rate Accelerations. Fetal heart rates accelerate above the baseline in response to fetal movement. Fetal heart rate accelerations during labor occur in early labor normally. They may also coincide with variable FHR decelerations. Fetal heart rate accelerations occurring in the antepartum period or in early labor represent intact neurologic functioning of the fetus. If they occur and are accompanied by a variable deceleration rate, they can indicate compression of the umbilical cord, causing decreased fetal cardiac output.

Fetal Heart Rate Decelerations. A decrease in the FHR below the baseline in response to uterine contractions is referred to as a FHR deceleration. Fetal heart rate decelerations may be classified according to their shape and their timing specific to the uterine contractions (*see* Figure 27-14). The following classification may be used[15]:

- *Uniform:* The FHR pattern relates to the uterine contraction. Subcategories would be early decelerations and late decelerations.
- *Variable.* There is no relationship between the uterine contraction and the FHR.

Early Decelerations. Early decelerations of the FHR have the following characteristics[15,34]:

1. The curve has a uniform shape that remains the same from contraction to contraction.
2. The pattern of the FHR is like that of the contraction.
3. The onset of the deceleration occurs early in the contraction.
4. The nadir of the deceleration occurs at the peak of the contraction.

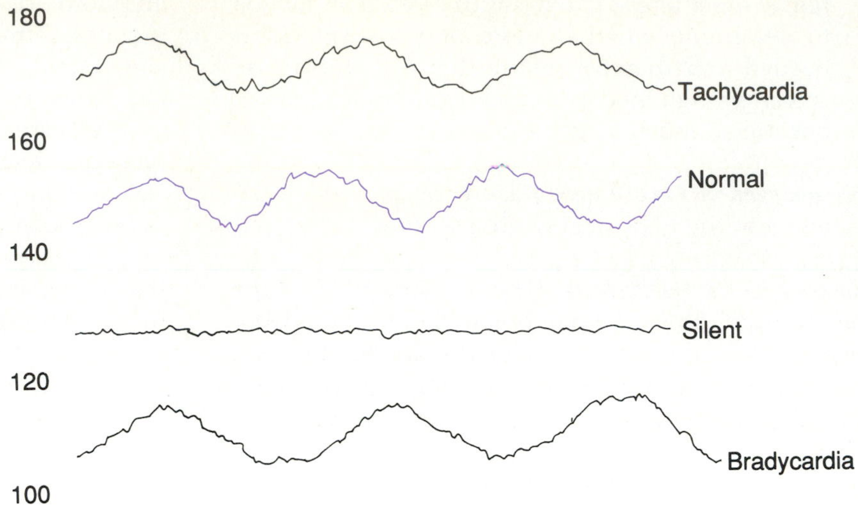

Figure 27–13. Fetal heart rate baselines and variability. (*Reproduced, with permission, from Oxorn H, ed.* Oxorn-Foote Human Labor and Birth. *5th ed. Norwalk, Conn: Appleton-Century-Crofts; 1986: 623.*)

5. The FHR returns to the baseline before the contraction ends.
6. The lowest amplitude is proportional to the strength of the contraction.
7. Baseline FHR usually does not fall below 100 beats per minute.
8. Baseline beat-to-beat variability is maintained.

Early decelerations are transient decelerations that usually occur in the later stages of labor and do not indicate fetal distress. They usually occur as a result of pressure on the fetal skull, and no treatment is indicated.

Late Decelerations. Late decelerations of the FHR are usually an ominous sign. Late decelerations have the following characteristics[15, 34]:

1. The curve has a uniform shape that remains the same from contraction to contraction.
2. The onset of the deceleration occurs late in the uterine contraction (after the acme).
3. The FHR does not return to baseline until after the uterine contraction ends.
4. The interval between the peak of the uterine contraction and the lowest level of the FHR is longer than 20 seconds.
5. The duration of the deceleration is proportional to that of the uterine contraction.
6. The amplitude of the deceleration is proportional to the strength of the contraction.
7. The pattern is repetitive and the deceleration is usually 20 to 30 beats per minute.

Late decelerations of the FHR may indicate uteroplacental insufficiency, which causes a reduction in the fetal Po_2. Uteroplacental insufficiency may be caused by maternal supine hypotension, maternal dehydration, hyperstimulation of the uterus with oxytoxic agents, fetal growth retardation, postmaturity, and abruptio placentae.

If late decelerations are noted, the nurse may turn the mother on her side and discontinue the use of oxytoxic agents for stimulation of labor. Administration of oxygen to the mother may also be helpful. The pattern of late decelerations should be reported. If they persist for over 15 minutes or are accompanied by decreased FHR variability, delivery may be indicated.

Variable Decelerations. Variable decelerations occur at any time during a contraction and may be associated with cord compression. Variable decelerations have the following characteristics[15, 34]:

1. The decelerations have variable shape and form that differ from one deceleration to the next.
2. The onset of the deceleration with regard to the contraction is variable.
3. The interval between the peak of the uterine contraction and the FHR at its lowest level is variable.
4. There is variability in amplitude and duration of the deceleration.
5. They do not have to be repetitive.
6. They are frequently followed by accelerations of the FHR.

Variable decelerations may be caused by cord compression as the fetus descends into the birth canal. They may be seen with breech presentations because of the possibility of prolapse of the cord. They may also be noted with occipitoposterior positions that are not accompanied by compression of the cord. The distinguishing feature between the two (cord compression and no cord compression) is that variable decelerations with cord compression are usually followed by FHR accelerations. Variable decelerations associated with occipitoposterior positions are usually benign. Other criteria that indicate that the variable deceleration is benign include an FHR deceleration lasting no longer than 45 seconds on a repetitive basis, an abrupt return of the FHR to the baseline, a baseline rate that does not increase, and a baseline variability that does not decrease.[15]

Management varies according to the interpretation of the cause of the variable decelerations and the stage of labor that the mother is in. If the mother is in early labor and the cause is thought to be cord compression, then delivery by cesarean section may be indicated, whereas the mother who is in the second stage of labor may be delivered vaginally. If the nurse suspects a prolapsed cord, the mother may be placed in a knee-chest position to take pressure off the cord, and administered oxygen until delivery can be accomplished (*see* Chapter 40 for further discussion). For variable decelerations that are considered benign, no treatment is indicated. Figure 27–14 illustrates deceleration patterns of the FHR.

Fetal Scalp pH Sampling

Indications. Fetal blood pH levels are obtained only when there are indications of fetal distress such as late or severe variable decelerations, bradycardia, tachycardia, loss of beat-to-beat variability, marked meconium staining, and previous pH levels of 7.20 to 7.25 (normal pH is 7.26 and above; pH levels 7.20 to 7.25 are borderline suspicious for acidosis; pH levels below 7.15 indicate acidosis).

Fetal scalp pH sampling is not done when the membranes are intact and the woman is not in active labor; when the FHR shows very ominous signs that do not respond to treatment; when placenta previa, abruptio placentae, or face presentation occurs; and when the woman refuses to have the procedure performed on her fetus. Some new fetal monitoring machines are being tested that perform continuous pH testing through the fetal scalp electrode.

Procedure/Nursing Care. For scalp pH sampling, the membranes must be ruptured and the cervix at least 1 to 2 cm dilated, with the presenting part at least at −2 station and readily available.

The nurse should have the following equipment available: rod with 2-mm blade, three heparinized long tubes, magnet, four internal magnetic string rods, sealing wax for tubes, conical endoscope with a light source, two long cotton swabs, appropriate-size sterile gloves for the practitioner, two pair of sterile ring forceps, five 4 × 4 sterile gauze sponges, sterile silicone ointment, small basin with ice, sterile towel on which to set the equipment, and transport tube.

The nurse sets up the equipment in a sterile manner, places the client in lithotomy or left lateral position, and continues to monitor maternal vital signs, contractions, and FHR throughout the procedure. The nurse also assists with handling the light source, capillary tubes, and transport tubing and ensures that the specimens get to the lab quickly.

Once the client is in position, the physician puts on sterile gloves and inserts the endoscope into the vagina, guiding it with his or her fingers. The fetal presenting part is cleansed with bactericidal solution and sterile 4 × 4 gauze sponges. Next, the physician applies silicone ointment to the area of choice, punctures the area with the sterile 2-mm blade, and collects blood samples with the long heparinized capillary tubes, sealing the end of the tube with wax or clay. The puncture site is then cleaned with sterile gauze on the ring forceps, and pressure is applied to the site for 2 minutes. After checking the puncture site for bleeding, the physician removes the endoscope.

The physician may also request that a sample of maternal peripheral blood be sent to the lab with the fetal blood to determine whether a base deficit exists. Throughout the procedure, the nurse explains to the woman and her support persons what is happening, and at the end returns the woman to a position of comfort.

Benefits. Scalp pH sampling is another tool that can be used in determining fetal well-being. It is used to confirm a diagnosis of fetal distress when other signs seem to point to that fact. It is a direct (via blood) rather than indirect (FHR) way to determine if the fetus is having difficulty. It can "buy" time for the practitioner to wait for a vaginal delivery if the fetus has an acceptable pH, but it may also indicate the need for immediate cesarean delivery.

It may be necessary to obtain several samples to determine if the pH is decreasing or remaining stable.

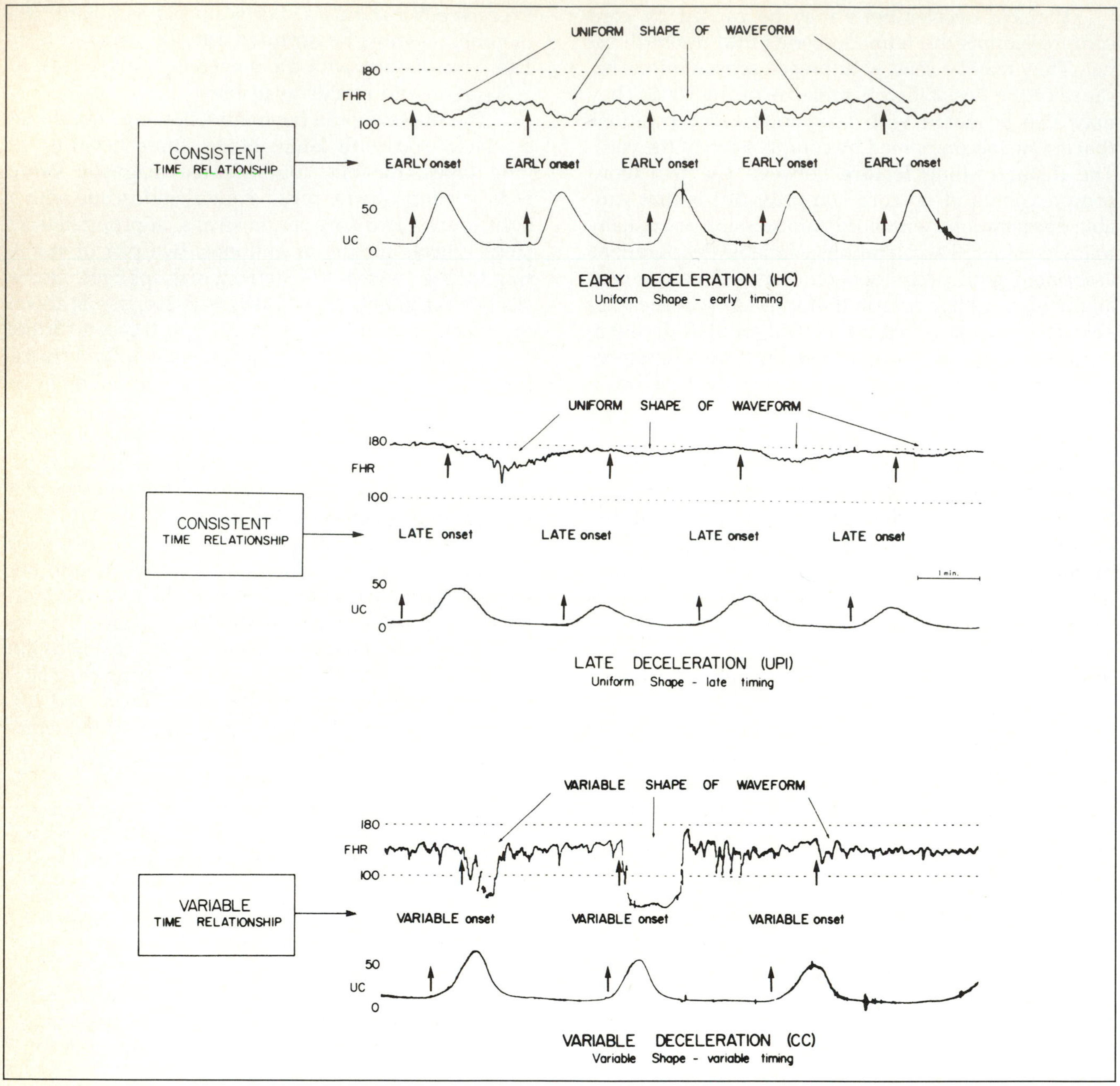

Figure 27–14. Fetal heart rate decelerations. (*Reproduced, with permission, from Hon:* An Atlas of Fetal Heart Rate Patterns. *New Haven, Conn: Harty, 1968.*)

It is also important for the hospital lab to report the pH levels quickly and accurately.

Risks. Fetal scalp pH sampling is an invasive procedure that requires a practitioner well trained in fetal blood scalp sampling technique, as well as quick laboratory results. The fetus faces the risk of excessive bleeding from the puncture site and the risk of infection, either at the puncture site or from the rupture of membranes.[7]

Induction or Augmentation of Labor

Indications. **Induction** is the process of starting labor artificially by the use of medications, primarily oxytocin (Pitocin) (Box 27–1). **Augmentation** is the

BOX 27–1. OXYTOCIN

Proprietary Names:
Pitocin (Park-Davis); Syntocinon (Sandoz); oxytocin injection, LypoMed (Wyeth-Ayerst).

Classification:
Ocytocic.

Action:
Synthetically produced hormone similar to endogenous hormone produced by the posterior pituitary gland. Stimulates contraction of the uterine smooth muscle. Also facilitates milk ejection in lactating women.

Indications:
Induction of labor in clinical situations where prolongation of labor may be harmful to fetus, mother, or both. Augmentation of contractions in first and second stages of labor if labor is prolonged or dysfunctional uterine inertia occurs. Management of postpartum bleeding.

Route and Dosage:
Administered intravenously or intramuscularly. Dosage determined by uterine response. *Induction of labor:* 1 mU/min and increased at 15-minute intervals by 1 mU/min until desired response. *Augmentation of labor:* 2 mU/min. *Postpartum bleeding:* 10–40 U added to 1000 mL nonhydrating diluent to control uterine atony.

Pharmacokinetics:
Absorption: Not absorbed orally. *Distribution:* Throughout extracellular fluid. Small amount distributes into fetal circulation. *Elimination:* Rapidly metabolized by liver and kidneys with half-life of 3 to 5 minutes.

Contraindictions/Precautions:
Contraindicated for induction of labor in cases of CPD, unfavorable fetal position, or uterine scarring from previous surgery or when vaginal delivery is contraindicated. Use caution in fetal distress, partial placenta previa, prematurity, overdistension of uterus, grand multiparity, or history of uterine sepsis of traumatic delivery.

Adverse Reactions:
Maternal: With large doses or in sensitive clients, hyperstimulation of uterus with strong and prolonged contractions, which could result in uterine rupture, postpartum hemorrhage, abruptio placentae, impaired fetal blood flow. Also, hypotension, tachycardia, cardiac arrhythmias. *Fetal:* With excessive maternal doses, sinus bradycardia, cardiac arrhythmias, brain damage, intraventricular hemorrhage, death from asphyxia.

Drug Interaction:
Cyclopropane or vasoconstrictive drugs: more pronounced hypotension and bradycardia.

Nursing Implications:

Labor and Delivery

- Assess and record maternal blood pressure and vital signs, intake-output ratio, nature of uterine contraction, FHR, and FHT.
- Careful control and monitoring of infusion is essential.
- Use Y-connection so that infusion with oxytocin can be discontinued while keeping vein open.
- If contractions occur at less than 2-minute intervals or last 90 seconds or longer, or if monitor records contractions at about 50 mm Hg, stop infusion to prevent fetal anoxia, turn client on left side, give oxygen if necessary, and report.

Postpartum

- During delivery, IV oxytoxin may be continued or IM oxytocin is easily injected deep into deltoid muscle; massage injection site for quick absorption.
- Fundus should be checked frequently during first few postpartum hours and several times daily thereafter.

General
Oxytocin administration should be supervised by persons having thorough knowledge of the drug and the skill to identify complications.

Nursing implications are adapted from Govoni LE, Hayes JE. Drugs and Nursing Implications. *6th ed. Norwalk, Conn: Appleton & Lange; 1988:885–886.*

stimulation of labor once natural labor has begun and can be done by means of oxytocin or breast stimulation.

Some practitioners also believe that amniotomy and enema stimulate labor. In the case of amniotomy, this has not been scientifically proven.[8] In the case of enema, the mechanism is not clear but may involve the release of prostaglandin or the irritated bowel may stimulate the uterus; however, neither of these mechanisms has been thoroughly investigated.

Procedure/Nursing Care. If the woman is being considered for induction the practitioner first determines whether the client is inducible. A scoring system, for example, the Burnett scale or Bishop score, is often used, noting cervical dilation, effacement, position of cervix, consistency of cervix, and station of fetal head, to determine whether the client's condition is favorable for induction. On the Burnett scale each item is rated from 0 to 2, with a total score of 0 to 5 carrying risk to mother and fetus, and 5 to 10 increasing chance of delivery within 6 hours if adequate oxytocin is given.

If induction is decided on, the membranes are ruptured, a fetal monitor is attached, and an intravenous infusion consisting of 1000 mL of Ringer's lactate or saline with 10 U of oxytocin diluted in it is set up. Ideally an internal electronic fetal monitoring system is used as soon as it can be safely applied. This is the only method that detects intrauterine pressure, which is necessary to determine if adequate or excessive oxytocin is being administered.

Two intravenous bottles are required, one containing the oxytocin and the other with no drug in it. The second bottle is needed in case the oxytocin must be stopped or other medications or blood need to be administered to the woman. The intravenous line attached to the oxytocin should be attached to an infusion pump to ensure that the correct amount of drug is administered to the woman. The bottle containing the oxytocin must be labeled with the name of the drug and the number of units.

The intravenous line should be inserted ideally in the forearm, using an angiocath or the like, approximately 18 gauge in size. This allows the client freedom of movement and, once inserted, is usually more comfortable and reliable than a plain needle.

If it is done artificially, augmentation is achieved using the same procedure described for induction, but without the need of the scoring system. Augmentation can also be done "naturally" by nipple stimulation, which is similar to the procedure used in the contraction stress test antepartally (*see* Chapter 22), except that in this case the stimulation is continued until a good labor pattern is established.

Benefits. Induction can be very helpful for women who are postdates; for women with pre-eclampsia, Rh incompatibility, or diabetes; and for fetuses who are intrauterine-growth-retarded, because in these cases the risk of induction is less than the problems associated with letting the pregnancy continue.

Augmentation has about the same benefits as induction, but additionally, because labor has already started, there is less probability of complications resulting specifically from the induction process. With augmentation through nipple stimulation there is also a decreased risk, as no drugs are involved.

Risks. Induction and augmentation are sometimes contraindicated when the mother has a contracted pelvis, scarred uterus, overdistended uterus (multiple fetuses or polyhydramnios), grand multiparity, prematurity, and acute fetal distress. Complications from these procedures include hypertonic uterus and hypertonic contractions, fetal distress, uterine rupture, iatrogenic prematurity of the fetus, and neonatal jaundice. In addition, breast stimulation as a form of augmentation has only recently been used on a large scale so that the best procedures, precautions, and risks are not well documented.

Rupture of the Membranes. Membranes may rupture as a normal, natural event during labor; thus, there are no "indications, benefits, or risks" to consider as there are with the other interventions. Nursing care, however, is involved.

Nursing Care. When the membranes rupture, a gush of amniotic fluid may soak the absorbent pads that have been placed beneath the woman's hips. The nurse should immediately take the FHT, note change in fetal station as described by the examiner, and note the color, quantity (estimated), and odor (or lack of it) of this fluid when rupture of membranes occurs.

The FHR is of primary concern. A forceful gush of amniotic fluid could permit a loop of umbilical cord to slide between the fetal presenting part and the maternal pelvis. Subsequent cord compression would compromise oxygenation of the fetus, resulting in fetal bradycardia.

In addition, the mother's wet bed linens and bed clothes need to be changed as quickly as possible. Charting involves the date and time at which the membranes ruptured, the color and consistency of the fluid, and the fetal heart rate. This information is placed on the client's chart and graph paper if the electronic monitor is used.

Amniotomy

Indications. Artificial rupture of the fetal membranes in labor is done to prevent the fetus from aspirating amniotic fluid with meconium at delivery (the exact mechanism or timing of this complication is not clearly known), to permit internal fetal monitoring, and to induce or augment labor. It is contraindicated when the presenting part is not engaged, when the woman is not in active labor (unless this is for induction), in funic (cord) presentation, or in placenta previa.

Procedure/Nursing Care. The purpose of amniotomy is to rupture the membranes without complications. The following equipment is needed: sterile gloves, bacteriostatic cleansing solution, bed pan, incontinent pads, fetoscope or fetal monitor, sterile gauze pads, and sterile Allis clamp or amniohook.

The nurse explains the procedure to the woman, listens to the FHTs, and puts the woman on the bedpan. After donning sterile gloves (a mask is worn as well for protection of health care staff against hepatitis and human immunodeficiency virus transmission as a result of fluid contact with the mucous membranes), the nurse washes the perineum with the bactericidal solution and then empties the bedpan (this ensures that the color of the cleansing solution does not interfere with color determination of the amniotic fluid). The physician or nurse-midwife performs a vaginal examination, and then ruptures the forewaters with the amniohook or Allis clamp, keeping the hand in the vagina and slowly letting the fluid out (Figure 27–15), while noting the color, consistency, and volume of fluid and ensuring that there is not a prolapse of the umbilical cord. If the electronic monitor is not already attached, the nurse listens to the FHT with a fetoscope or Doppler stethoscope. The nurse then cleanses and dries the woman, removes the bedpan, places an absorbent pad under her, and charts the date, time, and results of the procedure and the FHT before and after the procedure. If an electronic monitor has been used, the date, time, and results of the procedure should also be noted on the graph paper.

Benefits. Amniotomy allows internal electronic monitoring and scalp pH sampling and permits the practitioner to view the amniotic fluid directly to ensure there is no meconium, which might indicate fetal distress. Controversy exists about whether amniotomy actually quickens the pace of labor. One early study[35] and one more recent study[8] have shown variously that there is no effect and that the first stage of labor may be shortened by 61.5 minutes with early amniotomy.

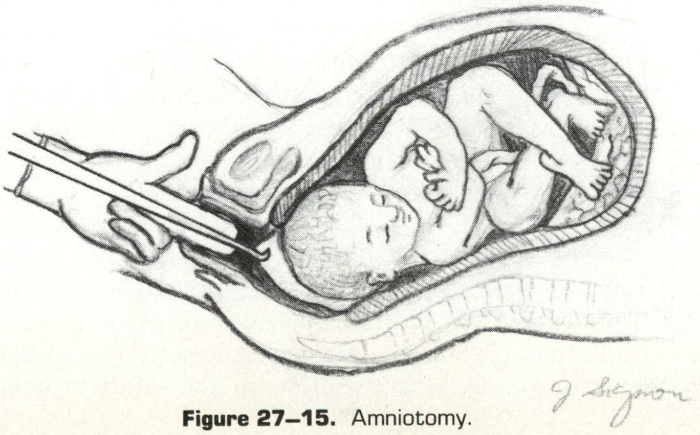

Figure 27–15. Amniotomy.

Risks. One drawback associated with amniotomy is that clients report these labors as more difficult and painful (they are sometimes called a "dry birth," which is a misnomer). Discomfort may be increased because the greater direct pressure of the presenting head against the cervix stimulates the Ferguson reflex (mechanical stretching of the cervix enhancing uterine activity, which stimulates uterine contractions[25]); the decreased volume shortens the myometrial fibers, which stimulates uterine activity; and the decreased uterine blood flow causes increased uterine activity.

Other risks include possible prolapse of the umbilical cord and infection. Once the membranes are ruptured the seal to the fetus and uterus from the outside world is broken and the risk of infection increases significantly after 48 hours. For this reason if the woman does not show adequate progress in her labor by 12 hours some practitioners may be very aggressive in stimulating contractions with oxytocin to ensure a delivery by 24 hours. If she does not deliver by then, the practitioner may perform a cesarean delivery. This aggressive approach is controversial and the protocols vary in different institutions.

The risk of infection increases significantly after 48 hours for both mother and baby and this type of infection can be extremely difficult to treat and dangerous for the mother. Some studies have also shown that early rupture of membranes can lengthen the labor, lower the fetal scalp pH, increase the number of FHR decelerations, increase caput succedaneum, and increase cranial bone disalignment.[8]

Positions for Labor and Birth. Nursing care of the mother during the intrapartum period also includes helping the mother assume positions for labor and birth.

Indications. The position that the woman takes for the labor and birth is determined by a number of factors: custom, comfort, fetal status, force of uterine contractions, and the need for the nurse to do certain procedures (eg, listen to FHTs). Earlier in this chapter it was pointed out that the woman should not lie on her back in labor for prolonged periods because of the negative effects of the supine hypotension syndrome on the mother and fetus. In terms of efficiency of uterine contractions and overall reported maternal comfort, the best positions for labor, in descending order, are upright, sitting, lying on left side, and lying on the right side.[11]

For delivery the woman should take the position that provides for the most comfort while working with the forces of gravity and labor. Effective positions for pushing include sitting up while pushing, lying on the left side with head elevated while pushing, on hands and knees or squatting, or even standing. Lying flat on the back is the least effective method.[36]

Procedure/Nursing Care. During labor the woman is encouraged to take the position of greatest comfort and not to feel confined to one position. During monitoring the woman could be in a sitting position in bed or in a chair near the bed. The electronic fetal monitor is adjusted to meet the client's comfort; the woman is not positioned to facilitate use of the machine. If monitoring is continuous the woman should still be able to move about in or around the bed or nearby chair. If internal electronic monitoring is used, the woman can be hooked up to telemetry so that she can also be walking. If the client is up walking in active labor she should be accompanied by a support person who can assist her during contractions.

Benefits. Allowing the woman to assume various positions of comfort, particularly positions in which she is up walking, increases the efficiency of uterine contractions leading to a shorter labor, while simultaneously providing more comfort and less need for pain medication. An upright position in labor has fewer side effects for the fetus; in fact, fetal complications such as hypoxia, bradycardia and acidosis are noted in the supine or dorsal positions but not as frequently in the upright position. The position for delivery must also be considered as well as the amount of maternal effort used in the second or pushing phase of labor. Left lateral, semisitting, or squatting are the best positions because they allow for the most efficient maternal effort with the fewest side effects to mother or fetus.[37,38]

Risks. The risks of various maternal positions depend on how physiologic and physically safe a position is to a woman at a particular phase in her labor. More research is needed regarding how positions influence the progress of labor, but it is known that lying flat in bed throughout labor is the least physiologic position in terms of fetal and maternal outcomes. Another risk factor involves how well-balanced a woman in advanced active labor can be in the upright position, that is, her risk of falling.

NURSING CARE DURING THE SECOND STAGE OF LABOR

Nursing management for the childbearing family during the second stage of labor involves support and care through the so-called expulsive stage and culminates with the long-awaited birth of the baby (Figure 27–16). As with the first stage of labor, certain procedures may (or may not) be performed, depending on the birth setting; the wishes/needs of the mother, fetus, and family; and the treatment modalities of the practitioner.

Maternal Physiologic Response

Contractions in the second stage are intense, strong, and frequent and may reach a maximum duration of 90 seconds. Occurring every 2 to 3 minutes, contractions typically last 60 to 90 seconds. Assessment of the intensity and duration of the contraction is accomplished with a monitor or through palpation. Use of the monitor tape alone is not sufficient, as the urge (involuntary) to bear down or push that accompanies second-stage labor may distort the tracing through artifacts (false markings on the tape) or positioning.

Bloody show increases as capillaries are torn during descent. It must be emphasized that a flow of blood, spurting blood, or clotted blood is not a normal finding and requires that the nurse further assess the client and report the findings.

As the fetal head compresses the rectum, the laboring woman perceives the pressure as an urge to defecate. If feces are present in the rectum and descending colon, defecation frequently occurs, which may embarrass the mother. She should be reassurred that defecation is a sign that her bearing down efforts are effective, and hygienic care and quick replacement of padding should be provided between contractions.

If one were to stand outside the labor room where a woman in the expulsive stage of labor was being coached, activity strongly (and correctly) would suggest an athletic event. Although former nursing practice held that detailed bearing down instructions be given to the mother, the developing trend is to allow the mother to set her own bearing down pattern. Current research is being directed to these practices (*see* the Research Abstract at the end of Chapter 25).

The support person alerts the parturient (who may be sleeping between contractions) to the onset of contraction. The mother may require physical support of her back as she grasps her legs (or one of her legs, in a side-lying position) in the effort to bear down. The coach or support person may also provide the verbal encouragement for a long and strenuous expulsive effort, coupled with the maintained inspiration or a quick emptying and refill of the lungs. The deep involvement of support persons in this final predelivery stage will carry over into delivery if the professional staff refrains from displacing or replacing these valuable participants.

As a general rule, when birth is to occur in a hospital delivery room, the primigravida is usually allowed to labor until the caput (fetal scalp) appears, whereas the multigravida is moved to the delivery room earlier. The physician or nurse-midwife may indicate the stage and station at which the woman choosing a delivery room birth is to be transported, or the decision may be at the discretion of the nurse attending the client. Most practitioners prefer that the multigravida be transferred to the delivery room before the second stage. When delivery is planned in a birthing room or in the setting where the client has labored, she is spared the stress of movement and transfer to a delivery table.

Fetal Physiologic Response

Assessment of fetal well-being during the second stage of labor is continuous. Labor represents a stressor to the fetus, and although the body of the fetus is generally well adapted to withstand this stress, a primary goal of those caring for mother and baby is to minimize intrapartum risk and maximize optimal health. This goal is successfully achieved when the caregivers have utilized every means available to ensure that no sign of distress, regardless of how fleeting, is ignored, and that the client remains alert and informed.

Procedures and Treatments

As in the first stage, not all procedures are done in all settings, or for all clients. Two procedures that may be done are the episiotomy and the forceps/vacuum extraction. The nurse provides continuity of care throughout the birthing process and during possible operative obstetric procedures. Materials that may be available for the birth include forceps, stirrups, anesthesia sets, infant warmer, intubation and resuscitation supplies, infant identification sets, clamps and bulb syringes, fetal monitoring equipment, delivery room garb, infant eye prophylaxis, infant wrappers, and other small sterile supplies (scissors and so on).

Episiotomy for Delivery of the Fetus

Indications. **Episiotomy** is an incision into the perineum and vagina to enlarge the vaginal opening for delivery of the fetus and to protect the surrounding muscle and fascia from tears. It is the second most common obstetric surgical procedure (cutting the umbilical cord is first). Episiotomy is indicated when the likelihood of a laceration is increased because of a large fetus, short perineum, weak scar tissue, or indication that a tear has begun (such as trickle of bright red bleeding or central bluish discoloration in a long perineum). Other indications are delivery of a premature, breech, or distressed fetus, protracted second stage with head on perineum, rigid perineum, and forceps delivery. Episiotomy is also performed for cardiac and pre-eclamptic clients to decrease bearing down efforts, which put stress on the heart and raise the blood pressure.

Procedure/Nursing Care. Two types of episiotomies are often used: midline and mediolateral (Figure 27–17). The incision for the midline episiotomy is made from the forchette straight down toward the rectum but *not* including it. The mediolateral episiotomy is either a right-angle or left-angle incision extending from the forchette at a 45° angle into the perineum. The mediolateral incision is designed to decrease the possibility that an extension of the incision will tear into the rectum. Figure 27–18 demonstrates repair of a median episiotomy. Figure 27–19 illustrates a healed episiotomy at the 6-week checkup.

Benefits. Many of the advantages to the episiotomy listed in medical textbooks are not documented with scientific evidence; in fact, there is growing evidence that routine episiotomy is not beneficial to the normal mother or baby. Gordon and Logue[39] showed that episiotomy did not assist with improving postpartum vaginal/perineal muscle tone; in fact, their study clearly demonstrated the role of exercise in muscle tone regardless of the woman's parity. Formato[40] demonstrated short-term and long-term good maternal and fetal outcome without routine episiotomy (*see* Research Abstract, p 659).

Benefits often listed as reasons for routine episiotomy include preventing trauma to the fetal head, shortening the second stage, preventing ragged lacerations, and avoiding third-degree and fourth-degree lacerations. The advantage in doing an episiotomy lies in the indications listed earlier. For example, if a tear is imminent, a straight cut is easier to repair; if the fetus is in distress, an episiotomy will speed delivery and this may help the fetus; if the mother's circulatory system is in jeopardy, any reduction in pushing will help; if more room is needed because of an abnormal presentation or because manipulation or forceps must be used, an episiotomy

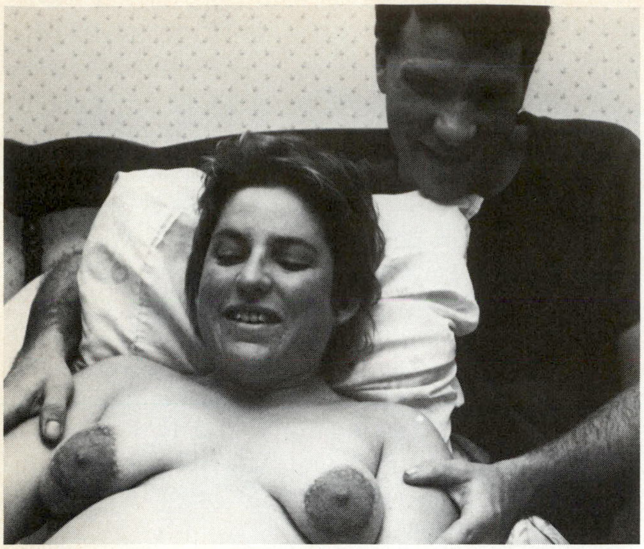

A

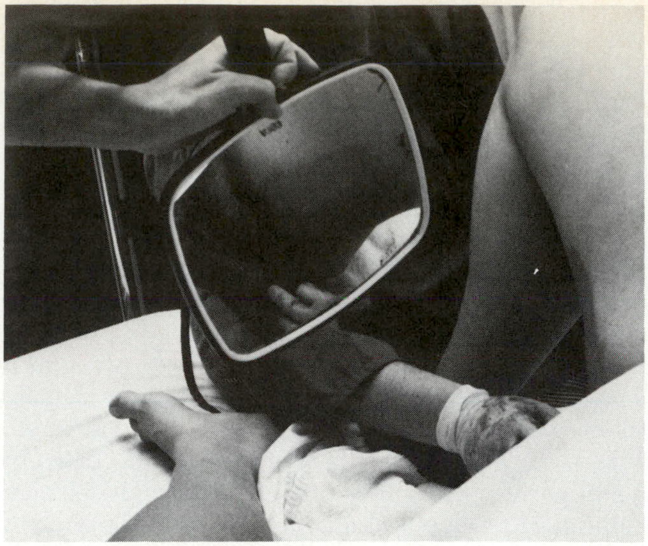

B

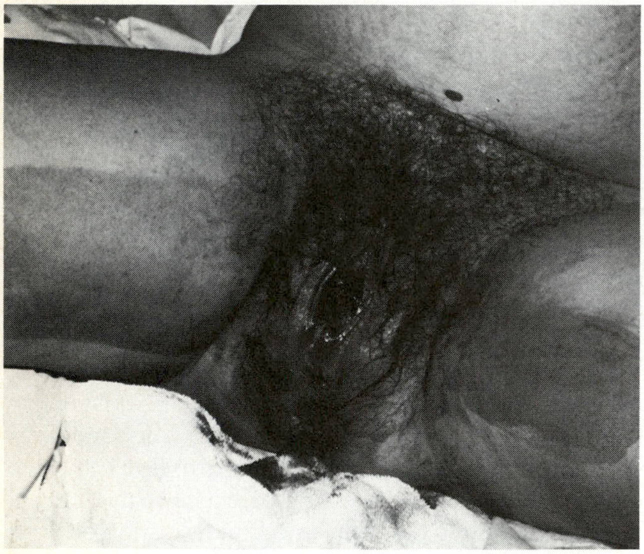

C

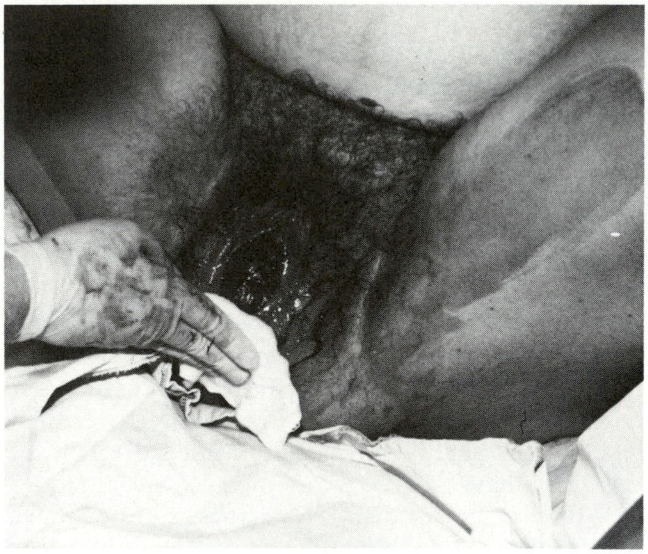

D

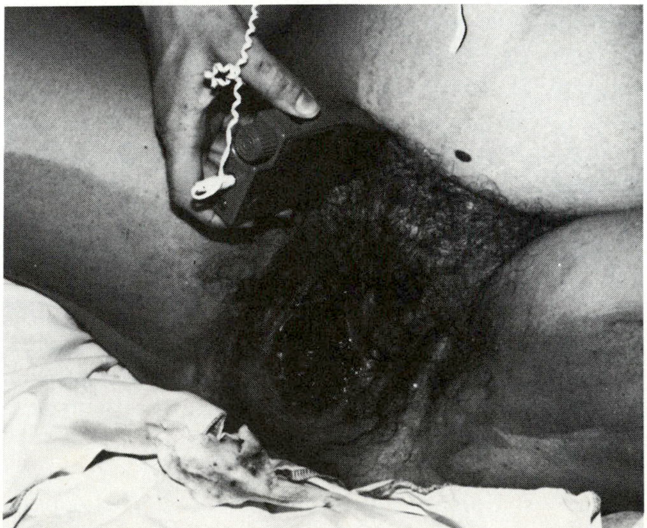

E

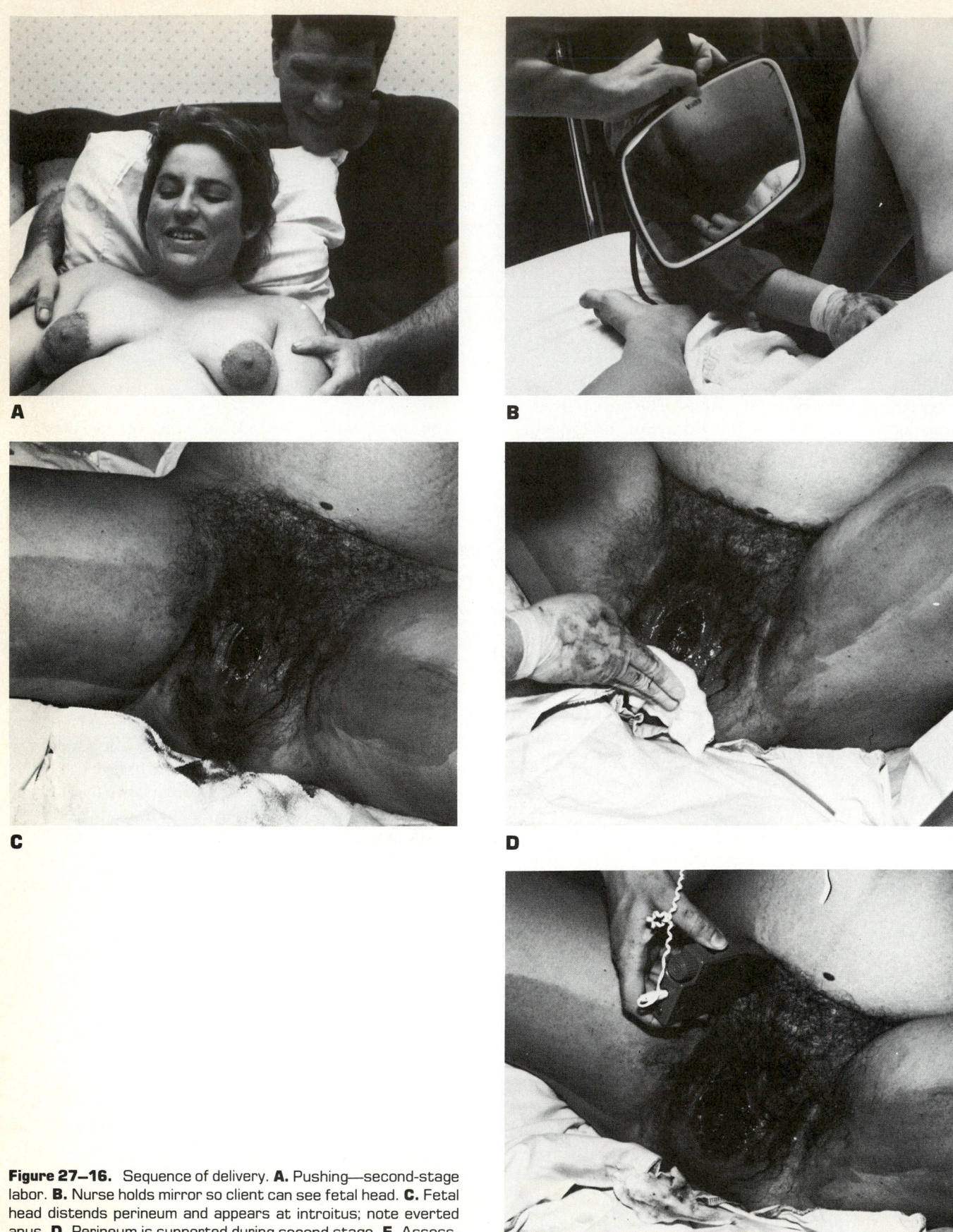

Figure 27–16. Sequence of delivery. **A.** Pushing—second-stage labor. **B.** Nurse holds mirror so client can see fetal head. **C.** Fetal head distends perineum and appears at introitus; note everted anus. **D.** Perineum is supported during second stage. **E.** Assessing for heart rate during second stage. (*Figure continues*.)

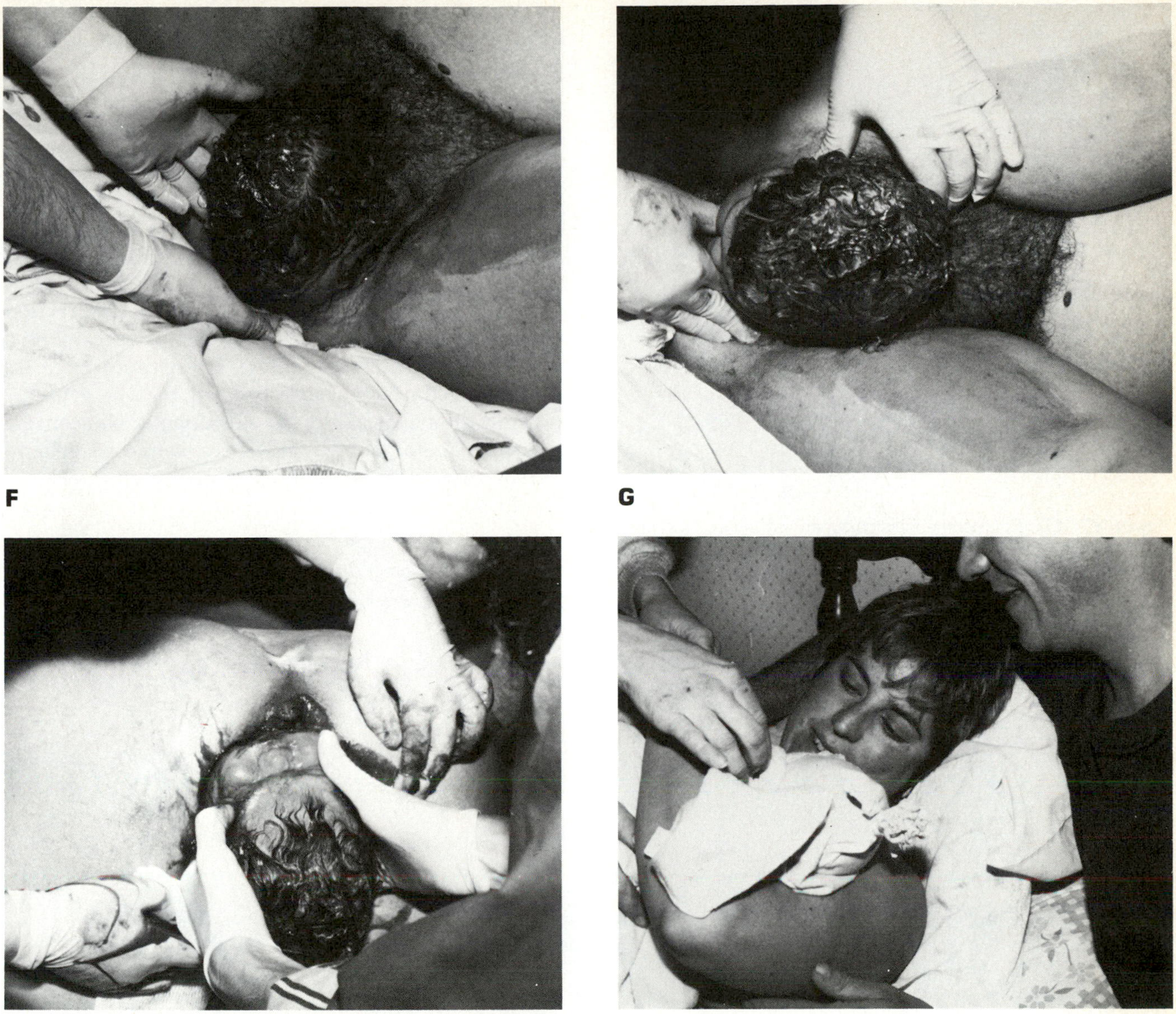

F G H I

Figure 27–16. (*Continued.*) **F.** Delivery of fetal head begun. **G.** Client lies on side for completion of delivery of fetal head. **H.** Delivery of shoulders. **I.** Mother and newborn after birth.

will give the practitioner more room to work for a better maternal-fetal outcome.[41]

There are also advantages and disadvantages to the types of episiotomies, and practitioners in different parts of the world have preferences. Most European practitioners prefer the mediolateral episiotomy; most American practitioners, the median episiotomy. The median has the advantage of being more anatomically sound in that the muscles are separated rather than cut across. A median episiotomy is easier to repair, healing is better, pain is less, dyspareunia is less common, and blood loss is less; however, the mediolateral episiotomy has fewer extensions into the rectum.

Risks. The disadvantages of episiotomy include pain during the procedure, its repair, and postpartum, and dyspareunia for months afterward. Dyspareunia may interfere with the maternal-infant relationship and damage the couple's sexual relationship. An emotional disadvantage is the feeling of being violated that women report.[42] In addition, episiotomies may extend, by laceration, into the anal sphincter (third degree) or rectum (fourth degree), and there is a risk

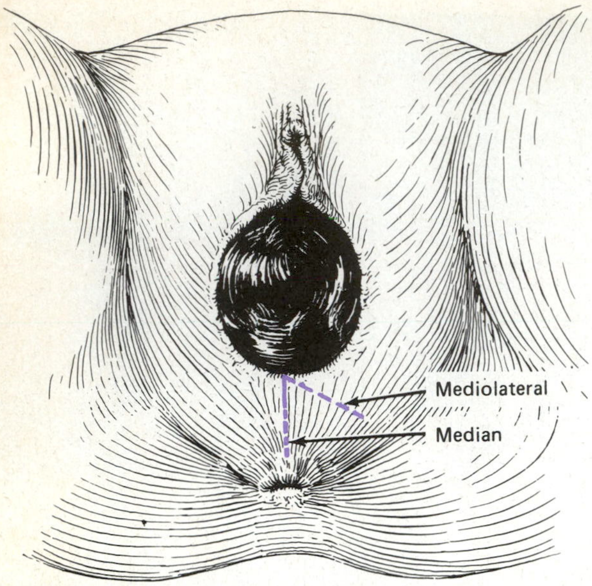

Figure 27–17. Episiotomy incision types. (*Adapted, with permission, from Benson RC.* Handbook of Obstetrics and Gynecology. *8th ed. Los Altos, Calif: Lange Medical Books; 1983:166.*)

of infection or possible loss of sphincter control or a fistula from the rectum into the vagina. These latter complications may occur from lacerations as well; however, many experts believe that if fewer episiotomies were performed there would be a lower incidence of related complications without the jeopardy that is presented in the literature.

Forceps/Vacuum Extraction

Indications. Whether **forceps** or **vacuum extraction methods** are used, the purpose is to extract the fetal head from the maternal pelvis. These procedures are done when the fetal head is arrested, for whatever reason, in the pelvis. They are not done to shorten the second stage of labor. Forceps are stainless steel and can be used for extraction but not rotation (Figure 27–20).

Procedure/Nursing Care. The need for the procedure must first be explained to the client. The woman is

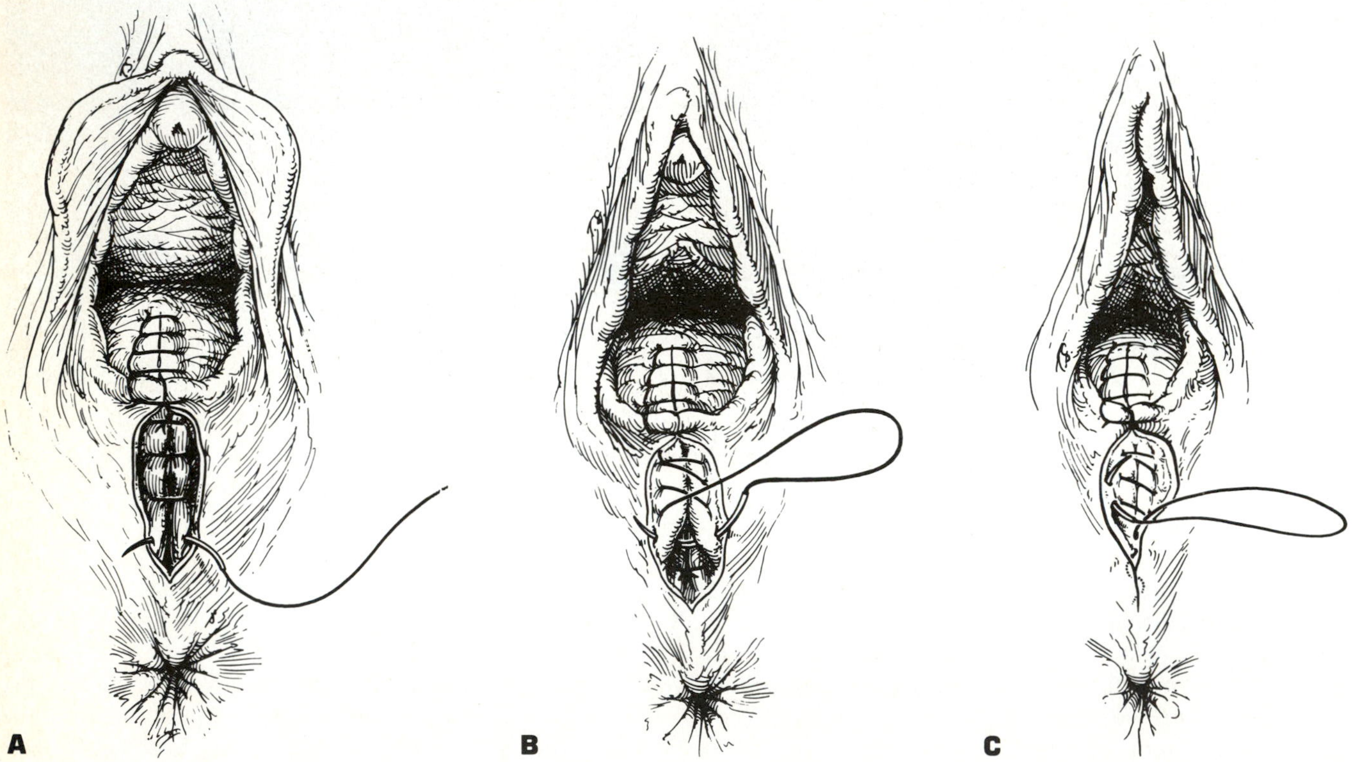

Figure 27–18. Median episiotomy repair. **A.** After closure of the vaginal incision and reapproximation of the cut margins of the hymenal ring, the suture is tied and cut. Next, three or four sutures are placed in the fascia and muscle of the incised perineum. **B.** A continuous suture is now carried downward to unite the superficial fascia. **C.** Completion of the repair. (Reproduced, with permission, from Cunningham FG, et al. *Williams Obstetrics.* 18th ed. Norwalk, Conn: Appleton & Lange; 1989:324.)

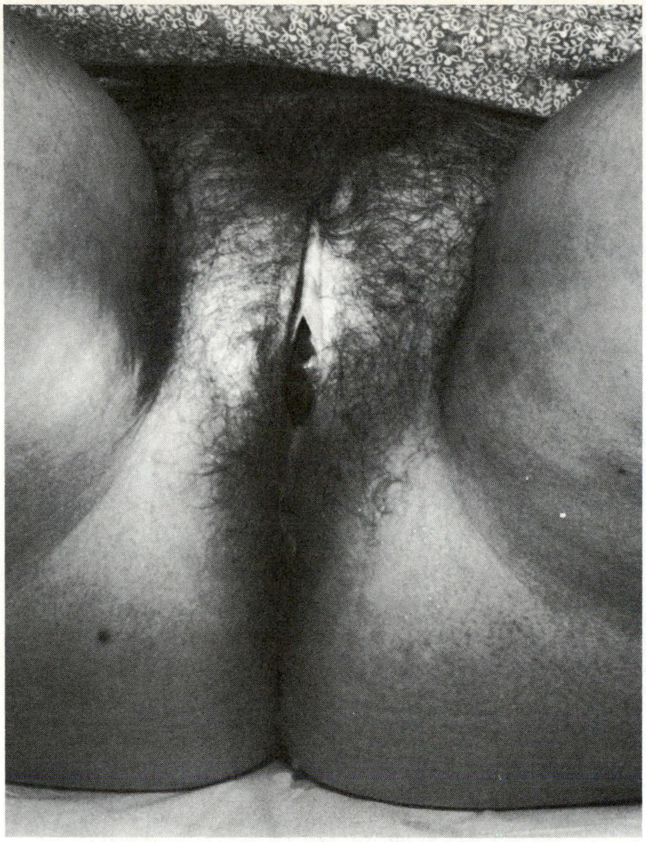

Figure 27–19. Healed episiotomy repair.

moved to the delivery room and placed in the lithotomy position. Then the nurse cleans the perineum and drapes the client. The nurse catheterizes the client to reduce bladder trauma on order of the physician. FHTs and uterine contractions are monitored throughout the procedure by the nurse.

The nurse passes the requested vacuum extractor or forceps and provides water-soluble lubricant to the physician for the forceps blades. With the forceps method, the physician places one and then the other blade of the forceps over the fetus's parietal bones and locks the blades together. Traction is applied during contractions until the head is low enough to permit an episiotomy. The episiotomy is done and forceps are removed when the biparietal bones pass through vulvar ring. With the vacuum method, the suction cup is placed on the fetal head over the bony area and suction is gradually applied (Figure 27–21). Suction is released when the fetal head is on the pelvic floor.

Benefits. Forceps or vacuum extraction is useful primarily with a vaginal delivery (to avoid cesarean delivery) when there is maternal exhaustion, fetal distress, undesirability of maternal pushing efforts (for example, the client with cardiac disease, hypertension, or tuberculosis), or failure to progress in second stage of labor.

Risks. These methods are difficult to learn, carry out, and apply properly. The physician must be sure that the woman has an adequate pelvis, the bladder and rectum are empty to avoid injury, an accurate diagnosis of fetal presentation and position is made, anesthesia is present and adequate, lacerations are kept to a minimum and repaired properly, and asepsis is maintained. The mother may develop bruising or a hematoma from the manipulation. In addition, the fetus may have soft tissue damage to the face, fracture of the skull, tentorial tears, shoulder dystocia, and brain hemorrhage.

Delivery of the Neonate

Once the fetal head has emerged, the clinician quickly explores the fetal neck to ensure that the cord has not become looped around the neck during labor. If this has occurred, the cord is either slipped over the head if length permits, clamped and cut to prevent tearing of the cord or rupture of the placenta, or manipulated over the fetal shoulders to permit delivery through the looped cord. The body of the neonate is delivered with the next one or two contractions. The mother is urged, during these final contractions, to pant rather than push to prevent fetal and maternal damage such as lacerations or damage to the fetal head. A gush of amniotic fluid follows the expulsion of the fetal body and limbs.

The neonate's nares and mouth may be suctioned as soon as the head emerges, particularly if the physician or midwife has time to wait for external rotation before delivery of the shoulders and body. It is very important to prevent neonatal aspiration of mucus, amniotic fluid (particularly if meconium stained), and debris which may occur with the first inspiration as compression of the rib cage by the birth canal is released by delivery. The umbilical cord is double clamped and cut between clamps. As the first cries of the neonate fill the delivery room, the second stage of labor ends.

On delivery of the infant, the parents are presented with the first opportunity for neonatal-parental attachment. The neonate may be placed on the mother's abdomen while the cord is cut. Skin-to-skin contact facilitates attachments as well as thermoregulation of the newborn.[43]

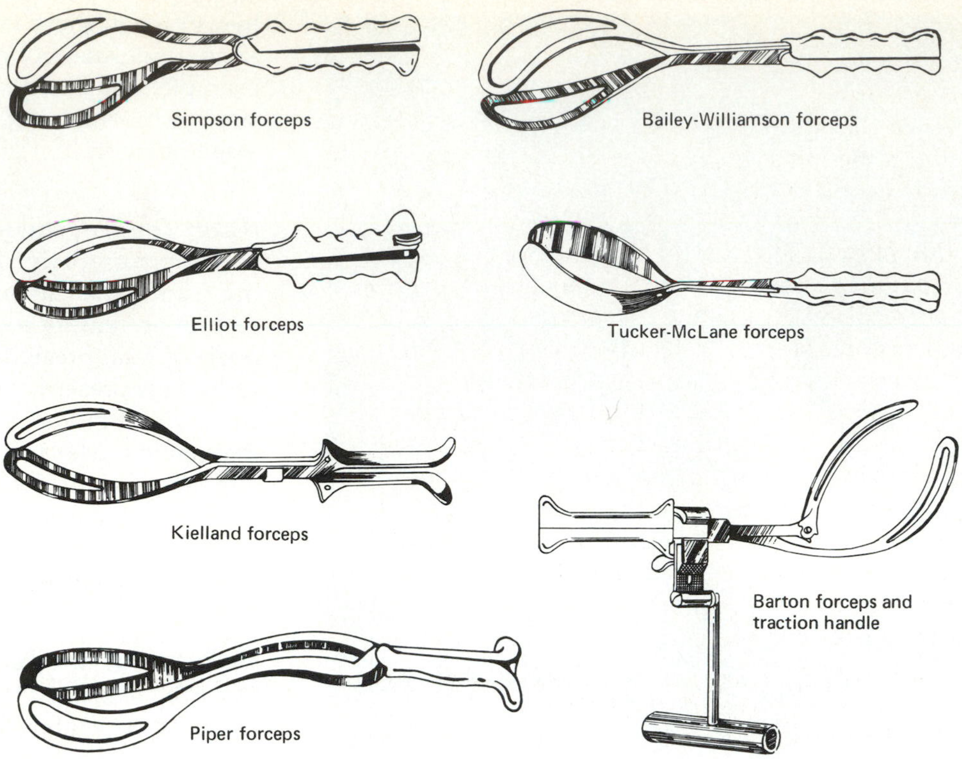

Figure 27–20. Commonly used forceps. (*Reproduced with permission, from Benson RC.* Handbook of Obstetrics and Gynecology. *8th ed. Los Altos, Calif: Lange Medical Books; 1983.*)

Birth of the baby culminates the long waiting period of pregnancy. The fantasized infant now becomes a reality. The nurse, as parent advocate, can ensure that parents have an opportunity for privacy in becoming acquainted with their new baby. Once neonatal respirations have been established, the many technical aspects of newborn care (eg, infant identification, eye prophylaxis, weighing) can be delayed until after this initial acquaintance period. (*See* Chapter 34 for further discussion of care of the infant immediately after birth.)

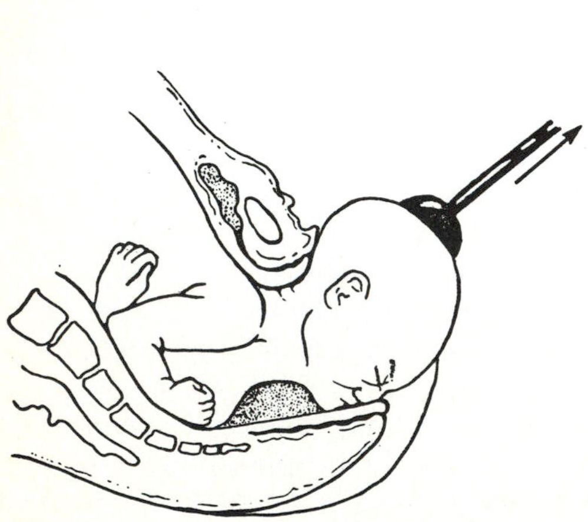

Figure 27–21. Vacuum extraction method. *Arrow* indicates direction of traction. (*Reproduced, with permission, from Benson RC.* Handbook of Obstetrics and Gynecology. *8th ed. Los Altos, Calif. Lange Medical Books; 1983:477.*)

NURSING CARE DURING THE THIRD STAGE OF LABOR

The third stage of labor is also called the placental stage. Nursing management entails care and support of the client during the delivery of the placenta.

After birth of the newborn, the placenta begins to separate from the uterine wall. Signs of placental separation include a change in the shape of the uterus from ovoid to globular; a trickle or gush of blood; lengthening of the umbilical cord; rise of the fundus, which occurs as the placenta descends; and failure of the cord to retract when the uterus is pushed upward (Brandt-Andrews sign).

The role of the nurse during the third stage is to ensure that the placenta is delivered intact. In addition, the nurse assesses the fundus for contractility, the vaginal discharge for evidence of excessive bleeding (eg, bright red blood gushing from the vagina), and the maternal vital signs.

After delivery, the placenta is carefully examined to ascertain whether any fragments have remained attached to the uterus. If deemed to be complete, the placenta is bagged in plastic and labeled according to protocol. The umbilical cord is inspected to ascertain placement, length, the presence of one vein and two arteries, and any evidence of a knot or bleeding within the cord. The presence of a cord abnormality directs the nurse to examine the neonate for defects or damage associated with the cord problem.

Pharmacologic Management

To facilitate contraction of the uterus during or after the third stage of labor, the practitioner frequently utilizes pharmacologic agents such as oxytocin (Pitocin), ergonovine (Ergotrate), and methylergonovine (Methergine) to promote the firm contractions that help to accomplish separation of the placenta while minimizing maternal blood loss. If the client has an intravenous line in place, the oxytocin can safely be added to a fresh liter of ordered intravenous fluid (D_5W, normal saline, or Ringer's lactate solution) because the safety precautions required by the intrauterine presence of the fetus prior to delivery are no longer in force. The dosage of intravenous oxytocin (10 to 40 U/1000 mL) is regulated to the lowest possible rate that will maintain contractility of the uterus. Before administration of the third-stage oxytoxics, the nurse palpates the uterus to ensure that an extra fetus is not present and assesses maternal blood pressure. Ergonovine and methylergonovine may also be ordered after delivery of the placenta to stimulate contraction of the uterus. Oxytocin alone must never be relied on to maintain contraction of the uterus, but in the third and fourth stages, it is always coupled with gentle, guarded fundal massage.

NURSING CARE DURING THE FOURTH STAGE OF LABOR

The fourth stage of labor is the period during which the mother's body systems stabilize, usually within 1 to 4 hours after the delivery of the placenta (*see* Chapter 29). The labor and delivery nurse monitors the beginning indicators of this stabilization.

During this stage, the cardiovascular system quickly adjusts to the loss of pressure from the gravid uterus, but the mother should be reminded not to rise too quickly from a supine to a sitting position, as hypotension and dizziness or syncope may result. A chill causing a brief episode of shivering is common in the fourth stage and appears to be the result of physical and emotional factors. It is hypothesized that loss of the fetal body heat, the relaxation of large pelvic blood vessels, and the sudden emotional "calm after the storm" cause this reaction. A warm blanket and a warm drink are usually sufficient to bring relief.

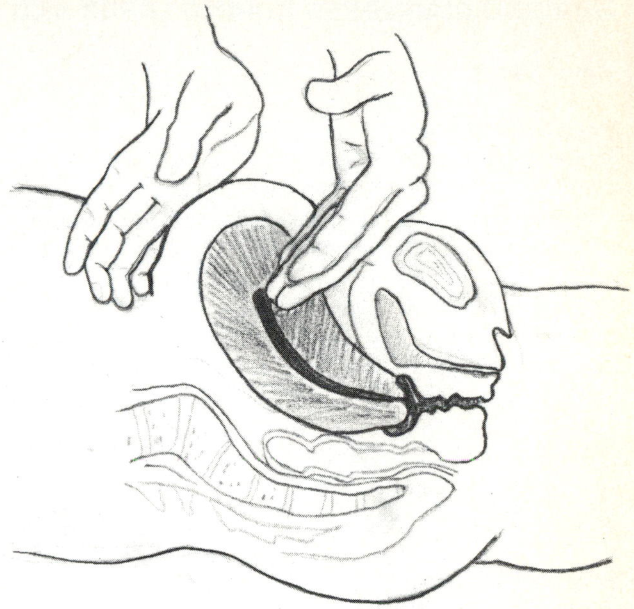

Figure 27–22. Fundal massage.

The fundus is palpated gently but firmly during the postdelivery period to assess firmness and to promote contraction (Figure 27–22). Unless relaxation of the uterus is a persistent problem, the nurse should refrain from expressing uterine contents forcefully, as such manipulation may disturb the clotting that is the beginning of placental site healing.

Lochia is assessed for color, odor, consistency, and amount. Maternal vital signs are taken every 15 minutes during the first postpartum hour until stable. It is during the fourth stage of labor that parental acquaintance with the newborn can continue. In addition, the individual who has supported the mother throughout labor and delivery may be encouraged to obtain food and rest at this time. (*See* Chapter 31 for additional management strategies during the postpartum period.)

NURSING DIAGNOSES

Nurses who care for families during the labor and delivery period make careful assessments of the physiologic and psychosocial needs of the woman and her fetus. Nursing diagnoses are made after comprehensive assessment. See the box on p 698 for examples of nursing diagnoses for the family during the labor and delivery process. The nurse is an integral member of the health team that manages the family during this critical time in the childbearing cycle.

NURSING DIAGNOSES DURING LABOR AND DELIVERY

Physiologic

Problem-Oriented

Impaired tissue integrity, related to episiotomy or laceration during delivery of a large infant

Pain, related to contractions, pressure of presenting parts against maternal nerves

Strength-Oriented

Normal progress during labor and delivery, related to positive health care practices during pregnancy

Asset in maternal and fetal health during intrapartum period, related to normal progression of labor as evaluated by Friedman's curve

Psychosocial

Problem-Oriented

Sensory perceptual alterations (visual, auditory and tactile), related to transitional stage of labor

Powerlessness, related to lack of preparation for labor or the effects of certain medications in labor

Strength-Oriented

Enhanced self-esteem, related to perceived control in labor and delivery and effective use of childbirth preparation techniques

Enhanced paternal self-esteem, related to active participation during labor and delivery

Cultural

Problem-Oriented

Potential self-esteem disturbance, related to incongruence between cultural beliefs and childbirth practices in health care settings in the United States

Strength-Oriented

Asset in maternal coping, related to presence of culturally appropriate labor social support

CASE STUDY/CARE PLAN: THE COUPLE EXPERIENCING ANXIETY IN CHILDBIRTH

Lisa and Frederick Kemler are expecting their first baby. Lisa is admitted to the labor and delivery unit and placed in the birthing room. Assessment reveals that she is in the latent phase of labor. Her cervix is completely effaced and 2 cm dilated. Membranes are intact. Her contractions occur every 5 minutes, last 40 seconds, and are moderate to strong in intensity.

During the latent phase of labor, the nurse caring for the couple notes that both Lisa and Frederick are anxious. Lisa is able to concentrate on her breathing with some, but not all, contractions. She continuously talks in a rapid manner, paces around the room between contractions, and aimlessly touches objects in the room. Frederick appears to be anxious as he observes Lisa pace. The nurse further notes that Frederick coaches Lisa only during some contractions. Lisa and Frederick attended Lamaze childbirth preparation classes. They have brought with them their wedding picture to focus on during contractions.

As the labor progresses, Lisa's contractions occur every 2 to 3 minutes, last 50 seconds, and are strong in intensity. Her membranes rupture spontaneously when her cervix is 6 cm dilated.

Supporting Assessment Data	Expected Client/Family Outcome	Nursing Action/ Intervention	Rationale	Criteria for Evaluation
Nursing Diagnosis: Anxiety, related to impending birth and entry into the health care institution				
Client is unable to concentrate on her breathing, continuously talks in a rapid manner; paces around room between contractions; aimlessly touches objects in room Client's husband appears anxious; unable to coach wife through contractions	By the end of the latent phase, the couple will: Demonstrate use of controlled breathing and concentration methods Exert a measure of control over the labor process Perceive the birth with low anxiety Demonstrate familiarity with the health care facility and team members	Review with couple their plans for this birth Ascertain cultural orientation to birthing. Assist with Lamaze relaxation techniques and breathing patterns. Remain with couple and allow them to vent feelings concerning impending birth. Maintain physical comfort of client. Change position of mother; keep upright and ambulate as long as possible. Offer ice chips. Keep linens clean. Support father in coaching role. Keep family informed about progress of labor. Orient couple to environment, staff, and procedures that may be used.	Stress reduction is facilitated by continuity of care. Knowledge and familiarity with situations reduce anxiety. Childbirth preparation assists in positive coping strategies to relieve stress and perceived control of behavior.	Couple will demonstrate less anxious behavior and begin concentrating on contractions. Couple state that they feel more confident about going through labor and delivery. The couple use resources in environment appropriately. The couple verbalize that staff is helpful to them during labor.
Nursing Diagnosis: Asset in fetal and maternal health during labor, related to maternal physiologic adaptation				
Client is in latent phase of labor; contractions occur every 5 minutes, lasting 40 seconds and are moderate to strong in intensity; fetal heart tones are heard in the left lower abdominal quadrant. FHR 120–124; occiput at zero station; cervix 2 cm. dilated and 100% effaced; maternal BP 120/70; P 80; R 16 (between contractions); T 99F	During the active phase of labor the mother and fetus will demonstrate normal progression as evidenced by: vital signs, Friedman's curve	Assess maternal temperature every 4 hours until membranes rupture, then every 2 hours. Assess maternal pulse and respirations between contractions every 2–4 hours. Assess maternal blood pressure between contractions every hour. Assess fetal heart every 30 minutes for rate, quality, and regularity. Locate where fetal heart tones are heard loudest. Assess contractions for interval, duration, and strength by placing fingertips over fundus.	Temperature is an important vital sign because it is an indicator of hydration and infection. Pulse and respirations are indicators of anxiety, hydration, infections and maternal exertion. Changes in blood pressure above the prepregnancy levels may indicate pregnancy-induced hypertension; a decrease in blood pressure may indicate shock. Fetal heart activity is an indicator of fetal well-being. Contraction patterns indicate progression of labor.	Temperature will remain within normal limits. Pulse and respirations will remain within normal limits. Systolic blood pressure does not rise 30 mmHg or more; diastolic blood pressure does not rise 15 mmHg or more. BP does not fall below 90/60. Fetal heart tones will remain within normal limits. Contraction pattern will follow Friedman's curve.

(continued)

CASE STUDY/CARE PLAN: The Couple Experiencing Anxiety in Childbirth (*continued*)

Supporting Assessment Data	Expected Client/Family Outcome	Nursing Action/ Intervention	Rationale	Criteria for Evaluation
Nursing Diagnosis: Diversional activity deficit, related to anxiety during labor				
Client is in latent phase of labor; exhibiting many signs of anxiety (pacing, talkativeness, aimless touching of objects) Contractions lasting 40 seconds occur every 5 minutes and are moderate to strong in intensity Couple attended Lamaze childbirth preparation classes; have their wedding picture to focus on during contractions Client's husband unable to coach	By the end of the latent phase, the couple will engage in diversional activities taught in childbirth preparation classes	Assist couple in anxiety reduction behaviors (*see* earlier Interventions). Review with couple the diversional activities suggested in the childbirth preparation classes (breathing, focusing on picture, walking, television, music, cards). Praise couple when they use diversional activities and concentration. Make sure diversional activities are available and meet the couple's needs and standards.	Anxiety will prevent use of diversional activities and interfere with the ability to focus. Diversional activities should be those with which the couple are familiar and comfortable. Concentration on a focal object (diversion) will allow couple to perceive some control over labor. Focusing on familiar, homelike surroundings and objects helps decrease anxiety.	Client will focus on wedding picture and use appropriate breathing techniques during contractions. Client will relate to the nurse the diversional activities that promote her comfort. Husband will support client's use of diversional activities and provide praise.
Nursing Diagnosis: Asset in maternal and fetal health during labor, related to normal progression of labor as demonstrated by Friedman's curve				
Client is in active phase of labor; contractions occur every 2 to 3 minutes, last 50 seconds, and are strong in intensity; spontaneous rupture of membranes; fluid clear with no evidence of meconium staining	During the transitional phase and second stage of labor, the mother and fetus will demonstrate normal labor progression as evidenced by: vital signs, Friedman's curve	Assess maternal temperature every 2 hours. Assess maternal pulse and respirations every 2 hours. Assess maternal blood pressure every hour. Assess fetal heart tones every 15 minutes between contractions for rate, quality, and regularity; assess fetal heart tones immediately following rupture of membranes.	After the membranes rupture, the potential for infection is greater than when the membranes are intact. Temperature, pulse, respirations, and blood pressure will elevate with infection. When the membranes rupture, the umbilical cord may prolapse causing irregularity in FHT and variable decelerations in the fetal heart rate.	Maternal vital signs will remain within normal limits. Fetal heart tones will be normal in rate, quality, and regularity.

SUMMARY

The nurse is an integral part of the delivery team, which may also include a variety of medical and nurse specialists. In this chapter, the approach has been to describe intrapartum management based on an understanding of the events of labor. Because nurses practice and clients deliver in a variety of settings, the description has been very broad. In some settings, the nurses act as primary care providers and the physician or nurse-midwife comes in only for the delivery. These nurses carry a great deal of responsibility and must be very knowledgeable about labor assessment and management.

Nursing care during the intrapartum period includes a comprehensive health history. The prenatal course for the mother and her family is an important predictor of risk during labor and delivery. Assessments of the mother include vital signs, maternal contraction patterns, estimation of dilation and effacement of the cervix, positions of the fetal presenting part, and psychologic and cultural influences. The fetus is assessed by monitoring fetal heart tones, estimating fetal age and weight, and determining fetal presentation.

The nurse should be aware of stimuli during labor and delivery that will affect the process of childbirth. These include the birthplace environment, support persons for labor, fatigue, nausea and vomiting, fear, and pain. Pain may be managed with non-pharmacologic or pharmacologic methods, including analgesia and anesthesia, or both. Assessing the method of childbirth education that the couple has had enables the nurse to support the couple in the techniques learned for labor and delivery.

Nursing care of the mother and fetus during each of the four stages of labor and delivery may include monitoring through various procedures. Some of these procedures are shaving of pubic hair, bathing in labor, fetal monitoring through auscultation or electronic methods, stimulation of labor, episiotomy, and forceps or vacuum extraction deliveries.

Conscientious nursing assessment and care is essential in facilitating an optimal labor and delivery outcome.

REVIEW QUESTIONS

1. Describe three ways to monitor fetal heart tones and patterns in labor.
2. Describe at least five different ways to determine the progress of labor.
3. Describe at least four different types of stimuli of labor and how they may affect maternal coping during labor.
4. Describe the drugs most commonly used in labor in terms of type, dose, indications, route of administration, and side effects.
5. For each of the elective procedures used in the first and second stages of labor, give the indications, pros, and cons to their use.

REFERENCES

1. Creasy R. Prenatal risk assessment and perinatal outcome. Quote from March of Dimes conference, November 24, 1986, New York City.
2. American College of Nurse-Midwives. *Definition of a CNM According to ACNM.* Washington, DC: American College of Nurse Midwives.
3. Oberle JC. If you want to specialize. . . . *RN.* 1984:55–67.
4. Poole C. Educating new labor and delivery nurses. *J Obstet Gynecol Neonat Nurs.* 1985;14:456–462.
5. Pernoll ML, Benson RC. *Current Obstetric & Gynecologic Diagnosis and Treatment.* 8th ed. Norwalk, Conn: Appleton & Lange; 1987.
6. Varney H. *Nurse-midwifery.* 2nd ed. Boston: Blackwell Scientific; 1987.
7. Whitley N. *A Manual of Clinical Obstetrics.* Philadelphia: JB Lippincott; 1985.
8. Rosen MG, Peisner DB. Effects of amniotic membrane rupture on length of labor. *Obstet Gynecol.* 1987;70:604.
9. Friedman EA. Assessing labor progression in Friedman EA (ed): *Obstetric Decision Making.* St. Louis, Mo: CV Mosby; 1982.
10. Blum M; Raff B, ed. *Selected Drugs Used During Labor and Delivery: Effects on the Fetus and Neonate.* 2nd ed. New York: March of Dimes Birth Defects Foundation; 1989.
11. Roberts J. Alternative positions for childbirth, part I: First stage of labor. *J Nurse-Midwifery.* 1980;24:11–18.
12. Cox S, et al. The natural history of preterm ruptured membranes: what to expect of expectant management. *Obstet Gynecol.* 1988;71:558.
13. Caldeyro-Barcia R. Some consequences of obstetrical interferences. *Birth Fam J.* 1975;2:34.
14. Lederman RP. *Psychological Adaptation in Pregnancy.* Englewood Cliffs, NJ: Prentice-Hall; 1984.
15. Oxorn H, ed. *Oxorn-Foote Human Labor and Birth.* 5th ed. New York: Appleton-Century-Crofts; 1986.
16. Morse JM, Park C. Home birth and hospital deliveries: a comparison of the perceived painfulness of parturition. *Res Nurs Health.* 1988;11:175–181.
17. Brown C. Therapeutic effects of bathing during labor. *J Nurse-Midwifery.* 1982;27:13–16.
18. Lowe NL, Roberts JE. The convergence between in-labor report and postpartum recall of parturition pain. *Res Nurs Health.* 1988;11:11–21.
19. Fridh G, et al. Factors associated with more intense labor pain. *Res Nurs Health.* 1988;11:117–124.
20. Wilkie DJ, et al. Use of the McGill pain questionnaire to measure pain: a meta-analysis. *Nurs Res.* 1990;39:36–41.
21. Morse JM, Park C. Differences in cultural expectations of the perceived expectations of parturition. In: Michaelson, ed. *Childbirth in America: Anthropological Perspectives.* South Hadley, Mass: Bergin & Garvey; 1988:121–129.
22. Gaston-Johansson F, et al. Progression of labor pain in primiparas and multiparas. *Nurs Res.* 1988;37:86–89.
23. Malinowski JS, et al. *Nursing Care During the Labor Process.* 3rd ed. Philadelphia: FA Davis; 1989.
24. Geden EA, et al. Effects of cognitive and pharmacologic strategies on analogued labor pain. *Nurs Res.* 1986;35: 301–306.
25. Cunningham FG, et al. *Williams Obstetrics.* 18th ed. Norwalk, Conn: Appleton & Lange; 1989.
26. Hazle N. Hydration in labor: is routine intravenous hydration necessary? *J Nurse-Midwifery.* 1986;31:171–176.
27. Odent M. The evolution of obstetrics at Pithivers. *Birth Fam J.* 1981;8:7–15.
28. Haverkamp AD, et al. A controlled trial of differential effects of intrapartum fetal monitoring. *Am J Obstet Gynecol.* 1979;143:399.
29. Klein M, et al. A comparison of low-risk pregnant women booked for delivery in two systems of care: shared-care (consultant) and integrated general practice unit. II. Labor

and delivery management and neonatal outcome. *Br J Obstet Gynaecol.* 1983;90:123.
30. Levenco KJ, et al. A prospective comparison of selective and universal electronic monitoring in 34,995 pregnancies. *N Engl J Med.* 1986;315:615.
31. McDonald D, et al. The Dublin randomized controlled trial of intrapartum heart rate monitoring. *Am J Obstet Gynecol.* 1985;152:524–539.
32. Gonzalez FA. Ultrasound. *J. Nurse-Midwifery.* 1984;29: 391–394.
33. Haire D. Fetal effects of ultrasound: a growing controversy. *J Nurse-Midwifery.* 1984;29:241–246.
34. Blank JJ: Electronic fetal monitoring: nursing management defined. *J Obstet Gynecol Neonat Nurs.* 1985;14:463–467.
35. Wetrich D. Effect on amniotomy upon labor. *Obstet Gynecol.* 1970;35:800–806.
36. Liu YC: The effects of the upright position during childbirth. *Image.* 1989;21:14–18.
37. Lehrman E. Birth in the left lateral position: an alternative to the traditional delivery position. *J Nurse-Midwifery.* 1985; 30:193–197.
38. Noble E. Controversies in maternal effort during labor and delivery. *J Nurse-Midwifery.* 1981;26:13–22.
39. Gordon H, Logue M. Perineal muscle function after childbirth. *Lancet.* 1986; 2:123–125.
40. Formato L. Routine prophylactic episiotomy: is it always necessary? *J Nurse-Midwifery.* 1985;30:145–148.
41. Gass MS, et al. Effect of episiotomy on the frequency of vaginal outlet lacerations. *J Reprod Med.* 1986;31:240–244.
42. Kitzinger S, Walter R. *Some Women's Experiences of Episiotomy.* London: National Childbirth Trust; 1981.
43. Hill ST, Shronk LK. The effect of early parent-infant contact on newborn body temperature. In: Sherwen LN, Weingarten CT, eds. *Analysis and Application of Nursing Research: Parent-Neonate Studies.* Belmont, Calif: Wadsworth Health Sciences Division; 1983.

The Cesarean Experience

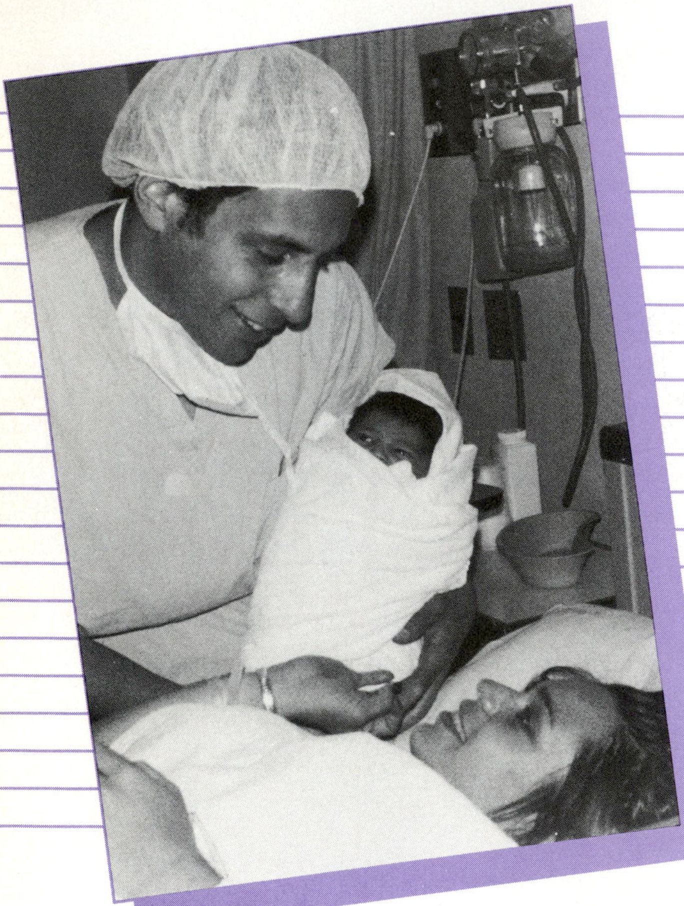

chapter 28

Key Terms

cesarean delivery
iatrogenic prematurity
vaginal birth after a cesarean (VBAC)

A **cesarean delivery** is a surgical procedure in which a fetus is delivered through an incision made through the abdominal wall and the uterus. Although cesarean section is a technically correct term for the operation, cesarean delivery, cesarean birth, and cesarean experience are currently used to highlight the importance of the birth event. As surgical and maternity clients, women who deliver in this manner present special challenges to the nurse. Cesarean clients are always considered to be high risk, because the cesarean procedure is regarded as major abdominal surgery; however, the degree of risk is related to the circumstances that led to the need for an abdominal birth. Nursing implications evolve from goals, such as early identification of high-risk conditions for which cesarean birth is indicated, implementation of strategies that will ensure safe, healthy delivery outcomes for mother and fetus, and the design of interventions that will promote an emotionally satisfying, family-centered birth experience.

BACKGROUND AND INCIDENCE

Cesareans are not new operations and were performed before the time of the ancient Romans. Unfortunately, client survival was a major problem, and cesarean delivery was done only in desperate situations; the procedure was also performed on dead women to separate the mother and fetus. The first professional cesarean delivery in the United States took place in 1827. During the next 50 years, there were only 71 cesarean deliveries in the United States, and the mortality rate was 52 percent, mostly from infection and hemorrhage.[1] Indeed, prior to 1882, the uterus was usually not sutured for several reasons including the belief that sutures were not necessary and served only to increase infection.

During the 20th century, dramatic technologic advances such as improved anesthetics, aseptic techniques, development of antibiotics, and refinement of surgical procedures greatly reduced the risk of cesarean delivery for the mother. As the likelihood of maternal survival increased and the professional attitude toward abdominal birth changed, cesareans were performed more frequently. By the 1950s the cesarean rate was about 3 to 4 percent; however, this rate continued to climb. At one time physicians had to justify why a cesarean was done. By the end of the 1970s, however, in a professional climate that focused on the pathologic aspects of childbirth, physicians often had to explain why a cesarean was not done.[2] Currently, cesarean rates have been noted to be above 20 percent nationally and as much as 30 percent or higher in some communities, although the women are not unusually high risk.[3,4]

At the same time that the incidence of cesarean births has increased, there has been a decrease in perinatal and maternal mortality.[3,5] Does a cause-effect relationship exist? This is a difficult and controversial question. According to data reviewed and presented in the National Institutes of Health's Consensus Development Statement on Cesarean Childbirth, cesarean birth may benefit maternal and neonatal outcome only in true obstetric emergency situations.[6] Porreco noted that such factors as better prenatal and neonatal care could also have contributed to improved perinatal and maternal status. In his prospective, comparative study of 969 pregnant clinic clients who received obstetric interventions aimed at decreasing the number of cesarean deliveries and of 2302 women who were managed at the discretion of their private physicians, the clinic group had one third the number of cesareans as did the private group. Yet, the perinatal outcome, defined by mortality rates and occurrence of low 5-minute Apgar scores, was identical for the two groups.[3] Bing also cautioned against the cheerful acceptance and marketing of major abdominal surgery for childbirth.[7]

It is difficult to specify what the cesarean birth rate should be. The complexity of the human birth experience necessitates that each client be evaluated on an individual basis. This is clearly a topic that needs careful professional assessment and continued research.

ISSUES AND CONTROVERSIES

Cesarean section today remains one of the most controversial topics in obstetrics. Although cesarean delivery carries higher morbidity and mortality rates than vaginal delivery and is considered to be major abdominal surgery, the rates of cesarean delivery are the highest in history.

1. As discussed in this chapter, vaginal birth after cesarean is supported by research studies and in theory by the American College of Obstetricians and Gynecologists, the Organization for Obstetric, Gynecologic and Neonatal Nurses, and other organizations; however, this birth option may be avoided in practice and remains controversial. The relationship between technology such as electronic fetal monitoring and the higher incidence of cesarean delivery also presents a major obstetric issue. To what extent does the immobility and restriction in maternal positions during labor contribute to the development of abnormal fetal heart patterns and the incidence of cesarean delivery? To what extent can fetal heart rate patterns in relation to maternal contractions be misinterpreted as fetal distress requiring emergency cesarean delivery?
2. Another major issue in obstetrics centers around the unnecessary use of technology and the practice of "defensive" nursing and medicine for the purposes of avoiding a malpractice suit or accruing data that could be used in the practitioner's defense should a malpractice suit arise.
3. A philosophic issue questions making cesarean delivery so family centered, pleasant, and routine that it may come to be used without the careful forethought necessary for major surgery. Conversely, it is not ethical to deny cesarean clients the opportunity to share delivery and have a family-centered birth experience.

INDICATIONS

Cesarean delivery is performed whenever it is unlikely that a safe vaginal delivery can take place or whenever it is judged that a delay in delivery would jeopardize the well-being of mother, fetus, or both.[5] Unfortunately, this sounds simpler than it is in clinical practice. Intrapartum complications can be complex, and it may be hard to determine whether an obstetric catastrophe will or will not take place if a cesarean is delayed. Careful client evaluation, clinical judgment, and collaboration among nurses, physicians, other health professionals, and clients themselves are important.

CONTRIBUTING FACTORS

One or more factors can contribute to the occurrence of cesarean birth:

1. Safety of the procedure. Although cesarean birth carries greater risks than vaginal delivery, the morbidity and mortality from cesareans have greatly decreased. Cesarean deliveries have been noted to result in fewer complications than any other type of abdominal surgery.[8] In addition, physicians practicing obstetrics or obstetric anesthesia are more skilled in the performance of this now common procedure.
2. Factors related to the health of the mother, such as severe pre-eclampsia, or pre-existing conditions, such as diabetes and heart disease. Certain health problems, for example, hypertension and uterine myomas, tend to occur in older women, and may contribute to the incidence of cesareans in older pregnant women, especially nulliparas.[9]
3. Factors related to fetal status, such as fetal distress, the most frequent reason for the increased cesarean rate, or maternal death.
4. Factors related to the interactions of maternal and fetal factors, such as uterine dystocia, failure to progress in labor, uterine rupture, placenta previa, abruptio placentae, prolapsed cord, fetal malpresentations (inability of the fetus to enter and pass through the birth canal), breech presentations (especially for primiparas), cephalopelvic disproportion, fetal distress related to decreased placental blood flow during contractions, and certain types of prenatally diagnosed congenital abnormalities (eg, spina bifida) in which vaginal delivery might injure the fetus.
5. Infections in the birth canal, such as active herpes lesions, because of the risk of the fetus' contracting the infection during the birth process. However, if membranes have been ruptured longer than 12 hours, the fetus has been exposed to the organism, and vaginal delivery becomes a possibility.
6. Previous cesarean or uterine surgery. Although the safety of vaginal birth after cesarean delivery has been demonstrated for women who meet certain criteria (*see* later text), Cregin's 1916 decree of "once a cesarean, always a cesarean" persists. During the early 1980s it was estimated that 98 percent of American women who had cesarean deliveries still elected to have subsequent children in that way.[10] By the late 1980s, about 90 percent of women who had previous cesarean deliveries elected to have repeat cesarean deliveries.[4] Cesarean delivery may also be considered if the woman has had previous uterine surgical procedures.
7. Multiple births. Many intrapartum problems, such as fetal malpresentations, abruptio placentae, and abnormal uterine contraction patterns, occur with greater frequency in pregnancies with multiple fetuses.[5] In uncomplicated, progressive labors, twins may be delivered vaginally; however, cesareans are nearly always done in the United States when more than two fetuses are present.
8. Technologic advances, such as electronic fetal monitoring, which have made early detection of fetal distress possible. The great emphasis that is placed on actual or suspected fetal distress has contributed to the increase in cesarean deliveries. Studies indicate that cesarean rates increase with continuous electronic fetal monitoring, although fetal outcome does not improve.
9. Professional concern over potential malpractice suits. Physicians may be more willing to perform a fairly safe surgical procedure than to risk an unfavorable outcome and a malpractice suit.[4]
10. Client request for cesarean delivery and the right of women to be actively involved in their own treatment decisions. Johnson and coworkers note that a physician can rightfully refuse a woman's request for intervention if the risk is very large. However, they observe that although cesarean delivery is always associated with some risk, the risk is similar to that taken by the healthy woman having elective gynecologic surgery. Results of their survey of 112 obstetricians in the United States indicated that some physicians considered the client's request in itself enough reason for cesarean delivery, although this practice is controversial.[11]
11. Evolving lack of physician experience in managing difficult deliveries. As more cesareans are done for complex births, there will theoretically be fewer physicians trained and experienced in management of problem vaginal deliveries. This factor is likely to have a large impact on the future practice of obstetrics.
12. Miscellaneous conditions, such as tumors in the birth canal, failed forceps delivery, and certain congenital anomalies.

BENEFITS

The main benefit of cesarean birth is that it is a lifesaving procedure in situations of obstetric emergency and in situations in which vaginal birth is not possible. Cesarean delivery has become safe enough so that nearly all clients can expect to recover. Women who know in advance of their elective cesarean delivery also have the advantage of being able to prepare for the birth. When the delivery is scheduled in advance, couples can attend cesarean education programs and plan for a family-centered birth experience. In addition, the delivery can be timed so that the health team and facilities necessary for the cesarean can be assembled without difficulty.

DRAWBACKS

There are several drawbacks related to cesarean delivery.

Despite increased safety of the surgery, maternal morbidity and mortality are higher for cesarean than vaginal births. Differences among studies and difficulties in compiling data, especially related to morbidity, make actual comparisons difficult. Mortality rates for cesarean delivery have been reported to be less than 1 death per 1000 births, with many of the deaths attributable to factors other than the cesarean procedure.[5,9] In one study of 10,231 consecutive cesarean deliveries, no maternal deaths occurred.[12] Cesarean delivery has been reported to have a two to four times larger maternal mortality risk than vaginal delivery.[9] The greatest risks for mortality are from anesthesia, severe infection, and thromboembolism. Risk of death related to aspiration pneumonia, once a major problem, has been decreased by the administration of a nonparticulate antacid such as sodium citrate and citric acid solution prior to the surgery.[6] Maternal morbidity has been estimated to occur with a frequency of 10 to 80 percent; clearly a broad range.[9] The exact incidence has been related to such factors as length of labor, rupture of membranes, and whether or not the cesarean was a repeat or primary operation. Infection, hemorrhage, and urinary tract injury are the leading reasons for maternal morbidity related to cesarean delivery.

The procedure itself can carry risks to the fetus. At times, miscalculation of fetal maturity has resulted in scheduling of a cesarean too early in gestation and delivery of a premature infant. This is called **iatrogenic prematurity,** because the prematurity results from inadvertent or erroneous treatment given by the physician. Careful client assessment using strategies to evaluate fetal maturity can minimize the likelihood of this event. Another risk to the fetus is accidental injury during the uterine incision, although this rarely happens. A very narrow uterine incision can also result in fetal trauma during delivery; however, there is greater chance of fetal trauma occurring during vaginal delivery.[5]

When done for medically or obstetrically high-risk clients, cesarean procedures can be complicated by pre-existing conditions. For example, diabetic women whose blood sugar levels are not monitored and controlled carefully may become hyperglycemic or hypoglycemic during or after surgery. This can lead to further complications such as fluid and electrolyte imbalance.

There is little choice in childbirth settings for cesarean clients. As a surgical procedure, cesarean delivery is always done in an operative environment within a hospital setting. Not every hospital that encourages family-centered, "homelike" birth practices for women with vaginal deliveries creates similar experiences for cesarean clients. Women who have cesareans can find themselves with a delivery experience very different from what they may have envisioned (eg, separated from their support partner, required to have general anesthesia because of a lack of available personnel qualified to administer regional anesthesia, or recovery in a general postoperative unit where maternal-infant contact is restricted).

Women who have emergency cesarean deliveries must deal with an unexpected outcome of their birth plan. This is especially problematic if a woman began labor and anticipated delivery in an out-of-hospital birth environment or in a hospital birthing room. Although some women feel relief at having a cesarean terminate labor,[13] others may have a sense of crisis and experience feelings such as disappointment, anger, confusion about the cesarean and loss of self-esteem.[13–14]

Women who deliver by cesarean have the simultaneous tasks of parenting a newborn and recovering from major abdominal surgery. Without help from family, friends, or hired assistants, this can be a difficult and exhausting problem.

Cesarean birth is more expensive than vaginal birth in terms of hospital fees for the procedure and lengthened hospital stay. Out-of-hospital costs include extended child care for children at home and the mother's needs for more assistance after discharge. In addition, the emotional cost of the cesarean to the client and her family must be considered.

Women who deliver by cesarean have a longer period of discomfort and restricted mobility than do women who deliver vaginally. Most cesarean clients require pharmaceutical assistance with pain control. It may take about a month before a woman who delivers by cesarean can move about with complete comfort. Such activities as driving a car (especially with manual transmission), changing positions (eg, from supine to sitting), or making any physical movements that require use of the abdominal muscles can be painful.

The presence of an abdominal scar may be upsetting to some women, especially if a vertical skin incision was used.

The likelihood of cesarean delivery for future pregnancies remains. Many women continue to have elective repeat cesareans, although an attempt at vaginal birth after cesarean would be considered safe in their situations. Even when women attempt vaginal delivery after a cesarean, delivery occurs in a setting where operative delivery is accessible, as ability to perform the cesarean within 30 minutes is one of the guidelines for a vaginal birth after a cesarean.[9] Delivery alternatives, such as the use of a birth center, are also restricted, because of licensing regulations, concerns for client safety, and other factors.

CONTRAINDICATIONS

The safety level of cesarean delivery has improved so that no absolute maternal contraindications to the procedure exist. If, however, maternal blood clotting ability is greatly compromised, vaginal delivery, if possible, is preferred because it presents less risk of bleeding. Cesarean delivery is not done when the fetus is thought to be too premature to survive.[5] This situation also raises moral and ethical questions.

TYPES

Definitions

A cesarean delivery may be primary (that is, a woman's first abdominal delivery) or repeat. A cesarean is called "repeat" when the woman has delivered at least once before in this manner. Both primary and repeat cesareans can be done on an elective basis or on an emergency basis. An elective cesarean is a planned abdominal delivery; the woman knows in advance that a cesarean birth will be performed. An elective cesarean may be done for a variety of reasons, including maternal diabetes, malpresentation of the fetus, placenta previa, and history of previous cesarean. Emergency cesareans are done for conditions in which prompt delivery is thought necessary to preserve the life or well-being of the mother, fetus, or both. Emergency cesareans can be performed for situations that require immediate delivery, such as abruptio placentae and acute fetal distress, or for situations in which a delay of an hour or two is unlikely to harm the mother or fetus, such as failure to progress in labor and prolonged rupture of membranes.

Incisions

Cesarean deliveries are done using two major incisional approaches: classic and low segment (Figure 28–1). With a classic cesarean incision, a midline incision is made vertically through the skin and subcutaneous tissues and vertically into the body of the uterus. The incision extends from above the lower uterine segment to the fundus of the uterus. Advantages of this type of incision are that it provides quicker access to the fetus in a true emergency, offers greater visibility of the pregnant uterus to the physician performing the surgery, and can readily be extended upward if more room for delivery of the fetus is needed. A classic incision is technically easier to do than a low-segment incision (described next) and therefore might be selected by an inexperienced physician handling an emergency delivery.

Several disadvantages are related to the classic cesarean incision. From a technical standpoint, there may be greater blood loss because of the location of the incision through the uterine muscles. A vertical skin incision leaves a midline abdominal scar, which many women consider cosmetically undesirable. In addition, the scar tissue that forms vertically along the muscles in the uterus presents a plane of weakness in this organ. Although the chance of uterine rupture is small during a future pregnancy or labor, there is greater likelihood of rupture with a vertical classic incision than with a horizontal, low-segment incision.[5]

Low-segment cesarean incisions are currently the incisions most frequently performed for cesarean delivery. With this approach, a low, transverse incision is made through the skin and subcutaneous tissue at the level of the pubic hairline. This is called a Pfannenstiel incision, after the 19th-century German gynecologist who pioneered the procedure. (The Pfannenstiel incision refers to the incision through the skin and subcutaneous tissue, but not to the type of uterine incision.) A popular term for this incision is "bikini cut," for the healed incision is most often contained within the pubic hairline, or bikini line.

Cosmetically, a Pfannenstiel incision is preferable to a vertical midline skin incision, because, after healing, the abdomen is not visibly marked with a pronounced scar, as with a vertical skin incision. In addition, the Pfannenstiel is a stronger incision, with less chance of wound opening or hernia development.[5] Disadvantages of the Pfannenstiel incision include less visibility of the uterus for the physician performing the surgery than with a vertical incision (especially in obese women) and difficulty in extending the incision, should the physician require more room to deliver the fetus. A greater amount of time,

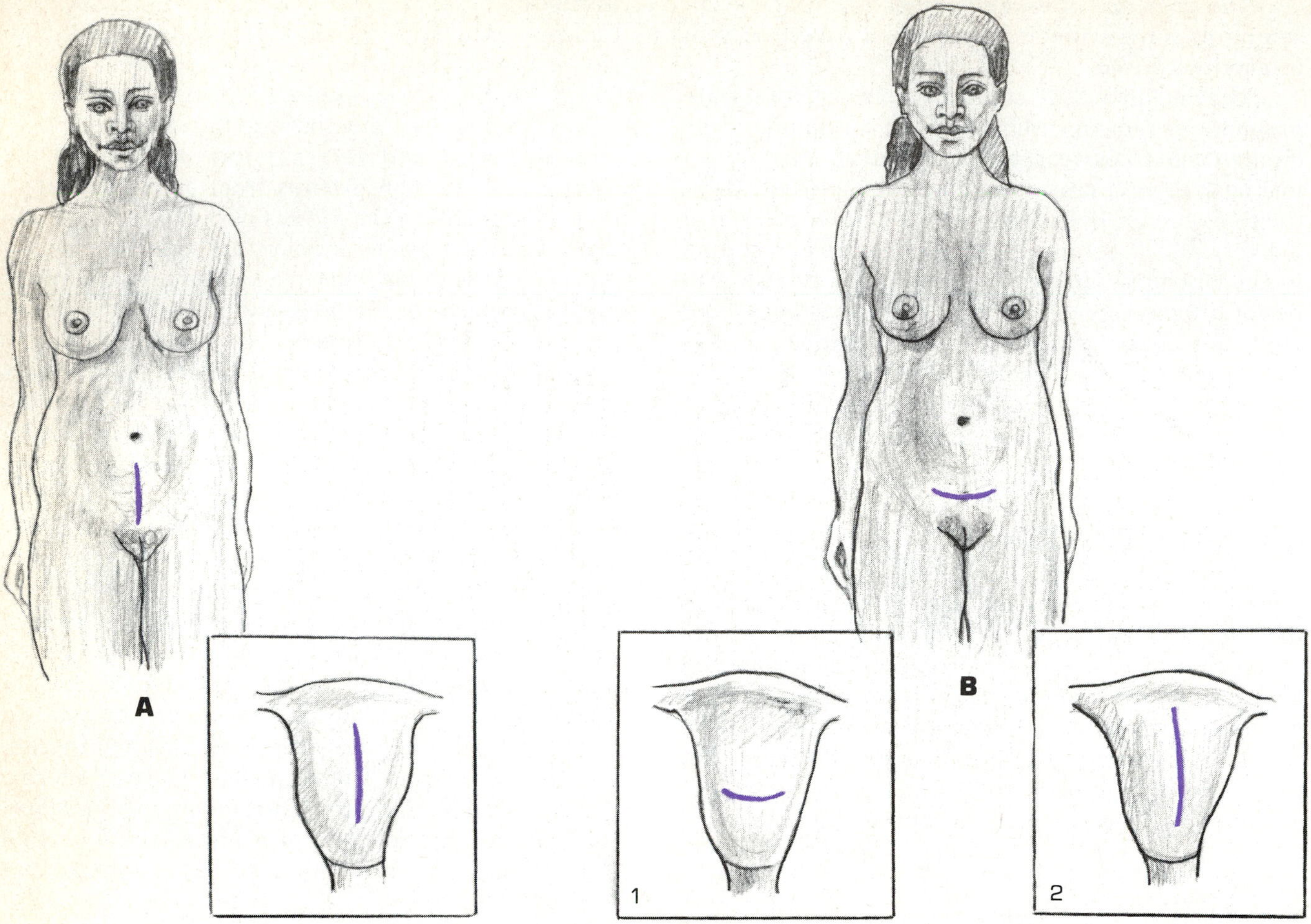

Figure 28–1. Types of uterine incisions. **A.** Vertical skin incision with vertical uterine incision ("classic" incision). **B.** Horizontal skin incision with (1) horizontal low-segment uterine incision or (2) vertical uterine incision ("classic" incision).

particularly during repeat cesarean, is required for this incision; this can be a threat to fetal well-being in some emergency cases.[5] A horizontal, low-segment uterine incision has the advantages of less associated blood loss, less likelihood of the development of adhesions of abdominal organs (such as the bowel) to the healed incisional line, and less chance of rupture in future pregnancy and labor.

Various combinations of skin and uterine incisions may be used according to the clinical situation. A horizontal, low-segment uterine incision and a vertical skin incision may be used for the very obese client, so that the skin incision does not lie directly within the deep skin folds of the obese abdomen. Occasionally, a vertical uterine incision may be accompanied by a Pfannenstiel incision. In situations such as prematurity, the lower uterine segment has not thinned as it does in late pregnancy, and this makes a horizontal incision more difficult. A vertical uterine incision may also be preferable when the fetus is in a breech position.

Skin and uterine incisions are separate. There is no way simply to look at a cesarean abdominal skin suture line or scar and identify the type of uterine incision used. This information, however, which is recorded by the physician in the client's chart immediately after the procedure is completed, is important. For instance, a client with a previous low-segment, transverse uterine incision and no other suspected recurrent risk conditions would be in an optimal situation in which to attempt a future vaginal birth.

Repeat cesareans are usually performed through the same incisions, even if the previous incisions were vertical. The scar tissue, if thick, is removed. In addition to the obvious cosmetic benefit of one rather than two types of skin and uterine incisions, scar tissue of a healed incision is a plane of weakness. It is therefore of physiologic advantage to minimize the number of incision sites into the uterus.

Cesarean hysterectomy, a surgical procedure in which the uterus as well as the fetus is removed, is performed as a last-resort measure during obstetric emergencies like uncontrollable uterine hemorrhage, severe uterine infection, and the presence of large uterine tumors. Obviously, sterilization results from removal of the uterus and is of great consequence to women who want future pregnancies. Women who do not desire more children may also have negative feelings related to the loss of a "feminine" body organ. Cesarean hysterectomy is not a recommended method of voluntary sterilization. This procedure entails more extensive, higher-risk surgery than tubal sterilization after cesarean delivery.

The type of cesarean procedure selected depends on the clinical situation, physician judgment, and client request. Nurses need to be able to provide knowledgeable information to women about cesarean procedures. Prenatally, nurses can provide teaching on this topic during prenatal visits or during prepared childbirth classes, as cesarean delivery is a potential method of delivery for all clients. Nurses can also encourage clients, as a means of participating in their own childbirth experience, to discuss this subject with their physicians or nurse-midwives prior to delivery. Although nurse-midwives do not perform cesareans, they educate clients prenatally about what to expect in case a cesarean becomes necessary. In many instances, the nurse-midwife remains with the client to provide support throughout the cesarean delivery. During the postpartum period, through interventions based on assessment of client and family responses to the cesarean, nurses can further promote client understanding of cesarean delivery.

ANESTHESIA FOR CESAREAN DELIVERY

Currently several anesthetic options, including various anesthetic agents and techniques, can be used for cesarean delivery. Selection of drugs to be used for anesthesia is made by the anesthesiologist or the certified nurse anesthetist in consultation with the anesthesiologist and is based on the unique needs of the client. Choice of a technique of anesthesia depends on factors such as the obstetric requirements, the judgment of the individual administering the anesthetic, and the desires of the client.[15]

The major anesthetic techniques used for cesarean delivery include general anesthesia and regional anesthesia. Table 28–1 presents advantages, limitations and potential complications of general and regional anesthesia.[15–24] Morbidity and mortality can be lower for regional anesthesia used for cesarean delivery. Regional anesthesia has also been used increasingly for cesarean birth because women are able to be awake for the birth of their infant.

General Anesthesia

During general anesthesia, the mother is not awake during the cesarean delivery, for loss of sensation is accompanied by loss of consciousness. The woman is always intubated during the procedure so that optimum respiratory status may be maintained.

Regional Anesthesia

With regional anesthesia, the client is awake during the cesarean delivery, and a "region" of the body is anesthetized. The two types of regional anesthesia used for cesarean delivery are spinal anesthesia and epidural anesthesia.

Spinal Anesthesia. With spinal anesthesia, an anesthetic drug is injected through the second, third, or fourth interspace of the lumbar vertebrae and into the subarachnoid space (Figure 28–2). Although the needle is inserted at this level, the effect of the sensory blockade is felt higher, to the level of the fourth thoracic dermatome (T4). The drug acts on the spinal nerve roots and prevents both nerve transmission and sensation of pain. The effect of the anesthesia begins with the toes, spreads to the perineum, and then includes the legs and abdomen.[25] The needle is inserted below the level of the spinal cord (not into the spinal cord, as some clients fear).

Epidural Anesthesia. Epidural anesthesia, also used for cesarean births, is a type of regional anesthesia in which an anesthetic drug is injected into the epidural space (*see* Figure 28–2). The terms *peridural*, *epidural*, and *extradural* are used interchangeably. The anesthetic is placed outside the dura and not in the subarachnoid space (where spinal anesthetics would be inserted). It may be recalled that the epidural space is a potential rather than an actual space, located between the dura, which is the fibrous membrane containing the spinal cord and cerebrospinal fluid, and the vertebrae. The epidural space holds blood vessels, lymphatics, areolar tissue, and an internal venous plexus. The anesthetic drug that is injected blocks the nerve fibers that transmit pain, as the nerves coming from the spinal cord leave the dura.[17]

Like spinal anesthesia, epidural anesthesia may be given in a "one shot" dose; however, it is frequently administered through a catheter placed by

TABLE 28–1. ADVANTAGES, LIMITATIONS, AND POTENTIAL COMPLICATIONS OF GENERAL AND REGIONAL ANESTHESIA FOR CESAREAN BIRTH

Advantages	Limitations	Potential Complications
General Anesthesia		
Pain free induction of anesthesia and delivery Can be induced rapidly; useful in emergencies requiring immediate delivery (eg, massive bleeding, severe fetal distress) Level of anesthesia readily controlled Associated with less hypotension and cardiovascular instability than regional anesthesia; better control of airway and ventilation Preferable in clients with such conditions as gross neurologic problems, infections, or blood clotting problems In all states can be administered by a nurse-anesthetist as well as by physicians; may be the only choice available in hospitals where staffing by anesthesiologists is limited May be preferred by some clients who do not want to be awake for abdominal delivery	Client is not awake for delivery; loss of experience of being aware of baby's birth; may be "groggy" in recovery room; possible delay in bonding In some settings, fathers not allowed in delivery room if mother not awake; thus, limitation of fathers' birth experience A less vigorous, sleepier baby at birth	Pneumonitis from aspiration of gastric contents (To minimize this, in emergency situations a clear, nonparticulate oral antacid can quickly increase gastric pH above 2.5. In elective cases, a histamine-blocking agent such as ranitidine may be given 2 hours before anesthesia induction to raise gastric pH above 2.5 and to decrease gastric volume. Metoclopramide, given 1 hour before induction, promotes gastric emptying, raises gastrointestinal tone, and lowers risk of reflux and regurgitation.) Potential respiratory depression Problems with accessing and maintaining patent airway Tension pneumothorax related to positive pressure ventilation Possible injury to teeth and mouth during intubation Neonatal depression
Regional Anesthesia: Spinal		
Client awake and able to experience delivery; able to share delivery with support person Pain-free delivery; mild discomfort when administered Client able to breathe on her own; Oxygen administered by face mask Avoids the risk of failed intubation, a complication related to general anesthesia Decreased risk of aspiration of gastric contents, as client remains awake Safer for emergency delivery if client has recently eaten Does not irritate respiratory system Less neonatal drug depression than with general anesthesia	Requires a skilled operator for administration (in many places, can be given by physicians only) Almost always given in single dose which produces 1½ to 4 hours of anesthesia; complications prolonging surgery may then necessitate general anesthesia Less likely to be given via spinal catheter than epidural because of greater risk of postspinal headache Requires slightly more time to establish than general anesthesia Contraindicated with local or certain systemic infections, coagulation defects, abnormalities of the vertebral canal; preexisting neurologic disease conditions of spinal cord or peripheral nerves are relative contraindications Nausea and shivering, related to the surgery, may be experienced during the cesarean delivery	Hypotension Hypovolemic shock Possibility of postspinal headache, which could last up to 4 days postpartum. (This may be related to leakage of cerebrospinal fluid following dural puncture for injection of the local anesthetic into the subarachnoid space; incidence of headache may be minimized by use of a high-gauge, small-bore spinal needle.) Postspinal backache or soreness at site of injection Total spinal anesthesia with respiratory paralysis; occurs rarely Vasopressor-induced hypertension from interaction of vasoactive drugs and ergot derivatives
Regional Anesthesia: Epidural		
Similar to advantages for spinal anesthesia Can be administered in single dose or repeated through catheter placed in epidural space; inserted at interspace between second, third, or fourth lumbar vertebrae; length of procedure with indwelling epidural catheter is not a problem Since epidural does not enter subarachnoid space, less incidence of headache; hypotension occurs less rapidly than with spinal level of anesthesia Easier to control than spinal Provides a route for administration of postpartum analgesics, such as the opioids	Similar to limitations for spinal anesthesia; time required to initiate epidural block and get effective analgesia	Hypotension Nausea, vomiting Accidental misplacement of anesthetic and overdose (eg, intravenously) can cause major problems such as cardiac arrest or convulsions; injection into the subarachnoid space may cause a total spinal and may be associated with permanent neurologic damage Specific complications relate to the drug used Epidural hematoma at site of injection Infection Nerve injury (rare, because any pressure on spinal cord or nerve roots would be so painful that it is unlikely the procedure would be done)

Source: References 15–24.

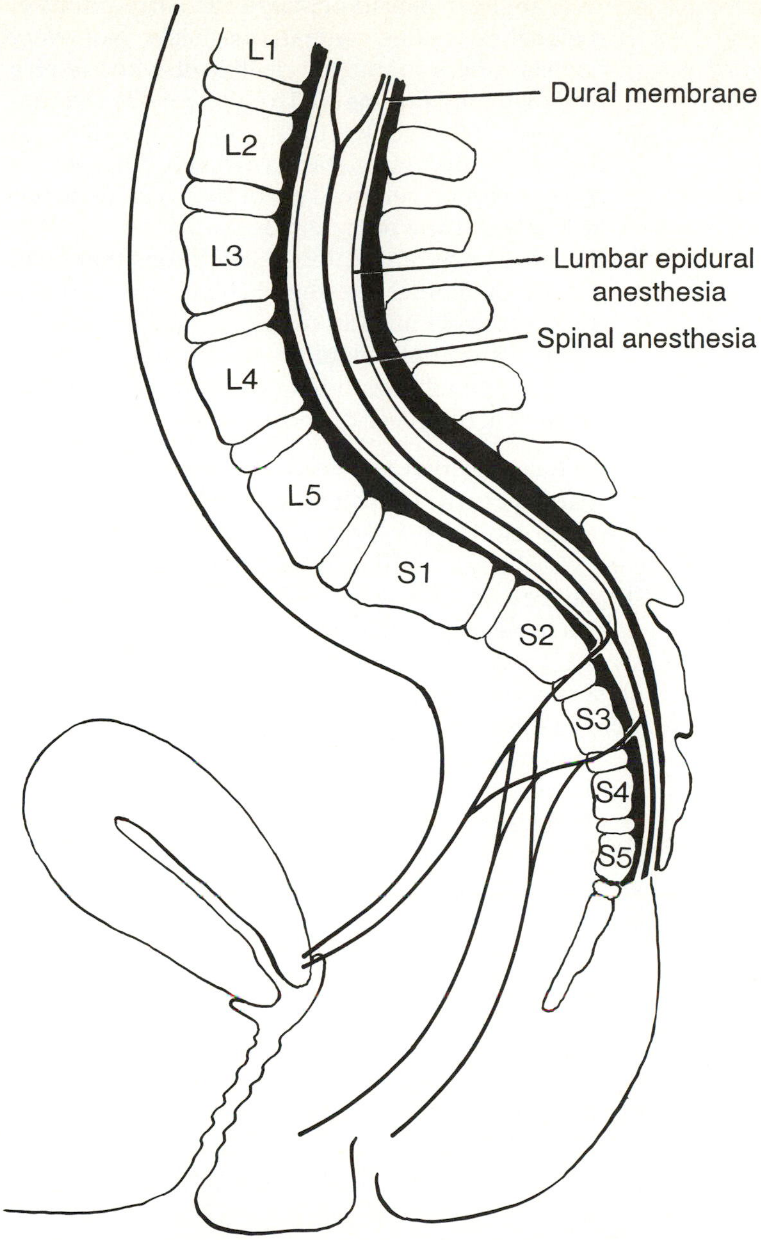

Figure 28–2. Placement of epidural and spinal anesthetics. (After Beischer NA, Mackay EV. *Obstetrics and the Newborn.* 2nd ed. Sydney: WB Saunders: 1986:358.)

the anesthesiologist into the epidural space prior to the cesarean delivery. Repeated doses of the anesthetic drugs can then be given to ensure a pain free surgery, regardless of the time needed to complete the delivery. Although most cesarean deliveries and abdominal repairs are completed in less than one and a half hours, complications can prolong the time needed for the surgery and, therefore, anesthesia. Continuous epidural anesthesia is frequently selected over continuous spinal anesthesia for cesarean delivery, because clients who receive spinal anesthesia are at greater risk of postspinal headache (possibly related to leakage of cerebrospinal fluid during instillation of anesthesia) and infection.

Prior to removal of the epidural catheter, the anesthesiologist may administer a narcotic through the catheter (*see* later discussion). This provides prolonged analgesia by interrupting opiate pain receptors at the level of the cord itself.

During cesarean delivery with successful regional anesthesia, the mother is awake and aware, yet feels no pain. Additional oxygen may be given by mask, but the woman is not intubated. An intravenous infusion is kept running for fluid and electrolyte therapy during surgery and as an available route for intravenous medications.

Occasionally, a woman may feel a sensation of pressure as the baby is being delivered or pressure and nausea as the uterus is manipulated. Some women feel cold during the procedure. Afterwards, shivering, possibly related to the loss of body heat from extensive sympathetic nerve blockade, may occur with greater frequency than after vaginal delivery.[17] (The use of warmed blankets on completion of the procedure can do much to promote client comfort.) In the recovery room, the woman will first be able to feel touch; motor function, position sense, temperature sensation, superficial pain, and autonomic activity then return.[25]

Other Techniques

Local infiltration anesthesia has been used for cesarean delivery in the past. Currently, local infiltration anesthesia is performed only in emergency situations where regional or general anesthesia is unavailable. Higher doses of drugs needed to produce anesthesia with local infiltration, longer time needed to ensure anesthesia, and the potential for greater client discomfort are among the reasons spinal, epidural, or general anesthesia are preferred to local infiltration.

On occasion, women may ask about other techniques of anesthesia, such as hypnosis or acupuncture. These are not considered to be standards of practice for cesarean delivery in the United States and therefore are not readily available. Further reports and research are necessary before these techniques can be recommended as anesthetic alternatives.

Decision on Type of Anesthesia

It is not possible to identify a perfect technique of anesthesia for all women having cesarean deliveries. The type of anesthesia used for a cesarean depends on several factors:

Whether the delivery is done on an emergency or an elective basis. Obstetric emergencies such as massive bleeding and severe fetal distress necessitate immediate cesarean delivery with the fastest mode of anesthesia, usually general anesthesia. In some situations, such as failure to progress in labor or failure of labor induction, immediate delivery is not crucial, and a choice between general and regional anesthesia is possible.[15]

Obstetric requirements.

Client preference. Some women do not wish to be awake during the surgery, whereas others do.

Judgment of the person administering the anesthetic.

5. Availability of skilled personnel able to administer regional as well as general anesthesia. Not every hospital offers round-the-clock staff who are able to provide regional as well as general obstetric anesthesia. In some settings, general anesthesia is the only option available to women who deliver by cesarean on certain days of the week or at certain times of the day.
6. Presence of certain maternal conditions that favor the use of general anesthesia (hemorrhagic disorders, hypovolemia, infection in the area where the regional anesthetic would be administered, and so on) or regional anesthesia (a difficult airway, just having eaten, obesity, and so on).

When maternal and fetal safety allows, families can participate in selection of type of anesthesia. Ideally, this would be a topic discussed prenatally with each client, just as the possibility of cesarean birth should be considered. In this way, women have a chance to determine whether they would want to be awake for delivery and have an opportunity to express any of their concerns related to anesthesia. In collaboration with the physician, the nurse can provide information about anesthesia and about anesthetic options available at local hospitals.

Nurses must be knowledgeable about these topics related to anesthesia, because there can be great variation among hospitals. For example, as noted earlier, regional anesthesia may not always be available at some hospitals. Some hospitals may allow a support person to be present whether or not a woman receives general anesthesia; many others will allow a support person to be present only if the woman is awake for delivery.

PREPARATION FOR CESAREAN DELIVERY

Before Pregnancy

Preparation for cesarean birth actually begins prior to pregnancy. Today, cesareans are common procedures. Many couples have friends or relatives who have had cesareans; some have had previous cesarean deliveries themselves. These experiences may or may not have been positive. Television, noted by Kalisch and Kalisch to be second in influence in the United States only to the White House,[26] radio, publications, and other media have also had great impact on public impressions of cesarean births. Such impressions can evolve from factually presented material or highly distorted approaches tailored to story lines.

An important nursing responsibility is to be aware of how cesarean births are being portrayed by the media, as well as the nature of client perceptions of this type of childbirth. In addition, the nurse needs to examine her or his own attitude toward cesarean births. Through roles as authors, speakers, and consultants, as well as in letters to the media, nurses can affect the accuracy of information presented to the public and can promote public awareness of options available to families regarding cesarean birth.

During Pregnancy

The topic of cesarean birth should be raised with all clients, regardless of risk status. Childbirth always carries an element of uncertainty; it is not possible—or prudent—to promise a low-risk vaginal delivery. During prepared childbirth classes or antenatal health visits or through work with the media, the nurse is in an unique position to provide information regarding cesarean birth and options available to clients in their local hospitals. The nurse also can encourage and facilitate discussion between the pregnant couple and their physician or nurse-midwife.

Currently, a number of hospitals and organizations offer childbirth education programs specifically for the couple who will have a planned cesarean delivery. The reasons for these classes are similar to the reasons for classes for couples expecting a vaginal delivery. Physical and psychologic preparation can help couples to integrate birth, whether vaginally or abdominally, into the cycle of life events, to maintain a sense of control, and to have an emotionally satisfying, safe delivery. In addition, a positive cesarean birth experience may facilitate the attachment process between parents and newborn.[27,28]

Many topics are covered during cesarean birth classes, for example:[27–29]

- Previous cesarean experiences, plans, and goals of expectant couples attending the classes
- Attitudes toward cesarean births
- Indications for cesarean birth
- Safety and risks of cesarean birth
- Tests for fetal well-being and maturity
- Importance of good maternal health during pregnancy
- Nutrition
- Physical conditioning—exercises for relaxation, exercises to promote comfort during pregnancy and postpartum
- Cesarean prevention, vaginal birth after cesarean
- Signs of impending labor and what to do if labor begins
- The hospital experience (tour of facility, description of admission procedures, hospital policies regarding cesarean deliveries, differences among local hospitals in policies regarding cesarean deliveries)
- Role of nurses and other health care personnel in care of the cesarean family
- Preparation for surgery, family concerns related to surgery
- Home arrangements (eg, child care for other children, advance preparation for help at home following discharge)
- In-hospital physical preparation (eg, blood tests, intravenous line insertion, vital signs, fetal assessment, urinary catheter, shave and scrub)
- Anesthesia options
- The cesarean procedure—what will be experienced before, during, and after the cesarean (films on cesarean birth may be shown)
- Role of the support person (what she or he will and will not be able to do, what the support person may experience)
- Appearance of the newborn and care in the delivery room
- Opportunities for parent-infant contact in delivery room and recovery area
- Recovery unit procedures and personnel; whether the client recovers in a maternity unit or in a general hospital recovery unit
- Recovery from anesthesia, pain and pain medications, relaxation exercises such as deep breathing and imagery
- Postpartum care in the recovery unit
- Postpartum care in hospital (pain management, positions and exercises to promote comfort in the first postpartum days, changing positions, ambulation, deep breathing, coughing, comfortable positions for infant care)
- Infant feeding choices, techniques, and positions
- Involution—physical and emotional changes in hospital and after discharge
- Diet and exercise
- Possibility of early discharge programs
- Managing at home after discharge (physical needs, integration of infant into family, special needs of cesarean parents)
- Emotional responses related to cesarean birth
- Value of cesarean support group

Role of the Nurse Preoperatively

Nurses in delivery room settings work with women who did not expect to have a cesarean, with women who knew in advance of their scheduled surgical birth, and with women who are planning a vaginal birth after a previous cesarean but who may undergo another cesarean if labor complications emerge. Whatever the situation, it is essential for the nurse to assess the client's level of knowledge and preparation and to provide clear, accurate information. The nurse must remember that most people have fears related to childbirth and to surgery, even if they do not initiate discussion of them. Calm, knowledgeable emotional support can do much to reduce the sense of crisis associated with cesarean birth (Figure 28–3). Strategies that enhance a sense of control and joy in the birth experience, such as actively encouraging the couple in the decision-making process and making the surgical birth as family-centered as possible, can do much toward fostering a sense of client-staff collaboration and toward ensuring a positive delivery experience for the woman.

Preoperative teaching should be done for clients whether or not they have attended prepared childbirth classes and regardless of their backgrounds. This includes physicians and nurses who have cesarean births. These individuals at times have been deprived of the quality of educational preparation offered to other clients, because staff assume that they already know "all there is to know."

The nurse has a broad and varied role in preoperative preparation of the client for cesarean birth. The importance of anticipatory guidance, teaching, and emotional support, noted earlier, remains constant throughout any nurse-client-family interactions. The actual sequences of preoperative events may vary according to the client's status and individual hospital, medical, or nursing policies.

Verification of client identification takes place as soon as the woman arrives on the unit. At this time an identification bracelet and anklet for the baby may be obtained and taped to the front of the mother's chart. This does not, however, absolve delivery room nurses from the responsibility of checking to make sure that the neonate's identification number corresponds to the mother's identification number before either leaves the delivery room.

Consent for the cesarean is obtained on admission to the unit or at the time that need for the cesarean has been determined. Although getting consent is within the role of the physician, in many hospitals the nurse may act as a witness to the consent. For ethical and legal reasons, the nurse should not sign any consent that he or she has not directly witnessed; for the same reasons, nurses are advised not to obtain consent for the cesarean. Nursing history and physical assessment are done, prenatal records are reviewed, and nursing goals, intervention strategies, and expected outcomes (nursing care plan) are developed.

Preoperative testing is performed. A urine specimen is sent to the laboratory for analysis; simple testing for glucose, acetone, and protein may be done on the unit.

Blood samples are drawn for complete blood count (CBC), electrolytes, and clotting studies (when indicated). A blood sample is also sent to be typed and cross-matched with available blood bank blood in case the woman requires transfusions. In some settings, the nurse performs the venipuncture and

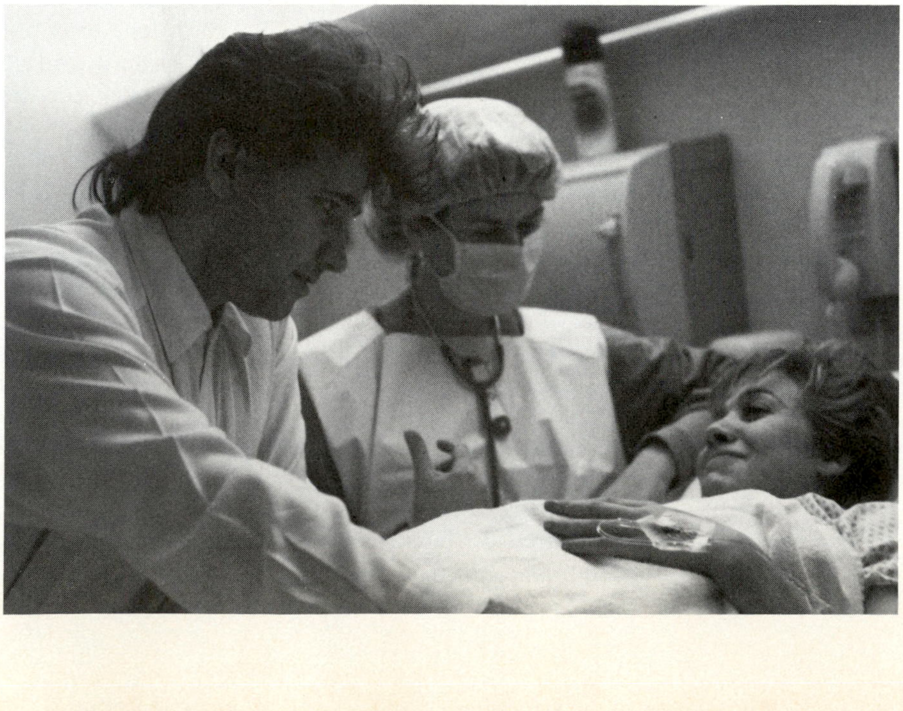

Figure 28–3. The nurse provides anticipatory guidance to the couple prior to cesarean birth.

obtains and sends the blood specimens. In other settings, technicians or house staff are available. Blood specimens must be clearly labeled and sent without delay for laboratory analysis, especially if the cesarean is being done on an emergency basis. In emergency situations, a staff member should notify the laboratory of the importance of prompt attention.

In some hospitals, scheduled elective cesarean clients may be preadmitted; that is, laboratory studies may have been done prior to their admission date. In this case, the results need to be recorded on the client's chart before the cesarean. Both physicians and nurses must know recent laboratory results for a client prior to any surgical procedure. In the interest of client well-being and in the spirit of professional collaboration, the nurse should make certain that the physician is aware of any abnormal values and that, whenever indicated, appropriate interventions have been initiated.

An intravenous line is inserted. In many labor and delivery units, this procedure is done by the nursing staff. An intravenous infusion is needed to provide ready intravascular access for medications, for fluid and electrolyte therapy, and for blood transfusions, if necessary. An intravenous catheter to avoid infiltration and a bore large enough for blood products (18 g) should be used. Small, "butterfly" needles are not used.

Prescribed medications are administered. For example, intravenous antibiotics may be given when the woman is thought to be at risk for infection (eg, prolonged ruptured membranes). A nonparticulate antacid may be administered 30 to 60 minutes before the surgery, along with the histamine blocking and gastric emptying agents.

The abdomen is shaved and scrubbed from the xiphoid to about 2½ in. below the pubic hairline. It is not necessary to shave the entire mons, although this is common practice in some hospitals.

An indwelling urinary catheter is inserted. In nonemergency cases, this can be done after establishing the regional block to avoid needless maternal discomfort. Continuous urinary drainage is established to keep the bladder decompressed during cesarean surgery and to lower the risk of surgical injury to the bladder. In women who have normal renal function and who are receiving intravenous fluid therapy, the bladder can quickly become distended during the surgery; this could also inhibit proper contraction of the uterus after delivery of the infant. Routine procedure in many hospitals calls for insertion of the catheter before the woman is brought to the delivery room. At best, this is a very uncomfortable procedure for the woman. The catheter can easily be inserted in the delivery room after the woman has been anesthetized, even when cesarean delivery is unplanned. (The nurse should be aware that diplomacy, especially in dealing with other nurses and with physicians, may be necessary in altering traditional routines.)

A histamine-blocking agent, such as ranitidine, may be given about 2 hours before elective use of general anesthesia to raise gastric pH above 2.5 and to decrease gastric volume.[24] Metoclopramide, which may be administered an hour before anesthesia is induced, promotes gastric emptying and raises gastrointestinal tone; this lowers the chance of reflux and regurgitation. Histamine-blocking agents need 60 to 90 minutes after administration for optimal effect. Therefore in emergencies or before regional anesthesia, a nonparticulate (clear) antacid (such as 30 mL of sodium citrate) may be given to quickly raise gastric pH for at least an hour. Traditionally, clients are kept NPO prior to general anesthesia; however, the amount of time between the last oral feeding and the induction of general anesthesia does not have much importance in identifying the client's actual chance of aspiration.[24]

The father, or other support person, is assisted in preparing for the cesarean. Appropriate clothing for the delivery room is given, as well as information about what he may expect, where he will be positioned during delivery, and what his role will be (Figure 28–4). Directions need to be clear and simply stated. The nurse needs to provide appropriate support, as an expectant father about to see his infant born by cesarean may be experiencing feelings ranging from excitement to terror.

To promote the client's safety, side rails need to be kept raised, and the woman should not be left unattended. The labor room nurse does not leave until the client has been transferred to the cesarean delivery room and until the nurses who will attend the cesarean have directly assumed responsibility for her care. In many units, the nurses who care for the client in the labor unit also assist at the cesarean delivery. A woman who has an unplanned cesarean may have had an epidural catheter placed while she was in the labor room. During transport and transfer to the operating table, special care needs to be taken so that the epidural catheter does not become displaced or that the woman does not sustain injury as a result of impaired sensory and motor functions of her lower extremities.

The nurse also makes certain that the cesarean delivery team has been notified of the impending birth. This includes the anesthesiologist, nursery

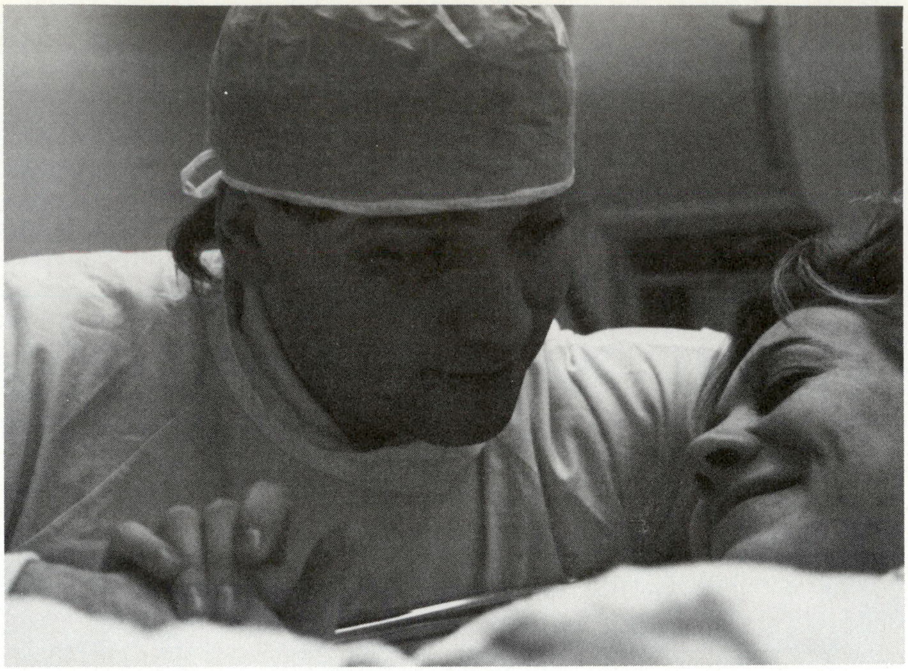

Figure 28–4. The couple remains together prior to planned cesarean birth.

nurses, and pediatrician, as well as the obstetrician or perinatologist. When problems are expected with the newborn, a special-care nursery nurse and a neonatologist, when part of the hospital staff, may also be called to attend the birth.

DELIVERY ROOM CARE

After the woman arrives in the cesarean delivery room (Figure 28–5), the obstetrician, medical assistants, anesthesiologist, pediatrician, and nursing staff

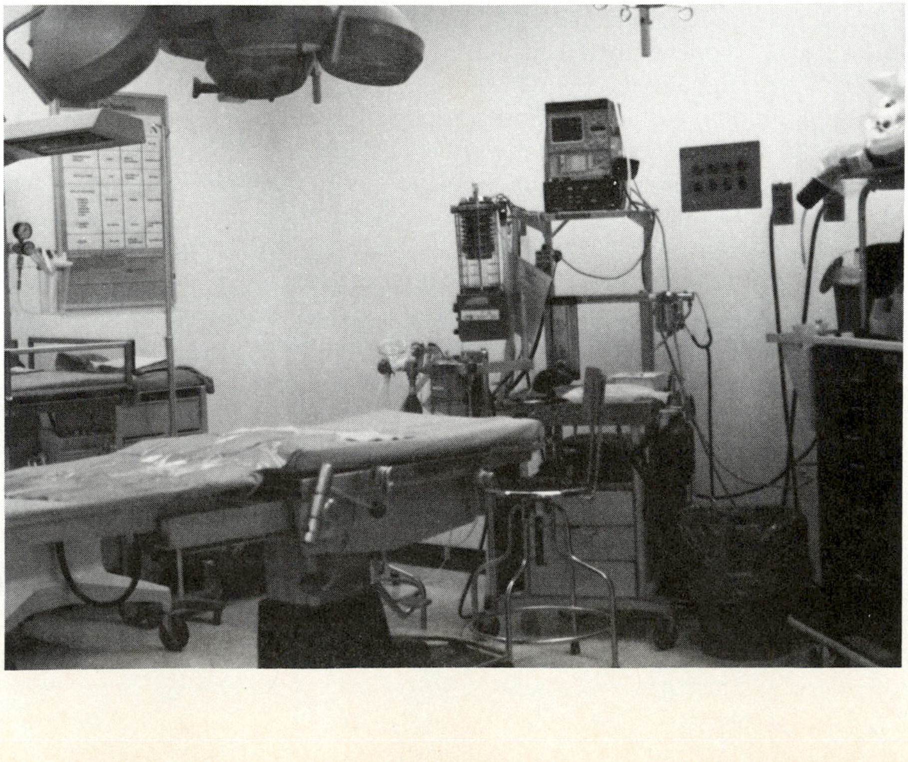

Figure 28–5. Cesarean delivery room.

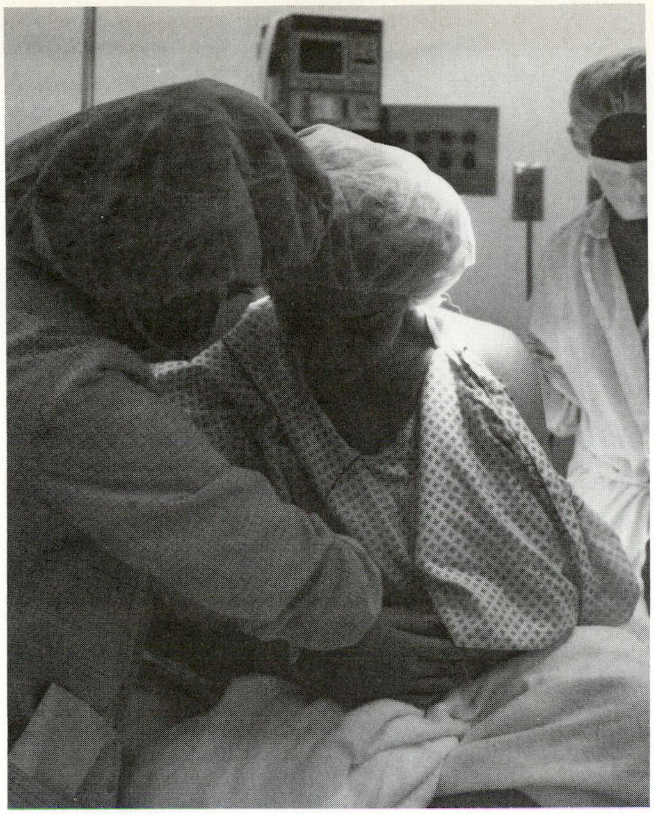

A

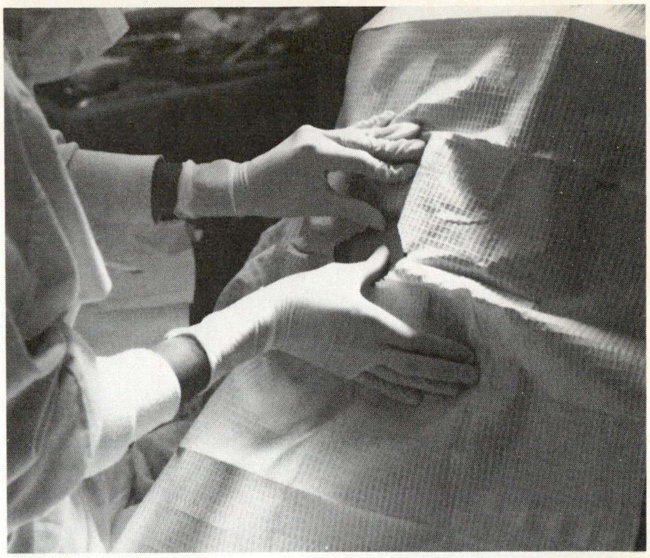

B

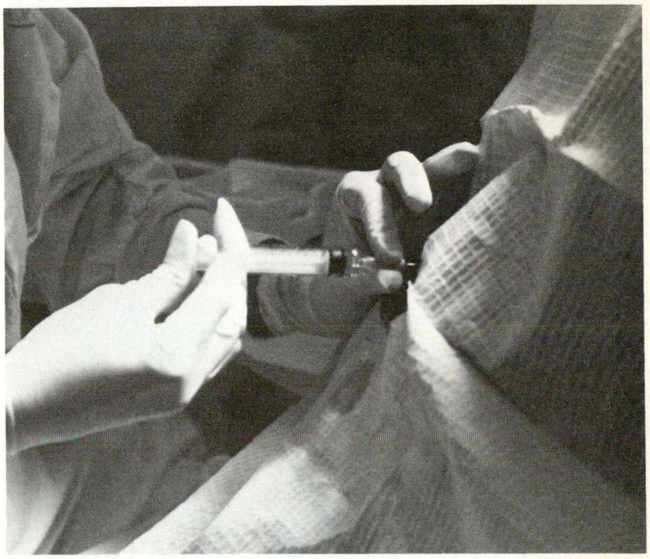

C

Figure 28–6. Regional anesthetic is given prior to cesarean delivery. **A.** The nurse comforts the client as she assists her into position for spinal anesthesia. Keeping the head bent and back arched forward widens the spaces between the vertebrae and facilitates placement of the spinal needle. The client's back is cleansed prior to administration of spinal anesthetic. **B.** The anesthesiologist then palpates prior to insertion of the spinal needle. **C.** Administration of spinal anesthetic; after return of spinal fluid through the needle hub indicated that the needle penetrated the spinal canal.

who will assist at the delivery assume responsibility for her and her baby. In some hospitals cesareans are performed in the general surgical suites by obstetricians or are assisted by operating room nurses who come to the maternity unit to attend the cesarean. In other hospitals, nurses who regularly work in labor and delivery may scrub and assist with the procedure. They may also circulate and assist with nonsterile functions that do not require a surgical scrub, such as aiding the anesthesia personnel, helping the scrub nurses and physicians dress in sterile attire, performing an antiseptic scrub of the operative area, verifying the initial and final sponge and instrument count with the scrub nurse, recording the time and nature of delivery room events, participating in immediate care of the neonate, and giving encouragement to the mother and her support person.

Normal maintenance of delivery rooms is in large part under nursing supervision. Rooms should be kept stocked with current equipment in good repair. Nurses attending cesarean deliveries must also know how to use the equipment properly and with ease. An actual delivery is not the time to find out there are no more sutures, that the suction machine does not work, or that the oxytocin has expired. An operative suite equipped for cesarean delivery always needs to be ready to receive a client, even on units where cesarean deliveries are not frequently performed.

Regional anesthesia is administered by the anesthesiologist prior to the staff's scrubbing and prior to the preparation of the surgical site (Figure 28–6). This allows time for the anesthesia to take effect. If general

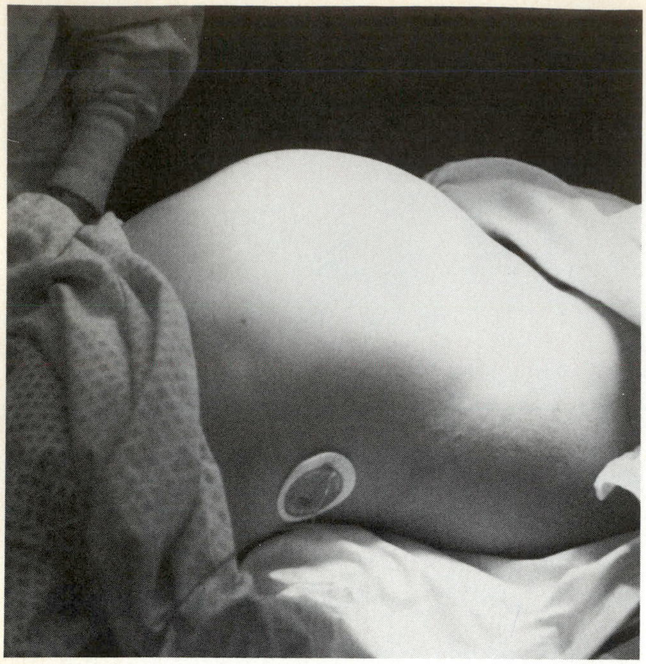

A

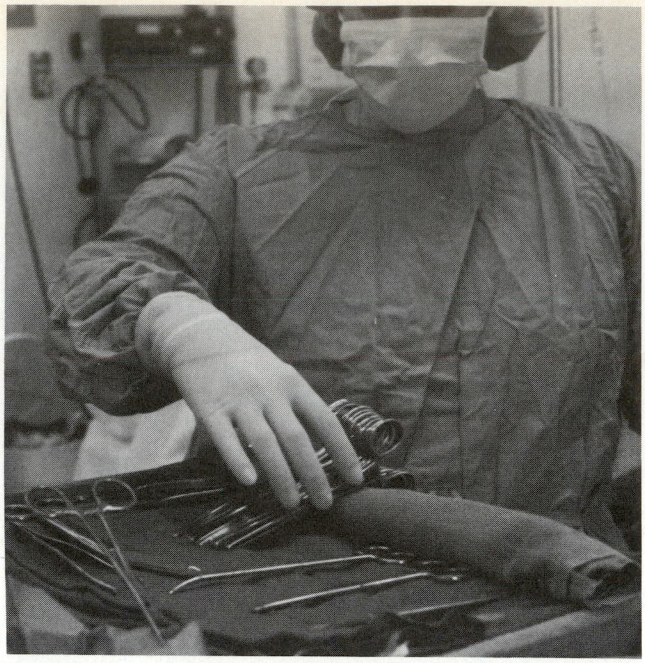

B

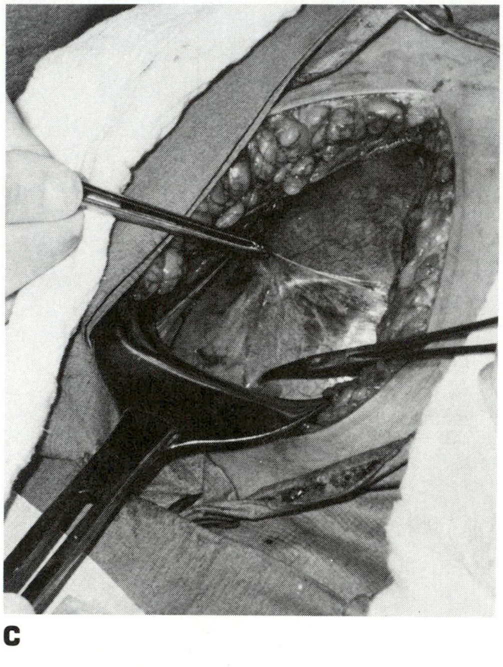

C

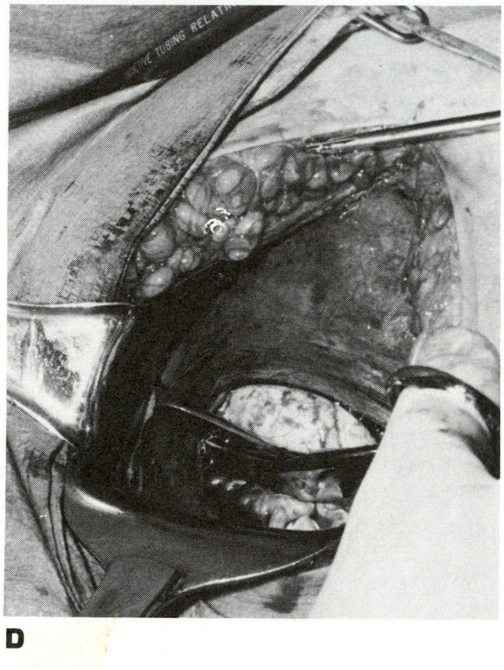

D

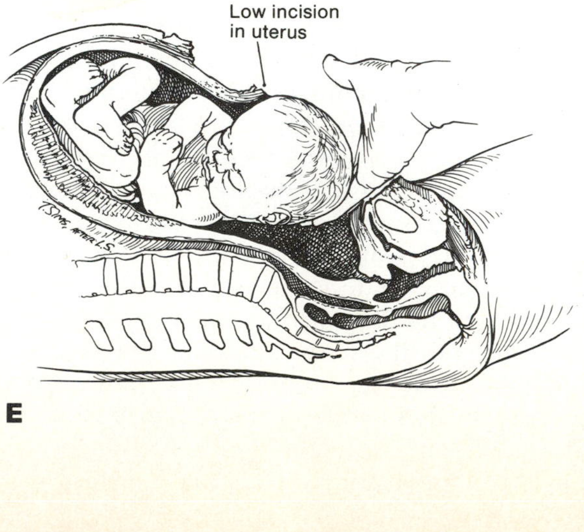

E

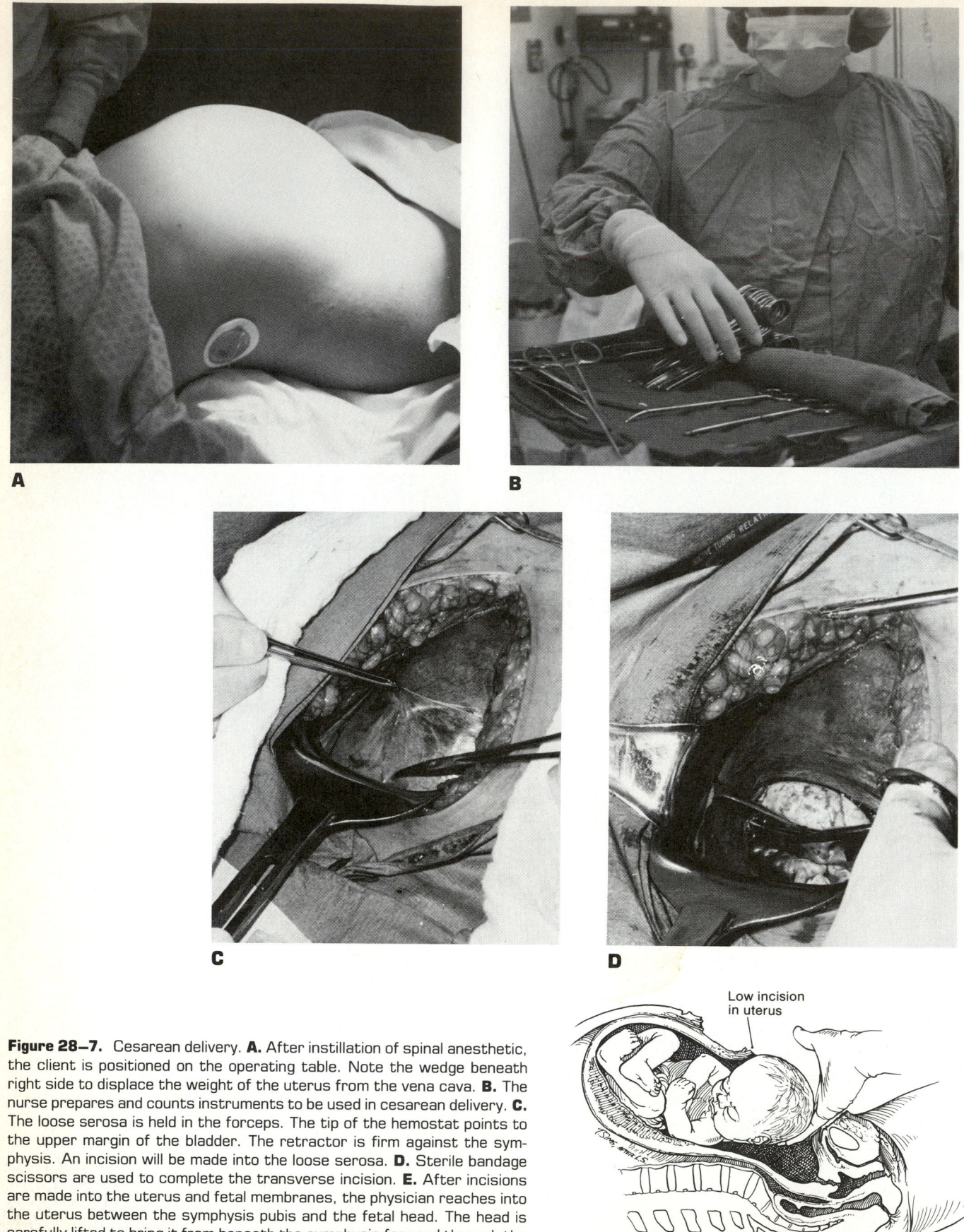

Figure 28–7. Cesarean delivery. **A.** After instillation of spinal anesthetic, the client is positioned on the operating table. Note the wedge beneath right side to displace the weight of the uterus from the vena cava. **B.** The nurse prepares and counts instruments to be used in cesarean delivery. **C.** The loose serosa is held in the forceps. The tip of the hemostat points to the upper margin of the bladder. The retractor is firm against the symphysis. An incision will be made into the loose serosa. **D.** Sterile bandage scissors are used to complete the transverse incision. **E.** After incisions are made into the uterus and fetal membranes, the physician reaches into the uterus between the symphysis pubis and the fetal head. The head is carefully lifted to bring it from beneath the symphysis forward through the uterine and abdominal incisions. (*Figure continues.*)

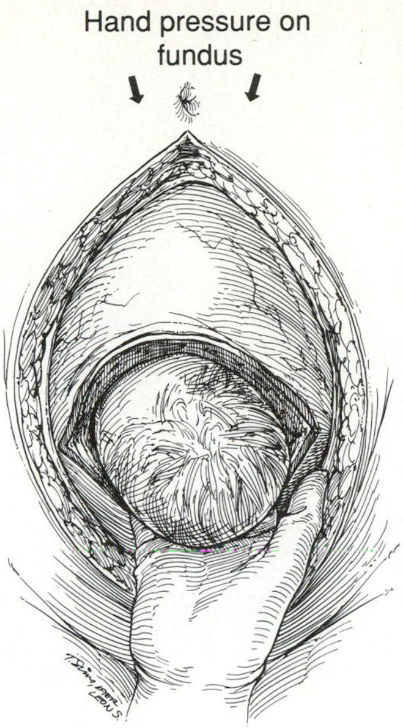

F

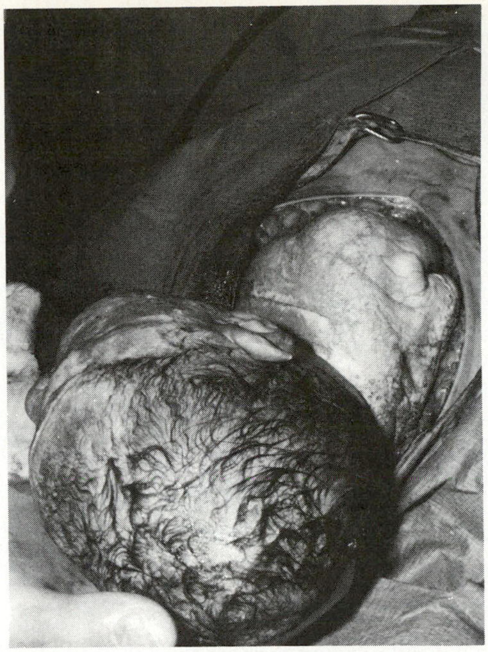

G

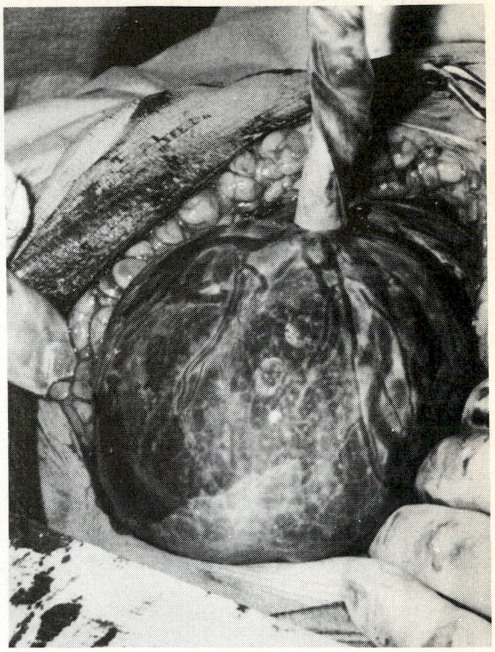

H

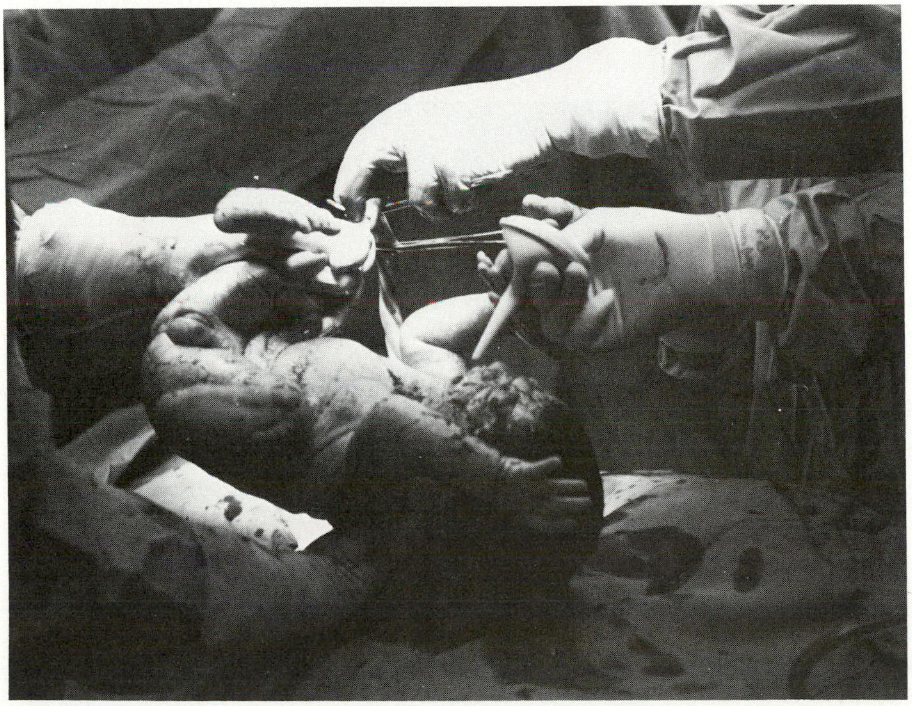

I

Figure 28–7 (continued). F. As the fetal head is lifted through the incision, pressure is usually applied to the uterine fundus through the abdominal wall to help expel the fetus. **G.** Just as the shoulders are delivered, intravenous oxytocin infusion is started. **H.** Placenta is bulging through uterine incision as uterus contracts. **I.** Immediately after delivery the infant's nose and mouth are suctioned; sterile hemostats are used to clamp the cord prior to cutting. (**C** *through* **H** *are reproduced, with permission, from Cunningham FG, et al.* Williams Obstetrics. *18th ed. Norwalk, Conn: Appleton & Lange; 1989:448–451.*)

anesthesia is to be used, the woman is completely prepared and the team is scrubbed and ready to begin the cesarean prior to the induction of anesthesia.[5]

After the operative area has been scrubbed with an antiseptic solution (ideally for the same amount of time as hands are scrubbed for surgery, ie, 10 minutes), an incision is made by the physician through the skin, subcutaneous tissues, and uterus. During the procedure, retractors are used to allow for visibility of the operative field (Figure 28–7). Suction is used to remove fluids from the operative area, and electronic cauterization of small blood vessels is done to

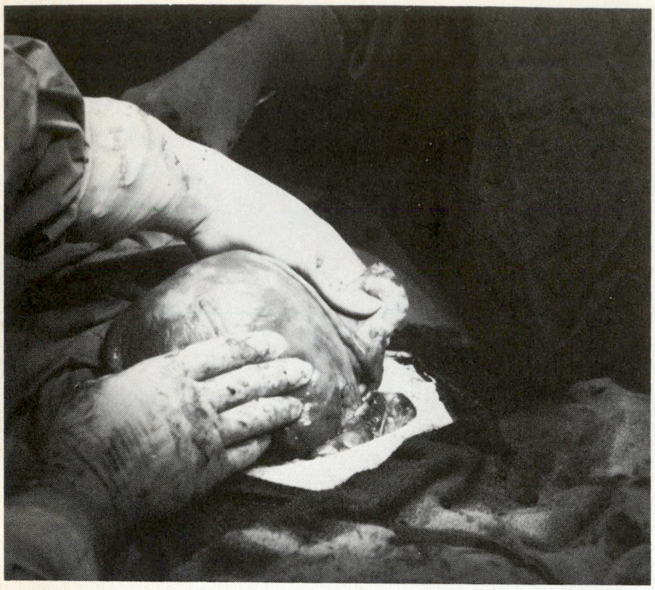
A

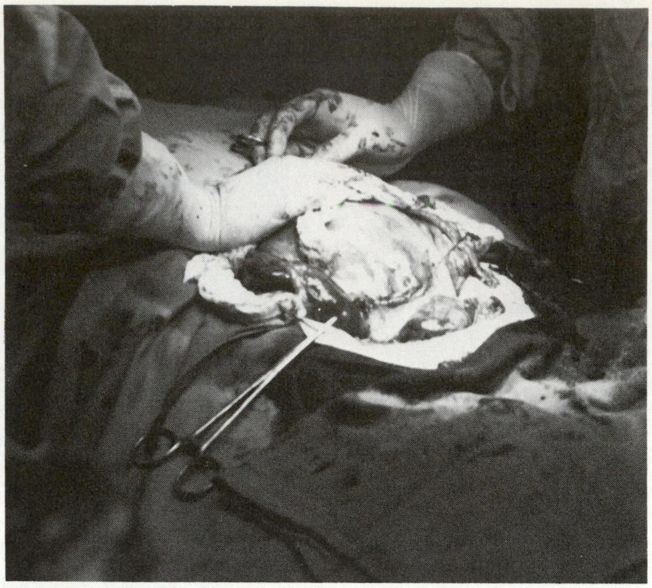
B

Figure 28–8. Uterine repair. **A.** The uterus is replaced after repair outside the body. Ovaries, uterus, and fallopian tubes are inspected. **B.** The uterine suture line is inspected prior to closure of the subcutaneous tissues and skin.

reduce bleeding. The infant is delivered through the incision, and the cord is clamped and cut. A sample of cord blood is taken from the cord. Cord blood studies are based on the client's unique needs and hospital protocol and may include analysis of bilirubin, type, Rh factor, and pH.

After delivery of the newborn, the physician manually removes the placenta, if it has not spontaneously separated. Intravenous oxytocin to stimulate uterine contraction and decrease bleeding is administered by the anesthesiologist after delivery of the fetal shoulders. The uterus is then repaired with nonremovable sutures (Figure 28–8). In one commonly used technique, the physician lifts the uterus through the abdominal incision, places it onto the sterile drapes covering the abdominal wall, and proceeds with the repair. Advantages of this include easy visualization of areas of uterine relaxation or bleeding and better visual exposure of the adnexa. Disadvantages of this technique include possible discomfort experienced by clients receiving spinal or epidural anesthesia and, occasionally, nausea and vomiting when the uterus is brought out or replaced.[5]

While the obstetric team is involved in surgical repair, the newborn, after initial assessment, can be wrapped in a warm blanket, shown to the mother, and held by the father or support person (Figure 28–9). In this way the attachment process can be facilitated within the cesarean room. This, however,

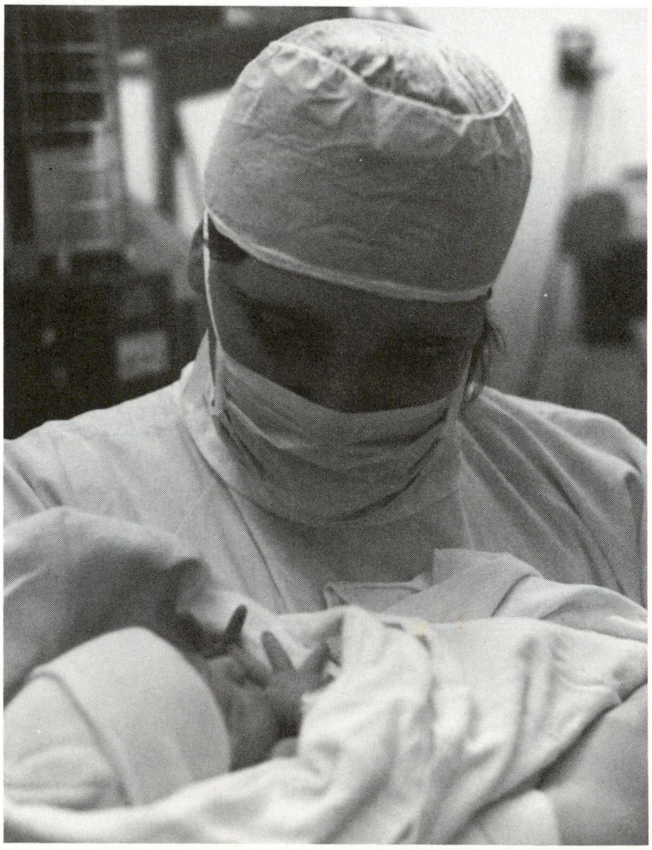

Figure 28–9. Father holds newborn in delivery room.

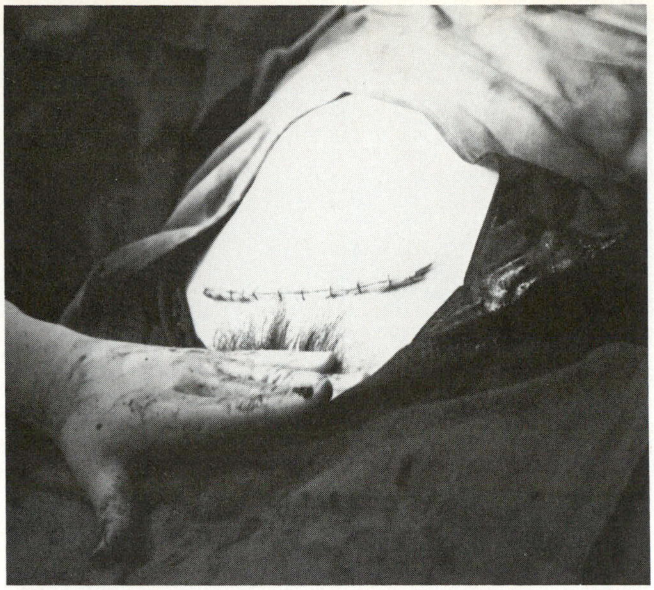

Figure 28–10. Repaired skin incision with staples used for closure. Note that pubic hair around the incision was removed; however, there is no reason for a complete pubic shave.

depends on the health status of the newborn and the type of anesthesia used for the mother.

After repair of the uterus, a final sponge and instrument count is taken and recorded before the abdominal wall is closed. The skin incision may be closed with sutures or with staples (Figure 28–10). A light dressing, for example three 4 × 4 sponges unfolded once and secured with tape, is applied to the skin incision. The woman is then transferred to a gurney and brought to the recovery unit.

When a woman who received regional anesthesia for her cesarean birth is moved to an obstetric recovery unit, the support person who has attended the delivery can usually remain with her, although hospital rules vary. In certain hospitals, the newborn, if healthy, may also stay with the couple. When recovery takes place in a general postoperative recovery suite, visitor presence may be restricted. For these reasons, prior to delivery, couples need to be aware of the policy at the hospital where they plan to deliver.

CARE OF NEWBORN IN DELIVERY ROOM

As a cesarean is considered a high-risk delivery, all neonates born in this manner are considered at risk and are examined carefully. Often, a member of the special-care nursery staff attends, along with a pediatrician or neonatologist. Indeed, all staff responsible for the newborn need to be skilled in neonatal resuscitation techniques as well as in the immediate care of a high-risk neonate.

A heated crib with resuscitative equipment is prepared prior to the cesarean and is considered necessary to any obstetric unit (Figure 28–11). The newborn is handed by the physician performing the cesarean to the nurse or pediatrician attending the newborn. The neonate is placed beneath the radiant warmer, suctioned, dried, and assessed. Apgar scores (*see* Chapter 32) are done at 1 and 5 minutes after birth. Identification bands with numbers corresponding to the mother's identification number are placed on the newborn's ankle and wrist, and footprints are taken. Antimicrobial eyedrops may be delayed to facilitate eye contact between the new parents and the baby. If the mother has not received general anesthesia, the baby is brought close to her,

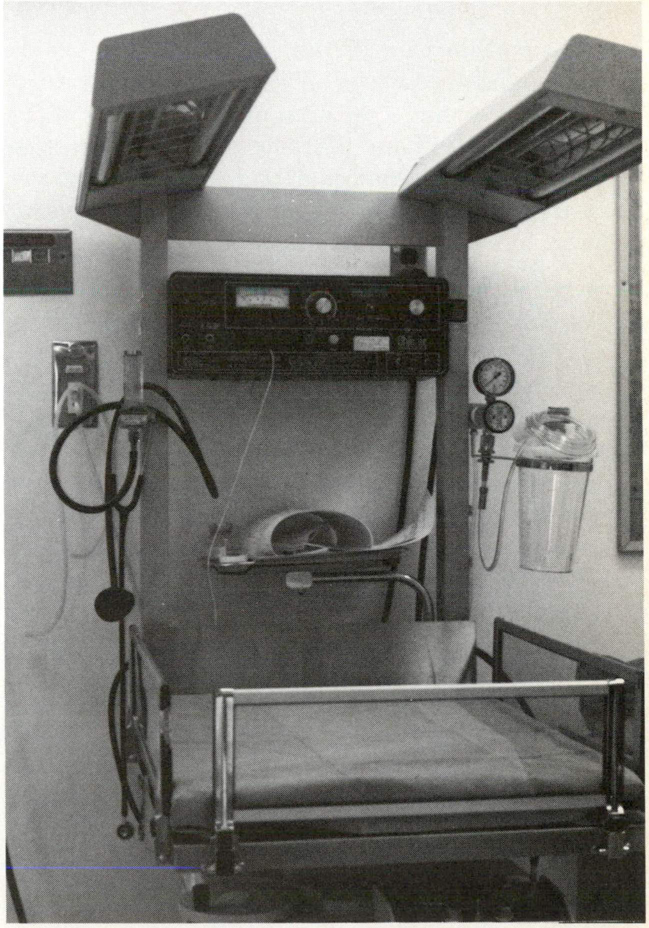

Figure 28–11. Infant warmer with resuscitation equipment.

so that she may see and kiss her newborn. If all is well, the baby, wrapped warmly and wearing a hat to conserve heat, may be given to the father or support person to hold within the mother's range of vision. As the surgery is completed, the new parents may interact with their newborn. If the baby's condition is unstable, however, he or she is brought at once to the special care nursery. The parents may be extremely distressed by their newborn's uncertain status; therefore, attention needs to be focused on providing emotional support to the parents during the cesarean, as well as afterward.

Ways in which parents may be supported during the remainder of cesarean delivery when neonatal outcome is poor should be discussed in staff planning meetings before crisis situations are encountered. In this way effective strategies that may be realistically implemented in a particular hospital setting can be developed.

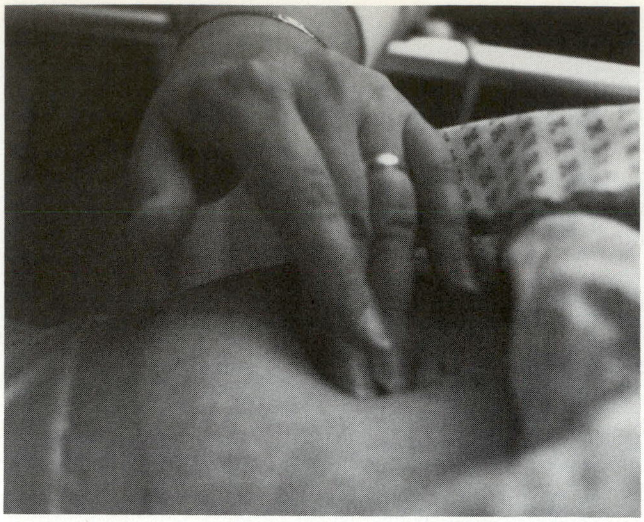

Figure 28–12. Height of fundus is palpated after cesarean delivery.

The postpartum care of the cesarean client blends principles and practices of surgical and obstetric nursing (*see* the Nursing Care Plan included in this chapter). The nurse will find that a systematic approach to the client provides a thorough and efficient method of assessment. Such an approach in the recovery unit includes three types of assessment:

Assessment of physical and physiologic parameters. Overall impression of the client, neurologic status, sensory and motor function (recovery from anesthesia), cardiovascular status (pulse, blood pressure, skin color), respiratory status, temperature (oral temperatures should be avoided unless the woman is completely awake), fundal height and degree of firmness (Figure 28–12), appearance of the abdominal dressing, amount and color of lochia, intravenous therapy and fluid intake, urine output and patency of catheter.

Assessment of pain and determination of need for analgesics as ordered. As the effects of anesthesia wear off, the woman may be increasingly aware of pain related to the surgery. Uterine palpation to ensure that the uterus remains well contracted can be an especially uncomfortable, although necessary part of postoperative care. Intramuscular analgesics, for example, meperidine, may be given when the woman is fully reactive from the anesthesia.[5] Epidural administration of a narcotic drug, such as morphine, has provided especially effective analgesia after cesarean delivery, and is becoming an increasingly widespread alternative to intramuscular analgesics in the immediate postoperative period. Table 28–2 summarizes information related to epidural analgesia.[30–34]

Assessment of psychologic parameters. The immediate response of the woman and her partner to the cesarean delivery, the woman's desire to be with her infant, the woman's beginning acquaintance with the infant.

Nursing strategies that may be undertaken to promote the client's comfort in the recovery room include providing warmed blankets (these may be applied when the woman is transferred from the delivery table to the gurney), mouth care, sponge bath, prompt administration of prescribed analgesics (unless epidural analgesia has been given), and assistance with positioning. Emotional comfort measures include orienting the woman and her support person to the recovery unit, providing reassurance that the cesarean is indeed over, and fostering opportunities for contact between the mother and her support person and between the couple and the newborn. The nurse needs to allow the mother and support person to express feelings about the delivery; the nurse also needs to accept these feelings as valid, whether they are positive or negative. If the newborn cannot be brought to the recovery unit, the delivery or recovery nurse, the special-care nurse, pediatrician, or neonatologist may provide information about the neonate's condition.

Several clients may be in the same recovery unit, especially if it is a general surgical recovery suite. Concern for the client's reactions to others who have just had surgery requires thoughtful placement of the client in the unit. Client privacy can be promoted by drawing drapes completely around the gurney whenever physical assessment and care are being undertaken.

Safety is a major priority within a recovery unit. Side rails remain raised at all times. In addition, whenever sensory or motor function has been altered, the nurse needs to take measures to protect the client against inadvertent injury. Although it is desirable to encourage early parent-newborn contact, the nurse should remember that the woman is also recovering from the effects of anesthesia and drugs that have muscle relaxant or sedative effects. Although the newborn may be held close to the mother by the nurse or the support person, the baby should not be placed unsupervised on the gurney.

Admission to Postpartum Unit

When the woman is recovered (ie, completely awake, and able to move independently, with blood pressure, pulse, and respirations stable, a well-contracted uterus, no excessive bleeding, and a urine output of at least 30 mL per hour), she is brought to the postpartum unit.[5] In addition to receiving the client and her chart, the postpartum nurse also takes an oral report of the woman's surgical and recovery experiences from the recovery nurse. An assessment of the client needs to be done on her admission to the postpartum floor and *before* the departure of the nurse from the recovery unit. At that time, the client's record should be reviewed to verify that all medications, fluids, physical signs, and other parameters have been documented.

Stay in Postpartum Unit

Care of the postpartum cesarean woman resembles nursing care for the woman who delivers vaginally, with the following important differences:

Cesarean clients are surgical clients with all the needs of women who have had major abdominal surgery. Although cesarean women do not have the perineal discomfort experienced by women who have delivered vaginally, they may realistically have considerable incisional pain, especially on the first postpartum day, unless epidural analgesia was administered. The nurse needs to anticipate this and to *offer* analgesics and other comfort measures. In some hospitals transcutaneous electrical nerve stimulation (TENS) units are used successfully to decrease the client's perception of pain. Some hospitals may use client-controlled analgesics, administered by intravenous pump according to the client's own perceived needs, but with a preset safety limit for dosage. Assessment of the uterine fundus will also be painful for the cesarean client, and the nurse can organize care so that the woman receives an analgesic prior to this.

Postoperative pain limits mobility. For 24 to 48 hours postpartum, the cesarean client will need encouragement and physical assistance, especially in changing positions, getting out of bed, and handling her newborn. Cesarean clients do need help with personal hygiene measures, such as sponge bathing hard-to-reach body areas. By the third postoperative day, showering is usually possible;[5] however, nursing assistance may be needed. The nurse should organize the environment surrounding the client so that call bell, telephone, personal items, and other items are within easy reach. A postpartum cesarean client should not have continuous rooming-in until she is able to ambulate and hold her newborn independently.

Postanesthesia effects on respiratory function necessitate that the nurse listen for breath sounds and supervise deep breathing and coughing exercises as well as early ambulation. As noted in Table 28–2, assessment of respiratory status is particularly important in women who have received epidural analgesia.

The intravenous infusion may remain for 24 to 48 hours, or until the client tolerates fluids well by mouth. In addition, some postcesarean clients retain intravenous access for continued antibiotic administration.

Nearly all women have indwelling urinary catheters inserted prior to the surgery to keep the bladder decompressed and out of the surgical field. The catheter may be removed the morning after the cesarean or sooner, depending on obstetric judgment. As in caring for any catheterized client, the nurse needs to check urinary output (eg, color, quantity) make certain that straight drainage is not impaired by "kinks" in the tubing, and minimize chance of infection through good hand washing and aseptic technique. In certain cases urine samples for urinalysis and culture may be taken before the catheter is removed; however, these tests are costly and are not routinely performed for all postcesarean clients. To prevent bladder distension and minimize the possibility of associated complications such as uterine hemorrhage and urinary tract infection, women should void spontaneously within 4 to 6 hours of removal of the catheter. Assisting the client into the bathroom, ambulation, running water in the sink, or pouring warm

TABLE 28–2. EPIDURAL ANALGESIA FOLLOWING CESAREAN DELIVERY

Purpose	Relief of postpartum pain after cesarean or difficult vaginal delivery.
Placement of epidural catheter	During labor; before cesarean delivery.
Administration of analgesic	Administered by clinician skilled in epidural management. One dose of epidural narcotic (eg, morphine 4 to 5 mg) is usually given to cesarean clients at the time the abdomen is being closed or before the epidural catheter is removed. Pain is minimized, because the effects of epidural analgesia take hold as the effects from the epidural anesthesia wear off.
Action	Thought to act directly on spinal cord opiate receptors; block pain sensation without impairing motor, sensory, or sympathetic function. Systemic absorption plays little role in analgesia.
Example of analgesics used	Preservative-free morphine (Duramorph). Drug choice is based on client assessment and is made by the anesthesiologist. The usual dose of epidural morphine is 4 to 5 mg; no more than 10 mg per 24 hours is recommended. No restriction in breastfeeding is necessary, because of the low dose of epidural morphine used.
Contraindications	Allergy to the analgesics used (absolute contraindication). *Epidural morphine should not be used when staffing is inadequate to provide careful monitoring of respiratory adequacy for 24 hours after administration.* All clients receiving epidural morphine analgesia are at risk for respiratory depression and *must* be evaluated closely and carefully for 24 hours after the last injection.
Effectiveness	Varies according to the analgesic used. Effects of epidural morphine begin within 30 to 60 minutes and may last through the first 18 to 24 hours. Postpartum pain is usually minimal. "Breakthrough" pain may occur in some clients. Reasons for breakthrough pain include administration of too little of the narcotic analgesic or local anesthetic dissipation before the onset of morphine analgesia. Administration of additional parenteral narcotics to relieve breakthrough pain can raise the chance of respiratory depression and other adverse effects.
Side effects	Respiratory depression (rate less than 12 per minute) or obstruction, occurring as early as 30 minutes or as late as 16 hours after administration of epidural morphine, is an uncommon but significant complication in healthy postcesarean clients. (Within the first 20 hours of epidural administration, the physician should evaluate any client before any more narcotics are given.) Pruritus (itching) is the most common side effect, occurring in about 50 percent of clients and usually experienced on face or upper body. Pruritus may start within 3 hours and last up to 24 hours after administration. In most cases it is not severe and can be treated with 0.1 to 0.2 mg naloxone. Urinary retention may occur in clients receiving epidural morphine. Usually it is not a problem, because the cesarean client has a Foley catheter in place after surgery. Nausea and vomiting have been noted to take place frequently in clients who received epidural morphine.
Nursing interventions	For clients receiving postcesarean epidural analgesics, such as epidural morphine[a]: Make certain that risks and benefits are discussed prior to the surgery. This is usually a physician's responsibility; however, nurses also need to be able to answer clients' questions, help clarify differences between epidural anesthesia and analgesia, and dispel misconceptions. After the cesarean, nurses may need to present information about epidural analgesia again and to advise clients to report side effects. Make certain resuscitation equipment is accessible and working; oxygen and suction materials should be at the client's bedside; keep naloxone available for management of narcotic complications; make certain a physician skilled in epidural analgesia and management of complications is readily available. Assess client's level of pain. Check respiratory rate, depth, and pattern for full minute every 15 minutes for the first hour, every hour for the next 24 hours, and then every 2 to 8 hours (close assessment for first 24 hours). Assess other parameters indicating respiratory status, such as level of alertness and agitation. If respirations are suppressed, inform physician without delay; give naloxone as ordered. Assist client to assume semi-Fowler position to minimize chance of respiratory depression. If appropriate, apply apnea monitor to aid nursing observations (however, apnea monitors curtail client movements, interfere with normal activities, tend to give many false alarms and can be a source of stress). Maintain intravenous infusions for 24 hours in case of need for resuscitation measures. Assess presence and degree of itching. Reassurance alone may be adequate for mild itching. Cool compresses may provide some relief. If severe itching occurs, naloxone and/or diphenylhydramine may be used for control.

TABLE 28–2. EPIDURAL ANALGESIA FOLLOWING CESAREAN DELIVERY *(continued)*

Nursing interventions	Observe for nausea and vomiting, which may occur in 12 to 50 percent of clients between 4 and 7 hours after administration. Droperidol (1.25 mg) or other anti-emetics given intravenously may decrease nausea, yet maintain analgesia. Maintain indwelling Foley catheter for 12 to 24 hours after cesarean to minimize complications related to urinary retention. Continue usual postcesarean care (turning, blood pressure assessments, fundal checks, and so on).
Benefits	Prolonged pain relief Early ambulation, better ability to turn, cough and deep breathe because of less discomfort; therefore, decreased risk of postoperative complications related to pain-induced restricted mobility (eg, atelectasis, pneumonia). Lower doses of narcotic are needed to control postcesarean pain when the epidural rather than systemic route is used. Decreased need for sedation or other analgesics. Potential benefits to attachment, related to greater feelings of maternal well being and ability to care for her newborn.
Drawbacks related to epidural morphine analgesia	Potential complications (see "Side Effects"). Need for careful, frequent monitoring, especially during first 24 hours. Need for adequate staffing and staff expertise to provide monitoring and to intervene appropriately should complications arise. Need for presence in the hospital of a physician, skilled in the management of epidural analgesia and its complications.

Source: *References 30–34.*
[a] Hospital protocols may vary.

water over the vulva may help clients void and avert the need for reinsertion of a catheter.

On the second and third postoperative days, gas pain related to incoordinate bowel action may become problematic. Strategies such as early ambulation can be helpful. A bowel movement usually provides relief, but may need to be induced with a rectal suppository or, if ineffective, an enema, as prescribed by the physician.

The abdominal incision site needs to be inspected and any redness, swelling, oozing, or separation reported to the physician and charted. After the surgical dressing has been removed by the physician, a light dressing, without heavy tape, may be used for protection, especially if a maternity belt holding a sanitary pad would come into contact with the wound. The presence of an abdominal incision, along with the circumstances that led to the need or diagnosis of the need for the cesarean, may put the cesarean client at higher risk for infection than the woman who delivers vaginally.

Cesarean clients whose skin incisions were closed with nonabsorbable materials such as metal skin staples will need these removed, usually by the fourth day. Some physicians may choose to close cesarean skin incisions with absorbable sutures that do not need removal; however, suture removal from the postcesarean skin incision is fairly swift and involves minimal discomfort.

Some cesarean clients fear they will not be able to breastfeed because of the cesarean. Cesarean mothers often have their first breastfeeding experience several hours later than mothers who deliver vaginally.[35] There is no reason, however, why a cesarean delivery alone should affect a mother's ability to breastfeed successfully. The nurse needs to identify cesarean-related fears about breastfeeding and to provide reassurance and assistance for the client who wants to breastfeed.

Discharge Teaching

Women with an uncomplicated postcesarean course may expect to go home on the fourth or fifth postpartum day. Frequently, women may be discharged earlier if all is well. The trend toward earlier discharge reflects such factors as the client's desire to minimize time away from her family and the ever-increasing costs of hospitalization. In some areas, the progress of an early-discharge cesarean client may be assessed through a home visit by a nurse.

Many aspects of discharge teaching, such as breastfeeding and sexuality, are similar for clients regardless of whether they deliver abdominally or vaginally. Teaching specific to cesarean mothers focuses on assisting the mother to continue to recover from surgery while adapting to the addition of the newborn to the family. Teaching should also include significant family members, as the client will need assistance with household responsibilities and with infant care.

On return home, the cesarean client may feel tired and should be encouraged to rest at intervals during the day. At least for the first week, the woman is advised to restrict her activity to caring for herself and, with help, her newborn.[5]

Although the acute pain related to surgery has subsided, activities such as rising from a supine to a sitting position may be painful and difficult, especially in the home setting where most people do not have hospital-style beds that can be raised and lowered. The woman may be advised to roll to her side and splint the incision with one hand as she gently pushes herself upward with the other hand. Heavy lifting or other activities that could potentially strain the healing wound should be avoided. Most women experience only minor physical discomfort, usually effectively controlled with mild oral analgesics, prescribed by the physician.

As part of discharge teaching, any medications to be used by the client are explained. The nurse makes certain the client has received appropriate prescriptions, for example, for pain control, and that she is able to obtain the medications. Women are advised against self-medication with aspirin-containing preparations, because aspirin may increase the risk of bleeding.

Prior to discharge, the cesarean client should be informed about danger signs, for example, infection (redness, swelling, discharge, or separation of the incision area; fever; foul-smelling vaginal discharge) and recurrent heavy bleeding, and advised to contact her health care provider if the signs appear. Exercises that can safely be performed at home are frequent topics of concern for cesarean clients. Exercises are recommended on the basis of each client's unique situation.

Discharge teaching includes emotional reactions to the cesarean on the part of the client and her significant others. The nurse can provide reassurance and anticipatory guidance about normal reactions. The nurse can also identify clients who are having difficulty in postpartum adaptation or in coping with the cesarean delivery and then make appropriate referrals for further evaluation. All clients should be informed of groups, such as Cesarean Support, Education, and Concern (C/SEC) that focus on the special needs of cesarean families. Nurses working with cesarean clients should be aware of such groups in their local communities, as well as the existence of national organizations.

Before discharge, the client makes an appointment for a follow-up postpartum, postcesarean examination. Clients who deliver vaginally are usually seen around 6 postpartum weeks. Cesarean clients are seen around 3 postpartum weeks, so that their recovery from surgery as well as their postpartum adaptation may be assessed.

Psychologic Responses

In the 1950s, cesarean and vaginal delivery clients were treated in a similar fashion. Childbirth was widely viewed as a pathologic event for which most people received general anesthesia and remained hospitalized for periods extending to 2 weeks. By the mid-1970s, however, prepared childbirth and family-centered, father-attended birth became widely publicized and available for women who delivered vaginally. As noted earlier, this did not happen for cesarean clients who continued, and who still continue in many places, to be denied a similar birth experience. From this, a body of literature evaluating client and family responses to cesarean delivery emerged.

Postpartum cesarean clients may undergo a psychologic experience potentially different from that of clients who deliver vaginally. Although some women feel joy and relief after the cesarean, others may feel anger and depression, a sense of failure, and a loss of self-esteem. Lipson and Tilden identified five phases that women may pass through as they assimilate the cesarean delivery[36]; these phases are similar to those of the grieving process. Austin applied these phases toward explication of the cesarean birth experience (Table 28–3).[10]

According to Sandelowski and Bustamante, much of the literature discussing undesirable psychosocial effects of cesarean birth focuses on the expectations and experiences of women who belong to the group valuing natural childbirth.[37] For these women, who tend to be from the middle classes, the birth experience is a goal in itself and cesarean delivery, which alters that experience, could present a devastating disappointment. Results from their study of women receiving care in a public hospital serving the medically indigent indicated that women from this socioeconomically deprived group did not display the same type of psychic wounding after cesarean birth that has been reported by natural childbirth followers.

Culp and Osofsky conducted a prospective study of primiparous, well-educated, middle-class married women and their husbands.[38] Data were collected, beginning in the second trimester of the women's pregnancies, continuing with observations

RESEARCH ABSTRACT

Kearney MH, et al. Cesarean delivery and breastfeeding outcomes. Birth. *1990;17:97–103.*

The effects of cesarean delivery on breastfeeding outcomes were explored in married primiparas. Subjects were recruited during prepared childbirth classes for participation in a larger study requiring prenatal commitment to breastfeeding for at least six weeks. Twenty seven (23 percent) of the women had cesarean deliveries and 97 delivered vaginally. Prenatally, subjects were interviewed and completed questionnaires. A postpartum home interview at one postpartum week was followed by weekly telephone interviews from two through six postpartum weeks and monthly telephone interviews from two through six postpartum months.

Cesarean mothers breastfed their newborns for the first time several hours after mothers who delivered vaginally were able to breastfeed their infants. In addition, cesarean mothers expressed less satisfaction with their labor and delivery experience than did mothers who delivered vaginally. No relationship was found, however, between the time of first breastfeeding and duration of breastfeeding, between delivery type and duration of breastfeeding, or pain or fatigue related to breastfeeding.

Comment:
Women who have cesarean deliveries frequently worry about their ability to breastfeed. This study supports the belief that a woman who is motivated can breastfeed successfully whether or not she delivers vaginally. Later first breastfeeding experience and less client satisfaction with labor and delivery have many nursing implications. Nurses should examine hospital policies which in themselves prolong first breastfeeding for the cesarean mother and encourage and assist cesarean mothers to breastfeed as soon as they are physically able. Working with physicians and other health care providers, nurses can also identify factors that prevent a satisfying labor and delivery experience for cesarean mothers and implement strategies in their own settings that can promote family-centered care regardless of the method of delivery.

of mothers in the hospital 2 days after delivery, and concluding with interviews and observations at 3 months postpartum when the infants were brought for well-baby examination. Twenty-four of the mothers had cesarean deliveries and 56 gave birth vaginally. The researchers concluded that cesarean delivery did not cause difficulties in infant development and did not alter patterns of parent-infant interaction or raise the risk of parental depression or marital difficulty among their study's subjects. They also indicated the need for further research to understand the social and behavioral impact of changes in care during childbirth.

Discrepant findings among studies focusing on comparisons of women who deliver vaginally and women who deliver by cesarean have been attributed to numerous factors[38,39]:

- The efforts of cesarean birth organizations which have sought to have family-centered care, including the participation of the father or significant other in the birth, instituted for cesarean clients
- Inclusion of content about cesarean preparation in prepared childbirth classes
- Changes over the past 10 to 15 years in public perceptions and attitudes toward cesareans
- The high incidence of cesarean birth, which may make women feel less different or abnormal
- Greater acceptance of the use of technology in childbirth and increasing emphasis on birth as more of a "high-risk" event; greater acceptance of cesarean birth as a viable method of delivery
- The methods used in the studies

Conflicting results could possibly be attributed to factors such as the nature of study designs, the type of questions asked, or the timing of the study after cesarean delivery.

Cultural background must also be considered in assessing the emotional responses of clients and families to cesarean birth in the United States. For example, results of a study of Mexican-American women illustrated ways that cultural beliefs and attitudes can affect a woman's perceptions of the childbirth experience.[40] Of the 518 women in the study, 58 delivered by cesarean. Cesarean birth was not found to be unsatisfying or psychologically negative for most of the women in the study. Eleven percent even reported feeling "lucky" to have the cesarean; however, 28 percent reported dissatisfaction with their cesarean experience. Feelings of fear, guilt, and failure were expressed.

Nurses must be able to identify the potentially wide variety of responses that clients may have toward abdominal birth and to realize that many complex variables may affect client and family responses. Culturally sensitive nursing interventions that foster family-centered personalized care for all clients, in addition to thoughtful assessment of psychologic aspects of this experience, can do much to ensure quality care regardless of the route of delivery.

TABLE 28–3. UNDERSTANDING THE CESAREAN BIRTH EXPERIENCE

Time Frame	Emotions	Observations	Nursing Interventions
Immediate postoperative hours First 21–24 hours	Feels "shocked numbness," flat affect, sense of suspended animation; is just coping; accepts that cesarean was necessary for the safety and welfare of herself and infant	Consciousness is clouded by anxiety, exhaustion, anesthesia, analgesia Repression and denial keep the stimuli of surgical birth within limits	Provide physical comfort and total nursing care Bring baby as soon as possible Involve partner and assist in touching, holding, examining, and feeding infant as mother desires (photos, if infant in special-care nursery)
Initial postpartum days Hospital stay 24 hours to 4–7 days	Feels disappointed over loss of anticipated natural delivery; feels relief, guilt, anger, or an envy of others who have delivered vaginally; possibly feels detachment or lack of enthusiasm for infant; may feel overwhelmed or have "blues," especially around third day	Psychic energy is channeled into early ambulation, pain control, elimination, eating, and attempting to sleep May need to adjust to birth events before moving to mothering tasks Infant care, breastfeeding begin	Give nonhurried, sensitive sympathetic support for physical needs Encourage to discuss birth experience Give instructional and anticipatory guidance in infant care and breastfeeding Give resource number to call if questions or problems Emphasize importance of help with laundry, meals, care of other children for 2–3 weeks
Emerging awareness Hospital discharge until about 8 weeks postpartum	Feels strong need to be taken care of, mothered, nurtured, and nourished; may be disappointed in mothering skills and blame cesarean for all difficulties; may have intense feelings of anger, stigma, and failure, as well as self-image problems	Feels conflict between 24-hour newborn care and demands of recovery from major surgery; fatigue and incisional discomfort may make breastfeeding more difficult, and slow mothering skills development Individual meaning of cesarean emerges; troubling questions arise, including facts about surgery and reasons for it Memories of or feelings associated with cesarean may emerge in dreams	Advise to ask for and accept help, rest when baby rests, maintain adequate rest and fluids, keep baby close by to avoid fatigue, feed baby in comfortable position, try heating pad if lingering incisional discomfort or backache occur, take time for herself daily, have contact with other new parents, contact professional/community resources as needed (eg, breastfeeding), make follow-up doctor appointments Give birth control information as needed
Intermediate resolution 2 months postpartum to end of first year	Returns to a feeling of strength and well-being; has increased confidence in mothering skills; intense feelings or memories of the cesarean begin to surface unexpectedly	Has intermittent struggle to accept and understand experience (a few cope with repression and denial) Individual coping mechanisms and support group are helpful in resolution Is passive or active in reworking memories and feelings Reconstruction of birth process increases; is able to fill in memory gaps and label feelings Group exposure helps put cesarean in broader perspective	Assist in reconstruction of the birth experience by listening and filling in the gaps Encourage attendance at a cesarean support group meeting

TABLE 28–3. UNDERSTANDING THE CESAREAN BIRTH EXPERIENCE *(continued)*

Time Frame	Emotions	Observations	Nursing Interventions
Resolution			
Beginning after 1 year (if it is a significant life event, complete and final resolution is rare)	Accepts cesarean; places it in perspective with the rest of her life; feels a need to have her cesarean experience "count"	Reconstruction continues Resolution is analogous to that of grieving Now is able to identify some item of positive evaluation about cesarean; frequently refers to health and welfare of child	Help to become informed health-care consumer Encourage participation in an appropriate prepared childbirth series for subsequent pregnancies

Based on Lipson J, Tilden V. Psychological integration of the cesarean birth experience. *Am J Orthopsychiatry.* 1980; 50;598–609. Reproduced, with permission, from Austin SEJ. Childbirth classes for couples desiring VBAC. *Am J Matern Child Nurs.* 1986; 11:250–255.

THE FATHER'S EXPERIENCE

Cesarean delivery presents a potential risk to the father's childbirth experience. Many hospitals currently encourage fathers to be present during the vaginal delivery of their babies. However, this policy does not automatically extend to cesarean deliveries. In some places, fathers are still regarded as intruders who have no business in an operating room; sets of institutional regulations may restrict paternal participation in cesarean delivery. Ironically, the arguments that were once used to keep fathers from attending vaginal deliveries have now been applied to fathers' attendance at cesarean deliveries: the infection rates may increase; the father would be in the way; the father could not "stand" to witness cesarean surgery. Neither research nor clinical reports have given evidence to substantiate barring fathers from cesarean deliveries.

At this time hospital policies regarding fathers' presence at cesarean deliveries vary. Some hospitals allow fathers to attend elective cesareans if they have gone to cesarean preparation classes. Some hospitals will not permit fathers into the cesarean room in any circumstances. Some hospitals allow fathers to attend whether the cesarean is being done on an emergency or an elective basis. Attitudes of obstetricians and delivery room nurses also determine whether a father can see his infant born. May and Sollid studied fathers' responses to unanticipated cesarean birth.[41] Fathers' negative reactions did not tend to focus on the cesarean itself, but on policies that set up barriers to their participation in the birth and on physicians' and nurses' behaviors that made them feel unsupported and excluded from the birth, regardless of whether they were actually present for the delivery.

Change in hospital practices has come about largely because there are so many cesareans being done and in response to consumer demand for a father-attended birth experience similar to that offered to women having vaginal deliveries. The media has done much to promote public acceptance of father-attended births, and many fathers look forward to this experience. Being denied access to the delivery can foster feelings of anger, frustration, and disappointment for fathers. At times they may blame staff or their partners. On the other hand, attendance and staff support can promote feelings of togetherness and common purpose. One study of fathers of infants born vaginally and fathers of infants born by cesarean found that a father's presence at delivery and early contact with his infant tended to predict his future involvement in infant caretaking activities.[42]

Nurses have major roles in care of the father experiencing cesarean delivery. Prenatally, nurses can encourage expectant fathers to discuss their plans, thoughts, and fears about cesarean delivery, and provide information about options, as well as restrictions, available at local hospitals. In their role as educators, nurses can develop and teach cesarean birth classes to expectant couples. Nurses can also encourage fathers to be present in the delivery room and to seek early contact with their infants. In the delivery unit, nurses can provide anticipatory guidance, even if the father has attended cesarean preparation classes, and advise the father in aspects of the cesarean experience such as how to don surgical attire, where to stand, what to expect, and what he may do. Nurses should also provide an opportunity for fathers to discuss their feelings about the cesarean delivery. In their roles as client advocates and health professionals, nurses can work toward the establishment of family-centered care that includes father-attended cesarean, as well as vaginal deliveries.

At times it may not be feasible for a father to be present for the cesarean delivery, or he may choose not to be present. In such cases, the reason why the father was not present should first be identified, as interventions may be affected by this reason, especially if the reason was hospital policy alone. Fathers who decline the invitation to be present for the cesarean should be treated with respect, and staff should not attempt to "force" them to see the delivery.

Nurses can promote paternal involvement by keeping the father informed about the progress of the cesarean, encouraging him to express his feelings about the cesarean, and offering emotional support; this is especially important when obstetric complications occur. In addition, there are several ways in which the nurse can facilitate early father-newborn attachment. For example, the nurse can invite the father to accompany the newborn to the nursery, to observe the nursery admission procedures, and to touch and hold the newborn.

VAGINAL BIRTH AFTER CESAREAN DELIVERY

Whether a woman who has at one time had a cesarean birth can safely deliver vaginally in the future has been a controversial issue in obstetrics. Early in the 20th century the idea of "once a cesarean, always a cesarean" took hold. Despite evidence to the contrary, the belief persists.

The argument against **vaginal birth after a cesarean (VBAC)** focuses on the possible occurrence of major and life-threatening complications such as uterine rupture. Fibrotic scar tissue from previous uterine surgery is not as strong as uncut muscle and forms a plane of weakness in the uterus. Distension of the uterus in a future pregnancy and the force of contractions during labor could theoretically exert enough pressure to split the uterus along the old incision line, although the actual incidence of this event is low. Professional fear of obstetric catastrophe has come to be the greatest reason for elective repeat cesarean birth.[43] Despite the concerns raised over the persistent high incidence of cesareans, it has been estimated that the repeat cesarean rate in the United States continues to be around 90 percent.[4] In addition, current professional worry about potential malpractice suits supports the notion of "once a cesarean, always a cesarean" and limits the option of VBAC.

Proponents of VBAC claim that cesareans pose greater risks than VBAC. Cesarean birth has been reported to carry twice the maternal mortality rate of vaginal delivery.[9] Pauerstein noted that the chance of maternal death resulting from rupture of a previous cesarean scar was one-fortieth that of a maternal death for elective repeat cesarean deliveries.[44] Miller and Sutter observed that "when concrete data are examined, concerns voiced over uterine rupture seem to be exaggerated and based more on history than the current clinical environment."[43] In several large studies, no maternal deaths occurred from trials of labor for women who wished to attempt VBAC.[45–47] Morbidity rates for elective repeat cesarean deliveries have also been reported to be higher than the 3 percent morbidity rate associated with vaginal delivery.[48, 49] Maternal and perinatal mortality rates for VBAC are not greater than those for repeat cesarean birth.[50] In addition, repeat cesarean delivery is financially and emotionally more expensive than VBAC. With physician consultation as indicated and with readily accessible hospital services, nurse-midwives may manage and deliver clients attempting VBAC, thereby adding the benefit of choice of caregiver to VBAC.[51]

Qualifications

Vaginal birth after cesarean has been noted to be a viable option to routine repeat cesarean by groups such as the Organization of Obstetric, Gynecologic and Neonatal Nurses (NAACOG), the American College of Obstetricians and Gynecologists (ACOG),[52] and the 19-member task force established under the auspices of the National Institute of Child Health and Human Development[48] to study cesarean childbirth. Third party insurers are recognizing VBAC as a reimbursible option. Vaginal birth after cesarean has been estimated to occur for about 50 to 80 percent of women who meet the criteria for VBAC.[50] Optimal candidates for VBAC are women who desire to avoid cesarean delivery and desire to experience labor and vaginal delivery, have access to a hospital and staff supportive of VBAC, had a previous cesarean for a problem that is unlikely to recur, are in good physical health and have had a healthy pregnancy with a fetus weighing less than 4000 g, and understand the risks and benefits of VBAC and the possibility of an emergency cesarean if labor does not progress smoothly.

Vaginal birth after cesarean would be contraindicated in any condition that of itself precludes vaginal birth (eg, complete placenta previa), difficult fetal presentations, situations where the woman does not want to try VBAC, and in facilities where women do not have access to emergency cesarean delivery should the need arise. Maternal history of more than one uterine incision has been considered to be a contraindication to VBAC; however, recent evidence has supported the safety of a trial of labor for women with previous cesarean deliveries. An overall success rate for vaginal delivery of 69 percent was found in one study of women who had two previous cesarean births.[53] Although a previous "classic" uterine incision is not a complete contraindicaion to VBAC, it does add to the risk of the delivery. Alternative birth settings that cannot provide prompt access to facilities for cesarean delivery, if needed, are not recommended for VBAC; however, VBAC could be attempted in a hospital birthing room.

Role of the Nurse

Nursing care of the woman attempting VBAC combines strategies for family-centered low-risk labor and delivery with strategies for care of the high-risk labor and delivery client. Ideally, the client would arrive in the labor unit with two birth plans: one for vaginal delivery and one in the event that cesarean delivery became necessary. In this situation, the client would have collaborated prenatally with her obstetric health care providers to ensure an optimal birth experience whether the birth occurred vaginally or abdominally. Support from nursing and medical staff promotes maternal confidence in attempting VBAC. During labor and delivery, careful monitoring of maternal and fetal status is essential. In addition, the unit should be readied in case an emergency cesarean becomes necessary. The nurse must be able to identify promptly deviations from normal labor progression, especially indications of uterine rupture (signs of hemorrhage, shock, subjective reports of a "ripping sensation" or of sharp uterine pain, abrupt cessation of contractions, a fetus that can be palpated with excess ease) and the onset of any fetal distress. Should a threat to maternal or fetal well-being arise during the course of labor, the nurse must promptly inform the physician and prepare for the possibility of an emergency cesarean.

Women who do have VBAC may experience pride, confidence, and excitement about achieving a personal goal. Feelings may not be completely positive, if the reality of a VBAC experience was not congruent with the client's expectations.

Nurses need to provide special support to the client who attempts VBAC but requires a repeat cesarean delivery. Some clients may equate VBAC with success as a woman and are at risk for feelings of failure and disappointment if VBAC does not become possible. During prenatal preparation, nurses need to avoid equating VBAC with "success" and to make certain that clients and families understand that VBAC cannot be guaranteed. Development of a prenatal alternative birth plan can help the client and her partner retain a sense of control over their birth experience and can promote a family-centered birth. Nurses should also anticipate negative client reactions and provide opportunity for the client and her family to express their feelings.

Nurses have an important role in helping to dispel the myth of "once a cesarean, always a cesarean." Nurses as well as other obstetric caregivers need to explore their own attitudes toward this practice, to review the professional literature about VBAC, and to assist colleagues in learning about VBAC. Prenatally, clients who could potentially attempt VBAC should be taught about this option and supported so they may attempt VBAC. Clients desiring VBAC may also have to contend with negative attitudes from family members who should also be included in VBAC teaching. Through roles as authors and consultants to the media, nurses can foster public perceptions of VBAC as a safe means of delivery for many women who have had previous cesarean childbirth.

CASE STUDY/CARE PLAN: CARE OF THE CLIENT IMMEDIATELY AFTER ELECTIVE CESAREAN DELIVERY

Jacky Vincent, G 2 P 1, 32 years old, is admitted to the delivery unit for a repeat cesarean birth. Her first child was born by emergency cesarean delivery four years ago as a result of failure to progress in labor and cephalopelvic disproportion.

Jacky is brought to the delivery suite at 8:00 A.M. She receives epidural anesthesia and is awake for the cesarean, with her husband Jim in attendance. The Vincent's newborn son weighs 7 lbs 4 oz. and has Apgar scores of 9 at one minute and 10 at five minutes. Following an uncomplicated 2 hour stay in the recovery room, Jacky is transferred to the postpartum floor. She receives 75 mg of meperidine, IM, for incisional pain. An indwelling catheter is in place and an intravenous drip of lactated Ringer's is running at 125cc per hour.

CASE STUDY/CARE PLAN: Care of the Client Immediately After Elective Cesarean Delivery (*continued*)

Supporting Assessment Data	Expected Client/Family Outcome	Nursing Action/ Intervention	Rationale	Criteria for Evaluation
Nursing Diagnosis: Asset in health, related to physiologic adaptation following cesarean delivery				
Blood pressure 110/70, pulse 72 and regular, respirations 17, temperature 98.2°F Dressing dry and intact Fundus firm, located at umbilicus Lochia rubra, moderate Urine clear and yellow and color	During the postpartum period, the client will maintain normal physiologic balance	Maintain continuous assessment (q 15 minutes in recovery room, on admission to postpartum floor, then q 4h or each shift as ordered) of: Neurologic status and progressive recovery from anesthesia Pulse, blood pressure, respirations Fundal height Lochia Incision/dressing Intravenous flow rate Patency of in-dwelling catheter; color and amount of urinary output	Assessment provides data about health status and recovery following cesarean delivery.	Client's postpartum hospital stay is without complications.
Nursing Diagnosis: Alteration in comfort: pain, related to cesarean delivery				
Client reports incisional pain; requires assistance to turn in bed	Client will report decreased discomfort related to incisional pain	Assess incision and dressing.	Pain in incision may indicate infection or separation, as well as normal postoperative discomfort.	Client will report decreased pain related to cesarean delivery.
		Administer pain medication as ordered.	Analgesic relieve postoperative pain.	
		Provide comfort measures: Prepared childbirth techniques of distraction, breathing, relaxation, imagery Turn and position as indicated Keep warm Provide sponge bath, mouth care, back rub	Comfort measures will assist client to relax, improving ability to cope with postoperative incisional pain.	
		Encourage husband to stay with client.	Promotes family-centered birthing experience.	
		Bring newborn to mother and father to see and touch after mother is made comfortable.	Promotes initial parent-infant attachment and provides alternate focus for attention.	
Nursing Diagnosis: Potential alteration in respiratory function, related to postoperative immobility and pain				
Client in pain, hesitant to deep breathe and cough or change position	By the first postoperative day, client will cough, deep breathe, and change position By the end of the first postoperative day, client will be out of bed with assistance	Administer pain medication as ordered. Assist client with change of position, coughing, deep breathing, and getting out of bed.	Client will tolerate deep breathing, coughing and mobility if made comfortable. Deep breathing, coughing, and early ambulation help to prevent postoperative respiratory complications.	By the end of the first postoperative day, client is performing coughing and deep breathing and is able to get out of bed with assistance.

SUMMARY

A cesarean delivery is a surgical procedure, in which delivery takes place following an incision through the abdominal wall and the uterus. Cesarean delivery is performed whenever it is unlikely that a safe vaginal birth can take place and whenever it is judged that a delay in delivery would jeopardize the well-being of mother, fetus, or both. A cesarean delivery may be primary or repeat and performed on an emergency or elective basis. When indicated, cesarean delivery can be a life-saving procedure; however, the surgery has drawbacks, such as a higher associated incidence of maternal morbidity and mortality than vaginal birth.

Cesarean delivery should be discussed with all clients during pregnancy because many primary cesarean deliveries are unplanned. Clients need to be aware of cesarean policies at the facility where they plan to deliver, as policies related to cesarean delivery may differ from those used for vaginal delivery. Clients who know in advance of their cesarean birth may attend cesarean childbirth classes.

Preoperative, operative, postoperative and postpartum care of the cesarean client combines principles of surgical and obstetric nursing. While the physiologic needs of the cesarean client are met, health care providers must also work together to promote a family-centered birth experience for cesarean clients. Clients who desire to breastfeed require encouragement and assistance to ensure a successful early breastfeeding experience. Paternal participation in cesarean birth should be fostered just as paternal participation in vaginal delivery is supported; however, health care providers should respect the choice of an expectant father who does not wish to be present. Nurses should anticipate a variety of emotional responses to cesarean birth on the part of clients and families. Although some clients accept the cesarean birth without difficulty, others experience depression, guilt and crisis.

General anesthesia, spinal anesthesia, and epidural anesthesia are the major choices of anesthesia for cesarean delivery. Every anesthetic method has advantages and limitations. With spinal or epidural anesthesia, the client is able to remain awake and interact with her newborn and support person. The epidural route allows for the administration of epidural analgesics which provide effective post-cesarean pain relief.

The old belief of "once a cesarean, always a cesarean" persists despite the support for vaginal birth after cesarean delivery (VBAC) from professional groups. When appropriate, VBAC is a safe and less costly alternative to cesarean delivery. Professional support for VBAC and public education about this alternative may help decrease the high rate of cesarean deliveries.

REVIEW QUESTIONS

1. Describe factors that contribute to the incidence of cesarean birth.
2. Discuss benefits and drawbacks of cesarean birth.
3. Identify nursing implications for care of a client who has received an epidural anesthetic for cesarean delivery, or an epidural analgesic after cesarean delivery.
4. Discuss psychologic reactions couples may have to cesarean birth.
5. Describe nursing care strategies for a couple who desire to attempt vaginal birth after cesarean delivery.

REFERENCES

1. Oxorn H, ed. *Human Labor & Birth.* 5th ed. Norwalk, Conn: Appleton-Century-Crofts; 1986.
2. Enkin M. Having a section is having a baby. *Birth Fam J.* 1977;4:99–104.
3. Porreco RP. High cesarean section rate: a new perspective. *Obstet Gynecol.* 1985;65:307–311.
4. Marieskind H. Cesarean section in the United States: has it changed since 1979? *Birth,* 1989;16:196–202.
5. Cunningham FG, et al. *Williams Obstetrics.* 18th ed. Norwalk, Conn: Appleton & Lange; 1989.
6. National Institutes of Health Consensus Development Conference. *Cesarean Childbirth.* Bethesda, Md: Office of Research Reporting, NIHCD; 1981.
7. Bing E. Correspondence. *Birth Fam.* 1978;5:105.
8. Affonso DD, Stichler JF. Cesarean birth: women's reactions. *Am J Nurs.* 1980;80:468–470.
9. Zuspan FP, Quilligan EJ. *Douglas-Stromme Operative Obstetrics.* 5th ed. Norwalk, Conn: Appleton & Lange; 1988.
10. Austin SEJ. Childbirth classes for couples desiring VBAC. *Am J Matern Child Nurs.* 1986;11:250–255.
11. Johnson SR, et al. Obstetric decision-making: Responses to patients who request cesarean delivery. *Obstet Gynecol.* 1986;67:847–850.

12. Frigoletto FD, et al. Maternal mortality rate associated with cesarean section: an appraisal. *Am J Obstet Gynecol.* 1980; 136:969.
13. Affonso DD, Stichler JF. Exploratory study of women's reactions to having a cesarean birth. In: Sherwen LN, Weingarten CT, eds. *Analysis and Application of Nursing Research: Parent-Neonate Studies.* Monterey, Calif: Wadsworth Health Sciences; 1983;171–177.
14. Marut JS, Mercer RT. The cesarean birth experience: implications for nursing. In: Lederman RP, Raff B, eds. *Perinatal Parental Behavior: Nursing Research and Implications for Newborn Health.* March of Dimes, OAS, XVII. New York: Alan R. Liss; 1981:129–152.
15. Schnider SM, Levinson G. Obstetric anesthesia. In: Miller RD, ed. *Anesthesia.* 2nd ed. New York: Churchill Livingstone; 1986: vol 3, 1681–1728.
16. Norheim A. Spinal anesthesia. *Nursing 86.* 1986;16:42–44.
17. Smith CM. Epidural anesthesia in labor: various agents employed. *J Obstet Gynecol Neonat Nurs.* 1984;13:17–21.
18. Avard D, Nimrod CM. Risks and benefits of epidural anesthesia: a review. *Birth.* 1985;12:215–225.
19. Nicolls ET, et al. Epidural anesthesia for the woman in labor. *Am J Nurs.* 1981;81:1826–1830.
20. Corke BC, Spirlman FJ. Problems associated with epidural anesthesia in obstetrics. *Obstet Gynecol.* 1985;65:837–839.
21. American College of Obstetricians and Gynecologists. *Obstetric Anesthesia and Analgesia.* Washington, DC: The College; 1988: Technical Bulletin 112.
22. McDonald JS. Obstetric analgesia and anesthesia. In: Pernoll ML, Benson RC, eds. *Current Obstetric & Gynecologic Diagnosis & Treatment.* 6th ed. Norwalk, Conn: Appleton & Lange; 1987: 456–480.
23. Nicholson C. Nursing considerations for the parturient who has received epidural narcotics during labor or delivery. *J Perinatal Neonatal Nurs.* 1990;4:14–26.
24. Gutsche BB. Obstetric anesthesia and perinatology. In: Dripps RD, et al (eds). *Introduction to Anesthesia.* 7th ed. Philadelphia: Saunders; 1988.
25. Miller RD. Anesthesia. In: Schwartz SI, et al, eds. *Principles of Surgery,* vol. 1. 5th ed. New York: McGraw-Hill Book Co; 1989:459–468.
26. Kalisch B, Kalisch P. Nurses on prime time television. *Am J Nurs.* 1982;82:264–270.
27. Hassid P. *Textbook for Childbirth Educators.* 2nd ed. Philadelphia: JB Lippincott; 1984.
28. Donovan B. *The Cesarean Birth Experience.* Revised ed. Boston: Beacon Press; 1986.
29. Fawcett J, Burritt J. An exploratory study of antenatal preparation for cesarean birth. *J Obstet Gynecol Neonat Nurs.* 1985;14:224–232.
30. Inturrisi M, et al. Epidural morphine for relief of postpartum, postsurgical pain. *J Obstet Gynecol Neonat Nurs.* 1988;17: 238–245.
31. Kotelko DM, et al. Epidural morphine analgesia after cesarean delivery. *Obstet Gynecol.* 1984;63:409–413.
32. Henrikson ML, Wild L. A nursing process approach to epidural analgesia. *J Obstet Gynecol Neonat Nurs.* 1988;17: 316–319.
33. Powell AH, Bova MB. How do you give continuous epidural fentanyl? *Am J Nurs.* 1989;89:1197–1200.
34. Mersmann CA. Nursing care following duromorph administration. Poster presentation, national meeting of the Organization for Obstetric, Gynecologic and Neonatal Nurses, St. Louis, Mo; March 1989.
35. Kearney, et al. Cesarean delivery and breastfeeding outcomes. *Birth.* 1990;17:97–103.
36. Lipson J, Tilden V. Psychological integration of the cesarean birth experience. *Am J Orthopsychiatry.* 1980;50:598–609.
37. Sandelowski M, Bustamante R. Cesarean birth outside the natural childbirth culture. *Res Nurs Health.* 1986;9:81–88.
38. Culp RE, Osofsky HJ. Effects of cesarean delivery on parental depression, marital adjustment and mother-infant interaction. *Birth.* 1989;16:53–56.
39. Shearer EL. Does cesarean delivery affect the parents? *Birth.* 1989;16:57–58.
40. Cummins LH, et al. Views of cesarean birth among primiparous Mexican women in Los Angeles. *Birth.* 1988;15:164–170.
41. May KA, Sollid DT. Unanticipated cesarean birth from the father's perspective. *Birth.* 1984;11:87–95.
42. Fortier JC. The relationship of vaginal and cesarean births to father-infant attachment. *J Obstet Gynecol Neonat Nurs.* 1988;17:128–134.
43. Miller CR, Sutter CS. Vaginal birth after a cesarean. *J Obstet Gynecol Neonat Nurs.* 1985;14:383–389.
44. Pauerstein C. Labor after cesarean section, from precept to practice. *J Reprod Med.* 1981;26:409–412.
45. Jarel MA, et al. Vaginal delivery after cesarean section: a five year study. *Obstet Gynecol.* 1985;65:628–634.
46. Merrill BS, Biffs CE. Planned vaginal delivery following cesarean section. *Obstet Gynecol.* 1978;52:50.
47. Morewood GA, et al. Vaginal delivery after cesarean. *Obstet Gynecol.* 1973;42:589–595.
48. Consensus Task Force on Cesarean Childbirth. *Cesarean Childbirth.* Bethesda, Md: US Department of Health and Human Services; 1981: NIH 82–2067.
49. Minkoff H, Schwartz R. The rising cesarean rate: can it safely be reversed? *Obstet Gynecol.* 1980;56:2135–2143.
50. Frigoletto FD, Little GA, eds. *Guidelines for Perinatal Care,* 2nd ed. Washington, DC: American Academy of Pediatrics & American College of Obstetricians and Gynecologists; 1988.
51. Hangsleben K, et al. VBAC program in a nurse-midwifery service: five years of experience. *J Nurse Midwifery.* 1989; 34:179–184.
52. Committee statement: guidelines for vaginal delivery after a previous cesarean birth. Washington, DC: American College of Obstetricians and Gynecologists; Jan 1982, Nov 1984.
53. Phelan JP, et al. Twice a cesarean, always a cesarean? *Obstet Gynecol.* 1989;73:161–165.

The Postpartum Period

unit 8

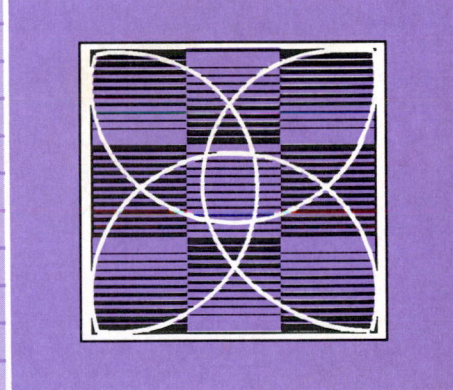

Physiologic Changes During the Postpartum Period

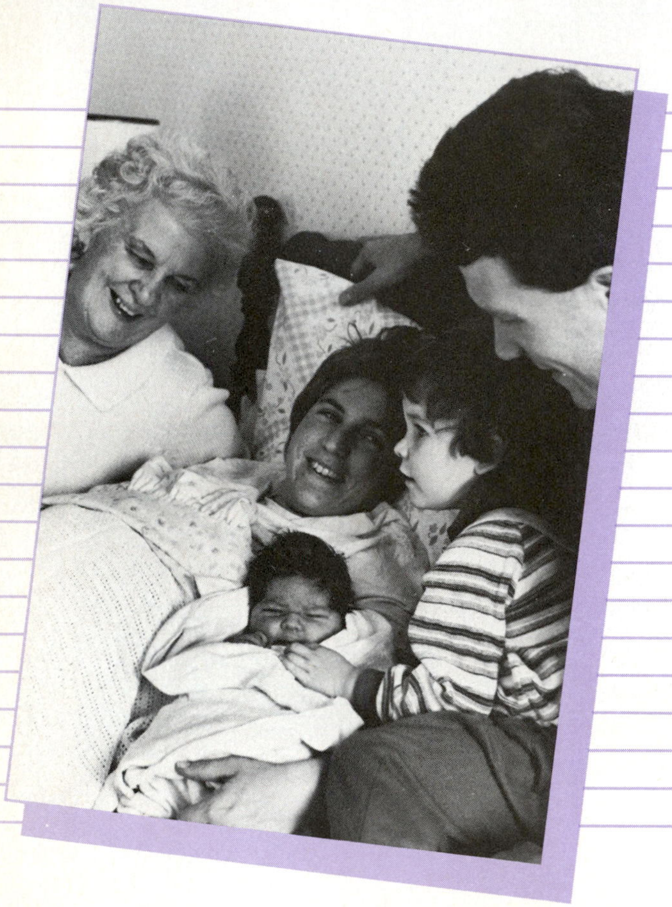

chapter 29

Key Terms

colostrum
exfoliation
involution
let-down reflex
lochia
postpartum period
puerperium

Traditionally, the first 6 weeks after giving birth, during which the woman's body undergoes multiple physiologic changes in response to childbirth, has been referred to as the **puerperium.** Thus, the puerperium refers primarily to the woman's physiologic restoration. Over the past two decades, however, health care professionals have come to believe that the period after giving birth is a time for both physical and psychologic restoration, and a time in which the parents develop a relationship with their infant.[1] As a result of this altered philosophy, many health care professionals view the first 6 to 8 weeks after birth as the **postpartum period,** and also label the first 3 months after birth as the fourth trimester.

CHANGES IN MATERNAL BODY SYSTEMS

Reproductive System

The return of the reproductive system to approximately prepregnancy size and function is termed **involution.** The process of involution takes about 6 weeks, with the exception of resumption of menses and ovulation. The most rapid changes of the reproductive system occur immediately after birth and within the first 3 to 4 days.

Uterus. Immediately after expulsion of the placenta the uterine fundus, now firmly contracted, assumes a position approximately midway between the umbilicus and symphysis pubis. The uterine walls, now paled as a result of compression of blood vessels, are thickened and in close proximity compared with the previous pregnant state.

By 12 hours postpartum, the fundus rises to the umbilicus or slightly above. Thereafter, the uterine fundus descends 1 to 2 cm, or one fingerbreath, per day, so that by the 10th day after delivery the fundus may no longer be palpated abdominally. By 6 weeks postpartum the uterus has assumed nearly a pregnancy size and shape (Figure 29–1).

At delivery the uterus weighs approximately 2.2 pounds or 1 kg. By 6 weeks after delivery the uterus weighs 60 to 100 g because of a reduction in cell size from autolysis of protein within the uterine wall cells.

Uterine ligaments are stretched and loose after delivery, and thus their ability to support the uterus is diminished. In particular, a full bladder's ability to displace the uterus is aided by the nonsupportive uterine ligaments. As uterine involution progresses, the ligaments regain tone.

Endometrium. With the delivery of the placenta and membranes, the underlying decidua, irregular in thickness and appearance, is filled with blood. At the placental site the tissue is raised and jagged and contains numerous thrombosed blood vessels.

During the first few days after delivery, the spongy layer of the decidua is discarded as a discharge called **lochia.** By 2 to 3 days, the basal layer of the decidua differentiates into two layers: (1) a superficial layer that, becoming necrotic, is cast off as lochia, and (2) a new basal layer adjacent to the myometrium that contains endometrial gland fundi and connective tissue, the precursors for the new endometrium. Regeneration of the endometrial tissue from the neoplacental decidua is achieved by proliferative and mitotic activity of the endometrial gland fundi and connective tissue. Within 7 to 10 days, epithelium lines the uterine cavity except at the placental site; and by 3 weeks the endometrial tissue is restored, although some leukocytes and hyalinized decidual remnants persist.[2]

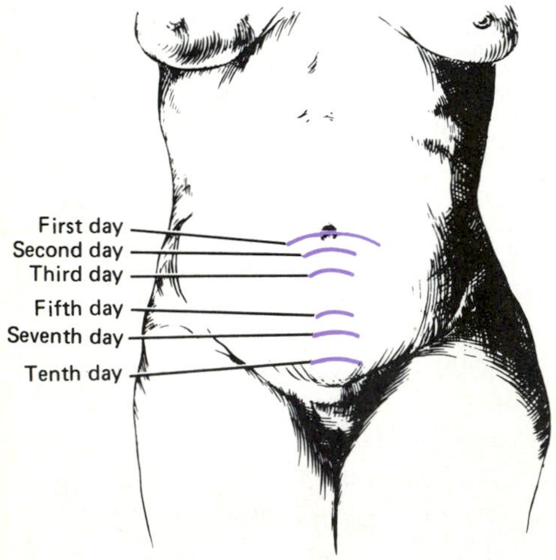

Figure 29–1. Uterine involution, showing changes in the height of the fundus and the size of the uterus during the first 10 days postpartum. (*Reproduced, with permission, from Pernoll ML, Benson RC, eds.* Current Obstetric & Gynecologic Diagnosis and Treatment. *Norwalk, Conn: Appleton & Lange; 1987:216.*)

In the initial postpartum, the uterine lochia is categorized according to color and content. During the first 2 to 3 days the lochia contains primarily decidual tissue, epithelial cells, red blood cells, white blood cells, some meconium, vernix caseosa, and lanugo; it is termed *lochia rubra* because it is red. By approximately the third day, *lochia serosa,* a pale serosanguinous discharge containing decidua, red blood cells, white blood cells, bacteria, and cervical mucus, is present. Lochia serosa continues until the tenth day after delivery and is followed by *lochia alba,* a creamy yellow discharge, which gradually ceases. Lochia alba is composed primarily of white blood cells, bacteria, some decidual cells, epithelial cells, fat, cervical mucus, and cholesterol. In general, by the time the cervix is fully closed at 2 to 3 weeks after delivery, the lochia has just about ceased. The presence of lochia past the third to fourth week after delivery warrants medical evaluation.

In the first hour postpartum, as much as 120 mL of lochia may be discharged with complete cardiovascular tolerance. Even the loss of 500 mL of blood after completion of the third stage of labor may be tolerated, although this amount of blood loss is traditionally classified as postpartum hemorrhage.[2] In general, a large peripad holds 60 to 100 mL of lochia when fully saturated. Saturation of more than one or two pads during the first hour postpartum or saturation of one pad within 15 minutes should be reported to the primary health care provider.

After the first hour postpartum, the amount of lochia discharged gradually diminishes in volume. The total volume of lochia discharged averages 255 mL.

Lochia may be altered by several factors. A greater amount of lochia is discharged when the woman is in of an upright position after long periods in a recumbent position. Lochia tends to pool within the uterus and vagina with inactivity. Accordingly, many women note that there is an increase in the

RESEARCH ABSTRACT

Tulman L, Fawcett J. Return of functional ability after childbirth. Nurs Res. *1988;37:77–81.*

This retrospective, exploratory study examined the recovery of functional ability after childbirth in a sample of women who had vaginal deliveries and cesarean sections. The subjects of the study were 70 women who had delivered full-term infants within the 5 years prior to data collection. Of these, 30 women (43 percent) had vaginal deliveries and 40 (57 percent) had cesarean deliveries. Further, 15 of the 30 women who delivered vaginally had vaginal births after previous cesarean deliveries.

The instruments used for the study were the Childbirth Impact Profile Form MQ (CIP-MQ) and a background data sheet. The CIP-MQ measures functional ability, and includes items regarding physical energy, household activities, and occupational activities. The background data sheet was used to collect data on demographic variables, type of delivery, parity, maternal and neonatal complications, and method of infant feedings. Fifty one percent of the women regained their usual level of energy by the end of the 6-week postpartum period: 72 percent of the women who delivered vaginally and 34 percent of the women who delivered by cesarean. Differences were noted between the two groups of women with respect to when household tasks, socializing with friends, and participation in religious organizations were resumed. There was also a difference between the two groups in the time they took to assume infant care responsibilities. The authors suggest that the traditional 6-week period of recovery from childbirth needs to be reconsidered, especially for women experiencing cesarean deliveries.

Comment:
Traditionally, the postpartum period is considered to last 6 to 8 weeks. As this study suggests, many women may not be fully recovered, particularly if they had cesarean deliveries. This study's results raise questions about such topics as the appropriate length of time for maternity leave after vaginal and cesarean births.

amount of lochia in the morning, after resting during the night. Concurrent with pooling of blood, women may note the passage of small blood clots after periods of rest. As long as the small clots are free of placental tissue, they are harmless. Retained placental tissue can produce large clots and hemorrhage. Persistent lochia or resumption of lochia rubra is indicative of subinvolution (failure of the uterus to return to its normal size) and postpartum infection. A sudden increase in physical activity in the early postpartum can cause an increase in uterine bleeding. Additionally, the presence of an infection within the uterus can produce foul-smelling lochia.

Placental Site Restoration. At the placental site, as necrotic tissue is sloughed off, endometrial restoration begins at the margins by extension and downward growth of tissue, as well as by proliferation of the endometrial fundi and connective tissue. This process, termed **exfoliation,** is thought to prevent the formation of scar tissue. Through exfoliation, the placental site decreases in size so that within 14 days the diameter of the site is approximately 3 to 4 cm, and by 42 days complete placental site involution has occurred.[2]

Lower Uterine Segment and Cervix. After delivery, the lower uterine segment, thin and flabby, readily collapses. The muscle tissue of the lower uterine segment contracts and retracts so that by 4 to 6 weeks postpartum, this structure is identifiable as the uterine isthmus.

The cervix, also flabby, thin, and collapsed after delivery, gradually contracts so that by 2 days postpartum, it is dilated 2 to 3 cm. By the seventh day postpartum, the cervix is nearly closed and thick.

During the delivery the external os is often lacerated and may be discernible later as depressions on the cervix. As the cervix involutes, the external os never regains the oval shape, but rather is identified as a wider, transverse slit with extensions (Figure 29–2). Unilateral and untreated lacerations of the cervix, like those of the vagina, can be the cause of prolonged continuous bleeding in the presence of a firmly contracted uterus.

Ovulation and Menstruation. Although ovulation and menstruation may occur by 6 to 8 weeks postpartum, considerable variation exists. Resumption of ovulation and menstruation differs between lactating and nonlactating women, and even within these two groups of women there are variations.

In nonlactating women, menstrual flow resumes in 6 to 8 weeks for 40 to 45 percent, and in 12 weeks for 65 to 70 percent. Almost all nonlactating women are menstruating by 6 months postpartum. Fifty per-

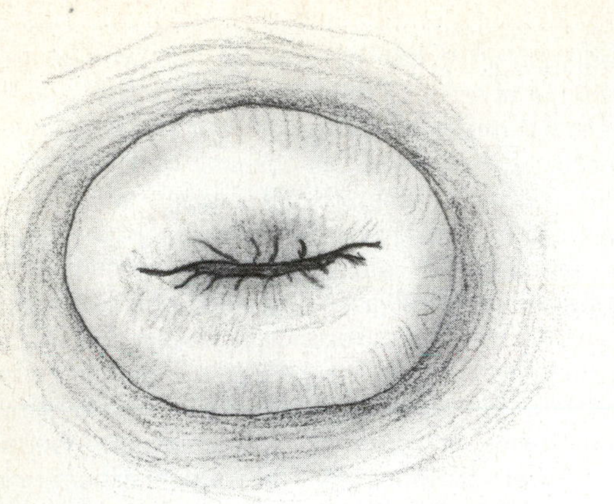

Figure 29–2. Multiparous cervix postdelivery.

cent of nonlactating women have an anovulatory menstrual flow for the first cycle. The average time for resumption of ovulation in nonlactating women is approximately 10 weeks after delivery.[4,5]

Lactating women often experience postpartum amenorrhea for a longer period compared with nonlactating women. According to one plausible explanation, the prolactin level, which is elevated during the initation of lactation, has an inhibitory effect on follicular development, resulting in a failure of the ovaries to respond to gonadotropins.[6] Menstruation resumes in 2 months in 26 percent of lactating women, by 3 months in 45 percent, and by 6 months in 90 percent. Approximately one third of lactating primiparas ovulate in 3 months, whereas multiparas are more likely to ovulate before 3 months. In general, postpartum amenorrhea in lactating women can range from 6 weeks to over 2 years.[6] This wide range is highly dependent on whether the woman breastfeeds continuously or breastfeeds with supplements. Through interpretations of endometrial biopsy, basal body temperature, vaginal cytology, and cervical mucus of 170 lactating women, Perez and associates[7] found in their classic study that 14 percent ovulated while fully breastfeeding, 29 percent ovulated while partially breastfeeding, and 57 percent ovulated when breastfeeding was discontinued. In this particular sample the first postpartum menstruation was ovulatory in 78 percent of these lactating women.[7]

Vagina and Vaginal Orifice. The vagina, vaginal outlet, and labia surrounding the outlet are stretched during delivery; rugae are obliterated. Gradually the vagina regains shape and tone. Although rugae reappear by 3 weeks postpartum, the increase in tone and reduction in size of the vagina and vaginal outlet generally require at least 6 weeks. Once the lochia has stopped, the vagina is dry, especially in the lactating woman. Lacerations of the vagina should be suspected if profuse bleeding occurs despite the presence of a firmly contracted fundus. The labia become progressively less flabby, but generally do not regain the nonparous tone.

In the delivery of the baby, the hymen is lacerated. The lacerated edges of the hymen heal as separate tags called caruncula myrtiformes.

Perineum. The perineal body is the tissue that lies between the vaginal introitus and the anus. As the anus is often affected by a vaginal delivery, discussion of the perineum includes content related to the anus.

The perineum and anus are often the site of puerperal discomfort for women who have delivered vaginally. The perineum is often edematous and ecchymotic. Perineal lacerations and episiotomies, which may extend into the anus, are additional causes of puerperal discomfort. The edges of the episiotomy and repaired lacerations should be approximated with sutures intact during the early postpartum. Generally, dissolvable suture is used to repair lacerations and the episiotomy. Within 1 to 2 weeks some women may find pieces of suture on the peripad. The presence of hemorrhoids adjacent to the perineal body may exacerbate discomfort.

Within a week perineal and anal discomfort begins to diminish. The perineal edema and bruising may resolve within the first postpartum week. Hemorrhoids usually reduce in size during the first few weeks after delivery, but for some women hemorrhoids may become a chronic problem. The episiotomy and repaired lacerations are usually healed within 2 to 3 weeks.

Breasts. Several changes occur in the breasts to prepare them for lactation during the postpartum period. (*See* the section on "Lactation" later in this chapter for a detailed discussion of these changes.)

Cardiovascular System

The cardiovascular system is greatly altered during pregnancy to meet the demands of gestation, labor, and delivery. During the postpartum, the cardiovascular system gradually resumes a nonpregnant state.

With delivery of the baby, the diaphragm is no longer pushed upward against the heart by the uterus and abdominal contents. Consequently, the heart, no longer displaced to the left and upward, resumes the nonpregnant position within the chest wall.

Cardiac Output, Pulse, and Blood Pressure. The increase in cardiac output induced by pregnancy and the first and second stages of labor is resolved shortly after delivery. Reflecting the diminished cardiac output, postpartum women experience bradycardia for the first 6 to 10 days after delivery. Pulse rates as low as 50 to 70 beats per minute are common and considered quite normal. Conversely, a rapid pulse rate during this period is indicative of postpartum hemorrhage, anxiety, fatigue, infection, fever, or cardiac disease.

Generally, the blood pressure during the postpartum does not differ from that in the nonpregnant state. Increased blood pressure suggests pregnancy-induced hypertension. Decreased blood pressure suggests uterine hemorrhage, orthostatic hypotension, or a physiologic response to diminished intrapelvic pressure.

Blood Volume and Concentration. Normally, pregnancy induces a marked increase in maternal blood volume. The blood volume undergoes considerable reduction during labor and delivery as a result of erythropoiesis, dehydration, and muscular activity. Hemoconcentration results. An additional reduction in blood volume occurs shortly after delivery. In the next few days, however, the blood volume remains fairly stable. By 1 week postpartum, the blood volume undergoes a further reduction and then stabilizes at levels that are nearly equivalent to nonpregnant levels.

During labor, erythropoiesis increases, and if accompanied by dehydration, the hemoglobin and hematocrit also increase. By 3 days postpartum the increased erythropoiesis observable during labor reverses and stabilizes.[8] As fluids are replaced and the fluid volume stabilizes the erythropoiesis, hematocrit and hemoglobin decrease[2,8,9] so that by 3 to 4 days postpartum, these values have stabilized.[9] Postpartum erythrocyte, hematocrit, and hemoglobin values below prelabor or early-labor levels indicate that the woman has sustained a significant blood loss. According to Taylor and Lind[9] hemoglobin levels on the second postpartum day best predict hemoglobin concentration by 6 weeks postpartum; thus, screening for anemia is best done on the second postpartum day. Women receiving intravenous solutions and oxytocin during labor can, however, have significantly reduced hemoglobin concentration in the first 4 days postpartum.[8]

Leukocytes are markedly elevated in the early postpartum. Levels as high as 25,000 mm^3, without an infection, have been reported[2,8] although the average is 14,000 to 16,000 mm.[2,9] Although postpartum leukocytosis is common, an increase of more than 30 percent over a 6-hour interval is considered suggestive of infection.[10,11]

Blood Loss. Blood loss during vaginal delivery of a single infant and in the first 24 hours postpartum amounts to approximately 500 to 600 mL.[9–11] Approximately 930 to 1000 mL of blood is lost with the delivery of twins or in a cesarean delivery.[2] Traditionally, a blood loss of more than 500 mL in the first 24 hours after delivery has been labeled postpartum hemorrhage; however, women can tolerate the loss of most of the blood added to the circulation during pregnancy without adverse effects.[2] Consequently, many health care professionals now consider that an estimated blood loss greater than 500 mL is a warning sign that hemorrhage may be imminent[2] and have labeled mild postpartum hemorrhage as blood loss of 750 to 1250 mL.[8,12] Women are at greatest risk of postpartum hemorrhage within the first 24 hours of delivery; however, late postpartum hemorrhage may occur during the seventh to tenth day after delivery when blood coagulation factors reach low levels.

Blood Coagulation. Clotting factors that increased during pregnancy tend to remain elevated during the initial postpartum period. Additionally, the level of protein C, a main coagulation inhibitor, decreases slightly after delivery.[13,14] By 3 to 5 days postpartum, protein C levels increase as compared with predelivery levels. Nonpregnant individuals with an inherited protein C deficiency frequently develop venous thromboembolic disorders.[14,15] Persistent elevation in clotting factors, the low level of protein C, diminished activity, infection, and injury predispose a woman to thromboembolism of the lower extremities and pulmonary embolism.

Varicosities and Edema. Lower extremity varicosities that developed during pregnancy because of an increase in blood volume and dependent venous stasis lessen in severity shortly after delivery. As the water metabolism of pregnancy is reversed, edema of the extremities, as well as of other parts of the body, diminishes.

Respiratory System

Respirations remain in the normal range during the postpartum period. As the abdominal organs resume their nonpregnant position, the respiratory diaphragm returns to its usual position. By 2 months postpartum, total pulmonary resistance increases by 50 percent as compared with pregnancy. Specific airway conductance, which increased during pregnancy, returns to the nonpregnancy level by 5 to 8 weeks after delivery. The changes in airway conductance may be caused by the decreased level of progesterone.

Generally, women who deliver vaginally do not complain of dyspnea. Women who deliver by cesarean, however, may experience abdominal pain when trying to deep breathe, and cough. Any woman complaining of dyspnea, regardless of the method of delivery, should be assessed for pulmonary embolism. As with any surgical client, woman who have been delivered by cesarean need to be assessed for respiratory status.

Urinary System

In the early postpartum, the ability of the bladder to eliminate urine warrants close attention. After an uncomplicated vaginal delivery, women may get out of bed to go to the bathroom. Although some women may have the urge to void spontaneously after delivery, many women experience diminished awareness of the need to urinate accompanied by difficulty with the first postpartum void. Perineal lacerations, hematomas, generalized swelling and bruising of the perineum and tissues surrounding the urinary meatus, physiologic and conductive anesthesia, and diminished sensation of bladder pressure impede urination after delivery.[15] Furthermore, the use of a bed pan may impede urination. The postpartum woman is subsequently at risk for urinary retention, bladder distension, urinary stasis, and urinary tract infection. Her risk of developing these conditions is further increased by the rapid filling of the bladder with body and intravenous fluids as the antidiuretic effect and level of labor-administered and endogenous oxytocin diminish. With bladder distension the postpartum woman is also at risk for uterine atony (inability of the uterine musculature to contract), resulting in hemorrhage. Specifically, as the bladder distends, the uterus is displaced and the ability of the uterus to contract is diminished. When the uterus fails to contract, cut blood vessels are free to bleed, and thus uterine hemorrhage may ensue.

Generally, within 4 to 8 hours of a vaginal delivery, women have a spontaneous urge to void. In the next 48 hours, women void frequently as the water metabolism of pregnancy is reversed and extracellular fluids that are no longer needed are excreted. This postpartum diuresis also causes rapid bladder filling and may contribute to bladder distension.

In the first 2 days after delivery, proteolytic enzymes promote self-digestion of protein substances from the uterine wall (autolysis). Mild proteinuria may occur as a result of this process. Pathologic conditions such as hypertensive disorders and diabetes may produce markedly elevated proteinuria and ketonuria. Urine may also test positive for acetone/ketones resulting from dehydration during a prolonged labor. Lactosuria may occur in breastfeeding women as a result of the lactation process.

Within a week of delivery, creatinine clearance, which is normally elevated during pregnancy, returns to a normal level. Blood urea nitrogen (BUN) increases in response to the autolytic process occurring within the uterus. By 4 to 6 weeks, kidney function is normal and the ureteral dilation of pregnancy has diminished.

Musculoskeletal System

With delivery of the placenta, the influence of progesterone on the woman's general muscle tone is removed. Consequently, restoration of muscle tone in the postpartum may proceed provided there is a balance of rest , activity, exercise, and diet. In particular restoration of tone in the rectus abdominis muscles, the pubococcygeal muscle, and the muscles of the lower extremities is often of concern to women during the postpartum period.

For most women the general shape and appearance of the postpartum abdomen cause much concern. The previously pregnant abdomen is now soft, flabby, and weak. The thick central abdominal muscles, the rectus abdominis muscles, are usually separated after the delivery, giving the abdomen the flabby appearance. The extent of the separation may be greater when there was previous muscle weakness, multiple gestation, polyhydramnios, excessive weight gain, and grand multiparity. Women need to be taught that with diet, exercise, and rest, the abdominal muscles can usually regain muscle tone. Although muscle tone may be regained in 6 weeks, some women need more time. The abdominal musculature in some women fails to regain maximum tone, despite exercise and diet.

Childbirth is accomplished with stretching and trauma to the pubococcygeal muscle, the major sphincter of the pelvis. The pubococcygeal muscle usually aids in maintaining bowel and bladder function, supports the contraceptive diaphragm, and may influence vaginal responses to intercourse.[16] Kegel exercises in the postpartum period may help to heal the muscle.

In the first 24 hours after delivery many women experience lower-extremity soreness and weakness as a result of the muscular tension and exertion experienced during labor and delivery. Women who have received regional anesthesia may experience decreased sensation in the lower extremities.[17]

Integument

The integument undergoes overt changes during the puerperium. As estrogen and progesterone levels decrease, the increase in pigmentation that was experienced during pregnancy, such as darkening of the areolae and nipples, facial chloasma (the "mask of pregnancy"), and linea nigra, gradually diminishes. Striae, the reddish purple marks that during pregnancy formed on the breasts, abdomen, and thighs as elastic skin fibers were stretched and ruptured, begin to fade and eventually appear as silver or white skin streaks. Spider angiomas and palmar erythema begin to disappear presumably in response to the diminished estrogen level.

During the early postpartum period, the integument also aids in ridding the woman of some excess water. Specifically, during the first week after delivery, women experience diaphoresis (profuse sweating) during the night. Diaphoresis may interrupt sleep and cause chilling and discomfort.

Many women experience mild and temporary alopecia, an increase in loss of scalp hairs, for several weeks to months after delivery. This postpartum alopecia reduces the number of growing scalp hair (anagens), which had increased during the last two trimesters of pregnancy in response to altered androgen levels. The alopecia usually ceases gradually without long-term effects. For most women, the loss of scalp hair is not noticeable to others, but merely identified by an increase in hairs lost after grooming or washing the hair.

Gastrointestinal System

Immediately after a vaginal delivery many women experience hunger and thirst. If there are no signs of nausea and vomiting, and general or regional block anesthesia was not used in labor and delivery, a light meal is appropriate. If anesthesia was given during labor and delivery, a light meal can be given 2 hours after delivery if the woman is stable.

Whether they deliver vaginally or by cesarean, women experience sluggish bowels for several days after delivery. Decreased peristalsis occurs in response to anesthesia, surgery, diminished intra-abdominal pressure, diminished muscle tone, lack of an appropriate diet, insufficient fluid intake, and a history of diarrhea or an enema while in labor. Additionally, pain and fear of harm from hemorrhoids, an episiotomy, or lacerations lead to a decreased willingness by the postpartum woman to exert pressure on the perineum. Constipation and gas pain may result.

Many women develop hemorrhoids during pregnancy and labor and delivery. Hemorrhoids, distended rectal veins with entrapped blood, result from pressure on the pelvic floor. As the woman strains, internal hemorrhoids may become external and bleed. Generally hemorrhoids are painful for a couple of days after delivery. They gradually decrease in size over the next several weeks; however, many women may experience mild chronic hemorrhoidal discomfort.

Endocrine System

Reproductive Hormones. With delivery of the placenta there is a rapid decline in human placental lactogen (hPL) or human chorionic somatomammotropin (hCS), human chorionic gonadotropin (hCG), estrogen, and progesterone. By 1 week postpartum, only estrogen may be discernible in plasma. Additionally, levels of follicle-stimulating hormone and luteinizing hormone are very low at 10 days postpartum.

In nonlactating women, estrogen levels begin to rise to follicular levels at approximately 3 weeks after delivery, followed by rising, but still low levels of progesterone. Frequently the first menses postpartum is anovulatory. Return to prepregnancy levels of estrogen and progesterone occurs at a more variable, slower pace in lactating women than in nonlactating women.

During pregnancy, the pituitary gland begins to secrete prolactin. As the levels of progesterone and estrogen rapidly decline after delivery, and lactation is initiated, the prolactin level rises. With increased breastfeeding, the prolactin level rises further.[18] (*See* section on "Lactation" later in this chapter.) In nonlactating women, the prolactin level declines and reaches the nonpregnancy level by 14 days.

Thyroid Hormone. Pregnancy-induced hyperplasia of glandular tissue, general increased vascularity, and increased iodine turnover in response to a higher glomerular filtration rate and renal iodine clearance[19] can cause slight, nonpathologic enlargement of the thyroid gland. Additionally, during pregnancy the thyroid gland may enlarge slightly and the basal metabolic rate increases. By 6 weeks postpartum the thyroid gland should return to the prepregnant state.

A small percentage of women develop puerperal thyroiditis, an autoimmune disease characterized by increased thyroid antibody titers, painless thyroid enlargement, and either hyperthyroid or hypothyroid symptoms.[19] In most cases puerperal thyroiditis is relieved with treatment. Occasionally, chronic thyroid disease and recurring, transient thyroid disease persist.

Psychoendocrine Relationships. Many women experience an emotional state known as "postpartum blues" 3 to 4 days after delivery. One explanation for postpartum blues suggests that changes in the levels of endogenous substances alter the emotional status of women. (*See* Chapter 41 for further discussion of postpartum blues.)

Changes in Metabolic Activity: Weight Loss

The immediate weight loss after delivery is approximately 10 to 12 pounds. This initial weight loss includes 1.5 pounds for the placenta, 2 pounds of blood and amniotic fluid, and the weight of the baby. Within the next 2 to 4 days, postpartum diuresis results in the additional loss of 5 pounds. With complete involution, 1.8 pounds will be lost. Additional weight is lost as a result of circulatory changes for several weeks.[20]

Traditionally, health care professionals have professed that if the total weight gained during the pregnancy is about 25 pounds, the woman usually will attain her prepregnancy weight by 6 weeks postpartum, but if more than 25 pounds is gained, the woman will retain more than 50 percent of the extra weight; however, a study by Olsen and Mundt[21] indicates that because the weight gained during pregnancy is extremely varied, return to prepregnancy weight is also varied. They report that although the average weight gain for 182 urban women was 27.8 pounds, the range was 3 to 82 pounds. Of these 182 women, only 28 percent returned to their prepregnancy weight or less by 8 weeks postpartum. The majority of the women retained an average of 5.9 pounds over their prepregnancy weight at 6 weeks postpartum. Primigravidas lost more weight and women of gravida 2 lost the least. Women who gained at least 40 pounds had more difficulty in losing weight.[21]

Mothers who bottlefed their infants tended to lose more weight than those who were breastfeeding at 6 weeks postpartum.[21] These differences in weight loss between bottlefeeding and breastfeeding women are expected because of the nutritional needs of the breastfeeding women.

By 3 months postpartum many breastfeeding mothers begin to notice additional weight loss, presumably as the fat stores of pregnancy are depleted for lactation. The bottlefeeding mother who has gained excessive weight during pregnancy tends to retain fat stores unless she exercises and diets appropriately.

During the puerperium, most women express concern about their figures and weight. Although they may be pleased with the initial weight loss, many women become discouraged with their weight and corresponding figures at 2 to 4 weeks postpartum. Fawcett,[22] studying body image during pregnancy and the puerperium, found that women perceived a decrease in body space after delivery but by the second postpartum month their perception of body space was increased. Fawcett interpreted these findings as reflective of women's displeasure with the pattern of weight loss in the puerperium.

LACTATION

Establishment and maintenance of lactation are the results of a highly integrated psychophysiologic process that occurs within the mother-infant dyad. Although, in reality this process is indivisible, the following discussion has been divided into three components—anatomic, physiologic, and psychologic—for conceptual ease.

Anatomy of the Breast

The mature human female breast is composed of glandular epithelial tissue embedded in adipose tissue and supported by fibrous connective tissue. Externally, in the center of each mature female breast is the areola, distinguished as the circular pigmented skin area that surrounds the nipple. Montgomery tubercles, small sebaceous glands of the areola, lubricate the nipples.

Each breast, known as a mammary gland, is organized into approximately 15 to 20 lobes. Each lobe, in turn, is divided into lobules. The lobules contain connective tissue that houses alveoli, the secretory cells of the mammary gland. Alveoli are clustered around ductules. These ductules unite to form a single excretory lactiferous (mammary) duct in each lobe. The lactiferous ducts enlarge slightly to form sinuses or ampullae behind the nipple and underlying the areola. Each lactiferous sinus terminates in a small opening on the surface of the nipple, called the mammary papilla. The nipple is well supplied with nerve endings that are particularly sensitive to touch. Each nipple contains bundles of smooth muscle fibers that stiffen to allow for better grasp by the breastfeeding infant.[23]

Physiology of Lactation

In preparation for lactation the human mammary gland undergoes physiologic changes during pregnancy and the early postpartum. These physiologic changes are accompanied by anatomic changes in breast tissue (Figure 29–3). Prenatally, estrogen stimulates the proliferation and differentiation of the ductal system of the breast. Progesterone increases the lobes, lobules, and alveoli. By the end of pregnancy, the anterior pituitary gland secretes increasing levels of prolactin, resulting in additional proliferation of epithelial cells in the mammary glands and in the production of a new group of enzymes involved with carbohydrate metabolism. Additionally, hPL stimulates the alveolar cells to begin lactogenesis, or milk production, so that by the third trimester the breasts may secrete **colostrum,** a yellow, premilk substance. Colostrum is high in protein and contains antibodies, particularly immunoglobulins G and A (IgG and IgA). The antibody-rich colostrum may act protectively in the newborn's gastrointestinal system. Colostrum production gradually diminishes after delivery. Occasionally, for some primiparous women, colostrum production may persist for a couple of weeks.[23]

As the production of true breast milk begins, the breasts become larger, firmer, heavier, and more tender. The breast veins distend and become more prominent. By 3 to 5 days after delivery, bluish white milk is produced. In some multiparous women breast milk production begins before 3 days postpartum. The bluish white breast milk is slightly lower in protein than colostrum. At the beginning of the feeding, the milk, known as fore milk, contains less fat and flows at a faster rate than at the end of the feeding. Toward the end of the feeding the hind milk is whiter and contains more fat calories. The higher fat content at the end of the feeding is believed to satisfy the infant and signal that the feeding should come to an end.

Lactation involves the synthesis of human milk by the alveolar cells, the release of milk into the alveolar lumen, and the ejection of milk through the ductal system. The first two phenomena constitute the secretion stage of lactation; the latter phenomenon is labeled the ejection stage.

Secretion Stage. Prolactin is the hormone primarily responsible for stimulating the synthesis of milk and the release of milk into the alveolar lumen. With

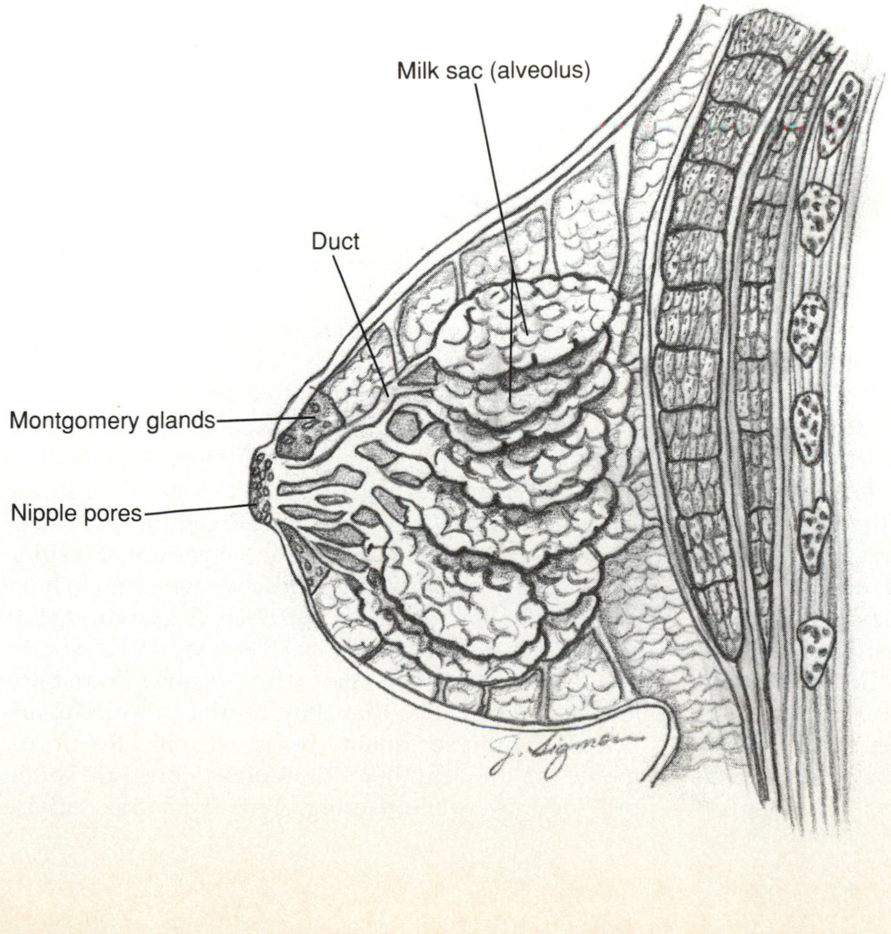

Figure 29–3. Human mammary gland during lactation.

delivery of the placenta, levels of progesterone and estrogen decrease, thus diminishing their probable inhibitory effect on prolactin production. Additionally, the hypothalmus no longer produces a prolactin-inhibitory factor after delivery. Consequently, with the removal of prolactin-inhibitory agents, the anterior pituitary gland's secretion of prolactin hormone increases soon after delivery and, within a few days, true human milk is produced.

Although prolactin is directly responsible for the secretion of human milk, other factors indirectly influence the process. Sufficient levels of growth hormone and adrenal corticosteroids are needed for the intiation of lactation. More importantly, the frequency and the length of time the infant suckles on the breasts influence the amount of milk secreted. In the first few weeks, the mother usually produces more milk than is actually required for her infant. As a result the mother's breasts are not emptied completely with each feeding. Gradually, the amount of milk produced is reduced to meet the amount demanded by the infant. In essence, the mother's supply of breast milk becomes synchronized with the infant's need and demand for milk. As the infant grows and demands more, the breasts produce more milk. Generally, the more frequent the feedings, the greater are the amounts of milk secreted. Incomplete emptying of the breasts usually results in diminished milk secretion.[24]

Prolactin acts on the alveolar cells to stimulate the synthesis of milk. Within the alveolar cells lactose, fat, casein, and some proteins are synthesized and combined with other proteins, vitamins, minerals, and water from maternal plasma to produce breast milk. The newly produced milk is then secreted into the alveolar lumen. The secreted milk remains in the alveolar lumen, awaiting ejection stimuli.

Ejection Stage. The ejection of milk through the ductal system is accomplished through a neurohormonal reflex commonly called the **"let-down reflex."** Primarily in response to the infant's sucking on the breast, the posterior pituitary gland secretes oxytocin. Under the influence of oxytocin, the myoepithelial cells surrounding the alveoli contract, propelling milk through the ductal system to the infant.

The let-down reflex may take several days to weeks to establish. Some women are not physically aware of the let-down reflex, but rather note their infant's behavior. At the beginning of the feeding, the infant in search of breast milk takes quick, short, almost frantic sucks. As the mother begins to feel a tingling sensation within her breasts, milk is propelled through the ductal system to the infant. As a result, the mother observes the infant taking longer, more relaxed sucks.

Psychologic Aspects of Lactation

Intricately woven and inseparable from the physiology of lactation is the psychology of lactation. Successful lactation is guaranteed only when both the physiologic and psychologic milieus of both the mother and infant are in synchrony. Despite the fact that almost all women are physiologically and anatomically capable of lactation, psychologic conditions may inhibit lactation.[25] Furthermore, the physiologic mechanism of lactation may stimulate sexual arousal, with psychologic implications for some women.

Psychologic Milieu. One of the most important factors contributing to the degree to which breastfeeding is successful is the mother's willingness to breastfeed. In particular, women who have a strong desire to breastfeed tend to continue to breastfeed longer than women who hold negative or ambivalent feelings toward breastfeeding. Women who have a strong desire to breastfeed frequently demonstrate more tolerance for breast discomforts, such as cracked or sore nipples or leakage of milk, and are more accepting of the need for more frequent feedings with infant growth spurts.

Not all women who have decided to breastfeed are eager to breastfeed. Many women do not feel comfortable exposing their breasts,[26] and in many cultures breastfeeding in public is not approved. Some women believe that breastfeeding interferes with their home and work routines, but decide to breastfeed out of guilt. Other women may have had a negative experience with breastfeeding in the past or simply lack the social milieu to support breastfeeding. These women often experience frustration and anxiety with breastfeeding.

Women who have negative or ambivalent feelings toward breastfeeding, as well as those who lack encouragement from significant others, tend to wean the infant from the breast whenever a problem arises, whether directly related to breastfeeding, for example, cracked nipples, or related to a variety of factors, for example, infant crying. These women tend to have more difficulty handling the normal growth spurts common in infants at 10 days, 3 weeks, and 3 months of age. Frequently, women with negative or ambivalent feelings believe that they cannot produce a sufficient quantity or quality of breast milk. Reinforcements of the mother's misconceptions are often provided by well-meaning, but erroneous, advice from significant others who are not knowledgeable about breastfeeding. As a result women may feel guilty and become anxious with feedings. If interventions are not instituted, the woman's beliefs become reality. The woman may become anxious, diminishing or even totally inhibiting the let-down reflex; the infant in turn becomes frustrated and increases the demand for milk.[24] If this cycle is not interrupted with effective interventions, the mother will eventually give up on breastfeeding (*see* Chapter 31).

Closely related to the woman's willingness to breastfeed is the timing of her decision to breastfeed. Gulick,[26] studying 88 primiparas, found that women who made the decision to breastfeed early in the pregnancy tended to be successful with breastfeeding. Conversely, women who made the decision to breastfeed late in their pregnancies were more likely to give up on breastfeeding by 1 month postpartum. Gulick's study indicates that making the decision to breastfeed early in the pregnancy may help to prepare the mother emotionally, cognitively, and physiologically for successful breastfeeding.

Psychologic Stimulation of the Let-Down Reflex. Although the primary stimulus for initiating the let-down reflex is the infant's sucking on the breast, several psychologically based stimuli can stimulate the reflex. A lactating mother will suddenly experience the let-down reflex, with leakage of breast milk, when she hears an infant cry, when she thinks about her infant, and when she anticipates a feeding. As the mother and infant become synchronized for feedings, the mother may experience a let-down at the precise moment the baby awakes for a feeding, even if she is not in the general vicinity of her infant.

Sexual Arousal and Sexual Activity. The physiologic responses of breastfeeding are closely tied to responses from sexual arousal.[27] The nipple becomes erect and lengthened during breastfeeding and sexual arousal. The release of oxytocin as the infant suckles on the breast causes the uterine muscle fibers to contract rhythmically as in sexual arousal. Many women do, in fact, become sexually aroused from breastfeeding and some may even experience an orgasm. For some women this instills feelings of guilt and may eventually lead to weaning of the infant. Nurses need to educate couples that sexual arousal is common with breastfeeding and is normal.

The physiologic similarities between breastfeeding and sexual arousal can affect sexual activity. In particular, during sexual intercourse, oxytocin is released. Accordingly, the lactating woman frequently experiences the let-down reflex with leakage of milk during intercourse. This can be disconcerting for couples who did not know this can happen.

Desire for sexual activity may be affected by lactation. Many lactating women experience a diminished sexual desire because their tactile needs are being fulfilled by holding and feeding the infant. Additionally, belief in cultural taboos that prohibit sexual intercourse for lactating mothers may decrease the couple's desire for sexual relations. Conversely, many couples experience an increased desire for sexual intercourse because of frequent nipple stimulation, as well as the belief that the chances of conception are diminished with lactation.

NUTRITIONAL REQUIREMENTS AND THE HEALING PROCESS

The postpartum woman requires adequate nutritional intake for physical and psychologic restoration after delivery. In particular, the nurse needs to ensure that the diet contains the appropriate amounts of protein and vitamin C, the two nutrients most involved in the promotion of healing. Amino acids, which are derived from proteins, are needed for restoring and maintaining tissues, enzyme formation, antibodies, hormones, and energy and controlling bodily processes.[23] Protein sources include milk, cheese, eggs, meat, grains, legumes, enriched breads, and nuts. Vitamin C is necessary to promote and maintain tissue formation and integrity and iron absorption, and acts as the cement substance in connective and vascular tissues. Sources of vitamin C include citrus fruits, berries, melons, tomatoes, chili peppers, green peppers, green leafy vegetables, broccoli, and potatoes.

Nutritional requirements for lactating women tend to be higher than those for nonlactating women. Generally, the nonlactating woman does not require vitamin or mineral supplements if dietary intake of nutrients is sufficient. Because maternal iron depletion can occur during the last two trimesters as the fetal stores of iron are increased, a woman with a pre-existing iron deficit or one who experiences a postpartum hemorrhage often requires iron supplements for at least 1 month after delivery. Women who are lactating usually continue to take prenatal vitamins to maintain good nutritional status for lactation. The reader is referred to Chapter 10 for discussion of nutritional requirements for the lactating woman.

SUMMARY

In the immediate postpartum period, the woman's body systems undergo physiologic changes. The most dramatic changes occur in the reproductive system. The uterine fundus descends 1 to 2 cm a day during the process of involution. The spongy layer of the decidua is also discarded; this discharge is referred to as lochia. Ovulation and menstruation may occur by 6 to 8 weeks postpartum in nonlactating women. Resumption of these functions takes longer in lactating women.

Other body systems that undergo major changes during the postpartum period are the cardiovascular system, respiratory system, urinary system, musculoskeletal system, integumentary system, gastrointestinal system, and endocrine system. Many women experience "postpartum blues" in the 3 to 4 days after delivery which may result from a drop in the level of hormones.

The process of lactation begins with delivery of the baby. To facilitate breastfeeding, the breasts undergo several physiologic changes involving proliferation and differentiation of the ductal system. Colostrum production, which may have begun in the third trimester, gradually decreases after delivery. Bluish white breast milk is produced within 3 to 5 days of delivery. Psychologic factors also influence lactation. The mechanism of lactation may be facilitated or hindered by psychologic conditions. Additionally, the woman may find that lactation stimulates sexual arousal or that sexual activity results in the letdown reflex and secretion of milk. Women and their partners need to be advised that this is a normal physiologic process.

Finally, nutrition plays an important role in promoting healing in the postpartum period. Women require additional nutritional intake during this period, and often also require continued iron supplementation after delivery. Women who are breastfeeding should continue to take prenatal vitamins to aid successful lactation.

REVIEW QUESTIONS

1. List the major body systems that undergo physiologic changes during the postpartum period and describe two adaptations of each system.
2. Identify hormones that are responsible for many of the physiologic changes of the postpartum period; describe how these hormones affect the emotional and physiologic status of the postpartum woman.
3. Describe two major physiologic processes of lactation.
4. Identify two psychologic factors that may affect the woman's ability to breastfeed.
5. Discuss resumption of ovulation and menstruation in lactating and nonlactating women.

REFERENCES

1. Mercer RT, Ferketich SL. Predictors of family functioning eight months following birth. *Nurs Res.* 1990;39:76–78.
2. Cunningham FG, et al. *Williams Obstetrics.* 18th ed. Norwalk, Conn: Appleton & Lange; 1989.
3. Jacobson H. A standard for assessing lochia volume. *Am J Matern Child Nurs.* 1985;10:174–175.
4. Perez A. Natural family planning: postpartum period. *Int J of Fertility.* 1981;26:219.
5. Lethbridge DJ. The use of breastfeeding as a contraceptive. *J Obstet Gynecol Neonat Nurs.* 1989;18:31–37.
6. McNeilly AS, et al. Release of oxytocin and prolactin in response to sucking. *Br Med Journal.* 1983:286;257.
7. Perez A, et al. First ovulation after childbirth: the effect of breast-feeding. *Am J Obstet Gynecol.* 1972;114:1041–1047.
8. McKenzie CA, et al. Comprehensive care during the postpartum period. *Nurs Clin North Am.* 1982;17:23–48.
9. Taylor DJ, Lind T. Puerperal haematological indices. *J Obstet Gynecol.* 1981;88:601–606.
10. Pritchard J. Blood volume changes during pregnancy and delivery. *Anesthesiology.* 1965;26:393–399.
11. Robson SC, et al. Haemodynamic changes during the puerperium. *Br Med Journal.* 1987:294;1065.
12. Danforth DN, Scott JR, eds. *Obstetrics and Gynecology.* 5th ed. Philadelphia: Lippincott; 1986.
13. Mannucci P, et al. Protein C antigen during pregnancy, delivery and puerperium. *Thromb Haemostas.* 1984;52:217.
14. Romem Y, Artal R. C-reactive protein in pregnancy and the postpartum period. *Am J Obstet Gynecol.* 1985;151:380–383.
15. Kerr-Wilson RJH, et al. Effect of labor on the postpartum bladder. *Obstet Gynecol.* 1984:64–115.
16. Henderson J. Effects of a prenatal teaching program on postpartum regeneration of the pubococcygeal muscle. *J Obstet Gynecol Neonat Nurs.* 1983;12:403–408.
17. Tulman L, et al. Changes in functional status after childbirth. *Nurs Res.* 1990;39:70–75.
18. Yuen BH. Prolactin in human milk: the influence of nursing and the duration of postpartum lactation. *Am J Obstet Gynecol.* 158;583.
19. Davies R, Cobin R. Thyroid disease in pregnancy and the postpartum period. *M Sinai J Med.* 1985;52:59–77.
20. Greene GW, et al. Postpartum weight change: how much of the weight gained during pregnancy will be lost after delivery? *Obstet Gynecol.* 1988:71:701.
21. Olsen LC, Mundt MH. Postpartum weight loss in a nurse-

midwifery practice. *J Nurse-Midwifery.* 1986;31:177–188.
22. Fawcett J, et al. Spouses body image changes during and after pregnancy: a replication and extension. *Nurs Res.* 1986;35:220–223.
23. Worthington-Roberts B, et al. *Nutrition in Pregnancy and Lactation.* St. Louis: Times Mirror Mosby; 1989.
24. Kearney MH, et al. Breastfeeding problems in the first week postpartum. *Nurs Res.* 1990;39:90–94.
25. Hill PD, Humenick SS. Insufficient milk supply. *Image.* 1989; 21:145–148.
26. Gulick E. Informational correlates of successful breastfeeding. *Am J Matern Child Nurs.* 1982;7:370–375.
27. Riordan J, Rapp E. Pleasure and purpose: the sensuousness of breastfeeding. *J Obstet Gynecol Neonat Nurs.* 1980;9: 109–112.

Psychologic and Sociocultural Dimensions During the Postpartum Period

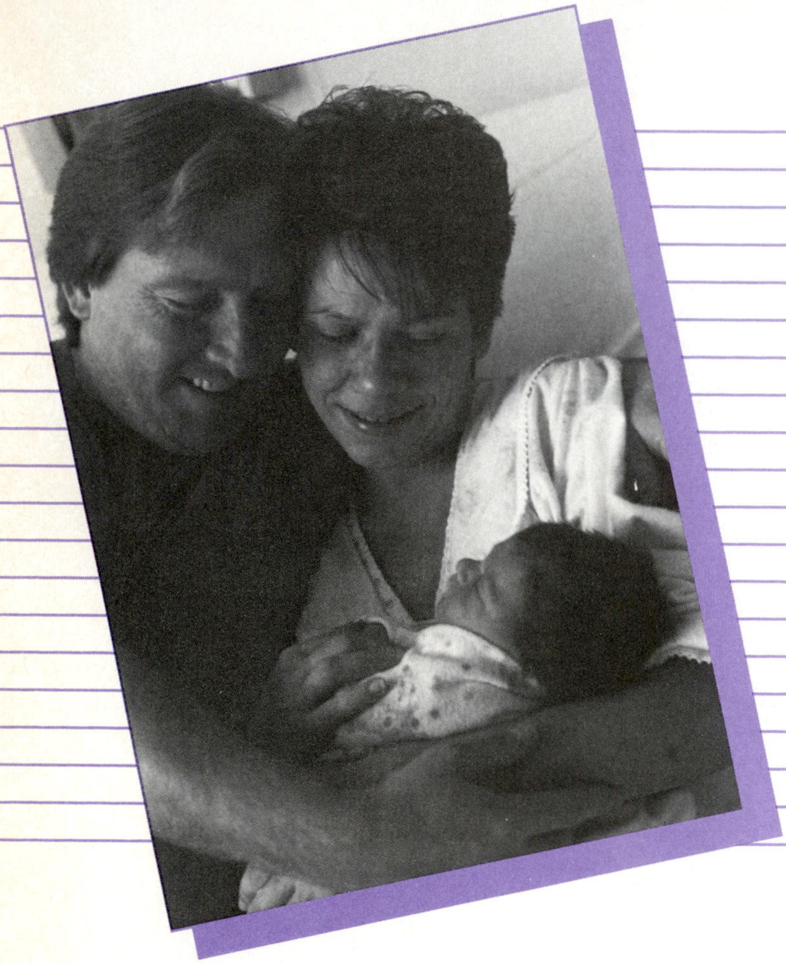

chapter 30

Key Terms

achievement phase
disruption phase
engrossment
maternal-infant dyad
physical recovery phase
reorganization phase
transitory depression

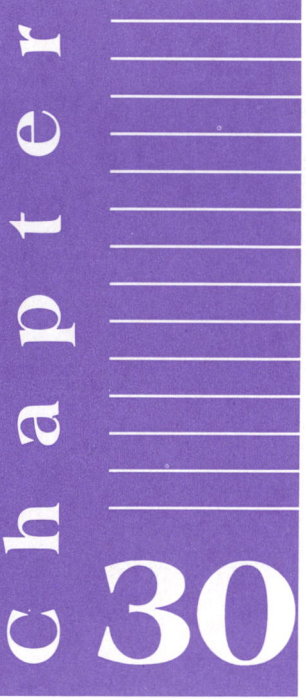

The postpartum period is not only the culmination of pregnancy, labor, and birth, it is also the beginning of the childrearing phase of the family life cycle. Structural and functional changes in the family system initiate patterns for healthy or altered family functioning in the future, including parent-child interactions.[1] Thus, nursing interventions at this time are crucial. Ensuring that the family and developing child establish a positive, health-promoting mode of interaction from the start is an important nursing goal and may well influence the future lives of parents and children.

Pregnancy and birth (adding a new member to the family system) produce great changes in the family system as discussed in Chapter 3. These events may be highly stressful to the family and its members. For example, Holmes and Rahe[2] rate pregnancy as the 12th most stressful life event for an adult, and gaining a new family member as the 14th. Such high-ranking stressful life events are believed to predispose individuals to stress-related problems including illness.

Children, too, experience stress when a new brother or sister is born. One modification of Holmes and Rahe's Social Readjustment Rating Scale ranks birth of a brother or sister as the 10th most stressful life event for a preschooler and the 17th most stressful event for a school-aged child.[3] Birth of a sibling thus may be seen as potentially contributing to the development of stress-related conditions in children.

Despite stresses, the postpartum is a time of family health and well-being. Nursing care is directed toward providing anticipatory guidance and support as the newborn is integrated into the family.

PARENTING AND THE FAMILY SYSTEM

Parents' expectations of what it will be like to have children, along with their perceptions of themselves as parents, have much to do with successful parenting. Several common expectations of parents have been described[4]:

1. Children may be seen as an extension of the valued aspects of parents. Parents may, however, be disappointed if their children do not fulfill their expectations.
2. Children may be seen as a "second chance." Parents may hope that their children will "make up"

for perceived deficiencies in themselves by achieving parental goals. They may thus pressure their children to achieve these goals without accepting the children for who they are.

3. Family life with children may be seen as always loving and peaceful. If problems develop, reason and love may be expected to solve all problems. Thus, if turmoil persists, something or someone "has gone wrong."

Nursing research has also demonstrated that several other factors affect success in parenting. These researchers suggest ways in which nurses and other health professionals may help parents refine their roles as parents to achieve greater parenting skill. Among the areas investigated are perceptions about the birth experience,[5,6] prenatal expectations about the infant,[6,7] postnatal expectations of the infant,[9–11] parents' perceptions of their parenting skills,[11] and the nature of parental concerns and their resolution.[13–15]

Parenting is a highly complex interaction. Despite continuing research by nursing and other disciplines in the area of parenting, it is likely that much will remain unknown. There can be no "how-to-do-it" recipe book for raising children; too many factors are involved, many far beyond the parents' or nurses' control.[4] Just as parents cannot control their children's lives, nurses cannot control what happens to the family; however, in collaborating with the family, nurses can foster postive parenting experiences.

Tasks and Transitions in Parenting

The transition to being parents is often a difficult period for the couple.[7] They may experience difficulty in adequately communicating their needs to one another.[16] The birth of an infant to first-time parents has also been demonstrated to result in (1) decreased expressions of affection between parents, (2) a major change in interdependency patterns between the partners, and (3) a great change in sexual interest in the postpartum period in women married less than 5 years.[17] Many of these changes experienced during the transition to parenthood can have a negative impact on the couple.

Several reasons have been suggested for the difficult nature of this transition[18, 19]:

- During this early period, an infant is completely dependent on parents for survival; thus, his or her need for them is absolute. This need can be overwhelming for new parents.
- There is still a certain amount of cultural pressure to assume the parenting role. Many couples become parents as a result of such pressure from family, friends, and societal expectations.
- A couple's assumption of the parental role may not be voluntary. Despite current contraceptive technology, many pregnancies are still unplanned and may result from unplanned sexual encounters. Abortion, although legal, is still an unacceptable and controversial alternative for many.
- Except in rare cases, parenthood is irrevocable and permanent. Parents cannot simply terminate the relationship with a child, especially a minor, in a manner similar to terminating a marriage.
- Despite current trends in education to "prepare" individuals for parenthood, there is as yet no standard method, during schooling or pregnancy, by which couples are prepared for the role of parent.

In addition, the change from a stable dyadic (two-person) relationship to a triangle (three-person) relationship or to a series of shifting triangles places great stress on family structure and function. In triangular relationships, someone is always, at least temporarily, the "isolate." Family members, especially the new father or an older sibling, may find themselves left out of the symbiotic mother-neonate dyad in the early postpartum.

Tasks of New Parents

In addition to the difficulties inherent in the transition to the parent role, new mothers and fathers face a variety of psychosocial tasks that go along with role assumption. A summary of these tasks for new parents is presented in Table 30–1. The resolution of these tasks is an added challenge for the family system that may already have its coping abilities stretched to the limit.[20]

Social Networks and the Transition to Parenthood

Studies of social network ties and support systems by many nurse researchers and behavioral scientists have identified the importance of these systems to the couples' transition to parenthood. Support from the parents' social network (ie, friends, relatives, coworkers, and so on) promotes the couple's physical and psychologic adaptation to pregnancy and the postpartum period.[21–23]

The birth of children also alters the parents' social network. For example, grandparents often increase contact with new parents after birth of the first baby.[24, 25] New fathers and mothers also have more contact with other parents of young children.[26] Especially for mothers, the old social networks of coworkers and friends who are not parents tend to wane

TABLE 30–1. TASKS FOR NEW PARENTS

- Attach to infant
- Plan activities to optimize the mother's physiologic restorative processes and lactation
- Reconstruct and review the birth experience
- Work through any losses associated with the childbirth experience or new parenthood (eg, pregnant body, ideal or perfect child, ideal birth experience, freedom, any role given up or changed, some of partner's attention)
- Develop infant caretaking skills
- Stimulate infant's growth and development
- Accept infant as a unique individual and encourage that individuality
- Develop a satisfactory relationship with partner that includes parenting
  - Maintain or improve the couple relationship (ie, emotional and sexual intimacy, intellectual exchange, recreational activities)
- Facilitate the partner's development as a parent
  - Wife—promote the father-child relationship from the beginning (bonding, caretaking, enjoying infant's growth and development): recognize and reinforce husband's growth as a father
- Husband—share parenting responsibilities; recognize and reinforce wife's growth as a mother: attempt to decrease stressors impinging on wife[a]
  - Develop view of infant as "ours"
- Develop mutual conceptions of major roles
- Allocate time and energy to all roles (wife, mother, worker, or professional; husband, father, worker, or professional)
- Maintain his or her own identity as an individual
- Develop a sense of being a family
  - Learn about new things to do and places to go as a family with an infant
- Adapt some of previous couple activities so that they can be done as a family with an infant (eg, biking, boating, camping)
  - Alter environment to meet needs of infant
  - Obtain supplies and needed equipment
- Provide for safety of infant
- Allow for infant's exploration as his or her locomotion begins
  - Plan for adequate income and housing to meet the needs of the expanded family
- Work out relationships with relatives
- Maintain relationships with friends
- Make decisions regarding having or not having another child; implement family planning method as indicated
- Improve strategies for dealing with conflict
  - Accept conflict as a part of life that is neither good nor bad, but neutral
- Learn more effective conflict resolution skills

[a] The terms *husband* and *wife* are used to simply and clearly distinguish between the roles of partner-mate and parent. The tasks are also applicable to unmarried couple living together as a family and, to some extent, to the single-mother family in which the boyfriend is somewhat involved.
Reproduced, with permission, from Newton LD. Fourth trimester. In: Sonstegard L, et al, eds. Women's Health: Childbearing. *New York: Grune & Stratton; 1983.*

after childbirth. Loss of this network is often painful for new mothers.[27]

Social networks are an important area for nursing assessment throughout the childrearing cycle, but especially during the postpartum period. Anticipatory guidance about some of the changes that parents may expect in their social contacts after birth may help both partners make the transition with less stress.

PSYCHOSOCIAL ADAPTATION OF THE MOTHER

Maternal Role Attainment

Previous chapters in this text have shown that the process of maternal role attainment begins long before the actual birth of the infant. Birth, however, ushers in a new phase in the development of the mother-infant relationship.

Several researchers have studied attainment of the maternal role after the birth of the infant. Maternal role attainment has been described as a process that continues over a 3- to 10-month period after the birth of the infant.[28, 29] Maternal tasks during this period include attaching to the infant by identifying, claiming, and interacting with the infant[30–32]; becoming competent in performing mothering behaviors[33]; and feeling gratification in the mother-infant interactions.[28]

Mercer identifies several variables in both the mother and the infant that affect attainment of the maternal role for a first-time mother.[28] These maternal factors and infant variables are discussed next. Other variables that indirectly influence attainment of maternal role include culture, socioeconomic status—especially educational level (*see* discussion later in this chapter), and marital status.[28]

Maternal Factors

Maternal Age at First Birth. Contrary to the generally held view, some teenage mothers and their children may not be at great risk for physical or psychologic problems. The more mature gravida and her child are often at greater physical risk. Additionally, although the older gravida often has more assets, a higher level of education, and more commitment to the mothering role, she may also experience more career-mother role conflicts.

RESEARCH ABSTRACT

Walker LO, Crain H, Thompson E. Maternal role attainment and identity in the postpartum period: stability and change. Nurs Res. *1986;35:68–71.*

This study examined stability and change in maternal identity and maternal role attainment among postpartum mothers. There were three study questions: (1) What changes occur in the level of maternal identity and maternal role attainment for primiparous and multiparous women during the postpartum period? (2) How stable are the phenomena? (3) What relationship do infant sex, maternal age, maternal education, and socioeconomic status have to maternal identity and maternal role attainment?

The sample consisted of 64 primiparous and 58 multiparous women (aged 17 to 41 years) who were predominantly white, married and had healthy pregnancies with no significant labor, delivery, or postpartum complications. Their infants were full-term singletons who were free of major congenital abnormalities or perinatal illnesses and who were largely breastfed.

The instruments used in the study included the Pharis Self-Confidence Scale to measure a parent's self-confidence in carrying out baby care; the Semantic Differential Scale SD-Self to evaluate the concept "myself as mother"; and the Semantic Differential Scale SD-Baby to evaluate the concept "my baby." Mothers were given the scales to complete 1 to 3 days postdelivery and 4 to 6 weeks later. Analysis of variance and product-moment correlations were used to analyze the data.

The results demonstrated that multiparas showed more positive attitudes toward themselves as mothers than primiparas, with attitudes toward themselves of both groups becoming more positive from the first to the second testing. It was also found that both groups' attitudes toward their infants became less positive at the time of the second testing. Sociodemographic variables had little to do with these results.

The investigators concluded that maternal role attainment may be of greater significance in the formation of a maternal identity among primiparas than multiparas. Maternal attitudes during the postpartum period demonstrated both change and stability. The mothers in the study became more self-confident and positive about themselves from birth to 4 to 6 weeks later. They also viewed their babies less positively at the end of the postpartum period than in the beginning.

Comment:
This study attempted to test the relationship of maternal role attainment to maternal identity. There appear to be differences between multiparas and primiparas in indicators of maternal role attainment and maternal identity. Additional research is needed to test the relationship of these concepts to actual parenting behaviors.

Maternal Perception of Birth Experience. Birth may be viewed as the first act of "motherhood" and is often seen by the woman as an indication of her possible capabilities as a mother. A woman's view of the birth process is related to her knowledge about childbirth; her expectations of what birth should be like; the presence or absence of her partner or other support persons; the type of birth experience (eg, vaginal or cesarean delivery); and the amount of control she maintains throughout labor and birth. Differences between a woman's expected and actual performance in labor may affect her self-esteem in the postpartum period.[34, 35]

Early Mother-Infant Separation. Although researchers[30] have associated early mother-infant contact with greater attachment behaviors, there are too many complicating variables (such as the type of delivery experienced and the condition of the infant) to be able to draw clear conclusions about effects of early contact and effects of separation.[28] (*See* Chapter 4 and later discussion in this chapter.)

Social Support. As discussed earlier, social networks are one source from which new parents receive support (Figure 30–1). For the new mother, in particular, the impact of postpartum stress can be reduced by her social support system. Several types of support may help the new mother[33]:

1. *Emotional support.* Feeling loved, cared for and understood.
2. *Informational support.* Receiving information useful in the problem/situation.
3. *Physical support.* Direct concrete (physical) help (eg, assistance with childcare).
4. *Approval support.* Information that will help the mother evaluate her performance.

Personality Traits. Innate personality traits (such as temperament) or socially acquired traits (such as empathy) may influence maternal role attainment. Sometimes a mother and her infant simply have incompatible personalities. For example, the mother and infant may have completely different sleep-wake

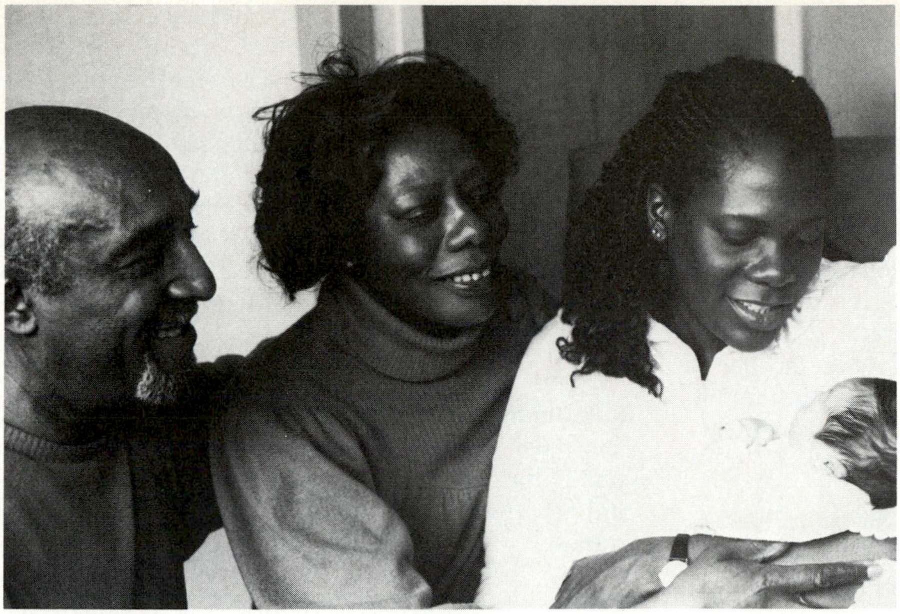

Figure 30–1. Social support promotes maternal role attainment.

patterns. When the mother is normally asleep, her infant may be awake and demand attention. In another example, the mother may be a quiet, placid individual and her baby may be highly active and irritable. A clue that the mother's personality traits are affecting role attainment can be obtained in such statements as "I always was a calm person, I can't understand how I got an irritable demanding baby!"

Self-Concept. Self-concept is defined as perception of self that includes self-satisfaction, self-acceptance, self-esteem, and congruence between the "real" and "ideal" self.[36] A positive maternal self-concept may help the woman relate positively to her infant. In turn, attainment of a positive (or negative) maternal role may increase (or decrease) the woman's self-concept.

Childrearing Attitudes. A woman's attitudes and beliefs about childrearing may affect both her child's socialization and how she fulfills the maternal role.

Health Status. Illness during pregnancy and the postpartum period may affect maternal attitudes about pregnancy and childbirth, and hence mothering behaviors. These behaviors affect the woman's attainment and performance of the maternal role. For example, a breastfeeding mother who develops mastitis may have symptoms of pain and fever that immobilize her. This may interfere with mother-infant interactions.

Infant Variables

Infant Temperament. An infant who is easy to care for and who demonstrates predictable behaviors increases parents' feelings of competence in their ability to deliver care. Parents may, however, perceive infant behavior differently based on previous experience caring for other infants.

Infant Health Status. A sick infant may affect the maternal attachment process and role attainment in several ways. After delivery, a sick infant is often separated from the mother, which may affect attachment. The mother may subsequently delay attaching to the infant because of her fears that the infant may die. Finally, because these infants require more complex care, mothers may not feel competent to deliver care to sick infants.

Phases of Maternal Role Attainment. The process of attaining the maternal role extends over the first year of the infant's life, at least for the first-time mother. This process is not an inevitable, step-by-step progression. Instead, there are peaks and valleys in behaviors that indicate maternal role attainment over the course of the year. The challenges of the infant's continuous and changing developmental behaviors almost invariably lead to the mother's feelings of role incompetency at different points in time (especially at the 8- and 12-month stages).[37]

Mercer describes four phases in the process of adaptation to the maternal role during the first year,[28] which she calls (1) the physical recovery phase (birth to 1 month), (2) the achievement phase (2 months to 4 or 5 months), (3) the disruption phase (6 months to 8 months), and (4) the reorganization phase (beginning after the eighth month and continuing after 12 months). This adaptation occurs at three interacting, interdependent levels: the biologic level, having to do with the mother's recovery from pregnancy and birth, and infant adaptation; the psychological level, having to do with the mother's emotional reactions to motherhood; and the social level, having to do with the mother's social context and lifestyle changes.[28,37]

Physical Recovery Phase (Birth to 1 Month). During the **physical recovery phase,** biologic adaptation dominates as the mother recovers from birthing and her infant makes the transition to the external world. Among various cultures this difficult biologic transition is readily acknowledged by the woman's social network, which offers much help.

Achievement Phase (2 Months to 4 or 5 Months). The **achievement phase** begins after the mother's physical recovery, at about the second month. As the mother now feels better, the psychologic and social levels of adaptation to the role, rather than the biologic level, dominate. The infant has now settled into a predictable routine, the mother generally feels competent in care of the young infant, and the infant's socialization skills (such as the spontaneous smile) make him or her a pleasure to care for at this point. Many mothers choose to return to work during this phase, increasing the complexity of the mothering role. This phase continues until about the fourth or fifth month, when the infant begins to be much more active.

Disruption Phase (6 Months to 8 Months). The **disruption phase,** which begins at about the fifth month, seems to peak at the eighth month after birth. The mother begins to feel stress at the social level of adaptation, as she tries to balance conflicting roles of work, mother, and wife. The infant's developmental changes and new-found mobility challenge the mother's skills and competence in mothering behaviors, making her question herself again. A clash may develop between the infant's evolving self and the mother's need to regain a sense of herself similar to her prepregnant state.

Reorganization Phase (Beginning After the Eighth Month and Continuing After 12 Months). During the **reorganization phase,** all levels of adaptation—biologic, psychologic, and social—are evident. Biologic changes occur as the infant continues to grow, develop, and master the environment, and as the mother begins to wean the infant. Psychologically, the mother becomes restless with the all-consuming nature of motherhood and the burden of responsibility for her infant. Socially, she wishes to be recognized in roles other than that of mother. She individuates herself more and more from her infant as she attempts to regain some of her prepregnancy activities.

Role Conflict and Transition to the Maternal Role. The transition to the maternal role can result in role conflict for contemporary women. Several factors including previous roles and relationships may affect a woman's sense of conflict in transition to the maternal role.[38,39] It is not at all clear whether having a career, in and of itself, produces role conflict. One researcher found that career women, perhaps experiencing greater self-fulfillment, actually experienced less role conflict than did noncareer women.[39]

The level of marital satisfaction may also contribute to a woman's transition to the maternal role.[40,41] One study found that marital satisfaction was positively related to ease of transition to the maternal role.[42] Conversely, marital discord after birth of an infant may produce additional conflicts for the mother as she attempts to adapt to the maternal role.

Attainment of the maternal role is a complex and long-lasting process. Nursing interventions such as discharge planning and telephone follow-up during the immediate postpartum period may help set the stage for a positive outcome to the woman's role attainment activities.

The Maternal-Infant Dyad

Immediately after birth, and for some time thereafter, the mother and newborn form what is called the **maternal-infant** (or child) **dyad.** The formation of the mother-infant dyad seems to be an important factor in the continued process of parent-child attachment. Indeed the formation of the new family is believed to depend, to a large extent, on the integrity of this dyad.[43] Maternal-infant "bonding," which has been described by Klaus and Kennel,[30] is a vital component of the attachment process that occurs in the immediate postpartum.

Bonding is only one necessary component of the parent-child attachment process. Although such intriguing empiric evidence seems to document negative effects of early maternal-infant separation,[30] bonding, as an isolated event, will neither doom nor ensure parent-child attachment and a healthy parent-child relationship. The attachment process is lengthy and complex, and requires positive outcomes at many phases.[31,32]

The process of attachment begins when the embryo/fetus is in utero. The mother and fetus share a special, intense type of closeness and communication. After birth, the closeness between mother and newborn is akin to the relationship that exists between the mother and fetus during pregnancy. Some researchers speak of the maternal-infant "common membrane,"[44] and others call this intense closeness "emotional symbiosis."[45]

Within the maternal-infant dyad, the behaviors of bonding occur, and the process of attachment continues to evolve during the postpartum period. At about 4 to 5 months, attachment behaviors between mother and infant are joined to beginning separation-individuation behaviors (*see* Chapter 4). These attachment and separation-individuation behaviors continue as parallel processes throughout the first 2 years of the mother-child relationship. Ideally, the outcome of these processes will be the individuation of the child and mother into two independent, autonomous individuals—a parent and child who have a healthy, loving relationship.[46]

Attachment (Bonding) Behaviors. Various behaviors assist the bonding between a mother and her newborn in the immediate postpartum period. These behaviors are reciprocal; that is, the mother's behaviors evoke certain responses from her newborn and the newborn's behaviors elicit responses from the mother. Several maternal and infant behaviors are recognized.[30] These are summarized in Table 30–2.

Identification of the Infant. Much of the early thought on the manner in which the new mother learns to identify her infant after birth came from observations made by Rubin.[43] Although more recent research has disproven some of this early theory, much of it has yet to be tested, and Rubin's ideas provide a good starting point for looking at this process.

Identification does not occur after a single contact with the infant, but with repeated contact, made most often during and after feeding.[43] Repeated exposures are necessary for the mother to observe characteristics of *her* infant. Rubin describes two forms of observations: tactile and visual identification.

Tactile Identification. New mothers have been observed to follow a sequence of tactile (using touch) identification of their infants. Early studies found that mothers progressively moved from touching the infants' periphery (ie, hands, feet) with the fingertips to touching the torso with the full palm[48] (newer

TABLE 30–2. MATERNAL-INFANT BONDING BEHAVIORS

Interactions Originating in the Mother That Affect the Infant	
Touch	Serves to bind mother and infant together in the early part of their relationship
Eye-to-Eye contact	Well-known and frequently observed "en face position;" mutual gazing (especially at about 9 to 10 in., the distance at which the neonate can best focus on objects) is a very powerful behavior for assisting maternal-infant attachment
Mother's voice	Mother's high-pitched voice tones fit the infant's auditory perception range
Entrainment	Rhythmic pattern of movements by which the infant responds to the mother's voice
Re-establishment of biorythmic cycles	Infant's intrauterine cycles (such as sleep-wake and rapid eye movement cycles) are disrupted at birth; mother's cycles and routines help the newborn to re-establish his or her daily cycles
Breast milk and bacterial nasal flora	Both are contributed by the mother and help to protect the newborn from the new extrauterine environment
Odor	By the fifth day, a breastfeeding newborn can distinguish his or her mother[30]
Heat	Mother provides reliable source of heat for her newborn[47]
Interactions Originating in the Newborn That Affect the Mother	
Eye-to-eye contact	The "other half" of maternal gazing (*see* above, for a description of the process)
Cry	Infant's voice also affects the mother; eg, breastfeeding mothers sometimes experience the let-down reflex when they hear their infants cry
Release of oxytocin and prolactin	Infant stimulates hormonal changes in the mother through suckling or other contact with the breast
Odor	By third or fourth day, mothers have been found to recognize the odor of their own infants
Entrainment	Infant responds to mother's voice with a "dance" or rhythmic movements

research, however, has called this sequence into question[49, 50]).

Although many questions remain about the process of tactile identification, the ability of a new mother to provide for both the physiologic and contact needs of her infant is important in providing an infant with tenderness[50] and in aiding the maternal-infant attachment process.

Visual Identification. Visual identification is part of the larger process called "claiming"[48] (Figure 30–2). In this process, the mother identifies features and characteristics of the neonate that are "like" those of other family members or like her own. Each aspect of the infant's appearance and behavior is linked in this way to the mother or members of the larger family system. Naming the child is an important part of the claiming process. By conferring a name, the mother and family affirm the infant's existence and belonging.

Finally, the way in which the mother and her infant interact affect the mother's identification of her newborn. The feeding relationship is especially important in establishing a harmonious maternal-infant interaction. These early feeding situations are often stressful for the mother as she attempts to prove herself a "good" mother as measured by the infant's response to feeding. A successful feeding relationship will not only help in a positive identification of the neonate, it will also increase the mother's self-esteem.

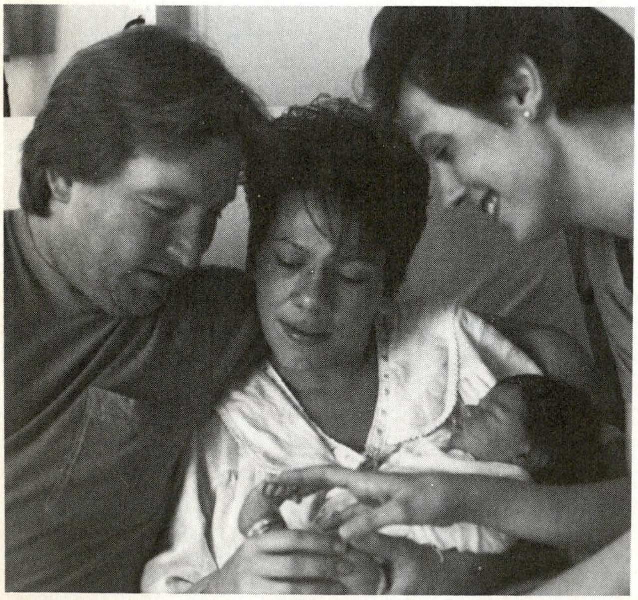

Figure 30–2. Tactile and visual identification of the newborn.

Maternal Body Image

The postpartum woman often expects her body to return to normal and to look like her prepregnant self. This is rarely the case.

Fawcett, who looked at changes in perceived body space for spouses during the eighth and ninth months of pregnancy and during the first and second postpartum months, found that women's perceived body space increased during pregnancy, decreased markedly during the first postpartum month, then increased during the second postpartum month.[51] By the second month, women realized that they were not as small as they would like to be.

Although the postpartum woman may feel somewhat better about her postpartum body image than about her pregnant body image, she feels more positive about her prepregnant body image than about her postpartum body image.[52] Achieving a return to the prepregnant figure is cited by most women as their primary postpartum concern.

Along with dissatisfaction about their postpartum body image, women also must adjust to a physical separation from the fetus/infant. Some women feel a sense of nostalgia for the intimate experiences of the fetus in utero and a sense of emptiness in the perceived body.

Maternal Concerns

Maternal concerns in the postpartum period were reported in one study to involve two main areas—the tasks of physical restoration and the tasks of adding a new family member.[53] As mentioned, the most frequently expressed concern of new mothers was a return to their prepregnant body proportions. Closely related to this were concerns about exercise and diet. Other concerns involved regulating the demands of housework, infant, and family; changes in relationship with the spouse; and worry about sexual relationships. Few concerns related directly to infant care were reported as primary preoccupations for the majority of mothers in this study.

In other studies, mothers indicated concerns about infant care by asking questions over the telephone. Questions about infant feeding—especially breastfeeding—were asked most frequently. Mothers also expressed concern about infant gastrointestinal problems (colic), infant skin problems, and infant sleeping and crying patterns.[54, 55]

Primiparous and multiparous women share many of the same concerns in the postpartum period; however, multiparas voice additional concerns about the strain that a new child places on the rest of the family[22] and about the new more complex structure of the family system. Multiparas cite meeting the needs of everyone at home as their most frequent area of concern.[56–58] Another primary concern of multiparas is allocation of insufficient time to meet the needs of the new infant and of other family members and manage a household.[58, 59]

New mothers often experience some degree of depression after delivery. This postpartum depression may be characterized as either **transitory depression** (also called "postpartum blues") or puerperal depression.[60] (*See* Chapter 41 for a detailed discussion of this condition.)

PSYCHOSOCIAL ADAPTATION OF THE FATHER

An important "discovery" of researchers and clinicians in recent years is that the neonate's experience extends beyond his or her relationship with the mother. Fathers (as well as siblings, substitute caretakers, grandparents, and others) are now acknowledged to be an integral part of the neonate's life.

Paternal Role Adaptation

Three areas appear to influence how the father will fulfill his new role and his behaviors in that role[61]: (1) the father's participation in childbirth, (2) the family role organization, and (3) the father's sex role identification.

Participation in Childbirth. Changes in childbirth practices now promote greater supportive involvement by the father during labor and delivery, and have increased the opportunity for direct paternal experience with the neonate. Some research suggests that participation in childbirth enhances subsequent father-infant interaction.[62, 63] Additionally, fathers who have immediate and extended contact with newborns after the birth demonstrate more en face behavior and talk to the neonate more during feedings.[64] For some men, participation in childbirth may affect their self-confidence and relationship with their spouse more than their early interactions with the infant.[65, 66] The father's participation in childbirth, through preparation and involvement in either vaginal or cesarean delivery, seems to foster more positive feelings about birth, and increases the opportunity for early contact and frequent interaction with the infant.[67–71]

Family Structure and Sex Role Identification. Two other aspects of modern life affect the nature of the role the father will play with his newborn. One is the organization of the family; the other is sex role identification.

Several studies indicate that in families in which both the mother and father are employed, fathers are more involved with childcare.[72, 73] Results, however, are not always consistent.[74] The level of father interaction with the baby in dual-earner families may be the result of the employed mother's need to have contact with the infant, the father's need for contact, and the mother's support of the father's interaction with the infant.

Psychologic androgyny is an emerging pattern in both male and female sex role identification. Men who have an androgynous identification (ie, a personality that combines both traditional masculine and feminine personality traits) behave in a more nurturant manner to their offspring.[75–78]

Father-Infant Relationship

Studies have documented the powerful impact on the father of seeing and holding his newborn immediately after birth.[79, 80] Fathers react to their infants with elation, relief that the infant is healthy, pride and increased self-esteem, and feelings of closeness when the infant opens his or her eyes.[80]

As with mothers, early contact between fathers and infants increases in face holding and play in the early weeks of the infant's life.[81] Fathers also display a progressive touch sequence with their infant over the first few days,[82] and both fathers and mothers appear equally sensitive to the newborn's behavioral cues in the early postpartum.[83]

Greenberg and Morris' classic study[84] describes the father's reaction or bond to the newborn as **"engrossment"** (Figure 30–3). Engrossment comprises seven aspects:

1. *Visual awareness of the newborn.* The father perceives the infant as attractive, pretty, or beautiful.
2. *Tactile awareness of the newborn.* The father has a desire to touch and hold the infant. This holding and touching are further perceived as very pleasurable.
3. *Awareness of distinct features of the newborn.* The father feels that he can distinguish his own infant from other infants.
4. *Perception of the newborn as perfect.* In spite of some unsightly aspects and awkwardness of the infant, the father sees the infant as the epitome of perfection.
5. *Strong attraction to the newborn.* The father focuses his attention on the infant.

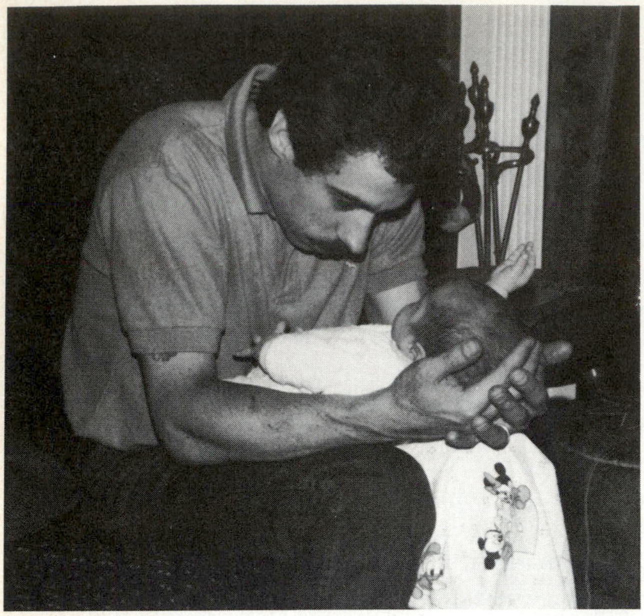

Figure 30–3. Engrossment behavior of a new father with his infant.

6. *Extreme elation.* The father describes a "high" after birth of his child.
7. *Increased sense of self-esteem.* The father describes himself as feeling proud, bigger, more mature, or older after seeing his infant for the first time.

The father's engrossment responses were further enhanced by behaviors of the newborn.[84] Greenberg and Morris believe that engrossment is a potential response for all fathers, and can be developed.

Infant's Attachment to the Father During the Early Months of Life

Health professionals have long felt that the mother is the most important figure in the child's life and that the child becomes attached to her first. This belief has not been supported by research.[85, 86] Instead, most infants seem to form attachments to both their parents at about the same time.[87, 88] In fact, by the second year of life, boys begin to show a preference for their fathers. Girls, however, show no consistent preference for either parent.[89] Under stress conditions, infants seem to prefer their mothers; a possible explanation for this preference is that in most families the mother is still the primary caretaker.[86]

There is no reason, either the father's ability to attach to and care for his infant or the infant's ability to attach to his or her father, for the father not to share equally in caretaking activities. Parental roles are most likely the result of culture and social conventions. New parents should therefore decide for themselves what is the most comfortable mode of interacting with their infants.

ADJUSTMENT OF SIBLINGS

Many places where birth occurs—be it at home, birthing center, or hospital—encourage sibling visitation and bonding with the newborn during the early postpartum (Figure 30–4). Indeed, some children are present at the birth and in the immediate postpartum period. Proponents of sibling visitation programs believe that lessening the separation of the older child from his or her mother and encouraging early sibling acquaintance and bonding will promote positive future interaction patterns between siblings and between each sibling and the parents.

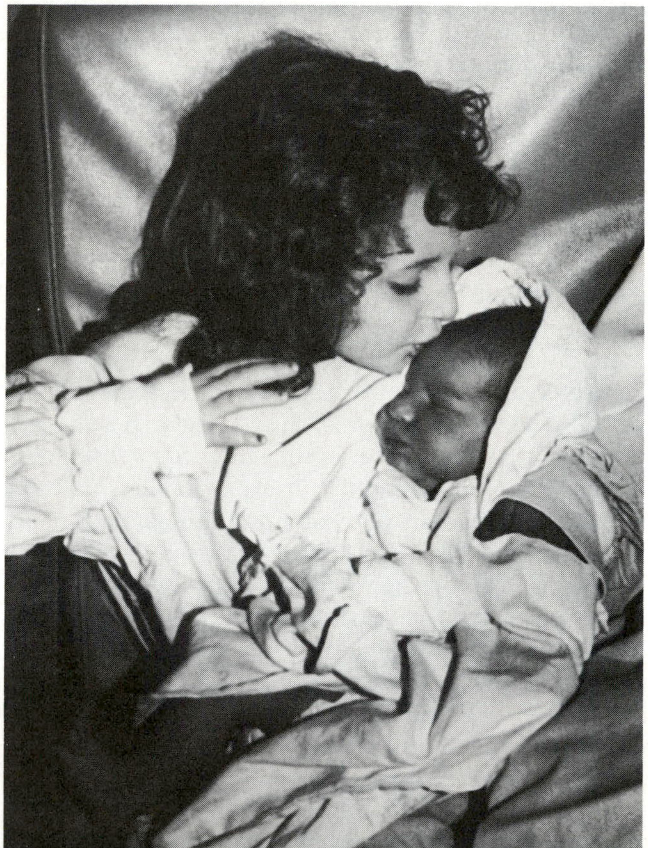

Figure 30–4. Early sibling acquaintance fosters sibling relationships.

Two factors seem to support the importance of fostering a good relationship between the newborn and older children.[90] First, siblings create environments for each other that seem to affect the future development of each child. Second, the view of the mother-infant dyad is really an oversimplification when considering the family system. Rather than a dyad, there are multiple shifting, interacting triangles. Thus, roles of parents evolve, in part, from complex interaction patterns with the older child(ren) and the newborn.

Sibling Reactions to the Newborn

Several factors tend to influence the older child-newborn interactions: the birth or ordinal position of each child, the age spacing between children, the sex of each child[90], the age of the older child at the birth of the newborn[91] (children under age 5 tend to become more upset than older children).

Although interaction patterns of siblings seem to be established during the infancy of the later-born child,[92] few studies actually document these older child-newborn interactions or the process of establishing a relationship. Observations of older siblings show that they tend to react to the newborn by demonstrating regressive behaviors, frequent crying, sleep disturbance, demanding behaviors, and other negative behaviors. While few observations to date show positive responses by older children to the newborn, older children are usually very interested in the new baby[92] (Figure 30–5).

Maternal Relationship to Older Children

Changes in the relationship between an older child and his or her mother would seem unavoidable after the birth of a new infant. The infant is totally dependent and requires much more attention—attention that was often directed exclusively to the older child. Research supports the reality of change in the mother-older sibling relationship. In general, the relationship is marked by a decrease in maternal attention and play between mother and older child and an increase in confrontations and maternal restraint.[93] Similar research is needed into patterns of father-older sibling interactions as well.

Two factors may help the sibling adjust to the birth of a brother or sister. The first of these is the child's personality.[91] Difficult, hard-to-manage children who have trouble with change react most negatively to birth of a sibling. The second factor is the parent-child relationship. A stable, supportive relationship between parents and the older child will facilitate the child's adjustment to the newborn.[92]

Nursing strategies to foster sibling adaptation to the newborn are discussed later in the chapter; however, it must be noted that few of these nursing strategies, such as sibling preparation classes, have been documented to make a difference in sibling adjust-

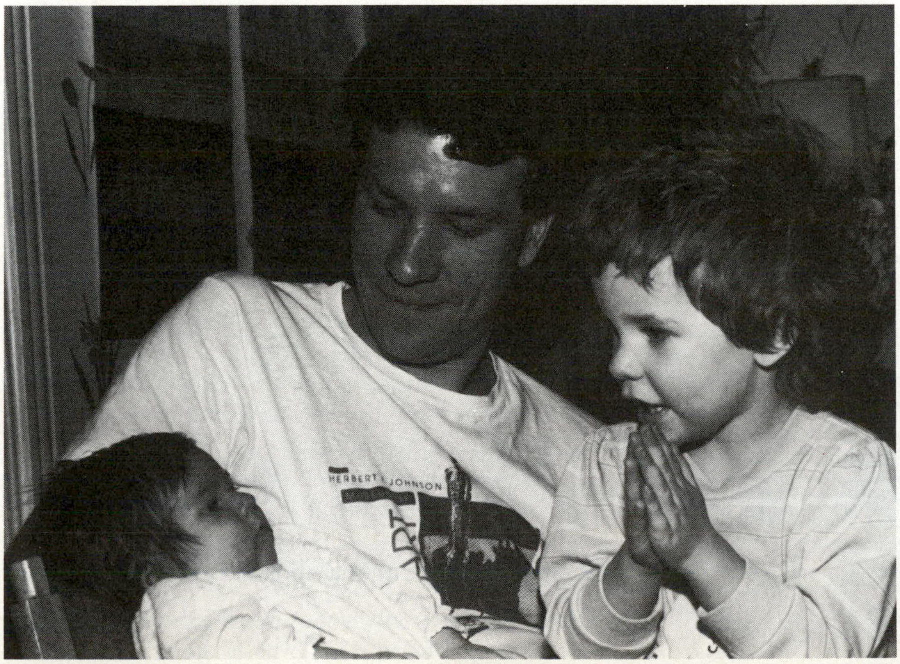

Figure 30–5. Sibling reaction to newborn.

ment. This is an area that would benefit from additional nursing research. Another related area for research involves the father's role as a support person for the older sibling.

ADJUSTMENT OF GRANDPARENTS

Birth of a first grandchild marks the development of a multigenerational family system made up of grandparents, parents, and children (Figure 30–6). Grandparents who are close to the new family are presented with two major themes in this multigenerational family pattern: the "spirit of change" and "the spirit of conservation."[94]

In the "spirit of change," the patterns of interaction that were used in the past are broken and new interpretations are brought to present events. A new mother may remember how her mother oriented her to a sex role (eg, by teaching her to cook and clean). She may resolve to orient her new daughter (or son) in a more androgynous pattern (ie, daughters may mow lawns and sons set tables). New parents reflect on their parent's childrearing and decide to "do it differently."

The "spirit of conservation," on the other hand, maintains the continuation of family patterns from one generation to the next. These patterns are family routines and rituals that are a fabric of everyday life and become enduring family events passed down to each succeeding generation. A Christmas or birthday celebration may become an enduring family ritual. Other examples include a variety of specific parenting patterns, such as reading bedtime stories to children. New parents often carry on these rituals in their own family. The spirit of conservation gives some stability to multigenerational families.

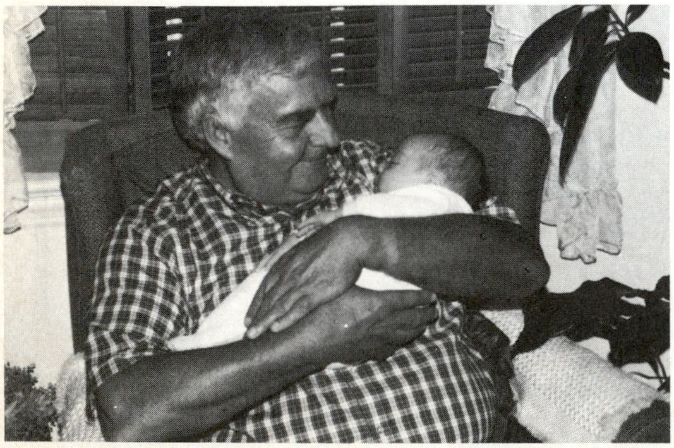

Figure 30–6. A grandfather with his new grandchild.

Parents and Grandparents: Role Models

The themes of change and conservation are mirrored in research concerning new parent's role models. One study showed that the majority of women name their mother as their principal role model during their first year of motherhood.[95] In addition, the majority of these new mothers rate themselves the same as their mothers in the area of childcare. Other similarities include judgment and use of physical discipline. Most new mothers do, however, see themselves as more lenient or fairer than their mothers had been with them. Thus, although women tend to mother as they were mothered, they may believe that they are more liberal and fairer than their mothers.[95]

The same findings seem to be true for fathers and the fathering role. One study found that a man's relationship as a child with his own father was very important in establishing a "father identity." Pleasant memories of being fathered or dissatisfaction with the relationship seem to motivate a new father either to repeat or to rework more successfully his own experiences of being parented in his own fathering behaviors.[96]

After the birth of an infant, the new parents' parents still are important role models in how they care for the new child. Thus, proximity, support, and advice from grandparents often play a vital role in the evolving parent-neonate relationship. The extent of the grandparent's role may vary among cultural groups; thus the nurse will need to ascertain the culturally appropriate role of grandparents for each individual family group.

Practical Grandparenting

What, then, are some helpful roles for grandparents in the early postpartum period? Several helpful (and some nonhelpful) role behaviors may be identified:

Helpful Grandparenting Behaviors

1. Supporting the new mother and father in parenting activities
2. Helping with the running of the household while the mother recuperates from childbirth
3. Providing additional attention to older children
4. Avoiding putting parents in conflicting situations concerning childcare advice
5. Passing on appropriate family rituals; eg, baptism or bris (ritual circumcision) traditions

Nonhelpful Grandparenting Behaviors

1. Assuming care of the newborn when the mother is capable of caring for him or her herself; however, this may be an acceptable pattern if the

mother is a young teen and the family pattern of coping with the situation is to raise mother and infant as "siblings"
2. Disagreeing with childcare methods and techniques advised by professionals or others and accepted by parents themselves
3. Being emotionally unavailable to parents
4. Being a burden, rather than a help, in the parent's household
5. Hindering father-neonate interactions; making the father an "isolate"

Although these behaviors are far from inclusive, they can serve as a guide to the nurse caring for a multigenerational family. Many more helpful and nonhelpful role behaviors of grandparents will also become apparent as the nurse interacts with families after the infant's birth.

SOCIOCULTURAL FACTORS

Sociocultural factors influence family members' interactions with the newborn during the puerperium. The family's cultural affiliations also affect the type of care given to the newborn and the mother. For example, Taiwanese women stay in the home for approximately 40 days after the delivery and have other caretakers for the infant. Several cultural groups have a "nurse" come into the home to care for the newborn while the mother regains her strength.

Another important aspect of culture during the puerperium is the rituals concerned with childrearing. For example, there are many religious rituals that introduce the newborn into the religious community (baptism, bris, and so on). Further, there are customs that family members adhere to based on their cultural background.

Chapters 13, 17, 21, and 26 focused on the black family, the Japanese-American family, the Chicano family, and the Puerto Rican family to illustrate cultural influences on pregnancy and delivery. This chapter discusses the Native American family and the way in which this cultural group traditionally perceives childbearing and childrearing. In addition, childbearing cultural practices of the previously mentioned groups are summarized with a focus on the postpartum period. Nurses must be aware of the cultural orientation of the childbearing family to understand their unique needs in the postpartum period. Nurses should also be aware of the influence of socioeconomic factors on the childbearing family in this period.

Socioeconomic Factors

The socioeconomic status of the family affects the manner in which the newborn is integrated into the family. It determines resources available to the family to care for the newborn; it may determine the person(s) who will care for the newborn; it may determine where the newborn will receive care; and it determines if the family will qualify for local, state, or federal assistance. The nurse must be aware of the socioeconomic status of a family so that discharge instructions can be delivered in an appropriate fashion.

The family structure in poor families, as well as families of other cultures, may differ from the middle-class norm of the nuclear family. The newborn may be entering into a family composed of various combinations of extended family members and friends. For example, a teenage mother may bring her newborn home with her to her own mother, who lives with a variety of children, grandchildren, aunts, uncles, or cousins. It will be important to include the grandmother in discharge planning sessions, as she may actually assume the role of "mother" for both her daughter and grandchild. The nurse must remain nonjudgmental in assessing family functioning in such alternate family structures. Different family structures, with several individuals fulfilling the role of "mother," may be an adaptive means of coping with a hostile environment.

Resources available for caring for the newborn also differ for families of differing socioeconomic status. The nurse may discuss appropriate toys and infant equipment that might be bought with middle-class parents; however, such toys and equipment may be inaccessible for parents who can barely feed their children. Parents who live in poverty can be helped to assess already existing furniture or objects in their homes that might be adapted for the newborn. For example, a dresser drawer might substitute for a bassinet, and a sink for an infant bathing tub (*see* Chapter 34). Families can be given information on local stores that sell second-hand cribs or infant clothes. The family's church might also supply some of the material things needed by the newborn. The nurse's creativity is needed to make substitutions for expensive equipment that the family who lives in poverty cannot obtain.

The person who assumes care of the newborn may vary depending on the family's socioeconomic status. The nurse should not assume that the mother will be the person responsible for care. Circumstances may dictate that the mother continue work or school. A variety of individuals may actually deliver care to the newborn. The nurse needs to ascertain who the caretakers will be, in preparation for the newborn's homecoming. For example, if the person who will be the caretaker is an aged grandmother who has limited mobility, the home might have to be adapted to facilitate infant care activities. Newborn safety needs must be met within the realities of the family's circumstances.

Sometimes, the newborn will not be cared for in the same dwelling that the mother inhabits. For example, if the newborn's parents are experiencing "hard times," they may give their newborn to a relative or close friend to raise until their economic status improves. This "informal adoption" is another means by which poor families cope with the environment of poverty.

Finally, the nurse must assess the socioeconomic status of families during the postpartum period to determine eligibility for public assistance programs. The nurse should know the eligibility criteria for the Special Supplemental Food Program for Women, Infants, and Children (WIC), Medicaid, and Aid to Families With Dependent Children (familiarly known as "welfare") in his or her state. In addition, families living in poverty might be referred to social service departments if appropriate.

Nurses who care for childbearing families in lower socioeconomic groups are challenged to be flexible, creative, and adaptive in their management strategies for discharge planning. Above all, they must remember that being poor does not, in and of itself, make a family dysfunctional. Many poor families cope well within the context of their difficult environments. The nurse should not assume that simply being poor places the newborn at risk. Poverty and high risk for developmental delay, however, often go hand in hand; therefore, careful nursing assessment of the family during the postpartum period is essential to identify potential newborns and families at risk.

Cultural Focus: The Native American Family

Perhaps more so than for any other minority group, it is difficult to discuss common cultural characteristics of Native Americans, a group that includes both American Indians and Alaska Natives. There are approximately 200 Indian tribes in the United States,[97] each with its own unique culture and customs. Health professionals who practice with Native Americans must therefore learn about the culture of the particular tribe from which their clients come.

Every Native American family should be assessed by the nurse individually to determine unique patterns and characteristics; however, identification of several broad cultural patterns and characteristics may help the nurse to understand the responses of Native American clients to the childbirth experience. These patterns, rather than specific cultural family structure and function, are the focus of this section.

Native Americans, indigenous and reservation populations, live predominately in 26 states,[98] mostly in the western part of the United States. They also live in upper New York State, Maine, Florida, North Carolina, rural Michigan, Minnesota, and Wisconsin.[98] States with the largest number of Native Americans are Oklahoma, Arizona, California, New Mexico, and Alaska.[99] Native Americans are also found in urban areas. Most major cities in the United States have populations of American Indians, Alaska Natives, or both. More than half of American Indians and Alaska Natives do not consider reservations to be their principal residence.[98]

During the forced westward migrations of Native Americans, as settlers colonized the United States, much of the Indian population died. (In fact, some authors consider the treatment of Native Americans by the dominant US culture to have been genocidal.[100] The 1980 US census indicated the Native American population was approximately 1.8 million.[98] Half of this population was under 20 years of age, and only 10 percent was over 55[98]; thus, large numbers of young families were expected in the childbearing/rearing phases of the life cycle.

Traditional Family Organization. Although families from different tribes take on very different organizational patterns, some commonalities are observed in Native American families.[98] In contrast to the modern "American" family, the three-generation extended family remains an ideal for many Native Americans.[98] Among the three generations, parental functions are often delegated among grandparents, aunts, and uncles. Traditionally, cousins were considered as close as siblings and incest taboos applied to even distant cousins. In earlier times, grandparents often had a major role in care of infants and young children, with parents responsible for economic matters of the family. Aunts and uncles often had particular disciplinary and teaching responsibilities toward children, freeing the biologic parents for more pleasurable interactions with children.[98]

In this structure, which was very child centered, children had ties from birth that allowed attachment to several parental figures. This provided the security of affection and a variety of role models for the developing child. This family structure is still a highly desirable ideal, and many Native American families strive to maintain these important ties.[98]

Role of Women. In most tribes, women are respected and influential. The woman is traditionally the most verbal family member and the member who holds the family together. Some tribes are matrilineal, so children "belong" to the mother's clan.[100]

Role of Children. Children are highly prized and desired in the Native American family.[100] The sex of the first-born child often does not seem to matter to parents. In a matrilineal clan, however, a girl is often desired. The child's upbringing is permissive, and physical punishment is rare. Children are allowed to unfold and develop naturally, at their own pace (eg, children wean and toilet-train themselves at their own rate with little interference from adults). Although limits are set concerning proper and life-threatening behaviors toward others, the child is free to choose whether and when to engage in a wide variety of behaviors. Consequences of behaviors, rather than parental direction, teach the lessons to children. Guilt is not a tool used to persuade Native American children to conform. These children often run into trouble in schools designed for children in the dominant culture.[100]

Cultural Characteristics. As mentioned earlier, although Native American families and individuals differ according to the specific culture of their tribes, several broad characteristics may be identified that will greatly influence the nurse-client interaction. These include orientation to time, relationship to the environment, orientation toward social relationships, noninterference, and perceptions of health.

Orientation to Time. The traditional Native American and Alaskan Native cultures are oriented in the present. To the Native American, however, "present" has a different meaning from the linear concept of present: here and now. The Native American's concept of present is geared to personal rhythms (eg, body needs) and seasonal rhythms, rather than to clock or calendar time.[98] Events in the life cycle, such as childbearing, are also rhythmic. At each stage of life, the focus is on the present with little concern for the next or succeeding stages. A pregnant Native American may thus focus only on her childbearing and give little thought to care of the infant.

Relationship to the Environment. Instead of a desire to control nature and manipulate others, which is a traditional orientation of the dominant Western culture, the Native American desires to understand and work in harmony with natural forces.[98] Submission, through acceptance of "overwhelming" natural events that cannot be controlled, is part of life for the Native American. Health professionals may be frustrated by this attitude, if, for example, it leads the pregnant mother with a high-risk condition to refrain from participating in a high-tech antenatal medical regimen.

Orientation Toward Social Relationships. Like the Asian-American cultural groups discussed in Chapter 17, Native Americans view the needs and goals of the group as more important than the needs and goals of the individual.[98] The group may be the tribe, band, family, or other identifiable cluster of people. Communal sharing of essentials such as food and clothing is an important element in the society of the Native American. Thus, it may be difficult to convince the pregnant woman on WIC to keep her milk and food for herself if there is need to share such essentials with other children and members of the extended family.

Noninterference. Although the group is of primary importance, the person is seen as having innate, individualized potential. Native Americans thus respect the autonomous, natural unfolding of the personality of each person—a concept labeled "noninterference." Direct confrontation with others related to control of behavior is limited to making sure the individual is aware of the consequences of behavior.[98] This attitude on the part of the family is often seen as "uncooperative" by health professionals.

Perceptions of Health. The traditional Native American believes that health is living in total harmony with nature.[99] Within this broad belief, each tribe has its own variations in belief of sickness and health (fate, evil spirits, and so on).[97]

Perhaps more than with any other group, the traditional healer or medicine person (shaman, spiritual leader) plays an important part in the health of the Native American family.[97,98] This medicine person is seen as wise in the ways of nature and the interrelationships beween humans and the environment. One author suggests that the relationship between the modern health provider and Native American medicine person should parallel the relationship between the provider and clergy. Further, medicine persons may be welcomed and necessary collaborators in health care of the Native American.[98] The traditional healer looks for the "spiritual" cause of a health problem in a culturally relevant manner. His or her purpose is seen as the cure of the whole person.

Health Care Problems. Several specific health problems affect the Native American. Spector ranks the five top causes of death of Native Americans as (1) accidents, (2) heart disease, (3) cirrhosis of the liver, (4) suicide, and (5)homicide.[97] Leading causes of morbidity include accidental injuries, cirrhosis, alcoholism, malnutrition, and deformities resulting from fetal alcohol syndrome.

The principal cause of death and illness is alcohol abuse, a widespread and severe problem in the Native American community. Two problems facing the nurse working with mothers and infants also stem from the problems of alcohol abuse: domestic violence and fetal alcohol syndrome.[97, 98]

Domestic Violence. Traditionally men and women are seen as harmonious parts of an ordered universe[97]; however, this pattern seems to be disintegrating among Native Americans under current economic pressures. Although women can market their housekeeping skills in modern society, many men, especially in urban settings, have nothing to market but physical strength.[98] This pattern often generates female-dominated households with poor male role models for boys and, coupled with alcohol abuse, makes women much more vulnerable to violence. Violence toward women may be a problem especially during pregnancy.[101]

Fetal Alcohol Syndrome. Fetal alcohol syndrome is a very difficult problem facing Native American parents, given the high value of children in this culture. The parents often deny the child's handicap. Media campaigns that focus on frightening parents into sobriety seem to provide little help, as they offer no hope to children already affected.[98]

Childbearing. Native American communities on or near reservations have the highest rate of population increase in the country,[100] with a birth rate almost twice the rate of the general population[97]; however, Native Americans also have the highest infant mortality rate in the United States. Although the neonatal death rate has been reduced, the postneonatal rate is 2.3 times that for infants of all other races.[97] The high rate is attributed to the high incidence of diarrhea in young infants and to the harsh environment in which most infants must survive.[97]

As noted earlier, the Native American philosophy views pregnancy as part of the rhythmic, cyclic pattern of life. Although childbirth is approached in a different manner by different tribal groups, several threads run through many tribes' beliefs about pregnancy and the puerperium[100]:

1. Childbrearing is seen as "healthy."
2. Mothers are encouraged to be happy throughout and to think happy thoughts.
3. The medicine person or folk "healer" is often quite involved in the care of the pregnant woman and the rituals of birth.

The postpartum is often highly structured by the particular tribal custom. For example, Farris describes postpartum customs among the Navajo Indians.[100] Traditional Navajo women still often deliver at home in the presence of a tribal midwife and the whole family. After the delivery, the placenta is buried (a fairly common traditional practice among Indian tribes). The postpartum woman is given a hot herbal tea to drink (perhaps to ensure that the uterus contracts),[97] and the infant is given an herbal emetic so that he or she vomits whatever was swallowed during birth. Traditional Navajo women breastfeed their infants, but do not begin immediately.[100] "Modern" Navajo women, on the other hand, go to the Indian Health Service for delivery by a physician or a midwife. Breastfeeding among these "modern" mothers is not as common.[100]

One postpartum/newborn tradition seen in many tribes is the use of a cradle board (or some variation) allowing the infant to be easily transported with parents as they move about (Figure 30–7). Each tribe has particular rituals and ceremonies connected to the cradle board, along with ritual ways of decorating the board.[100]

Strengths of the Native American Family. Many authors agree that a major strength of Native Americans is the desire to retain their heritage.[97–100] Families attempt to keep alive their tribal language, folkways, crafts, and values. As more and more Native Americans deliver in the manner of Western medicine, nurses will need to consider their specific cultural needs and design care that allows families to participate in the birth and postpartum period according to their beliefs.

The Postpartum Experience of Selected Cultural Groups

Families from many other cultural groups also have specific customs concerned with the postpartum. Among the families discussed here are the black American family, the Vietnamese American family, and the Chicano family. Table 30–3 provides a summary of some cultural practices of these groups.[102–104]

The descriptions given here are broad and should not be viewed as more than common threads within a cultural group. Individual differences exist within any cultural group; these differences are further ac-

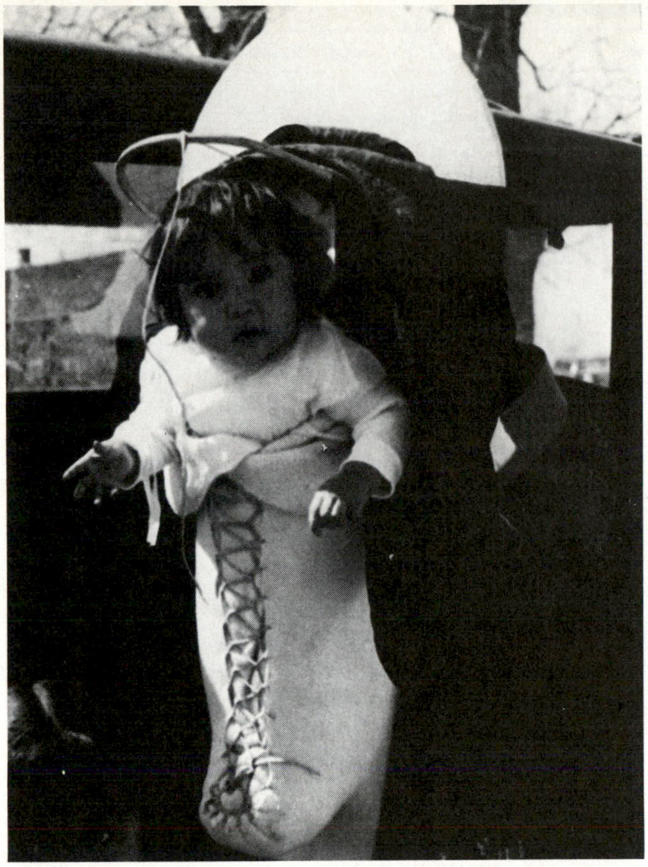

Figure 30–7. A Bannock Indian infant is carried in a traditional cradle board.

centuated by differing rates of acculturation into the predominant culture. Although the need for individualized assessment and care cannot be overemphasized, these descriptions of several cultural groups provide examples that should alert the nurse to the importance of providing culturally sensitive care for the childbearing family.

NURSING STRATEGIES FOR MANAGEMENT OF PSYCHOSOCIAL CONCERNS: FAMILY-CENTERED CARE

Psychosocial nursing care of the childbearing family during the postpartum period focuses on the establishment of an integrated, harmonious family unit. This concept is also the basis for programs of family-centered maternity care, which emphasize providing care that fosters family unity while maintaining safety. Family-centered nursing care is client-oriented care. Birth of an infant is a major life event to be shared by the family to the extent desired and within the context of the family's cultural value system.[105]

More than a system of nursing care delivery, family-centered maternity care is a philosophy.[105, 106] To be successful this attitude toward care must be valued by nursing staff. Family-centered maternity care, especially in the postpartum period, implies a philosophic orientation that values the family, however the client chooses to define that concept. The caregiver must respect the needs of the family, as a unit, and each of its members.[105]

McKay and Phillips outline several components that are central to family-centered care during the postpartum period.[106] These include providing a family-centered environment to foster attachment (rooming-in, flexible visitation, mother-baby nursing), teaching, and discharge planning.

Attachment

During the postpartum, the nurse is responsible for monitoring the developing attachment between all family members and the newborn. Attachment is monitored through observation, through efforts to promote and facilitate parental attachment behaviors, and through intervention and referrals to appropriate resources if attachment seems to be problematic.

Promoting Maternal Attachment. Nursing strategies for promoting attachment between mother and newborn include the following:

- Care for the mother's dependency needs, such as bathing, rest, and food.
- Allow the mother to discuss her labor and delivery experience. As the mother expresses her feelings about her experience, she can resolve and integrate the labor and delivery into her personal history. She will then move on and focus her attention on the newborn.
- Mobilize the mother's support systems, for example, infant's father, friends, parents. When the mother receives nurturing from others, she can better nurture her infant.
- Allow the mother to inspect her infant. Encourage her to take the infant out of the blanket and inspect the unclothed infant's toes, fingers, trunk, and so on. Inspection fosters identification and allows the mother to replace the "fantasized" infant with the real infant. It also allows the mother to note her infant's intactness. If the infant has an observable physical handicap, it allows the mother to realistically observe the extent of the handicap and begin to grieve. The mother will require preparation and support for this process.
- Encourage face-to-face and eye-to-eye contact. This activity is a priority in establishing mutual interactions between mother and infant. This can be ac-

TABLE 30–3. SELECTED CULTURAL PRACTICES DURING THE POSTPARTUM

Cultural Group	Practices Related to Postpartum	Practices Related to Newborn
Rural and southern black Americans[102]	Mother is considered sick when experiencing lochial flow Restrictions: tub baths, shower, shampooing hair Foods: avoid liver to decrease bleeding, drink sassafras tea to promote healing Female relatives, older children help with household chores Young children may be sent to extended family for care	Concerned with "spoiling" baby; mothers do *not* respond to every cry Demonstrate affection through feeding and caretaking Nickname baby Dress baby in excessive clothing to prevent chilling Use baby oil on skin and scalp Use "belly bands" to prevent hernia Celebrate baby's arrival and survival (4 weeks or more) at church
Chicanos[103]	Mother needs to convalesce after birth Restrictions: Should avoid exposure to air for 14 days Foods: avoid pork, chili, and tomatoes for 40 days; ingest chamomile tea, boiled milk, and toasted tortillas for first few days Mother's mother does housework Young children are cared for by mother-in-law	Breastfeeding begins after lactation; colostrum is "unclean" Meconium passage is stimulated by olive oil or castor oil Use belly bands Male infants generally not circumcised Girls have their ears pierced Infants may receive religious medal to wear Folk illnesses—*pujos* (grunting) caused by being held by menstruating woman; *mal ojo* ("evil eye") by somebody who desires to hold baby but cannot; cured by folk cures Coparent is named for baby and is in charge of the ritual baptism Extended family members may informally adopt some of the biologic family's children
Vietnamese-Americans[104]	Mother is kept warm by applying heat and being fed highly seasoned food Restrictions: cannot bathe or shampoo hair for a month after initial cleansing bath; wear elastic wrap around waist to reduce size Foods: avoid sour foods and cold liquids; ingest hot tea, soup, pork stew, and salty foods for regeneration Grandmother or older sibling cares for infant if mother works	Baby kept with mother continuously after birth; picked up immediately if cries Baby is considered 1 year old at birth

complished by teaching the mother to position the infant at an optimum gazing distance (approximately 9 to 10 in.), and teaching the mother to interact with the infant when the infant is awake and alert. The nurse should also ensure that the first interaction is during an infant's alert period (ie, immediately after delivery and the second period of reactivity; *see* discussion in Chapter 32.)

- Allow the mother to verbalize about the infant. Initially, in the process of resolving the discrepancy between the "real" and "ideal" infant, the mother may express some disappointment about appearance, sex, and so on. This should not be confused with deficits in attachment at this point. Verbalization about the infant also allows the mother to identify with the infant ("Look! he has his father ears").
- Encourage early and frequent feedings. Feeding is perceived as an act of mothering. Moreover, feeding is an opportunity for close interaction with the infant. The nurse should be present during feedings to assist the mother with breastfeeding and bottlefeeding interactions, so that the mother will begin to feel competent and successful.
- Encourage the mother to talk to her infant. The infant responds to the mother's voice by moving and looking at her. This type of interaction is a positive experience for both mother and infant.
- Describe to the mother the potential orienting responses and temperament of the infant. Parents need to understand that the manner in which the infant interacts with them depends in part on her or his own behavioral style (*see* Chapter 34).

Promoting Paternal Attachment. Many of the nursing strategies that are used in promoting maternal-newborn attachment are appropriate in promoting paternal-newborn attachment as well. Most of the described attachment behaviors are human behaviors and the same strategies work for both mother and father. Some specific strategies that focus on the father alone are allowing early and sustained contact with the infant, beginning in the delivery room, and fostering paternal engrossment with the newborn (*see* discussion early in this chapter). These might include encouraging the father to talk about the infant, allowing the father to have nonverbal time with the infant, allowing the father to inspect the infant, encouraging en face behavior, and allowing the father to express feelings, which are often intense.

Promoting Sibling Attachment. Although little is documented in relation to sibling attachment behaviors, clinical observations indicate that they may make a difference to family functioning. Certain strategies can foster sibling attachment:

- Allow the sibling to visit his or her mother at the birth site.
- Encourage parents to focus attention on the older child. For example, parents may present the child with a gift or toy or talk to and play with the child alone, without the new baby present.
- Allow the child to touch or hold the infant. Some institutions have sibling rooms to promote this experience.
- Counsel parents regarding expectations of sibling attachment in relation to the child's developmental level.
- Use dolls and play equipment to help the older child to express feelings about the new infant.

Promoting Grandparent Attachment. Promoting grandparent attachment is important in providing support for the family.

- Encourage involvement with the newborn. This may include holding, caretaking, and so on.
- Allow visitation of the parents' parents.
- Encourage grandparents to support and help parents in the parenting roles.
- Encourage the parents to support and help the grandparents in the grandparenting role.
- Allow grandparents to discuss their feelings about the new infant and their roles.

Several cautions are in order concerning observation of attachment behaviors. First, the nurse needs to know that forms designed to measure parental (most often maternal) "bonding" must not be used rigidly. They are simply guides to help the nurse focus on appropriate behaviors. The meaning and pattern of attachment behaviors must be assessed in the context of the total family system and environment. In particular, the family's cultural background must be considered.[105] Different cultural groups may demonstrate attachment to a newborn in different ways as shown by the examples of several groups discussed in the preceding section.

Promoting a Family-Centered Environment. Providing a nurturing environment for the developing family is an important nursing strategy. This is an environment in which the new family can be together in a homelike atmosphere, with sensitive interested caretakers available as necessary[106]; however, the environment away from the home is often not a place conducive to family interactions.

One creative nursing instructor had her students observe, without intervening, interaction behaviors in a hospital environment. The students noted the many extraneous environmental factors that may interfere with the mother-infant interaction, including hospital loudspeaker paging systems, traffic in and out of the room (dietary personnel, nurses, physicians, aides), noise from the television, conversations in the hall, telephones ringing at the nurses' station, and an assortment of other noises. It is easy to see how such a chaotic environment may have a negative effect on early family development. Indeed, the environment may be a reason why the mother goes home exhausted!

Rooming-In

With rooming-in, the mother and infant are in the same room for an extended period (such as 24 or 48 hours). Most birthing institutions still have a central nursery, and parents transport their infants back and forth between the nursery and room at will. In certain situations, all care for the infant is delivered in the room, by the parents, nurse, or both. In many situations, however, the infant returns to the nursery for special procedures such as examinations.

This component of family-centered postpartum care provides the parents and the infant with an opportunity to be together to the extent they desire during the postpartum period. This facilitates early and prolonged contact and self-demand feedings and helps the parents to get to know their newborn.[106]

The actual length of time spent with the newborn varies with the family. Caregivers and institutions should be flexible in structuring rooming-in so that each individual family's needs can be met. For example, some mothers may wish to have their infant with them for a full day; others may wish to return the infant to the nursery in the afternoon to take a nap.

Institutions should facilitate this type of parental decision making without being judgmental.

There are several strategies that the nurse can employ to foster a positive rooming-in experience for the family.

- Be available to the family as a consultant for newborn care
- Organize the room and supplies to facilitate family-centered care
- Keep unpleasant stimuli (eg, noise, traffic in the room) to a minimum
- Plan for flexibility in parents' participation in rooming-in

Rooming-in does not substitute for nursing assessments and interventions. The nurse should not assume that mothers who room-in, including multiparas, are either confident or independent. New mothers have many personal needs to be met and require nursing care. For example, mothers who have perineal discomfort may require time to take a sitz bath. A flexible rooming-in situation allows hospital staff to care for the infant while the mother's needs are being met.

Flexible Visitation

With flexible visitation programs, fathers are not considered "visitors" and have complete access to the mother and newborn. Other individuals in the family—siblings, grandparents, relatives, and friends—have more flexible visiting hours as well (each program will be specified by the birthing institution). Sibling visitation is often a feature of these programs, which allow older brothers and sisters to interact with the newborn and become acquainted with him or her.

The nurse can help ensure flexible visitation for childbearing families in his or her institution. Some strategies include: educating other health professionals concerning benefits of flexible family visitation, instituting flexible visiting policies for childbearing families in the birthing institution, and encouraging family members to establish a visiting pattern that meets their needs.

Mother-Baby Nursing

Mother-baby nursing is a form of care delivery vital to establishment of family-centered postpartum care; however, it is also one of the most problematic aspects of implementing a family-centered program. In this form of nursing care delivery, one nurse is assigned to complete care of a mother-infant dyad. "Complete care" includes physical care for both mother and infant, teaching, charting, reporting, and other aspects of implementing the nursing process.[106]

Nursing strategies relevant to mother-baby nursing include interventions already discussed in sections on "Attachment," "Rooming-in," and "Flexible Visitation." One of the major roles of the nurse in implementing mother-baby nursing is at the policy development level. Mother-baby nursing is a system of care delivery that requires that nurses have specific attitudes, values, and philosophies concerning birth and the new family. It does not matter if the infant is cared for in a central nursery or in the mother's room; the nurse regards the mother-infant dyad as "the client."

In a traditional hospital setting, nurses tend to work only with the healthy newborn or only with the postpartum mother. Many nurses are therefore uncomfortable in delivering care to a mother and infant dyad.

Teaching

Formal and informal teaching of the new family features flexibility, sensitivity to parental learning needs, and attunement to individual learning styles.[106] Methods usually include both group and one-to-one teaching techniques. Educational preparation during the childbearing cycle is discussed in depth in Chapter 24. In addition Chapter 34 discusses teaching needs of parents concerning the newborn.

Teaching in the postpartum period focuses on physiologic changes that occur in the mother, developmental aspects of the newborn, neonatal feeding and elimination patterns, activities of daily living, and restructuring of the family environment to include the new member, as reflected in these specific topics:[107, 108]

- Involution, including lochial changes, warning signs of infection, possible afterpains, perineal healing, and care of hemorrhoids
- Breast changes, including secretion of colostrum and breast milk, engorgement, care of the nipples (if breastfeeding), warning signs of infection, milk expression, comfort measures (eg, showers, supportive bra)
- Behavioral styles of the newborn, including temperament, orienting responses, sensory capabilities, and interactional responses (*see* Chapters 32 and 34)
- Neonatal feeding (breast and bottle) (Figure 30–8)
- Feeding patterns
- Introduction of solid foods
- Neonatal elimination patterns, including frequency and appearance of urine and feces
- Common variations in the newborn such as milia and mongolian spots (*see* Chapter 33)
- Developmental milestones
- Activities of daily living, including dressing the

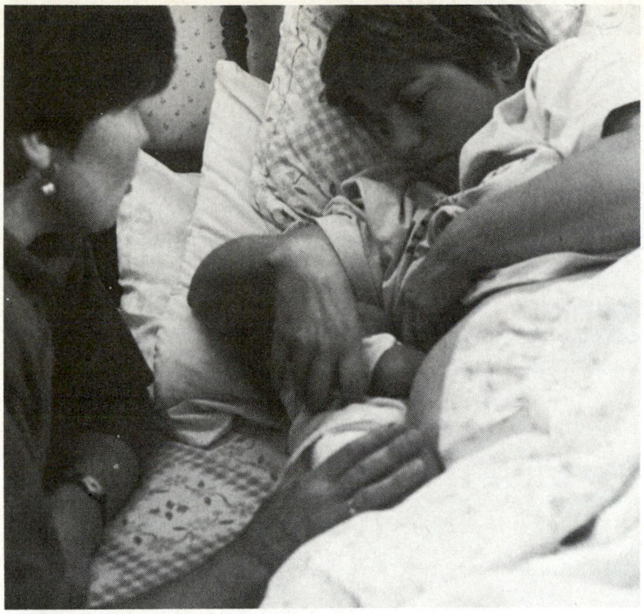

Figure 30–8. A nurse provides teaching during breastfeeding.

baby, taking the baby outside, and criteria for choosing a babysitter or childcare (*see* Chapter 34)

- Possible reactions of siblings
- Utilization of social support systems such as parents or friends
- Restructuring of living space and parental time to incorporate a new infant
- Career issues
- Financial issues
- Resources for supporting new parents in the community, such as women's health groups, pediatric nurses, and LaLeche league
- Immunization plans for the infant
- Family planning resources (*see* Chapter 9)
- Rest and sleep concerns of parents
- Resumption of sexual activity
- Exercises for the postpartum period (*see* Chapter 31)
- Physician's appointments for mother and baby
- Breast self-examinations (*see* Chapter 5)
- Information on car seats
- Nutrition for postpartum lactation

Discharge Planning

The final component of family-centered maternity care is attention to the family's discharge from the birth facility and return home.[106]

- Discharge instructions that reinforce teaching are given to family members by nursing staff (*see* the list of teaching topics in the preceding section).
- Parents are given the telephone number of the birth facility and told to call on a 24-hour basis as needed.
- The nurse who cared for the family makes a follow-up telephone call between 48 and 72 hours after the family returns home.
- Referrals to postpartum classes and self-help and support groups are made as needed.
- Home visits (either by a community nursing agency or by a nurse from the birthing facility) are arranged as needed.
- Referrals to other community sources of assistance (eg, WIC, Child Health Conferences, Aid to Families With Dependent Children) are made as needed.

Some interesting work has been done on supporting parents through telephone consultation. Investigators found that a telephone consultation service was able to provide information and emotional support to parents of children from birth to 5 years of age. They reported that the calls of parents for infants up to 1 month of age centered on infant feeding and complaints of infant fussiness. The next largest category of problems related to the mother, rather than the infant. Maternal concerns focused on depression and anxiety, physical problems, or requests for information, particularly information about parent support groups.[109]

Figure 30–9 is an example of a form for discharge planning/teaching. Figure 30–10 is a form for observing attachment to the newborn during the postpartum period.

Advantages of Family-Centered Postpartum Care

Family-centered nursing care has many advantages for both the birthing facility and the family.

Advantages for the Family

1. Care promotes the health and well-being of the entire family unit and members in an integrated fashion.
2. Individual client needs can be easily met with the flexibility inherent in the program.
3. Physical and psychologic safety are promoted.

Advantages for the Birthing Facility

1. The program can be tailored easily to each individual facility's existing structure, as family-centered postpartum care is more a philosophy of care delivery than a physical building.
2. The birthing facility, in meeting consumer demands for this type of birth, becomes competitive in attracting clients.
3. Care delivery is actually simplified,[105] as there is no need to make special arrangements for rooming-in mothers; each family chooses the pattern desired. (*Text continues on p 779.*)

DISCHARGE PLANNING/TEACHING FLOW SHEET

POSTPARTUM CARE

EXPECTED PARENT/FAMILY OUTCOMES	INITIAL TEACHING DATE/SIGNATURE	ASSESSMENT/ COMMENTS	OUTCOME ACHIEVED DATE/SIGNATURE
Verbalizes understanding of:			
____A. Unit structure/facilities			
____B. Medication regime			
____C. Routine checks			
____D. IV therapy (*give booklet*)			
____E. Catheterization/foley			
____F. Preeclampsia/eclampsia checks			
____G. Handwashing			
____H. Other			
Verbalizes understanding of physical care including:			
____A. Perineal care/incision care			
____B. Sitz baths (location, frequency, procedure)			
____C. Breast care (bathing, engorgement, support, nipple care)			
____D. Physical changes during involution (diaphoresis, lochia, afterpains, edema)			
____E. Nutrition			
____F. Elimination			
____G. Exercises (class and/or review *handout*)			
____H. Rho(D) immune globulin (*handout*)			
____I. Rubella (*handout*)			
____J. Other			

Figure 30–9. Discharge planning flowsheet. (*Figure continues.*)

DISCHARGE PLANNING/TEACHING FLOW SHEET

POSTPARTUM CARE Page 2

EXPECTED PARENT/FAMILY OUTCOMES	INITIAL TEACHING DATE/SIGNATURE	ASSESSMENT/ COMMENTS	OUTCOME ACHIEVED DATE/SIGNATURE
Verbalizes understanding or perceptions of post-partum psychological impact			
____A. Changes in body image			
____B. Changes in emotional state			
____C. Adjustments to parenting			
____D. Siblings			
____E. Grandparents/other support people			
Verbalizes understanding or perceptions related to postdischarge needs:			
____A. Rest/sleep			
____B. Physician appointment			
____C. Reportable S/S			
____D. Exercises/daily activity			
____E. Sexual activity			
____F. Contraception			
____G. Breast self-examination			
____H. Return to work			
____I. Community resources			
____ Parenting classes			
____ PHN			
____ LaLeche League			
____ Car seat rental			
____ Immunization sources (*handout*)			
____ ________________			

Figure 30–9 (continued). Discharge planning flowsheet.

ATTACHMENT ASSESSMENT FORM

Name__________ **Age**_____ **Marital status:** ***Single***____ ***Married***____ ***Separated***____

Gravida______ **Para** ______ **AB** ______ **Delivery Date** ______

Expected date of confinement ______ **Method of feeding** ______

Summary of labor and delivery (*anesthesia, complications, presence of a supportive person*):

____

____

____

____

____

DIRECTIONS: This form is provided to systematically assess and record the components of the attachment process based on information obtained from available records, observations, and interviews with the parent(s) and other health care providers.

PRENATAL

	Yes	No	COMMENTS
Planned the pregnancy	____	____	
Confirmed the pregnancy	____	____	
Accepted the pregnancy	____	____	
Received early prenatal care	____	____	
Described fetal movement	____	____	
Personalized the fetus	____	____	
Asked what the fetus was like in utero	____	____	
Attended prenatal classes	____	____	
Planned for infant's needs	____	____	

Figure 30–10. Attachment assessment form. (*Figure continues.*)

PRENATAL (*continued*)

	Yes	No	COMMENTS
Thought of possible names	_____	_____	_____
Client in good health	_____	_____	_____
Father of infant involved	_____	_____	_____

Areas of concern:

DELIVERY PERIOD (Birth through 4 hours)

	Yes	No	COMMENTS
Accepts sex of infant	_____	_____	_____
Calls infant by name	_____	_____	_____
Calls infant by affectionate terms	_____	_____	_____
Comments on beauty of infant	_____	_____	_____
Realistically appraises the physical appearance of the infant	_____	_____	_____
Looks and reaches out to infant	_____	_____	_____
Touches infant	_____	_____	_____
Smiles at infant	_____	_____	_____

Areas of concern:

Figure 30–10 (continued). Attachment assessment form. (*Figure continues.*)

POSTPARTUM PERIOD (From second day to 6 weeks)

	Yes	No	COMMENTS
Enjoys caring for intant	____	____	____
Holds infant close	____	____	____
Feels infant belongs to her	____	____	____
Feels infant notices her	____	____	____
When away, thinks about infant	____	____	____
Verbalizes warm comments about infant	____	____	____
Recuperates with little difficulty	____	____	____
Responds sensitively and appropriately to infant	____	____	____

Areas of concern:

Figure 30–10 (continued). Attachment assessment form.

4. Staff experience greater satisfaction and reward in caring for the family unit as a whole.
5. Nurses have the opportunity to deliver high-level nursing care and transcend an isolated approach to maternity and newborn care.[105]

Family-centered maternity care, in general, and family-centered postpartum care, specifically, have much to offer the client, the health professional, and the health care facility. Those planning to implement family-centered care need to assess the attitudes, values, and needs of the communities to be served.[106] Collaboration with consumer groups, as well as other health professionals, will promote family-centered maternity care based on the needs of the expanding family.

CASE STUDY/CARE PLAN: PROMOTING MATERNAL PSYCHOSOCIAL ADAPTATION IN THE EARLY POSTPARTUM PERIOD

Kalisha Allen is a 35-year-old gravida 3, para 3, who has just delivered her third son. She is 1 day postdelivery. The nurse brings her the infant and places him in her arms. Kalisha says, with a grimace, "Another boy! I wanted a little girl more than anything!" When the nurse asks Kalisha to continue, she admits that she only had girls' names picked out and could only fantasize of having a girl during pregnancy.

Kalisha further states that she did not get back into shape with her second pregnancy as easily as she did with her first pregnancy, "and this time it will be even worse!" "I wanted this to be my last pregnancy. I hate the way I look after having a baby."

Supporting Assessment Data	Expected Client/Family Outcome	Nursing Action/ Intervention	Rationale	Criteria for Evaluation
Nursing Diagnosis: Potential for ineffective family coping, related to possible alteration in attachment				
Gravida 3, para 3, three sons	Before discharge, client will:	Encourage client to grieve the wished-for fantasy girl	Client must resolve loss of wished-for infant before investing in the real infant.	Client demonstrates infant care and nurturing behaviors toward new son.
Client states: "Another boy! I wanted a little girl more than anything"	Begin to resolve the loss of the fantasized girl	Encourage client to verbalize her feelings about having another son.	Acting as a nonjudgmental support helps allay client's guilt over feelings and encourages further verbalization.	Client demonstrates eye-to-eye contact, en face position, talking to son, and other attachment behaviors.
Fantasized during pregnancy only of a girl; only girls' names picked for baby	Become acquainted with her new son and demonstrate beginning attachment behavior	Support client in a nonjudgmental manner.		
	Begin to nurture the infant	Use Brazelton tool in assessing infant; encourage client to watch and participate.	Demonstrating the infant's abilities to parent assists in fostering attachment.	Client selects name for her son.
	Begin to investigate boys' names and choose one for the infant	Reassess mother-infant interactions noting behaviors that indicate attachment or alterations in attachment (especially eye-to-eye contact, en face position, talking to infant, exploring infant, and so on).	Presence or absence of attachment behaviors indicates progression of process.	
		Refer client to parent support group and visiting nurses' association.	Potential for inadequate attachment necessitates further support and evaluation.	Client participates in support group.

(continued)

CASE STUDY/CARE PLAN: Promoting Maternal Psychosocial Adaptation in the Early Postpartum Period (*continued*)

Supporting Assessment Data	Expected Client/Family Outcome	Nursing Action/ Intervention	Rationale	Criteria for Evaluation
Nursing Diagnosis: Body image disturbance, related to normal body changes of pregnancy and postpartum				
Weight: 150 pounds, 20 pounds over prepregnancy weight Striae on abdomen, fundus firm 1 cm below umbilicus; lochia moderate rubra; abdominal muscle tone flabby Client states: "I hate the way I look . . ." indicates that she has found it more difficult to get back into shape with each successive pregnancy	By discharge, client will: Identify that her body is normal for this stage of the postpartum Identify self-care behaviors such as exercise and nutrition that will promote a return to prepregnancy body status and a positive body image.	Reinforce teaching about physiologic changes in the postpartum (fundus, lochia, breasts). Teach client new self-care behaviors and reinforce her existing positive self-care behaviors. Teach client about normal weight loss in the postpartum.	Knowledge of normal process of weight loss and physiologic changes in postpartum will help client accept her current body status and image. Participation in positive health care practices assists in promotion of positive self-concept. Self-care behaviors assist with postpartum weight loss and increased muscle tone.	Client identifies normal physiologic changes and status. Client makes positive statement about herself. Client describes her self-care regimen to the nurse. Client writes a plan for exercise, diet, rest, hygiene, and so on.

SUMMARY

Many psychologic changes occur in the childbearing family and its members during the postpartum period. Each member and the family as a whole are affected by the addition of a new member—the neonate.

Material tasks during the postpartum period include attachment to the infant through identification, claiming, and interaction with the infant. The mother needs to feel competent in performing mothering behaviors and feel gratification in the mother-infant interaction.

The new father also adapts to his new role and to the infant. Fathers display sensitivity to the newborn's behavioral cues. They also display a progressive touch sequence with their infants. Studies on fathers identify "engrossment" as the behavioral style of the father with his infant.

Siblings interact with the newborn in an effort to establish their relationship with him or her. Factors that influence sibling interaction include age of the sibling, developmental level, ordinal position in the family, and sibling visitation in the hospital.

Grandparents complete the task of moving up a generation. They are often important in the social support network of the new parents. Therefore, such nursing strategies as teaching grandparent classes facilitate role assumption activities of grandparents.

Cultural considerations are always important when caring for the postpartum family. The Native American family is presented as one example of how cultural practices may affect health care delivery to the childbearing family.

Nursing strategies emerge from the philosophy that the family is the appropriate client during the childbearing cycle. Strategies to promote family-centered care in the postpartum period include rooming-in, flexible visitation, and mother-baby nursing.

REVIEW QUESTIONS

1. Identify the maternal tasks during the postpartum period.
2. Discuss the paternal process of engrossment.
3. Describe the relationship of the mother to her older children during the postpartum period.
4. List two helpful and two nonhelpful grandparenting behaviors.
5. Discuss four advantages of family-centered maternity care.
6. List two nursing strategies to foster infant attachment with each of the following persons: mother, father, sibling, grandparent.

REFERENCES

1. Mercer RT, Ferketich SL. Predictors of family functioning eight months following birth. *Nurs Res.* 1990;39:76–82.
2. Holmes TH, Rahe RH. The social readjustment rating scale. *J Psychosomat Res.* 1967;11;213–218.
3. Coddington RD. The significance of life events as etiological factors in diseases of children. *J Psychosomat Res.* 1967;2:213.
4. Group for the Advancement of Psychiatry. *The Joys and Sorrows of Parenthood.* New York: GAP, 1973.
5. Hott J. Best laid plans: pre- and postpartum comparison of self and spouse in primiparous Lamaze couples who share delivery and those who do not. In: Sherwen N, Weingarten C, eds. *Analysis and Application of Nursing Research: Parent-Neonate Studies.* Monterey, Calif: Wadsworth Health Sciences; 1983.
6. Sunner G, Fritch J. Postnatal parental concerns: the first six weeks of life. In: Sherwen N, Weingarten C, eds. *Analysis and Application of Nursing Research: Parent-Neonate Studies.* Monterey, Calif: Wadsworth Health Sciences, 1983.
7. Humenick SS, Bugen LA. Parenting roles: expectation versus reality. *Matern Child Nurs J.* 1987;12:36–39.
8. Humenick S, Bugen L. Correlates of parent-infant interaction: an exploratory study. *Birth Defects.* 1981;17: 181–199.
9. Hall L. Effect of teaching on primiparas' perceptions of their newborn. *Nurs Res.* 1980;29;317–322.
10. Snyder C, et al. New findings about mother's expectations and their relationship to infant development. *Am J Matern Child Nurs.* 1979;4:354–357.
11. Ventura J. Parent coping behaviors, parent functioning and infant temperament characteristics. *Nurs Res.* 1982;31: 269–273.
12. Pridham K. Parents' beliefs about themselves as parents of a new infant: instrument development. *Res Nurs Health.* 1985;8:19–29.
13. Lovell M, Fiorino D. Combating myth. A conceptual framework for analyzing the stress of motherhood. *Adv Nurs Sci.* 1979;1:75–84.
14. Bull M. Change in concerns of first-time mothers after one week at home. *J Obstet Gynecol Neonat Nurs.* 1981;10: 391–394.
15. Sweeny SL, Davis FB. Transition to parenthood: a group experience. *Matern Child Nurs.* 1979;8:59–64.
16. Broom B. Consensus about marital relationship during the transition to parenthood. *Nurs Res.* 1984;33:223–228.
17. Scott-Heyes G. Marital adaptation during pregnancy and after childbirth. *J Reprod Infant Psychol.* 1983;1:18–28.
18. Newton LD. Fourth trimester. In: Sonstegard L, et al, eds. *Women's Health: Childbearing.* New York: Grune & Stratton; 1983.
19. Rossi A. Transition to parenthood. *J Marriage Fam.* 1968; 30:26–39.
20. LeMasters EE. Parenthood as crisis. *Marriage Fam.* 1957;19:352–355.
21. Norbeck JS, Tilden VP. Life Stress, social support, and emotional disequilibrium in complications of pregnancy: a prospective, multivariate study. *J Health Soc Behav.* 1983;24:30–46.
22. Cronenwett LR. Network structures, social support and psychological outcomes of pregnancy. *Nurs Res.* 1985;34: 93–99.
23. Cronenwett LR. Parental network structure and perceived support after birth of first child. *Nurs Res.* 1985;34:347–352.
24. Belsky J, Rovine M. Social network contract, family support and the transition to parenthood. *J Marriage Fam.* 1984;46:455–462.
25. Power TG, Parke RD. Social network factors and the transition to parenthood. *Sex Roles.* 1984;10:949–972.
26. Cronenwett LR. Parental network structure and perceived support after birth of first child. *Nurs Res.* 1985;34:347–352.
27. Russell CS. Transition to parenthood: problems and gratifications. *J Marriage Fam.* 1974;36:294–301.
28. Mercer R. *First Time Motherhood: Experiences from Teens to Forties.* New York: Springer Publishing Co; 1986.
29. Majewski JL. Conflicts, satisfactions and attitudes during transition to the maternal role. *Nurs Res.* 1986;31:10–14.
30. Klaus M, Kennell J. *Parent-Infant Bonding.* St. Louis, Mo: CV Mosby; 1982.
31. Walker LO. A longitudinal analysis of stress process among mothers and infants. *Nurs Res.* 1989;38:1339–1343.
32. Walker LO. Stress process among mothers of infants: preliminary model testing. *Nurs Res. 1989;38:100–116.*
33. House JS. *Work Stress and Social Support.* Reading, Mass: Addison-Wesley; 1981.
34. Lederman R. *Psychosocial Adaptation in Pregnancy.* Englewood Cliffs, NJ: Prentice-Hall; 1984.
35. Schroeder MA. Development and testing of a scale to measure locus of control prior to and following childbirth. *Matern Child Nurs J.* 1981;10:111–121.
36. Wylie RC. *The Self-Concept.* Lincoln, Neb: University of Nebraska Press; 1974.
37. Mercer R. The process of maternal role attainment over the first year. *Nurs Res.* 1985;34:198–204.
38. Harrison AO, Minor JH. Interrole conflict, coping strategies, and satisfaction among black working wives. *J Marriage Fam.* 1978;40:799–805.
39. Holahan CK, Gilbert LA. Interrole conflict for working women. *J Appl Psychol.* 1979;64:86–90.
40. Meyerowitz J, Feldnan H. Transition to parenthood. *Psychiatr Res Rep.* 1966;78:84–89.
41. Miller B, Sollie D. Normal stresses during the transition to parenthood. *Fam Relations.* 1980;29:459–465.
42. Majewski J, Feldan H. Conflicts, satisfactions, and attitude during transition to the maternal role. *Nurs Res.* 1986;35:10–14.
43. Rubin R. *Maternal Identity and the Maternal Experience.* New York: Springer Publishing Co; 1984.
44. Mahler M, et al. *The Psychological Birth of the Human Infant.* New York: Basic Books; 1975.
45. Benedek T. The psychobiology of pregnancy. In: Anthony E, Benedek T, eds. *Parenthood.* Boston: Little, Brown; 1970.
46. Sherwen L. Separation: the forgotten phenomenon of child development. *Top Clin Nurs.* 1983;5:1–11.
47. Hill S, Shronk L. The effect of early parent-infant contact on newborn body temperature. *J Obstet Gynecol Neonat Nurs.* 1979;8:287–292.
48. Rubin R. Maternal touch. *Nurs Outlook.* 1963;11:828–831.
49. Tulman L. Mothers' and unrelated person's initial handling of newborn infants. *Nurs Res.* 1985;34:205–210.
50. Tulman L. Initial handling of newborn infants by vaginally

and cesarean-delivered mothers. *Nurs Res.* 1986;35: 296–300.

51. Fawcett J. The relationship between identification and patterns of change in spouses' body images during and after pregnancy. *Int J Nurs Stud.* 1987;14:199–213.
52. Strang V, Sullivan P. Body image attitudes during pregnancy and the postpartum period. *J Obstet Gynecol Neonat Nurs.* 1985;14:332–337.
53. Gruis M. Beyond maternity: postpartum concerns of mothers. *Am J Matern Child Nurs.* 1977;2:
54. Sumner G, Fritsch J. Postnatal parental concerns: the first six weeks of life. *J Obstet Gynecol Neonat Nurs.* 1977;6:27–33.
55. Bliss-Holtz J. Primiparas' prenatal concern for learning infant care. *Nurs Res.* 1988;37:20–24.
56. Hiser P. Concerns of multiparas during the second postpartum week. *J Obstet Gynecol Neonat Nurs.* 1987;16: 195–203.
57. Mercer R. She's a multip . . . she knows the ropes. *Am J Matern Child Nurs.* 1979;4:301.
58. Larsen V. Stresses of the childbearing year. *Am J Pub Health.* 1966;56:32.
59. Grubb C. Perceptions of time of multiparous women in relation to themselves and others during the first postpartal month. *Matern Child Nurs J.* 1980;9:226.
60. Cunningham FG, et al. *Williams Obstetrics,* 18th ed. Norwalk, Conn: Appleton & Lange; 1989.
61. Pedersen F. Differentiation of the father's role in the infancy period. *Adv Family Intervention Assess Theory.* 1983;3:1985–208.
62. Peterson G, Mehl L, Luderman P. The role of some birth-related variables in father attachment. *Am J Orthopsychiatry.* 1979;49:330–338.
63. Entwisle D, Doering D. *The First Birth.* Baltimore, Md: Johns Hopkins University Press; 1981.
64. Kotelchuck M. The infant's relationship to the father: experimental evidence. In: Lamb M, ed. *The Role of the Father in Child Development.* New York: Wiley; 1976.
65. Cronenwett L, Knunst-Wilson W. Stress, social support and the transition to fatherhood. *Nurs Res.* 1983;5:29.
66. McBride AB. Differences in women's and men's thinking about parent-child interactions. *Res in Nurs and Health.* 1985;8:389–396.
67. Cain R, et al. Effects of the father's presence or absence during a cesarean delivery. *Birth.* 1984;11:10–15.
68. Pedersen F, et al. Cesarean childbirth: psychological implications for mothers and fathers. *Infant Ment Health J.* 1981;11:23–28.
69. Vietze P, O'Conner S. Mother to infant bonding: a review. In: Kretchmer N, Brasel J, eds. *Biomedical and Social Bases of Pediatrics.* New York: Masson; 1980.
70. Grossman F, et al. *Pregnancy, Birth and Parenthood.* San Francisco: Jossey-Bass; 1980.
71. Pedersen F, Robson K. Father participation in infancy. *Am J Orthopsychiatry.* 1969;39:466–472.
72. Fein R. Men's entrance to parenthood. *Fam Coordinator.* 1976;25:341–348.
73. Jordon PL. Laboring for relevance: expectant and new fatherhood. *Nurs Res.* 1990;39:11–16.
74. Pedersen F, ed. *In the Beginning: Readings in Infancy.* New York: Columbia University Press; 1982.
75. Bem S, Lenny E. Sex typing and the avoidance of cross-sex behavior. *J Pers Soc Psychol.* 1979;33:48–54.
76. Bem S, et al. Sex typing and androgyny: further explorations of the expressive domain. *J Pers Soc Psychol.* 1976; 34:1016–1023.
77. Russell G. The father role and its relation to masculinity, femininity, and androgyny. *Child Dev.* 1978;49:1174–1181.
78. Bem S. The measurement of psychological androgyny. *J Consult Clin Psychol.* 1974;42:155–162.
79. Yogman M. Observations on the father-infant relationship. In: Cath S, Gurwitt A, Ross JM, eds. *Father and Child.* Boston: Little, Brown; 1982.
80. Ferketich SL, Mercer RT. Men's health status during pregnancy and early fatherhood. *Res in Nurs and Health.* 1989; 12:137–148.
81. Earls F, Yogman M. The father-infant relationship. In: Howells J, ed. *Modern Perspectives in the Psychiatry of Infancy.* New York: Brunner-Mazel; 1979.
82. Abbott L. *Paternal Touch of the Newborn: Its Role in Paternal Attachment.* Boston: Boston University, School of Nursing; 1975. Master's thesis.
83. Parke R. Pespectives in father-infant interaction. In: Osofsky J, ed. *The Handbook of Infant Development.* New York: Wiley; 1979.
84. Greenburg M, Morris N. Engrossment: the newborn's impact upon the father. *Am J Orthopsychiatry.* 1974;44: 520–531.
85. Pedersen F, et al. Conceptualization of father influences in the infancy period. In: Lewis M, Rosenblum L, eds. *The Child and Its Family.* New York: Plenum; 1979.
86. Lamb M. *The Role of the Father in Child Development.* New York: Wiley; 1981.
87. Lamb M. Effects of stress and cohort on mother-and-father-infant interaction. *Dev Psychol.* 1976;12:435–443.
88. Lamb M. The development of parental preferences in the first two years of life. *Sex Roles.* 1977;3:495–497.
89. Lamb M. Father-infant and mother-infant interaction in the first year of life. *Child Dev.* 1977;48:167–181.
90. Kutzner S. Responses of siblings to pregnancy. In: Sherwen L, ed. *Psychosocial Dimensions of the Pregnant Family.* New York: Springer, 1987.
91. Dunn J, et al. The reaction of first-born children to the birth of a sibling: mothers' reports. *J Child Psychol Psychiatry.* 1981;22:1–18.
92. Dunn J. *Sisters and Brothers.* Cambridge, Mass: Harvard University Press; 1985.
93. Dunn J, Kendrick C. The arrival of a sibling: changes in patterns of interaction between mother and first-born child. *Annu Prog Child Psychiatry Child Dev.* 1981;36: 362–379.
94. Taylor D. Reflections on parenting: a multigenerational perspective. *Family Process.* 1983;22:341–346.
95. Mercer R. Predictors of maternal role attainment at one year post birth. *West J Nurs Res.* 1986;8:9–32.
96. Soule B, et al. Father identity. *Psychiatry.* 1979;42:255–263.
97. Spector R. *Cultural Diversity in Health and Illness.* 2nd ed. Norwalk, Conn: Appleton-Century-Crofts; 1985.
98. Attneane C. American Indians and Alaska Native families: emigrants in their own homeland. In: McGoldrick M, et al, eds. *Ethnicity and Family Therapy.* New York: Guilford; 1982.
99. Primeaux M. American Indian health care practices: a cross-cultural perspective. *Nurs Clin North Am.* 1977;12: 57.

100. Farris L. The American Indian. In: Clark A, ed. *Culture, Childbearing, Health Professionals.* Philadelphia: FA Davis; 1978.
101. Helton A. *Protocol of Care for the Battered Woman.* Houston: Texas Woman's University; 1986.
102. Carrington BW. The Afro-American. In: Clark A, ed. *Culture, Childbearing, Health Professionals.* Philadelphia: FA Davis; 1978.
103. Kay MA. The Mexican American. In: Clark A, ed. *Culture, Childbearing, Health Professionals.* Philadelphia: FA Davis; 1978.
104. Stringfellow L. The Vietnamese. In: Clark A, ed. *Culture, Childbearing, Health Professionals.* Philadelphia: FA Davis; 1978.
105. Hawkins J, Gorvine B. *Postpartum Nursing, Health Care of Women.* New York: Springer Publishing Co; 1985.
106. McKay S, Phillips C. *Family-Centered Maternity Care.* Rockville, Md: Aspen; 1984.
107. David JH, et al. A study of mothers' postpartum teaching priorities. *Matern Child Nurs J.* 1988;17:441–450.
108. Hampson SJ. Nursing intervention for the first 3 postpartum months. *J Obstet Gynecol Neonat Nurs.* 1989;18:116–121.
109. Elmer E, Maloni J. Parent support through telephone consultation. *Matern Child Nurs J.* 1988;17:13–23.

Assessment and Nursing Care of the Family During the Postpartum Period

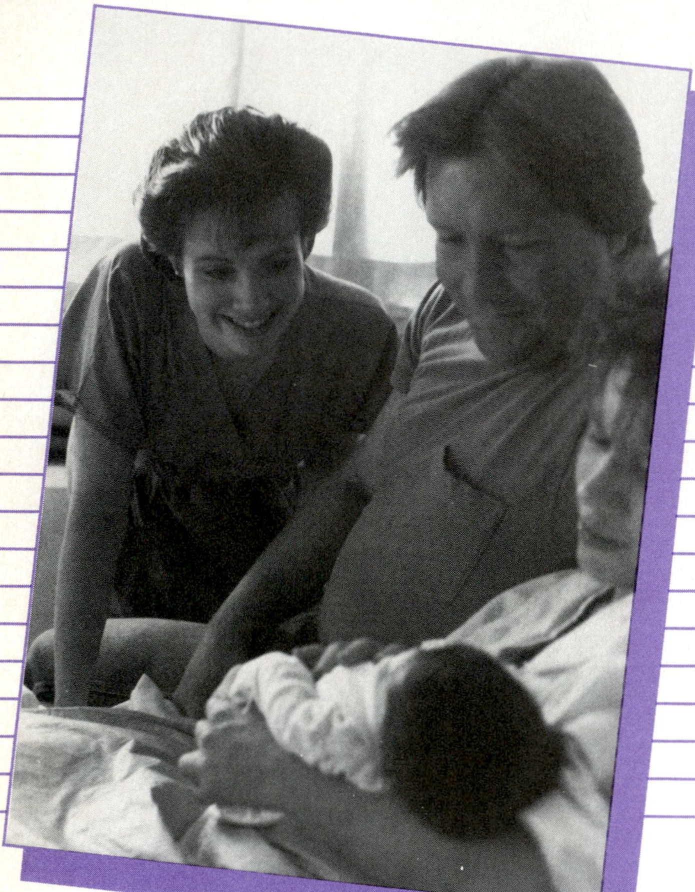

chapter 31

Key Terms

"afterpains"
engorgement
inverted nipples

The postpartum period is a time for maternal physical and psychologic restoration. Nursing care is a critical factor influencing the degree to which maternal restoration is achieved. To provide high-quality nursing care, each postpartum mother must be viewed as an individual. Sound nursing care is achieved when the nursing process is adhered to judiciously. In this chapter, nursing assessments of the major physiologic systems routinely appraised in the postpartum period, and the nursing care needed, are addressed. The reader is referred to Chapter 27 for a detailed discussion of nursing assessments and care during the fourth stage of labor, to Chapter 28 for an in-depth discussion of nursing care of the mother who has a cesarean delivery, and to Chapter 30 for nursing considerations related to the psychologic aspects of the postpartum period.

During the first few days of the postpartum period, the nurse plays a key role in the delivery of care that the postpartum woman receives. In planning and providing care, the nurse coordinates the care the woman receives from other health professionals. The nurse collaboratively works with nurse-midwives, physicians, dieticians, social workers, and other specialists.

The postpartum nurse is frequently the first health care professional to identify the physical, psychologic, and educational problems, needs, and assets of the postpartum family. As the nurse identifies the specific facets of care needed for a given woman and her family, she or he determines whether other health care professionals or laypersons are needed to provide care or support along with nurses. When other health care professionals are required the nurse and those health care professionals work collaboratively. Frequently, nurses make referrals to community resources such as parent or breastfeeding support groups.

In most institutions, nurses and physicians have developed a list of standing orders that have been found to be effective in treating many of the common physiologic problems encountered in the puerperium, for example, breast engorgement and postpartum pain. The nurse then has the responsibility of helping the woman select the appropriate treatments. If pathologic problems develop, for example, hemorrhage, the nurse notifies the physician, and a collaborative plan of care is formulated and implemented.

In those situations in which women opt for early discharge from the hospital, or when ongoing problems are identified, the hospital nurse identifies the ongoing needs of an individual family and makes referrals to the appropriate nursing agency for follow-up care in the home. In some settings a nurse may make a home visit to provide continuity of care.

THE DATA BASE

To formulate comprehensive care plans that yield desirable outcomes, the nurse needs to obtain pertinent subjective data with emphasis on the major systems that are affected in the puerperium. The initial subjective data base includes a review of systems pertinent to the puerperium. The subjective data collection also focuses on daily habits, past history, changes during pregnancy, perception of present status, and cultural and social expectations. Any current problem identified should have a complete symptom review exploring onset, duration, location, quality, quantity, precipitating factors, aggravating factors, alleviating factors, time-associated factors, and previous history of a similar problem. Subjective data should also include the mother's perception of her knowledge level concerning self-care, the puerperium, breastfeeding, bottlefeeding, infant care, and family dynamics. After the initial data base is collected, subsequent daily subjective data focus on present status and potential problems, needs, and assets.

Subjective data can be obtained prior to or along with the physical examination. As problems or needs are identified, the experienced nurse can incorporate the implementation of interventions into the time when the mother is physically assessed; for example, breast self-examination can be taught at the same time that the nurse examines the mother's breasts.

The objective data base includes the physical assessment data collected through the use of inspection/observation, palpation, percussion, and auscultation, as well as laboratory data. Physical assessment is usually performed from the general to the more specific, and in a cephalocaudal (or head-to-toe) manner. On postpartum units, the mother is given a postpartum physical, frequently referred to as a postpartum check, once a shift. In addition to the postpartum check, the nurse collects objective data related to the mother and infant on a 24-hour basis. A postpartum flow sheet, such as the one presented in Figure 31–1, can be helpful in delineating the routinely assessed systems.

Analysis of all data identifies physical, psychosocial, and educational problems, needs, and assets on which care plans are developed. As much of postpartum nursing care evolves around educating the mother, a postpartum flow sheet (Figure 31–1) delineating the knowledge area assessed, the education given, and the evaluation of the education can be helpful in documenting this facet of care.

ADMISSION TO THE POSTPARTUM UNIT

On the mother's admission to the postpartum unit, the admitting nurse is given a brief report from the recovery room or labor and delivery nurse. The report contains the the length of labor; type of delivery; status of fetal membranes and amniotic fluid; vital signs and status/progress of mother since delivery; medication, treatment, and other care since delivery; blood type of mother; laboratory data; prenatal risk factors and health problems; newborn status; and psychosocial responses of parents to the newborn. After receiving the report, the nurse needs to make certain that the mother has physically and psychologically tolerated the transfer to the postpartum unit. Consequently, an initial assessment of the mother's emotional status, vital signs, pain/discomfort level, fatigue, thirst, hunger, uterine fundus, bladder, perineum, and lochia is performed. If the mother is receiving intravenous fluids, the intravenous site, the tubing, and the amount of fluid left in the bottle are assessed. Those mothers who had received analgesia and anesthesia would be assessed for sensation level, ability to move body parts, and level of consciousness. Additional assessment made for mothers who have had a cesarean delivery includes appraisal of respiratory status, abdominal dressing/incision, urinary output via a Foley catheter, and ability to move and turn. An in-depth description of the physical assessment of the major systems appraised is provided under "Routine Assessments and Nursing Care."

Although most women are stable on transfer to the postpartum unit, the time may not be appropriate to obtain in-depth subjective data or to assess educational needs. The postpartum mother's need for rest, food, and fluid, her need to interact with significant others, her degree of pain and discomfort, and the effects from medications frequently de-

Client's Name ________________ **Gravida** ___ **Para** _____
Delivery Date ________

Physical Assessment

	Shift		Remarks
Vital Signs			
Blood pressure			
Pulse			
Respirations			
Temperature			
Fundus			
Condition			
Height and location			
Lochia/Vaginal Discharge			
Color			
Amount and condition			
Number of pads changed			
Breasts			
Breast or bottle feeding			
Engorgement			
Nipple tenderness			
Lactation suppression medication:	Yes ___No___	Name of medication	
Incision/Lacerations (REEDA)			
Perineum Episiotomy site Lacerations			
Abdominal incision Appearance Dressing change Wound irrigation			
Nutrition Diet Intake			
Fluids Type and amount IV solution, rate, site			
Elimination			
Voided Amount Any discomforts			
Bowel movement Number and type Constipation Treatments			

Figure 31–1. Postpartum flow sheet. (*Figure continues.*)

Physical Assessment			
	Shift		Remarks
Comfort Measures			
Rest			
Pain (type, location intensity)			
Homan's sign			
Interventions Sitz bath Witch hazel pads Surgigator Pericare Nipple shield Breast binder Benzocaine spray Analgesic (name, route, time) Other			

Psychosocial Assessment			
	Shift		Remarks
Coping Appearance, behavior			
Interactions Maternal/infant Paternal/infant Sibling visitation Grandparent Support systems			

Education			
Knowledge and Skills	**Date and Time**	**Present: Mother, Father, Other Supports**	**Outcome (Needs reinforcement, return demonstration, assessment)**
Postpartum Assessments			
Comfort Measures			
Sitz bath procedure and frequency			
Pedicare Medications			
Nutrition			
Elimination			
Exercises			
Preventive Measures Rh (D) immune globulin Rubella Breast self-examination Family planning Reportable signs and symptoms Physician/midwife appointment			

Figure 31–1 (*continued*). Postpartum flow sheet.

Education			
Knowledge and Skills	**Date and Time**	**Present: Mother, Father, Other Supports**	**Outcome (Needs reinforcement, return demonstration, assessment)**
Discharge Planning			

Rest/sleep
Exercises/daily activities
Sexual activity
Return to work
Infant care
  Appearance
  Senses and reflexes
  Temperature taking
  Sleep/wake cycles
  Stools
  Feeding
  Bathing
  Cord Care
  Circumcision Care
  Skin
  Handling
  Diapering
Community resources
  Parenting classes
  La Leche League
  Day care
  Car seat rental
  Child health clinics
  Referral			

Figure 31–1 (*continued*). Postpartum flow sheet.

termine the nature of nurse-client interactions. Nursing interactions at this time frequently involve orienting the mother to the room and to usual hospital procedures, providing the mother with food and fluids, making certain the mother is comfortable, and providing time for sleep, rest, or privacy. The nurse should explain that after the client's immediate needs are met, a nurse will further assess her status and develop an individualized plan of care. Prior to leaving the room, the nurse should caution the mother that she should not get out of bed unless assisted by the nurse at least for the first time and until she is physically stable.

About the time of admission to the postpartum unit mothers often have the urge to void. Women who deliver vaginally without anesthesia may be out of bed to void after the first hour postpartum provided that vital signs are stable and there are no signs of hemorrhage. Because of the rapid change in body posture on rising out of bed, many women experience hypotension when standing for the first time. Accordingly, the nurse needs to initiate preventive measures: the nurse carries spirits of ammonia to use if the client becomes faint; the client is instructed to dangle her feet over the side of the bed for a few minutes before rising; and the client is assisted with ambulation (Figure 31–2). When in the bathroom, the nurse needs to show the mother where the emergency call button is and how to use it in case of future problems. In many settings the mother is told that the first three voids will need to be measured to assess bladder elimination accurately. The nurse also instructs the mother on pericare, as outlined later under "Perineum." Provided the mother is not experiencing lightheadedness, the nurse can step outside of the bathroom to allow the mother some privacy; however, the nurse should remain near the bathroom, ready to assist the mother as needed. After using the bathroom, the mother is assisted back to bed. If the mother's first experience out of bed is uneventful, she may be permitted out of bed without assistance. The mother should be instructed to continue to dangle her feet before rising out of bed and to call for help if any signs of lightheadedness occur.

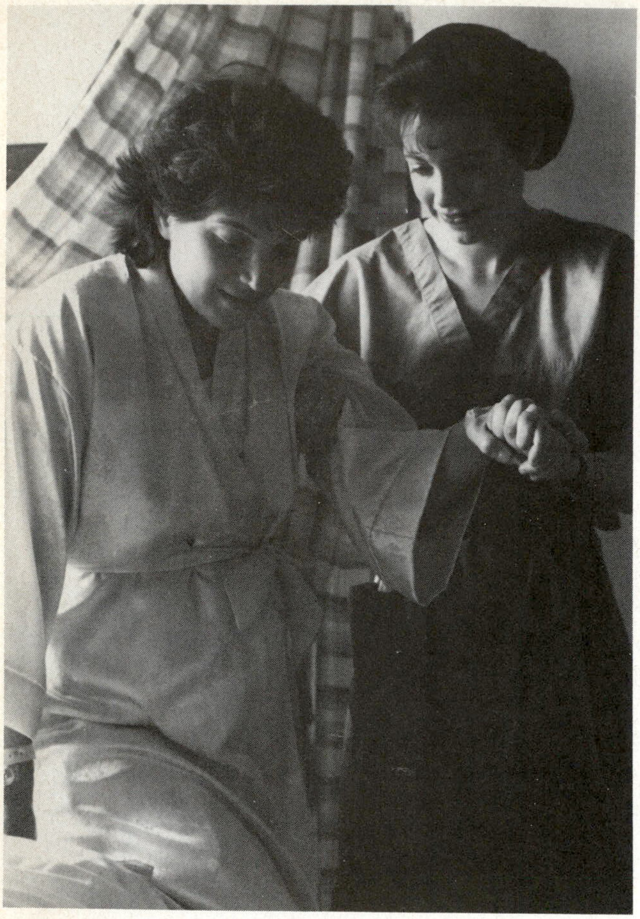

Figure 31–2. Nurse assisting client out of bed for the first time after delivery.

ROUTINE ASSESSMENTS AND NURSING CARE

General Data and Survey

Subjective data obtained daily focus on the mother's self-perception of her level of energy, a symptom review of pain, discomfort, and other problems, degree to which basic needs (such as sleep, hunger, and cleanliness) are met, ability to perform self-care, success of breastfeeding (if appropriate), emotions and feelings (about labor and delivery, the baby), and identification of areas of concern or education deficits. Additionally, the mother's ongoing evaluation of how successful interventions have been is needed.

The objective general survey of the postpartum mother includes skin color, facial expression, grooming, posture, motor activity, gait, personal hygiene, body odor, speech, level of awareness/consciousness, mood, and affect. Data collected from the general survey, when combined with the general subjective data, often determine the focus of immediate nursing care. Complaints of extreme fatigue, lack of energy, little sleep or rest, and a high degree of discomfort coupled with a depressed mood, slouched or bent posture, and inability to provide self-care alert the nurse that the needs for physical and psychologic restoration have not been fulfilled yet. If these needs are not met, the mother may be unable to fully interact with and assume complete responsibility for her infant. An extremely offensive, foul odor to the lochia alerts the nurse to a possible uterine infection. A teary-eyed or crying mother alerts the nurse to possible transitory or postpartum depression. Subsequent nursing assessments and care are then focused on the initial cues the nurse receives from the mother.

Vital Signs

During the first hour postpartum, the mother's pulse, respirations, and blood pressure are assessed every 15 minutes. If stable, pulse, respirations, and blood pressure are then assessed at half-hour intervals for 1 hour, followed by vital sign checks every 4 hours for 24 hours and thereafter every 8 hours. Temperature is assessed at the onset of the first hour postpartum. If the mother is afebrile, temperature may be reassessed every 2 hours for a minimum of two readings, followed by a check every 4 hours during the next 24 hours and thereafter every 8 hours.

A pulse rate of 50 to 70 beats per minute is quite common. Higher pulse rates may indicate hemorrhage, cardiac disease, infection, and anxiety. When the mother experiences tachycardia the nurse should immediately assess for hemorrhage by focusing on the blood pressure, uterine tone, quantity of lochia, and condition of the perineum or abdominal dressing/incision.

Blood pressure should be fairly consistent with prelabor measurements. A suddenly low blood pressure alerts the nurse to hemorrhage, orthostatic hypotension, and a possible adverse reaction to regional anesthesia (if hypotension occurs shortly after administration of regional anesthesia). A blood pressure elevated well above the mother's baseline blood pressure, or an increase of 30 mm Hg in systolic pressure, 15 mm Hg in diastolic pressure, or both, suggests pregnancy-induced hypertension. The nurse needs to assess for headaches, epigastric pain, edema, and hyperreflexia. The mother should be instructed to lie on her left side, and a physician should be notified. The nurse should be prepared to place the mother on seizure precautions should the hypertension persist.

During the first 24 hours, temperature is usually normal. Slight elevations in the temperature up to 38°C (100.4°F) suggest dehydration. Higher elevations during the first 24 hours or a temperature above 38°C after 24 hours is indicative of infection. Temperature will need to be assessed at least every 4 hours during the first 24 hours and then every 4 to 8 hours, unless elevated. The nurse should assess the mother for overt signs of puerperal infection, for example, foul lochia and inflamed incisional/lacerated areas with purulent drainage, as well as nonpuerperal infections, for example, respiratory infection as evidenced by cold symptoms and urinary tract infection with associated flank tenderness or pain and dysuria. The most likely areas for puerperal infection are the uterus, the bladder, any incision line or lacerated area (eg, an episiotomy or repaired lacerations), and the cesarean incision line. Lochia cultures, obtained from within the uterus, and urine cultures would usually be ordered.

Respirations generally are within normal limits in the puerperium. Slightly increased respirations may be present with anxiety and pain. A slightly diminished respiratory rate may be the result of analgesia and anesthesia. Respiratory depression secondary to narcotic administration is treated with a narcotic antagonist, for example, naloxone (Narcan), levallorphan (Lorfan), and nalorphine (Nalline).

Breasts

Subjective data from the mother are needed regarding the method of infant feeding; the mother's knowledge of breast care, lactation, and suppression of lactation; a history of breast disease or problems; and whether or not the mother practices breast self-examination. On a daily basis the nurse should ask the breastfeeding mother about the progress in breastfeeding and status/condition of the breasts. The bottlefeeding mother should also be asked about the status of her breasts and how successfully lactation has been suppressed.

Physical examination of each breast should begin with inspection. The nurse should first note if the mother is wearing a brassiere. Both breastfeeding and bottlefeeding mothers should be wearing a supportive brassiere; if not, the nurse will need to instruct the mother about the need for breast support. During the examination the brassiere should be removed or, for lactating women wearing a nursing brassiere, the cups can be opened. The breasts are inspected for shape, contour, general symmetry, direction of nipples, degree of nipple prominence, condition of nipples and areolae, areas of redness, venous distension, fullness, and leakage. The breasts may then be palpated to determine temperature, nodules, and degree to which they are filling with milk (Figure 31–3). As the nurse palpates the breasts, the mother is asked whether or not she is experiencing any discomfort or tenderness. The nurse completes palpation of the breasts, determining nipple erectility. Additionally, the breastfeeding mother may be asked to demonstrate manual expression of colostrum or milk from her breasts.

During the physical examination of the breasts, the nurse can reinforce general breast care. While performing a breast examination the nurse also has the opportunity to teach or reinforce breast self-examination.

Common Breast Problems

Engorgement. At 2 to 4 days postpartum, as the milk begins to fill the breast, many women experience engorgement as characterized by heat, tightness, pressure, and pain in the breasts. **Engorgement** is the normal swelling of the breasts that results from an increase in the blood and lymph supply to the breasts and the beginning of milk production. Engorgement is present when the breasts are extremely firm, frequently with areas of hardness, and warm to the touch; venous distension is pronounced; areas of redness are prominent; and there is leakage from the breasts. For the lactating mother, engorgement, although uncomfortable, is a positive sign that lactation is progressing. Engorgement, however, may also oc-

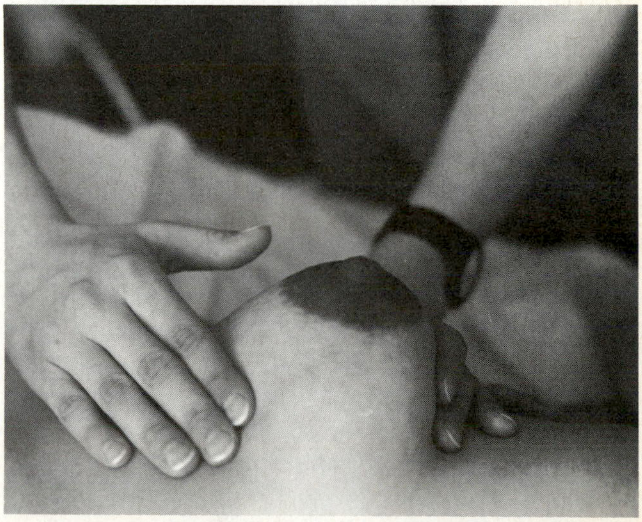

Figure 31–3. Nurse assessing woman's breasts.

cur with nonbreastfeeding mothers. Nursing interventions implemented to alleviate discomfort and resolve engorgement are dependent on whether the mother is breastfeeding or bottlefeeding her infant. With the appropriate interventions, acute discomfort resolves in about 24 hours; suppression of lactation in the bottlefeeding mother can require a week or longer; and full resolution of engorgement in the lactating mother occurs in a couple of weeks as milk supply and the demand for milk become synchronized.

Interventions for the Breastfeeding Mother. Soon after delivery, the mother is instructed to wear a well-fitting, supportive brassiere continuously during the early puerperium and for approximately one to two months. Thereafter the mother may be able to remove the brassiere at night, during sleep hours. The supportive brassiere minimizes the heavy feeling in the breasts that occurs with engorgement and also provides support.

To minimize discomfort and eventually resolve engorgement in the lactating woman the breasts need to be emptied regularly and frequently. With breast engorgement the most effective means of emptying the breasts is to encourage the infant to feed about every 2 hours for a maximum of 10 minutes on each breast. (Women not experiencing any breast discomfort need not limit the feeding time as long as feeding time is gradually built up.) The mother can further assist in emptying the breast during the feeding by massaging the breast, especially the tail and upper, outer quadrant, when she observes that the infant is no longer ingesting milk. As the milk drains from the alveolar lumina and arrives at the lactiferous sinuses, the infant's sucking will slow and become more rhythmic to withdraw the milk. If the infant does not drain the breasts or is unwilling to suckle, the mother can relieve engorgement by manual or mechanical expression of milk.[1]

With engorgement the lactating breasts become so filled with milk that the nipple and areola may not soften to allow the infant to grasp on for feeding. The mother may experience acute pain as the infant tries to grasp the nipple; in this situation a mild analgesic, administered before the feeding, is appropriate. Additionally, prior to the feeding the areola and nipple need to be softened by releasing some milk. A warm shower or application of warm compresses to the breast may provide enough stimulation to release some milk from the breasts. If not, the manual expression of some of the milk is indicated.

The breastfeeding mother who is experiencing extreme discomfort from engorgement can try applying ice to the breasts. As the infant is still stimulating the breast when feeding, the use of ice packs does not often result in an inadequate milk supply.

Interventions for the Bottlefeeding Mother. To effectively resolve engorgement in bottlefeeding mothers, lactation needs to be suppressed. Medications used to suppress lactation are discussed later, under "Pharmacotherapeutics." Lactation, however, can be suppressed and engorgement resolved without medication.[2,3] Minimizing stimulation to the breasts, wearing a support bra, wearing a compression binder, restricting fluid intake, and applying ice packs to the breasts reduce discomfort from engorgement and help to suppress lactation.[2] Brooten and colleagues[3] found that women using a compression binder experienced less leakage of colostrum and milk than women using a bra or restricting fluid.

To minimize stimulation to the breasts, mothers need to be cautioned that when showering, water should flow from the back over to the breasts. Additionally hot water should be avoided. Until lactation is fully suppressed stimulation of the breasts during sexual activity should be avoided.

Some bottlefeeding mothers believe that discomfort from engorgement can be relieved through the expression of colostrum or milk. Although this intervention may temporarily relieve breast pain, lactation may be inadvertently stimulated. If milk is expressed, ice packs should be applied immediately afterward to diminish blood flow to the breasts.

Cracked/Bleeding Nipples. On physical examination, the nurse may find that the breastfeeding mother's nipples are cracked and bleeding. Periodic observation of infant feedings is necessary to identify improper feeding techniques that lead to nipple trauma. Nipples tend to crack and bleed if the infant fails to take in the areola, if the nipple is improperly removed from the infant's mouth, and if nipple toughening is delayed. The nurse should make certain that the mother is offered assistance and guidance during the initial feedings. Frequently, mothers believe that they are expected to know how to breastfeed and thus are reluctant to ask for help. The nurse needs to dispel this belief and provide an atmosphere that encourages the mother to express concerns and needs. Much of the trauma to the breasts, and difficulty in breastfeeding in general, can be lessened with proper education. Measures used to treat cracked/bleeding nipples are listed in Table 31–1.

Women need to be made aware that if the nipples bleed they may find small amounts of blood in the infant's mouth or in regurgitated milk. These

TABLE 31–1. MANAGING CRACKED/BLEEDING NIPPLES

1. Manually express some milk before the feeding so the infant can latch onto the nipple easily and will not need to suck vigorously.
2. Take a mild analgesic before the feeding, if nipples are painful.
3. Offer the breast that is least sore first so that the more vigorous sucking is on the less sore nipple.[4]
4. Breastfeed no longer than 5 minutes on the sore breast; after the nipple has healed, increase the time gradually.[4]
5. Wear a nipple shield during the feedings, but cease using the shield as soon as possible so that infant does not become dependent on it; stop using the shield if discomfort increases.
6. Wash the nipples with water after feeding.
7. Expose the nipples to air for 10 to 20 minutes after washing them.
8. Apply either a light coat of lanolin or a wet tea bag to the nipples.

women can continue to breastfeed; however, they need to be aware of the potential for breast infection.

Inverted Nipples. Occasionally some mothers have **inverted nipples.** True inverted nipples remain flat or retract inward when stimulated (Figure 31–4). Often nipples appear inverted but can be drawn out manually. Infants have difficulty latching on to the breast with an inverted nipple. Nipple exercises and wearing a nipple shield prenatally may gradually stretch the nipple's attachment to the breast (Figure 31–5). If prenatal treatment was not instituted or was unsuccessful, the woman is counseled postnatally as outlined in Table 31–2.

Lungs

Generally, unless there are signs of respiratory infection, respiratory distress, or respiratory depression, the nurse does not need to routinely assess the lungs of a woman who has delivered vaginally. The nurse does, however, need to observe the quality and rate of respirations and to be alert for signs of respiratory difficulty, as some women are predisposed to embolic diseases. Sudden onset of unexplained dyspnea may be related to a pulmonary embolism. When hemoptysis and pleuritic chest pain accompany the sudden dyspnea, pulmonary infarction, resulting from an embolism, may have occurred.

Women who have delivered by cesarean, like other clients who have had major surgery, should be assessed daily for respiratory status. In particular, be-

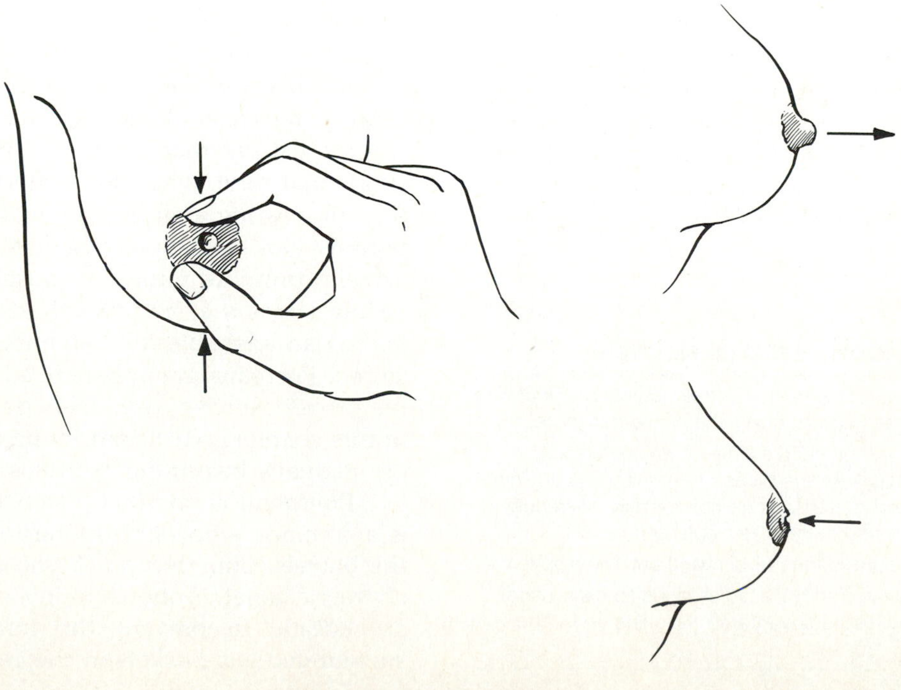

Figure 31–4. Inverted nipples.

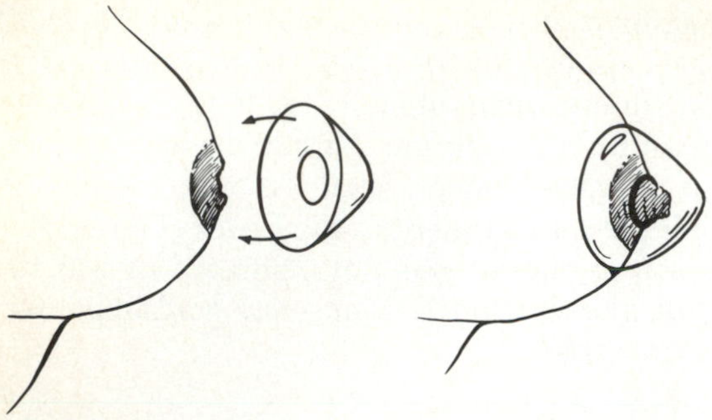

Figure 31–5. Nipple shield for inverted nipples.

cause of the anesthesia administered during delivery, impaired mobility resulting from surgery, and abdominal pain that restricts deep breathing and coughing, the woman who delivers by cesarean is prone to accumulation of mucus in the lungs with a potential for respiratory infection and atelectasis. The lungs should be assessed daily. The chest should expand symmetrically, even if the mother does not voluntarily allow full expansion because of abdominal pain. The nurse assesses for equal resonant percussion notes and clear lungs on auscultation. If adventitious sounds are auscultated, the nurse should ask the mother to take a few deep breaths and to cough. The lungs should then be reassessed. Frequently, coughing loosens and moves secretions up through the lung.

Deviations from the norms, for example, a deviated trachea, asymmetry of chest expansion, fremitus, or percussion notes, and the presence of persistent rales or rhonchi, should be reported to the physician immediately. A deviated trachea and unilateral dull area on percussion with diminished to absent tactile and vocal fremitus are suggestive of a collapsed or atelectatic lung and may occur secondary to a respiratory infection and mucus plugging of the bronchi.

TABLE 31–2. MANAGING INVERTED NIPPLES

1. Wear a breast shield (eg, Nesty Breast Shield or Woolwich Shield) between feedings to bring the nipple out more.
2. Exercise the nipple four or five times a day by placing thumbs or forefingers at the sides of the nipple and gradually pulling toward the areola edge horizontally; then position thumbs above and below the nipple and repeat.
3. Pump the breast as a means of drawing out the nipple.
4. Try holding the infant in different positions to determine which position facilitates the infant's latching on to the breast.

Measures to prevent respiratory stasis of mucus initiated immediately after surgery include deep breathing and coughing every 2 hours, use of incentive spirometry, turning every 2 hours, and early ambulation.

Abdomen

General Tone. The shape, appearance, and general muscle tone of the puerperal abdomen are often a source of concern for women. Postpartum women frequently express their displeasure with their flabby, still pregnant-looking abdomens. Subjective data focus on the individual woman's perception of self, her body image; knowledge of the gradual change in the shape and appearance of her body; and knowledge of exercises.

On physical assessment the puerperal abdomen, in the first week after delivery, looks about 5 months pregnant. The abdomen is frequently flabby, unless distended with flatulence. With trapped flatus the abdomen distends upward, as opposed to laterally, when the mother is lying down in the bed. A large, flabby abdomen indicates diminished muscle tone. Most often the rectus abdominis is separated, a condition termed *diastasis rectus abdominis* (Figure 31–6). To assess for diastasis of the muscles, the mother is instructed to lie flat and then raise her head, placing her chin on her chest. A visible pouching out of the abdomen running vertically from the xiphoid process to the symphysis pubis is found on inspection. On palpation the separation of the muscles is evident and may be measured.

Postpartum mothers often need information concerning the restoration of abdominal tone. Many women believe that wearing a girdle helps restore abdominal tone. The nurse should explain that although wearing a girdle may make the woman temporarily look like she is in better shape, it does not actually promote return of muscle tone. The nurse should stress that by properly exercising and maintaining an adequate diet, abdominal tone can be restored. Postpartum mothers need to be instructed on the proper exercises (*see* "Exercise and Activity" later in this chapter). Particular emphasis must be placed on gradually beginning exercises.

Puerperal abdominal distension from flatulence is a common sign of temporary diminished tone of the bowels. Simethicone (Mylicon), an antiflatulent chewable tablet, is often administered after meals and at bedtime to prevent the formation of mucus-surrounded gas pockets in the gastrointestinal tract.

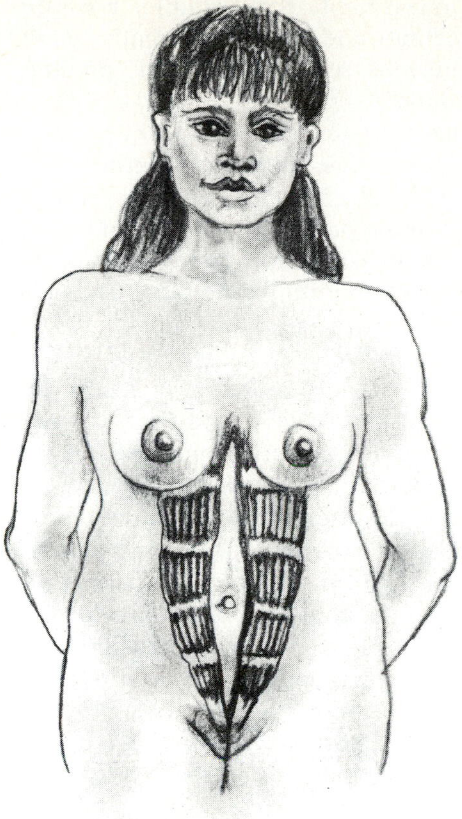

Figure 31–6. Separation of rectus muscles in the abdomen.

Additionally, interventions implemented to restore bowel functioning in the puerperium also promote the expulsion of flatus and restore general bowel and abdominal tone. Once bowel functioning is fully restored, abdominal distention from flatulence should be resolved.

Bowels. The nurse needs to take a history of bowel elimination. Emphasis is placed on obtaining data about bowel habits, quality and timing of last bowel movement, dietary and fluid intake, degree of ambulation, presence of perineal and rectal discomfort, and use of aids to promote bowel functioning. The nurse must elicit the information in terms of prepregnancy history, pregnancy history, intrapartum experience, and the postpartum.

In assessing bowel function, the nurse must also take into account any analgesics and other medications given to the mother. Codeine and codeine products may promote constipation.

To assess for bowel functioning the nurse first inspects for abdominal distension as discussed previously. Then the nurse auscultates the abdomen in all four quadrants. Further assessment of the abdomen is performed through percussion and palpation of the abdomen. Normal bowel functioning is characterized by bowel sounds, that is, clicks and gurgles, occurring at a rate of 5 to 34 per minute; generalized tympany and areas of dullness (caused by varying amounts of fat), with a prominent tympanic gastric bubble over the stomach; and a soft abdomen. High-pitched tinkling sounds are indicative of intestinal air and fluid under tension in the bowel. Sluggish bowels, characterized by abdominal distension, infrequent bowel sounds, generalized tympany of the bowels upon percussion, and a lack of bowel movements, are common in the first few days postpartum as a result of the common occurrences of loose bowel movements or an enema during labor, lack of food ingestion while in labor, and diminished activity level after delivery. Furthermore, in the first few days after delivery, especially while in the hospital, some women do not resume their usual dietary intake. If constipation occurs, the abdomen may be distended; increased bowel sounds may be heard with early obstruction, followed by decreased bowel sounds if bowel obstruction is prolonged; stool may be palpated within the bowels when the woman is examined abdominally.

As the postpartum woman's dietary intake of roughage and fluids increase, and as the effects from anesthesia, labor and delivery, or surgery diminish, peristalsis increases. For many women, bowel functioning is restored without the implementation of overt interventions. For some women with episiotomies, lacerations, and hemorrhoids, bowel functioning may be impaired out of pain and fear of further harm to the perineum. If interventions are not initiated constipation may ensue.

Interventions to alleviate or prevent constipation generally include drinking at least 6 to 8 glasses of fluid a day to keep stool soft and promote hydration, assuming renal function is normal; maintaining a diet that contains fresh fruits, raw vegetables, whole bran or whole grain cereals, and bread to provide fiber; and participating in daily exercises to promote peristalsis (eg, in the hospital, frequent ambulation). If no bowel movement occurs in 2 to 3 days, one of the following measures may be used: glycerine suppository, bisacodyl (Dulcolax) suppository, 30 mL of Milk of magnesia; or 50 mg of dioctyl sodium sulfosuccinate (Colace). If the woman does not have a bowel movement, another intervention such as an enema may be given.

Oral stool softeners and laxatives are frequently

given routinely to prevent constipation and are the treatment of choice for women with fourth-degree lacerations, as the administration of suppositories and enemas can rupture the sutures for extensive lacerations. Once the lacerations have healed, an enema, if needed, is permitted.

Uterus. During the early postpartum, the mother's knowledge about uterine involution, uterine massage, and reproduction should be assessed. Additionally, the nurse collects objective and subjective data concerning characteristics of lochia including amount, color, odor, and changes noted, as well as data pertaining to afterpains.

Uterine Involution. With each postpartum check uterine tone is assessed by palpating the uterine fundus. To assess the fundus, the postpartum mother is asked to lie with the bed flat. The nurse places one hand on the lower abdomen and, beginning a few centimeters above the umbilicus and moving downward, palpates with the other hand for the uterine fundus (Figure 31–7). Immediately after delivery, the fundus is approximately midway between the umbilicus and the symphysis pubis; by 12 hours after delivery the fundus rises to the umbilicus or slightly above; and thereafter the fundus descends 1 to 2 cm (approximately one fingerbreath) per day. The fundus should be in a contracted state and thus should be firm on palpation. Additionally, the fundus should be found on the midline of the abdomen. Various notations are used by nurses to record the fundal assessment. For example, a fundus that is firm, midline, and one fingerbreath below the umbilicus may be recorded as "FF1, midline" or "FF U/1, midline."

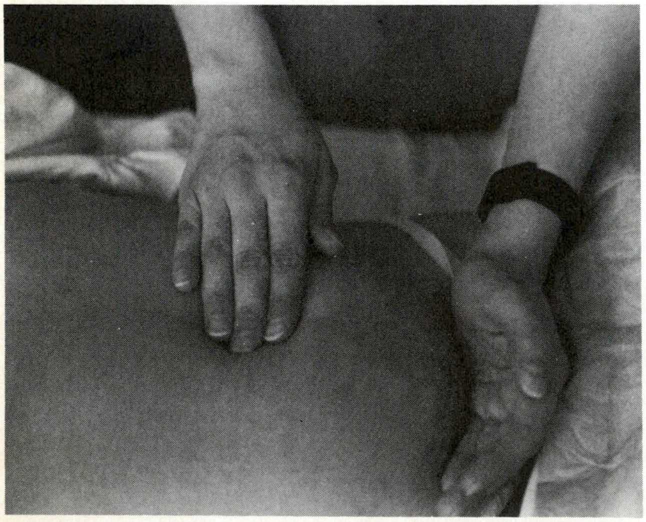

Figure 31–7. Nurse-midwife assessing fundal height.

While palpating the uterus, the nurse should assess for excessive uterine tenderness. Abdominal guarding, facial grimacing, and subjective verbalization of extreme pain are indicative of uterine tenderness and suggest an infection of the uterus. Medical follow-up and monitoring for signs and symptoms of infection are indicated.

Occasionally the nurse may find that the fundus is soft, boggy, and deviated to one side. The woman should be asked to void and then the uterus reassessed. To prevent uterine hemorrhage, fundal contraction should be stimulated by external fundal massage. If the uterine atony is due to a full urinary bladder, as the uterus is massaged and the fundus becomes firm, the distended bladder will protrude more into the abdomen than previously; furthermore, when the nurse stops massaging the uterus, the fundus will once again become soft, boggy, and displaced (*see* the section on the "Bladder"). If the uterine atony is due to retained placental tissue, the nurse may observe that as the fundus is massaged, blood clots with tissue are expelled from the vagina. If the uterine atony is due to infection, the lochia may have a foul odor. Whenever the nurse finds a soft and boggy fundus, the amount, the odor, and the quality of lochia should be assessed, recorded, and reported.

Women experiencing uterine atony as a result of urinary bladder distention should be asked to void. The uterus and the bladder should be reassessed. When the bladder is emptied fully the fundus should be firm and midline. The nurse should counsel puerperal women about the need to empty the bladder frequently.

The nurse should report to the physician or certified nurse-midwife if uterine atony persists after the bladder is emptied and if placental tissue is expelled and lochia is foul smelling or excessive. A postpartum dilation and curettage (D&C) is frequently indicated for retained placental tissue. Lochia obtained from within the uterus is collected for culture and sensitivity when an infection is suspected. Frequently, oxytocic agents such as methylergonovine maleate (Methergine), ergonovine maleate (Ergotrate), or oxytocin (Pitocin) are administered to stimulate uterine contractions.

In the first few days postpartum, women should receive information concerning normal uterine involution. Women should be taught how to feel for the fundus and how to perform fundal massage in case of excessive bleeding. The nurse should stress that a rapid increase in activity can produce an increase in uterine bleeding. Additionally, women should be counseled concerning ovulation, menstruation, sexual activity, and family planning, as discussed later in this chapter.

Lochia. The nurse routinely assesses the lochia for amount, consistency, color, and odor. Before physically assessing the lochia, the nurse should ask the woman when her peripad or sanitary napkin was last changed. Subjective data are needed regarding the amount of lochia, number of pads worn since the woman was last checked, and passage of any blood clots. In talking to the nurse, women often express concerns about the amount of lochia and seek reassurance that the lochia is normal.

To assess the lochia, the nurse removes the peripad for inspection and applies a new pad. Nurses should wear disposable gloves when inspecting the lochia and handling peripads as a precaution against possible transmission of bloodborne infections. In the first 3 days, lochia rubra is observed. Small clots without tissue may be present that represent pooling of blood during periods when the woman is inactive. Within 2 to 3 days the lochia turns pink and is termed lochia serosa. Lochia alba appears by the tenth day and can last until the third week postpartum. The lochia may have a slight fleshy odor, but the odor should not be foul or offensive.

The nurse estimates the amount of lochia by inspecting the drainage on the peripad. Jacobson[5] has developed the following standard to help nurses improve the accuracy of their assessments of peripad saturation: If the stain on the peripad is less than 1 in., the lochia is scant; if less than 4 in., the lochia is light; if less than 6 in., the lochia is moderate; and if the pad is saturated, the lochia is heavy. A fully saturated pad holds 60 to 100 mL of lochia. In general, saturation of one pad within a 15-minute period or saturation of more than one pad in 1 hour suggests hemorrhage. If the woman reports that her pads have been saturated in a short period, the nurse should place a clean peripad on the woman and monitor the amount of lochia during the following hour. Usually during the first few days, lochia is light to moderate, with four to eight pads used daily. As the lochia changes to serosa and then to alba, the amount continues to diminish.

Afterpains: Postpartum Contractions. During the first few days postpartum, uterine contractions, called **"afterpains,"** are frequently the source of abdominal discomfort. Multiparas, lactating women, and women who had a greatly distended uterus, for example, from twin gestation, large fetus, or polyhydramnios, experience more afterpains. The uterus of the multiparous woman goes through cycles of contracting and relaxing, whereas the primiparous uterus is more likely to remain contracted. Lactating women most frequently experience contractions while breastfeeding as a result of the release of endogenous oxytocin with the let-down reflex. The lactating multipara may experience strong contractions during infant feedings. Analgesics should be administered to the woman prior to the feedings to minimize maternal discomfort and produce sufficient relaxation. Women should be counseled to use breathing and relaxation exercises. In particular, the nurse should emphasize that breathing and relaxation exercises taught in childbirth preparation courses can be quite effective in dealing with afterpains. (*See* Chapter 24 for a discussion of childbirth exercises.)

Bladder. To assess accurately the urinary system and bladder functioning during the puerperium, data obtained from each woman should include history of usual elimination pattern; history of urinary tract infection; history of bladder distention or urinary retention; present ability to void; presence of urgency, burning, or frequency; quality of present voids, that is, amount, color, concentration, sense of emptying the bladder; and present ability to sense when the bladder is full. Additionally, general knowledge about hygiene and means to prevent urinary tract infections should be assessed.

A physical assessment of the bladder should be performed whenever the uterus is assessed and at least every 2 hours for the first 8 hours, then every 8 hours for the next 3 days. In some settings, the routine may be more intense, with bladder checks every 15 minutes for the first hour, every 30 minutes for the next 2 hours, every hour for the next 2 hours, every 4 hours for the next 24 hours, and thereafter every 8 hours.

With the woman lying flat, the nurse inspects the abdomen for bladder distention. An empty bladder will not be visible. As the bladder fills the surfaces become convex. When the bladder contains more than 500 mL of urine a bulging mass is visible in the lower abdomen. When the bladder is greatly distended, an ovoid mass well above the symphysis pubis is visible. If the bladder is greatly distended the uterine fundus will be soft, boggy, and often displaced to one side. For this reason, the client should be advised to void frequently.

To percuss or palpate the bladder the nurse starts about 2 in. (5 cm) above the symphysis pubis and moves downward. Percussion of a filling or full bladder will emit a dull sound. The bladder may be palpated when it contains at least 150 mL of urine. If the bladder contains a large amount of urine, the woman will experience a sense of pressure. The palpated bladder feels soft, fluid filled, and ballottable, that is, easily pushed about.

Generally within 4 to 8 hours of delivery women have regained their urge to void. In the next 48 hours the postpartum woman will frequently urinate, ridding her body of the large amounts of urine that accumulate as the water metabolism of pregnancy is reversed. As much as 3000 mL of urine per day, with 500 to 1000 mL of urine at one void, is possible during the second to fifth postpartum days. Women should be encouraged to void at least every 3 to 4 hours to prevent bladder distention. Women should be instructed that at least the first three voids after a vaginal delivery or after a catheter is removed must be measured to determine if the bladder is functioning properly. A measured void of less than 100 mL of urine is considered indicative of urinary overflow from a distended bladder.

Some women are unable to void initially after a vaginal delivery. To stimulate voiding several interventions can be employed (Table 31–3). If after the first void the bladder is still distended, the woman should be asked to void again in 1 hour. Usually after the second void the bladder is emptied. Again, if the bladder is not emptied and only a small amount of urine is excreted, the nurse should assess whether or not the urine was overflow from a distended bladder. If these interventions are not successful a straight catheterization is appropriate. When catheterizing a postpartum woman, the nurse needs to be aware of the condition of the perineum. As with any catheterization, aspetic technique must be used. Many health care professionals believe that removal of more than 1000 mL of urine could cause a shock reaction. It is recommended that the nurse only remove up to 1000 mL of urine via the catheter at one time. After a straight catheterization the woman should be assessed frequently for bladder filling and ability to urinate. Usually only one straight catheterization is necessary.

TABLE 31–3. MANAGING A FULL BLADDER

1. Run tap water.
2. Pour warm water over the vulva.
3. Encourage voiding in a sitz bath, followed by a shower.
4. Expose urinary meatus to fumes from peppermint spirits (2–3 drops in a bedpan causes relaxation of the urinary meatus).
5. Drink a warm beverage.

Because of their tendency to develop bladder distention in the early postpartum, women may develop urinary tract infections. As a precautionary measure, urine is frequently collected for culture and sensitivity within 48 hours of delivery. A urinalysis may be performed. Nurses can counsel women about drinking citrus juices and ingesting other vitamin C products, wearing cotton underwear, practicing proper care of the perineum, and urinating at least every 3 to 4 hours to prevent urinary tract infections.

Women who deliver by cesarean usually have an indwelling urinary catheter inserted before delivery that remains in place for 1 to 2 days. Strict monitoring of intake and output is needed for any postpartum woman with an indwelling catheter. Less than 600 mL of urine in 24 hours suggests kidney dysfunction. In the immediate postoperative period, women who deliver by cesarean should pass at least 30 to 60 mL of urine per hour via an indwelling catheter to demonstrate kidney functioning. Urine obtained from the catheter should be checked for glucose, acetone, protein, and specific gravity.

As an indwelling catheter places an individual at greater risk for a urinary tract infection, a sterile urine specimen may be collected prior to removing the catheter. After removal of the catheter, the first three voids should be measured. Women who deliver by cesarean frequently have difficulty urinating because of a decreased sensation of bladder filling and the reflex spasm of the meatal sphincter resulting from the indwelling catheter. Interventions, as described in Table 31–3, should be instituted to stimulate urination.

Abdominal Dressing/Incision. Ongoing subjective data collected from women after cesarean delivery focus on level of comfort/discomfort, perception of progress, and knowledge of self-care. Additionally, the woman's feelings about the surgery and her scar should be assessed.

Women who deliver by cesarean have an abdominal dressing in place for the first 24 hours. The dressing should be assessed for seepage or drainage. Overt signs of drainage should be recorded and reported to the physician in terms of quantity of drainage on bandage in a given time span. The dressing should be reinforced as needed. Excessive drainage necessitates immediate action and may indicate hemorrhage.

After the initial dressing is removed, the nurse should assess the incision every 8 hours. The incision and surrounding area are inspected for redness, edema, ecchymosis, discharge, and approximation or intactness. In the past mothers were not permitted to shower for several days after the surgery. Presently, however, many hospitals permit a shower if the original dressing has been removed and there are no signs of infection. Women are told to allow the incision to air dry, to avoid restricting undergarments, and to wear cotton undergarments.

Back

The postpartum woman should be asked about back pain or discomfort. In particular, the nurse assesses for costovertebral angle (CVA) tenderness. The costovertebral angles are those angles formed between the 12th ribs and the vertebral column. To assess for CVA tenderness the nurse places the palm of the left hand over a CVA and strikes that palm with the ulnar surface of the right fist. Normally no pain is elicited. Elicitation of pain suggests a kidney infection.

Perineum

Although the perineum refers to the area of tissue between the vaginal introitus and the anus, assessment of the perineum includes the anus as well. The nurse needs to assess the postpartum mother's comfort level relative to episiotomy, lacerations, and hemorrhoids. Included in this assessment is a complete symptom review emphasizing the conditions that lessen or worsen discomfort. Additionally, the nurse needs to assess if the postpartum woman has sufficient knowledge related to perineal care and sufficient knowledge to decide which of the interventions would best relieve her discomfort and at the same time promote healing of the perineum and anal area.

To physically assess the perineum, the woman is placed in the Sim's position, with the top leg flexed slightly. The upper buttock is lifted so that the perineum and anus are clearly visible. A penlight is often needed to provide proper lighting.

Episiotomy and Lacerations. Puerperal women often experience a considerable amount of discomfort from repaired perineal lacerations and episiotomies. The nurse assesses the perineum for signs of healing, trauma, and infection. Davidson[6] offers an acronym, REEDA, to evaluate postpartum healing of the episiotomy. It should be noted, however, that the acronym is applicable to any sutured line. Specifically, according to the REEDA method the episiotomy or sutured laceration would be assessed for *R*edness, *E*dema, *E*cchymosis, *D*ischarge, and *A*pproximation. Nurses need to describe and record the location and extent of redness, edema, and ecchymosis. Discharge, if present, should be described in terms of quality (ie, serous, serosanguineous, bloody, or purulent) and quantity. In terms of approximation, nurses need to note the degree to which the episiotomy or repaired laceration site is intact. Skin separations should be described in terms of extent and depth of separation, that is, the length of the separation and the layers of skin affected.

During the first day edema and redness are common, but the edges of the episiotomy or repaired lacerations should be intact and there should be no discharge. If the perineum was traumatized during the delivery, ecchymosis may be present. Severe redness, edema, ecchymosis, and the presence of discharge inhibit healing of the perineum. In particular, moderate to severe redness and edema and the presence of discharge are indicative of infection.

Nursing care of the perineum focuses on general pericare; use of Kegel exercises to strengthen the pubococcygeal muscle; interventions to reduce swelling, increase circulation, promote healing, and provide temporary relief from perineal discomfort; and ways to determine when the perineum has healed (*see* "Sexuality and Return to Sexual Activity" under "Sexual Issues and Family Planning").

General Pericare. The postpartum woman is taught to rinse the perineum from the front toward the back after each void or defecation. A peribottle filled with warm water is an efficient means of rinsing the perineum. Some hospitals have surgigators in the bathroom that spray an antiseptic or water, or both, onto the perineum. The perineum should be wiped from the front towards the back to prevent contamination of the vagina and urinary meatus with fecal material. A new peripad should be applied each time the woman urinates or defecates and at least every 3 hours.

Kegel Exercises. Kegel exercises in the postpartum period increase circulation to the pelvic floor and thus promote healing of the pubococcygeal muscle, an episiotomy, and a perineal laceration (*see* "Exercise and Activity").

Interventions to Reduce Swelling, Increase Circulation, Promote Healing, and Provide Temporary Pain Relief. In the first 8 to 24 hours, the nurse should apply an ice pack to the perineum to minimize swelling through vasoconstriction. The ice pack may be commercially prepared or the nurse may use a rubber glove filled with ice and wrapped with a wash cloth.

After the first 24 hours, a heat treatment may be used to increase circulation and thereby promote healing. Women should be counseled on the use of a sitz bath or perineal heat lamp as a means of providing a heat treatment. Prior to using a heat treatment the woman should cleanse the perineum with a peribottle, surgigator, or shower. In some cases, a cool water sitz bath may provide relief.

Sitz Bath. In the past hospitals used metal, portable sitz baths that were shared among many clients. Most institutions now provide individual plastic sitz baths that are taken home. The plastic sitz bath consists of a basin that fits into the commode or toilet with the seat lifted away. A plastic bag with tubing, similar to an enema bag, is filled with hot water and placed at a level above the basin (Figure 31–8). The tubing is then attached to the inside of the basin. The basin is filled with warm or cool water and the tubing is clamped off. The woman is instructed to sit in the bath with her gluteal muscles relaxed so that the perineal body can receive the treatment. For maximum effectiveness the woman should be instructed to maintain the water temperature at about 100°F. As the water in the basin cools, the woman should unclamp the tube and allow the hot water to rush into the basin; excess water will flow out through the back of the basin and down into the commode or toilet. Sitz baths are effective treatments when used for 20 minutes, two or four times a day.

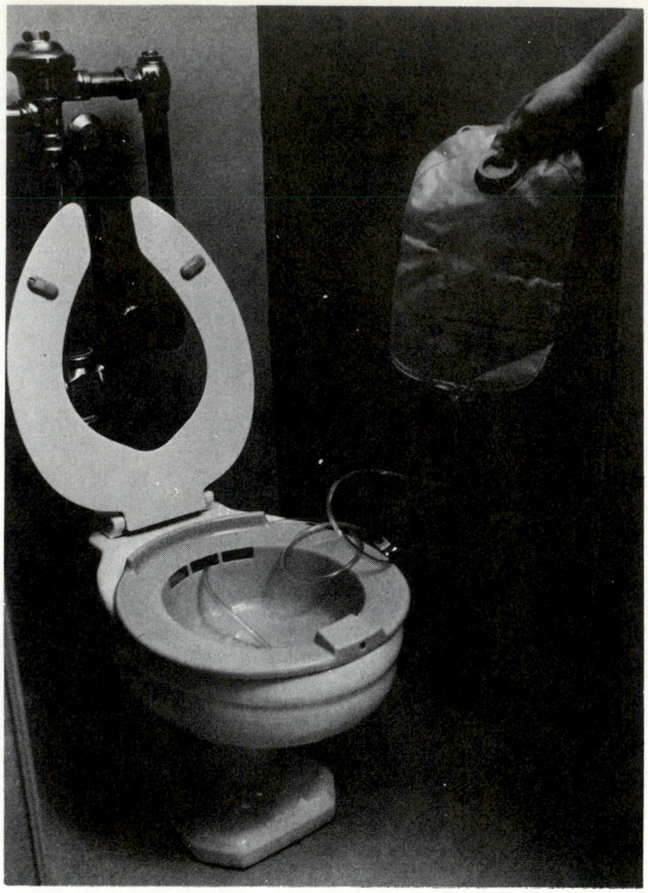

Figure 31–8. Plastic sitz bath.

Perineal Lamp. Occasionally while in the hospital a woman may be given a perineal heat lamp to stimulate perineal vasodilation. The perineal heat lamp, which contains a 30- to 40-W bulb, is placed approximately 12 in. away from the exposed perineum for 20 minutes, three times a day. Prior to use of the perineal lamp the perineum should be cleansed. The woman is placed in a dorsal recumbent position. A sheet is brought over the arch of the lamp to cover the woman. Perineal heat lamps are not routinely provided for home use.

Other Treatments. For temporary pain relief, oral analgesics such as acetaminophen (Tylenol) and oxycodone (Percodan, Percoset) may be offered. Many women need analgesics for the first few days. Application of local anesthetic sprays and ointment and witch hazel pads to the perineum also may provide temporary relief. Placing the woman in a knee-chest position, along with Kegel exercises and buttock tucks, can promote perineal healing, minimize pain, and reduce swelling. Some health care professionals advocate sitting on a hard surface for support.

Hemorrhoids. Hemorrhoidal discomfort often accompanies a vaginal delivery or a cesarean delivery after a long unsuccessful second stage of labor. Internal hemorrhoids may become external with the forces of labor. Both internal and external hemorrhoids may enlarge from the pressure exerted on the pelvic floor.

The anal area is examined for the presence of hemorrhoids. Hemorrhoids are described in terms of number, size, presence of bleeding, and degree of tenderness.

Interventions used to promote comfort and reduce hemorrhoidal size are similar to the interventions used in treating the episiotomy or lacerations. In the first 24 hours after delivery, ice packs may be applied to the perineum and anus to minimize swelling. Thereafter, moist heat, as provided by a sitz bath, can help to reduce swelling by increasing circulation. Cool witch hazel pads placed on the hemorrhoids or on an episiotomy are soothing, and help to relieve and prevent itching. Women can be taught to replace the hemorrhoid into the anorectal canal with a lubricated glove or finger cot, and then assume a knee-chest position for a short period.

Frequently women are afraid that bowel movements will exacerbate the hemorrhoids. These women need to be counseled that when they voluntarily inhibit bowel evacuation, constipation may ensue. The constipation, in turn, causes more pressure to be placed on the hemorrhoids. Measures must be initiated to prevent or alleviate constipation.

Hematomas. Occasionally postpartum women develop vulvar and vaginal hematomas, that is, masses that form when blood seeps into connective tissue beneath the vulvar skin and the vaginal mucosa. Women with hematomas often experience severe pain or rectal pressure. During a physical examination a vulvar hematoma is identified as a bulging mass covered by the vulvar skin or a mass bulging into the vaginal wall. Small hematomas may not be visible or palpable.

Hematomas may bleed, and if excessive the woman may hemorrhage. Bleeding may not be overt; therefore, signs of internal hemorrhage (eg, increased pulse, decreased blood pressure, pallor, clamminess, hypovolemia, and anemia) need to be assessed. The nurse should notify the physician or nurse-midwife of any hematomas so that prompt treatment, if needed, can be initiated. Medical treatment may involve incision and evacuation of the hematoma (*see* Chapter 41.)

Extremities

The nurse should assess the extremities of the postpartum woman every 8 hours while the woman is hospitalized. Objective and subjective data from the woman include history of venous disease, signs of swelling and pain in the extremities, and presence of varicosities.

Both the upper and lower extremities may be assessed for edema and vascular changes; however, the lower extremities must be routinely assessed for edema, venous disease, and reflexes. The nurse first inspects the extremities for skin color, overt varicosities, and swelling. Edema is assessed by pressing over a bony prominence such as the dorsum of the foot and pre-tibial area (Figure 31–9). If edema is present the nurse notes whether there is pitting. The extremities are compared for temperature on palpation. A localized area of redness, increased temperature, and tenderness over a vein, suggests thrombophlebitis (*see* Chapters 39 and 41).

In the past, Homan's sign was one test widely used to identify the presence of deep vein thrombosis. Calf pain on dorsiflexion of the foot was considered to be a positive Homan's sign. This test, however, has not proved to be a reliable indicator of deep vein thrombosis. In 50 percent of clients with actual deep vein thrombosis, overt clinical signs and symptoms may be absent.[7] A client's complaint of leg pain or tenderness should be reported to the nurse-midwife or physician for further investigation (Figure 31–10).

Women with edema and varicosities should be given support stockings to wear when ambulating. They should be encouraged to elevate the legs while lying supine. Women should be discouraged from crossing their legs as circulation tends to be impeded in this position. Ambulation should be encouraged to increase circulation and prevent the stasis of fluid and the possibility of venous complications. Women should be told that as the water metabolism of pregnancy is reversed, edema will diminish and varicosities may also lessen in severity.

Neurologic System

Reflexes are expected to be within normal limits. Women with hyperreflexia may be experiencing

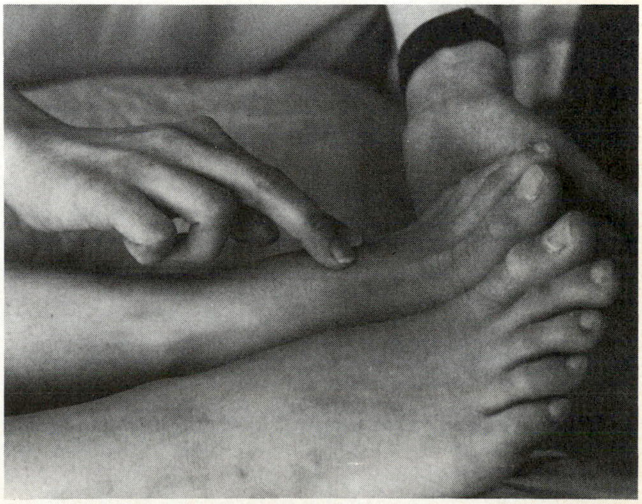

Figure 31–9. Nurse assessing client's feet for edema.

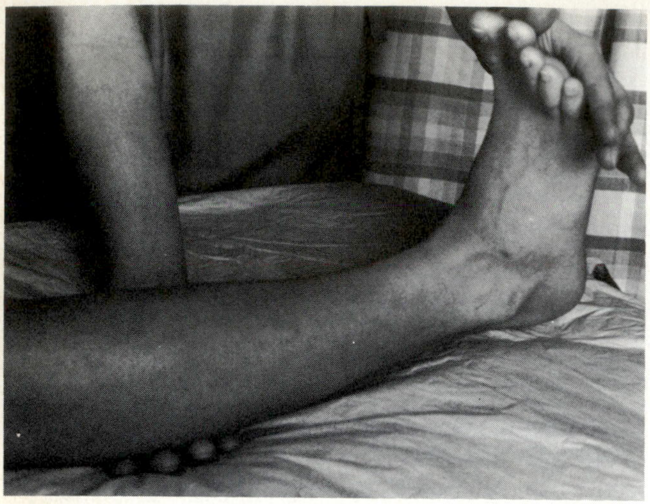

Figure 31–10. The nurse assesses the client's legs.

pregnancy-induced hypertension (PIH) with potential for a seizure. If hyperreflexia is present, the nurse should assess for other signs of PIH, for example, increased blood pressure, proteinuria, edema, epigastric pain, and headaches.

Table 31–4 summarizes selected clinical findings for the postpartum client.

IMMUNIZATIONS

Rubella

Because of the severe birth defects that can result when a pregnant woman contracts rubella, women are screened prenatally for antibody titers; however, rubella immunization must be deferred until the postpartum period. Consequently, during the early puerperium, the nurse identifies which women need rubella counseling and immunization (Box 31–1). Women should be advised to avoid becoming pregnant for 3 months after the immunization because of the potential risk to the fetus if exposed to rubella.[8]

Prevention of Rh Sensitivity

The most severe hemolytic disease of the newborn results from Rho(D) isoimmunization, which occurs when the Rh-negative woman possesses the antibody to the Rh factor, which destroys fetal Rh-positive red blood cells. If fetal/newborn red blood cell destruction is severe, death of the newborn may ensue.

Isoimmunization of the Rh-negative woman may occur from a previous pregnancy with a fetus having Rh-positive blood. As the placenta separates from the uterine wall, villi break and venous sinuses at the placental site become exposed. Fetal red blood cells containing the Rh factor, that is, Rh-positive cells, leak from the villi into the venous sinuses.[9,10] The Rh-negative mother lacking the Rh blood factor identifies and labels the Rh-positive fetal red blood cell as an antigen. Unless prevented, the mother produces antibodies to the antigen. A potentially dangerous situation now exists for future pregnancies in which there is maternal-fetal Rh incompatibility. Specifically, as the circulating maternal antibodies cross the placenta and come into contact with the fetal antigen, the fetal red blood cell is destroyed. Hemolytic disease of the fetus and newborn results. Isoimmunization can also result when a client is transfused with improperly matched blood, or when a woman has a spontaneous or induced abortion, an ectopic pregnancy, amniocentesis, manual removal of the placenta, or antepartum bleeding. Fortunately, Rho(D) isoimmunization is preventable during pregnancy and the early postpartum.

On admission to a hospital maternal blood is drawn for typing. Nurses are alerted for women with Rho(D)-negative blood type. Immediately after the delivery, cord blood is drawn to determine the newborn's blood type. If the newborn is Rho(D) positive, the nonsensitized mother is given an intramuscular injection of 300 μg of Rho(D) immune globulin (Box 31–2). Generally, the standard dose of 300 μg of Rho(D) immune globulin neutralizes 15 mL of packed cells, or 30 mL of whole blood.[9] However, in less than 1 percent of cases, there is a large fetomaternal hemorrhage requiring a larger dosage of the immune globulin. Conversely, only 50 μg of Rho(D) immune globulin is needed to isoimmunize after a first-trimester abortion. Usual protocol requires that postnatally Rho(D) immune globulin be administered within 72 hours of delivery; however, prevention of isoimmunization may still be effective if this immune globulin is administered up to 3 to 4 weeks after delivery.[9] The drug is considered to be a blood product.

Rh-negative women receiving Rho(D) immune globulin occasionally experience skin irritation at the injection site. If, inadvertently, an Rh-positive woman receives the immune globulin, a generalized reaction characterized by lysis of maternal red blood cells can occur. Careful adherence to precautions used when administering medications and blood products will prevent erroneous administration of Rho(D) immune globulin.

TABLE 31–4. SELECTED CLINICAL FINDINGS DURING THE POSTPARTUM PERIOD

Body System	Clinical Findings	Physiologic Changes	Nursing Assessment
Integument	Facial chloasma and linea nigra gradually diminish; striae fade; alopecia common for 3 to 6 months after delivery	Estrogen and progesterone levels decrease; hair growth enters resting phase	Assure mother of normalcy, especially of hair loss which may be a major concern.
Cardiovascular	Vital signs within normal limits, no evidence of vulvar or vaginal hematoma or bleeding	Cardiovascular system returns to normal in postpartum period	Assess blood pressure, cardiac sounds for rhythm, rate, murmurs; inspect perineal area for hematoma; observe for varicosities/venous disease.
Respiratory	Respirations within normal range; may increase slightly with anxiety and pain; may be slightly diminished secondary to narcotic administration	Respiratory diaphragm returns to normal position; anxiety and pain tend to increase respirations; narcotics can cause respiratory depression	Assess rate, rhythm of maternal respirations; ascultate breath sounds; assess maternal discomfort and anxiety.
Hematologic	Elevated white blood cell count (counts as high as 25,000/μL, average count 14,000 to 16,000/μL)	Healing process after labor and delivery	Monitor maternal physiologic processes; reassess white blood cell count if there are signs of infection.
	Hemoglobin and hematocrit levels stabilize to prelabor levels by 4 days postpartum; hgb and hct levels increase immediately postpartum when maternal dehydration is present	Erthropoiesis and hemoconcentration occur during labor and delivery; after initial reduction, blood volume stabilizes	Assess maternal hydration, hemoglobin and hematocrit (2 days postpartum), maternal blood loss and diet.
Gastrointestinal	Sluggish bowels for several days after delivery; decreased peristalsis; may experience discomfort related to hemorrhoids, constipation	Occurs in response to analgesia and anesthesia, diminished muscle tone, intraabdominal pressure, lack of appropriate diet; hemorrhoids may occur during pregnancy and as a result of straining during labor and delivery	Assess bowels and diet; encourage early ambulation; provide stool softener as ordered; encourage fluids and roughage in diet.
Musculoskeletal	Color, temperature, turgor of extremities within normal limits	Postdelivery, musculoskeletal system returns to normal	Assess extremities for skin color, edema, and temperature.
Urinary	Within 4–8 hours of delivery, the urge to void is regained; 2–5 days postpartum, as much as 3000 mL of urine is voided per day	Water metabolism is reversed	Assure mother of normalcy of frequency of urination. Assess urine for quantity and quality.
Reproductive	Fundus palpated midway between umbilicus and symphysis pubis immediately after delivery; by 12 hours, fundus rises to umbilicus; thereafter, fundus descends 1–2 cm per day; fundus firm, not boggy, found on midline of abdomen	Uterine involution related to contraction of uterus after delivery	Assess height and consistency of fundus.
	Lochia rubra first 2–3 days; lochia serosa 3–4 days; lochia alba 10th day; slightly fleshy odor	Uterine involution—shedding of decidua	Assess quantity, color, odor, and consistency of lochia.
	Possible repair of episiotomy and laceration; clean and dry incision; no redness or discharge	Healing process from repair of episiotomy and lacerations	Assess perineal area for healing, swelling, drainage, pain, or other signs of infection. Teach perineal comfort measures. Teach client to clean from vaginal area to anus after elimination.
	Colostrum secreted from nipple in first 24–48 hours, followed by breast milk; engorgement within 48 hours.	Process of lactation engorgement related to fluid retention and venous stasis	Counsel mother to wear supportive bra and to shower. Assure of normalcy.
	After pains (uterine contractions), especially in multiparas	Process of involution; also occurs in breastfeeding because of oxytocin secretion	Teach breathing and relaxation exercises. Assess fundus and lochia. Analgesics may be administered.
Neurologic	Normal reflexes in all four extremities	1^+ or 2^+ deep tendon reflexes indicate intact neurologic system	Assess deep tendon reflexes.

BOX 31–1. RUBELLA VIRUS VACCINE

Classification:
Attenuated live virus vaccine.

Actions:
Rubella virus vaccine live promotes long-term immunity to rubella by inducing production of specific antibodies in individuals over 12 months of age.

Indications:
To provide active immunity to rubella and therefore prevent intrauterine infection, which can result in miscarriage, abortion, stillbirth, and congenital rubella syndrome. The combination measles, mumps, and rubella virus vaccine live (MMR) is the vaccine of choice when rubella immunization is indicated and when the individual is also likely to be susceptible to measles, mumps, or both.Stability:

In lyophilized form, vaccines containing rubella virus should be refrigerated at 2–8°C but may be frozen. The vials containing diluent may be stored at room temperature. After reconstitution with the diluent provided by the manufacturer, the vaccines should be refrigerated at 2–8°C and discarded if not used within 8 hours. Both lyophilized and reconstituted vaccines should be protected from light.

Dosage and Route:
Rubella virus vaccine live is administered only by subcutaneous injection, preferably into the outer aspectof the upper arm. Vaccines containing rubella virus live are reconstituted by adding the entire amount of diluent supplied by the manufacturer to the corresponding vial of lyophilized vaccine and agitating the vial. Only the diluent provided by the manufacturer should be used.

Reconstituted vaccines containing rubella virus live should be inspected visually for particulate matter and discoloration prior to administration. The vaccine should be reconstituted and administered using sterile syringes and needles that are free of preservatives, antiseptics, and detergents, as these substances may inactivate live viruses; a 25-gauge, ⅝-in. needle is recommended for administration of the vaccine.

The dose of rubella virus vaccine live is the same for all individuals. The usual dose is 0.5 mL administered as a single dose. A booster dose of rubella vaccine is not needed. Children who received rubella virus vaccine live when less than 12 months of age should be revaccinated.

Adverse Reactions:
Incidence increases with age of vaccine. Symptoms associated with natural rubella infections including lymphadenopathy, rash, urticaria, fever, malaise, sore throat, and headache; nausea and vomiting occur occasionally in vaccinees. Symptoms may occur 11–20 days after vaccination and are usually mild and transient, generally persisting 1–5 days. Arthralgias and rarely transient arthritis may occur.

Burning and stinging of short duration may occur at the injection site because of the slightly acidic pH of the vaccine. Induration, erythema, tenderness or pain, and wheal and flare may occur occasionally at the vaccine injection site.

SLEEP/REST/COMFORT

During the normal process of labor and delivery maternal energy expenditure is high. As a result, most women are physically exhausted after delivery. Sleep, rest, and comfort measures are needed to replenish maternal energy.

Bed rest is usually maintained for at least the first hour postpartum or until the woman's status has stabilized. During this initial recovery period, a quiet, warm environment should be provided for the mother, father, and their newborn. If a private recovery room cannot be provided, the nurse should make certain that the curtains are drawn around the bed to ensure privacy. A portable air warmer may be placed over the mother and newborn to warm the immediate air temperature surrounding the mother and her newborn. Frequently, however, the skin-to-skin contact between mother and newborn, the use of a blanket over the dyad, or both measures may be sufficient. The nurse needs to help position the mother and her newborn to promote comfort and prevent undue stress on the already tired maternal muscles. In particular the use of supporting pillows behind the mother's head, back, and the arm that cradles the newborn minimizes the work that needs to be done by the mother's body, thus allowing for energy conservation.

As the initial recovery period comes to an end, the nurse helps the woman to sponge bathe or take a shower. Women, now feeling temporarily refreshed, are prepared for transfer to a postpartum unit.

The need for rest and sleep to restore maternal

Contraindications and Precautions:
No allergic reactions have been reported. The vaccine is contraindicated in individuals who have had an anaphylactic reaction to topically or systemically administered neomycin.

Replication of rubella vaccine virus may be potentiated in individuals with primary immunodeficiencies (eg, cellular immune deficiency, hypogammaglobulinemia) or with suppressed immune response resulting from leukemia, lymphoma, other malignancies affecting the bone marrow or lymphatic system, or blood dyscrasias, and vaccination with rubella virus vaccine live is contraindicated in these individuals. The vaccine should not be given to an individual with a family history of congenital or hereditary immunodeficiency until the immunocompetence of the individual has been documented. In the United States it is recommended that the vaccine not be given to individuals with symptomatic human immunodeficiency virus (HIV) infections but the vaccine is recommended for use in individuals with asymptomatic HIV infections.

Rubella virus vaccine live generally is contraindicated in individuals receiving immunosuppressive therapy (eg, corticosteroids, corticotropin, alkylating agents, antimetabolites, radiation therapy) although the manufacturer states that the vaccine is not contraindicated in individuals receiving corticosteroids as replacement therapy. Febrile respiratory illnesses or other active febrile infections are contraindications to receiving the vaccine, whereas a simple upper respiratory infection does not preclude vaccination. Pregnancy is a contraindication to receiving rubella vaccination for 3 months after vaccination.

Drug Interactions:

- Tuberculin: Rubella virus vaccine live has been reported to suppress temporarily tuberculin skin sensitivity; therefore, tuberculin tests should be done before, simultaneously with, or 6 weeks after administration of the vaccine.
- Vaccines: Rubella virus vaccine live may be administered simultaneously with an inactivated vaccine, poliovirus vaccine live oral, measles virus vaccine live, and mumps virus vaccine live. Incidence and severity of adverse effects may be increased by concomitant administration of live virus vaccines other than measles or mumps.
- Immunosuppressive agents: Possible diminished response to rubella virus vaccine live and replication of virus may be potentiated. Vaccination should be deferred until the immunosuppressive agent has been discontinued for approximately 3–12 months. Corticosteroids for replacement are not a contraindication.
- Immune globulins and blood products: Vaccination should be deferred in clients who have received blood, plasma, or more than 0.04 mL/kg immune globulin within the preceding 3 months, as these products contain antibodies that may interfere with the immune response to the vaccine. Rubella virus vaccine live should be given at least 14 days prior to or at least 6 weeks, preferably 3 months, after administration of an immune globulin.

Nursing Implications:

- Identify women who have low or zero antibody titer against rubella.
- Advise women to avoid becoming pregnant for 3 months after immunization.

energy is still paramount after the initial recovery period. Despite this need, many women experience euphoria after the first few hours postpartum. This euphoria, accompanied by an inability to rest, is often related to the woman's need to talk about her experience. Many women will readily accept telephone calls and will telephone friends and relatives as a means of verbalizing about their experience. The euphoria and inability to sleep usually end with the first evening after delivery as women go through their usual routines in preparation for bed. Thereafter, sleep and rest periods are most often controlled by hospital routines and newborn needs.

In the hospital nurses can plan time for care with each postpartum woman so that rest and sleep are not disturbed. If, during the night, the newborn is brought to the mother only for feedings, then night feedings should be based on newborn demands rather than on a predetermined feeding schedule. Many mothers, however, prefer to have their infants room-in. Often these mothers sleep better when their infant and, if possible, a support person are in the room. Conversely, nurses need to be aware that many times maternal exhaustion may be so great that a woman may be unable to provide 24-hour care for her newborn initially. This latter situation should not be viewed as a negative attachment behavior, but rather as a normal maternal need for physical restoration.

Once at home, the need for physical as well as emotional restoration is still a priority. Prior to discharge women need anticipatory guidance and education on how to obtain the needed rest and sleep and on how to care for the infant (Figure 31–11). Nurses provide instruction on return to physical ac-

BOX 31–2. RHO(D) IMMUNE GLOBULIN

Proprietary Names:
RhoGAM (Ortho), Gamulin (Armour), others.

Classification:
Immune globulin.

Action:
Suppresses antibody response and formation of anti-Rho(D) in Rho(D)-negative, D^u-negative individuals exposed to Rh-positive blood. The exact mechanism of the suppression is unknown, but it is thought that the immune globulin binds to the antigen and prevents stimulation of the primary immune response.

Indications:
To suppress the active antibody response and formation of anti-Rho(D) in the Rho(D)-negative, D^u-negative individual exposed to Rh-positive blood as a result of delivery of an Rho(D)-positive or D^u-positive infant, termination of pregnancy, amniocentesis or abdominal trauma during pregnancy, or transfusion with Rho(D)-positive or D^u-positive blood.

Dosage and Route:
Administered by intramuscular injection only (to the mother and not the infant) in the deltoid muscle. *Full-term delivery:* One standard dose vial (contains enough anti-Rho(D) to suppress the immunization potential of 15 mL of Rho(D)-positive or D^u-positive packed red blood cells) in divided doses at different sites within 72 hours of delivery. *Termination of pregnancy:* Up to 13 weeks of gestation, one microdose vial (contains enough anti-Rho(D) to suppress the immunization potential of 2.5 mL of Rho(D)-positive or D^u-positive packed red blood cells) within 72 hours. At 13 or more weeks gestation, one standard dose vial is given within 72 hours.

Contraindications and Precautions:
Use with caution in patients with history of allergic reactions to preparations containing human immune globulins, and in patients with thrombocytopenia or bleeding disorders. Contraindicated in Rho(D)-positive or D^u-positive individuals or in Rho(D)-negative individuals who have been sensitized to Rho(D) or D^u antigens and have anti-Rho(D) in their serum.

Adverse Reactions:
Most common: Discomfort at injection site, slight fever. *Less common:* Myalgia, lethargy, splenomegaly, elevated bilirubin, allergic reactions.

Nursing Implications:

- Assess blood group and presence of Rh factor (Rho(D)) in mother, father, and infant.
- Administer Rho(D) immune globulin within 72 hours of delivery when mother is Rho(D) negative and infant is Rho(D) positive.
- Inform Jehovah's Witnesses that drug is considered a blood product.
- Administer IM injection deep in muscle.
- Explain rationale for therapy to couple.

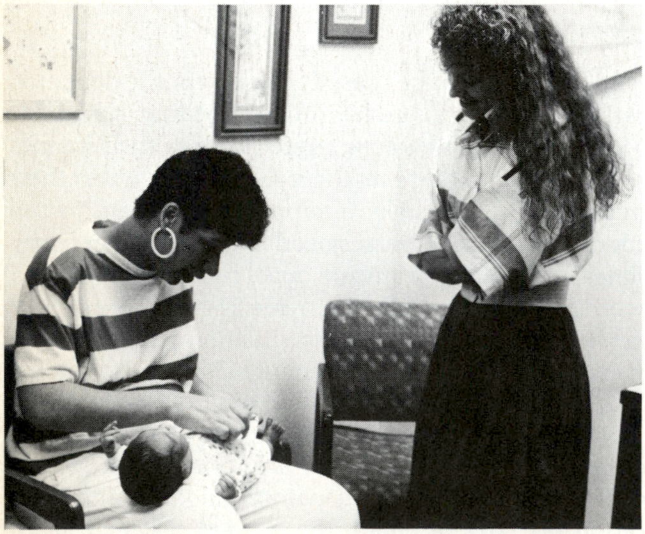

Figure 31–11. Nurse reviewing newborn care with the mother before discharge.

tivity, as described in this chapter. Included in the instructions given to postpartum women and their partners are suggestions on how to organize the necessary activities in providing newborn care as well as self-care for mothers. Guidance is provided on how to handle uninvited visitors at home. For example, couples are advised to tell visitors that the nurse or physician has said that the mother needs rest and should only have visitors for a short period; a note is placed on the door stating that mother and infant are sleeping; the mother is instructed to take the phone off the hook to prevent unwanted interruptions.

EXERCISE AND ACTIVITY

In the initial postpartum, the woman needs to restore her body's energy. Daily activities should be resumed and physical activity and exercise initiated gradually.

Ambulation

Although women who deliver vaginally without anesthesia may be out of bed after the first hour postpartum, provided vital signs are stable and there are no overt signs of hemorrhage, most women ambulate within 4 to 8 hours of delivery. Many women experience hypotension when standing for the first time; thus, extreme caution is needed. If the first time out of bed is uneventful, the woman can usually get out of bed as desired.

Women who deliver by cesarean are usually on bed rest at least 8 hours. They should be encouraged to turn at least every 2 hours. Within 24 hours of surgery, women who have a cesarean delivery should be out of bed with assistance. These women need to be encouraged to ambulate first within the room and then as tolerated.

Daily Activities and Care of Newborn

During the early postpartum, the woman is confronted with conflicting tasks. First is the task of physical and emotional restoration. Second is the need to assume complete responsibility for the newborn and resume previous activities and responsibilities.[11, 12] The need to complete these tasks can create undue physical and emotional strain. The nurse should provide anticipatory guidance and instruction concerning the woman's activities during the first few weeks postpartum. Light household chores such as dusting furniture or preparing a meal are appropriate physical activities for the first week postpartum. If feasible, women should enlist the aid of another adult to help with the cleaning and laundry for 1 to 2 weeks. Women who attempt to resume all previous household tasks and responsibilities at once or too early frequently experience an increase in uterine bleeding, with an increased risk for uterine subinvolution or hemorrhage. The woman should therefore be taught that increase in bleeding may mean she is doing too much. Household chores should be resumed gradually, by adding one chore a day. Lifting heavy objects should be postponed for about 6 weeks.

Return to occupational and educational settings is highly individualized and dependent on the nature of the activities involved. Generally, women who deliver vaginally can safely return to occupational and educational settings in 3 to 4 weeks provided the activities to be performed are not too strenuous. Women who deliver by cesarean section should wait at least 6 to 8 weeks before returning to work and school.

Many women want to know when they can resume driving a car. Generally women who have delivered vaginally resume driving within a week; however, women who have delivered by cesarean should wait until driving activities do not cause pain.

Postpartum Exercises

Studies show that women who have had vaginal deliveries have significantly less pelvic muscle strength than women who have had cesarean births.[13, 14] Muscle strength is improved by a moderate exercise program begun at home.[15] Any exercise program for postpartum women needs to include exercises that promote muscle tone of the pelvic floor and abdomen, as well as those that enhance circulation of the lower extremities.[16] A postpartum exercise program begins with one exercise. Each day another exercise is added. Ideally, exercises should be practiced at least twice a day. Except for the Kegel exercises, women should be instructed that in any exercise session, each particular exercise should be repeated four to five times for the first few days and gradually built up to repetitions of at least ten. Table 31–5 presents a 9-day schedule of exercises recommended for women who have delivered vaginally. Women who have delivered by cesarean section should delay the onset of exercises until after a physical examination by the physician several weeks after surgery.

More vigorous exercises such as situps and straight leg lifts may be started after the second postpartum week. Mothers should be cautioned not to proceed with postpartum exercises if vaginal bleeding reappears.

SEXUAL ISSUES AND FAMILY PLANNING

Sexuality and Return to Sexual Activity

As a result of the rapid physical and psychologic changes of pregnancy and the postpartum, as well as the need to assume a new or expanded role, the postpartum couple's sexual activity may be affected. In particular, sexual interest and response can be altered after the birth of a child.

Recommendations for Resumption of Sexual Activity. Historically, physicians advised couples to refrain from intercourse until 6 weeks postpartum. This recommendation was based on the belief that the perineum needs this time to heal and that the woman is subject to infection. Although the woman does need time to heal physically and to adjust psychologically to the multitude of changes she has undergone, there is no clear evidence suggesting that the couple must wait until 6 weeks postpartum before resuming inter-

TABLE 31–5. POSTPARTUM EXERCISES

DAY 1: Kegel Exercises	Henderson[17] found that postpartum regeneration of the pubococcygeal muscle is significantly improved if, prenatally, women are taught Kegel exercises. Kegel exercises can be initiated soon after a vaginal delivery to strengthen the pubococcygeal muscles and promote healing of the muscle and episiotomy.[15] Approximately 50 to 100 Kegel exercises a day are needed for effectiveness. To perform Kegel exercises, the woman tightens the perineal (pubococcygeal) muscle, starting at the anus and progressing toward the urinary meatus. Contraction of the perineal muscle is maintained for 5 seconds and then gradually relaxed. The woman can determine if she is doing the exercise correctly by trying the exercise while urinating. If she can stop the flow of urine, she is correctly performing Kegel exercises. Kegel exercises, however, should not be routinely performed when urinating because of the potential for urinary stasis, retention, and infection (Figure 31–12A).
DAY 2: Abdominal Toning Exercise 1: Deep Abdominal Breathing	The mother, lying supine, inhales slowly and deeply to expand the abdomen. Then, exhaling slowly by either hissing or blowing through pursed lips, she tightens her abdominal muscles (Figure 31–12B).
DAY 3: Abdominal Toning Exercise 2: Deep Breathing with Chin Flexion	In this modification of the deep abdominal breathing exercise, the mother slowly flexes her chin onto her chest as she inhales and lowers her head back to the floor as she exhales (Figure 31–12C).
DAY 4: Abdominal Toning Exercise 3: Arm Raises	The mother, lying supine with legs parted slightly, extends arms outward so that they are resting on the floor at right angles to the trunk of the body. The arms are gradually raised and the hands brought together. As the hands touch, the arms are then gradually lowered. Mothers should be instructed to breathe in as the arms are raised and to breathe out slowly as the arms are lowered (Figure 31–12D).
DAY 5: Abdominal/Back Toning Exercise: Pelvic Rocks	Lying supine with arms down at the sides, knees flexed, and feet firmly on the floor, the mother breathes in deeply and arches her back as she tightens the abdomen and buttocks. As the mother lowers her back and buttocks onto the floor, she exhales slowly (Figure 31–12E).
DAY 6: Abdominal/Buttock Toning Exercise	Lying supine with knees and hips flexed and feet firmly on the floor, the mother tilts her pelvis inward and tightly contracts her buttocks as she lifts her head. She then returns slowly to her original position and repeats the exercise, remembering to inhale at the start of the exercise (Figure 31–12F).
DAY 7: Abdominal and Thigh Tighteners	Lying with legs straight, the mother raises her head and slightly raises her right knee, as her left hand reaches toward (but does not actually touch) the right knee. The mother should then slowly return to her original position and repeat the exercise using her left knee and right hand.
DAY 8: Buttock, Thigh, and Abdominal Stretching Exercise: Modified Bicycling	The mother lies supine with arms at her sides and knees and hips flexed. She inhales slowly and raises one leg toward the abdomen, stretching out as if to bicycle. She returns her leg to the original position, as she exhales. The exercise is then repeated for the opposite leg.
DAY 9: Buttock, Thigh, and Abdominal Stretching Exercise: Modified Leg Lifts	The mother lies supine with arms at sides and legs straight. One knee and hip are flexed and brought toward the abdomen. The leg is then extended and slowly brought down straight (Figure 31–12G).

course. Additionally, despite the traditional recommendation, many couples resume intercourse by 3 weeks.[18,19]

In the last two decades, the traditional recommendation for an abstinence period of at least 6 weeks postpartum has been challenged by health care professionals and couples alike. Presently the recommended time frame for resumption of sexual intercourse varies greatly. The general rule is that intercourse can safely be resumed when the bleeding has stopped[19] and the episiotomy has healed.[20] These two conditions are generally met by 2 to 3 weeks postpartum. Nurses need to inform couples that postpartum sexual activity should be based on the couple's individual circumstances.[21] Women need to be able to recognize when they are physically able to tolerate penile penetration. Dyspareunia, pain during intercourse, is one of the most common problems en-

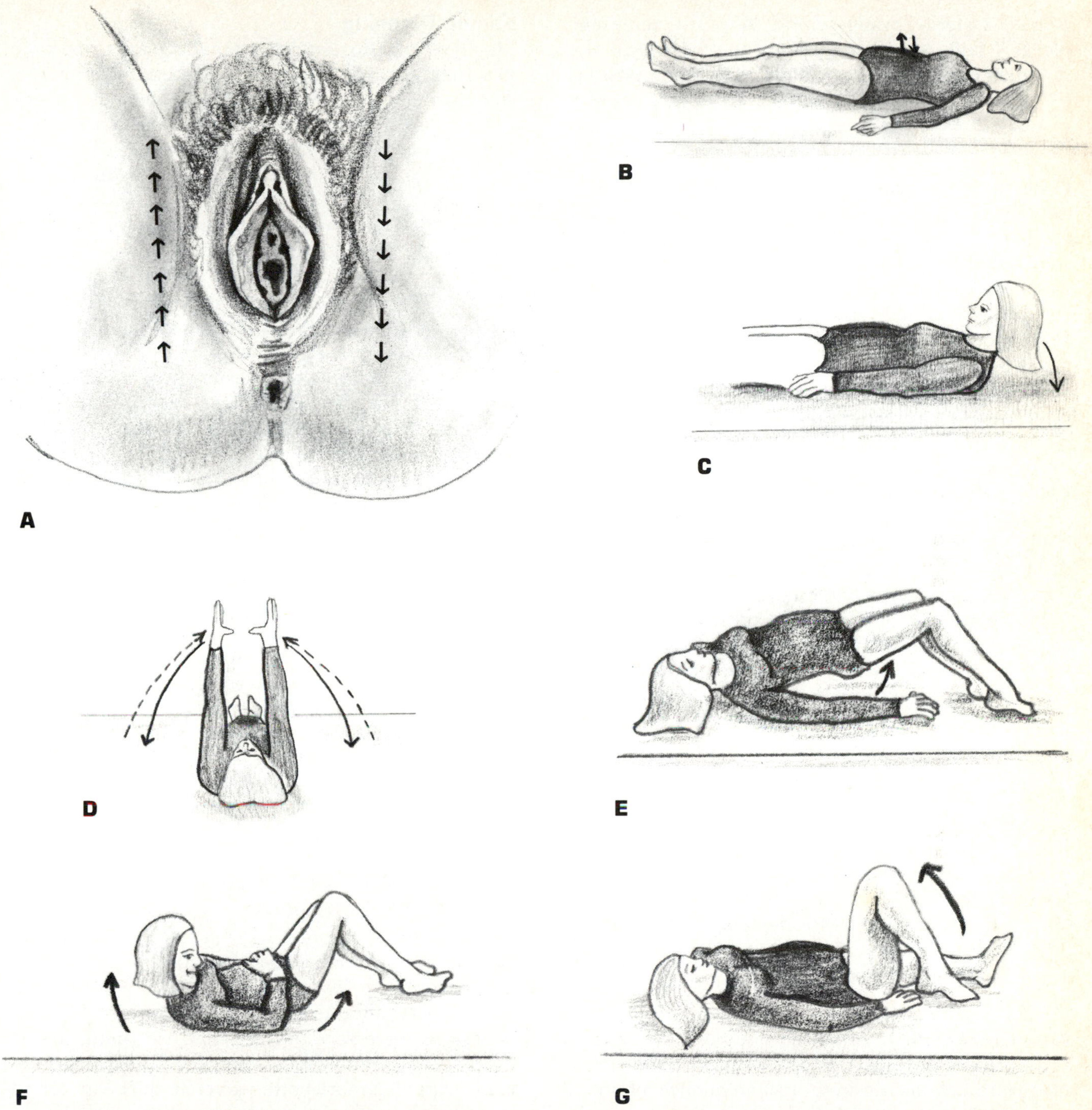

Figure 31–12. Postpartum exercises. **A.** Kegel—arrows indicate squeezing of pubococcygeal muscles during exercise. **B.** Abdominal toning No. 1. **C.** Abdominal toning No. 2—deep breathing with chin flexion. **D.** Abdominal toning No. 3—arm raises. **E.** Abdominal/back toning—pelvic rock. **F.** Abdominal/buttocks toning. **G.** Buttocks, thighs, abdominal stretching—modified leg lifts.

countered during postpartum intercourse because of perineal and vaginal tenderness, unhealed episiotomy, and lessened vaginal lubrication. To determine whether the woman can tolerate penile penetration, two fingers can be inserted into the vagina, and, if tolerated, three. The fingers are then rotated and possible areas of discomfort identified. If the woman can tolerate this procedure, she will probably tolerate intercourse. In addition, this procedure may help relax the pubococcygeal muscle. Prior to intercourse, a sterile, water-soluble lubricant, for example, K-Y Jelly, should be used. The woman can also diminish dyspareunia by using a side-lying position or a superior position, which allows for greater control of the depth of penetration.

Couples' Preferences for Resumption of Sexual Activity. The time preferred by postpartum couples for resumption of intercourse varies greatly; however, research indicates that a large number of couples resume intercourse before 6 weeks postpartum. Masters and Johnson[18] reported that despite physician recommendations for 6-week postpartum abstinence, many couples resumed intercourse by 3 weeks. In a sample of 19 primigravidas, Falicov[22] found that two thirds of the sample resumed intercourse within 2 months, with the majority resuming intercourse by 6 to 7 weeks. After reviewing the records of more than 800 women who delivered vaginally with an episiotomy, Richardson and coworkers[19] found that the majority of couples resumed intercourse with reasonable comfort and no adverse effects by 2 to 3 weeks postpartum. In a small sample of 26 couples, Hames[21] found that 62 percent resumed intercourse before 6 weeks, with a mean of 4.4 weeks. Ryding[23] reported that 12 percent of 50 women resumed intercourse during the first 4 weeks and 54 percent between 5 and 8 weeks; 16 percent had not resumed intercourse by 3 months postpartum.

Factors that prevent the resumption of sexual intercourse during the puerperium, as reported by both men and women, include fear of harm to the incision, fear of pregnancy, vaginal bleeding, physician's orders, and fear of infection.[21] Women frequently cite fatigue, soreness, or pain from the episiotomy[21,22] and tension[22] as reasons for delaying resumption of intercourse. Men often fear they will hurt their partner during puerperal intercourse.

Altered Sexuality. Although couples may resume sexual intercourse in the puerperium, their sexual responses, sexual desires, and frequency of intercourse are often altered. Several studies have indicated that women and men may experience lower levels of sexual desire after the birth of a child as compared to before the pregnancy,[18,23,24]; however, women may also experience heightened sexual desire after childbirth.[22] Some husbands of breastfeeding women have reported an increased sexual desire during the puerperium.[18] Return to prepregnancy sexual desire levels may occur any time starting in the early puerperium to more than 7 months postpartum.[25]

Family Planning

Most women do not intentionally plan to become pregnant again in the early puerperium; however, some women are pregnant again by their sixth week postpartum checkup. Lack of knowledge concerning resumption of ovulation and failure to use a contraceptive measure during intercourse are frequently the cause.

To prevent unwanted, unplanned pregnancies, women and their partners should be counseled about resumption of sexual activity and contraceptive use within a few days of the delivery. Education must include information about the variations in onset of ovulation and menstruation. Nurses should stress that ovulation frequently resumes before the first menses. The fact that ovulation can occur as early as 1 month after delivery indicates the need for early family planning counseling.

Women who do not intend to breastfeed may use oral contraceptives after delivery; however, oral contraceptives are contraindicated with breastfeeding, as the medication may cross through the breast milk. Diaphragm fittings, intrauterine device insertions, or cervical cap fittings are not performed until after 6 weeks postpartum to allow for complete reproductive involution and postpartum weight loss. The use of condoms, gel, or foam is recommended for women planning to use one of these mechanical contraceptive methods. Condoms are frequently provided before discharge. Breastfeeding mothers also are advised to use a condom, foam, or gel until a mechanical device can be used.

EDUCATIONAL PREPARATION FOR BREASTFEEDING

Education of the breastfeeding woman is necessary if lactation is to be successful. Gulick[26] found that prenatal education is a correlate to successful breastfeeding. Conversely, factors that are predictors of breastfeeding problems at one week postpartum include supplementary bottles given in the hospital and early maternal dissatisfaction with breastfeeding.[27]

In the postnatal period, nurses must reinforce and build on the knowledge that women have regarding lactation and breast care. The topics that generally should be covered in postnatal education are feeding schedules, anatomic and physiologic features of the infant that promote suckling, body positions of mother and infant, manual and mechanical expression of milk, signs and symptoms of successful lactation, management of breastfeeding and out-of-home responsibilities, care of the breasts, supplemental feedings, effects of drugs and other substances on breast milk, and treatment for common breast problems. Provision of supplementary bottles in the early postpartum period should be avoided, if possible, to avoid nipple confusion in the newborn.[28]

The reader is referred to Chapter 10 for nutritional information related to breastfeeding not covered in this section.

Feeding Schedules

Hospitals and birthing centers vary in their recommendations and practices concerning the first time the infant is placed on the breast, the frequency of feedings, and the duration of feedings. In general, successful lactation is promoted in those settings that provide for early initiation of breastfeeding and flexibility in feeding schedules.

Initiation of Breastfeeding. Providing that the mother and infant are healthy, the infant may be put to the mother's breast immediately after delivery.[30] The infant is alert within the first hour of birth and the sucking reflex is most intense during the first 20 to 60 minutes after delivery. Many health care professionals believe that this is the opportune time for the infant to accept the breast nipple. The early initiation of breastfeeding provides the infant with nourishing colostrum, stimulates the infant's digestive tract, and promotes lactation. Furthermore, initiation of breastfeeding in the immediate postdelivery period also benefits the mother by promoting uterine contractions through the release of oxytocin (Figure 31–13).

The mother needs to be made aware that the infant may not immediately take to breastfeeding. The infant should be allowed time to smell and lick the nipple when awake. The mother should not force the infant to take the nipple, for this will only frustrate the mother and the infant.

Frequency of Breastfeeding. In the early puerperium, breastfed infants require feedings every 1½ to 3 hours. The frequent feedings promote lactogenesis. For some infants, however, the need for sleep in the first few days after birth is greater than the need for nourishment, and thus an infant may refuse the breast at a given feeding. An infant's refusal of the breast is more likely to occur when hospital routines dictate a rigid "every 4 hour" feeding schedule. In general, a demand feeding schedule, that is, one in which the infant determines when to feed, is rewarding to both the mother and her infant.

As the mother's supply of milk becomes synchronized with the infant's demand for milk, the infant may begin to increase the interval between feedings, so that feedings are closer to every 3 hours and at times even less frequent. Additionally, some breastfed infants begin to sleep sporadically through the night at around 6 weeks of age, and thus do not require a night feeding.

During growth spurts at around 10 days, 3 weeks, and 3 months after birth, infants require more milk. As a result, infants will breastfeed more frequently for a day or two until the milk supply is once again synchronized with the demand. Many mothers are troubled by their infant's behaviors during growth

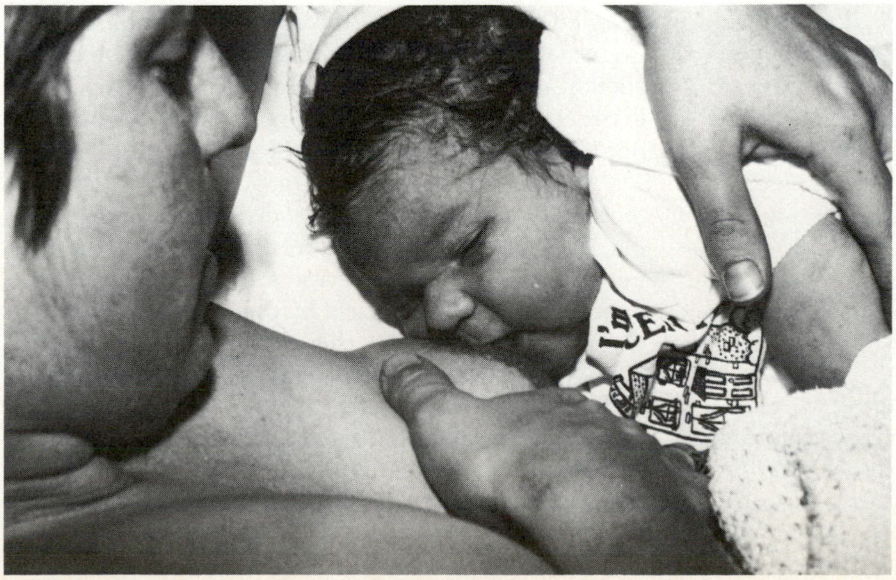

Figure 31–13. Many women wish to breastfeed immediately after delivery.

spurts, especially if they are unprepared for this phenomenon. In particular, the infant may sleep less, cry more often, respond less favorably to mother's cuddling attempts, and be less satisfied with suckling on the breast. In turn, the mother may feel she is inadequate to meet the needs of her infant and has an insufficient milk supply.[29] At the same time, well-meaning significant others, also erroneously interpreting the situation, often suggest that the mother supplement feedings with a bottle. Although a supplementary bottle may meet the immediate need of the infant, the need for increased stimulation of the mother's breasts is not met.

With anticipatory guidance from nurses, mothers can be prepared to deal effectively with the demands of growth spurts. Education should include discussion of infant behavior during growth spurts so that the mother can anticipate and correctly identify the behavior without developing feelings of inadequacy or experiencing high anxiety levels. The mother needs to be made aware of the need for increasing rest and fluid intake until feedings have stabilized again. The nurse should stress that although most women require increased fluids and rest during infant growth periods, the specific needs are highly individualized. Additionally, the mother needs to be reminded that a quiet, peaceful environment promotes the let-down reflex.

Duration of a Feeding. Usually on the first day, mothers are taught to allow the infant to suckle 5 minutes on each breast. Mothers are advised to gradually increase the time that the infant suckles on each breast by 2 to 3 minutes a day, until the infant is suckling at least 12 to 15 minutes on each breast per feeding. In addition, mothers are told to alternate the breast on which the infant suckles first at each feeding. This recommended pattern for feedings promotes lactogenesis and may prevent nipple soreness. In particular, lactogenesis is promoted through the emptying of the breasts. Generally, within the first 5 to 7 minutes of a feeding, most of the milk is ejected, and by 12 minutes the breast is emptied. As soon as the mother's nipples are toughened, she can allow the infant to suckle on her breasts longer then the amount of time needed to empty the breast so that the infant's oral needs are satisfied.

Infant Mechanisms to Aid in Feeding

The infant is born with several mechanisms to aid in breastfeeding. The less prominent lower jaw and the fat pads in the cheeks aid in sucking. The sucking and gag reflexes help to control fluid intake. The rooting reflex is particularly helpful in orienting the infant to the human breast. To use the rooting reflex, the mother should stroke the infant's cheek that is closest to the breast that she wants the infant to suck on first. The infant's head will then turn toward the breast and the mouth will open in search of the breast. The mother should be cautioned that only the cheek adjacent to the breast should be stimulated. Stroking the other cheek may only confuse and frustrate the infant.

Body Positions of Mother and Infant

Proper positioning of the mother and infant is essential for the promotion of successful breastfeeding and the prevention of related problems. Improper positioning of the mother places undue strain on maternal body parts and may subsequently make the mother tense and uncomfortable during the feeding. Improper positioning of the infant during a feeding can traumatize the mother's breasts, as well as frustrate the infant. With improper positioning, the infant is unable to draw the nipple and areola into the mouth fully and ends up gumming the nipple and parts of the areola without receiving milk. The nipples and parts of the areolae may become sore and cracked and may bleed. In addition, improper positioning may prematurely break the suction of the infant's mouth on the breast, thus traumatizing the nipple and frustrating the infant. If the nipple and areola are viewed as the face of a clock, soreness typically occurs in two areas: on the right breast between 10 and 12 o'clock and 4 and 6 o'clock; and on the left breast between 12 and 2 o'clock and 6 and 8 o'clock.[31]

Proper positioning enables the infant to latch onto the breast appropriately and effectively and promotes the mother's comfort during the feeding. Additionally, when the infant and mother are appropriately positioned the mother has the control to gently insert a finger into the side of the infant's mouth to break the suction at the end of the feeding. The mother will need instruction and assistance in positioning herself and her infant during the first few feedings.

In positioning the infant on the breast, the mother must take care to prevent trauma to the nipple. Specifically to prevent nipple trauma the mother needs to guide her nipple and areola straight into the infant's mouth. As much of the areola as possible should be taken into the infant's mouth (Figure 31–14). Some infants do not need assistance in drawing in the nipple and areola; however, many infants initially are unable to grasp the areola. In these latter situations, the mother should first reposition herself and the infant; then, with the areola compressed between her index and middle finger, she should guide the nipple and areola into the infant's mouth.

RESEARCH ABSTRACT

Chapman JJ, et al. Concerns of breast-feeding mothers from birth to four months. Nurs Res. *1985;34:374–377.*

This qualitative descriptive study investigated the concerns of 50 breastfeeding mothers. Subjects ranged in age from 18 to 35 years. Thirty-four were primiparas, one of whom had a history of breastfeeding an adopted child. Sixteen were multiparas, 15 of whom had breastfed previously. Six mothers stopped breastfeeding before 4 months, thus reducing the sample to 44. Eleven of the infants were preterm, ranging from 27 to 37 weeks of gestation; two of these infants remained hospitalized for 2 to 6 weeks.

The researchers defined "concerns" as the quality of breastfeeding experiences as reported by the mother. To assess the concerns of breastfeeding mothers, one of the researchers, the project nurse, recorded interactions that took place between the mother and this researcher at hospital visits, at home visits, and through telephone conversations.

Data were analyzed and grouped into three emerging themes: breast concerns, infant concerns, and postpartum concerns; a time reference was included to indicate the prevalence of these concerns. Mothers expressed breast concerns about adequate amount of milk through the second month; sore nipples for up to 3 months; frequency of breastfeeding for up to 63 to 111 days; infant preference for one breast up to 4 months; and pumping and saving milk through 4 months. Mothers expressed concerns about infant behaviors, for example, fussiness, sleepiness, and day-night confusion throughout the 4 months; infant rash during all 4 months; weight of infant throughout the 4 months; and responses of the infant beginning at 3 weeks, peaking during the second month, and lasting until the end of the study. Mothers expressed postpartum concerns about fatigue during all 4 months; adjustment of siblings an unspecified time; ambivalence about returning to work or school peaking at the fifth week and the third month; lack of weight loss during the second and third weeks, peaking at the end of the second and fourth months; and having a cold from 2 weeks to the end of the study. The authors conclude that because concerns persist throughout the 4 months, a professional needs to evaluate and assist breastfeeding mothers for at least 16 weeks.

Comment:
This study builds on previous studies that assessed concerns of mothers shortly after delivery and up to 1 month postpartum. The results of this study indicate that the early concerns expressed by mothers continue beyond the first month postpartum. The researchers aptly note that effective guidance and counseling must be timed and thus indicate that anticipatory guidance may not always be effective. Problems and or concerns that are expressed early in the puerperium may change in quality and characteristics, necessitating different interventions or reinforcement of counseling.

The mother often needs assistance in finding a comfortable position for breastfeeding. Mothers experiencing abdominal or perineal discomforts may be more comfortable lying on their sides. Using pillows for support, the mother should lie on her side in the recumbent position. The infant is then placed on a pillow or a rolled blanket in a side-lying position with the mouth parallel to the mother's nipple and the feet toward the mother's waist (Figure 31–15A).

If the mother experiences cracked or bleeding nipples, the infant's side-lying position can be altered so that her or his feet are near the mother's head. With this variation a different area of the nipple is stimulated.

Many mothers prefer to sit in a chair or in a bed while breastfeeding. Support to the mother's back and her arms is needed to provide comfort and reduce strain. A pillow under the mother's knees if she is in bed or a stool on which to rest her flexed legs if she is sitting in a chair provides additional support. Some mothers find that placing a pillow on the abdomen to rest the infant on helps to reduce strain (Figure 31–15B). Usually while in the sitting position, the mother cradles the infant's body; however, the infant can be placed in a football hold, especially if the mother has cracked or bleeding nipples. (Figure 31–15C).

Regardless of the position that the mother and infant assume, the mother needs to make certain that the infant's nares are not obstructed by the mother's breast. To accomplish this, the mother usually presses her breast away from the infant's nose with a finger from her free hand.

Signs and Symptoms of Successful Lactation

A major concern of breastfeeding mothers is how to know if the infant is receiving enough milk. The mother can be taught to observe for signs and symptoms that indicate successful lactation.

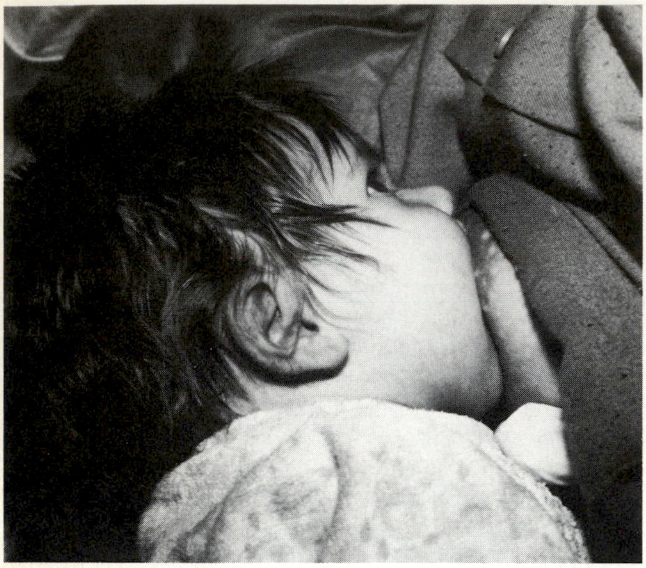

Figure 31–14. Proper positioning of the infant's mouth on the breast.

Within the first few days of birth colostrum provides sufficient nourishment to meet the infant's nutritional needs.[30] Mothers need to be taught that newborn infants do not require a large intake during the first few days after birth. Most often the infant's need for sleep is greater than the need for nutrition at this time. The small frequent feedings are all the infant requires initially. At about the same time that the mother's milk production begins, the infant's need for sleep diminishes. The mother will note that the infant demonstrates a desire to suckle for a longer period.

The mother can determine whether the infant is ingesting enough breast milk if the infant urinates pale straw-colored urine at least six to eight times a day. Bowel movements are not as indicative of sufficient intake of breast milk. Many breastfed infants will have a loose bowel movement with each feeding. Other breastfed infants may have a bowel movement every other day or even every third or fourth day.

Weight gain is obviously a sign that the infant is receiving enough milk; however, a newborn normally may lose up to 10 percent of the birth weight. Parents should be discouraged from purchasing a baby scale or from placing too much emphasis on the daily weight rather than the actual pattern of weight gain.

The mother can also determine if the infant is taking in sufficient quantities of milk if, during the feeding, the infant can be heard swallowing. Furthermore, if the infant is content after feedings, he or she most likely has ingested a sufficient quantity of milk.

Lactation and Responsibilities Out of the Home

Many lactating mothers decide to continue breastfeeding as they resume their roles outside of the home. Three main alternatives for continuing breastfeeding exist for the mother returning to work, school, and other out-of-home activities. The alternative selected depends on the mother's responsibilities outside of the home, the degree to which the mother can maintain lactation while separated from her infant, and the mother's physiologic and psychologic responses to assuming multiple roles.

Some mothers with flexible schedules who are generally in close proximity to the infant may opt to return to the infant for feedings. This option requires that the infant be on a feeding schedule so that the mother can plan, in advance, when she will need to return home.

Many mothers decide that they want their infant to receive breast milk from a bottle when they cannot be available for the feeding. To provide a supply of breast milk for bottlefeedings, the mother needs to manually express or pump her breasts at those feedings that she misses and to express any milk left at the end of each feeding. The mother will need information on the proper storage of milk.

As the amount of milk pumped or manually expressed is usually less than that obtained by an infant suckling, the mother needs to anticipate that the amount of milk she produces may gradually be diminished. At the same time, however, the mother will find that the infant may be independently weaning from specific feedings; for example, some 2- to 3-month-old infants no longer require a late evening feeding. The mother can express and store milk from those feedings that the infant no longer requires. This alternative for maintaining a supply of breast milk for bottlefeeding can be quite successful. Some women find that if they are physically or psychologically exhausted they cannot maintain a sufficient supply of stored milk and, as a consequence, may feel guilty. Nurses need to help the mother anticipate the possible problems encountered in trying to maintain an adequate supply of milk and handle the stressors produced from other responsibilities. Anticipatory guidance needs to include discussion of the alternatives available to the breastfeeding mother.

As a third alternative, the infant can be provided formula feedings when the mother misses a feeding. Essentially, the infant is weaned off breast milk for given feedings. This alternative works well for those mothers who are unable to pump their breasts on a regular basis. Initially, the mother may experience fullness in the breasts and leakage of milk when she

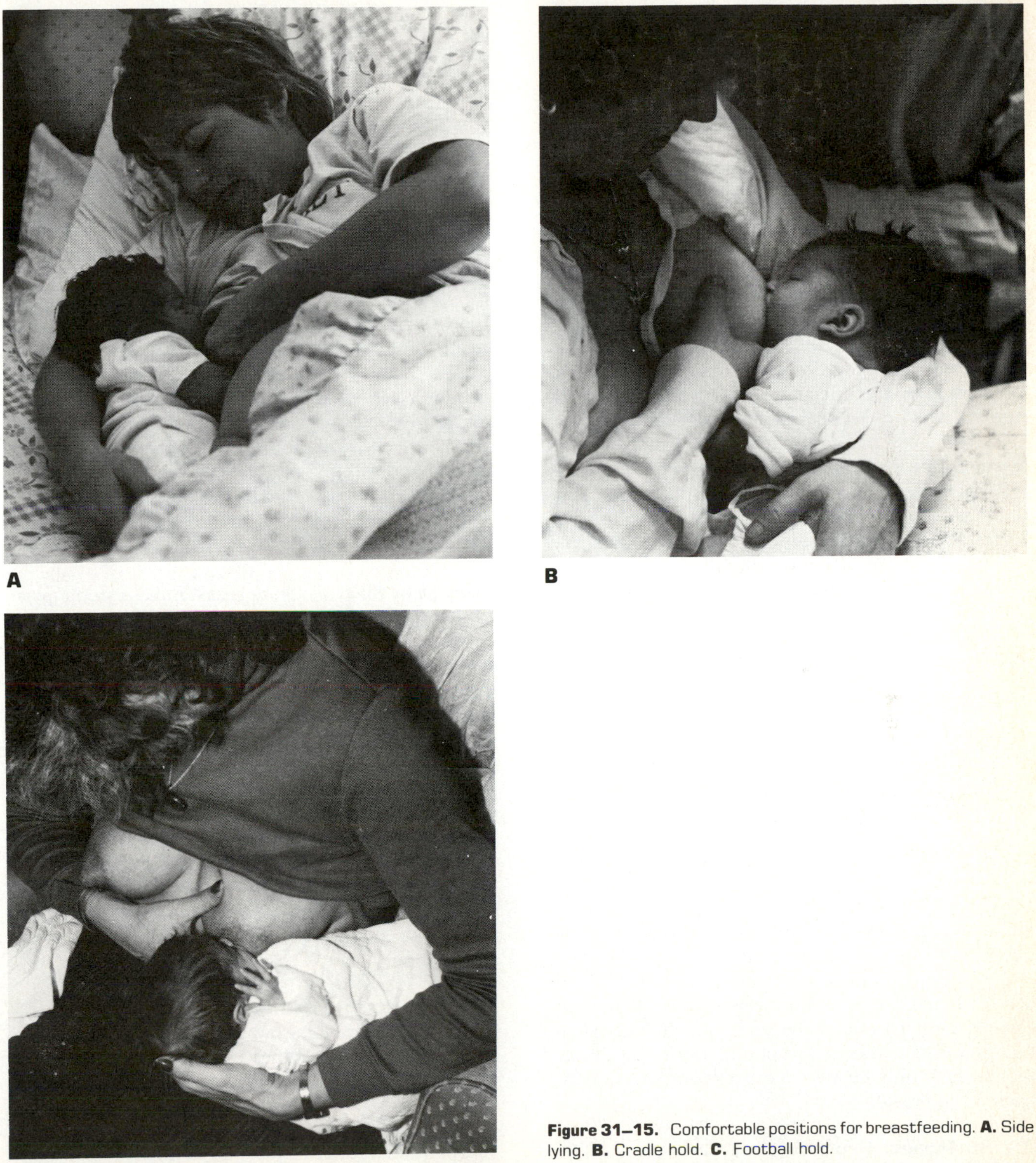

A

B

C

Figure 31–15. Comfortable positions for breastfeeding. **A.** Side lying. **B.** Cradle hold. **C.** Football hold.

misses a feeding. Wearing breast pads and tightly folding her arms across her nipples can control the leakage of milk temporarily. To relieve breast discomfort caused by missed feedings, the mother can try expressing some milk. Without sufficient stimulation, the breasts eventually cease lactation for those feedings from which the infant is weaned.

Manual and Mechanical Expression of Milk

All breastfeeding women should be taught how to express milk from their breasts and the proper method of storage. Expression of breast milk is needed to relieve breast engorgement, to maintain lactogenesis when the mother and infant are separated, and to provide human milk to the infant when conditions prevent the infant from breastfeeding.

Both manual and mechanical expression of milk begins with bringing the milk from the alveolar lumina through the ductal system toward the areola. Application of moist heat to the breasts in the form of a shower or compresses, followed by breast massage, promotes the initial release of milk through the ductal system. Breast massage may be accomplished by encircling the periphery of the breast and applying gentle traction toward the nipple. Breast massage may also be performed by supporting the breast with one hand and, with the flat surface of the other hand, firmly, repeatedly stroking the breast from the periphery toward the center until the entire breast is massaged. After breast massage, the milk is ready to be expressed. If the milk is to be saved and used later, a sterile container should be used to collect the milk.

To express milk manually, the thumb is placed on the upper outer edge of the areola while the fingers are placed on the lower edge. The thumb and fingers exert pressure back toward the chest wall and then are compressed together slightly in a downward direction. Initially a small amount of milk is secreted (Figure 31–16). After a few seconds, the mother experiences the let-down reflex; however, if the manual expression immediately follows a feeding, the let-down reflex may not be elicited.

The mother should be cautioned that the amount of milk expressed by hand rarely equals the amount of milk the baby obtains by sucking. Whereas an infant may obtain at least 3 oz of milk from a breast, the mother may only be able to express an ounce or two from a full breast.

Breast Pumps. Depending on the nature of the need for expression of milk, the mother may wish to obtain a breast pump. The nurse can help the mother decide on which type of pump will meet her needs and those of the infant. The LaLeche League, a support group for breastfeeding mothers, can also provide information on breast pumps.

All breast pumps consist of a glass or plastic funnel attached to a glass or plastic receptacle. Until recently, manual breast pumps (eg, Lloyd B pump) created suction by squeezing either a bulb or a handle attached to the funnel. With the Kaneson pump, however, suction is created by the mother's moving an inner cylinder funnel back and forth within an outer cylinder. These pumps are appropriate for mothers who want to maintain lactogenesis when temporarily separated from their infant. Additionally, these pumps may be sufficient to meet the needs of working mothers.

Mothers who need to collect milk for premature infants or for infants who cannot suck because of a health problem may want to rent an electric pump (Figure 31–17). When the infant cannot suck for an extended period, the electric pumps can best stimulate lactogenesis as well as empty the breasts completely. Mechanical pumping should be gradually increased and should not exceed 10 minutes per breast.

Breast pumps should be thoroughly cleaned after each use. The funnel and milk receptacle should be sterilized.

Storage of Milk. To store breast milk, a sterile plastic container is recommended. Immunoglobin present in breast milk tends to stick to glass bottles. At home, some mothers prefer to store milk in sterile plastic disposable bottle inserts. All milk stored in the hospital needs to be labeled with the mother's name, the date, the time, and the amount. All milk stored at home should be labeled with the date, time, and amount. Breast milk can be safely stored for 48 hours in the refrigerator and up to 2 months in the main storage area of the freezer of a two-door refrigerator.

Frozen milk should be defrosted by placing it in the refrigerator a few hours before the feeding. The bottle is then placed under warm tap water. As stored breast milk often separates, the bottle needs to be shaken.

Supplementary Feedings

Hospitals provide dextrose and water or plain water bottles for breastfeeding infants. Many lactating women, fearing that their infant is not receiving enough nourishment, are tempted to give their infant a supplementary bottle. Unfortunately, in the early puerperium, frequent bottle supplements tend to confuse the breastfed infant.[28] The sucking mechanism of breastfeeding differs from that needed with bottle-feeding in terms of effort exerted, use of muscles,

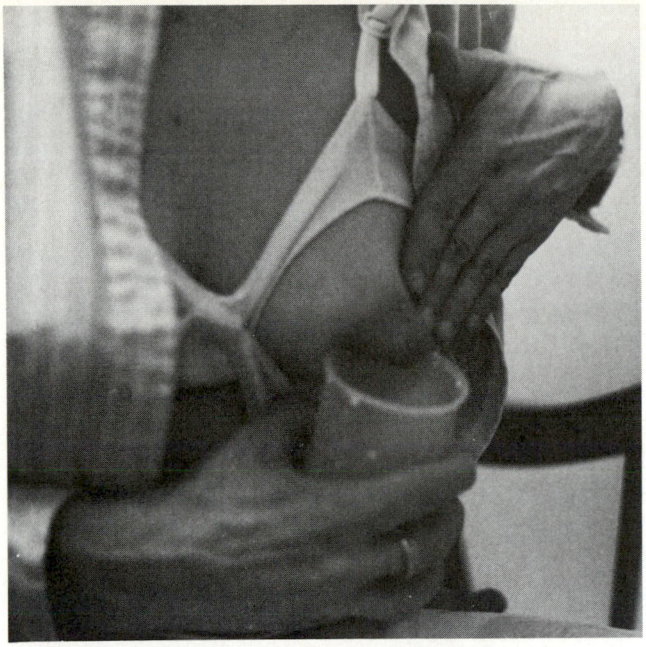

A

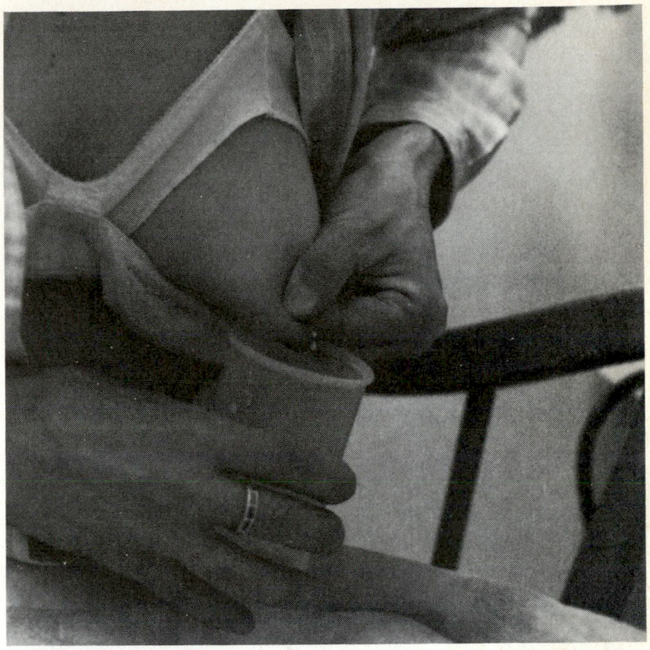

B

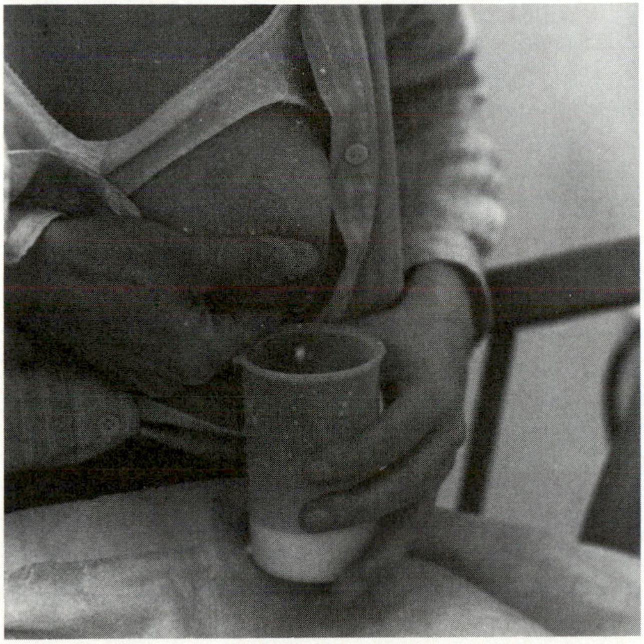

C

Figure 31–16. Sequence of manual expression of milk. **A.** Breast massage stimulates release of milk from the ducts. **B.** Initially only a small amount of milk is secreted. **C.** Within a few seconds the let-down reflex occurs.

amount of air taken in, and direction in which the tongue is thrust.

In breastfeeding, the infant must suck vigorously to stimulate the let-down reflex. Aided by facial muscles, the infant thrusts the tongue up and forward to grasp and draw the human nipple into the mouth and against the hard palate. The areola is compressed by the gums, limiting the amount of air swallowed. Accordingly, many breastfed infants do not need to be burped frequently.

With bottlefeedings, the facial muscles are relaxed as the tongue is thrust forward to control the flow of milk from the rubber nipple. Closure of the infant's mouth around the rubber nipple is incomplete, resulting in the ingestion of air and the need for frequent burping (Figure 31–18).

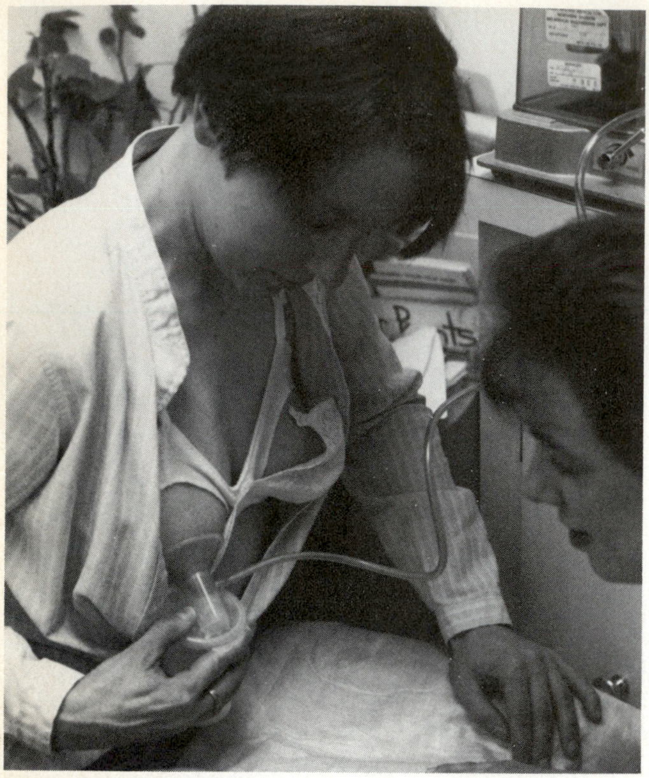

Figure 31–17. Nurse instructs mother in use of electric breast pump.

When offered a bottle, the breastfed infant may ingest too much fluid and regurgitate frequently in the early postdelivery period. If the breastfed infant receives a supplementary bottle frequently in the first few weeks of life, the infant is likely to refuse the breast out of frustration when the breast milk does not flow immediately as does formula. In general, supplementary bottles should be avoided until lactation is well established. When additional water is needed after breastfeeding in the early postdelivery period, a dropper or spoon instead of a nipple can be used to avoid nipple confusion. If after breastfeeding is established, supplementary bottles are needed, use of a Nuk nipple, which is shaped like the human nipple in the infant's mouth, or a nipple with a small hole is advised (Figure 31–19). Waiting until 2 to 3 weeks to give a supplementary bottle will provide enough time for the infant to master the sucking mechanism of breastfeeding, as well as to tolerate the altered rate of fluid flow from a bottle.

Mothers who have responsibilities out of the home, who are extremely tired and need a night's rest, or who would like the father or other persons to feed the infant occasionally may decide to have the infant bottlefed at times. If the mother knows in advance that she will miss a feeding she can express and leave breast milk for the infant. If the mother wishes to have the infant receive formula, a soy formula may be tried first because there is less chance of an allergic reaction to soy than to a formula based on cow's milk. (*See* Chapter 34 for additional discussion of infant formulas and bottlefeeding.)

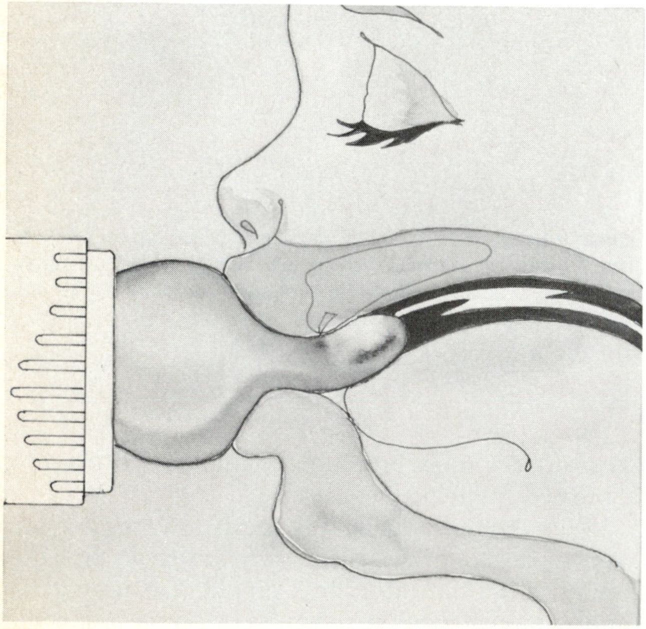

Figure 31–18. Sucking mechanism; infant's mouth sucking on bottle.

Care of the Breasts

Potential problems related to breastfeeding can be prevented through proper breast care. A well-fitted brassiere provides support. Many women find that until the milk supply matches the infant's demands, a brassiere needs to be worn 24 hours a day to minimize discomfort. Nursing brassieres have a hook or

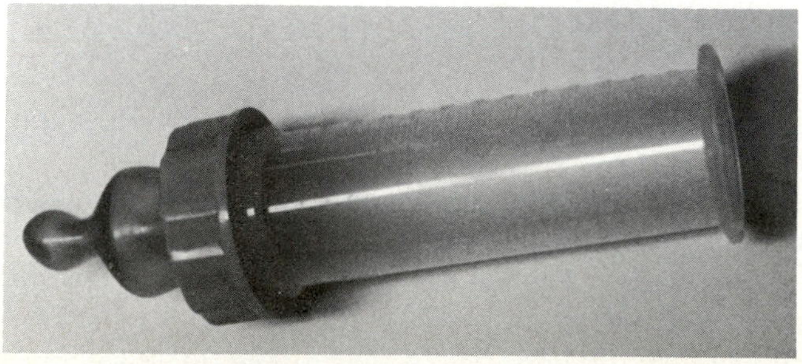

Figure 31–19. Bottle with Nuk nipple.

snap on top of each cup, so that the breast may be exposed without losing support. The mother should be cautioned to avoid nursing brassieres that have a plastic lining. Although plastic linings protect outer clothing from leakage of milk from the breasts, the nipples may become sore and prone to infection from trapped moisture. Disposable nursing pads can be used to protect clothing. Homemade pads from handkerchiefs and diapers are also useful.

Many hospitals advise that the mother wash her nipples with sterile water prior to the feeding. Most women forego this practice once at home without any adverse problems. After feedings, excess milk should be wiped off to prevent clogging of the nipples.

The nipples should not be washed with soap or dusted with powder as these agents dry the nipples. Nipples should be air dried. Lanolin cream may be applied to lubricate the nipples. Usually women do not require any nipple creams after a few weeks of breastfeeding. Any ointment used should be wiped off before the next feeding.

Effects of Drugs and Other Substances on Breast Milk

Drugs and other substances ingested by the mother may be transported to breast milk by diffusion through lipid membranes, diffusion through water-filled pores, and active transport.[32] Many drugs and other substances are potentially harmful to the infant. Consequently, mothers need to be educated about the potential danger to the infant. Nurses need to stress that the breastfeeding mother should always consult a health care professional before taking any medications. Appendix F lists the drugs that may pass through the breast milk and their effects on the infant. Nurses should point out that alcohol is also a drug. Mothers should also be advised that caffeine may be found in breast milk. High levels of caffeine may cause the infant to be restless.[33]

Nicotine from smoking can pass from the maternal blood system into the breast milk. Nicotine is thought to reduce the supply of breast milk.[33] Smoking during a feeding or when holding a baby is generally not advised because the infant may inhale the smoke.[33,34]

Effects of Environmental Pollutants on Breast Milk

In the past two decades much concern has been expressed about environmental pollutants contaminating the milk of breastfeeding women. Polychlorinated biphenyls (PCBs), polybrominated biphenyls (PBBs), and insecticides such as DDT and dieldrin have been found in relatively small amounts in breast milk and cow's milk. Governmental restrictions and prohibitions of these pollutants have reduced their levels in the environment within the United States. Although the levels of these pollutants in breast milk are not considered to be harmful, precautionary measures are advised. As these pollutants tend to be stored in fat, women should avoid foods high in butter fat and should remove the fat from meats and poultry. All fruits and vegetables should be washed well to remove insecticidal residue that may have accumulated. Both mother and infant should avoid places recently sprayed with insecticides.

NUTRITIONAL COUNSELING

Nurses, in collaboration with nutritionists, need to provide individualized nutritional counseling and education for postpartum women. Diet histories including present dietary intake, usual diet at home, maternal expectations and perceptions about body weight and configuration, knowledge of infant and maternal nutritional needs, and plans for dieting need to be assessed. The recommended dietary intake is based on a healthy, average woman. Breastfeeding women who are overweight and have excessive food intake should not increase consumption. Conversely, women who are underweight frequently need to increase their consumption of food. Breastfeeding women who are already drinking enough fluids need not be encouraged to drink more, but rather should be provided with encouragement for the desired behavior.

Nutritional education and counseling should include anticipatory guidance regarding weight loss. In the early postpartum period, many women are dissatisfied with their body weights and configurations. Despite the needs of lactation and the fact that fat stored during the pregnancy is used up within 3 months, many breastfeeding women place themselves on a reducing diet. Nurses need to help breastfeeding women plan appropriate, well-balanced diets that also allow for some weight loss.

PHARMACOTHERAPEUTICS

During the early postpartum period, pharmacologic agents may be used to suppress lactation, to promote uterine contractions so that uterine bleeding is minimized, and to relieve pain and discomfort from episiotomy, lacerations, abdominal incision, abdominal flatulence, nipple soreness, and afterpains. The nurse is responsible for monitoring the responses to pharmacologic agents.

Suppression of Lactation

Suppression of lactation through pharmacologic agents has been popular since the middle of the 20th century. Until recently, estrogens and estrogen-androgen preparations were widely used. Occasionally diuretics have been used to suppress lactation. The success rate, however, is low. Because of the known side effects of hormonal preparations, supporters of pharmacologic suppression of lactation have, for the most part, switched to a nonhormonal prolactin inhibitor.

Estrogen Preparations. Diethylstilbestrol (DES) and chlorotrianisene (Tace), synthetic estrogen preparations, have been used to suppress lactation. Usually diethylstilbestrol 5-mg tablets one to three times a day for a total of 30 mg, or chlorotrianisene 75-mg capsule twice a day for 2 days, is prescribed. Rebound breast engorgement frequently occurs when administration of these estrogen preparations ceases.[35]

Increased knowledge about the side effects from estrogen preparations and the Food and Drug Administration's mandate that all women receiving estrogen therapy be given written information regarding the side effects of these drugs have been cited as the reasons for the significant decline in the use of estrogen preparations to suppress lactation. Side effects from estrogen preparations are nausea, bleeding, and thromboembolic disease in postpartum women.[3] In particular, women already predisposed to thromboembolic disease during the postpartum period are at risk if they are given estrogen preparations.

Estrogen-Androgen Preparations. Deladumone (testosterone enanthate and estradiol valerate), a long-acting estrogen-androgen preparation, was widely used to suppress lactation prior to the 1980s. Immediately after delivery, 2 mL of Deladumone was injected intramuscularly. In addition to the side effects from estrogen, deladumone also has side effects from the androgen component, including virilization as manifested by hirsutism, hoarseness, and acne, and additional delay in resumption of menstruation.

Prolactin Inhibitor. Use of the prolactin inhibitor bromocriptine mesylate (Parlodel) has for the most part replaced hormonal preparations for suppression of lactation (Box 31–3). As a dopamine receptor antagonist, bromocriptine mesylate acts at the dopamine receptor sites of prolactin-secreting cells of the anterior pituitary gland to release prolactin-inhibiting factor, thereby preventing mammary secretion, engorgement, and pain resulting from lactogenesis. The usual dosage of bromocriptine mesylate is one 2.5-mg tablet twice a day with meals for 14 to 21 days. As bromocriptine mesylate can cause hypotension, the treatment should not be initiated until vital signs are stable and at least 4 hours have passed since delivery. Known side effects include nausea, headaches, dizziness, and hypotension. Brooten and colleagues,[3] comparing four different treatment groups, found that women receiving bromocriptine mesylate experienced significantly less breast engorgement, pain, and leakage of colostrum and milk than women treated with either a compression binder, a standardized support bra, or fluid restrictions. Regardless of the treatment, Brooten and coworkers[3] found that the highest incidence of breast pain occurred between the third and fifth postpartum days. Although this study indicates that a prolactin inhibitor may be more effective than any one nonpharmacologic measure, there is no indication of how a prolactin inhibitor compares in effectiveness to a combination of nonpharmacologic measures in suppressing lactation.

Promotion of Uterine Contractions

Oxytocin. Synthetic oxytocin (Pitocin) is commonly used in the immediate postdelivery period to stimulate uterine contractions as a means of controlling postpartum bleeding (*see* Box 27–1). Typically the dosage of oxytocin is 10 to 40 U/1000 mL of intravenous fluid, although the drug is available for intramuscular and buccal administration. Tetanic contractions may occur. Oxytocin is contraindicated in women with severe toxemia and hypersensitivity.

Ergonovine Maleate. Ergonovine maleate (Ergotrate) is administered as a 0.2-mg oral tablet every 6 to 12 hours to promote uterine contractions postpartum (Box 31–4). Within 6 to 15 minutes, and lasting for approximately 90 minutes, this drug produces firm tetanic contractions of the uterus. The tetanic contractions gradually change to more clonic contractions. Known side effects include hypertensive episodes, sudden allergic shock, nausea, and vomiting.

Methylergonovine Maleate. Methylergonovine maleate (Methergine) (Box 31–4) rapidly produces a sustained tetanic contraction to minimize blood loss

BOX 31–3. BROMOCRIPTINE MESYLATE

Proprietary Name:
Parlodel (Sandoz).

Classification:
Dopamine agonist.

Action:
This semisynthetic ergot alkaloid inhibits release of prolactin from anterior pituitary gland by dopamine agonist activity, by direct effect on pituitary, or by both. In women with amenorrhea secondary to hyperprolactinemia, it stimulates ovulation. Also suppresses physiologic lactation.

Indications:
Treatment of hyperprolactinemia and associated disorders, such as amenorrhea, infertility in women, and galactorrhea. Prevention of physiologic lactation after stillbirth or abortion or after parturition when the mother elects not to breastfeed or if breastfeeding is contraindicated.

Dosage and Route:
Administered orally only. *Hyperprolactinemic disorders:* Dose should be individualized for client. Starting dose is 1.25 to 2.5 mg daily. If needed, increase dose by 2.5 mg daily at 3- to 7-day intervals. Therapeutic dose generally ranges from 2.5 to 15 mg daily. *Prevention of lactation:* 2.5 mg twice daily for 14–21 days. Should be initiated no sooner than 4 hours after delivery and only after vital signs are stable.

Pharmacokinetics:
Absorption: Only 28 percent of dose is absorbed from gastrointestinal tract, but significant amounts first pass through the liver, reducing bioavailability to 6 percent. *Distribution:* Peak levels 1–1.5 hours after ingestion. Highly bound to albumin (90–96 percent). *Elimination:* Metabolized in liver and excreted in feces via biliary elimination with half-life of 45–50 hours.

Contraindications and Precautions:
Contraindicated in clients with pituitary tumors, uncontrolled hypertension, toxemia of pregnancy, and sensitivity to ergot alkaloids. Caution in renal or hepatic disease, with concurrent hypotensive agents, pre-existing psychiatric disorders, or cardiac arrhythmias. Safety not established in pregnant women or children under 15 years of age.

Adverse Reactions:
More common in doses ≥20 mg/day and in treatment of hyperprolactinemic disorders. *Most common:* Nausea, headache, dizziness, decrease in blood pressure (≥20 mm Hg systolic, ≥10 mm Hg diastolic) primarily in postpartum women but usually transient. *Less common:* CNS—drowsiness, fatigue, insomnia, confusion, hallucinations, seizures; CV—hypertension (mean onset 6 days postpartum), stroke (mean onset 13 days postpartum); GI—vomiting, anorexia, epigastric pain, diarrhea, constipation, peptic ulcer, GI hemorrhage; other—metallic taste, visual disturbances, urticaria; fetal—major anomalies have been reported after taken by mother during pregnancy, but incidence no higher than overall population.

Drug Interactions:

- Amitriptyline, butyrophenones, imipramine, methyldopa, phenothiazines, reserpine: May increase prolactin levels.
- Alcohol (ethanol): Decreased tolerance to alcohol with high doses of bromocriptine.
- Antihypertensive agents: Additive hypotensive effect.
- Oral contraceptives: May antagonize effects of bromocriptine.

Nursing Implications:

- Assess vital signs.
- Withold medication until vital signs are stable and at least 4 hours have passed since delivery.

CNS = central nervous system, CV = cardiovascular system, GI = gastrointestinal system.

after delivery. This medication is used in cases of subinvolution, that is, when the uterus does not reduce in size as expected. The usual oral dose is a 0.2-mg tablet three to four times a day, up to 1 week. If intramuscular injection is desired 1 mL containing 0.2 mg of the drug is administered every 2 to 4 hours. Intravenous administration of methylergonovine maleate is discouraged for routine usage because of the increased chance of sudden hypertension or cerebrovascular accident. Known side effects are nausea, vomiting, transient hypertension, headaches, dizziness, tinnitus, palpitations, diaphoresis, and dyspnea.

Relief from Pain and Discomfort

Pharmacologic therapy for pain and discomfort from episiotomy, lacerations, abdominal incision, or puerperal uterine contractions ranges from mild analge-

BOX 31–4. ERGONOVINE AND METHYLERGONOVINE MALEATE

Proprietary Names:
Ergonovine maleate—Ergotrate (Lilly); methylergonovine maleate—Methergine (Sandoz).

Classification:
Oxytocic.

Action:
Directly stimulates contraction of uterine and vascular smooth muscle. Also produces vasoconstriction, primarily of capacitance vessels.

Indications:
Prevention and treatment of postpartum and postabortion hemorrhage caused by uterine atony or subinvolution.

Dosage and Route:
Administered orally or IM (may be used IV if uterine bleeding is severe and it is given over more than 1 minute). *Oral:* 0.2–0.4 mg every 6–12 hours for 2–7 days. *IM or IV:* 0.2 mg every 2–4 hours as needed (maximum five doses).

Pharmacokinetics:
Absorption: Rapidly absorbed after oral administration. Onset of action 5–15 minutes after oral, 2–5 minutes after IM, and immediately after IV dose. *Distribution:* Limited data; detected in breast milk, but insufficient amount to affect infant. *Elimination:* Limited data, believed to be by nonrenal routes with half-life of 0.5–2 hours.

Contraindications and Precautions:
Use with caution in women with cardiovascular disease or hepatic or renal dysfunction.

Adverse Reactions:
Most common: Nausea, vomiting. *Less common:* CNS—headache, tinnitus, dizziness; CV—palpitations, chest pain, hypertension (especially after rapid IV administration); GU—hematuria.

Drug Interactions:

- Regional anesthesia: Increased risk of hypertension.
- Vasoconstrictors: Increased risk of hypertension.

Nursing Implications:

- Assess vital signs.
- Provide information regarding possible discomforts, such as cramping.

IM = intramuscular(ly), IV = intravenous(ly), CNS = central nervous system, CV = cardiovascular system, GU = genitourinary system.

sics to narcotics and includes combinations of a mild analgesic with a narcotic. These medications are usually available to women on an as needed (prn) basis, every 4 hours.

Analgesia. Acetaminophen, ibuprophen, and propoxyphene are effective for mild to moderate discomfort of the perineum and breasts and for uterine cramping. Acetaminophen also has antipyretic effects. In therapeutic doses acetaminophen usually does not produce side effects. In excessive amounts, acetaminophen can cause gastrointestinal irritability, nausea and vomiting, tachycardia, cyanosis, jaundice, anemia, and liver damage.

Ibuprofen (Motrin, Advil) is a non-narcotic analgesic that also has anti-inflammatory and antipyretic properties. The drug's actions include blocking prostaglandin synthesis. Ibuprofen is useful in the postpartum for relief of uterine cramping and episiotomy discomfort. The usual dosage ranges from 400 to 800 mg, 3 to 4 times per day, but not to exceed 3.2 g/day. Adverse effects include visual disturbances, renal function changes, and increased tendency for bleeding.

Given in excessive quantities, propoxyphene can cause sedation dizziness, paradoxic excitement, and weakness. It is slightly less potent than codeine.

Codeine. Codeine 30 to 60 mg orally is indicated for severe to moderate pain from abdominal incision, episiotomy, lacerations, and pharmacologically induced uterine contractions. Codeine can depress respirations; decrease gastrointestinal activity, resulting in constipation and decreased mobility of the bladder; produce euphoria; and induce nausea and vomiting.

Oxycodone. Oxycodone (Percodan, Percocet) is a derivative of morphine and is related to codeine. (Percocet combines oxycodone with acetaminophen.) Side effects are the same as those for codeine and morphine.

Simethicone. Simethicone (Mylicon) 40 to 80 mg is used to minimize gastrointestinal discomfort from entrapped flatus, especially after a cesarean delivery. For maximum effectiveness one tablet should be chewed after meals and at bedtime.

CARE AFTER DISCHARGE AND IN ALTERNATIVE SETTINGS

Care of the postpartum woman takes place in a variety of settings, for example, homes, birthing centers, and hospitals. Contemporary health care providers no longer view pregnancy and childbirth as illnesses, but rather as healthy phenomena. In accordance with this positive view of pregnancy and childbirth, most health care delivery settings now strive for early discharge of the healthy postpartum woman. Birthing centers, both within a hospital or in close proximity, may discharge women as early as 2 to 24 hours after delivery. Even within the traditional hospital setting, some women are discharged within 12 to 24 hours. Home births and early discharge from birthing centers and hospitals alter the role that nursing plays, foster self-care by the postpartum woman, and encourage family participation in postpartum care.

Discharge Teaching

Discharge teaching is one of the most important roles of the nurse in preparing the new family to return home. Planning for parent education begins with assessment of the mother's and other family members' learning needs and readiness to learn. A generalized teaching checklist may be individualized for each family. The following methods may be used by the nurse:

- Small group discussion
- Individualized teaching
- Use of audiovisual aids such as diagrams and pictures
- Return demonstration (for example, the nurse assessing a parent's bathing of the newborn)
- Development of written instructions to which the family can refer at home
- Postpartum educational classes after the mother is discharged
- Referral to appropriate community agencies, for example, LaLeche League
- Development of a list of community resources that the family can take home

Throughout the teaching-learning process, the nurse evaluates the strategies used and the family's comprehension. Included is the family members' ability to read and understand written teaching materials.[36]

Role of the Nurse

In discharge teaching the nurse's primary role is to educate the woman and her family. The nurse teaches the woman and her family how to perform pertinent assessments and what danger signs to note and report (Table 31–6). General postpartum education, as covered in Figure 31–1, must also be provided; however, some of the information may be provided in prenatal classes and on follow-up home visits.

When the delivery occurs at home or when the postpartum woman is discharged early from the hospital or birthing center, a nurse may be responsible for visiting the family within 24 hours of discharge and then again within 2 to 4 days. Additional visits and phone calls may follow. (*See* Chapter 44 for home care of the childbearing family.) In most health care systems, the postpartum woman is expected to return to the primary health care professional within 6 weeks after delivery. At this time, uterine involution, episiotomy healing, and postpartum adaptations are assessed (Figure 31–20).

TABLE 31–6. DANGER SIGNS IN THE POSTPARTUM PERIOD

Complication	Signs and Symptoms
Subinvolution (failure of the uterus to diminish in size)	Boggy, soft uterus that fails to contract when massaged; uterus remains at same height or rises
Uterine infection	Lochia has strong, offensive odor; blood clots with white tissue; uterine pain; fever
Hematoma (blood in tissue beneath skin of vulva or vaginal mucosa)	Bulging/swelling beneath skin of vulva and wall of vagina; excruciating perineal pain with profuse bleeding
Pregnancy-induced hypertension	Persistent headache; dizziness; blurred vision; spots before the eyes; muscular irritability; convulsions; edema/swelling of extremeties and face; epigastric pain
Pulmonary embolism (blood clot in the lung)	Chest pain; shortness of breath; air hunger; increased respirations; apprehension
Thrombophlebitis (blood clot in legs)	Pain in calves; localized heat, redness, swelling, and knot-like area on lower extremity
Hemorrhage	Profuse, bright red lochia; increased pulse
Urinary tract/kidney infection	Fever; pain/burning on urination; increased frequency of urination; decreased amounts of urine; spasms of urethral meatus; back pain
Disseminated intravascular coagulation; blood coagulation disorder	Increased bleeding; generalized tendency to bleed

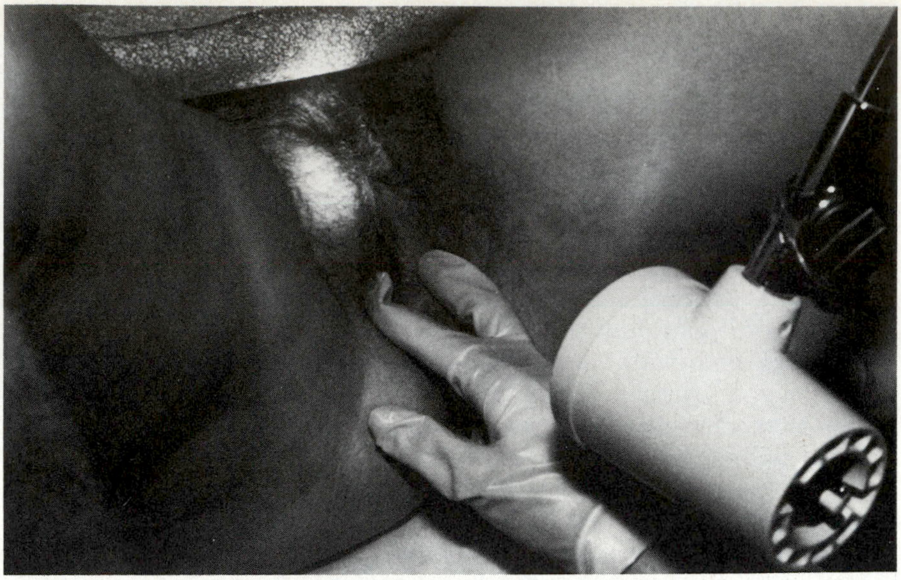

Figure 31–20. Assessment during the 6-week postpartum checkup includes examination of the vagina and perineum.

NURSING DIAGNOSES

Assessment in the postpartum period provides the nurse with data about the client and her family. Diagnoses can then be developed from the subjective and objective data. These nursing diagnoses allow the nurse to plan individualized care that reflects the client's healthy and unhealthy responses. See the box for examples of nursing diagnoses related to the postpartum period.

NURSING DIAGNOSES RELATED TO THE POSTPARTUM PERIOD

Physiologic

Problem-Oriented

Ineffective breastfeeding, related to pain of breast engorgement

Potential for infection, related to perineal laceration during labor and delivery

Constipation, related to low intake of roughage during the postpartum period

Strength-Oriented

Potential for successful lactation, related to positive health practices and desire to breastfeed

Asset in normal progress of involution, related to minimal trauma during labor and delivery and uterine contractility

Psychosocial

Problem-Oriented

Body image disturbance, related to changes of pregnancy in the maternal body

Strength-Oriented

Asset in sibling coping, related to early family interaction at sibling visitation in postpartum period

Asset in paternal-infant attachment, related to paternal engrossment behaviors

Cultural

Problem-Oriented

Ineffective coping, related to cultural conflicts between parents and relatives regarding newborn care

Strength-Oriented

Asset in integration of newborn in family, related to performance of cultural rituals (eg, baptism, naming ceremonies)

CASE STUDY/CARE PLAN: MANAGING MATERNAL PERINEAL DISCOMFORT

Linda Harris is a 24-year-old primiparous woman who delivered vaginally, with a midline episiotomy. She is presently 24 hours postpartum. The nurse enters Mrs. Harris' room to assess breastfeeding. On entering the room the nurse observes that Mrs. Harris is sitting awkwardly in bed, trying to breastfeed her son. The newborn latches onto the breast, taking in the nipple and areola without difficulty. Mrs. Harris uses her free hand to gently displace breast tissue away from her son's nose. As the newborn begins to suck, Mrs. Harris groans and, removing her hand from her breast and placing the hand on the bed, tries to change her position. The newborn loses hold of the breast and begins to cry. Mrs. Harris looks sadly at her son and cries, "We're not doing too well, are we? I'm not helping you to feed." At this point the nurse reaches out and touches Mrs. Harris' shoulder. Mrs. Harris looks at the nurse and cries, "It hurts so much that I can't even stay in one position long enough to feed him." The nurse asks Mrs. Harris to describe where the pain is. Mrs. Harris replies that "it hurts by my stitches."

Supporting Assessment Data	Expected Client/Family Outcome	Nursing Action/ Intervention	Rationale	Criteria for Evaluation
Nursing Diagnosis: Alteration in perineal comfort, related to episiotomy repair and manifested by edema				
Client complains of "stitches," throbbing	By 2 days postpartum, client will:			
Pain interferes with caring for newborn Unable to sit in a comfortable position Surgigator provides momentary relief Changes peripad every 1–3 hours	State the purpose of sitz bath, benzocaine spray, witch hazel pads, assumption of side-lying position, and resumption of Kegel exercises Verbalize decreased perineal discomfort with use of comfort measures	Teach client proper use and purpose of sitz bath, benzocaine spray, assumption of side-lying position, and resumption of Kegel exercises.	Education is needed to promote self-care; knowledge of purpose of a treatment aid or comfort measure can motivate client to use those treatments, aids, and measures.	Client can state purposes of sitz bath, witch hazel pads, benzocaine spray, side-lying position, and Kegel exercises. Client begins to use perineal treatments and comfort measures.
Did 100 Kegel exercises per day during third trimester; has not done Kegel exercise since before delivery	Demonstrate how to set up and use sitz bath	Teach client how to set up sitz bath; have client return the demonstration.	Return demonstration evaluates client education.	Sitz bath is set up and used appropriately by client.
Does not use benzocaine spray or sitz bath; does not know how to use sitz bath or its purpose	Use perineal aids and comfort measures	Assess client's responses to perineal aids and comfort measures.	To ensure health and safety of all clients, responses to all treatments, aids, and comfort measures must be assessed.	Client uses perineal aids and comfort measures appropriately.
Episiotomy red, moderate edema; approximated, no ecchymosis or discharge	By the 6 week visit postpartum, client's episiotomy site will be clean, dry, intact, and without redness, ecchymosis, or edema	Teach client self-assessment of episiotomy site. Advise client to call if problems develop.	Self-assessment promotes self-care, keeps client in control of her health, and allows for early interventions if problems develop.	Client reports episiotomy site is clean, dry, intact, with progressive signs of healing.
		Reinforce need to continue use of peribottle, changing pads every 3–4 hours, after each void and bowel movement.	Reinforcement is a means of promoting the continuation of appropriate client actions.	Client continues to carry out pericare with peribottle, and changes pads every 3–4 hours.

(continued)

CASE STUDY/CARE PLAN: Managing Maternal Perineal Discomfort *(continued)*

Supporting Assessment Data	Expected Client/Family Outcome	Nursing Action/ Intervention	Rationale	Criteria for Evaluation
	At telephone follow up, client will report progressive healing. At 6 weeks postpartum, client will report that she is free of perineal discomfort	Provide telephone follow-up support for client after discharge.	Client needs support after discharge to assist in self-care practices.	At telephone follow up client reports progressive healing. At 6 weeks postpartum client is free of perineal discomfort; perineum is healed.
Nursing Diagnosis: Ineffective breastfeeding, related to maternal perineal discomfort				
Client complains of discomfort while breastfeeding infant; states, "I'm not helping you to feed", "It hurts so much that I can't even stay in one position long enough to feed him" Client sitting awkwardly in bed while feeding newborn; newborn lost hold of breast and cries	By the next feeding, client will obtain temporary relief of perineal pain so that she may effectively breastfeed her newborn	Place client in lateral recumbent position when she is lying in bed or advise buttocks tightening prior to sitting.	Lateral recumbent position and buttocks tightening reduces pressure on perineum and anus, thus providing temporary relief.	Client assumes lateral recumbent position in bed and uses buttocks tightening before sitting; experiences a reduction in perineal discomfort. Client is able to resume breastfeeding her newborn comfortably.
		Offer analgesic before feeding newborn if perineal discomfort is severe.	If needed, oral analgesics should be offered before mother interacts with newborn so that medication can have time to act, thus enabling mother to be relaxed and free of pain when with newborn.	Client reports diminished perineal discomfort.
		Teach client to use sitz bath, and peribottle ½ hour before feeding newborn.	Sitz bath provides moist heat, which promotes circulation and reduces edema. Sitz bath, and peribottle clean perineum.	Client reports relief of perineal discomfort.
		Teach client to change peripad, apply benzocaine spray and witch hazel pads to perineum 15 minutes before feeding newborn.	Soiled peripads can irritate perineum and provide a medium on which microorganisms can grow. Benzocaine spray provides temporary anesthesia to perineum.	Client reports increasing comfort when breastfeeding newborn.

SUMMARY

A thorough assessment of the mother and her family provides the basis for development of all nursing interventions in the postpartum period. Interventions used to assist the healthy mother and family in resuming the level of prepregnancy function and incorporating a new infant into the family are varied.

Important nursing interventions include management of breastfeeding and associated problems (including suppression of lactation for the bottlefeeding mother); management of the process of resumption of normal bowel and bladder function; management of the process of uterine involution and stabilization of reproductive function; care of episiotomy and repaired lacerations; teaching of postpartum exercises; nutritional counseling; and, in general, assisting the new mother and her family to return to a state of equilibrium.

Other nursing interventions are directed at prevention of Rh sensitivity; maintenance of maternal sleep, rest, and comfort; and education regarding exercise and activity, resumption of sexual activity, and family planning. Finally, the nurse must be familiar with pharmacologic agents commonly used in the postpartum period. These include medications to suppress lactation, to promote uterine contractions (eg, oxytocin), and to relieve pain and discomforts.

Discharge planning is a vital component of nursing care during the postpartum period. Initial support of the family unit during this period will foster future successful family development.

REVIEW QUESTIONS

1. Identify the three most common breast problems that a woman may have during the postpartum period, and describe nursing interventions for each of these problems.
2. Explain the mechanism of Rh sensitization in the Rh-negative woman. How does Rho(D) immune globulin interrupt the development of antigens against Rh?
3. Develop an exercise plan for a woman during the first 9 days postpartum.
4. Identify three educational needs of the breast-feeding mother, and describe how you would meet these needs.
5. Describe the components of discharge planning during the puerperium.

REFERENCES

1. Storr G. Prevention of nipple tenderness and breast engorgement in the postpartal period. *J Obstet Gynecol Neonat Nurs.* 1988;17:203–209.
2. Wong S, Stepp-Gilbert E: Lactation suppression: non pharmaceutical versus pharmaceutical method. *J Obstet Gynecol Neonat Nurs.* 1985;14:302–310.
3. Brooten D, et al. A comparison of four treatments to prevent and control breast pain and engorgement in nonnursing mothers. *Nurs Res.* 1983;32:225–229.
4. De Bruyne LK, et al. *Life Cycle Nutrition: Conception Through Adolescence.* St. Paul , Minn: West Publishing Co; 1989.
5. Jacobson H. A standard for assessing lochia volume. *Am J Matern Child Nurs.* 1985;10:174–175.
6. Davidson N. Reeda: evaluating postpartum healing. *J Nurse-Midwifery.* 1974;19:6–8.
7. Strandness DE. *Duplex Scanning in Vascular Disorders.* New York: Raven Press; 1990.
8. Georges P, ed. *Report of the Committee of Infectious Diseases.* 21st ed. Elkgrove Village, Ill: American Academy of Pediatrics; 1988.
9. Cherry S. Current concepts of hemolytic disease and blood group incompatibility. *M Sinai J Med.* 1980;47:454–460.
10. Kelton JG, Cruickshank. Hematologic disorders of pregnancy. In Burrow GN, Ferris TF. *Medical Complications During Pregnancy.* 3rd ed. Philadelphia: WB Saunders, 1988; 65–92.
11. Tulman L, Fawcett J: Return of functional ability after childbirth. *Nurs Res.* 1988;37:77–89.
12. Tulman L, et al. Changes in functional status after childbirth. *Nurs Res.* 1990;39:70–75.
13. Sampselle CM, et al. Digital measurement of pelvic muscle strength in childbearing women. *Nurs Res.* 1989;38:134–138.
14. Samples, JT, et al. The dynamic characteristics of the circumvaginal muscles. *J Obstet Gynecol Neonat Nurs.* 1988; 17:194–201.
15. Dougherty M, et al. The effect of circumvaginal muscle (CVM) exercise. *Nurs Res.* 1989;38:331–335.
16. McKenzie CA, Canaday ME, Carroll E. Comprehensive care during the postpartum period. *Nurs Clin North Am.* 1982; 17:23–48.
17. Henderson J. Effects of a prenatal teaching program on postpartum regeneration of the pubococcygeal muscle. *J Obstet Gynecol Nurs.* 1983;12:403–408.
18. Masters W, Johnson V. *Human Sexual Response.* Boston: Little, Brown; 1966.
19. Richardson A, et al. Decreasing postpartum sexual abstinence time. *Am J Obstet Gynecol.* 1976;126:416–417.
20. Inglis T. Postpartum sexuality. *J Obstet Gynecol Nurs.* 1980;9:298–300.
21. Hames C. Sexual needs and interests of postpartum couples. *J Obstet Gynecol Nurs.* 1980;9:313–315.
22. Falicov C. Sexual adjustment during first pregnancy and postpartum. *Am J Obstet Gynecol.* 1973;117:991–1000.
23. Ryding E. Sexuality during and after pregnancy. *Acta Obstet Gynecol Scand.* 1984;63:679–682.
24. Ellis D, Hewat R. Mother's postpartum perceptions of spousal relationships. *J Obstet Gynecol Neon Nurs.* 1985;14: 140–146.
25. Mueller LS. Pregnancy and sexuality. *J Obstet Gynecol Neonat Nurs.* 1985;14:289–296.
26. Gulick E. Informational correlates of successful breastfeeding. *Am J Matern Child Nurs.* 1982;7:370–375.
27. Kearney MH, et al. Breast-feeding problems in the first week postpartum. *Nurs Res.* 1990;39:90–95.
28. Chapman JJ, et al. Concerns of breast-feeding mothers from birth to 4 months. *Nurs Res.* 1985;34:374–377.
29. Hill PD, Humenick SS: Insufficient milk supply. *Image.* 1989; 21:145–148.
30. Winick M. *Nutrition, Pregnancy, and Early Infancy.* Baltimore: Williams & Wilkins; 1989.
31. Riordan J, Countryman BA. Basics of breastfeeding, part IV: Preparation for breastfeeding and early optional functioning. *J Obstet Gynecol Nurs.* 1980;9:277–283.
32. Berglund F, et al. Drug use during pregnancy and breast-feeding. *Acta Obstet Gynecol Scand.* 1984:supple 126.
33. Lawrence RA. *Breastfeeding.* 2nd ed. St. Louis, Mo: CV Mosby; 1985.
34. Riordan J, Riordan M. Drugs in breast milk. *Am J Nurs.* 1984;84:328–332.
35. Blakemore K. Lactation suppression is a matter of choice. *Contemp Ob/Gyn.* 1986;28:39.
36. O'Hare PA, Terry MA. *Discharge Planning.* Rockville, Md: Aspen; 1988.

The Normal Infant

unit 9

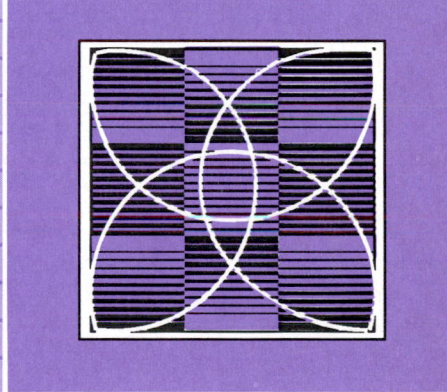

The Normal Newborn

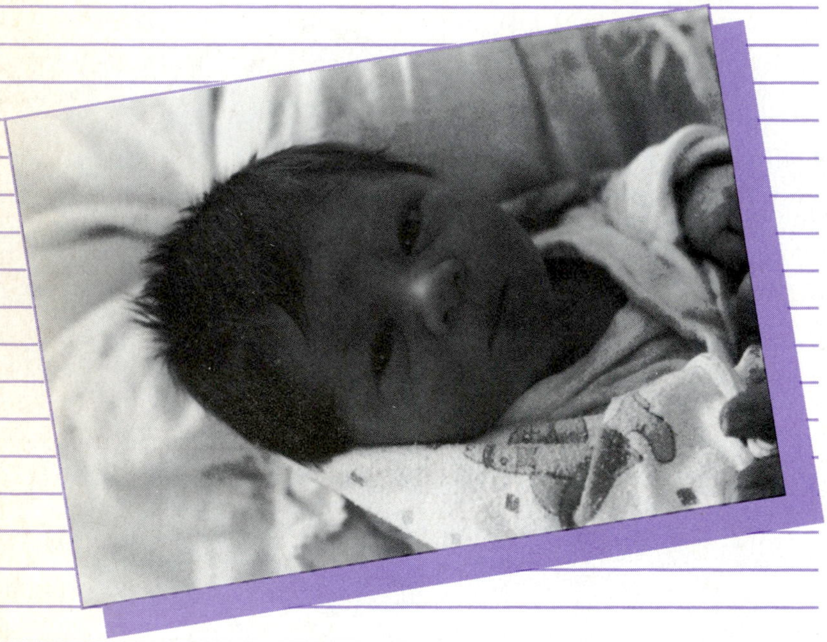

chapter 32

Key Terms

breast-milk jaundice syndrome
critical temperature
homoiotherms
meconium
milk stools
neonatal period
neutral thermal environment
nonshivering thermogenesis
passive immunity
physiologic jaundice
transitional stools

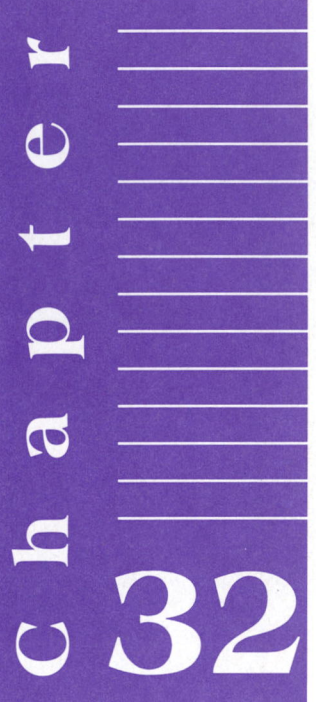

During the **neonatal period,** the first 28 days of life, family members change in response to the physiologic, psychologic, and developmental needs of the newborn. At the same time, parents and siblings have needs relative to their changing roles within the family system. Coping with these roles begins in the prenatal period when parents fantasize about their idealized infant; however, the birth of the newborn requires that family members become reality oriented as they focus attention on the care of the newborn.

The newborn has physical features that are much different from those of children and adults. The head is large in comparison to the rest of the body, the extremities are relatively short, and the abdomen is prominent. At birth, the newborn may show evidence of edema of the presenting part, or the head may be molded from the process of labor and delivery. The newborn also may have skin variations such as milia, mongolian spots, and Epstein's pearls in the mouth, which may be unfamiliar to parents. In short, the newborn's physical features may be different from those fantasized by the parents during pregnancy.

Birth requires that the newborn make several physiologic changes in adjusting to the extrauterine environment. The most critical adaptations involve the respiratory and cardiovascular systems. The newborn must also begin to regulate body temperature, an activity that was unnecessary for the fetus in utero. Several other systems also undergo major changes as the newborn moves from intrauterine to extrauterine life.

Behavioral responses of the newborn are predictable. The newborn is equipped with a repertoire of behavioral interactions that will elicit responses from caregivers. The nurse's role includes teaching parents about the normal characteristics of the newborn so that positive parent-newborn interactions can be facilitated.

PHYSIOLOGIC ADJUSTMENT TO EXTRAUTERINE LIFE

The transition from the intrauterine to the extrauterine environment is a critical period during which the newborn makes behavioral and physiologic adjustments to extrauterine life. Birth inititates a series of systematic physiologic events, including regulation of body systems, that will enable the newborn to adjust to the extrauterine environment.

The most important adjustments the newborn undergoes are respiratory (initiation of breathing), cardiovascular (circulatory system adjustments), and thermal (regulation of body temperature). Newborns who fail to make these vital adjustments are at serious risk for survival (*see* Chapters 42 and 43 concerning the high-risk newborn).

Respiratory Adjustment

Respiratory effort is perhaps the most critical adjustment that the newborn must make at birth. With the first breaths of air, the newborn initiates the following sequence of cardiopulmonary changes: (1) converting from fetal to neonatal circulation, (2) emptying the lungs of fluid, (3) establishing the characteristics of pulmonary function.[1]

The lungs of the fetus have developed systematically since conception. By 24 weeks of gestation, alveolar sacs in the lungs develop; by 28 weeks, the cells of the alveoli differentiate into type I and type II cells. Type I alveolar cells make gas exchange in the lungs possible. Type II cells allow for the production of surfactant, a surface-acting phospholipid, that prevents the alveoli from collapsing on expiration. By 36 weeks of gestation, the number of type II alveolar cells has increased concurrently with surfactant production.

During intrauterine life, exchange of oxygen and carbon dioxide occurs across the placenta from one fluid medium to another. After birth, this exchange occurs across the neonatal alveolar membrane between a gaseous medium (air in the alveoli) and a fluid one (blood in the alveolar capillaries). One of the most crucial adjustments that the newborn must make at birth is the adjustment of respiratory function to a gaseous environment.[2] Several factors are necessary before the neonatal lungs can maintain respiratory function, including initiation of respiratory movements, expansion of the lungs, establishment of functional residual capacity (retention of some air in the lungs at the end of expiration to prevent collapse of the lungs), and increase in pulmonary blood flow and redistribution of cardiac output.[2]

Initiation of Respirations. Many theories have been proposed regarding the initiation of respirations in the newborn. The theories focus on stimuli that interact to contribute to the respiratory effort. The newborn is subjected to a variety of stimuli that interplay to initiate respirations. They may be classified into mechanical, chemical, and sensory-proprioceptive stimuli. For purposes of discussion, they are presented separately, although they influence respiratory effort simultaneously (Figure 32–1).

Mechanical Stimuli. The fetus has made respiratory movements in utero in preparation for the initiation of breathing at birth. The lungs at birth are about half inflated with fluid derived from fluid secreted by the fetal lungs and the tracheal glands.[3, 4] The volume of this fluid is equal to almost one half of the

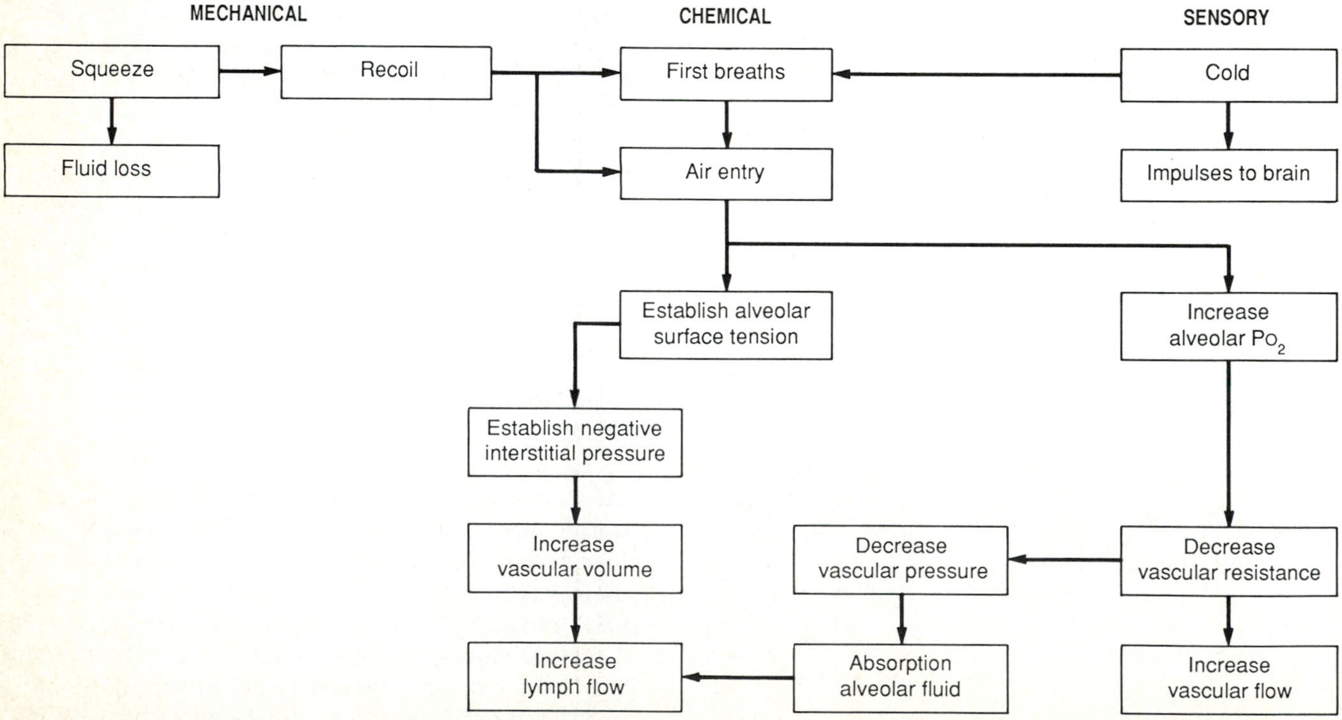

Figure 32–1. Stimuli influencing newborn respirations. (*Adapted, with permission, from Smith CA, Nelson NM.* Physiology of the Newborn Infant. *4th ed. Springfield, Ill: Charles C Thomas; 1976.*)

total lung capacity. The fetal lungs also have a high vascular resistance as a result of pulmonary arterial vasoconstriction.[5] The transition from the uterine to the extrauterine environment requires the immediate onset of breathing, the absorption of lung fluid, its replacement with air, and a rapid increase in the blood oxygen content.[6]

The primary mechanical stimulus that facilitates adequate neonatal respirations is the compression of the fetal chest during the delivery process. During delivery, the squeezing of the fetal thorax increases the intrathoracic pressure and expels 30 to 35 mL of fluid from the lungs. This represents one third of the total volume of fluid in the lungs of a 7½-pound neonate.[2] After delivery, the chest wall of the fetus recoils, creating a negative interstitial and intrapleural pressure. This recoil of the chest wall probably produces a small passive inspiration of air, forcing some of the air into the lungs and some blood into the pulmonary capillaries. An air-fluid interface is thus established within the larger airways. The alveoli would tend to collapse under these conditions were it not for the presence of surfactant.[1]

The newborn exhales, usually with crying; this activity expands the alveolar sacs by creating a positive intrathoracic pressure. At the same time, an adequate functional capacity (volume of air in the lungs at the end of expiration) is attained to prevent collapse of the lungs. The functional residual capacity of the lungs at 10 minutes after birth is the same as that found at 5 days postdelivery. One hour after birth, the distribution of air with each breath is similar to that observed in the young adult.[5] The functional residual capacity of air is maintained because the surface tension of the fluid in the lungs is reduced by surfactant. This reduction in surface tension allows the alveoli to remain expanded, and some air to remain in the lungs after expiration.

Pressure changes that take place during expiration are integral to the initiation of adequate respirations. With expiration, there is descent of the newborn's diaphragm, resulting in negative pressure. That is, pressure in the alveoli becomes considerably higher than pressure in the interstitial tissue, resulting in the flow of fluid from the alveoli to the interstitial space. From the interstitial tissue, the fluid is removed by the pulmonary capillaries and lymphatics.[4] With each successive breath, the pulmonary vascular resistance decreases and the remainder of the fluid is absorbed. Removal of fetal lung fluid thus occurs in two stages: (1) displacement of fluid from alveolar spaces to interstitial tissue, which occurs rapidly; (2) removal of fluid into lymph and blood vessels, which can take several hours.[2]

Problems can occur with the onset of neonatal respirations when surfactant is deficient because there will be no reduction in the surface tension of the fluid in the lungs, causing the alveoli to collapse on expiration. Preterm infants may have surfactant deficiency and, as a result, serious problems with respiratory effort. Newborns delivered by cesarean section also may have some difficulty with respiratory effort because they may have more fluid and less air in the lungs during the first 6 hours of life. This initial fluid retention is related to the lack of compression of the fetal chest during cesarean delivery.

Chemical Stimuli. Several chemical stimuli also contribute to the respiratory efforts of the newborn. Once the umbilical cord is cut, uteroplacental circulation ceases. The placenta has acted as the "fetal lung" during pregnancy. Carbon dioxide (CO_2) readily crosses the placenta so that there is equilibrium of Pco_2 on both the fetal and maternal sides of the placenta. Conversely, oxygen (O_2) transport is less efficient (maximum Po_2 in the fetus is 40 mm Hg). Yet despite the low Po_2, oxygen saturation in the fetal blood is approximately 80 to 85 percent.[6]

During the birth process, the uteroplacental circulation is compromised, resulting in an initial increase in the Pco_2 and a drop in the Po_2 (Pco_2 may rise to 80 mm Hg, and Po_2 may drop to 10 mm Hg).[7] These high carbon dioxide and low oxygen concentrations in the blood stimulate peripheral and central chemoreceptors, which in turn transmit impulses to the respiratory center of the brain. The respiratory center in the medulla then transmits impulses to stimulate the neonate's respiratory effort.

With the mechanical expansion of the lungs during the first breaths, the Po_2 rises, and the pulmonary vascular resistance decreases. This, in turn, increases pulmonary arterial blood flow that had previously bypassed the pulmonary circulation through shunts in the fetal circulation. Arterial Po_2 rises rapidly from less than 30 mm Hg to 60 mm Hg or more in the first minutes of life, demonstrating the efficiency of the lungs for oxygen exchange.[8]

Sensory-Proprioceptive Stimuli. The newborn is subjected to multiple sensory stimuli—thermal, proprioceptive (stimuli produced in body tissues), and tactile—at birth. These, combined with the mechanical and chemical stimuli, play a role in initiation of breathing in the normal newborn.

The relative cooling effect of the environment in the delivery room stimulates sensory impulses in the trigeminal area of the face. Impulses are then transmitted to the respiratory center of the brain to initiate respirations in the newborn. Cooling is probably an intense stimulus to breathing, and the response is immediate.[2]

Other stimuli, such as light, noise, and pain also probably play a role in the initiation of respirations.[1] The role of tactile stimulation is less clear and is probably of minor significance. For this reason, the slapping of the heels or buttocks of the newborn on delivery is discouraged because of the minimal effect on respiratory effort.[2]

The initiation of respirations in the newborn is thus an interaction of a barrage of mechanical, chemical, and sensory stimuli. These are summarized in Table 32–1.

Newborn Respirations. The respiratory rate of the newborn is between 30 and 60 breaths per minute. Newborns have higher respiratory rates when crying, and lower rates when sleeping. The pattern of respirations is characterized by shallow, irregular breathing, sometimes interrupted by short periods of apnea. Neonatal respirations are also abdominal in nature. By 1 month of age, full-term newborns have a mean respiratory rate of 38.5 compared with a mean of 45.1 at birth.[9]

Cardiovascular Adjustment

Important cardiovascular changes occur when the newborn emerges from the intrauterine to the extrauterine environment. Fetal circulation is discussed in detail in Chapter 11, and may be summarized as follows:

1. Oxygenated blood enters the umbilical vein and is mostly directed into the inferior vena cava through the ductus venosus.
2. The blood from the inferior vena cava flows into the right atrium, where most of the blood passes into the left atrium through the foramen ovale, bypassing the right ventricle and pulmonary circulation.
3. From the left atrium, the blood flows into the left ventricle and then to the aorta. This blood, with the highest oxygen content, nourishes the heart, brain, and upper extremities.
4. Blood returning from the brain and upper extremities enters the heart by way of the superior vena cava. This less oxygenated blood is directed into the right ventricle.
5. Most of the blood in the right ventricle bypasses the pulmonary circulation by being shunted into the descending aorta through the ductus arteriosus. This blood nourishes the trunk and lower extremities of the fetus. Because of the high pulmonary resistance in fetal circulation, only a small amount of blood from the right ventricle goes to the lungs.

In fetal circulation, the fetal placental vessels offer little resistance to the flow of blood. The placenta has a low-resistance circuit of vessels that eventually receives blood from the fetal aorta. In contrast to the low-resistance placental vessels, there is a high pulmonary vascular resistance to blood flow in the fetus. As a result, the fetal aortic blood pressure is lower

TABLE 32–1. MECHANICAL, CHEMICAL, AND SENSORY STIMULI THAT INITIATE NEONATAL RESPIRATIONS

Stimuli	Response
Mechanical	
Squeezing of fetal chest during delivery	Increases intrathoracic pressure; expels 30–35 mL fluid from lungs
Chest recoil	Produces small passive inspiration, forcing some of air into lungs; air-fluid interspace established
Exhalation, usually with crying (expiration)	Positive intrathoracic pressure established; adequate functional capacity attained; descent of the diaphragm, causing negative pressure; pressure in alveoli becomes higher than in the interstitial tissue, resulting in flow of fluid from alveoli to lymphatics
Chemical	
Cessation of uteroplacental circulation	Initial increase in P_{CO_2} and drop in P_{O_2}
Increase in P_{CO_2} and decrease in P_{O_2}	Stimulation of peripheral and central chemoreceptors, which transmit impulses to brain, stimulating respiratory effort
P_{O_2} rises, pulmonary vascular resistance decreases	Increase in pulmonary arterial blood flow
Sensory	
Cool environment in delivery room	Stimulates sensory impulses in trigeminal area of face; impulses transmitted to respiratory center of brain to initiate respirations
Light, noise, pain	Probably stimulate respirations; exact mechanism unknown

than the pulmonary artery pressure and little blood goes into the pulmonary circulation (lungs). At birth, changes occur in the pulmonary-systemic pressure relationships and in the right-to-left shunts[2] (foramen ovale, ductus arteriosus, ductus venosus).

Conversion of Fetal to Neonatal Circulation

Change in Pulmonary-Systemic Pressure Relationships. The two factors that are important in conversion of fetal to neonatal circulation are removal of the placenta and expansion of the lungs with air. Clamping the umbilical cord at birth removes the placental circulation, the component that offers the least resistance to the flow of blood. As a consequence, aortic blood pressure is raised and the return of blood from the inferior vena cava is reduced.[2]

With the newborn's first breaths, vasodilation of pulmonary vessels occurs, producing a significant decrease in pulmonary vascular resistance and an increase in pulmonary blood flow.[7] Neonatal lung expansion is important in stimulating pulmonary arteriolar relaxation (decreasing pulmonary artery blood pressure) and providing adequate oxygenation to the newborn. At the same time, systemic blood pressure (aortic blood pressure) increases because of the greater peripheral vascular resistance brought about by removal of the placental circulation. This reversal of pulmonary and systemic blood pressures, from fetal to neonatal circulation, affects the right-to-left shunts found in fetal circulation.[2]

Closure of Right-to-Left Shunts. The shunts in fetal circulation (foramen ovale, ductus venosus, ductus arteriosus) are termed right-to-left shunts because they shunt blood from the right side to the left side of the heart (foramen ovale, ductus arteriosus), or from the umbilical vein to the inferior vena cava (ductus venosus). At birth, changes occur in the shunts that alter neonatal blood flow.

Closure of the Foramen Ovale. The foramen ovale is an opening in the interatrial septum, which shunts blood from the right atrium to the left atrium, bypassing the right ventricle and the pulmonary circulation (Figure 32–2). In fetal circulation, the pressure in the right atrium is higher than in the left. Oxygenated blood therefore flows from the right to the left atrium (area of higher pressure to lower pressure), keeping the foramen ovale open.

At birth, the decrease in pulmonary vascular resistance, combined with an increase in peripheral vascular resistance, causes an increase in the amount of blood in the left atrium. This results in an increase in left atrial pressure and a decrease in right atrial pressure, causing the foramen ovale to close within minutes of birth.[1, 7] Some right-to-left shunting of blood may still normally occur for a few months after birth without causing problems for the neonate.

Closure of the Ductus Venosus. The ductus venosus, the fetal structure that shunts blood from the umbilical vein to the inferior vena cava, closes within 3 to 7 days of birth (Figures 32–2 and 32–3). After birth, umbilical venous return decreases so that very little blood flows through the ductus venosus. Although the mechanism is unknown, one possible explanation for the closure is that the ductus venosus becomes fibrotic (ligamentum venosus) from lack of circulation.

Closure of the Ductus Arteriosus. In fetal circulation, the ductus arteriosus shunts blood (right-to-left) into the descending aorta, bypassing the pulmonary circulation (Figures 32–2 and 32–3). With the onset of neonatal breathing, the pulmonary vascular resistance decreases, and the systemic resistance increases, causing a reversal of the shunting of blood through the ductus (left-to-right).

In utero, the ductus arteriosus remains open because of the vasodilating effects of prostaglandins E_1 and E_2 found in the ductal tissue. When the oxygen tension rises after birth, constriction of the ductus occurs. This constriction, combined with the left-to-right shunting of blood, promotes closure of the ductus arteriosus beginning 4 to 12 hours postnatally; the ductus functionally closes by the time the newborn is 24 hours of age. Fibrosis of the ductus arteriosus, which closes it permanently (ligamentum arteriosus), may take as long as 3 weeks to occur. Figures 32–2 and 32–3 describe the changes from fetal to neonatal circulation.

The interim period, before the ductus permanently closes, is termed the *transitional phase* of perinatal circulation.[1] If, during the transitional phase, the pulmonary vascular resistance should again increase to a level higher than the systemic resistance, a reversal from neonatal to fetal circulation will occur (eg, in a preterm newborn). During the transitional phase, left ventricular volume and pressure increase while right ventricular pressure decreases (ie, the left ventricle pumps twice the volume load of the right ventricle). This means that the newborn has unequal volumes in the left and right ventricles during this phase, in contrast to the equal volumes of blood found in the child and adult.

Constriction of the Umbilical Arteries and Umbilical Vein. The umbilical vein carries oxygenated blood to the fetus, and the two umbilical arteries remove de-

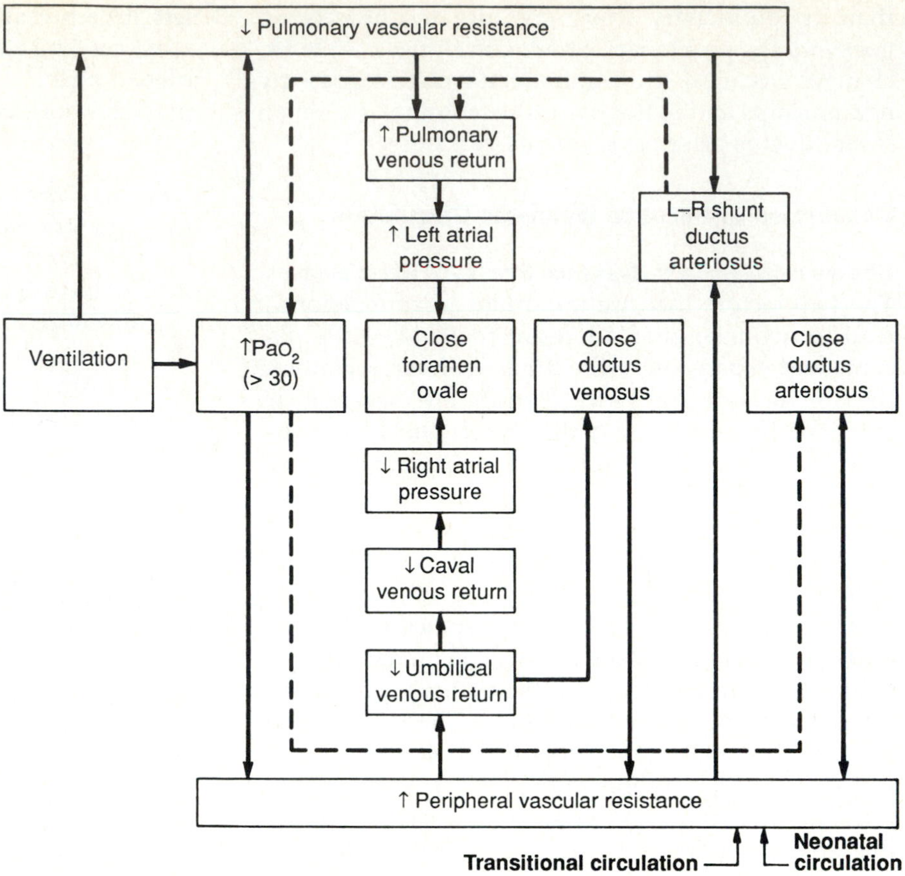

Figure 32–2. Conversion of the perinatal circulation after the onset of ventilation. (*Reproduced, with permission, from Smith CA, Nelson NM.* Physiology of the Newborn Infant. *4th ed. Springfield, Ill: Charles C Thomas; 1976.*)

oxygenated blood and waste materials from the fetal circulation. Constriction of the umbilical vein and arteries begins at birth, as a result of the increase in peripheral circulation and the removal of the placental circulation.

Summary of Cardiovascular Adjustments at Birth. To summarize, the major features of cardiovascular adjustment at birth are as follows:

- Decrease in pulmonary vascular resistance
- Increase in peripheral vascular resistance
- Increase in Po_2 (Pao_2)
- Increase in left atrial pressure and decrease in right atrial pressure, causing closure of the foramen ovale
- Decrease in umbilical venous return, causing closure of the ductus venosus
- Left-to-right shunting of the ductus arteriosus, causing closure of the ductus arteriosus
- Constriction of the umbilical vein and umbilical arteries
- Transitional increase in the workload of the left ventricle
- Transitional decrease in the workload of the right ventricle

Neonatal Heart Rate and Blood Pressure. The heart rate of the newborn ranges between 120 and 160 beats per minute. The heart rate may increase to as much as 180 beats per minute when the newborn is crying, and may decrease to a low of 70 to 100 beats per minute when the newborn is sleeping.

The mean heart rate for the normal full-term newborn is 116.3 beats per minute at birth. This increases to 141.3 beats per minute at 15 days postdelivery, and then drops to 136.2 at 4 weeks of age.[9] Transient functional cardiac murmurs may be heard in the neonatal period as a result of the changing dynamics of the cardiovascular system at birth.

During the first 12 hours of life, the mean blood pressure for a neonate weighing 3.5 kg (7.7 pounds) is 67/41. For a newborn weighing 3.6 kg (8 pounds), mean blood pressure is 80/58 during the same period.[10] The newborn's blood pressure is highest after birth and reaches a plateau at about 4 to 6 days after birth.

Hematologic Adjustment

At term, the placental vasculature contains 75 to 125 mL of blood, which represents one fourth to one third

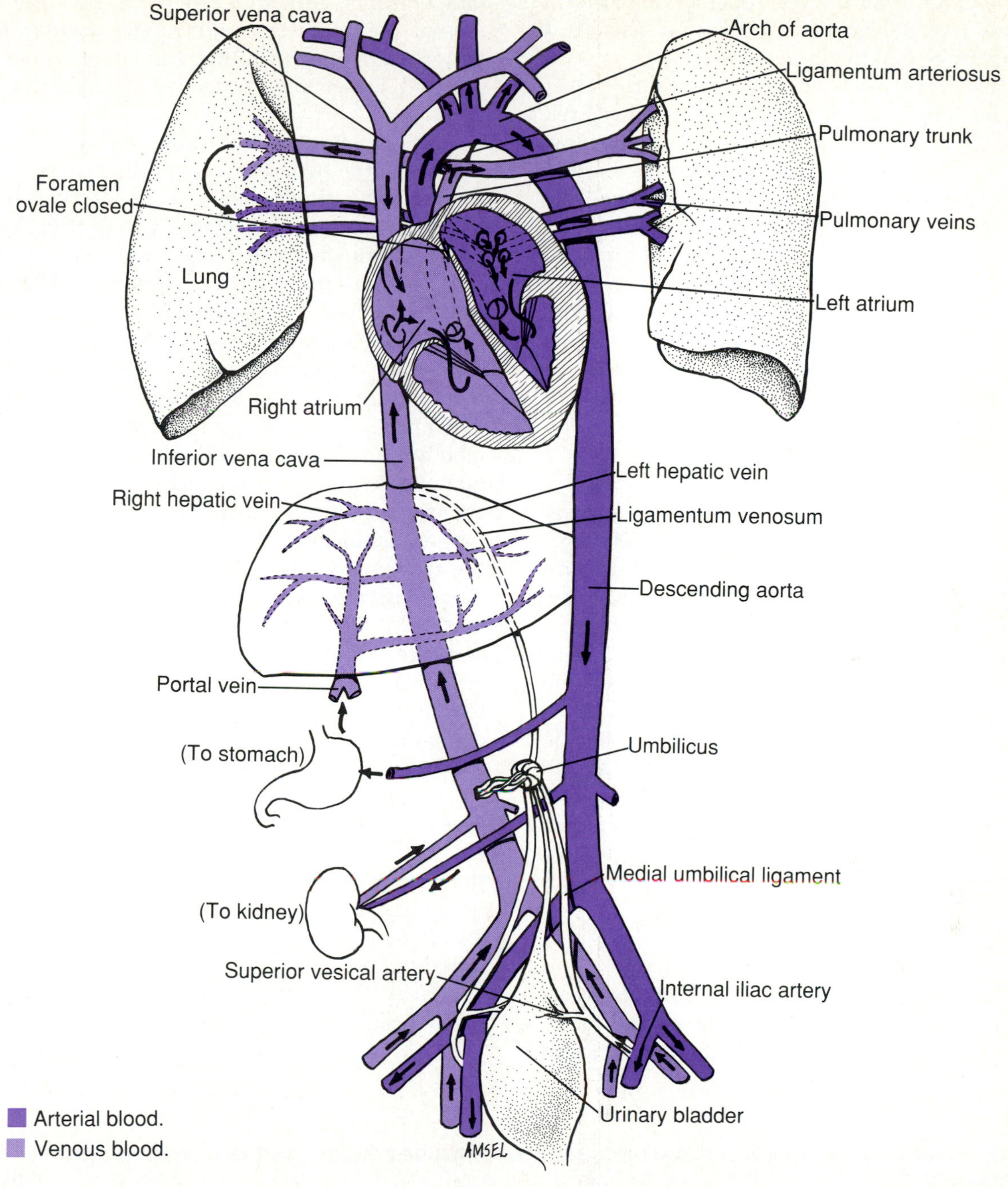

Figure 32–3. Major changes in the newborn's circulatory system.

of the total fetal blood volume. Blood volume in the newborn can be increased by 40 to 60 percent[4] if the newborn is held below the level of the placenta and clamping of the cord is delayed. This extra blood volume provides the advantage of increased oxygen and nutrients to the newborn.

Because the fetal circulation is less efficient at oxygen exchange than the lungs, the fetus needs additional red blood cells for transport of oxygen in utero. To meet this need, the fetal bone marrow becomes hyperactive and produces increased numbers of red blood cells (erythropoiesis). The hemoglobin concentration of the newborn at birth is therefore higher than that of the child or adult. The number of reticulocytes (the precursors to mature erythrocytes) is also higher in the circulating blood of the newborn than in the child or adult. The reticulocytes at birth range from 4 to 8 percent of red blood cells; at 4 weeks, the range is 0 to 0.5 percent.

After birth, more efficient oxygen exchange takes place in the lungs of the newborn, and fewer red blood cells are required. The bone marrow of the newborn becomes hypoactive, resulting in a decrease in the concentrations of hemoglobin. The average hemoglobin concentration is 14 g/100 mL at 4 weeks and 12 g/100 mL at 8 weeks. The hemoglobin of the newborn also converts from fetal hemoglobin (hemoglobin F), which provides greater oxygen carrying capacity needed in utero, to adult hemoglobin (hemoglobin A). By 8 to 12 weeks postdelivery, however, the bone marrow of the newborn is again stimulated to increase red cell production by the excretion of erythropoietin, a renal hormone. By 6 months of age, the hemoglobin of the infant begins to rise.

The white blood cell count of the newborn at birth is usually between 15,000/mm^3 and 25,000/mm^3. By the sixth day postdelivery, lymphocytes predominate (37 percent) and persist through the first 5 years of life.[7]

The platelet count in the neonatal period averages between 150,000/mm^3 and 250,000/mm^3, the same as that in the child and adult. Factors II, VII, IX, and X, found in the liver, are decreased during the first few days of life because the newborn is unable to synthesize vitamin K. (*See* discussion under "Role of the Liver in Coagulation," later in the chapter.) The newborn is thus susceptible to bleeding, a tendency that is reduced by administration of an intramuscular injection of vitamin K (0.5 to 1 mg) at birth.[7]

Thermal Regulation

Children and adults are considered **homoiotherms** because they can maintain a constant core body temperature regardless of a wide range of environmental temperatures. Although newborns have the capabilities of homoiotherms, the range of environmental temperatures to which they can adapt without being stressed is severely restricted compared with the adult.[11]

The newborn differs from the child and adult by having a large surface area in proportion to mass, less thermal insulation (subcutaneous fat), and relatively lower vasomotor control (ability to control skin blood flow). The newborn also has greater potential for heat loss than does the adult, and differs in mechanisms of heat production (thermogenesis).

All homoiotherms have a **neutral thermal environmental range,** that is, the range of environmental temperature in which an individual is able to maintain a normal internal temperature with minimal metabolism and oxygen consumption for heat production. Because the newborn differs from the adult in the proportion of surface area to mass, as well as in thermal insulation, the neutral temperature zone of the newborn is 32 to 34°C (89.6 to 93.2°F) as compared with the adult's neutral zone of 26 to 28°C (78.7 to 82.4°F). Below this range, termed the **critical temperature,** a metabolic response to cold is necessary to replace heat loss. The neutral range thus represents the thermal range of minimal stress.[11] Table 32–2 compares factors that contribute to temperature control in the newborn and older child/adult.

Mechanisms of Heat Transfer. In utero, the internal or core temperature of the fetus is slightly higher than that of the mother. At birth, the newborn's internal temperature may drop rapidly because the delivery room is usually 25 to 30°F lower than the maternal temperature.

Heat loss in the newborn is the result of four mechanisms: (1) evaporation, (2) radiation, (3) convection, (4) conduction. The heat transfer depends

TABLE 32–2. COMPARISON OF FACTORS INFLUENCING TEMPERATURE CONTROL IN THE NEWBORN AND OLDER CHILD/ADULT

Newborn	Older Child/Adult
Large surface area in proportion to mass	Smaller surface area in proportion to mass
Less thermal insulation (subcutaneous fat)	Mature deposits of subcutaneous fat providing thermal insulation
Some mature vasomotor control (ability to control skin blood flow)	Mature vasomotor control
Neutral temperature zone 32 to 34°C (89.6 to 93.2°F)	Neutral temperature zone 26 to 28°C (78.7 to 82.4°F)
Nonshivering thermogenesis in response to cold stress	Shivering thermogenesis in response to cold
Six times as many sweat glands as adults; but maximum response of each gland one-third that of adult	

on the temperature of the environment (air and walls), air speed, and water vapor pressure or humidity.[12]

Evaporation. Through evaporation, the water in the amniotic fluid that covers the newborn at birth escapes to the environment as vapor. The process of evaporative loss depends on air speed, the absolute humidity of the environment, or both.[11] The cool environment of the delivery room combined with the low relative humidity encourages heat loss by evaporation. It is thus important that the nurse dry the newborn at birth to prevent evaporative heat loss.

Radiation. Radiative heat loss occurs when heat from the newborn is transferred to cooler objects in the environment (walls of the incubator, air temperature of the room). In an effort to prevent heat loss through radiation, the nurse should wrap the newborn in warm blankets. Skin-to-skin contact with the mother also is very helpful. Radiant warmers are also used to prevent heat loss by radiation (*see* Chapter 34).

Convection. The air speed in the delivery room also contributes to heat loss in the newborn. Cool air passing over the newborn's body causes heat loss by convection. Along with radiation, convection is a major channel for heat loss in the newborn.[11] Infant warmers have been used to prevent heat loss by convection. Swaddling the newborn also helps prevent heat loss.

Conduction. Conductive heat loss is dependent on the thermal conductivity of objects in contact with the body. In other words, the neonate loses heat to cooler objects that come in contact with the body. Thermal exchange through this method is usually small because the newborn is usually placed on a warm mattress of low conductivity.[11] Contact with the mother also prevents this type of heat loss.

Heat Production (Thermogenesis) and Heat Retention. The newborn has the capability to produce and retain heat through various mechanisms. Mechanisms to produce heat include nonshivering thermogenesis, muscular activity, and positional changes. Vasomotor control is a mechanism that allows the newborn to retain heat.

Nonshivering Thermogenesis. The newborn increases heat production in a cool environment mainly through **nonshivering thermogenesis,** a complex process that increases the metabolic rate and rate of oxygen consumption in the newborn. More specifically, the process includes the metabolism of brown fat for heat production when the newborn is subjected to cold stress.

Brown fat cells begin appearing in the fetus by 17 to 20 weeks of gestation[12] (*see* Chapter 11). At term, brown fat accounts for 2 to 6 percent of the total body weight of the newborn. Brown fat is found at the nape of the neck, posterior to the sternum, surrounding the kidneys and adrenals, and in the perineal area.[12, 13] Brown fat is found for weeks after birth unless its stores are depleted from cold stress.

The cells in brown fat tissue contain numerous mitochondria and fat vacuoles, as well as an abundant blood and sympathetic nerve supply. When the newborn is subjected to cold, norepinephrine is released from the sympathetic nerve endings in the brown fat tissue. The norepinephrine stimulates brown fat metabolism by activating the enzyme lipase, which breaks down the fat to form triglycerides. The triglycerides are then hydrolyzed to form glycerol and free fatty acids; this process causes a heat-producing reaction. The heat that is produced is applied to the blood that nourishes the tissue mass.[2]

Changes in environmental temperature have the potential to disturb the core body temperature, with serious consequences to the newborn. Brown fat metabolism is activated in response to changes in environmental temperature that are perceived by the thermal sensors in the newborn's skin, even when the core temperature of the newborn is unchanged. The stability of the core body temperature is thus protected by the newborn's mechanisms of heat production.

Muscular Activity and Positional Changes. Although the newborn does not have the same capabilities as the adult to change position and increase muscular activity in response to cold, evidence suggests that these activities are important in maintaining core body temperature in cold surroundings.[11] When exposed to cold, the newborn may become restless and increase muscular activity. Moreover, the attitude of flexion (flexing the extremities and back) helps to decrease the amount of skin surface exposed to cold and conserve heat.

Vasomotor Control. In addition to mechanisms to produce heat, the newborn's body has the ability to retain heat by controlling skin blood flow. By constricting blood vessels in the skin, heat can be retained in the tissues, thereby helping to maintain the

RESEARCH ABSTRACT

Bliss-Holz J. Comparison of rectal, axillary and inguinal temperatures in full-term newborn infants. Nurs Res. *1989;38:85–87.*

This study compared rectal, axillary, and inguinal temperatures in full-term newborns aged 12 to 48 hours. The sample consisted of 62 female and 58 male newborns, ranging in gestational age from 36 to 42 weeks and weighing from 2570 to 4900 g.

The instruments used for the study included three mecury-in-glass thermometers with stubby bulb ends. The thermometers were shaken down below 90°F before insertion. Temperatures were read every 30 seconds and were discontinued when no change occurred for 90 seconds. Temperature stabilization was defined by the reseacher as the reading at which the mercury in a mercury-in-glass theromometer remained constant for a 90-second period.

The largest difference between mean maximum temperature readings occurred between rectal and inguinal temperatures (0.8°F); however, this pair of readings also had the highest correlation. The researcher concluded that the inguinal site may be more reflective of the rectal temperature.

Comment:
If axillary or inguinal temperatures are reflective of rectal temperatures as this study indicates, there is good rationale for using these routes rather than the rectal route, as the first two will decrease the energy expenditure of the newborn. As rectal temperatures may not be accurate in determining the core temperature, other measures of temperature observation also are necessary.

core temperature. The newborn's thermal insulation is, however, poor compared with that of the adult[11]; therefore, this mechanism, alone, is inadequate in maintaining the core temperature.

Hyperthermia. Hyperthermia develops more rapidly in the newborn than in the adult because of the larger surface-to-volume ratio of the newborn's body.[12] Although newborn infants have six times as many sweat glands per unit area as adults, the maximum response of each gland is only one-third that of the adult. Thus, when exposed to high temperatures the newborn is unable to sweat to lower the temperature. The risk of hyperthermia to the newborn is great when the environmental temperature is above the neutral temperature zone. Heat stress will cause the newborn to increase metabolic rate and respirations in an effort to control temperature because of the inability of the sweat glands to respond.[11]

Consequences of a Nonneutral Thermal Environment. The neutral thermal environment is the temperature range that results in minimal stress to the newborn. It is important to note that no single environmental temperature is best for all sizes and conditions of newborns. The environment that is appropriate for the normal newborn may be too cold for the preterm newborn. Conversely, the environmental temperature that is appropriate for the preterm newborn may be too warm for the full-term healthy newborn. Severe consequences may result when newborns are exposed to environmental temperatures above or below their neutral temperature zone.

Serious overheating of the newborn can cause cerebral damage from dehydration, heat stroke, and even death. Cold stress produces less obvious consequences, unless it is severe enough to cause neonatal cold injury. The newborn's need to increase heat production results in increased nutritional requirements, increased metabolic rate, and an increased need for oxygen.[11] In the case of cold injury, severe cooling may result in metabolic acidosis, a decrease in the arterial oxygen blood level, and hypoglycemia.[13] Further, fluctuations in environmental temperature can precipitate periods of apnea in the newborn.[13] (*See* Chapter 34 for methods of temperature control.)

Temperature of the Newborn. The axillary temperature of the newborn averages from 36.5 to 37°C (97.6 to 98.6°F). The temperature of a full-term healthy newborn should stablilize within 10 hours of birth. An axillary temperature greater than 37.2°C (99°F) may indicate that the environment is too warm or that the newborn is suffering from either dehydration or infection/sepsis. An axillary temperature below 36.1°C (97°F) may indicate a cold environment, which is subjecting the newborn to cold stress. It is important for the nurse to monitor the newborn's temperature and environment closely to prevent fluctuations in body temperature.

ADJUSTMENTS IN OTHER SYSTEMS

Respiratory and cardiovascular system adjustments and temperature control are crucial to the health of newborns as they emerge into the extrauterine environment. Adjustment of other systems also is necessary, as outlined in the following discussion.

Urinary System

The newborn's urinary system is structurally complete but physiologically immature at birth. The musculature of the bladder is underdeveloped, the epithelium of the kidney is thick, and reabsorption and filtration in the renal tubules are limited.

The primary roles of the kidneys are to maintain fluid and electrolyte balance and to filter waste materials from the blood. The kidneys help to maintain fluid balance through their ability to concentrate urine. The newborn, however, is unable to concentrate urine. Maximum urine concentration is only about one-half that of the adult under conditions of thirsting. Water losses are therefore greater in the newborn than in the adult, and water requirements per kilogram of body weight are greater in the newborn period than in any other period of the life cycle. The daily fluid requirement for the healthy full-term newborn is approximately 125 mL/kg in a 24-hour period; the preterm newborn needs 150 mL/kg per day.[7]

In the second week of life, the full-term newborn's need for water ranges from 125 to 150 mL/kg per day. Approximately one half of this is required for the formation of urine; the rest is needed to offset the insensible water loss by the lungs, skin, and other losses. The insensible water loss is directly related to the calories metabolized by the newborn (about 40 mL/100 cal).[14]

The ability of the newborn to handle high-osmolarity or high-acid loads is also limited. Most newborns, however, thrive despite a high protein and osmolar intake, probably because much of this intake is used for growth and is not passed on to the kidney for excretion.[7] The urine of the newborn may contain small amounts of proteins and excessive amounts of urates. The urates in the urine may stain the diaper pink in the first week of life. Parents should be given anticipatory guidance regarding this possibility as the discovery of pink stains (brick dust color) on the diaper may be quite disturbing. Reassuring parents that this is normal will help allay their anxiety.

Urea clearance is low in the newborn; therefore, a slight transient rise in the blood urea nitrogen may occur during the first days of life.[14] There also is limited production of ammonium ion. The urine in the neonate appears colorless and has an average specific gravity of 1.008.

The bladder capacity of the newborn is approximately 15 mL and emptying of the bladder occurs frequently. The newborn usually voids at birth, but will not void again for 12 to 24 hours. After this time, the newborn may void 20 or more times a day. Voiding is a good indication that the newborn is receiving adequate fluid intake. Parents often ask "how will we know the baby is getting enough fluid?" The nurse can reassure them by explaining that wet diapers are a sign of adequate hydration.

By 6 months of age, the urinary system becomes more efficient because of maturation of the renal tubules, thinning of the epithelium of the kidneys, and increased ability to concentrate urine. Reabsorption and filtration in the renal tubules are more efficient so that the infant responds better to the need for fluids and electrolytes than the newborn.

Integument

At birth, the full-term newborn's skin demonstrates good texture and tone. During the first week postdelivery, the skin may begin peeling because of the thinness of its layers and its sensitive nature. The extrauterine environment does not provide the same protection for the skin as did the intrauterine environment. Households that are dry may cause the newborn's skin to peel and crack. Lubricating the skin with nonperfumed lotions and humidifying the air sometimes help this condition. (*See* Chapter 33 for a full discussion of common skin variations in the newborn infant.)

Sebaceous glands are present at birth and may be found mostly on the face and scalp. The glands that produce sweat (exocrine glands) are immature at birth so that they respond little when the newborn is overheated. The exocrine glands begin maturing within a few weeks of birth.

Newborns are born with varying amounts of hair. The hair is usually silky to the touch. During the first few months after birth, newborns may begin losing their hair. The growth of new hair usually starts on the sides of the head, with the slowest growth at the crown.

Endocrine System

The endocrine system of the newborn is usually fully developed, but functionally immature. In utero, the adrenal cortex of the fetus is active in the production of maternal hormones (*see* Chapter 12). Because of this overactivity of the adrenals in utero, the fetal adrenal gland is extremely large during pregnancy. The adrenals rapidly involute at birth, but are still functional.[7, 15]

There is a greater secretion of adrenal androgens in the neonatal period than in later childhood. Adrenal androgens are not secreted in appreciable amounts again until puberty. The newborn also controls tissue concentrations of adrenocortical steroids by means of a hypothalamic-pituitary-adrenal homeostatic mechanism. The hypothalamus is sensitive to tissue levels of cortisol and contains an adrenocorticotropic hormone (ACTH)-releasing factor and corticotropin-releasing hormone. When cortisol levels are low, these factors stimulate the release of ACTH by the pituitary gland. Adrenocorticotropic hormone, in turn, stimulates cortisol biosynthesis. Increased levels of cortisol inhibit the production of ACTH.[15] The adrenals also secrete aldosterone in response to low sodium and potassium levels in the blood. This response assists the newborn in maintaining fluid and electrolyte balance.

In utero, the fetal thyroid begins functioning by 12 weeks of gestation, allowing the fetus to accumulate and concentrate iodine. By 14 weeks of gestation, synthesis of thyroxine (T_4) and triiodothyronine (T_3) is apparent.[15] At birth, the thyroid gland of the newborn is active. The amount of protein-bound iodine rises immediately after birth and remains elevated for several weeks.[7]

Thyroid function tests are elevated in the newborn and remain elevated for the first several months of life. They are lower in premature and sick newborns than in healthy term newborns. The T_4 level of cord blood ranges from 7 to 13 μg/dL, with a mean of 10.9 μg/dL. The T_3 level of cord blood ranges from 12 to 90 ng/dL, with a mean of 48 ng/dL. Thyroid function screening is important at birth because congenital hypothyroidism may lead to serious problems in growth and development, specifically in central nervous system functioning.[15]

Gastrointestinal System

The full-term neonate is born with the capacity to swallow, digest, metabolize, and absorb proteins and simple carbohydrates, and to emulsify fats. With the exception of pancreatic amylase, the characteristic enzymes and digestive juices are present even in low-birth weight neonates.[16]

The motility of the gastrointestinal tract and the newborn's sphincteric control are immature. As a result, symptoms such as regurgitation, gas distension, flatus, and a wide variety of stool patterns may be found in the newborn.[16]

Protein Digestion. The newborn efficiently digests proteins from the diet. Digestion of proteins is facilitated by rennin and then pepsin in the stomach, pancreatic proteases in the duodenum, and enteric proteases and peptidases in the intestines.[16] The infant adds approximately 3.5 g protein daily to the body during the first 4 months of life and about 3.1 g per day during the rest of the first year.[17]

Carbohydrate Digestion. The salivary glands do not begin functioning until 2 to 3 months of age, when drooling becomes quite evident; however, the salivary enzymes that are present are sufficient to handle simple carbohydrates in the neonatal period.

Carbohydrate digestion begins in the mouth with salivary amylase. The newborn is deficient in pancreatic amylase and thus has difficulty digesting complex carbohydrates such as starches (polysaccharides). The small intestine contains four enzymes: lactase, sucrase, maltase, and isomaltase. These enzymes convert the disaccharides lactose, sucrose, and maltose into the monosaccharides glucose, galactose, and fructose.[16]

The disaccharide lactose accounts for 38 to 40 percent of the calories in human milk. Lactose is usually well digested by the newborn, although cases of lactose intolerance have been documented.[16]

Fat Digestion. Fat digestion in the newborn is less efficient than in the older child and adult because of the relatively lower levels of pancreatic lipase enzyme and bile salts. The digestion of fats begins in the stomach, stimulated by lingual lipase derived from the glands in the tongue. Hydrolysis of fat continues in the duodenum and jejunum under the influence of pancreatic lipase, and bile salts further emulsify the fats.[16]

Fats are needed by the newborn to meet the high-energy requirements for growth and development. Approximately 45 to 50 percent of the calories in human milk and most formulas is provided by fat. Human milk supplies linoleate, an easily digested fat as 6 to 9 percent of its calories. Human milk fat is better absorbed by the newborn than cow's milk fat (butterfat). As a consequence, most commercial formulas are made with vegetable fat rather than butterfat.

Human milk contains significantly more cholesterol than commercial formulas. Although the desirable level of cholesterol is unknown, cholesterol is required for the synthesis of bile salts and the development of the central nervous system.[17] (*See* Chapter 34 for further information on breast milk and formula composition.)

The newborn excretes 10 to 20 percent of the dietary intake of fats, resulting in some steatorrhea (fatty stools). This does not produce a problem for the newborn; however, if the newborn is given fat-soluble vitamins, these may be excreted in the stool.

Stomach. The stomach of the newborn has a capacity of approximately 90 mL, with an emptying time of about 2½ to 3 hours. The pH of the stomach secretions is high (5 to 6) at birth, but falls to normal adult values within a few hours.[7]

Stools. In utero, the fetus swallows amniotic fluid, which contains skin cells, hair, and vernix caseosa. The first stool of the newborn (called **meconium**) contains these substances, as well as blood, mucus, and bile pigments. The newborn usually passes the meconium within 12 to 36 hours of birth. This first stool appears sticky and greenish black.

By the third day postdelivery, the newborn passes **transitional stools,** which appear watery or loose and greenish brown to yellowish brown. The change in stool color (and consistency) is a result of the newborn's ingestion of formula or breast milk. By the fourth day, the typical **milk stools** are observed. Milk stools vary according to the feeding method and the individual newborn. Breastfed newborns have stools that are yellow and pasty. Some breastfed newborns may have up to ten stools a day; others may have one stool every few days. Bottlefed newborns usually have fewer stools than breastfed newborns. Cow's milk formulas produce stools that are yellow brown and firmer than stools of breastfed newborns.

Hepatic Regulation

The liver of the newborn is immature, but has several important functions, among them the conjugation of bilirubin and a role in blood coagulation.

Conjugation of Bilirubin. One of the functions of the liver is the conjugation of bilirubin. As red blood cells die, heme, a component of hemoglobin found in red blood cells and other proteins such as myoglobin, is liberated. Heme is metabolized to unconjugated bilirubin (indirect bilirubin). The bilirubin is carried to the liver by albumin and other blood proteins. Within the liver cells, bilirubin is transported by ligandin (Y protein) to a site where conjugation occurs. The enzyme glucuronyl transferase is needed for the conjugation process. The conjugated bilirubin is transported into the bile which then enters the intestinal tract. Bacteria in the small intestine convert bilirubin into stercobilinogen, which is excreted from the body in the feces, and urobilinogen, which is excreted in the urine.

If the feces are not expelled, unconjugated bilirubin levels may again rise. As a result of factors such as the enzyme beta-glucuronidase, the conjugated bilirubin may be hydrolyzed to unconjugated bilirubin within the bowel lumen and reabsorbed, thereby again increasing overall unconjugated bilirubin levels and the potential for neonatal jaundice.

Neonatal Physiologic Jaundice (Icterus Neonatorum). Neonatal **physiologic jaundice** is defined as an unconjugated bilirubin concentration that peaks at less than 12.9 mg/dL with a rise in bilirubin levels of less than 5 mg/dL per day. Conjugated bilirubin levels remain less than 1.5 mg/dL. Bilirubin levels return to normal around 10 days after birth. Physiologic jaundice may result from an increased load of bilirubin on the liver cells or decreased bilirubin clearance from the plasma.[18] Physiologic jaundice is a common occurrence in healthy newborns.

Increased Load of Bilirubin on the Liver. An increased load of bilirubin on the liver is related to bilirubin production and enterohepatic circulation. It is estimated that the newborn produces 8 to 10 mg/kg bilirubin per day. This production is related to the newborn's high circulating red cell volume (per kilogram), the shorter mean red cell life span, and an early bilirubin peak in the blood. The production of bilirubin decreases with increasing postnatal age, but is still twice the adult production at 2 weeks of life. The newborn also absorbs larger quantities of unconjugated bilirubin (indirect) from the enterohepatic circulation (intestines, liver) than does the adult. Moreover, newborns have fewer bacteria in the small intestines and greater activity of the deconjugating enzyme beta-glucuronidase. As a result, conjugated bilirubin is hydrolyzed to unconjugated bilirubin, and the larger quantities of unconjugated bilirubin place additional stress on the newborn's immature liver, contributing to neonatal jaundice.[18]

Decreased Bilirubin Clearance from the Plasma. The decreased ability of the liver to clear bilirubin from the plasma is associated with decreased transport of bilirubin by ligandin in the liver cells and decreased conjugation. Uptake of bilirubin from the plasma takes place when the bilirubin binds to the proteins in the liver. The predominant bilirubin-binding protein ligandin is relatively deficient in the newborn liver for about the first 5 days after birth.[18]

ISSUES AND CONTROVERSIES

The neonatal period is a time of adjustment for all family members. One issue involves the parents' decision to breastfeed or bottlefeed. In their overzealousness to inform parents about the advantages of breastfeeding, health professionals sometimes covertly convey the message that this is the *only* way for parents to feed the newborn. Some mothers simply do not enjoy breastfeeding or may have other reasons for wanting to bottlefeed. Nurses should support mothers whatever their decision. Another issue is raised when the father wishes the mother to breastfeed but the mother may not want to do so. Whose choice should it be? How can the nurse help the parents resolve the conflict?

Conjugation of bilirubin also is impaired in the newborn. There is less glucuronyl transferase produced by the liver. At the same time, the newborn is breaking down red blood cells. The result is an increase in blood levels of unconjugated bilirubin. This, accompanied by the newborn's reabsorption of larger quantities of unconjugated bilirubin from the bowel, contributes to physiologic jaundice beyond the first 24 hours after birth.

In normal circumstances, the neonatal liver is capable of excreting bilirubin that has been conjugated (direct bilirubin). Thus, serum levels of conjugated bilirubin usually are not elevated in physiologic jaundice; however, the ability of the neonatal liver to secrete conjugated bilirubin is more limited than that of the adult. If there are significant increases in bilirubin levels, as in hemolytic disease, the ability to excrete conjugated bilirubin will be impaired. Elevated serum levels of conjugated bilirubin are thus indicative of nonphysiologic jaundice[18] (*see* Chapter 34).

Other Factors. Chilling, decreased fluid and calorie intake, and weight loss also may contribute to jaundice in the newborn.[19–21] Chilling can cause the newborn's core temperature to decline, precipitating metabolic acidosis. The state of acidosis, in turn, can reduce the capacity of bilirubin to bind to albumin, thereby causing an increase in the serum level of unconjugated bilirubin.[19]

Decreased fluid and caloric intake and weight loss have been associated with elevated bilirubin levels in the neonate. Early and frequent feedings reduce weight loss and promote adequate fluid and caloric intake. Such feedings also promote more frequent stools and a decrease in the enterohepatic circulation.[18] (*See* Chapter 34 for further discussion of management of physiologic jaundice.)

Breastfeeding Jaundice. Breastfed newborns sometimes have increased serum bilirubin concentrations. The bilirubin rises progressively from the fourth day of life, reaching a maximum level of unconjugated bilirubin of 10 to 30 mg/dL by 10 to 15 days of life. This condition, referred to as breast milk jaundice syndrome, is a relatively benign condition and there is no evidence to suggest that breastfeeding jaundice causes hemolysis of cells or bilirubin encephalopathy.[18]

Breastfeeding jaundice is thought to be caused by an unusually high lipoprotein lipase activity in the breast milk which liberates large quantities of unsaturated fatty acids in the newborn's bowel. Unsaturated fatty acids inhibit the conjugation of bilirubin, thereby increasing the serum bilirubin level.[22] In one study, serum bilirubin levels of breastfed newborns also were associated with the frequency of feeding in the first 3 days of life. Researchers found that newborns who nursed eight or more times a day had significantly lower bilirubin levels than those who nursed fewer than eight times in 24 hours.[23] Mothers should thus be encouraged to breastfeed early and frequently during this period. Feeding the newborn on demand will usually accomplish this goal. (*See* Chapter 34 for additional management strategies for breastfeeding jaundice.)

Some investigators believe that a double standard should be used in the classification of hyperbilirubinemia for bottlefed and breastfed infants. In a large study (2416 infants), it was found that the upper limit for bilirubin concentration for formula-fed infants was 11.4 mg/100 mL, and that for breastfed infants was 14.5 mg/100 mL. The investigators suggest that a diagnosis of jaundice, requiring further testing, may not be indicated unless the serum bilirubin exceeds 15 mg/dL in the breastfed infant or 12 mg/dL in the formula-fed infant.[24]

Another study suggests that hyperbilirubinemia caused by breastfeeding acts to compensate for the antioxidant deficiency found in normal newborns.[25] Although the results of this study need to be confirmed, the idea that increased serum bilirubin levels in the newborn may in fact be needed as a physiologic defense is an interesting notion. Breastfeeding may thus have benefits beyond those that have already been documented.

Role of the Liver in Coagulation. The liver plays an important role in blood coagulation as a source of coagulation factors II, VII, IX, and X. These coagulation factors, as well as prothrombin, are dependent on the synthesis of vitamin K. For the first few days of life, however, the newborn lacks the bacterial flora in the gastrointestinal tract necessary for vitamin K synthesis. Thus, during this period, the newborn may be deficient in prothrombin and other coagulation factors.

Bacterial colonization of the intestines occurs with the intake of formula or breast milk. Newborns are at risk for vitamin K deficiency when their mothers have taken anticonvulsant medications (eg, phenobarbital, dilantin) prenatally.[2]

Since 1961, it has been common practice to administer a prophylactic injection of vitamin K_1 (phytonadione, 0.5 to 1 mg intramuscularly) at birth to prevent hemorrhagic disease of the newborn. Although there has been some controversy about whether all newborns need vitamin K, research findings have documented vitamin K deficiency in the newborn and recommended prophylactic treatment.[26] For those infants who are especially at risk for hemorrhagic disease (those whose mothers have taken anticonvulsants), it is recommended that 1 to 2 mg of vitamin K be administered intravenously immediately at birth.[2] (*See* Chapter 34 for care of the newborn immediately after birth.)

Immunologic System

Newborns, especially full-term newborns, are born with the capability to combat some infections as a result of placental transmission of maternal antibodies. The newborn also has the potential for both cell-mediated and antibody-mediated immune responses.

Cell-mediated immunity depends on the T lymphocytes, which develop from stem cells in the embryonic mesenchyme and appear in the embryonic yolk sac. These T lymphocytes migrate to the fetal liver and then from the liver to the thymus where they differentiate into functional types. T lymphocytes are mediated by antigens, dividing and increasing their numbers at the site of an antigen reaction. They also play an indirect role in stimulating circulating antibodies. By 30 weeks of gestation, the number of T lymphocytes is similar to that of the adult.[2]

B lymphocytes also originate in the embryonic mesenchyme and mature in the fetal liver. B lymphocytes are differentiated into plasma cells in the bone marrow, lymph nodes, and spleen. They also differentiate into plasma cells in the presence of helper T lymphocytes. The function of the B cells is also antigen mediated, stimulating the production of antibodies. By 15 weeks of gestation, circulating B lymphocytes are found in the same numbers as they are found in the adult.

Antibody-mediated immunity depends on B lymphocytes' producing specific antibodies called immunoglobulins. The principal groups of immunoglobulins are immunoglobins G, M, and A.

Immunoglobulin G (IgG) readily crosses the placenta from the maternal to the fetal circulation. Placental transfer of IgG begins during the third month of gestation, but markedly increases in the third trimester. At term, the IgG level in the fetus is approximately 100 mg/dL.[2] The short-lasting immunity that the newborn receives from the IgG is called **passive immunity.**

Over the first 3 months of life, maternal IgG levels are depleted in the infant; however, the infant synthesizes IgG during the same period, partially making up for this depletion.[2] The newborn receives passive immunity to diseases for which the mother has developed specific antibodies. Among the diseases are diphtheria, tetanus, poliomyelitis, measles, mumps, and gram-positive cocci such as pneumococcus. The schedule of immunizations for infants is based on the premise that the infant receives only passive immunity from the mother and needs to develop his or her own antibodies for protection from some of the common childhood diseases.

As IgG is transferred in increased amounts during the last trimester, the premature newborn is at a deficit in combating infections. Moreover, all newborns, whether full term or premature, are not protected from gram-negative rods by maternal IgG.

Immunoglobulin M (IgM) is the immunoglobulin that contains antibodies to gram-negative bacteria as well as to blood group antigens and some viruses. Maternal IgM does not cross the placenta, although by 30 weeks of gestation, the fetus can produce IgM in response to exposure to infection. At birth, the normal serum IgM concentration is usually below 20 mg/dL, so that the newborn has increased susceptibility to infection with gram-negative bacteria such as *Escherichia coli.* The level of IgM increases rapidly during the first month of life, and is approximately one-half that found in the adult by 6 months of age.[2]

Immunoglobulin A (IgA) does not cross the placenta and there is no evidence that the fetus synthesizes this immunoglobulin in utero. It is found in two forms, circulating IgA and secretory IgA. Secretory IgA is found over secreting surfaces of the body, such as the intestinal and respiratory mucosa, the eyes, and the epithelium of the urinary tract. It resists destruction by pH and enzymatic sources.[2] Secretory IgA helps protect the newborn from infection on secretory surfaces. Breast milk, especially colostrum, contains a significant amount of secretory IgA, thereby providing the newborn with some passive immunity. IgA begins to be produced by the first month of life.

The full-term newborn is usually able to combat minor infections; however, there are deficits in the neonatal immune response. For example, the absence of IgM contributes to the increased susceptibility of the newborn to gram-negative bacterial infections. Newborns also have a diminished capacity to localize infections because they cannot clear bacteria from the blood as quickly as adults. Further, antibody production is dependent on exposure to antigens, which usually does not occur until after birth. The development of immunocompetence to such bacteria as *Hemophilus* does not occur until after the neonatal period.[2] Premature newborns, especially those less than 34 weeks of gestation, are especially prone to infections because of their immature immune response.

Neurologic System

The normal full-term newborn has an intact, although immature, nervous system. The development of the nervous system occurs in stages in utero. In the first stage, completed by midpregnancy, the fetus develops the actual number of nerve cells that will exist for the remainder of the lifespan. During the second stage, rapid growth of neurons occurs. In the third stage, beginning in the latter part of gestation and continuing through the fourth year of life, the number of glial cells and dendrites increases. Myelination of neurons begins at about the fourth month of gestation and continues through the fourth year.

Neurologic development follows cephalocaudal and proximodistal patterns. Myelin, which increases the speed and accuracy of nerve impulses, develops earliest in the transmitters of sensory impulses and the nerves of the brain stem. The newborn, therefore, has an acute sense of hearing, smell, and taste. The newborn also is able to survive by breathing and maintaining acid-base balance because of this early myelination.

Motor Behavior and Reflexes. Gross motor behavior begins with movements in the upper part of the body. The newborn is able to move her or his eyes and fixate on human faces. Newborns also are able to control their heads and make movements with their mouths. Fine motor behavior begins with purposeless flailing of the arms and progresses to purposeful movements during infancy, such as reaching for objects. As the infant grows and develops, sensorimotor coordination further develops, as evidenced by the ability to walk by 12 to 18 months of age.

Primitive reflexes also are found in the newborn. These reflexes assist the newborn's survival and safety. Among the primitive reflexes found in the newborn are the Moro, palmar and plantar grasp, tonic neck, sucking and rooting, swallowing, Babinski, stepping, Galant, crossed extension, magnet, traction, arm recoil, crawling, and glabellar reflexes (*see* Chapter 33). These primitive reflexes give way to righting reflexes (eg, righting of the neck and head) and protective reactions as the infant develops.

The Senses. The newborn is capable of responding to a variety of stimuli through his or her senses. These behaviors are related to the newborn's level of arousal and orienting response (*see* later discussion).

Visual Responses. At birth, the newborn is able to process complex visual information and track an object in space (Figure 32–4). Newborns also can defend themselves from unpleasant visual stimuli such as a bright light by blinking and withdrawing their heads. If repeated stimulation is presented to newborns, they have the ability to shut out these stimuli. This process of shutting out stimuli, referred to as habituation, enables newborns to free themselves to meet other physiologic demands[27] (*see* later discussion).

Newborns prefer complex visual stimuli. They are fascinated by geometric shapes, large circles, dots, and squares, and focus their attention on patterned objects rather than plain ones. They also prefer black-and-white contrasts (Figure 32–5).[28]

Research also indicates that newborns prefer a human face over other objects and will follow a drawing that resembles a human face 90° to 180°.[29] They also have the ability to scan the environment to focus on preferred stimuli.

Visual acuity is difficult to measure in the newborn, although it appears to be in the range 20/100 to

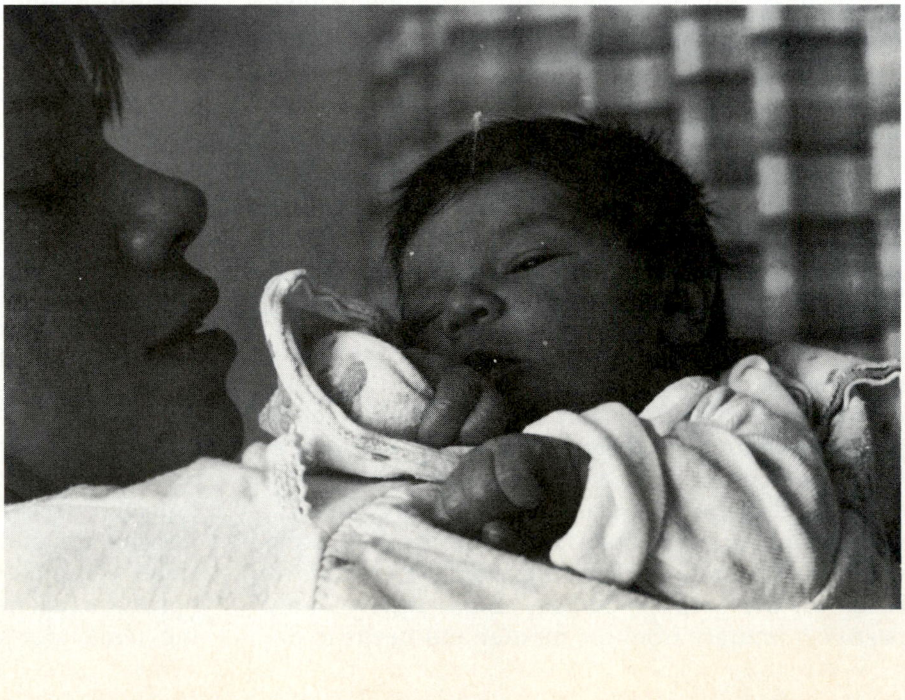

Figure 32–4. Newborn visual response.

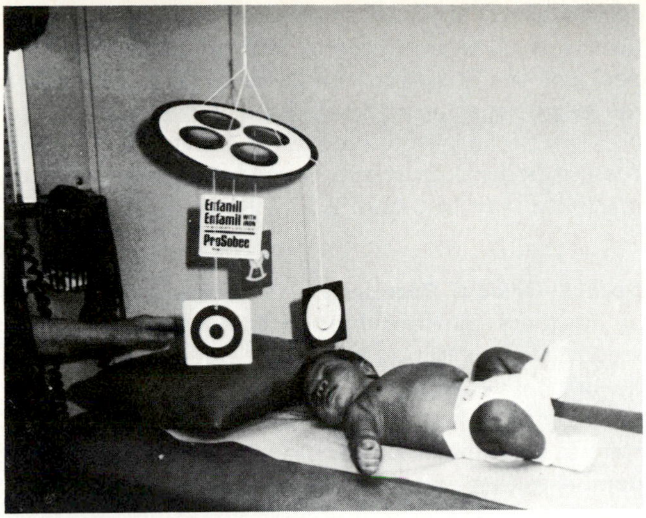

Figure 32–5. Mobile for newborn. Geometric shapes are interesting for the newborn.

20/400. Newborns, however, can define the edges of ⅛-in. and ¹⁄₁₆-in. strips at 9 in. and 12 in. and fixate on objects for 4 to 10 seconds. They can also refixate every 1.0 to 1.5 seconds.[28]

Brazelton[27] describes the optimal response to visual stimulation as an initial alerting, attention that increases, a gradual decrease in interest, and a final turning away from a monotonous stimuli.

Hearing. The anatomic structures of the ear are well developed at birth. The newborn's eustachian tube is shorter and wider than that of the adult. The newborn also has specific and well-organized auditory responses.

Brazelton[27] notes that when the newborn is presented with an interesting stimulus, such as a rattle, she or he will become alert, breathing will become irregular, eyes will open, and the newborn will scan the environment, turning toward the sound. As with visual responses, repeated auditory stimuli cause the newborn to shut out the stimuli, or habituate.

Newborns are able to discriminate between sounds, and seem especially responsive to the human voice in the range 500 to 900 Hz.[30] Low-frequency stimuli (25 to 40 dB) soothe the newborn; high-frequency stimuli (above 4000 Hz) produce an immediate response but may cause distress.[27] Research has shown that newborns as young as 3 days old can discriminate between their mother's voice and the voice of another woman.[31]

Olfactory Response. Newborns have a highly developed sense of smell. They prefer odors that are sweet, such as milk, to odors that are noxious, such as alcohol. Evidence has shown that a 5-day-old newborn can distinguish his or her own mother's breast pad from those of other mothers.[32] This highly developed sense of smell helps the breastfeeding infant root toward the nipple.

Taste. Newborns also have a discriminating sense of taste at birth. They prefer sweet fluids to unsweetened and salty fluids. When newborns are given a sweet fluid (eg, 15 percent sucrose), they suck more frequently and take shorter rest periods initially; however, they suck more slowly with increasing concentrations of sucrose.

When the newborn is fed cow's milk formula, she or he will suck continuously, pausing irregularly. If breast milk is then substituted, the newborn recognizes the change in taste, sucking in bursts with frequent pauses. The pauses are directly related to the taste of the breast milk, and the burst-pause pattern of the sucking is related to accommodation to a different stimulus.[27]

Response to Tactile Stimuli. Research has indicated that newborns respond to touch in a variety of ways. When newborns are upset, gentle, soothing patting or stroking appears to quiet them. On the other hand, when newborns are quiet, an intrusive tactile stimulus quickly brings them to an alert state and may cause distress. Moreover, it has been demonstrated that mothers use touch to quiet a distressed infant, and fathers use tactile stimuli to excite the infant.[27]

Newborns also respond to touch for purposes of survival. For example, stroking a newborn's cheek elicits the rooting and sucking reflexes that aid in feeding.

Periods of Reactivity in the Newborn. Within the first 24 hours of birth, newborns demonstrate predictable periods of reactivity: a first period of reactivity, a period of sleep or inactivity, and a second period of reactivity. These periods are characterized by physiologic adjustments and behavioral states of the newborn. The sleep-wake patterns and physiologic adjustments of newborns during the periods of reactivity are influenced by the difficulty of the labor and delivery and any medications that the mother may have received during the labor and delivery process.

First Period of Reactivity. The first period of reactivity occurs during the 30 minutes immediately after birth. In the initial phase of this period, newborns are in a state of quiet alertness. Their eyes are open and bright. They can focus attention on their parents' faces and attend to voices, especially those of their mothers. This phase lasts approximately 15 minutes and is followed by a phase of active alertness (Figure 32–6).

In the phase of active alertness, neonates have frequent bursts of movements, which may be accompanied by crying. They have a strong sucking reflex and appear to be hungry. This phase lasts approximately 15 minutes.

The first period of reactivity is characterized by physiologic as well as behavioral responses. During this period, neonates have rapid, shallow respirations, which may be accompanied by transient flaring of the nares, grunting, and retractions of the chest. The heart rate is rapid and irregular. Bowel sounds are absent and stools are present, although passage of meconium may or may not occur during this period.

Parent-newborn attachment can begin in the first period of reactivity. This can be facilitated by allowing the parents opportunities to hold and talk to their newborn. Eye-to-eye contact can be fostered by the nurse's delaying preventive eye treatment so that the newborn's eyes are open and alert. Because the newborn has a strong sucking reflex during this period, breastfeeding can be initiated if the mother wishes. This may promote immediate satisfaction of the mother with the breastfeeding experience.

Period of Sleep or Inactivity. After the first 30 minutes, newborns become drowsy and then fall asleep. During the sleep state, newborns are relatively unresponsive and difficult to awaken. Respiratory and heart rates slow and become more regular. The temperature of the newborn may drop. The posture of the newborn appears relaxed and bowel sounds are present. Because of the relative inactivity of the newborn, it is difficult to initiate feeding. This period of inactivity may last from 2 to 4 hours (Figure 32–7).

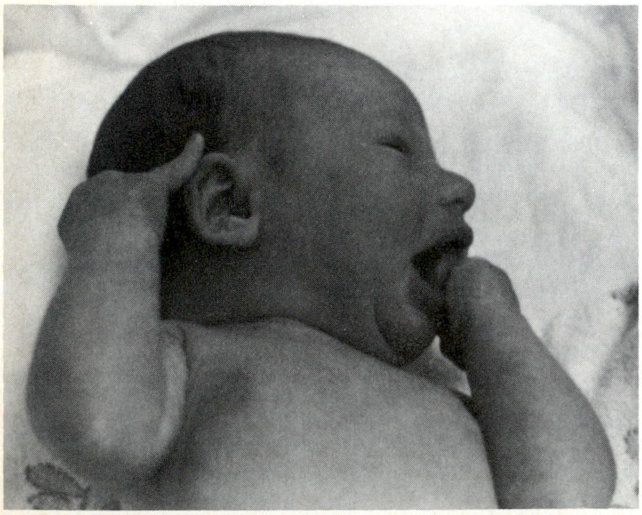

Figure 32–6. First period of reactivity.

Second Period of Reactivity. After the period of sleep or inactivity, newborns enter the second period of reactivity. This period may last from 4 to 6 hours in the normal newborn. The newborn is awake and alert during this period. The variability of the behavioral state of the newborn is apparent, with the newborn demonstrating states of quiet alertness, active alertness, and crying.

The newborn's physiologic responses also may vary during this period. Respiratory and heart rates may change rapidly. Newborns should be observed for tachypnea and apnea during this period. Newborns produce gastric and respiratory mucus, which may cause them to regurgitate and gag. They also may demonstrate changes in color, with transient phases of mild cyanosis. Bowel sounds increase during this period, and the newborn may pass the first meconium stool. The first voiding also may occur.

During this period, the nurse can provide the parents opportunities to begin attachment behaviors (*see* Chapter 34). Feeding also may be initiated if it was not initiated during the first period of reactivity. The neonate sucks, roots, and swallows during this second period of reactivity and becomes interested in feeding.

BEHAVIOR

Newborns respond interactively and reciprocally with their caregivers. These response characteristics, in turn, contribute to parent-newborn interactions.[33] In addition to interactive reponses, newborns also demonstrate several other characteristic behavioral responses. Among these are the levels of arousal of the newborn.

Behavioral State

Brazelton's[34] classic research on behavior and neurologic responses of the newborn was based on the description of the newborn's state of consciousness by Prechtl and others.[35] The newborn's behavioral state can be categorized into six levels of arousal:

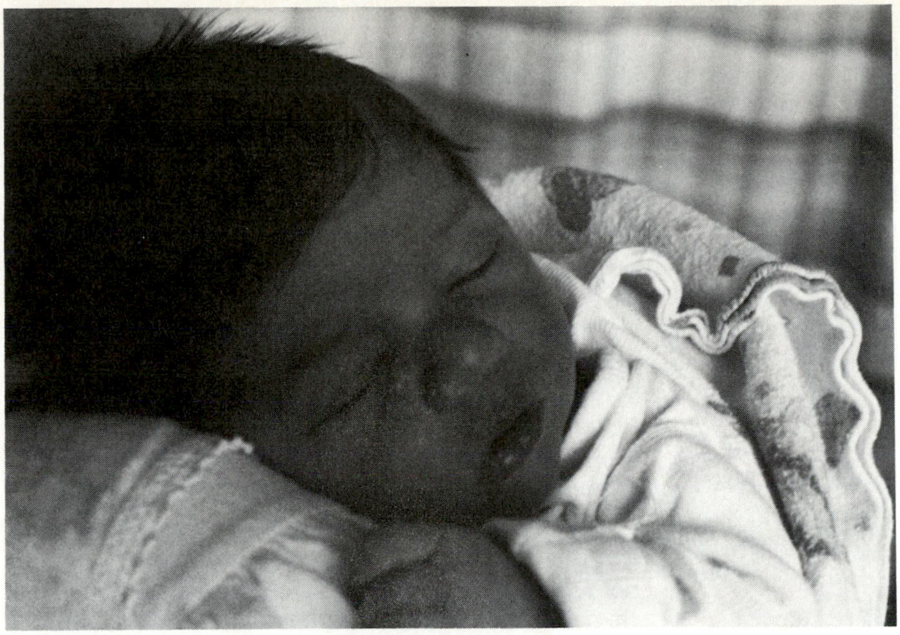

Figure 32–7. Period of inactivity.

1. *Deep Sleep.* The newborn's face appears relaxed, and the eyelids are closed and still with no movement. Breathing is regular and deep. There is little or no motor activity, with the exception of an occasional startle or fine mouth movements.
2. *Light Sleep.* The newborn's eyes are closed and rapid eye movements (REMs) occur. Occasional body activity, ranging from minor twitches to stretching of the extremities, can be noted. Breathing is irregular and more rapid than in deep sleep.
3. *Drowsiness or Semidozing.* The newborn's eyes may be open or closed. If open, the eyes have a glazed look and do not focus. There may be some motor activity, with an occasional startle. The respirations are fairly regular, but faster than in sleep states.
4. *Quiet Alert.* Newborns' eyes are open and appear bright and alert. They can focus on and follow appealing objects such as a red ball. They also are able to attend to auditory stimuli such as their mothers' voices.
5. *Active Alert.* Newborns experience frequent bursts of movement of the extremities. Their eyes are open, scanning the environment. This state is apparent when the baby is fussing or prior to feeding.
6. *Intense Crying.* Newborns have periods of motor activity, accompanied by continuous bursts of crying. This state helps newborns to shut out disturbing stimuli and also alerts the caregiver to hunger and discomfort of the newborn.

Sleep-Wake Cycle

Newborns appear to have individualized sleep-wake patterns. In general, sleep cycles (light REM sleep and deep sleep) at term occur in intervals of 45 to 50 minutes, with immature babies having shorter intervals. Rapid eye movement sleep, which occurs in the deep sleep state as well as the light sleep state, contributes to the growth and maintenance of neural structures.[27]

The newborn's sleep-wake cycles become patterned so that eventually diurnal patterns of daytime wakefulness and night sleeping occur. These diurnal patterns are influenced by appropriate feeding patterns, sufficient nurturing activities, and a fussing period prior to a long sleep.[27] Weight also influences diurnal patterns. When newborns reach a weight of approximately 12 pounds, they begin stretching their feeding times, and eliminating nighttime feedings.

Nurses have a role in educating parents about sleep-wake patterns in infants. Parents quickly become attuned to the needs of their own infants. They will be less anxious in their interactions with the infant when they are aware of these common sleep-wake patterns. For example, one mother informed the nurse that her infant had begun sleeping 8 hours during the night; however, the infant had a fussy period of about 45 minutes before going to sleep. This period was disturbing to the parents because it seemed that they could not console the infant. The nurse explained that a fussy period was common in infants before they went to sleep for long periods. This simple explanation helped to reduce the mother's anxiety so that she could try alternate approaches to console her infant.

Behavioral Responses

Newborns demonstrate several predictable responses when interacting with caregivers and when responding to environmental stimuli.[27] Brazelton's[34] early research demonstrates that newborns can be assessed for these responses, which vary depending on their behavioral state. For example, when newborns are in the deep sleep state, they respond only slightly to a moderately loud rattle. In the active alert state, on the other hand, newborns respond to the rattle by becoming quiet, alerting, and then turning to the rattle as if searching for it.[27] Brazelton[34] also found that newborns can be assessed for orienting response, habituation, consolability and self-quieting, cuddliness, and motor organization.

Orienting Response. The response of newborns to stimuli is called the orienting response. Research indicates that newborns become more alert when they sense a new stimulus, and less responsive when orienting to a repetitive stimulus.[33] This ability to respond less to repetitive stimuli is termed the response decrement. This phenomenon allows neonates to control their behavioral state. Overresponsive newborns are said to lack response decrement. They are easily aroused and tend to respond to many stimuli by crying. Unresponsive newborns are relatively inactive and difficult to arouse. Quiet alert newborns respond to stimuli with a normal response decrement.

Habituation. Habituation is the process whereby neonates shut out disturbing or overwhelming stimuli. This process allows the newborn to respond less to a repeated stimulus. Stimuli such as light, noise, or a pin prick to the heel will first alert the newborn to the stimulus. With repeated applications of the stimulus, however, the response of the newborn will diminish.[34] It is important that parents understand this concept. As one parent stated, "I was so worried that sometimes my baby could not hear. He seemed to startle and awaken when our dog barked when we first took him home. Now, he sleeps even when the dog is barking."

Along with habituation, newborns appear to have clear preferences for certain stimuli. They prefer female voices over male voices and human faces over other objects.[27]

Consolability and Self-Quieting Behavior. The consolability of the newborn, either by intervention of the caregiver or by self-consolation, is important to the success of parent-newborn interactions. Consolability refers to the way in which newborns are able to change from the crying to the active alert, quiet alert, drowsy, or sleep state. Parents who have success in consoling their newborns experience a sense of satisfaction. As one mother proudly noted, "When my baby is crying, it seems that only my husband or myself can quiet her." On the other hand, the inability to console may be very distressing to the parents.

Newborns also have the ability to console themselves. This is referred to as self-quieting behavior. Self-quieting or self-consoling behaviors include hand-to-mouth movements, sucking, alerting to external stimuli such as voices or faces, and motor activity.

Nurses can assist parents in identifying self-quieting behaviors of their newborn so that they will not feel they have to pick up the newborn as soon as she or he starts to cry. Nurses also should assist the parents in identifying behaviors that will help console the newborn, such as rocking, holding, and patting.

Cuddliness. Cuddliness is a response of the newborn to being held by the caregiver; specifically, it is the degree to which the newborn nestles into the contours of the caregiver's body. Many newborns cuddle, although some resist being held. Nurses can foster this behavior by advising parents to assume comfortable positions, and by explaining that newborns differ in this response.

Motor Organization. Motor organization refers to those activities that enable the newborn to control and coordinate movement. When stimulated, newborns with good motor organization demonstrate movements that are rhythmic and spontaneous. For example, when roused from sleep, they may initially startle and then attempt to bring their hands to their mouths. To bring the hand to the mouth, the newborn may turn the head to one side, thus displaying control of one side of the body. The newborn then extends and flexes the arm to enable the hand to reach the mouth. As the hand reaches the mouth, the newborn's body relaxes and the face softens as he or she attempts to insert the clenched fist. When these efforts are successful, the newborn maintains a quiet state of semi-alertness. Such motor behavior is a good indication of central nervous system organization in newborns.[27]

Chapter 33 provides further discussion of neonatal behavioral assessment. Parents can learn the specific individual responses of their newborn as they build their confidence as caregivers.

Attachment/Bonding

The newborn's behavioral state also affects the attachment behaviors of parents and infants. Theories of attachment and bonding have been presented in Chapters 4 and 31.

Parents must be knowledgeable about newborn behavior so that they can be sensitive to the cues of their newborn. Because parent-newborn interactions are reciprocal, both participants will modify their behaviors in response to one another. Two nursing researchers, Golas and Parks,[36] developed a teaching intervention based on a modification of the Brazelton Neonatal Behavioral Assessment Scale (BNBAS). An experimental group of 17 primiparous mothers received the teaching intervention representative of the behaviors identified by Brazelton[27] (eg, orientation, response decrement, consolability). A second group of 16 mothers completed a newborn information checklist 2 weeks postnatally. A third group of 13 mothers received neither the teaching intervention nor the checklist. The researchers found that at 4 weeks postpartum, the experimental group had more knowledge about newborn behavior than the other two groups; however, there were no differences among the groups of mothers regarding maternal confidence in interpreting behavioral cues of newborns. Confidence building is probably a developmental process that occurs over time with the aid of support people such as the nurse.

SUMMARY

The transition from the intrauterine to the extrauterine environment is a critical period for the newborn. At birth, a series of physiologic events occur that make this transition possible for healthy newborns. A successful transition to extrauterine life facilitates the newborn's future growth and development. In addition, interactional patterns initiated during this period form the basis for healthy family relationships.

Respiratory adjustment is probably the most critical transition that newborns must make. The first breaths of air establish the characteristics of pulmonary function and expansion of the lungs. Several theories have been proposed to explain the initiation of respirations in newborns. The neonatal respiratory effort is probably a combination of mechanical, chemical, and sensory-proprioceptive stimuli.

Cardiovascular adjustment also is necessary for the survival of newborns. The expansion of the lungs with air causes changes in the pulmonary-systemic pressure relationships and closure of the foramen ovale, ductus venosus, and ductus arteriosus. The hemoglobin, initially high at birth, decreases in response to the more efficient oxygen exchange of the lungs.

Newborns also must regulate their temperatures at birth. They lose heat through evaporation, radiation, convection, and conduction. Heat in the newborn is produced primarily through nonshivering thermogenesis. It is important that caregivers maintain a thermally neutral environment for newborns.

Other neonatal body systems that undergo adjustments at birth include the urinary, integumentary, endocrine, gastrointestinal, and neurologic systems. Adjustments also take place involving hepatic regulation and immune response.

Newborns are capable of seeing, hearing, smelling, and tasting. They also demonstrate characteristic behavioral states and behavioral responses, including orienting responses. Newborns interact with their caregivers in predictable ways, and this interaction is reciprocal. Parents need to be knowledgeable about the responses of their newborns. As a key member of the health care team, the nurse's responsibility includes providing parent teaching about these physiologic and behavioral responses.

REVIEW QUESTIONS

1. Identify mechanical, chemical and sensory stimuli that contribute to the onset of respirations.
2. List the changes that must occur in fetal circulatory shunts at birth.
3. Describe two ways in which the nurse can provide a thermally neutral environment for the newborn.
4. Describe the mechanism of physiologic jaundice in the newborn.
5. Discuss behavioral states and orientation responses of the newborn.

REFERENCES

1. Nelson NM. The onset of respirations. In: Avery G, ed. *Neonatology: Pathophysiology and Management of the Newborn,* 3rd ed. Philadelphia: JB Lippincott; 1987.
2. Korones SB. *High Risk Newborn Infants: The Basis for Intensive Care.* 4th ed. St. Louis, Mo: CV Mosby; 1986.

3. Moore KL. *The Developing Human: Clinically Oriented Embryology.* Philadelphia: WB Saunders; 1988.
4. Moore KL. *Before We Are Born.* 3rd ed. Philadelphia: WB Saunders; 1989.
5. Martin RJ, et al. Respiratory problems. In: Klaus MH, Fanaroff AA, eds. *Care of the High-Risk Neonate.* 3rd ed. Philadelphia: WB Saunders; 1986.
6. Hodson WA, Woodrum DE. Respiratory problems in the newborn. In: Kelly VC, ed. *Practice of Pediatrics.* Philadelphia: Harper & Row; 1987:vol 2.
7. Oliver TK. The newborn. In: Kelley VC, ed. *Practice of Pediatrics.* Philadelphia: Harper & Row; 1987:vol 2.
8. Truog WE. Care of the newborn in the delivery room. In: Kelley VC, ed. *Practice of Pediatrics.* Philadelphia: Harper & Row, 1987:vol 2.
9. Richards JM, et al. Sequential 22-hour profiles of breathing patterns and heart rate of 110 full-term infants during the first 6 months of life. *Pediatrics.* 1984;74:763–777.
10. Versmold HT, et al. Aortic blood pressure during the first 12 hours of life in infants with birth weight 610–4220 grams. *Pediatrics.* 1981;67:611.
11. Hey E, Scopes JW. Thermoregulation in the newborn. In: Avery GB, ed. *Neonatology: Pathophysiology and Management of the Newborn.* 3rd ed. Philadelphia: JB Lippincott; 1987.
12. Moore KL. *Before We Are Born: Basic Embryology and Birth Defects.* Philadelphia: WB Saunders; 1983.
13. Klaus MH, et al. The physical environment. In: Klaus MW, Fanaroff AA, eds. *Care of the High Risk Neonate.* 3rd ed. Philadelphia: WB Saunders; 1986.
14. Behrman RE, Vaughan VC, eds. *Nelson Textbook of Pediatrics.* 12th ed. Philadelphia: WB Saunders; 1983.
15. Moshang T, Bongiovanni AM. Endocrine disorders of the newborn. In: Avery G, ed. *Neonatology: Pathophysiology and Management of the Newborn.* 3rd ed. Philadelphia: JB Lippincott; 1987.
16. Avery GB, Fletcher AB. Nutrition. In: Avery GB, ed. *Neonatology Pathophysiology and Management of the Newborn.* 3rd ed.Philadelphia: JB Lippincott; 1987.
17. Robinson CH, et al. *Normal and Therapeutic Nutrition.* 17th ed. New York: Macmillan; 1986.
18. Maisels MJ. Neonatal jaundice. In: Avery GB ed. *Neonatology: Pathophysiology and Management of the Newborn.* 3rd ed. Philadelphia: JB Lippincott; 1987.
19. Cottrell BH, Anderson GC. Rectal or axillary temperature measurement: effect on plasma bilirubin and intestinal transit of meconium. *J Pediatr Gastroenterol Nutr.* 1984;3: 734–739.
20. Maisels MJ, et al. The yellow baby syndrome (or why babies get jaundiced). *Pediatr Res.* 1985;19:2407. Abstract.
21. Osborn LM, et al. Jaundice in the full-term neonate. *Pediatrics.* 1984;73:520–526.
22. Poland RL, et al. High milk lipase activity associated with breast-milk jaundice. *Pediatr Res.* 1980;14:1328–1331.
23. De Carvallo et al. Frequency of breast-feeding and serum bilirubin concentration. *Am J Dis Child.* 1982;136:737–738.
24. Maisels MJ, Gifford K. Normal serum bilirubin levels in the newborn and the effect of breast-feeding. *Pediatrics.* 1986; 78:743.
25. Stocker R, et al. Bilirubin is an antioxidant of possible physiological importance. *Science.* 1987;235:1043–1045.
26. Shapiro A, et al. Vitamin K deficiency in the newborn infant: prevalence and perinatal risk factors. *J Pediatr.* 1986;109: 675–680.
27. Brazelton TB. Behavioral competence of the newborn infant. In: Avery GB, ed. *Neonatology: Pathophysiology and Management of the Newborn.* 3rd ed. Philadelphia: Lippincott; 1987.
28. Ludington-Hoe SM. What can newborns really see? *Am J Nurs.* 1983;9:1286–1289.
29. Rantz RL. Visual perception from birth as shown by pattern selectivity. *Ann NY Acad Sci.* 1965;118:793.
30. Eisenberg RB. The development of hearing in man: an assessment of current status. *J Am Speech Hearing Assoc.* 1970;12:119–123.
31. De Casper A, Fifer W. Of human bonding: newborns prefer their mother's voices. *Science.* 1980;208:1174–1176.
32. MacFarlane A. Olfaction in the development of social preferences in the human neonate. In: *Parent-Infant Evaluation.* Ciba Foundation Symposium. New York: American Elsevier; 1975:vol 33.
33. Als H, Brazelton TB. A new model of assessing behavioral organization in preterm and full-term infants. *J Am Acad Child Psychiatry.* 1981;20:239.
34. Brazelton TB. *Neonatal Behavioral Assessment Scale.* National Spastics Foundation, No. 50. London: William Heinemann; 1973.
35. Prechtl H, Beintemia D. *The Neurological Examination of the Full Term Infant.* Child Development Series, No. 12. Philadelphia: Lippincott; 1975.
36. Golas GA, Parks P. Effects on early postpartum teaching on primiparas' knowledge of infant behavior and degree of confidence. *Res Nurs Health.* 1986;9:209–214.

Assessment of the Neonate

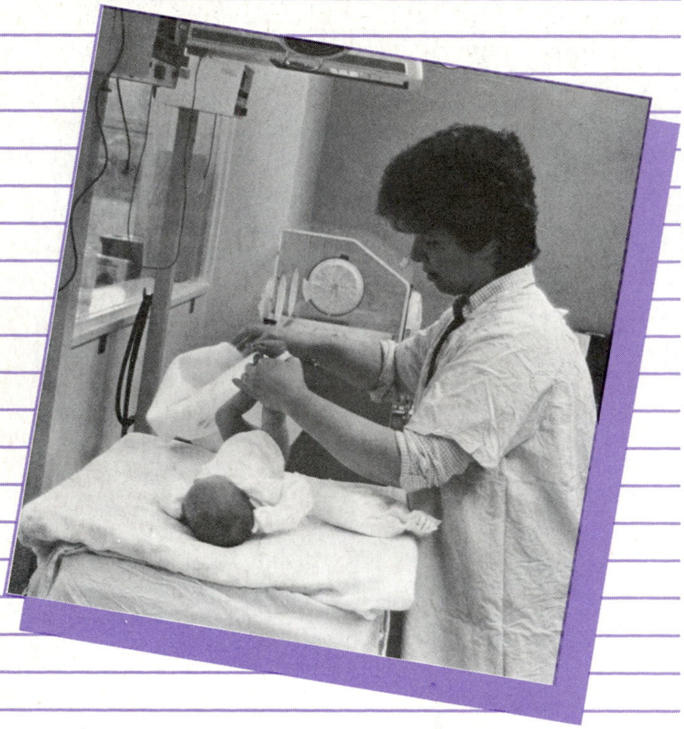

chapter 33

Key Terms

acrocyanosis
Apgar score
caput succedaneum
cephalhematoma
Epstein's pearls
Erb-Duchenne paralysis
erythema toxicum
Gallant's reflex
harlequin color change
hydroceles
milia
Mongolian spotting
Moro (startle) reflex
nevus flammeus
palmar grasp reflex
petechiae
placing reflex
plantar grasp reflex
polydactyly
rooting reflex
stepping reflex
stork bites
sucking reflex
swallowing reflex
syndactyly
tonic neck (fencing) reflex
trunk incurvation

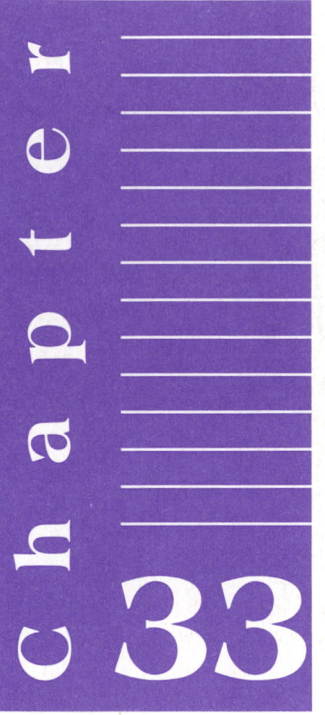

Assessment of the neonate is an ongoing process that involves the collection of physiologic and psychosocial data by the nurse. Immediately after birth, the nurse determines the newborn's Apgar score, which includes assessment of heart rate, respiratory effort, reflex irritability, muscle tone, and color. A variety of screening procedures may also be done in the early newborn period.

The nurse continues to provide ongoing assessment of the neonate and family after birth. This chapter emphasizes methods of assessment used by the nurse to identify potential and actual problems, strengths and weaknesses, and other variables that influence the neonate's well-being.

The health of neonates is related to the health of their parents, family, and environment. Factors that influence any one of these systems will certainly affect the neonate. The data base obtained by the nurse provides relevant information about the newborn against which later comparisons can be made. Thus, it is imperative that the initial data base be comprehensive and consider all of the facets that affect the newborn.

METHODS OF ASSESSMENT

Assessment of the neonate involves the collection of data about several different parameters of health and physiologic well-being. This ongoing process enables caregivers to compare initial assessment findings with those obtained at a later date. This has special significance for findings that may be considered normal at one period of life and abnormal at another. Knowledge of the changes that occur during the perinatal and postnatal periods assist the nurse in making the correct determination of a neonate's health status and, therefore, in planning the appropriate interventions. The information is gathered from a variety of sources: interviews of the parents; maternal and paternal records; prenatal and delivery room records; various assessment tools; and physical observation and assessment of the neonate individually and as a member of a family unit (Figure 33–1).

One of the first methods used to assess the neonate is the assignment of an Apgar score.[1] The score provides a reliable measurement of the physiologic status of the neonate and indicates the need for resuscitation. Other methods of assessment, performed after the initial assessment of the neonate, include screening procedures, a health history, a complete physical examination, and an assessment of gestational age.

APGAR SCORE

The **Apgar score** was developed in 1953 by Dr. Virginia Apgar to assess the neonate's condition at birth.[2] Five parameters are assessed at 1 minute and 5 minutes after birth: (1) heart rate, (2) respiratory effort, (3) reflex irritability, (4) muscle tone, and (5) color.

Heart Rate

The heart rate of the neonate should be counted for a full minute through auscultation or palpation. A score of 2 is given if the heart rate is over 100/min; a score of 1 is given if the heart rate is under 100/min; a score of 0 is given if the heat rate is absent.

Respiratory Effort

Respiratory rate of the neonate is assessed by counting the number of respirations for one full minute. Respirations may be assessed through observation or auscultation. A score of 2 indicates regular respirations or crying; a score of 1 indicates slow, irregular respirations; and a score of 0 indicates absent respirations (apnea).

Reflex Irritability

Reflex irritability is assessed by observing the neonate's response to a stimulus such as rubbing the back or gently flicking the soles of the feet. A score of 2 is given when the neonate responds to the stimulus by crying; a score of 1 is given when the neonate responds by grimacing or frowning; a score of 0 is given when the neonate has no response to the stimulus.

Muscle Tone

Muscle tone is assessed by observing the neonate's activity level, the level of resistance when the examiner extends the neonate's extremities, and the rapidity with which the extremities return to a state of flexion. A score of 2 is given when the neonate demonstrates good muscle tone, activity, and spontaneous flexion of the extremities; a score of 1 is given when there is some activity, some flexion of the extremities, and some resistance to extension; and a score of 0 is given when the neonate is limp or completely flaccid.

Color

The color of the neonate also is assessed at 1 and 5 minutes after birth. Most neonates are somewhat cyanotic at birth. With the onset of respirations, the skin becomes pink, but the extremities may remain cyanotic. A score of 2 for color is given when the neonate is completely pink; a score of 1 is given when the extremities are blue or pale and the body is pink; a score of 0 is given when the newborn is blue or pale.

Table 33–1 summarizes the Apgar score. The score assists caregivers in determining how much, if any, resuscitation the neonate will need. A total score of 7 to 10 indicates that the neonate is in good condition and will need only possible suctioning of the mouth and nose and observation. A score of 3 to 6 indicates a moderately depressed neonate who will need some resuscitation and close observation. A score of 0, 1, or 2 indicates a severely depressed neonate who will need resuscitation, possible ventilatory assistance, and intensive observation and care.

Neonates who are at term or close to term when delivered are more likely to have higher Apgar scores than those who are premature. Of the five categories of assessment, heart rate is the least affected by gestational age; muscle tone, reflex irritability, and respiratory effort increase with advancing gestational age. Color is the most unreliable parameter at any given gestational age.

SCREENING PROCEDURES

Screening procedures for the neonate may include determination of cord blood type, blood group, and Coombs' reaction; test for phenylketonuria (PKU); test for hypothyroidism; test for syphilis; and initial hearing screening.

Cord Blood Type, Group, and Coombs' Reaction

A sample of cord blood is collected in the delivery room and sent to the laboratory. The cord blood is tested for blood type and group. A Coombs' test should also be performed for neonates, especially for those whose mothers have type O or Rh-negative

DATE ______

NEONATAL ASSESSMENT DATA

	AT BIRTH	TODAY
NAME ______	WEIGHT ______	WEIGHT ______
BIRTHDATE ______	LENGTH ______	LENGTH ______
BIRTHTIME ______	H.C. ______	H.C. ______
RACE ______	CHEST ______	CHEST ______
SEX ______	BLOOD TYPE ______	
	APGAR 1 ______ 5 ______	

BIOGRAPHIC DATA

	MOTHER	FATHER	SIBLINGS
Name			
Age	______	______	______
Occupation	______	______	______
Religion	______	______	______
Insurance	______	______	______

FAMILY MEDICAL HISTORY

Heart Disease ______	Diabetes ______	Allergies ______
Hypertension ______	Arthritis ______	Migraines ______
Blood Disorders ______	Obesity ______	Other ______
Renal Disease ______	Mental Illness ______	
Cancer ______	Seizure Disorder ______	

GENOGRAM

MOTHER'S PRENATAL HISTORY G ______ P ______ A ______ SB ______

Date prenatal care started ______ Blood Type______

Medications ______ Vitamins ______ Nutritional Status: *good* ______ *fair* ______ *poor* ______

Alcohol Ingestion ______ Other Substances ______

Smoking ______ Exposure to Radiation______

Sexually Active Until ______ Month Gestation

Weight Gain ______pounds

Health Problems:

hypertension ______ bleeding ______ infection ______

diabetes ______ control: *diet* ______ *insulin* ______

accidents ______ other______

Childbirth Preparation Classes: ______ who attended ______

Figure 33–1. Sample neonatal assessment tool. (*Figure continues.*)

PRENATAL HISTORY

Delivery: *vaginal* ______ *forceps* ______ *vacuum extraction* ______
C/S ______ indication ______
anesthesia ______ medications ______
complications ______
Support system during L&D ______
Attachment experience immediately postdelivery ______

POSTNATAL HISTORY

Physical Abnormalities ______
Health Problems ______
Discharged With Mother ______

NUTRITIONAL STATUS

Breast ______ *Bottle* ______
Feeding: *well* ______ *fair* ______ *poor* ______
Tolerated: *well* ______ *fair* ______ *poor* ______
Breast: ______ min/breast frequency ______ hours
P.C. supplement: what ______ how often ______ how much ______
Formula: type ______ amount ______ oz frequency ______ hours
Vitamins: ______
Bowel movements: color ______ consistency ______ frequency ______ /day
problems ______
Urination: frequency ______ /day problems ______

DEVELOPMENTAL STATUS

Regards face ______ smiles responsively ______
Lifts head when prone ______

SOCIOCULTURAL STATUS

Primary caretakers ______

Grandparents:	MATERNAL	PATERNAL
supportive?	______	______
available?	______	______

Significant others
relationship ______
available ______

ENVIRONMENT/SAFETY

Safety seat ______ Use: *front* ______ *rear* ______ *both* ______
Smoke detectors ______
Smokers in home ______
Pets/animals in home ______
Number of residents in home ______
Water supply: city/flouride treated ______ well ______
Other:

Figure 33–1 (*continued*). Sample neonatal assessment tool. (*Figure continues.*)

PHYSICAL ASSESSMENT

T. ________ H.R. ________ R.R. ________ B/P________

General Appearance:

flexed ________ extended ________ symmetric________

if not, describe ________

muscle tone: WNL ________ hypotonic ________ hypertonic________

state of arousal: deep sleep ________ light sleep________

drowsy ________ quiet alert________

active alert ________ crying ________

strong/lusty________

high pitch/shrill ________

weak ________

tremors________

Other:

Skin: pink ________ meconium staining ________ turgor/ tenting Y ___ N___

dusky ________ petechiae ________ location________

cyanotic ________ rash ________ pustules ________ vesicles________

acrocyanosis ________ ecchymosis ________

pale ________

jaundice ________

beefy red ________

Other:

Head: fontanelles

soft/flat ________

depressed ________

bulging ________

sutures

WNL ________

open/wide space ________

closed ________

hair

silky smooth ________ wooly________

distribution WNL ________ *if not, describe* ________

Face: symmetric/proportional ________ *if not, describe* ________

Eyes: iris color

dark blue/gray ________

brown ________

true blue ________

pink ________

sclera color

white ________

jaundice ________

	R	L
blink reflex	________	________
pupillary reflex	________	________
red reflex	________	________

conjunctiva: pink ________ erythema ________ discharge ________ hemorrhages________

tears: present ________ not present ________ excessive________

Other:

Ears: position WNL ________ low set________

pinnae developed/firm ________ shapeless/floppy________

TMs color ________ boney landmarks ________ intact ________ mobile________

acoustic blink or startle reflex + ________ − ________

Other:

Figure 33–1 (*continued*). Sample neonatal assessment tool. (*Figure continues.*)

Nose: mucus: none ______ small amt. ______ mod.amt. ______ copious ______
appearance WNL ______ *if not, describe* ______
nasal flaring: Y ______ N ______

Mouth and Throat: symmetric ______ *if not, describe* ______
buccal mucosa/gingiva: pink ______ moist ______ lesions______
other ______
soft/hard palate: intact ______ jaundice ______
Epstein's pearls ______ other ______
mucus: none ______ small amt. ______ mod.amt. ______ copious ______
tongue: midline ______ symmetric ______
frenulum WNL ______ *if not, describe* ______
macroglossia ______ protruding ______ other ______
Other:

Neck: muscle tone WNL ______ *if not, describe*______
full range of motion ______ *if not, describe* ______
rigid ______ torticollis ______ webbing ______
masses ______ *if so, describe* ______

Chest: symmetric ______ *if not, describe* ______
clavicles intact ______
nipples WNL ______ *if not, describe* ______
breath sounds ______ bilateral ______
expiratory grunting ______
inspiratory wheeze ______
retractions ______ *if so, describe* ______
gasping ______ apnea >15 sec ______
Other:

Heart: location of PMI ______

pulses	FULL	SYMMETRIC
apical	______	______
femoral	______	______
dorsalis pedis	______	______
brachial	______	______

murmurs ______ *if so, describe* ______
Other:

Abdomen: symmetric ______ *if not, describe* ______
soft ______ tense ______ concave ______ distended ______
umbilical cord: on ______ off ______
number of vessels ______ arteries ______ vein
drying WNL ______ bleeding ______ discharge ______ other ______
bowel sounds regular ______ increased ______ decreased ______ absent ______
masses or organomegaly ______ *if so, describe* ______
liver edge felt ______ *if so, where* ______

Genitalia: WNL ______ *if not, describe* ______
male: circumsized ______ uncircumsized ______
meatal opening: tip of glans ______
hypospadias ______ *if so, describe* ______
epispadias ______ *if so, describe* ______
testes descended ______
hydrocele ______
age of 1st voiding ______ hrs ______
urinary stream: adequate ______ dribbles ______
Other:

Anus and Rectum: patent ______ + wink reflex ______ fissures ______
other ______
age when meconium first passed ______

Figure 33–1 (*continued*). Sample neonatal assessment tool. (*Figure continues.*)

Extremities: symmetric ______ *if not, describe* ______
full ROM ______ *if not, describe* ______
muscle tone: good ______ hypotonic ______ hypertonic ______

hip	R	L
Ortalani	______	______
leg length	______	______
creases	______	______
knee height	______	______

Other:

Spine: appears WNL ______ *if not, describe* ______

Reflexes:	PRESENT	ABNORMAL		PRESENT	ABNORMAL
Moro	______	______	placing	______	______
palmar	______	______	crossed extension	______	______
grasp	______	______	magnet	______	______
tonic neck	______	______	traction	______	______
sucking	______	______	arm recoil	______	______
rooting	______	______	crawling	______	______
swallowing	______	______	Galant's	______	______
Babinski	______	______	glabellar	______	______
stepping	______	______			

ASSESSMENT SUMMARY

Figure 33–1 *(continued)*. Sample neonatal assessment tool.

blood or for neonates who become significantly jaundiced.[1] The direct Coombs' test will determine if antibodies are present in the neonate's blood. (*See* Chapter 42.)

Test for Phenylketonuria

To test for phenylketonuria (PKU), a blood sample is taken from the heel after the neonate has ingested sufficient quantities of milk (24 to 36 hours of milk ingestion) (Figure 33–2). Phenylketonuria is an inborn error of metabolism in which the blood level of the amino acid phenylalanine becomes very high, resulting in mental retardation. This condition can be prevented through dietary control.

Screening for PKU is required by most states. Some practitioners require that the neonate's urine be tested for phenylalanine at 4 weeks of life as well as the initial screening. Retesting can be performed at 4 weeks using a phenistix, a litmuslike paper that turns dark green when the urine contains phenylalanine.

TABLE 33–1. DESCRIPTION OF THE APGAR SCORE

Sign	0	1	2
Heart rate	Absent	Less than 100/min	Greater than 100/min
Respiratory effort	Absent	Slow, irregular	Regular or crying
Reflex irritability	No response	Grimace, frown	Cry, cough
Muscle tone	Limp	Some motion, some flexion of extremities, some resistance to extension of extremities	Active, spontaneous flexion, good tone
Color	Cyanotic or pale	Body pink, extremities cyanotic	Completely pink

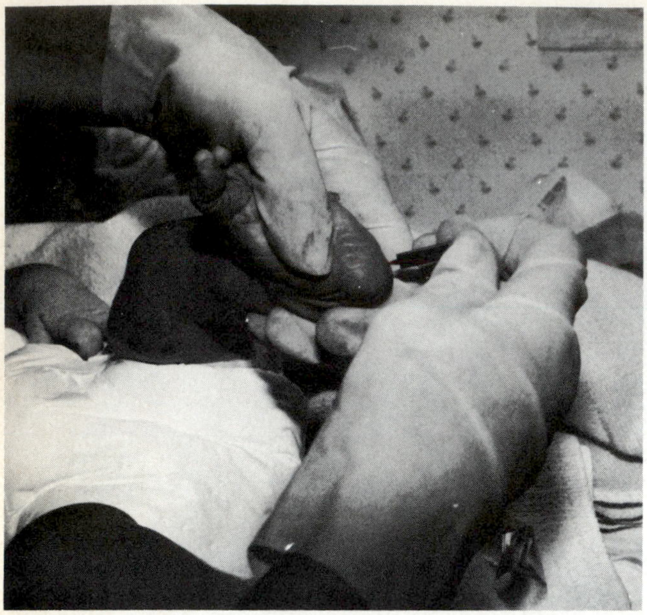

Figure 33–2. Heel stick test for phenylketonuria taken after newborn has ingested milk for 24 to 36 hours.

Test for Hypothyroidism

Mass neonatal screening for hypothyroidism also has been found to be cost-effective in preventing mental retardation caused by thyroid dysfunction in neonates. A sample of the neonate's blood is taken and usually sent to an outside laboratory. The incidence of hypothyroidism (1 in 4000) and efficacy of early replacement therapy in preventing mental retardation make this an appropriate screening test for neonates.[1]

Test for Syphilis

Because of the increase in syphilis seen in neonates, many institutions routinely test for this condition. Tests used are the Venereal Disease Research Labs (VDRL) test, or the Rapid Plasma Reagent (RPR) test.

Initial Hearing Screening

Hearing can initially be assessed when the neonate is in the quiet alert state. A hand clap or ringing of a bell near the ear will usually cause a startle or blink response. The neonate may also respond by alerting to the sound as he or she becomes more mature. If the neonate does not respond to the sound initially, the nurse should retest for hearing.

HEALTH HISTORY

Interviewing the parents is an important step in data gathering (Figure 33–3). This initial time is important for the development of a trusting relationship between parents and nurse. The nurse may begin with an introduction of self and conduct the interview in a relaxed, courteous, and unhurried manner. Confidentiality and privacy must be assured to place the parents at ease. Open-ended questions are helpful in obtaining the information sought, but the nurse must take care to guide the discussion to be most effective.

Parents may wonder about the need for the extensive questioning that accompanies the health history. Often, telling them that this information enables the health care providers to provide the most comprehensive care possible is enough reassurance.

The health history contains biographic data; present concerns of the caregivers, usually a brief comment set off in quotation marks; prenatal through postnatal history; family history; a family profile, which includes developmental, psychologic, sociocultural, and environmental aspects, and adaptation

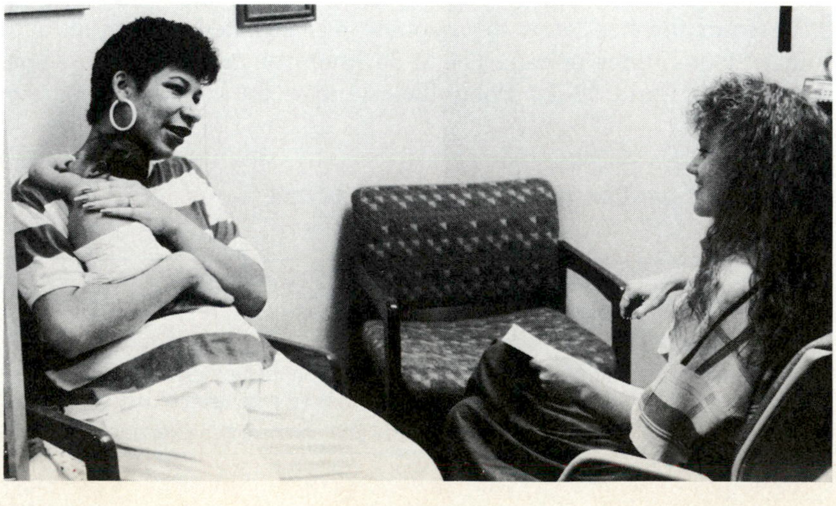

Figure 33–3. Nurse interviewing mother in quiet, relaxed atmosphere.

RESEARCH ABSTRACT

Maloni JA, et al. Validation of infant behavior by neonatal nurses. Nurs Res. *1986;35:133–138.*

Maloni and associates designed a study to determine if normal, healthy neonates identified by nursery nurses as acting differently from other neonates did indeed behave differently from the neonates whom the nurses described as normal. All neonates in the study were considered normal by pediatric examination. In addition, the reseachers used the Brazelton Neonatal Behavioral Assessment Scale (BNBAS) to assess all neonates. The nursery nurses were asked to identify any neonates in the unit about whom they were concerned. Each of the 55 "suspect" neonates was carefully matched with a control neonate. The BNBAS was administered by a trained examiner who had no prior knowledge of the group assignment.

The investigators found that the suspect group of neonates scored significantly lower on the BNBAS than did their matched controls. The interactive dimension was the most common area of concern regarding behavior, followed by state organization. In addition, although the groups were carefully matched, a significant difference was noted on two maternal variables. Mothers of suspect neonates were more likely to be gravida 4 or greater and more likely to have an abnormal medical history.

The investigators concluded that the nurses' empiric knowledge enabled them to identify problem neonates and that this knowledge could be measured and tested. The traditional neonatal assessments were not sufficient to identify suspect behavior, and the present medical model of neonatal assessment has its limitations.

Comment:
Maloni and associates have provided a valuable service to those who specialize in the care of the "normal" neonate. Their study was exploratory in nature, seeking to identify what it is that nurses observe and how this can influence client outcomes. Observation has been documented by the investigators as one of nursing's strengths. In this study, observation was enhanced by nursing activities. The discussion and conclusions of this research offer practice and possibilities for further research concerning parenting, development of more comprehensive means of neonatal assessment, and curriculum development for both undergraduate parent-child courses and continuing education for graduate nurses.

responses of the neonate (*see* Figure 33–1). The information obtained is time dependent and will vary with the age of the neonate at the time the data are collected. The form used to collect data may also vary from agency to agency depending on individual policies and procedures, but the information is generally standardized. The nurse should not feel limited to the form used, but could also expand to include information that is deemed relevant. The nurse may also want to construct a data collection tool that is tailored to present practice.

PHYSICAL EXAMINATION

As discussed in Chapter 32, the transition of the newborn from intrauterine to extrauterine life is accompanied by major physiologic adaptations. Throughout the immediate postnatal period the neonate continues to adapt to extrauterine life and to demonstrate changes in several physical and physiologic variables. For this reason, appraisals of the neonate should be dated and timed.

Timing and Setting of Examination

The first physical examination is performed at the time of delivery regardless of the setting. Coupled with the Apgar score, it attests to the general "wholeness" of the neonate. A more comprehensive examination is performed within the first 24 hours after birth. Another examination should be performed before the neonate is discharged from the hospital, and again at 2 and 4 weeks of age.

If possible, the neonate's parents should be present during the examination. Parental anxiety is often engendered by discovering small "imperfections" that health care providers regard as normal. Performing the examination with the parents in attendance affords an opportunity for the nurse to discuss the normal findings and point out the normal variations that can occur. The nurse can also answer any questions or allay any fears that parents might have. At the same time, the nurse can demonstrate techniques for handling the neonate as well as assess the parental responses to these interventions.

The physical examination should be performed with the neonate lying unclothed in a warm, well-lighted area. Radiant warmers often are used in the nursery for the initial examination. Careful handwashing and cleansing of the stethoscope and the other instruments used should precede the examination. In addition, the nurse should use universal precautions, especially as the newborn may still have some dried blood on the body or hair. The nurse should also obtain baseline data for analysis. These data include vital signs; weight; length; and head, chest, and abdominal circumferences, and may be obtained before or during the examination.

Baseline Data

Vital Signs. Temperature, heart rate, and respiratory rate are always obtained. Blood pressure may not be routinely assessed unless there is an indication, such as a suspected cardiac problem.

Temperature generally should be measured by the axillary route[3, 4] (Figure 33–4). The use of electronic thermometers has expedited the performance of this task, and affords a reading within one minute. Standard mercury thermometers should be held in place for 3 minutes.[5] Previously, it was recommended that the initial temperature be done by rectum to rule out imperforate anus. It is generally accepted that the observation of meconium passage is sufficient to validate a patent anus.

The normal axillary temperature averages between 36.5 and 37°C (97.6 and 98.6°F) with a range from 36.1 to 37.2°C (97 to 99°F). The temperature should be stabilized by 10 hours of age.

The normal neonatal heart rate can average from 120 to 160 beats per minute, ranging from as low as 70 to 90 while sleeping to as high as 180 while crying. The rate should be counted for a full minute to allow the nurse an appreciation of normal fluctuations and to detect abnormalities.

Respiratory rates will vary between 30 and 60 breaths per minute. Respirations are abdominal in nature and can be easily counted by observing the rise and fall of the abdomen. The neonatal respiratory pattern is characterized by shallow, irregular breaths, often interrupted by short periods of apnea from 5 to 15 seconds in length. An accurate appraisal of respiratory function is made by observing the breathing pattern for one full minute.

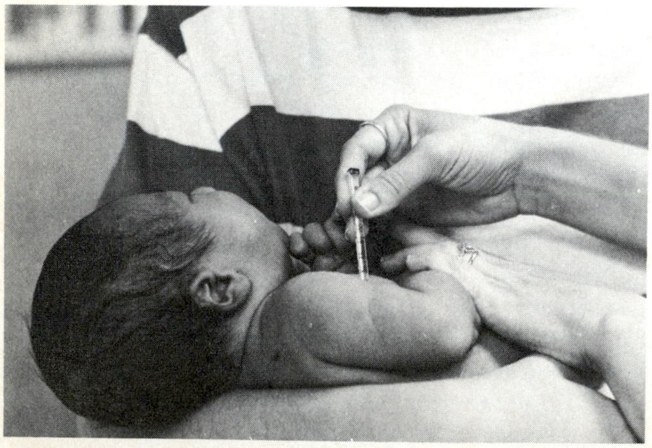

Figure 33–4. Nurse taking the neonate's axillary temperature with a standard mercury thermometer.

Recent data suggest that both heart and respiratory rates are affected by age. Full-term neonates will demonstrate a decrease in respiratory rate with a mean of 38.5 at 4 weeks of age compared with a mean of 45.1 at birth. Heart rate shows an increase from a mean of 116.3 at birth to 141.3 at 15 days, and then decreases to 136.2 at 4 weeks of age.[6] A racial difference in heart rate has been identified between black and white neonates of the same gestational age and socioeconomic class, with the black neonates averaging 8 beats per minute higher.[7]

Blood pressure is obtained using the Doppler method of electronic monitoring or ausculated with a stethoscope. A 1-in. cuff is used with the stethoscope placed over the brachial artery. Neonatal blood pressure has been found to be the highest immediately after birth, but falls to a minimum within 3 hours of birth. It then begins to rise steadily and reaches a plateau at about 4 to 6 days after birth. This measurement is usually equal to that of the immediate postpartum blood pressure. The average blood pressure in a neonate weighing more than 3 kg is 67/41 but the reading will vary with activity.[8]

Parameters of Physical Growth. Parameters of physical growth must be carefully assessed. As the progress of the neonate is validated by these parameters, it is important to measure them accurately and record them correctly. Serial measurements are used to determine the neonate's growth patterns. These can be recorded on growth charts and compared with the previous readings.

The following measurements are made each time the neonate is routinely assessed.

Weight. Neonates are usually weighed on admission to the nursery (Figure 33–5). The scale should be properly balanced and the neonate placed unclothed on the center of the scale. The examiner places one hand lightly over the neonate to prevent her or him from falling off the scale. The neonate is usually weighed at the same time every day while in the hospital. The weight is recorded in grams or kilograms but converted to pounds for the benefit of the parents.

The average neonatal birth weight is 3400 g, or 7 pounds 8 ounces. Weight ranges from 2500 to 4000 g, or from 5 pounds 8 ounces to 8 pounds 13 ounces. Neonates lose weight after birth, generally 10 percent of the birth weight or less, but regain their birth weight by 10 to 14 days of age.

Length. The average length of the newborn is 20 in., or 50 cm, with a range of 18 to 22 in. (45 to 55 cm). This

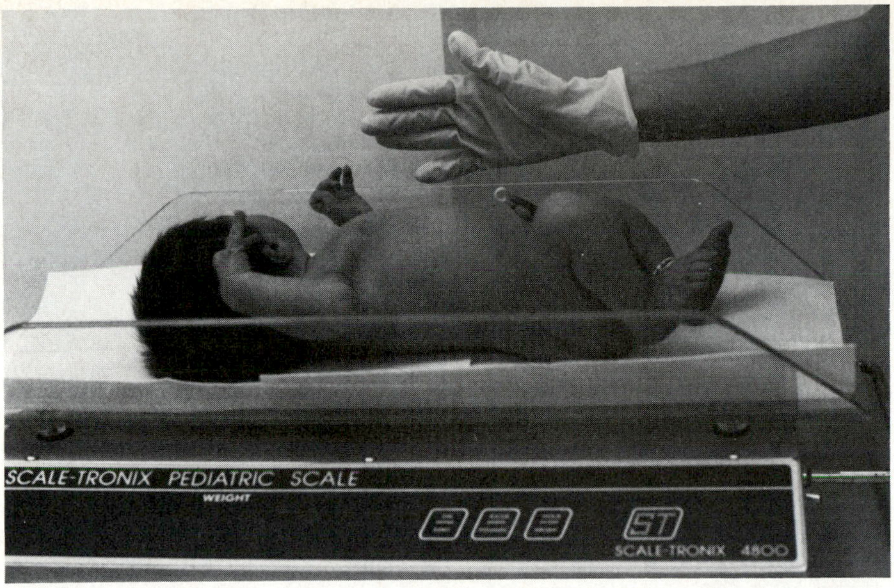

Figure 33–5. Weighing the neonate.

measurement is often difficult to obtain because of the position of flexion that the neonate assumes. The neonate should be flat on the back and the knees held in an extended position. The soles of the feet should be perpendicular to the surface. The examiner then measures using an accurate tape measure from the top of the head to the soles of the feet (Figure 33–6).

Head Circumference. Head circumference is measured at the widest diameter, which is the occipitofrontal diameter (Figure 33–7). The head may initially be misshapened as a result of molding, and therefore should be measured until it regains its original shape. This occurs within several days of birth. The average head circumference is 33 to 35 cm (13 to 14 in.).

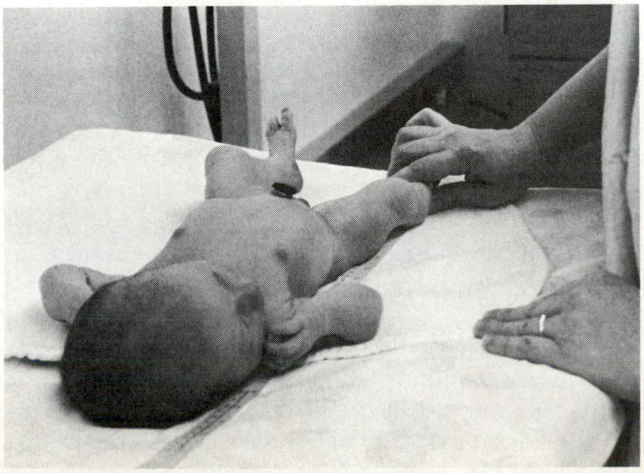

Figure 33–6. Measuring the length of the neonate.

Chest Circumference. The chest circumference is obtained by placing the tape around the chest at the nipple line (Figure 33–8). The chest circumference may be equal to the head circumference but should not exceed it. Generally, it is about an inch less.

Abdominal Circumference. Abdominal circumference is measured by placing the tape around the abdomen at the level of the umbilicus. Abdominal measurements are usually made when there is a suspicion of pathology that causes abdominal distension.

Table 33–2 presents a summary of the neonatal vital signs and measurements, as well as the findings on a complete physical examination.

General Appearance

The normal resting position of the neonate is one of flexion. Both the arms and legs are adducted and flexed. The head is large in proportion to body length, averaging about one fourth of the total. The umbilicus is the center of the neonate's body. The neck is short and the abdomen is prominent.

The nurse begins by noting the neonate's state of arousal and orienting response. These are described as follows: (1) deep sleep with eyes closed, regular breathing, and no eye movement; (2) light sleep with eyes closed, irregular breathing, and rapid eye movements; (3) drowsiness with the eyes either opened or closed, mild startles, delayed response to sensory stimuli, and smooth movements; (4) quiet alert with open eyes that may focus attention on a stimulus, minimum motor activity; (5) active alert with open eyes, movements of the extremities, in-

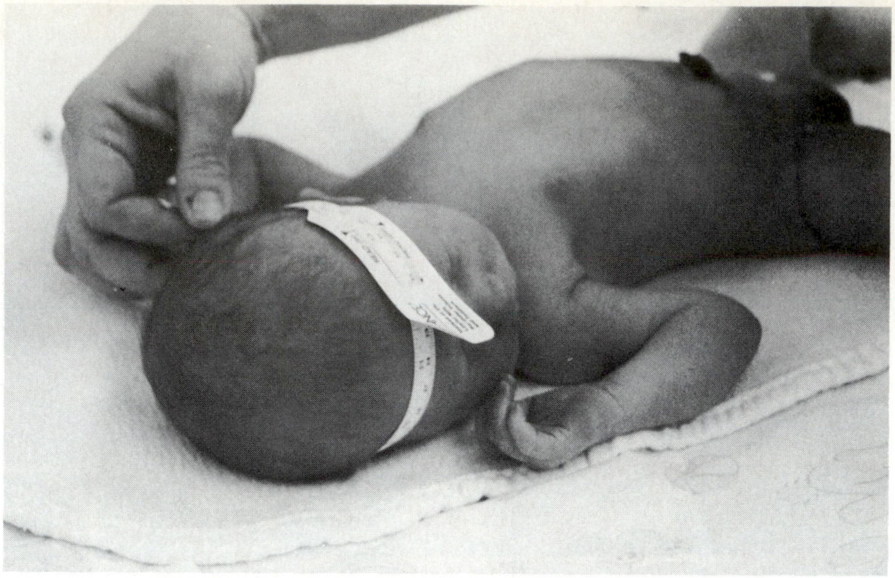

Figure 33–7. Measuring head circumference.

crease in startles, and a general high activity level; and (6) crying that is difficult to console.[9]

The examination is easiest to accomplish with the neonate in the quiet state. The characteristics of color, flexion, muscle tone, symmetry, obvious birth defects, respiratory patterns and body movements can then be noted. The neonate should have a strong, lusty cry that is neither high pitched nor shrill. The latter may indicate neurologic impairment.

Skin

The neonate's skin is observed for the following characteristics: color and color changes during activity, familial and racial features, rashes, milia, anomalies or deformities, birthmarks, jaundice, petechiae, forceps marks (Figure 33–9), tone, and hydration status. Any of these characteristics present should be noted and recorded.

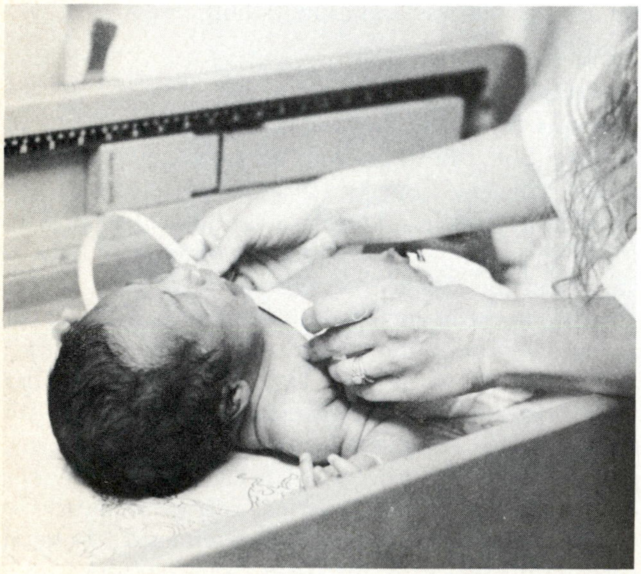

Figure 33–8. Measuring chest circumference.

Color may vary according to the racial background, pigmentation, and physiologic changes. The neonate is generally pink, but may become acrocyanotic if is chilled. **Acrocyanosis** is characterized by bluish discoloration of the hands and feet, and is caused by a normal condition of vasomotor instability and poor peripheral circulation found in the newborn. Acrocyanosis caused by vasomotor instability can be differentiated from true cyanosis by vigorously rubbing the sole of the foot. The sole will turn pink if the acrocyanosis is due to vasomotor instability.

The skin may be mottled, a color change that occurs in response to temperature changes. Occasionally a neonate may experience a **Harlequin color change** whereby one side of the body may develop a deep red color. This is in response to a normal vasomotor disturbance causing the blood vessels on one side of the body to constrict while those on the other side dilate. This change needs to be recorded and reported.

Other normal variations may include **petechiae,** which are found over the presenting part; **erythema toxicum** (Figure 33–10), a transient newborn rash characterized by white vesicles with a red macular base; and capillary hemangiomas (telangiectatic nevi), commonly called **"stork bites",** which are often present on the nape of the neck and on the bridge of the nose, the forehead, and eyelids. Stork bites on

TABLE 33–2. SUMMARY OF NEONATAL ASSESSMENT: USUAL FINDINGS, ACCEPTABLE VARIATIONS, AND ABNORMAL FINDINGS

Area Assessed	Usual Findings	Acceptable Variations	Abnormal Findings
Temperature	Axillary route preferable Averages between 36.5 and 37°C (97.6 and 98.6°F) Stabilized by 10 hours of age	Ranges from 36.1 to 37.2°C (97 to 99°F)	> 37.2°C (99°F) (may indicate excessively warm environment, dehydration, infection/sepsis, brain damage) < 36.1°C (97°F) (may indicate cold environment, infection)
Heart rate	Average apical pulse at rest 120–160 beats per minute Heart rate regular Increases with crying and movement Decreases with quieting and sleep	70–100 beats per minute sleeping 180 beats per minute crying Irregular heart rate for brief periods or after crying	Tachcardia: > 160 beats per minute awake and at rest Bradycardia: < 120 beats per minute awake and at rest Irregular heart rate
Respirations	Average 40 respirations per minute Abdominal breathing Quiet and shallow Irregular, periodic breathing	30–60 respirations per minute Cheyne-Stokes–type breathing without evidence of respiratory distress Transient tachypnea, especially in the newborn period Apnea lasting 5–15 seconds	Tachypnea: > 60 respirations per minute Bradypnea: < 30 respirations per minute Apnea lasting longer than 15 seconds
Blood Pressure	At birth Systolic 60–90 mm Hg Diastolic 40–60 mm Hg 0–6 months: Systolic 80–110 mm Hg Diastolic 45–60 mm Hg	Change in activity level will cause variations in readings	Hypotension (may indicate hypovolemia or shock) Hypertension (may be sign of coarctation of aorta, especially if there is a difference in blood pressure readings between the upper and lower extremities)
Weight	Full term (gestation 38–42 weeks), birth weight > 2500 g Full term, average weight 3400 g (7 pounds 8 oz) Preterm (gestation < 37 weeks), birth weight < 2500 g	Birth weight 2500–4000 g (5 pounds 8 oz to 8 pounds 13 oz) Approximately 10 percent weight loss after birth Will regain birth weight by 10–14 days of age	Weight loss > 10–15 percent Weight inappropriate for gestational age
Length	Average length 50 cm (20 in.)	45–55 cm (18–22 in.)	< 45 cm (18 in.) (may indicate congenital dwarf)
Head circumference	Average head circumference 33–35 cm (13–14 in.)	32.5–37.5 cm (12.5–14.5 in.)	Microcephaly < 32.5 cm > 37.5 cm (hydrocephalus should be considered)
General appearance	Normal resting position: flexion Good muscle tone Body size proportional Umbilicus center of body Body movement symmetric Strong, lusty cry	Jerky movements Tremors of arms, legs, and body with vigorous crying or at rest during the first 48 to 72 hours of life	Hypotonia Hypertonia Tremors Associated with hypoglycemia or hypocalcemia At rest at 4 days of age (may indicate central nervous system disease) Birth defects High-pitched or shrill cry (may indicate neurologic impairment) Weak or absent cry (indicates severe illness or mental retardation) Asymmetric body movement (may indicate central or peripheral neurologic deficits, birth injuries, or congenital anomalies)

(*continued*)

TABLE 33–2. SUMMARY OF NEONATAL ASSESSMENT ***(continued)***

Area Assessed	Usual Findings	Acceptable Variations	Abnormal Findings

Skin	Pink color (varies according to racial background)
	Nailbeds pink
	Familial and racial features
	Milia
	Good skin turgor, no tenting
	lanugo
	Vernix caseosa
		Desquamation
		Acrocyanosis
		Mottling
		Harlequin color change
		Petechiae over presenting part
		Erythema toxicum
		Capillary hemangiomas (telangiectatic nevi)
		Ecchymosis
		Mongolian spotting
		Physiologic jaundice
		  Formula: $<$ 12–13 mg/dL
		  Breast: $<$ 15 mg/dL
		Nevus flammeus
		Nevus vascularis
		Cavernous hemangiomas
			Jaundice after 24 hours of life
			Physiologic jaundice
			  Formula: $>$ 12–13 mg/dL
			  Breast: $>$ 15 mg/dL
			Cyanosis/duskiness
			Beefy red (may be associated with polycythemia)
			Petechiae on nontraumatized body areas
			Tenting (may indicate poor hydration)
			Generalized pallor (may indicate anoxia or anemia)
			Pustules, vesicles, rashes
			Meconium staining (indicates fetal stress)

Head	Anterior fontanelle
	  Diamond shape at junction of coronal/sagittal sutures
	  Soft/flat
	Posterior fontanelle: triangular shape at junction of sagittal/lambdoidal sutures
	Silky smooth hair distributed evenly over scalp
		Molding
		Fontanelle size (black infants may have larger fontanelles)
		Caput succedaneum
		Cephalhematoma
		Scalp abrasions, lacerations, punctures from forceps, scalp pH determinations, internal monitor probe, or delivery trauma
			Widely spaced suture lines (may indicate hydrocephalus)
			Closed suture lines (indicates synostosis)
			Very large anterior fontanelle (may indicate hypothyroidism)
			Bulging fontanelle (may indicate increased intracranial pressure)
			Depressed fontanelle (may be a sign of dehydration)
			"Woolly," fine hair found on premature neonates
			Unusual hair lines (may be associated with chromosomal disorders)

Face	Symmetric facial features well positioned and proportional Facial movement equal bilaterally Eyebrows, eyelashes, hairline present Receding chin	Small degree of asymmetry (may be the result of intrauterine positioning)	Facial palsy when neonate grimaces or cries (may be caused by intrauterine positioning, forceps, or birth trauma) Distorted facies (may be seen in newborns with chromosomal disorders)

Eyes	Symmetric in shape, movement, and placement
	Iris color
	  Dark blue (Caucasians)
	  Brown (dark-skinned infants)
	Positive blink reflex
	Tears may not be observed
	Conjunctiva pale pink
	Pupillary size and shape equal bilaterally
	Positive pupillary reflex bilaterally
	Sclera white with slight bluish tint
	Movement of eyeballs random and uneven
	Fixates momentarily
	May follow to midline
	Psuedostrabismus
	Doll's-eye phenomenon
	Positive red reflex
		Transient lid edema (may be caused by maternal hormones or eye prophylaxis)
		Subconjunctival hemorrhages
		Transient strabismus or nystagmus
		Brushfield's spots (may also be found in newborns with Down's syndrome or other conditions associated with mental retardation)
		Epicanthal folds in newborn of Oriental descent (may also be present in newborns with chromosomal disorders)
			Dacryostenosis
			Dacryocystitis
			Eye discharge related to bacterial infection or chemical conjunctivitis related to eye prophylaxis
			Sclerae yellowish (indicative of jaundice)
			Corneal opacities
			Ptosis
			Gross nystagmus
			Constant strabismus
			Coloboma
			Pink iris (albinism)
			True blue sclera (osteogenesis imperfecta)

TABLE 33–2. SUMMARY OF NEONATAL ASSESSMENT *(continued)*

Area Assessed	Usual Findings	Acceptable Variations	Abnormal Findings
Ears	Top of ear in alignment with inner and outer canthi of eyes Well formed with firm cartilage Patent ear canals Tympanic membranes Pearly gray Intact Translucent and bony middle ear landmarks visible Mobile Positive acoustic blink or startle reflex	Crumpled and flattened against side of head (as a result of intrauterine positioning) Vernix caseosa in ear canals Floppy if premature	Unilateral or bilateral preauricular skin tags Low-set ears (may indicate chromosomal aberrations) Malformations of the ear (may be associated with renal problems) Floppy if full term
Nose	Placement should be midline on face Nostrils patent Sneezing to clear nostrils Pink, moist, mucous membranes	Small amount of mucus Misshapened nose (may result from intrauterine positioning)	Copious mucus Flaring nostrils (indicates respiratory distress) Malformed or misshapened (may occur in chromosomal problems) Choanal atresia Deviated septum
Mouth and Throat	Lips and lip movement symmetric Lips pink and moist Tubercle on upper lip from sucking Buccal mucosa and gingiva pink and moist Edentulous Hard and soft palates intact Uvula midline Tongue freely moveable and symmetric in shape and movement Sucking pads No tonsilar tissue	Short frenulum without tongue tie Cysts in floor of mouth near frenulum Epstein's pearls	Precocious teeth Cleft lip, cleft palate, or both Protruding tongue (may be a sign of chromosomal problems) Macroglossia (may be early sign of hypothyroidism or may be caused by hemangioma) Micrognathia (associated with Pierre Robin or another syndrome) Short frenulum (tongue tie) Yellowish palate (indication of jaundice) Excessive saliva (may indicate tracheoesophageal fistula or atresia) Oral thrush Continuous inspiratory and expiratory stridor (may indicate small larynx or tracheomalacia)
Neck	Short, straight with many skin folds Trachea midline Full range of motion Adequate muscle strength Thyroid not palpable	Palpable cervical lymph nodes < 5 mm	Masses Rigidity/torticollis Webbing or abnormally short neck (may be associated with chromosomal disorders)
Chest	Symmetric in size, shape, and movement Cylindrical shape Circumference equal to or less than head circumference Nipples symmetric and developed Breath sounds clear and equal bilaterally	Xyphoid process may be prominent Ribs may be noted on deep inspiration Breast engorgement (caused by maternal hormones) Witch's milk Supernumerary nipples Transmitted upper airway sounds, should clear on crying	Asymmetric in shape and movement Funnel-shaped (pectus excavatum) Fractured clavicles Signs of respiratory distress Unequal chest expansion Decreased breath sounds Rales or adventitious sounds Expiratory grunting Retractions Nasal flaring Gasping Inspiratory wheeze Decreased, increased, or abnormal breath sounds

(continued)

TABLE 33–2. SUMMARY OF NEONATAL ASSESSMENT *(continued)*

Area Assessed	Usual Findings	Acceptable Variations	Abnormal Findings
Heart	Point of maximal impulse lateral to midclavicular line in third or fourth left intercostal space Femoral, dorsalis pedis, brachial pulses full and symmetric S_1 and S_2 clearly heard throughout the precordium S_2 splitting	Point of maximal impulse visible Functional heart murmur	Arrythmias Asymmetric femoral and apical pulse (may indicate cardiac anomaly) Heart sounds heard prominently on right instead of left side of chest with dextrocardia Murmurs associated with congenital defects
Abdomen	Prominent, cylindrical in shape, protrudes slightly Superficial abdominal veins Umbilical cord Two arteries and one vein Shrivels and blackens second or third day of life Bowel sounds present in all four quadrants Stomach percussion tympanic Liver and spleen percussion dull Liver Span 5.6–5.9 cm Palpated 1–2 cm below right costal margin Edge feels soft Spleen tip palpated under left costal margin Kidneys Palpated adjacent to vertebral column approximately 1–2 cm above umbilicus Lower half of right kidney and tip of left kidney palpable Meconium passed within 24 hours of delivery First voiding within 24 hours of delivery	Umbilical hernia reducible Irregular bowel sounds	Concave (may indicate diaphragmatic hernia) Distended or tense Increased, decreased, or absent bowel sounds Umbilical cord Single artery Granuloma Bleeding Infection Discharge Omphalocele Abdominal masses Organomegaly Inguinal hernias, male > female
Genitalia	Female Edematous clitoris and labia majora Increased pigmentation of external structures (as a result of hormonal influences) Whitish mucoid or psuedomenstruation (as a result of hormonal influences) Smegma under labia Male Foreskin not retractable if not circumcised Smegma under foreskin if not circumcised Meatal opening is a centrally located slit on tip of glans Strong, arching, urinary stream Penile erection when stimulated or with urination Scrotum; pink or dark brown depending on complexion, rugae (full term), both testes descended, positive cremasteric reflex Male and Female Uric acid crystals in urine	Female Vaginal/hymenal tags Fusion of labia minora Male Testes at junction of external inguinal rings Hydroceles	Female Ambiguous, hypertrophied, or underdeveloped genitalia Male Ambiguous, hypertrophied, or underdeveloped genitalia Hypospadias or epispadias Cryptorchidism Phimosis (usually not evident until infant is older)

TABLE 33–2. SUMMARY OF NEONATAL ASSESSMENT *(continued)*

Area Assessed	Usual Findings	Acceptable Variations	Abnormal Findings
Anus and rectum	Anus patent Good sphincter tone Positive wink reflex Passage of meconium within 24 hours	Meconium passage within 48 hours	Meconium present in other genital orifices Imperforate anus Anal fissures
Extremities	Symmetric and equal in size and movement Full range of motion Flexed position Good tone Nails present on fingers and toes Planter creases over anterior half of sole of foot Fat pads on feet give flat-footed appearance	Extended knees with breech presentation Misaligned position as a result of intrauterine positioning Absent plantar creases as a result of prematurity	Congenital dislocation of hip Positive Ortolani movement Unequal leg length Unequal thigh creases and gluteal folds Polydactyly Syndactyly Simian line (may indicate chromosome abnormality such as Down's syndrome) Erb-Duchenne palsy Talipes equinus (clubfoot) Metatarsus varus
Spine	Appears straight but can easily be flexed Can lift head and turn side to side when prone	Pilonidal dimple without tuft of hair or discharge	Pilonidal dimples with tuft of hair (may be associated with spina bifida occulta) Pilonidal cyst Myelomeningocele or meningocele Masses

the face commonly disappear by several months of age; those on the neck remain longer. **Milia** are small white papules caused by the plugging of sebaceous glands on the nose, face, forehead, and upper torso. They are approximately 1 mm in diameter.

Ecchymoses may be present as a result of birth trauma, use of forceps, or both. **Mongolian spotting,** large irregular darkly pigmented areas on the posterior lumbar region, is commonly found in neonates of black, Oriental, and Native American descent. It may

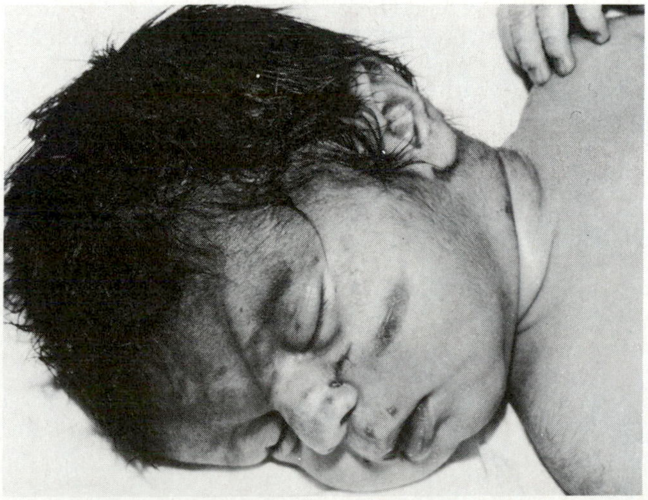

Figure 33–9. Forceps marks. (*Reproduced, with permission, from Rudolph AM, ed.* Pediatrics. *18th ed. Norwalk, Conn: Appleton & Lange; 1987:117*)

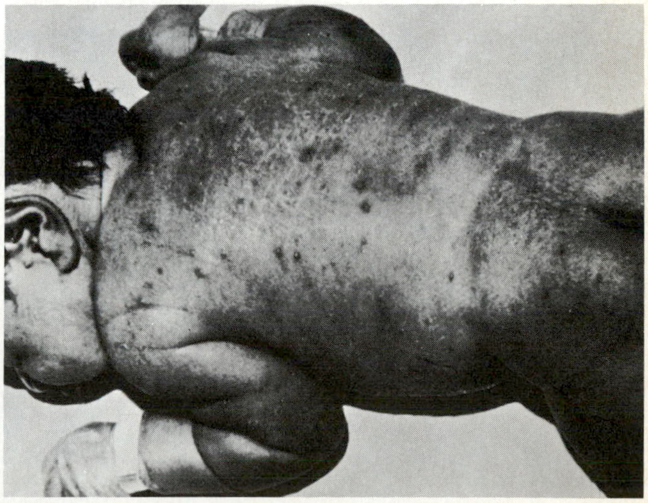

Figure 33–10. Erythema toxicum. (*Reproduced, with permission, from Rudolph AM, ed.* Pediatrics. *18th ed. Norwalk, Conn: Appleton & Lange; 1987:116.*)

also be found in white neonates who have dark complexions. The spotting may not disappear until 2 years of age.

The skin is covered at birth by vernix caseosa, a white cheesy substance that protects the skin in utero (Figure 33–11). Lanugo, the fine, downy hair that covers the infant in utero, may be present in varying degrees on the body but is most prevalent on the back, shoulders, pinna of the ears, and forehead.

Physiologic jaundice, a yellow discoloration of the skin that is caused by bilirubin metabolism, may appear after the first 24 hours of life. It can easily be identified by depressing the bridge of the nose and observing the color. Jaundiced neonates exhibit a yellow color when this is done. Jaundice occurring before 24 hours of age is considered pathologic. (*See* discussion in Chapters 34 and 42.)

The skin should also be inspected for birthmarks. The examiner notes the location, color, size, characteristics, and distribution of any of these marks. Hemangiomas or vascular tumors include **nevus flammeus** or port-wine stain, nevus vascularis or strawberry marks, and cavernous hemangiomas. Nevus vascularis and cavernous hemangiomas usually begin disappearing several weeks after birth, but may not completely disappear until 7 years of age. Nevus flammeus does not disappear with time.

The skin should also be palpated for texture and tone. The neonate's skin is very sensitive. The skin commonly desquamates during the first week or two of life. Skin turgor is checked by gently pinching the neonate's skin and noting the return to original position.

Head

The shape and symmetry of the neonate's head are greatly affected by the forces of delivery, a process known as molding. Head circumference is noted. The nurse should palpate the head, feeling for the fontanelles and the suture lines (Figure 33–12). In a vaginal delivery, the suture lines may be overriding, a condition caused by the shifting of the bony plates of the skull. This will usually correct itself after birth.

The condition of the suture lines should be noted. They should be palpable. Widely spaced suture lines may indicate hydrocephalus, an excessive accumulation of cerebrospinal fluid in the ventricles of the brain; closed sutures indicate synostosis, a premature closing of the skull that can prevent normal brain growth and development.

The fontanelles are palpated and measured. The anterior fontanelle is located at the junction of the sagittal and coronal sutures and is diamond-shaped. The fontanelle usually feels soft and the nurse may note pulsations. The posterior fontanelle, a triangular depression, is located at the junction of the lambdoidal and sagittal sutures. It is usually palpable in a neonate.

Fontanelles will vary in size. On average, the anterior fontanelle is 3 to 4 cm long by 2 to 3 cm wide, and the posterior fontanelle is between 0.5 and 1.0 cm; however, average fontanelle size has been shown to vary between black and white neonates, with black neonates having both larger anterior and posterior fontanelles than the white neonates.[10] In one study, the mean anterior fontanelle size of black neonates was 3.08 ± 0.80 cm, and the mean posterior

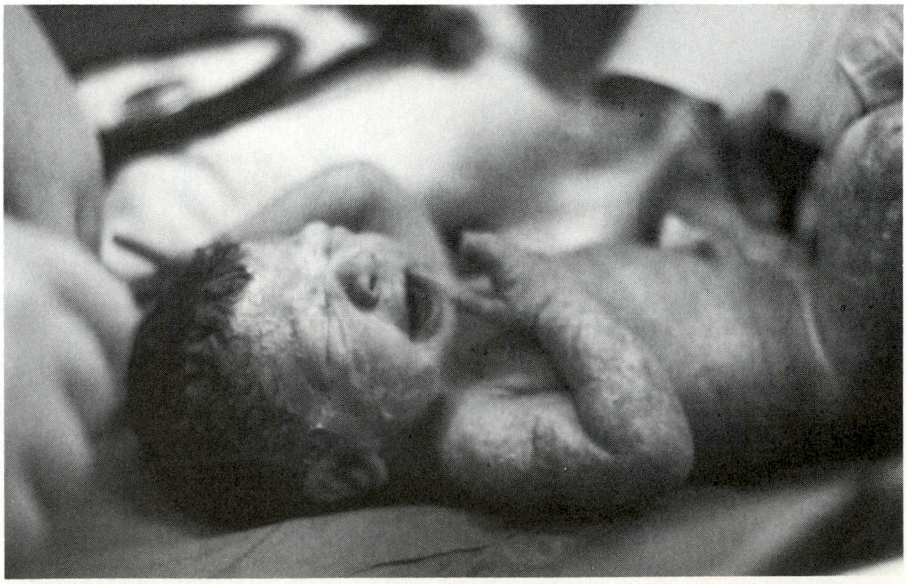

Figure 33–11. Newborn covered with vernix caseosa.

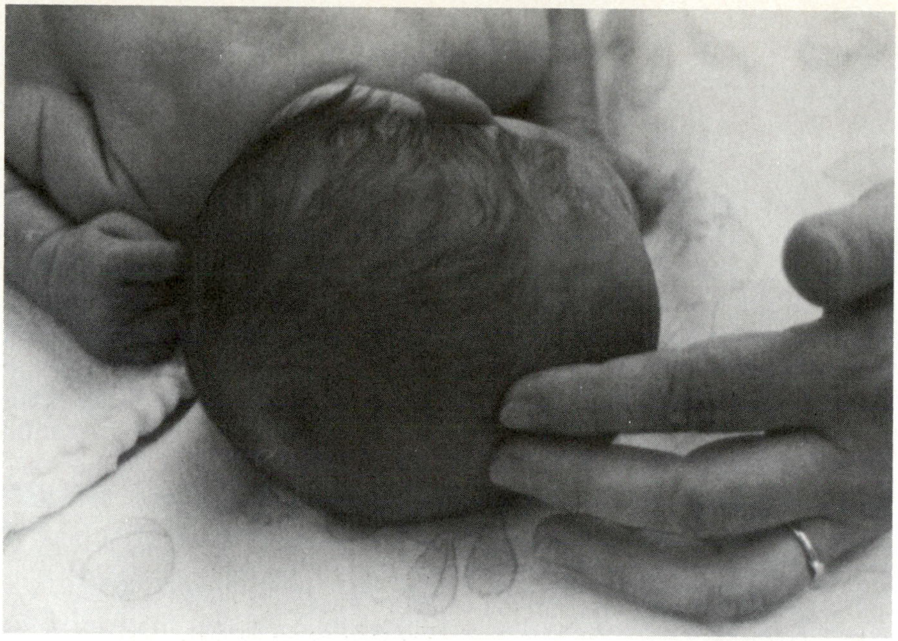

Figure 33–12. Nurse measures and palpates the fontanelles.

size was 0.70 ± 0.45 cm. White neonates had an anterior fontanelle of 2.67 ± 0.70 cm and a posterior fontanelle of 0.49 ± 0.22 cm.

Neonates whose anterior fontanelles are very large may be suspected of being hypothyroid. A tense or bulging fontanelle may indicate increased intracranial pressure. A normal fontanelle may appear slightly depressed, but one that is severely depressed indicates dehydration.

The scalp is also palpated for the presence of **caput succedaneum** (Figure 33–13), a soft tissue edema that occurs from the pressure of delivery. It crosses the suture lines and in this way can be distinguished from **cephalhematoma** (Figure 33–14), a subperiosteal hemorrhage that is limited to one side of the scalp. This condition may take several weeks to recede. Occasionally a neonate may have bilateral cephalhematomas, or cephalhematoma and caput succedaneum.

The scalp is also inspected for the presence of abrasions or lacerations that may occur as a result of forceps use. The insertion site for the internal monitor probe should be located and inspected until it heals, as it may be a potential source for infection and abscess formation.[11]

The texture and distribution of hair are noted.

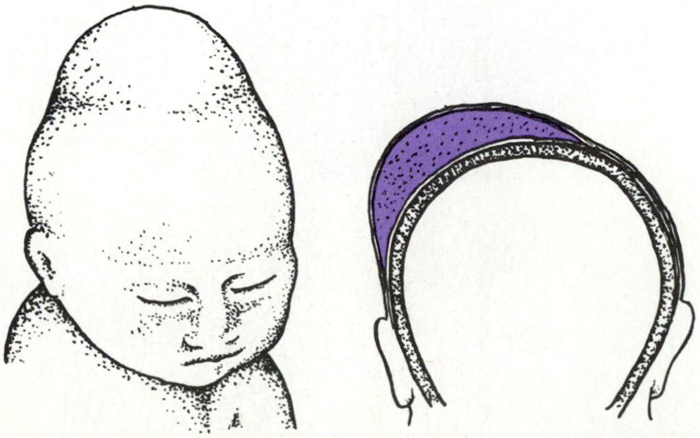

Figure 33–13. Caput succedaneum is a soft tissue edema that crosses the suture lines.

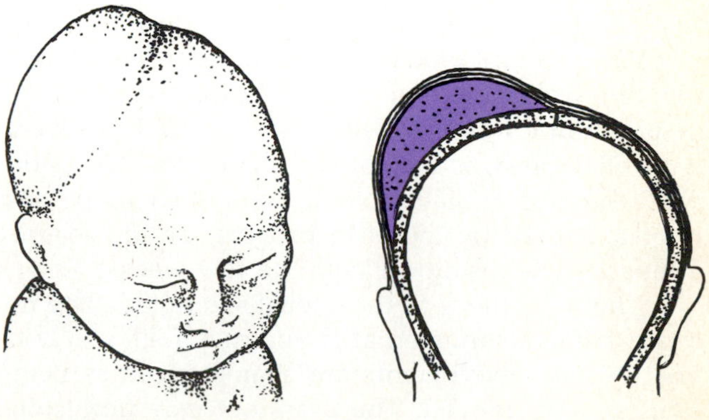

Figure 33–14. Cephalhematoma is bleeding between the bone and periosteum limited to one side of the head. Note that bleeding is not into the brain.

The amount and color will vary and are dependent on genetic factors. The neonate's hair is usually silky and smooth. Unusual distribution or texture should be noted.

Face

The overall appearance of the neonate's face is noted. The face should be symmetric, with the facial features well positioned and proportionate. Eyebrows, eyelashes, and hairline should be present. Facial movement should be equal bilaterally. The chin appears to recede. The neonate may have a small degree of asymmetry as a result of intrauterine positioning. Facial palsy, resulting from use of forceps or intrauterine positioning, is evident when the neonate cries or grimaces.

Eyes

The neonate's eyes are observed for symmetry and placement on the face. They are usually dark blue in color but will be brown in dark-skinned neonates. Eyelids should move easily with eyelashes present on both the upper and lower lids. The lids should blink when a light is directed to the eyes. This is known as the blink reflex. Tears may not be observed as the tear ducts and lacrimal glands are not completely functional for at least a month after birth.

Silver nitrate application may cause some transient lid edema. Neonates who have been given prophylactic silver nitrate also may experience some eye discharge. To avert this, many hospitals use erythromycin ointment or drops instead of silver nitrate. Dacrocystitis, "blocked tear ducts," also can cause eye discharge.

The conjunctiva should be pale pink. Pupillary size and shape are noted. The pupillary reflex is elicited by shining a bright light into the eyes and noting for equal constriction of the pupils.

The color of the sclerae is noted. The sclerae usually have a slight bluish tint. Sclera that have a definite blue color are abnormal and can indicate osteogenesis imperfecta. A yellowish hue, noted several days after birth, is indicative of jaundice. Occasionally, the nurse may note subconjunctival hemorrhages, caused by the birth process, on the sclerae. These usually disappear within a few weeks.

The movement of the eyeballs is noted. The neonate can focus momentarily and may follow to midline, but eye movements are characterized as being random and uneven. The examiner may note some transient strabismus or nystagmus resulting from immature neuromuscular control. This may last for up to 4 months. When the neonate's head is rotated from side to side the eyes do not follow in response to head movement but move in the opposite direction. This is known as the "doll's-eye" phenomenon and is usually present for about 10 days after birth. The "setting sun sign," in which the eyes gaze downward allowing visualization of the sclera above the pupil, may briefly be seen in some normal newborns. Its presence, however, often indicates hydrocephalus.

The neonate's corneas should be observed for opacities. The nurse uses an ophthalmoscope to elicit the red reflex, caused by the light of the scope falling on the retina (Figure 33–15). It is easiest to perform if the neonate is held in a semiupright position or upright position, so that the eyes automatically open.

Brushfield's spots, black and white specs around the periphery of the irises, may be seen in some normal neonates, but are more often seen in neonates with Down's syndrome. Coloboma, absence of a part of the iris, may be noted.

Neonates of Oriental descent normally have epicanthal folds, vertical folds of skin that cover the inner canthus of the eye. These folds also may be present in non-Oriental infants who have chromosomal disorders.

Ears

The neonate's ears are examined for size, shape, and position on the head. The top of the ear should be in alignment with the inner and outer canthi of the eyes. The ears may appear crumpled and flattened against the side of the head, but should be well formed, with firm cartilage. Occasionally, preauricular skin tags are present, either unilaterally or bilaterally.

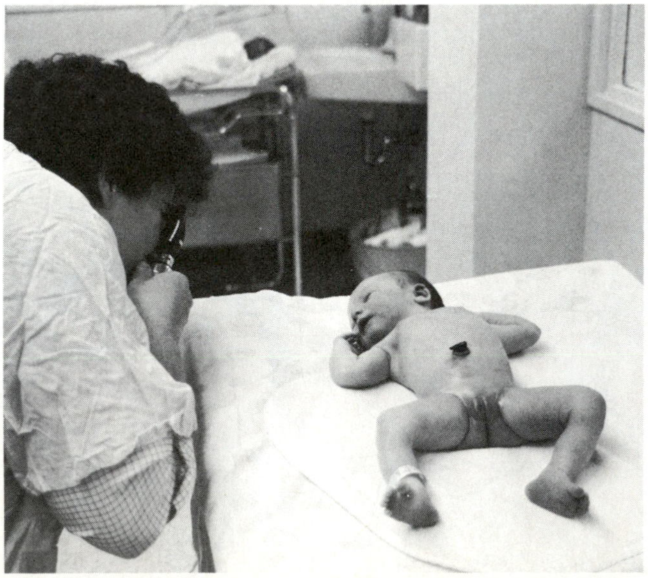

Figure 33–15. Assessing the eyes for the red reflex with an ophthalmoscope.

Low-set ears may indicate a variety of syndromes and chromosomal aberrations. Malformations of the ear may also be associated with renal problems.

The ear canal should be inspected for patency. Vernix caseosa may be present in the canals for several days after birth and may make visualization of the tympanic membranes difficult. To facilitate visualization of the inner ear, the neonate should be examined in a prone position. The nurse stabilizes the neonate's head and pulls the pinna of the ear up and back using one hand. The otoscope is then inserted using the other hand (Figure 33–16). The tympanic membrane is observed for color, translucency, and landmarks. The neonate's head is then turned to the other side for inspection of the other ear.

Hearing can be assessed by clapping the hands or ringing a bell near the neonate's ear. The normal response is a startle or blink response.

Nose

The neonate's nose is examined for size, shape, patency of the nostrils, mucous membrane integrity, and discharge. The placement of the nose should be midline on the face. Neonates are obligatory nose breathers, and use sneezing as a mechanism to clear partially obstructed nares. The mucous membranes are pink and moist and may have a small amount of mucus but no copious drainage. Flaring of the nostrils indicates obstruction of the nares as well as respiratory distress. A malformed or misshapened nose may occur in certain chromosomal abnormalities. Inability to pass a small catheter through each nostril may indicate choanal atresia.

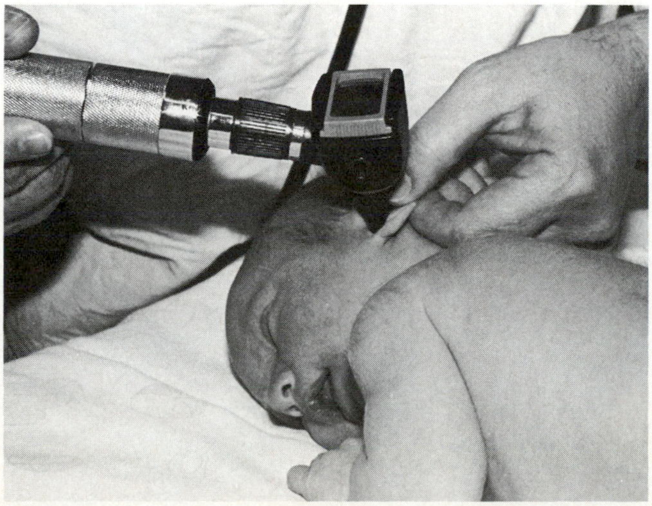

Figure 33–16. Assessing the tympanic membrane with an otoscope.

Mouth and Throat

The mouth is inspected and palpated. Symmetry of the lips and lip movement, as well as the internal structures of the mouth, is noted. The lips are pink and moist. Most neonates develop a tubercle in the middle of the upper lip from sucking.

The buccal mucosa and gingiva should be pink and moist. Normally, the neonate is edentulous (without teeth); however, some neonates are born with precocious teeth. These teeth are usually pulled if they are loose, as they present a hazard to the neonate. Both the hard and soft palates are inspected for the presence of cleft palate. The shape of the palate is noted. The uvula is midline.

The size and placement of the tongue are noted. The tongue should be freely movable and symmetric both in shape and in movement. The characteristics of the frenulum should be checked. Occasionally, a neonate may have a shortened fibrous frenulum (tongue tie), but as long as the tongue can extend to the alveolar ridge, there is no indication for intervention.

Frequently, the nurse will note the presence of **Epstein's pearls,** small white epithelial cysts on the hard palate and on the gums. Sucking pads can be palpated inside the cheeks. To elicit the sucking reflex, the examiner places a finger inside the neonate's mouth. The rooting reflex can also be elicited at the same time by stroking the neonate's cheek; this causes the neonate to turn toward the source of the stimulus.

The posterior pharynx should be visualized. It is easiest to see when the neonate is crying (Figure 33–17). Saliva is usually scant, because the salivary glands are immature. The presence of excessive saliva in a neonate should alert the nurse to the possibility of tracheoesophageal fistula or atresia.

Neck

The neck of the neonate is short and straight with many skin folds. To inspect the neck, the examiner holds the neonate's shoulders and head in one hand and gently extends the neck. The neck should be held in the midline and moved symmetrically from side to side.

The position of the trachea is palpated. The thyroid is usually not palpable in the neonate. The nurse also feels for masses. Palpable cervical lymph nodes are usually small, less than 5 mm in diameter. Muscle strength can be assessed by palpation.

Chest

Assessment of the neonate's chest involves inspection, palpation, and auscultation. Percussion is of lim-

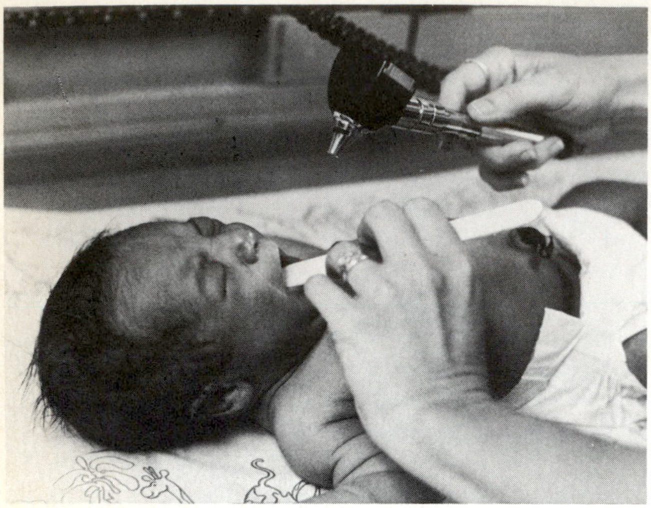

Figure 33–17. The mouth is assessed using a tongue blade and light.

ited value because of the size of the chest. The chest is observed for symmetry, size, shape, and respiratory movements. It is cylindrical in shape, with the circumference equal to or less than the head circumference. The xyphoid process is frequently seen under the skin because of the thinness of the chest wall. The ribs may also be noted on deep inspiration.

The breasts in both male and female neonates may be engorged because of the influence of maternal hormones. This condition usually regresses by the end of the second week of life. Occasionally, a whitish secretion is noted from the nipples. This discharge, known as witch's milk, is also the result of maternal hormones. The nipples should be symmetric on the chest. The nurse should palpate the breast nodule and note the size; this is part of the gestational age assessment. Some neonates may also have supernumerary nipples, located below the true nipples along the nipple line. These do not contain breast tissue.

The examiner should palpate the clavicles for any fractures. These can occur during delivery and can impair the neonate's arm motion.

The character of the respiratory cycle is noted. In the neonate, respiratory movements are abdominal in nature. The rate and rhythm of respirations as well as the quality are noted. The movement of the chest should be equal throughout the cycle.

Breath sounds are auscultated in both the anterior and the posterior lung fields. The neonate's breath sounds are normally bronchial in nature, because the chest cavity is short and the chest wall is thin. Occasionally, transmitted upper airway sounds are heard, but these generally clear with crying.

The nurse also notes the presence of any signs of respiratory compromise. These include unequal chest expansion, decreased breath sounds, rales or any adventitious sounds, grunting, retractions, and nasal flaring. Intercostal retractions frequently may be seen during crying; however, the presence of subcostal or supraclavicular retractions indicates a severely compromised neonate.

Heart

The neonate's circulatory system is dependent on the integrity of the heart and its ability to function normally. The neonate is first inspected for skin color as well as color of the mucous membranes, lips, and nailbeds, which are pink. Apical pulsation, or the point of maximal impulse (PMI), may be visible, usually lateral to the midclavicular line in the third or fourth interspace.

The nurse should palpate the PMI and note its presence. The neonate's other pulses (femoral, dorsalis pedis, and brachial) should be palpated. The pedal pulses may not always be palpable, so their absence is not necessarily abnormal. Absence of the femoral pulses is always abnormal and indicates decreased aortic blood flow caused by coarctation of the aorta. It is best to use light palpation with the index finger and simultaneously feel the bilateral pulses to assess their equality and fullness.

Auscultation of the heart involves the use of both the bell and the diaphragm of the stethoscope (Figure 33–18). It may take the nurse a few moments of careful listening to distinguish between breath sounds and heart sounds. The heart should be auscultated at all four areas—aortic, pulmonic, tricuspid, and

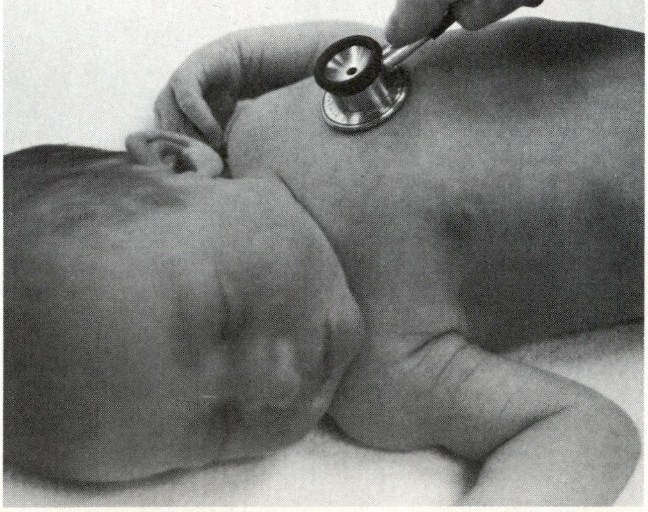

Figure 33–18. Auscultation of the heart.

mitral—and, in addition, below the left axilla and posteriorly below the left scapula. Both S_1 and S_2 heart sounds should be clearly heard. S_1 is the first heart sound and is caused by closure of the mitral and tricuspid valves. It is best heard at the apex where it is the loudest. S_2, the second heart sound, is best heard at the upper sternal border. It is caused by closure of the aortic and pulmonic valves. S_2 splitting, a normal finding, may be difficult to appreciate because of the neonate's rapid heart rate. It is also important to note the side of the chest in which the heart sounds are heard. If the neonate has dextrocardia, the presence of the heart on the right side of the chest as opposed to its normal position, the sounds will be heard on the right instead of the left.

The nurse also notes the presence of heart murmurs. Some murmurs may be functional and occur as the result of the changing hemodynamics of birth. Others may occur as the result of congenital defects. The location, quality, timing and loudness of murmurs should be noted. In addition, the appearance or disappearance of murmurs over time is important in identifying their significance.[12]

Abdomen

The neonate's abdomen is prominent in appearance. It is cylindrical in shape and protrudes slightly. Shape, contour, respiratory pattern, and presence of defects should be noted. Superficial abdominal veins are a normal finding.

The presence of the umbilical cord is noted, and in the early neonatal period, the vessels should be counted. The umbilical cord normally contains two arteries and one vein. The cord begins to dry several hours after birth, and shrivels and blackens by the second or third day of life. The umbilicus should be inspected frequently for signs of infection (foul odor, redness, and or purulent drainage), granuloma (small, red, raw-appearing polyp where the umbilical cord separates), bleeding, and discharge. The cord normally falls off by 2 weeks after birth. By the time the neonate is a month old, the umbilicus should be healed.

Umbilical hernias are a common problem and are easily visualized when the neonate is crying. The size and characteristics of hernias should be noted. They are caused by a persistent separation of the rectus muscles (diastasis recti) and may self-correct by the age of 1 year.[13]

The abdomen should be observed for signs of distension or gross bulging, which may be due to obstruction, infection, or a solid mass. The presence of visible peristaltic waves and upper left quadrant distension suggests pyloric or duodenal obstruction, especially if accompanied by vomiting. Serial abdominal circumference measurements are valuable in documenting the progress of abdominal distension.

Auscultation of the abdomen should be performed before palpation and percussion. The nurse listens for peristaltic sounds in all four quadrants. The sounds are usually present within 1 to 2 hours of birth, and may be irregular.

The abdomen is percussed over the stomach, liver, and spleen. Liver and spleen percussion produces a dull sound; stomach percussion results in a tympanic sound.

Palpation of the abdomen is accomplished using both light and deep techniques. The neonate's knees are flexed to relax the abdominal muscles. The liver of the average neonate spans 5.6 to 5.9 cm, and can be felt 1 to 2 cm below the right costal margin.[14] Normally, the liver edge feels soft (Figure 33–19). The spleen tip can be felt just under the left costal margin.

The kidneys are best palpated within the first 6 hours of birth before the abdomen becomes distended with air and feedings. The kidneys can be felt adjacent to the vertebral column, approximately 1 to 2 cm above the umbilicus. Normally, the lower half of the right kidney and the lower tip of the left kidney are felt. The nurse should place one finger under the neonate's flank and press upward. The other hand then presses downward. The kidney should be felt as a firm oval structure.

The passage of meconium is noted. The neonate's bowels can occasionally be palpated. The two areas easiest to feel are the cecum, located in the lower right quadrant, and the sigmoid, located in the lower left quadrant.

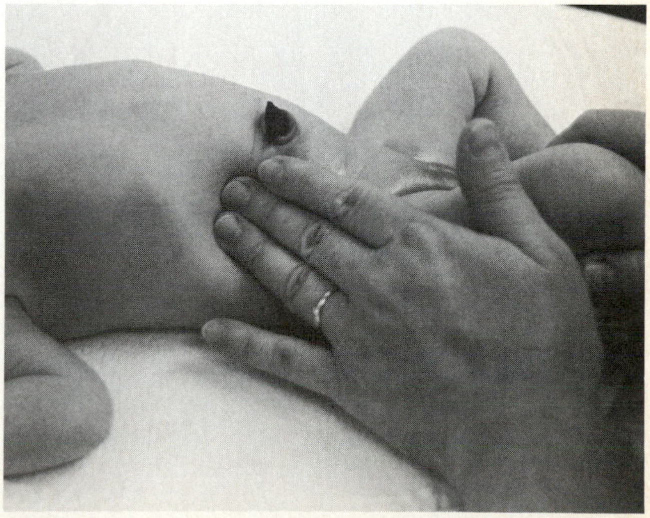

Figure 33–19. Abdomen: palpating the liver border.

The bladder may be percussed just above the symphysis pubis. The presence of urine will produce a tympanic sound. The time of the first voiding should be noted.

The presence of superficial abdominal reflexes should be noted. The nurse should lightly stroke each of the four quadrants around the umbilicus. Using the index finger, diagonal strokes are made in the form of a diamond. The abdominal muscles and umbilicus should move in the direction of the quadrant that is assessed.

The presence of masses in the lower abdominal area should be noted. Inguinal hernias are a common finding in neonates, and are more prevalent in males than females. Palpable inguinal nodes are a common benign finding in the neonatal period.[15]

Genitalia

Assessment of the genitalia involves both inspection and palpation. The nurse notes the color, size, shape, and position of the various structures of both the male and female organs.

The female neonate usually has an edematous clitoris and labia majora (Figure 33–20A). The clitoris appears large and may be sensitive to touch. Increased pigmentation of the external structures as a result of hormonal influences is often evident. The labia majora are drawn slightly apart to inspect the labia minora. The vaginal opening is observed. Vaginal or hymenal tags may be observed (Figure 33–20B). These often disappear within a few weeks of birth. The nurse may also note a whitish mucoid or blood-tinged vaginal discharge resulting from the withdrawal of maternal hormones. The bloody discharge is known as psuedomenstruation. A white cheeselike substance called smegma may be found under the labia. The internal structures of the female genitalia are not routinely assessed.

In the male neonate, the nurse examines both the penis and the scrotum. The penis should be intact with no additional orifices on the ventral surface (hypospadias) or dorsal surface (epispadias). The foreskin of an uncircumcized neonate may not be retractable (Figure 33–21). Circumcision removes the foreskin and exposes the glans penis. The meatal opening should be seen as a slit centrally located on the tip of the glans. The nurse should note the adequacy of the urinary stream. The penis may become erect when stimulated or just before urination.

The color of the scrotum is assessed. It may vary from pink in light-skinned neonates to dark brown in darker-complexioned neonates. Rugae, or wrinkle formations, are noted on the surface of the scrotum in full-term neonates. The testicles should be compared. In many neonates, they are not fully descended and can be felt just at the junction of the external inguinal ring. The nurse uses the thumb and forefinger to assess testicular size. Using the first two fingers of the other hand, gentle pressure can be exerted on the inguinal canal in a downward position to keep the testicles from retracting. **Hydroceles,** caused by an accumulation of fluid around the testes, are a common finding. They can easily be transilluminated with a light and will usually decrease in size. The

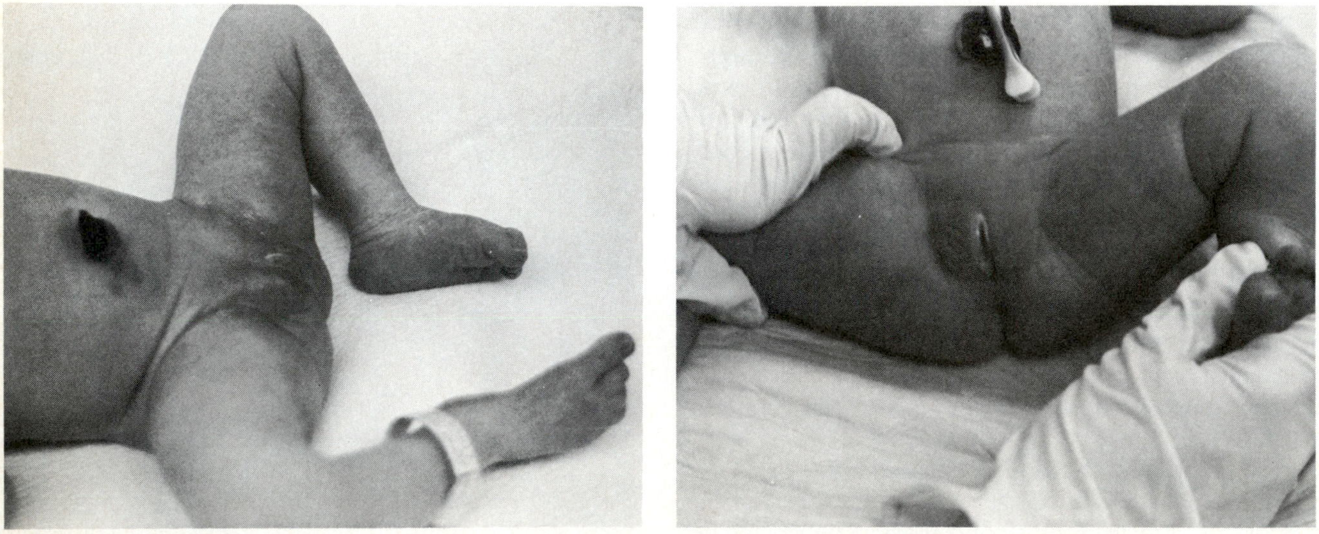

A B

Figure 33–20. Female genitalia. **A.** Hypertrophied. **B.** Note the hymenal tag and clamped cord treated with triple dye.

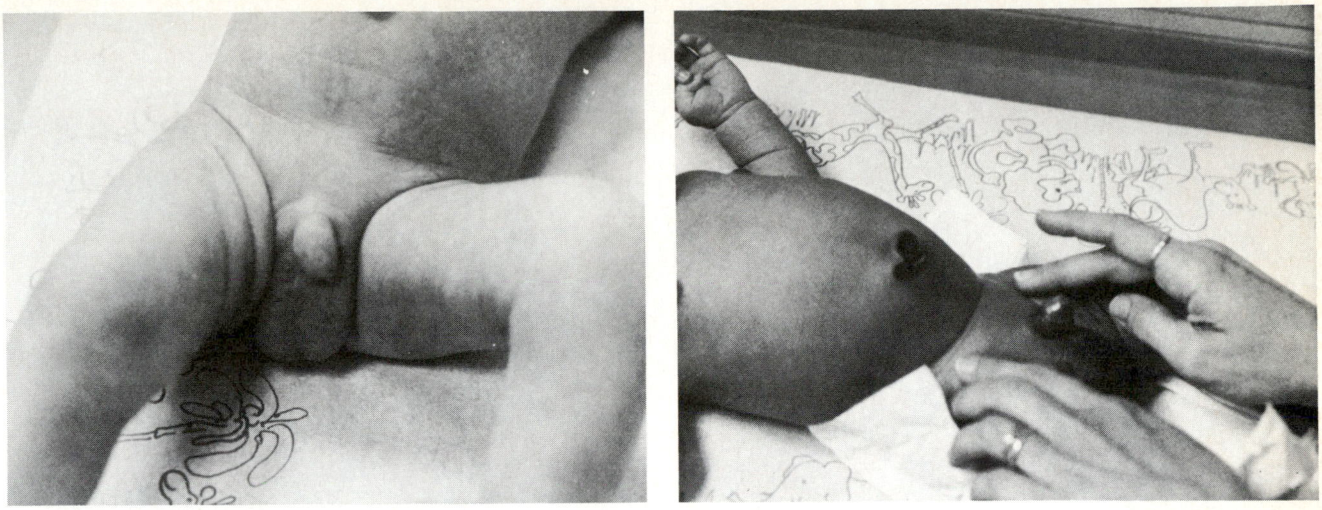

A B

Figure 33–21. **A.** Uncircumcised male neonate. **B.** Circumcised male neonate.

nurse can elicit the cremasteric reflex by stroking the inner thigh and observing the bilateral retraction of the testes.

The gender of the neonate is assigned at birth. Occasionally, abnormalities in genital development occur. Organs may appear hypertrophied, underdeveloped, or ambiguous. If there is a question about the true gender of the neonate, gender is not assigned until a diagnosis is made through buccal smear for karyotype and blood tests for ketosteroids. This is usually done within the first 3 days of life.

Another common finding in neonates is the presence of rust-colored (brick dust) stains on the diaper. This is caused by the presence of uric acid crystals in the urine and may resemble blood spots.

Anus and Rectum

The position of the anus in relation to the genitalia is noted. The passage of meconium from the rectum should be recorded, as this assures the patency of the anus. The presence of meconium in other genital orifices should be noted as this is an abnormal finding. The anus should have good sphincter tone as noted by observation. The wink reflex, or contraction of the anal sphincter, can be elicited by gently stroking the perianal area.

Extremities and Spine

The extremities and spine may be assessed in conjunction with the neurologic examination. For the purposes of this discussion, the two examinations are presented separately.

The extremities are inspected for symmetry, equality, muscle tone, and range of motion. The newborn position of flexion may make it difficult to assess the extremities by inspection alone. The nurse examines the neonate for any gross abnormalities or the presence of extra digits. Movement of the extremities should be symmetric and subject to the full range of motion.

The hands and arms are inspected. Arm length should be equal. The fingers and toes are counted. Nails should be present. Extra digits (**polydactyly**) are sometimes found on either the hands or the feet. Fingers or toes may be fused (**syndactyly**). The palms of the hands are inspected for creases. The simian line, a single palmar crease, is often found in Down's syndrome.

Movement of the arms should be assessed. Occasionally, trauma to the brachial plexus during a difficult delivery will result in brachial palsy. The most common type of palsy involves the fifth and sixth cervical nerve roots (**Erb-Duchenne paralysis**). In this condition, the affected arm is held in a position of tight adduction and internal rotation at the shoulder. Although the grasp reflex on the affected side may be intact, the Moro reflex cannot be elicited. Restoration of function is dependent on the degree of injury. With treatment, most neonates have complete recovery.

Leg length is assessed by extending both legs simultaneously. They should be equal with symmetric skin folds. The nurse inspects the legs in both the prone and supine positions. A neonate who is delivered in a breech presentation may have extended knees. Hip integrity is assessed by using the Ortolani movement. The index and middle fingers of each

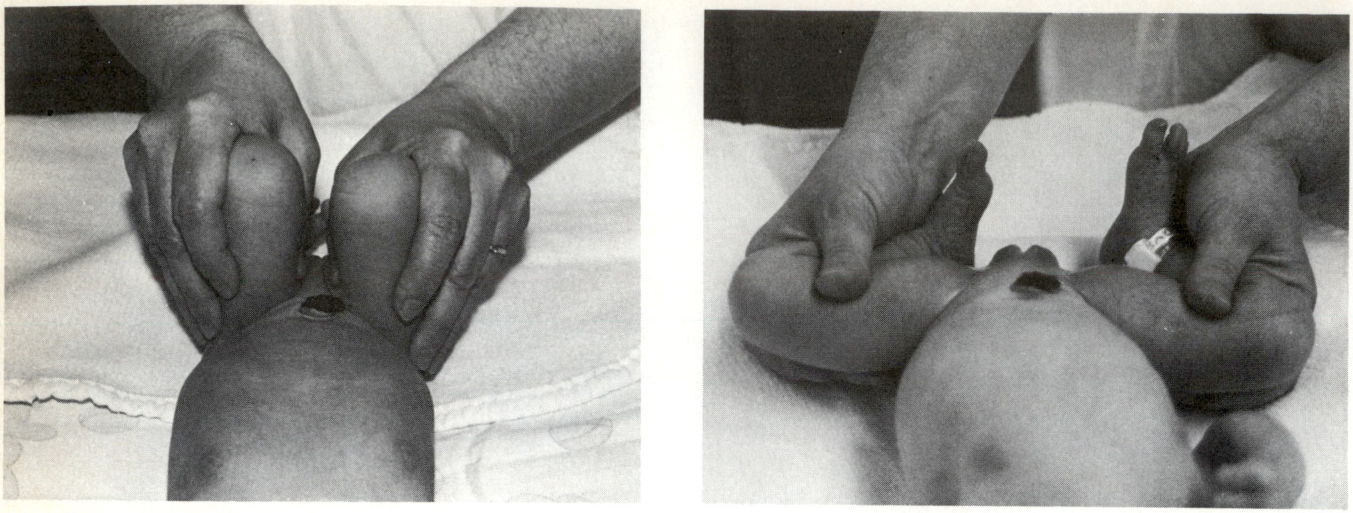

Figure 33–22. Examination of the hip.

hand are placed over the greater trochanters of the hips at the same time. Downward pressure is exerted on the hips while the neonate's knees are flexed. The hips are abducted at least 70° and then adducted (Figure 33–22). The motion should be smooth without any unusual clicks felt. Presence of a click, unequal movement, or extra skin folds is considered a positive response, indicating that the hip is dislocated, and that the neonate should be referred for further assessment.

The legs are assessed for evidence of clubfoot (talipes equinus). Both feet are put through range of motion, as feet that appear to be misaligned may result from intrauterine positioning.

The soles of the feet are inspected for creases (Figure 33–23). Premature newborns have absent creases. The fat pads of the feet give the neonate the appearance of being flat-footed.

The neonate's spine is examined for any obvious defects. The spine appears straight but can easily be flexed. The neonate is able to lift the head and turn from side to side when prone. The nurse should be able to palpate the vertebrae and note any abnormalities. The presence of a pilonidal dimple should be noted. Dimples containing a tuft of hair are often associated with spina bifida occulta.

Neonatal Reflexes

The neurologic system of the neonate is examined by assessing the presence of reflexes and neuromuscular movement. Throughout the course of the examination, the neonate is constantly observed for movement and symmetry. As the nurse conducts the examination, specific reflexes are identified and tested. Many of these reflexes are present at birth and are retained as the neonate matures; others disappear within the first weeks to the first year of life. These reflex behaviors are necessary for the neonate's survival and safety. The absence of reflexes may indicate central nervous system (CNS) damage. Persistence of reflexes beyond the time they normally disappear may also indicate CNS problems.

Moro Reflex. **Moro (startle) reflex** (Figure 33–24) is elicited holding the neonate in a semisitting position and allowing the head and trunk to fall backward a few centimeters. It may also be elicited by striking a flat surface adjacent to where the neonate is lying supine. The neonate should abduct and extend the arms symmetrically. The fingers will fan out, with

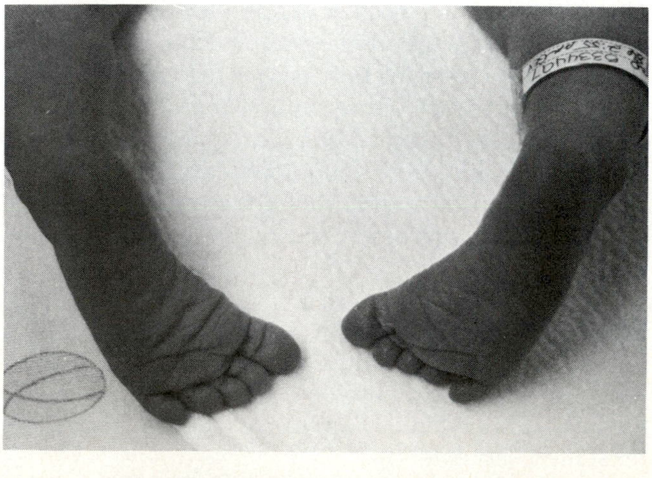

Figure 33–23. Inspection for sole creases.

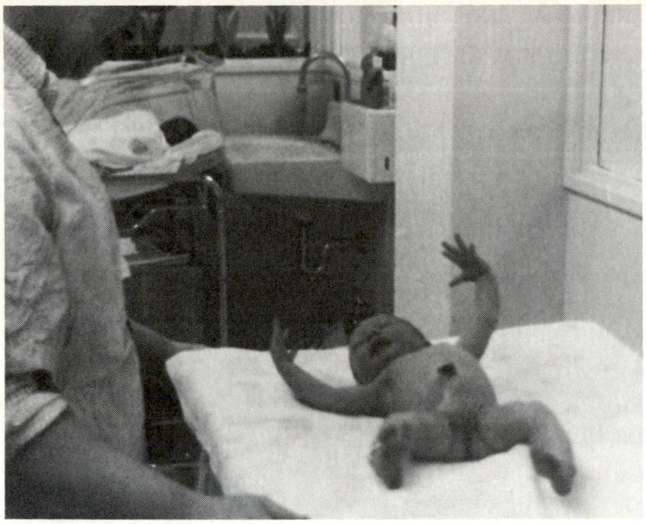

Figure 33–24. Moro reflex.

the thumb and forefinger forming a "C". The arms then adduct in an embracing movement and return to their relaxed position. The legs may also follow in a similar motion. The Moro reflex should be present at birth and usually disappears by 3 to 4 months of age. Persistence of the reflex beyond 6 months of age warrants further assessment.

Palmar and Plantar Grasp Reflexes. To elicit the **palmar grasp reflex,** the nurse places a finger in the neonate's palm approaching from the ulnar side (Figure 33–25). The neonate's fingers will curl around the nurse's finger with a firm grasp that enables the neonate to be lifted from the supporting surface. This reflex disappears by 2 to 4 months of age.

The nurse elicits the **plantar grasp reflex** by placing his or her thumbs at the base of the neonate's toes. The toes curl downward in response (Figure 33–26). This reflex diminishes by 8 months of age.

Tonic Neck Reflex. The **tonic neck (fencing) reflex** is elicited by quickly turning the neonate's head to one side while she or he is lying on the back. The extremities on that same side extend and those on the opposite side flex, giving the neonate the appearance of a "fencer." The reflex usually fades by 3 to 4 months, although some children may assume this position during sleep as late as 2 to 3 years. Persistence of this reflex in an alert infant beyond 4 months of age may indicate cerebral palsy.

Sucking and Rooting Reflexes. The **sucking reflex** and **rooting reflex** are elicited by touching the neonate's cheek, lip, or corner of the mouth with a nipple or other stimulus. The neonate responds by turning in the direction of the stimulus, opening the mouth, and beginning to suck. These reflexes usually disappear by 7 months of age.

Swallowing Reflex. The **swallowing reflex** can be observed during the act of feeding. Fluid should be ingested easily without gagging, coughing, or vomiting. Swallowing may be poorly developed in a premature newborn or in a newborn with a neurologic defect.

Babinski Reflex. To elicit the **Babinski reflex,** the nurse strokes the lateral aspect of the sole upward across the ball of the foot with an object. The neonate responds by hyperextending the toes and dorsiflexing

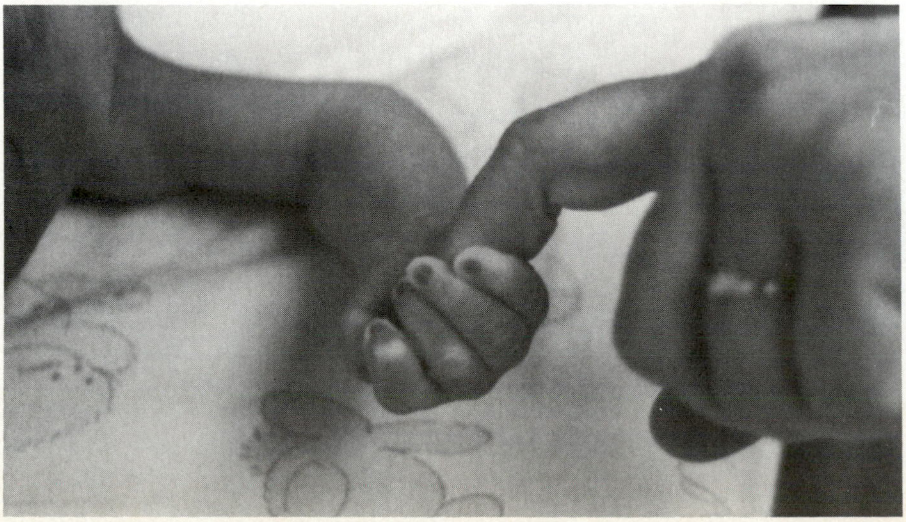

Figure 33–25. Palmar grasp reflex.

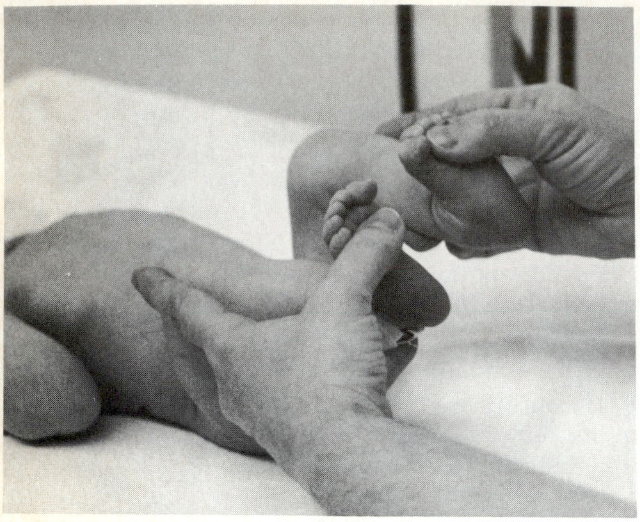

Figure 33–26. Plantar grasp reflex.

the great toe. The Babinski reflex disappears after 1 year of age.

Stepping and Placing Reflexes. The **stepping reflex** is elicited by holding the neonate in an upright position and allowing one foot to touch a flat surface (Figure 33–27). Alternate stepping movements that stimulate walking are observed. To elicit the **placing reflex,** the neonate is positioned upright, with the dorsal surface of the feet placed against the edge of the table. The neonate responds by flexing the knees and hips and moving the legs up to the table surface. These reflexes usually disappear by 4 months of age.

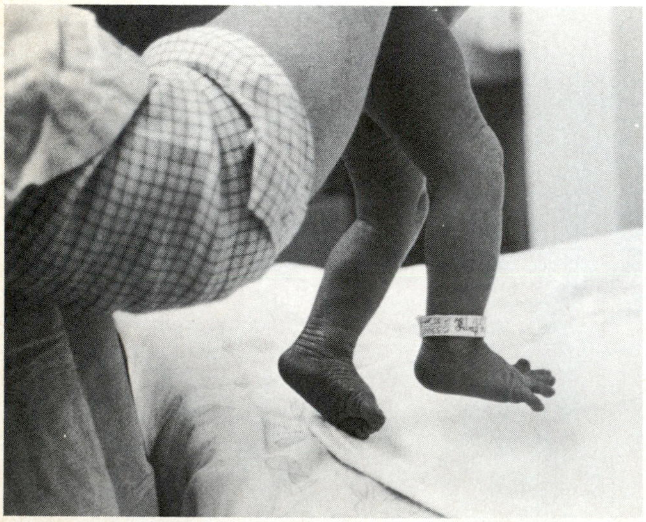

Figure 33–27. Stepping and placing reflexes.

Galant's Reflex. **Galant's reflex (trunk incurvation)** is elicited by placing the neonate in a prone position. The nurse firmly strokes the back about 5 cm (2 in.) from the spine in a downward motion (Figure 33–28). The neonate responds by curving the body to the side of the stimulus. The opposite side is then checked. This response diminishes by 2 to 3 months of life.

Crossed Extension. With the neonate lying on the back, the nurse extends one leg, pressing the knee down to the surface of the examining table. The foot of the extended leg is stimulated. The opposite leg responds by flexing, adducting, and extending.

Magnet Reflex. The neonate is placed on the back. The nurse partially flexes both legs, applying gentle pressure to the soles of the feet. The neonate responds by extending both legs against the source of pressure.

Traction Reflex. The nurse pulls the neonate up by the wrists from a supine position. Head lag is noted first; the neonate then responds by lifting the head and holding it upright before allowing the head to fall forward on the chest. The amount of head lag noted depends on the maturity and muscle tone of the neonate.

Arm Recoil. Both arms are extended together by pulling them down by the wrists. Brisk flexion of the elbows is noted when the arms are quickly released.

Crawling Reflex. The neonate should make crawling movements when placed in a prone position. This usually disappears by 6 weeks of age.

Glabellar Reflex. With the neonate's eyes open, the nurse taps lightly over the forehead or bridge of the nose. The neonate responds by blinking for the first four or five taps. Continued blinking with repeated taps may indicate an extrapyramidal disorder.

GESTATIONAL AGE ASSESSMENT

The practice of assigning gestational age on the basis of the maternal menstrual cycle and expected date of confinement (EDC) is inadequate for assessing neonatal outcome. Neonatal size and weight may also

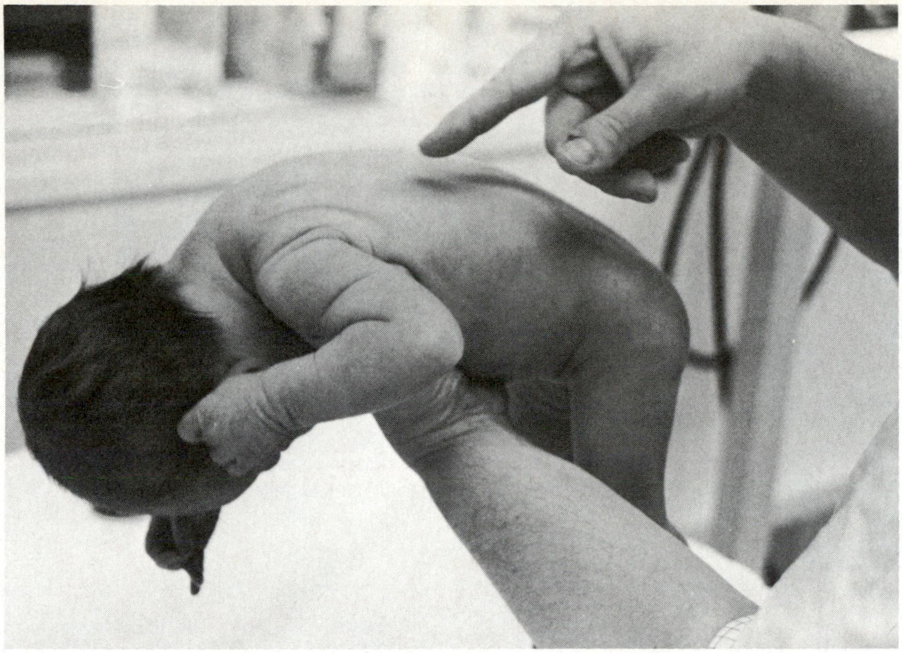

Figure 33–28. Trunk incurvature.

combine to confuse the examiner about expected behavioral patterns and physical appearance.

Neonates can be designated according to birth weight as being small for gestational age (SGA), average for gestational age (AGA), or large for gestational age (LGA) (Figure 33–29). This classification is valid whether the neonate is preterm (before 38 weeks), term (between 38 and 42 weeks), or postterm (after 42 weeks).[16]

The gestational age assessment tool devised by Dubowitz and coworkers is used to determine the appropriate gestational age of the neonate regardless of birth weight. Research focusing on the characteristics and neurologic development of neonates began about 1950. Dubowitz and coworkers subsequently synthesized the findings of earlier investigators and, with some modifications, developed a reliable method of assessment.[17] The tool is most reliable when used on neonates between 28 and 43 weeks of gestation.

Gestational age of the newborn is predicated on neurologic signs including posture and primitive reflexes, which vary with gestational age, and both external and superficial characteristic of the newborn, which change with gestational maturity. This assessment is reliable immediately after birth and within the first 24 hours. According to the authors, it may be used up to 3 to 5 days after birth, but then becomes unreliable because of the maturational changes that occur.

The tool contains 21 criteria (10 neurologic criteria and 11 superficial or external criteria) and takes approximately 20 to 25 minutes to implement. The method was designed for use by those who have direct care of the neonate. As nurses care for neonates around the clock, the tool is an easy and accurate way for them to assess gestational age and identify potential problems on the basis of their findings.

The neurologic criteria cover assessment of complete body posture; square window flexion of the wrist (Figure 33–30), arm recoil, ankle dorsiflexion, leg recoil, popliteal angle, heel-to-ear placement, scarf sign of the arm and shoulder (Figure 33–31), head lag, and ventral suspension of the body. The superficial or external criteria cover inspection of the neonate for the presence of edema, skin texture, skin color while quiet, skin opacity of the trunk, presence of lanugo on the back; plantar creases, nipple formation, breast size, ear formation, ear firmness, and genital development. Each category is scored, and the scores added to produce a total score. Total scores can range between 0 and 69, indicating gestational ages between 26 and 46 weeks.

Ballard and coworkers have modified the Dubowitz tool to allow quick assessment. The Ballard tool deletes head lag, ventral suspension, and leg recoil, criteria that are difficult to assess in a neonate who is on a respirator or has monitoring equipment and intravenous catheters in place.[18] The scoring method is similar to that for the Dubowitz tool and it can be completed in less time (Figure 33–32). Each category is given a value and a total score is computed. The maximum score is 50, which equals a gestational age of 44 weeks.

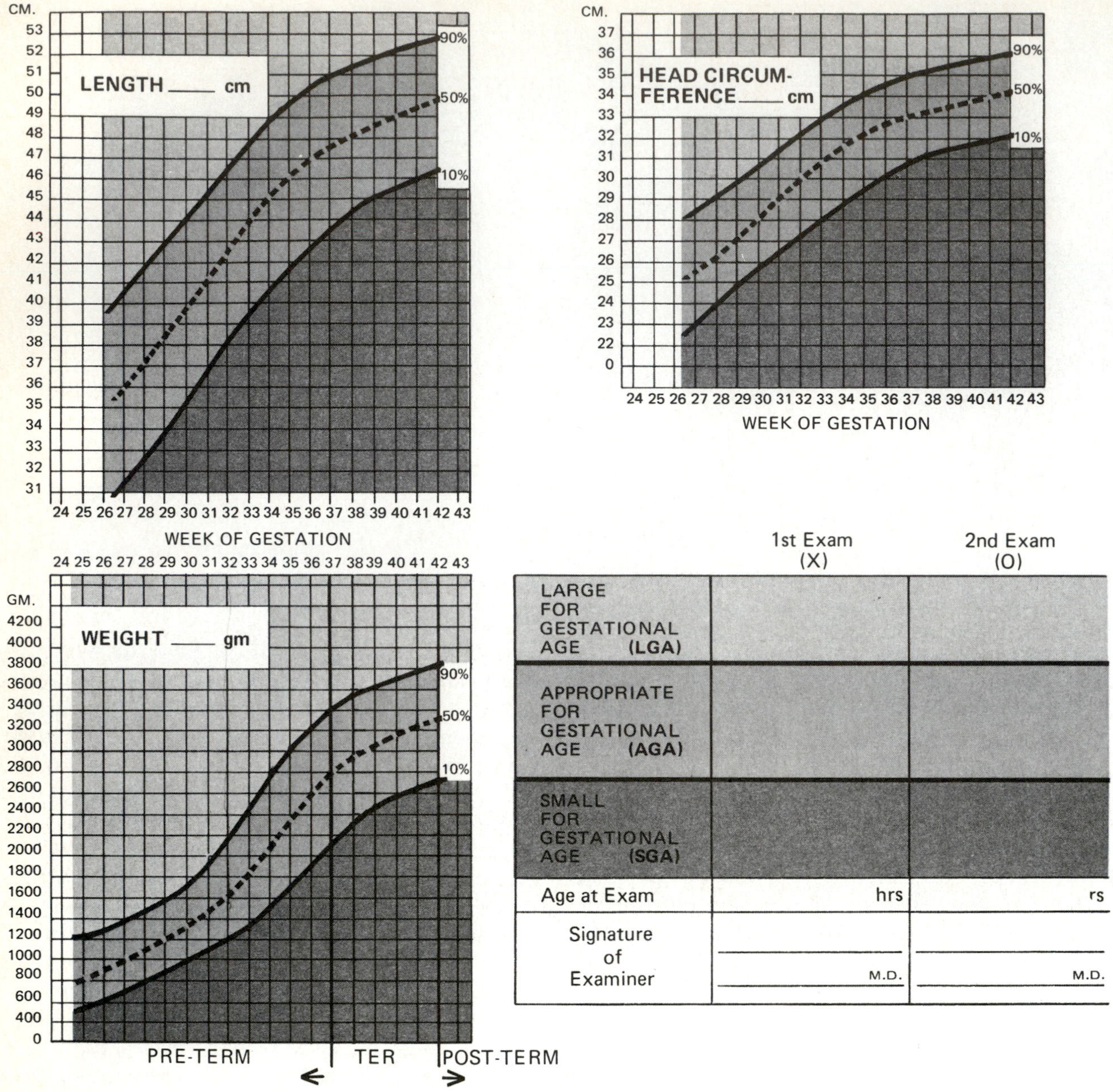

Figure 33–29. Gestational age assessment tool. (*Reproduced, with permission, from Battaglia FC, Lubchenco LO. A practical classification of newborn infants by weight and gestational age.* J Pediatr. *1967;71:159–163.*)

BEHAVIORAL ASSESSMENT

Several tools can be used to assess the neonate's behavioral responses and predict maternal-neonate interactions. These include the Neonatal Perception Inventory developed by Broussard and Hartner[19] and the Brazelton Neonatal Behavioral Assessment Scale.

Neonatal Perception Inventory

The Neonatal Perception Inventory (NPI) is used to assess maternal perception of certain neonate behaviors and may predict the behavioral interaction between mother and newborn. The inventory consists of two similiar instruments, administered on the first or second postpartum day and repeated when the neonate is 1 month old. Crying, feeding, spitting up, sleeping, elimination, and predictable patterns of eating and sleeping are addressed. The mother is asked to compare her concept of the "average" newborn with her perceptions of her own newborn at two different points in time. This inventory assists the nurse to identify potential problems in the interaction between mother and neonate.

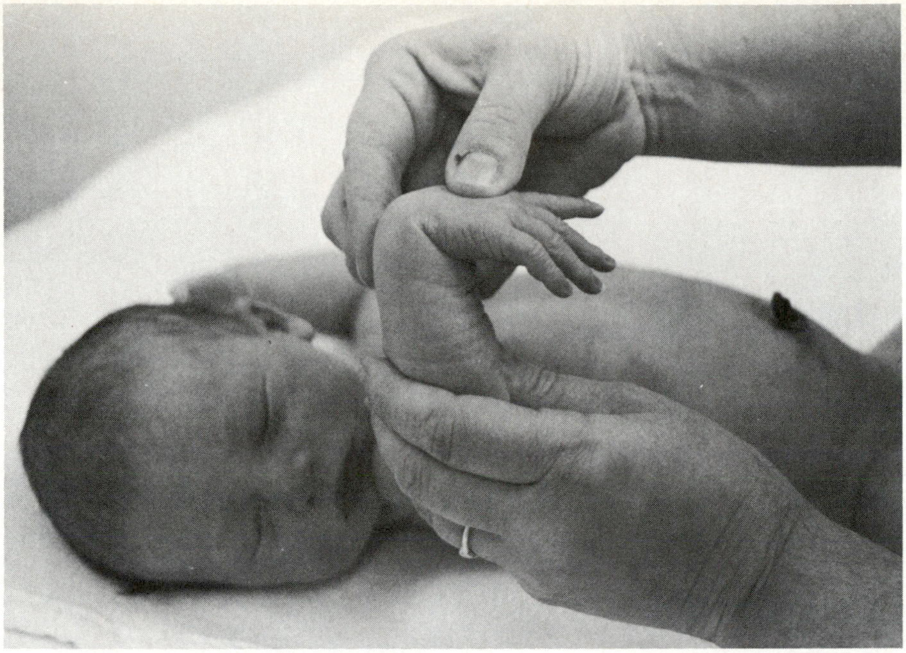

Figure 33–30. Square window flexion of the wrist.

Brazelton Neonatal Behavioral Assessment Scale

The Brazelton Neonatal Behavioral Assessment Scale (BNBAS) was devised by Brazelton[20] to assess newborn behavior and neurologic integrity. Neonates are equipped with a marvelous repertoire of behaviors and neurologic responses that allow them to control their responses to the environment. The BNBAS evaluates the neonate's state and response to stimulation by assessing interaction with the environment, motor processes, defensive reactions, and organizational processes. The neonate's state of consciousness is an important factor when interpreting the reactions to stimuli, as reactions will depend on the neonate's state at the time of testing.

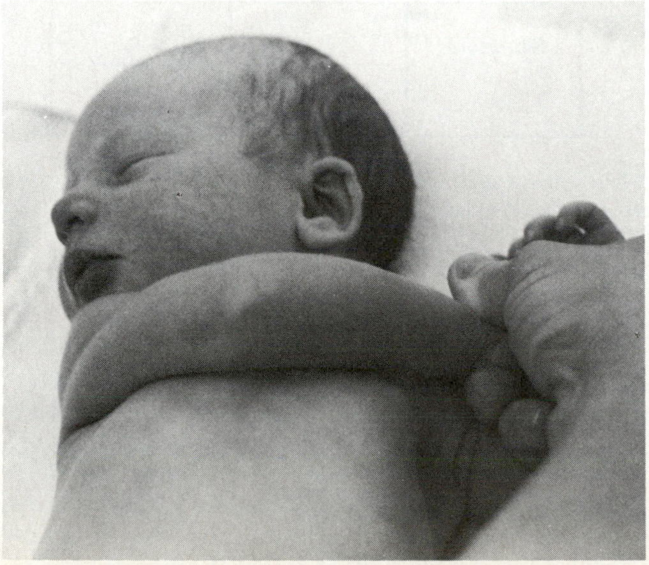

Figure 33–31. Scarf sign.

Brazelton's research was based on the description of the neonate's states of consciousness by Prechtl and coworkers.[9, 20] These include (1) deep sleep, (2) light sleep, (3) drowsiness or semidozing, (4) alert, (5) active alert (eyes opened with increased motor activity), and (6) crying. The neonate is assessed on 28 behavioral items that are scored on a 9-point scale. In addition, the examiner elicits 18 neurologic responses that are scored on a 3-point scale. The various criteria are tested as the neonate proceeds from one state to the next in a sequential order. The midpoint of most of the scales is considered the norm. As labor, delivery, and medication use influence neonatal reactions, the behavior on the third day of life is considered the expected mean. The neonate is scored on the best, not average, behavior.

The assessment is conducted in a quiet, dimly lit environment to avoid distractors. It takes approximately 30 minutes to complete. At present, special training is needed to use the BNBAS with a high degree of reliability and test validity; however, the information obtained has several benefits. It can assist the nurse in developing a more comprehensive care plan for the neonate and family, promote parents' understanding of their newborn's unique capabilities,

NEUROMUSCULAR MATURITY

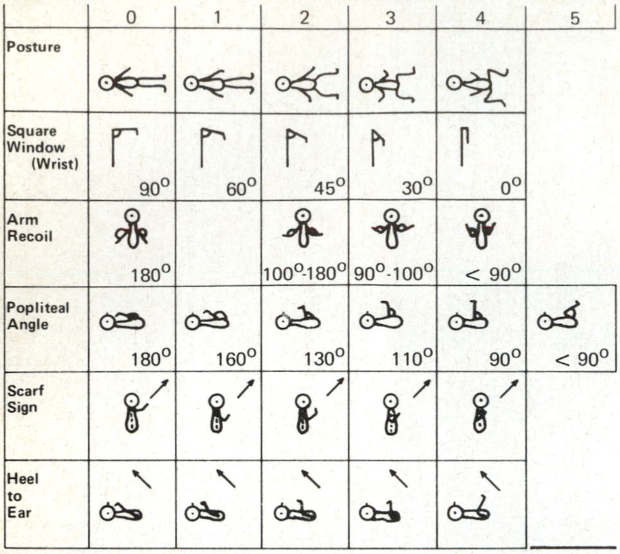
0
1
2
3
4
5
Posture
Square Window (Wrist)
90°
60°
45°
30°
0°
Arm Recoil
180°
100°-180°
90°-100°
< 90°
Popliteal Angle
180°
160°
130°
110°
90°
< 90°
Scarf Sign
Heel to Ear

PHYSICAL MATURITY

	0	1	2	3	4	5
SKIN	gelatinous red, trans-parent	smooth pink, visible veins	superficial peeling &/or rash, few veins	cracking pale area, rare veins	parchment, deep cracking, no vessels	leathery, cracked, wrinkled
LANUGO	none	abundant	thinning	bald areas	mostly bald	
PLANTAR CREASES	no crease	faint red marks	anterior transverse crease only	creases ant. 2/3	creases cover entire sole	
BREAST	barely percept.	flat areola, no bud	stippled areola, 1–2 mm bud	raised areola, 3–4 mm bud	full areola, 5–10 mm bud	
EAR	pinna flat, stays folded	sl. curved pinna, soft with slow recoil	well-curv. pinna, soft but ready recoil	formed & firm with instant recoil	thick cartilage, ear stiff	
GENITALS Male	scrotum empty, no rugae		testes descend-ing, few rugae	testes down, good rugae	testes pendulous, deep rugae	
GENITALS Female	prominent clitoris & labia minora		majora & minora equally prominent	majora large, minora small	clitoris & minora completely covered	

Gestation by Dates ______________ wks

Birth Date ____________ Hour ____________ am / pm

APGAR ____________ 1 min ____________ 5 min

MATURITY RATING

Score	Wks
5	26
10	28
15	30
20	32
25	34
30	36
35	38
40	40
45	42
50	44

SCORING SECTION

	1st Exam=X	2nd Exam=O
Estimating Gest Age by Maturity Rating	______ Weeks	______ Weeks
Time of Exam	Date ______ Hour ______ am / pm	Date ______ Hour ______ am / pm
Age at Exam	______ Hours	______ Hours
Signature of Examiner	______ M.D.	______ M.D.

Figure 33–32. Ballard tool for gestational age assessment. (*Reproduced, with permission, from Ballard JL, et al. A simplified score for assessment of fetal maturation in newly born infants.* J Pediatr. *1979;95:769–774.*)

and decrease parents' anxiety through improved understanding of newborn behavior.

During the behavioral assessment, the nurse notes how well the neonate tolerates the various stimuli. This informs parents whether their newborn quiets easily when stimulated or is able to shut out external noise. An example of shutting out stimuli was noted by one mother who stated that she could vacuum a room while the newborn was sleeping without disturbing him.

The neonate's visual and auditory alertness is noted. This attribute is extremely important if the parents are to attach in a positive way with the newborn. The ability to look at the mother's and father's faces, to self-alert to their vocal interaction, and to follow their voices is necessary to establish interactive communication patterns. One mother who had complications after an emergency cesarean delivery noted that her son's ability to look and "seem to listen" to her made such an impression that she tended to forget the tubes and drains she had in place. The fact that the newborn was so alert every time she held and fed him overshadowed her discomfort. The nurse needs to identify neonates who may not be as alert so that potential problems with attachment and relationships may be averted through specific interventions.

The nurse notes muscle tone and motor maturity. These are best observed while the neonate is being handled, turned, and lifted. Movements should be smooth. The neonate's cuddliness while being held is noted. This is important in assisting parents to find satisfactory ways to soothe and quiet the neonate when she or he is distressed.

The neonate's ability for self-quieting behavior when distressed also is noted. Often parents feel that they have to rush to the newborn the moment crying begins; however, many newborns fuss for a short time but then are able to settle down either by sucking their fingers or a pacifier or by being patted. Others may have to be held and rocked to be quieted. The nurse can assist parents in identifying which method is best for their newborn. This also helps new parents establish self-confidence in their caregiving abilities.

NURSING DIAGNOSES

Based on the data from the delivery record and comprehensive assessment of the neonate after birth, nursing diagnoses are developed. See the box for examples of nursing diagnoses for the neonate.

NURSING DIAGNOSES FOR THE NEONATE

Problem-Oriented

Potential for injury, related to parents' lack of knowledge of infant safety in car

Potential impaired physical mobility, related to musculoskeletal injury at birth

Sensory perceptual alteration, related to use of medication for prevention of ophthalmic infection

Strength-Oriented

Effective breastfeeding, related to good sucking and rooting reflexes

Positive attachment behaviors, related to parent-neonate eye-to-eye contact, parent touching, enfolding, touching behaviors

Asset in nutritional status, related to appropriate intake of nutrients and fluid

CASE STUDY/CARE PLAN: NEONATAL ASSESSMENT

Melissa Lee is a 2-day-old newborn of Chinese-American parents, Steven and Kimberly Lee. Steven is 26 years old and is a manager of a bookstore. Kimberly is 24 years old and is a student at a nearby community college. They have been married for 3 years and are renting a two-bedroom apartment. Melissa is their first child. The health history reveals no parental or family health problems. Steven smokes cigarettes in the home and car.

Melissa was delivered vaginally with low forceps after approximately 9½ hours of labor without complication. Mother had an epidural block but no other medications were used during labor or delivery. Father was present during labor and delivery. Parents and Melissa spent approximately one-half hour together in the delivery room afterwords.

Melissa had no problems at birth and had Apgar scores of 9 at 1 minute, 9 at 5 minutes. Her birth weight was 7 pounds 2 oz and her blood type O+. Melissa has been breastfed since birth. She is now 2 days old and weighs 6 pounds 8 oz. Melissa is rooming-in with her mother. The parents are concerned about Melissa's weight loss, the color and consistency of her stools, and "bruising" on her back.

(continued)

CASE STUDY/CARE PLAN: Neonatal Assessment (*continued*)

The results of a physical examination are:
Age: 2 days
Weight: 6 pounds 8 oz (25th percentile)
Length: 19 in. (25th percentile)
Head: 34 cm (25th percentile)
Chest: 33.5 cm
VS: 98.2°F, HR: 130, RR: 40

General appearance: Neonate is a content, alert, responsive female who appears in no apparent distress.

Skin: Pink; mongolian spot at posterior lumbar region approximate 2 × 3-cm area; milia on nose; good turgor; no rashes, petechiae, or lesions; nails pink with rapid capillary refill.

Head: Round, anterior and posterior fontanelles soft and flat; anterior fontanelle 1 × 1 cm; posterior fontanelle ½ cm; suture lines palpable within normal limits; no caput succedaneum or cephalhematoma; no abrasions, lacerations, or lesions; full head of black silky hair.

Face: Symmetric with Oriental features; movement equal bilaterally.

Eyes: Sclera clear; conjunctiva clear and pink; bilateral epicanthal folds, no ptosis, lid lag, or deformity; eye movements random without psuedostrabismus; positive blink reflex; cornea and lens clear; positive red reflexes bilaterally; irises dark gray/black; no coloboma or Brushfield's spots.

Ears: Pinnae well formed and firm with instant recoil; normal alignment with eyes; no preauricular skin tags; auditory canals patent bilaterally; tympanic membranes translucent, mobile with normal light reflex; responds to bell.

Nose: Symmetric, patent without septal deviation, mucosa pink without discharge; no flaring of nostrils.

Mouth and Throat: Lips symmetric and pink without lesions; gums and mucosa pink, moist without lesions; tongue midline, symmetric; Epstein's pearls noted midline on hard palate; soft and hard palate intact without lesions; saliva within normal limits; uvula midline.

Neck: Supple with full range of motion; trachea midline; no masses or lymphadenopathy.

Chest: Symmetric without masses or tenderness; nipples symmetric without supernumerary nipples; clavicles within normal limits; breath sounds clear and equal bilaterally without rales, rhonchi, or wheezing; no retractions or grunting.

Heart: Pulse regular; PMI, left fourth intercostal space at midclavicular line, diameter 1 cm; femoral, dorsalis pedis and brachial pulses full and equal throughout; S_1 and S_2; no murmur, gallop, or extra sounds.

Abdomen: Symmetric, rounded, soft, nontender without masses or organomegaly; umbilical cord attached with application of triple-dye stain, umbilicus healing without signs of infection, or bleeding, discharge; no umbilical or inguinal hernia; bowel sounds active in all four quadrants; superficial abdominal reflexes within normal limits.

Genitalia: External female genitalia within normal limits without erythema, rash, or discharge.

Anus and rectum: Anus midline, patent; adequate sphincter tone with positive wink reflex; no fissures, bleeding, or rashes.

Extremities and spine: Extremities symmetric in movement and appearance; normal muscle tone; full range of motion throughout; hips abduct normally with negative Ortolani movement; no polydactyly or syndactyly; creases within normal limits; spine straight, flexible without deformities; no pilonidal dimple.

Neonatal reflexes: Primitive reflexes normal. Positive Moro, palmar and plantar, tonic neck, sucking, swallowing, rooting, Babinski, stepping and placing, Galant's, crossed extension, magnet, traction, arm recoil, crawling, and glabellar reflexes.

Supporting Assessment Data	Expected Client/Family Outcome	Nursing Action/ Intervention	Rationale	Criteria for Evaluation
Nursing Diagnosis: Parental knowledge deficit, related to normal newborn characteristics and variations				
Well 2-day-old Oriental female neonate Weight loss in normal range; stools of breastfed infant; Mongol spot present Parents are concerned about neonate having lost weight, and about "diarrhea", and "bruising" on her back	By the third postpartum day, parents will verbally express understanding of selected normal newborn characteristics, including: Weight loss Bowl and bladder elimination Skin variations	Encourage parents to be present at physical examination so that newborn characteristics can be demonstrated and explained, including voiding and stool patterns for breastfed neonates and skin features. Teach parents physiologic reasons for weight loss and normal patterns of weight gain in neonates. Give parents written literature about newborn characteristics to reinforce verbal explanations. Provide anticipatory guidance to parents about resources for concerns and questions.	Uncertainty increases anxiety. Increased knowledge tends to decrease anxiety. Anticipation of parents' concerns will help decrease fears of the unknown.	When asked, parents describe characteristics and patterns of weight gain in the neonate.
Nursing Diagnosis: Susceptibility to hazard, related to father's smoking in the home and car				
Father smokes cigarettes in the home and car	By the first well-child visit, neonate's environment will be smoke free	Provide parents with information about passive smoking and increased risk for respiratory disease when exposed to cigarette smoke. Assist parents in developing a plan to maintain a "smoke-free" environment for neonate both at home and in car. Refer father to a smoking cessation program. Specialized strategies and support may be necessary to eliminate smoking habit. Provide anticipatory guidance about fire safety in home: Smoke detectors Fire extinguishers Plan for escape from home Home fire drills Easy access to phone numbers for fire department Tot-finder labels for windows and doors	Passive smoke inhalation increases the risk of respiratory disease. Knowledge assists parents in making decision about positive health practices.	At first well-child visit, parents describe measures instituted to provide smoke-free environment for neonate. At the first well-child visit, parents describe safety features that have been instituted in the home.

SUMMARY

Immediately after birth the nurse assesses the neonate's adjustment to the extrauterine environment. The Apgar score, one of the first methods used to assess the newborn, provides a determination of physiologic status and the need for possible resuscitation. Screening techniques, including tests for phenylketonuria, thyroid function, and hearing, are also performed.

Comprehensive neonatal assessment is essential in establishing a healthy and supportive beginning for the neonate's care. This assessment includes physiologic, psychologic, developmental, and sociocultural parameters of health. Assessment begins with a thorough history that allows the nurse to gain a complete picture of the neonate and family. The first physical examination of the newborn is performed at delivery. This is followed by a more comprehensive examination within the first 24 hours. The nurse should ensure that parents are present during this examination, if possible, as this promotes parents' understanding of normal findings and helps to allay fears about normal neonatal variations. The nurse also plays an important role in assisting parents' transition to their new roles.

Comprehensive assessment includes gestational age and behavioral assessments. Various tools can be used by the nurse when examining the neurologic and behavioral responses of the neonate, including the Neonatal Perception Inventory and the Brazelton Neonatal Behavioral Assessment Scale. Based on data from neonatal assessment, the nurse develops nursing diagnoses and plans comprehensive care for the neonate and his or her family.

REVIEW QUESTIONS

1. Describe the assessment parameters of the Apgar score.
2. Discuss the importance of performing a physical examination with the neonate's parents in attendance. How would the nurse use the findings of the examination to promote parent-newborn interaction?
3. What is the relationship between gestational age and weight?
4. Discuss how the Brazelton Neonatal Behavioral Assessment Scale can assist the nurse in the care of the neonate and family.
5. Discuss the role of the nurse who cares for neonates and their families. What are the responsibilities the nurse assumes by virtue of this role?

REFERENCES

1. Kraybill EN. Needs of the term infant. In: Avery G, ed. *Neonatology, Pathophysiology and Management of the Newborn.* 3rd ed. Philadelphia: JB Lippincott; 1987.
2. Apgar V. A proposal for a new method of evaluating the newborn infant. *Curr Res Anesth Analg.* 1953;July/Aug: 260.
3. Bliss-Holz J. Comparison of rectal, axillary, and inguinal temperatures of full-term newborn infants. *Nur Res.* 1989;38: 85–87.
4. Mayfield SR, et al. Temperature measurement in term and preterm neonates. *J Pediatr.* 1984;104:271–275.
5. AAP Committee on Fetus and Newborn and ACOG Committee on Obstetrics. *Guidelines for Perinatal Care.* Evanston, Ill: American Academy of Pediatrics; 1983.
6. Richards JM, et al. Sequential 22-hour profiles of breathing patterns and heart rate in 110 full-term infants during their first 6 months of life. *Pediatrics.* 1984;74:763–777.
7. Schacter J, et al. Heart rate and blood pressure in black newborns and in white newborns. *Pediatrics.* 1976;58: 283–287.
8. Smith CA, Nelson NM. *The Physiology of the Newborn Infant.* 4th ed. Springfield, Ill: Charles C Thomas; 1976:162–163
9. Prechtl H, Beintema D. *The Neurological Examination of the Full Term Infant.* Child Development Medical Series. Philadelphia: Lippincott; 1975:vol 12.
10. Faix RG. Fontanelle size in black and white term newborn infants. *J Pediatr.* 1982;100:304–306.
11. Okada DM, et al. Neonatal scalp abscess and fetal monitoring: factors associated with infection. *Am J Obstet Gynecol.* 1977;12:185–189.
12. Freed MD. Disorder of the cardiovascular system. In: Avery ME, Taeusch HW, eds. *Schaffer's Diseases of the Newborn.* 5th ed. Philadelphia: WB Saunders; 1984:part 4.
13. Avery ME, Taeusch HW, eds. *Schaffer's Diseases of the Newborn.* 5th ed. Philadelphia: WB Saunders; 1984:ch 40.
14. Navah Y, Berant M. Assessment of liver size in normal infants and children. *J Pediatr Gastroenterol Nutr.* 1984;3: 346–348.
15. Bamji M, et al. Palpable lymph nodes in healthy newborns and infants. *Pediatrics.* 1988;78:573–575.
16. Battaglia FC, Lubchenco LO. A practical classification of newborn infants by weight and gestational age. *J Pediatr.* 1967;71:159–163.
17. Dubowitz LM, et al. Clinical assessment of gestational age in the newborn infant. *J Pediatr.* 1970;77:1–10.
18. Ballard JL, et al. A simplified score for assessment of fetal maturation in newly born infants. *J Pediatr.* 1979;95:769–774.
19. Broussard ER, Hartner MS. Further considerations regarding maternal perception of the first born. In: Hellmuth J, ed. *Exceptional Infant: Studies in Abnormalities.* New York: Brunner/Mazel; 1971:vol 2, 432–439.
20. Brazelton TB. *Neonatal Behavioral Assessment Scale.* 2nd ed. Philadelphia: JB Lippincott; 1984.

Nursing Care of the Neonate and Infant in the First Year

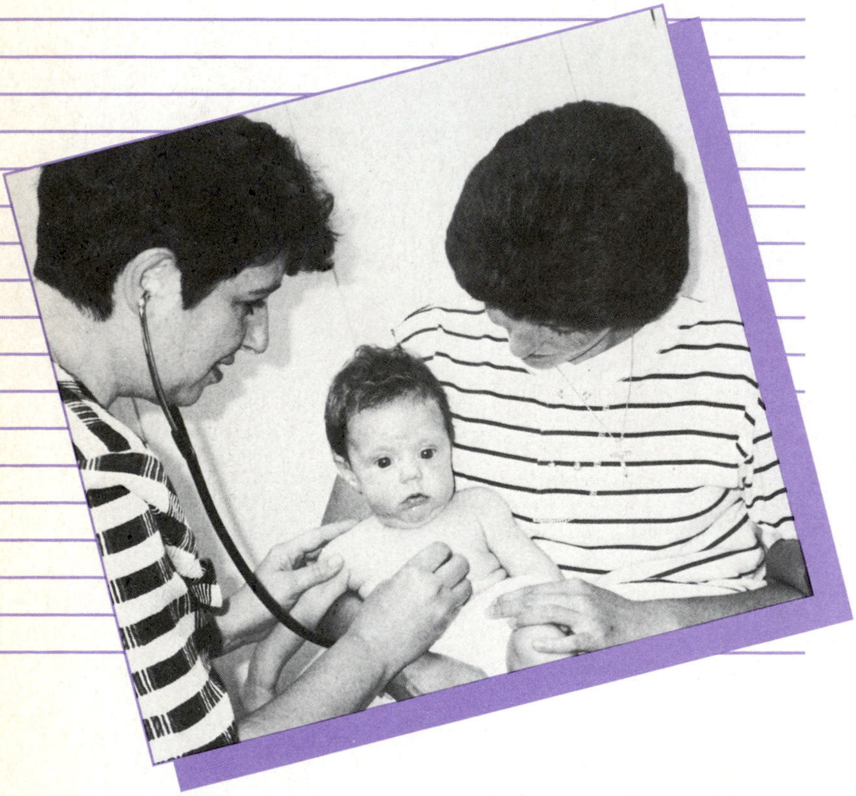

chapter 34

Key Terms

active immunity
cephalocaudal
clubfoot
colic
cradle cap
diaper dermatitis
fever
irritability
passive immunity
proximodistal
temperament
thrush

Physical and psychosocial adjustment to extrauterine life begins in the immediate newborn period. Maturation of body systems and sensory functions continues throughout infancy and into childhood. The first year of life lays the foundation for growth and development throughout childhood. Interaction between the infant and the environment, physical status, genetic endowment, and responses of caretakers are major determinants of the extent to which growth and development occur.

The period of infancy begins in the neonatal period and is characterized by rapid biologic, psychologic, social, cognitive, and verbal development. There is no other comparable period in the life cycle of human beings. During the first year, the infant increases in weight three-fold, makes the transition from relative immobility to a predictive progression of stages that result in the ability to walk independently, and metamorphoses into a socially responsive being with clearly identifiable personality traits.

Nursing care begins in the newborn period and focuses on preventive measures that protect the infant. Promotion of parent-newborn attachment begins at birth and continues throughout the first year. Discharge planning is important in anticipating needs of families and their newborns.

This chapter discusses goals of nursing care and selected parental concerns during the neonatal period and the first year of life. Maternity nurses coordinate care with community and pediatric nurses in an effort to provide continuity and holistic nursing services to families and their newborns. Nurses assist family members to promote the health and well-being of the neonate and infant, and educate parents about normal growth and development parameters and care of common problems that may occur during infancy.

NURSING CARE OF THE NEONATE

The immediate neonatal period is usually a time of joy and relief for parents. They usually are also somewhat apprehensive about the well-being of their newborn and their new roles as parents. Nursing care in the immediate neonatal period focuses on assisting the newborn to adjust to his or her environment and assisting family members to adjust to their new roles. Several goals guide nursing care of the newborn in this period, including: maintenance of a patent airway, promotion of thermoregulation, prevention of hemorrhage, prevention of infection, promotion of initial parent-newborn attachment, identification of the newborn, promotion of nutritional well being, and meeting the educational needs of parents. Through discharge planning, the nurse ensures follow-up care for the newborn and family after they leave the health care facility.

Maintenance of a Patent Airway

Immediately after delivery, the newborn may need suctioning to remove fluid from the mouth and nares. Suctioning should be done gently with a bulb syringe or other neonatal suction, removing fluid first from the newborn's mouth and then from the nares (Figure 34–1). If the nares are suctioned first, the newborn may be stimulated to develop an inspiratory gasp which may cause aspiration of fluid into the lungs.

The newborn with good respiratory effort and heart rate needs little suctioning beyond that done initially with the bulb syringe. Excessive suctioning may produce trauma, with mucosal swelling and partial occlusion of the airways.[1] Drainage can be facilitated by placing the newborn in a side-lying position. A bulb syringe should be placed by the crib in the event that further suctioning is necessary.

Adequacy of respiratory effort is determined by observation and auscultation of breath sounds and heart rate. If the pulse rate is over 100 beats per minute and respiratory movements are observed, or if the newborn is crying, the transition from intrauterine to extrauterine life is assumed to be progressing normally. Close observation of the newborn, however, is still essential during the first days of life.

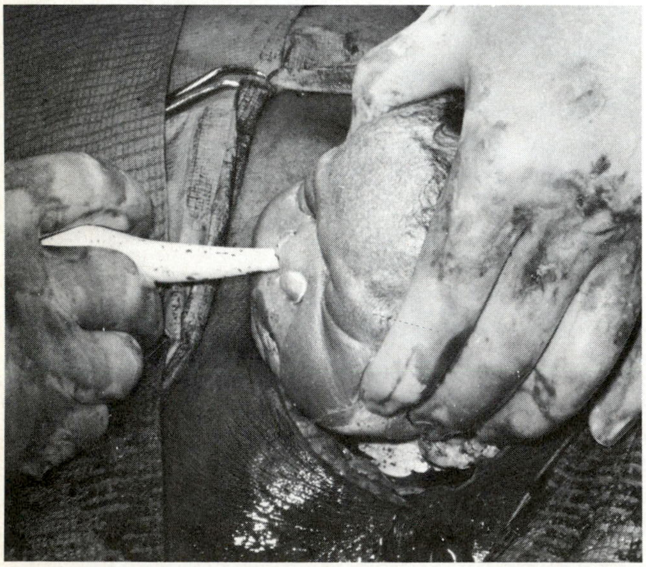

Figure 34–1. Immediately after delivery the newborn's nose and mouth are suctioned. (*Reproduced, with permission, from Cunningham FG, et al.* Williams Obstetrics. *18th ed. Norwalk, Conn: Appleton & Lange; 1989:236.*)

Promotion of Thermoregulation

Newborns lose heat through radiation, evaporation, conduction, and convection when exposed to cold (*see* Chapter 32). Initial nursing care thus includes maintenance of a neutral thermal environment for the newborn. Table 34–1 summarizes principles guiding management of thermoregulation in the newborn.

Several methods are important to achieving and maintaining thermoneutrality in the newborn. They include drying the newborn's body at delivery; the use of servocontrolled heaters, incubators, and overhead radiant heaters; and cot nursing. The warm body of the mother also plays a significant role in achieving thermoneutrality.

Drying the Newborn's Body. The decrease in core and skin temperatures is most rapid immediately after birth. A substantial amount of heat is lost through evaporation from the wet body of the newborn. Newborns who remain wet in a delivery room have a mean decline in rectal temperature of 2.1°C (3.8°F) and a mean decline in skin temperature of 4.6°C (8.3°F) within 30 minutes of birth. In contrast, newborns who are dried and placed under a radiant heater experience a decline in core temperature of only 0.7°C (1.3°F) and a decrease in skin temperature of 0.8°C (1.5°F).

TABLE 34–1. PRINCIPLES GUIDING MANAGEMENT OF THERMOREGULATION IN THE NEWBORN

The goal of temperature control for the newborn is thermoneutrality.
Stability of body temperature causes minimal stress to the newborn.
The neutral thermal environment is the environment in which a newborn with a normal body temperature has minimal oxygen consumption and nutritional requirements associated with heat production.
Below the neutral thermal range (also termed the critical temperature range), a metabolic response to cold is necessary for heat production.
Above the neutral thermal range, the newborn may become hyperthermic.
Newborns lose heat by radiation, conduction, convection, and evaporation.
Evaporative heat loss may occur rapidly from the newborn's moist body at delivery. Drying the newborn immediately on delivery is thus very important.
Newborns produce heat when under cold stress, mainly through nonshivering thermogenesis.
No single environmental temperature is appropriate for all sizes of newborns (full term, preterm).

Simply drying and wrapping the newborn in a warm blanket also diminishes heat loss considerably.[2] The importance of drying the newborn cannot be overemphasized. A family-centered approach to care includes drying and wrapping newborns and giving them to their mother and father to cuddle.

Servocontrolled Heaters. Because the newborn has a narrow optimal temperature range, some institutions use servocontrolled heaters to regulate incubator temperatures. A sensing thermistor is placed on the newborn's abdomen; this adjusts the incubator air temperature to the temperature of the newborn.

Disadvantages of servocontrolled devices are that they can cause fluctuations in incubator temperatures when the position of the sensor changes as a result of handling or movement. Further, these fluctuations can subject the newborn to overheating and cold stress.[3] Also, is not clearly documented that these devices are useful in managing the newborn's temperature.

Incubators. Incubators are one of the most commonly used devices for heating the newborn. In an incubator, the newborn is heated by convection; however, because temperature of the walls of the incubator cannot be controlled, the newborn may lose heat through radiation (warm skin of the newborn to the cool walls of the incubator). In an effort to prevent radiant heat loss in incubators, some incubators are equipped with clear cylindrical plastic heat shields. Radiant losses are diminished by the use of the shield because the warm incubator air heats the shield to the same temperature as the air within the incubator. The newborn radiates heat only to the plastic shield instead of to the cooler walls of the incubator.[4]

Radiant Heaters. Radiant heaters (Figure 34–2) are warming panels that are placed above the newborn in an effort to prevent heat loss through radiation. These devices provide heat from infrared energy. Under the radiant heater, radiant losses are reduced; however, convective and evaporative losses are markedly increased because of the increased insensible water loss. Perspex heat shields have been used in an effort to prevent this evaporative water loss. Although radiant heaters are generally more convenient in intensive-care situations, well-humidified incubators may provide a more stable thermal environment.[3]

Cot Nursing. *Cot nursing* is the term used when caring for the newborn in a dressed, rather than naked, state. Lightly dressing the newborn minimizes the effects of fluctuations in environmental temperature and maintains thermoneutrality.[4] Further, some studies have found that placing a hat of wool and gauze on the newborn's head will prevent heat loss from the head and help control the thermal environment.[5]

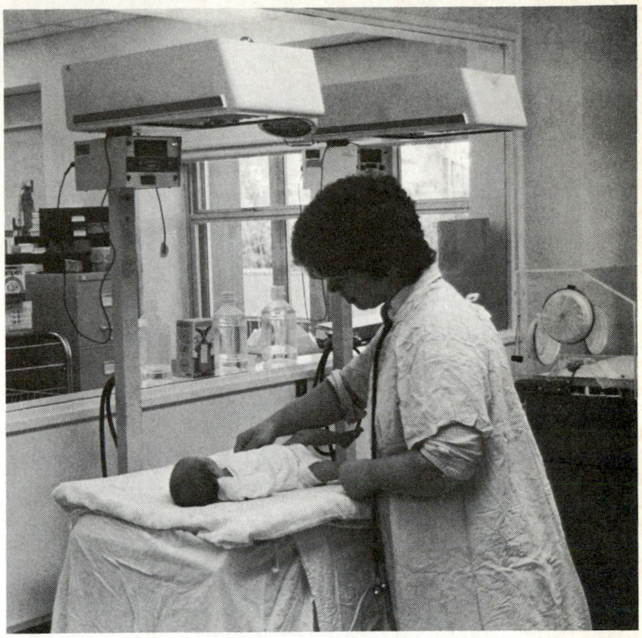

Figure 34–2. Nurse assessing newborn in a radiant warmer.

Parent-Newborn Contact. Early parent-newborn contact is a principle of a family-centered approach to care. Research has shown that contact with one or both parents in the delivery room is a method for controlling the newborn's temperature.[6,7] Hill and Shronk[6] found that when newborns were properly dried and wrapped and given to one or both of their parents, their temperatures were similar to those of newborns who were immediately placed in a heated transporter. This inexpensive way to regulate the newborn's temperature has the added benefit of promoting parent-newborn attachment in the delivery room.

Prevention of Hemorrhage

Newborns have a deficiency of vitamin K–dependent factors, which places them at risk for bleeding. A prophylactic injection of vitamin K (phytonadione) is therefore given to prevent neonatal hemorrhagic disease (Box 34–1).

Prevention of Infection

Preventing infection is important in the neonatal period. Scrupulous handwashing by health care workers is probably the single most important factor in preventing infections in the nursery. Some birthing institutions require that health care workers perform a 3 to 5 minute scrub of the hands and arms before

BOX 34–1. PHYTONADIONE (VITAMIN K)

Proprietary Names: Mephyton (MSD), Aqua-Mephyton (MSD), Konakion (Roche).

Classification:
Vitamin.

Action:
Same activity as naturally occurring vitamin K, which is required in the synthesis of blood coagulation factors II, VII, IX, and X in the liver.

Indications:
Prophylaxis and treatment of hemorrhagic disease of the newborn.

Dosage and Route:
Administered orally, IM or IV. *Hemorrhagic disease of newborn*: 0.5–1.0 mg IM immediately after delivery and repeated after 6–8 hours if necessary. Alternatively, 1–2 mg may be given orally immediately after delivery and repeated after 12–48 hours if necessary.

Pharmacokinetics:
Absorption: Absorbed from gastrointestinal tract after oral ingestion only in the presence of bile salts. *Distribution*: Concentrates in liver. Crosses the placenta in only limited amounts, and distributes into breast milk. *Elimination*: Limited data.

Contraindications and Precautions:
Caution when given IV because of risk of anaphylactic-type reaction. Use only in emergency situations.

Adverse Reactions:
Relatively nontoxic. *IV administration-related*: Cardiac irregularities, chest pain, cyanosis, convulsive movements, dulled consciousness, flushing of face, circulatory collapse, bronchospasm, rapid and weak pulse, shock, and death. *IM administration-related*: Pain, swelling, tenderness at injection site.

Drug Interactions:
Warfarin: Vitamin K antagonizes anticoagulant activity.

Nursing Implications:

- Injected IM into the lateral aspect of the thigh.
- Observe injection site for hematoma, redness, and nodule formation.
- Store in light-resistant containers as light will destroy medication.

IM = intramuscular(ly), IV = intravenous(ly).

entering the nursery at the beginning of the shift. At the least, health care workers should wash their hands with soap and water before caring for each newborn. In addition, health care workers who have infections should not care for newborns.

In the United States many birthing institutions also have specific regulations aimed at preventing infections in the nursery. They require that special clothing be worn by health care workers and those visiting the nursery. A scrub gown is usually worn by nurses and other health care workers and a cover gown by those visiting the nursery such as the father of the newborn or the physician or nurse-midwife. In addition, health care workers use universal precautions to protect against spread of HIV and other blood-borne or body fluid–borne infections. Newborns have their own equipment and cribs in an effort to prevent infection. Other measures implemented to prevent infection in the newborn include neonatal eye care and cord care.

Eye Care. The most common organism causing neonatal ophthalmia in the United States today is chlamydia. The incidence of gonococcal ophthalmia is approximately 0.04 percent in comparison to chlamydial ophthalmia, which is 0.4 percent.[8]

Prenatal care should routinely include culturing maternal cervical secretions for gonococci and treatment of women who are infected. Even when this is done, the routine use of a prophylactic agent in the newborn's eyes is recommended to prevent infection with *Neisseria gonorrhoeae* (ophthalmia neonatorum, which can cause neonatal blindness).

Prophylactic agents that are currently recommended for instillation into the newborn's eyes to prevent gonococcal ophthalmia include: erythromycin, 0.5% ophthalmic ointment or drops in single-dose tubes or ampules; tetracycline, 1 percent ophthalmic ointment or drops in single-dose tubes or ampules and 1 percent silver nitrate solution in single-dose ampules (Box 34–2). One of these agents is instilled into the eyes of the newborn shortly after birth. It is recommended that the agent not be flushed from the eyes after the application.[9]

The nurse instills the medication by pulling down on the lower eyelid and instilling drops or ointment into the lower conjunctival sac (Figure 34–3). The eyes are then closed so that the medication can permeate the eyes. The medications, especially silver nitrate, can cause mild conjunctivitis which may interfere with the quiet alert state of the newborn. For this reason, eye prophylaxis is often delayed up to an hour to facilitate initial interactions between parents and their newborns.

BOX 34–2. SILVER NITRATE ($AgNO_3$)

Proprietary Names:
Dey-Drop, Dey (Lilly).

Classification:
Anti-infective ophthalmic.

Action:
Silver ions combine with chemical groups on the surface of the bacteria causing substantial changes in the cell wall and membrane, precipitating bacterial proteins.

Indications:
Prophylaxis of gonococcal ophthalmia neonatorum.

Dosage and Route:
Administered topically only, after delivery. After the newborn's eyes have been cleaned, 2 drops of 1 percent solution are instilled into lower conjunctival sac of each eye. Eyelids should be elevated from the eyeball to allow the solution to come into contact with the entire conjunctival sac and eye for 30 seconds.

Pharmacokinetics:
No significant absorption occurs.

Contraindications and Precautions:
Avoid contact with skin or other surfaces because of possible irritation and stain.

Adverse Reactions:
Mild chemical conjunctivitis during first 6 hours after application, but resolving by 24 hours. Solutions more concentrated than 1 percent may cause serious damage to the eye.

Nursing Implications:

- Puncture container; instill 2 drops in subconjunctival area after lowering lid; close newborn's eyes.
- Caution should be taken to avoid contact with skin.
- Delay instilling drops in eyes until parents have had opportunity for eye-to-eye contact.
- Observe for chemical conjunctivitis.

Silver nitrate is inexpensive and has a long record of providing good protection against gonococcal infections. It does not, however, protect the newborn from ophthalmic infections caused by chlamydia.[8]

In contrast, treatment to prevent chlamydial ophthalmia aims at detection and treatment of the condition in the pregnant woman. If the newborn becomes infected, the treatment of choice is orally administered erythromycin, 50 mg/kg/day in three or four divided doses for 10 to 14 days. Topical therapy of the newborn's eyes has been associated with a 60 to 80 percent failure rate,[8] as compared to a 10 to 20 percent failure rate for systemically administered erythromycin.

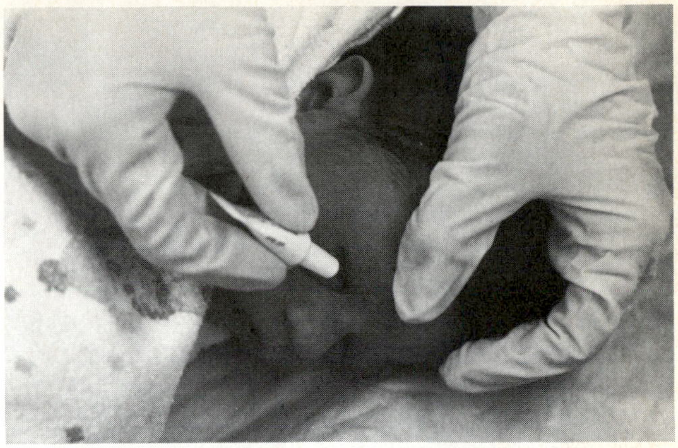

Figure 34–3. Eye prophylaxis using erythromycin ointment.

Cord Care. The cord is clamped in the delivery room and the clamp remains in place at least 24 hours (Figure 34–4). Some nurseries apply an aseptic solution such as triple-dye, erythromycin solution, or alcohol to the cord to prevent infection. Triple-dye causes the cord to turn dark blue. The nurse explains this procedure to parents, and assures them that this is a normal reaction.

The nurse observes the cord for signs of hemorrhage or infection. If bleeding is noted, a second clamp is applied and the physician notified.

Promotion of Initial Parent-Newborn Attachment

The nurse can help to promote initial parent-newborn attachment by enabling the parents to hold and touch their newborn in the delivery room, if the parents so desire. As described in Chapter 32, all newborns experience a quiet-alert period (termed the first period of reactivity) during the 30 minutes immediately after birth. This is followed by a period of sleep or inactivity, lasting from minutes to 2 to 4 hours, and a second period of reactivity, lasting 4 to 6 hours. Table 34–2 outlines the newborn's physiologic and behavioral responses and related nursing care during these periods.

During the first and second periods of reactivity, the nurse can promote attachment behaviors between newborns and parents. Because the newborn demonstrates good sucking reflexes during the first period of reactivity, if the mother wishes to breastfeed she

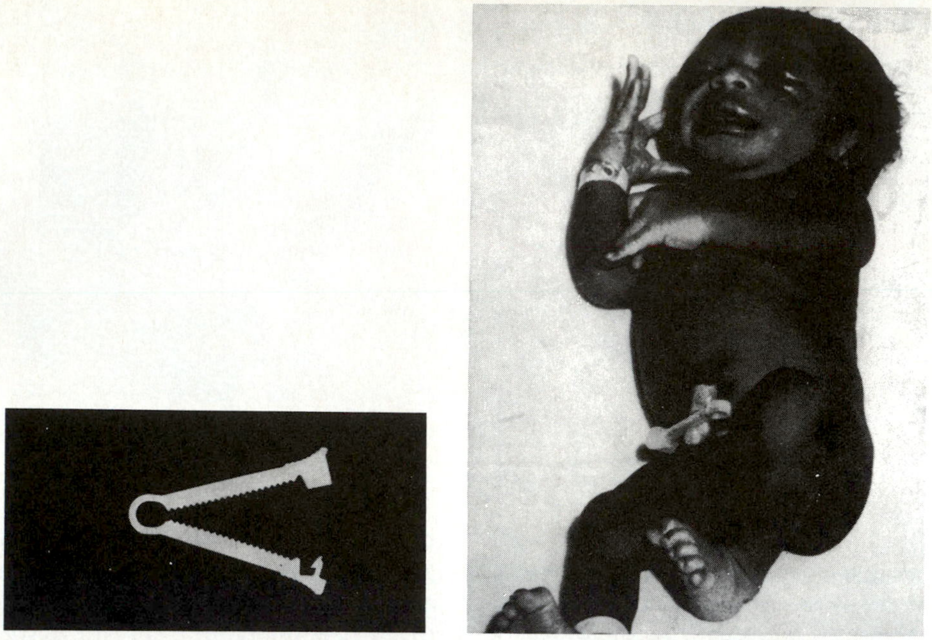

Figure 34–4. Plastic cord clamp. These clamps lock in place and cannot slip. They are removed on the second or third day by simply cutting the loop, or they can be allowed to drop off with the cord. *(Reproduced, with permission, from Cunningham FG, et al.* Williams Obstetrics. *18th ed. Norwalk, Conn: Appleton & Lange; 1989:319.)*

can be encouraged to put the newborn to breast at this time. Eye prophylaxis should be delayed to promote newborn-parent attachment through eye-to-eye contact and routine newborn care provided in a manner that will not interfere with this initial acquaintance period.

Identification of Newborn

Identification of the newborn usually is done using ankle and wrist bracelets for the newborn and a wrist bracelet for the mother. The same information is placed on each bracelet and includes mother's name, sex of newborn, hospital number, and date and time of delivery. The nurse prepares and places the identification bracelets on the mother and newborn before they leave the delivery room. Some states require footprinting of the newborn (Figure 34–5), although this is probably not a reliable method of identification (a perfect print of the great toe would have to be made to reliably identify the newborn).

Promotion of Nutritional Well-Being

One of the first acts of parenting is feeding the newborn. Parents, especially mothers, tend to judge their parenting skills by how well the newborn feeds on the breast or bottle and how much weight the newborn is gaining. If problems occur with the feeding experience, parents often become frustrated and their confidence as caretakers may be affected.

Nutritional Needs of the Newborn/Infant. The Food and Nutrition Board bases its recommended dietary allowances for infants during the first 6 months of life on the nutrients in human milk and the amount of that milk ingested by healthy infants of well-nourished mothers.[10] The Recommended Dietary Allowances (RDAs) are used as a guide in predicting the nutritional requirements for each infant.

Infants need the same nutrients as older children and adults; however, a larger quantity of each nutrient is needed per unit of infant body weight. For example, the infant needs 115 kcal/kg body weight during the first 6 months of life as compared with the adult female, who needs 36 kcal/kg body weight. The infant's kilocalorie need per unit of weight is therefore more than three times that of the adult.[11] Table 34–3 identifies the RDAs for normal infants from 0 to 6 months and 6 months to one year.

Energy Needs. Immediately after birth, the newborn's energy requirement is approximately 120 kcal/kg per day, and for the next 6 months of life, ranges from 95 to 145 kcal/kg per day. From 6 months to 1 year, infants require from 70 to 135 kcal/kg per day, with an energy requirement of 100 kcal/kg per day at the end of the first year. The RDA for energy is 115 kcal/kg per day (52 kcal/pound) during the first 6 months and 105 kcal/kg per day (47 kcal/pound) during the second 6 months.[10]

TABLE 34–2. PHYSIOLOGIC AND BEHAVIORAL RESPONSES OF NEWBORNS DURING THE PERIODS OF REACTIVITY

Period	Behavioral Response	Physiologic Response	Nursing Intervention
First period of reactivity (first 30 minutes after birth)	Quiet alertness, followed by active alertness; eyes are bright and open; attention focused on the environment, especially human faces and mother's voice; active alertness is accompanied by bursts of movement of the extremities; strong sucking reflex is evident	Respirations are shallow and rapid (may be as high as 80/min); transient flaring of nares may be present, as well as grunting and retractions of the chest; heart rate is rapid and irregular (range 120 to 150 beats per minute); bowel sounds are absent	Assess vital signs. Maintain patent airway. Dry newborn immediately at birth and maintain a neutral thermal environment. Provide opportunities for parent-newborn attachment (holding, talking to newborn, eye-to-eye contact). Delay prophylactic eye treatment so that newborn can focus on parents' faces. Assist in putting newborn to breast if desired by mother.
Period of sleep or inactivity (follows first period of reactivity and may last minutes to 2 to 4 hours)	Relatively unresponsive; difficult to awaken; shows no interest in sucking	Respiratory and heart rates return to baseline; posture relaxed; bowel sounds present; temperature may drop	Assess vital signs. Maintain a neutral thermal environment. Provide opportunities for parents to hold newborn. Explain difficulty in initiating feeding during this state.
Second period of reactivity (begins after sleep period and may last 4 to 6 hours)	Awake and alert; varies from quiet alertness to active alertness and crying	Respiratory and heart rates may change rapidly; periods of tachypnea and apnea may occur; may produce gastric and respiratory mucus; may regurgitate and gag; may have transient color changes; bowel sounds increase; sucking; rooting, and swallowing apparent	Assess vital signs, activity, color and tone. Maintain patent airway by positioning newborn on side and possibly suctioning nasal and oral cavities. Assist mother to begin feeding. Promote attachment behaviors by allowing parents to hold and talk to newborn.

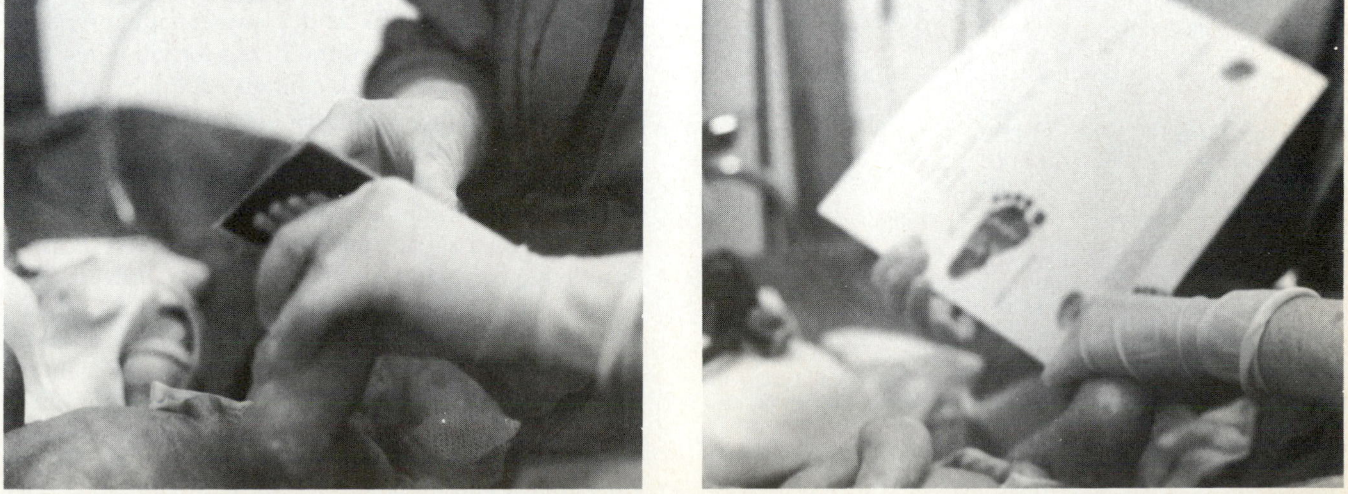

Figure 34–5. Footprints may be taken before the newborn leaves the delivery room.

About one half of the total energy expenditure is accounted for by the basal metabolism of the infant. The basal metabolic rate (BMR) in infancy is high because of the need to regulate body temperature and maintain high levels of metabolic activities. Another one third of the total energy expenditure is accounted for by the normal rate of growth during the first 4 to 5 months. For the remainder of the first year, about one tenth of the energy requirement is needed for growth, whereas an increasing amount is needed for activity. Infants who are quiet and placid require less energy than those who are active and crying.[12]

Human milk and most commercially prepared formulas supply approximately 20 kcal/oz. The kilocaloric requirements of the infant are met by protein, carbohydrates, and fats.

TABLE 34–3. RDAS FOR NORMAL INFANTS DURING THE FIRST YEAR

	0-6 months	6-12 months
Weight		
kg	6	9
pounds	13	20
Height		
cm	60	71
inches	24	28
Nutrient	**RDA**	
Protein, g	13	14
Vitamin A, μg RE[a]	375	375
Vitamin D, μg[b]	7.5	10
Vitamin E, mg TE[c]	3	4
Vitamin K, mg	5	10
Ascorbic acid, mg	30	35
Thiamine, mg	0.3	0.4
Riboflavin, mg	0.4	0.5
Niacin, mg NE[d]	5	6
Vitamin B_6, mg	0.3	0.6
Vitamin B_{12}, μg	0.3	0.5
Folacin, μg	25	35
Calcium, mg	400	600
Phosphorus, mg	300	500
Magnesium, mg	40	60
Iodine, μg	40	50
Iron, mg	6	10
Zinc, mg	5	5
Selenium, μg	10	15

[a] Retinol equivalents. 1 retinol equivalent = 1 μg retinol or 6 μg betacarotene.
[b] As cholecalciferol. 10 μg cholecalciferol = 400 IU of vitamin D.
[c] Alpha-tocopherol equivalents. 1 mg d-alpha-tocopherol = 1 alpha-TE.
[d] 1 NE (niacin equivalent) is equal to 1 mg of niacin or 60 mg of dietary tryptophan.
Source: *Food and Nutrition Board.* Recommended Dietary Allowances. *Revised 1989. 10th ed. Washington, DC: National Research Council-National Academy of Sciences; 1990.*

Protein. During the first 4 months of life, infants add about 3.5 g of protein daily to their bodies. From age 4 months to 1 year, they add 3.1 g of protein daily. The increase in body protein in the first year ranges from 11 to 14.6 g.[10,12]

Human milk provides the infant with about 2.2 g protein per kilogram per day during the first month of life. By the sixth month, protein in breast milk has fallen to 1.5 g/kg per day. The RDA for protein for the first 6 months is 13 g per day, and during the second 6 months, 14 g per day.[10]

Carbohydrates. Lactose accounts for about 40 percent of the calories in human milk. The lactose content of human milk is higher than that of cow's milk. For this reason, lactose or other simple carbohydrates are added to commercial formulas. Several carbohydrates, including sucrose, dextrose, destrin, maltose, and corn syrup solids, are added to commercial formulas to modify flavor. Other carbohydrates that are added to formulas to modify consistency are arrowroot starch, cornstarch, and tapioca starch.[11] The Food and Nutrition Board does not include a recommended daily carbohydrate allowance for infants.

Fats. Fat is needed during infancy to meet the high energy requirements of growth and development. Approximately 45 to 50 percent of the calories in human milk and most formulas is provided by fat. The fat linoleate supplies 6 to 9 percent of the calories in human milk. Formulas that furnish 3 percent of the calories as linoleic acid will meet the infant's needs.[10]

Low-fat formulas for infants are contraindicated because it is difficult to achieve sufficient caloric intake for weight gain and brain development without sufficient intake of fats.[12]

Vitamins. Human milk and commercially prepared formulas furnish most of the RDAs for vitamins. Human milk and cow's milk contain adequate amounts of A and B-complex vitamins; however, although human milk also meets the ascorbic acid (vitamin C) needs of the infant, cow's milk does not. Thus, most commercial formulas are fortified with ascorbic acid. If the formula is not fortified with ascorbic acid, a supplement should be given. The RDA allowance for ascorbic acid is 30 mg per day for the first 6 months of life,[10] and 35 mg per day for the second 6 months.[10]

The only vitamin that is somewhat deficient in human milk is vitamin D. The RDA for vitamin D is 10 μg (400 IU) per day during the first year of life. Commercial formulas are fortified with vitamin D. Breastfed infants can obtain the required vitamin D through exposure to sunlight, a good source of the vitamin.

Vitamin K is deficient in the newborn at birth. The synthesis of vitamin K is delayed for several days after birth because the newborn lacks the necessary intestinal bacterial flora. An intramuscular injection of 0.5 to 1.0 mg of vitamin K (vitamin K_1) is therefore recommended at birth to prevent neonatal hemorrhage.

Minerals. Human milk and commercially prepared formulas fulfill most of the RDAs for minerals. Ensuring adequate iron intake probably requires the most attention in infancy. The iron stores of a healthy infant of a well-nourished mother are adequate for the first 4 to 6 months of postnatal life. The average need of the infant for iron is 1.5 mg/kg per day. The RDA for iron is 6 mg daily for the first 6 months of life and 10 mg daily for the next 6 months.[10]

Although the iron content of breast milk is low, about one half of the iron present in breast milk is absorbed by the infant. Contrast this with the 10 percent rate of iron absorption from formulas.[12]

Breastfed infants obtain 60 mg calcium per kilogram body weight. The RDA for this mineral is 60 mg/kg per day.[10] Breastfed infants retain about 50 to 60 percent of their total calcium intake. Bottlefed infants, on the other hand, retain only 25 to 30 percent of the total calcium intake from cow's milk formula; however, as formulas contain a higher proportion of calcium than breast milk, the net retention is the same.[12]

The RDAs for salt, magnesium, zinc, and iodine are met by both breast milk and formulas. Many pediatricians and nurse practitioners recommend fluoride supplementation for infants who are breastfed (as little fluoride is transmitted in the breast milk) and for infants who live in areas where the fluoride concentration in the water supply is low (Box 34–3). Fluoride is needed to prevent dental caries. There is, however, still some controversy over whether fluoride should be added to water supplies or supplemented in the diet.

Water. An infant requires more water relative to body weight than an adult because the infant's kidneys are unable to concentrate waste efficiently. An infant therefore excretes more water to carry off wastes than an adult. Daily water excretion of the infant is high, about 15 percent of the body weight. The RDA for water is about 150 mL/100 kg body weight.

The water needs of the infant are usually met by

BOX 34–3. FLUORIDE

Proprietary Names:
Pediaflor Drops (Ross), Karidium Liquid (Lorvic), Luride Drops (Colgate-Hoyt), Flura Drops (Kirkman), many others.

Classification:
Fluoride supplement.

Action:
Is incorporated into and stabilizes apatite crystal of teeth and bone, and increases the resistance to acid dissolution and formation of dental caries.

Indications:
Provides protection against dental caries, particularly in areas where the fluoride concentration in drinking water is 0.7 ppm or less.

Dosage and Route:
Administered orally. *Oral supplement*: If fluoride in drinking water is < 0.3 ppm: 0–2 years old, 0.25 mg/day; 2–3 years old, 0.5 mg/day; 3–13 years old, 1 mg/day. If fluoride in drinking water is 0.3–0.7 ppm: < 2 years old, none; 2–3 years old, 0.25 mg/day; 3–13 years old, 0.5 mg/day. Oral solutions may be mixed with foods or juices.

Pharmacokinetics:
Absorption: Completely absorbed from gastrointestinal tract after oral administration. *Distribution*: Distributes primarily into bone and teeth. Crosses the placenta and into breast milk. *Elimination*: Rapidly excreted by kidneys.

Contraindications and Precautions:
Contraindicated in areas where fluoride ion in drinking water is greater than 0.7 ppm.

Adverse Reactions:
Result from overdosage. *GI*—hypersalivation, salty taste, nausea, vomiting, abdominal pain, diarrhea; *MS*—muscle weakness; *CNS*—tremors, seizures; *CV*—shock, death; *other*—urticaria, dehydration.

Nursing Implications:

- Assess level of fluoride in drinking water and whether parents will be using water to prepare formula.
- Teach parents how to administer drops (aim dropper toward side of cheek, slowly administer).
- Teach parents warning signs of overdosage.

GI = gastrointestinal system, MS = musculoskeletal system, CNS - central nervous system, CV = cardiovascular system.

breast milk and properly prepared formulas, containing 5 to 10 percent sugar and enough water to make the concentration 65 to 70 kcal/dL.[11] Infants may need additional water if dehydration is a possibility, for example, when the infant is exposed to high environmental temperatures or suffers from vomiting and diarrhea.

Differences Between Human Milk and Cow's Milk. The most balanced food available for the infant is human milk. The nutrients found in human milk are more easily digestible than those contained in cow's milk or artificial formulas. Moreover, the relatively high lactose level, relatively low protein and phosphorus levels, and high vitamin C level of human milk facilitate increased iron absorption.[13]

Sixty percent of the protein in human milk consists of lactalbumin, which has an amino acid composition very similar to that of human body tissues. In contrast, only 15 percent of the protein in cow's milk is lactalbumin. The higher percentage of lactalbumin in human milk makes it more easily digestible than cow's milk or artificial formulas. The remaining protein in both human and cow's milk is primarily casein. As whey is easier to digest, the increased whey-to-casein protein ratio in human milk, along with the zinc-binding proteins, also make the absorption and utilization of human milk higher than that of cow's milk or artificial formulas.[13]

Human milk contains a large amount of unsaturated fatty acids. The level of linoleic acid is higher in human milk than in cow's milk. In addition, newborns absorb about 95 to 98 percent of the fat because of the high lipase activity present in human milk, which is not heat treated. Only about 80 percent of the fat from a milk-based formula is absorbed by the neonate.[12]

Although human milk and cow's milk are both low in iron, the iron in human milk is absorbed better than the iron in cow's milk. Cow's milk contains higher levels of calcium, phosphorus, sodium, and potassium than human milk; however, more calcium is retained from human milk than from cow's milk. Also, the balance of minerals in human milk is sufficient to meet the newborn's needs.

Human milk furnishes the ascorbic acid needs of the infant, whereas cow's milk does not. There is also more vitamin A in human milk than in cow's milk. Both milks are deficient in vitamin D. Additional components present in human milk include folate and thyroid hormone. These are important for DNA synthesis and growth.[14]

Formulas

Commercially Prepared Formulas. Commercially prepared formulas (eg, Enfamil, Similac, SMA) are patterned on the nutrient content of human milk, although none of the formulas is identical to human milk. Many of the commercially prepared formulas are based on cow's milk, using nonfat dry milk. There are several adaptations[12]:

- Protein content is decreased; protein is treated to produce a fine, flocculent, easily digested curd
- Butterfat is removed, and vegetable oils, such as corn oil, are substituted to increase the lineoleic acid content
- Cholesterol content is reduced
- Lactose or other carbohydrates are added
- Levels of calcium, phosphorus, and other minerals are reduced by dilution
- Vitamins A, C (ascorbic acid), D, and E are added
- Iron may be added because of the infant's need for iron in the first year of life

Other formulas such as soy-based formulas are available instead of milk-based formulas for infants who have an intolerance to milk-based formulas. Soy-based formulas also are fortified with iron. Table 34–4 compares the constituents of several commercial formulas.

Commercially prepared formulas are available as liquid concentrates or powders or in ready-to-use forms. Parents should be taught about the different types of formulas and the appropriate method of preparation for each.

Evaporated Milk. Formulas prepared in the home usually use evaporated milk as the base. Whole milk or skim milk is not appropriate for the infant in the first year of life. Moreover, generic evaporated milk (not diluted with water) should be avoided.

In preparation of an evaporated milk formula, strict sanitary conditions as well as proper measurements are essential. The evaporated milk formula should be prepared fresh each day, and kept no longer than 24 hours to prevent contamination of unused milk. The ingredients are evaporated milk, 1 can (13 oz, 390 mL); water (18 oz, 540 mL); and corn syrup, 2 tablespoons. The evaporated milk preparation is then divided into the number of bottles that will be needed for 24 hours.

As the infant grows, the amount of evaporated milk in the formula is increased. By 4 to 6 months, equal amounts of water and evaporated milk are used. Honey should never be used in the preparation

TABLE 34–4. CONSTITUENTS OF SEVERAL COMMERCIAL FORMULAS[a]

	Infant Formulas					Soy Protein Formulas			
	Human Milk	SMA[b]	Similac w/FE[b]	Enfamil w/Fe[b]	Whole Cow Milk	Nursoy[b]	Isomil	Prosobee	I-Soyalac
Protein (W/V)[c]	1.2%	1.5%	1.5%	1.5%	3.4%	2.1%	1.8%	2.0%	2.1%
Casein	40%	40%	82%	40%	82%	—	—	—	—
Whey protein	60%	60%	18%	60%	18%	—	—	—	—
Fat (W/V)[c]	3.6%	3.6%	3.6%	3.8%	3.4%	3.6%	3.7%	3.6%	3.7%
% Polyunsaturated	14.2	14.5	41.2	31.8	4.0	14.5	37.1	28.9	60.5
% Monounsaturated	41.6	41.2	14.7	16.9	30.5	41.2	17.1	15.4	23.9
% Saturated	44.2	44.2	44.1	51.2	65.5	44.2	45.7	55.6	15.6
Vitamin E IU/L	3.4	9.5	20	21	1.3	9.5	20	21	16
Minerals (mg/100 mL [mEq/liter])									
Total (ash)	210	250	330	300	740	350	380	400	400
Na	15 (7)	15 (7)	22 (10)	18 (8)	51 (22)	20 (8.7)	32 (14)	29 (13)	28.5 (12)
K	55 (14)	56 (14)	81 (21)	72 (18)	157 (40.2)	70 (18)	95 (24)	78 (20)	79 (20)
Ca	34 (17)	42 (21)	51 (25)	46 (23)	123 (61.2)	60 (30)	71 (35)	63 (32)	69 (35)
P	14 (9)	28 (18)	39 (25)	32 (21)	96 (61.9)	42 (27)	51 (33)	50 (32)	48 (31)
Cl	37 (11)	37.5 (11)	51 (15)	42 (12)	96 (27.1)	37.5 (11)	44 (12)	55 (16)	53 (15)
Iron (per L)	0.8 mg	12 mg[d]	12 mg[d]	12.6 mg[d]	0.5 mg	11.5 mg	12 mg	12.7 mg	13 mg
Carbohydrate (W/V)[c]	7.2% (lactose)	7.2% (lactose)	7.2% (lactose)	6.9% (lactose)	4.8% (lactose)	6.9% (sucrose)	6.8% (corn syrup solids, sucrose)	6.8% (corn syrup solids)	6.8% (sucrose, tapioca dextrins)

[a] All data for competitive products derived from product labels, *Physicians Desk Reference*, or analyses.
[b] Concentrate with iron (standard dilution).
[c] W/V = weight per volume.
[d] SMA lo-iron, Enfamil, and Similac contain 1.4 mg iron per quart. Infants fed these formulas should receive supplemental dietary iron from an outside source to meet daily requirements.
Courtesy of Wyeth Labs, Philadelphia, PA; © 1986.

of the formula because of the possibility of infant botulism.

Safety of Formulas. The American Academy of Pediatrics, in 1976, proposed minimum levels for essential nutrients in infant formulas.[14] In 1980, the Infant Formula Act was passed by the federal government. This legislation requires that the Food and Drug Administration regulate the composition of all infant formulas so that safety and wholesomeness are ensured. Manufacturers of formula must keep accurate records, and notify the Food and Drug Administration about any proposed changes in composition of their products.

Safety also can be taught to parents with regard to formula preparation. Labels should be carefully read so that infants are not inadvertently given concentrated formula for ready-to-feed formula. Parents also should be taught sterilization techniques if these are deemed necessary (*see* later discussion).

Volume and Frequency of Feeding. Healthy newborns, whether breast or bottle fed, should be fed on a demand basis. They will regulate their feedings to their needs.

To calculate the amount of breast milk or formula needed by the infant, the following rule of thumb can be used:

Based on a kilocalorie need of 115 kcal/kg body weight, a 7 pound (3.18 kg) newborn should receive 115 kcal × 3.18 kg, or 365.6 kcal, daily. As breast milk and formulas contain 20 kcal/oz, the newborn requires 365.6 kcal divided by 20 kcal, or 18.28 oz of breast milk or formula.

Breastfed neonates will nurse between six and ten times a day. If they seem satisfied after nursing, urinate at least six times per day, and gain weight after the initial weight loss, they are receiving an adequate supply of milk.

Formula-fed neonates may feed six to eight times per day. They can usually go longer between feedings because formula is digested more slowly than breast milk thereby causing the neonate to feel satisfied longer. Formula-fed infants can be assessed for adequate intake by noting the number of bottles, and the amount of formula in each bottle consumed in a 24-hour period. Assessing the weight gain and the number of wet diapers also gives an indication of the nutritional status of the formula-fed newborn.

Initial Feeding. The breastfed newborn may be put to breast immediately after delivery or during the first period of reactivity if the mother so desires. Breastfeeding of newborns soon after birth promotes mother-newborn interaction. During the first period of reactivity the newborn is awake and alert and tends to latch onto the breast. The mother will have a sense of accomplishment if the newborn nurses even for a short period of time. An additional benefit of early breastfeeding is stimulation of lactation. If the newborn seems to have difficulty feeding, a sterile water feeding may be given to allow the nurse to assess for potential feeding problems.

Newborns who are bottle fed and those who have not nursed early may also be given sterile water. An initial feeding of a few milliliters of sterile water allows the nurse to assess the newborn's sucking, swallowing, and gag reflexes. Sterile water is used instead of glucose water or formula because if the newborn should aspirate the feeding the sterile water will be absorbed by the lungs and cause no lung damage. On the other hand, glucose water and formula, if aspirated, are not absorbed by the lung tissue and can cause damage.

During the initial feeding the nurse can assess the newborn for symptoms such as regurgitation and cyanosis that may point to complications. These symptoms may indicate the presence of tracheoesophageal fistula (an abnormality in which the esophagus is connected to the trachea by an opening) or esophageal atresia. In this latter condition, the esophagus ends in a blind pouch instead of in the stomach. As the pouch fills with fluid from the feeding, regurgitation of the fluid results. If there is a question as to the patency of the esophagus or to the possibility of tracheoesophageal fistula, assessment of the gastrointestinal tract is performed.

The initial formula feeding for the bottle fed newborn may occur after the newborn has ingested sterile water for one to two feedings, usually according to the protocol of the birthing institution. Newborns will usually consume one-half to one ounce during this feeding. Newborns who breastfeed will also consume one-half to one ounce after nursing actively 3 to 5 minutes on each breast during the initial feeding.

Meeting Parental Educational Needs

Parents have many educational needs that can be met prior to discharge from the birthing institution. Common parental concerns in the neonatal period focus on handling and positioning the neonate, nasal and oral suctioning, circumcision care, cord care, bathing and skin care, sucking needs, feeding and elimination patterns, bottle sterilization procedures, diapering, and clothing and wrapping the neonate. These concerns can be priorities of the nurse during discharge planning from the birthing facility.

Handling and Positioning. Parents can be taught various positions in which to hold the neonate including the cradle hold, the football hold, and the upright position (Figure 34–6). The parents and the neonate should feel comfortable in whatever position is chosen. It is important to teach parents to support the neonate's head and neck in the various positions.

In the cradle hold, the parent cradles the neonate in the arm against the chest. This is the position often used by parents for feeding. The advantages of this hold is that it permits parents to use the other hand, it provides a sense of security to the neonate, and allows the parent to look at the neonate when feeding.

In the football hold, the parent holds the neonate's head in the palm of the hand, and the rest of the body straddles the forearm. This position allows the parent to hold the neonate while keeping the other hand free to perform such tasks as washing the neonate's hair, walking up steps, or holding another child's hand.

In the upright position, the parent holds the neonate upright with both hands so that the neonate's head rests on the parent's shoulder. This position is often used for burping the neonate.

Parents should also be taught neonatal positions for sleeping. The neonate can be placed on the right side with a rolled blanket to the back for support. This position is particularly beneficial after feeding to allow for drainage of any regurgitated milk. After the cord falls off, neonates may also be placed lying on the abdomen. Neonates in this position will turn the head to the side; thus parents can be reassured that suffocation will not occur.

When picking the neonate up out of the crib, the parent is taught to place one hand under the neck

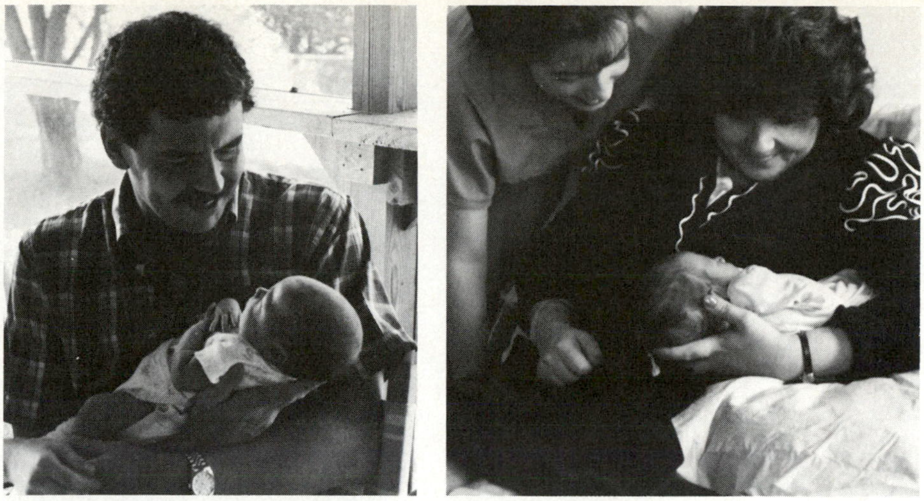

A B

Figure 34–6. Positions for holding the neonate. **A.** Cradle hold. **B.** Football hold.

and shoulders and the other hand under the buttocks. With a slow, smooth motion, the neonate is then lifted from the crib. Another technique is to swaddle the neonate in a blanket before picking up the neonate, again with two hands.

The nurse demonstrates the different positions for handling and holding the neonate to the parents. The parents should return the demonstration by handling and holding the neonate in various positions. Parents should feel comfortable in handling and holding the neonate; positions that are comfortable for some parents may not be comfortable for others.

Nasal and Oral Suctioning. Many parents are concerned that they will need to know how to intervene if the neonate "chokes" or has difficulty breathing. Neonates are compensatory nose breathers and at times may sound as if they are nasally congested when in fact they are not. The neonate may sneeze to clear the nasal passage; this does not indicate an upper respiratory infection. At times, however, excess mucus or regurgitated milk may need to be cleared from the oral and nasal passages. The nurse should therefore teach the parents to use a bulb syringe.

The parents are taught to place the neonate in a football hold, leaving one hand free to manipulate the bulb syringe. The bulb of the syringe is compressed and the tip placed in the neonate's mouth. (Placing the syringe in the mouth first prevents an inspiratory gasp that might occur if the syringe were placed in the nasal passage, instead.) The tip of the syringe is aimed at the side of the mouth and the parents slowly release the compression of the bulb to draw in the secretions (Figure 34–7A); the tip of the syringe is then removed from the mouth and the secretions released into a tissue. This procedure is repeated in the nares (Figure 34–7B). After use, the bulb syringe should be washed with soap and water and stored near the neonate. A return demonstration by the parents will evaluate their knowledge of the procedure. The bulb syringe should be used judiciously, as overuse can inflame the mucous lining of the neonate's nares.

Circumcision Care. Circumcision is the surgical removal of the foreskin, exposing the glans penis. The philosophy of practitioners concerning circumcision has varied greatly in the past several years. In 1975, the American Academy of Pediatrics, altering a long standing position recommending circumcision for male infants, took a position of not recommending routine circumcision. At that time, the Academy stated that there was no medical indication for routine circumcision. In 1989, however, the Academy again changed its position, advising that circumcision may have medical benefits, as well as risks. Benefits of circumcision, according to the Academy, include possible prevention of diseases such as urinary tract infection and cancer of the penis. Risks, on the other hand, include potential postprocedure bleeding and infection.[15] It is likely that routine circumcision will remain controversial for some years to come. Some parents choose to have their male newborns circumcised for a variety of reasons, including religious or cultural ones.

The circumcision procedure is performed in the birthing facility or, in the Jewish culture, in a home or synagogue. In the birthing facility, the nurse obtains

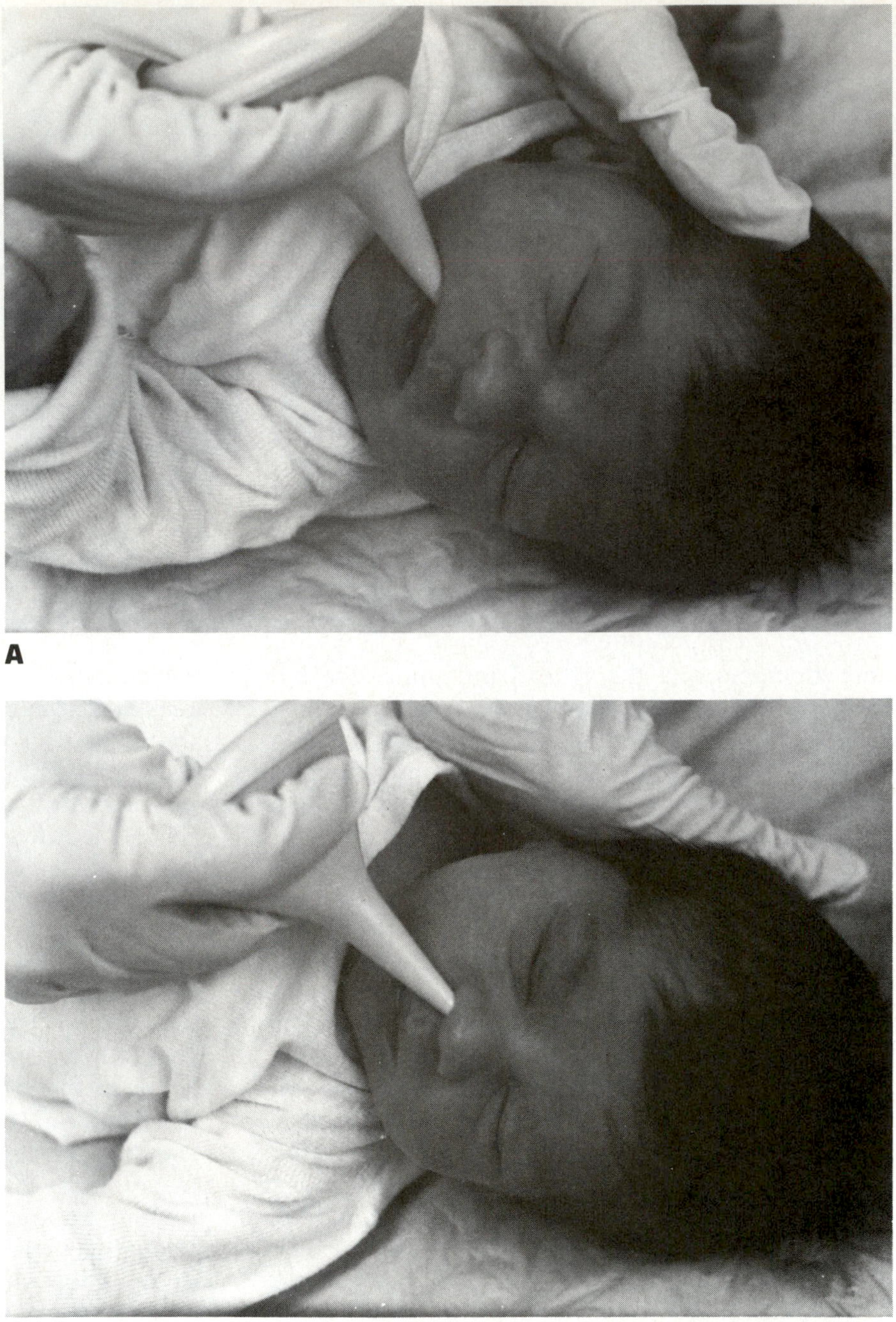

A

B

Figure 34–7. Parents should be taught how to suction the neonate's mouth and nose using a bulb syringe. **A.** Oral suctioning. **B.** Nasal suctioning.

an informed consent from the parent or parents. The neonate is restrained on a circumcision board, draped with sterile towels, and the penis is cleaned with soap and water. The physician uses sterile technique to remove the foreskin.

Equipment for the procedure may include a scalpel, Gomco clamp, or a Hollister plastibell. The clamp or plastibell, a bell-shaped plastic device, is used to minimize bleeding during and after the procedure. When the Gomco clamp is used, the prepuce is first separated from the glans penis with a sterile probe and stretched over a metal cone. The Gomco clamp is applied and after 4 to 5 minutes the prepuce above the clamp is removed with a scapel. The Gomco clamp is removed immediately after the procedure. If the plastibell is used, the prepuce is separated from the glans penis with a probe. The plasitibell is then placed over the glans and a suture is tied around the prepuce that is located at the rim of the plastibell. The prepuce above the tied area is then removed by a scalpel. The plastibell will stay in place for three or four days and then fall off. If the plastibell fails to fall off, the parents are instructed to call their physician who will manually remove it.

After the procedure, the nurse observes the neonate at the site for bleeding and normal voiding. A dressing of petroleum gauze may be placed loosely around the penis (Figure 34–8). Vitamin A and D ointment may also be used to prevent friction from the diaper. The diaper is then placed loosely around the neonate. The neonate should be given to the mother or parents as soon after the procedure as possible to allay their anxiety and for his comfort. The neonate should be kept off his abdomen for 12 hours after the circumcision to prevent irritation of the wound by friction.

No special care of the circumcision is required at home. The nurse teaches the parents to observe the penis for signs of bleeding and normal healing. A small yellow exudate may be seen on the second day after circumcision. This is part of the healing process and should not be removed by the parents. Tub baths should be avoided until the circumcision is healed. As circumcisions may be done after the neonate has left the birthing institution as part of religious rituals, these parents will also need information related to circumcision care prior to discharge.

Cord Care. Parents should be advised that the cord will dry and fall off in approximately 5 to 10 days. The application of aseptic solutions such as triple-dye to the cord should also be discussed with parents. Parents are taught signs of infection (that is, redness, swelling, and drainage) that should be reported to the physician. Cord care is also taught to the parents. This may include applying alcohol to the cord 2 to 3 times per day to help it dry. Parents are taught to diaper the neonate with the diaper folded down away from the cord to prevent rubbing and to expose the cord to the air. Sponge bathing is recommended until the cord falls off. Parents may ask the nurse about the use of bellybands. In some cultures the use of bellybands is thought to prevent umbilical hernias. The nurse should explain to the parents that bellybands do not prevent umbilical hernias and in fact may delay drying of the cord.

Bathing. The newborn is given an initial bath after the vital signs have stabilized. The nurse uses mild soap and water or plain water and observes the newborn throughout the bathing procedure for signs of physiologic and behavioral adaptations. The purpose of the initial bath is to remove blood, especially from the face, neck, and head. Care must be taken to keep the newborn thermally neutral during the initial bath.

A bath demonstration by the nurse teaches the parents techniques of bathing the neonate. The parents can return the demonstration to ensure their comfort with bathing. Both sponge bathing and tub bathing are taught to parents.

Before the bath begins, all the necessary equipment should be gathered. This includes towels, washcloths, mild soap, mild shampoo, baby lotion, vitamin A and D ointment or petroleum jelly, diapers, clothing, and blankets. The water should be a safe temperature, approximately 98°F (37°C). Parents

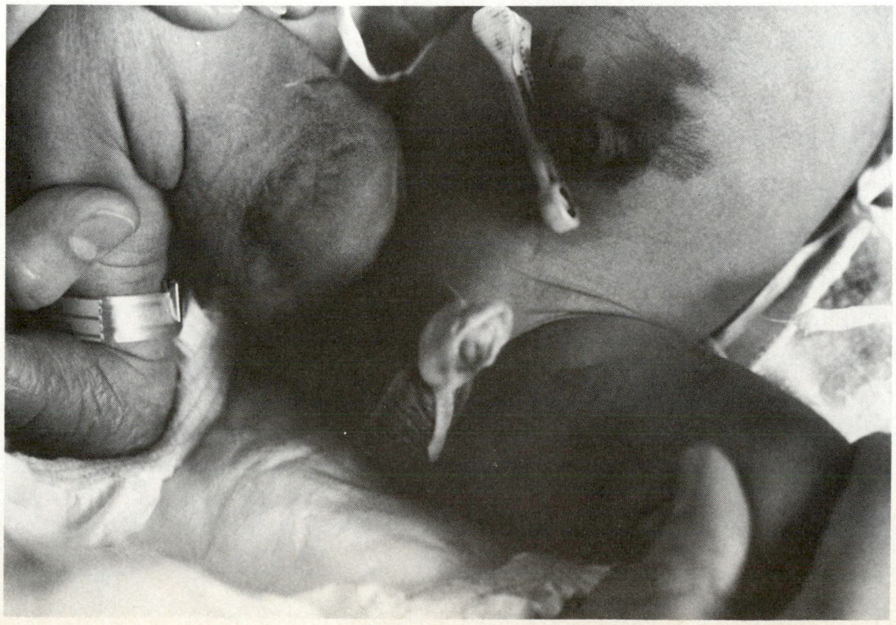

Figure 34–8. Newly circumcized neonate with vaseline gauze dressing in place. (Note cord clamp and presence of triple-dye on cord and abdomen.)

should test the water temperature with a thermometer or on their own skin by inserting the elbow into the water. The water should feel warm, but not hot. The room where the bath will be given should also be warm and free from drafts. The neonate should be washed from head to toe, with the diaper area bathed last because this is the area that is most soiled. Bathing time should be enjoyable for both neonate and parents. The neonate should be bathed when he or she is not fussy and preferably before meals.

The bath is a time when parents can inspect their newborn to see that he or she is healthy. The nurse can also point out common variations in the newborn such as molding to reassure parents of the newborns normalcy.

Sponge Bath. Until the cord drops off, parents and other caretakers should sponge bathe the neonate. The part of the neonate being bathed is exposed while the rest of the body is dressed or covered. Bathing begins with the eyes which are washed with a cotton ball or washcloth and clear water. Each eye is wiped from the inner to the outer corner. A new cotton ball or portion of the washcloth is used for each eye to prevent cross-contamination. The nares are observed and any crusted material wiped with the washcloth or a tissue. The ears are then washed by twisting the washcloth around the finger and washing around the pinna and in the area behind the ears. Cotton-tipped swabs should not be inserted into the nares or ear canals. They can cause injury to the nasal mucosa and tympanic membrane. The parents should be taught that the eventual development of cerumen in the external ear canal is normal. Swabs should not be placed in the ear canal to rid the canal of cerumen as they can cause the cerumen to become packed in the ear canal, resulting in discomfort to the neonate. After washing the ears, the rest of the face is washed with warm water.

While the neonate is still dressed the hair may be cleansed with water or shampooed with a mild shampoo. To shampoo the hair the neonate is placed in a football hold over a basin of water. The scalp is wiped or lathered and rinsed with warm water. Parents sometimes worry that they will injure the "soft spot" when washing the hair. They should be reassured that the head may be washed over the fontanelle without causing any injury. The hair is then towel dried and brushed with a soft brush.

The neonate's shirt is then removed and the folds of the neck, the arms, axillae, chest, back, and abdomen are washed with a mild soap and rinsed with a wet washcloth. The cord is kept dry during the bath. The skin is then thoroughly dried and the upper part of the body wrapped with a blanket to prevent chilling. The neonate's legs and feet are then unwrapped and washed with mild soap and water and dried thoroughly.

The genitalia and buttocks are washed last with mild soap and water. Cleansing of the female genitalia is done from the front to back to avoid contamination of the urethra and vagina with fecal material. The scrotum and the penis in the male are also washed with mild soap and water. Uncircumcised males do not have to have the foreskin retracted for cleansing. Forcibly retracting the foreskin may cause edema and constriction of vessels. The penis of the circumcised male is also washed gently with soap and water and dried. The buttocks and anal area are then washed thoroughly with soap and water. The genitalia, buttocks and anal area should also be washed after each diaper change to prevent skin irritation.

Lubricants such as unperfumed lotions, vitamin A and D ointment, and petroleum jelly can be used effectively for skin care. Powders and oils are not recommended for the neonate's skin. Oils may clog the pores, and the small particles of powders may be inhaled by the neonate, causing respiratory difficulty.

Tub Baths. After the cord falls off, tub bathing of the neonate is possible. Parents do not need to buy an expensive infant tub. The kitchen sink is a satisfactory infant tub; however, certain safety precautions are necessary for parents who bathe the neonate in the sink. The sink should be cleaned before the neonate is bathed. Cold water should be run through the faucet before the neonate is placed in the bath and the faucet should be turned away from the neonate to prevent accidental burns.

As with the sponge bath, parents should have all the equipment for the bath prepared and available before beginning the bath. Two or three inches of water should be placed in the tub or sink and the water temperature tested for comfort.

The neonate's eyes, nose, ears, and face are washed as in the sponge bath. The head is washed in the same manner. The neonate is then placed in the tub. While the parent supports the head and neck, the body is washed (Figure 34–9). The neonate may also be lathered sparsely with soap and then placed in the tub or sink for rinsing. Parents may wish to place a towel on their arm and then cradle the neonate in the towel when placing the neonate in the tub. This provides additional traction to help prevent slipping in the tub.

Neonates do not have to be completely bathed every day, although the diaper area is cleansed at each changing. The parents or other caretakers should schedule the bath at a time that is convenient for them.

Care of Nails. Parents are often concerned about how to cut the neonate's nails. The best time to cut

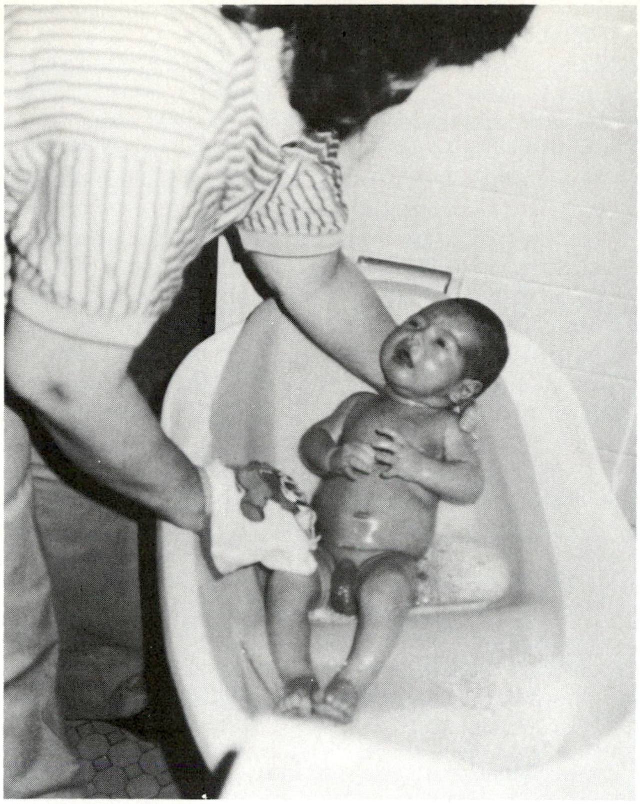

Figure 34–9. Bathing the neonate in an infant tub.

the nails is when the neonate is sleeping. The parent should use an infant scissor and cut the nails straight across if the nails are long and the neonate is scratching himself or herself. The fingernails and toenails may sometimes grow inward and adhere to the skin. Parents should be reassured that this is normal and should not attempt to cut the nails in this case because in doing so they may cut the skin.

Infant Sucking Needs. Neonates may have a variety of sucking needs beyond those needed for feeding. Nurses should assess the parents' likes and dislikes regarding the use of pacifiers. For the neonate who needs additional sucking, pacifiers may be used if the parents wish. Neonates who thumb suck usually have begun this behavior in utero. Thumb sucking may continue into the preschool years (*see* later discussion of thumbsucking).

Feeding and Elimination Patterns. Feeding the neonate is one of the first acts of parenting. The nurse should support the parents' decision about whether to breastfeed or bottlefeed. Healthy newborns should be fed on a demand basis. The parents are taught that neonates and infants also experience growth spurts during which they need to be fed more frequently. Growth spurts occur at about 10 days, 3 weeks, and 3 months after birth. Parents should feed the neonate or infant on demand during these times. Growth spurts last for several days and are self-limiting. Anticipatory guidance by the nurse will help parents deal effectively with their neonate's or infant's demands during these times. Breastfeeding mothers often feel that they have an insufficient milk supply and that is why their infants are waking more frequently. Bottlefeeding mothers often feel that the formula is not satisfying the infant and solid foods should be added. Parents should be reassured that the infant's needs can be met by either the breast or bottle during growth spurts without supplementary solid feeding.

During the first year of life infants have changing needs related to breastfeeding or bottlefeeding. Table 34–5 provides a guide related to the frequency and ounces per feeding in the first year. Breastfed infants will usually nurse more frequently than bottlefed infants because breast milk is more easily digested than formula. Parents are also taught that the infant will usually sleep through the night when he or she has reached 12 pounds or in about 8 weeks. This is highly individualized for each infant.

Patterns of Breastfeeding. Parents should be informed that the mother's milk supply will become synchronized with the neonate's demand for milk. On the first day, the mother is taught to allow the neonate to suckle 5 minutes on each breast and then gradually increase the suckling time on each breast by 2 to 3 minutes per day until the neonate is suckling approximately 12 to 15 minutes on each breast. The neonate usually empties the breast within 12 minutes. (*See* Chapter 31 for a complete discussion of educational preparation for breastfeeding).

Patterns of Formula Feeding. Parents are taught that formula-fed neonates will take about 2 to 3 oz per feeding or 12 to 15 oz in the first week of life. Neonates will increase their consumption of formula at each feeding as their stomach capacities increase. Another rule of thumb that can be taught to parents is that neonates will initially consume 2½ oz per pound of body weight in the first weeks of life. If, for example, the neonate weighs 8 pounds, he or she will consume 20 oz in a 24-hour period. If the 20 oz is consumed in eight feedings, the neonate will take 2.5 oz per feeding; if taken in 6 feedings, the neonate will take 3.3 oz per feeding.

Techniques for Bottlefeeding and Formula Preparation. Parents and other caretakers should be taught to hold the neonate in a comfortable position when bottlefeeding. The bottle should be held upright so that

TABLE 34–5. SCHEDULE FOR MILK FEEDINGS DURING THE FIRST YEAR

Age	Number of Feedings per 24 Hours	Amount per Feeding (oz)	Total amount per 24 Hours (oz)
1 week	6	2–3	12–18
2–4 weeks	6	3–5	18–30
2–3 months	5	4–6	20–30
4–5 months	5	5–7	25–35
6–7 months	4	7–8	28–32
8–12 months	3	8	24

Reproduced, with permission, from Lewis CM. Nutrition and Nutritional Therapy in Nursing. *Norwalk, Conn: Appleton-Century-Crofts; 1984.*

milk and no air is in the nipple and neck of the bottle. This prevents the neonate from swallowing air that may cause discomfort from gas. Several different types of bottles and nipples are sold. The opening in the nipple should allow a steady flow of formula but should not be too large as it will cause the neonate to swallow too much liquid and regurgitate the formula.

Commercial formulas are sold in concentrated liquids, powders, ready-to-feed, and prepackaged ready-to-feed formula in bottles. The concentrated liquids and powders require mixing with water. Equal amounts of water and concentrated formula should be mixed when preparing the formula. For example, if the can of formula has 13 oz of concentrated liquid, it should be mixed with 13 oz of water. Powders should be mixed according to the directions on the can. The concentrated formulas and powders are less expensive than the ready-to-feed formulas.

Parents should be taught to carefully read the labels on commercially prepared formulas. Inadvertent use of concentrated formula without dilution can cause metabolic problems and dehydration in the neonate. Formulas should be prepared for a 24-hour period if concentrated liquid is used. Once prepared, they should be stored in the refrigerator for no longer than 48 hours. The bottle may be taken out of the refrigerator one-half hour before use or run under warm water to take the chill out of the formula. Powders and ready-to-feed formulas may be prepared for each feeding. Once the can of ready-to-feed formula is opened, it should be refrigerated and discarded if not used within 48 hours. The can of powdered formula may be stored at room temperature, once opened, for a period of 3 weeks.

Parents are cautioned to avoid propping the bottle. The neonate may regurgitate and aspirate the formula when the bottle is propped. Neonates who nurse from propped bottles are also prone to bottle-mouth syndrome (*see* later discussion).

ISSUES AND CONTROVERSIES

Reciprocal attachment of the parent or parents to the infant is vital and provides the basis for what Erikson refers to as the "sense of trust." The first year of life is a critical time during which a secure parent-infant relationship is established. Parents learn about the infant. They recognize the infant's alert moments, readiness for interaction, rhythms that produce responses, and ways of playing and interacting. Brazelton recommends that the primary caregiving parent remain at home during the first four months to get to "know" the infant.[a] When there is a choice, it is believed that the longer a parent can remain to care for her or his own infant, the more intimacy and attachment will be shared.

Brazelton's recommendations are controversial and raise the following issues related to parent-infant attachment:

1. Is it necessary for individuals with careers or economic needs to remain home with an infant for a number of months after birth?
2. Many state governments are considering parental leave acts. Should businesses be forced to provide parental leaves?

Other issues that arise during the first year of the infant's life include:

1. Current research indicates that parents cannot "spoil" an infant; however, some cultural groups adhere to the belief that infants should not be held each time they cry or have every need met. How would the nurse incorporate the cultural beliefs of the family into the plan of care while ensuring that the infant's needs are met?
2. Colic may be a problem for infants during the first 3 months of life. There is some indication that colic may be related to infant temperament. The common practice is to change infant formulas in response to the symptoms. Is this always necessary? How would the nurse differentiate between colic caused by infant state and colic caused by milk intolerance?

[a] *Brazelton B.* Working and Caring. *Reading, Mass: Addison-Wesley; 1985.*

Bottle Sterilization. Parents and other caretakers are taught that the bottles and nipples should be washed with soap and water. The dishwasher may be used effectively to wash the bottles. If the water supply is not purified or if there is a question about the cleanliness of the water supply, sterilization procedures are taught to parents.

When bottle sterilization is indicated, two methods may be used: the terminal method and the aseptic method. For either method, the first step is to wash the bottles (other than bottles that use liners to hold the milk), nipples, and bottle caps in soapy, warm water.

Terminal Method. After the equipment is washed, the formula is prepared according to the directions on the can. The bottles are filled with the formula and the nipples are inverted into the bottles with the caps loosely applied. The bottles are placed in a large kettle in 2 or 3 in. of water or, alternately, in a bottle sterilizer. The kettle or sterilizer is covered and the bottles are boiled for 25 minutes. The bottles remain in the sterilizer until cool. They are then removed, the lids are tightened, and the bottles stored in the refrigerator.

Aseptic Method. After the equipment is washed, it is placed in a large kettle or sterilizer and boiled for 5 minutes. The amount of water needed to mix concentrated formula is boiled separately for 5 minutes. The bottles, caps, and nipples are removed with tongs from the sterilizer or kettle. A sterilized measuring pitcher is used to measure the appropriate amount of water and formula into each bottle. Bottles are refrigerated until needed.

Burping. Neonates and infants should be burped at least twice during a feeding. Parents are taught to recognize their neonate's signals related to burping: the neonate will stop sucking when he or she needs to be burped; if the neonate does not burp after several minutes, he or she probably does not need to burp. The neonate can be burped in the upright position on the parent's shoulder by gently patting the back. Alternately, the neonate may be placed in a sitting position with one hand holding the chin for head support and the other hand gently patting the back. This position allows the parent to watch the neonate during burping (Figure 34–10).

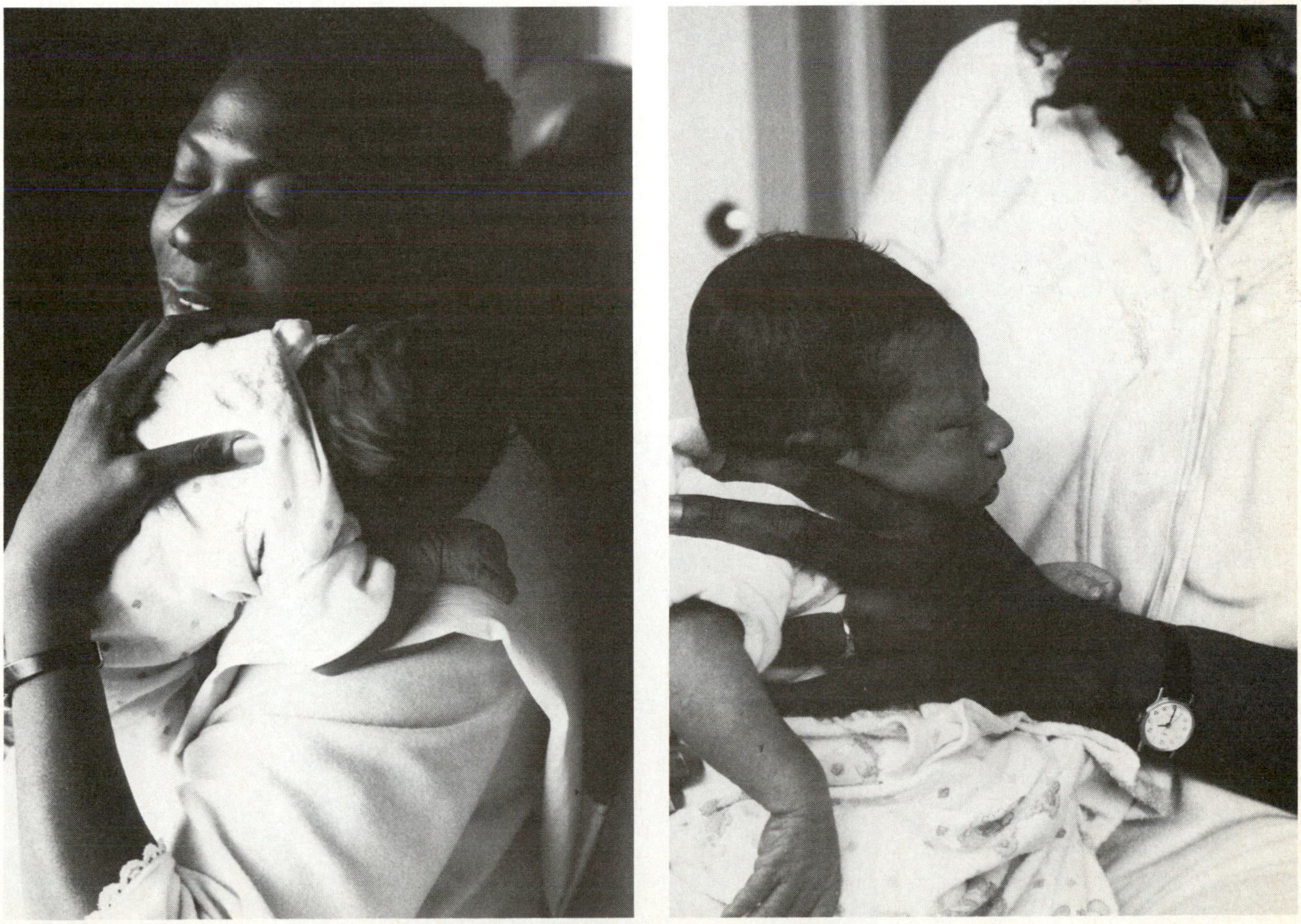

A **B**

Figure 34–10. Positions for burping the neonate. **A.** Upright. **B.** Sitting.

Elimination Patterns. Parents are often concerned about elimination patterns of their neonates. Breastfed neonates will have stools that are watery and yellow after the initial meconium and transitional stools. They may pass stools up to ten times a day or go several days without a stool. Formula-fed infants have stools that are firmer than breastfed neonates and yellow-brown in color. Soy-based formulas produce stools that are greenish brown in color and pasty.

The neonate may void 20 or more times a day. Parents and other caretakers are taught that voiding is a good indication that the neonate is receiving adequate fluid intake.

Diapering. Parents and other caretakers should be informed about the various types of diapers available and the techniques for diapering the neonate (Figure 34–11). Diapers may be disposable or cloth. Disposable diapers are prefolded, with differing construction for girls and boys. The diapers for girls have extra padding toward the back of the diaper because this is where the diaper will become most wet. Diapers for boys have extra padding in the front because this is the portion of the diaper that requires the most absorbency. Disposable diapers are costly and are not biodegradable, yet many parents choose to use them.

Cloth diapers should also be placed on the neonate according to the needed level of absorbency; that is, they should be folded with extra padding toward the back for girls and extra padding in the front for boys. Parents are taught to wash the diapers in mild soap and water, rinsing the diapers twice so that soap residue will be removed. Commercial diaper services may also be used.

Clothing and Wrapping. Parents and other caretakers have many concerns about the proper clothing for neonates. They should be taught to dress the neonate for comfort. In general, neonates should wear a T-shirt, diaper, and light- to medium-weight sleeper that covers the neonate from neck to toe. The neonate should not be dressed too warmly in warm temperatures or too sparsely in cold temperatures. If the neonate is in an air-conditioned room, a blanket may also be used over the clothing to avoid chills.

The neonate's head should be covered with a hat when outdoors in the sun or when the temperature is cool. The skin should also be protected from the sun as the skin is sensitive and easily burns. The neonate should not be placed directly in the sun. Some sunscreen products made specifically for the neonate's sensitive skin may also be used.

Parents are taught to launder the neonate's clothing and cloth diapers separately from other clothing. A mild detergent should be used and the clothing should be rinsed thoroughly to avoid any residue that might cause irritation. Laundering the clothes with fabric softeners may also cause irritation of the skin.

The nurse should also teach parents how to wrap their newborn. A baby blanket is placed on a flat surface with one corner of the blanket at the top. The neonate's head is placed at the top corner and one side of the blanket is wrapped under the opposite side of the neonate. The bottom corner of the blanket is then placed upward toward the neonate's chest

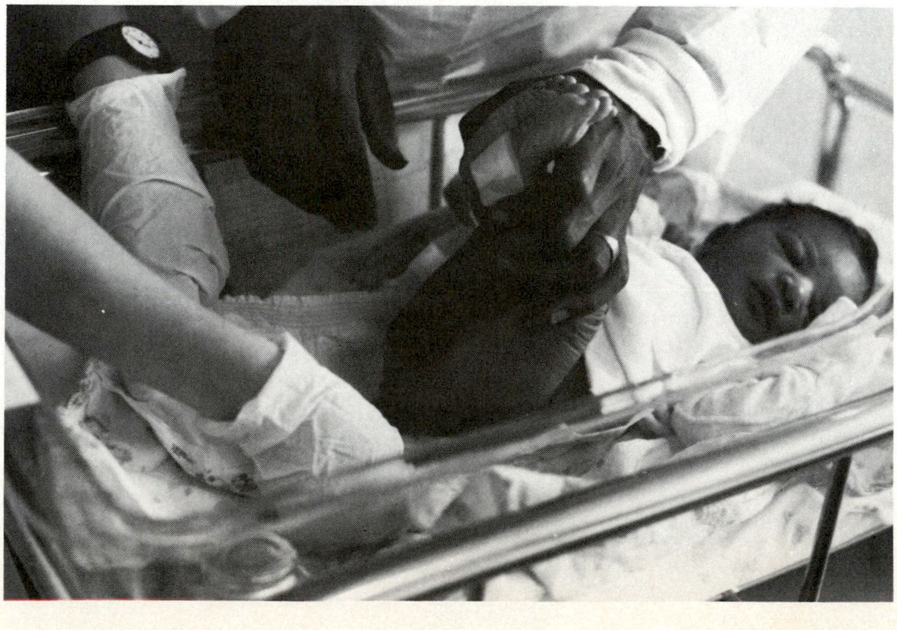

Figure 34–11. The nurse assists a new father as he learns to change his newborn's diaper.

and the other side of the blanket is wrapped around the opposite side of the neonate. Wrapping the neonate in this manner provides security and allows the parent to cradle the neonate with confidence.

Discharge Planning

Prior to discharge the nurse anticipates parents' and other caretakers' concerns by educating them about infant care. The nurse will also want to obtain information that assures the neonate's continued well-being. It is important to find out if the parents have made plans for the health maintenance of the neonate. If they have not made plans for follow-up either with a physician, nurse practitioner, or clinic facility, the nurse can assist them to make an appointment to ensure health promotion.

NURSING CARE OF THE INFANT IN THE FIRST YEAR

The rapid growth rate and developmental changes of the infant require careful assessment and management during the first year of life. Settings for infant health care include physician's offices or health clinics. The primary caregiver in these settings may be a physician or nurse practitioner. The schedule for infant visits may vary from setting to setting. The infant may visit the health setting at 2 weeks and one month, and thereafter once a month during the first year of life. A variation of this schedule is for the infant to visit the setting at 2 weeks, one month, two months, four months, six months, nine months, and one year.

A thorough health history is taken by the nurse when the infant is brought for the first child care visit. The health history provides general information, assists the nurse in identifying health needs, and provides subjective data about the infant that supplements objective data obtained during the health visit. The subjective data obtained from the health history should be documented and updated at each child health visit. Health teaching and anticipatory guidance should be based on the gathered data.

The traditional techniques of inspection, palpation, percussion, and auscultation are used in physical examination of the infant. The physical examination provides the nurse with information about the infant's health status, general appearance, level of activity, responses to others, and developmental skills. At each health visit a complete physical and developmental assessment is done.

The role of the nurse, no matter what the setting, is to anticipate the needs of caretakers and to assist them in effectively using skills necessary for care of the infant. The goals of nursing care for the infant include promotion of growth and development, promotion of nutritional well-being, prevention of communicable diseases, prevention of accidents, and parent education.

Promotion of Growth and Development

Growth is a product of the continuous and complex interaction of heredity and environment.[16] Why growth occurs in certain progressive patterns is not known; however, it is known that although growth rate may vary, the patterns of growth remain stable. Growth is one of the phenomena that constitutes development and can be defined as one of the units acquired in the course of development. It is quantitative; that is, it can easily be observed and objectively measured.[17,18] An important part of the infant assessment is measurement of height, weight, and head and chest circumference. The infant's growth is charted during health care visits to identify and monitor the progress and pattern of growth.

The infant's physical appearance during the first year of life clearly reflects changes in height, weight, and body proportions. After the neonatal period the infant doubles his or her birth weight during the first 5 or 6 months and triples it by the end of the first year. The infant should gain an average of 140 g (5 oz) per week during the first 5 months of life and 105 g (3¾ oz) thereafter. On the average, the infant's length increases by 50 percent (9 to 10 in.) by the end of the first year. In addition, the trunk grows rapidly, making the extremities appear very short. The head still appears proportionately large in comparison with the body. The abdomen is rounded and protuberant; thus, the infant appears to consist mostly of head and abdomen.[17]

Development is an interaction of the processes of physical growth, learning, and heredity. Development is a qualitative continuous process that begins at conception. Developmental changes are the products of maturation and experience, so intricately intertwined that their contributions to, or effects on, development cannot be separated for analysis.[19] Development of locomotion skills and cognition is the result of an interaction between maturation and learning. Regardless of how much practice is provided, an infant cannot walk until myelination occurs and a certain level of maturity is reached. The cognitive, sensory, and motor development that occurs prior to this developmental milestone is a contributory factor. Although the processes underlying growth and development are complex, general principles govern how development proceeds:

1. Growth and development are orderly and usually do not vary. Throughout infancy definite patterns

in motor, physical, cognitive, and psychosocial growth can be observed. Although the time at which these occur may vary, there are definite periods when behaviors are expected to emerge. All early physical and motor development is "directional." Development is **cephalocaudal** (head-to-toe). The maturation process of the central nervous system is similar; the cervical area of the spinal cord matures earlier than the lumbar and sacral areas. Thus, infants are able to lift their heads before they can lift the thoracic area and they can sit before they stand. Development also has a **proximodistal** dimension. Development proceeds from the central axis of the body and moves outward toward the extremities. Infants are able to use their fingers as a unit before they are able to control finger movements and they are able to gaze at items before they can reach out and grasp them.

2. Behavior becomes more versatile as development proceeds. There is greater elaboration and a greater repertoire of behaviors in the spheres of fine motor, social, and cognitive areas with an increase in age. For example, infants communicate their needs through crying. Communication progresses to cooing, babbling, and single words in infancy to the ability to express complex thoughts and feelings during late childhood and adolescence. All behavior is influenced by genetics and environment. The time at which behaviors occur can vary within limits and under a variety of environmental conditions.[20]
3. Development is patterned and continuous, but it may be stable at one time and labile at another. There may be acceleration of development in one area with a lag in another. For example, an infant's motor ability may progress rapidly while speech progresses more slowly.
4. There is continuing interaction between a changing organism and a changing environment. Responses of the infant to the environment produce changes in the infant so that later responses to similar or other events in the environment differ from earlier behaviors. For example, infant sucking patterns become modified with practice and the infant develops the ability to differentiate between nutritive and nonnutritive sucking and modify her or his modes of sucking.

Although development is patterned and predictable, it cannot proceed without appropriate stimulation. Kaye and other investigators have validated that infants have learning abilities as early as the first days of life; they conclude that the infant's abilities are more sophisticated and organized than was formerly

RESEARCH ABSTRACT

Blank DM. Relating mother's anxiety and perception to infant satiety, anxiety, and feeding behavior. Nurs Res. *1986;35: 347–351.*

This study explored the relationship of mother's anxiety and perception to changes in infant satiety, anxiety, and feeding. The sample consisted of 65 healthy mother-infant couples. Of these 30 were primiparous mothers and 25 multiparous mothers. All infants were bottle-fed with 30 calories per ounce formulas and their age at time of entrance into the study ranged from 45 to 76 hours.

Instruments used to measure maternal variables included the Blank Infant Tenderness Scale (BITS). This scale was developed by the researcher to measure mothers' perceptions of infant tenderness needs, which included both physiologic and contact requirements. The State-Trait Anxiety Inventory was used to measure maternal anxiety.

Infant variables were measured by infant serum glucose, infant serum cortisol, and Brazelton's level-of-consciousness criteria of measurement of infant state. Infant serum glucose assessed degree of satiety. Infant serum cortisol was used to assess degree of anxiety. Because it has been documented that cortisol can fluctuate with infant state, state behavior was assessed before and after feeding. Infant blood samples were obtained just before and 60 minutes after feeding for assessment of glucose and cortisol.

The findings demonstrated that maternal state-trait anxiety was associated with infant glucose, cortisol and formula consumption. More specifically, mild maternal prefeeding state anxiety was related to lower infant cortisol difference scores, and extremely low maternal prefeeding anxiety was related to higher infant cortisol difference scores. Mild maternal feed state anxiety also was related to greater infant formula consumption, and extremely low maternal feed state anxiety was related to lower formula consumption.

The investigator concluded that mothers' anxiety is related to their infants' satiety and anxiety levels and feeding behavior. The data appear to indicate that mild maternal anxiety at feeding time increases infant consumption of formula and lowers infant anxiety as measured by cortisol levels. Conversely, extremely low maternal anxiety is associated with low infant formula consumption and increased cortisol and anxiety levels.

Comment:

This well-controlled study adds knowledge to the nursing literature about psychophysiologic reactions in mother-infant couples. More research is needed on physiologic as well as behavioral variables so that a better understanding of the interactions between mothers and their infants can be developed.

believed.[21] This knowledge of infant behavior can help the nurse provide guidance to parents. Effective teaching dictates that the nurse have knowledge in the areas of infant growth and development, psychosocial theory, psychosexual development, cognitive growth, and separation-individuation.

By understanding the role of experience in infant growth and development, the nurse can assist parents in planning care that will nurture or foster each developmental stage. Such caretaking behaviors as cuddling, talking, eye-to-eye contact, and providing nutrition stimulate attachment and auditory, visual, and physiologic progress in the infant.

One of the most important factors in infant development is the quality of caretaking. All infants must establish a trusting relationship with at least one caretaker who will meet their needs. The mutual, reciprocal interaction that occurs contributes to the infant's gratification and growing sense of expectancy that specific behaviors will elicit positive responses from his or her caretakers. Spontaneous nurturing and parenting stimulate the development of language, social skills, and learning that are the foundation for further achievement.

Language, cognitive, social, and motor skills can be developed if the primary caretakers respond to the appropriate infant cues at the appropriate time. For example, the best method for teaching language is to talk to the infant and respond to his or her crying, cooing, and babbling.

The ability of the nurse to provide anticipatory guidance to parents is based on thorough knowledge of the timing and significance of the developmental milestones. Table 34–6 outlines language, cognitive, social, and motor development in the first 12 months of life.

Knowledge about newborn abilities has resulted in the growth of an industry devoted to parents who are interested in using tools that stimulate and educate infants. Toys, self-help books for parents, exercises, swimming classes, and learning programs have been designed to promote cognitive skills and motor abilities during infancy and toddlerhood. Nurses must have information about these programs and their advantages and disadvantages. Setting unrealistic goals and pushing infants and children into precocious achievements can stifle the infant's natural curiosity and interfere with opportunities for play.[22]

Development will occur as a natural process in all infants according to their potential as long as they have a variety of experiences in which they actively participate. The quality and quantity of development are influenced by temperament, readiness, and mastery of previously developed skills.

Temperament. **Temperament** is the behavior that the infant uses to cope with environmental demands. Thomas and Chess'[23] research on temperament differences among infants and children identified nine factors that can be used to assess infant temperament:

1. *Activity level.* Level of activity of the infant
2. *Rhythmicity.* Regularity of schedule the infant has for feeding, sleep, or bowel movements
3. *Approach-withdrawal.* Infant's response to a new stimulus
4. *Adaptability.* Ease with which the infant adapts a routine to fit a new situation
5. *Mood.* Amount of happy versus unhappy behavior
6. *Threshold.* Amount of stimulation required before the infant reacts to a given situation
7. *Intensity.* Degree to which the infant expresses herself or himself
8. *Attention-persistence.* Length of time a given activity is pursued by the infant.
9. *Distractability.* Ease with which the infant's attention can be diverted

Thomas and Chess[23] also described variable patterns of infant/child behavior, including (1) the easy-child pattern, in which the infant shows high rhythmicity, positive mood, positive approach, high adaptability, and high intensity; (2) the difficult-child pattern, in which the infant displays low rhythmicity, negative mood, withdrawal, low adaptability, and high intensity; and (3) the slow-to-warm pattern, in which the infant exhibits low activity, withdrawal, low adaptability, negative mood, and low intensity. As these differences in temperament appear to be present from birth, children in the same family may have different temperaments. As one mother noted, "My first child was so easy; my second was so difficult that I probably would not have had another if he had come first!"

The nurse can provide parents with information about the differing temperaments of infants. Care should be taken to avoid placing qualitative tags on temperament, for example, "easy" children are "good," "difficult" children are "bad." Parents who recognize their infant's temperament can begin to use caretaking approaches that will meet their own and their infant's needs.

Irritability. **Irritability** is another behavior demonstrated by infants.[24] Irritability is related to the sensory threshold of the infant. Some infants respond to a stimulus by crying and seem to become upset when even small amounts of the stimulus are present.

TABLE 34–6. DEVELOPMENTAL MILESTONES DURING THE FIRST YEAR

	Birth	1	2	3	4	5	6	7	8	9	10	11	12
LANGUAGE	Responds to stress by crying			Coos and babbles; "talks" when spoken to; squeals with pleasure			Babbles; makes sounds to inanimate objects			Imitates sounds			Vocalizes some words (eg, "mama," "dada")
COGNITIVE	Exhibits inborn primitive reflexes; becomes efficient at sucking	Can repeat reflexes spontaneously (eg, moves hands to mouth)			Exhibits coordination between motor skills and vision				Exhibits object permanence; distinguishes self from others				
SOCIAL	Follows objects with eyes; responds by crying	Has social smile					Laughs aloud; may show preference for usual caretakers			Cries and becomes tense in strange situations and with strange people (stranger anxiety)			Responds to "no"; understands names of objects
MOTOR	Lifts head while lying on abdomen; holds hands in fixed position			Able to lift head 90°; supports weight on forearms; clasps and unclasps hands voluntarily; turns head toward moving objects		Turns over	Transfers objects from hand to hand; sits with support			Sits without support; crawls; pulls self to standing position; uses pincer grasp			May begin to walk

Birth 1 2 3 4 5 6 7 8 9 10 11 12 13

Age (months)

One researcher has proposed that irritable infant syndrome may be the proper term for infant colic, a condition in which a well-fed infant has attacks of crying, fussing, and irritability that may last up to 3 hours.[25] Keefe[25] postulates that infant colic is best termed irritable infant syndrome because it is a dysfunction in behavioral state regulation. That is, infants with this syndrome may actually be demonstrating difficulty in moving from a crying state to a sleep state. Although this hypothesis has not been validated, the nurse who considers an infant's behavioral state in assessing for such problems as colic may reassess the tendency to blame the condition on breast milk or formula (*see* later discussion of colic).

Promotion of Nutritional Well-Being

Adequate nutrition is considered the single most important factor affecting infant physical growth and development.[26] The first 4 to 6 months constitute the most rapid period of growth for the infant. Because requirements for nutrition are most critical during this period, nutritional deficiencies can have long-term effects on growth and development.[27] Food provided to the infant must be nutritionally sound, must provide energy, must be digestible, must be adapted to renal capacity, and must be able to sustain the rapid growth rate of the first year of life.

Infants double their birth weight by the fifth month and triple it by the twelfth month. In addition, length usually increases by 50 percent. These large increments require a consistent and adequate food supply. An inadequate diet during the first year cannot support optimal growth and nutrient storage. Nutritional status on entry into the toddler and preschool period might be characterized by deficits in physical growth, symptoms of nutritional deficiency, and susceptibility to infection.[27]

Deficiencies in nutrition have their most profound effect on the cellular development of the brain and adipose tissue. Brain cell multiplication and differentiation increases from conception to 12 to 15 months of age. After this period there is an increase in brain mass and body cell mass. Studies of childhood obesity indicate that children with excess cell mass from excessive caloric intake develop adult fat cells early in life. Subsequently, fat stores continue to increase because of increases in the number of fat cells.[28]

Human milk or infant formula alone provides the best nutrition for infants in the first 4 to 6 months of life. The full-term infant has iron stores in the body that are estimated to be adequate until 4 to 6 months. After this time exogenous iron should be added to the diet to decrease the risk of development of iron-deficiency anemia.[27] Iron-fortified dry infant cereal is an excellent low-cost source of iron for infants.

Individual custom, beliefs, and practices may dictate when parents decide to introduce solid foods into the infant's diet. The American Academy of Pediatrics Committee on Nutrition[28] recommends that solid foods not be introduced before 4 to 6 months of age. By 16 weeks of age infants have developed a more mature sucking pattern; they can move the tongue back and forth and hold the head more erect and in the midline. Hand-eye coordination is also developing; by 24 weeks the infant can grasp an object in sight and place it in the mouth. Chewing movements begin between the 24th and 28th weeks. All of these developmental achievements indicate that infants are ready to feed finger foods to themselves.[29] Physiologically, the gastrointestinal tract has matured and is producing the digestive enzymes necessary for absorption and metabolism of fats, protein, and starches. The excretory capacity of the kidneys also has adapted to larger osmolar loads.[28]

Parents should be taught to introduce solid foods slowly. A single-grain, ready-to-serve iron-fortified dry cereal is usually the first solid food offered to the infant. Rice is the least allergenic of the cereals and is recommended as the first cereal to be introduced. Cereal is followed by fruits and juices and pureed yellow and green vegetables. Pureed meats do not need to be added until 9 months of age. Foods should be introduced one at a time and fed to the infant for one week or longer. In this way if food intolerance or allergy develops, the allergen can be readily identified. Once a variety of foods have been introduced, foods can be combined and new textures and flavors introduced. As food intake increases, milk intake should decrease; however, breast or formula feedings are still important to supply nutrients needed by the infant.[29]

In providing guidance to parents, the nurse must consider several variables that directly influence eating patterns. Cultural practices, socioeconomic status, parental knowledge, and readiness to modify the diet must be explored and discussed. The most important goal of the nurse and parents should be to provide the infant with a nutritious, adequate diet that is low in salt, glucose, and cholesterol and meets dietary needs. As the nurse provides guidance there must be acknowledgment that a wide variety of foods can meet these criteria. Alterations must be made for infants who have food sensitivities or strong food dislikes. Consultation with a nutritionist will assist the nurse in providing expert guidance to the parents.

The transition to solid foods offers an excellent opportunity for parents or other caretakers to set the stage for healthy eating habits. Acquired tastes for salts, sugars, and empty caloric foods may be established at this time. Effective teaching techniques and a sound knowledge base in nutrition and infant growth and development can serve as effective tools for the nurse in providing anticipatory guidance about infant nutrition.

Prevention of Communicable Diseases

Immunization against communicable disease is an important aspect of disease prevention and health promotion throughout childhood. Communicable diseases among infants and children are some of the oldest known public health problems. Sustained public concern and scientific discovery have resulted in successful development of many effective and powerful immunizing agents that are readily available to children.[30]

The American Academy of Pediatrics' Committee on Infectious Disease[31] recommends that immunizations be initiated at 2 months of age. Before this time the immaturity of the infant's immune system

BOX 34–4. DIPHTHERIA AND TETANUS TOXOIDS AND PERTUSSIS ADSORBED (DTP)

Action:
DTP promotes immunity to diphtheria, tetanus, and pertussis by inducing production of specific antitoxins and antibodies. Diphtheria toxoid component provides protection only against the exotoxin caused by *Corynebacterium diphtheriae;* local infection of the respiratory tract or skin with *C. diphtheriae* occurs occasionally in immune individuals. Primary immunization with four doses of DTP in susceptible individuals is needed to induce production of antitoxin levels that result in immunity to diphtheria and tetanus in more than 90 percent of vaccinees and induces immunity against pertussis in 75–85 percent of vaccinees. Administration of the first three doses of DTP (at 2, 4, and 6 months of age) reportedly provides protection against diphtheria, pertussis, and tetanus; the doses at 18 months and 4–6 years of age enhance protection through the preschool and early school years. Immunity to diphtheria and tetanus has been reported to persist at least 10 years after primary immunization with four doses of DTP. Pertussis immunity begins to decrease approximately 4–6 years after primary immunization with four doses of DTP.

Indications:
DTP is the preparation of choice to provide active immunity to diphtheria, tetanus, and pertussis in infants and children 6 weeks through 6 years of age. Infants in whom pertussis vaccine is contraindicated should still receive the diphtheria and tetanus toxoids adsorbed. Individual antigens should be used only when there is a contraindication to the other two components in DTP.

Stability:
DTP is a turbid, whitish suspension that may have a faint odor. DTP should be stored at 2–8°C and should not be frozen. If DTP is exposed to temperatures less than 2°C or greater than 25°C for 24 hours or longer, resuspension of the antigen may be difficult. Expiration date is 18 months after date of issue from manufacturer's cold storage. DTP should be free from clumps after vigorous shaking and should not be used if suspension cannot be achieved.

Dosage and Route:
DTP is administered only by deep injection, preferably into the midlateral muscles of the thigh or deltoid, with care to avoid major peripheral nerve trunks. The same muscle should not be used more than once during the course of primary immunization. Containers of DTP should be shaken vigorously prior to withdrawal of a dose.

DTP is administered in 0.5-mL doses. For primary immunization of infants 6 weeks through 6 years of age DTP is given in a series of four doses. The first three doses should be given at 4- to 8-week intervals (usually 2, 4, and 6 months of age) and the fourth dose should be given approximately 1 year after the third dose (usually at 18 months of age). Interruption of the recommended immunization schedule does not interfere with final immunity achieved and it is not necessary to give additional doses or start the series over. Schedule can be adjusted during pertussis epidemics, where the DTP can be initiated as early as 2 weeks of age and the first three doses can be given as frequently as 4 weeks apart. At 4–6 years of age or just prior to entry into school, children who received the fourth dose of DTP at ages younger than 4 years of age should receive a fifth dose of DTP. All individuals who received primary immunization with DTP should receive routine booster doses of tetanus and diphtheria toxoids adsorbed for adult use, not DTP, every 10 years to maintain adequate immunity against diphtheria and tetanus. It is recommended that children with symptomatic or asymptomatic human immunodeficiency virus infections receive immunization against diphtheria, tetanus, and pertussis according to the normal recommended schedules.

DTP may be administered simultaneously with an inactivated vaccine, poliovirus vaccine live oral, measles vaccine live, mumps virus vaccine live, and rubella virus vaccine live.

makes it unlikely that antibody production could occur. Also, the transfer of antibodies via maternal-fetal circulation provides **passive immunity** for the infant. The infant is protected against any diseases for which the mother has antibodies for approximately 6 months to 1 year.

Active immunity is conferred when toxoids or vaccines are given at 2, 4, and 6 months of of age. Diphtheria and tetanus toxoids combined with pertussis vaccine (DTP, Box 34–4) is administered by injection. Trivalent oral polio vaccine (OPV, Box 34–5) is administered orally (Figure 34–12), and additional immunizations are scheduled through adolescence. The schedule is flexible; immunity is achieved whether the intervals between doses are short or long. The important factor is that the correct number of repeat doses be administered. Table 34–7 provides the recommended schedule for active immunization of normal infants and children.

Immunizations are contraindicated when there is an acute illness accompanied by fever and severe reactions to pertussis vaccine (eg, convulsions and high

Contraindications and Precautions:
DTP should not be administered to individuals 7 years of age or older because of the increased incidence of adverse reactions to preparations containing pertussis vaccine or more than 2 Lf units of diphtheria. Children with a proven or suspected underlying neurologic disorder should be evaluated before receiving DTP or DT before the child's first birthday.

Local Reactions:
Frequent: 40–70 percent of vaccinees experience mild to moderate local reactions at the injection site (tenderness, erythema, swelling, induration). A nodule may be palpable at the injection site for a few weeks. *Less Common:* Localized hypersensitivity reaction, characterized by severe local reactions that usually begin 2–8 hours after injection have occurred in individuals who have received prior booster doses of DTP.

Systemic Reactions:
Frequent: Mild to moderate fever, chills, and malaise occur frequently within several hours of administration of DTP and persist approximately 2 days. Fever and other systemic effects occur more frequently after administration of DTP than after preparations not containing pertussis vaccine. *Rare*: Serious, sometimes fatal reactions presumably caused by the pertussis component have occurred rarely. This reaction consists of fever (39°C or higher), irritability, screaming, episodes characterized by prolonged crying during which the child cannot be comforted, vomiting, seizures, infantile spasms, transient shocklike state, excessive somnolence, encephalopathy, and other symptoms. Neurologic reactions have occasionally been followed by permanent CNS damage. Reactions usually occur within 24–48 hours but have been reported up to 7 days after DTP. Hypotonic, hyporesponsive episodes lasting 10–36 hours have rarely occurred. Incidence of seizure may be higher in individuals with underlying seizure disorders. Generalized urticaria and anaphylaxis have occurred rarely after administration of DTP. Cochlear lesions, brachial plexis neuropathies, paralysis of radial or recurrent nerves, EEG disturbances and dysphagias have been reported with preparations containing tetanus toxoid. If severe reactions (collapse or shock, persistent screaming episodes, temperature of 40.5°C or greater, seizures, severe alterations of consciousness, systemic allergic reactions) occur, future doses of DTP are contraindicated. Immunization with diphtheria and tetanus toxoids adsorbed should be used to complete the course. Lesser reactions do not preclude further use of DTP. Subsequent use of a preparation containing pertussis vaccine is contraindicated in individuals who have experienced severe reactions and neurologic changes with a dose of DTP. Some manufacturers state that DTP is contraindicated during an outbreak of poliomyelitis and in individuals with a personal or family history of CNS disease; this is not considered absolute. Pertussis-containing vaccines are contraindicated in individuals with a progressive or evolving neurologic disorder (eg, progressive encephalopathy), as well as in individuals with acute or active infections. Minor illness such as an upper respiratory infection, a stable neurologic illness (cerebral palsy, mental retardation), or a family history of CNS disease does not preclude immunization.

Drug Interactions:
Immunosuppressive agents (eg, corticosteroids, corticotropin, alkylating agents, antimetabolites) may diminish immunologic response to DTP; therefore, DTP should be deferred until 1 month after the immunosuppressive is discontinued. If immunosuppressive therapy is likely to continue, routine immunization with DTP should be initiated.

Nursing Implications:

- Shake vial vigorously before each dose is withdrawn.
- Inject via deep intramuscular route, preferably into the lateral thigh muscles.
- Teach parents about possible side effects (eg, fever).
- Provide parents with immunization record.

CNS = central nervous system.

BOX 34–5. POLIO VACCINE LIVE ORAL (OPV, SABIN VACCINE)

Classification:
Live attenuated vaccine.

Action:
Promotes immunity to poliomyelitis by inducing production of specific antibodies. OPV induces antibody formation in the lymphatic tissues surrounding the intestinal tract as well as inducing humoral antibodies. Intestinal immunity may reduce the number of temporary carriers and reduce dissemination of wild poliovirus. After administration of OPV, live attenuated polioviruses multiply in the gastrointestinal tract where they persist for 4–6 weeks. Antibody response to OPV occurs within 7–10 days of ingestion and peaks 21 days later. Primary immunization induces immunity to all three serotypes of poliovirus in more than 95 percent of vaccinees.

Indications:
To provide active immunity to poliomyelitis caused by poliovirus types 1, 2, and 3 in immunocompetent individuals 6 weeks to 17 years old.

Stability:
OPV is usually clear and red or pink because of the presence of phenol red as a pH indicator. OPV requires storage at less than 0°C and has an expiration date not exceeding 1 year after date of manufacture. If frozen, the vaccine must be completely thawed prior to use. It may be thawed and refrozen up to 10 times. If the vaccine is thawed for more than 24 hours it must be stored at 2–8°C and used within 30 days. Color changes that occur during storage or thawing have no importance provided the vaccine remains clear.

Dosage and Route:
OPV is administered orally. The vaccine must not be given parenterally. OPV may be administered into the mouth with the single-dose pipette supplied by the manufacturer; mixed with distilled or chlorine-free water, syrup NF, or milk; or administered adsorbed on bread, cake, or cube sugar.

For primary immunization, OPV is administered in a series of three doses to ensure seroconversion to all three sterotypes of poliovirus. Interruption of immunization schedule does not interfere with final immunity achieved nor does it necessitate additional doses or starting over.

The first dose of OPV should be given at 2, 4, and 5–18 months of age but not less than 6–8 weeks should lapse between the first two doses. An additional dose at approximately 6 months of age is recommended in areas where there is substantial risk of exposure to poliomyelitis. At 4–6 years of age or before entering school, children should receive an additional dose of OPV unless the third primary dose was administered on or after the fourth birthday.

When primary immunization with OPV is indicated in older children and adolescents through 17 years of age, two doses of OPV should be given not less than 6

fever). The common cold and upper respiratory infections usually are not contraindications; however, this guideline can be confusing and may cause parents to delay further immunizations until respiratory symptoms disappear.

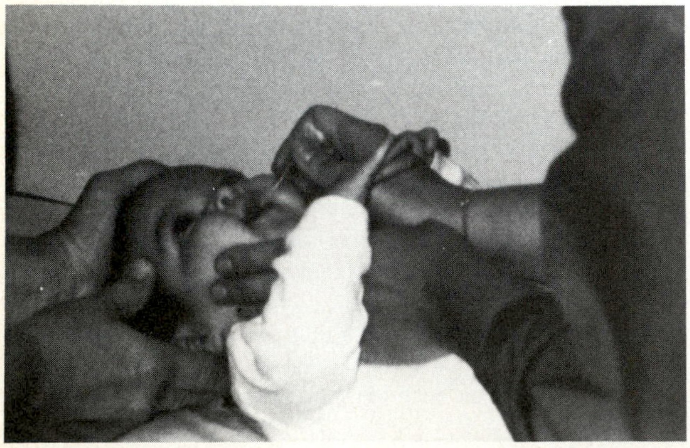

Figure 34–12. Administration of oral polio vaccine.

The nurse involved in health care of infants must be an effective teacher who can provide, interpret, and reinforce information given to parents. In addition, the nurse must be knowledgeable about the infectious process and understand antigen-antibody relationships and immunization schedules and procedures.[32]

The nurse should discuss the benefits and risks of immunizations with parents and ask them to sign an informed consent prior to the administration of immunizations to the infant. An immunization record is then given to the parents and updated as additional immunizations are provided.

Prevention of Accidents

Home safety and accident prevention are integral components of health maintenance and should be instituted during the childhood of every individual. Accidents are one of the leading causes of death in the first year of life.[33, 34] Perhaps the only positive aspect of this statistic is the knowledge that most accidents to 8 weeks apart, and the third dose should be given 6–12 months after the second dose. Adults at increased risk of exposure to poliomyelitis should receive primary immunization with poliovirus vaccine inactivated (IPV) whenever possible. When less than 4 weeks are available before prevention against poliomyelitis is required in unimmunized adults 18 years of age or older, a single dose of OPV should be administered. If the adult remains at increased risk of exposure, the second dose of OPV should be given at least 6–8 weeks after the first dose, and the third dose should be given at least 6 weeks, preferably 8–12 months, after the second dose.

Individuals with symptomatic and asymptomatic human immunodeficiency virus (HIV) infections should receive IPV, not OPV.

Contraindications and Precautions:
Vaccination with OPV should be postponed in individuals with persistent vomiting and diarrhea. OPV is contraindicated in individuals with primary immunodeficiencies (eg, cellular immune deficiency, hypogammaglobulinemia, dysgammaglobulinemia) or in individuals with suppressed immune response resulting from HIV infections, leukemia, lymphoma, other malignancies affecting the bone marrow or lymphatic system, certain blood dyscrasias, or therapy with immunosuppressants, as replication of polioviruses may be potentiated. OPV should not be used in close household contacts of individuals with primary immunodeficiencies or suppressed immune response. If immunization is necessary in these contacts IPV should be used.

Vaccination during pregnancy should be avoided unless immediate protection against poliomyelitis is needed because of imminent exposure.

Adverse Effects:
Rare: Paralytic poliomyelitis primarily in unimmunized young adult household contacts of vaccinated infants and clients with primary immunodeficiency.

Drug Interactions:

- Tuberculin: OPV has been reported to suppress tuberculin skin sensitivity temporarily, therefore, tuberculin test should be done simultaneously with or 6 weeks after administration of vaccine.
- Immunosuppressive therapy: Individuals receiving immunosuppressive therapy may have a diminished response to OPV and replication of the virus may be potentiated.
- Immunoglobulins: Administration of immunoglobulin within 3 months preceding administration of OPV may block the antibody response to the vaccine. Immunoglobulin should not be given until 2 weeks after administration of OPV.

Nursing Implications:

- Administer by oral route.
- Inform parents that vaccine should not be given if child is in contact with individuals with immunodeficiencies (eg, individuals on chemotherapy).
- Provide parents with immunization record.

can be prevented.[35,36] Parents must be made aware of the extent of accidental death and provided with an effective accident prevention plan.

Research indicates that both infant stage of development and maternal (or primary caretaker) factors influence infant accident rates.[37,38] Mothers whose infants are at the highest risk for accidental death are young and poorly educated women who have more than one child.[38] Limited access to health care and poverty are variables that are not infrequently associated with poor education and teenage pregnancy; the infants of these young women are at a particularly high risk for accidental injury and death.[38]

The infant is totally dependent on parental care and supervision for the prevention of accidents. One can easily understand how the overextended mother with several children, the young mother who has developmental needs of her own, and the poorly educated mother who has limited problem-solving skills or little knowledge of infant development could easily overlook or fail to recognize the safety needs of her infant.

An effective accident prevention plan must take into consideration the needs and development of both infants and caretakers. It is not too early to begin discussing newborn safety during the prenatal period, with reinforcement sessions at each well-child and postpartum visit. Nurses who work with infants and caretakers, whether it be in hospitals, clinics, physicians' offices, or home visiting agencies, are in a position to play an active role in accident prevention. The U.S. Consumer Product Safety Commission, Washington, DC 20207, is an excellent source of information and teaching materials that may be shared with parents and primary caretakers.

Knowledge about infant abilities at specific ages and developmental stages is the basis of every accident prevention plan. Health care providers are encouraged to share pamphlets in the caretaker's language and articles concerning normal infant development along with any accident prevention information

TABLE 34–7. RECOMMENDED SCHEDULE FOR ACTIVE IMMUNIZATION OF NORMAL INFANTS AND CHILDREN[a]

Recommended Age	Immunization	Comments
2 months	DTP, OPV	Can be initiated as early as age 2 weeks in areas of high endemicity or during epidemics
4 months	DTP, OPV	2-month interval desired for OPV to avoid interference from previous dose
6 months	DTP	A third dose of OPV is not indicated in the United States but is desirable in geographic areas where polio is endemic
15 months	MMR	MMR preferred to individual vaccines; tuberculin testing may be done at the same visit
18 months	DTP,[b,c] OPV,[d] PRP-D	See footnotes
4–6 years	DTP,[e] OPV	At or before school entry
14–16 years	Td	Repeat every 10 years throughout life

DTP = diphtheria and tetanus toxoids with pertussis vaccine; OPV = oral poliovirus vaccine containing attenuated poliovirus types 1, 2, and 3; MMR = live measles, mumps, and rubella viruses in a combined vaccine; PPR-D = *Haemophilus* b diphtheria toxoid conjugate vaccine; Td = adult tetanus toxoid (full dose) and diphtheria toxoid (reduced dose) for adult use.

[a] For all products used, consult manufacturer's package insert for instructions for storage, handling, dosage, and administration. Biologics prepared by different manufacturers may vary, and package inserts of the same manufacturer may change from time to time. Therefore, the health professional should be aware of the contents of the current package insert.

[b]Should be given 6 to 12 months after third dose.

[c]May be given simultaneously with MMR at age 15 months.

[d]May be given simultaneously with MMR at 15 months of age or any time between 12 and 24 months of age.

[e]Up to the seventh birthday.

From: Committee of Infectious Diseases, American Academy of Pediatrics. Report of the Committee of Infectious Diseases. *21st ed. Elkgrove Village, Ill: 1988.*

that may be disseminated. And, as with all educational efforts, the needs, abilities, and environment of the learner cannot be overlooked.[39]

Table 34–8 outlines accident prevention information for the following types of accidents: aspiration, suffocation, strangulation, falls, motor vehicle, poisoning, burns, and bodily injury (lacerations and punctures). Accident prevention information is most useful when taught alongside the developmental activities and abilities that place the infant at risk for a particular accident given the infant's stage of development.

Parents and primary caretakers must be impressed with the necessity and importance of accident prevention. Simply mentioning accident prevention is not sufficient. Despite all the public awareness campaigns, it is not uncommon to observe infants and children out of car safety seats.[40] Parent education is the only manner in which this problem can be addressed.

Numerous films and teaching materials are available in a variety of languages for use in prenatal classes and clinics, well-child clinics, physicians' offices, daycare centers, and other facilities in which parents, infants, and primary caretakers may be encountered (Figure 34–16). Parents and primary caretakers must be made active participants in recognizing the dangers in their own automobiles and homes and the methods by which those dangers can be eliminated.[40–49]

Meeting Parental Educational Needs

Parenting is a developmental process that requires specific information that enhances knowledge, builds skills, and changes behavior as needed. Health promotion during infancy thus focuses on anticipatory guidance. Parents identify many concerns during the period of infancy. Among these are weaning and the introduction of solid foods, teething, infant sleep patterns, fever, thumbsucking, sibling rivalry, and consequences of working parents on infant development.

Weaning and Introduction of Solid Food. Weaning usually occurs between 6 months and 1 year of age and should be instituted gradually. One recent study of breastfeeding mothers investigated patterns of weaning that could be chosen by mothers. Three patterns were found: gradual weaning, minimal breastfeeding, and sudden severance. The mothers who chose gradual weaning replaced total breastfeeding with cow's milk or formula and/or solid foods over a period of one to eight weeks. Mothers who chose minimal breastfeeding gradually reduced the number of feedings until the infant was breastfeeding only twice a day; thus, when the mother wished to terminate breastfeeding completely, only two feedings needed to be eliminated. In the third pattern, sudden severance, the breastfeedings were totally eliminated in one day.[50] The investigators concluded that gradual weaning was preferable.

TABLE 34–8. ACCIDENT PREVENTION DURING THE FIRST YEAR

Developmental Ability	Preventive Behaviors
Birth to 2 Months Weak gastroesophageal sphincter: vomits and regurgitates easily Only beginning head and neck control Engages in movement that may propel or project the infant Kicks legs Rolls from side to supine Lifts head momentarily Rotates and extends head Has grasp reflex Moves arms and hands	**Aspiration** Hold infant 15 to 30 minutes after feeding to prevent vomiting. Place infant in prone position with head to side. Do not offer solid foods. Pacifiers should be of one-piece construction with a large shield to prevent entry into mouth.
	Suffocation Never leave infant alone in any amount of water. Avoid sleeping with infant. Avoid the use of plastic of any sort; discard plastic bags immediately. Crib slats should not be more than 2⅜ inches apart. Cover crib slats with bumpers. Remove unnecessary pillows, blankets, and stuffed toys from crib.
	Strangulation Avoid use of necklaces, straps, ties, or cords around neck or near crib. Do not hang pacifier around infant's neck. Remove bibs for naps. Be cautious of any toys with straps or cords.
	Falls Never leave infant unattended on high surfaces (place infant on floor if need be). Supervise toddlers and young children around infant. Avoid placing infant in high chairs or grocery carts until the infant can sit well. Use security straps in infant seats and strollers.
	Motor Vehicles *Always* use an infant seat, even with premature infants.[40] At this age place infant seat facing rear of car (Figure 34–13). Never leave infant unattended in carriages or strollers. Never leave infant unattended in cars.
	Burns Check surface temperature of car seats and belts. Avoid smoking around infant. Expose to direct sunlight only for brief periods. Cover infant's head when in sun; head is largest body surface of infant. Check bath and formula temperatures carefully. Avoid drinking or pouring hot liquids while holding infant. Keep infant away from hot objects. Avoid use of hot-mist vaporizers.
	Bodily Injury Always close safety pins. Avoid sharp objects or toys. Be careful with sharp jewelry or clasp pins for jewelry.
3 to 6 Months Places everything in mouth Regards tiny objects Can grasp and actively reaches for and manipulates objects Recovers objects Rolls over Wriggles free of straps Sits up	**Aspiration** Remove any small objects from reach: buttons, beads, screws, jewelry, candy, nuts, small toy parts. Chop or mash solid food finely. Do not permit infant to play with baby powder container. Avoid small removable toy parts, whole hot dogs, popcorn, balloons, and pieces of raw vegetables.
	Suffocation Follow instructions for previous months.
	Strangulation Follow instructions for previous months. Restrain in high chair using straps between legs as well as waist strap; infant may slide down and strangle on waist belt if center strap is not used to hold infant in place.

(continued)

TABLE 34–8. ACCIDENT PREVENTION DURING THE FIRST YEAR (*continued*)

Developmental Ability	Preventive Behaviors
3 to 6 Months (*continued*)	**Falls** Follow instructions for previous months. Elevate crib rails at all times. Do not leave on bed or in infant seat unattended. **Motor Vehicles** Follow instructions for previous months. **Poisons** Elevate or hang plants and discard any poisonous plants. Evaluate house, toys, and furniture for lead paint. Lock away or elevate to high cabinet all toxic substances (Figure 34–14). Do not store toxic substances near food. Discard all toxic substance containers immediately. Do not use food containers to store toxic substances. Know and post local poison information center number. **Burns** Follow instructions for previous months. Do not allow infant to play with faucets during bath. Be particularly careful to avoid drinking hot beverages or smoking near infants. Cover electrical outlets. **Bodily Injury** Follow instructions for previous months. Do not allow infant to play with fork or knife while being fed. Continue to examine toys and environment for sharp edges. Use nonbreakable and splinterproof eating utensils.
6 to 9 Months Puts everything in mouth Uses sense of smell to explore environment Interested in sounds that objects make Rolls supine to prone Begins to stand holding on Pulls to standing Crawls Manipulates objects freely Secures tiny objects Begins to crawl up stairs Looks for hidden objects Beginning to poke with index finger	**Aspiration** Continue to examine toys for loose parts. As solid food is offered avoid peanuts, popcorn, candy, bones, raw vegetables, and whole hot dogs. Keep floors and reachable surfaces clear of small objects. **Suffocation** Follow instructions for previous months. Discard plastic bags immediately. Do not permit infant to play near gas jets or floor heaters. Do not allow infant to play with balloons or pieces of balloons. Keep bathroom door closed. Do not allow infant to play near buckets, toilet, wading pool, or swimming pool unsupervised. Keep trunks, refrigerators, dishwashers, front-loading washers or dryers, and ovens securely closed. Discard old appliances or remove doors. **Strangulation** Follow instructions for previous months. Be sure that child cannot reach curtain or window blind cords or mobile cords from his or her crib or playpen. Keep electrical cords out of reach. Do not permit infant to play with "pull toys" while unsupervised. **Falls** Follow instructions for previous months. Use portable fence or gate to keep infant away from stairs or in same room as caretaker (Figure 34–15). **Motor Vehicles** Follow instructions for previous months. Do not permit infant to crawl or play around cars. **Poisons** Follow instructions for previous months.

TABLE 34–8. ACCIDENT PREVENTION DURING THE FIRST YEAR (*continued*)

Developmental Ability	Preventive Behaviors
6 to 9 Months (*continued*)	**Burns** Use guards in front of fireplaces, heaters, floor furnaces, and so on. Do not allow infant to play or crawl around stove or oven. Keep matches, candles, lighters, and any other hot objects out of reach. Remove or secure tablecloths. Cover electrical outlets with plastic caps. Keep electrical cords out of reach. Do not allow infant to play with electrical appliances. **Bodily Injury** Follow instructions for previous months. Store all sharp objects out of reach. Keep portable fans or air conditioners out of reach or safely guarded. Store soda bottles or any type of glass out of reach. Tack down small rugs or remove them altogether.
9 to 12 Months Puts everything in mouth Crawls expertly Stands holding on Walks holding onto furniture and other objects Crawls up stairs and backs down stairs Throws objects Stoops and recovers objects Overcomes obstacles to obtain desired object Pokes with index finger Uses neat pincer grasp Takes objects out of a container Puts objects into containers Looks for hidden objects Unwraps paper and lifts covers Removes pieces from toy puzzles and takes toys apart Some infants begin to walk Trys to drink from any cup or glass	**Aspiration** Follow instructions for previous months. **Suffocation** Follow instructions for previous months. When around pools, keep child in eyesight at all times. **Falls** Follow instructions for previous months. Supervise closely when around stairs or windows. **Motor Vehicles** Follow instructions for previous months. Lock car doors. Hold or restrain infant while in parking lots or around cars. **Poisons** Follow instructions for previous months. Do not tell infant that medication is candy. Be sure that all cabinet doors are secure. Use childproof caps on all medication. Store all medications immediately after use. Do not permit infant to play with adult handbags that may contain medications. **Burns** Follow instructions for previous months. Do not allow infant to play in kitchen during cooking times. Keep all hot beverages out of reach. Keep infant out of kitchen while oven is on. Turn pan handles in so that they cannot be pulled down or knocked over.

The transitions from breast to bottle, from breast to cup, or from liquids to solids all describe weaning. Improved hand-eye coordination, attempts to hold the bottle, decreased interest in breastfeeding or bottlefeeding, and an interest in chewing are signs that the infant is ready to respond to feeding changes. Many parents and health professionals feel that this is an appropriate time to introduce solids. At the same time, the amount of milk and the number of feedings should be reduced (*see* earlier discussion).

Weaning to the cup should be attempted when the infant is ready. The infant's age, signs of readiness, number of milk feedings per day, ability to use a cup, and way in which sucking needs are met should be assessed prior to counseling parents.

Teething. Primary tooth eruption begins at about 6 months of age, with teeth erupting approximately every 2 months until 2 years of age. Teething can occur with or without pain. Painful teething causes discomfort, irritability, crying, restlessness, drooling, and rubbing of the gums. The gums appear red and swollen. Parents should be informed that discomfort can often be relieved by giving the infant hard, clean objects to chew on (such as teething rings, teething beads or hard bread). Rubbing the gums with teeth-

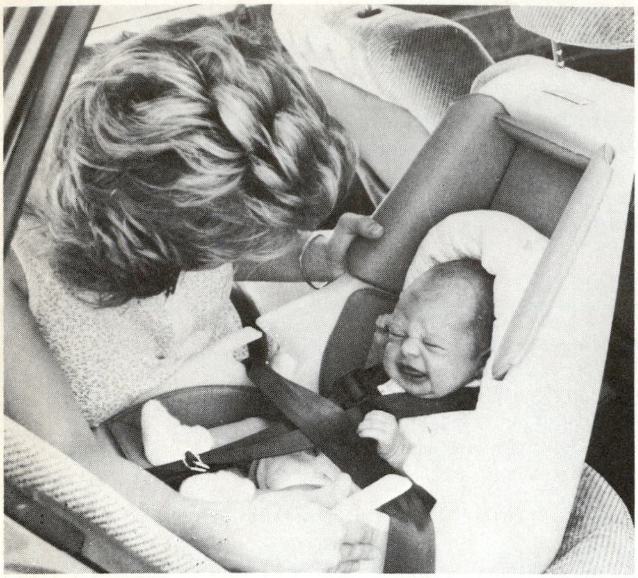

Figure 34–13. Mother secures infant in car seat.

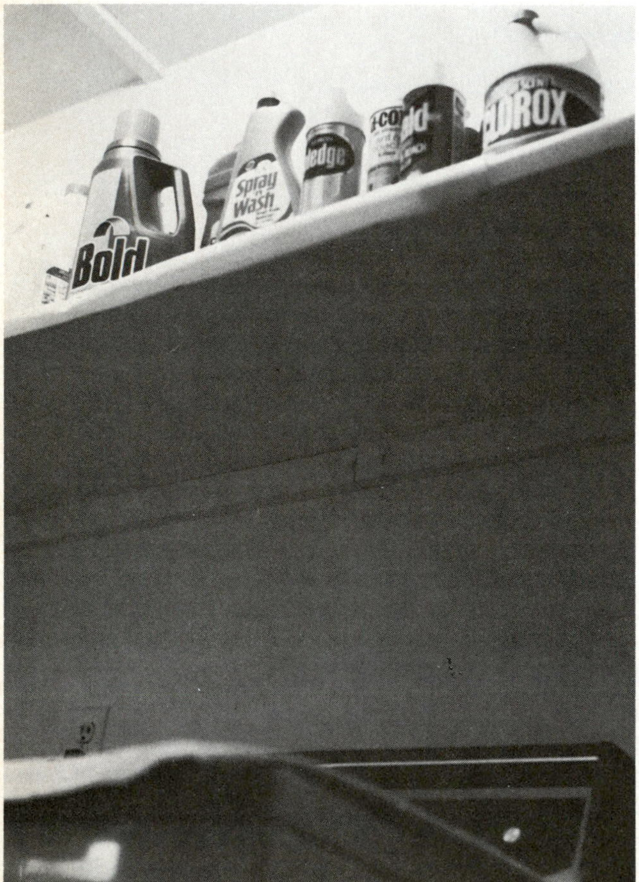

Figure 34–14. Many common household products are poisonous; they should always be kept in locked cabinets or out of the reach of children.

ing lotions is a treatment that is frequently recommended. Contrary to popular belief, fever is not always a manifestation of teething and warrants further investigation.[51]

Sleep Patterns. The majority of childcare experts agree that sleeping patterns vary among infants and change with maturation. Generally speaking, infants between 2 and 6 weeks of age show a great variation in sleep patterns but gradually phase into a diurnal cycle.[52] In the first 2 weeks of life, most newborns sleep the same number of hours during the day as they do during the night. By 5 weeks of age, 66 percent of infants begin to sleep longer at night, and by 3 months of age, 98 percent of infants sleep longer at night. The pattern that is established by 4 to 5 months of age is usually one of 2- to 4-hour naps after feedings and 6 to 7 hours of sleep through the night. At about 6 months of age, the nap periods shorten to a morning and afternoon nap after meals and sleeping through the night. It is not uncommon for night awakening to occur at about 7 months of age, when infants begin to experience separation anxiety. By 1 year of age some infants discontinue the morning nap, sleep longer in the afternoon, and sleep through the night.[52] The variability of infant sleep patterns cannot be overemphasized, and as with almost all other infant activities, sleep is influenced by the environment.[53, 54]

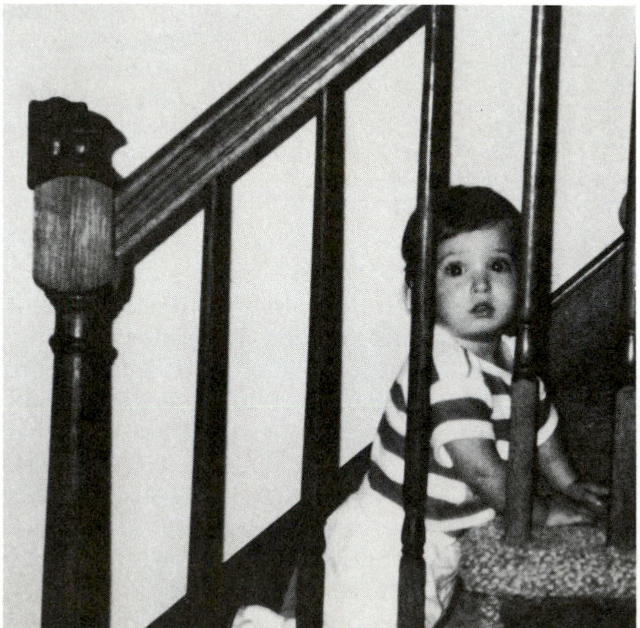

Figure 34–15. Infants should be prevented from climbing stairs, for example with a portable gate.

Sleep problems, particularly not sleeping through the night, may cause a great deal of stress to families and create problems of sleep deprivation, exhaustion, and irritability for caretakers. Awakening in the night in and of itself is not considered a problem; rather, awakening and then crying and not returning to sleep is what is defined as a problem by parents.[53] New, young, inexperienced parents or parents lacking an experienced and knowledgeable support system may have more difficulty than their experienced counterparts.[52,53,55] Problems may arise when parents do not understand normal infant sleep behaviors and view the sleepless, crying infant as a sign of their incompetence as a parent, or view the sleepless crying as an attempt by the infant to manipulate the parent.[52] More commonly, parents have difficulty with the night awakening because they are exhausted the next day and find it problematic to meet the demands and obligations of managing a home, job, and personal and professional relationships.[53]

The age of the infant when sleep problems are reported will influence the management of the problem. There is so much variation among infant sleeping patterns in the first 6 weeks of life that parents must be educated to the fact that a "normal" infant sleeping pattern does not exist. Parents may require instruction as well as emotional support during this period. To gather accurate information about the infant's sleeping, waking, and crying times, parents are instructed to keep a record during two or three 24-hour periods. Most young infants sleep 15.4 hours in 24 hours (although how those 15.4 hours are spread throughout the 24-hour period may vary) and cry 1½ to 3½ hours per day. Parents may just need to understand that their infant is behaving normally. Nurses should not overlook the fact that when parents are complaining of a sleep problem in their young infant, they may actually be having difficulty with the infant's crying and not his or her awake state. Education of the parent as to individual temperamental traits and interventions for excessive crying (discussed later under "Colic") may help the parent cope with this early period.[52]

Awakening and crying during the second half of the first year are not uncommon and are thought to be related to separation anxiety. The infant usually awakens and cries after 2 hours of sleep and responds to being brought to the parents' or older siblings' bed.[52,53,55] As most parents do not wish to establish this habit, it is best left unpracticed. Results from one study indicate that other successful measures are rocking the infant back to sleep, staying with the infant until he or she returns to sleep, and performing consistent bedtime routines.[53] Interestingly, a method that is commonly recommended in childcare literature, letting the infant cry until she or he falls asleep, was not found to be successful by some mothers in this sample.[53] This particular study, as many before it, found that successful measures for coping with night waking are as varied as infant sleeping patterns.[53]

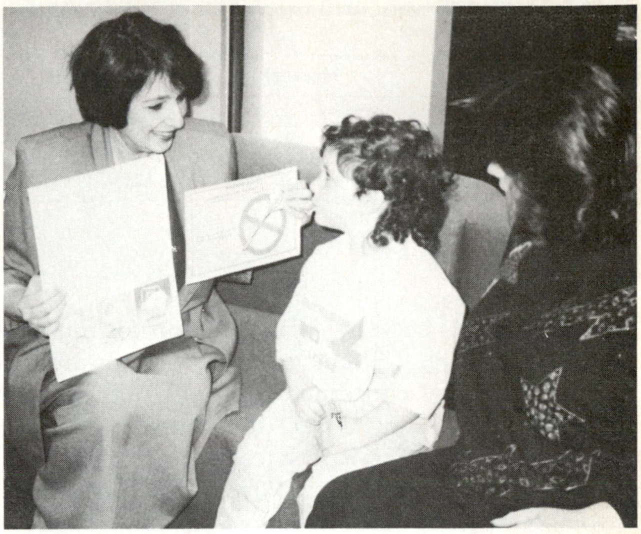

Figure 34–16. Nurse teaching a pregnant woman and her child about safety.

Other strategies useful in coping with night waking include the following:

1. When both parents work outside the home they may find it helpful to alternate night care of the infant so that they can be assured of a good night's sleep at least every other night.
2. Parents who have the means or support system may have a babysitter care for the infant in the evening or morning while they "catch up" on their sleep.
3. Caretakers who remain home with the infant should take advantage of the infant's day nap to take a nap themselves.

Parents, in particular first-time parents, may require anticipatory guidance regarding sleep behaviors and developmental variations of infants. Nurses, before giving advice about infant sleep problems, are encouraged to investigate the infant's individual waking, sleeping, and crying pattern, as well as to explore the temperament of the infant and the environment that influences the infant.

Fever. A **fever** is a body temperature elevated above normal (Table 34–9). Fever is the most common rea-

TABLE 34–9. NORMAL AND ELEVATED TEMPERATURE VALUES OF INFANTS

	Normal	Elevated
Rectal temperature	99.6°F (37.6°C)	> 101°F (38.3°C)
Oral temperature	98.6°F (37.0°C)	> 100°F (37.8°C)
Axillary temperature	97.6°F (36.5°C)	> 99°F (37.2°C)

Source: *Reference 56.*

son the parents seek medical attention for their infants and children.[56] Many of these parents are unduly anxious and concerned as a result of a lack of knowledge regarding fever in infants and young children.[57] Parents' greatest fears are that children will develop neurologic problems such as seizures, mental retardation, and learning problems.[57]

Parents often lack knowledge not only about fever, but about the measurement and management of fever as well.[58–60] It is not uncommon for parents to be unnecessarily aggressive or inappropriate in the management of fever.[60] Casey and others were able to document this knowledge deficit even among well-educated parents who were attuned to their infants' needs. It is a problem that must be addressed at all educational and socioeconomic levels.[60]

Many of the problems and anxieties concerning fever could be allayed with infant education during discharge planning and well- and sick-child visits to health care providers. Studies have shown that parents rely on physicians and nurses to be their main source of information about fever[57] and that educational efforts in which parents are active learners can result in decreased medication errors by parents and reduce needless physician contacts.[60]

Although some fevers caused by focal infections and a few caused by bacteremia must be treated, 60 to 70 percent of all fevers are caused by respiratory tract infections, 90 percent of fevers are of a viral nature and require only supportive therapy, and the majority of fevers are mild and self-limiting.[56, 58, 61]

Neonates (infants under 29 days of age) may not necessarily exhibit an elevated temperature during illness. During this period, parents are encouraged to report any behavior that is different or unusual for their infant. Examples of unusual behavior would be a change in level of activity (either very sleepy or lethargic or overly fussy and agitated), not looking at objects or people, not responding to stimuli, and not taking feedings as usual. It is important for parents to know age-appropriate behavior so that they can recognize when their neonate or young infant is acting out of the ordinary.[56, 62] Any fever during the neonatal period should also be reported.

Medications are another source of problems for parents. The overly aggressive treatment of fever by parents may result in overdosage and all its accompanying dangers.[63] Parents must receive clear written instructions on the dosage and administration of antipyretics (eg, Tylenol) and be warned against the use of aspirin in children who have viral flu symptoms. Aspirin is not recommended for use in children because of the risk of Reye's syndrome.[56]

To be reliable partners with health care providers, parents must know normal and elevated temperature values (*see* Table 34–9), know how to take a temperature and to reduce a fever, be able to follow orders and administer medications safely, and know when to seek further assistance from health care personnel. Refer to the Case Study/Care Plan for fever management at the end of the chapter. A high fever in a child is defined as a temperature over 105°F (40.5°C), and some researchers feel that fevers do not cause harm until they reach 106°F (41.6° to 41.7°C). It must be remembered, however, that the rapid ascent of a temperature is what triggers a seizure, not the degree of fever; therefore, careful and frequent (every 1 to 2 hours) temperature readings must be taken. When a fever is above 103°F, the health care provider should be contacted. Sponging with tepid water for ½ hour every 2 hours is recommended. The nurse should validate that parents know how to correctly take an axillary or rectal temperature and read a thermometer (*see* the Case Study/Care Plan for fever management at the end of the chapter).

Thumb Sucking. During infancy, thumb sucking is considered a normal phenomenon. Parents often become disturbed with the activity because they fear that it will develop into a habit that not only interferes with the normal alignment of teeth, but is poorly received socially. Thumb sucking is not indicative of an emotional disorder in and of itself, even when chronic in nature; it is a habit or learned response that like many rhythmic patterns feels good or provides self-nurturance.

Restriction of thumb sucking is not necessary in the first year of life, nor is it suggested by most authorities during the preschool years. Left to their own accord, most children lessen their thumb sucking by age 6 and stop completely by age 11.

Parents who fear that their infant will turn into a thumb sucker can be advised that a supportive, loving, and stress-reduced environment may diminish the development of tension-reducing behaviors such as thumb sucking. There are also confirmed orthodontic reports that properly designed bottle nipples and pacifiers provide sensory gratification and may provide a deterrent to thumb and finger sucking. Pacifiers, if they are to be successful in preventing thumb sucking, must be used before the thumb sucking becomes a habit.[52] As the infant becomes mobile, the pacifier will gradually be forgotten, but some young children may require weaning from the pacifier. Parents are discouraged from hanging the pacifier around the neck of an infant or young child. Not only is the practice unsafe (strangulation may result), but it serves to replace thumb sucking with pacifier sucking as a habit.

Sibling Rivalry. Sibling reactions to a newborn vary depending on the age, parent-child interaction, feelings of security, presence or absence of other siblings, and preparation for the addition to the family (*see* Chapter 26 for additional discussion). Whatever the older child's responses, they are intended to regain or maintain parental attention that has been lost with the changing family structure.[64] Studies have identified common behaviors in siblings of a newborn, including increased demands for parental attention, changes (usually regressive) in toilet habits, demands to resume bottlefeeding or breastfeeding, clinging and other displays of anxiety, "baby talk," increased confrontations, and aggression.[65, 66]

Discussions with parents during the antepartum and postpartum periods should include anticipatory guidance about sibling rivalry. The nurse should emphasize to parents that birth of a sibling represents a crisis for the older child or children that can increase psychologic vulnerability or provide an opportunity for further maturation. Parents' readiness to recognize its existence and their willingness to be available to the child can help resolve the crisis. Nursing intervention should include teaching the parents and child new coping patterns aimed at helping the child. For example, parents can be advised to set aside individualized "child's time" during which the child receives undivided parental attention. The child can be encouraged to verbalize feelings rather than "act out" and to continue to use age-appropriate rather than regressive behavior to get parental attention.

Positive attitudes toward a sibling that are established at birth might lay the foundation for positive relationships later in life. Parental guidance by the nurse and parental support for the child may decrease difficulty in adapting to a new baby.

Working Parents. Concern about parental absence and its effect on the infant has always existed. That concern has escalated with the number of families where both parents work outside the home. As the number of dual-income couples has grown, more infants are being cared for by other adults in home settings and daycare centers.

The number of women with young children tripled between 1970 and 1976 and has continued to increase annually. By 1985, one half of all women with children under three years of age were employed outside the home. Demographic data indicate that as dual-earner families continue to increase, mothers of young children will continue to enter the work force in large numbers.[67]

Attention must be directed toward a better understanding of how two-income and single-parent families provide child care for their infants. The selection of caretakers and their characteristics can have serious implications for the psychologic well-being of parents and their children.

Most children in daycare spend more than 30 hours per week with a caretaker other than the parents. Whether or not the alternate caretakers are able to do so, they must assume primary responsibility for all aspects of the infant's care during the parents' absence. They provide for the infant's social, emotional, and cognitive development, as well as meet the infant's more basic needs.[68]

Whether mothers of infants should work is no longer debatable. The reality is that many do and more will work in the future. Realistic questions center on when they should return to work and the infant's response to maternal absence, paternal absence, or both. In addition, an important issue of concern to working parents is obtaining affordable, appropriate childcare.

Owen and colleagues studied the parent-child relationships in 59 dual-income families and their infants.[69] The quality of the mother-infant attachment did not decrease when the mother returned to work. No overall differences were observed in father-infant interaction where the mother worked. Whether the mother returned to work when the child was an infant or toddler did not seem to affect the stability or quality of development.

Careful assessment of the infant's level of development and parent-infant attachment are important factors to be considered when a parent returns to work. The time spent with the infant should provide nurturing care that promotes cognitive, emotional, and social growth.

SELECTED NEONATAL AND INFANT STRESSORS

The neonate and infant possess unique physiologic capabilities to adapt to stress, both internal and external. Occasionally, however, interventions are necessary to ensure or facilitate a return to wellness. Many stressors identified during the neonatal and infant periods can be managed through nursing interventions or through joint protocols developed in conjunction with medical and other health professional colleagues. This section discusses nursing care of physiologic jaundice, musculoskeletal impairment, obstruction of the lacrimal ducts, skin problems, thrush, feeding problems, colic, and tooth decay.

Physiologic Jaundice

Physiologic jaundice is a common condition in the early neonatal period, occurring in approximately 50 percent of term infants during the first week of life, usually on the second or third day. (*See* discussion in Chapter 32 under "Hepatic Regulation.") The condition most often occurs when the neonate's immature liver is unable to handle the breakdown of protein, resulting in hyperbilirubinemia, an excess of bilirubin in the blood. This process is considered a normal finding in most neonates who are otherwise healthy; however, jaundice present at birth or within the first 24 hours is always considered pathologic. Table 34–10 lists several criteria that may be used to differentiate between physiologic and nonphysiologic (pathologic) jaundice.[70] Further assessment is usually needed if the newborn meets any of these criteria, as discussed in Chapter 32.

Several mechanisms, individually or in combination, contribute to the development of physiologic jaundice: bilirubin overproduction, defective uptake and transport of bilirubin within the liver cells (hepatocytes), impaired bilirubin conjugation, impaired bilirubin excretion, and increased bilirubin reabsorption from the intestinal tract.[71]

A serum bilirubin level of 2.0 mg/dL or greater is a common finding in neonates during the first week of life. Usually jaundice does not become visible until the serum concentration exceeds 7.0 mg/dL. The peak level for physiologic jaundice in normal neonates has traditionally been considered to be 12.9 mg/dL.

Several studies have shown differences in peak bilirubin levels between breastfeeding and bottlefeeding infants. In one sample, breastfeeding was the factor that most predicted hyperbilirubinemia of greater than 12.0 mg/dL. The jaundice resolved in 10 days for breastfed infants, compared with 7 days for formula-fed infants.[72] Another study found that serum bilirubin levels in breastfed infants were still elevated at 21 days.[73] These findings have led some clinicians to suggest that the peak level for hyperbilirubinemia be changed. The new suggested standards would be 13 mg/dL for bottlefed neonates and 15 mg/dL for breastfed neonates.[74]

TABLE 34–10. CHARACTERISTICS OF NONPHYSIOLOGIC JAUNDICE

Clinical jaundice in the first 24 hours of life
Total serum bilirubin concentration increasing by more than 5 mg/dL per day
Total serum bilirubin concentrations exceeding 12.9 mg/dL in a full-term neonate or 15 mg/dL in a premature neonate
Direct serum bilirubin concentration exceeding 1.5 to 2 mg/dL

Jaundice can be detected by blanching (pressing) the neonate's nose, palms, or soles of the feet. If the skin blanches yellow, the neonate is considered to be jaundiced. In many instances, the sclerae of the eyes will also be yellow tinted. Neonates of dark-skinned or olive-complexioned parents may appear to be jaundiced when in actuality they are not.

Although serum bilirubin levels have been the traditional method used to screen for hyperbilirubinemia, many institutions now employ noninvasive, transcutaneous bilirubinometry methods. One methods uses an icterometer, an inexpensive Plexiglas strip on which are painted five yellow transverse stripes that are precisely colored. The Plexiglas strip is pressed against the neonate's skin and the color of the skin is compared with the color on the stripes. A jaundice score is then assigned. Another method uses a jaundice meter that measures the intensity of the yellow color in the skin through spectrophotometry. The jaundice meter is placed against either the neonate's forehead or sternum and a reading is taken. Both methods are considered appropriate in screening for jaundice,[75] and decrease the number of times serum samples must be taken for analysis. If bilirubin levels exceed acceptable levels, phototherapy will be instituted. (Acceptable levels may vary from institution to institution.) Chapter 42 discusses treatment for jaundice in the neonate.

Nursing care of the newborn with physiologic jaundice centers on providing clear and appropriate explanations to the parents. Too often the newborn is taken for a blood test with the explanation that a "bilirubin level" is needed. Even the most knowledgeable of parents may have little understanding of the meaning of such a test. Clear and concise explanations of the physiology and purpose of testing can do much to allay parents' anxieties.

Protocols for treatment of breastfeeding jaundice vary. If the mother continues to nurse, elevated levels of bilirubin may persist, reaching normal values by 3 to 12 weeks of age. If breastfeeding is interrupted, serum bilirubin levels decline within 48 hours and bilirubin levels rise only about 1 to 3 mg/dL after nursing is resumed. Some investigators conclude that when the serum bilirubin concentration approaches

17 mg/dL, breastfeeding should be interrupted for 48 hours, at which time nursing can be resumed.[70] If this protocol is chosen, the nurse needs to support the mother and allay any fears she may have that there is something wrong with her milk or that she is doing harm to the newborn by breastfeeding. The nurse should also assist the mother to maintain lactation through the use of manual expression and breast pumps.

Other practitioners have attempted to supplement breastfed newborns with glucose water. This practice does not reduce the serum bilirubin level. In fact, using glucose water may increase the level of bilirubin and be potentially harmful to the newborn.[70] Supplementing with plain water is thought to have no effect on the bilirubin concentration.[76]

One study of bottlefed and breastfed infants found a greater excretion of bilirubin in those who had a greater stool output. Bottlefed infants were found to have more frequent stools, whereas breastfed infants experienced a greater weight loss in the immediate neonatal period. It was suggested that hyperbilirubinemia in breastfed infants could be minimized by earlier stimulation of intestinal motility.[77] Nurses can support this by explaining the benefits of early rooming-in, and frequent nursing to reestablish hydration as well as promoting the early onset of milk supply, and by encouraging nonnutritive sucking with a pacifier. If the mother does not desire to have the newborn room-in, every effort should be made to bring the newborn to her when hungry, instead of waiting for the routine hospital schedule.

Musculoskeletal Impairment

Hip Dysplasia. Physical assessment of the neonate's hips may occasionally produce a palpable Ortolani click, an indication of hip dysplasia (subluxation of the joint). Complete dislocation of the hip at birth or within the neonatal period is rare.

Hip dysplasia has an incidence of approximately 4 to 7 per 1000 live births, affecting females more than males in an 8 to 1 ratio. The greater incidence among female neonates is felt to be the result of production of relaxin by the fetal uterus, a condition that affects the tensile strength of the hip ligaments adversely. The joint is not fully ossified, having a shallow acetabulum and a soft and less elastic capsule. There may also be a genetic predisposition toward dysplasia.[78]

The condition may not be present at birth, and may not manifest itself for several months. For this reason, assessment of the hip joint is an important part of the physical examination until the age of 2. The affected limb appears to be shortened. The nurse can identify a shortened limb by holding the pelvis straight and pressing the knees flat against the table top; inequality in the position of the soles of the feet will be apparent. There may also be asymmetry of thigh creases or an extra fold of skin present on the shortened thigh. The nurse should be able to abduct both thighs equally while in a flexed position. Inability to do so indicates the presence of subluxation. X-rays of the affected hip reveal upward and outward malposition of the femoral head.

Treatment is designed to keep the affected hip in an abducted position with the hip flexed and externally rotated, maintaining the head of the femur in contact with the acetabulum. This is accomplished by using one of the following methods: (1) the Frejka pillow splint, which is applied over the diapers and must be removed and reapplied with each diaper change; (2) triple or quadruple diapers, which when applied maintain the hip in the desired position; or (3) the Pavlik harness, a device that holds the hip in the desired position but allows limited range of motion at the hip joint, thereby preventing the problem of avascular necrosis of the femoral head. Extreme cases of hip dysplasia may require casting with a hip spica cast and, possibly, surgery. Ultrasonography has been successfully used in the continued evaluation of infants with hip dysplasia, providing the clinician with accurate assessments even for the infant who is in a cast, brace, or harness.[79]

Clubfoot/Talipes Equinovarus. "Clubfoot" is a pathologic deformity in which the leg and foot resemble a clubbing instrument. It occurs in two forms, talipes equinovarus and talipes calcaneovalgus, and may be unilateral or bilateral.

Talipes equinovarus is the more severe form in which there is inversion of the heel and forefoot, adduction of the forefoot, and plantar flexion of the entire foot. Less severe is talipes calcaneovalgus in which the heel and forefoot are everted, the forefoot is abducted, and the entire foot is dorsiflexed.

Both forms of clubfoot occur in approximately 1 out of every 200 live births. Fifty percent of cases are bilateral, affecting boys twice as frequently as girls. An infant born with a clubfoot is referred to an orthopedic physician for treatment and follow-up. Further treatment may involve casting and, possibly, surgery.

Often the position of neonates' feet may suggest a problem with clubfoot, but actually the problem is due to intrauterine positioning. In this case, the apparent deformity can be easily brought into a normal position by gentle manipulation of the feet. If this occurs, parents can be taught exercises to gradually return the infant's feet to a normal position.

Obstruction of the Lacrimal Ducts

Many new mothers may be concerned about constant tearing and a mucoid discharge from either one or both of the neonate's eyes. Lacrimal outlet obstruction or dacryostenosis occurs in more than 50 percent of neonates in the first week of life. Usually the nasolacrimal ducts will spontaneously open by 3 months of age. Parents can be taught to massage the ducts to promote mucous drainage. Massage is accomplished by firm pressure in a small circular motion along the side of the nose toward the eye and the opening of the lacrimal duct at the inner canthus. The drainage is then cleared away with a cotton ball and warm water, wiping from the inner to the outer canthus. This process is repeated three to four times a day in the affected eye.

Rarely does acute infection (dacryocystitis) occur. This is characterized by purulent discharge, swelling in the inner canthal region, and tenderness and redness over the area. Topical and systemic antibiotics are usually indicated for dacryocystitis. Eye hygiene is the same as for dacryostenosis.

Skin Problems

It has been estimated that 20 to 30 percent of all children brought for health care services have either a skin complaint or skin finding.[80] One study revealed that the primary problem of 4.4 percent of infants under the age of 1 year who sought medical services was a skin problem.[81]

Numerous skin diseases and problems may be noted in infancy. Fortunately, the most common are also usually the most benign. The common skin problems of infants include cradle cap, which is a form of seborrheic dermatitis, and diaper dermatitis, which includes contact, ammoniacal, and fungal diaper rash.

Cradle Cap. **Cradle cap** is a form of seborrheic dermatitis that results from a buildup of sebaceous matter on the scalp, usually over the anterior fontanelle. It differs from more severe and chronic forms of seborrheic dermatitis because it is easily treated with proper washing of the scalp. Infants with cradle cap have the characteristic yellow, crusty, waxy patches restricted to the anterior scalp. Infants with other, more severe forms of seborrheic dermatitis express the lesions on the eyebrows, behind the ears, on the eyelids, chest, cheeks, neck, and axilla, as well as on the scalp.[80]

A shampooing should be demonstrated to the mother or caretaker, who often is surprised that the scalp can be vigorously scrubbed without causing damage. Baby oil may be massaged into the scalp 15 to 30 minutes prior to shampooing; then with gentle but firm rubbing with a dry washcloth or combing with a finetooth comb, some of the crusty patches can be lifted from the scalp. The scalp and hair may then be washed with a mild shampoo and rinsed well with tepid water. The mother or primary caretaker is instructed to repeat this procedure daily until the cradle cap is removed.

In more severe cases of cradle cap, an antiseborrheic shampoo may be indicated.[82] It should also be noted that secondary infections can develop on the scalp that may require antimicrobial treatment.[80]

Diaper Dermatitis. **Diaper dermatitis** is a general term for numerous and distinct skin irritations and inflammations that may occur in the diaper area. The specific causes may vary and require different treatments. It has been estimated that 10 percent of all infants acquire some form of diaper dermatitis before the age of 2 years, with the peak age of incidence being 7 to 9 months.[83,84]

Contact Diaper Rash. The most frequently observed diaper dermatitis is a contact diaper rash, which is due to friction and contact irritation. The infant diaper area is repeatedly subjected to moisture from frequent urination and friction from the diaper itself. Infrequent diaper changes result in excessive hydration and maceration of the skin from prolonged contact with moisture; the least amount of friction will irritate or break down the skin, or both. Overzealous cleanliness in which the diaper area is cleansed too frequently, too harshly, or with soaps or other agents that are irritating to infant skin may also cause contact dermatitis.[85]

Other causes of contact diaper rash are laundry soaps and additives, plastic or rubber pants used over cloth diapers, disposable diapers in infants who are intolerant of them, and diarrhea.[86]

Skin affected by contact diaper rash is characterized by erythematous shiny patches on the convex skin surface (buttock, lower abdomen, upper thighs, and genital area); the skin-fold areas are not usually involved. When diarrhea is the cause of a contact diaper rash the area around the anus, perineum, and buttock will appear irritated and inflamed.

The goal of treatment is to determine the cause of the rash and to keep the diaper area clean, dry, and aerated without causing additional trauma or irritation. The nurse should provide reassurance to the mother or primary caretaker as she or he often feels ashamed and at fault for the problem. Further information can be given to parents during discharge planning in an effort to promote health and prevent the problem. The nurse can provide written instructions and demonstrations of skin care if needed, including the following points:

1. Check and change both cloth and disposable diapers frequently so that urine and feces are not in prolonged contact with the skin.
2. Avoid the use of baby wipes that may not adequately cleanse the skin.
3. Rinse the diaper area with tepid water after each voiding and use a mild soap and tepid water rinse after each bowel movement. Gently dry the skin thoroughly.
4. Expose the skin to air for approximately 10 minutes before reapplying diaper.
5. Avoid plastic and rubber pants as they permit excessive moisture buildup. Use a thick two- to three-layer diaper and place the infant on a covered changing mat to avoid constant wetting of bed linen.
6. When disposable diaper intolerance is suspected, try cloth diapers. Some infants may simply be sensitive to the elastic or plastic used on some disposable diapers and a simple change in the type or brand of diaper may be all that is needed.
7. Wash cloth diapers with a mild soap and rinse twice, using one-half cup of either vinegar or bleach in the last rinse. Clothes softeners usually contain perfumes and chemicals that may be irritating to infant skin. Machine-drying cotton diapers at a high temperature destroys organisms and softens cotton without the use of a softener. If a commercial diaper service is used, parents should inquire about their methods of diaper washing.
8. For infants with a diarrhea-induced rash, apply A&D ointment, Desitin, or zinc oxide to the cleaned, irritated skin to provide a protective barrier against the diarrhea. Gently cleanse the skin with a mild soap and tepid water after each bowel movement, gently pat dry, and reapply the ointment.[85]
9. Treat severe irritant dermatitis with 1 percent hydrocortisone as prescribed.[86]
10. Avoid the use of powders or lotions when the skin is inflamed or broken.

Ammonia Diaper Rash. Research studies seem to indicate that there is no evidence that the ammonia in an infant's urine is sufficiently concentrated to cause or initiate a diaper dermatitis. What has been found, however, is that the ammonia in an infant's urine can exacerbate an already existing skin eruption, irritation, or rash.[87,88]

The erythema, papulovesiculation, and ulceration that is found on the convex surfaces of the diaper area[82,86] is in all likelihood an exacerbation of a preexisting contact rash or irritation. The strong ammonia odor that is given off is more often the result of infrequent diaper and clothes changes and inadequate bathing and laundering than an indication of overly concentrated urine.

The diaper area should be examined well to determine the extent of skin damage and to rule out skin infections. If cloth diapers are used, a history of the care of the diapers should be obtained. A complete history of the rash and method of skin care is also obtained.[86] Proper bathing and diaper area cleansing should be demonstrated to the primary caretaker. The recommendations described under "Contact Diaper Rash" may be used.

Fungal Diaper Rash. As with ammonia diaper rash, some diaper dermatitis attributed to *Candida albicans* can be a result of aggravation or invasion secondary to a preexisting skin irritation. There is, however, evidence that *C. albicans* can be a primary invader in diaper dermatitis.[85] Furthermore, there is a significant correlation between the content of *C. albicans* in the stool and the severity of diaper dermatitis caused by *C. albicans*.[89]

The lesions of candidal diaper dermatitis are well circumscribed, have a characteristic vivid or "fire engine" red color, and are pustulovesicular in appearance. Satellite lesions may appear in the inguinal creases, on the lower abdomen and suprapubic area, and on the upper thighs.[85,86]

The nurse should encourage the primary caretaker to follow the skin and diaper cleansing recommendations suggested under "Contact Diaper Rash." Topical nystatin should be applied two to three times daily. Severe cases may also respond to the application of topical 1 percent hydrocortisone. A protective ointment or powder may be used after the infection subsides. Caldesene, Zeasorb, and Desitin are medicated powders that have mild antibacterial and antifungal properties.[86]

Diaper dermatitis, whatever the cause, can usually be easily resolved if recognized and treated early. Unfortunately, the longer the skin irritation persists, the more likely a secondary infection will result. *Staphylococcus aureus* has been found to occur frequently as a secondary invader in severe cases of inflamed diaper dermatitis, particularly in the presence of pustules. Topical antibiotic therapy is required in such cases.[88]

Thrush

Thrush is an oral infection by the fungus *Candida albicans*. The infection usually results from contact with an infected vaginal canal during delivery. Other sources of contamination include hands, feeding equipment, breasts, or bedding.

The peak incidence is usually around the second week of life, long after the neonate has been discharged from the hospital. Thrush may also occur after antibiotic therapy, as the medication destroys the normal flora and allows opportunistic organisms to flourish.

The infection appears as white patches in the mouth, which the mother may at first interpret as milk curds. The lesions can be present on the buccal mucosa, the gums, the tongue, and the hard and soft palate. The nurse can attempt to remove some of the lesions by gently rubbing the area with a cotton-tipped applicator. Removal of the lesions will cause bleeding. Some neonates may experience sucking difficulties if the involvement is extensive.

Oral thrush can easily be treated with a course of nystatin suspension. The medication is administered four times a day for up to 2 weeks. The mother can be taught to instill a dropperful of medication into the side of each cheek, and then "paint" the lesions with a cotton-tipped applicator. Gentian violet 1 to 2 percent dye is also used to treat thrush. This method costs less than nystatin and may be preferable for families of low income. The parents will have to be cautioned that gentian violet stains the neonate's mouth and clothing, and they may want to take precautions while the neonate is being treated.

Cleanliness of everything that comes in contact with the neonate's mouth must be stressed. Bottle nipples and pacifiers should be boiled after use. Handwashing is imperative. The mother should be encouraged to change the crib sheets and pads frequently. If the mother is breastfeeding, her nipples may become sore from the infection. The breasts may be treated with topical nystatin to avoid a cycle of reinfection.

Feeding Problems

The most common feeding problems encountered in the first year of life are underfeeding, overfeeding, regurgitation, and colic.[90] Feeding and food consumption in infancy have far greater implications than the obvious provision of nutrients for energy, maintenance, and growth. Feeding is usually the first and perhaps the most important sharing behavior that is experienced between the infant and the primary caretaker. It is a function necessary for sustaining physical life that has far-reaching effects on the psychosocial well-being of both infant and parent.[91]

Underfeeding. The underfed infant usually eats all the food, formula, or breast milk that is offered, but has a history of inadequate weight gain, irritability, and fussing between feedings. On occasion, underfeeding may result when the infant refuses feedings that are offered.[91,92]

The underfed infant is not an infant with organic or systemic disease. Rather, the problem is one of the infant not being offered adequate nutrition or there being some mechanical or feeding technique problem that prohibits the adequate intake of nutrition. There may be a psychologic component such as a problem with mother-infant attachment, but more commonly there is a lack of knowledge on the part of the mother or primary caretaker.[90,92,93] Some mothers may be inexperienced and lack an effective support system in the home; other mothers may be concerned with obesity, overfeeding, or spoiling the child by feeding on request. Still other mothers may be responding to pressures in the home from family members who have their own ideas about infant feeding. Finally, in conjunction with other indicators, underfeeding may signal child neglect or abuse. The health care provider is cautioned to assess for other signs before drawing this conclusion on the basis of underfeeding alone.

A complete and thorough feeding history must be obtained. The mother or primary caretaker must be instructed in every aspect of infant feeding, including calorie and ounce requirements, formula preparation, proper holding of the infant, effective breastfeeding and bottlefeeding techniques, and adequate eructation (or "burping") of the infant. Bottles and nipples should be examined for air leaks and appropriate nipple hole size.[90]

The mother's attitude, expectations, ideas, and desires about infant feeding as well as those of other significant family members are also explored. Any conflict or stress that may be affecting the feeding of the infant must be addressed and settled. Lastly, the mother or primary caretaker and significant others may be made active members in the solution of the underfeeding problem. Growth charts and desired outcome goals may be shared with these individuals as the infant is followed closely to ensure adequate weight gain. In some cases, after a careful assessment, referral to social or legal agencies may be appropriate.

Overfeeding. Most authorities agree that it is seldom the breastfed infant who has a problem with overfeeding and subsequent problems such as regurgitation, vomiting, and obesity.[86,90,94] The feeding practices most frequently associated with overfeeding are bottlefeeding, excessive amounts of formula, overly concentrated formula, and the early introduction of nonmilk solids.[86,93,95]

Bottlefed infants tend to be overfed because parents expect the infant to empty the bottle at each feeding and persist until the infant does so,[86] and because the bottle may be offered by some parents whenever the infant makes any demand of his or her environment. The parent misreads the need for play, stimulation, attention, affection, or some other need as a need for food.[92] Parents may also use the bottle simply to keep the infant quiet.[95]

Overly concentrated formulas are usually the result of errors in preparation rather than the makeup of the formula itself. For this reason, formula preparation cannot be taken for granted, either during discharge planning or at well-infant visits, and should be reviewed with all mothers who use formula and in particular when diarrhea or loose stools are noted in the neonate[90] or excessive weight gain is noted in the older infant.[94] (*See* earlier discussion of "Techniques for Bottlefeeding and Formula Preparation.")

Nonmilk solids are not required by an infant until 6 months of age. Prior to this age the infant is neither physiologically nor developmentally ready to begin semisolid feedings nor does he or she have a need for them[86]; however, findings in the United States reveal that many infants are consuming strained foods by 4 weeks of age and that many parents offer their infants these feedings for a variety of reasons, including family, friend, and peer pressure.[86]

Management focuses on the following recommendations[86, 93, 94]:

1. Encourage breastfeeding until at least 3 months of age if possible as breastfeeding infants seldom have problems with overfeeding.
2. Instruct parents to avoid feeding their infants sweeteners, sugar, and solids. Semisolid foods may be introduced at 5 to 6 months of age.
3. Use growth charts to help parents understand normal growth in height and weight.
4. Review calorie and ounce requirements of the infant at each health visit and discourage parents from forcing infants to empty every bottle.
5. Review the correct mixing and concentration of formulas when the infant is bottlefed.
6. Encourage parents to read solid food labels and avoid those high in carbohydrates.
7. Instruct parents that when solid foods are started, they should avoid mixed dinners and use plain vegetables and meats, as these contain fewer additives and carbohydrates.
8. Review with parents the cues that infants use to indicate hunger and satiety.
9. Present information so that the parents can make informed decisions and choices. Remember that some cultures value "plump" babies.

Regurgitation. Regurgitation is the effortless bringing up of a small amount of formula (usually one or two mouthfuls) and does not lead to nutritional deficiency. In lay terms, regurgitation is known as "spitting up."[92]

Regurgitation is extremely common and is believed to be caused by an immature lower esophageal sphincter. The condition is self-limiting and, in most infants, resolves within the first 6 months of life[86]; in the remainder, the problem is corrected within 3 months of the time the infant begins walking.[96]

Regurgitation is most common in infants who are overfed; a full stomach will easily overflow an immature sphincter. Regurgitation and rapid weight gain are both indications of overfeeding. An infant who tends to regurgitate should be given his or her calorie and ounce requirements in smaller, more frequent feedings. A minimum of 2½ hours should elapse between feedings to permit the stomach to empty completely.[96]

Excessive air swallowing (or aerophagy) may also increase the incidence of regurgitation. Prolonged crying, as is seen in underfeeding and delayed feeding, improper nipple hole size, or sucking on an empty bottle, results in air swallowing. A nipple hole should be large enough to permit milk to drip out at a constant pace when the bottle is inverted. A nipple hole that permits formula to stream out or, conversely, not drip continuously is respectively too large or too small. During feeding pauses, the infant should be held in an upright position and gently patted to produce an eructation (burp).

Improper positioning of the infant may also induce regurgitation. Parents should be instructed to avoid added pressure on the infant's stomach. For example, they should not allow the infant to double over at the waist while sitting, double up the infant's legs when changing diapers, use tight diapers or clothing, position the infant too high on the caretaker's shoulder so that there is pressure directly on the stomach, or lay the infant down too soon after a feeding.

The infant should be fed only in areas that are easily cleaned and away from valued furniture, carpeting, and clothing. Bottle-fed infants may be offered commercial formulas instead of cow's milk. The butterfat in cow's milk has a much stronger odor when exposed to normal stomach acids than does the vegetable oil in commercial formulas.[96]

The infant may be positioned in an infant seat that is angled at 50° to 60° for ½ to 1 hour after each feeding. The infant seat should be made comfortable so that the infant may nap or play without difficulty.

Feedings may be thickened with infant cereal (1 tablespoon of cereal to 4 ounces of formula) to help the formula remain in the stomach. Parents must be closely instructed on the calorie and fluid requirements of the infant.[96] The nurse should reassure parents that the condition is due to an immature lower esophageal sphincter and that the problem is usually corrected by 6 months of age and at the latest by walking age.

Colic

Colic and paroxysmal fussiness are terms used for unexplained crying. The infant cries suddenly, loudly, and continuously for no apparent reason; sometimes the crying lasts hours. Other signs that may be observed include a flushed face; distended, tense abdomen; legs drawn to the abdomen; cold feet; and clenched fists.[86, 96]

Colic is seen in approximately 10 percent of all infants. There is no proven organic basis. The crying episodes begin early, often in the first weeks of life, and continue until approximately 3 months of age. Infants with sensitive or vigorous temperaments and infants who seem to need less sleep than the norm tend to be colicky. The crying also tends to occur at the same time each day, usually late in the afternoon or early evening or during the busiest time of the day.[86, 90]

Although the exact cause of colic is not known, overfeeding, primary caretaker anxiety, milk allergy, excessive air swallowing, formulas with a high carbohydrate content, intestinal allergy, immaturity of the digestive system, and tension in the household may all contribute to the crying episodes.[86, 90, 96, 97]

The goal of management is to determine, if possible, the factors that contribute to an episode of colic in the individual infant, to provide support for the parents, and to provide relief for the infant. No one method of treatment seems to consistently provide relief. Parents are taught numerous possible interventions to allay the infant's crying and discomfort.

Infants should not be overfed or offered food every time they cry. The nurse should review overfeeding, calorie and ounce requirements, formula preparation, and feeding techniques with the primary caretaker.

Prior to an anticipated episode, the infant should be dressed warmly and comfortably, with socks or booties. Some infants respond to being wrapped snugly in a blanket. The infant should be engaged in a rhythmic, soothing activity, as can be achieved in an automatic swing, a back or chest carrier, vibrating mat or chair, a rocking cradle or chair, a ride in the stroller or car, or by a gentle massage. Some infants are soothed by a pacifier or by thumb sucking.

Some infants respond to warmth, as provided by a warm bath or placement on a well-covered, partially filled hot-water bottle or heating pad at the lowest setting. Extreme caution should be exercised to avoid burning or overheating the infant. Lying prone on a hard surface such as a parent's knees or a firm mattress may provide relief.

A reduction in activities, tension, and noise during the time that the crying episode occurs may also soothe the infant. (This will require a cooperative spouse and family.) Soft, continuous or monotonous music or sound helps some infants. Two ounces of sweetened, noncaffeinated peppermint tea has been found useful by some parents.

Parents should avoid becoming fatigued or exhausted. The nurse should explore possible options with the parents. The unrelenting crying can lead to child abuse and poor parent-infant attachment. (In this instance, support services for the parents should be provided.) If all else fails, the parents should ensure that the infant is safe, fed, and dry; position the infant in the crib or rocking cradle in a different room; and let the infant cry until he or she falls asleep. Some parents play music as distraction from the crying. If this suggestion sounds particularly unkind, the reality of an infant who cries for periods of 2 hours or longer should be considered. Although not an ideal alternative, it is better than parents striking the infant.

In severe cases, mild sedatives may be prescribed to be administered prior to the crying episode. Parents must be given instructions so as to avoid overdosage. In extremely severe cases the infant may be hospitalized for observation and to permit the parents to rest and avoid physical exhaustion.

The nurse should encourage the parents to be loving, kind, and supportive with the infant. The infant does not have control over the discomfort.[97–100]

Tooth Decay

In the first year of life the oral cavity is routinely examined during visits to the well-child clinic. To avoid the high incidence of dental problems that continue to plague children in our society, early teaching of parents concerning proper dental care should be instituted at the first well-child visit. The primary teeth usually do not begin to erupt until approximately 5 months of age, but dental care initiated prior to this time will establish healthy dental habits for the child later in life.

Dental caries (or tooth decay) has been reported in as many as 5 percent of children at the age of 1 year, and by age 5, the incidence of tooth decay has been reported to increase to 75 percent. Dental caries is the most common oral problem encountered in children.[81, 100, 101]

In the first year of life tooth decay can be prevented by omitting added sugar and other sweeteners from formula or water. Water may also be offered after breastfeeding or bottlefeeding to cleanse milk from the gums and erupting teeth. Most children are not able to manage a tooth brush before 18 months of age, but an infant's caretaker can cleanse the gums and developing teeth by wrapping a thin layer of fine mesh gauze around the little finger and gently "sweeping" the gums and teeth to remove milk and food residue. The earlier this procedure is initiated, the more receptive the young child will be to the experience. The gauze may be moistened with water if desired. Care must be taken not to gag the infant or young child or in any other way make the procedure uncomfortable.[86, 102]

To prevent the development of "nursing bottle mouth syndrome," parents should be discouraged from giving the infant and young child a bottle at bedtime or naptime. Although this condition is not seen until 18 months or later, the habit of sleeping with a bottle is established in early infancy. The continuous bathing of the teeth with carbohydrate liquids such as milk, juices, and sugar water, for prolonged periods, is the primary cause of nursing bottle mouth syndrome.[86, 103, 104]

The use of fluoride to prevent tooth decay, although controversial, has been proven to be effective and is recommended by the Committee on Nutrition of the American Academy of Pediatrics and the Council on Dental Therapeutics. To be most effective, fluoride must be introduced in infancy and continued throughout the period of tooth development well into the 16th to 18th year of life.[105]

CASE STUDY/CARE PLAN: PARENT TEACHING—FEVER

Stephen and Amy Hirschburg delivered Sara, their first baby, 2 months ago. Today, they have taken her to the pediatrician's office for a physical and the first diphtheria/pertussis/tetanus (DPT) and polio immunizations. The nurse teaches Stephen and Amy about the immunizations and possible side effects. Both parents explain to the nurse that they are very anxious about the possibility of Sara's getting a fever. They further state: "We don't even know how to take her temperature, much less what we should do if she gets a fever!"

Supporting Assessment Data	Expected Client/Family Outcome	Nursing Action/ Intervention	Rationale	Criteria for Evaluation
Nursing Diagnosis: Parental knowledge deficit, related to fever measurement and management in an infant				
Parents anxious regarding care of infant if fever should occur; state: "We do not even know how to take her temperature, much less what we should do if she gets a fever"	By end of visit, parents will: Identify normal and elevated temperature values Demonstrate correct temperature assessment in an infant Demonstrate correct reading of mercury thermometer Verbalize correct method for reducing fever Identify situations in which medical intervention should be sought	Teach parents/primary caretakers normal and elevated temperature values.	Information on temperature decreases undue anxiety over minor elevations and provides knowledge base for caretaker.	Parents state the normal and elevated temperature values for infants.
		Teach parents/primary caretakers how to read a mercury thermometer.	Liquid strip thermometers are easier to read but have been proven to fail to detect an elevated temperature.[196]	Parents read the mercury thermometer correctly.
		Teach parents/primary caretakers how to take a temperature in an infant.	Knowing how to take the infant's temperature decreases feelings of inadequacy and dependence, and provides accurate information regarding temperature.	Parents demonstrate on infant the correct procedure for temperature assessment.

(continued)

CASE STUDY/CARE PLAN: Parent Teaching—Fever (*continued*)

Supporting Assessment Data	Expected Client/Family Outcome	Nursing Action/ Intervention	Rationale	Criteria for Evaluation
		A rectal temperature is usually recommended for infants.	Oral temperatures cannot be safely measured in an infant. Axillary temperatures may be done but take longer.	
		Shake thermometer down; lubricate bulb with Vaseline or lubricating jelly.	This procedure ensures that the correct temperature is measured and allows for ease in insertion of thermometer into rectum.	
		Separate buttocks, visualize anus, insert bulb of thermometer into rectum, and hold in place 3 minutes.	This procedure ensures accurate and safe placement and measurement.	
		Teach parents/primary caretakers how to reduce a fever.	Increasing the knowledge base reduces unnecessary anxiety, reduces overmedication errors, and reduces unnecessary visits and calls to health care providers.	Parents describe the methods that can be used to reduce fever.
		When temperature increases to 101°F to 102°F:		
		• Give acetaminophen every 3 to 4 hours only as directed. Do not medicate neonates without physician's approval. Do not medicate with aspirin.	Overdosage is common and can be deadly. Fever in a neonate should always be reported. Aspirin may cause Reye's syndrome in a neonate/infant/child.	
		• Offer infant plenty of fluids in the form of Jello water, water, clear fruit juices, and noncarbonated soft drinks.	An elevated temperature causes fluid loss and dehydration.	
		• Remove any blankets or heavy clothing; dress in light T-shirt and diaper only.	Light bed and body clothing allows body heat to escape.	
		If temperature increases to 103°F: • Contact the health care provider if the temperature reaches 103°F.		
		• Bathe infant in lukewarm water for 15 to 30 minutes or until temperature decreases. Do not use ice water or alcohol.	Excessively cold water is not only uncomfortable but may cause chills, which will further elevate temperature. Alcohol may be toxic.	

Supporting Assessment Data	Expected Client/Family Outcome	Nursing Action/ Intervention	Rationale	Criteria for Evaluation
		• Continue to check temperature every 1 to 2 hours.		Parents contact the health care facility when the infant has fever.
		Teach parents/primary caretakers when it is appropriate to seek medical intervention for a fever. If a fever cannot be reduced in 24 hours. If the infant has vomiting or diarrhea or is not taking in fluids. If the infant is sleepy, lethargic, or not easily aroused. If the infant is excessively restless and agitated. If spots, discolorations, or rashes of any sort are noted. If the infant has tremors, shivers, or any type of seizure activity. As stated earlier, when a fever of 103°F cannot be brought down with medication and bathing.	Knowing when to seek medical intervention decreases chance that a very ill infant will not be brought to medical attention when needed, and decreases unnecessary calls and visits to a health care provider.	

SUMMARY

Growth and development of the infant during the first year are influenced by the infant's interaction with caretakers and the environment. As the infant grows and develops, family members also develop in their new roles and relationships with the infant. It is important for nurses who care for childbearing families to have knowledge about physiologic and psychologic developmental parameters of the infant so that they can prepare new parents for these changes.

Nursing care for the infant begins in the neonatal period and focuses on protection of the neonate from infection and injury. Assessment of the neonate and infant is an ongoing process, and visits to health care providers should be scheduled regularly over the course of the first year. The infant's growth is charted during the health care visits to identify and monitor the progress and pattern of growth. Infant developmental ability is also monitored.

Care of the infant in the first year is focused on ensuring that the infant's nutritional needs are being met, promoting growth and development, promoting health through a schedule of immunizations, and counseling parents on accident prevention. Assessing parental knowledge of infant abilities, needs, and care and providing necessary teaching are important nursing roles.

Major concerns of parents during the neonatal period include positioning and handling of the neonate, nasal and oral suctioning, bathing and skin care, infant sucking needs, feeding and elimination patterns, diapering, and clothing and wrapping the neonate. Concerns of parents during infancy include weaning and introduction of solid foods, teething, infant sleep patterns, fever, thumbsucking, sibling rivalry, and the consequences of working parents. Nurses can provide anticipatory guidance for these common concerns as well as offer support and counseling to parents beginning in the prenatal period and in the early days and months of the infant's life.

Several stressors may affect the neonate and infant in the first year. These include physiologic jaundice, musculoskeletal impairment, obstruction of the lacrimal ducts, feeding problems, and tooth decay. Nursing care includes helping parents prevent problems through discharge planning and assists families to cope with these stressors in a manner that facilitates the infant's return to health.

REVIEW QUESTIONS

1. Describe the three goals of nursing care during the neonatal period.
2. Discuss the differences between breast milk and commercial formulas.
3. Identify at least three common concerns of parents in the infant's first year of life.
4. List three stressors of neonates and infants and discuss the nursing care involved in dealing with each.
5. Identify three reasons why nurses concerned with childbearing families should have knowledge about infants in the first year of life.

REFERENCES

1. Nelson NM. The onset of respirations. In: Avery G, ed. *Neonatology: Pathophysiology and Management of the Newborn,* 3rd ed. Philadelphia: JB Lippincott; 1987.
2. Korones SB. *High Risk Newborn Infants: The Basis for Intensive Care.* 4th ed. St. Louis, Mo: CV Mosby; 1986.
3. Hey E, Scopes JW. Thermoregulation in the newborn. In: Avery GB, ed. *Neonatology: Pathophysiology and Management of the Newborn.* 3rd ed. Philadelphia: JB Lippincott; 1987.
4. Klaus MH, et al. The physical environment. In: Klaus MW, Fanaroff AA, eds. *Care of the High Risk Neonate.* 3rd ed. Philadelphia: WB Saunders; 1986.
5. Stothers JK. Head insulation and heat loss in the newborn. *Arch Dis Child.* 1981;56:530.
6. Hill ST, Shronk LK. The effect of early parent-infant contact on newborn body temperature. In: Sherwen LN, Weingarten CT, eds. *Analysis and Application of Nursing Research: Parent-Neonate Studies.* Belmont, Calif: Wadsworth Health Sciences Division; 1983.
7. Gardner S. The mother as incubator after delivery. *J Obstet Gynecol Nurs.* 1979;8:174–176.
8. Hammerschlag MR. Medical progress: chlamydial infections. *J Pediatr.* 1989;114:727–734.
9. Kraybill EN. Needs of the term infant. In: Avery G, ed. *Neonatology, Pathophysiology and Management of the Newborn.* 3rd ed. Philadelphia: JB Lippincott; 1987.
10. Food and Nutrition Board. *Recommended Dietary Allowances.* 10th ed. Revised 1989. Washington, DC: National Research Council-National Academy of Sciences; 1990.
11. Lewis CM. *Nutrition and Nutritional Therapy in Nursing.* Norwalk, Conn: Appleton-Century-Crofts; 1984.
12. Robinson CH, et al. *Normal and Therapeutic Nutrition.* 17th ed. New York: Macmillan; 1986.
13. Gulick EE. The effects of breast-feeding on toddler health. *Pediatr Nurs.* 1986;12:51–54.
14. Committee on Nutrition, American Academy of Pediatrics. Commentary on breast feeding and infant formulas, including proposed standards for formulas. *Nutr Rev.* 1976;34:248–256.
15. American Academy of Pediatrics. Report of the task force on circumcision. *Pediatrics.* 1989;84:388–391.
16. Tanner J. *Education and Physical Growth.* London: University of London Press; 1966.
17. Nelms B, Mullins R. *Growth and Development: A Primary Care Approach.* Englewood Cliffs, NJ: Prentice-Hall; 1982.
18. Fong B, Resnick M. *The Child Development Through Adolescence.* Menlo Park, Calif: Benjamin Cummings; 1980.
19. Hinde R. Ethology and child development. In: Mussen P, ed. *Handbook of Child Psychology.* 4th ed. New York: Wiley; 1983.
20. Gottlieb G. The psychobiological approach to developmental issues. In: Mussen P, ed. *Handbook of Child Psychology.* 4th ed. New York: Wiley; 1983:vol II.
21. Kaye K. *The Mental and Social Life of Babies.* Chicago: University of Chicago Press; 1982
22. Winn M. *Children Without Childhood.* New York: Penguin Books; 1983.
23. Thomas A, Chess S. *Temperament and Development.* New York: Brunner/Mazel; 1977.
24. Als H, Brazelton TB. A new model of assessing behavioral organization in preterm and full-term infants. *J Am Acad Child Psychiatry.* 1981;20:239.
25. Keefe MR. Irritable infant syndrome: theoretical perspectives and practice implications. *Adv Nurs Sci.* 1988;10:70–77.
26. Horowitz F. The first two years of life: factors related to thriving. In: Moore G, Cooper C, eds. *The Young Child: Reviews of Research.* Washington, DC: National Association for the Education of Young Children; 1982:vol 3, 22.
27. Beal V. Nutrition of infants and young children. In: Wallace H, et al, eds. *Maternal and Child Health Practices.* New York: Wiley; 1982.
28. American Academy of Pediatrics, Committee on Nutrition: Toward a prudent diet for children. *Pediatrics.* 1984;73:876.
29. Pipes P. *Nutrition in Infancy and Childhood.* St. Louis, Mo: CV Mosby; 1983.
30. Wallace M. The status of immunization in the United States. In: Wallace H, Gold E, Oglesby A, eds. *Maternal and Child Health Practices.* New York: Wiley; 1982.
31. Georges P, ed. *The Report of the American Academy of Pediatrics Committee on Infectious Disease, 21st ed.* Elkgrove Village, Ill: American Academy of Pediatrics; 1988.
32. Waechter E, et al. *Nursing Care of Children.* New York: JB Lippincott; 1985.
33. Agran PF. Motor occupant injuries. *Pediatrics.* 1981;67:838–840.
34. Department of Health, Education and Welfare. *Young Children and Accidents in the Home.* Publ. No. 79-30034.

Washington, DC: US Government Printing Office; October 1979.
35. Feldman KW. Prevention of childhood accidents: recent progress. *Pediatr Rev* 1980;2(3):75–82.
36. Kravath RE, et al. Prevention of childhood accidents by eliminating the agent of injury. *J Pediatr.* 1981;99:575–576.
37. Freidman AS, Freidman DB. Parenting: a developmental process. *Pediatr Ann U.* 1977;6:10–22.
38. Wicklund K, et al. Effects of maternal education, age and parity on fatal infant accidents. *Am J Public Health.* 1984;75:1150–1152.
39. Shamansky S, ed. *Primary Healthcare Handbook: Guidelines for Patient Education.* Boston: Little, Brown and Co; 1984.
40. Bull MJ, Stroup KB. Premature infants in car seats. *Pediatrics.* 1985;75:336–339.
41. Player C. A mother's guide to coping with accidents. *Your Life Health* 1984;99:10–13.
42. Nachem B, Bass RA. Children still aren't being buckled up. *Am J Matern Child Nurs.* 1984;9:320–323.
43. Krozy RE, McColgan JJ Jr. Auto safety: pregnancy and the newborn. *J Obstet Gynecol Neonat Nurs.* 1985;14:11–15.
44. Righi FC, Korzy RE. The child in the car: what every nurse should know about safety. *Am J Nurs.* 1983;83:1421–1424.
45. Kraus JF. Effectiveness of measures to prevent unintentional deaths of infants and children from suffocation and strangulation. *Public Health Rep.* 1985;100:231–240.
46. Thomas KA. Evaluation of group well-child care for improving burn prevention practices in the home. *Pediatrics.* 1984;74:879–882.
47. Kravath RE. A lethal pacifier. *Pediatrics.* 1976;58:853–855.
48. King K, et al. Heat stress in motor vehicles: a problem in infancy. *Pediatrics.* 1981;68:579–582.
49. Feldman KW. Prevention of childhood accidents: recent progress. *Pediatr Rev.* 1980;2:75–82.
50. Williams KM, Morse JM: Weaning patterns of first-time mothers. *Am J Matern Child Nurs.* 1989;14:188–192.
51. Chow M, et al. *Handbook of Pediatric Primary Care.* 2nd ed. New York: Wiley; 1984.
52. Edelman C, Mandle C. *Health Promotion Throughout the Lifespan.* Princeton, NJ: CV Mosby; 1986.
53. Edgil AE, et al. Sleep problems of older infants and preschool children. *Pediatr Nurs.* 1985;11:87–89.
54. Richman N. A community survey of characteristics of 1 to 2 year olds with sleep disorders. *J Am Acad Child Psychiatry.* 1981;20:281–291.
55. Osternholm P, et al. Sleep disturbances in infants age 6 to 12 months. *Pediatr Nurs.* 1983;9:269–271, 301.
56. Cushing A. Fever diagnosis at your fingertips. *Emerg Med.* 1984;16:58–64, 66.
57. Schmitt B. Fever phobia: misconception of parents about fever: *Am J Dis Child.* 1980;134:176–181.
58. Scholefield JH, et al. Liquid crystal forehead temperature strips: a clinical appraisal. *Am J Dis Child.* 1982;136:198–201.
59. Weiss J, Herskowitz DO. House officer management of the febrile child. *Clin Pediatr (Philadelphia).* 1983;22:766–769.
60. Casey R, et al. Fever therapy: an educational intervention for parents. *Pediatrics.* 1984;73:600–605.
61. Atkins E. Fever: its history, cause and function. *Yale J Biol Med* 1982;55:283–289.
62. McCarthy PL, et al. Diagnostic styles of attending pediatricians, residents, and nurses in evaluating febrile children. *Clin Pediatr.* 1982;21:534–537.
63. Weiss CF, ed. Acetaminophen: potential pediatric hazard. *Pediatrics.* 1973;52:883.
64. Karmel M, Karmel L. *Growing and Becoming: Development from Conception Through Adolescence.* New York: Macmillan; 1984.
65. Dunn J, Kendrick C. The arrival of a sibling: changes of patterns of interaction between mother and first-born child. *J Child Psychiatry Psychol.* 1980;21:119–132.
66. Stewart R, et al. The firstborn's adjustment to the birth of a sibling: a longitudinal assessment. *Child Dev.* 1987;58:341–355.
67. Department of Commerce, Bureau of Census. *Households, Families, Marital Status and Living Arrangements, Current Population Reports.* Series p-2, No. 202. Washington, DC: US Government Printing Office; March 1985.
68. Schindler P, et al. Time in day care and social participation of young children. *Dev Psychol.* 1987;23:255–261.
69. Owen MT, et al. The relation between maternal employment status and the stability of attachment to mother and father. *Child Dev.* 1984;55:1894–1901.
70. Maisels MJ. Neonatal jaundice. In: Avery GB, ed. *Neonatology, Pathophysiology and Management of the Newborn.* 3rd ed. Philadelphia: JB Lippincott; 1987.
71. Oski FA. Physiologic jaundice. In: Avery ME, Taeusch HW, eds. *Schatter's Diseases of the Newborn.* 5th ed. Philadelphia: WB Saunders; 1984:ch 69.
72. Adams JA, et al. Incidence of hyperbilirubinemia in breast- versus formula-fed infants. *Clin Pediatr.* 1985;24:69–73.
73. Kivlahan C, James EJ. Natural history of neonatal jaundice. *Pediatrics.* 1984;63:364–370.
74. Maisels MJ, Gifford K. Normal serum bilirubin levels in the newborn and the effect of breast-feeding. *Pediatrics.* 1986;78:738–743.
75. Schumacher RE, et al. Transcutaneous bilirubinometry: a comparison of old and new methods. *Pediatrics.* 1985;76:10–14.
76. De Carvallo M, et al. Effects of water supplementation in physiological jaundice in breast-fed babies. *Arch Dis Child.* 1981;56:568–569.
77. De Carvallo M, et al. Fecal bilirubin excretion and serum bilirubin concentrations in breast-fed and bottle-fed infants. *J Pediatr.* 1985;107:786–790.
78. Fraser CF. Congenital defects involving joints. In: Avery ME, Taeusch HW, eds. *Schaffer's Diseases of the Newborn.* 5th ed. Philadelphia: Saunders; 1984:ch 94.
79. Boal D, Schwenkter E. The infant hip: assessment with real-time US. *Radiology.* 1985;157:667–672.
80. Hayden GF. Skin diseases encountered in a pediatric clinic: a one-year prospective study. *Am J Dis Child.* 1985;139:36–38.
81. Hoekelman RA, et al. A profile of pediatric practice in the United States. *Am J Dis Child.* 1983;137:1057–1660.
82. Duberley J. Common skin disorders: infancy, childhood, adolescence. *Nursing (Oxford).* 1983;2:271–272.
83. Grant WW, et al. Diaper rashes in infancy. *Clin Pediatr.* 1973;12:714.
84. Weston WL, et al. Diaper dermatitis: current concepts. *Pediatrics.* 1980;66:532.
85. Leyden JJ. Diaper dermatitis. *Pediatr Dermatol.* 1986;4:23–28.
86. Chow MP, et al. *Handbook of Pediatric Primary Care.* 2nd ed. New York: Wiley; 1984:242–243.

87. Leyden JJ, et al. Urinary ammonia and ammonia producing microorganisms in infants with and without diaper dermatitis. *Arch Dermatol* 1977;114:1678.
88. Leyden JJ, Kligman AM. The role of microorganisms in diaper dermatitis. *Arch Dermatol.* 1978;114:56.
89. Reborah A, Leyden JJ: Diaper dermatitis and gastrointestinal carriage of *Candida albicans. Br J Dermatol.* 1981; 165:551.
90. Behrman RE, Vaughan VC, eds. *Nelson Textbook of Pediatrics.* 12th ed. Philadelphia: WB Saunders; 1983:1751–1753.
91. Pipes PL. Nutrition in infancy and Childhood. In: Steffe WP, Krey S, eds. *Primary Care: Nutrition in Primary Care.* Philadelphia: WB Saunders; 1982:vol 9, 497–510.
92. Rudolph AM, Hoffman JIE, eds. *Pediatrics.* 17th ed. Norwalk, Conn: Appleton-Century-Crofts; 1982:594–595, 900–901.
93. Lawrence RA. Approach to breastfeeding. In: Walker WA, Watkins JB, eds. *Nutrition in Pediatrics: Basic Science and Clinical Application.* Boston: Little, Brown and Co; 1985:829–846.
94. Taitz LS. Obesity in pediatric practice: infantile obesity. *Pediatr Clin North Am* 1977:24,107–122.
95. Whitfield M. Nutrition in infancy and childhood. In: Hart C, ed. *Child Care in General Practice.* New York: Churchill Livingston; 1977:227–229.
96. Schmitt BD. *Pediatric Telephone Advice.* Boston: Little, Brown and Co; 1980:136–139, 228–229.
97. Crawshaw JP. The fussy infant: dealing with colic. *Patient Care.* 1985;19:93–96, 99, 102.
98. Dicyclomine for infant colic-toxic double dose. *Nurses Drug Alert.* 1984;8:83–84.
99. Questions and answers about colic . . . patient education aid (teaching materials). *Patient Care.* 1985;19:108–109.
100. Kempe CH, et al, eds. *Current Pediatric Diagnosis and Treatment.* 8th ed. Los Altos, Calif: Lange Medical; 1984: 267–271, 276–277.
101. Luce M, Sande D. Oral health in children: prevention of dental caries. *Nurs Pract.* 1983;8:43, 47, 49.
102. Riley HD Jr, Berney J. Preventive dental care. *Am Baby.* 1981;43:45.
103. Deely WS. The slow spoiler . . . the dangers of nursing bottle mouth syndrome. *Am Baby.* 1980;42:24.
104. Holst HP. Help for victims of nursing bottle syndrome. *Am Baby.* 1981;43:14.
105. Rebich T Jr, et al. Fluoride programs in the school setting: preventive dental health. *J Sch Health.* 1982;52:14–16.

High-Risk Maternal-Fetal Nursing

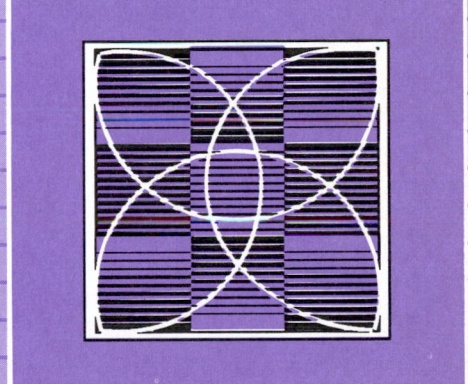

unit

10

The Perinatal Perspective

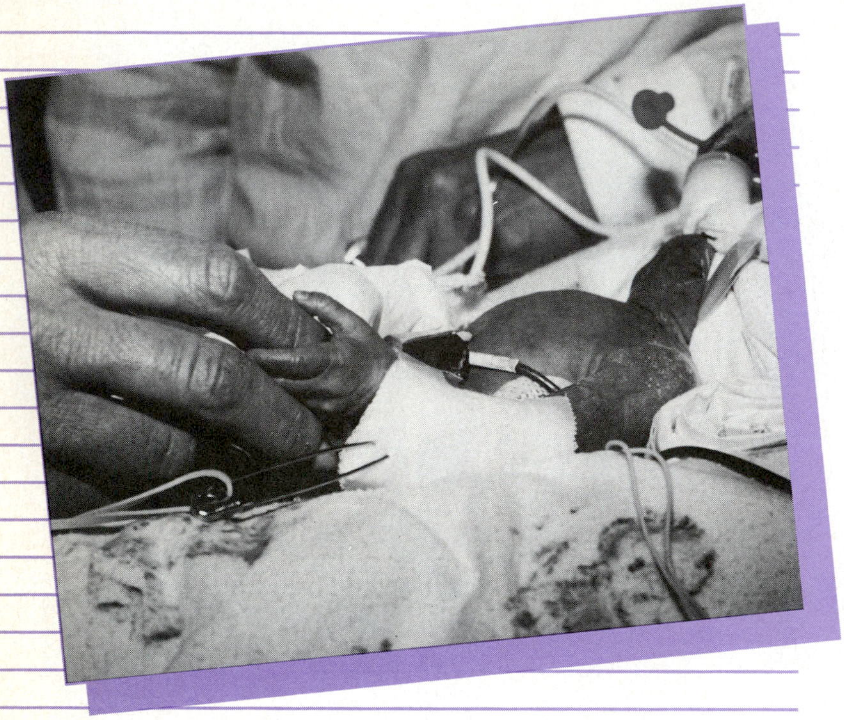

chapter 35

Key Terms

high-risk perinatal nursing
maternal transport
neonatology
neonatal transport
perinatal nursing
perinatal period
perinatology
point of viability
regionalization

The perinatal period spans the developmental stages of fetal and neonatal life whether the pregnancy is considered high risk or low risk. The concept of the perinatal period is important because many of the stresses and hazards that affect the fetus have either a direct or an indirect effect in the neonatal period. Moreover, jeopardy to life is greater during this period than at any subsequent time in the person's life cycle. Of the deaths occurring in the first year of life, about 70 percent occur in the first 28 days. If fetal loss is added to this statistic, then the perinatal period is the greatest threat to life for a given time interval.[1]

This chapter provides an overview of the perinatal perspective, including factors influencing care of low-risk, moderate-risk, and high-risk childbearing families. A framework of perinatal nursing is presented, describing the components of care for the low-risk, moderate-risk, and high-risk client. Perinatal care is, by nature, collaborative. Thus, the framework for perinatal nursing presented in this chapter emphasizes collaborative care, but structures this care in a manner that parallels the steps of the nursing process. A model for interdisciplinary team development is also presented, with an emphasis on the need for role flexibility, mutual cooperation, and communication in achieving truly collaborative interdisciplinary care.

Several historical trends in perinatal care, most importantly regionalization and transport, have contributed to a decline in perinatal mortality over the past 40 years; however, continued improvement is needed. The perinatal nurse will play an important role in achieving improved birth weight and access to care for members of lower socioeconomic groups, who are particularly at risk for poor perinatal outcome.

Regardless of whether nurses practice with healthy or compromised childbearing clients and neonates, identification of risk status is an inherent part of the nursing process. Thus, all maternity nurses will need to maintain the perinatal perspective.

PHILOSOPHY OF PERINATAL CARE

Although there is nothing inherent in the term *perinatal care* to indicate that it concerns high-risk or low-risk mothers, fetuses, and neonates, in practice the concept deals with identification of risk factors on a continuum from low to high risk. What does it mean to classify a mother, fetus or neonate as "high risk" or "low risk" and to include them in a system of perinatal care delivery? Nurses and other health professionals assess and screen mothers, fetuses, and neonates throughout pregnancy and the neonatal period. They assess for physiologic and psychologic strengths of the family, as well as possible vulnerabilities and problems. In other words, they determine the risk status of the woman and family, be it low or high.

Within this broad perspective, probable and definite risk factors are identified as early in the pregnancy as possible. For example, adolescents or women over age 35 may be identified as being at risk for problems in the perinatal period. In addition, some women enter the childbearing cycle with a condition such as diabetes, which might profoundly affect the course of the pregnancy for both mother and fetus. Similarly, some neonates are born with inherent problems, such as prematurity, which may produce a poor reproductive outcome for mother and neonate in certain circumstances and may affect their subsequent development and well-being. These families would be considered to be at moderate or high risk; however, problems can be prevented or treated if childbearing families are assessed early and risk factors identified.

Timely intervention, made possible by careful monitoring of "high-risk" mothers, fetuses, and neonates, helps to optimize reproductive outcome for all involved. The goals of high-risk and low-risk maternity care are identical: optimum well-being for mother, neonate, and family. Identification of the risk status of the childbearing family alerts the health team to problems that may emerge during the course of the pregnancy or the neonatal period. Interventions can thus be initiated in the most timely fashion to prevent or minimize a poor reproductive outcome.

DEFINITION OF TERMS

Although authorities agree that the **perinatal period** spans fetal and neonatal life, there is disagreement as to when this period begins. Some authorities say that the perinatal period begins as early as conception; others say it begins as late as 28 weeks of gestation. The confusion rests on the lack of knowledge of when the fetus can reasonably survive outside of the uterus, that is, the **point of viability.** The estimate that is given as the lowest point of viability is 20 weeks of gestation, with some states using 24 or 28 weeks as the point of viability for statistical purposes. For clarity, 20 weeks of gestation will be used as the point of viability. Thus, the perinatal period is defined as the period from 20 weeks of gestation through the 28th day of neonatal life for purposes of reporting outcomes of low-risk and high-risk pregnancies.

Perinatal nursing is broader by definition than those definitions used for statistical purposes. Because risk status should be identified early in the pregnancy or even in the preconception period, and because the nurse cares for the childbearing family throughout the span of gestation and the neonatal period, perinatal nursing is defined as the practice of professional nursing in response to the needs of the high-risk or low-risk family throughout the antepartum, intrapartum, postpartum, and neonatal periods. **High-risk perinatal nursing** is the practice of nursing of childbearing families who have an increased probability of either psychosocial or physical illness, disability, or death, that is, the nursing care of childbearing families assessed to have a moderate-risk or high-risk status.

Other terms relevant to perinatal care are defined in Chapter 1 and in Table 35–1.

CONCEPTUAL FRAMEWORK FOR PERINATAL NURSING

Perinatal nurses structure their care delivery for families in various states of risk using the nursing process. In addition, they must tailor their care to complement care delivered by other members of the interdisciplinary team. Figure 35–1 provides a framework that identifies the components that form the basis for perinatal nursing. These components parallel the steps of the nursing process. They are nursing assessment of reproductive and developmental competence, the decision-making process and nursing diagnoses, collaborative planning and intervention, and evaluation and revision of outcome criteria.

Several factors are associated with the expertise of perinatal nurses. These include their educational preparation, personal and professional experience, and the attitudes, beliefs, and values that make up their personal philosophies regarding perinatal care.

Nursing Assessment of Reproductive and Developmental Competence

As a member of the health team, the perinatal nurse systematically assesses the expectant parents, fetus, neonate, family, and environment. The expectant parents are assessed for physiologic, sensory, motor, language, cognitive, educational, self-help, and emotional/behavioral factors. Physiologic parameters are

TABLE 35–1. DEFINITIONS RELEVANT TO PERINATAL NURSING

Term	Definition
Stillbirth rate	Number of stillborn infants per 1000 population
Neonatal death	Death of an infant before 29 days of life
Neonatal period	First 28 days of life; the period of greatest mortality in childhood, with the highest risk occurring in the first 24 hours of life
Perinatology	Specialty of obstetric medicine devoted to care of the high-risk mother and fetus
Neonatology	Specialty of pediatric medicine devoted to care of the high-risk neonate; if the infant remains hospitalized for several months after birth, the neonatologist often provides care for that infant beyond the age of 28 days
High-risk pregnancy	Pregnancy in which the woman has an increased chance of developing a psychosocial or physical illness or dying; or a pregnancy in which the fetus has an increased chance of developing an illness or dying; or both
High-risk neonate	Infant who has an increased possibility of developing a psychosocial or physical illness or disability or of dying at birth or in the near future
High-risk postpartum client	Woman who has, during the first 6 weeks after delivery, an increased chance of developing a psychosocial or physical illness or dying as a result of the childbearing process
High-risk father	Male partner of a woman or parent of a fetus/neonate who is at risk during the prenatal, intrapartum, or neonatal period, or a father who experiences psychologic or physiologic stress related to the responsibilities associated with the childbearing process, or both

assessed in the fetus. Assessment of the neonate includes the same factors assessed in the expectant parents, with the added dimension of neonatal temperament. The family is assessed for structure and dynamics. Assessment of the environment includes assessments of the home, community, work, and school environments. The cultural affiliation of the family is also assessed.

Assessment of these parameters provides the nurse with the data base from which decisions and nursing diagnoses are made relative to the health status of the perinatal family. Assessment concepts significant to both reproductive and developmental parameters of the childbearing family are also included.

The Decision-Making Process and Nursing Diagnoses

The framework for nursing assessment, as well as nursing decisions, is a health-risk-illness continuum. Assessment about health provides the basis for decisions about client/family strengths and resources; assessment related to risk provides the basis for decisions about vulnerabilities; and assessment related to illness provides the basis for decisions about both acute and chronic health deviations or problems.

Data collected during the initial assessment and on subsequent visits are used to formulate nursing diagnoses and direct the collaborative development of goals and objectives on which the plan of care (including diagnostic, therapeutic, and client education interventions) is formulated.

Planning and Collaborative Goal Setting

Nursing assessment and diagnoses concerning the family are pooled with data gathered by other professionals on the interdisciplinary team. Nursing and other data form the basis of collaborative goals for the family and will direct the management plan and interventions developed by the team. Goal planning is accomplished through team discussion and sharing of discipline-specific perceptions; the process of negotiation will determine the plan and the coordinated, collaborative interventions of team members.

Collaborative Intervention

Collaborative intervention is an important dimension of the framework for perinatal nursing outlined in Figure 35–1. The nurse collaborates with other members of an interdisciplinary team to promote health, prevent complications, and restore the client to a level of health care that will promote well-being for the childbearing family.

Decisions about health care for the client and the family require the integration of information from a variety of sources. Although the health-illness continuum is used within this framework, nurses must recognize that perinatal families have dynamic and changing health states. Thus, the high-risk client may become a low-risk client with comprehensive interventions. Similarly the adolescent mother may be considered at moderate risk because of age, but healthy self-care practices may produce a good reproductive outcome for mother and neonate. Strengths

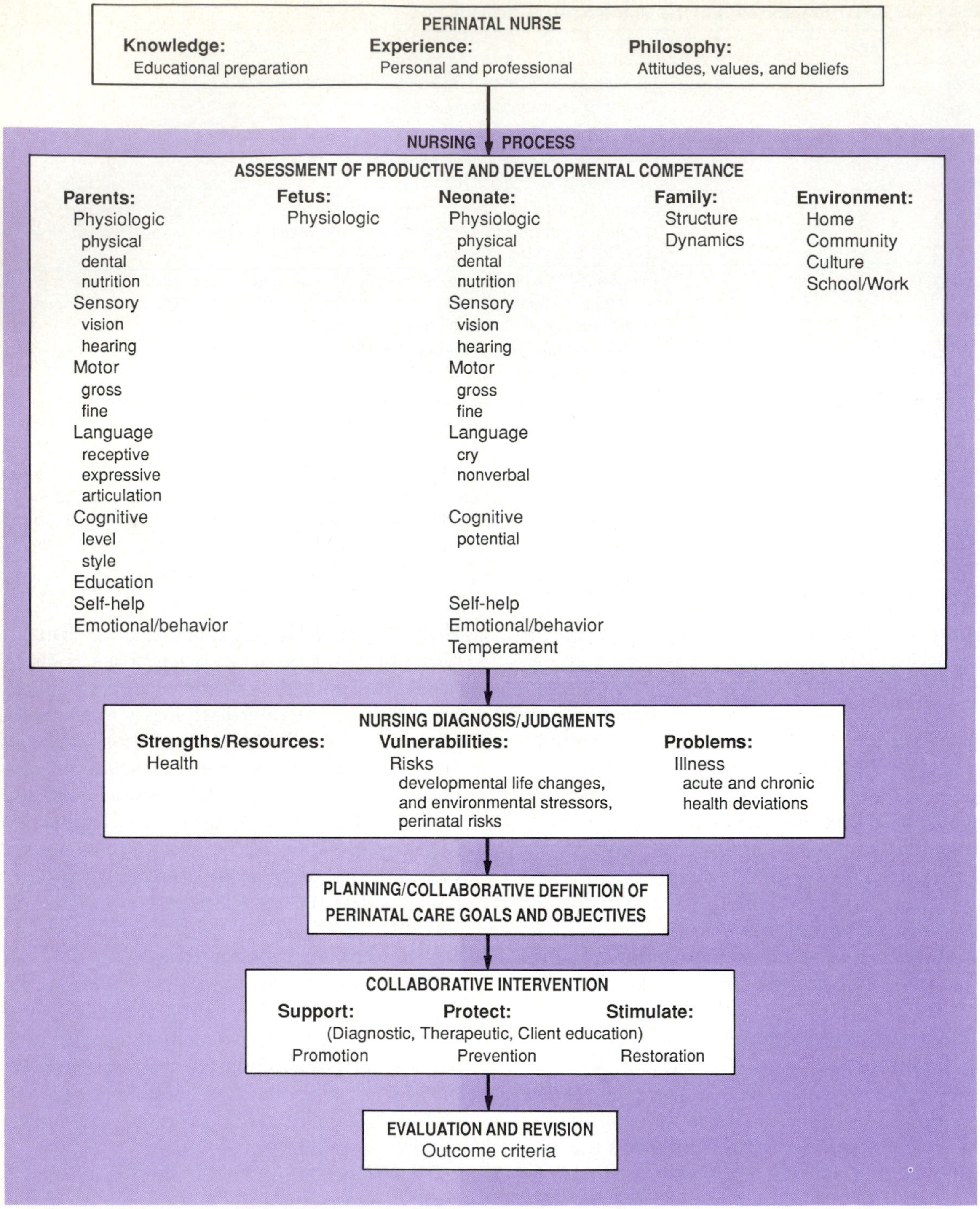

Figure 35–1. Conceptual framework for perinatal nursing.

RESEARCH ABSTRACT

Brooten D, et al. A randomized clinical trial of early hospital discharge and home follow-up of very-low-birth-weight infants. N Engl J Med. *1986;315:934–939.*

The purpose of this study was to determine the safety, efficacy, and cost savings of early discharge of very-low-birth-weight infants. The sample consisted of 79 infants. Forty infants weighing approximately 2200 g were randomly assigned to a control group who were discharged according to routine criteria. Thirty-nine infants were discharged before reaching this weight after meeting a set of conditions; these infants were discharged 11 days earlier and were 2 weeks younger than the control infants. Families of infants in the early-discharge group received instruction, counseling, home visits, and daily on-call availability of a nurse specialist for 18 months. The costs for the two groups were determined. The groups were compared relative to number of rehospitalizations, number of acute care visits, and measures of physical and mental development.

The investigators concluded that the mean hospital charge was 27 percent less for the early-discharge group than for the control group. The mean physician's charge was 22 percent less for the early-discharge group. The two groups did not differ in number of rehospitalizations, number of acute care visits, or measures of physical or developmental growth.

Comment:
This study addresses a major problem in perinatal health care today: cost. The risks associated with growth and development of high-risk infants, the high cost of long hospital stays for these infants, and alternatives to standard nursing practice are all considered. Brooten's team designed an alternative nursing intervention using clinical nurse specialists that resulted in decreased costs without compromising the quality of the outcome for these infants.

The methodology used, a randomized, controlled clinical trial, was optimal. It served as a means to judge the results of the intervention program with minimal bias.

This study is an example of nursing research at its finest. It is a well-designed evaluation of an innovative nursing intervention in an area of perinatal care of concern to the nation. The findings will have an impact on the delivery of perinatal care and nursing practice, as well as allow those infants at risk to join their families sooner at home.

and resources exist at the same time as problems and vulnerabilities. Care for the perinatal family should therefore include three types of intervention:

1. *Health promotion.* Activities that support existing strengths and resources.
2. *Prevention.* Activities that protect the family from stressors.
3. *Restoration.* Activities that stimulate the family's ability to adapt.

Evaluation and Revision of Outcome Criteria

The final phase of the framework of perinatal nursing includes care and revisions based on these evaluations. Because the nursing process is cyclic, the nurse reassesses the perinatal family on an ongoing basis.

Concept of Risk: Developmental and Reproductive Risk

In practice it is common to categorize perinatal risk as either low, moderate, or high. Butnarescu and associates[2] define these three levels as follows:

- *Minimal (low) risk* exists whenever there is a potential for little or no damage to the mother and fetus. Should damage occur, it is of short-term duration or does not interfere with optimal long-range functioning. Residual damage is absent. Examples of minimal risk include such conditions as mild maternal anemia, a nonsensitized Rh woman, and a nondiabetic neonate with transitory hypoglycemia.
- *Moderate risk* is the concept used to describe an increase in the number or complexity of variables that combine to require increased perinatal supervision, education, and therapy to maintain or restore the health of the mother and fetus. Examples of moderate risk are maternal age under 19 years, maternal obesity, mild maternal hypertension, and transient tachypnea in the neonate.
- *Maximal (high) risk* refers to an increase in the number and complexity of variables of such magnitude that here is a real likelihood of damage or death of the mother, fetus, or neonate. Extensive therapy is needed to restore a functional level, there is often residual damage, and long-term follow-up is usually needed. Examples are maternal diabetes, severe maternal hypertension, and neonatal respiratory distress syndrome.[2]

Perinatal clients may be at risk both reproductively and developmentally. These risks may be viewed on a continuum as depicted in Table 35–2.

TABLE 35–2. REPRODUCTIVE AND DEVELOPMENTAL RISK CONTINUUM AND NURSING ACTIONS

Type of Risk	Health →	At Risk →	Illness
Reproductive	Assess client for change to at-risk/ill status Educate client about childbirth, self-care, infant care and management, nutrition, and resources	Assess client for risk and treat/monitor Educate client about at-risk status management, outcomes, and resources	Assess client for change in status Educate client about illness, possible deviations from normal
Developmental	Assess mother/family for developmental tasks Educate mother/family about parenting, infant stimulation, milestones	Assess mother/family for developmental/situational crises Educate mother/family about resources, support groups, classes, and financial aid	Assess mother/family for change in status Educate mother/family about disability, rehabilitation, and financial aid

This table also provides examples of representative nursing actions in the appropriate columns below the components of the continuum.

Many factors may influence the maternal-fetal status and the status of the neonate.[3] Chapters 14, 18, and 22, which provide a detailed description of assessment during pregnancy, identify these factors. Other factors that influence risk status are prepregnancy factors such as genetics and medical history. Prepregnancy counseling and education have the potential to reduce the reproductive and developmental risks associated with these factors.

Identification of perinatal clients at risk begins ideally before pregnancy or at the first prenatal visit and continues throughout the perinatal period. Several scoring systems to assess the risk to the fetus/neonate have been developed, including the tools by Goodwin,[4] Hobel,[5] and Coopland[6] and their colleagues. The Coopland scoring system, which is the least complicated and easiest to use, is shown in Figure 35–2. Once the nurse-midwife, nurse practitioner, obstetrician, perinatologist, or perinatal team identifies the woman or fetus at risk, collaborative management by the perinatal team is initiated.

The initial visit for all childbearing families is essentially identical (*see* Chapter 14). Screening tools and routine procedures are used to identify families and individuals at risk. Once risk status is identified, plans for monitoring and intervention are made by members of the interdisciplinary team in collaboration with the family. For example, the presence of certain risk factors may prevent the family from delivering in the chosen birth setting because of a lack of specialized personnel and equipment. Therefore, the family and caregivers must collaborate to develop a plan for delivery that will meet both the needs of the situation and the family.

Subsequent chapters of this text will describe specific conditions that place the family, mother, and fetus/neonate at moderate or high risk. These chapters discuss nursing and collaborative management strategies designed to accomplish the best possible reproductive outcomes for the family.

HISTORICAL FACTORS AND TRENDS IN PERINATAL CARE

The realization that certain situations in the prenatal, intrapartum, postpartum, and neonatal periods can have an adverse effect on maternal and fetal/neonatal outcome is not new. It was not, however, until the 1950s that health care providers began to focus on the relationship between specific factors and their outcomes. A study in 1951 identified cerebral palsy as being linked to high-risk factors during the childbearing cycle.[7] By the 1950s, a number of states developed maternal mortality committees. These committees gathered data that were used to direct activities designed to reduce maternal mortality. The decade of the 1950s thus became the age of neonatal awareness among health care providers.[8]

During the 1960s and 1970s, further investigations contributed to the knowledge of risk factors associated with morbidity and mortality. The 1960s has been termed the decade of fetal medicine, and the 1970s, the decade of perinatal medicine.[8] In the 1980s, the concept of perinatal medicine grew to include management of childbearing families by interdisciplinary teams, on which nurses became important members.

In the 1960s, 1970s, and 1980s the emphasis on fetal and perinatal health care played a major role in the decline of mortality rates for mothers and neonates. Tables 35–3 and 35–4 show this decline in mortality rates.[9] Table 35–3 reflects the wide disparity between mortality rates for whites and other ethnic groups. Blacks, in particular, have a much higher mortality rate. This disparity is of great concern to perinatal caregivers and results from many factors,

HIGH-RISK EVALUATION FORM

Name ____________ Age ______ Gravida ______ Para ______ Aborta______

LMP ____________ EDC ________ EDC by ultrasound ____________

Reproductive History

Age: <16	= 1	
16–35	= 0	
>35	= 2	____
Parity: 0	= 1	
1–4	= 0	
>5	= 2	____
Two or more abortions or history of infertility	= 1	____
Postpartum bleeding or manual removal	= 1	____
Child >9 lb	= 1	____
Child <5 lb 8 oz	= 1	____
Toxemia or hypertension	= 2	____
Previous cesarean section	= 2	____
Abnormal or difficult labor	= 2	____
COLUMN TOTALS		____

Medical or Surgical Associated Conditions

Previous gynecologic surgery	= 1	____
Chronic renal disease	= 1	____
Gestational diabetes (A)	= 1	____
Class B or greater diabetes	= 3	____
Cardiac disease	= 3	____
Other significant medical disorders (*score 1 to 3 according to severity*)	=	____
COLUMN TOTALS		____

Present Pregnancy

Bleeding		
<20 weeks	= 1	____
>20 weeks	= 3	____
Anemia (<10 g%)	= 1	____
Postmaturity	= 1	____
Hypertension	= 2	____
Premature rupture of membranes	= 2	____
Polyhydramnios	= 2	____
IUGR	= 3	____
Multiple pregnancy	= 3	____
Breech or malpresentation	= 3	____
Rh isoimmunization	= 3	____
COLUMN TOTALS		____

Total Scores (Sum of the three columns) ________

Low risk = 0–2
High risk = 3–6
Severe risk = ≥ 7

Figure 35–2. The Coopland High-Risk Evaluation Form. (*Reproduced, with permission, from Coopland AT, et al. A simplified high-risk pregnancy screening form: statistical analysis of 5459 cases.* Can Med Assoc J. *1977;116:999.*)

including socioeconomic status, that are not readily changed.

Socioeconomic status is associated with hygiene, living standards, nutrition, and education. Poverty brings with it poor health care practices, overcrowding, malnutrition, and low educational status. These factors are related to perinatal mortality and morbidity. Because there are more poor individuals from minority groups, such as blacks as compared with whites, the risks to mothers, fetuses, and neonates associated with poverty are more apparent in these groups.

Regionalization

The progress that has been made in reducing mortality is, to a great extent, due to the regionalization of perinatal care. The concept of regionalization had its roots in the period 1964–1968 when studies were undertaken in Massachusetts, Wisconsin, and Arizona to analyze causes of neonatal morbidity and mortality. As result of these studies and the subsequent implementation of their recommendations, mortality rates were markedly reduced.[10]

According to Fanaroff and colleagues[10] three additional factors facilitated the movement toward regionalization: (1) the study and report of the Joint Committee of the Society of Obstetricians and Gynecologists of Canada and the Pediatric Society, entitled *Regional Services in Reproductive Medicine*; (2) the adoption of a statement on regionalization of perinatal care by the American Medical Association; and (3) the report of the Joint Committee on Perinatal Health of the American Medical Association, the American College of Obstetricians and Gynecologists, the American Academy of Family Physicians, and the American Academy of Pediatrics, entitled *Toward Improving the Outcome of Pregnancy*.[11]

Two private foundations, the Robert Wood Johnson Foundation and the March of Dimes Birth

TABLE 35–3. MATERNAL MORTALITY IN THE UNITED STATES, 1935–1985

Maternal Deaths		Rate Per 100,000 Live Births		
Year	Number	Total	White	Other
1935	12,544	582.1	530.6	945.7
1940	8,876	376.0	319.8	773.5
1945	5,668	107.2	172.1	454.8
1950	2,960	83.3	61.1	221.6
1955	1,901	47.0	32.8	130.3
1960	1,579	37.1	26.0	97.9
1965	1,189	31.6	21.0	83.7
1970	803	21.5	14.4	55.9
1975	403	12.8	9.1	29.0
1980	334	9.2	6.7	19.8
1985	295	7.8	5.2	18.1

Reproduced, with permission, from Cunningham FG, et al. Williams Obstetrics. *18th ed. Norwalk, Conn: Appleton & Lange; 1989:3.*

Defects Foundation also have added impetus to the perinatal movement and regionalization.

In the mid-1960s leaders in the delivery of perinatal care at the national level, including obstetricians, neonatologists, and pediatricians, recognized that a change in the way perinatal health services were delivered was necessary to dramatically improve the reproductive and developmental outcomes for families at risk. The new way of organizing services was called **regionalization.** As described in *Toward Improving the Outcome of Pregnancy*, regionalization refers to "The development, within a geographical area, of a coordinated cooperative system of maternal and perinatal health care in which, by mutual agreements between hospitals and physicians and based upon population needs, the degree of complexity of maternal and perinatal care each hospital is capable of providing is identified so as to accomplish the following objectives: quality care to all pregnant women and newborns, maximal utilization of highly trained perinatal personnel and intensive care facilities, and assurance of reasonable cost effectiveness."[11]

The basic premise of regionalization is that there should be a single standard of care for all perinatal clients. Any mother and her fetus/neonate/infant should have equal access to whatever aspect of perinatal care they need. To provide the best care in a cost-effective manner, all perinatal care institutions in a given region are organized so that three levels of perinatal care are available to a perinatal client in that geographic area. Perinatal care institutions are designated by each state and are categorized as level I, II, or III facilities according to the following criteria.[12]

- *Level I facilities.* These maternity facilities manage normal pregnancy, labor and delivery, and postpartum care. They also identify high-risk pregnancies and neonates and refer them to level II and III facilities. Level I facilities have competent personnel to provide for unanticipated obstetric or neonatal emergencies and are located within small community hospitals.
- *Level II facilities.* Level II maternity facilities offer more high-risk perinatal services than level I facilities and are often located in urban and suburban communities. They have personnel and equipment to manage most maternal and neonatal complications, as well as uncomplicated childbearing. Level II facilities have the capability of providing continuing and intermediate care to mothers and newborns

TABLE 35–4. PERINATAL MORTALITY IN THE UNITED STATES, 1950–1985

	Perinatal Deaths[a]		Fetal Deaths[b]		Neonatal Deaths[c]	
Year	Number	Rate[d]	Number	Rate[d]	Number	Rate[e]
1950	141,117	39.0	68,262	18.8	72,855	20.5
1960	148,213	34.3	68,480	15.8	79,733	18.7
1970	109,240	28.9	52,961	14.0	56,279	15.1
1975	70,212	22.1	33,796	10.6	36,416	11.6
1980	63,971	17.5	33,353	9.1	30,618	8.5
1983	57,259	15.6	30,752	8.4	26,507	7.3
1985	55,840	14.7	29,661	7.8	26,179	7.0
1987	—	—	—	—	—	6.5[f]

[a]Perinatal Definition II is used, which includes fetal deaths of 20 weeks' gestation or greater and infant deaths of less than 28 days.
[b]Fetal deaths of 20 weeks' gestation or more.
[c]Deaths of neonates less than 29 days.
[d]Rate per 1000 live births and fetal deaths.
[e]Rate per 1000 live births.
[f]Provisional data based on a 10 percent sample of US death certificates.
From the National Center for Health Statistics, Vital Statistics of the United States, vol II: Mortality, 1985, *and unpublished data courtesy of Dr. Harry Rosenberg and Dr. Marian MacDorman of the National Center for Health Statistics. Reproduced, with permission, from Cunningham FG, et al.* Williams Obstetrics, *18th ed. Norwalk, Conn: Appleton & Lange; 1989:5.*

ISSUES AND CONTROVERSIES

Several issues arise in the discussion of perinatal services and care:

1. Is it better to spend federal and state dollars on preventive services rather than on high-risk services? Studies need to be done documenting the benefits of prevention as a basis for health policy decisions. It is much more cost effective to ensure a healthy birth outcome through prenatal care, which will prevent illness, than to treat a sick neonate or mother.
2. Is it ethical for level II institutions to treat acutely ill high-risk neonates in their own facility rather than transport those neonates to level III facilities? Regionalization of perinatal services has the potential to improve care delivered to low-risk and high-risk childbearing families. Because of competition among institutions for maternity clients, however, some level II institutions retain clients who should be transported. This can result in duplication of services and lower quality care to clients.

at risk, and may additionally provide intensive care to some mothers and newborns.

- *Level III facilities.* These maternity facilities manage the most complex maternal and neonatal problems. They have a health care team of highly specialized personnel that are able to provide comprehensive, sophisticated intensive care to acutely ill mothers and newborns. Moreover, some level III facilities are designated as regional centers for a particular geographic area. The regional center has the responsibility of providing coordination and continuing education programs for personnel in level I and II and other level III facilities. Some states require that the interdisciplinary team of such a facility include a masters-prepared clinical nurse specialist in a maternal/neonatal specialty area.

These level I, II, and III designations do not necessarily indicate quality of care delivered by the institution. They refer only to the extent of care provided by the facility.[13]

Theoretically, regionalization should provide quality services and the appropriate level of care to all perinatal clients without duplication of services.[14] Further, the designation of level I, II, or III should inform the consumer of the specific type of services available at various institutions; however, a recent study indicates that in reality, there is a blurring among services offered at each level, especially between the level II and III facilities. Thus, level II institutions may treat acutely ill neonates or mothers in their own facilities rather than transfer them to level III facilities.[15]

A more important point made by the same study is the general failure of regionalization to provide universal prenatal care and to identify and manage high-risk mothers more successfully.[15] In the ideal situation, a regional perinatal network would ensure that the following objectives are met:[15]

1. Clients are monitored during pregnancy to prevent or manage any health problems.
2. Clients are referred for prenatal care and delivery to a site that provides a level of care appropriate to their needs.
3. Specialized facilities are available for managing pregnant clients and newborns known to be at high risk.
4. Quality of care is improved and costs are reduced by avoiding duplication of facilities.

Figure 35–3 provides a conceptual model of a regional perinatal system.[16] As this figure indicates, all perinatal clients should be assessed for risk factors and transported if indicated; thus, all clients would have access to the same quality of perinatal care. This concept of regionalized perinatal care is an excellent one; however, the current system is still inadequate. Many women in the United States, especially those who are poor and black, are still without perinatal health care services of reasonable quality. This is even more apparent when considering access to prenatal care (*see* later discussion).

Transport

If the perinatal client requires a level of care different from that the hospital can provide, the client is transported to another hospital with more appropriate resources. If the caregivers predict that the neonate will require neonatal intensive care, every effort is made to transport the woman before delivery. Transfer of the pregnant woman to another perinatal center is referred to as **maternal transport**; transfer of a neonate is referred to as **neonatal transport**.

When a nurse practitioner, nurse-midwife, obstetrician, or family practice physician determines that transport is required, the appropriate level perinatal care center in that geographic location is called and advised that a transport is needed. When the "receiving" perinatal center ascertains that transport is indicated and when a bed is available for the mother and neonate, the transport is arranged. Prior to transport, the "sending" agency must stabilize and support the perinatal family to reduce the possibility that emergency situations will develop in the transport vehicle.

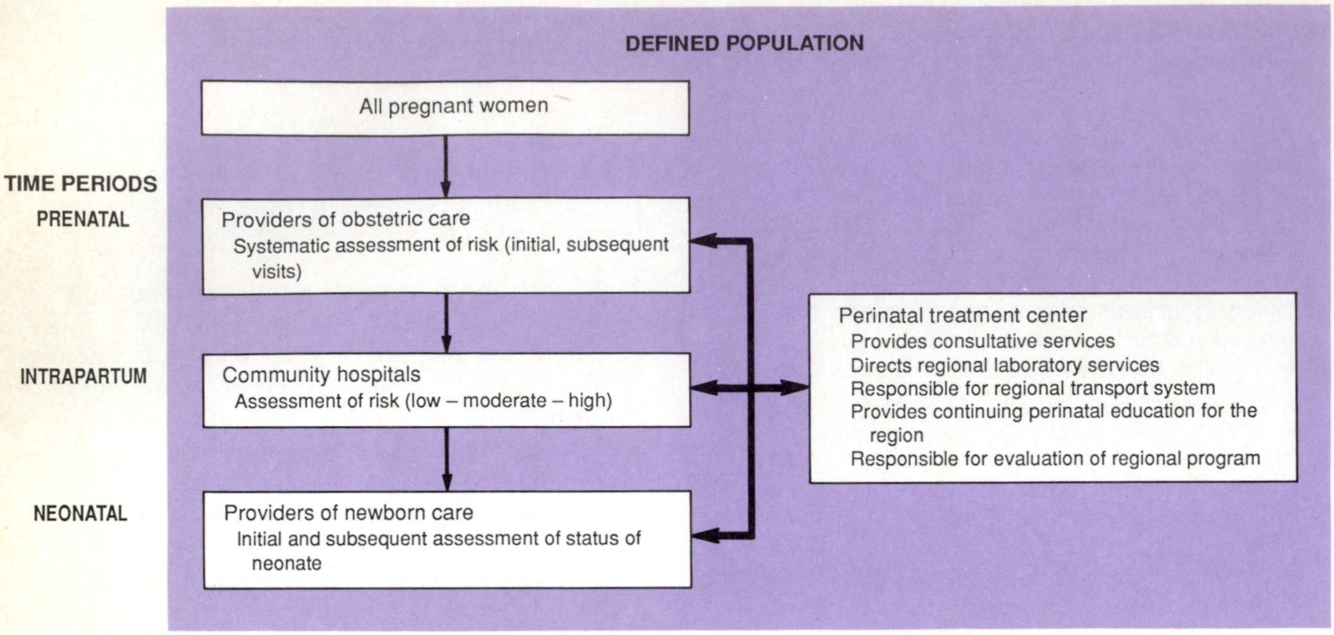

Figure 35–3. Conceptual model of a regional perinatal system within a defined geographic area. (*Reproduced, with permission, from Merkatz I, Johnson K. Regionalization of perinatal care for the United States.* Clin Perinatol. *1976;3:272.*)

The transport vehicle is usually a privately owned ambulance, ambulance helicopter, or fixed-wing aircraft that is under contract for transport purposes. The transport team may be a group of nurses, a group of paramedics especially trained for perinatal emergencies, or an obstetric resident or a respiratory therapist and nurse. Most of the supplies and equipment available in the intensive care unit are carried in the transport vehicle (Figure 35–4).

Before departing from the "sending" hospital, the transport team assesses the client, provides treatment as needed, instructs the client and family about the transport procedure and the location of the "receiving" agency, and then proceeds with the transport. If the individual to be transported is the neonate, parents are provided an opportunity to see the neonate prior to transport.

On arrival at the receiving agency, the client and family are assisted in their adaptation to the emergency situation and transfer. If the client's condition warrants a transfer back to the original agency, a transfer is then made back to the sending hospital or other appropriate facility. The transport "road" is a two-way street.[17] This is in keeping with the goal that the appropriate level of care should be provided as close geographically to the client's home as is possible.

Access and Barriers to Prenatal Care

As described in Chapters 1 and 43, low birth weight in infants is one of the most devastating high-risk problems during the perinatal period. It is also believed to be one of the primary factors related to infant mortality in the United States today. Low birth weight has been linked directly to lack of prenatal care.[18–21] The lack of access to prenatal care appropriate to risk status is one of the failures of the current system of regionalized perinatal care. One of the primary concerns, then, of nurses and other health care professionals involved in perinatal care must be to improve access to prenatal care, thus helping to reduce low birth weight and decrease infant mortality. Equal access to prenatal care is a prerequisite for successful regionalization. Reduction of barriers to quality prenatal care for all pregnant women must be a national priority.

In 1986, four regional consensus conferences on access to prenatal care and low birth weight were held by the American Nurses' Association.[19] These conferences were designed to build on the 1985 Insti-

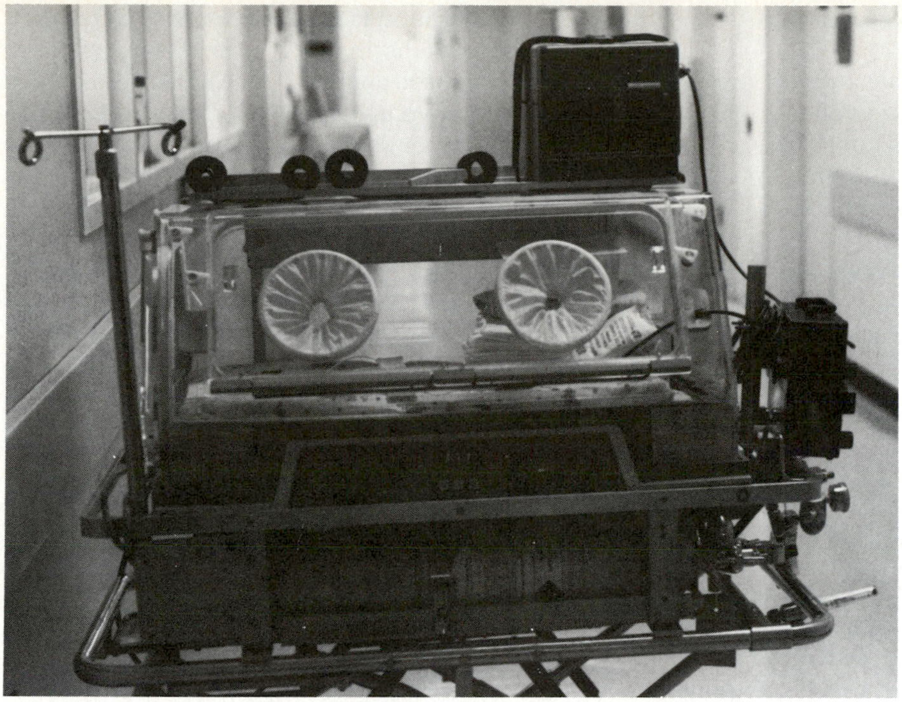

Figure 35–4. Infant transport equipment.

tute of Medicine Study on low birth weight.[18] The conferences focused on three issues: nonfinancial barriers to prenatal care, components of prenatal care most effective in reducing low birth weight, and recommendations for health policy needed to reduce low birth weight.

Nonfinancial Barriers to Prenatal Care. Three categories of nonfinancial barriers to prenatal care were identified: (1) public policy/system barriers (inconvenient locations and hours of service, inadequate support and use of nurse-midwives, maldistribution of providers, lack of transportation, and multiple eligibility requirements for benefits); (2) provider barriers (negative behavior characteristics, inadequate education regarding psychosocial and cultural aspects of care, and communication problems between providers); and (3) client barriers (lack of knowledge about the importance of prenatal care, fear of the system and health care providers, denial and ambivalence about pregnancy, and lack of incentives to seek care).[19] These areas must be addressed through greater public awareness and action in order to improve access to care for low-risk and high-risk women of all socioeconomic levels.

Components of Prenatal Care. Seven categories of prenatal care were identified as most effective in reducing the incidence of low birth weight: (1) initial and ongoing risk assessment, (2) individualized care based on case management, (3) nutritional counseling, (4) education to reduce or eliminate unhealthy habits, (5) stress reduction, (6) social support services, and (7) health education.

Prenatal care should be individually tailored to each woman's needs, degree of risk present, and mutually determined goals. Low-risk mothers require only selected categories of components and a minimal number of visits; women at high risk require almost all of the components and frequent visits.[19]

Recommendations for Health Policy. The major overall recommendation of the Consensus Conference is that "A national system of public maternity financing be developed, financed through a combination of federal and state revenues, administered by states, and implemented at the community level."[19] Other recommendations follow:

- Funding for the community and migrant health centers programs and the Title V maternal and child

health block grant programs be increased and targeted for perinatal health services
- Nutrition assistance and other public support programs be broadened for pregnant women
- All health professional schools be required to incorporate into their curricula theory and practice related to health education, counseling, and the social and cultural aspects of care
- Eligibility for all federal public assistance programs required by pregnant women operate on the basis of identical eligibility criteria that measure only financial need
- Reimbursement under Medicaid, Title V, and other public and private programs be based on uniform standards to ensure that women receive all necessary components of care
- An equitable system of malpractice compensation be maintained
- Federal and state governments and the private sector launch a national effort to educate the public, policymakers, and pregnant women about the importance and cost-effectiveness of timely, high-quality maternity care
- State nursing practice laws be unified to permit practice to the maximum extent possible by certified nurse-midwives and nurse practitioners
- Federal tax laws be amended to require all employers to furnish prenatal leaves to employees[19]

Much remains to be accomplished to ensure quality care for all childbearing women, regardless of socioeconomic circumstances or risk status. Nurses have an important role in fostering successful regional systems of care.

CAREGIVERS IN PERINATAL CARE

The practice of having a single health care provider attend to the needs of the perinatal client has all but disappeared from today's health care system.[12] Obstetricians rely on consultation from pediatricians, and appropriate therapeutic decisions cannot be made without information from the nurse at the bedside. Perinatal clients with complications require the coordinated, sophisticated interaction of allied health professionals and a myriad of multidisciplinary specialists, as well as physicians and nurses, to ensure quality care.[20]

Collaboration as a Basis for Perinatal Care

Collaboration means working with other individuals or groups of individuals to achieve a goal. In perinatal settings, collaboration is multidisciplinary, interdisciplinary, and intradisciplinary; it is a team effort to provide the highest quality of perinatal health care.

In collaborative management, the role of a given team member depends on that person's expertise and relationship with the client and family. A factor that never changes is the need for all team members to value one another's contributions and to work together as a team to achieve the best possible outcome. The continued reduction of infant mortality and morbidity will not occur through further development of technology alone. In the future emphasis must be placed on the development of approaches to prevent high-risk births, principally prenatal care. This will require additional nursing resources as well as the efforts of the entire perinatal team.

The Interdisciplinary Team

An interdisciplinary approach to the provision of perinatal care is no different than the team approach required for the delivery of any other type of health care today. Perinatal team members may include social workers, chaplains, nutritionists, laboratory technicians, respiratory therapists, physical therapists, transport team members, obstetricians, perinatologists, neonatologists, and nurses.

Perinatal neonatal nurses provide care in a variety of settings including outpatient and inpatient settings, staff development departments, perinatal outreach programs, and maternal and neonatal transport teams. As in any nursing situation, roles and tasks vary from time to time. For example, the nurse in the neonatal intensive care unit may have primary responsibility for care of the neonate. On the other hand, clinical nurse specialists may have the responsibility of coordinating care for the neonate, mother, and family in high-risk situations.

A Model for Interdisciplinary Care

Challela[21] describes a model that can be used to guide the development of an interdisciplinary team. In this interdisciplinary model (IDM), the responsibility for assessment, decision making, delivery of service, and evaluation is shared by the different disciplines constituting the team. The philosophy supporting the model is "one of providing service to clients through a shared commitment to group goals, achieved through interdisciplinary team planning."[21] Challela identifies several factors that have the potential to influence the development of interdisciplinary teams and their effectiveness: philosophy, professionalism, territoriality, communication and influence, role identity, and development.[21]

Philosophy. Commitment of the team members to collaboratively determined priorities is essential to the development of an effective team. A commitment must be made to the client's and family's needs rather than to a professional's ego.

Professionalism. The behavior acquired by the team members during their disciplinary educational program affects how each member will function within the interdisciplinary team. Nurses have traditionally functioned under the direction of the physician. As a member of the interdisciplinary team the nurse must assert autonomy and exhibit expertise in professional nursing in a manner that "complements but does not threaten either the physician or other professionals."[11,21] Often nurses experience conflicts related to authority and territoriality that have developed through their socialization during the nursing educational program and practice.

Nurses who are just beginning their practice often experience significant frustration. They have the ability to provide competent care to childbearing families, but probably need a period of 6 months to a year and continuing education to function efficiently on a high-risk interdisciplinary team.[22]

Territoriality. All members of the interdisciplinary team rely on basic knowledge from the physical, natural, behavioral, nursing, and medical sciences and from the humanities. Although nursing focuses on the whole person and the family, "other professions have more precisely delineated territory."[21] Within the interdisciplinary team conflict emerges where there is an overlap into others' territory. Boundaries must be negotiated between team members and it takes time for norms to be established within the group. Problems often develop in settings where there are frequent personnel changes. The overall effectiveness of the team is dependent on the capabilities of the individual members to collaborate, cooperate, communicate, and interact as an interdependent group of individuals (Figure 35–5).[23]

Communication and Influence. Influence may be defined as any interpersonal interaction with psychologic effects.[24] Each member of the team must acquire influence. Challela suggests that it should be acquired within the team through emulation (attainment of equality through the achievement of success by methods similar to those used by other team members), suggestion (direct suggestion of an idea to the team), and persuasion (application of force to achieve a goal).[21] Nurses develop influence through the succinct articulation of suggestions and demonstration of expertise in the nursing role.

Role Identity. Effective team members are able to give and take and perform a variety of roles within the team dependent on what is needed to meet client needs. According to Challela, to become a member of the interdisciplinary team, the nurse must (1) define the nursing role, (2) recognize the overlap between the disciplines, (3) learn what other disciplines can do and be aware of the territoriality issues and bound-

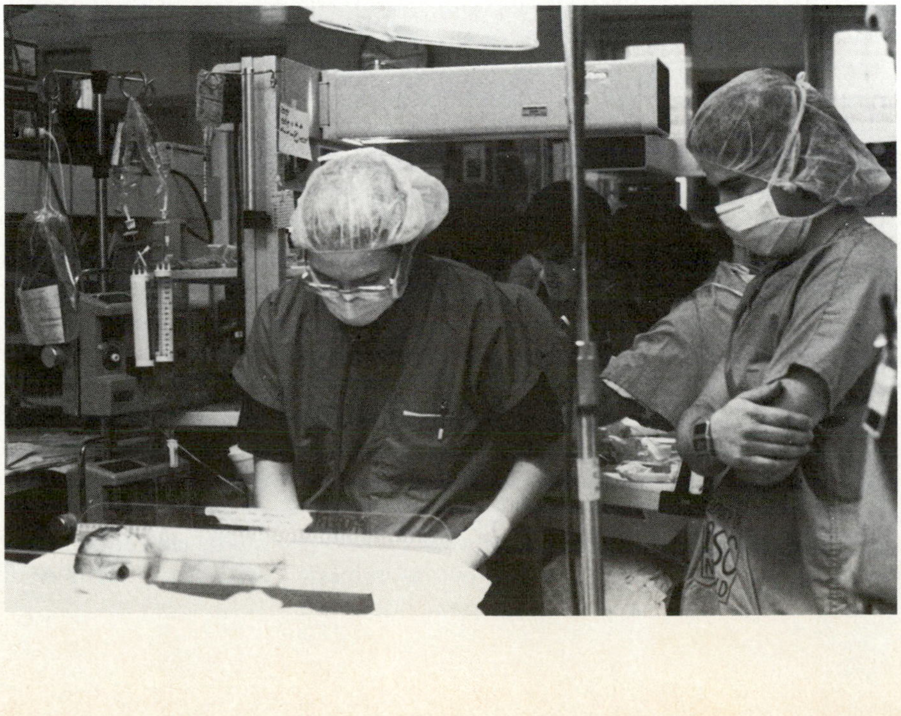

Figure 35–5. Teamwork in the neonatal intensive care unit (NICU). In the foreground, a neonate is weighed on admission by the NICU staff members who attended the delivery. In the background, a nurse and physician work together to provide care to a critically ill neonate.

aries, and (4) develop influence and share in the distribution of power.[21]

The components of the nursing role are often difficult to specify. Different settings and client populations demand different nursing activities. The conceptual framework for perinatal nursing illustrated in Figure 35–1 describes the nursing role as supportive, protective, and stimulative. These activities may be refined further within the specific perinatal health care setting. There are specific nursing responsibilities common to all perinatal care settings:

1. *Promotion and maintenance of health.* Identification of the particular needs of the perinatal client that interfere with functioning (problems, acute or chronic health deviations), as well as vulnerabilities (aspects of health promotion relative to potential health problems).
2. *Facilitation of growth and development.* Anticipatory guidance, childbirth education, labor support.
3. *Supportive counseling.* Providing or referring the family for genetic, grief, or supportive counseling.
4. *Teaching.* Teaching self-care skills, strategies to promote development and minimize risk.[21]

Team Development. Development and administration of this complex team are best accomplished through on-the-job, simultaneous teaching of all the specialized team members, as a collective group. The new graduate of a nursing program requires at least a 6-month orientation before he or she can become an integral member of the team.[25] Neonatologists must complete a minimum of a 1-year "hands-on" clinical fellowship training program following a pediatric residency before being able to function as a capable team member. Table 35–5 provides a model describing the components of such an orientation program.

Even in the community hospital, perinatal care relies on an interdisciplinary philosophy. The team may contain fewer specialists, but nursing, medicine, and other support disciplines are still represented. The need for on-site training is as essential in the community-based nursery as it is in a level III care center.

Team members must be able to relate what they learn to the specific resources of their unit. Thus, the majority of the activities directed at developing a perinatal interdisciplinary team should occur in the setting in which care is to be provided.[26]

The educational program must also be directed toward the same interdisciplinary group that will be involved with providing care in the clinical setting. Thus, specialists in obstetric and pediatric medicine as well as nurses from both of these practice areas must be included in the program.

TABLE 35–5. A MODEL FOR ORIENTATION OF THE PERINATAL INTERDISCIPLINARY TEAM

Site	Provide program in actual setting in which care is to be provided.
Planning	Involve all team members in program planning. Involve learners in the definition of learning needs.
Implementation	Involve all team members in the teaching of the program. Involve the learners in the conduct of the program when possible.
Evaluation	Use both learner-focused and client-focused outcome criteria to evaluate the impact of the program. Involve all team members in the evaluation of the program.

The orientation program will be most effective when it is provided by other members of an interdisciplinary team. Team members integrate content more readily when there is another specialist in their discipline to relate to on the faculty. Appropriate orientation into the role of interdisciplinary team member therefore requires the efforts of all of the members of the perinatal team.

High-Risk Maternal-Fetal-Neonatal Assessment

As described earlier in this text (*see* Chapter 14), initially all childbearing women and their families are assessed and screened for possible factors that indicate risk. If one or more risk factors are identified in this initial screening, further assessment with specific risk-oriented assessment tools is conducted to clarify the nature of the risk factors.

Figure 35–6 is a case summary tool that incorporates the concepts in the assessment framework described earlier in this chapter (*see also* Figure 35–1).[27] The information collected by the nurse is summarized on the case summary form along with information supplied by the other members of the perinatal team. Some assessment may require more expertise than that possessed by a beginning-level professional nurse; however, the advantage of providing care through an interdisciplinary team is that if one team member is unable to obtain the needed information it becomes the responsibility of another team member to obtain it. The best qualified team member should obtain the most essential information. Several assessment tools that may be of use to the perinatal nurse are listed in Table 35–6. Subsequent chapters in this unit discuss the assessment and care of clients with specific high-risk conditions.

Name ______________________ Date of Initial Evaluation ____________ Evaluator's Name______________

I. Assessment (Judgments)	**Nursing Problems and Vulnerabilities**	**Nursing Strengths and Resources**	**Objectives** (Goals)	**Recommendations** (Diagnostic, Therapeutic, and Educational)
A. Physiologic 1. Physical 2. Dental 3. Nutrition				
B. Sensory 1. Vision 2. Hearing				
C. Motor 1. Gross 2. Fine				
D. Language 1. Receptive 2. Expressive 3. Articulation				
E. Cognitive				
F. Academic 1. Reading 2. Arithmetic 3. Spelling				
G. Self-Help 1. Feeding 2. Toileting 3. Dressing 4. Bathing				
H. Emotional / Behavioral / Social				
I. Family 1. Structure 2. Dynamics				
J. Environment 1. Home 2. School 3. Community 4. Culture				

II. Evaluation and Revision

III. Case Summary

A. Acute Health Deviations

B. Developmental Life Stages

C. Chronic Health Deviation

D. Cultural /Environmental Stressors

Figure 35–6. Case summary tool. (*Adapted from the faculty of graduate programs of the University of Indiana School of Nursing, Indianapolis, Indiana.*)

TABLE 35–6. SELECTED ASSESSMENT TOOLS USED IN PERINATAL NURSING

Family	FACES: Family dynamics assessment based on cohesion and adaptability. Mountain K; Humerick S, ed. *Analysis of Current Assessment Strategies in Health Care of Young Children and Childbearing Families.* Norwalk, Conn: Appleton-Century-Crofts; 1982.
Home	Caldwell assessment of the home environment. In: Powell M. *Assessment and Management of Developmental Changes and Problems in Children.* St. Louis, Mo: CV Mosby; 1981.
Fathering behavior	Assessment of fathering behaviors. In: Johnson S. *High Risk Parenting: Nursing Assessment and Strategies for the Family at Risk.* Philadelphia: JB Lippincott; 1979.
Assessment of mother-child interactions	Amis: Assessment of maternal interaction sensitivity. Price G. *Infant Behavior and Development.* 1983;6:353–359.
	Maternal-infant play interaction scale. Walker L, Thompson H; Humerick S, ed. *Analysis of Current Assessment Strategies in Health Care of Young Children and Childbearing Families.* Norwalk, Conn: Appleton-Century-Crofts; 1982.
Infant behavior	Infant temperament scale. Brewer J; Humerick S, ed. *Analysis of Current Assessment Strategies in Health Care of Young Children and Childbearing Families.* Norwalk, Conn: Appleton-Century-Crofts; 1982.
	Denver Developmental Screening Test. WK Frankenburg, MD; 1978.

CASE STUDY/CARE PLAN: MATERNAL TRANSPORT FOR PRETERM DELIVERY

Karen Blake is a 16-year-old high school student who is now 29 weeks pregnant. Karen lives with her mother, Ms Blake, who works as a secretary to support her single-parent family. Ms Blake's insurance pays for Karen's medical care, but will not provide for the infant's care.

At 29 weeks of gestation, Karen is admitted to a level I suburban hospital with frequency, urgency, dysuria, and uterine contractions. Shortly after Karen is admitted to the labor and delivery unit, her membranes rupture spontaneously. Karen's obstetrician performs a vaginal examination and determines that Karen's cervix is 80 percent effaced and 3 cm dilated. Her contractions are mild to moderate in strength, 4 minutes apart, and 40 seconds in duration. Karen's obstetrician advises Karen and her mother that delivery of the 29-week infant is imminent and that arrangements will be made for Karen to be transported to a level III hospital. Karen and her mother begin to cry when they realize they will have to leave their trusted obstetrician and move to a strange and distant hospital. Ms Blake also expresses concern about paying for the infant's long-term and expensive care.

The Blake's are reassured that they can maintain telephone contact with their family obstetrician. In addition, the perinatal nurse in the level I hospital gives Ms Blake a map of the route to the level III hospital as well as a diagram of the hospital. She also informs Ms Blake about state money available to help pay for the infant's hospital expenses. Karen's obstetrician then arranges for Karen's transport to the level III hospital by the level III hospital transport team. When the level III team arrives, they estimate that the 45-minute trip to the level III center can probably be made before delivery of Karen's infant. They review with Ms Blake instructions on how to reach the new hospital and then proceed with the transport.

Supporting Assessment Data	Expected Client/Family Outcome	Nursing Action/ Intervention	Rationale	Criteria for Evaluation
Nursing Diagnosis: Anxiety, related to transport to unfamiliar birth setting				
Client transported to level III agency; client and family receiving care from unfamiliar members of interdisciplinary team; client and her mother cry when they leave their trusted obstetrician	Client and her mother will use hospital resources with relative ease	Orient client and her family to agency, including neonatal intensive care unit.	Lack of familiarity with level III facility will foster client/family anxiety.	Client is oriented to environment. Client's mother visits cafeteria.
	Client and her mother will maintain contact with familiar obstetrician and nurse at level I agency	Arrange phone call with level I team. Encourage client and her mother to express feelings. Facilitate the presence of client's mother with client at level III facility.	Client/family need to maintain relationship with familiar caregivers at level I agency who have been identified as a support. Social support helps to alleviate anxiety.	Client's mother talks with team at level I agency. She is present with client at level III institution.
Nursing Diagnosis: Anxiety, related to anticipated high cost of neonatal care				
Client's mother states "How will we pay for the baby's hospital bill?"	Client's mother will talk with social worker about financial aid	Arrange for a social worker to meet with family and discuss financial needs.	Social worker is appropriate member of interdisciplinary team to arrange financial assistance via state funding.	Client's mother talks with social worker and states "She thinks we can get state money."

SUMMARY

Perinatal nursing is the practice of professional nursing in a variety of settings in which families seek assistance in maintaining health, preventing health problems, or restoring health around the time of birth. Optimally the practice of perinatal nursing occurs within the context of an interdisciplinary health care team. Collaborative assessment of the holistic needs of the perinatal family by the team results in the identification of strengths and resources to be supported, vulnerabilities or risks that the perinatal family should be protected against, and problems or illnesses that require intervention.

Regionalization of perinatal health care services has become an increasingly important means of achieving improved cost-effective reproductive and developmental outcomes. Competition for perinatal clients and lack of equitable compensation for medically underserved and indigent clients has resulted in an unwillingness on the part of some physicians and institutions to provide an integrated, leveled system of care. National initiatives are currently under way to resolve the problems associated with the delivery of perinatal care, but the problems are far from resolved.

For most families the chance of having a healthy infant has improved greatly in the past decade, in large part because of the increased sophistication of perinatal nurses and other professionals. Yet, many problems continue to plague the delivery of perinatal care services. Rates of neonatal mortality and morbidity across age, racial, geographic, and socioeconomic groups are disturbing. Significant improvements could occur by increasing access to prenatal care, developing better means of identification of high-risk pregnancies, and increasing availability of intensive perinatal services for families that need them. Perinatal nurses will continue to have a role in management of these families and in the political solutions needed to resolve these problems.

Perinatal nurses have the opportunity to make autonomous nursing decisions within the interdisciplinary perinatal team and to interact with colleagues in a broad variety of disciplines. Nursing actions involve teaching, promotion, and maintenance of health, facilitation of growth and development, provision or support and counseling, assessment of risk, and management of complex sophisticated technology. Nurses are vital members of the interdisciplinary team because of their holistic perspective of the childbearing family. They also must be involved in decisions that influence public policy.

REVIEW QUESTIONS

1. Differentiate among low-risk, moderate-risk, and high-risk pregnant families.
2. Define the concept of regionalization. Discuss two strengths and two weaknesses of regionalization for perinatal care.
3. Provide a description of the services in level I, level II, and level III centers for maternity care.
4. List three barriers to obtaining perinatal care. List three factors that facilitate access to perinatal care.
5. Discuss the nurse's role as a member of the interdisciplinary team; include the concept of territoriality.

REFERENCES

1. Pernoll ML, Benson RC, eds. *Current Obstetrics and Treatment.* 6th ed. Norwalk, Conn: Appleton & Lange; 1987.
2. Butnarescu GF, et al. *Perinatal Nursing, Volume II.* New York: Wiley; 1980:17–18.
3. McKenzie CM, Vestal K. Perinatal crisis. In: Kinnedy M, ed. *AACN's Clinical Reference for Critical Care Nurses.* New York: McGraw-Hill Book Co; 1981.
4. Goodwin JW, et al. Antepartum identification of the fetus at risk. *Can Med Assoc J.* 1969;101:458.
5. Hobel CJ, et al. Prenatal and intrapartum high-risk screening. *Am J Obstet Gynecol.* 1973;117:1.
6. Coopland AT, et al. A simplified antepartum high-risk pregnancy screening form: statistical analysis of 5459 cases. *Can Med Assoc J.* 1977;116:999.
7. Knuppel RA, Drukker JE. *High-Risk Pregnancy.* Philadelphia, Pa: WB Saunders; 1986.
8. Queenan JT, ed. *Management of High-Risk Pregnancy.* 2nd ed. Oradell, NJ: Medical Economics Co, Inc; 1985.
9. Cunningham FG, et al. *Williams Obstetrics.* 18th ed. Norwalk, Conn: Appleton & Lange; 1989.
10. Fanaroff AV, et al, eds. *Behrman's Neonatal-Perinatal Medicine.* 3rd ed. St. Louis, Mo: CV Mosby; 1983.
11. National Foundation-March of Dimes, Committee on Perinatal Health. *Toward Improving the Outcome of Pregnancy: Recommendations for the Regional Development of Maternal and Perinatal Health Services.* White Plains, NY: March of Dimes Birth Defects Foundation; 1977.
12. Brann AW, Cefalo RC, eds. *Guidelines for Perinatal Care.* Evanston, Ill: American Academy of Pediatrics and American College of Obstetricians and Gynecologists; 1983.
13. Korones SB. *High-Risk Newborn Infants.* 4th ed. St. Louis, Mo: Mosby; 1986.
14. Cordero L, et al. Appropriateness of antenatal referrals to a regional perinatal center. *J. Perinatol.* 1989;9:38–42.
15. *The Perinatal Partnership: An Approach to Organizing Care in the 1990's.* Providence, RI: National Perinatal Information Center, Inc; 1989.
16. Merkatz I, Johnson K. Regionalization of perinatal care for the United States. *Clin Perinatal.* 1976;3:272.
17. Finsterwald W. Neonatal transport: communication—the essential element. *J Perinatol.* 1988;8:358–360.
18. The Institute of Medicine. *Preventing Low Birthweight* Washington, DC: National Academy Press; 1985.
19. Report of Consensus Conferences on Access to Perinatal Care and Low Birthweight. Pub. No. MCH-16. Kansas City, Kans: American Nurses' Association; 1989.
20. Kattiwinkel J, et al. The team approach to outreach perinatal education. In: Raff BS, ed. *Perinatal Outreach Education: Methods, Evaluation and Financing.* White Plains, NY: March of Dimes Birth Defects Foundation; 1981.
21. Challela M. The interdisciplinary team: a role definition for nursing. *Image* 1979;11:9–15.
22. Perez RH. *Protocols for Perinatal Nursing Practice.* St. Louis, Mo: CV Mosby; 1981.
23. Rubin I, Beckhard R. Factors influencing effectiveness of health teams. *Milbank Fund Quart.* 1972;50:317–344.
24. Katz D, Kahn R. *The Psychology of Organizations.* New York: Wiley; 1966.
25. Sherwen LN. Maternal-infant competencies for new nurses: a joint effort by educators and practitioners. *J Perinatol.* 1989;9:173–177.
26. Sherwen LN. Interdisciplinary collaboration in perinatal/neonatal health care: a worthwhile challenge. *J Perinatol.* 1990;10:1–2.
27. Perez-Woods RC, et al. *A Perinatal Assessment Tool.* Indianapolis: Indiana University/Seattle: University of Washington; 1985.

Psychosocial Concerns of the High-Risk Childbearing Family

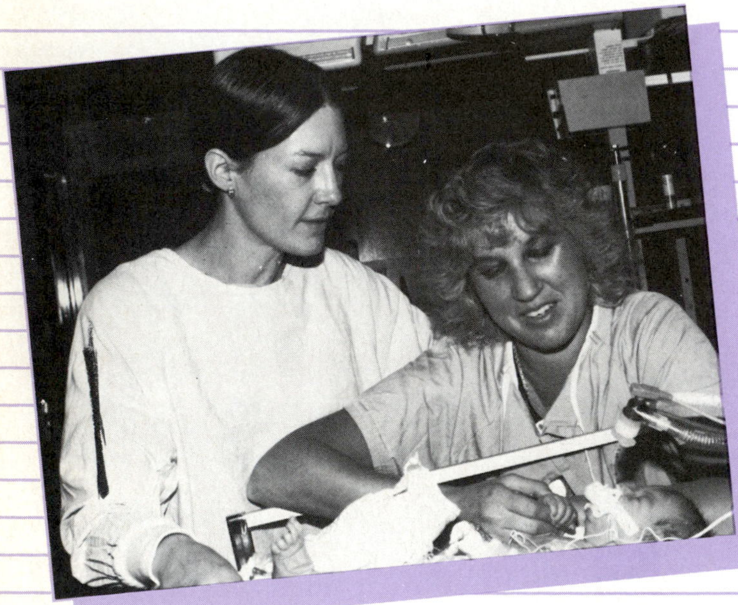

chapter 36

Key Terms

battering
high-risk clients
substance abuse

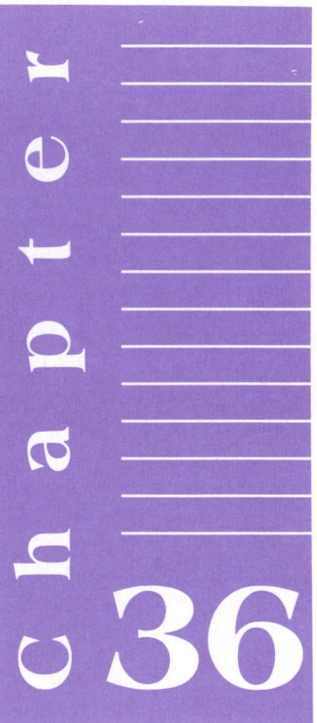

High-risk childbearing families are those whose physical, emotional, or social situations threaten their health, well-being, and development during the childbearing year. Every high-risk condition has broad and complex psychologic implications. Meeting the psychosocial needs of high-risk childbearing families requires strategies evolving from and understanding of crisis, grief, and mourning. Although high-risk conditions can have far-reaching negative psychologic effects on the childbearing family, they can also have positive, growth-producing outcomes. A unified, consistent, and interdisciplinary approach among multiple health care providers promotes adaptation to childbearing and parenthood for high-risk clients. By providing education, culturally sensitive support, and appropriate referrals, nurses can help clients and their families understand and cope with high-risk conditions.

Every nurse working with childbearing families will encounter clients who become high risk, even in wellness settings such as birth centers. Nurses therefore need to be prepared to deal with high-risk situations, if only on a temporary basis prior to a client's transfer.

THE CONCEPT OF HIGH RISK

High-risk clients are those whose physical, emotional, or social situations present some threat to their health, well-being, or development. In its broadest sense, the concept of high risk extends throughout the childbearing year from preconception through the postpartum/neonatal period. Some high-risk conditions, such as diabetes, chronic substance abuse, or a turbulent marriage, may have existed before conception. Others, such as the onset of premature labor, stillbirth, or the birth of an infant needing neonatal intensive care, may occur suddenly or without known cause. Many high-risk conditions, such as cesarean delivery and the birth of a very premature infant, have implications that extend beyond the childbearing year. Clients may be high risk for one or more reasons.

The High-Risk Client/The High-Risk Family

Any high-risk condition affects the entire family. In every high-risk situation, the ability of individuals to function appropriately within the context of their family unit or everyday activities becomes threatened in some way. Childbearing and early parenthood involve stress and role transition in the best of circumstances; however, high-risk parenting brings additional pressure and the need for more complex role changes.[1] In addition, such situations as the loss of an infant or the need for neonatal special care affects both parents simultaneously. The support system available to each partner can be jeopardized, as both parents are grieving.[2] If not dealt with successfully, these stresses can result in abnormal developmental processes and the breakdown of the family unit.[1] Any high-risk situation should therefore immediately classify the family, and not simply the client, as high risk.

Through their contact with clients in prenatal, intrapartum, postpartum, and neonatal settings, nurses are able to aid in high-risk identification, assessment, interventions, and follow-up. Working with high-risk clients requires the ability to blend scientific and technologic expertise with compassion and skill in interpersonal relationships. Nurses need to be aware of ways in which the client's cultural background may affect adaptation to high-risk status or behaviors in crisis and grief. For example, a client may be greatly distressed but may not openly cry because of cultural emphases on self-discipline and control. Clients from certain Asian cultures may not initiate questions for fear of insulting the health care provider. In addition, nurses are challenged to help clients develop confidence in their own ability to cope and to assist the high-risk family to develop joy and skill in beginning parenthood. Implementation of quality care also involves a collaborative approach that includes other health care professionals, such as physicians, social workers, and pastoral care representatives.

THEORETICAL BASES OF HIGH-RISK CARE

Crisis

Crisis theory presents a general model that readily applies to clients across the life span and in just about every type of clinical setting. Crisis is a state of upset or disequilibrium in which a person struggles with a situation that she or he perceives to be temporarily beyond personal ability to comprehend or to control.[3] A crisis forces a person to readapt his or her view of self, of his or her environment, or both.[4,5] This change in pattern of expectations evolves feelings of anxiety that can become so severe that the person is immobilized. A sense of crisis can persist days or weeks until the person is able to work out ways of dealing with the current predicament and adapting to possible future life changes.

During the course of a lifetime, nearly everyone can expect to encounter several crises. Some may be maturational or developmental crises, that is, broad life changes that occur during growth and development, such as the transition to parenthood. Others may be situational crises, that is, crises occuring in relation to particular and unexpected circumstances, such as having an infant admitted to a neonatal intensive care unit. Situational crises may or may not occur along with developmental crises.[5]

Not every new life event is accompanied by a crisis. The term *crisis* refers to a state or to an individual's *reaction* to a potentially threatening event and not to the specific event itself.[6] Crisis is therefore a manifestation of a person's unique perception. The degree to which a person experiences crisis depends on the following factors:[7]

1. *The event itself.* The event that elicits a crisis reaction has usually held great importance for the client and family; furthermore, the situation often cannot be readily resolved by the client's usual coping patterns. For example, a woman who prides herself on her good health and looks forward to a healthy pregnancy may experience crisis when told of the development of a high-risk condition such as gestational diabetes.
2. *The client's and family's perceptions of the event as a crisis or not as a crisis.* Certain events, such as the sudden death of a loved spouse, may be expected to result in family crisis for most people. Other types of events may precipitate crises for some people but not for others. For example, one couple may view the birth of twins as a wonderful way to have two children with one pregnancy. On the other hand, another couple may feel overwhelmed and unable to cope with the prospect of caring for two infants at once.
3. *The client's and family's resources.* The presence of supportive resources, such as close and loving family members, adequate finances, experience with successful resolution of previous crises, and

access to professionals skilled in crisis intervention, has several benefits. According to Caplan, a person in crisis has an increased need to be nurtured and may become more open to the influence of others.[3] The kind of support the person is able to get from significant others helps her or him to handle problems and to emerge from the crisis with greater mental and physical health, rather than with greater susceptibility to mental and physical illness. The crisis of a high-risk condition requiring bed rest may be complicated if a pregnant woman does not have financial support for high-risk care, as well as family or friends to help her manage household tasks.

Crisis resolution, for situational as well as developmental crises, may evolve in a healthy direction, with the client and family learning new adaptive responses and actually evolving toward a higher level of functioning; however, a crisis that is poorly resolved or dealt with in a maladaptive manner can become prolonged or result in a lower level of functional ability for the client and family. As Baird noted, the Chinese character representing crisis means both "danger" and "opportunity."[7] The potential threats presented by a crisis are accompanied by opportunities for the client and her family to grow, develop new life patterns, and become better able to deal with future problems.

Loss, Grief, and Mourning

Feelings of loss emerge when a person perceives that something of value has gone or been taken away. Grief comprises the emotional and physical responses to loss.[8] Mourning is the process of grieving and working through grief. Grief-producing situations in parent-neonate nursing range from inability to have a vaginal delivery to dealing with a stillbirth or the birth of an infant with a severe congenital anomaly. As with feelings of crisis, the nature of grief depends on the individual's unique perception. Perception, in turn, evolves from the complex interplay of many factors, for example, the client's cultural and religious background, presence of other family members, support (or lack of support) from significant others, previous life experiences, and physical status. Both crisis and grief are accompanied by emotional upheaval; indeed, grief may follow crisis, especially situational crises. Table 36–1 summarizes nursing strategies used with clients experiencing crisis and grief.

Much has been written on the topic of loss and grief, especially with reference to death and dying and birth of an abnormal infant. Researchers and clinicians have identified a predictable emotional pattern of grieving responses among adults.[9–11] Variation in the number of stages or phases defining the grieving process exists among theorists; however, the emotional processes they describe are similar. In working with high-risk families, the nurse needs to understand crisis, grief, and mourning and to be prepared to deal with clients' psychologic and psychosomatic reactions. Concepts related to grief and mourning are discussed next.

TABLE 36–1. NURSING STRATEGIES FOR WORKING WITH CHILDBEARING CLIENTS EXPERIENCING CRISIS AND GRIEF

Anticipate the potential for crisis and grief. For example, clients who receive news of a high-risk condition, particularly a condition requiring a change in lifestyle or having long-term implications, may be expected to experience crisis.
Assess the event itself and its implications for the client's health and well-being.
Assess the client's and family's responses in light of their religious and cultural backgrounds.
Provide an atmosphere of privacy and confidentiality to encourage the client to express feelings.
Allow adequate time to discuss the high-risk condition and the family's feelings. Listen carefully, but do not make unrealistic promises, such as "Everything will turn out fine." Having another nurse temporarily "cover" other clients can allow the staff nurse the uninterrupted opportunity to talk with a client in crisis.
Help clients identify physical, emotional, and behavioral responses related to crisis and grief. Reassure clients when responses are normal. Promptly enlist the assistance of mental health resources if clients' responses pose a threat to the health or safety of themselves or others.
Ensure that the client receives support in coping with crisis and grief. Assist the client in identifying sources of support within her own network of family and friends. Offer to speak with significant others if the client so desires. Provide the client with referrals, for example, for appropriate support groups, for telephone "hot line" assistance, for relevant counseling, or for appropriate financial aid services. Make certain that a plan for follow-up of the client experiencing crisis and grief is implemented—for example, telephone contact at intervals or home visits if appropriate.
Communicate with other health care providers directly involved in the family's care so that a consistent and supportive approach may be implemented.
Provide a mechanism to deal with tension on the part of health care providers, such as interdisciplinary staff conferences, so that staff members can discuss their own feelings related to working with clients in crisis and grief.

Shock and Disbelief. During this stage the client reacts to the news of the high-risk condition, which is interpreted as a loss. The client may be stunned and unable to concentrate or to make decisions, but may appear outwardly calm. Health care providers may mistakenly interpret this reaction as the client's handling the situation without difficulty. Somatic symptoms, such as lightheadedness, sweating, palpitations, and gastrointestinal discomforts, may accompany shock and disbelief. Clients may also try to avoid or to deny the high-risk condition and its impact.[12] "It could not be true" and "This can't be happening to me" are common statements.

Anger. Many clients express anger, which may be directed against staff, other family members, or themselves. In addition, they may express anger by blaming themselves or others (eg, "Why me?"), quarrel or fight with other family members, or find fault with nursing and medical care.

Bargaining. When a high-risk condition exists that is perceived as a loss, clients may seek to bargain in the hope that if they do or do not behave in a certain way all will be well. For example, they may promise to attend religious services, to be a "better" person, or to donate to charities. Through bargaining, clients try to attain some control over a difficult situation.

Development of Awareness of the Loss and Acute Mourning. During this stage the person becomes acutely aware of the loss. Feelings of helplessness, hopelessness, depression, and guilt may emerge. The individual may be unable to sleep, yet feel exhausted; somatic symptoms such as shortness of breath, lack of muscular power, and intense subjective distress may be experienced. Lindemann noted that acute symptoms of somatic distress related to mourning tended to occur in waves lasting from 20 to 60 minutes at a time.[9] From her study of mothers who lost a child through death, Wong observed that the phase of developing awareness evolves into a period of yearning and pining for the dead child.[11] During this time mothers often become irritable as they evaluate the relationship they had with the child. They also experience feelings of anger, guilt, and bitterness at everyone, including themselves.

Guilt. "Why didn't I take better care of myself during my pregnancy?" "Why did I continue to clean house by myself?" "Why didn't I come to see my baby more often in the special care nursery?" "Why wasn't I kinder to my wife when she was pregnant?" These are among the feelings that may be experienced, although not verbalized, by clients. In cultures that view death or illness as punishment for sin, guilt becomes an especially difficult burden. Many high-risk conditions, such as the development of preeclampsia, are beyond parental control; however, others, such as drug and alcohol abuse, do have negative effects on the developing fetus and do compromise the health of the newborn. A major challenge is to assist clients in acknowledging that being at risk or having an infant at risk does not mean they are "bad" or "undeserving" of good health or health care. Clients need to understand conditions over which they had no control and to receive anticipatory counseling about guilt feelings. Staff may become angry with clients whose behaviors, such as drug abuse or sexual promiscuity, injured the fetus or newborn; however, little is gained by moralistic scolding.[13] With relatively few exceptions, infants are discharged to the custody of natural parents or close family members. Health care providers therefore need to focus first on their own feelings of working with these parents to develop therapeutic plans of care. A forward-looking approach, focusing on present and future goals, is most fruitful. Feelings of guilt make clients vulnerable to comments of staff and family members. Dealing directly with the potential for guilt is a goal that is facilitated by collaboration among nurses, physicians, social workers, and chaplains involved in client care.

Estrangement. In a study of grieving families, Wong noted that communication between husband and wife tended to lessen after the death of a child, because each partner tried to avoid hurting the other with talk of their loss. This fear of upsetting each other extended to relationships with other children. A "detachment" process seemed to occur within the family and could be manifested either by emotional distancing or by absence from the home.[11]

Acceptance of the Loss.[9] During this phase the person begins to be less preoccupied with memories of the loss and is able to think more realistically about the event. The client is able to resume normal activities and develop new interests. Time, thought, and sufficient mourning need to take place before the client can arrive at this stage. Health care providers should not confuse the calm outward appearance the client may display in reaction to a recent loss with acceptance of the loss.

PREPREGNANCY CONCERNS OF THE POTENTIALLY HIGH-RISK COUPLE

Certain physical conditions place a couple at risk for poor pregnancy outcome or threat to maternal well-being. These conditions can be as varied as heart disease, diabetes, collagen diseases, and habitual spontaneous abortions. For the couple, the desire to have a child is accompanied by fears about what pregnancy would entail, whether the health of the mother would be jeopardized, and whether the birth of a healthy infant would be possible. Previous high-risk obstetric history, neonatal intensive care experience, or loss of a pregnancy or infant can also have strong emotional impact on the couple.

Nurses have important roles in education and support of couples contemplating a high-risk pregnancy. Nurses can be helpful in identifying the risks pregnancy poses to mother and fetus. Nurses can discuss the nature of the high-risk care that will be required and help clients in identifying life pattern changes that will evolve with the high-risk pregnancy. Nurses can help dispel misconceptions, provide emotional support, and also serve as sources of referral for couples in need of in-depth counseling.

For certain clients, such as those with severe diabetes or heart disease or those who are infected with the human immunodeficiency virus, pregnancy at any time is not advised. Not only do clients need to be informed of these situations, but opportunities for emotional support thereafter should be provided.

Ultimately, the decision to become pregnant or not to become pregnant is made by the client or the couple. The nurse has important roles in providing information that will help clients make their own decisions about pregnancy and in making certain that clients' fears and concerns are adequately addressed.

A normal human reaction is to want to reassure couples that the availability of high-risk technology and staff can help them have a healthy infant. Health care expertise can assist many couples in meeting these goals. Nevertheless, some high-risk clients will not be able to achieve pregnancy or birth of a healthy child. Health care providers therefore need to use a hopeful, yet realistic approach when counseling the high-risk client and family. For example, a nurse counseling a couple with an infertility problem cannot assure the couple that intercourse around ovulation will result in pregnancy.

Successful outcome of a high-risk pregnancy often depends on a close working relationship among the client, nurses, and other health care professionals. A haphazard or uncoordinated approach on the part of various health care professionals can add to the client's stress and prevent the establishment of a trusting relationship. Nurses therefore need to collaborate with other members of the interdisciplinary team in developing an organized approach to the high-risk client.

PSYCHOSOCIAL CONCERNS DURING HIGH-RISK PREGNANCY

In nearly every high-risk situation there is potential for an emotionally unhealthy situation to develop, as well as for the family to develop new and effective ways of coping. As discussed earlier, an understanding of the concepts of crisis, grief, and mourning is important in working effectively with the high-risk pregnant family. Nevertheless, these concepts must be tailored to specific client situations. The nurse needs to realize that high-risk conditions are accompanied to some degree by special emotional needs on the part of clients and families. The nurse must be prepared to anticipate problems, undertake interim crisis intervention, collaborate with other health care professionals, and make appropriate referrals.

Maternal Tasks During High-Risk Pregnancy

An individual evolves through different developmental stages during the life process. Successful achievement of expected life tasks at various stages leads to further emotional maturation and ability to deal successfully with future tasks. Developmental theory applies well to pregnancy, because a woman normally faces certain stages or tasks during transition to the motherhood role. These maternal tasks, according to Rubin, are safe passage for the woman herself and her fetus, acceptance by others, binding-in to the child, and giving of oneself (*see* Chapter 17).[14,15]

There is little research documenting comparative similarities and differences between high-risk and low-risk pregnant clients in their ability to meet developmental tasks of pregnancy. High-risk pregnancy, however, may alter this process. For example, uncertainty over her health and that of the fetus and anxiety related to the outcome of pregnancy can hamper a mother's ability to feel she has mastered the task of safe passage. Feelings of guilt or rejection over the high-risk condition can prevent a woman from feeling accepted by significant others. Abused women, already feeling rejected and fearing for their safety, are at great risk.

Prenatal attachment to the fetus has been noted to be a task accomplished by high-risk as well as low-risk women;[16] however, the high-risk mother who feels she may lose the fetus or newborn or who is very ill may avoid the task of binding-in to the fetus.[16] A woman may also become "desperate" to produce a child and anxiously aware of any indication of fetal life. The high-risk mother must often make greater changes in lifestyle than the healthy pregnant woman, especially when bedrest or hospitalization is required. The high-risk mother who has a normal infant and returns to good health may take pride in her "sacrifices"; the mother who suffers a perinatal loss may feel that her efforts have produced nothing but sorrow.

The great variation among etiology, course, and outcomes that constitute maternal-fetal risk make identification of a model for developmental tasks during high-risk pregnancy difficult. The ability of the high-risk client to meet tasks of pregnancy depends on the reason for the high-risk status and the quality of support she receives to help her meet the tasks of pregnancy. Nursing interventions regarding maternal tasks during high-risk pregnancy evolve from assessment of unique high-risk client needs in relation to normal developmental tasks of pregnancy. Certainly, this topic warrants further research.

Threats to Self-Image

High-risk pregnancy poses several threats to a client's self-image. Three of these sources are the client herself, the client's significant others, and health care providers.

Pregnancy is a womanly process. Many cultures, including traditional U.S. society, define success of a marriage in terms of ability to produce healthy offspring. In being considered high risk, a woman may feel that she is in some way lacking in a basic feminine ability to reproduce. Her concept of herself and her own worth may be compromised, especially if she comes from a background that places high value on reproduction.

High-risk pregnancy often means that the client must look to others for advice and assistance. This may foster an uncomforable sense of dependency. When hospitalization is required, the client is removed from the home environment. Away from her everyday roles in familiar surroundings, she may experience additional changes in self-image. As one client stated, "Suddenly I felt as if I had lost control of my body and could no longer do anything right. I was going to be a failure at the one thing all grown up women are supposed to be able to do."

Pregnancy is a time of emotional vulnerability, even for a low-risk client. A sizable literature documents the importance of social support, especially support from the infant's father, on a woman's transition to parenthood.[14–21] The high-risk client has potentially greater needs for approval and support, because of the existence of a problem or problems that may jeopardize her well-being. When hospitalization is necessary, strategies that foster self-confidence and feelings of being loved and valued assume additional importance. For example, the nurse can reinforce the positive aspects of the client's participation in her own care during hospitalization.

At times, a turbulent family background can be the source of risk as well as a major threat to self-image (*see* "The Battered Client"). Nurses frequently identify high-risk social situations. Providing immediate emotional support as well as referral to social service or mental health specialists can help clients through difficult psychosocial situations.

As previously noted, anger and blame can be direct or indirect manifestations of crisis and grief. Frequently, these emotions are expressed within the high-risk family, regardless of the reasons for high-risk status. The pregnant client may be the focus of the anger or blamed for the high-risk condition, further compromising her self-image. Anger and blame may be manifested physically, by verbal abuse, and by alteration in communication patterns.

Nurses and other health care providers can have a major effect on client self-image and willingness to continue with care. At times a client's lifestyle is responsible for a high-risk condition. Examples include substance abuse and sexually transmitted diseases. The client may face threats to self-image because of disapproval from health care professionals. Staff need to assess their own feelings about working with these high-risk clients and to develop therapeutic, nonjudgmental strategies aimed both at dealing with the high-risk situation and at promoting client self-image. Strategies such as staff meetings focusing on such topics as reactions to working with clients with high-risk behaviors and use of clinical consultants, can be of assistance. Prejudicial remarks directed toward clients because of their high-risk status are always to be considered inappropriate and unprofessional.

Health care providers direct much effort toward promoting, maintaining, and restoring the health of the physically ill client and fetus. The "high tech" approach can have a negative effect on a client's self-image, if the emotional aspects of high-risk care are not considered. As one client summarized, "After a while I began to feel like a scientific oddity. Doctors and nurses kept coming to examine me, but so few seemed to care about who I was . . . after a while I just wanted to cry, 'I'm a real person with an address and a family and a job and a life outside this pregnancy!' " In describing ways in which nurses and physicians helped her through a high-risk pregnancy, another client stated, "I came to feel that they cared so much for me personally. The nurses and doctors always seemed to make time to listen to me and to help me to feel good about myself, even though I was so ill."

Psychologic Impact of Prenatal Diagnosis

Clients at risk for abnormalities that can be identified through diagnostic techniques, such as chorionic villus sampling or amniocentesis, may refuse to accept the pregnancy until normal test results are known. Clients who might consider abortion of an abnormal fetus and clients who fear the possibility of raising an abnormal child may experience anxiety and guilt.

According to Zuskar, the opportunity to prepare emotionally for the birth of an abnormal infant could also be accompanied by acute crisis and by a long period of prenatal distress.[22] This could be particularly problematic in situations in which the extent of the abnormality is uncertain. Nursing strategies that can help families prepare for the birth of an abnormal infant are summarized in Table 36–2.

Implications of High-Risk Pregnancy

For many previously healthy women, high-risk status is a condition that occurs only with pregnancy. For example, women who become severely pre-eclamptic might have enjoyed active healthy lives prior to their pregnancies. Being classified as high risk can precipitate feelings of crisis in these clients and their families. Will I be all right? Will I live through delivery? Will I give birth prematurely? Will I have a handicapped child? Who will take care of my family if I have to be hospitalized? These are frequent concerns of the high-risk client. High-risk status has many implications for childbearing. Maternal or fetal outcome may be uncertain. More frequent and intensive assessment is needed during pregnancy. The potential for extended hospitalization exists. In addition, clients may have to relinquish the opportunity to select birth options. (Although secondary to physical well-being, this can compound feelings of loss and disappointment during childbearing.) In some cases, clients and their families must be transferred for care to high-risk hospital centers that may not be geographically close to their homes. This is especially problematic when hotel bills for family members add to financial burdens and when the client has other children who may greatly miss their mother's presence in the home. High-risk pregnancies can always be expected to test a family's resources and to require health care supportive interventions.

Psychologic reactions to a high-risk pregnancy are also affected by the level of the client's physical wellness. In certain high-risk conditions, such as severe pre-eclampsia, hyperemesis gravidarum, or human immunodeficiency virus infection, the client may be ill. In multiple gestation, the client may be uncomfortable at all times, especially as pregnancy progresses. Feelings of anguish and anxiety can further compromise physical well-being. Nurses need to plan care that integrates assessment of physical well-being with strategies for emotional support.

TABLE 36–2. NURSING STRATEGIES TO HELP FAMILIES PREPARE FOR THE BIRTH OF AN ABNORMAL INFANT

Accept the family's decision to have an abnormal child; avoid imposing one's personal values or opinions.
Identify the potential for crisis related to birth of an abnormal infant, even in the best of circumstances.
Make certain that a consistent collaborative approach is used among all health care providers. When possible, minimize the number of different health care providers who work with the client, so that an emotionally supportive relationship can be established between the client and caregivers and the client is not continuously interacting with strangers.
Make certain that the client is well educated about the potential status of the infant.
Assist clients in identifying ways in which they will inform others about the infant.
Help clients to identify ways they will cope with the infant.
Provide referrals to counseling and to support groups, such as parents of children with Down's syndrome.
Make certain that preparations are made prenatally, if the infant's condition may be expected to require specialized equipment and services.
Discuss realistically the positive aspects of the expected infant. Assist the parents to have the best delivery and early parenting experience possible.

Pregnancy After Previous Pregnancy Loss or Death of a Child

Little research has been done on the topic of prenatal parental responses in clients who have previously lost a pregnancy or a child. Even when physically normal during a subsequent pregnancy, these clients must be considered at risk for increased anxiety and for potential alterations in prenatal attachment. Carroll studied ways in which the previous death of an infant affected potential parents' feelings about a current pregnancy.[23] From exploratory interviews with pregnant couples who had lost infants between 6 months and 3 years earlier, Carroll was able to identify five emotional themes:

1. *Need for self-protection and protection of spouse.* A process of emotional distancing from significant others was frequently used, as the current pregnancy heightened feelings about the pregnancy that produced the infant who died.
2. *Need for information and support.* Current and anticipatory reassurance was needed from health care

providers. Reassurance was required for problems that were only imaginary, because past experiences intensified the couple's fears about what could be possible.

3. *Need to be in control.* According to Carroll, a need to alter patterns of behavior from the earlier pregnancy was shown by attempts to change health care providers or hospitals or simply to do things differently.
4. *Need to reaffirm the existence of the infant who died.* Couples in Carroll's study tried to keep alive the memory of their dead child; however, friends and family members tended to avoid mentioning that infant or the death. Attempts by others to avoid this topic or to encourage the couple to forget the past created conflicting feelings and resentment in the couple.
5. *Need for dialogue between spouses.* In Carroll's study verbal communication became extremely important, although spouses could recognize they expressed their grief in different ways.

Maternity nurses frequently care for pregnant couples who have experienced prior loss of a pregnancy or a child. Nurses need to anticipate that parents might experience residual or rekindled feelings of grief and loss, no matter how healthy or desired the current pregnancy. As Carroll noted, "healing after loss comes through time, experience and grief work, not through forgetting, ignoring or replacing the lost infant."[23]

Offering pregnant clients opportunity and encouragement to verbalize feelings about previous loss should be part of any nursing care plan dealing with this subject; however, this topic is often difficult and uncomfortable for health care providers. There may be a tendency to focus on the current pregnancy and to give the impression that it is somehow inappropriate to recall painful past experiences. In reality, although the nurse may find it easier to say "but you are now having a healthy pregnancy" and "your bad experience is in the past," this approach carries little therapeutic value. As the first level of care planning, nurses need to evaluate their own feelings about this subject and to seek consultation with colleagues whenever necessary.

Prenatal Hospitalization

Prenatal hospitalization indicates that a client is ill enough or potentially ill enough to warrant close and continuous professional attention that cannot currently be provided in the home setting. Conditions requiring prenatal hospitalization include severe preeclampsia, uncontrolled diabetes, premature labor, various infections, and fetal surgery. Hospitalization may be for a few days or for several months. All clients hospitalized prenatally are considered to be at high risk. A major benefit of hospitalization is that outcome may be improved for both mother and fetus.[24]

Prenatal hospitalization plucks the client from a lifestyle routine and superimposes the specter of illness on the transition to parenthood. Several stresses are associated with hospitalization:

- Separation from family members; loneliness and concern over household maintenance
- Alteration in family patterns, evolving from need of other family members to maintain the household without the client present; potential for anger and blame directed toward the client by the client herself or family members
- Worry about other children and the impact of separation from their mother; concern over childcare, especially when family members cannot stay in the client's home and the spouse has to work
- Realization that hospitalization means the client is at very high risk; potential threats to self-image and attainment of developmental tasks, such as safe passage and fetal attachment
- Need to conform to a hospital routine
- Need to undergo uncomfortable procedures, such as fetal monitoring or frequent blood studies
- Difficulty resting related to round-the-clock interruptions
- Concern over health care bills that may not be completely covered by third-party reimbursement; lack of insurance to cover even basic costs
- Fear of loss of a job, school, or work opportunity related to premature and prolonged hospitalization

Few hospitals have enough high-risk pregnant clients who need inpatient care to justify individual prenatal hospitalization units. Prenatal clients are therefore often hospitalized on postpartum units. Most units are still composed of semiprivate rooms. Private rooms are much more expensive and are covered by insurance only when "medically" justified. Unfortunately, promotion of mental health is usually not considered by insurance companies or entitlement programs to be reason enough for a pregnant client to be assigned to a private room. Although attempts may be made by staff to keep prenatal clients together, prenatal clients frequently share rooms with postpartum mothers. Given that the routine low-risk postpartum hospital stay is 2 to 3 days, it is possible that a pregnant client may have more than 20 different roommates during her stay. Some prenatal clients may welcome the chance to room with someone who is well and who has had a healthy infant. Other clients, however, may feel additionally stressed and upset about their own inability to be healthy or to go home. The presence of an infant in the room and hospital restrictions on visitors when infants are with their mothers may compound these feelings. Nurses therefore need to discuss reactions with the hospitalized pregnant client and, when possible, to work with members of the admitting department to make room arrangements that promote mental health.

The hospitalized pregnant client requires special psychosocial nursing strategies that extend beyond physical care expertise (Table 36–3). Nurses need to reinforce the positive aspects of the client's decision to be hospitalized and the potential contributions she is making to her infant. Because of hospitalization during an emotionally vulnerable transition to parenthood, the client may come to include staff among her significant others and to build a strong working relationship with certain staff members (Figure 36–1). Primary nursing or patterns that foster continuity of care by certain staff members can help to establish a sense of trust. Conversely, an everchanging stream of unfamiliar faces can contribute to client stress and despair. In some obstetric units, nursing staff rotate between labor and delivery and postpartum settings. Nurses who have cared for the prenatal client during her hospitalization may therefore work with her during her labor and delivery. As one client reported, "After 6 weeks in the hospital, I was frightened about how the baby would actually be. But I had so much faith in the nurses and doctors caring for me that I knew I wouldn't be abandoned. Whatever happened, I felt they would help me have courage."

TABLE 36–3. PSYCHOSOCIAL NURSING STRATEGIES FOR THE HOSPITALIZED HIGH-RISK PREGNANT CLIENT

Make certain the client and family are informed about her condition, her treatment plan, and her progress.
Provide time to talk with the client about herself, her fears, and her expectations. Identify ways in which hospitalization is and is not congruent with the client's expectations for her pregnancy. Identify the client's and the family's reactions to hospitalization. Assist the client and family in designing ways in which the family can manage at home during the woman's hospitalization.
Reinforce the positive aspects of the client's participation in her own care through hospitalization.
Whenever possible, encourage the client to help in the design of her care schedule.
Encourage the client to wear her own clothes if she so desires and to have mementos of home brought to the hospital, especially if hospitalization will be prolonged.
Adapt hospital routines whenever possible to allow for a more "normal" lifestyle, despite hospitalization.
Promote emotional, as well as physical, comfort measures. Help clients cope with boredom. Encourage visits from hospital personnel, such as volunteers and the librarian, when appropriate. Have television connected; seek charitable sponsorship if clients cannot pay for television. When possible, participate in the roommate selection process; at times, hospitalized antenatal clients may receive much support from each other.
Identify the importance of spiritual needs during high-risk prenatal hospitalization. If the client desires, refer her to the hospital chaplain, encourage visits from members of the client's spiritual community, and make certain she can attend religious services in hospital if she is physically able. Make certain that religious dietary practices, eg, kosher diet, can be maintained.
Be flexible with regard to visiting hours and visitors, including client's other children, to allow her to be with significant others.
Make certain that the client and family are able to receive childbirth preparation within the hospital setting, eg, through hospital or individual teaching sessions and videotapes shown on hospital video player.
With client, develop plan for ongoing emotional support after discharge.

Staff can do much to promote a family-centered experience despite hospitalization. A first step is evaluation of unit policies, such as restrictive visiting, that work against family-centered childbearing. In what ways can rigid policies be modified to promote a family-centered experience for the hospitalized client? This type of planning and implementation can also benefit postpartum clients. Other strategies include encouraging family members to visit and to bring pictures or other personal items to make the hospital room more homelike, providing for visits by the client's other children when feasible, and making time to listen to concerns of family members.

Nurses can help minimize feelings of dependency inherent in hospitalization by encouraging the client to participate in plans for her own care.[24] In addition, collaboration with other members of the interdisciplinary team, such as physical therapists who can design appropriate exercise programs, nutritionists who can work with the mother to plan a medically and culturaly acceptable diet, and chaplains who can assist with spiritual needs, is necessary. Contributions from volunteers are also important, as boredom presents a major stress during prenatal hospitalization.

Childbirth Education for the High-Risk Pregnant Client

Lack of access to childbirth education programs is a problem for the high-risk client who is hospitalized or at home on bedrest. In addition to missing content related to labor and delivery, clients and their families lose the often exciting and enjoyable experience of attending a childbirth education program together.

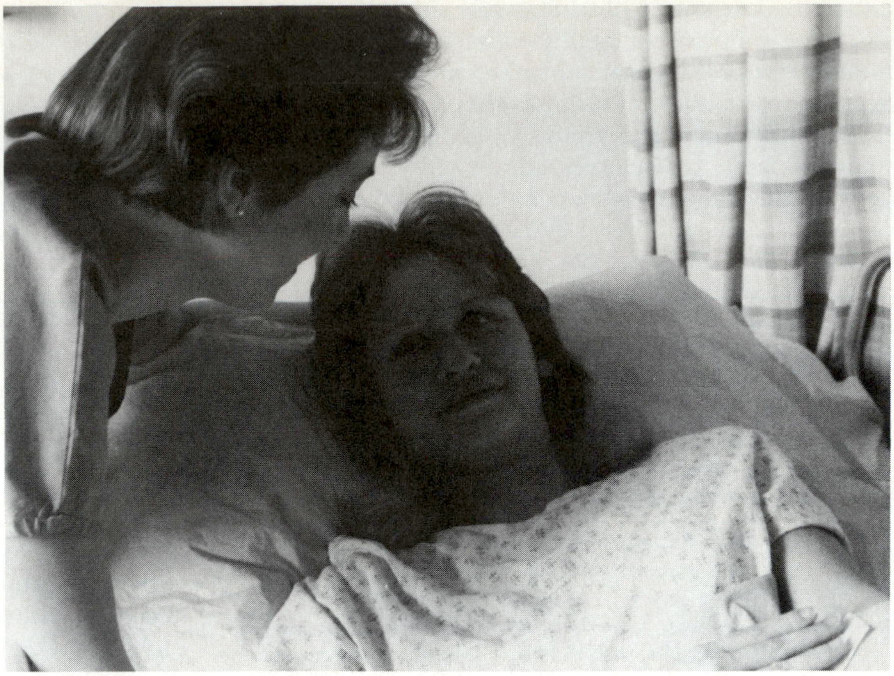

Figure 36–1. The nurse provides support and encouragement to a hospitalized pregnant client.

Traditionally, teaching for these clients has been done on a one-to-one basis that has focused on high-risk issues and has done little to foster a family-centered delivery experience.

Avery and Olson presented a model for childbirth education of the hospitalized pregnant client.[25] They suggested that classes be offered in the hospital setting for any high-risk clients and families able to attend. Avery and Olson felt that the course should be taught by a registered nurse childbirth educator who was certified by a national organization such as the International Childbirth Education Association and who also had a background in high-risk obstetric care. Use of a special instructor might ensure that all clients receive expert teaching, as staff nurses may not have the time or background to conduct this type of program. The childbirth educator would thus become a part of the interdisciplinary perinatal team.

According to Avery and Olson, content for the high-risk classes could include much of the material provided in standard childbirth education.[25] Content areas specific to the needs of high-risk pregnant women, such as techniques of anxiety reduction and relaxation, cesarean delivery, and bonding, could be expanded. Avery and Olson forecasted benefits of childbirth education for the hospitalized pregnant client to include reduced anxiety, increased attachment to the fetus, and an improved relationship for the expectant couple; however, because these classes were not generally available, they identified a need for research to document actual outcomes of the program for the expectant family.

In settings where childbirth education classes are not available for the hospitalized client and family, one-to-one teaching between the nurse and the couple, the use of videotapes, or both can promote learning.

The High-Risk Client on Bedrest at Home

Women at risk for conditions such as preterm labor may be prescribed bedrest at home. Home care has many psychosocial advantages. For example, the client remains in her own home and does not have to be separated from her family, a particularly difficult situation when the client has other children. The client, rather than a hospital's staff, has control over schedules and visits from significant others. Financial costs are much lower.

Although the client may welcome the opportunity to be self-reliant, she may nevertheless be anxious about successful management of her condition away from the constant surveillance that hospitalization provides. This can be problematic, especially when bedrest is first begun and the client lacks self-confidence. In many cases, clients spend weeks or months in bed as pregnancy progresses. Worry over the pregnancy, sleep interrupted by a round-the-clock schedule of tocolytics, shortness of breath and other uncomfortable side effects related to tocolytics, the need to depend on family and friends to assume tasks usually performed by the client, and loss of time or opportunities related to school or work are emotional burdens.[26] Boredom and lack of activities or companionship during working hours for family members makes pregnancy seem endless and the woman feel isolated. Like the hospitalized high-risk client, the client on bedrest at home is usually deprived of the educational and social benefits of childbirth preparation classes.

Periodic telephone calls by nurses to clients at home on bedrest can allay anxiety as well as assess client status. Nurses who work in home care monitoring settings can provide emotional support as well as teaching through their reegular telephone contacts or home visits. Childbirth educators may be available to offer individualized prepared childbirth programs in the client's home; however, these services can be expensive. Videotapes on various aspects of childbirth preparation can be purchased or developed by health care providers and lent to high-risk clients on bedrest at home as an economic alternative. The client may also be put in touch with organizations such as "The Confinement Line" of the Childbirth Education Association that offer services such as emotional support, advice on daily management of bedrest, contact with other women on bedrest, and details about other services (see Appendix F). If clients are to come for clinic or office evaluation, nurses can minimize their stress by making certain they are seen without delay and that any testing is performed at the same visit. By encouraging clients and family members to verbalize their feelings and by providing teaching and support, the nurse can promote emotional health during this stressful time.

The High-Risk Client During the Intrapartum Period

A client's perception of her labor and delivery experience has been noted to be an important factor in her transition to motherhood and postpartum adaptation.[27,28] Inability to have an anticipated birth experience has been described as a crisis and has been a source of grief for clients and their spouses. The high-risk intrapartum experience superimposes the challenge of ensuring a safe delivery on the challenge of promoting a family-centered birth experience.

Clients who are at high risk during the intrapartum period have either been considered at risk during their pregnancies or become high risk during the intrapartum period as a result of problems with the passenger, passage, powers, or psyche (*see* Chapter 40). Ideally, health care professionals have had opportunities to provide anticipatory guidance and support in advance of labor and delivery for those clients who were at risk. In these situations, nurses need to orient the client to the high-risk unit and to review teaching relevant to aspects of high-risk intrapartum care. Although a high-risk client may have had extensive prenatal care, nurses in the labor and delivery unit should not simply assume that she and her family are well informed. Assessment of level of knowledge and reaction to the high-risk condition is of primary importance before interventions can be undertaken.

As discussed in Chapter 40, a client with a healthy prenatal history may become high-risk during labor and delivery. Suddenly staff may begin to rush, uncomfortable procedures may be undertaken, and high-risk equipment may be used. In some cases, the client is physically prepared for emergency cesarean delivery. The client may experience a sudden crisis, accompanied by feelings of unreality, fear, and panic. High levels of anxiety can further complicate the intrapartum process.[28]

A major concern during high-risk pregnancy is that the fetus may be born abnormal or nonviable. In many cases, diagnostic fetal tests cannot predict with certainty whether an infant will be born normal; however, birth of the infant is still a future occurrence.

Labor brings the stress of knowing that answers to questions about fetal anomalies and status may soon be apparent. High-risk clients may therefore be especially anxious during their stay in labor and delivery units. Although some potential abnormalities turn out to be minor or nonexistent, many present real current and future problems. Despite advance preparation, clients experience shock and crisis even in the delivery room. The use of general anesthesia postpones but does not "spare" the mother grief. The father frequently has to deal with this information by himself until the mother recovers from anesthesia, thus potentially reinforcing a sense of family isolation during crisis.

Some clients, such as severely pre-eclamptic clients, may feel ill as a result of their high-risk status. In cases where fetal status is potentially in jeopardy, analgesic medications may be restricted. When possible, alternative strategies such as back rubs, assistance with position changes, guided imagery, and attentive labor coaching can promote relaxation and comfort.

Improving outcomes for high-risk clients has sparked the development of much obstetric technology. When used judiciously, such technology is able to provide information about maternal and fetal well-being during labor and delivery. Despite the most skillful technical care, the nurse needs to remember that high-risk equipment and procedures are new and frightening for most clients and that sudden transition to high-risk status can be terrifying. The nurse's ability to remain calm, to provide understandable explanations to the client and her family, to collaborate smoothly with other health care providers, and to blend a compassionate approach with technical expertise are essential to effective high-risk care.

As discussed throughout this text, the focus of care needs to be the family as well as the client. The nurse must remember that the father or significant other who accompanies the high-risk client during labor and delivery is also at risk for crisis. The presence of a loving and familiar person can be important to the client. Welcoming the presence of the support person when feasible, including the support person in client teaching, making it possible for couples who planned to share delivery to remain together, and being willing to listen to the fears and concerns of family members can promote psychologic health for the high-risk family during the intrapartum period.

Much has been done to ensure family-centered care for low-risk clients during labor and delivery. Unfortunately, the pathologic condition of the high-risk client is often focused on to the exclusion of family-centered care. Nurses should evaluate current practices and policies regarding the high-risk client and judge whether restrictions are outmoded traditions or truly in the client's best interests.

Birth of a Healthy Infant After a High-Risk Pregnancy

A healthy new mother and infant are goals of high-risk as well as low-risk care. Frequently, health care professionals are able to assist clients to meet these goals through careful monitoring and judicious interventions during the prenatal, labor, delivery, postpartum, and neonatal periods. Relationships with health care professionals may become an important part of the client's social network, especially as the client tries to negotiate the task of safe passage for herself and her fetus. In addition, much of the client's energy and thought may be devoted to the high-risk condition.

A "return to normal" in itself may be a situational crisis of sorts for clients and their families. After the stress of being high risk, the client and her family may have difficulty resuming a low-risk lifestyle. For example, clients may be extremely anxious about going home after delivery. They may have much need for reassurance about their own or their infant's health status, and worry whether common variations, such as sleepiness during initial feeding, are signs of pathology. According to Jones, parents who do not become increasingly secure in handling their child after about a week at home can be at risk for developing maladaptive parenting patterns.[24]

Nurses can do much to ease transition for a previously at-risk client and her family. Nurses can continue to regard these families as potentially at risk for anxiety related to their childbearing experience. Anticipatory guidance should include feelings related to high-risk status and should be offered prior to discharge. Postdischarge follow-up may take the form of the client's attendance at office or clinic sessions and home visits or telephone calls at periodic intervals. Clients experiencing acute or prolonged emotional difficulty related to the high-risk experience should be referred for counseling.

Birth of an Abnormal Infant

All parents of infants born with abnormalities are considered at psychosocial risk. When parents know about the abnormality prior to childbirth, they have opportunity to receive support and to begin to prepare for their infant; however, many abnormalities are not known until the infant is born. Both situations are accompanied by crisis. As summarized in the box, many complex and interrelated factors determine how well parents are able to cope with their infant's abnormality. A consistent, unified team approach helps parents deal with the birth of an infant with an abnormality. Health care providers need to under-

FACTORS RELATED TO PARENTAL ADAPTATION TO BIRTH OF AN INFANT WITH AN ABNORMALITY

The nature and extent of the abnormality; the degree of mental or physical impairment
Whether and to what degree the abnormality can be corrected through growth and development and medical or surgical means
The extent of cosmetic disfigurement
The nature and extent of the infant's acute and chronic needs
The amount of disruption in the family related to the infant's condition (eg, need for a parent to stop work or round-the-clock care required for the infant)
The nature of specialized care and costs
Religious and cultural views about the abnormality
Previous experience with individuals with similar abnormalities
Support from significant others; willingness of significant others to accept the situation and show love for the parents and the infant

stand that parents may not only grieve for their infant's condition but also for the loss of their fantasized infant and, in some cases, their dreams for the infant. Many of the strategies summarized in Table 36–2 are also applicable to parents after the birth of an abnormal infant. Individualized support, encouragement, referral to organizations and support groups focusing on children with similar abnormalities, and strategies that reinforce the parents' self-confidence and focus on the positive aspects of the infant help parents to build hope and love during a difficult transition to parenthood.

PSYCHOLOGIC ASPECTS OF CARING FOR PARENTS OF A HIGH-RISK NEWBORN

Every infant admitted to a neonatal intensive care unit (NICU) has or is at risk for pathology. Infants in a NICU are observed or treated for life-threatening or disabling conditions. With few exceptions, families of infants in NICUs are considered to be at risk for parenting. Families experience crisis and grief, although these feelings vary. Parents further have lost the opportunity for a healthy, low-risk neonatal experience. Some infants are taken immediately from the delivery room to the NICU. Others are transferred from a low-risk delivery setting to a tertiary-care hospital that has an NICU. Some infants are initially admitted to a well-baby nursery, but later transferred to an NICU because of the diagnosis of a high-risk condition.

Certainly, nurses working in NICUs need to be skilled in the physical care of the high-risk newborn (*see* Chapters 42 and 43) and in the psychologic aspects of working with frightened, grieving families; however, all labor-and-delivery nurses, well-baby nursery nurses, and postpartum nurses will at some point work with parents of a high-risk newborn. Mothers of infants in NICUs are cared for on postpartum units. No matter how well prepared a mother is prenatally for the possible birth of a high-risk infant, the reality of having an infant in the NICU is a shock. Nurses must therefore be able to understand the psychologic dimensions of parenting the high-risk infant and be prepared to implement strategies that will help inform and support new parents during such a difficult time in their lives.

Obstacles to Parenting Within the Neonatal Intensive Care Unit

Several factors related to neonatal intensive care can present obstacles to parenting and have major psychologic impact on the family.

Prevention of Extended Contact. A high-risk delivery experience and the physical status of the infant may prevent the extended contact desirable during and immediately after birth.[29] At times the unstable condition of the newborn may require rapid transfer to an NICU for intensive care support. The mother's physical condition may prevent her from seeing her newborn that day or for several days. In cases where the newborn is transferred to another hospital, the mother may not see her newborn until after her own discharge. (Although some hospitals are able to transfer both mother and infant, this is not done in all situations.) When the father accompanies the infant to the NICU, the mother is then left without her main support person.

Barriers Between Parents and Their Newborns. The neonatal intensive care unit with specialized equipment such as isolettes and rules for gowning and handwashing can serve as a barrier between parents and their infants.[30]

Reminders of the High-Risk Status of the Newborn. The presence of skilled personnel necessary for infant care and high-risk procedures such as frequent monitoring of vital signs and laboratory studies are further reminders of the high-risk status of the infant.[30] Some parents are terrified at the sight of monitors attached to their infant or by the realization that their infant is in need of such technical support. In addition, several authors have described parental reactions of disappointment, grief, horror, self-doubt, and worry over the infant's normal development.[29, 31–34]

Lack of Privacy. Lack of privacy within the NICU can have a mixed impact on parenting. The continuously visible presence of skilled personnel may be comforting to the parents, especially if the infant is ill or unstable. Yet, the lack of privacy can impede parental reactions and may not satisfy the need for family members to be alone together with the infant, away from the illness atmosphere of the NICU.

Newborn's Appearance and Ability to Interact. The newborn's appearance and ability to interact can have an impact on the developing parent-infant relationship.[35, 36] The weak, debilitated, premature, or sedated infant differs greatly from the alert, term infant. In addition, a physician's pessimistic view of the infant's chances for a healthy survival could negatively affect the mother's perception of and attachment to her infant.[30, 37]

Restrictive Visitation Policies. Neonatal intensive care units have restrictive visitation policies that can impede the acquaintance process among family members. Although many NICUs no longer restrict parental visiting, visitation rights are not always extended to other relatives or family friends. Because of concerns over childborne infections such as chicken pox, sibling visitation in NICUs is often restricted to a "special occasion" within the unit or viewing through the glass windows of a nursery. Ironically, almost any curious nursing or medical student can visit an infant in an NICU, but visitation by family members and their friends may be restricted.

Concerns Related to Prematurity

Each year in the United States, a quarter million infants are born at some degree of prematurity.[38] This represents 6 to 8 percent of all births, making prematurity one of the largest problems facing nurses, physicians, and parents today.[39] Depending on the degree of prematurity and the extent of associated complications, the premature infant could be hospitalized in a special care nursery for a few days or for several months (*see* Chapter 43). Despite advancements in technology and expertise that have improved survival and physical outcome for premature infants, there has been limited progress in the prevention of premature births or the ability to predict accurately whether a pregnancy will end prematurely.[40,41]

Premature birth cuts short the psychologic developmental processes that occur during the third trimester and superimposes a situational crisis on the normal developmental processes of pregnancy and childbirth.[7,42,43] Mothers of premature infants often report "not being ready" for the infant or "still feeling pregnant." A less than optimal delivery experience and the physical status of the infant may prevent the extended contact desirable during and immediately after delivery.[29] In addition, the NICU obstacles described earlier can further separate parents from their premature infants. The parents must deal with the reality of an infant whose appearance and ability to function may differ markedly from those of a full-term infant, although the degree of difference is related to fetal growth, actual maturity of the infant at birth, and the physiologic problems of prematurity.

Prematurity recurs in the literature in association with parenting difficulties, ranging from emotional problems of parents and infants to child abuse.[43] Although premature birth occurs in all groups of women, the incidence of prematurity is higher among women who are already physically, emotionally, or socioeconomically stressed. It is difficult to conclude from current research that the premature birth in itself directly causes parenting problems; however, poor resolution of crisis and grief contributes to the complexity of difficulties surrounding premature birth. Conversely, a supportive environment can foster positive perceptions of the premature infant.[18,43]

RESEARCH ABSTRACT

Weingarten CT, et al. Married mothers' perceptions of their premature or term infants and the quality of their relationships with their husbands. J Obstet Gynecol Neonat Nurs. *1990;19:64–73.*

This descriptive, comparative study used a questionnaire method to investigate perception of infant in 37 mothers of term infants and 28 mothers of premature infants at 2 to 4 days postpartum and at 6 to 8 weeks postpartum. It also sought to determine if there is an association between maternal perception of quality of relationship with husband and maternal perception of infant. The subjects were well-educated, Caucasian, married women who had a singleton infant in the well-baby or neonatal intensive care nursery of the same suburban community hospital. A parent-centered approach was used in these units.

Preterm mothers who compared their infants to an average premature infant were more positive in their perceptions of their infants than were term mothers who compared their infants to an average term infant. Results indicated, however, that new mothers tend to view their infants positively, whether or not the infants are premature. Although no relationship was found beween positive perception of infant and positive relationship with husband, mothers with negative perceptions of their marriages also tended to have negative perceptions of their infants. The study also found that early maternal perceptions of postpartum adaptation tended to persist, at least through the end of the postpartum period.

Comment:
This study highlights the importance of family-centered teaching to promote postpartum adaptation in mothers of premature infants and in mothers of healthy term infants. The observation of negative perceptions of husband and negative perceptions of infant in both groups is similar to the literature and point to potential family problems. Study results also reinforce the importance of nursing assessments prior to clients' discharge, so that problems in postpartum adaptation and parenting may be identified at a time when mothering patterns are being developed or refined and when clients are in contact with health care providers.

Almost all surviving premature infants are eventually discharged home to their parents. A major nursing challenge is to assist these parents of premature infants to develop joy and skill in beginning parenthood in the context of an intensive care setting. The extended periods premature infants may spend in the NICU and continued postdischarge contacts provide much opportunity for nurses to educate the family about prematurity, to address prematurity-related concerns, and to foster the development of attachment between parents and their premature infants (Figure 36–2).[43, 44]

Intensive Care/Expensive Care

Neonatal intensive care *is* expensive care. From a financial viewpoint, the daily charge for stay in an NICU is substantially higher than for care in a well-baby nursery. In addition, infants in an NICU are hospitalized longer then well infants who may be discharged on the second or third day after birth. Parents of infants in an NICU may not be covered by insurance for all expenses, especially if the infant has a prolonged stay and potential for chronic problems. Even with various public assistance or special care funds, families often must deal with the real financial stress of astronomic bills that can drain their economic resources.

The emotional impact of having an infant in an NICU cannot be measured in dollars. The anxiety that parents experience over the present and future health of their infants can be far reaching. Certain handicapping conditions, such as some types of cerebral palsy or learning disabilities, do not become apparent until the infant grows into childhood. Some parents may continue to harbor concerns related to their NICU experience until developmental milestones of childhood are met. As one mother of an infant who had been evaluated in an NICU for potential seizures and then discharged as "normal" stated: "The words 'probably fine' and 'wait and see how he grows' remained in my mind after we took him home from the NICU. Like a dark cloud they would sometimes float across my mind. It wasn't until five years later, as my son 'graduated' from kindergarten, that I could realize he was just as normal as the other kids."

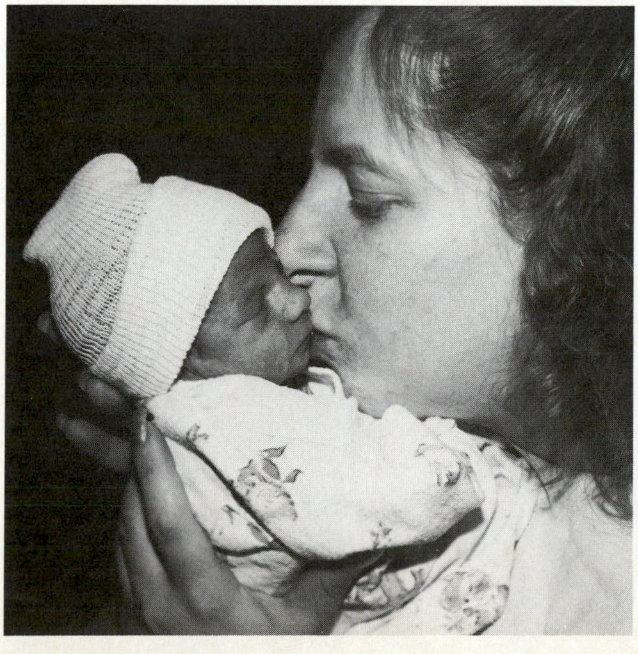

Figure 36–2. Mother with premature infant.

For some parents, having an infant in an NICU is a social stigma. Some parents feel they are the objects of pity or blame among their significant others, especially if the infant has a condition requiring chronic care. High-risk social behaviors and turbulent home situations are further complicated by a sick infant who requires special and attentive care from already stressed parents.

Nurses must *always* be aware of the broad costs of intensive care. Infants should *never* be admitted for casual reasons or simply because the well-baby nursery staff would feel "safer" if an infant were transferred. One way to minimize the risk of unnecessary NICU admissions is for well-baby nursery nurses to be skilled in assessment and normal varations of the newborn.

Nursing Strategies to Promote Parenting Within the Neonatal Intensive Care Unit

The influence of the earliest parent-infant perceptions and interactions on the developing parent-infant relationship has been an important topic of research and discussion.[18] Nurses can promote parenting of infants in the NICU in several ways by:

1. Expecting parents with an infant in an NICU for any reason to face a potential crisis.
2. Evolving strategies for emotional support from a team approach, including such professionals as physicians, other nurses, social workers, and pastoral care representatives.
3. Discussing with parents the infant's physical condition and reason for stay in the NICU. Has the infant been admitted for observation? Have health problems already been diagnosed? What is the likely prognosis? What current and future plans for the infant have been made?
4. Maintaining a collaborative team approach when providing information to parents. Joint meetings

and daily interdisciplinary rounds help staff members provide consistent, supportive care to parents of infants in an NICU (Figure 36–3).

5. Anticipating and identifying potential parental reactions to the NICU environment and to the physical condition of the infant. Parents visiting their infants for the first time should be accompanied by a member of the NICU staff who is able to orient them to their infant, to their infant's care routine, and to the NICU. This should also be done if there is a significant change in the infant's condition. Some infants, such as those born very prematurely or those with pronounced congenital anomalies, may look different from the standard of a healthy term infant. Anticipatory guidance must be given to parents prior to their seeing the infant.
6. Promoting the infant's appearance. Infant appearance can have an effect on parental perceptions, and nurses can do much to present infants in an optimal fashion. Infants need to be kept clean and in a well-organized environment. Whenever feasible, procedures should be undertaken with sensitivity to parental feelings. For examples, infants' heads should *never* be routinely shaved. One mother described her reaction to her infant's head being shaved: "She was born with a head full of thick hair. When I saw her in the NICU, they had half shaved her head; to me that white scalp looked disfigured. The staff tried to tell me that it was done 'just in case' she needed a scalp vein for an IV, which she never did. It took 9 months for the hair to grow in. People would stare at her on the street; every time I looked at her I was reminded of their thoughtlessness."
7. Facilitating contact between parents and infant. This can be done in several ways:
   - Discussing with parents the importance of their visits, not only for the infant, but also for their own development as parents.
   - Instituting policies, such as unrestricted visiting for parents and for significant others of the parents' choosing. (Parents should not be considered visitors, but integral members of the caregiving team.)
   - Assisting parents to come to visit. (Transportation can be a problem for families who do not have access to cars or who live far from the NICU. Although providing transportation for these families is not within the role of the nurse, relaying this information to social service can possibly help families receive transportation assistance. Hospital auxiliaries or other charitable groups may be willing to contribute either money or services to help these families with transportation.)
   - Providing telephone (or letter) updates to parents unable to visit. (This is especially important for mothers who are hospitalized elsewhere or for parents who live far from the NICU.)

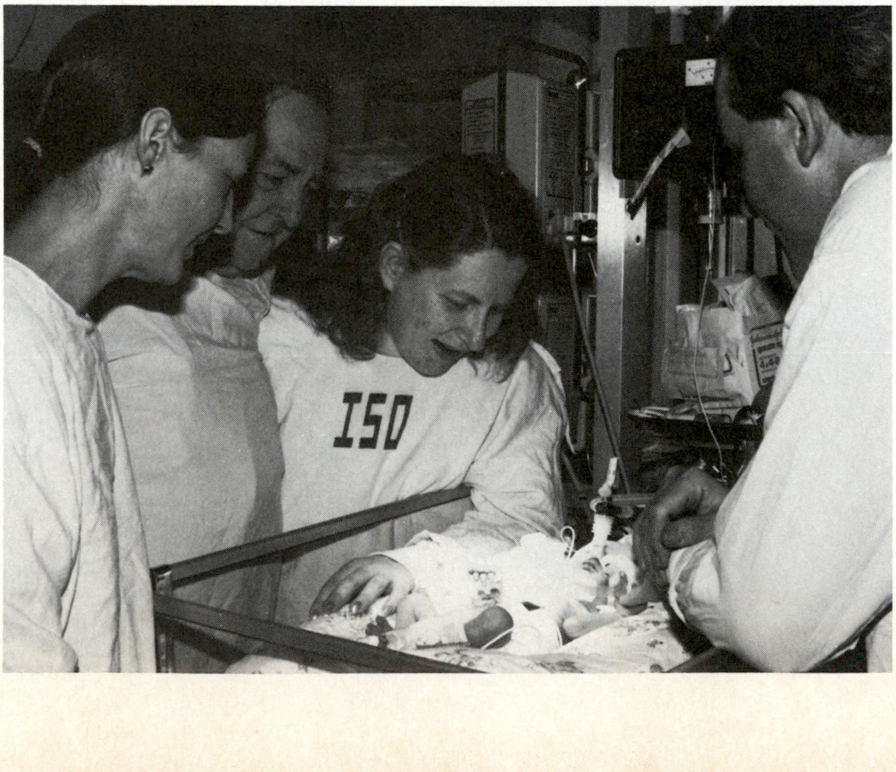

Figure 36–3. Interdisciplinary rounds in the neonatal intensive care unit.

- Assisting parents to participate in caring activities such as touching, holding, and feeding the infant if possible (Figure 36–4).
- Encouraging parents to bring in pictures of family members for use in the infant's crib as focal points. (Some families may also want to send in tapes to be played for the infant or clothing for the infant to wear.)

8. Providing opportunities for the family to ask questions and to express their concerns.
9. Providing privacy for parents and the infant whenever possible and appropriate. Some units have special "bonding" rooms where parents can be alone with their infants. When this is not possible, the use of removable screens placed around the parents and isolette is helpful.
10. Providing ongoing assessment of development of parenting behaviors and arranging for prompt counseling intervention for parents identified as having difficulty in developing attachment to their infants.[18]
11. Encouraging parents to express concerns about siblings and other family members and provide anticipatory guidance dealing with sibling and family responses to the high-risk neonate.
12. Providing for parental support from other sources, such as support groups for parents of infants in special care. Parents may also receive comfort from being introduced to other parents who have coped with an infant with a similar condition, for example, myelomeningocele. Parents of infants who require surgical repair of congenital anomalies may appreciate seeing photographs of infants who have had successful repair of these types of anomalies.

Nursing Strategies for Care of Parents of a Newborn Transferred to a Regional Neonatal Intensive Care Unit

The preceding discussion refers to almost all parents of infants in NICUs. Parents of a newborn transferred to an NICU from another birthing site have additional, unique needs.

In many states, neonatal intensive care has been concentrated in certain high-risk (level III) centers. Theoretically, this allows for the development of specialty units staffed by health care professionals skilled in the care of critically ill neonates and able to offer the latest in sophisticated technology. Most childbearing families are not at high risk and do not have infants who require intensive care. Birth in wellness-oriented, low-risk childbearing settings is appropriate. Indeed, childbearing in a high-risk center may place the healthy client at risk for complications arising from the often liberal use of obstetric interventions in these facilities.[45] Many hospitals have no

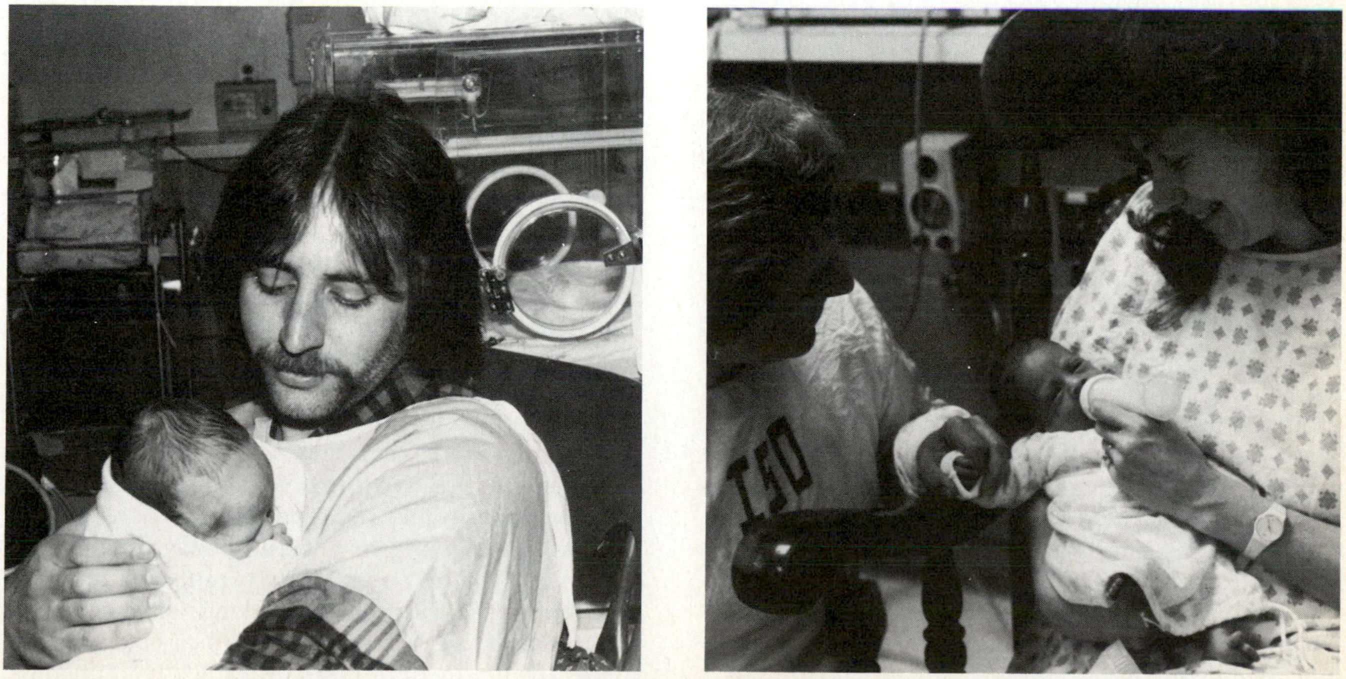

Figure 36–4. Family attachment is promoted when parents are encouraged to hold and feed the high-risk infant in the neonatal intensive care unit.

need to create high-risk units because they do not serve a large high-risk population. In addition, an NICU is an enormously expensive unit to maintain; many hospitals cannot afford its upkeep.

Although the regional model of care may decrease neonatal mortality and morbidity, there can be a negative impact on the parents of the transferred infant. Ideally, mother and infant would be transferred together. In many situations, however, a newly delivered mother remains in one hospital while the infant is transferred to the level III regional center. The regional center may be a few blocks or a few hundred miles away. In every case, the stress of having an infant who needs an NICU is compounded by maternal-infant separation and the often unexpected reason for transfer. In addition, parents may know the level III regional center only by reputation; they are compelled to rely on strangers who have not previously been involved in their care.

When the father accompanies the infant on the transport, the mother is left without her significant other. The father is also divided between two hospitals and may feel an additional burden of "having to be strong" for the mother. Concern over being separated from her infant may prompt a mother to make her own health secondary. For example, women who have delivered by cesarean may leave the hospital early and go directly to the NICU, rather than paying attention to their own physical needs for rest and recovery.

In a classic study of parents whose critically ill newborns survived after referral to a regional NICU, Benfield and colleagues found that most parents experienced grief reactions similar to those whose newborns had died.[46] Parents grieved deeply regardless of the severity of the infant's illness. The investigators noted that fathers reported dramatic changes in their daily patterns while their wives and infants were in separate hospitals; they also took on a central role in stabilizing the family during this time.

In working with parents of transferred infants, nurses must be aware of the nature of the family's birth experience (*see* the Case Study/Care Plan). Prior to the transfer, the mother should see and touch her infant, whenever possible. Any positive comments about the infant may also be appreciated and remembered by the mother.[18] On transfer, efforts must be made to orient the family to the facility as well as to the NICU. When the mother is in another hospital, telephone calls can be an important way to keep her informed about her infant's status. Neonatal intensive care units that regularly expect transfers can create areas where exhausted postcesarean or postpartum parents can rest.

Some NICUs restrict visiting to only biologic parents. Staff need to realize that supportive friends or relatives are important to the mental health of the father whose wife remains in another hospital. There are few circumstances critical enough to warrant exclusion of a significant other. Frequently, a mother is comforted by knowing that someone she loves and trusts will accompany her husband on her behalf, especially during such a stressful experience. The practice of having a father sit alone with his critically ill infant while a close relative is restricted to an outside waiting room is not therapeutic.

Staff need to realize that transfer of a child to a regional NICU brings other family burdens. Long distances between the NICU and the clients' home and threat of loss of work income may make it difficult for parents to visit. The high costs of hotels and restaurant meals are not covered by health insurance and may deeply affect a family's budget. The needs of siblings and problems associated with finding childcare, especially if overnight stays are involved, are additional concerns of parents of the transferred infant. Further, for families living in poverty, such arrangements might not be an option. These social problems deeply affect the emotional well-being of parents of an infant transferred to an NICU and are reasons for referral for social service assistance. In addition, local religious groups may be of assistance through provision of lodging and hospitality to parents of infants in NICUs. Nurses must realize that such problems pertain to parents from all types of social and economic backgrounds.

NURSING STRATEGIES FOR CARE OF SIBLINGS OF A NEWBORN IN THE NEONATAL INTENSIVE CARE UNIT

In the best of circumstances, the birth of an infant is a stressful event for siblings. When the new infant requires prolonged and intensive parental attention, siblings may feel resentful and anxious. Parents in crisis may seem to place other children "second" in their concern for the sick neonate. The children's lives and schedules may be greatly altered, especially if the parents are gone from the home for long periods, if the siblings are sent to stay with others, or if new arrangements for childcare are made. At times, parents may not be able to attend special sibling events, such as school plays, or to host holiday celebrations. Children also worry about their parents' distress. The actual response of the sibling depends on such factors as the child's age, the number of other siblings in the home, the nature of pre-existing family relationships, and the amount of change in daily routine related to

CASE STUDY/CARE PLAN: SUPPORTING PARENTS OF A NEONATE TRANSPORTED TO A REGIONAL NICU

Mary and Mark Mendez, both 28 years old, experienced a low-risk, uncomplicated pregnancy and planned to deliver at their local community hospital. Mary looked forward to breastfeeding. After 18 hours of labor, however, Mary had an unexpected cesarean delivery for fetal distress. Her membranes had spontaneously ruptured 36 hours prior to delivery.

Baby James, 40 weeks' gestation, had Apgar scores of 8 and 9 and at first appeared well, but one day after birth he was noted to have difficulty maintaining normal body temperature. After a seizure was observed, plans were made for Baby James to be transferred to the neonatal special care nursery at the level III regional center 20 miles away. His admitting diagnosis was to be "possible sepsis," and intravenous antibiotic therapy was begun. Mary was to remain in the community hospital where she delivered; her husband would accompany the transport team. Although the transfer was to take place during the night, Mary called her mother, sister, and brother-in-law who came immediately to the hospital. Mary and Mark responded to the news of the transfer in a frightened, tearful manner. Mary seemed unable to stop crying and asked her sister to "go in my place for the baby."

Supporting Assessment Data	Expected Client/Family Outcome	Nursing Action/ Intervention	Rationale	Criteria for Evaluation
Nursing Diagnosis: Fear, related to transport of neonate and potential threat to physical well-being of neonate				
Emergency cesarean delivery for fetal distress; neonate to be transported to NICU 20 miles away Neonate's diagnosis: "possible sepsis" Parents visibly upset and tearful	Prior to transport: Parents will be able to identify reason for neonate's transfer Parents will maintain contact with the neonate Supportive family members will be included in transport preparation	Assess parents' understanding of reason for transport and response to impending transport. Describe the transport and the NICU where neonate will be sent.	Clients may not ask yet still worry about what will happen to neonate and what NICU will be like, especially if they are unable to accompany neonate.	Prior to transport, parents are able to explain in their own words reason for transport, and to describe the transport and NICU.
		Assist mother to nursery; provide opportunity for parents to see and touch neonate. While providing realistic information about neonate, identify positive aspects of neonate's physical status.	Contact with neonate facilitates parent-neonate attachment and enables parents to begin grieving process.	Prior to transport, parents see and hold the neonate.
		Provide opportunity for mother's sister and brother-in-law to see and if possible, touch neonate.	Allowing sister and brother-in-law to see and touch neonate fosters initial family attachment and supportive behavior.	Prior to transport, family members see the neonate.
		Encourage one family member to stay with mother while one goes with father to NICU.	Support of significant others is needed during periods of crisis.	During transport, one family member stays with mother and another accompanies father.

(continued)

CASE STUDY/CARE PLAN: Supporting Parents of a Neonate Transported to a Regional NICU (*continued*)

Supporting Assessment Data	Expected Client/Family Outcome	Nursing Action/ Intervention	Rationale	Criteria for Evaluation
Nursing Diagnosis: Grief, related to separation from neonate and concerns for well-being of neonate				
Parents appear frightened; mother unable to stop crying	After transport, mother will be able to express her grief over ill neonate	Provide privacy for mother.	During vulnerable periods, clients need to be able to express feelings without presence of curious onlookers.	Mother is provided with privacy.
		Encourage mother to express feelings; assist her to talk about her concerns and fears; identify her grief reaction as normal.	The ability to express feelings freely is necessary for healthy crisis resolution.	Mother expresses feelings to staff and progresses through grief process.
		Encourage mother to call NICU for information about neonate; clarify information received.	Uncertainty can cause additional stress; clarification of information assists client in processing information.	Mother calls NICU and realistically describes information received.
Nursing Diagnosis: Potential for ineffective breastfeeding, related to mother's separation from neonate				
Mother planned to breastfeed; describes disappointment about inability to breastfeed because of neonate's transport to NICU	After transport, client will continue with plans to breastfeed by learning use of breast pumps or manual expression of milk	Encourage mother's breastfeeding plans; teach use of breast pump and how to manually express milk.	Lactation can be established even when neonate is separated from mother.	Mother is able to use breast pump or manual expression technique to provide breast milk for neonate.
		Assist mother in bottling, labeling, and storing milk to be brought to neonate in NICU by her family.	If mother does not initiate and maintain lactation, her ability to breastfeed may be compromised. Ability to provide milk for neonate enhances mother's feelings of successful parenting.	Relates sense of accomplishment in being able to provide for neonate.

the infant's hospitalization. It may be helpful for the nurse to discuss with the parents of the infant in an NICU the following strategies, which focus on siblings:

- Siblings should be told about the infant in language they can understand. In addition, parents should tell the siblings what their own feelings are and why.[47] Parents also need to make certain that the child has understood what they were trying to say. The type of explanation should be based on the developmental level of each child. Toddlers, as well as preschool-aged or school-aged children, are in need of information.
- Parents should be encouraged to keep siblings within their own home and not to send them to live with friends or relatives. Although parents may intend to "protect" their children from emotional crisis at home, children may cope better when they remain in their own household. As Trause and Irvin noted, children may be distressed by separation from their parents; they may suffer more from imagining what has gone wrong than by experiencing the real problem; and they may feel that they are being sent away because they are a burden or have little to contribute.[47] When distance and childcare problems necessitate that children be sent away, parents need to take care to keep them informed about their own health status and the infant's progress. Parents should be advised to try to maintain usual family routines and standards.
- Parents need to allay siblings' fears that their thoughts or actions caused the infant to be sick or, in cases of perinatal death, to die. Nurses should encourage parents to speak directly to siblings about this topic. Siblings normally have ambivalent feelings about a coming infant. Birth of a high-risk infant or death of the infant may make the siblings

feel responsible. In a culture where the media can make anything seem real, sibling guilt feelings need to be addressed.

- Siblings continue to have needs relevant to their own developmental level and social network. Parents need to be encouraged to provide special time alone with the siblings to show the sibling he or she is loved and valued.
- Children often have fears about their own health or the health of their parents. Nurses can help parents of a high-risk infant to anticipate these feelings and to reassure the siblings that they are healthy.
- Just as parents may grieve the loss of the fantasized infant, siblings may grieve the loss of the expected brother or sister and may also feel ashamed of the infant's high-risk status. Siblings also may grieve the loss of parental attention.[48]
- Nurses can encourage parents to bring siblings to visit their brother or sister in the NICU, especially if hospitalization is prolonged. Such visits may help siblings to understand more about the infant and to feel a part of the family (Figure 36–5). (Even in units that do not yet have sibling visitation programs, the sibling may be assisted to view the infant through nursery windows.) Many children handle such visits well; others, however, may be overwhelmed by the NICU and their infant brother or sister. Nurses can advise parents to anticipate a short initial stay with the older child or to bring other adults who can leave the unit if the child becomes overwhelmed.[47]
- Nurses can be instrumental in developing sibling orientation and visitation programs within the NICU. In this way care can focus on all family members, regardless of their youth. Troy and associates described a successful sibling visitation program in which staff received inservice education to help them work with parents and siblings, developmentally based teaching tools were created to help parents explain their infant's condition to siblings, and sibling visits were welcomed in the NICU.[49] Traditional problems such as fear of infection were handled by a physician or nurse assessing siblings for infection prior to their entering the NICU; a playroom, staffed by a volunteer, was available for childcare for siblings who were not able to stay as long as their parents in the NICU. Although most children were more curious than frightened by the NICU, staff were prepared to refer siblings to a child therapist, when necessary.
- During pre-discharge and post-discharge teaching sessions with parents, nurses need to include the topics of siblings and sibling responses.
- Nurses can develop or participate in development of learning materials that can promote children's understanding of high-risk infants and NICUs.

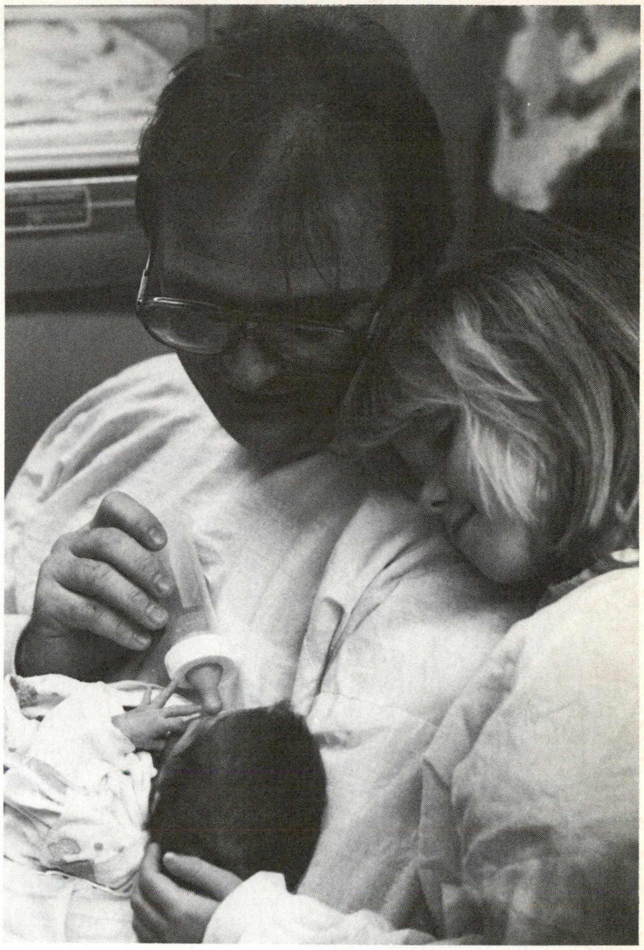

Figure 36–5. Father and sibling with newborn in the neonatal intensive care unit.

NURSING STRATEGIES FOR CARE OF GRANDPARENTS OF A NEWBORN IN THE NEONATAL INTENSIVE CARE UNIT

Grandparents are often deeply affected by the birth of an infant who requires neonatal intensive care. Concern for the current and future health of the infant is accompanied by feelings of anxiety, worry, and sadness about seeing their own child in distress. Extensive changes have taken place in neonatal intensive care since most grandparents were new parents, and these may be overwhelming to grandparents. Nevertheless, grandparents can potentially provide much support to parents in crisis. Nursing strategies for care of grandparents of an infant in a NICU include welcoming and orienting grandparents to the NICU and to the infant; encouraging grandparent participation in infant care, especially if grandparents will be caretakers after discharge; discussing the nature and importance of support needed by the parents of the infant; providing specific examples of ways in which grandparents can be helpful such as care of other children; dispelling myths; and discussing concerns of grandparents. Inclusion of grandparents or any significant others is done with the parents' permission.

NURSING STRATEGIES FOR CARE OF FAMILIES OF A NEWBORN WHO DIES

Nursing Strategies for Care of Parents

Miscarriages, stillbirths, and deaths during the neonatal period are referred to as perinatal deaths.[50] Despite advances in obstetric and neonatal care, it has been estimated that 2 of every 100 pregnancies ends in stillbirth and that 40,000 neonates die each year in the United States.[50] Stillbirth or death of a neonate is an event that can be accompanied by intense feelings of crisis, grief, and loss, especially on the part of the parents.

In the past, perinatal death was treated as a "nonevent," with staff, family, and friends trying to avoid the topic or distract the parents. Parents were given little opportunity to discuss their feelings. Often, well meaning staff isolated mothers on the postpartum unit or moved them to rooms on another floor; the mothers would then be discharged with plans only for physical follow-up.

Death is a topic that is poorly dealt with or avoided in U.S. society. Nevertheless, in life's natural order, a person is expected to progress from child to adult and in time to be buried by a member of the younger generation. The parent who experiences a perinatal death has a very different, yet intense experience. As Kirk noted, instead of being able to mourn a child she remembers, the mother of a stillborn infant mourns a person she has not known, cannot recall, and yet may not be able to forget.[8] Parents who have other children are faced with the demands of trying to function in the role they are trying to grieve.[2]

Parents of an infant who dies after birth have had some opportunity for contact with the "real" infant; however, interactions have frequently taken place within the high-risk hospital environment. Although some infants who die may have had a poor prognosis from birth, others may have progressed well, then died after experiencing an unexpected complication. Parents must deal not only with loss of the fantasy child, but also with the termination of hopes for infant recovery.

In addition to feelings of crisis, grief, and loss, the parents may feel cheated because of not being able to have a living child after the pregnancy. According to Furman, after a normal birth the infant may still be perceived by the mother as part of her bodily or mental self.[51] Death during the perinatal period may then represent loss of a part of the self, just as loss of a body part is perceived. This "injury to the self" may be accompanied by intense feelings of failure, helplessness, and loss of self-esteem as a parent. Klaus and Kennell felt that this perception of an infant as still a part of the mother accounted in part for the intense need of mothers to be close to their transported infants, even when the infants were doing well.[18] Anger may be directed toward family members, self, or staff members for not preventing the death. Negative parental reactions may also be intensified when staff are unwilling to address the loss and emotionally "abandon" the client. As Kirk observed, such abandonment could take the form of routine postpartum care without discussion of the infant or the pregnancy.[8]

As discussed earlier, maternal attachment to the fetus takes place in high-risk as well as low-risk pregnancies.[16] The stillborn infant at one time had a very real presence and relationship, especially with the mother.

Nursing strategies for care of parents experiencing a perinatal death require a compassionate, knowledgeable approach. Nurses should realize that grieving parents in crisis may not know about or think of even basic care options. Nursing strategies to assist parents experiencing perinatal loss are discussed in this section. Nursing diagnoses for parents experiencing perinatal loss are provided in the box.

Use Knowledgeable, Consistent Approaches and Unhurried Explanations. Most parents have a great need to learn why their infant died. Often, this may be the first question asked. Staff need to be well informed about the client's individual situation and to have collaborated on a team approach for working with the family. In beginning to resolve grief, parents need to have a trusting relationship with their caregivers. Haphazard, inconsistent responses from health care personnel can add to parental anxiety and distrust. Clients who know in advance that the fetus has died or that their infant is dying should be cared for by the same nurse from admission through delivery, whenever possible.

Staff need to be prepared to answer all questions

NURSING DIAGNOSES RELATED TO PARENTS EXPERIENCING PERINATAL LOSS

Problem-Oriented

Spiritual distress, related to:

- Death of infant
- Problems in grief resolution

Altered thought processes, related to death of infant

Sleep pattern disturbance, related to grief over loss of infant

Potential for social isolation, related to inability to share grief over infant's loss with others

Defensive coping, related to comments from others that deny the infant existed

Strength-Oriented

Asset in grief resolution, related to

- Seeing and holding infant who dies
- Comfort derived from religious and spiritual beliefs

in an honest, direct manner. When no apparent reason for the infant's death can be identified, staff should share this information. Bilingual interpreters should be sought for any clients who do not speak the same language as health care providers.

Information may be presented privately by the physician and reinforced later by the nurse or presented by a small interdisciplinary group. Members of this group might include the physician, nurse, bereavement social worker, and chaplain. Staff need to select a private setting that will allow for expression of personal feelings and to plan ample time for discussion with the parents. Communication strategies such as eye contact and touch are necessary. Staff members may also express their own sadness or empathy with the parents' situation.[52] Klaus and Kennell described intense, persistent anger toward health personnel whom parents perceived as being abrupt or as rushing through explanations to obtain autopsy permission. They also noted that parents felt greatly comforted by the nurses or physicians who expressed sadness or empathy with their situation.[53]

Avoid Comments That Deny the Existence of the Infant. "You can always have another baby." "Things are better off this way." "You already have children." "You didn't have the chance to really know the baby." Such comments deny the existence of the reason for the client's grief and should be avoided.

Thoughtfully Select the Environment for Care. The obstetric environment can present additional stresses for the grieving client. Letting the client decide whether to stay on the postpartum unit and making certain that the client experiencing fetal or neonatal death does not have to room with a postpartum mother who has a healthy neonate can foster the nurse-client relationship and help clients have some control during a difficult time.[54] Alerting all personnel to the client's condition can help minimize pain related to thoughtless remarks, such as "I'm sorry, I thought you had a baby."

Encourage Parents to See and to Handle the Infant. Frequently, parents conjure monstrous images of what they fear their infant was like. After viewing the infant, however, many feel a sense of relief and peace, even if a congenital anomaly was present. Actually seeing and holding the dead infant may help the couple in the grieving process. Parents should be prepared for the sight of the infant. Simple explanations of what they will see (for example, "the baby is very small and she is bluish but otherwise she looks like a baby is expected to look") may be given.[55] Even when severe congenital anomalies exist, parents should make their own decisions as to whether or not they will see the infant.

Arrangements should be made for the parents to view or hold the infant in an unhurried, supportive manner. In addition, the infant may be wrapped, garbed, or arranged in a manner that will soften his or her appearance. Parents may or may not wish to be alone with their infant or may wish to see their infant on more than one occasion. Some parents may want other family members to see the infant. Parents also benefit from knowing that the nurse will be nearby, should they not want to continue to be alone with their infant.

Be Respectful. Nurses need to treat the dead fetus or infant with the same respect that would be shown if he or she were alive. This is especially important when a fetus has died and the mother undergoes labor and delivery. The infant should be presented to the parents in a dignified manner, that is, cleansed, if possible, and wrapped in an infant blanket. Respectful care includes understanding and support for cultural traditions related to grief and death of an infant. For example, some cultural groups, such as Chicanos, may respond demonstratively to death, whereas others, such as certain Native Americans, may express grief in a more quiet manner. Certain Southeast Asian groups may show grief and depression in the form of somatic complaints, because mental illness is regarded as a disgrace.[56] Supportive, culturally sensitive family-centered nursing care, as well as attention to the way in which the dead infant is presented, can comfort parents during a difficult and vulnerable period.

Help Parents to Make Memories. Parents of a stillborn infant will have no memories of the infant alive after birth; however, the need to validate that the infant did live persists. Parents should be encouraged to name the infant and to baptize the infant if appropriate to their religion. Nurses and other health care workers can help to create memories by taking a footprint and handprint of the infant or by providing a lock of the infant's hair, the identification band worn by the infant, or the blanket in which the infant was wrapped.[50, 57]

A photograph of the infant contributes to memories. At times, parents elect not to see the infant, but later regret their decision. A photograph, kept by the perinatal staff until requested by the parents, can be a source of comfort and relief. Parents who have seen and held their infants may later treasure any photograph taken.

Facilitate Burial Arrangements and Other Options. Parents have the right to arrange for a private burial for their infant or to have the hospital dispose of the infant's remains. Representatives from the hospital pastoral care program or from the parents' congregation may be asked to conduct a simple service either on the unit or elsewhere. Nurses should know what the policies and possibilities are in the facilities where they work (whether cremation is routinely used, common burial with other infants, and so on). The perinatal social worker frequently assists parents in making such arrangements. Burial choices also depend upon the client's cultural and religious background.

Anticipatory Guidance for Parenting Siblings

Despite perinatal death, clients who have other children are faced with continuing demands of parenthood.[2] Grieving parents also have to deal with children in crisis. In trying to handle competing tasks of parenting children and relinquishing a parenting role, parents may try to distance themselves from their other children. The children may feel excluded as family members or guilty for in some way having caused parental grief; at times, they may manifest aberrant attention-getting behaviors. Anticipatory guidance can do much to assist grieving parents in dealing with their other children.

Many of the strategies discussed previously for care of siblings of an infant in an NICU apply to siblings of the infant who dies. As noted, interventions need to be based on understanding of the sibling's developmental level, as well as on such factors as family background. Siblings need to be told simply and directly about the death of the infant. Although they may not verbalize their feelings, children are aware of parental anguish; talking with siblings helps the entire family move through the grieving process.

Euphemisms such as "passed away" and "lost" are frequently used for "death." Parents need to take care not to use terms that can confuse or potentially be distressing to children. For example, telling siblings that the infant "went to sleep" or that the "baby was so good that the Lord came for him" will not help a sibling deal effectively with the death, but could contribute to fears about sleep or fears that the Lord will come to take the sibling.[12]

At times parents may feel too upset to answer their children's questions; however, sharing that feeling with the siblings and reassuring them of their willingness to talk together when they are able are important.[47]

Finally, attendance of siblings at the infant's funeral is a decision to be made by each family.

Nursing Strategies for Care of Grandparents

Anticipatory guidance about the grieving process needs to be given to grandparents. The parents' desire to hold a dead infant, arrange for a burial, and retain tangible mementos of a fetus who was not born alive may be considered abnormal and "weird" by their significant others. When families are already financially stressed, any money spent for these reasons may be questioned by family members. Indeed, the old idea that a stillborn is not really an infant may compound parental grief and isolation. Nurses and other health care workers need to assure grandparents and significant others that such behavior related to the stillborn infant is normal and a therapeutic part of the couple's being able to talk about the loss and not "just try to forget about it." Grandparents should be encouraged to express their own feelings. Many have difficulty dealing with their own grief at the loss of the desired infant and with the sight of their own child in emotional pain. Grandparents may benefit from referral to support groups for bereaved families.

Nursing Strategies for Care of Parents Experiencing Death and Survival of Infants of Multiple Gestation

Conflicting and complex feelings of joy and grief are experienced when one or more infants in a multiple gestation survives and one or more infants in the same gestation dies.[58] Contrary to myth, parents do not grieve less or simply forget about the loss of one infant in their happiness to have another living infant. According to Johannsen, parents faced with the death of an infant from a multiple gestation have special concerns[58]:

A more acute sense of loss; having "aching arms" despite an infant or infants to hold

Grief not only for the lost child but also for the loss of prestige and attention associated with a multiple birth

Fears about the health of the surviving infant(s), especially if ill

Inability to grieve adequately for the dead infant, because of concerns and responsibilities for the living infant(s)

Potential problems in attachment to the surviving infant(s); concern that their grief will in some way affect the surviving infant(s)

Worry that the surviving infant(s) will always be a reminder of the dead infant

Feelings of guilt, failure or low self-esteem, related to loss of the infant, for example, the perception that the infant's death represented inability to handle multiple children or had some connection to personal thoughts and preferences

Table 36–4 summarizes nursing strategies for care of parents experiencing death and survival of one or more infants of a multiple gestation.

TABLE 36–4. NURSING STRATEGIES FOR PSYCHOSOCIAL CARE OF PARENTS EXPERIENCING DEATH AND SURVIVAL OF ONE OR MORE INFANTS OF A MULTIPLE GESTATION

Anticipate complex feelings of joy and grief and identify the parents' responses to the loss and survival of the infants.
Ensure that parents are informed about the causes of the infant's death, if known, and about the health status of the surviving infant(s).
Anticipate that the grieving process can extend longer than 6 months beyond the expected year of grief usually felt by parents who lose a singleton infant.
Validate the reality, normality, and importance of the parents' feelings. Provide an atmosphere of privacy and enough time for parents to express conflicting feelings, such as concerns over bonding with the surviving infant and comparing the infant who survived with the infant who died. Provide anticipatory guidance about conflicting responses that may normally be experienced on anniversary dates, such as birthdays and holidays.
Encourage parents to verify which infant lived and which died. Assist parents in their progress through the grieving process, eg, in holding the dead infant and in gathering mementos, although they still have a living infant(s).
Remind parents of the importance of sharing feelings with each other.
Avoid actions and words that negate or minimize the loss of the infant. Educate parents, their significant others, and health care providers about the negative effects of comments that deny the loss of the infant, eg, "you're better off with one" or "you should be happy that you do have a baby."
Encourage parents to seek help with childcare for the surviving infant without feeling guilty.
Encourage parents to speak freely about the dead infant and also to inform the survivor as she or he gets older. Caution the parents about idealizing the dead infant to the survivor in ways that would make the survivor feel inadequate.
Refer parents to support groups and to counseling as appropriate.

Source: *Reference 54.*

Nursing Strategies for Discharge of Bereaved Parents

Discharge from the hospital can be painful after perinatal death. Although the mother physically goes through postpartum changes, she has no infant to bring home with her or she may bring home only the survivor(s) of her multiple gestation. Parents face mourning rather than the celebration usually accompanying homecoming after childbirth. Nurses can facilitate discharge for parents by providing anticipatory guidance and by asking questions that may help parents cope with their feelings. As Estok and Lehman suggest, nurses can help parents deal with potential questions such as, "How will you tell your friends and neighbors that your baby died?" and "How do you think you will feel when you're discharged and must leave with no baby to take home?"[59]

Physical wellness promotes emotional health during grieving. Discharge teaching should include the importance of healthy, healing lifestyle practices such as well-balanced diet, avoidance of substances such as tobacco, alcohol, and mind-altering drugs, daily exercise, and adequate rest, even if the parents are unable to sleep.[60] The couple should be advised to have a physical examination about 4 months after discharge, because of the potential risk for developing illness during intense grief. Keeping a journal, writing to or about the infant, and reading on grief-related topics may provide comfort. Nurses may also advise couples to postpone major life decisions, if possible, as decision processes can be affected by grief. The importance of sharing feelings with significant others and reaching out for help should be emphasized.

Prior to discharge, clients may be referred to bereavement support groups, available in many communities. These support groups are often organized by parents who have had children in an NICU or who have experienced perinatal death. They may meet regularly and offer a parent-to-parent support network, usually without charge. Support groups frequently work closely with NICU staff; group members may also be available to meet individually with parents within the NICU setting.

Follow-Up Nursing Care for Bereaved Parents

Ensuring client follow-up is an essential staff responsibility prior to discharge. Follow-up can take many forms. Telephone calls and home or office visits may take place through social service or through a home nursing service. In traditional settings, staff nurses usually do not provide postdischarge follow-up care. It is, however, appropriate for staff who have cared for the client during her hospitalization to call to express concern for her postdischarge progress. When available, interdisciplinary grief support teams may begin work with the client at the time of diagnosis or delivery and continue contact after discharge and toward resolution. Their goals may include providing ongoing comfort and support, encouraging grief expression, and promoting the mourning process.[57,60,61]

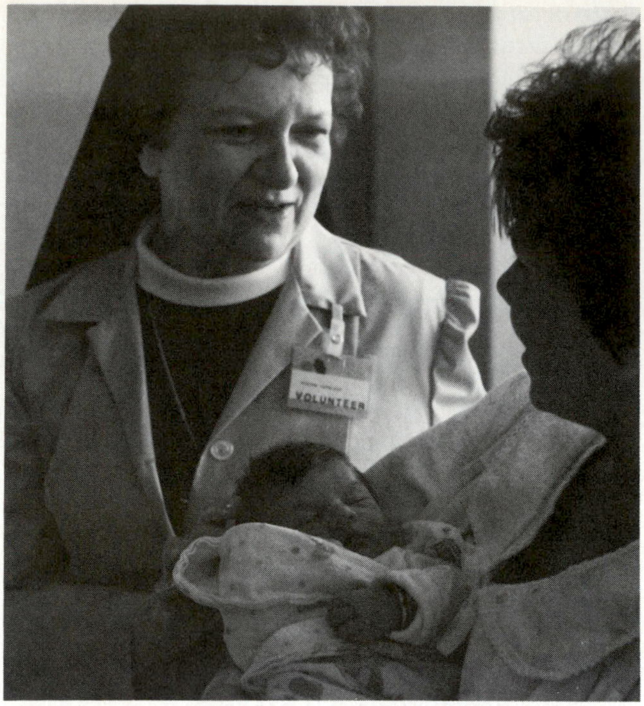

Figure 36–6. A representative from pastoral care meets with a client before her discharge.

SPIRITUAL SUPPORT OF THE HIGH-RISK CHILDBEARING FAMILY

Throughout life, the spiritual dimension of health care can help clients find comfort, strength, and perseverance to cope with crisis. Spiritual support can be especially important to the high-risk childbearing family. Families do not need to consider themselves "religious" to benefit greatly from spiritual assistance during crisis and mourning.

Many hospitals, especially those with religious affiliations, have pastoral care programs through which chaplains or other pastoral care representatives visit hospitalized clients. Local churches and synagogues may also have individuals available on an "on call" basis (Figure 36–6). Frequently, these people are skilled in crisis intervention and in dealing with grief and loss. Although representatives from pastoral care routinely meet with clients from their own religion, they can meet with clients regardless of background. As one mother recalled, "We were crying in the back of the unit when the nurse brought the Catholic chaplain to us during rounds. Although we are Jewish, she talked with us privately for over an hour. She was so caring and calm that she helped us to find the spiritual strength to somehow face what we had to. I'd like nurses to know that sorrow is sorrow, not Jewish, Catholic, Protestant or other sorrow."

Nurses working with the childbearing family need to know about spiritual resources available at their own hospitals and in their own communities. Whenever possible, nurses should meet their representatives and learn about the services offered. Pastoral care should be regarded as an integral part of the care of the high-risk childbearing family.

At times, clients may request the nurse to pray with them. Joining clients in prayer is appropriate, if the nurse is comfortable with this role; however, nurses should not insist that clients pray or attempt to influence clients with their own religious beliefs.

NURSES' RESPONSES TO CARE OF HIGH-RISK FAMILIES AND ETHICAL DILEMMAS

High-risk conditions bring clients into frequent and extended contact with nurses in clinic, office, hospital, and home visit settings. In situations where primary care is practiced, nurses assume ongoing responsibility for client care planning and delivery. Neonatal special care nurses may work with families for prolonged periods. Nurses and other health care providers may form close professional relationships with clients as they strive together to maintain a pregnancy, ensure a healthy birth, and work toward the discharge of an infant.

As noted previously, every nurse working with childbearing families will at some point come into contact with obstetric calamity. Psychologic stress for staff may be expected, because of close involvement with emotionally draining client situations. Dealing with expected or unexpected high-risk conditions makes parent-child nursing sometimes painful and frustrating, yet also immensely challenging and satisfying.[62]

One of the old-time myths is that health care providers should not become emotionally involved with client situations. By the nature of professional nursing and the amount of time devoted to the care of high-risk clients, nurses *are* involved. Client perception of being cared about is important to the establishment of a therapeutic relationship. As summarized by one mother who gave birth to a healthy infant after extended hospitalization, "My sanity was saved, my spirits always aimed upward, because I was secure in the knowledge that the nurses taking care of me *really do care*."

When a high-risk pregnancy is completed with safe delivery of a healthy and wanted infant, staff members share in the joy and satisfaction. Despite the best and most intensive caring efforts, there are times when adverse maternal, fetal, or neonatal outcomes occur. Severe social problems may result in parents' being unwilling or unable to care for their infant. Situations such as a lost pregnancy, stillbirth, or a sick infant who dies after a prolonged intensive care stay are stressful for all staff members who have worked closely with the clients. Further, delivery of care in high-risk situations often generates ethical dilemmas for staff. These difficult conflicting situations produce great stress. A variety of ethical dilemmas are included in Issue and Controversy boxes throughout this and later chapters.

There are times when the magnitude of client hardship does not seem "fair." Staff as well as family members may grieve, experience crisis, and question whether or not they did all that could be done for the client.[62] In addition, staff members may be caught in a variety of ethical dilemmas related to care, for example, do not recussitate orders for a neonate. Over time, "burnout" may occur. Staff may respond by emotionally distancing themselves from coworkers, by manifesting a "short temper," or by initiating conflicts with other staff members, or they may feel depressed. Frequent staff turnover is another manifestation of stress in high-risk client care settings.

Strategies for Dealing With Stress Among Staff Members Caring for High-Risk Clients

One way to promote excellent high-risk client care is to undertake strategies to help staff emotionally prepare for and deal with these situations. Every unit caring for the childbearing family needs to have staff able to attend to the emotional as well as physical needs of clients, even if the clients are to be transferred to another facility. It is no longer considered revolutionary to acknowledge stress reactions among staff members. Experiencing stress related to client care is not "weird" or "crazy," but rather an expected outcome of interactions with other human beings.

Staff planning conferences can explore potential staff reactions and appropriate interventions, should a high-risk condition emerge. In addition, staff planning conferences supply a forum to explore ethical conflicts related to care. These conferences should not be limited to nurses, but should include all personnel working closely with the high-risk client. When a high-risk client has been cared for, unit conferences that focus on staff members' positive and negative feelings about the client and situation can do much to promote feelings of support, sharing, and teamwork among staff. In high-risk units, staff meetings can be a regularly scheduled event, with time allocated to discussion of staff feelings. One-to-one talks among staff members can be informally helpful, as can the assignment of two staff members to give direct care to difficult infants, such as those with fatal anomalies.[62]

Strategies dealing with stressful staff reactions to work with high-risk clients or ethical dilemmas in care delivery include the expertise of mental and spiritual health colleagues and ethics specialists. In some settings, clinical nurse specialists in psychology, psychiatric social workers, psychologists, psychiatrists, or ethicists, are available to meet with unit staff members as a group or individually. These individuals may also be available as paid or volunteer consultants to facilities that do not regularly employ such specialists. Nurses can also rely on representatives from pastoral care for help in dealing with feelings about high-risk clients. As noted earlier, these individuals are skilled in crisis intervention and grief counseling and can be sources of comfort and support to staff regardless of religious affiliation. Some ongoing staff programs are regularly attended by an interdisciplinary group of nurses, physicians, social workers, psychologists, ethicists, and pastoral care representatives.

Adequate staffing, accepting lunch periods and short breaks as emotional necessities rather than luxuries, and avoidance of long work stretches or mandated double shifts are stress relief strategies that are not limited to high-risk situations. Recognition of staff efforts and definition of success in terms of quality care, rather than happy client outcome, are also important. In addition, nurses need to become skilled in recognizing care-related stress and ethical dilemmas among colleagues.

PSYCHOSOCIAL CONCERNS RELATED TO THREE MAJOR HIGH-RISK SITUATIONS

This chapter so far has dealt with psychosocial aspects of caring for clients with high-risk conditions specifically related to childbearing; however, clients can be at risk for many other reasons. Three major high-risk situations—the battered client, the infected client, and the substance-abusing client—are described in this section. An enormous amount of current literature exists on each of these subjects, and the reader is encouraged to pursue in-depth explorations in specialty sources.

The Battered Client

Definition. Battering is the repeated beating of or use of force on a person without regard to personal rights. There are several types of battering[63]: physical (eg, slapping, punching, kicking, use of weapons); sexual (eg, forced sexual relations, frequently after other types of abuse); economic (eg, threatened or actual destruction of property or removal of source of support, threat of deprivation of home or clothing); and psychologic/social (eg, threats to self-esteem, mental cruelty, threats of harm). It has been estimated that 95 percent of battering assaults are committed by men.[63]

Incidence. In the United States, battering occurs in families of all religious, racial, educational, and economic backgrounds. It occurs among political leaders, health care providers, teachers, and the unemployed. Helton noted that some sort of wife battering occurs at least once in two thirds of all marriages; afterward, a pattern increasing in severity can evolve.[63] Although battering is recognized as a far-reaching, widespread health problem, the exact incidence is unknown. The actual incidence of abuse is hard to identify, because it is underreported, is underrecognized, and takes place within the privacy of home and family.[64] Many of the studies that exist have been conducted with women in shelters, crisis centers, and hospitals. Unless battering takes the form of physical violence, it may not be recognized at all by health care professionals.

Battering has been discussed specifically in association with childbearing.[63–65] No clear-cut pattern, however, can be identified. For example, the pattern of battering could exist prior to pregnancy or occur for the first time during the pregnancy. As Hillard observed, battering could increase during pregnancy, with the confirmation of the pregnancy precipitating a violent attack for some women.[64] Conversely, battering could decrease during pregnancy, and may therefore be a reason why a woman would want to become pregnant again. From her study focusing on the extent of physical abuse in pregnancy, Hillard also noted that adolescent mothers still living at home could be abused by their own parents, despite their pregnancy. The topic of abuse during pregnancy thus extends from the possibilities for continued child abuse to abuse by the woman's husband or partner.

Battering Behaviors—A Cyclic Pattern. Battering behaviors are thought to occur in a three-phase pattern often referred to as a "cycle of violence."[63] During the first phase, as tension builds, the batterer may argue, insult, blame, or become angry. During the second phase, the batterer displays violent behaviors such as beating or kicking. This is followed by acts of remorse and kindness, or simply the absence of violence, in the third phase.[63] The phases do not have particular time limits. For example, the violent behavior may be over quickly or go on for hours. Without interventions, the cycle rarely is broken. Over time, the cycle of violence can become increasingly complex, with the woman potentially assuming an ever more submissive role to avoid being victimized.

Characteristics of Batterers. Batterers have been described as being jealous and possessive, having low self-esteem and a need to control, being resentful of the fetus during pregnancy, and tending to behave aggressively or violently outside the home.[65] Abusive behaviors may, however, be confined to the home environment; to "outsiders" some batterers may appear as exemplary citizens who are incapable of violence.

Why Women Stay in a Battering Relationship. Why women remain in a battering relationship is a complex issue. They may fear additional abuse if attempts to leave are thwarted, be concerned over not being able to survive economically, lack a place to go to or supportive people to turn to, lack confidence, feel that they are the cause of the abuse, believe that life circumstances can change, and love the man and the "good" parts of the relationship. Increasing feelings of vulnerability and dependency, characteristic of normal pregnancy, may also make women reluctant to leave any relationship during this period of transition.[64, 65]

Impact of Battering During Pregnancy. Battering during pregnancy can have many interrelated effects. Trauma related to physical abuse can result in life-threatening and pregnancy-threatening injuries to the woman and her fetus, who may subsequently be born prematurely or dead. Referring to a "battered fetus," Morey and coworkers noted trauma as a possible cause of stillbirth.[66] In addition, the stress of abuse has been linked to low birth weight of the newborn, as well as substance abuse in the pregnant woman.[63] Battering has also been described as contributing to alcohol or drug abuse in the pregnant woman.

Research has indicated an association between quality of relationship with partner and quality of relationship with infant. Women who have a history of being abused as children or adults may in turn be at risk for becoming abusing parents.[67] In addition, children of parents in an abusive relationship may be at high risk for development of emotional problems and illness,[63] as well as physical injury directed toward them or inadvertently sustained in the midst of violent episodes between parents.[67]

Nursing Strategies for Identification and Care of the Childbearing Client at Risk for Being Battered. Because of the nature and magnitude of abuse, all pregnant women need to be screened during routine prenatal care.[63] Nurses should be alert to signs of potential abuse such as prenatal depression or anxiety, low self-esteem, substance abuse, alteration in appointment patterns (missing appointments or making extra appointments for vague physical complaints), client reports of abusive behavior, fear of partner or family members, history of previous abuse, and bodily evidence of abuse and patterns of abuse observed at health care visits and prenatal classes. Although fathers should routinely be welcomed at prenatal visits, questions about abuse (eg, "Do you feel that anyone is threatening your health or safety?") should be addressed in private to the woman and never with any family members present. A woman may be ashamed or afraid to admit the problem with family members present, whereas she may confide in the nurse privately. As with any emotionally difficult topic, good communication skills and a nonjudgmental, sensitive approach need to be used by the nurse.

Table 36–5 summarizes nursing interventions for the battered pregnant client. Nurses must realize that battering is a brutal manifestation of disturbed interpersonal relationships. However, it is a problem that can be treated. At times, the greatest "success" comes from the termination of the abusive relationship. Often, counseling and support for both the victim and the batterer can be effective. Abusive patterns do not spontaneously disappear without help. The potential for major, long-term mental and physical difficulties related to abuse necessitate that this problem be a priority for health care professionals working with the childbearing family.

TABLE 36–5. NURSING STRATEGIES FOR CARE OF THE BATTERED PREGNANT CLIENT

Identify clients who are battered. Screen all pregnant clients, regardless of their socioeconomic background.
Provide privacy and ensure confidentiality to encourage battered clients to share their problem.
Teach pregnant clients at risk for battering about the cycle of violence. Reinforce that abused women do not deserve to be victims and they can make choices.
Identify clients whose health or safety is in jeopardy. Arrange emergency placement if appropriate. Provide referrals in the community for counseling and other assistance.
Document evidence of battering, health care teaching, and other interventions in the client's chart. This may be essential if legal proceedings occur.
Collaborate with the media to present public education programs on the widespread problem of battering, alternatives, and sources of help to pregnant women.

Source: *Reference 63.*

Battering is a community health problem; as such, it may be addressed from the perspective of primary prevention (before the problem arises), secondary prevention (screening for battering), and tertiaryprevention (dealing with clients who are the victims of battering). According to Helton and Snodgrass, primary prevention strategies include community education programs on abuse and domestic violence, legislative changes that increase penalties for battering and protection of abuse victims, development of programs for clients at risk of abuse, and the design of research projects focusing on abuse.[65] Helton and Snodgrass included among secondary strategies routine screening of clients for abuse and discussing abuse with clients. Tertiary prevention strategies encompassed the referral of battered women to shelters; conferring with family members, legal groups, and police departments; counseling for victims of abuse and their families; and follow-up care and advocacy for the abused woman in court proceedings. Appendix F lists resources available for battered clients.

The Infected Client—Psychologic Perspectives

Infections occur in individuals throughout the life process. Many are curable. Some have persistent, but minor effects; others, such as herpes in the newborn, can cause devastating acute or chronic problems. Still other infectious disease processes, such as human immunodeficiency virus (HIV) infection, result in incurable deterioration and death. Infected clients can range from being seemingly asymptomatic and feeling fine, to being uncomfortable, to being very ill or dying.

The infected client suffers from more than the physical effects of microorganisms. Family, other clients, and staff may be fearful of the implications of the disease or worried about contracting the disease. Historically, infections are potential occupational hazards; at times staff have contracted diseases, such as hepatitis, from clients. Staff or family members may avoid contact with the client or treat the client in a punitive manner. How the client is treated depends on several factors: such as:

- The client's background
- The type of infection
- How ill the client is
- Whether the client is expected to recover
- Whether the client is expected to require prolonged care in hospital or at home
- How contagious the infection is perceived to be, which may or may not be based on a real understanding of the infection
- Whether the infection is related to socially unacceptable behavior, for example, drug abuse, prostitution, and homosexuality (clients are at risk for being treated as if they "deserved what they got" and for being denied respectful and compassionate care)
- Availability of effective treatment for the infection
- How much of a family burden the illness is perceived to be
- Availability of financial or emotional support resources to help the family deal with the infected client
- Family's or staff's perceived abilities to care for a client and infant with the infection

ISSUES AND CONTROVERSIES

Many issues and controversies are related to care of the high-risk childbearing family. The importance of meeting psychological needs has been accepted; however, just how those needs are met and the nature of staffing required to meet those needs have not yet been established. Additionally, staff are faced with working not only with clients who will eventually have a healthy child, but with clients who face negative obstetric and neonatal outcomes.

Caring for infected clients remains a difficult area. Should clients be routinely screened for infections such as HIV? Should staff and roommates of clients at risk be informed if clients are HIV positive? How can the psychosocial needs of infected clients be adequately met in childbearing settings?

Care of pregnant substance abusers raises special ethical and legal dilemmas. For example, recent charges brought against pregnant women for endangering their fetuses through substance abuse are supposed to deter and punish high-risk behavior and hold pregnant women accountable for their actions. For pregnant women unable or unwilling to control drug use, however, the fear of criminal charges may discourage honesty or attendance at prenatal visits.

Psychosocial Implications of Human Immunodeficiency Virus. In modern times, no disease has had greater impact on health care practices than HIV infection. Human immunodeficiency virus infection has become prevalent enough to be regarded as an epidemic. To date, however, there is minimal evidence of transmission of HIV to health care providers purely as a result of employment or of transmission of HIV infection to family members simply through nonsexual household contact with the HIV-infected client.[68] The few individuals believed to have contracted HIV infection at work all had blood contact with an infected client.[69] To date there have been no occupationally related cases of HIV infection in nurses using recommended barrier precautions. Yet, HIV infection remains an incurable, contagious disease with devastating effects on clients and families. At present it is not known how many people infected with HIV will remain asymptomatic or will develop HIV disease or AIDS, the terminal stage of HIV infection.

An epidemic of fear has evolved along with the widespread daily media coverage of HIV infection. As Durham and Cohen noted, media reports about HIV infection (or AIDS), "combined with the public's perception that AIDS results from 'deviant' behaviors, has fueled a national paranoia."[70] As a result, clients who are HIV positive (ie, have HIV infection) have been treated as outcasts. In certain instances, they have lost jobs, had homes burned, or have been forced to relocate to other communities. Afraid for their own health or for community reprisals, families have been reluctant to adopt or provide foster care for infants at risk for HIV infection. Some of these children have spent the first years of their lives as "boarder" babies within hospitals, regardless of their level of wellness.

Emotional Concerns of Human Immunodeficiency Virus Infection and the Childbearing Client. It has been estimated that 80 percent of the cases of HIV infection in children occur in infants of parents who have or are at risk for the disease.[71] As Boland observed, parents may have been asymptomatic and identified as carriers only after the child was diagnosed as having HIV infection.[71]

Being HIV positive has major implications for the reproductively capable client. The HIV-infected woman is advised to avoid pregnancy, because the fetus would be at risk of contracting HIV in utero from his or her infected parent, although the exact degree of risk remains unclear (it is currently estimated that between 20 and 60 percent of infants born to HIV-positive mothers will become infected). In addition, the mother's own physical health is uncertain. The effects of pregnancy on the progression of HIV infection remain unconfirmed. Adoption of a child by the HIV-positive client is not usually an option, as the potential for development of HIV infection and death makes such clients unlikely candidates, if this information is known. The HIV-positive client who becomes pregnant also may be confronted with a choice between continuing and terminating the pregnancy. Not only does the HIV-positive client have to deal with the probability of never having a child, but she faces the possibility of catastrophic illness and death for herself and her partner. Although the nonpregnant client with AIDS may be too ill to consider childbearing among future plans, the client who is otherwise well may be greatly distressed by this information which affects all aspects of her life, including marital plans. Women who choose to become pregnant regardless of HIV infection may be shunned by lay persons and health professionals alike. The pregnant client with HIV infection may be realistically anxious about her infant's health and future placement. The need to avoid breastfeeding because of possible transmission of HIV is another distressing problem related to this disease.[72]

Concepts of crisis, grief, and loss apply to the client with or at risk for HIV infection. The far-reaching psychosocial implications of HIV infection extend beyond the scope of this chapter. Providing effective support requires a coordinated interdisciplinary team effort focusing on the entire family.

Educational Approach in the Care of Infected Clients. Clients have the right to competent and compassionate care whether they have HIV infection or any other type of health care problem. In addition, they have the right to privacy and confidentiality of all information, other than that required by law as reportable.[73] Programs directed toward health care providers at all levels and toward the general public can do much toward allaying fears about disease and toward presenting realistic ways to protect against disease transmission.

Concern regarding transmission of HIV has resulted in development of infection control policies applicable to all clients (*see* Appendix E). As Jackson and associates noted, the majority of people who may harbor infectious agents can be missed when isolation precautions are used only for those with diagnosed diseases.[74] All blood and body substances, such as urine, feces, and oral secretions, should therefore be regarded as potentially infectious. An infection control policy that emphasizes thorough handwashing, protective barriers to prevent direct contact with body fluids, measures to avoid injury from sharp objects such as needles, and proper disposal of items contaminated with body fluids can be important in reducing the spread of infections and in building staff confidence in working with these high-risk clients. Such an approach may foster high-quality delivery of care to the client with or at risk for infectious disease.

Nursing educators, nursing students, and graduate nurses must become knowledgeable about infection control policies. Hodges and Poteet note the importance of teaching and laboratory practice of skills prior to initial client contact.[75] In this way safe, yet thorough, learning experiences and confidence in client care can be fostered.

Nursing Strategies and Psychosocial Support of the Infected Client. Nursing care strategies used to provide psychosocial support for the infected client depend on who the client is (ie, pregnant woman, newborn, sexual partner of an infected person), the type of infection, the client's state of wellness or illness, the short-term and long-term implications of the infection, and the resources available to support and treat the client. A trusting relationship between health care providers and the family of the infected client is essential, not only for the provision of effective psychosocial support, but also to encourage the client to undertake treatment to cure or control the disease. An ongoing supportive relationship is needed to assist the client in changing social behaviors that may spread disease to others, for example, for individuals who are HIV positive. Several nursing strategies are used to provide psychosocial support for the infected client:

- Assessing the client's and family's level of understanding of the infection, including transmission and how to prevent spread of infection
- Assessing the client's and family's reaction to the infection, including fears about the client, the family's feelings about the client's acquiring the infection, and the current and future implications of the disease process for the client and family
- Teaching the client and family about the infection;

the importance of treatment; the types, possible side effects, and effectiveness of treatment; the sources and costs of treatment; the need for follow-up; the possibility of recurrence, and so on

- Discussing fears related to the infection and dispelling myths
- Assisting the family in planning for continued care of the infected client in the home setting, when necessary
- Teaching the family about the importance of screening other family members for the disease, for example, tine testing family and friends of a client with tuberculosis, and providing referrals so that screening may take place
- Ensuring that the family has continued care and making certain that clients are never denied care because of inability to pay
- Referring the client and family to support groups, counselors, or chaplains who specialize in helping clients and families deal with the effects of infections such as HIV
- Ensuring that confidentiality is maintained and that care is provided in a nonjudgmental manner
- Making certain that staff members are well informed about providing psychosocial support to infected clients and that universal precautions are always practiced
- Participating in public education campaigns that include the importance of compassion and understanding for people afflicted by infectious disease

Substance Abuse, Addiction, and the Pregnant Family

Substance abuse has been defined as compulsive and repetitive use of a chemical substance "despite detrimental social, physical, and psychologic effects."[76] This complex and increasingly widespread problem affects people from all racial, socioeconomic, and cultural backgrounds. Many women of childbearing age are using drugs, particularly cocaine, which has special harmful effects on pregnancy and the newborn.[77–79] Substance abuse during pregnancy presents special problems because of the subtle to severe negative effects on the progress of pregnancy and the development of the fetus and newborn. A person may abuse substances only on occasion, for example, smoking marijuana during a party or consuming too much alcohol on one holiday; however, a person may also be addicted and have a continuing and irresistible urge for a substance such as cocaine or crack[78,80,81] (*see* the box).

The effects of substance abuse on pregnancy and pregnancy outcome depend on the type and amount of substance abused. For instance, all pregnant clients should be advised to avoid alcohol; however, the client who has one glass of wine once during her pregnancy would be unlikely to have an infant affected by the drink. Unfortunately, a pregnant woman who uses cocaine even on one occasion could be at risk for major complications such as abruptio placentae. In a study of pregnant cocaine users, Chasnoff and colleagues found that women who stopped using cocaine during their first trimester did have improved obstetric and neonatal outcome[82]; however,

COCAINE AND CRACK

Cocaine

Cocaine, a white powder, is derived from the leaves of the coca plant, which grows in South America. Cocaine is referred to as "coke," "C", "snow," "The Lady," "toot." Cocaine is classified as a stimulant and gives the user a temporary high with a feeling of great power and energy. Cocaine is available in a variety of forms. Crack is one form of cocaine.

Crack

Crack, an alkaloid form of cocaine, is a combination of baking soda and cocaine. The mixture is heated together to convert cocaine into a chemical "base," as opposed to an acid or a salt.[80] The crack is therefore considered to be in the category of cocaine called "freebase." Crack is sold in several ways—as lumpy little "rocks"; in 3-in. ridged sticks, called "french fries" or "teeth"; and, according to some reports, as pills. The rocks are smoked in a pipe.[78] Crack is inexpensive and therefore available to many people from low socioeconomic groups, however, effects are short-lived. Crack has also been reported to be 10 to 20 times stronger than cocaine and much more addictive.[78] The rapid "high" of crack is followed by a deep, low feeling; the user is left wanting more crack. This need for a continuing drug effect contributes to the use of other substances along with cocaine, for example, alcohol.

Physical Signs and Symptoms

"Cold" symptoms, for example, runny nose, dilated pupils, chest pain, irregular pulse, heart failure (including people under age 30), seizures, strokes related to sudden hypertensive effects of cocaine, weight loss, poor nutritional status.[80, 81]

Psychologic Signs and Symptoms

Personality changes, impaired thinking, confusion, anxiety, depression, low self-esteem, memory loss, changes in financial or social status, feelings of panic, angry outbursts, becoming extremely suspicious of others regardless of relationship, departure from reality.

infants of women who used cocaine only in the first trimester, as well as those of women who used cocaine throughout pregnancy, showed significant impairment in orientation, motor ability, and number of abnormal reflexes, whereas infants of women who were drug free throughout pregnancy did not evidence these problems.

Substance abuse encompasses both legal and illegal materials. For example, alcohol, nicotine, airplane glue, mothballs, and cleaning fluid are commodities that can be purchased legally; all of these products have been known to be excessively ingested or inhaled during pregnancy or used in ways unintended by their manufacturers. Drugs such as diazepam (Valium) are available by prescription, whereas cocaine, marijuana, and heroin are illegal. However, these drugs are readily available "on the street" in most communities, regardless of the socioeconomic status of the residents.

Numerous theoretic models have been developed in attempts to describe why substances are abused. Naegle summarized several categories of theoretic models of substance abuse[76]:

- *Genetic and biologic models* that look for physiologic predispositions to substance abuse
- *Models that consider the abusing pattern,* such as alcoholism, as a disease
- *Psychologic theories,* for example, models in which substance abuse is considered a manifestation of a disturbed personality
- *Family models,* for example, models that consider substance abuse within the context of family interaction patterns
- *Social psychologic models,* which focus on social forces, social learning, role modeling, and the nature of a person's adaptation
- *Interactive models,* which tend to view substance abuse as behavior evolving from the complex interaction between the total individual and the total environment

All theories of substance abuse have limitations in clinical application. Many differ in concepts such as the definition of substance abuse. To date, no one theory adequately explains the complexity of substance abuse or why some family members abuse substances and others do not.

In the past, substance abuse was viewed as the excess consumption of an unhealthy or harmful substance and addiction referred to physical or psychologic dependence on substances such as narcotics and alcohol. Currently, addiction has also been noted to include such behaviors as compulsive eating and bulimia, gambling, and sex. All addictive behaviors affect not only the client, but also the family. When substance abuse or behavioral practices unsafe during pregnancy are used, the client and her family often have to deal with the consequences of addiction, such as spontaneous abortion, prematurity, stillbirth, maternal physical illness, mental and behavioral changes, risk of bloodborne or sexually transmitted diseases, inability to function as a parent, potential death, incarceration, and financial stress. Nurses need to realize that substance abuse is one category of addiction. An enormous body of literature exists on the topics of substance abuse and addiction; in-depth discussion of these subjects is beyond the scope of this book.

Nursing Strategies for Working With the Pregnant Family Involved With Substance Abuse. All pregnant women who are substance abusers are considered high risk, although the degree of risk depends on the type and extent of substance abused. Pregnant women who have a family member(s) who is a substance abuser are also at high risk for the following reasons:

1. Some substances, such as the smoke produced by crack, do affect the pregnant woman who is in the same room with the substance abuser.
2. Women whose sexual partners share needles when intravenously using drugs are at high risk of contracting bloodborne and sexually transmitted diseases, including HIV infection.
3. Such problems as financial burdens, altered interpersonal relationships, and legal difficulties present great psychosocial stress to all family members of substance abusers. As discussed in the chapters dealing with psychosocial adaptation, childbearing women normally need support from significant others, particularly the baby's father. Substance abuse frequently makes this support unlikely and, indeed, may produce turbulence and violence within the family.

Working effectively with pregnant substance abusers and their families is a challenge to nurses and other health care providers because of the complexity of the problem and social attitudes toward substance abusers, especially during childbearing. Dilemmas in practice also arise when women abusing drugs during pregnancy are criminally charged because of the effects of the drugs on the fetus. This may discourage women from returning for prenatal care or speaking honestly with health care providers. Several nursing strategies are available for working with pregnant substance-abusing clients:

- *Employ a patient, understanding, and caring approach.* A supportive, trusting relationship can assist the client in seeking treatment for the abusive patterns and in continuing with her prenatal care.
- *Encourage early and ongoing prenatal care.* For example, research indicates that comprehensive prenatal care may improve the outcome in pregnancies where the expectant mother used cocaine; however, comprehensive care cannot eliminate perinatal mortality if the mother continues to take cocaine.[83] By establishing an ongoing nurturing relationship nurses may provide support needed for clients to try to change behaviors.
- *Take a thorough history during client visits,* identifying the type, amount, route, and frequency of substance(s) taken. Whether substances are taken by the client alone, with others, or by others with whom the client associates provides important information.
- *Test urine for the presence of drugs* when appropriate.
- *When possible, refer to social service and to special counseling programs,* specifically programs focusing on substance abuse during childbearing (*see* Appendix F) and including a family focus.
- *Screen for, treat, and counsel about disease* related to intravenous drug use during pregnancy.
- *Carefully document substance abuse and interventions.*
- *Prepare for foster care of the infant* if the client is unable to control substance abuse and conditions potentially threaten health and safety of the newborn.
- *Institute a mechanism for support of staff* providing care to substance abusers during the childbearing process. Nurses and other health care providers may be expected to experience negative feelings such as anger toward a woman who would knowingly take harmful drugs during pregnancy, frustration at working with clients who continue to abuse drugs, and, at times, a sense of uselessness, particularly if clients ignore teaching at prenatal sessions. The psychologic changes that accompany use of drugs such as cocaine can make clients suspicious of and verbally abusive to staff. Mechanisms for interpersonal support for staff, such as conferences and counseling sessions, help staff members to share problems and feelings, to minimize their own burnout, and to remember that clients can sometimes conquer their addictions.

SUMMARY

Psychosocial concerns during high-risk pregnancy include potential alteration in maternal tasks, threats to self-image, problems related to the impact of prenatal diagnosis, and adapting to the implications of having a pregnancy at high risk. Clients who have previously experienced pregnancy loss or the death of a child may be anxious and have special emotional needs related to their prior loss. Prenatal hospitalization adds to the emotional burden of high-risk pregnancy, despite physical benefits related to physiologic interventions. Childbirth education programs need to be designed for the high-risk client who is hospitalized or at home on bedrest; these clients frequently receive little or no content related to labor, delivery, and early parenting and also miss the social benefits of childbearing classes.

The high-risk intrapartum experience superimposes the challenge of ensuring a safe delivery on the challenge of promoting a family-centered birth experience. Clients may experience crisis related to unexpected high-risk conditions or the outcome of an uncertain pregnancy. Clients who give birth to an infant with an anomaly require a unified, collaborative approach that assists them to maintain their self-esteem, to deal with the loss of their fantasized infant, and to develop a positive relationship with their infant who has special needs.

Every infant admitted to neonatal intensive care has or is at risk for pathology. All families of these infants are at emotional risk. In providing compassionate care, nurses need to be aware of obstacles to parenting within the NICU as well as the financial and emotional costs to the family. Specific strategies can be developed to promote parenting within the NICU and nurses should routinely attempt to facilitate contact between parents and their infant.

Parents of an infant transferred to the NICU from another birthing site have unique problems that include hospitalization of mother and infant in different facilities, division of the family, financial burdens related to visiting at long distances, and receiving care in unfamiliar surroundings. Nurses need to deal with the grief related to the transport; support services to foster family visiting and family integrity should be contacted. Nursing strategies for families of infants in a NICU include the emotional needs of siblings and grandparents.

All nurses in childbearing settings encounter perinatal death. Parents experiencing death and survival of infants of multiple gestation have conflicting feelings related to the surviving infant as well as to the infant lost. Discharge teaching for parents experiencing perinatal loss needs to include anticipatory guidance about ways to cope with personal feelings and interpersonal interactions. Staff responsibility also includes plans for follow-up care.

High-risk families have much need for spiritual support, regardless of whether they previously considered themselves "religious." Nurses can ensure that spiritual dimensions are included in care of the high-risk family and can collaborate with appropriate representatives from pastoral care to meet the needs of these families.

High-risk care can have an emotional impact on staff members and can result in stress and potential burnout among nursing staff caring for the high risk family. In addition, staff may be faced with a variety of ethical dilemmas during delivery of care to high-risk clients. Strategies to deal with stress among staff members should be implemented in every NICU.

Clients are at emotional risk for conditions that occur not only during childbearing. Battering, infection, and substance abuse are three problems that also have profound effects on childbearing. Nurses must not only recognize the physical manifestations of these problems but must help develop interventions that provide support, anticipatory guidance, and emergency assistance when appropriate.

REVIEW QUESTIONS

1. Discuss concepts of crisis, grief and mourning in relation to childbearing families.
2. Discuss nursing strategies to help parents, grandparents and siblings cope with an infant in neonatal intensive care or with perinatal loss.
3. Identify barriers to care of high-risk families during childbearing.
4. Identify ways in which health care providers can deal with stress related to care of high-risk childbearing families or ethical dilemmas.
5. Discuss psychosocial nursing implications related to high-isk conditions such as battering, infection and substance abuse during childbearing.

REFERENCES

1. Johnson SH. Introduction. In: Johnson SH. *Nursing Assessment and Strategies for the Family at Risk: High Risk Parenting.* 2nd ed. Philadelphia: JB Lippincott; 1986:1–11.
2. Rando TA. The particular difficulties of bereaved parents: unique factors and treatment issues. *Newsletter: Forum for Death Education and Counseling.* 1983;6:1–3.
3. Caplan G. Foreward. In: Infante MS, ed. *Crisis Theory: A Framework for Nursing Practice.* Reston, Va: Reston Publishing Co; 1982.
4. Parad H, Caplan G. A framework for studying families in crisis. In: Parad H, ed. *Crisis Intervention: Selected Readings.* New York: Family Services Association of America; 1969.
5. Sherwen LN. The pregnant family: structure and function. In: Sherwen LN, ed. *Psychosocial Dimensions of the Pregnant Family.* New York: Springer Publishing Co; 1987:17–30.
6. Infante MS. Crisis theory and its complementary concepts. In: Infante MS, ed. *Crisis Theory: A Framework for Nursing Practice.* Reston, Va: Reston Publishing Co; 1982:11–45.
7. Baird SF. Crisis intervention strategies. In: Johnson SH, ed. *Nursing Assessment and Strategies for the Family at Risk: High Risk Parenting.* 2nd ed. Philadelphia: JB Lippincott; 1986:361–378.
8. Kirk EP. Psychological effects and management of perinatal loss. *Am J Obstet Gynecol.* 1984;149:46–51.
9. Lindemann E. Symptomatology and management of acute grief. *Am J Psychiatry.* 1944;101:141–148.
10. Kubler-Ross E. *On Death and Dying.* New York: MacMillan; 1969.
11. Wong DL. Bereavement: the empty mother syndrome. *Am J Matern Child Nurs.* 1980;5:385–389.
12. Kushner HS. *When Bad Things Happen to Good People.* New York: Avon Books; 1981.
13. Mitchell CE. The substance abuse parent. In: Johnson SH, ed. *Nursing Assessment and Strategies for the Family at Risk: High Risk Parenting.* 2nd ed. Philadelphia: JB Lippincott; 1986:295–307.
14. Rubin R. *Maternal Identity and the Maternal Experience.* New York: Springer Publishing Co; 1984.
15. Sherwen LN. Maternal role attainment. In: Sherwen LN, ed. *Psychosocial Dimensions of the Pregnant Family.* New York: Springer Publishing Co; 1987:85–108.
16. Kemp VH, Page CK. Maternal prenatal attachment in normal and high risk pregnancies. *J Obstet Gynecol Neonat Nurs.* 1986;16:179–184.
17. Cranley MS. Social support as a factor in the development of parents' attachment to their unborn. In: Raff BS, Carroll P, eds. *Social Support and Families of Vulnerable Infants.* White Plains, NY: March of Dimes Birth Defects Foundation; 1984:vol 20,100–124.
18. Klaus MH, Kennell JH, eds. *Parent-Infant Bonding.* 2nd ed. St. Louis, Mo: CV Mosby; 1982.
19. Lederman R, ed. *Psychosocial Adaptation in Pregnancy: Assessment of Seven Dimensions of Maternal Development.* East Norwalk, Conn: Appleton-Century-Crofts; 1984.
20. Kutzner SK. *Adaptation to Motherhood from Postpartum to Early Childhood.* Ann Arbor: University of Michigan; 1984. Doctoral dissertation.
21. Richardson P. Women's perceptions of change in relationships shared with their husbands during pregnancy. *Matern Child Nurs J.* 1983;12:1–19.
22. Zuskar DM. The psychological impact of prenatal diagnosis of fetal abnormality: strategies for investigation and intervention. *Women Health Rev.* 1987;12:91–103.
23. Carroll RM. Subsequent pregnancy after loss: An exploratory study. Unpublished paper available from author, College of Nursing, Villanova University, Villanova PA; 1990.

24. Jones MB. The high risk pregnancy. In: Johnson SH, ed. *Nursing Assessment and Strategies for the Family at Risk: High Risk Parenting.* 2nd ed. Philadelphia: JB Lippincott; 1986:111–128.
25. Avery P, Olson IM. Expanding the scope of childbirth education to meet the needs of hospitalized, high risk clients. *J Obstet Gynecol Neonat Nurs.* 1987;16:418–420.
26. Koehl L, Wheeler D. Monitoring uterine activity at home. *AJN.* 1988;88:200–203.
27. Lederman R, et al. The postpartum self-evaluation questionnaire: measures of maternal adaptation. In: Lederman R, Raff BS, eds. *Perinatal Parental Behavior: Nursing Research and Implications for Newborn Health.* New York: Alan R. Liss; for the March of Dimes, Birth Defects: Original Article Series 17, 1981:201–223.
28. Lederman R, et al. The relationship of psychological factors in pregnancy to progress in labor. *Nurs Res.* 1979;28:94–97.
29. Kennell JH. Parenting in the intensive care unit. *Birth Fam J.* 1978;5:223–226.
30. Valentin L. Problems of grief and separation in the special care baby unit. *Nurs Times.* 1981;77:1942–1944.
31. Blake A, et al. Parents of babies of very low birth weight: long term follow-up. In: *Ciba Foundation Symposium: Parent-Infant Interaction.* London: Associated Scientific Publishers; 1975:271–280.
32. DuHamel TR, et al. Early parental perceptions and the high risk neonate. *Clin Pediatr.* 1974;13:1052–1056.
33. Johnson SH, Grubbs JP. The premature infant's reflex behaviors: effect on the maternal-child relationship. *J Obstet Gynecol Neonat Nurs.* 1975;4:15–20.
34. Seashore M, et al. The effects of denial on mother-infant interaction on maternal self-confidence. In: Schwartz JL, Schwartz LH, eds. *Vulnerable Infants: A Psychosocial Dilemma.* New York: McGraw-Hill Book Co; 1977:136–149. (Original work published in 1973.)
35. Boukydis Z. Adult perception of infant appearance: a review. *Child Psychiatry Hum Dev.* 1981;11:241–254.
36. Jeffcoate JA, et al. Disturbance in parent-child relationship following preterm delivery. *Dev Med Child Neurol.* 1979;21:344–352.
37. Klaus MH, Kennell, JH. Mothers separated from their newborn infants. In: Schwartz JL, Schwartz LH, eds. *Vulnerable Infants: A Psychosocial Dilemma.* New York: McGraw-Hill Book Co: 1977:113–135. (Original work published in 1970.)
38. Ballard R. Foreward. In: Harrison H, ed. *The Premature Baby Book.* New York: St. Martin's Press; 1983:ix–x.
39. Harrison H, ed. *The Premature Baby Book.* New York: St. Martin's Press; 1983.
40. Brooten D. Issues of research on alternative patterns of care of low birth weight infants. *Image: J Nurs Scholarship.* 1983;15:80–83.
41. Nance S. *Premature Babies: A Handbook for Parents.* New York: Arbor House Press; 1982.
42. Johnson SH. The premature infant. In: Johnson SH, ed. *Nursing Assessment and Strategies for the Family at Risk: High Risk Parenting.* Philadelphia; JB Lippincott; 1986:129–156.
43. Weingarten CT, et al. Married mothers' perceptions of their premature or term infants and the quality of their relationships with their husbands. *J Obstet Gynecol Neonat Nurs.* 1990;19:64–73.
44. Brooten D, et al. Clinical specialist pre- and postdischarge teaching of parents of very low birthweight infants. *J Obstet Gynecol Neonat Nurs.* 1989;18:316–322.
45. Tew M. Do obstetric interventions make birth safer? *Br J Obstet Gynecol.* 1986;93:659–674.
46. Benfield DG, et al. Grief response of parents after referral of the critically ill newborn to a regional center. *N Engl J Med.* 1976;294:975–978.
47. Trause MA, Irvin NA. Care of the sibling. In: Klaus MH, Kennell JH, eds. *Parent-Infant Bonding.* St. Louis, Mo: CV Mosby; 1982:110–129.
48. Wacht MA. The mentally disabled child. In: Johnson SH, ed. *Nursing Assessment and Strategies for the Family at Risk: High Risk Parenting.* 2nd ed. St. Louis, Mo: CV Mosby; 1986:172–183.
49. Troy P, et al. Sibling visiting in the NICU. *Am J Nurs.* 1988; 88:68–70.
50. Bruhn DF, Bruhn P. Stillbirth: a humanistic perspective, *J Reprod Med.* 1984;29:107–112.
51. Furman EP. The death of a newborn: care of the parents. *Birth Fam J.* 1978;5:214–218.
52. Read-Sisti D. A dream dies. *Am J Matern Child Nurs.* 1990; 15:258.
53. Klaus MH, Kennell JH. Caring for the parents of a stillborn or an infant who dies. In: Klaus MH, Kennell JH, eds. *Parent-Infant Bonding.* St. Louis, Mo: CV Mosby: 1982: 259–292.
54. Whitaker CM. Death before birth. *Am J Nurs.* 1986;86: 157–158.
55. Kowalski K, Osborn MR. Helping mothers of stillborn infants to grieve. *Am J Matern Child Nurs.* 1977;2:29–32.
56. Lawson LV. Culturally sensitive support for grieving parents. *Am J Matern Child Nurs.* 1990;15:76–79.
57. Lake M, et al. The role of a grief support team following stillbirth. *Am J Obstet Gynecol.* 1983;146:877–881.
58. Johannsen L. As birth and death coincide. *A J Matern Child Nurs.* 1989;14:89–92.
59. Estok P, Lehman A. Perinatal death: grief support for families. *Birth.* 1983;10:17–25.
60. Nuss S. Nursing care to ease parents' grief. *Am J Matern Child Nurs.* 1989;14:84–89.
61. DesRosiers MB. Taking a baby. *Am J Nurs.* 1988;88:67.
62. Hawkins JW. Did we do all we could? *Am J Nurs.* 1986;86: 158.
63. Helton AS. *Protocol of Care for the Battered Woman.* White Plains, NY: March of Dimes Birth Defects Foundation; 1987.
64. Hillard PJA. Physical abuse in pregnancy. *Obstet Gynecol.* 1985;66:185–190.
65. Helton AS, Snodgrass FG. Battering during pregnancy: intervention strategies. *Birth.* 1987;14:142–147.
66. Morey MS, et al. Profile of a battered fetus. *Lancet.* 1981; 2:1294.
67. Kauffman DK, et al. The abusive parent. In: Johnson SH, ed. *Nursing Assessment and Strategies for the Family at Risk: High Risk Parenting.* 2nd ed. St. Louis, Mo: CV Mosby; 1986:276–294.
68. Lubowitz RE. Infection control measures in institutional settings. In: Durham JD, Cohen FL, eds. *The Person with AIDS.* New York: Springer Publishing Co; 1987:81–94.
69. Clinical News. *Am J Nurs.* 1987;87:903.
70. Durham JD, Cohen FL, eds. Preface. In: *The Person With AIDS.* New York: Springer Publishing Co; 1987;xiii–xiv.
71. Boland MG. The child with AIDS. In: Durham JD, Cohen FL, eds. *The Person With AIDS.* Springer Publishing Co; 1987: 192–210.
72. Becker L, Lagomarsino W. Isolation guidelines for perinatal

patients: creating a new protocol. *Am J Matern Child Nurs.* 1987;12:400–404.
73. *Pennsylvania Medical Society's Policy on AIDS: The Person With AIDS.* Harrisburg: Pennsylvania Medical Society; 1987.
74. Jackson MM, et al. Why not treat all body substances as infectious? *Am J Nurs.* 1987;87:1137–1139.
75. Hodges LC, Poteet GW. The tragedy of AIDS: a new trial for nursing education. *Nurs Health Care.* 1987;565–568.
76. Naegle MA. Theoretical perspectives on the etiology of substance abuse. *Holistic Nurs Pract.* 1988;2:1–13.
77. Lewis, AD, et al. The care of infants menaced by cocaine abuse. *Am J Matern Child Nurs.* 1989;14:324–329.
78. Caring for cocaine's mothers and babies. *NAACOG Newslett.* 1989;16:1, 4–6.
79. Zarkowski L. Cocaine abuse threatens pregnancy & newborns. *NJ Nurse.* 1988;18:9.
80. Office for Substance Abuse Prevention, National Clearinghouse for Alcohol and Drug Information. *Cocaine/Crack: The Big Lie.* Washington, DC: US Department of Health and Human Services; 1988:DHHS publication No. (ADM) 88–1427.
81. Vandegaer F. Cocaine: the deadliest addiction. *Nursing.* 1989;19:72–73.
82. Chasnoff IJ, et al. Temporal patterns of cocaine use in pregnancy. *JAMA.* 1989;261:1741–1744.
83. MacGregor DN, et al. Cocaine abuse during pregnancy: correlation between prenatal care and perinatal outcome. *Obstet Gynecol.* 1989;74:882–888.

Age-Related Concerns in Pregnancy

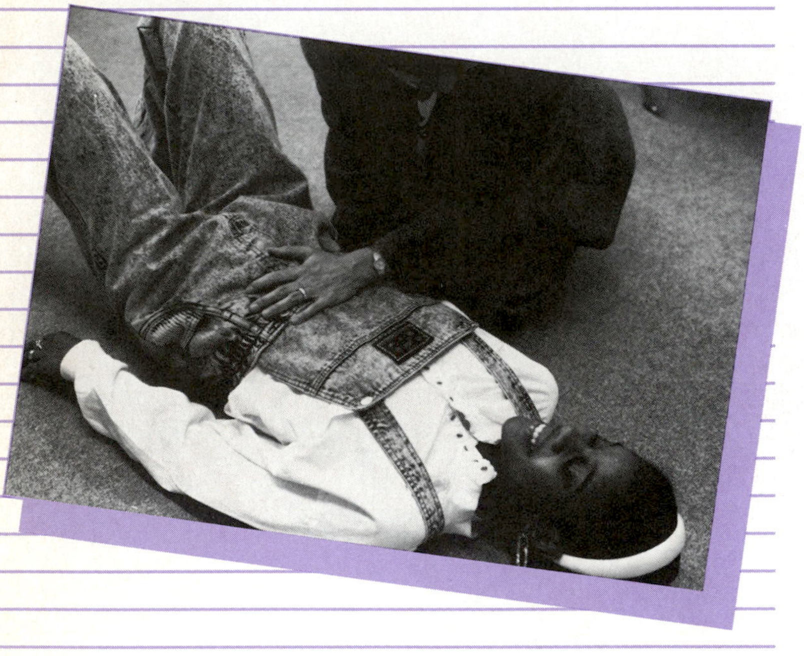

chapter 37

Key Terms

adolescence mature gravida

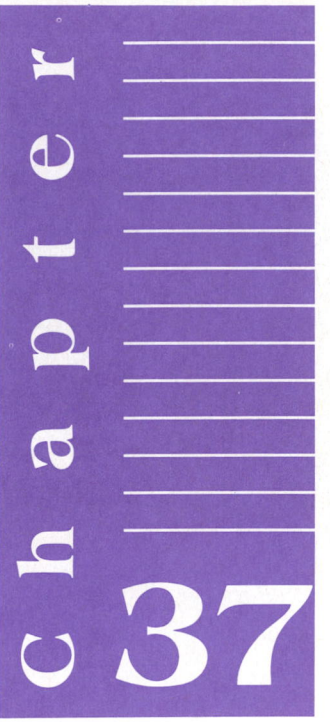

Childbearing and childrearing are events that have traditionally been included in the developmental tasks of young adults. Young women in their twenties were considered to be of "prime" childbearing age, and many of the resources available to expectant and new mothers are geared toward this age group. Societal roles and values are changing, however, and the number of women under 20 and over 30 who are giving birth is increasing each year. These women have unique needs that require alterations in the traditional care that has been provided for pregnant women and new mothers.

Adolescence is a time of struggling to develop a self-identity, and for most adolescents pregnancy is an unplanned, unwanted event that compounds this struggle. The nurse can make a valuable contribution in this situation. The choices that the adolescent makes regarding her pregnancy will have a profound effect on her future. The nurse can assist the pregnant adolescent in making these difficult decisions, and provide support and resources.

For the older woman, pregnancy may be a planned, desired occurrence; however, the older mother may be at increased risk for complications because of pre-existing health care problems or because of unresolved conflicts about incorporating the parenting role into her professional lifestyle.

Providing nursing care for women of diverse age groups can be challenging, yet rewarding. Both of these populations provide the nurse with the opportunity to develop and implement innovative plans of care. Alternate strategies are needed with each population. The nurse must provide education, resources, and support appropriate for each group.

This chapter examines the reasons for the increasing pregnancy rates for these diverse groups and explores the needs and requirements that are unique to the adolescent and older mother. The nurse's role in enhancing the positive aspects of childbearing and childrearing for such nontraditional mothers, and specific strategies for supporting them, are also explored.

ADOLESCENT PREGNANCY

Adolescent pregnancy is a major problem that is receiving increasing attention in the United States. It is estimated that one out of every ten female adolescents will become pregnant before the age of 20.[1]

Many of these adolescents will become high school dropouts and will be forced to seek public assistance to survive.

Comprehensive health care is needed early in pregnancy to decrease the risk to the adolescent mother and her child. The nurse can play an important role in providing this care. When the pregnant adolescent enters the health care system, nursing care should be focused on helping the adolescent to make decisions regarding her pregnancy based on the adolescent's goals and aspirations. To provide comprehensive care for the pregnant adolescent, principles of adolescent growth and development must be understood by the nurse and incorporated into the nursing care plan.

Adolescent Growth and Development

Adolescence spans the growth period between childhood and adulthood. The number of years required for completion of this period is determined individually because each youth progresses through this period at a unique pace. The onset of adolescence, puberty, is a time of rapid physical, psychologic, and social development that leads to maturity. These are years of confusion, years in which the adolescent vacillates between accepting the rights and responsibilities of adulthood and fleeing to the safety and security of childhood.

As hormonal influences become apparent, the adolescent may feel that he or she is locked into a stranger's body that changes daily in appearance and function. Labile emotions result, complicating the youth's struggle with such issues as identity development, value formation, and decision making. The manner in which adolescents confront these issues, along with their genetic potential and life experiences, will determine the complexity of this period for the youth and the family. Adolescence must be completed before the status of adult can be attained.

Developmental Tasks of Adolescence. Adolescence can be subdivided into three stages: early, middle, and late adolescence.[2] Age ranges are assigned to each stage, but these are arbitrary, as each adolescent progresses through these stages at a different rate[2] (Table 37–1).

Early Adolescence. Early adolescence begins with puberty, which usually occurs between 10 and 14 years of age.[2] During this stage, rapid physical growth and development occur (*see* Figures 6–8 and 6–9). Menarche occurs in girls[3] and sperm are found in the ejaculant of boys[4]; both sexes are theoretically capable of reproduction.[3]

Adolescents in this age group are concerned with their changing body images.[2] Preoccupation with questions of their sexual "normalcy" arises, and interest begins in members of the opposite sex.[2] These changes may result in sexual experimentation. Close friendships are usually of the same sex.[5] This age group is "now" rather than future oriented and seeks immediate gratification. As hormonal changes occur, new sexual urges may lead to unprotected sexual intercourse, resulting in unwanted pregnancies. Parents are no longer seen as infallible, and the adolescent may begin to question parents and other authority figures.[6]

Middle Adolescence. The years from 14 to 17 are considered middle adolescence.[2] Physical growth and development are nearly complete and psychosocial concerns move to the forefront. Emancipation from parents becomes central for these adolescents.[2,7] Peer relationships are strong and may temporarily replace

TABLE 37–1. STAGES OF ADOLESCENCE

Stage	Age	Physiologic Changes	Pyschologic Changes
Early adolescence	10–14	Rapid physical growth, menarche in girls, ejaculation in boys	Preoccupied with changing body image Concerned about being normal "Now" orientation Same-sex friendship Parents and authority figures seen as fallible
Middle adolescence	14–17	Slowing of physical growth	Strong peer relationships Emancipation from parents is central focus Friendships include opposite sex Magical thinking is common
Late adolescence	17–19 May last until early twenties	Physical growth is completed	Develops a unified self Involved in intimate relationships outside of family Improved relationships with parents

the role parents previously played in the lives of the adolescent.[4] Friendships broaden to include members of the opposite sex, and may become intense as the adolescent seeks the answers to such questions as "Who am I" and "Am I desirable?" (Figure 37–1). Magical thinking, illustrated by such statements as "All I have to do is carry my lucky penny and nothing can hurt me," is common,[2] and is reflected in the lack of concern over possible consequences of impulsive decisions such as unprotected sexual activity.

Youths in this stage are able to reason and conceptualize thoughts.[8] These abilities result in adolescent egocentrism, which is reflected in an inability to differentiate between one's own thoughts and the thoughts of others.[6] This self-centeredness results in the belief that "everyone is observing the adolescent's appearance and behavior." The adolescent responds by constantly acting and reacting to an "imaginary audience."[6] The imaginary audience has the ability to confirm feelings of unattractiveness or to support feelings of great importance.[9]

Belief in this imaginary audience can affect the adolescent's response to sexual encounters. If "everyone" knows or can observe the actions of the adolescent, visible means of contraception such as cervical devices may be shunned. On the other hand, this belief may explain the necessity of the adolescent male to brag about his sexual conquests.[9]

A complement to the construct of the imaginary audience in the thought processes of the adolescent is the personal fable.[9] Because of their feelings of self-importance, adolescents regard their emotions as being special and unique. No one else can feel such joy or pain! Corresponding to these feelings of uniqueness are feelings of invulnerability and immortality. Adolescents feel that tragedy can happen only to others; it cannot touch them. Thus, the adolescent girl believes that sexual activity without protection carries no risk; only the other girls will get pregnant or contract a venereal disease. Once pregnant, prenatal care is not a priority to the pregnant adolescent; she believes her pregnancy will be uncomplicated and her baby perfect.

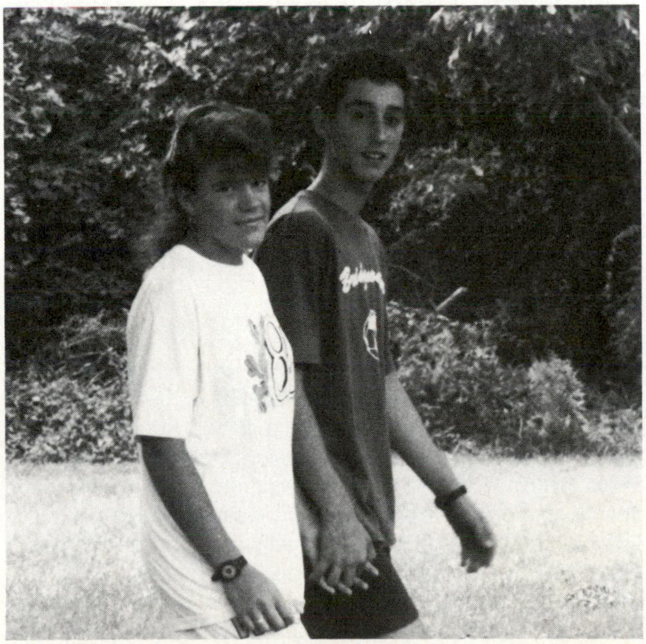

Figure 37–1. The middle adolescent's peer relationships begin to include members of the opposite sex.

Late Adolescence. Late adolescence starts with the completion of physical growth and is finished when the individual develops a unified self-identity.[2] Although often viewed as lasting until age 19, this period of "finding oneself" may extend into the early or middle twenties. The late adolescent has resolved the emancipation crisis and achieved some sense of self-identity.[2] This individual is ready for intimate relationships outside the family,[7] and there is a lessening of tensions between parents and the adolescent. The late adolescent has more realistic answers to the question "Who am I?" and "Where am I going?"

The transition from child to adult does not simply occur with the passage of years. The youth must develop mature ways of evaluating problems and arriving at solutions. Thus, reliance on chronologic age alone is not a valid basis for a plan of care; the nurse must assess individually each adolescent's developmental stage.

Adolescent Sexual Development

Factors Influencing Adolescents to Become Sexually Active. The incorporation of a sexual identity into an emerging personality is one of the greatest challenges facing the adolescent. Table 37–2 outlines several fac-

TABLE 37–2. FACTORS INFLUENCING ADOLESCENTS TO BECOME SEXUALLY ACTIVE

Earlier onset of physical maturity
Influence of media; sexuality portrayed as desirable
Hormonal changes
Desire for reassurance that they are sexually "normal"
Rebellion from family
Peer pressure
Desire to belong to a group

tors that may influence adolescents to become sexually active.

Adolescents today live in a world where sexuality is used to imply maturity and the adult status that adolescents are so eagerly seeking. Sexual overtones are everywhere, and adolescents may be confused by conflicting messages. The media portray the sophisticated adult as one who uses sexual expressions effectively; yet when adolescents attempt to imitate this behavior they are reminded of their young age and told to ignore the signals being sent by their maturing bodies. Sexual feelings become stronger during adolescence,[3] however, and may lead to premature sexual activity as a way to relieve sexual tension.

Statistics show that adolescents are becoming sexually mature at an earlier age. The age of menarche has been decreasing about 4 months each decade for the last century, with the average age being 12.5 years for girls in the United States.[10] Although most adolescent females are anovulatory for the first 2 to 3 years after menstruation starts, this is not an absolute, and many girls do conceive during this period.[11] If teenagers have not been forewarned about the normal physiologic occurrences of puberty, they may experience alarm or even terror when these changes take place. A girl not anticipating menstruation may fear she is dying from a terminal disease; a boy experiencing nocturnal emissions may think he is suffering from an abnormality.

All adolescents, even those prepared for the physiologic changes, have many questions about their sexual "normalcy" and may become preoccupied with these concerns. The onset of sexual activity may be hastened so that the adolescent can confirm that he or she is normal.[6] As the adolescent's sexual feelings become stronger, she or he must develop ways to release sexual tension. Hormonal changes and the resulting sexual urges encourage sexual experimentation.[3] Masturbation, leading to orgasm, remains the primary means of sexual expression for the majority of boys and for many girls during adolescence.[10]

Sexual intercourse may also be used as a method of communicating with members of the opposite sex.[3] Girls who fear that they are unattractive or undesirable may use sexual availability to gain the attention they so desire, providing sexual favors in return for affection.[9]

As the adolescent's need for independence from the family increases, rebellion against the parents and their values and beliefs frequently results.[3] For many adolescents, engaging in a sexual relationship outside of marriage may be one way of demonstrating independence. A girl may flaunt her sexual activities as a way of "getting back" at her parents. A boy may make insinuations about sexual conquests to his father or brothers to establish his manliness.[12]

Often, adolescents are pressured into becoming sexually active by their partners.[3] Peer pressure is also a major influencing factor on the onset of sexual activity.[3,9] Adolescents, especially males, brag about their sexual conquests. An adolescent may not want to carry the stigma of being the only virgin in the group. As inexperienced adolescents listen to the tales of sexual adventures, they have no way of knowing that many stories are invented to impress the listener; thus many become sexually active, not from sexual desire, but from the need to belong to the group.

The increase in sexual activity among adolescents also has been attributed to societal and cultural changes in the United States.[10,13] One of the most significant changes is the increasing number of single-parent families in the country. It is estimated that one out of every two marriages will end in divorce and that, on the average, the children of these relationships will live 6 years with only one parent.[14] Mothers are usually awarded custody of the children, and the majority of divorced mothers are compelled to work outside the home. Adolescents frequently assume duties previously held by adults in the family, thus increasing their feeling of maturity. In addition, many adolescents spend long periods in unsupervised situations, which increases the opportunity for sexual activity. Zelnik[15] reported that 80 percent of the adolescents who engaged in sexual activity stated that a home was the most frequent site of their first sexual encounter. The younger the girl was when sexual activity began, the more likely that the first experience occurred in her home or the home of a relative. With older adolescent girls, the partner's home was the most frequent location.

Contrary to popular belief, most adolescent sex-

ISSUES AND CONTROVERSIES

Many controversial issues relate to the rights of adolescents and to adolescent parenting. Some states have proposed that if an adolescent boy fathers an infant, his parents should be financially liable for that infant. Can parents be held legally responsible for the sexual activities of their teenagers? Similarly, do the parents of a pregnant adolescent have the right to know if she seeks an elective abortion? Should parents have to sign a consent before the adolescent's abortion can be performed?

ual relationships are not casual. In a study by Zelnik,[13] 80 percent of sexually active adolescent girls stated that they were "going steady or dating" their first sexual partners. Nine percent were engaged. Simens and Branzel[3] reported that many sexually involved adolescents have a monogamous relationship that lasts for an extended period.

Socioeconomic status and culture also influence when sexual activity will begin. There has been an upward trend in early sexual activity reflected in all racial, socioeconomic, and ethnic groups.[15–18] Some studies have indicated, however, that black adolescents initiate sexual activity earlier compared with white adolescents. This may be related to the larger number of black families living in poverty and the shortened life cycle of these families (*see* Chapter 3 for additional discussion).

In contrast, other studies indicate that although blacks are 40 percent more likely than whites to be sexually active as adolescents, the percentage of whites becoming sexually active as adolescents is leveling off, whereas the percentage for blacks is decreasing.[15,17] It is difficult to generalize about initiation of premature sexual activity in adolescents, regardless of socioeconomic or cultural background.

Contraceptive Use by Adolescents. Despite the increase in sexual activity among adolescents, only about 30 percent of those who are sexually active use some method of contraception, and those who do often use it sporadically or incorrectly.[15] As, statistically, 90 percent of couples who are sexually active on a regular basis will conceive within 1 year, it is easy to understand the increasing number of adolescent pregnancies. Studies show that, on the average, adolescents do not seek contraceptive information until they have been sexually active for at least 1 year.[19]

Many reasons are cited by adolescents for not using contraception, the two most common being lack of knowledge about the methods available and difficulty in obtaining the supplies.[19,20] For adolescents who are unable to discuss sexual topics such as contraception with parents, the peer group is the source of information. Often this information is misleading at best.[3,21]

Several common fallacies are perpetuated by adolescents:

1. Pregnancy never occurs "the first time"
2. Douching with Coke is a good method of birth control
3. The safest time to have sex is in the middle of the menstrual cycle
4. Jumping up and down after intercourse will make the sperm fall out

Many adolescents state that they would use contraception, but are afraid to visit a physician's office or clinic. They are concerned that their parents will be notified or that the staff will think they are immoral. Others fear the discomfort of a vaginal examination, or do not wish to handle their genitalia to insert a diaphragm or a vaginal suppository. In adolescents unsure about their sexuality, contraception is shunned because the spontaneity of the sex act is lost. For these adolescents, unplanned sex that "just happens" in the heat of passion is acceptable, but planned sexual relations are morally wrong.[3]

Sex Education for Adolescents. Many adolescents are not able to communicate with their parents about sexual topics. Research shows that only about 10 to 15 percent of young adults have ever discussed contraception or sexual intercourse with their parents.[22] The responsibility for discussing information and values about sexuality is frequently left to the schools. Although this is not ideal, research shows that incorporation of sex education into the curriculum may be successful in delaying the onset of sexual activity and reducing the number of pregnancies in adolescents who take these courses.[22] Research results, however, are mixed concerning outcomes of sex education for adolescents. It is generally concluded that creative educational methods and strategies need to be devised to better reach adolescents with an appropriate message concerning sexual behavior.[23]

In addition to the traditional sex education classes, several school districts across the country have opened clinics located on the school grounds. These clinics provide primary health services for the school population, and also provide sexual counseling services.[22,24,25] Some institutions actually dispense contraceptive devices.[22]

The advantages of these clinics are many. Students are able to receive the services they need in familiar surroundings. The services are convenient and confidential. Peers use the clinic so the adolescent feels "safe" seeking information. In addition, because adolescents are the only population served, staff working in the clinic are well-informed about adolescent growth and development.[25]

Alternatives Available to the Pregnant Adolescent

Currently, one out of every ten adolescents in the United States will become pregnant before the age of 20.[1] In 1983, there were 1,039,610 pregnancies in the age group 15 to 19, which resulted in 489,286 births. Legal abortions accounted for 411,330 of these pregnancies; the remainder ended in spontaneous abortions. In the group of adolescents 14 years or younger, 29,690 pregnancies occurred, resulting in 9752 births and 16,350 legal abortions.[26] The United States has the highest adolescent pregnancy rate among the Western nations.[27] Since 1960, the number of out-of-wedlock births to adolescents has risen, with the trend toward a decline in the number of births to older adolescents and an increase in pregnancies to girls under the age of 15. The pregnancy rate has remained constant among minorities, but has increased among white middle-class females.[28]

When an adolescent girl becomes pregnant, she has several alternatives: she can get married, have an abortion, place the infant for adoption, rear the child alone, or allow her parents or other family members to rear the child. Prior to the 1960s, the majority of adolescents either married or placed the infant for adoption after a "hush-hush" pregnancy. The legitimacy of the birth and the reputation of the adolescent and her family were of primary concern.

The 1960s marked the beginning of a sexual and cultural revolution that changed societal norms. Today teen idols such as actresses and rock stars openly discuss the advantages of single parenthood. Adolescents may follow their example, not considering that these famous women have resources far beyond the adolescent's resources that can facilitate raising a child alone.

In the period from 1960 to 1970, the birth rate for single women aged 15 to 19 increased by 76 percent, with a decrease in the number of infants placed for adoption.[29] In a 1976 survey of unmarried women who had delivered a child, 93 percent reported that the infant lived with them. This was a 7 percent increase from 1971.[29] This trend increased during the 1980s, when a variety of pro-life organizations emerged and offered supportive services for single adolescent mothers who wanted to keep their infants.[30]

Many adolescents terminate their pregnancies by abortion. More than 400,000 legal abortions are performed on adolescents each year,[29, 31] accounting for one third of all the legal abortions in the United States.[25, 31] Fifty percent of all pregnant females aged 10 to 14 elect to terminate their pregnancies by legal abortions.[28]

For most young women, abortion is not an easy decision.[32] Adolescents are aware of the conflicting views held by the members of society about the morality of abortion and are influenced by these ideas. An adolescent whose religious beliefs condemn abortion as murder may experience guilt if she elects to terminate her pregnancy. Many adolescents do not know where to seek services or lack a means of transportation to the facilities. Others do not have the money or resources needed for an abortion; still others deny the possibility of pregnancy until abortion is no longer a safe or legal alternative.[32]

Statistically, the mortality rate for women aged 15 to 19 is higher for pregnancy and delivery than for a first-trimester abortion. Tietze[32] reported the maternal mortality rate for adolescents aged 15 to 19 who underwent pregnancy and childbirth to be 11.1/100,000 compared with a mortality rate of 1.2/100,000 for legal abortions. Many adolescents delay the decision to terminate the pregnancy until the second trimester because of denial or ambivalence about the pregnancy.[33] For these adolescents, the morbidity and mortality rates for abortion are increased because of their advanced stage of pregnancy.[34]

Health care providers have been concerned about potential psychiatric problems in the young women who are having abortions. Although some cases have been reported in the literature, the majority of research indicates that adolescents do not experience long-term problems.[25, 35] Close followup and counseling is important for these clients.

Some adolescents choose to marry after the pregnancy is confirmed, although this option is becoming less favored. Two factors appear to influence whether or not a couple elects to marry: age and the cultural expectation.[2] The older a young woman is when she conceives, the more likely she is to marry. Socioeconomic status and culture also influence whether a couple marries or not; whites marry more often than blacks.[2]

The adolescent's search for independence is often stifled by an early marriage, as financial concerns may force the young couple to live with family members.[2] Although this arrangement provides tangible support for the couple, such as room, board, and perhaps infant care, it may prevent the young couple from developing an independent marital relationship. The adolescents may continue to rely on parents or other adults to make their decisions or may be forced to accept outside opinions because of their continuing dependent status. Different cultural groups, however, perceive this arrangement in a more positive manner. In family structures where boundaries are more flexible, a young couple may be easily incorporated into the system.

If the couple decides to set up a separate household, financial difficulties and problems stemming from emotional immaturity are common. Table 37–3 lists the principal effects of early childbearing on adolescents. Adolescent marriages are two to four times more likely to end in divorce than adult marriages.[35]

Some adolescents make the decision to keep their

TABLE 37–3. PRINCIPAL EFFECTS OF EARLY CHILDBEARING ON ADOLESCENTS

Decrease in satisfactory job opportunities
Increase in high school dropouts
Delayed independence from parents
Increased divorce rates
Larger family size
Increased reliance on public assistance

infant by default rather than by choice. Often adolescents do not accept the fact that they are pregnant until the fetus becomes active, and they can no longer deny the physical changes. Other adolescents enter emergency rooms in the acute discomfort of labor, denying the possibility of pregnancy.

Although there is a scarcity of infants available for adoption, placing the infant for adoption is an alternative that fewer young women are selecting. As cultural taboos against out-of-wedlock births have been lifted, more adolescents are choosing to have the child and raise her or him alone or with the help of family members.

If the adolescent does elect to place the infant for adoption, several organizations can be of assistance to her. Each state has an adoption agency as do many church affiliations. Private adoptions are also becoming more common. In this situation an attorney is usually the intermediary betweeen the couple seeking an infant to adopt and the young mother. The couple usually pays the mother's medical expenses and often supplements her living expenses for the last few months of her pregnancy. Although this adoption option is becoming more common, it is important that the laws of each state be known, as some states frown on such agreements and the legality of the adoption could be placed in question.

The adolescent who does elect to place her infant for adoption has made a very difficult decision and requires tremendous support from the health care team and her family members. The adolescent should be encouraged to see and spend time with the infant, if she so desires. Many mothers who place their infants for adoption state that they use this time to say goodbye to their child.[36]

The adolescent may also decide to keep the infant. Electing to keep the infant greatly affects the life options of the adolescent mother. She may be forced to leave school before completing her education. Returning to school or acquiring an equivalency degree is not a simple task. By the mid-twenties, half of adolescents who left high school due to pregnancy had not completed their education. Lack of a high school education severely limits the type of job available to single mothers.[37] Sixty-six percent of all adolescent mothers receive welfare at some point during their lives.[31]

The young mother's relationships with her friends and peers may be affected. Her responsibilities as a parent lessen her ability to participate actively in social functions with others of her age group. Additionally, the adolescent mother's friends may not relate to topics that are now of concern to her, such as which formula is best or whether she should use cloth or disposable diapers.

In some situations the grandmother takes on the mothering role. The adolescent mother, experiencing normal mood fluctuations, may vacillate between being grateful for her mother's help and feeling resentful for her intrusion. This can lead to conflict and confusion in the family. The infant may experience confusion as the mothering roles are divided. In some cultural groups, however, the adolescent mother and her infant are easily incorporated into the extended family system. The grandmother raises the adolescent mother and her child as siblings. (*See* Chapter 3 for further discussion.)

Effects of Early Childbearing on Adolescent Development

The Adolescent Mother. A major developmental task for the nonpregnant adolescent is acceptance of a changing body image.[2–4] Pregnancy compounds this task as the adolescent is experiencing changes that she may perceive as ugly and unattractive. She may feel ashamed or embarrassed about her protruding abdomen and enlarging breasts. If she experiences chloasma, she may wear excessive makeup in an attempt to hide the hormonal changes of pregnancy.

Pregnancy is viewed as a crisis by most adolescents. As physiologic changes reduce the adolescent's feeling of self-control, fear of the unknown may intensify her emotions, and she may act "tough" to mask her terror. The health care professional must provide adequate time to teach the adolescent about the changes that she is experiencing, and answer her questions honestly. Procedures must be explained beforehand, and the nurse should provide comfort and support during uncomfortable or embarrassing examinations. The adolescent must be included in the planning of her care, as her input will enhance compliance. Confrontation, power struggles, and patronization are ineffective communication techniques when working with adolescents.[7]

RESEARCH ABSTRACT

Ruff CC. How well do adolescents mother? Am J Matern Child Nurs. *1987;12:249–253.*

The purpose of this study was to analyze adolescent maternal behavior that would identify maternal-infant dyads who were at risk for maladaptation. The sample was limited to African-American mothers, aged 15–19, who had delivered their first infant. A total of 100 adolescents participated in the study. The educational level of the participants ranged from seventh grade through one year of college, with a mean grade level of 10.45. Almost 79 percent of the deliveries were vaginal; the remainder were cesareans.

Maternal behavior was measured by observing and rating an entire feeding event during the first week after delivery and when the infant was 12 weeks old. The Nursing Child Assessment Feeding Scale (NCAFS), with proven reliability and validity, and a demographic data questionnaire were used to collect data. The NCAFS examined four parental and two infant behaviors. The parent behaviors included sensitivity to cues, social-emotional growth fostering, cognitive growth fostering, and distress. Clarity of cues and responsiveness to parent were the infant behaviors.

In data analysis the Pearson correlation was used to calculate the identity relationship between demographic variables and maternal behavior. A paired *t* test was used to determine the significance of change in maternal behavior over time.

The mothers' scores were related to their age and grade in school. Initially, there were deficiencies in behaviors that fostered the newborns' cognitive, social, and emotional growth; however, these behaviors improved significantly in the first 6 to 12 weeks.

Comment:

This study gives some credence to the widely held belief that the younger adolescent may have some initial problems in relating to a newborn and supports the notion of nursing care focused on education and support. As the investigator used only one ethnic group, the findings of this study cannot be generalized to all adolescent mothers. Future research might compare adolescent mothers from different ethnic groups or adolescent mothers with older mothers to see if maternal-infant behavior patterns differ.

Ideally, the parents of the pregnant adolescent should be included in the plan of care; however, parents of adolescents who become pregnant respond in many ways to this news. Some are very angry and disappointed, feeling that their daughters have failed them. Others are more accepting. Some are hostile and force the adolescent from the home, believing that "she has made her bed and now she can lie in it." Others blame the father of the infant, believing that he took advantage of their daughter, and may forbid their daughter to maintain contact with him. The nurse caring for the pregnant adolescent can provide a support system for the family in turmoil. This is especially important as the decisions that the adolescent makes during her pregnancy will affect the remainder of her life.

Adolescents need to be presented with all the available options in a neutral, nonjudgmental manner, and should be offered help in realistically appraising the situation. Questions to be asked include the following: Does the adolescent want to continue her education? How much does it cost to raise a child? If she found a job, who would babysit? Could she get a job with her present level of education? In making decisions, the adolescent should consider the answers to such questions. Support services should be offered for whatever decision she makes and may include referrals for abortion services, adoption agencies, and social services. In addition, community nursing agencies, parenting education groups, and alternative educational or residential education programs may be suggested.

The amount of education that a young woman receives often will determine her socioeconomic status in the future.[1] Women who have children while they are adolescents are less likely than their peers who delay childbearing to enter the job market.[38] If they are employed, their work is frequently menial, low paying, and unrewarding.[39] In 1976, Title IX of the 1972 Education Amendments was implemented, making it illegal for public schools to expel students because of pregnancy or motherhood.[39] Although schools can set up separate programs for adolescents who are pregnant or who have children, attendance cannot be forced and the quality of education must be comparable to that in a regular classroom.

Adolescents should be encouraged to continue their education, and nurses should provide help for the family who may be too shocked or angry about the pregnancy to recognize this. On the average, women who begin childbearing at 17 years or younger complete only 10.8 years of school: women who are 18 to 19 when they become parents complete, on the average, 11.5 years of school.[39] Mott and Maxwell reported that women who do not attend or plan to attend college are more likely to bear a child in high school or soon after.[39] Pregnancy is the most common reason that adolescents cite for dropping out of school.[35]

Parenthood delays the adolescent's transition to a state of emotional, financial, and social independence. Zuckerman and colleagues[35] found that 88 percent of pregnant adolescents live with their parents during the pregnancy; 77 percent are still living at home when the child's first birthday occurs; 52 percent of adolescent mothers remain with their parents when the child is 3 years old; and 46 percent are not yet independent when their child is 5 years old.

Women who become mothers as adolescents tend to have large families, averaging 3.4 children.[40] The younger a woman is when she gives birth to her first child, the more likely she is to have another child while still an adolescent.[40]

Research has shown that perinatal risk increases when adolescents have subsequent pregnancies.[41,42] The perinatal death rate of the first infant born to an adolescent mother is 6/1000. This increases to 71/1000 with the second child. With the third child born to an adolescent mother, the infant mortality rate rises to 143/1000.[35]

The Adolescent Father. Despite the increase in research on adolescent pregnancy in recent years, few studies have focused on adolescent fathers. Much of the information that is reported is gained from the adolescent mother and is biased at best; however, it has been documented that in the majority of cases adolescent males do not intend for pregnancy to occur.[43]

Boys, on the average, become sexually active earlier than girls.[44] Research reports that 20 to 30 percent of adolescent males aged 15 or younger have had intercourse; by high school graduation, 30 to 50 percent have engaged in coitus; and by the time they are college age, 50 to 60 percent have been sexually active.

The onset of sexual activity by an adolescent male is influenced by his degree of independence from the family and the attitude of the peer group.[44] Males who are more autonomous are less influenced by family beliefs and values, and more likely to be sexually active.

The adolescent female and her partner are usually involved in a meaningful relationship when the pregnancy results. They usually have similar socioeconomic backgrounds, common educational achievement, and are within 3 to 4 years of each other in age.

There is a dearth of information about the long-term involvement of adolescent fathers with their infants. It has been reported that 50 percent of these fathers maintain some degree of contact with the mother and infant during the first and second year of the infant's life.[43] After the second year, the number of fathers involved with the adolescent mother and child substantially decreases. Outside influences often affect the father's involvement with his family. For example, government regulations concerning payment of welfare and Aid to Families with Dependent Children may force the father to live elsewhere. In some states, if a male admits to fathering a child born to a mother less than 16 years of age, he can be charged with rape.

Some young men are following role models when they father illegitimate children.[45] In a study by Robbins and Lynn, it was found that unwed fathers frequently were illegitimate themselves or had an illegitimate sibling or a sibling with an illegitimate child, and that their attitude toward adolescent sexual activity was permissive.[45]

Nurses working with pregnant adolescents should recognize that the degree of a father's participation in the pregnancy is usually determined by the wishes of the mother and by the relationship of the couple. Some fathers may desire to marry the mother; others deny responsibility for the pregnancy; still others do not wish to marry the mother, but want to participate in the pregnancy and rearing of the child. When the couple desires, the father can be encouraged to attend prenatal visits and classes, serve as the labor coach, and assume partial responsibility for childcare. The participation can result in a bonding between the father and his unborn child that may enhance the father's desire to remain a part of his child's life. For the adolescent mother, the father's participation may increase her feelings of self-esteem, resulting in better mothering behaviors.

Societal Costs of Adolescent Pregnancy

A variety of authors cite the high cost of adolescent pregnancy to society at large.[37] Childbearing adolescents are said to have problems which incur costs including additional health care expenses, such as NICU care for low-birth-weight infants; entitlement programs such as WIC, Medicaid, or Aid to Families with Dependent Children; and loss of a potentially productive, contributing member of society. Other studies, however, indicate that adolescent pregnancy alone may not be the culprit. It is hard to separate effects of adolescence, poverty, and lack of prenatal care on pregnancy outcome. All of these risk factors go together.

Risk Factors of Adolescent Pregnancy

Studies before the 1970s reported an increase in the morbidity and mortality of infants born to adolescent mothers. Prematurity and low birth weight were two common outcomes of pregnancies of young mothers.[46] In these reports, however, little attention was paid to contributing factors such as the amount of prenatal care a mother received, the prepregnancy maternal weight, antepartum weight gain, medical complications, and maternal smoking.[47] In many reports, black adolescents who were at increased risk for these factors, particularly nutritional deficiency and substance abuse, accounted for a large proportion of the population studied and affected the results.

More recent research has shown that the increased morbidity and mortality frequently seen in adolescent pregnancies are related more to socioeconomic factors than to the girl's age at conception.[48,49] With these variables controlled, there appears to be no biologic disadvantages unique to the adolescent based on age. When socioeconomic factors are accounted for, the primary cause of the poor outcomes associated with adolescent pregnancy is inadequate prenatal care.[48] The health of the infant has also been shown to relate to these factors rather than just maternal age.[44] Studies show that when adolescents, even those younger than 15, receive comprehensive prenatal care, the morbidity and mortality, for the first pregnancy, are no greater than those of older adolescents or of adult women of similar race, socioeconomic status, and marital status.[48,50]

Recent surveys show that 50 percent of pregnant adolescents receive no prenatal care during the first trimester, and 16 percent receive no care in the second trimester.[51] Without early and adequate antepartum care, adolescent pregnancies pose a greater risk for spontaneous abortion, abruptio placentae, placenta previa, low-birth-weight infants, perinatal mortality, pregnancy-induced hypertension, iron deficiency anemia, stunted bone growth, and prolonged labor.[51] The risk of maternal death is 60 percent higher for pregnant females under 15 years of age than for women in their twenties when prenatal care is not received.[51] Other factors influencing the outcome of adolescent pregnancy are smoking, alcohol and drug use, and sexually transmitted diseases.[51,52]

Many adolescents who have poor prepregnancy nutritional status and inadequate prenatal care do give birth to high-risk infants, with preterm deliveries, sepsis, birth trauma, and fetal morbidity and mortality frequently occurring.[47] Sudden infant death syndrome occurs more often in the second or third child of mothers 20 years of age. The reason for this increased incidence is unknown.[47]

The long-term consequences to children born to adolescent mothers also depend on socioeconomic factors. In situations where the young mother is raising her child alone, an increase in physical and developmental problems is frequently seen. When the mother has family support, either from her parents or a husband, the incidence of these problems decreases.[53] Socioeconomic factors, rather than just the age of the mother, seem to be the variables influencing the long-term outcome of children born to adolescent mothers.[48]

Statistically, the mortality rate for infants born to adolescent mothers varies with the age of the mother.[54,55] The mortality rate for white infants born to mothers younger than 15 is 48/1000 compared with 28/1000 for mothers aged 15 to 19. The rate drops to 22/1000 for mothers aged 20 to 24, but remains higher at all ages for nonwhite infants. The importance of early comprehensive antepartum care cannot be stressed too greatly. Health care for the pregnant adolescent should be provided with a team approach, with nurses, physicians, nutritionists, social workers, and school counselors playing vital roles.

Nursing and Collaborative Assessment

The adolescent may deny that she is pregnant until the physical symptoms are obvious and the reality of the pregnancy unavoidable. Where she turns for help will depend on her relationships with her sexual partner, her family, her peers, her teachers, and her school counselors. The school nurse may be the first person the young girl approaches for help, or she may confide in her boyfriend or her peers. Ideally, her family would provide support. It is uncommon for an adolescent fearing she is pregnant to make the initial contact at a health care facility alone. Her first interaction with health care providers will greatly influence her carrying out the health care plan.[7]

Providing health care for pregnant adolescents requires time, effort, and understanding by the health professional.[7] If an adolescent senses that the nurse is rushed or that she considers the adolescent just another "case," the atmosphere needed to build trust and rapport will not exist. Continuity of staffing also needs to be provided in subsequent visits to maintain this trusting relationship. The nurse must have knowledge and understanding of the normal growth and development of adolescents so that the vacillating emotions and moods of the adolescent will be accepted for what they are, a normal part of the teenage years.

In addition to normal adolescent growth and

development, the nurse needs to be aware of several other facts in order to support the adolescent as she makes her decisions. Psychosocial problems increase with the number of children a young mother bears. Adolescent mothers who have several children are less likely to finish school, develop a vocation, or hold a job than those having only one child.[39] The possibility of having a child born with complications increases with the number of children an adolescent has. The needs of a high-risk neonate may shatter an already fragile relationship between the young mother and father and burden the mother with a lifelong financial debt.

If the adolescent elects to remain pregnant, the nurse should work closely with the physician or nurse-midwife to provide comprehensive antepartum care. A detailed health history should be taken at the first visit and updated subsequently. If the adolescent is accompanied by a parent or other authority figure, more accurate answers may be obtained if the assessment is taken with only the client present. In particular, if the adolescent has been sexually abused by a family member, privacy is essential to obtain an accurate health history.

As many adolescents do not seek health care until pregnancy is advanced, it is important to establish baseline assessments at the first prenatal visit. Urine should be checked at each visit for the presence of glucose, protein, or ketones. The adolescent's weight should be recorded carefully. It may be helpful to note the type of clothing the adolescent is wearing so that questionable weight changes can be accurately assessed.

The anatomic and physiologic changes of pregnancy should be explained in terms that the adolescent can understand. As adolescents are "now" oriented, they will be most responsive to information that they perceive as important to them at that time.

Nursing Diagnoses

Several nursing diagnoses may be developed based on the assessment of the pregnant adolescent (*see* the box).

Nursing and Collaborative Management

A plan of care should be developed by the nurse and the adolescent that ensures appropriate rest, diet, and exercise (*see* the Case Study/Care Plan). Fetal growth and development should be explained, and the risk of smoking, alcohol, and drug use should be correlated with this so that the adolescent understands the rationale for not using these substances. Avoidance

NURSING DIAGNOSES RELATED TO AGE CONCERNS IN PREGNANCY: ADOLESCENT PREGNANCY

Problem-Oriented

Personal identity disturbance, related to premature childbearing and maternal role demands

Altered nutrition: less than body requirements, related to adolescent dietary patterns

Social isolation from peers, related to impending motherhood and feeling different than peers

Strength-Oriented

Progressive individual coping, related to social support during pregnancy

Enhanced self-esteem, related to paternal involvement in pregnancy

of over-the-counter medicines, such as aspirin and cold remedies, should also be stressed.

Information about substance use should be presented in a factual manner without using scare tactics. Nurses providing care for adolescents should be knowledgeable about the signs and symptoms of substance abuse, for example, "track" marks on the arms, ankles, or between the toes or fingers; inappropriate hyperactivity or sleepiness; dilated or constricted pupils. When working with an adolescent with a history of substance abuse, the nurse must remain nonjudgmental to keep the lines of communication open. An accurate drug history will be important to those caring for the infant in the neonatal period.

Educational Preparation. The adolescent's knowledge of labor and delivery should be assessed. Often "horror" stories are passed along by friends and relatives, and the adolescent may have many misconceptions about what labor will be like. These should be dispelled and replaced with accurate information. The pregnant adolescent should be encouraged to take part in childbirth classes. Learning about fetal growth and development, viewing childbirth films, learning relaxation techniques, and becoming aware of the analgesic and anesthetic methods available can reduce fear and anxiety. The adolescent should have a reliable support person willing to serve as the labor coach. This may be a friend, the expectant father, or a parent. In situations where no one is available, the nurse can serve in this capacity.

Parenting classes, which are especially important for adolescent parents, should also begin in the antepartum period.[56] It may be helpful for the pregnant adolescent to meet with other pregnant adolescents to explore her feelings and fantasies about infants and parenting. Many young women have never been exposed to small children, and their perception of parenting is based on television commercials, where the infant never cries, is cute, and is always well behaved. More experienced adolescents can share the realities of infant characteristics and infant care. Information that is obtained from peers is usually considered more reliable by adolescents than information shared by adults. The nurse can serve as a resource person in these groups, dispelling myths and correcting inaccurate information.

Health care professionals should begin to discuss future methods of planning a family with the pregnant adolescent long before the first infant is born. If contraceptive failure resulted in the first pregnancy, the nurse and client should explore the possible reasons for this occurrence. An assessment should be made of the adolescent's future aspirations and goals and her present lifestyle; contraceptive selection should be made on the basis of these factors. By discussing this information before delivery, the adolescent is able to consider her future sexual activity realistically, and to make plans to space her children.

Nutritional Counseling. An integral part of the prenatal care for the pregnant adolescent is ensuring that she receives adequate nutrients for her growth and the growth of the fetus. During adolescence, 50 percent of the adult weight and 15 percent of the adult height are obtained, accounting for the increased nutritional needs of the nonpregnant adolescent.[52] The younger the woman is at the time of conception, the greater her nutritional needs.[54] The prepregnancy weight and nutritional status of the young woman, in addition to her weight gain during pregnancy, are factors that influence whether the infant will be of normal or low birth weight. A thorough nutritional assessment should be completed at the first prenatal visit to determine the adolescent's present eating habits. It is estimated that pregnancy requires an additional 75,000 calories over the 9-month period, with the majority needed during the second and third trimesters.[54]

Many adolescents are concerned with maintaining a thin figure or hiding the evidence of a pregnancy, and restrict their diets accordingly. This can lead to acetonuria, which has been correlated with an increase in fetal and neonatal deaths.[54] Urine and weight gain should be monitored closely at each prenatal visit, and adolescents should understand the rationale for eating a well-balanced diet.

Depending on the pregnant adolescent's age, she will need between 2400 and 2700 calories a day to ensure an adequate growth rate for both herself and the fetus.[52, 54] It is essential that she eat well-balanced meals, increasing her protein intake to 76 to 78 g per day and her calcium to 1200 to 1600 mg per day.

Although a dietary supplement for many nutrients is not necessary if a varied, balanced diet is eaten daily, it may be difficult for the health care provider to be certain that the adolescent's diet contains the essential nutrients. In particular, the additional iron needed during pregnancy cannot be supplied without a supplement.[52, 54] The fetus requires 250 mg of iron, which will be obtained at the mother's expense if her iron stores are low. An increase in maternal red blood cells and the growing placental tissue require another 500 mg, for a total increase of 750 mg of iron for the pregnancy. Because much of the iron ingested in the diet is excreted unused by the body, supplementation of the diet with ferrous sulfate is usually necessary.[52]

Recent research has demonstrated that adequate folacin levels necessary for nucleic acid synthesis and amino acid metabolism are often deficient among pregnant adolescents; supplements of 200 to 400 mg per day are thus recommended. For these reasons prenatal multivitamins are usually prescribed for the pregnant adolescent.

To enhance adherance to the nutritional plan, the adolescent should understand the various nutrients and why they are important. She should be taught to take the supplement with food to minimize gastrointestinal upsets. A nutritionist can help develop a nutritional plan that will meet the needs of the pregnant adolescent. The plan should take into account her food likes and dislikes and her socioeconomic status.

When counseling the adolescent about nutrition, the nurse should teach her ways to increase the nutritional content of preferred foods. For example, pizza with extra cheese provides many needed nutrients. If a glass of milk instead of soda is added to a pizza meal, the teen will receive additional protein, phosphorus, and calcium. Adding lettuce, tomato, and cheese to a hamburger greatly enhances the nutritional value of this "fast food" item. (*See* Chapter 10 for a further discussion of fast food alternatives during pregnancy.)

Cultural beliefs about food must also be considered when planning nursing care. For example, Chicano women may avoid drinking milk during pregnancy to prevent having a large infant and a difficult delivery; black American women may limit "acid" or "strong" foods to prevent having an infant who is difficult to manage.[33] Adherance to the plan of care will be enhanced when the nurse assesses carefully for such food beliefs.

CASE STUDY/CARE PLAN: ADOLESCENT PREGNANCY

Melinda, age 15, arrives at the clinic with amenorrhea of 3 months, breast tenderness, and excessive fatigue. Her boyfriend, age 16, is with her. When talking with the nurse both refuse to make eye contact and instead look at the floor. They occasionally hold hands and glance at each other briefly. Melinda bites on her fingernails and plays with her long hair.

When questioned, Melinda states that she and her boyfriend have been sexually active for 6 months about twice a week. Withdrawal has been the only form of birth control used. She denies any alcohol, tobacco, or drug use, and reports that she has been trying to diet for the last 2 months. She states that she is afraid that she is pregnant and begins to cry. She has not told her parents about her fears. A physical examination shows changes consistent with a 12-week pregnancy, and her pregnancy test is positive.

Supporting Assessment Data	Expected Client/Family Outcome	Nursing Action/ Intervention	Rationale	Criteria for Evaluation
Nursing Diagnosis: Alteration in body image, related to physical changes of advancing pregnancy				
Client slumps when she walks, and wears baggy clothes Client states that she does not want a "big belly" and that she feels ugly	Client will demonstrate acceptance of her changing body image as evidenced by: Verbalizing positively about her changing body Gaining adequate weight each month Standing straight and wearing appropriate clothes.	Encourage client to wear comfortable clothing that makes her feel attractive. Discuss the need for adequate hygiene to keep her hair pretty and her complexion clear. Encourage client to attend peer support groups so that she can share her feelings.	Adolescents believe in the imaginary audience. If they feel unattractive, they are certain that everyone agrees with their assessment. Peer support is very important to adolescents.	Client wears attractive, comfortable clothes. Client's hair and face are clean. Client stands straight and tall, and no longer tries to hide her pregnancy. Client talks positively about her pregnant body. Client gains appropriate weight each month.
Nursing Diagnosis: Potential altered nutrition related to pregnancy and adolescence				
Client is tall (5′8″) and thin (118 lbs.); her hair is long and shiny Client states that she has been dieting so that the pregnancy would not show; she has lost 3 pounds in the last month; she does not like breakfast foods	Client will consume the essential nutrients as evidenced by: Weight gain of approximately 35 pounds No acetone in the urine	Check and record weight at each prenatal visit. Note the type of clothing client is wearing. Check urine at each visit.		Client is gaining weight, and not spilling acetone in the urine.
	Food diary reflecting foods from the basic food groups	Take a diet history at the first prenatal visit, and encourage client to keep a food diary. Explain why she needs the various nutrients, stressing their importance to her health as well as to fetal growth. Help client and her mother plan meals that include the basic food groups and avoid foods that the client dislikes.	Adolescents have specific food likes and dislikes and eat trendy foods. Many of their favorite foods, such as pizza and hamburgers, do contain essential nutrients, and can be supplemented to ensure sufficient intake of the needed nutrients.	Client's food diary reflects a variety of foods from the basic food groups.
	Reports of taking multivitamin suplements each day	Teach client how to take her vitamin and mineral supplements.	Vitamin and mineral supplements can meet nutritional needs during pregnancy.	Client reports that she is taking her multivitamin supplements daily.

(continued)

CASE STUDY/CARE PLAN: Adolescent Pregnancy *(continued)*

Supporting Assessment Data	Expected Client/Family Outcome	Nursing Action/ Intervention	Rationale	Criteria for Evaluation
Nursing Diagnosis: Potential for alteration in family system, related to premature pregnancy				
Client cries when talking about telling her parents that she is pregnant Client states that she is afraid to tell her parents that she is pregnant; her parents do not like her boyfriend	Client's parents will demonstrate acceptance of the pregnancy as evidenced by: Supporting client's decision to remain pregnant Allowing client to remain at home during her pregnancy Providing emotional support Attending prenatal visits	Support client's decision to tell her parents about the pregnancy. Allow client to role-play possible parental responses.	Parents of pregnant adolescents frequently react with anger and express disappointment that the pregnancy occurred. Pregnancy is a crisis situation, regardless of a woman's age, and requires physical and emotional support. If the adolescent is made to feel that her pregnancy is "bad" or "dirty," the attachment process with the infant after birth will be affected.	Client's parents can verbalize their feelings about the pregnancy. Client's mother comes to each prenatal visit with her, offering support. Client's boyfriend is allowed to visit her. Client's parents are helping her make plans for the infant, and her mother has agreed to babysit so that client can return to school. Client's mother attends prenatal visit with her.
		Counsel the parents about the expected changes of pregnancy and the danger signals. Encourage family counseling if the parents are unable to accept the pregnancy.	Role playing allows the client the opportunity to rehearse possible responses to her parent's reactions.	
Nursing Diagnosis: Knowledge deficit, related to physical and psychosocial changes of pregnancy				
Client states she knows very little about pregnancy and childbirth	Client will demonstrate knowledge of pregnancy as evidenced by: Asking appropriate questions Making and keeping prenatal appointments Following the plan of care developed with the health care team Reporting any danger signals to the health care team promptly	Determine client's present knowledge level about pregnancy and childbirth; build on this knowledge base in terms that client can understand, at each visit, by providing information about the physical, social, and psychologic changes of pregnancy, and fetal growth and development. Answer all her questions. Explore danger signals and the appropriate responses to these signals.	Adolescents are self-centered and "now" oriented, and health teaching should focus on the adolescent and current expectations. Explaining why changes are occurring and what to expect next enhances the acceptance of these changes. Talking about the growth and development of the fetus makes the pregnancy more real, and encourages prenatal attachment.	Client makes and keeps clinic appointments. Client verbalizes her concerns and fears. Client can discuss the expected changes of pregnancy, and fetal growth and development. Client keeps prenatal appointments. She also asks questions that reflect understanding of why procedures are being done.
		Explain why vital signs, urine, and weight gains are monitored.	Explaining why procedures are carried out will help client understand the importance of prenatal visits.	
		Encourage client to participate in prenatal and childbirth classes, especially one designed for adolescents, if available.	Attending classes with peers provides client with peer support and gives her the chance to share her fears and concerns with others her age who are also pregnant.	Client attends prenatal and childbirth classes regularly.

Supporting Assessment Data	Expected Client/Family Outcome	Nursing Action/ Intervention	Rationale	Criteria for Evaluation
Nursing Diagnosis: Alteration in adolescent development, related to premature pregnancy				
Age 15 years Amennorrhea 3 months Positive pregnancy test Increased uterine size Client states that she would like to keep her infant	Client will demonstrate acceptance of the pregnancy as evidenced by: Making an informed decision about the continuation of the pregnancy Seeking and participating in comprehensive antepartum care, if she elects to continue the pregnancy	Explore with client her goals and future aspirations. Provide factual information about the alternatives available.	Adolescents seldom have factual information about options like abortion or adoption. They have heard "scare stories," but have no realistic expectations of either alternative.	Client makes an informed decision about continuation of her pregnancy based on her future goals and aspirations. Client is able to discuss the options available to her, and to consider the pros and cons of each.
		Refer client to the appropriate agencies for support of her decision.	Pregnant adolescents need to be referred to a social worker for help with financial and educational concerns, if they elect to continue the pregnancy.	Client reports that she has initiated contact with appropriate referral agencies.

DELAYED PARENTING

Although traditionally women in their twenties have been considered to be of prime childbearing age, changes in societal and cultural values have resulted in a breaking away from traditional patterns. This is reflected in the emerging trend of delaying childbearing until after age 35. These **mature gravidas**[57] may have postponed the decision to have children for a variety of reasons, but all have been aware of the "biologic clock" signaling the end of their reproductive years. Their decision to parent is usually not a hasty one, and their approach to mothering is often more mature than that of their younger counterparts. Each mature gravida brings to motherhood an accumulation of life experiences that often enhances her mothering ability.

Factors Influencing Delayed Parenting

Women give many, diverse reasons for delaying childbearing and childrearing. A major influence has been the increase in job opportunities for women as societal restrictions have been lifted. A young woman's dreams are no longer solely oriented to thoughts of finding a husband and having children. Today, young women are entering diverse fields and professions, many of which were closed to women of previous generations. Many young women enter the work force or the university setting seeking skills for a career, not merely a job. Hard work and advanced degrees offer unlimited possibilities for the young woman of today.

The years from 20 to 30 are often critical in establishing oneself in a profession. The option of taking time out to search for a partner or start a family is often not available to the woman who wants to advance in a career. Once a woman is successful in her field, the decision to alter her status by adding the mothering role may require much thought and introspection.[58]

Late and second marriages also are given as reasons for delaying motherhood. Teenage marriages in the United States have been declining since 1956.[59] As more and more youths elect to attend college, the attraction of early marriages has diminished. When young adults do marry as students, they are often forced to hold down full-time jobs, as well as fulfill their educational responsibilities. This fast-paced lifestyle places stress on budding marriages and divorce is common.[59]

Many young women who marry while in school are forced to drop out to support their partner in his academic pursuit. This may result in feelings of hostility on the part of the women, placing additional strain on the developing relationship.[59] This is one reason many women delay choosing a partner until their education is completed. Starting a family is often then postponed while the couple adjusts to their developing relationship.

As societal bans on divorce have been lifted, the number of second marriages has increased. Most women take some time out after a failed first attempt to determine the qualities that they are seeking in a partner and a relationship. As a result, the average

age of women entering into a second marriage is 30; for a man, it is 35.[60] These couples may need time to establish their identity as a couple and often further delay childbearing for several years.

Improved contraceptive methods have allowed the postponement of childbearing during the "prime" childbearing years; however, some women discover that they have paid a price for this freedom. The prolonged use of oral contraceptives and intrauterine devices has resulted in the inability of some women to become pregnant when they so desire. Help may be needed from an infertility specialist to repair damaged fallopian tubes or regulate disrupted hormonal cycles, adding weeks, months, or even years to the desired age of childbearing.[60–62]

The natural aging process also affects the ability of women over 35 to become pregnant. It has been shown that 86 percent of women in their late teens and early twenties who are sexually active on a regular basis and not using contraceptives will become pregnant within 1 year. This percentage is reduced to 52 percent in women aged 35 to 39, and declines still further after age 40.[63] This reduced rate of pregnancy is related to the normal aging of the reproductive system and an increased incidence of reproductive tract disorders, with pelvic inflammatory disease a major factor.[50]

Advantages of Delayed Parenting

The decision to have a child after the age of 35 is one that is seldom made without thought. Although women describe being aware of the ticking of the biologic clock, the determining factor is usually not based on physiology alone. Most women who decide to become parents consider the options carefully, weighing the pros and cons.

Many women reach this period in their development having accomplished the professional goals that they set while in their early twenties. Although they are successful in their chosen careers, many state that they are left with the feeling that something is missing from their lives. They have a sense of being unfulfilled, and believe that having a child will fill this void.[57] These feelings are quite different from those of the immature adolescent who may be searching for someone to love her. The woman in her thirties is usually mature and independent, with high self-esteem and strong role identification.[64] She has a strong sense of identify and established life goals. Having a child is not seen as a way to obtain security, but as an opportunity to provide security to another.

Unlike the woman giving birth in her twenties, the mature gravida usually is financially stable. Because of her years in the work force, she has a higher salary level, and is a better money manager. If she decides to give up her career to be a full-time mother, she often has savings and investments on which to rely. The income of her partner is also usually sufficient to meet the needs of the growing family.

If the mature gravida desires to combine her career with motherhood, her employer may often be more likely to make concessions to keep a valuable employee. If she has demonstrated her worth to the company, she may receive special benefits as incentives to continue working. These may include more flexible working hours and additional vacation benefits.[58] Because of her financial status, she may also be able to have household help that younger women cannot afford, which eases the strain of combining working and parenting.

The older mother usually has the maturity to sustain complex interpersonal relationships and has demonstrated this skill in her private life as well as in the workplace. She is more realistic about parenting and what to expect from the mothering role.[58] She may also, however, be concerned about performing the maternal role perfectly or in a well organized fashion.

She brings to the mothering role the strengths that she has developed throughout her lifetime and is able to recognize her limitations and to set priorities. Many times, work has been her only responsibility, and she looks forward to adding an additional challenge to her life.[58, 65]

Disadvantages of Delayed Parenting

Society, in the United States, values youth and the activities that go with youth. Individuals spend millions of dollars yearly on health clubs and diet plans to present a youthful facade. Some women elect to become mothers after age 35, believing that having small children will keep them young.[58] In reality childbearing and childrearing are stressful events. Children have unlimited energy sources; most women over 35 do not. Rearing small children at an older age may be emotionally and physically draining.[66]

For the career woman continuing to work, pregnancy may be a difficult period. In these days of "dressing for success," it may be difficult to find maternity fashions that reflect the corporate image. Coworkers may be uncomfortable as the woman's pregnancy becomes obvious. Women cite incidences where they are excluded from business lunches or work-related social events as their pregnancy becomes more pronounced.[58]

It may be difficult for the professional who is

experiencing pregnancy and continuing to work to get adequate rest, exercise, and nutrition. If she is accustomed to working long, uninterrupted hours, perhaps "sending out" for coffee and a sandwich, she may have to alter her schedule to allow times for walking, napping, and eating well-balanced meals. This disruption in the daily schedule may be frowned on by her coworkers.

If the woman's profession requires long hours, she may feel guilty about the time spent away from her child. If she cuts short her working time to be at home, she may find that her coworkers no longer perceive her as being professionally competent.[66] Feelings of stress and guilt may affect her relationships at work as well as at home as she struggles to meet all her responsibilities.

The older mother may also find it difficult to find peer group support throughout childbearing and childrearing. Most women in her age group have completed their families and often have grown children. Her peers have difficulty relating to the mature gravida about such concerns as treatments for morning sickness or finding reliable childcare. These issues are more relevant to the woman of "prime" childbearing age. Yet, the mature gravida often has difficulty relating to the woman in her twenties who is struggling to pay monthly bills or to complete her education while mothering small children.[58, 66]

If the mature gravida chooses to give up her career and devote her time to raising her child, she may experience difficulty adapting to full-time motherhood. Boredom and lack of stimulation are two complaints ofter voiced by these women.[58] Finding private time may also be especially difficult for the older woman who is unaccustomed to children requiring constant attention.

Pregnancy Outcome and the Mature Gravida

Statistics show that the first-birth rate for women over age 35 has increased dramatically since 1970.[67] In 1970 7.3 of 1000 live births were to women 35 years of age or older. By 1979 this number had increased to 12.1 per 1000 live births.[68] In 1983 the National Center for Health Statistics reported that since 1972, the first-birth rate for women aged 30 to 34 had risen 4 percent. For women aged 35 to 39 the rate had risen 8 percent, and for women aged 40 to 44, the rate had risen 33 percent.[67] It is estimated that as the average age of the population shifts in the next two decades, this trend will increase.[67]

Although there are many advantages to delayed childbearing, there are some additional risks that are inherent in the aging process. The woman who elects to delay childbearing needs to be aware of these risk factors.

Recent studies have confirmed that there is a slight but significant decrease in the conception rate for women over age 30. This rate markedly decreases after age 35.[69] Along with the possibility of diminished fertility, there is an increase in certain types of birth defects resulting from chromosomal abnormalities.[68] Down's syndrome is one example. The risk of a woman giving birth to an infant with Down's syndrome at age 30 is 1 in 885 live births. By age 35 the risk is 1 in 365 live births. This number increases to 1 per 109 live births when the mother is age 40, and soars to 1 per 32 live births when the woman is 45.[68]

Other chromosomal defects, such as trisomies 13 and 18, are more common in infants of women of advanced maternal age. Although the number of infants born with defects does increase when the mother is over age 35, the risk is even more pronounced when women give birth after age 40.[70]

Another factor complicating childbearing after age 35 is pre-existing diseases. Studies have shown that diabetes, hypertension, and genital herpes are more prevalent in women over the age of 35.[57] Each of these conditions increases the risk to the mature gravida and her infant.

Although earlier studies correlated advanced maternal age with an increase in premature births and low-birth-weight infants, such variables as smoking, increased parity, low socioeconomic status, and pre-existing conditions most likely confused the outcomes.[70] More recent studies in which these factors were controlled have not supported the previous studies.[70] In previous decades the older woman giving birth was often stunned to find that she was pregnant. The pregnancy was often neither planned nor desired. Maintaining optimal health during the gestational period may not have been a major concern to this woman. Many times, pre-existing conditions were superimposed on the pregnancy, making this a high-risk situation. With the changing characteristics of today's mature gravida new research should be undertaken to determine if the previous findings hold true.

The woman over age 35 giving birth for the first time is twice as likely to deliver by cesarean than is the younger primigravida.[71] The reason for this increase is not understood. Complications of pre-existing conditions such as diabetes and hypertension are seen more commonly in older mothers; however, this does not explain this significant increase. Some authorities question whether the increased cesarean rate is due to the physician's belief that the mature gravida is automatically at risk because of her age regardless of her health status. As the number of healthy women over age 35 giving birth increases, further research needs to be conducted in this area.

Although the research on healthy women giving birth after 35 is not extensive, recent studies tend to show that if the woman is in good health and seeks and follows a comprehensive prenatal program, pregnancy after age 35 does not impose major risks.[72] Diagnostic tools such as ultrasound, amniocentesis, and chorionic villis sampling can be used to reassure the practitioner and the mature gravida that the pregnancy is advancing without complications.

Nursing and Collaborative Assessment

The type of care needed by the woman experiencing a pregnancy after age 35 depends on many assessment variables. Assessment data should include a comprehensive health history, physical examination, and information about socioeconomic status and support systems available to the family.

Previous health problems can be intensified as a result of the pregnancy. For example, a woman who has a pre-existing cardiac condition will require the care of a variety of health care professionals during her pregnancy. The family's socioeconomic status will provide the nurse with information about economic assistance that the family may need, as well as the woman's intention to return to work after the birth of the infant. Support systems play an important role in the family's transition throughout pregnancy. For example, the mature gravida and her partner who have friends or family who are eager to help during the childbearing and childrearing processes should have an easier transition into their parenting roles. On the other hand, if their support system is weak, they may need additional nursing time or a social service referral.

Chorionic villis sampling (CVS) or amniocentesis is usually recommended for the woman over 35 who is pregnant. These tests can provide information about whether the fetus is genetically normal, and offers the client and her partner the opportunity to decide about continuing the pregnancy if defects are present. Couples who do not believe in abortion on ethical or moral grounds may decide against undergoing CVS or amniocentesis or may elect to have these tests. Results can offer reassurance or time to prepare for a special needs infant. In any case, the nurse still can encourage these clients to verbalize any concerns and fears that they may have about the health of their infant.

NURSING DIAGNOSES RELATED TO AGE CONCERNS IN PREGNANCY: MATURE GRAVIDA

Problem-Oriented

Parental role conflict, related to incompatibility between parent and career roles

Anxiety, related to testing for genetic abnormalities

Fear, related to potential cesarean delivery

Strength-Oriented

Potential asset in parenting, related to maturity and planned pregnancy

Nursing Diagnoses

Examples of nursing diagnoses that may be developed for the mature gravida are provided in the box.

Nursing and Collaborative Management

The care of the mature gravida with previous health problems requires a team effort. The care of the mature gravida who has no pre-existing condition can safely be undertaken by the nurse-midwife with medical backup available only as needed. In these instances, professionals from other disciplines, such as social workers or nutritionists, would become involved only if consultation was desired.

Nurses play an important role in the care of the mature gravida and her family, with the need for nursing care often beginning with confirmation that pregnancy has occurred. If the woman and her partner are not expecting this announcement, shock and disbelief may be their initial response. Although the trend to have children at later stages of life is increasing, not all couples in this age group view pregnancy as a wanted occurrence. If the woman (or her partner) is uncertain about continuing the pregnancy, the nurse may provide education about the possible alternatives. The nurse must avoid interjecting personal values into the decision-making process, and should remain nonjudgmental regardless of the decision made. The nursing role should be to help the client and her partner make their own decisions based on an assessment of life desires and expectations rather than emotion.

For the woman and partner who are eager for parenthood, the nurse can provide the information needed by the couple as the woman undergoes the physical and psychologic changes of pregnancy. Research shows that older women who are pregnant will go to great lengths to educate themselves about preg-

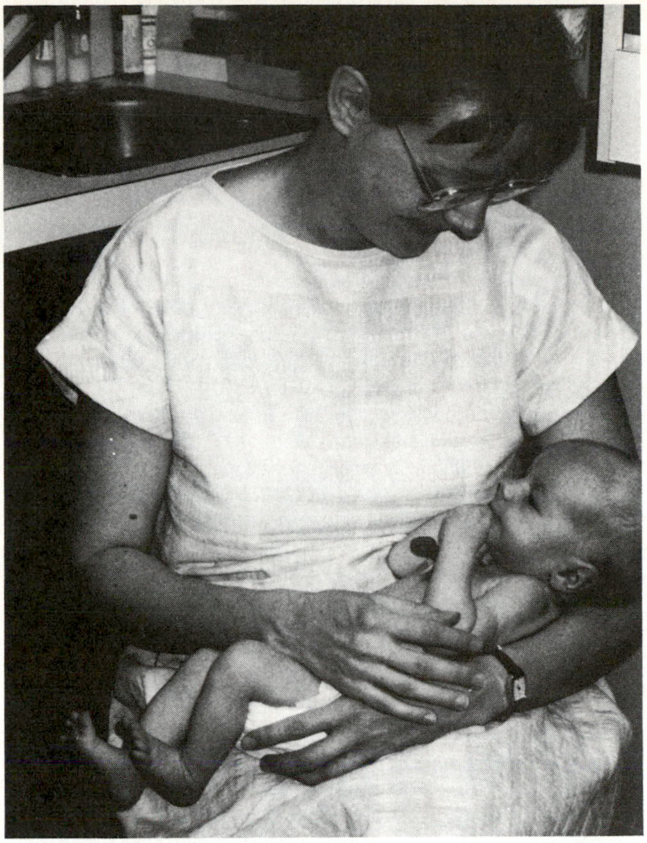

Figure 37–2. A healthy mature mother and newborn.

nancy, childbirth, and parenting.[73] The nurse's role is to facilitate this learning process.

One way in which the nurse can enhance the education of the mature gravida is by arranging special childbirth classes for women and couples of this age group. This allows for interaction among individuals at the same growth and developmental level, and encourages the client and her partner to discuss concerns without feeling that because they are older they should already have the answers to questions.

If the mature gravida elects to have the CVS or amniocentesis, the nurse should serve as a support person. The clinician performing the procedure is responsible for explanations; however, the nurse should assess the client's level of understanding and clarify any misinformation. For staff working with high-risk obstetric clients, these tests are routine procedures. The nurse caring for a client must remember that these procedures are not routine to the client. Each step of the procedure should be explained before it occurs so that the client will know what to expect. Even the abdominal scrub can be a frightening event to a woman unprepared for it. (*See* Chapters 15 and 18 for a detailed discussion of the advantages and risks of CVS and amniocentesis.)

If an amniocentesis has been elected, a period of time is required before the test results are known. During these days or weeks of waiting, the nurse should remain in touch with the expectant woman and her family. A short telephone call to ask how the woman is feeling or to keep her informed that the test results are not yet available can alleviate anxiety and establish rapport. When the results are received, the nurse should make sure that the information is relayed to the client and her partner quickly regardless of the outcome.

If the results of the genetic testing show that the fetus is not developing normally, the nurse can help the woman and partner explore all options available to them. Any decision made will be a difficult one, and the nurse should serve as a resource as the couple explores the alternatives. The nurse must remain neutral as the options are considered.

Although much attention has been given to the risks for older mothers, the majority of pregnancies in clients over age 35 progress without complications and the outcome is a healthy mother and infant (Figure 37–2).

SUMMARY

Traditionally, the twenties have been viewed as the ideal time for childbearing and childrearing. Developmental tasks for the young adult have included selecting a partner and starting a family. Yet societal and cultural values have changed and today women under 20 and over 35 are routinely bearing a first child.

Currently the number of births to women in these age groups is increasing. Each of these populations presents diverse and unique challenges to the nurse providing care for them during their childbearing and childrearing experiences. Their needs, although similar, are also different from those of their counterparts who are considered of "prime" childbearing age. Both the physical and psychosocial components of their pregnancies may be complicated by their age variations.

An adolescent's future will be profoundly affected by the decisions she makes about her pregnancy. The nurse can play a supportive role in helping the pregnant adolescent to evaluate her life goals and make decisions about the pregnancy based on these goals. Socioeconomic and cultural factors, family and peer support, and comprehensive health care play major roles in determining the pregnant adolescent's current and future well-being. The nurse can influence the course of the adolescent's pregnancy by providing education, support, and a guide to resources.

For the mature gravida, pregnancy may be complicated by pre-existing health problems and an aging reproductive system. These may influence the outcome of the pregnancy. Delayed parenting also has several advantages. The mature gravida is usually secure in her self-identity. She is more likely to be financially secure, and may have met her career goals. Having a child is usually a well thought out decision. The mature gravida chooses to have a child to enhance her life, but has other goals and interests as well.

Nurses play an important role in providing comprehensive health care to both adolescents and mature women. Traditional plans of care may have to be altered to meet the needs of the women in these diverse age groups. Providing nursing care that results in a successful childbearing and childrearing experience for these women and their families is most rewarding.

REVIEW QUESTIONS

1. Discuss the long-term effects of premature parenting on the adolescent.
2. Discuss the role of the adolescent father in parenting an infant.
3. Identify the educational needs of the pregnant adolescent.
4. Identify and describe the risks and benefits involved in delayed childbearing.
5. Compare the role of the professional nurse when providing care for the pregnant adolescent and the mature gravida.

REFERENCES

1. *The Problem That Hasn't Gone Away.* New York: Alan Guttmacher Institute; 1981.
2. Sahler OJ. Adolescent mothers: how nurturing is their parenting? In: McAnarney ER, ed. *Premature Adolescent Pregnancy and Parenthood.* New York: Grune & Stratton; 1983: 219–230.
3. Simens S, Branzel RC. *Sexuality: Nursing Assessment and Interventions.* Philadelphia: JB Lippincott; 1982.
4. Lawton JT. *Introduction to Child Development.* Dubuque, Iowa: William C. Brown; 1982.
5. Ripple RE, et al. *Human Development.* Dallas: Houghton Mifflin; 1982.
6. Elkind D. *Children and Adolescents: Interpretive Essays on Jean Piaget.* New York: Oxford University Press; 1974.
7. Handwerker LB, Hodgman CH. Approaches to adolescents by the perinatal staff. In: McAnarney ER, ed. *Premature Adolescent Pregnancy and Parenthood.* New York: Grune & Stratton; 1983:311–328.
8. Maier HW. *Three Theories of Child Development.* New York: Harper & Row; 1969.
9. Kriepe RE. Prevention of adolescent pregnancy. In: McAnarney ER, ed. *Premature Adolescent Pregnancy and Parenthood.* New York: Grune & Stratton; 1983:37–60.
10. Santrock JW. *Adolescence: An Introduction.* Dubuque, Iowa: William C. Brown; 1981.
11. Taylor HC. *Human Reproduction: Physiology, Population, and Family Planning.* Cambridge, Mass: MIT Press; 1976.
12. Lowry L, McGinnis D. Intergenerational education in human sexuality. *Am J Matern Child Nurs.* 1989;14:341–345.
13. Condom use among teens. *NAACOG Newsletter.* 1990;17: 16.
14. Hetherington EM: Divorce: a child's perspective. *Am Psychol.* 1979;34:851–858.
15. Zelnick M. Sexual activity among adolescents: perspectives of a decade. In: McAnarney ER, ed. *Premature Adolescent Pregnancy and Parenthood.* New York: Grune & Stratton; 1983:21–33.
16. Hollingsworth DR, Felice M. Teenage pregnancy: a multiracial, sociological problem. *Am J Obstet Gynecol.* 1986;155: 741–746.
17. Hofferth, Kahn J, Baldwin W. Premarital sexual activity among U.S. teenage women over the past three decades. *Fam Plan Perspect.* 1987;19:46–53.
18. Panzarine S, Gould C. Knowledge about contraceptive use and conception among a group of urban, black adolescent mothers. *J Obstet Gynecol Neonat Nurs.* 1988;17:279–282.
19. Greydanus DE. Alternatives to adolescent pregnancy. Review of the contraceptive literature. In: McAnarney ER, ed. *Premature Adolescent Pregnancy and Parenthood.* New York: Grune & Stratton; 1983:61–101.
20. Adler ES, et al. Educational policies and programs for teenage parents and pregnant teenagers. *Family Relations.* 1985;34:183–187.
21. Meeks LB, Heit P. *Human Sexuality: Making Responsible Decisions.* Philadelphia: WB Saunders; 1982.
22. Schoemaker D. The dissemination of family planning services and contraceptives in public schools. *J Leg Med.* 1987;8:587–611.
23. Murray V, et al. Reducing adolescent pregnancy through school and community-based education. *JAMA.* 1987;257: 3382–3386.
24. Levy SR, et al. Adolescent pregnancy process and educational interventions: a research synthesis and review. *J Roy Soc Health.* 1983;103:99–103.
25. Kirby D. Comprehensive school-based health clinics: a growing movement to improve adolescent health and reduce adolescent pregnancy. *J School Health.* 1986;56(7):289–291.
26. Henshaw SK. *Adolescent Pregnancy and Abortion.* New York: Alan Guttmacher Institute; 1987.
27. Baldwin W. Trends in adolescent contraception, pregnancy, and childbearing. In: McAnarney ER, ed. *Premature Adoles-*

cent Pregnancy and Parenthood. New York: Grune & Stratton; 1983:3–19.
28. Greydanus DE. Abortion in adolescence. In: McAnarney ER, ed. *Premature Adolescent Pregnancy and Parenthood.* New York: Grune & Stratton; 1983:351–371.
29. Kreipe RE, et al. Early adolescent childbearing: a changing morbidity. *J Adolescent Health Care.* 1981;2:127–131.
30. Smith D, Sherwen LN. *Mothers and Their Adopted Children: The Bonding Process.* 2nd ed. New York: Tiresias; 1988.
31. *Teenage Pregnancy Issues: Hearings on Teenage Pregnancy Before the Subcommittee on Public Assistance and Unemployment Compensation.* 99th Cong, 1st Sess (1985).
32. Tietze C. New estimates of morbidity associated with fertility control. *Fam Plan Perspect.* 1977;9:74–76.
33. Auvenshine MA, Enriquez MG. *Maternity Nursing: Dimensions of Change.* Monterey, Calif: Wadsworth Health Sciences Division; 1985.
34. Nadelson C. Abortion counseling: focus on adolescent counseling. *Pediatrics.* 1974;54:765–769.
35. Zuckerman BS, et al. Adolescent pregnancy: biobehavioral determinents of outcomes. *J Pediatr.* 1984;105:857–863.
36. Ritchie CW. Adoption: an option often overlooked. *Am J Nurs.* 1989;89:1156–1158.
37. Blum R. Contemporary threat to adolescent health in the United States. *JAMA.* 1987;24:3390–3401.
38. McCarthy J, Radish ES. Education and childbearing among teenagers. *Fam Plan Perspect.* 1982;14:154–155.
39. Mott FL, Maxwell NL. Schoolage mothers 1969–1979. *Fam Plan Perspect.* 1981;13:278–281.
40. McAnarney ER, Theide HA. Adolescent pregnancy: what have we learned during the 1970's and what remains to be learned. In: McAnarney ER, ed. *Premature Adolescent Pregnancy and Parenthood.* New York: Grune & Stratton; 1983: 375–395.
41. Horton BK, Strobino DM, MacDonald HM. Adolescence and pregnancy outcome. *Am J Obstet.* 1983;146:444–449.
42. Hollingsworth DR, et al. Impact of gynecological age on outcome of adolescent pregnancy. In: McAnarney ER, ed. *Premature Adolescent Pregnancy and Parenthood.* New York: Grune & Stratton; 1983:169–190.
43. Earls F, Siegel B. Precocious fathers. *J Orthopsychiatry.* 1980;50:469–480.
44. Elster AB, Panzarine S. Adolescent fathers. In: McAnarney ER, ed. *Premature Adolescent Pregnancy and Parenthood.* New York: Grune & Stratton; 1983:231–252.
45. Robbins MMB, Lynn DB. The unwed father: generation recidivism and attitudes about intercourse in California Youth Authority wards. *J Sex Res.* 1973;9:334–341.
46. Makinson C. The health consequences of teenage fertility. *Fam Plan Perspect.* 1985;17:137–139.
47. Lawrence RA, Merritt TA. Infants of adolescent mothers: perinatal, neonatal, and infancy outcomes. In: McAnarney ER, ed. *Premature Adolescent Pregnancy and Parenthood.* New York: Grune & Stratton; 1983:149–168.
48. Makinson C. The health consequences of teenage fertility. *Fam Plan Perspect.* 1985;17:132–139.
49. Carey WB, et al. Adolescent age and obstetric risk. In: McAnarney ER, ed. *Premature Adolescent Pregnancy and Parenthood.* New York: Grune & Stratton; 1983:109–118.
50. Shapiro S, et al. Relevance of correlation of infant morbidity for significant morbidity at one year of age. *Am J Obstet Gynecol.* 1980;136:363–373.
51. Miller KA, Field CS. Adolescent pregnancy: a combined obstetrics and pediatric study. *Family Planning Perspectives.* 1984;16:52–62.
52. Jacobson MS, Heald, FP: Nutritional risks of adolescent pregnancies and their management. In: McAnarney ER, ed. *Premature Adolescent Pregnancy and Parenthood.* New York: Grune & Stratton; 1983:119–135.
53. Baldwin W, Cain VS. The children of teenage parents. *Fam Plan Perspect.* 1980;12:34–43.
54. Bailey LB, et al. Folacin and iron stores in low income pregnant adolescents and mature women. *J Clin Nutr.* 1980;38: 1997–2001.
55. Spiro PS, Wang L. Short pregnancy intervals, low birth weight, and sudden infant death. *Am J Epidemiol.* 1975; 104:15–21.
56. Degenhart-Leskosky S. Health education needs of adolescent and nonadolescent mothers. *J Obstet Gynecol Neon Nurs.* 1989;18:238–243.
57. Price J. *You're Not Too Old to Have a Baby.* New York: Farrar, Straus, & Giroux; 1977.
58. Duvall EM. *Marriage and Family Development.* New York: Harper & Row; 1977.
59. Speroff L, et al. *Clinical Gynecologic and Endocrinology and Infertility.* Baltimore: Williams & Wilkins; 1981.
60. Blankstein J, et al. *Ovulation Induction and in Vitro Fertilization.* Chicago: Year Book Medical Publishing; 1986.
61. Menken J, Larsen U. Fertility rates and aging. In: Mastroianni L Jr, Paulsen CA, eds. *Aging, Reproduction and the Climacteric.* New York: Plenum Press; 1986.
62. DeVore NE. Parenthood postponed. *Am J Nurs.* 1983;83: 1160–1163.
63. Robinson GE, et al. Psychological adaptation to pregnancy in childless women more than 35 years old. *Am J Obstet Gynecol.* 1987;156:328–333.
64. Rubin SP. *It's Not Too Late to Have a Baby.* Englewood Cliffs, NJ: Prentice Hall; 1980.
65. Fabe M, Wikler N. *Up Against the Clock.* New York: Random House; 1979.
66. Resnik R. Age related outcomes in gestation and pregnancy. In: Mastroianni L Jr, Paulsen CA, eds. *Aging, Reproduction, and the Climacteric.* New York: Plenum Press; 1986.
67. Federation CECOS, et al. Female fecundity as a function of age. *N Engl J Med.* 1982;306:404–406.
68. National Center for Health Statistics. *Monthly Vital Statistics Report.* 32 (9), Supp. Dec. 229, 1983; 1982.
69. Hansen JP. Older maternal age and pregnancy outcome: a review of the literature. *Obstet Gynecol Surv.* 1986;41:726–742.
70. Stein A. Pregnancy in gravidas over age 35 years. *J Nurse Midwifery.* 1983;280:17–20.
71. Martel M, et al. Maternal age and primary cesarean section rates: a multivariate analysis. *Am J Obstet Gynecol.* 1987; 156:305–308.
72. Buehler JW, et al. Maternal mortality in women ages 35 years or older: United States. *Obstet Gynecol Surv.* 1986; 41:349–351.
73. Winslow W. First pregnancy after 35: what is the experience? *Am J Matern Child Nurs.* 1987;12:92–96.

Maternal Conditions in the First Trimester

chapter 38

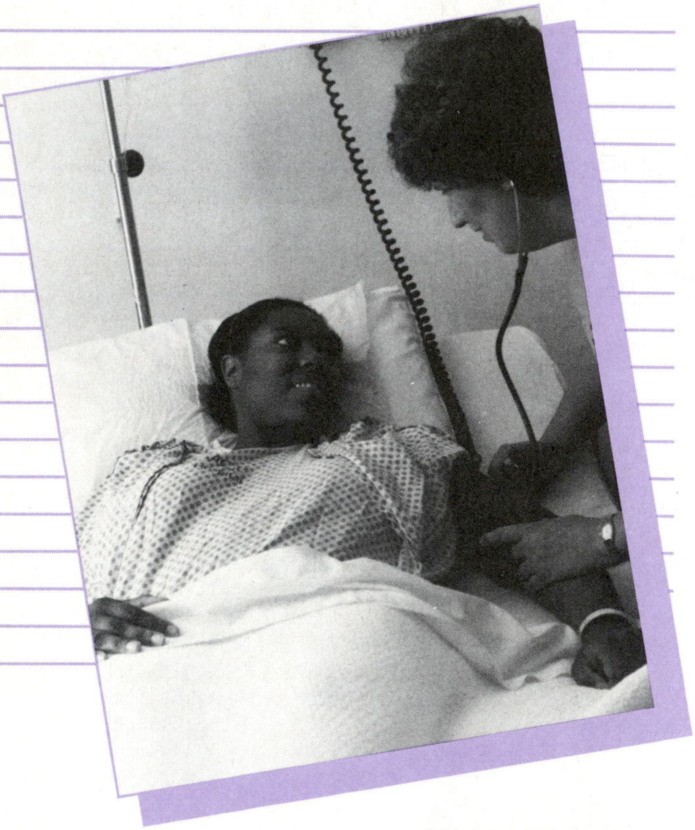

Key Terms

abortion
anemia
complete abortion
culdocentesis
ectopic pregnancy
habitual abortion
hemoglobin C disease
hemoglobinopathies
hyperemesis gravidarum
incompetent cervix
incomplete abortion
induced abortion
inevitable abortion
missed abortion
sickle cell anemia
spontaneous abortion
thalassemia
threatened abortion

During the first trimester of pregnancy, a woman's body undergoes many physiologic changes as the embryo grows and develops into a fetus. At the same time psychologic changes are occurring as the reality of approaching motherhood is validated.

Complications occurring in the first trimester of pregnancy are often approached differently from complications ensuing in subsequent trimesters. Many women may not realize that they are pregnant when help is sought for a health care need. As a result they often do not present themselves in a maternity or obstetric setting and may be quite amazed to learn of the diagnosis of pregnancy.

If problems are so severe that viability of the embryo or first trimester fetus is questioned, very little can usually be done. Perinatal medicine has not advanced to the point where treatment in such situations is definitive. A waiting and watching approach may develop. Sometimes, symptoms may be so severe that the mother's life is endangered and the pregnancy termination is elected. When medical conditions exist prior to the pregnancy, the mother's symptoms often become increasingly critical as the pregnancy progresses. For these clients, however, the first trimester often is relatively free of problems compared with later trimesters.

For these reasons it is somewhat difficult to characterize specific conditions as complications that occur during the first trimester of pregnancy. Many conditions that occur in the first trimester continue into the second and third trimesters. Two categories of conditions that occur during the first trimester are discussed in this chapter: hemorrhagic conditions, specifically spontaneous abortion and ectopic pregnancy; and metabolic conditions, including hyperemesis gravidarum, anemia, and thyroid disorders.

The nurse can play an important role in assisting the client and her family to deal with such complications in a positive manner. The nurse's ability to make clinical judgments is crucial, as care derived from such judgments may be lifesaving. Assessment skills are important in providing data on the nature and extent of the problem, so that appropriate care can be planned, implemented, and evaluated for effectiveness. Both physical and emotional supportive measures are needed to assist the pregnant woman and her family in understanding and coping with the high-risk condition that may be occurring during the first trimester.

HEMORRHAGIC CONDITIONS

Vaginal bleeding during pregnancy, except for very light spotting, is a serious complication that demands immediate attention. The two major causes of bleeding in early pregnancy are spontaneous abortion and ectopic pregnancy. These complications are more serious than many problems experienced early in pregnancy.

Spontaneous Abortion

Abortion is the termination of a pregnancy before the fetus is viable. A fetus of less than 20 weeks' gestation or weighing less than 500 g is considered an abortus, even though the exact age when a fetus is sufficiently developed to survive is very difficult to determine.

The term *abortion* may be used by health care personnel to describe either a spontaneous or an induced event. A **spontaneous abortion** is one that naturally occurs through its own accord. **Induced abortion** is one that is artificially initiated for therapeutic or personal reasons. Lay people, however, commonly use the word *miscarriage* to describe a spontaneous abortion and may become upset at the use of the word *abortion* to describe an event over which they had no control.[1]

As many as one in five pregnancies ends in a spontaneous abortion. Many pregnancies may not be identified before the abortion occurs, however, so the rate may actually be higher. Most occur during the first 12 weeks of gestation. The incidence decreases to about 3 percent by the 20th week.[2]

Types. The types of spontaneous abortion include threatened, inevitable, complete, incomplete, missed, and habitual. See Table 38–1 for symptoms and collaborative management of spontaneous abortion.

Threatened Abortion. A **threatened abortion** is suggested when the pregnant woman experiences vaginal spotting or bleeding early in pregnancy (Figure 38–1). Uterine cramping and backache often but not always accompany this form of abortion. The bleeding is usually slight in amount, but may continue for several days or weeks. No cervical dilation or effacement is present. Threatened abortion is estimated to occur in 10 to 30 percent of all diagnosed pregnancies. Of this percentage, approximately half abort.[3] In the other half, the pregnancy continues to viability.

Inevitable Abortion. The term **inevitable abortion** describes termination of a pregnancy that cannot be prevented. Although tissue may not have been passed, an abortion is determined to be inevitable when the cervix has begun to dilate, uterine contractions result in discomfort, and vaginal bleeding increases in amount. The membranes rupture as the process proceeds. Ultrasound may reveal the gestational sac in the dilated lower uterine segment.

Complete Abortion. In a **complete abortion** all of the products of conception are entirely expelled. A dilation and curettage is usually not necessary. There are very few physical complications with a complete abortion, but emotional support is necessary.

Incomplete Abortion. An **incomplete abortion** occurs when cervical dilation results in only partial expulsion of the products of conception; some products are retained in the uterus (*see* Figure 38–1). The placenta is more likely to be retained after the tenth week of pregnancy than prior to this time. When tissue remains in utero, the uterus is unable to contract completely. Blood vessels leading to the placenta are not

TABLE 38–1. SYMPTOMS AND COLLABORATIVE MANAGEMENT OF SPONTANEOUS ABORTION

Type	Symptoms	Collaborative Management
Threatened	Slight vaginal bleeding, mild cramping, backache	Maintain bed rest. Advise client to avoid stress and intercourse.
Inevitable	Moderate vaginal bleeding, moderate cramping, cervical dilation, backache	Give physical and emotional support. Assess for hemorrhage. Inspect clots and tissue for intactness.
Complete	Slight vaginal bleeding, mild cramping	No further physical intervention is necessary. Assist the parents to grieve the loss.
Incomplete	Heavy vaginal bleeding, moderate to severe cramping, cervical dilation	Dilation and curettage is performed to complete the pregnancy termination. Assist the parents to grieve the loss.
Missed	Slight vaginal bleeding, possible weight loss and decrease in uterine size	Wait up to 1 month for spontaneous evacuation of uterus. If this does not occur, pregnancy must be terminated. Be alert for problems of hemorrhage. Provide emotional support.
Habitual	Loss of three or more consecutive pregnancies	Surgical repair may be necessary to reinforce the cervix with sutures.

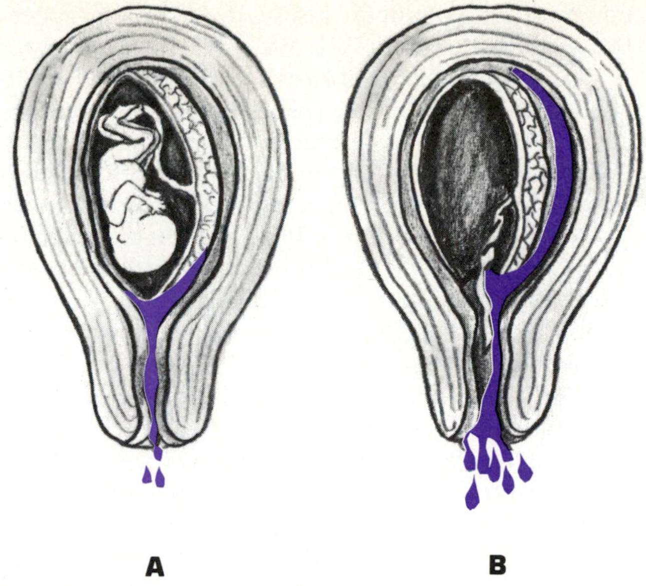

Figure 38–1. Types of spontaneous abortion. **A.** Threatened abortion. **B.** Incomplete abortion.

adequately compressed by the uterine muscle fibers. Excessive vaginal bleeding then results. Retained tissue also increases the risk of infection.

Missed Abortion. In a **missed abortion,** the fetus dies but continues to be retained in the uterus 8 weeks or longer after it is no longer viable. Clinical assessment indicates that the uterus has stopped enlarging and may become smaller as amniotic fluid is absorbed and degeneration of the fetus occurs. The pregnant woman loses a small amount of weight and experiences a brownish vaginal discharge. Subjective pregnancy symptoms such as nausea and breast tenderness disappear. A positive pregnancy test may become negative as gonadotropin production by the placenta ceases. Fetal heart tones remain absent or, if previously noted, disappear. An infrequent hemorrhagic complication is the development of a coagulation defect called disseminating intravascular coagulation (DIC) (*see* Chapter 39 for discussion). Rarely, the fetus is retained long enough to "mummify," or undergo calcification.

Habitual Abortion. **Habitual abortion** describes a situation in which a pregnant woman has had three or more spontaneous abortions consecutively. This is an extremely distressing experience for the woman and her family. Suggested causes include chronic pelvic infections, reproductive hormonal imbalances, inherited chromosomal anomalies, and structural defects of the reproductive tract. The most common structural defect predisposing to spontaneous abortion is an **incompetent cervix.**[4] This is defined as an anatomic defect of the cervix resulting in painless dilation without uterine contractions usually occurring between the 16th and 20th weeks of gestation. Incompetent cervix is fully discussed in Chapter 39.

Etiology. The majority of spontaneous abortions, approximately 60 percent, result from chromosomal abnormalities in the embryo or fetus.[3] Numerous factors predispose to chromosomal anomalies.[5] The age of the ova or spermatozoa may result in abortion. Guerrero and Rojas[6] found an increased incidence of abortion when intercourse occurred more than 4 days before or 2 days after ovulation. Radiation also causes damage to chromosomes. This fact has been widely recognized and was validated in a report by the Committee on the Biological Effects of Ionizing Radiation.[7] Drugs and environmental chemicals are responsible for some abortions (*see* Chapter 11). Recent studies link exposure to antineoplastic drugs[8] and paternal exposure to a wastewater treatment plant at the time of conception[9] with spontaneous abortion. Operating room nurses and anesthetists also have a high rate of abortion.[3] Any potential environmental exposure during pregnancy should not be taken lightly until its relationship to fetal loss and fetal development can be discovered.

Often the cause of a spontaneous abortion is not known. Cunningham and coworkers[2] describe a variety of maternal conditions that have been suspected as causes, but for which evidence is not totally convincing. These include congenital anomalies of the uterus, debilitating systemic disease such as metabolic disorders and severe nutritional deficiencies, psychologic stress, and physical trauma. Excessive physical activity and sexual intercourse are not causes of spontaneous abortion in normal situations. Rommey and others[3] report that infections and viruses such as herpes, rubella, syphilis, and cytomegalovirus cause developmental abnormalities in the fetus, but again there is no convincing evidence that they relate to chromosomal abnormalities or abortions. Lind and McFadyen[10] investigated human pregnancy failure at a preconception clinic. Their data indicate that a large proportion of women who miscarry have never achieved a living fetus and their spontaneous abortion reflects a feature of general reproductive difficulty.

Nursing and Collaborative Assessment. Assessment of spontaneous abortion includes observations of signs and symptoms. For all spontaneous abortions, the classic symptom is vaginal bleeding, which may begin as dark spotting and progress to frank, bright red bleeding.

RESEARCH ABSTRACT

Wall-Haas CL. Women's perceptions of first trimester spontaneous abortion. J Obstet Gynecol Neonat Nurs. *1985;14:50–53.*

Most first-trimester spontaneous abortions are not life threatening and medical treatment is relatively simple. The woman experiencing an abortion may, however, view the situation much differently. The purpose of this study was to investigate women's emotional responses to first-trimester spontaneous abortion. A group of nine women, aged 18 to 30, were asked to complete a short questionnaire describing their experiences surrounding their miscarriage. It consisted of demographic inquiries, questions concerning the participants' obstetric history, and fill-in or multiple-choice questions concerning the miscarriage. Subjects were also encouraged to include additional comments. Findings were presented in a tabular form. No further analyses were done due to sample size.

The most common behavioral experiences occurring after the miscarriage for this sample included episodes of crying, praying, experiencing depression and disbelief, not wanting to be left alone, and feeling closer to their husbands as a result of the miscarriage. Additionally, women indicated that they felt sad, preoccupied, angry, or irritable. They reported fantasizing about the lost baby.

The anecdotal remarks demonstrated the complexity and diversity of the women's feelings. For example, the women's feelings after miscarriage ranged from relief to profound loss. Some women reported a supportive response from family and friends; others felt the loss was minimized by the same group.

Comment:

The results of this study are important because emotional upheaval does occur after spontaneous abortion. It is important that the psychologic needs of women experiencing spontaneous abortion be recognized and that health care providers help them cope with their loss. The very small sample size limits the extent to which these findings can be generalized. Additional research should continue adding to the data base of the study. With further research on this topic, a therapeutic approach to encourage coping can be developed.

Careful assessment is required to determine whether the cause of the bleeding is a threatened abortion. It must be differentiated from other possible causes of bleeding such as cervical polyps, hydatidiform mole, ectopic pregnancy, carcinoma of the cervix, and normal implantation of the blastocyst.[11]

Assessment to differentiate spontaneous abortion from other possible causes is done through speculum examination to inspect the cervix and vagina for polyps; Pap smear to determine presence of carcinoma of the cervix; ultrasound examination to rule out an ectopic pregnancy and note the presence of an intrauterine gestational sac; serial ultrasounds to determine lack of fetal growth; and serial radioimmunoassay tests to determine the level of human chorionic gonadotropin (hCG). If the hCG level drops significantly before 100 days of gestation or if it is absent prior to this time, fetal death usually has occurred.[11]

Additional assessment includes signs of cervical dilation, which are noted through a pelvic examination, and signs and symptoms of intrauterine infection, which include fever greater than 100.4°F (38°C), white blood cell count greater than 16,000, foul-smelling vaginal discharge, general malaise, and urinary urgency or frequency. Other blood values, including hemoglobin and hematocrit, are obtained to assess for anemia resulting from blood loss.[11] In general, anemia in women is considered to be a hemoglobin less than 12.0 g/dL in the nonpregnant state and less than 11.0 g/dL during pregnancy. (*See* discussion on anemia later in this section.)

The nurse will want to ask the mother experiencing vaginal bleeding how many weeks pregnant she is; the onset, duration, intensity, and type of bleeding; whether any tissue or amniotic fluid is accompanying the bleeding; and what other symptoms are present, for example, cramps and abdominal pain. The nurse will also want to determine the mother's and father's response to the vaginal bleeding. Are they sad or frightened? Do they blame themselves or each other?[11]

Nursing Diagnoses. Nursing diagnoses are made after careful assessment of the woman to determine the cause of vaginal bleeding. See the box for examples of nursing diagnoses for the woman with spontaneous abortion.

NURSING DIAGNOSES RELATED TO SPONTANEOUS ABORTION

Problem-Oriented

Dysfunctional grieving, related to inability to express feelings for lost pregnancy

Situational low self-esteem, related to perceived inability to carry a fetus to term

Strength-Oriented

Asset in grieving, related to ability to express feelings concerning pregnancy loss to significant others

Nursing and Collaborative Management. The severity of symptoms experienced by the client determines the aggressiveness of the treatment for vaginal bleeding. Once symptoms are identified, the woman is usually advised to stay in bed. Intercourse or orgasm should be avoided for 2 weeks after any bleeding. If pain accompanies bleeding, the prognosis is less hopeful, although the circumstances may still resolve without any additional threat of abortion.

If symptoms persist, the woman may be advised to resume normal activities in an attempt to hasten the process of abortion. As most abortions result from fetal abnormalities, many clinicians question whether any attempt should be made to retain a pregnancy once symptoms of abortion are present.

If the abortion proceeds, it is important that all of the products of conception be expelled from the uterus. Intravenous oxytocin (Pitocin) in solution may be given. Prostaglandin E_2 vaginal suppository or gel may be used instead of oxytocin; however, prostaglandins are not used in combination with oxytocin.[11] If these are ineffective, surgical removal of the products of conception is necessary. A uterine curettage is done most often. Inspection for complete expulsion of the products of conception is important. The client, whether at home or hospitalized, should also be instructed to save all clots and tissues passed for inspection.

Nursing interventions for the woman experiencing spontaneous abortion are based on the prognosis of the pregnancy and the nursing diagnosis (*see* the Case Study/Care Plan). When bleeding occurs, the woman should contact her health care provider. Watching and waiting is a general guide to care if vaginal examination determines that the cervix remains closed. If the pregnant woman is at home, physical activity will often be restricted. Bed rest may be helpful in maintaining the pregnancy, and intercourse or orgasm should be avoided. The nurse explains that ultrasound reliably establishes the presence of a gestational sac. This method of assessment will be done regularly to help determine the pregnancy's continuing viability.

Inevitable and incomplete abortions require prompt nursing action. Hemorrhage is a priority concern. Vital signs are monitored frequently and the amount and character of vaginal bleeding continue to be assessed. The color of the blood is noted: Is it dark brown or bright red? Is bleeding heavy, moderate, or light? The woman must be observed carefully and treated for signs of shock, such as dizziness, lightheadedness, decreased blood pressure, and increased pulse. All clots and tissues should be saved for examination whether the client is at home or hospitalized. Rho(D) immune globulin must be given within 72 hours of delivery if the mother's blood type is Rh negative. Continued observation for and reporting of signs of infection are also nursing responsibilities. Symptoms of infection include an elevated temperature, foul-smelling vaginal discharge, general malaise, and urinary urgency and frequency.

CASE STUDY/CARE PLAN: SPONTANEOUS ABORTION

Susie Ottosen is 25 years old and pregnant for the first time. At 9 weeks of gestation, she notices a small amount of dark brown vaginal spotting about the size of a dime. By 11 AM the next day, the vaginal bleeding is bright red and the size of a half dollar. Susie immediately calls her obstetrician's office. About 3 hours later, mild cramping begins. The cramping becomes increasingly uncomfortable.

This planned pregnancy has been without complication to this point. Susie has been married for 4 years and conceived 6 months after she stopped taking birth control pills. She had experienced some minor discomforts of pregnancy including sore breasts, fatigue, and urinary frequency. There is no family history of spontaneous abortion. She has taken no medication since stopping her birth control pills. Susie is employed as a retail clerk in a woman's clothing store.

Susie calls her obstetrician and describes the classic symptom of threatened spontaneous abortion—vaginal spotting. She is told to stay in bed and avoid intercourse or orgasm; however, the spotting rapidly increases in amount as the day goes on, and cramping begins. She again calls her obstetrician, who suggests that she be hospitalized.

On admission to the hospital, Susie's bleeding and cramping increase, and she experiences a spontaneous abortion. Blood tests indicate that she is RH negative; she reports that her husband is RH positive.

(continued)

CASE STUDY/CARE PLAN: Spontaneous Abortion (*continued*)

Supporting Assessment Data	Expected Client/Family Outcome	Nursing Action/ Intervention	Rationale	Criteria for Evaluation
Nursing Diagnosis: Alteration in tissue perfusion, related to uterine cramping and bleeding				
Vaginal bleeding at 9 weeks of gestation; uterine cramping Client's blood reveal that she is Rh negative; she reports her husband is RH positive	During hospitalization: Client's vital signs will remain within normal range Client will: Maintain bed rest Report any increase in amount of vaginal bleeding	Assess history of present pregnancy; health status, infections, activities; and vital signs.	History may provide clues to possible cause of abortion.	Vital signs remain within normal limits.
		Encourage bed rest. Monitor blood loss. Note amount and character of blood loss.	Decreased physical activity may help to maintain the pregnancy.	Client maintains bed rest.
		Observe for signs of shock: decreased blood pressure, rapid pulse, low urine output, cool and clammy skin, dizziness.	Amount of blood lost is used to assess for hypovolemic shock and monitor extent of bleeding.	Blood loss is accurately assessed. Client reports any signs of increased bleeding. No additional signs of shock are apparent.
		Obtain hematocrit, hemoglobin, and blood type.		
		Encourage client to ingest iron supplements as prescribed.	If anemia occurs after abortion, iron stores need to be rebuilt.	Blood values remain within normal limits.
		Administer Rho(D) immune globulin.	If sensitization is possible in the Rh-negative client, Rho(D) immune globulin should be given. Leakage of fetal blood into the maternal circulation is possible.	Rho(D) immune globulin is given if client is Rh-negative and if father's blood type is Rh-positive or unknown.
		Save all tissue and clots for inspection.	Determination must be made as to whether all of the products of conception have been expelled.	Embryo/fetus and membranes have been passed or client has been prepared for dilation and curettage.
		Prepare client for possible dilation and curettage.	If products of conception are not completely expelled, medical intervention to remove them is necessary.	
Nursing Diagnosis: Alteration in comfort, related to uterine cramping				
Uterine cramping, which becomes increasingly uncomfortable	During hospitalization: Client will use controlled breathing and relaxation techniques Client copes effectively with discomfort until relief is achieved	Maintain calm, supportive approach. Remain with client or ensure that significant other is present.	Stress, anxiety, and fear produce muscle tension, adding to pain's discomfort, and should therefore be reduced.	Client is not left alone.
		Explain what to expect with a threatened abortion.	Explanations reduce anxiety related to uncertainty.	Appropriate explanations are given.
		Teach relaxation techniques and controlled abdominal breathing.	Relaxation techniques help relieve discomfort.	Client demonstrates relaxation and breathing techniques.
		Include client and family in decision making.	Informed decision-making keeps client and family in control.	Relevant participation by client and family is achieved.
		Administer analgesics as prescribed.	Analgesics reduce discomfort.	Pharmacologic agent is administered as needed.

Supporting Assessment Data	Expected Client/Family Outcome	Nursing Action/ Intervention	Rationale	Criteria for Evaluation
		Encourage position changes. Administer back rubs as needed.	Comfort measures provide non-pharmacologic relief of discomfort.	Client indicates a reasonable degree of comfort.
Nursing Diagnosis: Grieving dysfunction, related to loss of desired pregnancy				
Spontaneous interruption of first pregnancy; pregnancy is planned	Prior to discharge:	Determine personal meaning of this pregnancy to client and her family.	Such information provides insight into the extent of the loss.	Client and her family are able to talk about her feelings.
	Client and family will initiate grieving process	Accept feelings as client and family experiences them.	Attachment begins early in pregnancy.	Grief is resolved as evidenced by continuation of normal activities and family's statements.
	Client identifies support system (both personal and professional)	Facilitate client and family grieving.		
	Client maintains positive self-image	Offer information concerning the miscarriage.	Grieving is a natural phenomenon after such a loss.	
		Contact clergy, social worker, or other support people as appropriate.	Professional support people are trained to help women and families work through losses.	Professional support people or family are available for client and her significant others.
		Arrange for products of conception to be baptized and buried if client wishes.	Spiritual needs of family and client must be met.	Spiritual needs of client and her family are met concerning the abortion.
		Ensure that future childbearing potential is discussed.	Client and her family must be realistic in planning future pregnancies.	Future childbearing possibilities are clearly discussed by client and her family.
			Knowledge helps with grief resolution and reduces anxiety, guilt, and blaming.	
Nursing Diagnosis: Potential for infection, related to uterine cramping and bleeding				
Client has suffered spontaneous abortion	During hospitalization and after discharge:	Assess for symptoms of infection and treat appropriately:	Infection can readily occur after abortion.	No signs of infection are apparent:
	Client will show no evidence of infection	Temperature elevated over 100°F Foul-smelling vaginal discharge Urinary urgency and frequency.	Careful assessment of symptoms can allow for early detection of infection.	Temperature is within normal range Vaginal discharge is without foul odor No urinary frequency or urgency is experienced.

Uterine cramping is uncomfortable to the woman experiencing an abortion. The nurse's calm, supportive approach may be helpful in promoting relaxation. Slow, rhythmic back rub and abdominal breathing also promote relaxation. The nurse can provide support by reassuring the woman that she is managing well. Comfort measures—ice chips if allowed, cool, smooth linens, and comfortable positioning—may all prove helpful. Analgesics may be prescribed to lessen the discomfort.

Nursing management must also be directed toward the psychologic needs of the family experiencing a spontaneous abortion. Vaginal bleeding after the confirmation of pregnancy is frightening for the woman and her family. Waiting and watching is often difficult, although it may be the only treatment suggested by the clinician. As many, if not most, women and their significant others experience some ambivalence at the diagnosis of a pregnancy, loss of the pregnancy may cause significant guilt. Before they have accepted being pregnant, the pregnancy is lost. The guilt is often expressed in terms of wishing and wondering if the mother should have done things differently. Should I have eaten better? Did playing tennis or jogging cause the abortion?

It is now accepted that both fathers and mothers attach to their fetus prenatally.[12] Chodorow[13] describes the mothering relationship as very specialized and developing from the woman's relationship with her own mother. This relationship between a pregnant woman and her mother provides background for the relationship between a pregnant woman and her fetus[12] and subsequent attachment. Fathers also initiate a relationship with the fetus early in pregnancy.

Anger and disappointment are often common emotions expressed after a spontaneous abortion. This is particularly true when the pregnancy is planned. Often a woman prepares for pregnancy long before it occurs. She may begin paying close attention to her diet, drinking more milk, and eating fresh vegetables. She stops taking all prescription or over-the-counter drugs and stops smoking. To this woman, the fetus is much more than a mass of cells. It is already an infant to whom definite attachment has begun.

Nursing reasearch[14–17] has explored responses of women and their families to spontaneous abortion. These studies show that all mothers mourn the involuntary loss of a pregnancy, but with varying degrees of intensity. The fetus has not yet taken on specific physical characteristics or gender for the family. They must, therefore, grieve for their fantasies of the unseen, unborn child. The significance of the loss may be unrecognized by the woman as well as her family. Grief may last from 6 months to a year, or even longer. Husbands generally move through the grieving process more quickly than their wives.[17]

Feelings of anger, disappointment, and sadness are commonly experienced by the couple. They may want to express these feelings, but may feel that family, friends, and often health care personnel are uncomfortable or unable to provide emotional support after a spontaneous abortion. No societal customs, such as a funeral or period of mourning, exist to acknowledge the loss.

Swanson-Kauffman[15] identifies five categories of caring for women who experience miscarriage. These categories serve as an organizing framework for initiating nursing care:

- *Knowing* recognizes the woman's need to be understood about the personal meaning of the loss experienced. The nurse must attempt to see the miscarriage through the woman's eyes rather than basing care on previously preconceived ideas about spontaneous abortion. Women who experience spontaneous abortions frequently report receiving unhelpful comments from family, friends, and health care professionals. These comments seem to stem from a lack of empathetic listening.
- *Being with* goes further than knowing, to actually feeling with the woman who miscarried. Swanson-Kauffman indicates that for health professionals, this means "dropping the professional facade and willingly entering into an emotion-laden, person-to-person relationship."[15]
- *Doing for* relates to a woman's need to have others do things for her during this difficult time. The woman would care for herself were she able, but at this time she is not. Thorough, professional nursing care is expected. Comfort, protection, and health promotion must be included. Needs should be anticipated.
- *Enabling* facilitates the woman's ability to grieve. It takes on a variety of forms depending on the specific situation. Health care professionals are most successful in this category when they give information to woman and families. Being told what to expect decreases anxiety.
- *Maintaining belief* stresses the significance of others' belief in the woman to make it through the loss and ultimately give birth. It is important that others not lose sight of the woman as a capable, functional human being, even if right now she is having difficulty viewing herself in this way. Women expressed comfort in being assured that another pregnancy is a possibility. On the other hand, if the woman decides not to try again, she needs others to support her in that decision.

Once a woman has experienced an abortion, her attitude toward subsequent pregnancies changes.[18, 19] She may delay verifying the pregnancy or seeking prenatal care until the first trimester has passed. She may not tell her family or friends about the pregnancy to avoid "jinxing" the outcome. There is detachment from the fetus in an attempt to prevent hurt if the pregnancy should be lost again.[20]

The nurse can play an important role in helping the woman who has experienced a spontaneous abortion deal with her feelings and grief. Open-ended questions and active listening are helpful in initiating the emotional healing. The nurse should recognize that a range of feelings are commonly experienced by women after spontaneous abortion and should allow opportunities for the client to acknowledge and deal with her feelings. Empathetic listening is an essential therapeutic intervention.

Often restlessness, malaise, insomnia, and a general feeling of dissatisfaction follow a miscarriage. Women need to know these feelings do occur and that they are not abnormal for experiencing them. Support groups are available in various parts of the country to help women cope with miscarriage. If grieving is unresolved over a long period or dealing with the abortion is particularly traumatic, counseling services may be suggested.

The woman's partner and other family members also may be experiencing grief as they too have lost a potential child. Acknowledging and expressing their feelings are important, especially if they are to serve as a source of support for the primary client.

The importance of advising the client about what to expect with regard to medical intervention, pelvic examination, and laboratory testing cannot be overstated. Spontaneous abortion is a frightening experience; however, the client can be helped to regain a sense of control by understanding the expected sequence of events and the prognosis for future pregnancies.

Ectopic Pregnancy

An **ectopic pregnancy** is any pregnancy that occurs outside of the uterine cavity. This results when the fertilized ovum implants in tissue other than the lining of the uterus. Ectopic pregnancy is classified as tubal, ovarian, cervical, or abdominal, depending on the implantation site. The majority of ectopic pregnancies, close to 95 percent, implant in the fallopian tube. Rare sites of implantation include the abdomen (0.75 to 1 percent) ovary (1 percent), and cervix (less than 1 percent) (Figure 38–2). This section focuses on tubal ectopic pregnancies, as they are by far the predominant form.

Ectopic pregnancy is a serious problem that accounts for 14 percent of maternal mortality.[2] The reported rate in 1985 was 14 ectopic pregnancies per 10,000 females, although statistics vary across the United States.[2] Some large urban centers cite rates as high as 1 in 80 pregnancies.[21]

The incidence of ectopic pregnancy has almost tripled in recent years. This is attributed primarily to the growing number of women of childbearing age who are experiencing pelvic inflammatory disease and endometriosis, who use intrauterine devices, or who have had tubal surgery.[2] Other causes include congenital tubal anomalies such as diverticula, accessory tubes and excessively long tubes, and tubal tumors. Infertile women treated with human gonadotropins also experience an increased incidence of ectopic pregnancy.[22] Fortunately, the rise in incidence has been offset by decreases in morbidity and mortality because of improved diagnostic techniques and better access to health care.

Only the uterus is theoretically capable of sustaining the implantation of a fertilized ovum and then growing and nourishing it. Rarely are pregnancies carried to term in the abdomen. Other sites of implantation eventually rupture. The timing of the rupture depends on the implantation site. In the fallopian tube, the specific site's stretchability determines the rupture's timing. The ampulla of the fallopian tube is the most common site of an ectopic tubal pregnancy and usually ruptures between 6 and 12 weeks of gestation (Figure 38–3). The second most common site, the isthmic portion of the tube, generally ruptures during the first 6 weeks of the pregnancy. The rupture occurs as the fertilized ovum erodes and de-

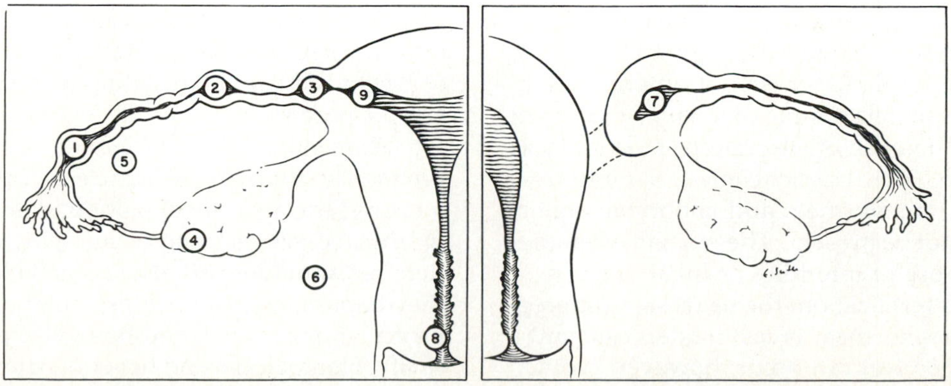

Figure 38–2. Implantation sites of ectopic pregnancy, in order of frequency: (1) ampulla of tube, (2) remainder of tube, (3) interstitial portion of tube, (4) ovary, (5) broad ligament (intraligamentary), (6) surface of peritoneum (abdominal), (7) rudimentary horn, (8) cervix, (9) tubouterine junction (angular). *(Reproduced, with permission, from Zuspan FP, Quilligan EJ.* Douglas-Stromme Operative Obstetrics. *5th ed. Norwalk, Conn: Appleton & Lange; 1988:204.)*

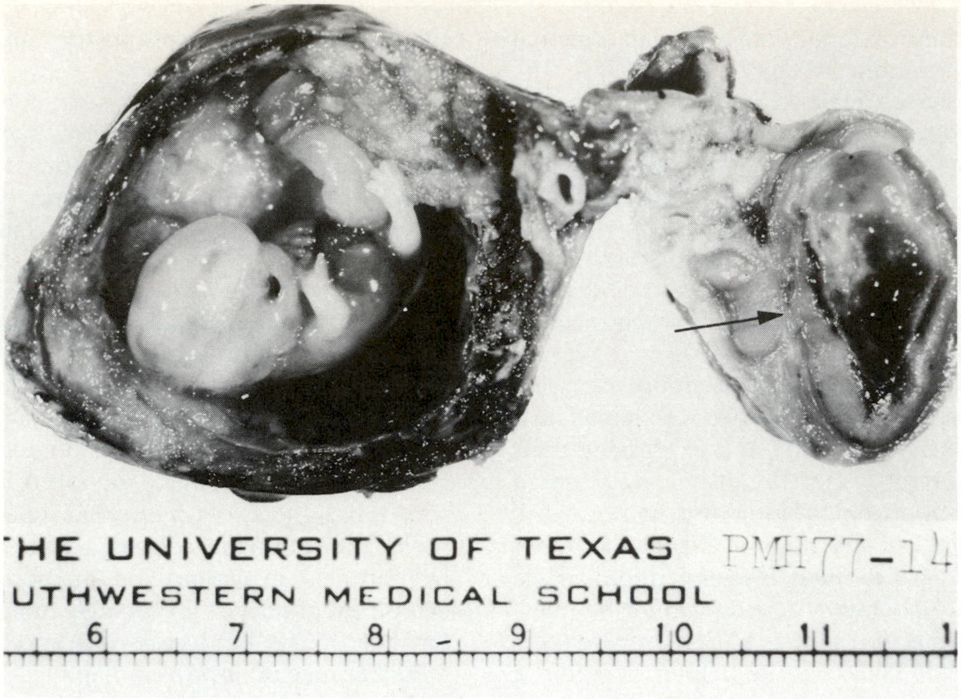

Figure 38–3. Right oviduct containing a fetus and placenta in the ampullary portion, and right ovary with corpus luteum of pregnancy (*arrow*). The woman had experienced vaginal spotting and intermittent dull pain for nearly a month. (*Reproduced, with permission, from Cunningham FG, et al.* Williams Obstetrics, *18th ed. Norwalk, Conn: Appleton & Lange; 1988:524.*)

generates the tube at the site of the placental insertion. The erosion of blood vessels results in bleeding that ranges from scanty bleeding to frank hemorrhage. Nourishment for the embryo's development is also severely limited. Any stress such as intercourse, straining at a stool, or a vaginal examination further weakens the structure. Eventually, however, as a result of overdistension, the tube ruptures spontaneously. Hemorrhage is internal.

Nursing and Collaborative Assessment. Unfortunately, many diagnoses of ectopic pregnancy are not made prior to rupture because the indications are not that different from those of an intrauterine pregnancy. Osguthorpe calls ectopic pregnancy the "great masquerader"[23] because of the variety of symptoms that may occur. The classic clinical symptoms—abdominal pain, amenorrhea, and abnormal vaginal bleeding—may not be present. The woman often presents with a history of infertility or tubal surgery.

Initially after fertilization, the usual signs of pregnancy such as amenorrhea, breast tenderness, and a positive pregnancy test can occur; however, women with irregular menstrual periods may not recognize any abnormality or delay in their menstrual periods. The more common signs of pregnancy, such as breast enlargement and nausea, may not be present because of the early stage of gestation and lower production of hCG, estradiol, and progesterone.[24] Thus, many women do not even recognize that they are pregnant.

Pain is the most common complaint and a valuable diagnostic clue. The pain usually occurs early, probably as a result of distension of the fallopian tube. Pain may be experienced for a week or longer but some clients report acute pain of less than 1 day's duration. The pain often is described as vague, colicky, or cramping. Frequently it is localized to the right or left pelvic area.[23] Intermittent vaginal spotting also may occur as the uterine decidua is sloughed off. The discharge is generally dark in color. Profuse or bright red vaginal bleeding is uncommon with an ectopic pregnancy.

More notable symptoms develop if the ectopic pregnancy ruptures. Characteristically these symptoms include abdominal pain, unilateral palpable pelvic mass, dizziness, and ensuing hypovolemic shock. Referred shoulder pain may occur if blood pools under the diaphragm. Vaginal examination may be very painful if extensive blood has collected in the vaginal cavity. Hemoglobin and hematocrit levels may be low. If rupture and subsequent bleeding are more gradual, the client may present with vague signs such as abdominal discomfort or fullness, nausea, vomiting, and diarrhea. This makes diagnosis somewhat difficult.

Other disorders with similar presenting symptoms include salpingitis, uterine abortion, ruptured corpus luteum cyst, appendicitis, twisted ovarian cyst, gastrointestinal disturbance, and discomfort from an intrauterine device. It is important that the diagnosis be accurately differentiated from other disorders. This is further complicated by the fact that the client may present at a variety of health care locations, unaware of the real cause of her symptoms. Table 38–2 summarizes problems that may be confused with ectopic pregnancy.

The combined use of ultrasound technology and radioimmunoassay of the beta subunit of human chorionic gonadotropin (beta-hCG) is increasingly helpful in early diagnosis of an ectopic pregnancy.[24] A positive pregnancy test (beta-hCG) rules out other conditions and helps narrow the focus of investigation. The accuracy of diagnosis of ectopic pregnancy via ultrasound alone varies from 70 to 92 percent;[25] however, diagnosis by ultrasound has improved with use of the transvaginal approach. With a normal pregnancy a gestational sac in the uterus is visible 5 to 6 weeks after the last menstrual period. A positive pregnancy test and the inability to visualize an intrauterine gestation by ultrasound lead to a presumptive diagnosis that is close to 100 percent accurate.[24]

Hemoglobin, hematocrit, and leukocyte values may also be useful in diagnosing suspected ectopic pregnancies. Hemoglobin and hematocrit values may show a slight reduction after the hemorrhage that accompanies the rupture of the ectopic pregnancy. After the first few hours, the hemoglobin and hematocrit may drop significantly because of acute hemorrhage. In about half the women with ruptured ectopic pregnancies, the leukocyte count is normal. In the other half, leukocytosis of up to 30,000 μL may be encountered.

Prior to instituting specific diagnostic procedures, a routine pelvic examination is performed. Because the procedure may be painful, the client must be prepared and the examination done with care.

Culdocentesis may be used to confirm ectopic pregnancy, especially when ultrasound is not available. In culdocentesis, the physician inserts a needle through the posterior vagina wall into the cul-de-sac of Douglas (a section of the peritoneal cavity behind the uterus) and aspirates fluid. Aspiration of nonclotting blood may indicate a ruptured ectopic pregnancy. Clear fluid rules out a ruptured ectopic pregnancy. Lack of fluid does not provide diagnostic data.[23]

A laparoscopy may be performed if a definite diagnosis cannot be made using other methods. A laparoscopy is a surgical procedure in which a small abdominal incision is made and a laparoscope is inserted to visualize the peritoneal cavity and organs (*see* Figure 9–5). Figure 38–4 describes a protocol for diagnosis of suspected ectopic pregnancy. Table 38–3 summarizes assessment techniques for ectopic pregnancy.

Nursing and Collaborative Management. Once the medical diagnosis is determined, surgical removal of the products of conception is initiated. Sometimes the affected tube must be removed, although there may be an attempt to save it by resection to maintain fertility.

Salpingostomy may be performed to remove a small ectopic pregnancy. A linear incision is made over the site of the ectopic pregnancy and the products of conception are carefully removed. In another technique, salpingotomy, a longitudinal incision is made in the fallopian tube and the products of conception are removed with forceps or gentle suction. These procedures are usually recommended with unruptured ectopic pregnancies and in women with no

TABLE 38–2. DIFFERENTIAL DIAGNOSIS OF ECTOPIC PREGNANCY

Problem	Symptoms
Salpingitis	Spotting, bilateral pain and tenderness, temperature exceeding 100.4°F (38°C), negative urinary pregnancy test, negative serum hCG
Abortion	Uterine bleeding more profuse, pain generally less severe, cramps likely to be rhythmic and located in middle of abdomen
Ruptured corpus luteum and follicular cyst	No chorionic gonadatropin, diagnosis frequently made during laparoscopy
Appendicitis	Signs and symptoms of pregnancy lacking, pain localized higher in abdomen, pain during vaginal manipulation of cervix less severe
Twisted ovarian cyst	No signs of pregnancy, mass more discrete
Gastrointestinal disturbances	Nausea, vomiting, diarrhea, abdominal pain without pregnancy present (If pregnancy symptoms are present, investigate further.)
Intrauterine device discomfort	Very difficult to differentiate as cramping, bleeding, pelvic pain (often unilateral) are common in both ectopic pregnancy and discomfort from an intrauterine device (Use of an intrauterine device does *not* prevent tubal pregnancy.)

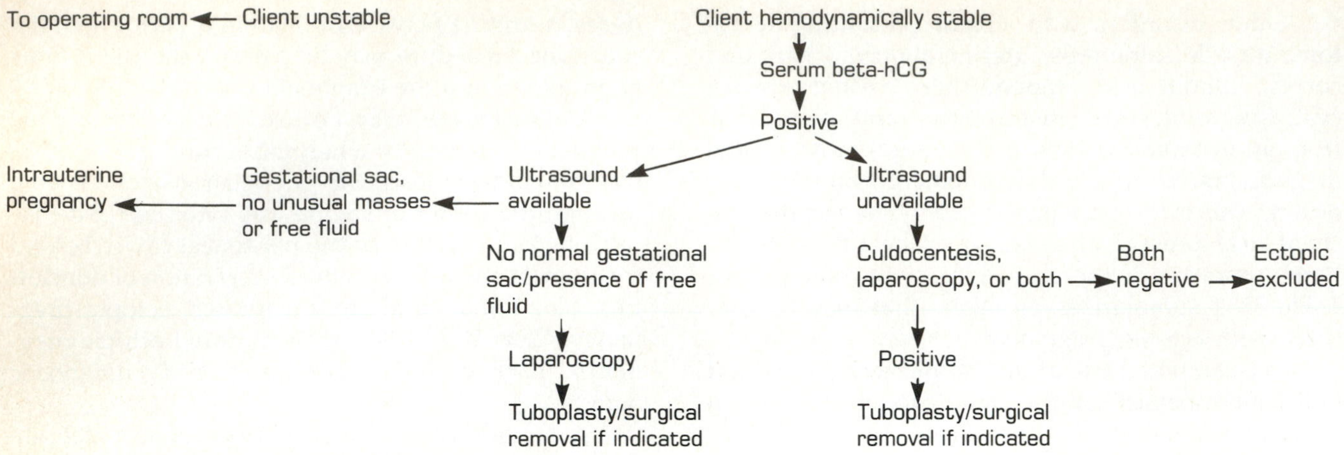

Figure 38–4. Protocol for diagnosis of suspected ectopic pregnancy. (*Reproduced, with permission of Aspen Publishers, Inc., from Patrick J. Ectopic pregnancy.* Top Emerg Med. *1985;7:30.*)

previous salpingitis and the desire to have another pregnancy.[2]

Tanaha,[26] and Ory,[27] and their colleagues have used methotrexate as a noninvasive treatment for early ectopic pregnancy to try to produce absorption of the products of conception. Use of this potent antieoplastic drug remains controversial, however, as it may be toxic to the woman and may damage the tube.

Ectopic pregnancy has become the primary cause of maternal mortality in the first trimester of pregnancy, and accounts for roughly 12 percent of all maternal deaths in the United States. Approximately 85 percent of these deaths are the result of blood loss. Infection accounts for approximately 5 percent of all deaths and complications of anesthesia account for 2 percent. The remaining deaths occur from a variety of causes including pulmonary edema, transfusion reactions, and air embolism.[28]

The large number of deaths resulting from ectopic pregnancy reinforces the necessity of "thinking ectopic." The diagnosis must be expeditiously sought every time it is suspected. Women at increased risk must be educated to seek care promptly when symptoms are present. Education and prompt action by health professionals should aid in reducing the mortality from this dangerous complication of pregnancy.

The main concern with ruptured ectopic pregnancy is hemorrhage. Blood transfusions and intravenous therapy are necessary to replace fluid loss. A central venous line may be used to monitor the extent of blood loss along with frequent assessment of vital signs and monitoring of skin color and urinary output. Some moderate vaginal bleeding is expected. A pad count must be initiated to determine the extent of vaginal bleeding. Maintaining bed rest is essential.

Postoperative nursing care after surgery for a ruptured ectopic pregnancy is similar to nursing care for any client experiencing abdominal surgery. The incision must be assessed for redness, edema, discharge, and intactness. The physician generally will prescribe broad-spectrum antibiotics prophylactically. Steroids are frequently administered to decrease inflammation so that adhesions do not develop.[23] Pain medication is needed to control discomfort.

Early ambulation and adequate rest should be encouraged. To prevent paralytic ileus, oral intake

TABLE 38–3. ASSESSMENT TECHNIQUES FOR ECTOPIC PREGNANCY

Technique	Purpose
Pelvic examination	Palpation of pelvic mass and state of cervix; determination of presence of pain and location
Abdominal palpation	Palpation of pelvic mass and enlargement of uterus; determination of presence of pain and location
Radioimmunoassay (hCG)	Determination of positive pregnancy test
Ultrasound	Visualization of gestational sac to rule out intrauterine pregnancy
Laparoscopy	Visualization of peritoneal cavity and organs
Culdocentesis	Aspiration of fluid from peritoneal cavity to rule out ruptured ectopic pregnancy
Hemoglobin, hematocrit	Determination of anemia resulting from blood loss
Leukocyte count	Determination of elevated white blood cell count (leukocytosis)

should be avoided until bowel function has returned to normal. If the client is Rh negative and has not been previously sensitized, she should receive Rho(D) immune globulin, as isoimmunization may follow an ectopic pregnancy. Reconstructive tubal surgery is an option once the woman's condition is stable.

Rupture of an ectopic pregnancy can be an overwhelming event to the childbearing family because of the often terrifying and life-threatening circumstances surrounding the woman's admission and surgery. Not only does the woman undergo surgery, but she also loses a baby and her fertility status may be altered permanently, especially if the other fallopian tube is not intact. The couple need time to sort out what has happened and work through grief.

Many couples develop attachment to their babies very early and experience much sadness even after a young embryo is lost. The nurse can encourage the client and her family to verbalize their feelings by asking open-ended questions. The couple should be assured that their grief is normal and also be allowed to grieve privately. The nurse can help to decrease feelings of guilt or blame by empathetically explaining the causes of ectopic pregnancy. Often couples may view the ectopic pregnancy as punishment for prior sexual behavior or some wrongdoing.[29,30] Support groups can offer ongoing help to the family. Particular attention should be paid to the husband's or significant other's concerns. Many men are likely to experience the same reactions to ectopic pregnancy as their female partner, but feel that their role is to "be strong."

Couples also need information about their chances for a subsequent successful pregnancy. The success of future pregnancies depends on the specifics of the woman's reproductive history and whether at least one fallopian tube remains available to transport a fertilized ovum to the uterus.

Additionally, couples need specific information during the recovery period. The couple can be advised that intercoure may be resumed once the incision has healed. It will probably be 6 to 8 weeks before a normal menstrual period occurs. The couple are advised to use contraceptives for at least three menstrual periods before attempting another pregnancy.[29]

METABOLIC CONDITIONS

Few metabolic conditions completely prevent pregnancy, but many can complicate its course. An understanding of the interaction of pregnancy and the specific disease state is essential to nursing care of the high-risk pregnant woman. Interdisciplinary collaboration also is required to provide optimal care of the woman experiencing a complication of pregnancy.

This section discusses several metabolic complications of pregnancy that require observation or intervention during the first trimester, specifically hyperemesis gravidarum, anemia and hemoglobinopathies, and thyroid disorders. Although management of these conditions is included as a part of first-trimester concerns, treatment of these conditions continues throughout the period of gestation.

Hyperemesis Gravidarum

Hyperemesis gravidarum, also called pernicious vomiting of pregnancy, is severe vomiting during pregnancy that results in maternal dehydration and nutritional deficiencies. It begins most frequently during the first trimester of pregnancy.[31]

Nausea and vomiting are fairly common during early pregnancy. Although troublesome and distressing, these symptoms usually respond to such measures as eating small, frequent meals and avoiding strong odors. Hyperemesis is vomiting that persists beyond the first trimester or excessive vomiting. Fortunately, hyperemesis develops in only a small fraction of pregnancies, affecting about 1 of every 1000 women, and the incidence is decreasing.[31] The condition appears to repeat itself in subsequent pregnancies and is more common in women who previously have suffered a spontaneous abortion or in multifetal pregnancies.[17] Other women at risk for hyperemesis include young women (under 20 years), primigravidas, and women who are overweight.[31]

The etiology of hyperemesis gravidarum is not well understood. It is likely that the true cause of this complication is a combination of factors already or yet to be identified. Much attention has been given to the increased level of hCG in women with this condition. This is especially apparent in molar pregnancies when hyperemesis gravidarum also exists; however, dehydration from the excessive vomiting may play some role in the elevated hCG levels. Additionally, more recent studies[31,32] have not confirmed a relationship between hCG levels and nausea and vomiting.

Another potential cause of hyperemesis is the high levels of estrogen secreted by the placenta in early pregnancy. Depue and colleagues[31] conducted a serum hormone study in 35 matched pairs. Their findings support the hypothesis that elevated estrogen levels in early pregnancy are a major cause of hyperemesis gravidarum. This result is also clinically supported by the observation that initial administration of estrogen also produces nausea and vomiting in clients.

The involvement of psychologic factors, particularly stress, rejection of pregnancy, and an unconscious wish to expel the child, is also cited as a possible etiology.[33] Psychologic causes are given some credence, especially as more is learned concerning the relationship of other eating disorders to emotional causes.

Nursing and Collaborative Assessment. The clinical picture of a pregnant woman suffering from hyperemesis gravidarum varies based on the severity of the complication. The condition begins with nausea, which progressively worsens and may persist all day so that eventually nothing can be retained by mouth. Weight loss results, along with stomach pain and heartburn. Dehydration and starvation eventually occur. Symptoms include fluid and electrolyte imbalance, hypotension, elevated hematocrit, hypokalemia, and decreased urine output. Eventually protein and vitamin deficiencies become apparent. These symptoms should be differentiated from other causes of nausea and vomiting such as hepatitis, gastroenteritis, cholecystitis, and pancreatitis. Left untreated, hyperemesis gravidarum can be fatal, although symptoms may cease at any point and health be restored. Interestingly, the disease is not associated with increased incidence of spontaneous abortion, prematurity, or low-birth-weight infants,[31] although the unfavorable uterine environment might be expected to lead to such complications. In fact, a lower incidence of fetal loss has been documented in women experiencing nausea and vomiting during pregnancy.[33]

Nursing Diagnoses. Several nursing diagnoses may apply to the woman with hyperemesis gravidarum. See the box for examples.

Nursing and Collaborative Management. Care of the client experiencing hyperemesis begins after other causes of nausea and vomiting are diagnostically ruled out. Once this is done, the following principles of care are stressed:

NURSING DIAGNOSES RELATED TO HYPEREMESIS GRAVIDARUM

Problem-Oriented

Potential fluid volume deficit, related to persistent vomiting

Altered nutrition for mother and fetus: less than body requirements, related to persistent vomiting

Altered oral mucous membranes, related to dehydration

Strength-Oriented

Potential asset in resolution of vomiting, related to home management of hyperemesis gravidarum

1. Hospitalization is often required. This may be necessary to change the woman's environment and institute a course of treatment. A change in the woman's environment is sometimes necessary if psychosocial factors in that environment contribute to the condition. Also, hospitalization may be required if the woman is severely dehydrated and needs fluid replacement; however, many women with hyperemesis gravidarum currently are being managed successfully at home.
2. Intravenous therapy is initiated to treat dehydration. Generally, the woman will receive approximately 3000 mL intravenously in the first 24 hours. The addition of glucose, vitamins, and electrolytes to the intravenous solution helps to restore electrolytes and nutrients that have been lost by the body. Intake and output need to be carefully monitored as the body's depleted fluid reserves are restored. Adequacy of hydration is assessed through measurement of urinary output; 1000 mL in each 24 hours is desired.
3. The woman begins small frequent feedings as tolerated. Usually this is possible within 48 hours of admission. Special attention should be paid to how the food is served, being sure it is arranged attractively and that cold food is cold and hot food is hot. Options other than oral food intake consist of high-calorie tube feedings or, in severe cases, hyperalimentation. Mouth care is also important, as the mouth may be very dry.
4. Sedatives may be given to relax the hyperactive gastrointestinal tract.

Supportive, therapeutic measures to deal with the emotional component of the disease are helpful. A therapist or counselor will often be involved in this process. The nurse, however, can offer an unhurried willingness to listen and do much to maintain a relaxed, nonstressful environment. The pregnant woman's acceptance of her situation and the pregnancy itself is essential to a favorable outcome of the condition. Assisting the woman in problem-solving and coping with a new child may be an effective strategy.

Anemia

Anemia is a decrease in the circulating red blood cell mass that results in a decrease in the capacity to carry oxygen to vital organs of the mother and the fetus. Although a minor increase in the oxygen-carrying ability of each cell is possible in response to this decrease in red blood cell mass, this compensatory mechanism is soon overwhelmed. Cardiac output must then increase to maintain adequate oxygen delivery to the tissues.

Anemia may be caused by the pregnancy, as with iron deficiency anemia, or it may be a pre-existing condition of the pregnant woman. Sickle cell anemia, for example, is a hereditary condition that may result in severe complications for the pregnant woman and her fetus.

As previously described in Chapters 12, 16, and 20, both red blood cell and plasma volume increase during pregnancy. The plasma volume begins to increase during the third month and continues until term. Around the sixth month of gestation, the red blood cell volume also begins to increase; however, this increase is not as great proportionately as the expansion of plasma volume. The result is a fall in the hematocrit and hemoglobin of a pregnant woman. Because the magnitude of this plasma volume change varies among pregnant women, a range of hemoglobin levels is seen during pregnancy. In addition, altitude may cause a variation in hemoglobin level. For example, women residing at sea level would be considered anemic if their hemoglobin is below 12 g/dL in the nonpregnant state or less than 11 g/dL during pregnancy or the puerperium. Finally, the stage of pregnancy may affect hemoglobin level.[2, 34]

The hemoglobin level of most iron-sufficient pregnant women is usually 11 g/dL or higher.[2] The incidence of all types of anemia during pregnancy is variable, depending on whether supplemental iron or other supplements are taken during pregnancy. Table 38–4 describes common assessment findings in iron deficiency anemias and hemoglobinopathies.

Iron Deficiency Anemia. The majority of women who develop anemia during pregnancy acquire iron deficiency anemia. This accounts for more than 75 percent of all anemia during pregnancy. A woman needs a total of about 1100 mg of iron during her pregnancy. This includes the amounts necessary for increasing maternal blood volume (approximately 800 mg) and for fetal development (approximately 300 mg).[2]

Fortunately, the body is more capable of absorbing iron during pregnancy because of its improved iron-binding capacity (approximately three times that in the nonpregnant state). Despite the intake of 18 mg or more iron daily and the increased iron-binding capacity of the body, the balance between iron need and availability is tenuous. This is especially true during the second half of pregnancy, when the need for iron is the greatest. Unfortunately, many women begin pregnancy in an anemic state and their situation is even more tenuous. Those particularly at risk include adolescents, the poorly nourished, followers of fad diets, and women whose pregnancies are closely spaced. The dietary habits of such women rarely include amounts of iron adequate for pregnancy.

Nursing and Collaborative Assessment. Assessment of iron deficiency anemia begins with a systematic health history that includes a record of hematologic diseases and a dietary history. The family's socioeconomic status is also assessed, as well as eating habits, pica practices, and any history of dieting.

A nutritional history is helpful in identifying the pregnant woman at risk for developing anemia during pregnancy. The use of lay terminology, for example, "thin blood" and "low blood," may help the nurse identify a previous history of anemia. In clients with mild to moderate anemia, symptoms are generally not detectable except by hemoglobin and hematocrit tests. Severe anemia may be more apparent.

In a method commonly used to provide an overview of the woman's dietary patterns, the woman recalls foods consumed during the previous 24 hours. She should be encouraged to list everything ingested at mealtime and between meals. The 24-hour recall is evaluated to determine usual variations in food intake throughout the week (*see* Chapter 10).

Other important information to gather includes general food habits, preparation methods, size of portions, seasonings used, and general likes and dislikes. The woman's usual ingestion of foods rich in iron, including liver, red meat, legumes, green vegetables, and shellfish, should be assessed (Table 38–5).

Craving for and ingestion of nonfood substances, termed *pica*, should also be assessed. Approximately 25 percent of pregnant individuals with iron deficiency and anemia are found to practice pica.[35] Substances frequently ingested by women practicing pica include dirt, clay, and laundry starch. Other substances include ice, wall plaster, cigarette ashes, coffee grounds, and burnt matches. Because of the high rate of iron deficiency among individuals who practice pica, it is recommended that health care providers screen for pica if the individual is anemic, and screen for anemia if the individual practices pica.

As iron deficiency anemia may result from decreased intake of necessary nutrients, the food consumed should be compared with intakes recommended during pregnancy to determine any area of deficiency in amount or quality of nutrients. The total intake of calories and protein can also be determined using standard nutritional guides.

The woman with iron deficiency anemia usually comes to the health care provider with skin pallor and complaints of fatigue, listlessness, weight loss, and weakness. The classic symptom of pallor may, however, be absent because of the hyperemia of the skin that is normally seen during pregnancy.[36] Other physical signs of iron deficiency anemia include infections due to a decrease in immunocompetence, which occurs in severe anemia, and changes in the structure and function of epithelial tissues.

Laboratory data include a blood count, which

TABLE 38–4. COMMON FINDINGS IN THE PREGNANT WOMAN WITH ANEMIA

	Common Findings in Deficiency Anemias	Common Findings in Hereditary Hemoglobinopathies
Subjective		
Family origin	Worldwide	Africa, Mediterranean, eastern hemisphere
Family health history	Anemia, cultural practices related to poor nutrition or pica	Hemoglobinopathy, family members with joint pain or crises
Psychosocial factors	Poverty, adolescence, food fads, listlessness, poor attention span, irritability	Variable
Nutrition	Diet deficient in sources of protein, iron, folate, vitamins, and calories	Fava beans trigger anemia in glucose-6-phosphate dehydrogenase deficiency
Pica	Clay, starch, ice, salt, cravings, and others; cultural variations	May experience pica
Medications	Noncompliance with iron, vitamin, and folate therapies	Degree of compliance with folate therapy
Systems review of past and current complaints		
Muscoloskeletal	Weakness, chronic fatigue	Joint and muscle pain
Integument	History of bleeding or bruising, paresthesias	Sensitivity to cold
Sensory	Visual disturbances	May have visual disturbances if severe
Gastrointestinal	History of nausea, vomiting, heartburn, epigastric pain, diarrhea, dark or bloody stools, malabsorption syndrome	Right upper quadrant pain, eructation, flatulence (because of common occurrence of cholelithiasis), abdominal and epigastric pain or tenderness
Urinary	Dysuria, hematuria, frequency in excess of normal pregnancy, urgency, history of repeated urinary tract infections	History of repeated urinary tract infections, dysuria, frequency, urgency, cloudy, dark, or bloody urine, flank pain
Cardiorespiratory	Palpitations, shortness of breath, chest pain	Chest pain, dyspnea, history of respiratory infections
Reproductive	History of heavy or abnormal menstrual bleeding or bleeding during pregnancy, past use of intrauterine device for contraception	History of infertility, spontaneous abortions, stillbirths, or low-birth-weight infants
Objective		
Musculoskeletal system		Long, thin extremities and digits; edema of hand or foot
Integument	Pallor of conjunctiva, skin, mucous membranes, nail beds, bruising	Pallor, jaundice, leg and ankle ulcerations, edema
Gastrointestinal system	Stomatitis	Rebound tenderness of abdomen, enlarged liver and spleen or nonpalpable spleen resulting from repeated infarctions
Cardiorespiratory system	Tachycardia, heart murmur, fever	Tachycardia, cardiomegaly, silent areas in lung, rales and rhonchi in pneumonia or pneumonitis

Reproduced, with permission, from DeWees CB. Hematologic disorders in pregnancy. Nurs Clin North Am. *1982:64–65.*

identifies the woman with low hemoglobin and hematocrit levels so that further testing may be done and treatment initiated. If the hemoglobin level is below 11 g/dL or if the hematocrit is below 32 percent, the woman is determined to be anemic. A complete blood count and total iron-binding capacity test also may be performed to further confirm the diagnosis.

With severe deficiencies, the red blood cells become microcytic and hypochromic, and the serum iron level decreases.[37] A decrease in transferrin saturation is also noted. Serum ferritin values offer a fairly

TABLE 38–5. IRON CONTENT OF SELECTED FOODS

Food	Serving Size	Iron (mg/serving)
Oysters	¾ cup	10.0
Beef liver	3 oz	8.0
Pinto beans	1 cup cooked	6.1
Navy beans	1 cup cooked	5.1
Lentils	1 cup cooked	4.2
Spinach	1 cup	4.0
Chipped beef	3 oz	4.0
Clams	3 oz	3.5
Lean beef, pork, lamb	3 oz	3.0

precise measurement of the available iron stored. These values should be obtained at 6- to 8-week intervals.[36]

Nursing Diagnoses. Several nursing diagnoses can be made after comprehensive assessment of the client with iron-deficiency anemia. See the box for examples.

Nursing and Collaborative Management. Oral iron supplements, such as ferrous sulfate 0.3 g two to three times per day, are successful in treating most iron deficiency anemias during pregnancy. In cases of severe anemia or when the oral iron supplements cause vomiting, diarrhea, or other side effects the pregnant client cannot tolerate, parenteral iron supplements (eg, Inferon) are available.

Because of the increased iron requirements during pregnancy and the fact that most women enter pregnancy with low iron reserves, most pregnant women receive prophylactic iron supplementation throughout their pregnancy (*see* Chapter 10). This treatment is somewhat controversial, however, especially because deleterious effects of mild anemia have not been documented.[3,38] Infants of mothers with iron deficiency seldom are iron deficient themselves or develop any other medical problems. Although the exact mechanism is unclear, anemic clients with proven iron deficiency do have an increased incidence of infection, postpartum hemorrhage, and pregnancy-induced hypertension.[39]

The nurse can assist the client in devising a dietary plan as rich in iron as possible. The diet should include foods known to be high in iron, taking into consideration the preferred foods of the client. Iron-fortified foods, especially cereals, may be an economic way of further fortifying the diet with iron.

NURSING DIAGNOSES RELATED TO IRON DEFICIENCY ANEMIA

Problem-Oriented

Alteration in nutrition: less than body requirements, related to inadequate iron in maternal diet

Constipation, related to oral supplementation of iron

Alteration in nutrition: less than body requirements, related to pica practices during pregnancy

Strength-Oriented

Potential asset in progressive family coping, related to consumption of ethnic foods high in iron

Potential asset in correcting inadequate iron intake, related to adequate public resources

Diet therapy alone is generally not sufficient to meet the iron needs of women experiencing iron deficiency anemia. Ingestion and absorption of amounts of iron adequate to overcome the deficit are difficult; however, most anemic clients respond readily to iron therapy. Oral administration is preferred because of its simplicity and safety. The nurse can be instrumental in encouraging the client to take the iron supplements as prescribed. Ingesting the iron with beverages high in vitamin C, such as orange juice, is known to improve absorption.[39]

Gastrointestinal side effects such as nausea, vomiting, constipation, and diarrhea are common with iron supplementation. The higher the dosage, the more likely that problems may occur. Because of these side effects, many women tolerate oral supplements poorly, especially in early pregnancy when a tendency for nausea already exists. Taking the iron preparation with or shortly after meals or before bedtime may minimize the nausea; the client may also benefit from a reduced dosage. The client should be advised that some iron in the pills will not be absorbed in the gastrointestinal tract and the woman's stools may turn dark green or black as a result. If constipation is a problem, the client should increase the amount of fluids and fiber in the diet to increase stool bulk and facilitate its passage. Exercise is also beneficial in preventing constipation.

Folic Acid Deficiency Anemia (Megaloblastic Anemia). During pregnancy, increased maternal red blood cell production and fetal demands can result in folic acid or folacin deficiency. Folic acid is a coenzyme necessary for the synthesis of nucleic acids. Nucleic acid and nucleoprotein synthesis are required for the production of red blood cells. Folic acid deficiency is the most common cause of megaloblastic anemia during pregnancy.[36] Megaloblastic anemia is a disorder of red blood cell production that demonstrates as an alteration in cell morphology. Besides anemia, other symptoms include a sore tongue, stomatitis, anorexia, nausea and vomiting.[2]

Folic acid plays an additional role in pregnancy that at present is not entirely understood. Many complications including abruptio placentae, spontaneous abortion, and pregnancy-induced hypertension have been related to folic acid deficiency, although evidence at present is not conclusive. Fetal growth and development do not appear to be affected by maternal folate deficiency.[2]

Nursing and Collaborative Assessment. Assessment for folic acid deficiency focuses on nutritional assessment of the mother, maternal signs and symptoms related to folate deficiency, and laboratory values.

Nutritional Assessment. Assessment of the mother's diet includes a 24-hour dietary recall and investigation of ways in which the mother prepares her food. Overcooking with large volumes of water and canning destroy as much as 80 percent of the available folic acid in food substances. Further, microwave cooking destroys more folic acid in foods than conventional cooking.

Signs and Symptoms of Folate Deficiency. Along with assessment of the nutritional status, the nurse also explores signs and symptoms related to folate deficiency. These may include nausea, vomiting, pallor, anorexia, soreness of the tongue, and stomatitis.

Laboratory Values. Laboratory values include hemoglobin, hematocrit, red blood cell indices such as mean corpuscular volume, peripheral blood smears, and serum folate levels. (*See* Appendix C for normal laboratory values during childbearing.) The mean corpuscular volume may be elevated. Smears of the peripheral blood will demonstrate macrocytes (an immature form of the red blood cell). A folate level less than 5 mg/mL is indicative of folic acid deficiency.[2,36]

Nursing and Collaborative Management. During pregnancy, the recommended daily dietary allowance for folic acid doubles from 400 to 800 μg because of the increased production of red blood cells.[2] Treatment for a deficiency consists of oral folic acid supplementation of 0.5 to 1.0 mg per day beginning in the second trimester.[36] Clients respond readily to therapeutic dosages.

Dietary instruction on the inclusion of foods containing high levels of folic acid in the diet is also important. Good sources of folic acid include green leafy vegetables, fish, meat, poultry, eggs, milk, and legumes. Cooking habits should be explored as part of the nutritional history. Excessive cooking of vegetables is common in some groups. The nurse should encourage the client to steam vegetables in small amounts of water to ensure retention of both folic acid and essential vitamins. Augmentation of iron intake is usually recommended to coincide with folic acid augmentation, as iron deficiency anemia is often found with folic acid deficiency.

Hemoglobinopathies. **Hemoglobinopathies** or abnormal hemoglobin conditions, are hereditary disorders that eventually produce signs and symptoms of disease. There are several specific types of hemoglobinopathies, including sickle cell anemia (hemoglobin S disease), hemoglobin C disease, thalassemia, and glucose-6-phosphate dehydrogenase deficiency. *See* Table 38–4 for common findings in these hemoglobinopathies.

Hemoglobin is an iron-containing protein molecule containing iron that is produced by red blood cells. The primary physiologic function of hemoglobin is to transport oxygen in arterial blood. In its predominant form, a molecule of hemoglobin (hemoglobin A) consists of four globulin chains: two alpha and two beta chains. Variations in the structure of hemoglobin also exist. For example, fetal hemoglobin, which is normally present in the fetus and in early infancy, consists of two alpha chains and two gamma chains (rather than beta chains); in addition, there are delta chains which may combine with alpha chains. Variations in the sequencing and varieties of amino acids in the protein strand result in great differences in the physiologic functioning of the hemoglobin.[40] For example, alterations of the amino acids on the beta chains may cause hemoglobin S and C diseases. Thalassemias, in contrast, are characterized by normal globin chains, but a decreased rate of chain synthesis. Any of the abnormalities can alter oxygen-carrying capacity and the impact on pregnancy can be fatal.[36]

Sickle Cell Anemia. **Sickle cell anemia** is the most common hemoglobinopathy in the United States. It is caused by the substitution of valine for glutamine at position 6 on the beta chain. The disease is genetically transmitted as a recessive trait almost exclusively in blacks to their offspring.

In the heterozygous form, known as sickle cell trait, the person is a carrier of the disease. Even though approximately 25 to 50 percent of the hemoglobin is abnormal, enough normal hemoglobin is produced to compensate for the defect and signs and symptoms do not present. Approximately 8 percent of black Americans are heterozygous carriers of the disease. The homozygous form of the disorder, sickle cell anemia, occurs in 0.7 percent of black Americans.[41]

ISSUES AND CONTROVERSIES

Ethical issues that may be engendered by high-risk conditions of the first trimester include:

1. Should a woman with sickle cell anemia become pregnant? If she does, when does concern over her health take precedence over fetal well-being?
2. If after a reasonable period of bed rest a pregnant woman threatening to abort is still experiencing vaginal bleeding, cramping, or both, should she be encouraged to become more active in an attempt to speed up the abortion?

These ethical dilemmas will likely be faced by the nurse who practices with childbearing families. The current climate of balancing maternal and fetal rights will give rise to far more such difficult situations.

Sickle cell anemia results in defective hemoglobin molecules. The red blood cells become elongated and crescent-shaped, and interlock with one another in the presence of decreased oxygenation. Their shape is distorted into a sickled or holly leaf–shaped cell. Small blood vessels become clogged by these sickle cells, and blood supply to various parts of the body is compromised. Infections and dehydration greatly increase the chances of sickling. When sickled red blood cells obstruct blood flow to tissues, further hypoxia and the resultant sickling occur. In addition, these sickled red blood cells have a life span of 15 to 20 days, in contrast to the normal life span of 120 days of most red blood cells. Decreased serum values for red blood cells result. The disease is inherited at birth but does not become apparent until about 4 months of age when fetal hemoglobin has been replaced by the abnormal adult hemoglobin.[42]

The course of the disease is one of episodes of acute crisis. These episodes may follow infections causing dehydration, respiratory infections resulting in hypoxia, or strenuous exercise causing hypoxia. Air pollution and anesthesia are other causes of inadequate oxygenation that may result in crisis. In some situations, no specific cause can be found. Symptoms of a crisis include pain in the extremities, acute abdominal pain, hepatomegaly, and splenomegaly. The symptoms result from pooling of sickled cells in blood vessels and subsequent tissue hypoxia.

Heterozygous carriers with sickle cell trait generally experience very few problems and are able to lead fulfilling, productive lives. Women with sickle cell trait may have an increased incidence of urinary tract infections during pregnancy[38]; however, there is no increased incidence of fetal problems.[43] Three maternal deaths associated with sickle cell trait have been reported in the literature.[44] All of these clients had severe complications (eclampsia, pulmonary embolism, and peripartum cardiomyopathy) and the presence of sickle cell trait may have merely been coincidental. Sickling was apparent with severe hypoxia, however, so that further research is indicated to determine the complete effect of sickle cell trait in pregnancy. Routine iron and folic acid supplementation should be given to women with sickle cell trait during the pregnancy to stimulate red blood cell production. The fetal cord blood should be checked for the presence of sickle cell trait or sickle cell anemia.

Women with sickle cell anemia experience a variety of problems beginning in early infancy. As medical and nursing treatment has improved, however, an increasing number of adults are surviving the disease and are reaching reproductive age. During pregnancy, both mother and fetus are at risk. Maternal complications include urinary tract infections, pneumonia, postpartum infections, anemia, congestive heart failure, and pregnancy-induced hypertension.[45] A maternal mortality rate of 20 percent suggests the serious consequences of pregnancy to the client with sickle cell anemia. The risk to the fetus is even greater, with perinatal mortality rates ranging from 23 to 52 percent.[39] This fetal wastage is due to increases in the numbers of spontaneous abortions, stillbirths, and low-birth-weight infants. Uterine hypoxia resulting from slow circulation of sickled red blood cells in the uterine blood vessels is cited as a cause.

In the past decade, the risks associated with pregnancy for mothers with sickle cell disease and their infants have decreased significantly. In a 1986 study by Powars and coworkers,[46] the maternal mortality rate among 79 women was 1.7 percent. Infant, fetal, and perinatal death rates decreased to 22.7 percent. These positive results are attributed to improved perinatal care.

Genetic Considerations. Genetic counseling is invaluable to couples at risk for passing the sickle cell trait to their offspring. If one parent is known to carry the trait, the other should also be screened for its presence. The parents' chances of producing a normal offspring need to be accurately determined and explained. If both parents carry the sickle cell trait, the child has a 25 percent chance of having sickle cell disease and a 50 percent chance of being a carrier of the disease. If one parent has sickle cell disease, the child will be a carrier or have the disease, depending on the other parent (Figure 38–5).

The fetus' genotype can be determined through chorionic villi sampling or amniocentesis. The results determine whether the fetus is unaffected, a carrier, or affected. If it is determined the fetus is homozygous and has sickle cell anemia, the partners should be counseled concerning the child's condition and resultant handicaps. The parent's beliefs and values must be the priority as decisions concerning carrying the pregnancy to term are made.

The nurse can serve as a support person to couples trying to sift through the information given to them by the genetic counselors. Often, the parents need additional emotional resources as the reality of the situation becomes apparent.

Because of the severe complications pregnancy superimposes on a woman already debilitated from sickle cell anemia, additional pregnancies are often not recommended. Sterilization may be considered or a very reliable method of birth control used. The methods recommended are a progestin-only oral contraceptive or a barrier contraceptive, such as the diaphragm or condom.[47] An intrauterine device is not recommended as it would increase the risk of infec-

Heterozygous

Parent HbA_1/S (columns); HbA_1/S (rows)

Gametes	A_1	S
A_1	A_1A_1 Normal	A_1S Carrier
S	A_1S Carrier	SS Affected

Homozygous/Heterozygous

Parent Hb S/S (columns); HbA_1/S (rows)

Gametes	S	S
A_1	A_1S Carrier	A_1S Carrier
S	SS Affected	SS Affected

Homozygous

Parent Hb S/S (columns); HbA_1/A_1 (rows)

Gametes	S	S
A_1	A_1S Carrier	A_1S Carrier
A_1	A_1S Carrier	A_1S Carrier

Figure 38–5. Genetic transmission of sickle cell trait.

tion. Oral conceptives containing estrogen also are contraindicated because sickle cell anemia already predisposes the client to heart disease, and vascular occlusion may be intensified by the estrogen.

A better prognosis resulting from increasingly individualized, comprehensive prenatal care will give these clients more alternatives with respect to childbearing decisions. In the past, recommendations for terminating the pregnancy might have been made to protect the mother's life and health. With the newer perinatal perspective, however, these high-risk mothers are identified and managed early and comprehensively. The possibilities of good outcomes for mother and infant are increasing with this type of meticulous management.

Nursing and Collaborative Assessment. The health history is an important assessment tool in caring for pregnant women with sickle cell anemia. Complications that the client has experienced should be documented in the history. During prenatal visits, the nurse should carefully investigate all problems that have arisen. Review of old information or new teaching concerning the disease is important to establish the client's knowledge. The client also should be assessed for nausea and vomiting, which may result in dehydration.

The nurse assists in many diagnostic tests and often may interpret the results of the test to the client. In most instances, the diagnosis of sickle cell anemia will have been made prior to pregnancy. A sickling test or Sickledex is commonly used for screening purposes. If the test is positive, hemoglobin electrophoresis is necessary to differentiate between the homozygous and heterozygous forms of the disease and to determine the percentage of abnormal hemoglobin.

Throughout the pregnancy, maternal and fetal assessments are made frequently. Urine cultures should be obtained monthly even if the mother is asymptomatic because of her predisposition to urinary tract infections. Fetal well-being must be assessed frequently to identify any difficulties. The nonstress test is a convenient and accurate technique to assess fetal well-being in this situation. A nonreactive stress test indicates the need for further evaluation. Placental function tests such as serum estriol levels may be indicated. Placental dysfunction resulting from placental infarction is common in clients with sickle cell anemia. Placental infarction can result in stillbirth and preterm labor.

The problems associated with sickle cell anemia may be exacerbated by the stress of labor. The increased need for oxygen by the cells may increase the risk of a painful sickle cell crisis. Determination of hemoglobin and hematocrit levels is important to the accurate assessment of this situation. The hemoglobin level should not be allowed to drop below 7 g/dL or the hematocrit level below 20 percent.[48] These women are also at risk for congestive heart failure because of numerous occlusions of pulmonary arteries by sickled cells. Cardiac enlargement often results.[49] Vital signs should be assessed, along with signs of dyspnea, cyanosis, and edema.

The risk of infection for the client with sickle cell anemia is increased in both the intrapartum and postpartum periods. Anemia results in improper oxygenation of tissues, allowing bacteria to become established. The client should be assessed for urinary tract infections, pyelonephritis, and pneumonia, which are frequently complications of sickle cell anemia.

During the postpartum period, the nurse should also carefully assess for thrombophlebitis, which may result from the increased viscosity of sickle cells. Each leg should be checked for Homan's sign and the calves assessed for reddened areas.

Nursing and Collaborative Management. One of the first concerns of management is counseling of the pregnant family. Counseling includes emphasizing the importance of attending all prenatal visits. It also focuses on optimal nutrition and the need for rest. The nurse should teach the mother the importance of avoiding symptom-relief measures that are generally acceptable to sickle cell clients except during pregnancy. In particular, pain medications must be prescribed by a physician; home or over-the-counter remedies should not be used.

Folic acid supplementation is needed because of the greatly increased production of red blood cells during pregnancy. Iron therapy may not be prescribed as iron deficiency is not characteristic of the disease. Careful monitoring for infection is of utmost importance because infection is a stressor leading to vascular stasis. Fluid intake should be encouraged to prevent dehydration. If a crisis occurs, immediate hospitalization is generally required to reduce the risk of morbidity.

Prophylactic exchange transfusion of red blood cells to prevent maternal and fetal complications remains controversial. This technique results in withdrawal of 75 to 85 percent of the recipient's blood and injection of an equal amount of donor blood. The end result is a decrease in the concentration of hemoglobin that sickles. The pregnant client exists on normal transfused cells rather than her own abnormal hemoglobin. Severe complications can occur, however, incuding maternal and neonatal hepatitis, hemolytic disease of the newborn, and sensitization of the mother. At present, it appears that this treatment is best reserved for clients with worsening anemia, infection, or cardiovascular insufficiency rather than for prophylactic use.[46, 50]

The anemia associated with sickle cell disease often results in a painful labor.[51] Support provided by the nurse or significant other in constant attendance by the bedside is important. Use of psychoprophylactic techniques to cope with contractions is helpful. Use of analgesics also may be indicated to decrease discomfort. An epidural can be offered in most situations. Oxygen is given continuously to decrease any risk of hypoxia to the fetus. The client should also be adequately hydrated with intravenous solutions. Blood should be typed and cross-matched in advance so that transfusions are available as needed. Strict aseptic technique must be used during delivery to prevent infection. Broad-spectrum antibiotics often are given prophylactically. The pediatrician or neonatologist and high-risk nursery should be notified when labor commences so that they are available if problems develop.

The mother is monitored during the postpartum period because recovery is often prolonged. The risks of further pregnancies also must be explained to the woman and her partner.

Hemoglobin C Disease. Other hemoglobinopathies may result in complications during pregnancy. This is particularly a problem if the hemoglobinopathy is combined with sickle cell trait. In **hemoglobin C disease,** lysine replaces glutamine at position 6 on the beta chain. As a result, the amount of normal hemoglobin is reduced. Rarely does a woman inherit two genes for hemoglobin C production. In about 1 in 2000 pregnancies, however, a black woman inherits sickle cell hemoglobin C disease.[2]

As with sickle cell anemia, this condition increases the rate of perinatal mortality resulting from spontaneous abortion and pneumonitis caused by embolization of necrotic bone marrow. Successful pregnancy outcome in women with sickle cell-hemoglobin C disease increases significantly with individualized prenatal care.[52]

Thalassemia. **Thalassemia** is a form of anemia that results from an alteration in the gene that normally controls the rate of the polypeptide chain synthesis. Either alpha or beta chains may be involved, leading to alpha or beta thalassemia. A hypochromic, microcytic anemia results.[37] Symptoms vary significantly depending on whether the homozygous or heterozygous form is present. Individuals who are heterozygous for alpha or beta thalassemia are said to have thalassemia minor. Individuals who are homozygous for alpha or beta thalassemia are said to have thalassemia major. Persons of Mediterranean, Central African, or Asian descent are most frequently affected.

The most commonly encountered thalassemia condition is sickle-beta thalassemia, in which sickle cell trait is combined with an underproduction of normal beta chains of hemoglobin. Clinical manifestations of this disorder vary depending on the differing proportions of sickle cell trait and the beta chains. The course of this condition in pregnancy is similar to that of sickle cell-hemoglobin C disease.

Homozygous alpha thalassemia is generally not compatible with life and results in intrauterine death. Homozygous beta thalassemia (Cooley's anemia) is a severe form of anemia, and persons with this condition rarely survive to the reproductive years. Pregnancy in such women has not been reported as those who do survive to the reproductive years are usually sterile.

Heterozygous thalassemia of either the alpha or the beta type is not a serious condition. Affected clients have no unusual fertility problems and their pregnancies follow a normal course.[38] Heterozygous beta thalassemia is the form of thalassemia most commonly found in pregnant women. For this reason, assessment and management for heterozygous beta thalassemia are discussed here.

Nursing and Collaborative Assessment. The client is assessed for an increase in hemoglobin A_2 and in hemoglobin F. Hemoglobin A_2 increases 3.5 percent above normal and hemoglobin F increases 2 to 5 percent with heterozygous beta thalassemia. A mean corpuscular volume less than 80 indicates that the client should be further assessed through electrophoresis. Prenatal nutritional assessment also is important for these clients, as they are at risk for iron deficiency.[36]

Nursing and Collaborative Management. Mothers with heterozygous beta thalassemia are considered low- to moderate-risk depending on the degree of anemia present. They are managed similarly to all normal pregnant women. When placed on iron supplementation, clients with anemia caused by beta thalassemia do not respond to the supplementation. This is one way in which heterozygous beta thalassemia is differentiated from other anemias. Hemoglobin A_2 levels should be rechecked again in 2 to 4 weeks.[36]

Thyroid Disorders

Thyroid disease is quite common in women. Estimated prevalence rates for hyperthyroidism and hypothyroidism approximate 1 to 2 percent for both conditions.[53] When caring for pregnant clients with thyroid disease, the following principles should be kept in mind:

1. Signs and symptoms of a diseased thyroid can be mimicked by the pregnancy itself.
2. Pregnancy alters standard thyroid function tests.
3. Placental transfer of most thyroid hormones is minimal.
4. Antithyroid drugs are easily passed to the fetus.

Hyperthyroidism. Hyperthyroidism is the second most common endocrine disorder in pregnancy next to diabetes. It occurs in approximately 1 in every 1500 pregnancies. Assessment of thyroid function is somewhat difficult during pregnancy as the pregnancy itself results in physiologic changes indicative of hyperthyroidism. The gland enlarges by about 50 percent during the prenatal period. Other changes include increased basal metabolic rate. By term, the pregnant woman's basal metabolic rate has increased by approximately 25 percent.[54]

In severe cases, hyperthyroidism causes anovulation and infertility. As the woman's metabolism increases with hyperthyroidism, so does metabolism of secreted sex hormones. Additionally, excessive synthesis of a globulin that binds the sex hormones eventually decreases blood concentrations of these hormones and, therefore, their availability.[40] In milder cases, hyperthyroidism increases the incidence of premature delivery and postpartum hemorrhage as all metabolic processes are increased. Burrow[55] also documents the increases in number of low-birth-weight infants and in neonatal mortality in pregnant women with hyperthyroidism.

Nursing and Collaborative Assessment. Symptoms of hyperthyroidism indicate the need for further diagnostic assessment. These symptoms include tachycardia, weakness, increased appetite, heat intolerance, sweating, enlarged thyroid, exophthalmos, increased nervousness, weight loss, and fine tremors. The woman may also demonstrate pronounced palmar erythema and resting pulse rate greater than 100 beats per minute, a wide pulse pressure, and atrial arrhythmias. Radioactive iodine cannot be used in testing or as a therapeutic agent because it may affect the functioning of the fetal thyroid gland. Laboratory tests will indicate an increased basal metabolic rate and increased serum thyroxine level. Laboratory analysis for hyperthyroidism includes measurement of circulating levels of T_4 (thyroxine) and resin T_3 (triiodothyronine) uptake to obtain a rough estimate of the metabolically active T_4. The normal value for free thyroxine index is 3 μg/dL (range: 1.8 to 4.2 μg/dL).[56]

Nursing and Collaborative Management. Hyperthyroidism in pregnancy can be treated with antithyroid drugs or surgery. With either method of treatment, the client's condition must first be controlled with medical therapy to avoid any risk of thyroid storm.[55] Thyroid storm is a rare occurrence in which the client presents with an extremely high fever, severe dehydration, sweating, tachycardia, and possible heart failure. Further, the woman may appear confused and disoriented. The drug of choice during pregnancy is propylthiouracil (Box 38–1) rather than methimazole, another drug commonly used to treat hyperthyroidism. Some evidence links methimazole with aplasia cutis (defective development of the scalp) in the newborns of treated women. Propylthiouracil crosses the placenta less readily than methimazole.[57] As a result, fewer problems with hypothyroidism would be expected in the fetus.

Fetal hypothyroidism is the major concern in managing the pregnant hyperthyroid client, as it is possible that the antithyroid drugs will cross the placenta and block the development and function of the fetal thyroid gland. At present, the best method to prevent this occurrence seems to be maintenance of

BOX 38–1. PROPYLTHIOURACIL (PTU)

Classification:
Antithyroid agent.

Action:
Inhibits synthesis of thyroid hormones by interfering with incorporation of iodine; has no effect on hormone already formed.

Indications:
Palliative treatment of hyperthyroidism.

Dosage and Route:
Administered orally only. *Initial dose:* 300–450 mg divided three times daily for 2 months. Clients with severe disease may require 600–1200 mg per day. *Maintenance dose:* 100–150 mg divided three times daily. *Thyrotoxic crisis:* 200 mg every 4–6 hours on Day 1; then gradually reduce dose to maintenance level.

Pharmacokinetics:
Absorption: Rapidly absorbed from GI tract after oral ingestion, with peak serum concentrations occurring 1–1.5 hours after the dose. *Distribution:* Highly concentrated in thyroid gland. Crosses the placenta and small portion of dose distributes into breast milk. *Elimination:* Metabolized in liver and excreted in urine with half-life of 1–2 hours.

Contraindications and Precautions:
Use with caution in clients older than 40 and with other drugs known to cause agranulocytosis. May induce goiter and hypothyroidism in fetus; thus value of drug therapy should be evaluated in pregnancy. Breastfeeding not recommended while on propylthiouracil therapy.

Adverse Reactions:
Most common: Rash, urticaria, pruritis, hair loss, skin pigmentation. *Less common:* GI—nausea, vomiting, loss of taste; MS—arthralgia, myalgia; CNS—drowsiness, vertigo; hematologic—agranulocytosis, granulocytopenia, thrombocytopenia, hypoprothrombinemia; other—drug fever, lupuslike syndrome.

Drug Interactions:
Warfarin: Propylthiouracil may potentiate its effect.

Nursing Implications:

1. Teach client to administer drug at the same time each day relative to meals.
2. Drug may be withdrawn 2 to 3 weeks before delivery to prevent excess drug passage across placenta.
3. Monitor neonatal thyroid function closely if mother breastfeeds.

GI = gastrointestinal, MS = musculoskeletal, CNS = central nervous system.
Nursing Implications are adapted from Govoni LE, Hayes JE. Drugs and Nursing Implications. *6th ed. Norwalk, Conn: Appleton & Lange; 1988:1007–1008.*

the client on as low a dosage of antithyroid medication as possible, so that thyroid function values are in the lower range of what is considered normal for a nonpregnant woman.[58] Newborns of hyperthyroid mothers should undergo thyroid screening to diagnose and treat any hypothyroidism. Monitoring the cord blood of these newborns is a means of quickly obtaining results.

Another concern for the fetus is hyperthyroidism. This occurs in about 1 percent of fetuses whose mothers experience hyperthyroidism.[55] Hyperthyroidism occurs as a result of the transfer of high titers of thyroid-stimulating immunoglobulins from mother to fetus.[59] Again, thyroid function tests should be performed on the newborn immediately after birth and if clinically indicated by the observation of irritability or tachycardia in the neonate over the next several weeks.

A subtotal thyroidectomy to remove part of the woman's malfunctioning thyroid may also be initiated for treatment of hyperthyroidism. The surgery removes the need for propylthiouracil drug therapy but does present some problems of its own. First, surgery is always a risk to an individual, but the risk is compounded by the presence of a fetus.[60] Second, risks associated with subtotal thyroidectomy, such as laryngeal nerve paralysis and hypoparathyroidism, are rare but disabling. Burrow[55] suggests that surgery be reserved for those instances of hypersensitivity to antithyroid drugs or cases in which drug therapy is ineffective. After surgery, the client must be carefully assessed for hypothyroidism. If laboratory values indicate the presence of decreased thyroid functioning, thyroxine replacement therapy should begin.

The literature[61–63] discusses a syndrome of transient postpartum hyperthyroidism followed by transient hypothyroidism with spontaneous recovery in most instances. A Japanese survey[62] found this to occur in 5.5 percent of the postpartum population. Interestingly, women experiencing this syndrome may have been misdiagnosed as having postpartum depression or excessive anxiety. A physical examination during the hyperthyroid stage reveals a small goiter in about 50 percent of the cases and laboratory tests reveal elevated thyroid hormones. Both stages usually last 1 to 2 months although the hyperthyroid phase occasionally is longer. Sometimes, drug therapy is required. Surgery should be avoided because of the transient nature of the illness.[55]

Antithyroid drugs are transferred to the infant through breast milk. Although less propylthiouracil appears to transfer than does methimazole,[64] breastfeeding while on antithyroid medication is controversial and most practitioners are against it. A recent study by Lamberg and others[64] concluded, however, that breastfeeding can be allowed if the client is maintained on a low dosage of propylthiouracil and neonatal thyroid function is closely monitored.

Hypothyroidism. Hypothyroidism in pregnancy is quite rare as this condition generally results in infertility until treated. The general metabolic depression characteristic of hypothyroidism affects the reproductive system, resulting in anovulation. In milder forms of the condition, however, conception can occur.

Consequences of maternal hypothyroidism include a higher-than-expected incidence of spontaneous abortion and stillbirth. An increased frequency of congenital anomalies also has been suggested, but this is not universally accepted. The reason for any increased perinatal mortality or fetal anomalies is unclear, because the fetal thyroid functions independently of the maternal system and transfer of thyroid hormone through the placenta is minimal. Fetal effects include spontaneous abortion, fetal goiter, cretinism, and fetal anomalies. Newborns are now routinely screened to detect low thyroxine levels.

The usual symptoms of hypothyroidism may be difficult to distinguish from physiologic changes in pregnancy. Typical symptoms include fatigue, weight gain, dry skin, constipation, and cold intolerance. If these clinical signs are present or the maternal history is suggestive of hypothyroidism, thyroid function studies should be done. These include T_4, T_3, and thyroid-stimulating hormone levels. The laboratory diagnosis of hypothyroidism is made if the T_4 level is between 4 and 8 μg/dL, like that found in the normal nonpregnant woman. The hypothyroid pregnant woman also demonstrates a reduction in T_3 resin uptake (less than 20 percent) to a level lower than that found in the normal pregnant woman. The thyroid-stimulating hormone level is higher than normal.[56] Testing to determine uptake of radioactive iodine is contraindicated, as radioactive iodine is also taken up by the fetal thyroid and may cause fetal anomalies.

Nursing and Collaborative Management. Treatment of hypothyroidism consists of supplemental hormone replacement. Serum levels of thyroid hormones should be restored to normal. (*See* Appendix C for normal values.) There is no evidence to suggest that replacement therapy with thyroid medication suppresses fetal thyroid function. Most evidence indicates that thyroid hormones do not cross the placenta in significant amounts.[38]

In general, infants of hypothyroid mothers are born healthy, without evidence of thyroid dysfunction; however, congenital hypothyroidism should be assessed during the neonatal period, as it may result in mental retardation.[65]

A woman receiving thyroid replacement therapy can still breastfeed, as only minimal amounts of thyroid hormone are passed to the infant through breast milk. These minimal amounts have little effect on the infant.

SUMMARY

Several high-risk maternal conditions are of particular concern during the first trimester of pregnancy. Some of these conditions may arise during the first trimester; others may have existed before pregnancy and first come to the attention of the nurse in risk assessment during the first trimester.

Hemorrhagic conditions include spontaneous abortions and ectopic pregnancy. Spontaneous abortions may be threatened, inevitable, complete, incomplete, missed, or habitual. Management will depend on the type of abortion. Ectopic pregnancy is a leading cause of maternal mortality during pregnancy. The majority of ectopic pregnancies occur in the fallopian tube, which may rupture with possible severe hemorrhage. Pain and bleeding or spotting are common findings, but many women with ectopic pregnancies are asymptomatic until rupture.

Metabolic conditions during the first trimester include hyperemesis gravidarum, anemia, and thyroid disorders. Hyperemesis gravidarum refers to excessive and prolonged vomiting and is marked by its severity as different from routine nausea and vomiting of pregnancy. Whereas hyperemesis may be life threatening to the mother, the fetus seems not to be affected.

Anemic states during pregnancy are of two types: deficiency anemias, such as iron deficiency anemia or folic acid deficiency anemia, and hemoglobinopathies, which are hereditary in nature. The latter include sickle cell anemia, hemoglobin

C disease, and thalassemia. Genetic counseling is a component of management of hemoglobinopathies.

Hyperthyroidism or hypothyroidism also may occur during the first trimester. Hyperthyroidism occurs in approximately 1 in 1500 pregnancies, but is difficult to diagnose as symptoms mimic signs of pregnancy. Hypothyroidism, on the other hand, is rare during pregnancy, as women with this condition are generally infertile.

REVIEW QUESTIONS

1. Define and describe three types of spontaneous abortion.
2. Describe two symptoms that are indicative of an ectopic pregnancy.
3. Discuss four principles guiding nursing care for a client experiencing hyperemesis gravidarum.
4. Describe three nursing considerations for a pregnant woman with sickle cell anemia.
5. List three effects on the fetus of maternal hyperthyroidism during pregnancy.

REFERENCES

1. Beard R, et al. Miscarriage or abortion. *Lancet.* 1985;2:1122–1123.
2. Cunningham FG, et al. *Williams Obstetrics.* 18th ed. Norwalk, Conn: Appleton & Lange; 1989.
3. Rommey S, et al. *Gynecology and Obstetrics: The Health Care of Women.* 2nd ed. New York: McGraw-Hill; 1981.
4. Strobino B, et al. Characteristics of women with recurrent spontaneous abortions and women with favorable reproductive histories. *Am J Public Health.* 1986;76:986–991.
5. Zacharias JF. The new genetics. *J Obstet Gynecol Neonat Nurs.* 1990;19:122–131.
6. Guerrero R, Rojas O. Spontaneous abortion and aging of human ova and spermatozoa. *N Engl J Med.* 1975;293:573.
7. Committee on the Biological Effects of Ionizing Radiation. *The Effects on Population of Exposure to Low Levels of Ionizing Radiation.* Washington, DC: National Academy Press; 1980.
8. Selevan S, et al. A study of occupational exposure to antineoplastic drugs and fetal loss in nurses. *JAMA.* 1985;313:1173–1179.
9. Morgan R, et al. Fetal loss and work in a waste treatment plant. *Am J Public Health.* 1984;74:499–501.
10. Lind T, McFadyen I. Human pregnancy failure. *Lancet.* 1986;1:91–92.
11. Gilbert ES, Harmon JS. *High Risk Pregnancy and Delivery.* St. Louis, Mo: CV Mosby; 1986.
12. Gaffney KF. Prenatal maternal attachment. *Image.* 1988;20:106–109.
13. Chodorow N. *The Reproduction of Mothering.* Berkeley: University of California Press; 1978.
14. Wall-Haas C. Women's perceptions of first trimester spontaneous abortion. *J Obstet Gynecol Neonat Nurs.* 1985;14:50–53.
15. Swanson-Kauffman K. Caring in the instance of unexpected early pregnancy loss. *Top Clin Nurs.* 1986;8:37–46.
16. Hardin S, Urbanus P. Reflections on a miscarriage. *Matern Child Nurs J.* 1986;15:23–30.
17. Hutti M. An exploratory study of the miscarriage experience. *Health Care Women Int.* 1986;7:371–389.
18. Gardner S, Merenstein G. Perinatal grief and loss: an overview. *Neonat Network.* Oct 1986:7–15.
19. Wilson AL, et al. The next baby: parents' responses to perinatal experiences subsequent to a stillbirth. *J. Perinatol.* 1988;8:188–192.
20. Stephany T. Early miscarriage: are we too quick to dismiss the pain? *RN.* 1982;49:89.
21. Lavy G, DeCherney A. Identifying tubal ectopic pregnancy. *Hosp Med.* 1987;23:23–38.
22. Gemzell C, et al. Ectopic pregnancy following treatment with human gonadotropins. *Am J Obstet Gynecol* 1982;143:761–765.
23. Osguthorpe N. Ectopic pregnancy. *J Obstet Gynecol Neonat Nurs.* 1987;16:36–41.
24. Patrick J. Ectopic pregnancy. *Top Emerg Med.* 1985;7:27–31.
25. Weeks LR. Ectopic pregnancy: current clinical trends, a fifteen year study. *J Natl Med Assoc.* 1981;73:823–833.
26. Tanaha T, et al. Treatment of interstitial ectopic pregnancy with methotrexate: report of a successful case. *Fertil Steril.* 1982;37:851–852.
27. Ory S, et al. Conservative treatment of ectopic pregnancy with methotrexate. *Am J Obstet Gynecol.* 1986;154:1299–1303.
28. Dorfman S, et al. Ectopic pregnancy mortality, United States 1979 to 1980: clinical aspects. *Obstet Gynecol.* 1984;64:386–390.
29. Kuczynski HJ. Support for the woman with an ectopic pregnancy. *J Obstet Gynecol Neonat Nurs.* 1986;15:306–310.
30. Devore N, Baldwin K. Ectopic pregnancy on the rise. *Am J Nurs.* 1986;86:674–678.
31. Depue RH, et al. Hyperemesis gravidarum in relation to estradiol levels, pregnancy outcome, and other maternal factors: a seroepidemiologic study. *Am J Obstet Gynecol.* 1987;156:1137–1141.
32. Soules MR, et al. Nausea and vomiting of pregnancy: role of human chorionic gonadotropin and 17-hydroxyprogesterone. *Obstet Gynecol.* 1980;55:696.
33. Wolkind S, Zajicek. Psychosocial correlates of nausea and vomiting in pregnancy. *J Psychosomat Res.* 1978;22:1–5.
34. Lugo E, Tominey T. The adverse effects of utilizing altitude-inappropriate fetal growth curves. *J Perinatol.* 1989;9:147–149.
35. Winick M. *Nutrition, Pregnancy, and Early Infancy.* Baltimore: Williams & Wilkins; 1989.
36. Angelini DJ, et al. *Perinatal/Neonatal Nursing: A Clinical Handbook.* Boston: Blackwell Scientific; 1986.
37. Bullock B, Rosendahl P. *Pathophysiology: Adaptations and Alterations in Function.* 2nd ed. Boston: Little, Brown; 1988.
38. Abrams RS, Wexler P, eds. *Medical Care of the Pregnant Patient.* Boston: Little, Brown; 1983.

39. Queenan J, ed. *Management of High-Risk Pregnancy.* Oradell, NJ: Medical Economics; 1985.
40. Groer MW, Shekleton ME. *Basic Pathophysiology: A Conceptual Approach.* 2nd ed. St. Louis, Mo: CV Mosby; 1983.
41. Danforth DN. *Obstetrics and Gynecology.* 4th ed. Philadelphia: Harper & Row; 1982.
42. Whaley LF, Wong DL. *Nursing Care of Infants and Children.* 3rd ed. St. Louis, Mo: CV Mosby; 1987.
43. Blattner P, et al. Pregnancy outcome in women with sickle cell trait. *JAMA.* 1977;238:1392.
44. Pastorek JG, Seiler BS. Maternal death associated with sickle cell trait. *Am J Obstet Gynecol.* 1985;151:295–297.
45. Jennings JC. Hemoglobinopathies in pregnancy. *Am Fam Physician.* 1977;15:104–110.
46. Powars DR, et al. Pregnancy in sickle cell disease. *Obstet Gynecol.* 1986;67:217–228.
47. Webb JB. Sickle cell disease in obstetrics. *Practitioner.* 1982;226:89–94.
48. Ship-Horowitz L. Nursing care of the sickle cell anemic patient in labor. *J Obstet Gynecol Neonat Nurs.* 1983;12: 381–386.
49. Karayalcin G, et al. Sickle cell anemia—clinical manifestations in 100 patients and review of the literature. *Am J Med Sci.* 1975;269:51–65.
50. Miller J, et al. Management of sickle hemoglobinopathies in pregnant patients. *Am J Obstet Gynecol.* 1981;141:237–241.
51. Richardson EA, Milne LS. Sickle cell disease and the childbearing family: an update. *Am J Matern Child Nurs.* 1983; 8:417–422.
52. Milner PF, et al. Outcome of pregnancy in sickle cell anemia and sickle cell-hemoglobin C disease. *Am J Obstet Gynecol.* 1980;138:239–245.
53. Gleicher N. *Principles of Medical Therapy in Pregnancy.* New York: Plenum Medical Books; 1985.
54. Guyton AC. *Textbook of Medical Physiology.* 7th ed. Philadelphia: WB Saunders; 1986.
55. Burrow GN. The management of thyrotoxicosis in pregnancy. *N Engl J Med.* 1985;313:562–565.
56. Pernoll ML, Benson EC, eds. *Current Obstetric & Gynecologic Diagnosis and Treatment.* Norwalk, Conn: Appleton & Lange; 1987.
57. Rosen H. Treatment of thyrotoxicosis in pregnancy. *N Engl J Med.* 1986;314:849.
58. Momotani N, et al. Antithyroid drug therapy for Graves' disease during pregnancy. *N Engl J Med.* 1986;315:24–28.
59. Zakarija M, McKenzie JM. Pregnancy-associated changes in the thyroid-stimulating antibody of Graves' disease and the relationship to neonatal hyperthyroidism. *J Clin Endocrinol Metab.* 1987;57:1036–1040.
60. Burrow GN. Thyroid diseases. In: Burrow GN, Ferris TF. *Medical Complications During Pregnancy.* 3rd ed. Philadelphia: WB Saunders; 1988:224–253.
61. Gossain VV, et al. Recurrent transient hyperthyroidism and hypothyroidism associated with pregnancy. *South Med J.* 1983;76:808–810.
62. Amino N, et al. Transient recurrence of hyperthyroidism after delivery in Graves' disease. *J Clin Endocrinol Metab.* 1977;44:130–136.
63. Ginsberg J. Walfish PG. Postpartum transient thyrotoxicosis with painless thyroiditis. *Lancet.* 1977;1:1125–1128.
64. Lamberg B, et al. Antithyroid treatment of maternal hyperthyroidism during lactation. *Clin Endocrinol.* 1984;21:81–87.
65. American Academy of Pediatrics. Newborn screening for congenital hypothyroidism: recommended guidelines. *Pediatrics.* 1987;80:745.

Maternal Conditions in the Second and Third Trimesters

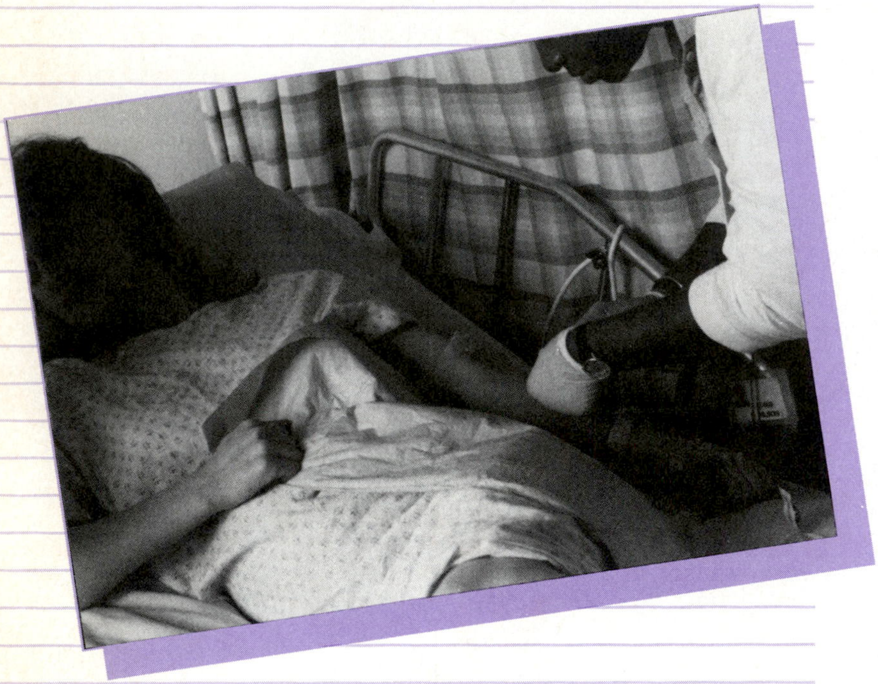

chapter 39

Key Terms

abruptio placentae
cerclage
chorioamnionitis
Couvelaire uterus
deep venous thrombosis
disseminated intravascular coagulation
eclampsia
HELLP syndrome
hydatidiform mole
incompetent cervix
placenta previa
polyhydramnios
pre-eclampsia
pregnancy-induced hypertension
preterm birth
preterm labor
proteinuria
postterm pregnancy
oligohydramnios
Rh isoimmunization
superficial thrombophlebitis
uteroplacental apoplexy

Most women experience normal pregnancy, deliver healthy infants, and suffer no ill effects. Pregnancy is, nonetheless, a period of heightened vulnerability. All body systems are affected by pregnancy. Nurses working with prenatal clients should know the signs and symptoms associated with low-risk pregnancy and recognize those outside the range of normal. Table 39–1 lists the common danger signs of pregnancy that nurses and their clients need to know. Once conditions are recognized, nurses are involved actively in their management.

Numerous high-risk maternal conditions are associated with adverse fetal and maternal outcomes. Some are associated with pregnancy—for example, pregnancy-induced hypertension, bleeding disorders in pregnancy, premature labor, intrauterine growth retardation, multiple gestation, and postmaturity. Others result from concurrent medical problems—for example, all types of infection, chronic hypertension, cardiac disease, and diabetes mellitus, though diabetes may only emerge during pregnancy. In general, the nurse must remember that pregnant women can experience the same medical or surgical problems as their nonpregnant agemates. In such cases fetal well-being is potentially in jeopardy.

Under optimal conditions pregnancy is a period of psychologic upheaval, taxing the woman's and her family's ability to adapt.[1] Every high-risk condition has psychosocial implications for the client and her family. The client's high-risk status can affect her lifestyle, her stress level, and the status of the newborn. In addition, the frequent assessments necessary in high-risk pregnancy are constant reminders that problems exist. The nurse can assist the family to adapt to the high-risk situation and to participate in therapies that will promote a positive outcome for mother and neonate.

Nursing strategies always include an emphasis on psychosocial as well as physiologic aspects of client care. For conceptual ease, specific high-risk conditions occurring during the second and third trimesters of pregnancy are discussed in this chapter. Psychosocial implications of high-risk pregnancy are discussed in Chapter 36.

HYPERTENSIVE DISORDERS

Hypertensive disorders of pregnancy are the leading medical causes of maternal deaths in the United

TABLE 39–1. SIGNS AND SYMPTOMS THAT INDICATE THE DEVELOPMENT OF COMPLICATIONS DURING PREGNANCY

Burning on urination, flank pain
Hematuria
Chills, fever, or other signs of infection
Serous, bloody, or malodorous vaginal discharge
Genital lesions
Vomiting that persists beyond the first trimester or is severe
Visual disturbances
Edema of face or hands
Pedal edema on arising
Severe, frequent, or persistent headache
Epigastric or right upper quadrant pain
Unusual abdominal tenderness
Absence or slowing of fetal movements after quickening
Dyspnea
Hemoptysis
Seizures

States and Great Britain.[2,3] Approximately 10 percent of Americans have chronic hypertension. The incidence among blacks is two to three times that among whites. Hypertensive disorders of pregnancy may be pregnancy-induced; however, pregnancy may aggravate or be complicated by pre-existing hypertension.

Determining the Presence of Hypertension

Hypertension is operationally defined as a diastolic blood pressure of at least 90 mm Hg, a systolic pressure of at least 140 mm Hg, a rise in diastolic blood pressure of at least 15 mm Hg, or a rise in systolic pressure of 30 mm Hg. The change in blood pressure must be observed twice at least 6 hours apart.[2] Systolic pressure greater than 140 mm Hg is generally regarded as cause for concern.[2] Mean arterial pressure (MAP) is an indicator of cardiac work, because it measures the resistance against which the heart works. The MAP is calculated with the formula

$$MAP = DP + [(SP - DP)/3]$$

where SP refers to systolic pressure and DP refers to diastolic pressure. A rise in MAP of 20 mm Hg is ominous and a MAP of 100 is abnormal. A MAP of 105 indicates hypertension.[4] These determinations depend on a knowledge of baseline levels. The MAP decreases from the 8th through the 30th weeks of gestation. For that reason, baseline blood pressure should be established early in the first trimester.

Pregnancy-Induced Hypertension

Pregnancy-induced hypertension (PIH) refers to conditions characterized by an abnormal rise in blood pressure during pregnancy. The three categories of PIH are[5]:

1. Hypertension alone.
2. **Pre-eclampsia,** a disorder defined by pregnancy-induced hypertension, proteinuria, and/or generalized edema. Pre-eclampsia may be mild or severe, although there is no exact distinction between the two conditions. What appears to be mild pre-eclampsia can swiftly become a critical condition. The severity of PIH reflects the frequency and intensity of signs and symptoms summarized in Table 39–2.
3. **Eclampsia,** a critical condition in which pre-eclamptic signs are accompanied by convulsions precipitated by the PIH.

The categories of PIH range in severity from least to most severe, with the greatest morbidity and mortality associated with eclampsia. Historically, PIH has been referred to as "toxemia of pregnancy," reflecting a belief that it was caused by circulation of unknown toxins released by the products of conception. For decades the terminology used to refer to hypertensive disorders in pregnancy has been unclear. In 1972 the Committee on Terminology of the American College of Obstetricians and Gynecologists set forth a nomenclature, which has now become widely recognized (Table 39–3). More recent terms that are gaining popularity include gestational edema-proteinuria hypertensive disorders (GEPH) and EPH gestosis, which also refers to the three cardinal signs of pre-eclampsia: *e*dema, *p*roteinuria, and *h*ypertension.

TABLE 39–2. INDICATORS OF SEVERITY OF PREGNANCY-INDUCED HYPERTENSION

Abnormality	Mild	Severe
Diastolic blood pressure	< 100 mm Hg	110 mm Hg or higher
Proteinuria	Trace to 1+	Persistent 2+ or more
Headache	Absent	Present
Visual disturbances	Absent	Present
Upper abdominal pain	Absent	Present
Oliguria	Absent	Present
Convulsions	Absent	Present
Serum creatinine	Normal	Elevated
Thrombocytopenia	Absent	Present
Hyperbilirubinemia	Absent	Present
SGOT elevation	Minimal	Marked
Fetal growth retardation	Absent	Obvious
Hyperreflexia	Absent	Present

SGOT = serum glutamic-oxaloacetic transaminase.
From Cunningham GF, et al. Williams Obstetrics. *18th ed. Norwalk, Conn: Appleton & Lange; 1989:655.*

TABLE 39–3. CLASSIFICATION OF HYPERTENSIVE DISORDERS IN PREGNANCY

Gestational edema	General fluid accumulation in the tissues with 1+ edema after 12 hours in bed, or weight gain of 5 pounds in 1 week of pregnancy or postpartum
Gestational proteinuria	Presence of proteinuria during pregnancy or postpartum in the absence of edema or other pathology
Gestational hypertension	Development of hypertension during pregnancy or early postpartum in a normotensive woman, in the absence of pre-eclampsia or hypertensive vascular disease; normotensive values are restored within 10 days of delivery
Pre-eclampsia	Development of hypertension with proteinuria, edema, or both during pregnancy or postpartum; occurs after the 20th week of gestation, but in the event of trophoblastic disease, it may occur sooner
Eclampsia	Occurrence of one or more convulsions in a woman with pre-eclampsia, in the absence of other central nervous system pathology
Superimposed pre-eclampsia or eclampsia	Development of pre-eclampsia or eclampsia in a woman with chronic hypertensive, vascular, or renal disease
Chronic hypertensive disease	Persistent hypertension before pregnancy, before the 20th week of gestation in the absence of trophoblastic disease, or after the 42nd postpartum day
Unclassified hypertensive disorders	Disorders in which too little information is available to make a classification

Reproduced, with permission, from Page EW, Christianson R. Influence of blood pressure changes with and without proteinuria upon the outcome of pregnancy. Am J Obstet Gynecol. *1976;126:821.*

Pre-eclampsia complicates 6 to 8 percent of all pregnancies in the United States.[3] Twenty-five percent of pregnant women with chronic hypertension develop pre-eclampsia.[2] Among women of low socioeconomic status giving birth in public or teaching hospitals, the incidence of pre-eclampsia is 15 percent. Pre-eclampsia occurs most often among women with a predisposition for chronic hypertension. Blacks are affected more frequently than whites.

Pre-eclampsia is important because it is a major cause of perinatal and maternal mortality; it is often associated with intrauterine growth retardation; it is associated with an increased tendency toward mental retardation in surviving offspring[2]; and if detected and managed early, its negative impact may be minimized or avoided.

Theories of Causation. Over the years, numerous theories for the etiology of PIH have been proposed. Theories have attributed PIH to abnormal immunologic responses of the woman, hereditary factors, overall physiologic and psychologic stress, placental parasites, nutritional excesses or deficiencies (especially protein deficiency) and endocrine disturbances. To date, the actual cause of PIH remains unknown.[2,3,5–11]

Pathophysiologic Processes of Pregnancy-Induced Hypertension. Decreased levels of prostaglandins, unusual sensitivity to angiotensin II, impaired glomerular perfusion, and decreased uteroplacental perfusion are evident in pre-eclampsia. It is by no means clear in what sequence these processes take place.

The characteristic lesion in pre-eclampsia is a renal glomerular endothelial cell swelling with fibrin deposits. Glomerular capillary lumens become narrowed. Glomerular filtration is reduced. Renal tubules demonstrate ischemia and deposition of protein materials. Serum blood urea nitrogen (BUN) and creatinine levels rise, sodium is retained, and urine output decreases. The sodium retention may contribute to the increased sensitivity to angiotensin II that is observed and the increased extracellular fluid volume. In severe cases arterial thrombosis can lead to renal cortical necrosis. The glomerular lesions usually heal once the pregnancy ends, but some clients demonstrate glomerular damage even years later.[2]

Vasospasm, which disrupts circulation by alternating constriction and dilation, is basic to the disease process of pre-eclampsia and accounts for the development of arterial hypertension. Vasospasm takes place throughout the arterial system, including the arteries of major organs, such as the uterus and placenta. Over time the vascular walls are damaged. In clients experiencing PIH, angiotensin II, which normally is increased during pregnancy, but to which these individuals are more sensitive, makes intravascular endothelial cells contract, creating leaks through which platelets and fibrin pass to be deposited subendothelially. Injury to the blood vessels thus may decrease platelet and fibrinogen levels. Red blood cells may be damaged or destroyed as they move through narrowed parts of blood vessels.[12] Vascular changes and local tissue hypoxia account for the lesions, hemorrhage, infarction, and necrosis that have been observed in many organs throughout the body including the ocular retinas, the placenta, the liver, the lungs, and the brain. The progression of pre-eclampsia to eclampsia may be caused by the formation of cerebrovascular occlusion by these lesions. This can lead to cerebrovascular accident (stroke). Vascular damage accounts for the presence of abnormally high levels of protein in urine of clients with pre-eclampsia.

As in any hypertensive state, the workload of the heart is increased. Clients with pre-eclampsia do not demonstrate the typical pregnancy-related 2000-mL increase in blood volume, probably because of the contracted vascular bed and the increased vascular permeability and extravasation of fluid into the extravascular compartment. They experience hypovolemia and hemoconcentration. Feedback from pressoreceptors in the vital organs demands increasing cardiac output to ensure maintenance of homeostasis.

The presence of generalized edema reflects vascular damage, decreased glomerular filtration, and hypertension. Implications include the development of increased central nervous system irritability reflecting cerebral edema, the onset of retinal edema, the development of dyspnea related to pulmonary edema, and the onset of congestive heart failure. Right upper quadrant pain reflects liver distension resulting from obstructed blood flow.

Probably because of the leakage of blood components into the extravascular space, a consumptive coagulopathy similar to disseminated intravascular coagulation may be observed. This contributes to a heightened vulnerability to hemorrhage.

In severe PIH there may be an alteration in liver function. Hepatic edema, subcapsular edema, or hemorrhage may account for the right upper quadrant or epigastric pain in severe pre-eclampsia. This pain may indicate that convulsions are about to occur.[5] Placental vasospasm and the development of infarcts can result in intrauterine growth retardation and fetal hypoxia. Vasospasm of cerebral vasculature probably accounts for the persistent headaches or visual disturbances associated with severe pre-eclampsia.

Sequelae of PIH represent serious threats to maternal and fetal well-being. They include abruptio placentae, retinal detachment, acute renal failure, cardiac failure, cerebral hemorrhage, maternal death and fetal growth retardation, hypoxia, and death. About 70 percent of fetal deaths are due to large placental infarcts, markedly small placental size, and abruptio placentae.[12]

Symptoms subside as soon as the placenta is delivered. The vascular bed will dilate in early postpartum and the hematocrit will fall. These clients are unusually sensitive to blood loss at delivery.[5] It is important to note that pre-eclampsia as well as eclampsia can emerge intrapartally or postpartally, even if there were no evidence of symptoms prenatally. The first 48 hours after delivery is a period of great risk.

HELLP Syndrome. In some cases of pre-eclampsia, the client's course is complicated by a potentially fatal syndrom of *h*emolysis, *e*levated *l*iver enzymes, and *l*ow *p*latelet count, called the **HELLP syndrome.**[9,13,14] Its pathophysiology is depicted in Figure 39–1. Arteriolar vasospasm is the underlying factor in the sequence of events. The precise cause of hepatic failure is unknown, but it may be the formation of microemboli in the hepatic vasculature, causing ischemia and tissue damage. Delivery is the only definitive treatment for HELLP syndrome; however, the symptoms may persist for several days after delivery. Management of the altered hemodynamic status and clotting represents the major challenge in medical management of the HELLP syndrome.

Risk Factors. Several risk factors for PIH have been identified[3]:

1. *Parity.* Nulliparas are eight times more susceptible to pre-eclampsia than multiparas.
2. *Family history.* A 49-year prospective study demonstrated that there was a 38 percent incidence of PIH in sisters of women with PIH, a 25 percent incidence in daughters, and a 16 percent incidence among granddaughters.
3. *Multiple fetuses.* There is a fivefold to sixfold incidence of PIH in association with multiple fetuses.
4. *Diabetes.* Women with diabetes have an increased incidence of PIH.
5. *Trophoblastic disease.* Women with trophoblastic disease, for example hydatidiform mole, have a tenfold increase in risk of PIH.
6. *Fetal hydrops* (profound fetal edema reflecting fetal-maternal blood incompatibility). This is associated with a tenfold increase in incidence of PIH.
7. *Chronic hypertension and renal disease.* These increase risk of PIH and cause it to occur earlier than usual.
8. *Age.* Women younger than 16 or older than 35 are at increased risk.
9. *Malnutrition.*[11]

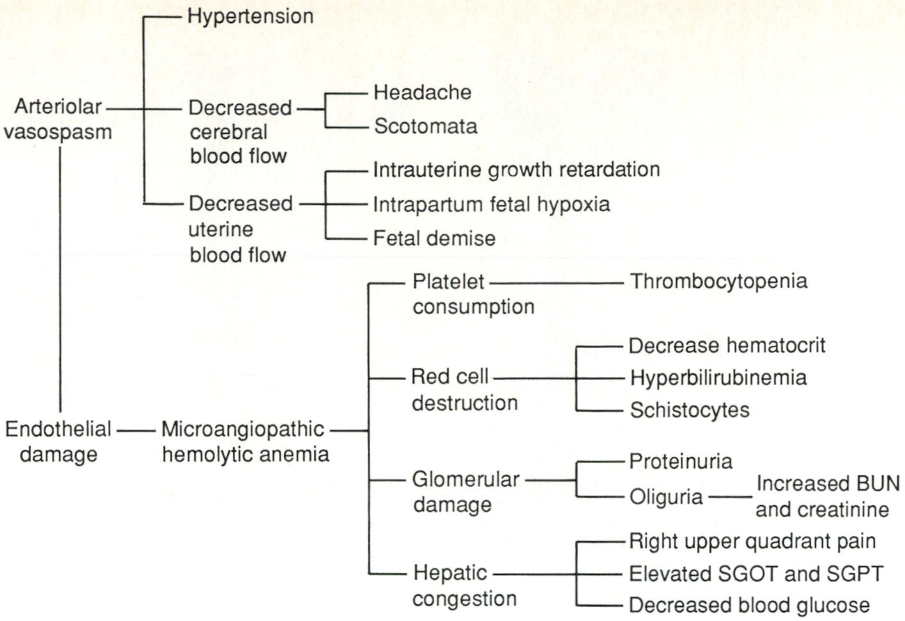

Figure 39–1. Physiologic alterations occurring in the HELLP syndrome. SGPT = serum glutamic-pyruvic transaminase. (*Reproduced, with permission, from Whittaker AA, et al. Hemolysis, elevated liver enzymes, and low platelet count syndrome. Nursing care of the critically ill obstetric patient.* Heart & Lung. *1986;15:402–408.*)

No body type or socioeconomic stratum is more likely to develop PIH, although poor women tend to experience pre-eclampsia of greater severity.[11]

Signs and Symptoms. Assessment is based on understanding of signs and symptoms of PIH. Signs and symptoms of PIH include the following parameters.

Blood Pressure. Identification of blood pressure elevation was described earlier.

Edema. Most pregnant women experience edema, even in their hands and faces; however, the degree of edema is not clearly associated with perinatal morbidity or mortality. About 85 percent of women develop some generalized edema during pregnancy, but only about 15 percent develop pre-eclampsia. Edema that occurs in association with hypertension or proteinuria indicates the pathophysiologic processes that are occurring.[2] The degree of edema does not correspond to the severity of pre-eclampsia. The criteria for assessing edema in pre-eclampsia, however, include the presence of dependent edema on arising, inability to remove rings from the fingers, and a weight gain exceeding 1.5 kg per month during the second trimester or 0.5 kg per week during the third trimester (Figure 39–2). Edema is described on a scale of 1+ to 4+, as explained in Table 39–4.

Proteinuria. Proteinuria is defined as the presence of 300 mg or more of protein in a 24-hour urine collection or a concentration of 1 g/L or more in at least two random samples collected at least 6 hours apart.[12] This is reflected in a 1+ to 2+ result with the standard turbidimetric (dipstick) method of testing. In contrast, trace protein in urine in the absence of hypertension, edema, or both represents a normal physiologic adaptation to pregnancy and is not a cause for concern. Proteinuria is a late sign in the course of the disease and its presence represents an increased risk of fetal mortality.

Impending Eclampsia. Pre-eclampsia may progress to eclampsia, a convulsive state. In severe cases clients may experience headache that is not relieved by analgesics, visual disturbances, right upper quadrant or epigastric pain, or vomiting, and may exhibit hyperreflexia, irritability, onset of fever, cyanosis, pulmonary edema, or oliguria.[2,5] These symptoms herald the progression of pre-eclampsia to eclampsia. Table 39–5 depicts common findings in impending eclampsia. As many as 25 percent of women developing seizures have demonstrated only so-called mild or even barely detectable symptoms of pre-eclampsia prior to the first convulsion; up to 14 percent of these women subsequently die. Additionally, 10 percent of eclamptic women have been reported to have their first seizure before proteinuria appears.[3] Detection is more difficult in adolescent clients because their blood pressure is normally lower than that of adult women, and they often delay prenatal care so that an early pregnancy baseline value cannot be established. A reading of 120/85 could actually be high in an adolescent.

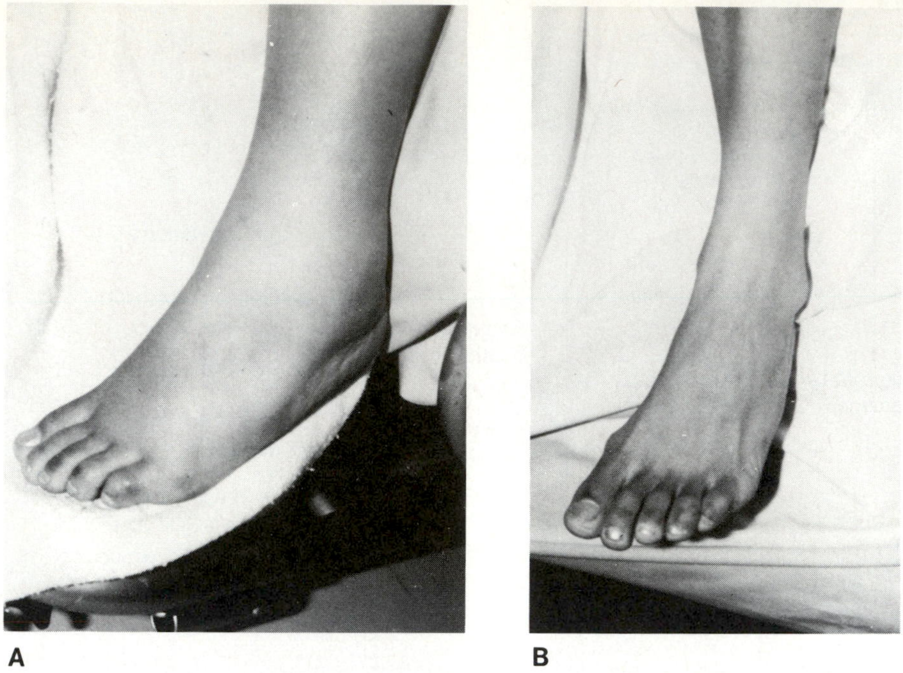

Figure 39–2. **A.** Severe edema in a young primigravida with antepartum eclampsia and a markedly reduced blood volume compared with normal pregnancy. **B.** The same woman 3 days after delivery. The remarkable clearance of pedal edema, accompanied by diuresis and a 28-pound weight loss, was spontaneous and unprovoked by any diuretic drug therapy. (*Reproduced, with permission, from Cunningham GF, et al.* Williams Obstetrics. *18th ed. Norwalk, Conn: Appleton & Lange; 1989:678.*)

Nursing and Collaborative Assessment. All clients are screened for signs and symptoms of pregnancy-induced hypertension at each prenatal visit, especially during the second and third trimesters. Chapters 14, 18, and 22 outlined routine assessment parameters during prenatal visits.

In assessing the client with pre-eclampsia, attention is focused on comparison of current blood pressure with previous blood pressure readings (repeat readings may be taken 15 minutes apart when elevated), the presence of protein in urine, presence and degree of edema (*see* Figure 39–2), pattern of weight gain, deep tendon reflexes, fetal growth, activity and heart rate, and presence of warning signs such as headache, visual disturbances, and right upper quadrant or epigastric pain. Serum glucose may be assessed, as diabetic clients have a higher incidence of pre-eclampsia than nondiabetic clients. Complete blood chemistry, serum liver and renal function tests, 24-hour urine collection for protein and creatinine clearance, and serial hematocrit levels are obtained. Screening for the presence of disseminated intravascular coagulopathy is also done. Blood specimens are sent for determination of prothrombin time, partial thromboplastin time, platelet count, fibrinogen levels, and the presence of fibrin split products. Laboratory findings in PIH are summarized in Table 39–6.

If the pre-eclamptic client is hospitalized, her sensorium and affect, vital signs, including blood pressure, pulse, respirations, and deep tendon reflexes, are assessed and recorded every 4 hours or more frequently if she is unstable. Fetal heart rate is recorded at the time maternal vital signs are assessed.

TABLE 39–4. ASSESSMENT OF PITTING EDEMA

1+	Edema is minimal at pedal and pretibial sites
2+	Edema of lower extremities is marked
3+	Edema is evident in face, hands, lower abdominal wall, and sacrum
4+	Generalized massive edema (anasarca) is evident with ascites (abdominal distension resulting from the accumulation of fluid in the peritoneal cavity)

TABLE 39–5. SIGNS AND SYMPTOMS OF IMPENDING ECLAMPSIA

Frontal or sometimes occipital headache unresponsive to analgesia
Epigastric or upper right quadrant pain
Nausea
Blurred vision; visual spots or "floaters" (perceived particles floating across the range of vision); other visual disturbances
Hyperirritability
Altered sensorium

TABLE 39–6. LABORATORY FINDINGS IN PREGNANCY-INDUCED HYPERTENSION

↑ Serum uric acid
↑ Blood urea nitrogen
↑ Serum creatinine
↓ Serum albumin
↓ Globulin
↑ Hematocrit
↓ Platelets
↑ SGOT (serum glutamic-oxaloacetic transaminase)
↑ SGPT (serum glutamic-pyruvic transaminase)
↑ Serum bilirubin
+ Burr cells (fragmented red blood cells)

Continuous fetal monitoring may be used to assess fetal status. The maternal lungs are assessed for rales, indicating pulmonary edema. Nail beds are assessed for cyanosis. The client is asked if she experiences any of the symptoms of pre-eclampsia, described previously. If the client is stable, a late night assessment may be eliminated in order not to interrupt her sleep.

Prior to term, fetal assessment for the pre-eclamptic client may include evaluation of fetal activity records, nonstress tests, contraction stress tests; ultrasound with Doppler studies of the placenta and fetal blood vessels; and biophysical profile. Tests for fetal maturity, such as amniocentesis for lecithin: sphingomyelin ratio and phosphatidylglycerol, may be performed in order to plan delivery. Some centers may still use serum or urinary estriol levels as indicators of fetal well-being, although most no longer use these tests.

Nursing and Collaborative Management. Early detection and management of PIH are associated with the greatest success in reducing risks and progression of this condition. Delivery is the most effective treatment for PIH. Management goals focus on maintaining pregnancy until the fetus is mature. In cases of severe pre-eclampsia or eclampsia, however, an immature neonate who receives excellent neonatal intensive care may have a better chance of survival than if not delivered.

Once the diagnosis of pre-eclampsia is confirmed, hospitalization is usually advised as pre-eclampsia can progress quickly. In some cases home management may be possible if a client is able to participate responsibly in her care and if she has a mild condition, eg, minor elevations of blood pressure, absence of proteinuria, disease that does not increase in severity, and no suspicion of fetal growth retardation.[5] The client and her family must understand the need for bedrest as indicated, must be able to recognize and report symptoms related to progression of the disease process, and must make certain that the client is assessed by her health care providers weekly, twice weekly, or as appropriate.

Modified bedrest in the left lateral position may be advised for the client with mild to moderate PIH. This position decreases pressure on the vena cava and is believed to improve venous return and placental and renal perfusion. With increased renal perfusion, excess fluid is mobilized, urine output increases, and blood pressure may stabilize or decrease. Dietary restrictions are no longer advised, and the client may follow a regular, well-balanced diet as tolerated.

Clients who have more than mild signs and symptoms of pre-eclampsia are hospitalized. Clients with severe pre-eclampsia are very ill and require careful observation. The client is kept on bedrest, although whether or not bedrest is complete will depend on her actual situation. The client is protected from central nervous system stimuli such as loud noise and bright light, which may aggravate central nervous system irritability. In some facilities the client is sedated; however, sedatives do not prevent seizures, can complicate assessment of the client's status, and, if oversedation occurs, can further compromise the fetus.[2]

Magnesium sulfate is the treatment of choice to prevent convulsions (Box 39–1).[15] Reflexes are assessed and blood levels of magnesium sulfate monitored to ensure that the therapeutic level is not exceeded. The client's respiratory status is monitored, as magnesium sulfate in excessive amounts can suppress respirations. The drug is usually withheld if the client's respiratory rate is less than 12 per minute.

When magnesium sulfate is prescribed, calcium gluconate must be available at the bedside to counter potential toxic effects. Maternity units are equipped with a "toxemia kit" containing medications, an airway, a suction catheter, and possibly a Foley urinary catheter kit to enable accurate measurement of intake and output in the event that seizures develop. This kit must be close at hand. It is checked and stocked as necessary each day. Likewise, the emergency cart and defibrillator are close at hand and checked daily.

If diastolic pressure exceeds 110 mm Hg, an antihypertensive drug, such as hydralazine, may be administered intravenously to lower diastolic pressure

BOX 39–1. MAGNESIUM SULFATE (EPSOM SALT, $MgSO_4$)

Classification:
Miscellaneous anticonvulsant.

Action:
Excess magnesium appears to decrease the amount of acetylcholine released by the motor nerve impulse, thereby depressing the CNS and producing anticonvulsant effects. It also acts peripherally to produce flushing, sweating, and decreased blood pressure.

Indications:
Prevention and control of seizures in severe pre-eclampsia or in eclampsia, control of seizure disorders associated with low plasma concentrations of magnesium, control of seizures and hypertension in children with acute nephritis.

Dosage and Route:
Administered IV or IM. For IM use, concentration should be 250 mg/mL or 500 mg/mL. For IV use, concentration should not exceed 200 mg/mL and rate should not exceed 150 mg/min. Severe pre-eclampsia or eclampsia (various doses have been used): 4 g in 250 mL 5 percent dextrose by IV infusion followed by 4–5 g IM into each buttock, and 4–5 g IM into alternate buttocks at 4-hour intervals as needed. Alternatively, after the initial IV dose, constant IV infusion of 1–2 g per hour can be used. Total dosage should not exceed 30–40 g daily. Serum and urine magnesium concentrations should be obtained to assess therapy.

Pharmacokinetics:
Absorption: Onset of action after IM administration occurs in about 1 hour and duration of action is 3–4 hours. *Distribution*: Crosses the placenta and into breast milk. *Elimination*: Excreted renally.

Contraindications and Precautions:
Use with caution in clients with impaired renal function. Contraindicated in clients with heart block or myocardial damage.

Adverse Reactions:
Result from magnesium intoxication (overdose). Flushing, sweating, hypotension, depressed reflexes, flaccid paralysis, hypothermia, circulatory collapse, depression of cardiac function, CNS depression, fetal respiratory paralysis.

Drug Interactions:

- Barbiturates, opiates, general anesthetics, and other CNS depressants: additive central depressant effects.
- Neuromuscular blocking agents: additive neuromuscular blocking effect; use concomitantly with extreme caution.

Nursing Implications:

- Assess for magnesium toxicity: absent or weak patellar reflex, respirations below 12 per minute, urinary output of 25–30 mL/per hour.
- Assess blood pressure and pulse every 15 minutes.
- Assess fetal heart rate every 15 minutes.
- Place resuscitation equipment in room.
- Place calcium gluconate or calcium gluceptate in room to be readily available if client displays magnesium toxicity.

CNS = central nervous system, IV = intravenous(ly), IM = intramuscular(ly).

to between 90 and 100 mm Hg. This is a short-term intervention. In PIH, placental perfusion is already compromised. Decreasing maternal blood pressure can further reduce placental perfusion and stress the fetus.[3] Fetal heart rate is monitored during therapy. Maternal blood pressure is assessed every 2 to 3 minutes after the initial dose and every 5 to 10 minutes during therapy. Maternal tachycardia is an unpleasant side effect; for this reason, the client's pulse is assessed whenever her blood pressure is determined.

Intravenous routes are maintained, and fluid therapy is designed to avoid cardiac overload. Ringer's lactate is often used. The client's intake and output are monitored and daily weights are recorded to assess fluid retention. Hemodynamic monitoring with a central venous pressure line or, more commonly, pulmonary artery (Swan-Ganz) catheter may be performed.

If pre-eclampsia is severe, the decision may be to deliver the client as soon as she is stabilized. If clinically indicated, vaginal delivery may be attempted through induction with intravenous oxytocin. Cesarean delivery is performed if induction is unsuccessful. Indications for delivery despite fetal prematurity include rapid weight gain on bedrest, elevation of blood pressure on bedrest, premonitory symptoms of eclampsia, increasing proteinuria, thrombocytopenia, impaired liver function, and intrauterine growth retardation with lung maturity.[2]

Nursing care for a client with PIH is outlined in the Case Study/Care Plan. Nursing strategies are based on several client needs:

CASE STUDY/CARE PLAN: PREGNANCY-INDUCED HYPERTENSION

Janet Orson, age 33, gravida 2 para 1, is 28 weeks pregnant. She and her husband, Steven, have a healthy two-year-old son, Jason. Her current obstetric history was normal, but it took 2 years to conceive this pregnancy. At 5 ft. 2 in., Janet weighed 132 pounds prior to pregnancy. She has gained weight appropriately. On her most recent prenatal visit her blood pressure was 122/78, her urine was negative for protein, and her 1+ pedal edema was relieved by elevation. One day in the 28th week, after walking two blocks, Janet suddenly experienced extreme edema of the lower extremities, dyspnea, "heartburn," and headache. The next morning in her obstetrician's office, her blood pressure was 240/170 and her urine was 4+ for protein. She has gained 10 pounds within two weeks. On immediate admission to the perinatal center, vital signs were blood pressure 252/178, temperature 36.5°C, pulse 94, and respirations 18. Fetal heart rate was 136. The fetus was active. Admission weight was 161 pounds. Pretibial edema was marked. Her face was swollen. Janet was apprehensive, complained of headache, and said "everything looks so dark." She had not voided since arising other than 15 mL in her obstetrician's office on the day of admission.

Supporting Assessment Data	Expected Client/Family Outcome	Nursing Action/ Intervention	Rationale	Criteria for Evaluation
Nursing Diagnosis: Alteration in safety of mother and fetus, related to abnormal cardiovascular adaptation, as evidenced by elevated blood pressure, proteinuria, edema and related symptoms				
Sudden onset of hypertension accompanied by edema, proteinuria, headache, epigastic pain, visual changes, low urine output BP = 252/178 Urine = 4+ protein T = 36.5°C P = 94 R = 18	Client will demonstrate stabilized cardiovascular status prior to delivery Client will experience decreased blood pressure, decreased edema, and increased urine output within 48 hours of delivery Client's pre-eclampsia will not progress to eclampsia. Client will demonstrate normal blood pressure by sixth postpartum week	Maintain client on bedrest in left lateral position.	Left lateral position enhances circulation.	Client remains stable until delivery.
		Assess vital signs, level of consciousness, and skin temperature and moisture every 30 minutes until stable.	Status can change quickly. Fever and altered sensorium can precede convulsions.	Client experiences reduction in blood pressure and return to normal within 12 hours. Client experiences no response to medication.
		Review laboratory data: CBC with platelets PT PTT Ca SGOT BUN.	Pre-eclampsia is associated with consumptive coagulopathy. Intravenous $MgSO_4$ is treatment of choice for prevention of convulsions.	Client demonstrates return to normal blood pressure on her six week postpartum visit.
		Initate intravenous route.		
		Maintain intake and output record.	All clients with IVs and all clients who are critically ill require assessment of intake and output.	
		Administer $MgSO_4$ as ordered.		
		Administer antihypertensives as ordered.	Elevation in blood pressure is responsible for many of the complications accompanying PIH.	
		Assess patellar reflexes every 2 hours, respiratory status every 30 minutes.	Mg^{2+} toxicity is evidenced by respiratory and neurologic depression.	

(continued)

CASE STUDY/CARE PLAN: Pregnancy-Induced Hypertension (*continued*)

Supporting Assessment Data	Expected Client/Family Outcome	Nursing Action/ Intervention	Rationale	Criteria for Evaluation
		Keep calcium gluconate at bedside.	Calcium gluconate is the antidote for excess $MgSO_4$.	
		Keep emergency cart and airway at bedside.	Respiratory depression may require emergency resuscitation.	
		Assess lungs, mucous membranes, neck veins, and presence of edema for evidence of cardiac failure.	Hepatomegaly can lead to congestive failure.	
		Briefly explain the nature of the disease process, purpose of treatment, and the symptoms that should be reported immediately.	Understanding promotes client cooperation and reduces stress. If the client reports evidence of a change in status, prompt intervention is possible.	
Nursing Diagnosis: Alteration in activity status, related to an increase in edema on exertion				
	Client will avoid activity until postpartum recovery is evident Client will demonstrate stabilized or improved pattern of urine output prior to delivery	Monitor respiratory status and maintain client on strict bedrest in left lateral position as described above. Explain need for restrictions and position call bell and table with oral fluids within client's reach. Advise client to call for bedpan to maintain bedrest.	This regimen minimizes cardiovascular and neurologic stress and promotes uteroplacental perfusion.	Client carries out regimen of rest until evidence of postpartum recovery allows increased activity.
Nursing Diagnosis: Altered tissue perfusion, related to pathophysiology of PIH, as evidenced by weight gain, proteinuria, pitting edema				
	Client will demonstrate output commensurate with intake and reduced pretibial edema 48 hours after delivery	Implement strict intake and output (indwelling catheter may be used). Record weight daily. Monitor BUN, creatinine, uric acid. Monitor urine protein every 4 hours. Adjust fluids based on output. Use Ringer's lactate for intravenous infusions.	With evidence of proteinuria and oliguria indicative of renal damage, and liver involvement that restricts circulation, fluid overload is a possible sequela.	Fluid load does not increase prior to delivery. Fluid balance restoration starts by 48 hours postpartum. Renal function is within normal limits by sixth postpartum week.
		Instruct client to salt food to taste and to include high-protein, low-fat, $FeSO_4$-rich foods in diet.	Protein, which is lost in urine, is needed for fetal growth and healing of tissue damage.	
Nursing Diagnosis: Potential for maternal and fetal hypoxia and injury, related to maternal convulsions and decreased uteroplacental perfusion				
	During hospitalization: Client will not experience seizure or cerebrovascular accident	Assess fetal heart rate every 30 minutes until client's vital signs are stabilized.	Fetal hypoxia may accompany seizures.	Client does not experience convulsions.

Supporting Assessment Data	Expected Client/Family Outcome	Nursing Action/ Intervention	Rationale	Criteria for Evaluation
	Fetus will not demonstrate ominous fetal heart rate	Prepare client for fetal electronic monitoring; assess baseline variability and fetal heart rate pattern with uterine contractions.	If fetal status deteriorates, immediate delivery is often needed.	Fetus does not demonstrate ominous fetal heart patterns.
		Prepare client for immediate delivery if fetal status deteriorates.		
	Client will deliver a viable neonate.	Administer nonstress tests twice daily until delivery.	Tests provide information on fetal well-being.	Client delivers a viable neonate.
		Take kick counts every shift.		
		Determine presence of meconium with rupture of membranes.		
		Assess client's level of consciousness, deep tendon reflexes, affect, headache, and reports of visual changes every 4 hours.	Neuorologic signs may herald eclamptic convulsions. Convulsions can be triggered by neurologic stimuli.	
		Place client in a dark, quiet room		
		Plan nursing activities with minimal disturbance.		
		Sedate client as ordered; remove prostheses.		
		Restrict visitors.		
		Remove telephone from room.		
		Keep bed at lowest level. Siderails should be up and padded.	In a safe environment the client will not incur trauma should convulsions occur.	Client does not sustain trauma.
		Keep emergency oxygen kit, and suction set at bedside; test equipment each shift.	Progression of preeclampsia requires treatment as an emergency.	
		Treat fetal bradycardia with O_2 and left lateral position.	Oxygen and maternal position will prevent fetal deterioration.	
		Give client brief, clear rationales for actions.	Understanding can reduce stress and promote rest.	
		Assess client for and teach her signs of labor.		
		Assess client for hemorrhage and evidence of abruptio placentae during labor.	Abruptio placentae is a complication of PIH.	

(continued)

CASE STUDY/CARE PLAN: Pregnancy-Induced Hypertension (*continued*)

Supporting Assessment Data	Expected Client/Family Outcome	Nursing Action/ Intervention	Rationale	Criteria for Evaluation
Nursing Diagnosis: Alteration in anxiety level, related to sudden development of threat to fetal well-being.				
	During hospitalization: Client will experience reduction in anxiety with orientation to unit and information about her condition and that of her fetus. Client will form a positive relationship with her primary nurse.	Assess sensorium, hyperirritability, hyperreflexia, and clonus. Determine client's level of comprehension of explanations. Address specific concerns of client. Explain procedures prior to implementation. Provide anticipatory guidance with respect to NICU. Assess sources of support. Advise family to contact clergyman.	Agitation may accompany PIH. Understanding the situation will foster relief of anxiety which will promote physical relaxation. Anticipation and understanding of events decrease their fears. Mobilization of support can reduce anxiety.	Child(ren) at home is cared for. Family member stays with client. Client develops rapport with primary nurse. Client becomes familiar with procedures. Client uses hospital resources, eg, social services, and chaplain, as needed. Client understands that health care team is prepared to support preterm infant.
Nursing Diagnosis: Potential for altered self-concept, related to obstetric emergency				
	During hospitalization and at the six week postpartum check up: Client will verbalize belief that she acted appropriately regarding this complication Client will grieve loss of expected pregnancy, labor and delivery experience appropriately	Assess client's beliefs about her condition; clarify reality. Observe family interactions. Provide positive reinforcement for client's prenatal course and actions. Help couple reconstruct experience during postpartum. Help client talk to older child on telephone daily.	High-risk clients may blame themselves or each other for the threat to their fetus. Couple needs to incorporate the experience into their life. Satisfying interaction with other child(ren) promotes positive self-concept as mother.	Client expresses satisfaction that she acted appropriately. Family members, especially husband, are supportive. Client grieves her high risk experience appropriately.

CBC = complete blood count, PT = prothrombin time, PTT = partial thromboplastin time, SGOT = serum glutamic-oxaloacetic transaminase, BUN = blood urea nitrogen.

- *Need for information about PIH.* If the client and her family have a clear understanding of the condition, they are more likely to carry out the prescribed regimen. The client and her family are instructed about PIH, the need to recognize and to report signs and symptoms of PIH, and the success expected from available treatments. Information is also provided about assessments of fetal well-being.
- *Need for rest.* The client must follow the prescribed regimen of rest which may minimize effects of the disease. The client is instructed to rest in the left lateral position to facilitate placental and renal perfusion, increase urine output, and reduce blood pressure. The amount of prescribed bedrest depends on the client's actual status. The client will need assistance in planning necessary activities around a schedule of rest.
- *Need to adapt to psychosocial impact of high-risk pregnancy and restricted activity.* The psychosocial impact of high-risk pregnancy and bedrest is discussed in Chapter 36. In addition to the emotional stress of pre-eclampsia, the client may not feel well. The client also may be justifiably anxious about her own well-being or the well-being of the fetus. The client needs to know that her fetus may be born early; a discussion of the neonatal inten-

sive care unit, its location, and parental involvement in the care of infants in the neonatal intensive care nursery may reassure the client and her support person.

- *Need to maintain adequate nutrition.* In the past, various dietary strategies were used in management of pre-eclampsia. Clients need to be educated about the importance of a well-balanced diet, as they may erroneously believe that substances such as salt should be restricted because of PIH.
- *Need to maintain safety.* Prevention of progression of pre-eclampsia and the development of convulsions is a goal of care of the client with PIH. Prompt identification of worsening signs and symptoms is essential. The nurse monitors the client's status at weekly or twice-weekly outpatient contacts or through frequent contacts with the hospitalized client. The nurse administers the appropriate medications as ordered and assesses any untoward responses to the medications. The nurse ensures that oxygen and suction apparatus is accessible and in working order. Clients on bedrest should have the siderails raised.
- *Need for a subdued environment to avoid excess stimuli.* The client should be placed in a quiet, darkened room. Disturbances must be minimal, and nursing activities should be organized accordingly. Even the sound of a telephone ringing at the bedside could trigger convulsions in a severe pre-eclamptic client. Siderails should be kept up if the client's PIH is severe, particularly if the client is sedated. A soft gag should be at the bedside and siderails should be padded to prevent injury if convulsions develop.

Eclampsia

Eclampsia represents the convulsive phase of PIH and occurs in about 5 percent of pre-eclamptic women. Although eclampsia most often occurs during pregnancy, it can also occur up to 48 hours or more after delivery. Eclampsia is rare among women in whom pre-eclampsia is promptly diagnosed and treated. The most dreaded maternal complication of eclamptic seizure is cerebral hemorrhage, which occurs when the blood pressure is not controlled.[2] Cerebral hemorrhage is often heralded by a loss of vision, which is usually temporary. The fetus of an eclamptic mother is at risk for hypoxia. Placental abruption occurs more commonly in this group of women than in the general population because the intervillous space is reduced as a result of vasospasm.

Signs and Symptoms. Eclampsia is marked by the occurrence of tonic-clonic seizures or vascular collapse. In the event of seizures, the following signs are observed: a prodromal facial twitching lasting only a few seconds, a tonic contraction of the entire body lasting about 20 seconds, and a convulsion lasting about a minute. During this time, the client may not breathe. After the convulsion, the client may fall into a coma lasting minutes or hours. *Eclampsia is an obstetric emergency;* the physician needs to be notified at once and management begun at once.

Nursing and Collaborative Assessment. If eclampsia occurs, the nurse notes the onset, course, and duration of the convulsions. Vital signs are monitored every 5 minutes until stable and every 15 minutes afterward. The client's lungs are checked for pulmonary edema. Blood is obtained for typing and cross-matching. Studies are the same as for severe pre-eclampsia. Fetal heart rate is determined and continuous fetal monitoring is initiated.

Nursing and Collaborative Management. Client safety is a primary concern during seizures. The nurse should remain with the client and summon help. A plastic airway or soft gag may be inserted into the client's mouth to keep her from biting her tongue. Siderails need to be up and padded to prevent injury. The nurse can gently try to position the client to prevent her from throwing herself out of bed or banging her head during a convulsion. The nurse needs to note the timing and sequence of events and record the episode as soon as possible. After seizure activity has ceased, the nurse assesses the client's airway and suctions secretions as needed. Oxygen is administered by mask.

The following management regimen is one approach that has been successful in treating eclampsia.[16] Magnesium sulfate is administered. Hydralazine is given if diastolic pressure exceeds 110 mm Hg. Labor is induced or a cesarean delivery is performed as soon as the client is conscious and oriented. No diuretics or sedatives are used; however, meperidine and promethazine may be given in labor. Hypertonics, plasma expanders, and heparin, a medication commonly used in consumptive coagulopathy, are avoided because of the rapid change in status that occurs once the placenta is delivered. If convulsions persist despite treatment with magnesium sulfate, sodium amobarbital may be used; however, this drug is avoided if delivery is expected within 1 to 2 hours because of its depressant effect on the fetus. In general, vaginal delivery presents a lower risk than cesarean delivery.

The client is positioned for postural drainage of secretions to prevent aspiration. A nasogastric tube may be inserted and 30 mL of antacid instilled. Stimuli such as light and noise are minimized. Fetal heart rate is assessed frequently as are signs of labor in the antepartum woman. The client and fetus are also monitored throughout labor and delivery and the nurse prepares for delivery of the neonate as determined by the interdisciplinary perinatal team.

Hypertensive Cardiovascular Disease

Hypertensive cardiovascular disease is marked by the formation of fatty deposits within the arterial walls. This increases vascular resistance to the flow of blood and increases the work of the heart. Tissue perfusion throughout the body is diminished as a result, and over a period of years all organs will be adversely affected. Hypertensive cardiovascular disease is a continued elevation of blood pressure of 140/90 or higher before pregnancy or before the 20th week of gestation in the absence of trophoblastic disease.[12]

Many factors are associated with the development of hypertensive cardiovascular disease. Major factors include family history of hypertension, race (increased prevalence among blacks), a sedentary lifestyle, use of tobacco, excessive use of alcohol, obesity, a diet high in cholesterol and triglycerides, a stressful lifestyle and inappropriate means of coping, and a history of PIH. The client with chronic hypertension may have an underlying predisposing condition such as renal disease.

It is difficult to distinguish chronic hypertension from pregnancy-induced hypertension, particularly in a woman who has not received early prenatal care. Because blood pressure may normally decrease in the first and second trimesters, blood pressure measurements for the woman with chronic hypertension may appear normal. Typically, as pregnancy progresses the blood pressure returns to its hypertensive state.

Nursing and Collaborative Assessment. Chronic hypertensive disease, in contrast to pre-eclampsia, is suggested by the observation of hemorrhages and exudates in the optic fundi; plasma creatinine concentrations greater than 1 mg/dL; plasma urea nitrogen concentrations greater than 20 mg/dL; and the presence of other predisposing chronic diseases such as diabetes, connective tissue disease, or renal disease.[2]

Complications of chronic hypertension in pregnant women include abruptio placentae, intrauterine growth retardation, and superimposed pre-eclampsia.

Nursing and Collaborative Management. Some experts believe that chronic hypertension is best left untreated during pregnancy unless diastolic pressure exceeds 110 mm Hg. Otherwise, treatment could mask the onset of pre-eclampsia until that disease process is well advanced. Furthermore, control of chronic hypertension does not seem to reduce the client's risk of developing PIH.[3,5]

According to a different perspective, the client with chronic hypertension should be treated during pregnancy just as she would be routinely.[2] Blood pressure is evaluated weekly. Tests to assess fetal well-being are performed (*see* Chapters 18 and 22).

Medications used to maintain blood pressure in the normal range are summarized in Table 39–7. If chronic hypertension is severe, alpha-methyldopa may be the preferred drug. If response is not satisfactory, hydralazine can be added to the regimen or substituted. The woman remains at home as long as her blood pressure is controlled; hospitalization is indicated when better control needs to be established.

The nurse needs to review the client's regimen for maintenance of her condition with her, including explicit teaching about the medication regimen and observation of untoward effects. Reinforcement and clarification are provided as needed. Blood pressure is carefully assessed at each contact. The nurse carefully observes the client for the development of superimposed pre-eclampsia and for evidence of fetal distress. The client is instructed to contact her health care provider without delay if any of the warning signs of pregnancy occur (*see* Table 39–1).

Pregnancy is not the appropriate time to undertake a weight control program, but moderation in sodium intake is appropriate, as is elimination of such hazardous substances as smoking and alcohol. Relaxation techniques can be taught. The client's life situation may be reviewed to identify ways in which overall stress can be reduced. Moderate exercise such as walking can be undertaken in the absence of pre-eclampsia.

The client and her partner need reassurance that, with good control of her hypertension, pregnancy can progress normally. They can exercise many options in planning their childbirth education and the delivery itself.

Superimposed Pre-eclampsia. The client with chronic hypertension is assessed carefully for the development of superimposed pre-eclampsia, which occurs in 25 percent of cases. She is maintained on her antihypertensive medication. If progression of the disease is observed, hospitalization may be warranted. If the pre-eclampsia worsens during a course of bedrest, the fetus may need to be delivered without delay.

HEART DISEASE

Types of Heart Disease

About 1 percent of pregnant women have heart disease. Formerly, most cases involved rheumatic heart

TABLE 39–7. MEDICATIONS USED IN THE TREATMENT OF HYPERTENSION OF PREGNANCY

Medication	Purpose	Nursing Implications
Thiazide diuretics, eg, hydrochlorothiazide (HydroDiuril, HydroChlor) chlorothiazide (Diuril), spironolactone (Aldactone)	Treatment of profound edema	Risk of decreased uteroplacental perfusion, fluid and electrolyte imbalance, and decreased renal perfusion. Monitor blood pressure and fetal heart rate. Prepare client for possibility of nonstress testing and contraction stress testing. Encourage client to eat potassium-rich foods.
Phenobarbital	Sedation	Risk of fetal depression, neonatal bleeding, and delay of lung maturation. Counsel client to adhere to medication regimen. Monitor neonate for withdrawal symptoms, respiratory effort, and bleeding.
Diazepam (Valium)	Sedation and control of eclamptic seizures; less effective than $MgSO_4$	Risk of fetal depression if administered within 24 hours of delivery. Monitor fetus and neonate for depression.
Hydralazine (Apresoline)	Treatment of marked hypertension in pre-eclampsia and eclampsia	Risk of hypotension when given with diuretics. Risk of increased fetal heart rate and decreased blood pressure. Potential for neonatal hypothermia. Monitor maternal blood pressure and fetal heart rate. Monitor neonatal temperature and provide a warm environment.
Glucocorticoids	Enhancement of fetal lung maturation	Monitor fetal heart rate.
Calcium gluconate (Kalcinate)/calcium gluceptate	Antidote to toxic level of $MgSO_4$	Medication should be kept at the bedside whenever $MgSO_4$ is used.
Diazoxide (Hyperstat I.V., Proglycem)	Potent antihypertensive	Side effects are more serious than those of hydralazine, including arrest of labor; retention of water, sodium, and uric acid; hyperglycemia; potentially lethal hypotension. Monitor blood pressure and fluids and electrolytes.
Sodium nitoprusside	Potent short-acting antihypertensive	Crosses placenta and may cause cyanide poisoning in the fetus and increase intracranial pressure in the mother. Monitor maternal and fetal vital signs.
Alpha-methyldopa (Aldomet, MSD)	Treatment of pregnant women with chronic hypertension if diastolic pressure exceeds 110 to partially reduce blood pressure	Use with care to avoid masking signs and symptoms of pre-eclampsia. Risk of maternal orthostatic hypotension and bradycardia. Risk of decreased systolic blood pressure of newborn 2–3 days after delivery. Monitor maternal, fetal, and newborn vital signs. Monitor client for signs of pre-eclampsia.

disease. Rheumatic fever is quite rare in the United States, although there is some evidence that it is on the rise. Currently, most maternal heart disease is congenital in origin.[17,18] Mitral valve prolapse is observed among as many as 10 percent of women of childbearing age. It involves elongation of the chordae tendinae, which allow the mitral valve leaflets to prolapse into the right atrium during ventricular systole. Other cardiovascular disorders can be observed in pregnant women, but they are uncommon. Rarely an idiopathic cardiac decompensation associated with late pregnancy is observed. The condition tends to recur in subsequent pregnancies.

The New York Heart Association has classified individuals with heart disease on the basis of past and present disability. *See* Table 39–8 for a description of the classes.[5]

The woman with heart disease may not be able to adapt to the physiologic demands of pregnancy. This is a risk that young women with congenital heart disease must take into consideration when they contemplate pregnancy. In some cases maternal death oc-

TABLE 39–8. NEW YORK HEART ASSOCIATION CLASSIFICATION OF FUNCTIONAL CAPACITY IN INDIVIDUALS WITH HEART DISEASE

Class I	*Uncompromised:* These individuals have no symptoms of cardiac insufficiency or anginal pain. Physical activity is not restricted.
Class II	*Slightly compromised:* These individuals with cardiac disease experience discomfort in the form of fatigue, palpitation, dyspnea, or angina if they undertake ordinary physical activity. Physical activity is slightly limited.
Class III	*Markedly compromised:* These individuals experience fatigue, palpitation, dyspnea, or angina when they undertake less than ordinary activity. Physical activity is markedly restricted.
Class IV	These individuals are unable to perform any physical activity without discomfort. Symptoms of cardiac insufficiency or angina may occur even at rest.

curs, though it is unusual. In one study of 542 pregnant women with heart disease, 10 of the women died.[19] Still, heart disease is the major nonobstetric medical cause of maternal death.[17]

Pregnancy Risks for Mother and Infant

The likelihood of a favorable outcome for the mother with heart disease and her fetus depends on the functional capacity of her heart, the presence of other complications during pregnancy and postpartum, the quality of care, her ability to rest, and the presence of psychologic, social, and economic support.[5]

Because of increasing sophistication in the repair of congenital heart defects, the number of women of childbearing age with a history of congenital heart disease is growing. Risk for the mother with congenital heart disease is related to the degree of cyanosis. If they do not have congestive heart failure or major venous thromboses, women with acyanotic conditions are not at appreciably increased risk during pregnancy.[17] Women who underwent early corrective surgery for congenital heart disease are at less risk in pregnancy than those who did not, although even they have more complications than women who did not have congenital heart disease. If the surgical repair of the defect was successful, the woman usually will experience a normal pregnancy.

Prophylactic antibiotic therapy is recommended to prevent subacute bacterial endocarditis. If repair was incomplete or not undertaken at all, the woman is at risk for cardiac decompensation during pregnancy.

Maternal and perinatal mortality is most likely if the mother has cyanotic heart disease, particularly with pulmonary hypertension. Women with pulmonary hypertension have about a 20 to 30 percent risk of major pulmonary thromboembolism during pregnancy or the early puerperium.[17]

Risks to the fetus include spontaneous abortion, intrauterine growth retardation, premature delivery, and intrauterine death. Whittemore and associates identified a fetal loss rate of 36 percent in pregnancies of mothers with hypoxic congenital heart disease.[20] If hypoxia is so intense that it stimulates a rise in hematocrit to 65 percent or more, pregnancy loss is nearly 100 percent.[5] An additional risk to the fetus is inheritance of congenital heart disease.[17]

Signs and Symptoms

Signs and symptoms of cardiac decompensation among nonpregnant individuals include systolic murmurs, edema, changes suggestive of cardiac enlargement and rotation, dyspnea, and fatigability (Table 39–9). Unfortunately these characteristics are often present during a normal pregnancy. One of the following confirms the presence of heart disease in pregnancy: a diastolic, presystolic, or continuous heart murmur; unequivocal cardiac enlargement; a loud, harsh systolic murmur especially if accompanied by a thrill; and severe arrhythmia.[5] Additional observations may include distended neck veins and pulmonary rales.

Cardiac decompensation, or congestive heart failure, occurs when the heart cannot keep up with the load placed on it. Normal homeostatic mechanisms, such as increasing heart rate, are mobilized without success. Venous blood backs up into the general circulatory system and into the pulmonary circulation. This accounts for the observation of progressive symptoms including generalized edema, distension of neck veins, dyspnea, pulmonary rales, and frequent moist cough. Heart rate increases to the extent that the electrical conduction system develops irregularities. The woman experiences palpitations, and ectopic beats can be observed on cardiac monitoring.

TABLE 39–9. SIGNS AND SYMPTOMS OF CARDIOVASCULAR DISORDERS

Symptoms	Signs	Diagnostic Tests
Shortness of breath	Cyanosis	Chest x-ray
Angina	Cardiac arrythmias	Electrocardiogram
Palpitations	Abnormal heart sounds	Echocardiogram
Syncope	Cardiomegaly	
	Hepatomegaly	
	Neck vein distension	
	Peripheral edema	

Collaborative Assessment and Management

Cardiac status is assessed carefully at each prenatal visit to identify signs of cardiac compromise. Although pregnant women with congenital heart disease are counseled to avoid weight gain in excess of 28 pounds, actual recommended weight gain depends on the woman's health status. Abnormal edema and the development of anemia are carefully assessed and promptly treated. Anemia triggers a homeostatic response to increase cardiac output. In these clients, the heart cannot accommodate an increased demand. These clients are carefully screened for PIH, which is more serious than usual when superimposed on heart disease. Women with heart disease are therefore counseled to report the earliest symptoms to their obstetrician. Hypotension is also undesirable, especially in women clients with shunting conditions, because of the difficulty in withstanding additional cardiac stress.

Clients with class I or II heart disease usually are able to complete pregnancy. They require intensive prenatal supervision. In one study of women who developed frank cardiac failure in pregnancy, 39 percent were class I.[21]

The physician assesses vital capacity at each visit. When anticoagulation therapy is indicated, heparin is used because of its minimal fetotoxic effects (Table 39–10 and Box 39–2). The woman may require diuretic, glycoside, and antiarrhythmic therapy. She will likely be hospitalized before delivery.

Vaginal delivery is preferable and strategies that avoid cardiac strain are used. Analgesia is important in labor and delivery for these women. Epidural anesthesia has the advantage of not depressing vital functions, but the risk of hypotension is potentially lethal. If the cervix is fully dilated and the fetus is engaged, prompt forceps delivery is indicated unless an easy, spontaneous vaginal delivery is imminent.[2] Medications that may be used include intravenous morphine, rapidly acting digitalis, and a potent diuretic such as furosemide.

Women with class III heart disease are generally advised not to become pregnant because of the risk to their lives presented by the physical stress of pregnancy. If they do become pregnant and desire to continue the pregnancy, they must understand the serious risk they will incur. Management of these clients includes bedrest throughout pregnancy. Hospitalization is usually required to achieve this. Vaginal delivery is preferred because of the additional stress presented by surgery.

Women with class IV heart disease are essentially in failure, and the focus of their care is medical rather than obstetric. Delivery for any woman in frank failure carries with it a high mortality rate.

TABLE 39–10. MEDICATIONS COMMONLY USED IN CARE OF THE PREGNANT WOMAN WITH HEART DISEASE

Medication	Purpose	Nursing Implications
Cardiac glycoside: digoxin (Lanoxin, Lanoxicaps)	Increases cardiac output	Assess apical pulse rate for 1 full minute and withhold medication if heart rate is less than 60. Monitor for presence of arrhythmias. Provide foods rich in potassium. Withhold medication if gastrointestinal disturbances develop.
Thiazide diuretic: hydrochlorothiazide (HydroDiuril, Hydrochlor)	Treatment of edema associated with congestive heart failure	Encourage client to eat potassium-rich foods. Record weight daily. The client may experience photosensitivity. Last daily dosage should be no later than 3 PM to avoid nocturia. Medication should be taken after meals to reduce gastric irritation.
Anticoagulant: heparin	Anticoagulant	Medication is incompatible with most antibiotics. Assess for evidence of hemorrhage. Rotate subcutaneous injection sites.
Antibiotic prophylaxis: benzathine penicillin, ampicillin, or gentamycin	Prevention of valvular infection for women with rheumatic heart disease	Antibiotics can cause local or generalized hypersensitivity response. Gentamycin is incompatible with other drugs in solution. Client should be questioned regarding medication allergies.
Iron supplement: $FeSO_4$	Prevention of anemia	Dietary fluids and roughage will prevent constipation.

BOX 39–2. HEPARIN

Proprietary Names:
Many.

Classification:
Anticoagulant.

Action:
Acts as a catalyst to accelerate the rate at which antithrombin III neutralizes thrombin and activates factor I. Inhibits thrombus formation when stasis is induced. Full-dose therapy may prevent extension of existing thrombi. Cannot lyse existing thrombi.

Indications:
Prophylaxis and treatment of venous thrombosis. Prophylaxis and treatment of pulmonary embolism. Treatment of atrial fibrillation with embolization. Diagnosis and treatment of disseminated intravascular coagulation. Treatment of peripheral arterial embolism.

Dosage and Route:
Administered by IV infusion, intermittent IV injection, or deep SC injection for full-dose therapy and deep SC injection for low-dose therapy. *Full-dose therapy: IV infusion:* Initial bolus dose of 5000 U by direct IV, then 20,000–40,000 U in 1000 mL isotonic sodium chloride solution over 24 hours. *Intermittent IV injection:* Initial dose of 10,000 U followed by 5000–10,000 U every 4–6 hours. *Deep SC:* Initial dose of 10,000–20,000 U IV, usually preceded by bolus dose of 5000 U IV, then 8000–10,000 U every 8 hours or 15,000–20,000 U every 12 hours. Follow PTT for adjustment of doses in all regimens. *Low-dose therapy:* 5000 U SC every 8–12 hours. *Disseminated intravascular coagulation:* 50–100 U/kg by IV infusion or IV injection every 4 hours. If no improvement after 4–8 hours, heparin therapy should be discontinued.

Pharmacokinetics:
Absorption: Not absorbed orally. Onset of activity after deep SC injection generally 20–60 minutes. *Distribution:* Does not cross the placenta or distribute into breast milk. *Elimination:* Appears to be removed from the circulation by reticuloendothelial system. Plasma half-life directly proportional to dose and is approximately 1–2 hours.

Precautions and Contraindications:
Use with caution in cases in which the risk of hemorrhage is increased, such as dissecting aneurysm; ulcerative GI lesions; diverticulitis; hemorrhagic blood dyscrasias; menstruation; ovulation; threatened abortion; subacute bacterial endocarditis; increased capillary permeability; arterial sclerosis; severe hypertension; renal, hepatic, or biliary disease; eye, brain, or spinal cord surgery; continuous tube drainage from any orifice; and spinal tap or spinal anesthesia.

Adverse Reactions:
Most common: minor bleeding. *Less common:* CV—major hemorrhage; hematologic—thrombocytopenia, localized or disseminated thromboses (white clot syndrome); GI—elevated liver enzymes; local reactions—with deep SC injection, local irritation, erythema, mild pain, hematoma, ulceration, or cutaneous and subcutaneous necrosis; other—hypersensitivity reactions, osteoporosis, and spontaneous fractures in clients receiving ≧ 10,000 U/day for 3 or more months.

Drug Interactions:

- Aspirin, nonsteroidal anti-inflammatory agents, dipyridamole: inhibit platelet function and may increase risk of hemorrhage.
- Streptokinase, urokinase: may increase risk of bleeding.
- Dihydroergotamine: may potentiate antithrombogenic effects of heparin.
- IV nitroglycerin: may antagonize anticoagulant effect of heparin.

Nursing Implications:

- Assess blood coagulation studies. If not within therapeutic range, contact physician.
- Assess for signs of bleeding (eg, epistaxis, blood in urine, ecchymosis).
- Observe needle sites for hematoma, swelling, heat, redness, and pain.
- Teach client and her partner the signs of hemorrhage and the rationale for the treatment.

IV = intravenous(ly), SC = subcutaneous(ly), PTT = partial thromboplastin time, GI = gastrointestinal, CV = cardiovascular.

Nursing Assessment

Assessment for signs and symptoms of cardiac decompensation is an essential aspect of nursing care. At each prenatal visit blood pressure, pulse, respirations, weight, and fundal height are measured. The client is assessed for evidence of generalized and pulmonary edema. Heart sounds are auscultated. Screening for evidence of PIH is conducted. The nurse reviews prescribed medications with the client so that side effects can be detected or misunderstandings clarified.

Nursing Diagnoses

Examples of nursing diagnoses for the client with heart disease are presented in the box.

NURSING DIAGNOSES RELATED TO HEART DISEASE

Problem-Oriented

Decreased cardiac output, related to heart disease during pregnancy

Activity intolerance, related to compromised cardiac status during pregnancy

Altered family processes, related to pregnant cardiac client's inability to care for family

Fear: client and family, related to maternal and fetal outcome complicated by cardiac disease during pregnancy

Strength-Oriented

Potential asset in maintenance of cardiopulmonary functioning during pregnancy, related to functional ability of heart

Nursing Management

The client is instructed to seek health care promptly if she experiences dyspnea, fatigue on mild exertion, edema, coughing, hemoptysis, tachycardia, or other evidence of progression of her disease.

Rest. The nurse instructs the client to get at least 10 hours of rest per night and to avoid exertion, including heavy housework and lifting children.

Nutrition. Clients with heart disease are instructed to follow a diet that is adequate in protein and that contains not more than 2 to 3 g of sodium. The caloric content will be appropriate for normal pregnancy, with modification as needed to accommodate the reduced activity level. Clients are instructed to rest one-half hour after meals in a semi-Fowler's position to reduce esophageal reflux and the sensation of heartburn. Nutrition planning also needs to be based on the client's cultural food preferences.

Infection. Infection can precipitate cardiac failure. The nurse carefully instructs clients with heart disease on the avoidance of situations where they may contact respiratory infection. Clients who suspect that they have contracted an infection must inform their physician immediately.

Preparation for Labor. The nurse must be sensitive to the anxiety of the woman and of her partner as they approach labor and delivery. Preparation for childbirth is especially important for this couple. They need to be oriented to the setting in which the woman will deliver and to the equipment and procedures to which they will be exposed. The importance of providing support is critical as anxiety can increase the demand of the adrenergic nervous system on the heart. Breathing and relaxation techniques, soothing music, massage, and an atmosphere of professional calm and competence will contribute to the physical as well as emotional well-being of the client.

DIABETES MELLITUS

Diabetes mellitus is regarded as a major health care complication of pregnancy. Diabetic mothers, especially those whose disease is uncontrolled, are subject to increased morbidity and mortality. Overall maternal mortality is about 0.5 percent, and perinatal mortality averages about 10 percent. Two to three percent of pregnancies are complicated by overt diabetes mellitus.[22] In 90 percent of these cases the diabetes arises as a result of the metabolic changes of pregnancy; this is termed *gestational diabetes.* In only 10 percent of cases does the diabetic condition precede pregnancy. The finding of pregnancy complicated by diabetes was quite rare before the discovery of insulin, as most diabetic women were infertile.[5] Among those who conceived, 25 percent of mothers and half of fetuses died.

During the last 10 years significant technologic advances have almost eliminated maternal mortality and markedly reduced maternal mobidity. The perinatal mortality rate for women with pregestational diabetes mellitus approaches the rate for women who are not diabetic when strict euglycemic control is maintained throughout pregnancy.

Effect of Pregnancy on Carbohydrate Metabolism

Even in a nondiabetic mother, pregnancy causes alterations in carbohydrate metabolism that serve to ensure satisfactory growth of the fetus and establish a maternal energy store. In a normal pregnancy, maternal sparing of glucose and increasing oxidation of fat occur to ensure nourishment of the fetus. The demand for insulin increases in response to this greater turnover of fats. If the insulin supply is insufficient, rapid lipolysis and gluconeogenesis result in ketoacidosis. Insulin production increases severalfold, but because of the effects of the placental hormone lactogen, resistance to insulin also increases. Despite the rise in insulin production, maternal glucose homeostasis is maintained at normal levels.[22,23] Fat deposition is promoted and glucose is directed toward the fetus. Cardiac output and glomerular filtration increase throughout the first two trimesters of pregnancy. The renal thresholds for glucose and ketones are lowered. Glucosuria and occasional slight ketonuria are found in nondiabetic women during pregnancy.[24]

Pregestational Diabetic Conditions

Pathophysiology. Diabetes mellitus is a complex syndrome a major feature of which is impaired carbohydrate metabolism. This manifests as hyperglycemia. In the face of excess serum glucose the body is actually starving, as the problem lies in the transport and utilization of carbohydrate molecules. The pancreatic hormone insulin effects this activity. In diabetes, insulin production is impaired, and many diabetic people are dependent on exogenous insulin. Use of fat and protein stores for energy in the absence of carbohydates leads to a state of ketoacidosis. Because of increased serum osmolality with increased glucose levels, fluids are drawn from cells and the interstices into the vascular bed. Because of the osmotic pressure exerted by glucose in the urine, polyuria is a prominent feature. With intercellular dehydration the individual experiences profound thirst.

Diabetic individuals have accelerated atherosclerotic microvascular disease in which capillary basement membranes thicken. Neuropathy is a serious complication as the disease progresses. With a higher level of glucose in the extracellular fluid, which is conducive to the growth of microorganisms, diabetic individuals are prone to infection. Decreased capillary exchange makes healing difficult. Neuropathy decreases the sensation of peripheral trauma. As a result, undetected skin wounds can quickly lead to gangrenous conditions that may require amputation.[25]

There are two types of diabetes: type I (or insulin-dependent) and type II (non–insulin-dependent). Also, in 1978, the National Diabetes Data Group of the National Institutes of Health developed a uniform classification system for diabetes mellitus.[26] Taken together, these terms and definitions are accepted as standard (Table 39–11).

In type I diabetes, the pancreatic beta cells in the islets of Langerhans are smaller and fewer than normal and they produce virtually no insulin. The etiology is unknown, but onset is often sudden. Genetic, environmental, and autoimmune factors may play a role in its development. In type II diabetes, the pancreas is unable to meet increased demands for insulin over time, as is the case in obesity-related type II diabetes, or pancreatic function diminishes over time. There is a familial tendency for type II diabetes.

TABLE 39–11. NATIONAL DIABETES DATA GROUP CLASSIFICATION OF DIABETES MELLITUS

A. Insulin-dependent type (type I)
B. Non–insulin-dependent type (type II)
   1. Nonobese
   2. Obese
C. Other types (diabetes occurring as a result of other conditions)
   1. Pancreatic disease
   2. Hormonally induced
   3. Chemically induced (caused by certain drugs or other chemicals)
   4. Insulin receptor abnormalities
   5. Certain genetic syndromes
   6. Others
D. Impaired glucose tolerance (subclinical diabetes)
E. Gestational diabetes (pregnancy-induced glucose intolerance)

Reprinted, with permission, from National Diabetes Data Group. Classification of diabetes mellitus and other categories of glucose intolerance. Diabetes. *1979;28:1039.*

With insulin deficiency, glucose is not transported from the extracellular into the intracellular compartment, and the cells must oxidize fats and proteins for energy. This results in tissue wasting. As serum glucose level rises, cellular water is pulled into the blood. The hyperosmotic pressure of glucose in the urine accounts for decreased renal tubular resorption of water. Extracellular dehydration develops. The four cardinal symptoms of diabetes, in response to these processes, are polyphagia, polyuria, polydipsia, and weight loss.[27,28]

Impact of Pregnancy on Pre-existing Diabetes. In addition to the classification system developed by the National Diabetes Data Group, there is a classification system (White's classification) for diabetes that complicates pregnancy. White first classified diabetes in pregnancy in 1949, but revised her classification system in 1978.[29] The system was adapted for clarification of the relation of diabetes and pregnancy by the American College of Obstetricians and Gynecologists[30] (Table 39–12).

The normal changes in carbohydrate metabolism that occur during pregnancy (described earlier) make control of pre-existing diabetes more difficult. Insulin resistance increases. Nausea and vomiting increase the risk of hypoglycemia and insulin shock. Ketoacidosis develops more easily. Any infection can lead to the rapid onset of ketoacidosis. It does not seem that pre-existing complications of diabetes are worsened by pregnancy. Retinopathy present prior to pregnancy may worsen, but this change regresses postpartally.[24]

TABLE 39–12. CLASSIFICATION OF DIABETES COMPLICATING PREGNANCY

	Pregestational Diabetes				
Class	**Age onset**		**Duration (years)**	**Vascular Disease**	**Therapy**
A[a]	Any		Any	None	A-1, diet only
B	> 20		< 10	None	Insulin
C	10–19	or	10–19	None	Insulin
D	< 10	or	> 20	Benign retinopathy	Insulin
F	Any		Any	Nephropathy	Insulin
R	Any		Any	Proliferative retinopathy	Insulin
H	Any		Any	Heart disease	Insulin

	Gestational Diabetes		
Class	**Fasting Plasma Glucose**		**Postprandial Plasma Glucose**
A-1	< 105 mg/dL	and	< 120 mg/dL
A-2	> 105 mg/dL	and/or	> 120 mg/dL

[a]Chemical diabetes.

Reprinted, with permission, from the American College of Obstetricians and Gynecologists. Classification of diabetes in pregnancy. ACOG *Technical Bulletin No. 92. Washington, DC: ACOG, 1986.*

Pathogenesis of Gestational Diabetes

Gestational diabetes occurs when the pancreas cannot meet the added demands of pregnancy. Factors indicating risk for gestational diabetes include prior gestational diabetes; prior delivery of or current evidence of a macrosomic infant (greater than 90th percentile weight for gestational age); family history of diabetes; unexplained stillborn; prior delivery or current evidence of an infant with a congenital anomaly; maternal obesity, hypertension, or glycosuria; polyhydramnios; recurrent urinary tract infection or vaginitis; and large or poor weight gain during pregnancy. Half of women who develop gestational diabetes exhibit none of these risk factors.[31] For that reason the American Diabetes Association advocates universal screening by means of an oral carbohydrate load followed by assessment of serum glucose level.[32]

Diabetic Emergencies

Ketoacidosis. The development of ketoacidosis is associated with a fetal mortality rate of 50 to 90 percent. It develops over hours or days when insulin levels are inadequate. As fats are metabolized for energy, ketones are produced faster than the body can catabolize them. Metabolic acidosis occurs and, in severe cases, results in diabetic coma. The need for insulin is increased by such factors as pregnancy, trauma, infection, development of insulin resistance, and psychologic stress. Women treated for premature labor with beta-sympathomimetic drugs may develop ketoacidosis.[33] Signs and symptoms of early and late ketoacidosis are presented in Table 39–13.

Hypoglycemia. Hypoglycemia is the most common cause of coma in diabetic clients; nearly all insulin-dependent diabetic clients experience hypoglycemia at some time. It is especially likely when a woman is trying to maintain strict euglycemic control during pregnancy. Onset is rapid, occurring in minutes. Hypoglycemia may result from decreased food intake, vomiting, increased exertion, or modification of insulin dose. Change to a more purified form of insulin or to human-derived insulin can result in hypoglycemia. Signs and symptoms are listed in Table 39–13.

Effects of Diabetes on Maternal-Infant Outcomes

There are numerous adverse effects of diabetes on pregnancy. Among diabetic women, there is about a 25 percent incidence of PIH.[34] The risk of hypertensive complications is particularly pronounced among women of White's classes F, D, and R. Infection is more frequent and more severe, and these women are at higher risk for urinary tract infection than nondiabetic pregnant women. There is an increased risk of cesarean delivery because of dystocia. Polyhydramnios plus a larger-than-usual fetus can lead to cardiopulmonary symptoms in the mother. Diabetic women demonstrate less of the normal increase in cardiac output that normally accompanies pregnancy.[35] This may contribute to the diminished uteroplacental perfusion observed in diabetic women, and to decreased fetal oxygenation. Diabetic women also demonstrate a greater incidence of postpartum hemorrhage.[5] Women with gestational diabetes are more likely than the general population to have glucose intolerance 3 years later,

TABLE 39–13. SIGNS AND SYMPTOMS OF HYPOGLYCEMIA AND KETOACIDOSIS

		Signs and Symptoms	
	Onset	**Early**	**Late**
Hypoglycemia	Rapid, within minutes	Tachycardia Diaphoresis Tremor Hunger Pallor Dizziness Irritability Nausea Headache Paresthesia	Confusion Strange behavior Stupor Convulsions Stroke syndrome Coma
Ketoacidosis	Slow, over hours or days	Polyuria Polydipsia Malaise	Rapid, deep breathing Hypothermia Acetone breath Nausea and vomiting Abdominal pain Coma Death

and many go on to develop type II (or non–insulin-dependent) diabetes.[36]

In addition, diabetes has adverse effects on the fetus. If the disease is not well controlled the fetal death rate is significantly higher than among the general population. Sutherland and Pritchard reported a twofold increase in the incidence of spontaneous abortion among diabetic women when other demographic and obstetric factors were controlled.[37] Infants of diabetic mothers are subject to a higher-than-usual morbidity rate. This may result from birth trauma because of their tendency toward macrosomia, or it may result from respiratory distress or metabolic imbalance disorders such as hypoglycemia and hypocalcemia.[5]

Women with vascular complications that compromise uteroplacental blood flow may have small-for-gestational age infants.[34] Infants of diabetic mothers are born prematurely more often than the general population. There is an increased incidence of fetal distress during labor among infants of diabetic mothers. Tachypnea, polycythemia, and hyperbilirubinemia occur more frequently than in the general population. These infants have an increased incidence of respiratory distress syndrome even at term. Infants of diabetic mothers are more likely to suffer from congenital anomalies, particularly neural tube defects, caudal regression syndrome (hypoplasia of the sacrum and lower extremities), and cardiac and other vascular defects. Neurologic symptoms such as seizure activity are observed in children of diabetic women more often than among the general population. Finally, the children of diabetic mothers are at increased risk of developing obesity and diabetes.[5] (*See* Chapter 42 for further discussion of the effects of diabetes on the newborn.) Problems related to maternal diabetes can be minimized in the newborn if maternal glucose levels are well controlled prior to and throughout pregnancy.

Collaborative Assessment

Controversy exists regarding the best assessment tests for gestational diabetes.[5] The American Diabetes Association now recommends screening of all pregnant women between the 24th and 28th weeks of pregnancy using a 50-g oral glucose load.[32] Plasma glucose level is then measured 1 hour later. Precise timing is, however, essential to avoid inaccurate interpretations of test results.[38] If the test is given without regard for the fasting state, 140 mg/dL is the upper limit of normal. If the test is given when the woman is in the fasting state, the upper acceptable limit is 135 mg/dL. If the upper limit of normal is exceeded, a 100-g oral glucose tolerance test is indicated. If the screening value exceeds 200 mg/dL, a fasting blood sugar should be done prior to a glucose tolerance test; if it is significantly abnormal the diagnosis of diabetes is confirmed.[32]

In the 100-g oral glucose tolerance test, the woman consumes 200 g of carbohydrates per day for 3 days. She then fasts for 10 to 16 hours prior to the test. A fasting serum specimen is drawn. She ingests 100 g of carbohydrates and specimens are drawn at 1, 2, and 3 hours. If any two readings exceed the upper limit of normal, a diagnosis of gestational diabetes is made. The normal plasma glucose levels (mg/dL) are 105 (fasting), 190 (1 hour), 165 (2 hours), and 145 (3 hours).

A useful way to assess the degree of glycemic control for the preceding 4 to 8 weeks is to measure hemoglobin A_{1c}, or glycosylated hemoglobin. During the lifetime of a red blood cell, glycolysation occurs in proportion to the average plasma glucose concentration to which the cell is exposed. The lower the value, the stricter the glycemic control that was maintained over the previous 1 to 2 months, and the better the indication.[39] Assessment of hemoglobin A_{1c} is particularly useful when the woman is planning to conceive.

On a daily basis, home monitoring of serum glucose level has replaced urine testing for glucose, as home urine testing for glucose is unreliable in diabetes. Home serum glucose monitoring involves obtaining a capillary sample on a test strip by fingerstick and use of a reflectance meter. Some brands of test strip can be read by comparison with a color chart. Accuracy of the reading depends on cleanliness of the fingerstick site and timing of the procedure. The best site is the midlateral aspect of a large finger pad. This procedure may be done as many as eight to ten times per day. Both pregestational and gestational diabetic clients monitor serum glucose levels. In addition, urine is tested at home daily for the presence of ketones by use of reagent strips.

Fetal well-being is assessed by fetal activity surveillance by the expectant mother, serial ultrasonography for assessment of fetal growth, nonstress tests weekly or twice weekly during the third trimester, contraction stress tests, and fetal biophysical profile. Near term, tests for fetal maturity, such as amniocentesis for phosphatidylglycerol and lecithin:sphingomyelin ratio, may be performed. Ominous developments in the diabetic pregnant woman include urinary tract infection with fever exceeding 39°C, diabetic acidosis, development of PIH, and neglect of the diabetic condition or inability to manage the disease.[34]

Collaborative Management

The objectives of management are to avoid the increased risk of intrauterine death in late pregnancy, to minimize the risk of complications in the mother,[40] and to educate the mother in self-care practices regarding nutrition, glucose testing, and treatment. Abnormal carbohydrate metabolism must be detected precisely, serum glucose level must be carefully regulated, the woman must be educated in self-care practices, and the woman and her neonate must be cared for by a skilled, experienced team.

Diet. Usually gestational diabetes can be controlled by diet alone; however, insulin treatment also may be needed to gain control of serum glucose levels. Excess weight gain must be avoided. Optimally, ideal weight is attained prior to conception. Although an adequate weight gain for the diabetic client is as important as for the nondiabetic client (*see* Chapter 10), the diet of the pregnant diabetic is more carefully controlled.[41] Optimal outcomes are observed with a total gain of 25 to 30 pounds. In obese women, a gain of 15 to 16 pounds is associated with the best outcomes; in underweight women, a gain of 30 pounds is associated with the best outcomes.[42]

Total caloric intake is the same in the first trimester as in the nonpregnant state. During the second and third trimesters, the woman needs 15 kcal per pound of ideal body weight plus 300 kcal. The Recommended Dietary Allowances for the pregnant diabetic woman are similar to those for women who are not diabetic.[41]

The primary goal of diet therapy is to promote normal blood glucose levels while meeting the elevated nutrient requirements of pregnancy. Specific dietary recommendations are based on the classification of the disease; however, general recommendations are outlined in Table 39–14. Currently, a low-fat, high-fiber, high complex carbohydrate diet is gaining favor.[40] Ten percent or less should be simple carbohydrates and the remaining carbohydrates should be from complex carbohydrate food sources; 12 to 20 percent of the diet should be in the form of protein, and the remainder should be provided by fats.[41] Use of polyunsaturated and monounsaturated fats instead of saturated fats is preferred. Foods high in cholesterol should be avoided.

Alcohol should be avoided because of its teratogenic effects. Alcoholic beverages contain only a trace amount of nutrients and alcohol itself can interfere with normal nutrient digestion, absorption, and metabolism. Saccharin is avoided; aspartame and caffeine intake should be limited because these products

TABLE 39–14. NUTRITIONAL RECOMMENDATIONS FOR THE PREGNANT WOMAN WITH INSULIN-DEPENDENT DIABETES MELLITUS, NON–INSULIN-DEPENDENT DIABETES MELLITUS, OR GESTATIONAL DIABETES

Weight gain	25–30 pounds
Kilocalories	300 kcal above normal requirements
Carbohydrates	
Total	55–60%
Complex	45–50%
Simple	10% or less
Protein	60 g/day or 12–20%
Fat	30%
Alcohol	None
Concentrated sweets (candy, cakes, pies, soda)	Restrict
Vitamin/mineral supplement	Yes

can affect glucose metabolism and make its regulation more difficult.[43]

Insulin-Dependent Diabetes Mellitus. For the pregnant woman with insulin-dependent diabetes mellitus (IDDM), adequate nutritional care should begin before conception. Because of the need for rigid control of blood glucose levels, the diabetic diet during pregnancy may be more restrictive than the diet to which the client was previously accustomed. In particular, special attention must be paid to the blood glucose fluctuations that occur during pregnancy.

Daily energy requirements to achieve the recommended weight gain according to the RDA are 300 kcal per week. To obtain an accurate estimation of the client's kilocalorie requirements, the nurse conducts a thorough nutrition assessment. Once the diet has been prescribed, weight gain and blood glucose levels are carefully monitored to determine whether the diet meets the individual's energy needs.

The balance of nutrients should follow the recommendations of the American Diabetes Association[41] for nutritional management of diabetes mellitus. To avoid fluctuations in blood glucose levels, food intake should be in balance with exercise and insulin intake. Five to six meals per day, or three meals with two to three between-meal snacks, are usually recommended. The bedtime snack should include complex carbohydrate and protein to avoid overnight hypoglycemia and ketosis. The American Diabetic Association exchange lists for meal planning can be used to plan diets (Tables 39–15 to 39–18).

Non–Insulin-Dependent Diabetes Mellitus. Pregnant women with non–insulin-dependent diabetes mellitus (NIDDM) ideally have been adhering to a diabetic diet prior to conception. Like clients with IDDM, clients with NIDDM should be re-educated about the need for more rigid control of blood glucose levels during pregnancy. The dietary principles are the same as those outlined for the individual with IDDM.

TABLE 39–15. AMERICAN DIABETES ASSOCIATION DIET

Food Group	Number of Exchanges per Day
Milk	4
Fruit	4
Vegetable	4
Bread	10
Meat	6
Fat	4

TABLE 39–16. EXAMPLES OF FOODS IN EACH DIABETIC EXCHANGE LIST

Milk	1 cup lowfat milk 1 cup plain skim milk yogurt
Fruit	1 small apple 1 small banana ¾ cup strawberries ½ cup orange juice
Vegetable	½ cup asparagus, beets, cauliflower, rhubarb, green beans, carrots, tomato juice
Bread	1 slice whole wheat bread, ½ cup unsweetened cereal, 6 Saltine crackers, ½ cup peas, 1 small corn on the cob, 1 small potato, ½ cup pasta
Fat	1 teaspoon margarine, 1 teaspoon mayonnaise, 1 teaspoon oil, 1 tablespoon salad dressing (oil-based)
Meat	1 oz lean beef, pork, lamb, poultry (without skin); 1 oz fish, 1 oz skim or part skim cheese

Gestational Diabetes. In gestational diabetes, adequate blood glucose control is essential to avoid the need for insulin. The nurse must carefully provide dietary instruction to the woman with gestational diabetes, who often has no prior knowledge of the diabetic diet. The diet composition is the same as that for the individual with IDDM (*see* earlier text).

Activity. Along with dietary management, physical activity is increased as tolerated to promote improved carbohydrate transport and metabolism. The most desirable activities are aerobic: three times per week, about 20 minutes per session. Walking at a rate of 2 miles per hour for 30 minutes is an appropriate form of exercise. Activity is not promoted if serum glucose levels exceed 300 mg/dL. Hypoglycemic reactions can result if an increase in activity is not accompanied by an increase in carbohydrate intake. Additional food, equivalent to a bedtime snack, is a good estimate of what is needed.

TABLE 39–17. GRAMS OF CARBOHYDRATE, PROTEIN, AND FAT FOR ONE PORTION OF EACH EXCHANGE LIST

Exchange List	Carbohydrate	Protein	Fat	Kilocalories
Lowfat milk	12	8	5	120
Lean meat	0	7	3	55
Fat	0	0	5	45
Vegetable	5	2	0	25
Fruit	15	0	0	60
Bread	15	3	trace	80

1 g carbohydrate = 4 kcal, 1 g protein = 4 kcal, 1 g fat = 9 kcal.

TABLE 39–18. SAMPLE MEAL PLAN FOR A 2200-KCAL DIABETIC DIET

Food Group	Breakfast	Snack #1	Lunch	Snack #2	Dinner	Snack #3
Milk	1		1		1	1
Fruit	1	1	1		1	
Vegetable			2		2	
Bread	2		2	2	3	1
Meat			1		3	1
Fat	1		1		2	

Insulin. If dietary management and increased activity are not adequate to bring about a normal serum glucose level, insulin is prescribed (Table 39–19). Gaining favor during pregnancy is the administration of smaller, more frequent dosages of insulin or even continuous infusion via a small, portable insulin pump in cases in which control is particularly difficult, such as during superimposed illnesses.[44]

Careful management can minimize the risk to the infant of a diabetic woman. In one study, infants of diabetic mothers who maintained their fasting serum glucose levels at less than 100 mg/dL and their postprandial levels at less than 140 mg% had no greater incidence of respiratory distress syndrome, one of the risks, than did infants of nondiabetic mothers.[45] Women are taught how to adjust insulin dosage on a day-to-day basis in accordance with their serum glucose levels. Pregnant women are switched to insulins that are more highly purified or are human in origin, because, over time, antibodies develop to porcine or bovine insulin. These antibodies render the drug less effective and higher dosages are needed, making it

TABLE 39–19. NURSING CONSIDERATIONS WHEN USING VARIOUS TYPES OF INSULIN

Type	Peak Effect (Duration)	Pregnancy Considerations	Nursing Implications
Regular insulin: Bovine Porcine Concentrated	1–2 hours (5–6 hours)	Insulin requirements decrease in first trimester, then increase to two to three times prepregnancy dose. Postpartum requirements drop drastically for 48 hours. Use of insulin in gestational diabetes reduces macrosomia. Insulin does not cross placenta.	Client may experience allergic reaction. Resistance to insulin with foreign protein contaminants is possible. Breastfeeding is safe. Neonate must be assessed for hypoglycemia. Drug must be refrigerated. Check expiration date. Establish site rotation chart. Regular, intermediate, or long-acting insulin can be mixed if in the same concentration. Regular insulin may be given intravenously.
Prompt Insulin Zinc Suspension (Semilente)	2–8 hours (12–16 hours)		
NPH (Isophane Insulin Suspension)	6–12 hours (24–28 hours)		
Insulin Zinc Suspension (Lente), Globin Zinc, Protamine Zinc Insulin Suspension, Extended Insulin Zinc Suspension	6–12 hours (24–28 hours)		
Human insulins: Actrapid Velosulin Monotard Insulatard (NPH)	 2½–5 hours (8 hours) 1–3 hours (8 hours) 7–15 hours (24 hours) 4–12 hours (24 hours)	Human insulins may lead to hypoglycemic response in same dosages as porcine or bovine products because of absence of allergic resistance.	Instruct women on need to increase serum glucose surveillance when changing from porcine or bovine to human-origin or purified insulins.

difficult to achieve the strict control needed for a good pregnancy outcome. Changing the type of insulin places the pregnant woman at risk of developing hypoglycemia, as the purified or human-origin insulin is pharmacologically more active at smaller doses (Table 39–19). The risk of hypoglycemia is intensified because the range of control during pregnancy is narrow; 60 to 100 mg/dL in the fasting state, not to exceed 120 mg in the postprandial state.

Many congenital anomalies in fetuses of diabetic women are believed to be preventable if diabetes that is overt prior to pregnancy is well controlled before conception.[46] Women whose disease is being managed with oral antidiabetic medications such as tolbutamide should be switched to insulin as soon as pregnancy becomes a possibility. The oral medications have been found to be teratogenic in research animals. Moreover, there is increasing advocacy of prescribing insulin more liberally among women with gestational diabetes when the serum glucose ranges described earlier are exceeded, to minimize teratogenic effects of the disease.[32,47]

Hospitalization. Hospitalization is required whenever strict glycemic control is not maintained.[48] Other indications include hyperemesis gravidarum, development of hypertension, any evidence of infection, ketoacidosis, onset of labor, or evidence of fetal distress.

Preparation for Delivery. In the past, induced or cesarean delivery at 37 weeks of gestation was routine because there was an increased incidence of late fetal demise among infants of diabetic mothers. This practice contributed to the higher-than-usual incidence of prematurity among infants of diabetic mothers. Now, with greater capabilities to monitor fetal well-being, a pregnancy without complications is allowed to continue to 38 or 39 weeks. If labor does not start, artificial rupture of membranes may be implemented. If this is not successful, oxytocin is administered if there is no evidence of fetopelvic disproportion; the cervix is soft, effaced at least partially, and dilated at least partially; and the fetus is engaged and the presentation is vertex. If labor does not progress, a cesarean delivery is performed.

Fetal monitoring is necessary during induction, and fetal distress is an indication for a cesarean delivery. On the basis of these criteria, as many as two thirds of diabetic women may deliver vaginally.[49] A neonatologist should be present at the delivery. Prenatally, a woman with diabetes may be referred to a level III regional perinatal center for delivery if good neonatal care is not available in her community birthing facility.

The metabolic changes that occur during delivery are dramatic. A small proportion of the woman's usual daily insulin dosage is administered in the form of NPH insulin the morning of delivery, and followed by intravenous or subcutaneous supplements of regular insulin as indicated by hourly serum glucose testing. Intravenous glucose can be used to achieve normal serum glucose levels. Dehydration must be avoided.

The woman may need no more insulin the rest of the day. Her serum glucose level may be high during the recovery phase, but may drop spontaneously later. During postpartum recovery, the parameters of glycemic control can be relaxed.

On the day after delivery one-half of the prepregnancy dosage of insulin in the form of NPH can be given, with supplements of regular insulin if the serum glucose level exceeds 200 mg/dL. Each day the dosage of NPH can be adjusted upward gradually as needed.

Breastfeeding is safe for diabetic women and their infants. The prenatal diet should be continued. Insulin requirements of nursing women are greater than their prepregnancy dosages.[22] Infection must be avoided and treated promptly when it occurs.

Nursing Assessment and Management

The nurse who has contact with pregnant clients must be knowledgeable about gestational diabetes, including risk factors and laboratory values. In a woman with pre-existing diabetes, assessment includes the onset, duration, and course of diabetes; the presence of diabetic complications of vital organs, peripheral nerves, or vasculature; the prepregnancy treatment regimen for diabetes, including a review of how insulin is administered and how glucose and ketone levels are monitored; prepregnancy weight; obstetric history of past and current pregnancies and history of infertility; nausea and vomiting; socioeconomic constraints on the therapeutic regimen; recent hypoglycemia or ketoacidosis; history of infections; and, for later reference, contraceptive history.

Physical assessment includes, in particular, pulse, respirations, and blood pressure; fetal heart rate; evidence of PIH; weight; pedal pulses; skin integrity at injection sites; vaginal bleeding or abdominal tenderness; and vaginal discharge suggestive of monilia.

The pregnant woman with diabetes has several specific needs:

- *Need to perform continued self-assessment.* The nurse instructs the client on the danger signs of pregnancy that require immediate attention. Nausea and vomiting can result in hypoglycemia. Evidence of infection such as burning on urination, fever, vaginal discharge or pruritis, and a cough can herald ketoacidosis. If the woman has decreased peripheral sensation, she must inspect her feet each day for lesions that can become infected. Vaginal bleeding or abdominal pain can signal abruptio placentae. Signs and symptoms of PIH are assessed. The client is instructed on early signs and symptoms of hypoglycemia and ketoacidosis. Using the woman's equipment, the nurse should review assessment of serum glucose level and of urinary ketone level by demonstration and assessment of return demonstration. After quickening occurs, the nurse will instruct the woman on surveillance of fetal activity.
- *Need to meet nutritional requirements of the disease and of pregnancy.* The nurse reviews dietary habits with the client and assesses food preferences, for example, ethnic food customs. The nurse also initiates a referral for dietary counseling. As a team, the client, the nurse and the nutritionist can plan a diet that meets American Diabetes Association criteria and is also sensitive to the client's preferences. On each contact between the nurse and the client there may be a need for dietary review and for clarification as to how the exchange lists are used in planning meals and snacks. Particularly for the woman with gestational diabetes, a large amount of material must be learned fairly quickly so that strict euglycemia can be maintained. Literature that is accurate, clear, and in the client's first language, preferably, will reinforce the nurse's teaching.
- *Need for initial instructions in the administration of insulin.* Insulin requires refrigeration. It is injected subcutaneously, and the sites are rotated to prevent skin toughening, which impairs absorption. Sites include the hips, thighs, abdomen, upper arms, and subscapular areas. Most insulin preparations are available in a concentration of 100 units/mL, and insulin syringes are calibrated in units. The nurse instructs the woman in drawing up the proper dosage and in self-administration.
- *Need of both the client and her family to know how to prevent and recognize hypoglycemia and ketoacidosis early, and what to do should these conditions arise.* Hypoglycemia is best prevented by compensating for activity by increasing food intake and by eating one or two evening snacks. Ketoacidosis develops more slowly. The client is taught to prevent ketoacidosis by diligently monitoring her serum glucose level and adjusting the insulin dosage accordingly. If ketoacidosis develops, emergency care is required to find and treat the cause.
- *Need to understand the tests she will undergo throughout her pregnancy.* The client will be expected to undergo testing for fetal well-being once or twice per week, or even daily in some instances. The nurse can explain the procedures and their rationales. If the client understands the need for careful fetal monitoring for an optimal outcome, she is more likely to value the benefits of frequent testing than be frightened by it.
- *Need of both the woman and her partner for support throughout the pregnancy.* Diabetic individuals are susceptible to "burnout" because of the unrelenting need to carry out a tedious health maintenance regimen.[50] The pregnancy complicated by diabetes is characterized by vulnerability and uncertainty. Scare tactics are counterproductive in motivating diabetic clients. More effective strategies include helping the woman to identify support people in her network of social contacts and support services whose assistance she may need, for example, a 24-hour telephone contact with a nurse who can provide guidance when urgent questions arise about her diabetes management regimen. Praise from the nurse for her self-care is highly motivating.[51]
- *Need for a sense of mastery.* Rather than being controlled by her disease, the pregnant diabetic woman needs to have her autonomy enhanced. The nurse can facilitate this by fully incorporating the woman into the planning of her care. A diabetic self-care regimen is a way of life; as such, it must be comfortable to the individual. This is particularly critical with diet planning, as food has other psychosocial meanings.
- *Need of both woman and her partner to deal with anxiety.* Past coping patterns may be useful now. Support groups for couples experiencing high-risk pregnancies or close friends as well as the nurse may support expression of feelings by the couple. Familiarity with the facility in which she will give birth and childbirth preparation appropriate to high-risk parents can allay fear of the unknown. The nurse can encourage relaxation strategies, such as diversional activities or meditation. See the Case Study/Care Plan for an outline of nursing management of the diabetic client.

CASE STUDY/CARE PLAN: GESTATIONAL DIABETES MELLITUS

Rasheeda Desmond, age 37, gravida 3 para 0, experienced three spontaneous abortions within the past 1½ years. She is now in the 26th week of pregnancy. In the third month she had a urinary tract infection. Rasheeda's 100-g oral glucose challenge test result was high, and a 3-hour oral glucose tolerance test confirmed that she has developed gestational diabetes. A dietary trial did not achieve euglycemic control. Rasheeda has been admitted to the hospital for regulation of insulin level. On admission the nurse notes that Rasheeda is crying. She states "My husband will be so worried. He really wants this baby."

Supporting Assessment Data	Expected Client/Family Outcome	Nursing Action/ Intervention	Rationale	Criteria for Evaluation
Nursing Diagnosis: Alteration in nutritional status, related to obesity and intracellular starvation secondary to insufficiency of insulin				
Client's own birth weight > 9 pounds History of urinary tract infections Positive obstetric history of spontaneous abortions of no known etiology Maternal family history positive for diabetes Blood pressure 132/84 Urine was protein negative Prepregnancy weight 165 pounds, Height 5 ft 7 in. Current weight 190 pounds Fundal height is AGA No abdominal tenderness or vaginal bleeding Urine culture + for bacteria Urine 1+ ketones Serum blood sugar 180 mg Nonstress test reactive	Client will gain 22–27 pounds by term Client's serum glucose level will remain at 120–160 mg throughout pregnancy	Record weight daily Instruct client about exercise and nutritional needs and encourage to follow prescribed diabetic diet. Teach client to use home serum glucose monitor. Instruct client on use of algorithm for determining insulin dosages throughout the day.	A balanced combination of a diabetic diet, insulin, and exercise are the pillars of euglycemic control and attainment of near-normal fetal outcomes. Fatty tissue is insulin resistant. Pregnancy RDAs are the same as those for nondiabetic women. Home monitoring allows for timely adjustment and insulin does and gives client a sense of control. Small frequent dosages of short-acting insulin allow for adjustments in dosage as needed. This permits stricter euglycemic control. Insulin requirements vary over the course of pregnancy.	Client maintains a food diary for 24 hours. Client gains 22–27 pounds by delivery. Client maintains her serum glucose level between 120 and 160 mg.
Nursing Diagnosis: Potential alteration in maternal-fetal safety, related to pathophysiology of gestational diabetes				
	During hospital stay, client and her partner will articulate early signs and symptoms as well as interventions for hypoglycemia and ketoacidosis	Teach couple early detection of hypoglycemia and intervention with oral complex carbohydrate and protein.	Early detection protects against neurologic damage to fetus.	Client experiences no episodes of severe hypoglycemia throughout pregnancy.

Supporting Assessment Data	Expected Client/Family Outcome	Nursing Action/ Intervention	Rationale	Criteria for Evaluation
	Client will not experience episodes of hypoglycemia or ketoacidosis throughout this pregnancy	Teach client and partner intramuscular glucagon administration.	Glucagon stimulates gluconeogenesis.	Client and her partner demonstrate correct technique administration of intramuscular glucagon.
		Teach early detection of ketoacidosis and its prevention.	Acidosis threatens fetal survival.	Urine tests no more than trace positive for ketones throughout pregnancy.
	Client will avoid infection during pregnancy	Instruct client on health maintenance measures and avoidance of urinary, genital tract and other infections.	Infection can lead to rapid onset of ketoacidosis.	Client remains free of infection throughout the remainder of pregnancy.
	Client will use aseptic technique when administering insulin	Instruct client on treatment for asymptomatic bacteriuria Teach client and partner to properly administer insulin	Correct aseptic technique in administering infection will reduce infection.	Client and partner demonstrate appropriate technique for insulin infection.
	Client will articulate danger signs of pregnancy and need for prompt medical attention should they occur	Instruct client on signs and symptoms of complications of pregnancy.	Knowledge enables the mother to participate in her care and to seek help before problems become life threatening.	If complications arise, the client seeks prompt treatment.
	Client will conduct fetal surveillance activities as instructed throughout pregnancy	Explain fetal surveillance regimen: why tests are done, what procedures are involved, where and when client is tested, fetal activity monitoring.	An understanding of the regimen increases a client's ability and motivation to participate fully.	The client participates in fetal surveillance regimen until delivery.
	Client's condition will not be complicated by PIH during pregnancy Fetus will demonstrate reactive nonstress tests throughout pregnancy Fetus will be delivered at term and will be AGA	Monitor for onset of PIH.	Diabetic women are at risk for PIH.	If PIH develops it is attended to promptly.
Nursing Diagnosis: Potential knowledge deficit, related to maternal learning needs about gestational diabetes				
Tests confirm diagnosis of gestational diabetes	Client will participate effectively in the therapeutic regimen throughout pregnancy Client will maintain a serum glucose level of 120–160 mg throughout pregnancy	Using demonstration/return demonstration strategy instruct client on: Types of insulin Storage of insulin Measurement of dose Rotation of sites Subcutaneous injection Asepsis Exercise as tolerated Snack before exercise ADA exchange diet Home serum glucose and urinary ketone measurement.	Client must master large amount of material quickly so that strict euglycemic control is achieved and maintained.	Client demonstrates correct injection technique, ability to plan appropriate menus, and use of glucose monitor and urine dipsticks.

(continued)

CASE STUDY/CARE PLAN: Gestational Diabetes Mellitus (*continued*)

Supporting Assessment Data	Expected Client/Family Outcome	Nursing Action/ Intervention	Rationale	Criteria for Evaluation
Nursing Diagnosis: Potential alteration in family function, related to stress on the couple (perceived threat to pregnancy)				
Client crying on admission. States that husband will be worried about pregnancy.	Prior to discharge: Couple will identify ways to reduce stress Couple will express satisfaction that they managed high-risk pregnancy well	Assess family coping patterns, refer to support group or high-risk childbirth classes, assess lifestyle and support available, mobilize client support network.	High-risk pregnancy is a situational crisis superimposed on a developmental crisis. The threat of fetal loss can be stressful. Diabetes requires unrelenting health maintenance behavior. Support systems and appropriate coping patterns help family manage gestational diabetes.	Client and partner meet others with gestational diabetes. Client is able to carry out the therapeutic regimen successfully, with support from partner and family.

AGA = average for gestational age, ADA - American Diabetic Association.

BLEEDING DURING THE SECOND AND THIRD TRIMESTERS

Second- or third-trimester vaginal bleeding complicates an estimated 3.8 to 4 percent of pregnancies.[52,53] Bleeding may vary from a small amount to hemorrhage. Hemorrhage continues to be a major reason for maternal deaths, because of the need for prompt blood replacement. Hemorrhage during the second and third trimesters jeopardizes maternal and fetal well-being and more than quadruples the rate of premature delivery and perinatal mortality.[54] In addition, maternal isoimmunization can occur as a result of bleeding (*see* later discussion in this chapter).

Five conditions most often account for second-trimester or third-trimester bleeding: abruptio placentae; placenta previa; uterine rupture; disseminated intravascular coagulation; and gestational trophoblastic disease. Each is considered in turn. Major signs and symptoms of each condition are compared in Table 39–20. Placental bleeding, for example abruptio placentae or placenta previa, is the most common source of heavy bleeding.[52]

Abruptio Placentae

Abruptio placentae is premature separation of the placenta from the uterine wall prior to delivery. It accounts for about 30 percent of cases of third-trimester bleeding. The incidence of abruptio placentae has been reported to be 1 in 250 deliveries. Of these deliveries, from 1 in 250 to 1 in 750 ends in fetal death.[55] In the remaining deliveries complicated by abruptio placentae in which the infant survives, there is an increased incidence of neurologic damage to the infant. This is related to the cause of the abruption or to fetal anoxia resulting from the abruption. Abruptio placentae can occur in the second trimester with equally grave implications.

Abruptio placentae can be complete or partial. The risks to the woman and her fetus are associated with such factors as the severity of hemorrhage, the extent of separation of the placenta, and the overall maternal and fetal health status prior to abruption.

Frank vaginal bleeding will not be seen if the margin of the placenta remains completely attached to the uterine wall or if the fetal head is tightly engaged. This is referred to as concealed hemorrhage (Figure 39–3A). Vaginal bleeding will be detected if some of the bleeding occurs external to the amniotic membranes. This is called external hemorrhage (Figure 39–3B). A hematoma forming in the decidua compresses the adjacent placenta, destroying placental function locally. This causes further separation of the placenta. Sometimes the hematoma is due to rupture of a decidual artery. The gravid uterus is unable to contract to stop the bleeding. The separation starts locally, but spreads by means of the process just described. Most often bleeding continues until the fetus is delivered or the mother dies.[5]

Often, the cause of abruption is not known. Predisposing or related factors include trauma, a short umbilical cord, the presence of a uterine tumor or anomaly, uterine pressure on the vena cava, smoking, ethanol consumption, or use of cocaine.[54,56–58] Abruptio placentae may also follow sudden decompression of the uterus as when membranes rupture in the case of polyhydramnios, precipitous delivery, or the birth of the first of twins. As many as half of all

TABLE 39–20. SIGNS AND SYMPTOMS IN FIVE HEMORRHAGIC CONDITIONS OF PREGNANCY

Abruptio Placentae	Placenta Previa	Uterine Rupture	Disseminated Intravascular Coagulation	Hydatidiform Mole
Onset sudden	Bleeding frank, bright red	Rapid onset of symptoms of shock	Petechiae	Brown vaginal spotting over several weeks
Dark vaginal bleeding possible	Spontaneous cessation of bleeding possible	Frank or concealed vaginal bleeding possible	Prolonged oozing from puncture sites	Vaginal expulsion of vesicles
Extreme abdominal tenderness possible	Abdominal pain infrequent	Bright red bleeding	Bruising	Onset of anemia
Rigid, boardlike abdomen possible	Anemia possible	Fetal distress	Bleeding from mucous membrane	Fundal heights exceeding norm for gestational age
Abdominal distension possible	Fetal distress possible	Parts of fundus not palpable in complete rupture	Alteration in laboratory indices of clotting ability	Absent fetal movement, heart sounds
Fetal distress possible	Shock possible	Cessation of contractions in complete rupture		Nausea
Hypovolemic shock possible				Onset of PIH
Occurrence in presence of PIH possible				Possible discomfort from uterine overdistension; rarely, rupture

cases occur in women with hypertension, either chronic or pregnancy induced. Once women have experienced an abruption, they have a 10 to 15 percent chance of experiencing its recurrence in a subsequent pregnancy.[59,60]

Disseminated intravascular coagulation (DIC) is a consumptive coagulopathy that is a serious consequence of abruptio placentae. The blood clotting process is triggered intravascularly and retroplacentally. Diffuse fibrin deposition takes place. Plasminogen is activated, which lyses the microemboli of fibrin and thereby maintains patency of the microcirculation. Because clotting factors are used up in this manner, they are not available for the control of bleeding sites. Furthermore, bleeding across mucous membranes may be observed. This process is discussed in greater detail below in the discussion of disseminated intravascular coagulation.

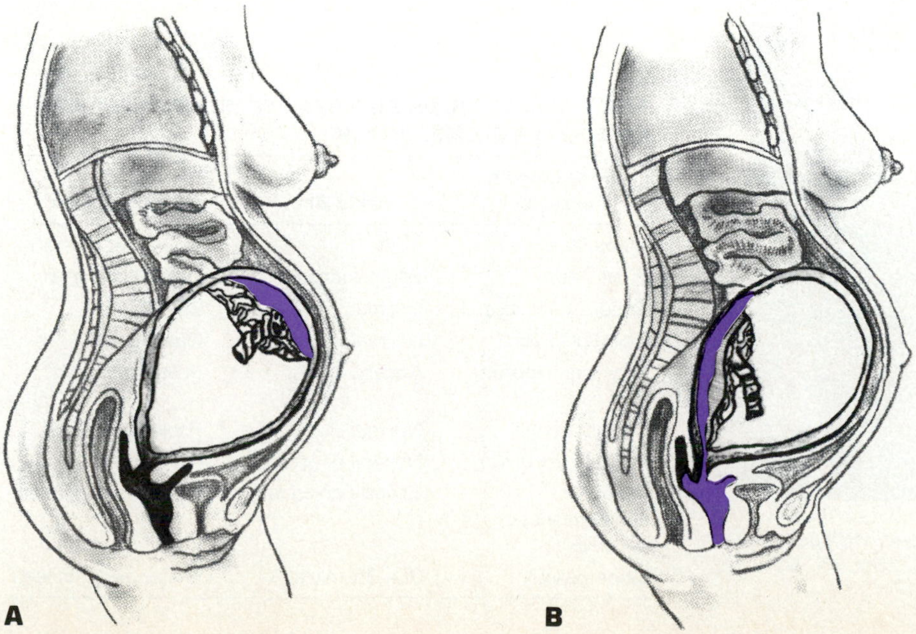

Figure 39–3. Abruptio placentae. **A.** Total abruption with concealed hemorrhage. **B.** Placental abruption with external hemorrhage.

Renal failure can occur in severe cases of abruptio placentae when hypovolemia is not aggressively treated. Renal cortical or cortical necrosis results from hypoperfusion of the kidneys.

Uteroplacental apoplexy, or **Couvelaire uterus,** occurs in severe abruptio placentae when blood extravasates into the uterine musculature, beneath the uterine serosa, into the connective tissue of the broad ligaments, and even into the peritoneal cavity (Figure 39–4). Formerly it was believed that Couvelaire uterus required hysterectomy to prevent postpartum hemorrhage because such a uterus would be unable to contract. Now, with suturing followed by administration of intravenous oxytocin postpartally, hemorrhage and the need for hysterectomy are rare.

Collaborative Assessment. Signs and symptoms can vary markedly in abruptio placentae and do not reliably indicate the degree of danger to the fetus. Commonly observed signs and symptoms include vaginal bleeding; uterine tenderness; back pain; stress; increased frequency of contractions; uterine hypertonicity and rigidity; premature labor; abnormal blood coagulation studies; fetal distress; and fetal death.[5,52]

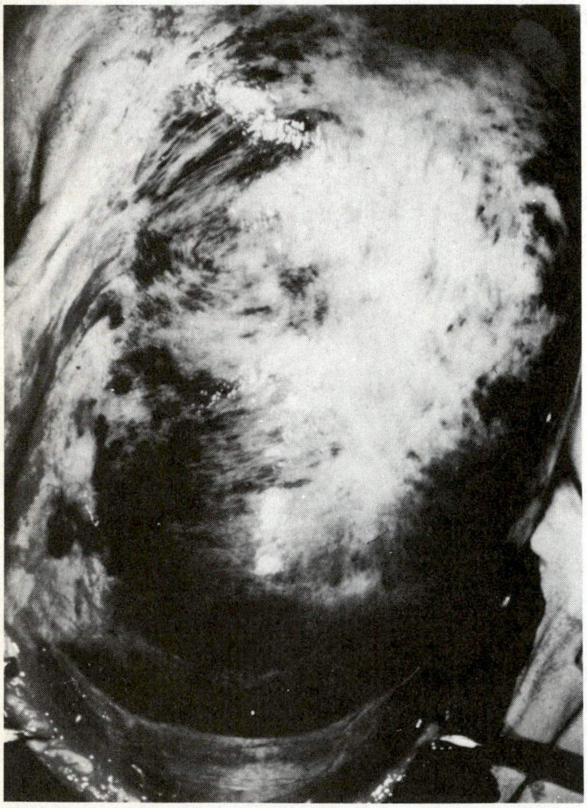

Figure 39–4. Couvelaire uterus. (*Reproduced, with permission from Cunningham FG,* Williams Obstetrics. *18th ed. Norwalk, Conn: Appleton & Lange; 1989:707.*)

Hemorrhagic shock depends on the degree of blood volume loss.[61] Signs and symptoms of early and late shock are contrasted in Table 39–21. The heart rate increases and the pulse becomes thready. Blood pressure remains normal until hypovolemia is severe, at which time a dropping blood pressure is observed. A drop of 20 mm Hg in systolic pressure or an increase of 20 beats per minute in heart rate generally signifies a 20 percent blood loss. Other signs include pallor, diaphoresis, and orthostatic hypotension. Individuals in hypovolemic shock experience a sense of foreboding or anxiety. With significant blood loss oliguria develops because of a decrease in renal perfusion. Postpartum pituitary necrosis (Sheehan's syndrome) may follow hypovolemic shock as a result of pituitary ischemia. This may be evidenced by lack of postpartum milk production.

Abruptio placentae usually occurs in relation to labor and delivery, but it can occur in the second trimester or during the third trimester. Cocaine use is also associated with this condition.[61] Any bleeding in the latter half of pregnancy must be evaluated by inspection, assessment for possible hemorrhage, and by such studies as ultrasound. Contrary to a popular belief, pain is not totally reliable as a means of differentiating betwen abruptio placentae and placenta previa.[5] Pain is more commonly associated with abruption and less commonly associated with placenta previa, but exceptions occur. Pain is more likely with concealed abruption as there is no relief of the pressure exerted by the entrapped blood.

TABLE 39–21. SIGNS AND SYMPTOMS OF EARLY AND LATE HYPOVOLEMIC SHOCK

Assessment Parameter	Early Shock	Late Shock
Blood loss	15%	30–40% or more
Pulse rate	Slight increase	> 120 or higher
Respiratory rate	Normal	30–40
Blood pressure	Normal	Decreased
Postural hypotension	Absent	Present
Capillary refill	Normal	Prolonged
Pulse pressure	Normal or widened	Narrowed
Level of consciousness/behavior	Slightly anxious	Agitated/confused
Urine output	30–35 mL/h	5–15 mL/h or less

Collaborative Management. Treatment depends on the status of the mother and fetus. If the bleeding is heavy, blood and intravenous fluid replacement is started immediately. Oxygen is administered. An indwelling catheter is inserted to assess urinary output.[52] Central venous pressure may be measured. Fetal monitoring is initiated and the fetus is delivered as soon as possible. Screening for consumptive coagulopathy is conducted. Heparin is used to block the action of thrombin in the clotting cascade, if consumptive coagulopathy is evidenced.

If blood loss is minimized and the fetus is immature but stable, close observation while the mother is hospitalized on bedrest may be prescribed. The mother and fetus are carefully monitored, and the possibility of an emergency cesarean delivery is continuous.[5]

Nursing Assessment and Management. The nurse assesses the client with respect to the following: risk factors such as cocaine use; amount and nature of bleeding (dark red vaginal bleeding); blood pressure, pulse, respirations; fundal height, which is marked with a pen (increasing size indicates bleeding); reports of uterine pain; uterine contractions or tonus; fetal heart rate patterns and fetal activity; evidence of coagulopathy; intake and output; reaction to blood products; and reaction of the client and her partner to this emergency.

The woman with abruptio placentae has specific needs that require nursing action:

- *Need for restoration of blood volume.* An intravenous route with a large-gauge (18 g) needle is established. Blood and fluid replacement is started. Intake and output are monitored. Urine output must exceed 30 mL per hour to avoid renal necrosis from hypoperfusion.
- *Need for oxygen.* The nurse positions the woman on her left side. Oxygen is administered by mask as needed.
- *Need for safety in preparation for delivery.* The physician is notified immediately of the woman's condition. The delivery room is set up for an assisted vaginal delivery and for cesarean delivery with possible hysterectomy. No vaginal or rectal examination is performed until the location of the placenta is known. Fetal monitoring is initiated with an external monitor until placenta previa is ruled out. Position of the fetus is assessed. If surgery is likely the woman is placed on NPO (nothing by mouth) status and the neonatal interdisciplinary team is contacted. Blood samples are obtained for typing and cross-matching and for evaluation of clotting status.
- *Need for support.* The family may be very anxious during this emergency. There may not be time to provide lengthy explanations of procedures or to encourage expression of feelings; however, the staff can allow the woman's husband or other support person to remain with her as much as possible. Procedures can be simply explained. A calm manner communicates competence. Continuity of nursing care throughout the experience promotes security. Touch communicates caring. False reassurance that everything will be just fine is to be avoided, because an emergency delivery attended by a neonatal interdisciplinary team clearly demonstrates that a serious, potentially life-threatening condition exists.[62]

Placenta Previa

Normally the placenta implants in the upper body of the uterus. In **placenta previa,** the placenta implants over or very near the cervical os.[5] Placenta previa is described by degree:

1. Total placenta previa exists when the placental totally covers the os (Figure 39–5).
2. Partial placenta previa exists when the placenta partially covers the os (Figure 39–5).
3. Marginal placenta previa exists when the edge of the placenta is at the margin of the internal os.
4. Low-lying placenta is the designation when the placenta is implanted in the lower uterine segment close to the internal os. Up to half of pregnant clients may have a low-lying placenta before 30 weeks; however, in many cases this does not become a clinical problem, because the placenta migrates away from the internal os as the cervix enlarges.[62]

The degree of placenta previa changes as cervical dilation progresses, influencing assessment of the problem. Cervical softening and dilation causes the cervix to pull away from the placenta. This results in bleeding and potential jeopardy to the fetus. The lower segment of the uterus is unable to contract effectively to compress the torn vessels. Because of this, low-lying placentae in general are also associated with increased risk of postpartum hemorrhage.

Placenta previa is reported to occur in 1 in 167 to 260 deliveries.[5] About 20 percent are complete placenta previas. Factors associated with placenta previa include multiparity; advanced maternal age; uterine anomaly; history of placenta previa; history of cesarean delivery or other uterine surgery; intrauterine growth retardation; placenta accreta (a con-

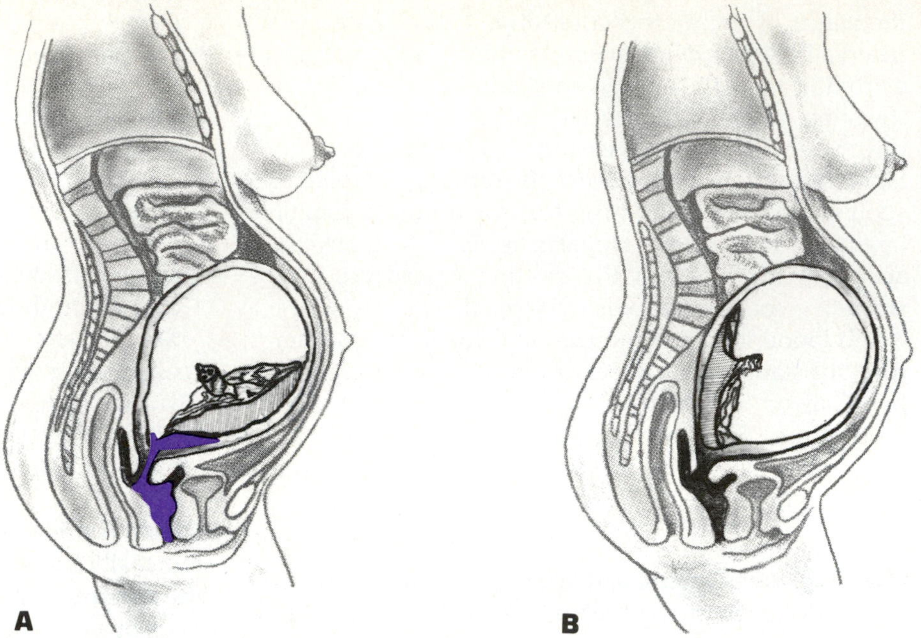

A B

Figure 39–5. Placenta previa. **A.** Partial placenta previa with external hemorrhage. **B.** Total placenta previa.

dition in which the placenta invades the myometrium and cannot easily be separated); breech and transverse lie; and large placenta (produced in such conditions as multiple gestation and fetal erythroblastosis).

The etiology of placenta previa is unknown. If the decidua does not have an adequate vascular supply, as a result of inflammatory or atrophic changes, placenta previa may develop. Additionally, a large placenta, as is found in multiple fetal gestation or fetal erythroblastosis may cover the internal os.[5]

Collaborative Assessment. Collaborative assessment focuses on identification of signs and symptoms that indicate placenta previa. The most characteristic observation is the sudden onset of bright red bleeding, generally in the third trimester. The woman may discover heavy bleeding by awakening in a pool of blood. Usually this bleeding is painless and may or may not be accompanied by contractions. The initial bleeding may stop spontaneously but suddenly resume later. Sometimes, hemorrhage does not occur until labor begins.[5] Women are assessed for signs and symptoms of hemorrhage (*see* Table 39–20), the nature of apparent bleeding, and the time of onset. Women with total placenta previa tend to bleed earlier and more severely during pregnancy.

In general, vaginal examinations are avoided in women with vaginal bleeding.[63] If placenta previa exists, vaginal examination could cause further separation of the placenta from the cervix, lacerate the placenta, and result in more bleeding.

Ultrasound is used to confirm placenta previa. If this is not possible, then careful vaginal examination is done in the delivery room. A double setup, that is, a setup for the vaginal examination and for cesarean delivery, is used in case hemorrhaging occurs and immediate cesarean birth is required.

Placenta previa is rarely complicated by consumptive coagulopathy. Cesarean delivery and blood replacement have reduced the incidence of shock and its sequelae in the event of placenta previa. The major cause of perinatal death is prematurity. The death rate and incidence of congenital anomalies are higher among these infants than in the general population, even when gestational age is taken into account.[5]

Collaborative Management. The goals of collaborative management are to minimize effects of blood loss, to deliver a healthy newborn, and to treat emotional crisis in the client and her family.

Cunningham and colleagues identify four groups of women with placenta previa, each of whom is managed differently[5]:

1. Women whose fetus is premature but the condition of mother and fetus is stable
2. Women who are within 3 weeks of term
3. Women who are actually in labor

4. Women who are hemorrhaging so extensively that they must be delivered despite fetal immaturity

For the first group, close observation and a regimen of restricted activity and bedrest are often enough. The woman may be hospitalized for observation until bleeding has stopped for 24 hours even after ambulation. The woman is instructed to avoid sexual intercourse. She is instructed on symptoms that necessitate immediate intervention, and her proximity to emergency care and transportation is evaluated.

When bleeding is heavy, blood is replaced to maintain an adequa e hemoglobin level. Women in the first group who ıave less than 30 percent previa may delivery vaginally, with constant monitoring. If bleeding is controlled and there is no fetal distress, women who are preterm and not in labor may be managed with bedrest until the fetus is mature. Preterm labor in the woman who is otherwise stable may be managed with tocolysis to suppress contractions and betamethasone to promote fetal lung maturity.[52]

For the other three groups, cesarean delivery is indicated, even when the fetus is dead, because of the potential danger to the mother of hemorrhage. With blood replacement and cesarean delivery the maternal mortality rate in placenta previa is low.

Nursing Assessment. The nurse assesses the onset, duration and amount of bleeding; vital signs and other evidence of hypovolemic shock; presence of pain; uterine contractions or tonus; fetal heart rate; fetal lie; length of gestation; laboratory values, including hemoglobin and hematocrit and clotting factors; and maternal understanding of the problem and coping behaviors.

Postpartally the nurse pays particular attention to assessment of postpartum hemorrhage. Contraction by the uterus is less effective than usual in compressing uterine vessels exposed at the placental site. In addition, the woman with placenta previa is more prone to intrauterine infection.

Nursing Diagnoses. Nursing diagnoses for the woman with partial placenta previa include, but are not limited to, those listed in the box.

Nursing Management. Nursing management addresses the following client needs:

- *Need for safety.* The woman is given nothing by mouth until it is determined that immediate delivery is not necessary. Enemas, rectal or vaginal examinations, and the insertion of any object into the vagina are prohibited unless a double setup is prepared. The nurse prepares the client for ultrasonography. The interdisciplinary neonatal team is contacted when delivery is imminent. If delivery is not indicated and the woman is discharged, the nurse reinforces teaching about the signs and symptoms that require immediate attention as well as the client's access to transportation and emergency care.
- *Need for rest.* The nurse explains the role of bedrest in the treatment of placenta previa. Resting in a semi-Fowler's position allows the fetus to act as a tamponade, thereby slowing bleeding. For the client who is discharged prior to delivery, health care providers must consider whether the woman's life circumstances permit adequate rest at home. If there are other children, another caretaker needs to be identified.
- *Need for alleviation of stress.* The woman realistically may be worried about such problems as her own health, the health of her fetus, and the implications of being on bedrest. The nurse can help the client identify sources of support and strategies that have helped her cope with stressors in the past. Accurate information about the situation, how it is usually handled, and access to health care experts can help the woman further deal with her concerns. It is true that the fetus is in greater-than usual jeopardy, and false reassurance must be avoided.

NURSING DIAGNOSES RELATED TO PARTIAL PLACENTA PREVIA

Problem-Oriented

Altered tissue perfusion, related to partial placenta previa

Anxiety, related to vaginal bleeding during third trimester

Fear of death, related to third-trimester bleeding

Strength-Oriented

Asset in physiologic integrity, related to minimal blood loss from partial placenta previa

Uterine Rupture

Rupture of the uterus is an uncommon emergency and is associated with high rates of maternal and perinatal mortality. Without immediate surgical intervention, as many as three fourths of all infants may die from hypoxia. Maternal deaths are most often due to hemmorhage.[5] In rare cases, severe hemorrhage does not occur if major arteries are not involved and the uterus contracts well after fetal expulsion into the peritoneal cavity. Uterine rupture is usually associated with prior uterine surgery, cesarean delivery, or abdominal trauma, but it can also be caused by inappropriate use of the drug oxytocin to stimulate or augment uterine contractions.[62–64] Other associated factors include prolonged labor, multiparity, polyhydramnios, macrosomia, fetal anomalies, a transverse fetal position, obstetric trauma, development of a pathologic uterine retraction ring, and overdistension of the lower uterine segment.

Nursing and Collaborative Assessment. Rupture occurs most often during labor but it has been known to occur spontaneously during pregnancy. The client is assessed for signs and symptoms of complete rupture, which include the following:

- Profuse bright red bleeding into the vagina (not universal, as covert bleeding into the peritoneum may occur)
- Sharp abdominal pain (related to covert bleeding into the peritoneum)
- Palpation of the fundus, which is firm and rounded, alongside the fetus
- Rapid onset of hypovolemic shock
- Rapid onset of fetal distress or cessation of fetal heart tones
- Cessation of regular contractions

If the rupture is incomplete, the following signs and symptoms are observed:

- Abdominal tenderness and pain that progresses (however, a great deal of pain may not always be present)
- Small amount of vaginal bleeding, although this is not universal
- Development of a palpable retraction ring across the lower uterine segment
- Distension of the lower uterine segment
- Failure of labor to progress even though contractions continue
- Early evidence of the onset of hypovolemic shock, such as maternal anxiety

These signs and symptoms may indicate impending uterine rupture:

- Severe lower abdominal pain
- Failure of labor to progress
- Formation of a retraction ring
- Palpable or visible distension of the lower uterine segment
- Uterine tetany

Collaborative Management. Uterine rupture necessitates emergency cesarean delivery and, frequently, hysterectomy. Antibiotics are administered. Packed red blood cells are infused as quickly as possible, with Ringer's lactate solution for fluid replacement via a second infusion system. Intravenous oxytocin may be administered to contract the uterus until it is removed.

Nursing Management. It may well be the nurse who observes the preceding signs and symptoms of impending or actual uterine rupture. Immediate action to stabilize the woman is mandatory. The nurse initiates notification of obstetric and neonatal medical staff and calls for assistance to obtain a large supply of blood. Blood and fluid replacement is started immediately. Surgical setups for cesarean delivery and hysterectomy are readied. Vital signs and evidence of shock are monitored every 2 to 3 minutes. Fetal monitoring is initiated, if not established prior to the emergency.

Because time is crucial to survival in this emergency, explanations are given succinctly and without delay. Continuity of nursing care can promote security in a crisis situation. Afterward, the woman and her close family members will need support and counseling to help them cope with the emergency events they have experienced, particularly if fetal impairment or loss or hysterectomy occurred.

Disseminated Intravascular Coagulation

Disseminated intravascular coagulation (DIC) is a complex condition in which the formation of blood clots and the lysis of clots are triggered throughout the vascular bed. When the coagulation mechanism is deranged in this manner, the risk of obstetric hemorrhage is increased.

The mechanism of normal clot formation is summarized in Figure 39–6. Pregnancy normally induces a state of hypercoagulability. Coagulation factors I (fibrinogen), VII, VIII, IX, and X and plasminogen are increased. This alteration prepares the woman for hemostasis during labor and delivery. All pregnant women are at some increased risk for DIC.

Conditions such as abruptio placentae, fetal demise, endotoxemia, hydatidiform mole, PIH, sepsis, hemorrhage, and saline abortion increase the potential for DIC to occur.

The coagulation mechanism is activated by the release of thromboplastin at sites of tissue destruction. Fibrinogen is converted to fibrin, causing a state of hypofibrinogenemia (depletion of fibrinogen). Platelets and fibrin are consumed by the formation of large numbers of microemboli, which are tiny clots, throughout the vascular bed. Clots are lysed (or dis-

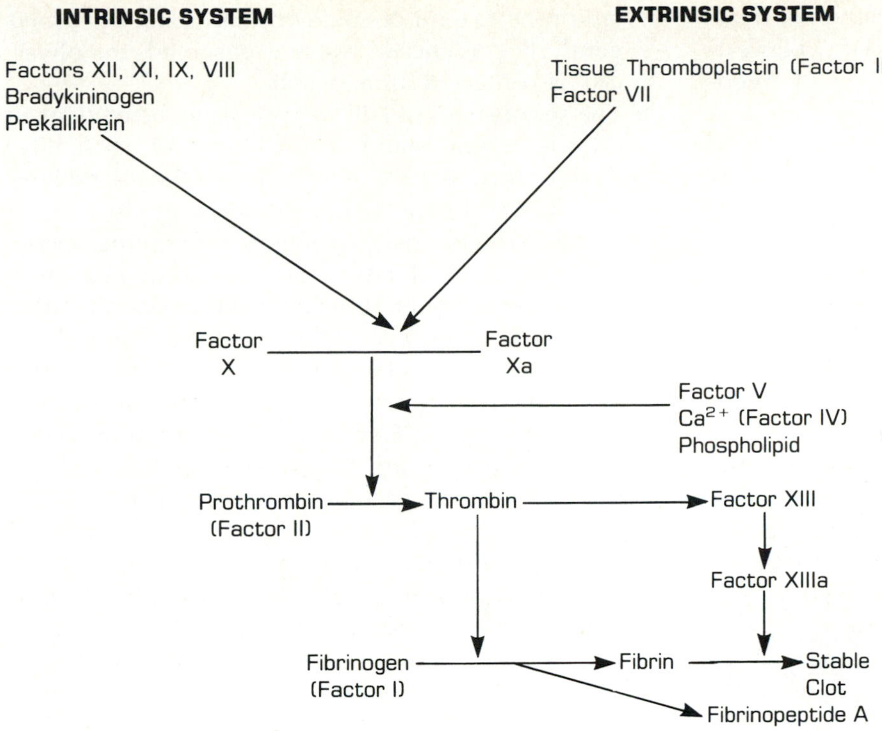

Figure 39–6. The clotting cascade under normal conditions.

solved), resulting in increased levels of fibrin split products. Fibrin split products have anticoagulant properties. The increase in fibrin split products, decrease in number of platelets, and reduction of fibrinogen combine to result in generalized hemorrhage. The woman may bleed extensively, for example, from venipuncture sites, and she may demonstrate petechiae and oozing from mucous membranes and gums. Hematomas may develop. The disseminated microemboli can cause ischemia of vital organs, resulting in any number of organic dysfunctions.[65]

Collaborative Assessment. Women at risk for DIC are assessed for signs and symptoms of generalized bleeding and screened periodically for its development. Table 39–22 summarizes blood tests which are commonly used to assess for DIC. In areas where laboratory analysis is readily available, clotting time and bleeding time tests have been widely replaced by the determination of the prothrombin time, partial thromboplastin time, the platelet count and measurement of products of fibrin degradation (fibrin split products).

TABLE 39–22. LABORATORY FINDINGS IN DISSEMINATED INTRAVASCULAR COAGULATION (CONSUMPTIVE COAGULOPATHY)

Test	Normal Nonpregnancy Value	Normal Pregnancy Value	Value in DIC
Platelets	130,000–400,000	75,000–320,000	Reduced
Burr cells	Absent	Absent	Present
Prothrombin time	9.5–11.3	Normal	Prolonged
Partial thromboplastin time	60–70 s	Shortened	Prolonged
Activated partial prothrombin time	25–45 s	Shortened	Prolonged
Bleeding time	7–8 min	Normal	Prolonged
Clotting time	6–12 min	Normal	Normal
Thrombin time	15–20 s	Shortened	Prolonged
Total bilirubin	0.2–0.9 mg/dL	Slightly increased	Increased
Fibrin split products	Absent	Absent	Present
Fibrogen	150–400 mg/dL	Slightly increased; 400–500 mg/dL	Decreased

Source: *References 7, 9, and 61.*

Collaborative Management. The objectives of treatment include prompt identification of DIC, elimination of the causative factor, stabilization of hypovolemic shock, and treatment of the DIC.

Whole blood or blood components are administered. Fresh whole blood contains all factors. Fresh-frozen plasma contains all factors except platelets. Platelets can be administered separately. Cryoprecipitate contains fibrinogen and factors VIII and XIII.[65] Heparin is sometimes administered because it blocks the activation of thrombin. This is controversial, as the risk of postpartum hemorrhage is increased. Salicylates are contraindicated because they promote bleeding.

Complications of DIC, for example, acute renal failure and infarction of other vital organs, must be diagnosed and treated promptly. The neonate may be compromised if hypoxia is experienced in utero.

Nursing Assessment. The nurse screens the client for factors indicating risk and presence of DIC; monitors laboratory data (*see* Table 39–22); observes for petechiae, gingival bleeding, oozing of blood caused by the pressure exerted on the arm when the blood pressure is taken, excessive bleeding after injections or venipuncture, and bruising; records intake and output and assesses for edema; auscultates the lungs and notes respirations; assesses the client's level of consciousness; checks urine and stool for the presence of blood; takes the vital signs every 2 hours when the client is stable; and looks for signs of early shock, such as tachycardia, central venous pressure, diaphoresis, and anxiety.

Nursing Management. Nursing care focuses on the following parameters:

- DIC is a grave obstetric emergency necessitating intensive care by the interdisciplinary team. If DIC is demonstrated and bleeding occurs, oxygenation is maintained by positioning the woman on her left side and administering oxygen by mask. The nurse administers blood products as prescribed by the physician. A large (16- or 18-gauge) needle or catheter is used. If hemorrhage has occurred, lactated Ringer's solution is usually given intravenously in addition to blood products. The client is observed for signs of cardiac overload as well as transfusion reactions.
- Activities that might cause bleeding are modified. The nurse instructs the client to use a soft-bristle toothbrush or even gauze sponges, rather than a regular toothbrush, to clean her teeth. The blood pressure cuff is inflated no more than 20 mm Hg above expected systolic pressure. Women with DIC are prone to skin breakdown, and must be turned gently. If evidence of shock is observed, the physician is contacted immediately.
- The seriousness of DIC will probably be evident to the client, who may be gravely ill, and her family. Fear for the sake of the woman and fetus, and anxiety related to the whole situation can be anticipated. Women may experience emotional crises related to the high-risk condition and to their pregnancy (*see* Chapter 36). The client needs adequate opportunities to express these feelings. She and her partner need to understand her condition, the tests, her inability to prevent DIC, and its tendency to resolve over time. Family members can be involved in the woman's care. This client is never left unattended by health care providers when she is in labor or when actively bleeding. After the birth, the nurse can promote family integrity to the extent that the woman and her newborn can tolerate it. If the newborn should not survive, family members will need to express their grief (*see* Chapter 36 on family response to neonatal death).[65]

Gestational Trophoblastic Diseases

Trophoblastic diseases originate in the fetal chorion. There are three categories of gestational trophoblastic disease[66]:

1. *Hydatidiform mole.* **Hydatidiform mole** is a benign abnormality of the chorionic villi characterized by trophoblast proliferation and edema of the villous stroma. The fluid-filled villi form grapelike clusters for which the condition is named. Moles may be complete or partial (Figure 39–7).
2. *Invasive mole.* The abnormal trophoblastic tissue

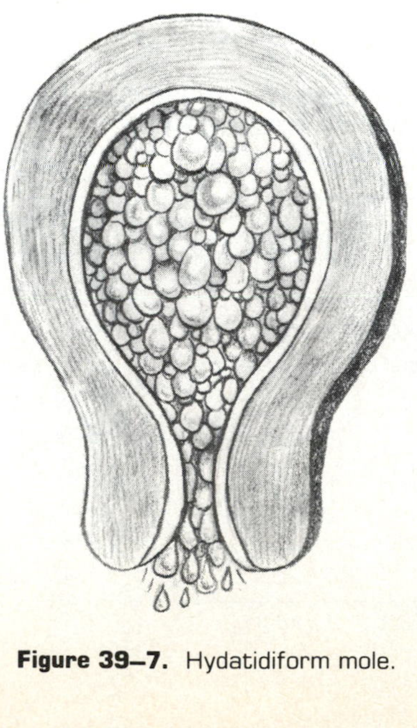

Figure 39–7. Hydatidiform mole.

found in hydatidiform mole may invade the uterus, adjacent structures, or distant sites.

3. *Choriocarcinoma.* In 10 to 20 percent of cases, the tissues described in the two preceding conditions undergo malignant transformation. Spread is rapid, and may be local or diffuse.

A complete hydatidiform mole is believed to arise from fertilization of an ovum in which the chromosomes are absent or inactivated by a haploid (46, XX) sperm. Other variations have been observed.[5] In the partial mole the karyotype is typically triploid, with the usual maternal genetic contribution but double the usual paternal contribution. Complete moles have a greater propensity than partial moles to transform into choriocarcinoma. The ratio of complete to partial moles is 1 to 2. Partial moles may occur in conjunction with twin pregnancy; a fetus may be present with a partial mole.

Hydatidiform mole occurs once in 1500 to 2000 pregnancies in the United States and Europe; in Asia, hydatidiform mole occurs 10 times more frequently than in the United States. The incidence among women over 45 is 10 times greater than that among women aged 20 to 40. There is a slightly increased incidence of hydatidiform mole among women who have had a molar pregnancy. Maternal mortality in hydatidiform mole is virtually zero when prompt diagnosis and appropriate therapy are carried out. In only a few recorded cases has a live fetus survived a partial molar pregnancy.

Invasive mole occurs in about 10 to 15 percent of women who have had a primary molar pregnancy.[67] It is a locally invasive neoplasm that can metastasize to other areas of the body. It occurs with about the same frequency as choriocarcinoma, 1 in 7500 to 20,000 pregnancies in the United States.

Choriocarcinoma may follow hydatidiform mole, abortion, ectopic pregnancy, or normal pregnancy. It is rare, occurring in an estimated 2 to 5 percent of gestational trophoblastic neoplasms,[67] and the etiology of the malignant transformation of the trophoblast is unknown. Choriocarcinoma is characterized by a rapidly growing mass invading uterine muscle and blood vessels, causing hemorrhage and necrosis. Sepsis may develop. The most common sign is irregular bleeding associated with uterine subinvolution. Complaints associated with pathologic changes at metastatic sites may precede identification of the choriocarcinoma. The growth may perforate the uterus, leading to peritoneal hemorrhage.

Nursing and Collaborative Assessment. Typically, molar pregnancy becomes evident later in the first trimester or in the second trimester.[5] Assessment for molar pregnancy includes the following observations.

- Uterine bleeding is the most outstanding sign of molar pregnancy. Marked hemorrhage can occur, but more typically dark brown spotting occurs for weeks or months. Iron deficiency anemia commonly accompanies this bleeding.
- Uterine size is an important index. In a molar pregnancy, the fundal height often exceeds that expected for the date.
- Fetal activity and fetal heart tones are usually absent.
- Molar pregnancy may be accompanied by hyperemesis gravidarum.
- Pregnancy-induced hypertension often accompanies a molar pregnancy, and in this one exception it develops earlier than the usual 24 weeks of gestation.
- Very high serum hCG levels may be noted 100 days or more after the last menstrual period.
- Pulmonary embolism may occur if trophoblastic material escapes the uterus in the venous outflow. Death and even local infarct are rare, but the tissue can establish itself and proliferate in this distal site as invasive mole or choriocarcinoma.
- Plasma thyroxine levels may be elevated.
- The grapelike vesicles may be passed vaginally, especially around the fourth month of pregnancy.
- Ultrasound confirms the diagnosis of molar pregnancy.

Assessment for metastatic disease may include a pre-evacuation chest x-ray. Computed tomography or magnetic resonance imaging may be performed, if indicated. Many women have not heard of molar pregnancies. Clients may react with horror, fear, or grief. The nature and extent of psychologic reactions to this condition will need to be assessed.

Nursing and Collaborative Management. Management addresses the objectives of immediate evacuation of the mole and follow-up for the prevention or early detection of malignant transformation.

Most often, vacuum aspiration performed by the physician is the method used to evacuate the mole. General anesthesia is used and the cervix is dilated. Two to four units of packed red blood cells are available, and an intravenous line is inserted using an 18-gauge needle. Oxytocin is administered intravenously to contract the uterus during the procedure. Curettage follows the evacuation, and the tissue obtained is submitted for histologic evaluation. Occasionally, hysterotomy is the method selected for evacuation. Oxytocin is infused and curettage follows the evacuation.

Hysterectomy may be elected, especially if the woman is over 40 or desires no more children. Choriocarcinoma is a more likely sequela among older and high-parity women.

In rare cases in which a fetus and placenta exist with a mole as a result of twinning, the pregnancy may be allowed to progress; however, the eventual risks to the mother and health of the infant have not been confirmed.[5]

The follow-up protocol is of critical importance for women experiencing molar pregnancy. Serum chorionic gonadotropin levels are assayed every 1 to 2 weeks until normal nonpregnancy levels are achieved. The assay is repeated monthly for 6 months and then every 2 months for 1 year. A rise or a plateau in the chorionic gonadotropin level necessitates further diagnostic assessment and usually treatment.

Pregnancy should be avoided during the 1-year follow-up period. Pregnancy would obscure the evidence of choriocarcinoma. Low-dose oral contraceptives prevent pregnancy, but they also suppress pituitary luteinizing hormone, which can confound assays for chorionic gonadotropin.

In addition, a baseline x-ray of the lungs is obtained postpartally and compared to the pre-evacuation x-ray.[5] If chorionic gonadotropin levels plateau or rise, the x-ray is repeated. Some protocols call for repeat chest x-rays every 2 months for 1 year.

If chorionic gonadotropin levels do not regress normally, curettage or hysterectomy is performed. If that does not effect a cure or if there is evidence of metastasis to the lungs, chemotherapy is initiated. Commonly used antineoplastic agents include methotrexate and actinomycin D. These may be used in combination with other antineoplastic agents.

The nurse addresses client needs that are similar to those observed in other hemorrhagic conditions. The client is prepared for the diagnostic and therapeutic procedures she is about to undergo. She needs education and support to participate in the year-long follow-up protocol.

Unique to gestational trophoblastic disease is the concept that pregnancy was associated with something other than a fetus and that cancer may result. Depending on the explanation of molar pregnancy provided by health care professionals, the woman's self-esteem can suffer from the awareness that the products of conception were so abnormal. The nurse can reassure the woman and her partner that this condition cannot be prevented, given current knowledge.

If the woman initially became aware of the disease because she passed a vesicle, the nurse needs to be sensitive to what a frightening or startling event this can be. A couple may have objections to abortion; therefore they need to understand that the life of a fetus is not at stake. If contraception during the 1-year follow-up protocol is objectionable, the nurse can emphasize that future reproductive integrity as well as preservation of the woman's life is the goal of follow-up care. In addition, ethicists from a religious background similar to that of the client may be consulted.

INFECTIONS

Infection can affect the progress and outcome of pregnancy. Specific effects depend on type of organism, body systems involved, and severity of infection. Infection places the fetus at risk for sepsis, low birth weight, prematurity, congenital anomalies, or death. Implications of various infections for pregnancy are summarized in Table 39–23.

Infection of the Urinary Tract

During pregnancy, anatomic and physiologic changes in the urinary tract predispose the woman to urinary tract infection (*see* Chapters 12, 16, and 20). Under the influence of elevated serum progesterone levels the renal pelves and ureters dilate. Peristalsis decreases, allowing urinary stasis. Increased uterine and vaginal secretion promotes leukorrhea, harboring gram-negative coliform microorganisms near the urethral meatus.[68] As the uterus expands, the ureters may be compressed. Torsion on the bladder makes it more susceptible to injury. These changes mean that pregnant women are at greater risk for bacteriuria. Ascending infection of the urinary tract develops more easily in pregnant than nonpregnant women.

Ascending urinary tract infection results in acute pyelonephritis, which is one of the most common medical complications of pregnancy and affects about 2 percent of pregnant women.[69] This condition is occasionally associated with septic shock, spontaneous abortion, fetal death, premature delivery, and stillbirth. Repeated episodes can result in chronic renal impairment.[68]

Asymptomatic bacteriuria occurs in as many as 12 percent of all pregnant women. It is most common among economically disadvantaged, multiparous, minority women, especially those with sickle cell trait, but it can be observed in any woman.[5,70]

Nursing and Collaborative Assessment. Infection is confirmed if there are more than 100,000 organisms of the same type per milliliter of a clean-catch midstream urine specimen. Because of the prevalence of

TABLE 39–23. IMPLICATIONS OF MATERNAL INFECTIONS FOR PREGNANCY AND THE NEONATE

Infection	Agent	Implications for Pregnancy
Asymptomatic bacteriuria, cystitis, acute pyelonephritis	Commonly *Escherichia coli, Proteus, Klebsiella*	Maternal hormones relax urinary tract, making ascent of bacteria easier. Risk of premature delivery. Sulfonamides in late pregnancy may cause hyperbilirubinemia and kernicterus in the neonate. Breastfeeding safety depends on drug therapy used.
Human immunodeficiency virus	Human immunodeficiency virus (HIV)	Transplacental infection may occur. Infant develops failure to thrive, hepatosplenomegaly, interstitial pneumonia, recurrent infections, and neurologic abnormalities. Infants are often SGA and may evidence Epstein-Barr virus. Neonatal/infant motality rate 81%. Breastfeeding is contraindicated except in Third World countries. Mother must learn appropriate, sometimes complex, infant care.
Bacterial vaginitis	*Gardnerella vaginalis*	Ampicillin or sulfa-containing vaginal creams may be used. Breastfeeding safety depends on particular drug therapy.
Chlamydia	*Chlamydia trachomatis*	Infants may develop conjunctivitis or pneumonia. Prematurity and fetal demise may occur. Breastfeeding safety depends on particular drug therapy.
Chorioamnionitis	Diverse organisms	Fetus can be severely compromised. Preterm labor may occur. Breastfeeding is safe when woman is febrile, depending on the drug therapy used.
Condyloma accuminata	A papovirus	Podophyllin, which is used in nonpregnant women, may be teratogenic. Local treatment such as laser or cyrosurgery may be used. Neonatal infection is possible. There are no restrictions on breastfeeding.
Cytomegalovirus	Cytomegalovirus	Neonate may develop learning disabilities, mental retardation, cerebral palsy, and deafness as well as anemia and hyperbilirubinemia. Breast milk should be pumped and discarded during infectious period.
Gonorrhea	*Neisseria gonorrhoeae*	Infection at birth may cause ophthalmia neonatorum and subsequent blindness in the neonate. Breastfeeding safety depends on particular drug therapy.
Hepatitis B	Hepatitis B virus	Infection of the fetus can result in prematurity and chronic liver disease. Breast milk should be pumped and discarded during infectious period.
Herpes	Herpesvirus type 2	Infection is contracted by the neonate during vaginal delivery. May cause death or neurologic damage. Primary infection, especially in the third trimester, may cause intrauterine growth retardation or prematurity. Breastfeeding is safe with good maternal handwashing.
Moniliasis	*Candida albicans*	An infant who comes into contract with the microorganism in the birth canal may develop oral thrush.
Rubella	Rubella virus	Early in pregnancy neonatal infection may result in such anomalies as congenital heart disease and cataracts, intrauterine growth retardation, mental retardation and cerebral palsy, diabetes, deafness, glaucoma, and a progressive encephalitis. Breast milk should be pumped and discarded during the infectious period.
Syphilis	*Treponema pallidum*	Disease may be transplacentally passed to the fetus. Result may cause second-trimester abortion, stillborn term infant, or a congenitally infected infant. Breastfeeding is safe after treatment.
Toxoplasmosis	*Toxoplasma gondii*	Infection is associated with increased incidence of abortion, prematurity, stillbirth, neonatal death, and severe congenital anomalies involving convulsions, coma, microcephaly, hydrocephalus, blindness, deafness, and severe retardation. Breastfeeding safety depends on particular drug therapy.
Trichomoniasis	*Trichomonas vaginalis*	The most commonly used drug, metronidazole, is potentially teratogenic. Breastfeeding safety depends on particular drug therapy.
Tuberculosis	*Mycobacterium tuberculosis, M. africanum, M. bovis*	Congenital infection can occur. The focus of fetal infection is the liver or lymph nodes. Mother and infant must be separated until treatment begins. Mother and baby must be strictly isolated. The pregnant woman taking INH must take pyridoxine. Breast milk should be pumped and discarded during infectious period. Breastfeeding during INH therapy is controversial.
Varicella	Human alpha herpes virus 3 (varicella zoster virus)	Infection can cause teratogenicity, fetal death, abortion. Varicella zoster immunoglobulin is recommended for the high risk infant after exposure. Breast milk should be pumped and discarded during infectious period.

bacteriuria among pregnant women and the grave implications of pyelonephritis for the fetus, a urine culture for screening purposes may be performed at the first prenatal visit. Urine cultures at least once per trimester may be recommended for high-risk clients. Even in the absence of symptoms bacteriuria is potentially harmful: in many women it persists past delivery and is often associated with the development of chronic lesions in the urinary tract.[5]

Signs and symptoms of cystitis, or bladder infection, include urinary frequency, urgency, dysuria, hematuria, and pyuria. In ascending urinary tract infection, and even occasionally in cystitis, flank pain or costovertebral angle tenderness is a prominent feature. When the kidneys are palpated, the individual experiences sharp, intense pain. Signs and symptoms of cystitis are discussed further in Chapter 41, along with preventive measures.

The woman with acute pyelonephritis experiences fever and chills or hypothermia, lumbar pain, anorexia, nausea, and vomiting. Tachycardia and hypotension may occur if bacteremia or bacterial toxemia has developed.

Assessment parameters also include temperature, pulse, respirations, blood pressure, and intake and output. Fetal monitoring is performed. Pyelonephritis can be confused with conditions such as chorioamnionitis and preterm labor; therefore, careful assessment is necessary.

Nursing Diagnoses. After careful assessment, nursing diagnoses related to urinary tract infection may be developed (*see* the box).

Nursing and Collaborative Management. Pregnant women should be instructed routinely about strategies that can lower their risk of urinary tract infection. Such strategies include use of cotton-crotch undergarments; avoidance of chemical irritants such as feminine hygiene sprays and bubble bath; adequate fluid intake; frequent urination; and urination after sexual intercourse. Women who are pregnant are instructed to seek health care immediately if burning occurs on urination.

As many as 40 percent of women with asymptomatic bacteriuria develop pyelonephritis, or infection of the kidney.[71] This can be prevented by the treatment of bacteriuria with antibiotics. Asymptomatic bacteriuria can be effectively treated in 75 to 80 percent of cases by a single dose of sulfisoxazole, nitrofurantoin (Box 39–3), or ampicillin. If infection persists, a 10-day course of antibiotic may be prescribed.[5] Symptomatic bladder infections are treated in the same manner; treatment is initiated with the development of symptoms, as drug sensitivity, or the appropriateness of the drug in treating the particular microorganism, is predictable. Most of the time the cause is *Escherichia coli, Proteus,* or *Klebsiella.* Nitrofurantoin produces high antibiotic urinary levels with little systemic effect. The medication can be changed if needed when urine culture and sensitivity results are available.

Women with cystitis and pyelonephritis are advised to increase their intake of clear, noncaffeinated fluids to 16 cups per day. Cranberry juice is often used to acidify the urine, making it less habitable to microorganisms.

Women who develop pyelonephritis are often hospitalized during the acute phase of the illness. Dehydration is treated with intravenous fluids. Blood is available and an 18-gauge intravenous line ensures access in the event of shock. Acetominophen may be prescribed to lower fever and a cooling blanket may be applied to reduce high fevers. Analgesics are used to relieve pain. If the client is not febrile, a heating pad may provide some topical pain relief.

Intravenous therapy with medications such as ampicillin or cephalosporins may be initiated. Changes in antibiotics are made if culture and sensitivity results indicate a need to do so. Intravenous antibiotic therapy for 72 hours should result in abatement of the woman's symptoms. At that time, oral antibiotics can be used and the client continues her treatment for 14 days. The urine should be recultured at the end of her course of medication. Cultures must be negative to consider the problem resolved. The client is instructed on the importance of continuing treatment for the prescribed period, although she may begin to feel well. Failure to complete antibiotic treatment can lead to recurrent infection and growth of antibiotic-resistant organisms.

NURSING DIAGNOSES RELATED TO URINARY TRACT INFECTIONS

Problem-Oriented

Altered patterns of urinary elimination, related to cystitis

Pain, related to pyelonephritis, cystitis

Potential for injury to urinary tract structure and function, related to infection

Strength-Oriented

Potential for continued positive role performance, related to relief of discomfort from urinary tract infection

BOX 39–3. NITROFURANTOIN

Proprietary Names:
Macrodantin (Norwich Eaton), others.

Classification:
Urinary anti-infective.

Action:
Generally bacteriostatic, but may be batericidal if high enough concentrations are reached at the site of action. Although the mechanism of action has not been clearly defined, it is thought to inhibit several bacterial enzyme systems. Spectrum of activity includes many gram-negative bacteria (*E. coli, Enterobacter, Klebsiella, Salmonella, Shigella, Citrobacter*) and some gram-positive bacteria (*Staphylococcus aureus, S. epidermidis, Streptococcus faecalis*).

Indications:
Treatment of initial or recurrent urinary tract infections caused by susceptible bacteria. Not effective for infections outside the urinary tract.

Dosage and Route:
Administered orally only and should be taken with food. Usual adult dose: 50–100 mg four times daily for at least 1 week.

Pharmacokinetics:
Absorption: Readily absorbed from the small intestine after oral administration. Macrocrystals are absorbed more slowly than products containing microcrystals. Food increases the extent of absorption. *Distribution:* Distributes into breast milk and crosses the placenta. *Elimination:* 30–50 percent of dose is excreted unchanged in the urine, with the remainder metabolized in the liver. Peak urinary concentrations are obtained about 30–60 minutes after ingestion of dose in adults with normal renal function. Plasma half-life is about 20 minutes.

Precautions and Contraindications:
Use with caution in clients with diabetes mellitus, vitamin B deficiency, electrolyte disturbances, anemia, and renal impairment because of increased risk of developing peripheral neuropathy. Also use with caution in clients with G6PD deficiency. Contraindicated when creatinine clearance <40 mL per minute.

Adverse Reactions:
Most common: Nausea, vomiting, anorexia. *Less common:* GI—diarrhea, abdominal pain; CNS—peripheral polyneuropathy, headache, dizziness, drowsiness, retrobulbar neuritis, trigeminal neuralgia; pulmonary—acute, subacute, or chronic pulmonary reactions; hematologic—hemolytic anemia, agranulocytosis, leukopenia, granulocytopenia, thrombocytopenia, megaloblastic anemia; dermatologic—exfoliative dermatitis, erythema multiforme, urticaria, transient alopecia; other—dark yellow or brown urine, photosensitization, anaphylaxis; fetal—potential for hemolysis in G6PD-deficient infants if used near term.

Drug Interactions:

- Probenecid: May inhibit renal excretion and increase serum concentrations of nitrofurantoin.
- Magnesium trisilicate antacids: Inhibit oral absorption of nitrofurantoin.
- Nalidixic acid, norfloxacin, ciprofloxacin: Nitrofurantoin may antagonize antibacterial effects.

Nursing Implications:

- Assess for foul-smelling, milky urine and perineal irritation, which may indicate urinary tract superinfection.
- Assess whether client has experienced allergic reaction to medication prior to administration.
- Teach client to take medication with food or milk to decrease gastrointestinal distress.
- Teach client possible adverse reactions to medication and to report reactions immediately.

G6PD = glucose-6-phosphate dehydrogenase, GI = gastrointestinal, CNS = central nervous system.

Chorioamnionitis

Chorioamnionitis is infection of the chorion, amnion, amniotic fluid and, by association, the fetus. Normally a mucous plug in the cervix protects the uterine contents from infection, and amniotic fluid has some bacteriostatic properties. But in as many as 1 percent of pregnancies, chorioamnionitis is a complication.[72]

The infection is often caused by bacteria that normally inhabit the genital tract. Commonly identified microorganisms include *E. coli*, group B beta-hemolytic streptococci, anaerobic streptococci, and *Bacteroides;* however, *Neisseria gonorrhea, Listeria monocytogenes,* herpes simplex virus, cytomegalovirus and *Candida albicans* also have been implicated.[71,73]

Factors associated with chorioamnionitis include poor maternal nutrition, socioeconomic disadvantage, amniocentesis, repeated vaginal or rectal examinations, vaginitis, cervicitis, and cervical cerclage. There is a relationship between chorioamnionitis and sexual intercourse when membranes are ruptured late in the third trimester.[74] Chorioamnionitis might be a secondary infection occurring because of organisms transported via the circulation from a distantly located maternal primary infection site. As many as one fourth of women with premature rupture of membranes develop this problem, and, conversely, premature rupture of membranes may follow the onset of infection.

Chorioamnionitis more often necessitates cesarean delivery than usual circumstances dictate. This reflects the need, if labor is not imminent or if the degree of illness is more than mild, to deliver the fetus as soon as possible. Postpartally, the mother who has undergone cesarean delivery faces greater risk of developing peritonitis, thrombophlebitis, and septicemia. For this reason, prior to cesarean delivery oxytocin induction or augmentation may be attempted. The infant is at great risk for central nervous system and respiratory infection.

Nursing and Collaborative Assessment. Early signs and symptoms may be nonspecific, including fever and tachycardia. Preterm labor is a possible manifestation of chorioamnionitis. Later, uterine tenderness develops, and may be accompanied by malodorous discharge. When the membranes rupture, the amniotic fluid is cloudy and foul smelling.

Nursing and Collaborative Management. Delivery of the infant and intravenous antibiotic therapy for the mother and, if needed, for the infant are the major medical interventions.[5] Cesarean delivery is performed when the fetus is stressed, or if an effective labor pattern cannot be achieved. But surgery in the presence of infection is always more dangerous than usual in terms of wound healing, abscess formation, secondary infections, and septicemia.

Antibiotic therapy is instituted. Broad-spectrum antibiotics, for example, cefoxitin, are effective against gram-negative and gram-positive aerobic and anaerobic bacteria. These drugs cross the placenta and achieve peak levels an hour after parenteral administration to the mother.[71]

Common interventions when preterm labor is present include administration of tocolytic agents and corticosteroids. Steroids can intensify infectious processes. It may be useful to perform amniocentesis for culture and sensitivity before attempting to halt preterm labor so that infection can be treated if it is the cause.

Nursing responsibilities include administration of antibiotic therapy as ordered and assessment of the woman's response, promotion of generous fluid intake, continual assessment of maternal and fetal status, and consideration of the infant's high-risk status. Specific observations include vital signs, intake and output, intactness of the intravenous infusion system, and symptoms of drug toxicity. Oxytocin may be used to induce labor; otherwise, the nurse prepares for cesarean delivery if indicated.

TORCH Infections

TORCH is an acronym for a variety of organisms, most of which can cross the placenta and damage the fetus. It stands for *t*oxoplasmosis; "*o*ther" infections (including type B hepatitis virus, coxsackie B virus, mumps, poliovirus, rubeola, varicella, *Listeria gonorrhea,* streptococcus, and treponema); *r*ubella; *c*ytomegalovirus; and *h*erpes.[75] Herpes rarely crosses the placenta.[76]

Toxoplasmosis. Toxoplasmosis occurs in about 0.5 percent of pregnancies.[77] Toxoplasmosis occurs wherever humans and their domestic animals are found.[78] It is caused by a protozoan and can be transferred hand to mouth after handling cat feces or contaminated soil and by consuming undercooked meat. The infection can also be transmitted transplacentally. The embryo or fetus is affected if the woman contracts the disease during her pregnancy.

There is a direct relationship between the time in pregnancy at which the mother becomes infected and the incidence of fetal infection. If the woman is infected in the first trimester, the chance of fetal infection occurring is 15 percent. This rises to 60 percent in the third trimester. The most severe infection occurs before the sixth month; however, the severity of infection for the fetus diminishes throughout pregnancy.[78] The perinatal mortality rate in maternal toxoplasmosis is 10 to 15 percent, but 85 percent of infants who survive show psychomotor retardation by age 4. Half have visual problems within the first year.

Nursing and Collaborative Assessment. Assessment for risk of toxoplasmosis may be done with a blood test to identify the presence of antibodies, for example immunoglobin G against *Toxoplasma* and immunoglobin M, which is usually encountered within the first month of acquired infection. Ideally, serologic assessment would be performed prior to pregnancy to distinguish women who are already immunized against the disease from women who remain at risk. Serial surveillance with blood tests around 8 weeks, 6 months, and at delivery may be done for women who live in areas where there is a high incidence of toxoplasmosis.[78] Serial blood testing is done for women who are assessed for the first time during pregnancy and have positive serologic results in order to identify whether a new infection occurred or whether test results reflected immunity from an old infection.

Nursing and Collaborative Management. Women with toxoplasmosis who are not pregnant are advised to avoid pregnancy for 1 year. If the woman is already pregnant, the health care provider discusses the options for treatment and, if infection occurred in the first trimester, for termination of the pregnancy. If the woman chooses to continue the pregnancy, treatment is oral sulfadiazine for 28 days. Pyrimethamine, a folic acid antagonist, is contraindicated during the first trimester because it is teratogenic. In the second and third trimesters, sulfadiazine is administered in conjunction with pyrimethamine. Folic acid is given concurrently to prevent bone marrow suppression.[71]

The nurse instructs the woman about her medication regimen, including timing and dosage, storage of the drugs, side effects to observe, and duration of treatment.

Preventive teaching of pregnant women includes advising them to cook meat thoroughly, freezing meat prior to cooking for 24 hours at 20°C to kill cysts, washing fruits, and vegetables thoroughly before eating them, avoiding cat litter boxes or wearing protective gloves to do this chore, and wearing gloves when gardening. In addition, good handwashing before and after food preparation and high-risk behaviors is an important preventive measure.

Other Infections

Hepatitis. The "other" category includes hepatitis B virus (HBV). Hepatitis B virus occurs in up to 3 percent of pregnancies. It is rarely transmitted to the fetus before delivery. Individuals at risk for HBV include parenteral drug abusers or their sexual partners, women in sexual relationships with bisexual men, women with multiple sexual partners, clients and staff in institutions for the mentally retarded, clients and employees in dialysis centers, and other health care professionals who handle blood or body fluids in any setting. Outbreaks have occurred in relation to tattoo and acupuncture.

Infection is more likely during delivery or in early postpartum. But if HBV is transmitted to the fetus, the risks of prematurity and perinatal morbidity are increased.[79] Infants who subsequently test positive for HBV surface antigen are rarely symptomatic. If acute hepatitis does develop its course is usually benign. Such infants may be chronic antigen carriers.

Signs and symptoms of hepatitis B include jaundice, lethargy, anorexia, vomiting, and fever. Intervention is supportive. No antiviral treatment exists at this time.

Women in the high-risk group should be screened early in pregnancy. An effective vaccine exists for HBV and it is recommended that individuals at risk be immunized; however, vaccination during pregnancy is avoided. On exposure, clients should be offered hepatitis B immunoglobulin prophylaxis. Infants of women who test HBV antigen positive should be given a dose of hepatitis B immunoglobulin immediately after birth and three doses of vaccine within the first week of life and at 1 and 6 months of age.

A mother who tests positive for HBV should not breastfeed, as transmission can occur via this route. She can handle her infant, but must be taught careful handwashing. The infant should be isolated from other infants. Rooming-in is an appropriate isolation strategy.

Varicella. Varicella is also one of the "other" TORCH infections. The occurrence of varicella zoster viral infections such as shingles and chicken pox during pregnancy can result in congenital malformations of the infant's skin, peripheral nervous system, autonomic nervous system, and musculoskeletal system. The infant can develop encephalitis. If the infection occurs after the 21st week of pregnancy, herpes zoster may be a problem in the neonatal period.[80]

Maternal signs and symptoms include eruption of vesicles along nerves arising from posterior ganglia. There is regional itching and pain. Malaise and gastrointestinal distress may occur before outbreak of vesicles. Varicella zoster immunoglobulin may prevent or modify disease if administered within 72 hours. Newborns of women who develop chicken pox within the 5 days preceding or the 2 days following delivery should receive prophylaxis. There is no evidence that prophylaxis is effective in protecting the fetus if administered to the mother earlier in pregnancy. Drugs used against herpes zoster include vidarabine and acyclovir. Safety of these drugs for use by pregnant women has not been established. Chicken pox vaccination has received approval for testing in the United States and is currently in trial stages.

Syphilis. Syphilis, another infection in the "other" TORCH category, is a sexually transmitted disease caused by the spirochete *Treponema pallidum* (*see* Chapter 8). In the United States, syphilis is most prevalent among individuals of reproductive age. If a pregnant woman with syphilis is untreated, the chance of her fetus dying in utero is 25 percent, the chance of neonatal death is 30 percent, and the chance of a surviving infant developing late syphilis is 40 percent. Lesions associated with congenital syphilis include interstitial changes in the lungs, liver, spleen, pancreas, and long bones.[75] Because of the severe effects of untreated syphilis on the developing fetus, as well as on the woman, a blood test to screen for this disease is performed at the first prenatal visit.

Rubella. Rubella is decreasing in incidence in the United States. Since the early 1960s, infants have been immunized routinely around 15 months of age. Women in the health care professions are screened and immunized. Despite these efforts, about 15 percent of women are susceptible to rubella. During epidemics rubella can infect as many as 4 percent of pregnant women; only 0.1 to 0.2 percent are infected under usual conditions.[75] Rubella titers ideally should be part of initial well-woman assessment. Immunizations should be offered to nonpregnant women who are not immune, along with counseling to avoid pregnancy for 4 months.

Pregnant women who are not immune should be advised to avoid, when possible, travel to areas where people are not routinely immunized and to avoid contact with infected individuals. For example, a pregnant nurse who is not immune should not care for a newborn with congenital rubella. In the early postpartum period, prior to discharge, immunization should be offered to women who are not immune.

The effect of maternal rubella on the fetus can be serious, depending on gestational age at the time of the infection. Rubella during the first month of pregnancy causes severe defects in about half of the embryos, not including those that spontaneously abort. The rate after a second-month infection is about 25 percent, and infection during the third month results in a rate of anomaly formation of about 12 percent. By the fifth month of pregnancy exposure to rubella carries no risk to the fetus.

The most common anomalies include defects of the eyes, heart, ears, and central nervous system; intrauterine growth retardation; hematologic deficits; hepatosplenomegaly; chronic diffuse interstitial pneumonitis; osseous changes; and chromosomal abnormalities (Table 39–24).[5]

TABLE 39–24. COMMON FINDINGS IN NEONATES WITH CONGENITAL RUBELLA[a]

Eye lesions
Cataracts
Glaucoma
Necrophthalmia
Other abnormalities
Heart lesions
Patent ductus anteriosus
Septal defects
Pulmonary artery stenosis
Auditory defects
Central nervous system defects
Mental retardation
Cerebral palsy
Small for gestational age
Hematologic deficits
Thrombocytopenia
Anemia
Liver alterations
Hepatosplenomegaly
Jaundice
Hyperbilirubinemia
Chronic diffuse interstitial pneumonia
Osseous changes
Chromosomal abnormalities
Elevated rubella immunoglobulin M antibody titer

[a]Infants born with congenital rubella can be contagious to susceptible adults, infants, and children. They may shed the virus for several months after birth.

Reproduced, with permission, from Cunningham GF, et al. Williams Obstetrics. *18th ed. Norwalk, Conn: Appleton & Lange; 1989;616.*

Nursing and Collaborative Assessment. Rubella serum antibody levels are routinely assessed at the first prenatal visit so that immunization status can be determined. If, after exposure to rubella, the levels rise in 3 to 4 weeks, the woman has been infected. Symptoms are absent in a third of infected women. One symptom that may occur is a mild rash with posterior auricular adenopathy.[81]

Nursing and Collaborative Management. There is no treatment for rubella. The dilemma faced by women who know that they have been exposed during the first trimester is whether or not to terminate the pregnancy. There is currently no method for early assessment of the extent of damage to the fetus, and although half of fetuses infected in the first month are seriously damaged, half are *not.* First-trimester rubella has been considered an indication for therapeutic abortion, but the decision depends on other factors in the woman's situation. She and her partner need complete information about the implications of rubella for her pregnancy. If she decides to continue the pregnancy her decision may be negatively regarded by some health care professionals. Whatever the woman and her partner decide, they need support and acceptance by professional nurses throughout their experience.

Cytomegalovirus. Cytomegalovirus (CMV) is usually asymptomatic in healthy people (*see* Chapter 8). It is estimated that 55 percent of young adults have CMV antibodies.[82] In one sample of 20,000 women, 108 were first infected with CMV during pregnancy. Half of the mothers who were first infected during pregnancy gave birth to infected infants, but only 5 percent of infected infants manifested the disease clinically. Reactivation can occur in some women who were infected prior to pregnancy, enabling them to transmit the disease to their infants.

Neonatal effects of CMV may be transient, as in patent ductus arteriosus. They may be reparable, as in hypospadias; however, they may constitute major handicaps. All infected infants need to be followed, as sensorineurologic problems can arise as much as 7 years later.[75,83] The degree of damage is not related to gestational age at the time of infection.

Prenatal screening is not cost effective as there is no treatment or vaccine. Abortion is not an appropriate measure after CMV infection because the risk of fetal infection and the severity of fetal illness or its sequelae are not predictable. Strategies for the prevention of this disease have not been devised, although it is common practice in neonatal intensive care units to avoid assigning pregnant nurses to care for CMV-infected infants. Because of the prevalence of CMV and the rarity of symptoms there is no way to identify and break the chain of transmission. Treatment and vaccination are in the research stage.

Herpes Simplex. All herpetic infections are potentially life threatening to neonates. Herpes simplex, particularly genital herpes, has reached epidemic proportions in the United States (*see* Chapter 8). The incidence of herpes simplex in pregnancy is 1 percent or less. The incidence in neonates is 1 in 7500.[84] Of these, half die and the majority who survive sustain permanent eye or central nervous system damage.

Herpes transmission occurs as the infant travels through the birth canal of an infected mother, either during active primary or recurrent infection; less commonly, the virus ascends the vaginal canal and cervix after rupture of membranes. Transplacental transmission can occur but rarely does. In some cases asymptomatic women shed herpes virus, placing their infants at risk.[85] For mothers who have had active herpes in the last month of pregnancy, cesarean delivery is common practice. Even with positive cultures or visible lesions, however, a woman with premature rupture of membranes is allowed to deliver vaginally if a length of time identified by the institution has passed. The rationale is that after 8 or 12 hours the fetus cannot be protected from the virus by cesarean delivery, so there is no point in subjecting the woman to abdominal surgery. Women who do not test positive for herpes or demonstrate lesions during the last month of pregnancy can deliver vaginally.[71]

Signs and symptoms of herpes include aches; chills or fever; localized itching; pain; cervical, vaginal, vulvar, or perineal ulcers; inguinal lymphadenopathy; and watery vaginal discharge. The first episode of this chronic illness is generally more severe and longer lasting than are recurrent episodes.

Women who know they have herpes should see their health care provider for culturing as soon as symptoms recur. Cultures from the lesion are performed weekly from the 32nd week of pregnancy, but the emergence of clinical symptoms supersedes a recent negative culture in determining activity of the disease.[86] If a woman's sexual partner has recurrent genital herpes, precautions should be taken particularly during the last 6 weeks of pregnancy so that the woman does not acquire a primary infection close to delivery. Primary infections are more easily contracted by neonates. This means that the couple should use condoms during sexual activity and abstain when his disease is active.

Primary herpes infection has been associated with spontaneous abortion and premature birth. Thirty to fifty percent of infants exposed to active herpes during vaginal delivery contract the disease. Neonatal herpes is usually disseminated, affecting the liver, adrenals, and central nervous system. As many as 90 percent of neonates with disseminated herpes die.

There are potential implications for nursery personnel who have chronic herpes infections, such as genital herpes or recurrent cold sores. Results are not clear on their likelihood of infecting neonates, but rotation to other settings may be advisable during active phases of the disease.[87] Herpes simplex infection is discussed further in Chapter 8.

Chlamydia trachomatis

Chlamydia trachomatis is the most prevalent sexually transmitted organism in the United States today. Infection tends to be asymptomatic. Chlamydial infection accounts for a tenfold increase in risk of fetal loss. Seventy percent of exposed infants develop congenital chlamydia, and 40 percent of these develop pneumonia. When the organism is transmitted to the eyes by flies, especially in Third World countries, by venereal transmission, or by fetal descent through the birth canal of an infected woman, a keratoconjunctivitis called trachoma may develop. Trachoma is the leading cause of preventable blindness in the world. Inclusion conjunctivitis develops by 5 to 12 days after birth. Infants at risk should be followed for 3 weeks. The organism is sensitive to systemic erythromycin and to tetracycline. Eye prophylaxis such as silver nitrate or erythromycin ointment is not effective in preventing trachoma. Any woman with sexually transmitted disease and her sexual partner should be screened for chlamydia, and treated if necessary.[88] (*See* Chapter 8 for further discussion.)

Candida albicans

Candida, or yeast infection, is commonly transmitted to the fetus during descent through the birth canal. The infant may develop oral thrush or yeast infection of the diaper area. Treatment with nystatin suspension or ointment is indicated, but this problem is generally minor.[89] Vaginal yeast infection is fostered by physiologic changes of pregnancy, and is discussed in Chapter 8.

Tuberculosis

Tuberculosis results from infection by *Mycobacterium tuberculosis*. Transmission is by droplets. Tuberculosis generally, but not always, involves the pulmonary system. In women, infection of the genital tract may result from blood transmission from the pulmonary tract. The gastrointestinal tract may also be the portal of entry, and lymphatic dissemination can occur. Congenital infection is rare but it may occur in the event of maternal bacillemia.

Pregnant women with tuberculosis may be asymptomatic. Symptomatic individuals may demonstrate malaise, fatigue, loss of appetite, weight loss, and 103 to 104°F fever. Body temperature tends to increase in the afternoon, and night sweats are characteristic. Production of blood-streaked sputum is a later-stage development.

Tuberculosis screening of antenatal women is routine. If the screening test is positive, chest x-ray may be done to confirm the presence of active tuberculosis. The pregnant woman's abdomen and pelvis must be well shielded by lead aprons when the chest x-ray is performed. If active tuberculosis is established or strongly suspected, isoniazid (INH) and ethambutol are administered daily.[71] Isoniazid is associated with an increase in fetal malformations, particularly neurotoxicity. Pyridoxine should be administered simultaneously to prevent their development.[90] Prophylactic chemotherapy is not administered until after delivery.

Human Immunodeficiency Virus

Human immunodeficiency virus infection is a condition of immune system suppression caused by the human immunodeficiency virus (HIV) (*see* Chapter 8). The disease remains dormant in cells of the immune and other systems for a period of months to years after infection. Currently there is no proven cure for HIV infection. HIV infection is both an acute and chronic disease, which eventually progresses to death in virtually every case.

Perinatal transmission of HIV infection is a major and growing problem, especially in populations where high-risk behaviors such as intravenous drug use or sexual relationships with multiple partners occur. About 10,000 to 20,000 children were estimated to be infected by 1991.[91] An infected woman has a 20 to 60 percent chance of passing the infection to her child.[92,93]

Although research findings are not uniform or conclusive, there is concern that the expression of HIV symptoms may be increased during pregnancy. Thus, pregnancy itself for a seropositive woman (a woman who carries the HIV antibody) may be risky.

All mothers who are seropositive passively transfer the HIV antibody to their fetus or neonate. In addition, neonates can be infected by the mother with HIV infection during the perinatal period. Although all fetuses receive HIV antibodies from their mother, it is not known why or how some of these fetuses actually become infected with HIV and some do not. Experts believe that the passively transferred maternal HIV antibody could persist in the infant for up to 15 months of life. At this point, infants who are not truly infected will convert to a seronegative status. Infants who are HIV infected will remain seropositive, and may begin to manifest symptoms of HIV disease, progressing eventually to AIDS (acquired immunodeficiency syndrome). Thus, infants who are seropositive perinatally should be tested at regular intervals for persistence of antibodies or any other abnormalities associated with HIV infection.[94] An infant who does not have symptoms and who has converted to a seronegative status can be considered unlikely to be infected with HIV.

Perinatal transmission can occur transplacentally, during the birth process, or through breastfeeding.[95] All newborns born of HIV infected mothers will test positive for the HIV antibody at birth. In some centers, assessment of HIV status by viral culture is available; however, this is an expensve, difficult, and insensitive test.[96] Although research is underway, there is currently no readily available method to determine whether the antibodies in the neonate are maternal or indicative of true infection.

Zidovudine (AZT) is a drug that has been approved for treatment of HIV infected adults and children. It prevents replication of HIV and slows the disease process; however, it does not cure the infection. AZT is being used experimentally with HIV-positive pregnant women to determine whether the drug can prevent the spread of the infection to the fetus. In addition, clinical drug trials with other retroviral agents, such as ddI, are currently underway.

Additional Nursing Management Considerations in Perinatal Infection

Women with perinatal infections need emotional support and physical assistance. The woman needs to understand her illness and its implications. In some cases, she must be isolated from her neonate. In some instances the course of pregnancy is markedly altered by development of an infection, as when herpes necessitates a cesarean delivery.

Nurses are becoming increasingly aware of the need for asepsis in practice. The Centers for Disease Control advocate universal precautions in all client care settings (*see* Appendix E). Rooms must be thoroughly cleaned after use by an infected woman. Ideally, a woman with a perinatal infection would labor, deliver, and recover in the same room, for the protection of other clients.

Specific isolation practices may be necessary. For example, enteric precautions are implemented when a client has hepatitis, and respiratory isolation is necessitated by tuberculosis. Isolation can be perceived by the client as alienation, particularly during such a social life event as birth. If possible, the infant of a woman with an infection should be isolated with her. If the infection or severity of maternal or neonatal illness necessitate separation of mother and infant, other family members can be encouraged to visit and handle the infant as appropriate.

Anxiety often develops when expectant mothers learn that they are carriers of disease, or if, after delivery, the infant is discovered to have acquired one. Before birth there may be constant worry that the infant will be ill. If the infant is ultimately found to have been infected, with negative consequences, the family can experience feelings of guilt, recrimination, and hopelessness.

Nurses can provide instruction on points identified earlier, with the goal of prevention. They can teach women the signs and symptoms they should report to their health care providers throughout pregnancy. For a number of the TORCH infections, however, there is little beyond general hygiene measures that an individual can do to control transmission. The family, particularly the woman, needs continual reassurance that they have responded appropriately to the threat of infection. Women with chronic viral infections do need to understand potential risks and what can be done to minimize them before they undertake pregnancy.

ABNORMALITIES OF AMNIOTIC FLUID PRODUCTION

Polyhydramnios

Polyhydramnios, or hydramnios, is an excessive quantity of amniotic fluid. This has arbitrarily been defined as more than 2000 mL.[97] Normally the amount of amniotic fluid is believed to increase steadily until 33 weeks of gestation, and then to decrease progressively to term.[98] During the last half of pregnancy amniotic fluid is produced by amnionic and fetal skin transfer of water and other molecules. During the second trimester, the fetus swallows, urinates, and inspires amniotic fluid. These processes probably regulate the amniotic fluid volume.

Polyhydramnios occurs in 0.4 to 1.5 percent of pregnancies, and is associated with various maternal and fetal complications of pregnancy, such as diabetes, multiple gestation, anencephaly, and esophageal atresia.[99] It has been observed that when fetal swallowing is impaired, as in esophageal atresia, polyhydramnios develops. In anencephaly and spina bifida it may be that there is increased transfer of fluid across exposed meninges.[5] Anencephalic fetuses lack antidiuretic hormone, so that they urinate excessively; this also contributes to polyhydramnios.[100] In twin pregnancy, one fetus is thought to have benefit of more of the fetal circulation than the other, and to have increased urine output. The relationship of polyhydramnios to maternal diabetes is not understood.[5] Increased placental weight may contribute to the development of polyhydramnios through the influence of increased prolactin output.[101]

Nursing and Collaborative Assessment. Signs and symptoms of polyhydramnios include a sensation of pressure, maternal dyspnea, and vulvar edema. Assessment includes vital signs, especially presence of respiratory difficulty; weight gain; measurement of uterine size; fetal heart rate, lie, and activity; evidence of uterine compression on venous return; and possible ultrasound assessment of amount of amniotic fluid.[98] Acute polyhydramnios is associated with a twofold increase in the incidence of premature labor.[5] The client is also assessed for signs and symptoms of maternal hazards, including preterm labor, abruptio placentae, uterine dysfunction, uterine rupture, and postpartum hemorrhage.

Nursing and Collaborative Management. Mild or moderate polyhydramnios is not treated. In severe cases, marked by maternal dyspnea, amniocentesis can relieve maternal distress. An 18-gauge intravenous catheter is placed abdominally under local anesthesia. Sonographic visualization guides the procedure so that the placenta or the fetus is not punctured. Removal of up to 1500 to 2000 mL of fluid usually relieves symptoms temporarily. Amniocentesis can be repeated as maternal discomfort dictates. The risks associated with this procedure include chorioamnionitis, abruptio placentae, initiation of preterm labor, and puncture of a fetal vessel.[97]

The nurse needs to understand and clarify for the client that restriction of salt or fluid intake or the use of diuretic drugs plays no known role in the prevention or relief of polyhydramnios.[5] The nurse answers the woman's questions about the condition and teaches her the changes to observe, including uterine hyperirritability, dyspnea, vaginal bleeding, and abdominal pain. Rest in the left lateral position may be advised to promote the client's comfort; however, bedrest does not usually decrease polyhydramnios.[5]

Oligohydramnios

A lower-than-normal volume of amniotic fluid is termed **oligohydramnios.** Operationally, this is defined in accordance with gestational age of the fetus. The average amount of amniotic fluid at 40 weeks is 800 mL. At 42 weeks, the average is 350 mL. Complications of oliguria arise most commonly when there is less than 200 mL of amniotic fluid.[102]

Oligohydramnios is associated with postmaturity and may occur in conjunction with congenital obstruction of the urinary tract or renal agenesis. It may be associated with a slow leak in the chorionic membranes. When that occurs, premature labor usually follows.

Fetuses born with renal agenesis have an array of characteristics referred to as "Potter's syndrome," including flat nose, recessed chin, flattened ears, pulmonary hypoplasia, and limb positional defects such as talipes equinovarus (club foot). These symptoms all reflect fetal compression by the uterus and, possibly, the lack of a growth hormone in amniotic fluid. Adhesions also can form between the fetus and the membranes.

Oligohydramnios may also be associated with pulmonary hypoplasia because inspiration of amniotic fluid is normally associated with alveolar maturity and with chest wall expansion. The development of oligohydramnios may reflect a lung defect or the failure to excrete fluid that contributes to total volume.

In addition, oligohydramnios is associated with umbilical cord compression because, normally, amniotic fluid cushions the cord from the pressure of the fetus's body.

Severe oligohydramnios is characterized by sonographic evidence of no echo-free space between fetal limbs and the uterine wall, or by the inability to identify more than two pockets of amniotic fluid at least 1 cm in diameter. Nuclear magnetic resonance imaging has also been useful in assessment (*see* Chapter 22). Because of the association of fetal distress from umbilical cord compression and oligohydramnios, a few perinatal centers have attempted to treat prolonged deceleration of fetal heart rate by instilling sterile saline into the uterus.[102] This is not a standard protocol, and the risk of sepsis cannot be ignored. There is no general treatment approach in oligohydramnios.

When amniotic membranes rupture, the birth attendant attempts to estimate total volume to anticipate special needs of the neonate. This infant needs careful assessment and monitoring.

SPONTANEOUS ABORTION/ INCOMPETENT CERVIX

Unplanned labor and parturition before the age of viability or before 20 weeks of gestation is termed *spontaneous abortion. Miscarriage* is the term often used by clients to avoid confusion with elective abortion, the process in which pregnancy is voluntarily terminated (*see* Chapters 9 and 38). During the second trimester spontaneous abortion may occur as a result of incompetent cervix.

Incompetent cervix is the most common structural defect predisposing to spontaneous abortion, although it does not occur often. **Incompetent cervix** is defined as an anatomic defect of the cervix resulting in painless dilation without uterine contractions. The membranes may prolapse through the opened cervix and into the vagina. The membranes may also rupture, and delivery may ensue so prematurely that the infant does not survive. Cervical dilation usually occurs between the 16th and 20th weeks of gestation, although the condition may take place earlier or later. The condition tends to recur in future pregnancies.[5]

Incompetent cervix may be caused by cervical trauma. The woman frequently has a past history of a traumatic delivery, dilation and curettage, or cervical biopsy conization. Abnormal cervical development may also play a role. For example, exposure to diethylstilbestrol (DES) is related to abnormal cervical development. Increasing weight and pressure of the uterus during advancing pregnancy result in dilation of the incompetent cervix. This dilation usually does not clinically occur until at least 16 weeks of gestation, when the products of conception are large enough to efface and dilate the cervix. Spontaneous abortion occurring as a result of incompetent cervix differs from first-trimester spontaneous abortion in causative factors (incompetent cervix results from a structural defect); signs and symptoms (*see* Chapter 38 for assessment of spontaneous abortion resulting from incompetent cervix); much less frequent occurrence; and different treatment (discussed next).

Treatment for incompetent cervix occurring between 14 and 20 weeks entails suturing of the cervix to prevent opening. This surgical approach, called

cerclage, is performed by a physician if the cervix is less than 4 cm dilated and no signs of other high-risk conditions, such as bleeding, ruptured membranes, and uterine contractions, are present. Ideally, the sutured cervix then remains closed until near term, when the sutures are removed in preparation for vaginal delivery or when cesarean delivery takes place. In some cases, cerclage may be considered a risk to induce preterm labor or rupture of membranes, especially in more advanced pregnancy. Bedrest, rather than cerclage, may then be used, particularly beyond 20 weeks of gestation. Successful cerclage has been reported in women who were between 21 and 24 weeks of gestation and who presented with advanced cervical changes.[103]

Prior to cerclage, vaginal examination and ultrasound are done to assess the degree of cervical effacement and dilation and to confirm the presence of a living fetus with no major anomalies. In addition, cervical smears are done to make certain that cervical cells are normal and that no infection, such as chlamydia or gonorrhea, is present. The client is advised not to have vaginal intercourse at least 1 week before and after cerclage; however, restrictions on sexual activity are based on the client's individual condition.

The McDonald technique and the Shirodkar technique are two surgical procedures currently performed by physicians to treat incompetent cervix. Both entail reinforcement of the cervix with an encircling pursestring suture. The McDonald procedure, shown in Figure 39–8, is technically simpler and has fewer complications such as bleeding. After the McDonald procedure, the suture must be removed at term to allow for vaginal delivery. If sutures from the Shirodkar technique remain intact, a cesarean delivery may be performed at term, so that future pregnancies will be possible without further surgical interventions of the cervix. Sutures can also be removed by the physician for vaginal delivery.

Postoperatively, the most common complications are rupture of the membranes and uterine contractions. Bedrest for 24 hours and close monitoring to detect uterine contractions are recommended. If the membranes rupture, the physician must be notified. The sutures must be removed by the physician and the woman delivered because of the risk of sepsis. If uterine contractions begin and the membranes remain intact, the woman is placed on bedrest and medication may be prescribed to arrest preterm labor.

During labor, a woman who has had cerclage may at first progress slowly as a result of the fibrotic changes that take place after the procedure in the cervix. This may be followed by a sudden delivery. Postdelivery, the client is assessed for cervical lacerations, as this is a common complication.

Incompetent cervix, by its very name, suggests that the client is less than adequate in her ability to carry a pregnancy to term. This negative connotation reinforces the tendency of the woman to feel she is a failure, especially if the fetus was otherwise normal. The situation is particularly difficult if a previous pregnancy ended because of incompetent cervix.

Although success rates of 85 to 90 percent have been achieved with cerclage, clients may be anxious about the outcome of their pregnancy and the sudden transition to high-risk status. Restrictions of daily activities may be a burden, especially for the employed woman. Family concerns are similar to those experienced by women after spontaneous abortion, for example, grief over loss of the pregnancy, worry over future pregnancies, desire to identify reasons why the condition existed.

The nurse's role includes anticipatory guidance and support of the client undergoing this high-risk procedure. In addition, careful physical assessment and prompt reporting of complications are necessary.

PRETERM LABOR AND BIRTH

Any true labor experienced before the end of the 37th week of gestation and after 20 weeks is called **preterm labor. Preterm birth** is delivery after the age of viability or potential for survival but before completion of 37 weeks of gestation. The age of viability is difficult to define, because technology and expert care have made survival of younger and sicker infants possible. The incidence of prematurity in the United States is about 8 percent of live births and accounts for over 75 percent of total perinatal deaths.[104] Despite technologic advances, the incidence of preterm births in the United States has not decreased.[105]

Preventing Prematurity

Prevention of preterm labor entails early assessment and management of predisposing conditions, including prompt detection of cervical changes. Preventive care includes nutrition counseling, assessment of fetal growth and development, screening for complications of or concurrent with pregnancy, instruction of women on health maintenance and symptoms of preterm labor, and identification of potential risks during pregnancy.

The problem of preterm labor is complex. A wide array of efforts is needed, for example, prevention of teenage pregnancy, access to and use of prenatal services early in pregnancy, screening and early inter-

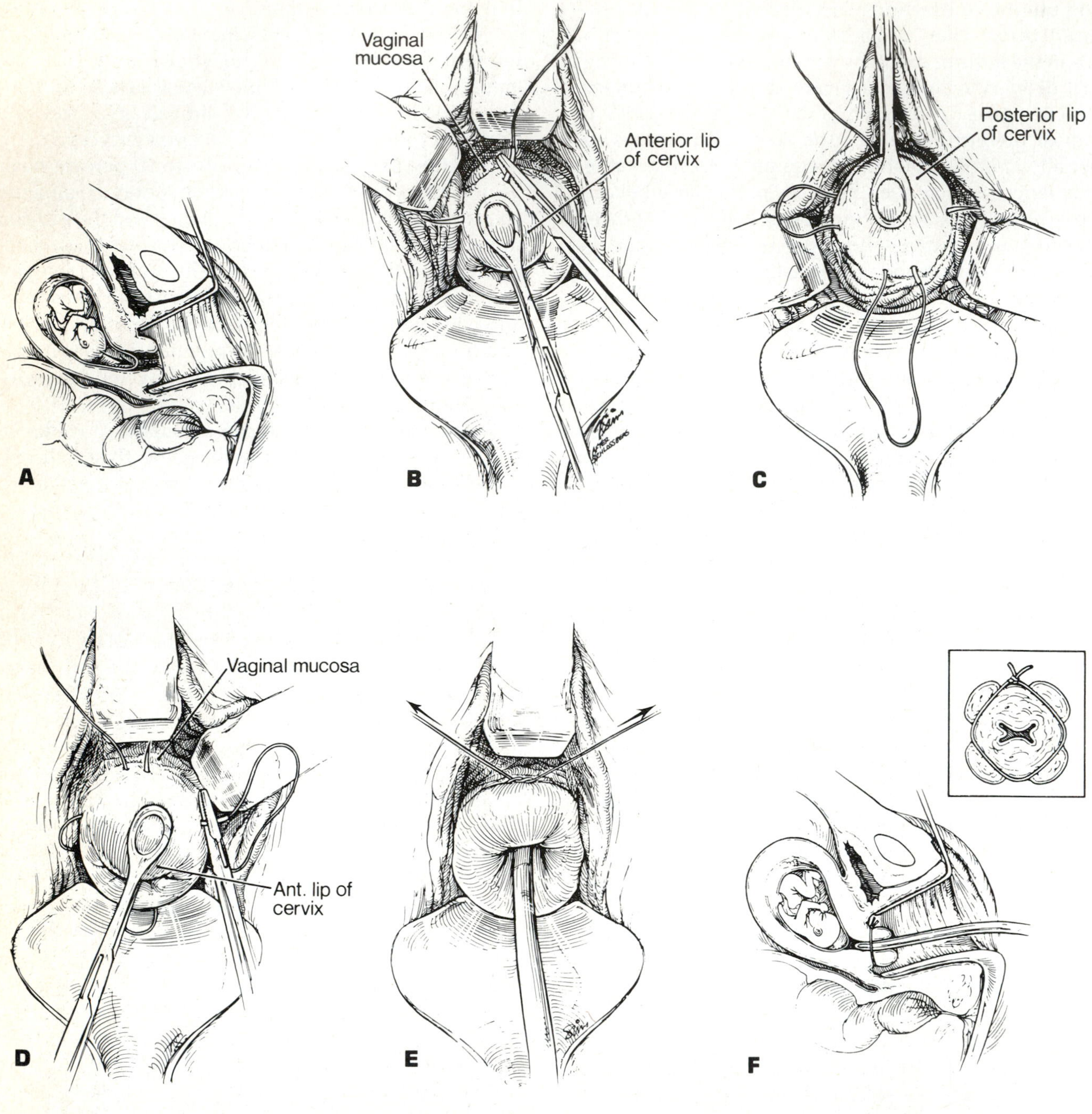

Figure 39–8. Correction of incompetent cervical os: McDonald procedure. **A.** Somewhat dilated cervical canal and beginning prolapse of membranes (*arrow*). **B.** Start of the cerclage procedure; a suture is being placed superiorly in the body of the cervix very near the level of the internal os. **C.** Continuation of the placement of the suture in the body of the cervix so as to encircle the os. **D.** Completion of encirclement. **E.** The suture is tightened around the cervical canal sufficiently to reduce the diameter of the canal to 5–10 mm and is then securely tied. **F.** The effect of the suture placement on the cervical canal is apparent. (*Reproduced, with permission, from Cunningham FG, et al.* Williams Obstetrics. *18th ed. Norwalk, Conn: Appleton & Lange; 1989:500.*)

ventions in such conditions as gestational diabetes and pregnancy-induced hypertension, and health education focused on decreasing the incidence of infectious diseases. Pregnant women need nutrition education early in pregnancy. Some need, and are eligible for, nutritional supplementation programs such as the Special Supplemental Food Program for Women, Infants, and Children (WIC) (*see* Chapter 10). Midwifery practices have demonstrated decreased incidence of prematurity and low birth weight among traditionally underserved populations, reflecting the benefit of client teaching and supervision for prevention of problems associated with preterm labor.

Nursing and Collaborative Assessment

All prenatal clients are assessed for factors indicating risk for preterm labor (Table 39–25), as well as for signs and symptoms of preterm labor (Table 39–26). Preterm labor is often difficult to distinguish from false labor before significant cervical effacement and dilation have occurred.

TABLE 39–25. ASSESSMENT OF RISK FOR PRETERM LABOR[a]

1 point each for	Parity of 2 or greater, low socieconomic status, work outside home, history of one early abortion, less than 1 year since last birth
2 points each for	Age less than 20 or over 40, single parent, history of two early abortions, smokes more than half a pack per day, weight gain less than norm, evidence of PIH, bacteriuria
3 points each for	Height less than 152 cm or weight less than 45.5 kg, history of three early abortions, heavy work, long commute, uterine fibroids, weight loss during this pregnancy, febrile illness, head engaged by 32 weeks
4 points each for	Age 18 or under, pyelonephritis, vaginal bleeding after first trimester, more than 50% effacement, dilation, uterine irritability
5 points each for	Cone biopsy, uterine anomaly, history of one second-trimester abortion, placental previa, polyhydramnios
10 points each for	Diethylstilbestrol exposure of this woman as a fetus, history of preterm delivery, history of two second-trimester abortions, preterm labor, multiple pregnancy, abdominal surgery during this pregnancy, cervical surgery during this pregnancy

[a]Score of 10 or more indicates risk.
Based on Creasy RK, et al. Systems for predicting spontaneous preterm birth. Obstet Gynecol. *1980;55:692.*

TABLE 39–26. SYMPTOMS OF PRETERM LABOR

Uterine contractions, 5–8 minutes apart or less; pain may or may not be present; contractions are unrelieved by rest
Low backache or pain, unrelieved by rest
Pelvic pressure; discomfort may radiate to inner thighs
Menstrual-type cramps
Intestinal cramping, with or without indigestion or diarrhea
Alteration in usual nature of vaginal discharge, particularly the onset of mucoid, watery or blood tinged discharge
Gush or trickle of fluid from vagina (ruptured membranes)

Source: *References 5, 104, 105, 110, 111.*

In addition, there are ethnic differences in average duration of pregnancy that do not reflect socioeconomic inequities alone; for example, black women tend to experience shorter pregnancies. Seasonal variations have been observed in the incidence of preterm labor, with the smallest number occurring in May and the greatest number in September. This may reflect seasonal trends in allergies and infectious diseases.[106–108] In 70 to 80 percent of cases of preterm labor, no risk factors can be identified.[109]

If the client has signs and symptoms of preterm labor, physical examination includes assessment of any cervical changes. Cervical effacement greater than 60 percent or dilation greater than 20 percent indicates actual preterm labor, although uterine irritability occurs sooner.[5] In this situation, monitoring with external electronic tocography may be performed to assess uterine activity.

Preterm labor generally involves hospitalization for monitoring, hydration, and pharmacologic therapy. Once the client has been stabilized, assessment of uterine activity may be done while the client is maintained on therapy at home. For clients able to participate responsibly in their own care, home therapy is much less financially and emotionally expensive than hospitalization. Clients may be taught to assess their own uterine contraction patterns and advised to contact their health care provider if contractions increase in frequency or intensity or if other signs of preterm labor emerge.

When indicated, perinatal nursing services may be employed to assess uterine activity while the client remains in her home. Nurses with special background in antenatal testing or labor and delivery remain in telephone contact with clients on a daily or more frequent basis. In addition to assessing a client's reports of her condition and responses to therapy, the nurse evaluates tracings of uterine activity.

The client who is managed at home is provided with a tocodynamometer, which is an electronic instrument that records uterine activity. She is in-

RESEARCH ABSTRACT

Loos C, Julius L. The client's view of hospitalization during pregnancy. J Obstet Gynecol Neonat Nurs. *1989;18:52–56.*

The purpose of this study was to explore the meaning of hospitalization during the prenatal period among high-risk women. This phenomenologic study attempted to describe the holistic aspects of the women's experiences for the synthesis of common themes. The study was conducted in Canada and a convenience sample of 11 prenatal clients hospitalized more than 5 days was selected. The women ranged in age from 17 to 35 years; the gestational ages of the fetuses ranged from 26 to 38 weeks. The at-risk diagnoses of the women included twin pregnancy (n = 3), threatened premature labor (n = 4), and antepartum bleeding (n = 4).

The investigators developed a questionnaire that included four elements:

1. *Human biology.* All aspects of health, both physical and mental.
2. *Environment.* All matters related to health that are external to the human body.
3. *Lifestyle.* All of the decisions made by individuals that affect their health.
4. *Health care organization.* Quantity, quality, arrangement, nature, and resources in the provision of health care.

Two open-ended questions were also asked to tap other feelings or perceptions of the women.

Themes uncovered by the investigators were loneliness, boredom, and powerlessness. In addition, women expressed concern for the fetus, finances, and lack of privacy. The investigators concluded that prenatal women in this study had certain psychosocial needs that were not being addressed during hospitalization.

Comment:
Hospitalization of high-risk pregnant women may control the physiologic aspects of the disease condition. A woman, however, is more than a fetal incubator. Loneliness, boredom, and powerlessness can contribute to an adverse pregnancy outcome for the whole family, even though the woman's medical condition is corrected. Nurses are in a position to devise care for all aspects of the client's life. Such findings provide the basis for nursing interventions.

structed how and when to record uterine activity; for example, 1 hour each morning and evening, or whenever uterine activity increases. The client fits the speaker part of her telephone onto a device on the recorder. She pushes a button which swiftly transmits the data to the antenatal testing center, and prints it for the nurse to read at once. The nurse then can provide counseling to the client, confer with the physician at the testing center on interpretation of strips, and refer the client to her obstetrician if nonreassuring patterns are identified.[110]

At times, antenatal testing for clients being treated for preterm labor may be done by the nurse through home visits. Although home monitoring services are much less expensive than hospitalization, clients may have problems in securing approval for reimbursement from certain insurance sources.

Nursing and Collaborative Management

As described previously under assessment, care of the client at risk for preterm labor requires collaboration and a close working relationship among health care providers, the client, and her family. The client at risk for preterm labor is instructed on surveillance for and prevention of labor.[111] She is taught to monitor uterine activity for an hour, while at rest in the left lateral position, once or twice daily. Teaching also focuses on reducing risk factors such as smoking.

The nurse instructs the woman to limit activity, for example to avoid active sports, heavy housework or lifting children, and to increase daytime rest to 2 to 3 hours or more if uterine activity does not abate. She is instructed to drink 8 to 10 cups of nonalcoholic, noncaffeinated beverages per day and to urinate every 2 hours. Additional amounts of fluids may be prescribed if contractions occur. Sexual arousal and breast or nipple manipulation are contraindicated because these activities affect the release of oxytocin. Clients who are not on prescribed bedrest may attend prepared childbirth classes, but are advised to participate only in breathing exercises.

If the above measures are ineffective in preventing increased uterine activity, the woman is hospitalized. Bedrest, hydration and pharmacologic intervention may be prescribed by the physician.

Tocolytic therapy, or the use of medication to decrease or stop uterine contractions, has an estimated 50 percent success rate in reducing preterm births.[112] Successful tocolytic therapy is defined as the reduction of contractions to less than 3 per hour. Tocolytic therapy, however, is contraindicated in the presence of fetal complications; premature rupture of membranes, although there are exceptions if the woman is hospitalized for strict supervision; hemorrhage; severe maternal illness that is progressing during pregnancy; and severe pregnancy-induced hypertension.

Ethanol, which inhibits the release of endogenous oxytocin, was used in the past to stop preterm labor; however, metabolic side effects of this drug were serious and included vomiting, fetal hypoxia and after-effects of intoxication. Ethanol has been replaced in current practice by other drugs.

Intravenous administration of magnesium sulfate is a method still in use in some settings. Magnesium sulfate is thought to control myometrial contractions by blocking the function of calcium. The client must be observed closely for signs and symptoms of magnesium toxicity, particularly absence of the patellar reflex and respiratory depression (*see* Box 39–1 on page 1060). The effect of magnesium sulfate on blood pressure, heart rate and cardiac output is less than that of the beta-sympathomimetics.

Currently, the drugs of choice for tocolytic therapy are ritodrine hydrochloride and terbutaline sulfate (Brethine). Ritodrine hydrochloride, a beta-sympathomimetic, is used for the arrest of preterm labor. Ritodrine is described in Box 39–4. Other beta-sympathomimetic drugs, including terbutaline sulfate, are also used to stop preterm labor. Cardiovascular side effects are similar throughout this drug category.

Progestins are another category of drugs that have been used in tocolysis. Long-term risks have not been evaluated, and caution is advised in administration of sex hormones to a fetus. If other options are contraindicated, this choice may be used.

Various strategies for management of preterm labor exist. In one approach, the woman in preterm labor is admitted to the hospital, hydrated, and stabilized on parenteral magnesium sulfate, ritodrine hydrochloride, or terbutaline sulfate.[113] She is then weaned to oral ritodrine or terbutaline and may be discharged for home care and continued follow-up as described above. The client may remain on the medication until 36 weeks of gestation; however, the beta receptors in the body may become desensitized after prolonged and continous high-dose therapy. Increased uterine activity may then recur. Administration of terbutaline subcutaneously by pump has been used to decrease the amount of desensitization.[113] Pump therapy delivers continuous low dose and intermittent bolus doses which can be timed according to specified periods of increased uterine activity. By this method, the client receives an average of 3 to 4 mg of terbutaline daily rather than the 30 to 60 mg required by daily oral dosages. The client may be taught to insert the infusion set and to receive pump therapy at home.

Bedrest may be prescribed for the client who experiences preterm labor; however, the amount and effectiveness of bedrest in treatment of preterm labor are controversial. In addition, women on prolonged bedrest for weeks or months have been theorized to undergo physiologic changes related to bedrest and to experience difficulty in being upright and mobile once bedrest is no longer indicated, for example at term or after delivery. Research is currently in progress to determine the physiologic impact of prolonged bedrest in pregnancy.[114]

The client being treated for preterm labor needs much support. She may require guidance in planning for outside assistance in maintaining her home and tending to the needs of her family. Furthermore, she needs assistance in dealing with boredom and social isolation that occur during weeks or months of inactivity.

The anticipation of delivery of a premature infant can be frightening for the couple. If bedrest is not prescribed, clients can be referred to high-risk childbirth education programs. A tour of the neonatal intensive care unit at the hospital in which she will deliver may prove reassuring; however, restricted activity often prevents attendance.

Women in preterm labor may feel emotionally unprepared, as they have not completed psychologic processes of the third trimester. Assessment and management focus on anticipatory guidance and teaching, should preterm delivery take place.

Preterm Delivery

In the case of preterm labor and delivery, the more immature the fetus, the greater the risks of labor and delivery. The blood vessels within the preterm infant's head are fragile and intracranial hemorrhage is a risk when the infant is exposed to pressure changes during labor and birth or to hypoxia. Some perinatal centers perform cesarean deliveries of all fetuses below an established gestational age to avoid head trauma. If delivery will be vaginal, labor must not be forceful. Oxytocics are generally contraindicated.[5] Continuous electronic monitoring is performed. Trauma, such as tugging on the infant in either vaginal or cesarean delivery, is avoided. If the infant is born vaginally, a liberal episiotomy further reduces head trauma. An interdisciplinary neonatal team should be on hand to resuscitate the infant if necessary. The infant will probably be placed in special care nursery for observation and treatment as needed. (Premature infants are at risk of developing complications, which are discussed in Chapter 43.)

Nursing care includes determining what premature delivery of the infant means to the woman and

BOX 39–4. RITODRINE

Proprietary Names:
Yutopar (Astra), others.

Classification:
Sympathomimetic.

Action:
Stimulates beta-adrenergic receptors, causing relaxation of smooth muscles of uterus, resulting in decreased frequency and intensity of uterine contractions. During IV infusion, transiently increases maternal and fetal blood glucose concentrations and maternal plasma insulin concentrations.

Indications:
To inhibit uterine contractions in preterm labor to prolong gestation. Efficacy and safety of use before 20th week of gestation or in advanced labor have not been established.

Dosage and Route:
Administered IV (via infusion pump) or orally. For IV use, should be diluted in 5 percent dextrose to a concentration of 300 μg/mL (ie, 150 mg in 500 mL 5 percent dextrose). Usual IV dose: 50–100 μg/min, and increased by 50 μg/min every 10 minutes until desired effect obtained. Infusion should be continued for at least 12 hours after cessation of uterine contractions. Maintenance dose: Approximately 30 minutes prior to stopping IV therapy, oral therapy should be started. Usual dose: 10 mg orally every 2 hours for first 24 hours followed by 10–20 mg every 4 to 6 hours. Total oral dosage should not exceed 120 mg per day.

Pharmacokinetics:
Absorption: Only 30 percent of oral dose is bioavailable. *Distribution:* Approximately one third of drug is bound to albumin. Crosses the placenta but whether it crosses into breast milk is not known. *Elimination:* Metabolized in liver and excreted in urine with a half-life of 10–20 hours.

Contraindications and Precautions:
Contraindicated in pregnant women before the 20th week of gestation, and in conditions in which continuation of pregnancy is hazardous, such as antepartum hemorrhage, eclampsia and severe pre-eclampsia, intrauterine fetal death, fetal anomaly incompatible with life, chorioamnionitis, abruptio placentae, and placenta previa. Also contraindicated in the following conditions in the mother: hypovolemia, cardiac disease, cardiac arrythmias, pulmonary hypertension, uncontrolled hypertension, pheochromocytoma, hyperthyroidism, uncontrolled diabetes mellitus.

Adverse Reactions:
Dose related and more severe with IV administration. *Most common:* increase in maternal and fetal heart rate, widening of maternal pulse pressure, palpitations, elevated blood glucose in mother and fetus, elevated insulin concentrations in mother. *Less common:* CNS—tremor, headache, nervousness, restlessness, anxiety; GI—nausea, vomiting, epigastric distress, impaired liver function, hepatitis; CV—tachycardia, cardiac arrythmias; other—anaphylactic shock, rash, sweating, chills.

Drug Interactions:

- Corticosteroids: Concurrent administration has rarely resulted in pulmonary edema.
- Other sympathomimetic agents: May result in increased incidence of side effects, particularly cardiac effects.
- Beta blockers: Antagonize effects of ritodrine.

Nursing Implications:

- Assess uterine contractions, maternal blood pressure, maternal pulse pressure, fetal heart rate.
- Assess for adverse reactions: maternal palpitations, elevated blood glucose levels, tachycardia, cardiac arrhythmias, headache, restlessness, gastrointestinal distress. Assess newborn for hypoglycemia.
- Place client on left side when administering drug IV to reduce potential for hypotension.

IV = intravenous(ly), CNS = central nervous system, GI = gastrointestinal, CV = cardiovascular.

her partner, how they perceive the events that led up to the delivery, what role in this sequence the woman ascribes to herself, what blaming behaviors are going on in the family system, how the family has coped with crises in the past, and what resources, particularly in the form of support persons, they can identify (*see* Chapter 36).

Where parents' perceptions of events surrounding the birth are inaccurate, correct information is required. The woman may feel guilty that she could not protect her infant or carry out her reproductive role, or that she does not have her fantasized infant. Nursing care that provides education and support can promote positive maternal perceptions despite prematurity.[115] Clients may also be referred to support groups (*see* Appendix F). Sensitivity is needed when assigning these women to rooms after preterm delivery.

Nursing care for the prevention and management of preterm labor is described in the Case Study/Care Plan.

CASE STUDY/CARE PLAN: PRETERM LABOR

William and Missy Trevor are expecting their first baby. At 25 weeks of gestation, Missy begins having uterine contractions. In the emergency room, she is found to have 2 cm cervical dilation and 50 percent effacement. History reveals that Missy has had a recurrent urinary tract infection throughout the pregnancy. Ultrasound confirms that Missy is 25 weeks pregnant. The physician determines that Missy is at risk for preterm labor, but that she can be managed at home, on modified bedrest and tocolytic therapy, with weekly antenatal visits. Three weeks later, Missy is readmitted with lower backache, ruptured membranes, and mild uterine contractions every 10 minutes lasting 30 seconds. Tocolytic therapy is initiated.

Supporting Assessment Data	Expected Client/Family Outcome	Nursing Action/ Intervention	Rationale	Criteria for Evaluation
Nursing Diagnosis: Knowledge deficit, related to client's lack of awareness of signs of preterm labor				
Presence of risk factors in nursing history: Urinary tract infection Cervical dilation 2 cm Effacement 50% in 25-week pregnancy	Client will identify onset of preterm labor promptly	Teach client signs and symptoms of preterm labor: cramps, pelvic pressure, backache, vaginal discharge, rupture of membranes, diarrhea.	Many women do not know the signs and symptoms of labor. If early treatment is sought, it may be possible to stop labor.	The client articulates signs and symptoms for which she will observe. The client seeks prompt attention for preterm labor.
Nursing Diagnosis: Potential asset in ability to prevent preterm labor, related to knowledge concerning reversible risk factors				
	During home management:			
	Client will seek prompt attention for reversible risk factors, such as urinary tract infection	Obtain urine specimen for urinalysis, culture and sensitivity.	Urinary tract infections increase uterine irritability.	The client receives prompt treatment for urinary tract infection.
	Client will fully participate in preventive treatment regimen	Explain the need for client to be followed at weekly antenatal visits.	Uterine activity and cervical status can be assessed for evidence of progression.	The client participates in surveillance regimen.
		Instruct client to avoid exertion or lifting of heavy objects, including children.	Understanding the reason will increase client's likelihood of participation in surveillance regimen.	The client does not engage in heavy lifting or exertion.
		Instruct client to rest 2 to 3 hours per day, midday, in the left lateral position.	Exertion may stimulate uterine contractions.	The client experiences decreased uterine activity and pregnancy is maintained.
		Instruct client to curtail or stop working (medical leave).	Periods of inactivity decrease uterine activity and increase uteroplacental perfusion.	The client reduces her workload or takes a medical leave.
		Instruct the couple to avoid sexual stimulation and stimulation of nipples as in breastfeeding preparation.	Sexual activity and nipple stimulation induce oxytocin, which stimulates uterine contractions.	The client can state that she has avoided sexual and nipple stimulation as instructed.

(continued)

CASE STUDY/CARE PLAN: Preterm Labor (*continued*)

Supporting Assessment Data	Expected Client/Family Outcome	Nursing Action/ Intervention	Rationale	Criteria for Evaluation
		Counsel client regarding diet, iron supplementation, avoidance of infection, and good hygiene.	Good nutrition enhances fetal oxygenation and maturation. Infection can precipitate preterm labor.	Twenty-four-hour diet recall indicates RDAs are met. The client develops no infections.
		Advise client to be prepared for sudden onset of labor: pack bag for hospital, do not travel from home area, make plans for transportation to hospital if necessary, ask family members to apprise one another of whereabouts.	Interventions may not successfully prolong the pregnancy to 36 weeks and preterm delivery may occur.	The client and her partner demonstrate preparedness for early delivery.
		Prepare client for possible referral to a level III regional perinatal center.	The type of health care facility required by the client depends on the stage of pregnancy at which labor starts.	The client knows where to go if preterm labor starts.
Nursing Diagnosis: Potential asset in positive coping with preterm labor, related to understanding the regimen and positive attachment to the fetus.				
	During surveillance regimen:			
	Client will verbalize her fears/stress	Provide an opportunity for client to verbalize fears.	Listening is often an effective comfort measure.	Client verbalizes fears and anticipates events appropriately.
	Client will demonstrate positive coping behaviors Client will identify sources of assistance during periods of bedrest or hospitalization	Assess usual coping responses, sources of support, and assistance available to client on bedrest for preterm labor.	The client may have a pattern of successful coping during crisis; if not, the nurse can make appropriate recommendations or referrals. Relaxation promotes rest.	Client and her partner demonstrate positive coping. Social support system is mobilized; household and other responsibilities are addressed.
	Client will demonstrate understanding of progression of events	Explain what is likely to happen throughout the course of treatment; arrange for the couple to tour level III high-risk perinatal centers.	Anticipation of events often reduces their fearsomeness.	The couple becomes familiar with the level III perinatal center.
		Include client and partner in planning care as much as possible.	Participation in planning of care can enhance client's and partner's autonomy and self-esteem.	
	Client will express satisfaction that she acted in the best interest of her fetus	Give client rationales for interventions or avoidance of certain interventions.	Knowledge increases client's motivation to participate in therapeutic regimen and reassures client that all that can be done for her is being done.	Client is able to participate fully in therapeutic regimen.
		Provide diversion for client on bedrest.	Sensory deprivation leads to boredom and distress.	Client is able to carry out bedrest regimen. Client expresses satisfaction for each week pregnancy is prolonged.

Supporting Assessment Data	Expected Client/Family Outcome	Nursing Action/ Intervention	Rationale	Criteria for Evaluation
				Client experiences intact self-esteem if pregnancy terminates early.
Nursing Diagnosis:	Potential asset in prevention of preterm birth, related to safe, effective management of preterm labor			
Backache Progressive uterine contractions—every 10 minutes, 30 seconds duration, mild intensity Cervical dilation 2 cm Cervical effacement 50% Spontaneous rupture of membranes	During hospitalization: The client's labor will be stopped; delivery will be postponed.	Initiate bedrest on admission.	Bedrest promotes uterine relaxation.	Uterine activity is halted. Client does not develop sequelae from tocolytic or steroid therapy. Client does not develop infection.
		Notify medical staff.		
		Test vaginal discharge for presence of amniotic fluid.	The presence of amniotic fluid confirms spontaneous rupture of membranes and preterm labor.	
		Initiate fetal monitoring.	Fetal distress may necessitate prompt delivery.	
		Initiate intake and output.	Good hydration contributes to uterine perfusion.	
		Encourage oral fluid intake.		
		Perform cervical examination on admission, then only as needed.	Frequent examinations can lead to infection.	
		Arrange complete blood count and urinalysis, as ordered.	Complete blood count and urinalysis assist in detection of infections and other complications.	
		Prepare the client for other tests as needed, eg, amniocentesis, ultrasound.		
		Initiate tocolytic therapy, as ordered.	Tocolytic therapy relaxes the uterus.	
		Obtain baseline electrocardiogram.	Cardiac arrhythmias may develop from tocolytic therapy.	
		Initiate steroid therapy, as ordered.	Steroid therapy is used to enhance fetal lung maturation.	
		Observe for adverse effects of medications.	Adverse effects may necessitate cessation of therapy.	
		Monitor vital signs every 15 minutes during loading dosage and every 1 hour during maintenance intravenous therapy. Note evidence of sepsis.	Side effects of steroid therapy include cardiovascular alterations. Infection may be a sequalae of symptoms.	
		Monitor uterine contractions.	Dosage and effectiveness of tocolytic therapy are determined by frequency and strength of contractions.	

(continued)

CASE STUDY/CARE PLAN: Preterm Labor ***(continued)***

Supporting Assessment Data	Expected Client/Family Outcome	Nursing Action/ Intervention	Rationale	Criteria for Evaluation
		Regulate intravenous infusion with infusion pump.	Infusion pump helps prevent exceeding therapeutic levels.	
		When contractions are halted, instruct client on self-administration of oral tocolytic therapy at home: dosage schedule, side effects to report promptly.	Oral tocolytic maintenance is implemented after successful intravenous initiation of tocolysis. Teaching is focused on signs and symptoms of complications.	Client articulates side effects that require prompt medical attention. Follow-up indicates client maintains appropriate dosage schedule, blood levels, and continuation of pregnancy.
		If tocolysis is contraindicated or is not effective, notify medical, obstetric, neonatology staff and other members of interdisciplinary team; follow protocols for preterm delivery.		Client experiences safe delivery of viable neonate.

RH ISOIMMUNIZATION

Rh isoimmunization is a hemolytic disease arising from incompatibility of the Rh factors of maternal and fetal blood. It is the result of an antigen-antibody reaction. Sensitization usually occurs when an Rh-negative woman is pregnant with an Rh-positive fetus. When the fetus is delivered, fetal erythrocytes enter the maternal circulation. The mother forms antibodies to the Rh complex of antigens. With subsequent pregnancies of Rh-positive fetuses, Rh antibodies from the sensitized woman's circulation cross the placenta and enter the fetal circulation. They cause the destruction of fetal red blood cells (Figure 39–9). Fetal anemia results, and can be fatal (*see* Chapter 42 for effects on the fetus and newborn). Sensitization can also result from other situations, such as transfusion of an Rh-negative woman with Rh-positive blood.

An individual's Rh type is genetically determined. The designation Rh stands for several factors,

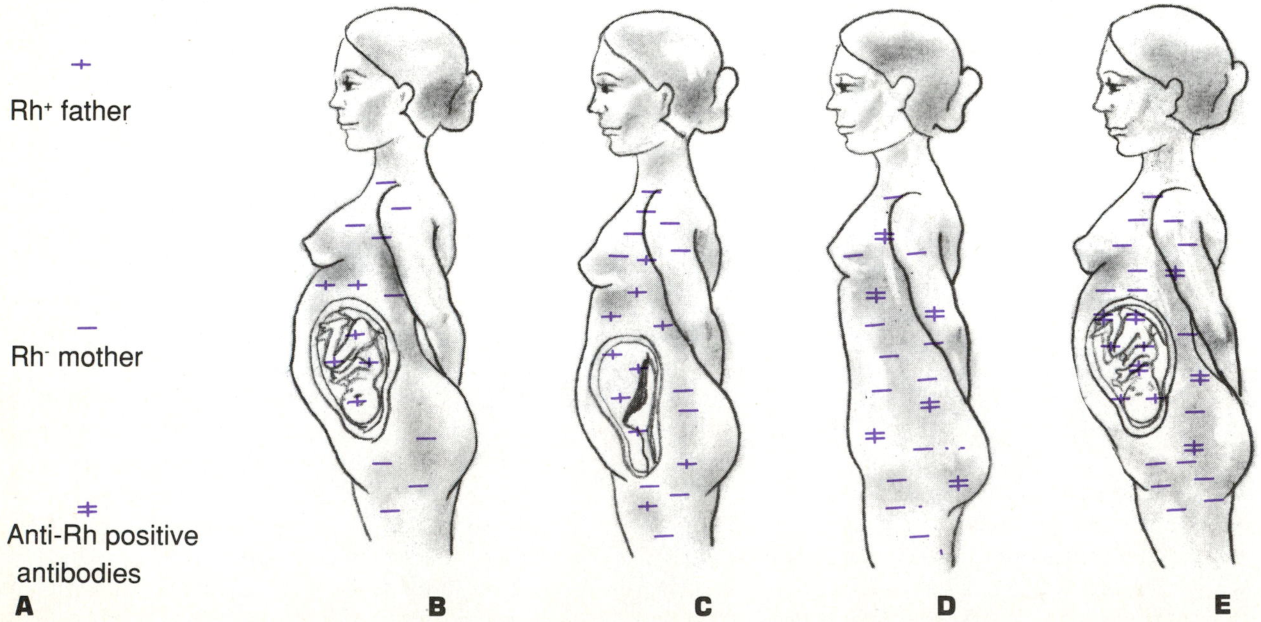

Figure 39–9. Rh isoimmunization process. **A.** Condition results from Rh-positive father and Rh-negative mother. **B.** Initial exposure, with possible mixture of some maternal and fetal blood—Rh-negative mother and Rh-positive fetus. **C.** Further mixture of maternal and fetal blood with placental separation. **D.** Sensitization—mother forms anti–Rh-positive antibodies. **E.** Antibody response on subsequent pregnancies with Rh-positive fetus—maternal antibodies cross the placenta and destroy fetal red blood cells.

namely, D,C,E, c, e, and d, occurring on the red blood cell. Of this complex, D is the most clinically important. Rh type is either homozygous (*DD*) or heterozygous (*Dd*). If two Rh-positive parents produce a child, the child can be either Rh positive or Rh negative, but the mother will not develop sensitivity to the fetal erythrocytes. If two Rh-negative parents produce a child, the child will be Rh negative, and again, the mother will not develop sensitivity to the fetal erythrocytes. If an Rh-positive mother and an Rh-negative father produce a child, the fetus is in no danger from maternal antibodies. If, however, an Rh-negative woman and an Rh-positive man produce a child, the child can be either Rh negative or Rh positive. There is no problem if the child is Rh negative. Rh blood incompatibility arises only if the child is Rh positive.

In the United States, 85 percent of the population is Rh positive. Hemolytic disease of the fetus or newborn occurs in 1.5 percent of pregnancies, and this particular blood incompatibility accounts for 75 percent of all maternal-fetal incompatibilities.

The incidence of Rh isoimmunization has been reduced drastically in the United States since the availability of Rho(D) immune globulin (RhoGAM). Rho(D) immune globulin is administered to the Rh-negative client within 72 hours of maternal exposure to antigens, specifically, after abortion, transfusion, premature separation of the placenta, amniocentesis, ectopic pregnancy, or birth of an Rh-positive infant. RhoGAM is also used prophylactically in an unsensitized woman at 28 weeks gestation.

Failure to eliminate the problems associated with Rh incompatibility results from previous occurrence of missed abortion; transplacental hemorrhage early in pregnancy; use of Rho(D) immune globulin that is not fully potent; and use of dosages that are too small.

Collaborative Assessment

Maternal history of Rh isoimmunization or contributing conditions is essential to assessment. Various tests are used to determine the presence of antibodies in the mother, including saline agglutination, albumin agglutination, and antiglobulin testing (indirect Coombs' test). The indirect Coombs' test is most commonly used to in clinical practice. This test can measure the number of antibodies in the maternal blood. A sample of maternal blood is diluted with a specific quantity of known washed Rh-positive RBCs. Antihuman globulin from animal sources is added. If the woman's serum contains antibodies, the Rh-positive RBCs will clump. The dilution at which the Rh-positive RBCs clump gives the titer of maternal antibody.[116]

Negative titers are accurate indicators that a fetus is not at risk. Positive titers are not as reliable. Other assessments of fetal well-being in high-risk pregnancy, such as serial ultrasonography, nonstress and oxytocin challenge testing, and biophysical profiles, are used simultaneously.

Titers are determined monthly through the second trimester and biweekly through the third trimester for Rh-negative women at risk. If titers exceed a laboratory's own critical titer, then spectrophotometric analysis of amniotic fluid for the presence of bilirubin is the most sensitive index of severity of fetal hemolysis.

One test for the detection and quantification of transplacental hemorrhage is the Kleihauer-Betke test. Fetal red blood cells (RBCs) can be distinguished from maternal RBCs on smear. The fetal/maternal hemorrhage per total estimated maternal blood volume is in the same ratio as the number of fetal RBCs to maternal RBCs on the smear.[116] Other tests used to detect fetal/maternal hemorrhage include the Fetaldex test, the alpha-fetoprotein test, the microscopic Du test (Du is one component of the Rh factor complex), the Rho(D) immune globulin cross-match test, and the enzyme-linked antiglobulin test (ELAT).

Rh isoimmunization results in erythroblastosis fetalis, or the destruction of RBCs, in the fetus (*see* Chapter 42). The destruction of RBCs releases bilirubin into the amniotic fluid, which can be used to assess severity of the condition. Erythroblastosis fetalis can cause severe fetal illness or death.

Collaborative Management

The objectives of medical management are the delivery of a mature fetus and the avoidance of erythroblastosis fetalis. Early detection of this complication is critical in meeting these objectives. All women are tested for blood type at their initial prenatal visit. Rh-negative women are tested serially, as described earlier. Some practitioners advocate administering Rho(D) immune globulin in the 28th week to all pregnant Rh-negative women.

If Rh sensitization has occurred, pregnancy is prolonged as long as possible by intrauterine transfusion to correct the anemia that results from fetal RBC hemolysis. Under the guidance of sonography, and using fluoroscopy, an 18-gauge catheter is inserted into the fetal peritoneal cavity. A volume equal to gestational age $-$ 20 $\times$ 10 mL of O-negative packed RBCs is infused into the fetus. The procedure is repeated in 10 days and then every 4 weeks until delivery. Percutaneous umbilical blood sampling (PUBS) is a newer technique that provides direct access to the fetal circulation. Not only does PUBS permit sampling of fetal blood, but it also allows for administration of transfusions.

Maternal risks from these procedures include local abdominal infection, placental injury leading to disseminated intravascular coagulation, or premature rupture of membranes and chorioamnionitis.

Fetal risks include trauma and graft-versus-host reaction. The overall survival rate for the fetus is greater than 90 percent.[116]

Ideally, fetal maturity of 36 to 37 weeks is achieved before delivery. Management during delivery depends on the status of the fetus.

Nursing Assessment and Management

Nursing assessment includes careful inquiry during the initial prenatal history regarding the woman's blood type, her reproductive and obstetric history, her medical and surgical history, and prior treatment with Rho(D) immune globulin. The nurse prominently notes the blood type throughout client records and verbally informs the medical staff if laboratory results differ from the woman's own report.

The woman needs instruction about when and why Rho(D) immune globulin is administered. It will be her responsibility to apprise health care providers of her need for Rho(D) immune globulin after exposure to the Rh-positive antigen for the rest of her childbearing years.

To participate successfully, the woman needs to understand the regimen of testing she will undergo. The woman and her partner will need psychosocial support throughout the regimen of monitoring and treatment of erythroblastosis fetalis. Serial amniocentesis and intrauterine transfusion are stressful. This couple requires childbirth education appropriate for high-risk pregnancy, and they may appreciate the opportunity to become familiar with the neonatal intensive care unit (NICU) and the NICU personnel in the center where the woman will deliver.

ABO Incompatibility

ABO incompatibility can also arise, but it rarely causes severe fetal hemolysis. It most typically results when a type O woman is pregnant with a type A or B fetus. The first fetus can be involved, and there is no relationship between the occurrence of the disease in the current pregnancy and subsequent pregnancies. Antenatal treatment is not warranted.[116] The neonate is monitored for the development of hyperbilirubinemia (*see* Chapter 42).

THROMBOPHLEBITIS AND DEEP VEIN THROMBOSIS

Superficial thrombophlebitis is an inflammatory process involving clot formation within a superficial vein. **Deep venous thrombosis** (DVT), a clot in the deep veins, does not involve an inflammatory process. The incidence of superficial and DVT in pregnancy has been estimated to be 1 in 70 pregnancies.[116] The risk is three times greater postpartally than antenatally. Factors associated with increased risk during pregnancy include maternal age greater than 35, obesity, immobilization, cardiopulmonary disease, diabetes mellitus, and prior history of thromboembolism. During the postpartum period, method of delivery is a factor, with cesarean delivery being associated with a three times greater risk than vaginal delivery. Deep venous thrombosis is less common than superficial vein involvement.

During pregnancy venous stasis tends to occur in the lower extremities and groin as a result of compression by the gravid uterus. The coagulation system, the fibrinolytic system or both may be activated as described earlier in the discussion of disseminated intravascular coagulation.

Signs of superficial thrombophlebitis include tenderness, redness, and induration directly over the superficial vein. Signs of DVT include calf tenderness, particularly on ambulation; swelling, confirmed by calf measurements or swelling of one leg in relation to the other; redness and warmth; pain in the back of the calf, elicited with dorsal flexion of the foot (termed Homan's sign). In 50 percent of clients with confirmed DVT, however, all of the preceding signs and symptoms may be absent.

The diagnosis of both these conditions may be confirmed by noninvasive tests or invasive tests.

Noninvasive Tests

1. *Duplex scanning.* Duplex scanning involves a combination of ultrasound imaging and Doppler analysis of blood flow. Ultrasound is used to visualize veins and to detect their compressibility. If a vein cannot be compressed when the transducer of the duplex scanner is pressed against the skin, thrombosis is likely.
2. *Impedance plethysmography (IPG).* The rate of emptying of the deep veins in the calf is measured after occlusion of the deep veins in the thigh by inflation of a thigh cuff. A clot in deep veins above the knee will cause obstruction of outflow of venous blood from the affected calf. Venous emptying time of the calf veins thus increases.
3. *Phleborrheography (PRG).* This test measures normal venous flow in the leg during the respiratory cycle and the changes that occur in this cycle as a result of the presence of a clot in the vein.

Tests such as IPG and PRG are useful only if there is complete occlusion of the deep venous system above the knee. These tests will not detect nonocclusive clots in the deep venous system or clots in the veins of the calf. Such limitations decrease accuracy of the tests. In pregnancy, compression of the deep venous system by the gravid uterus makes the tests more technically difficult to perform and more prone to error. Duplex scanning has replaced these older noninvasive tests in most vascular noninvasive laboratories.

Invasive Tests

1. *Venography.* Radiopaque dye is injected into a vein in the foot. The dye is then followed by x-ray as it travels through the deep veins of the leg into the pelvis. Clots in deep or superficial veins may be directly seen. This method is less popular during pregnancy because of exposure of the fetus to radiation.
2. *^{125}I-fibrinogen scan.* A radioactive tracer compound is injected and becomes incorporated into the clot. A "hot spot" can then be visualized. This method of testing is contraindicated during pregnancy and also has a high false-positive rate.

A major complication of DVT is pulmonary embolism. Clot fragments from deep veins may break off, travel up the inferior vena cava to the right side of the heart, and then proceed into the lungs. The clot may block or reduce the flow of blood from the right side of the heart into that part of the lung. This condition is called a pulmonary embolism. The client may not be able to maintain adequate oxygen levels in the blood because of poor perfusion of the affected part of the lung. If the clot is large enough, the client may go into sudden right-sided heart failure.

Signs of pulmonary embolism include dyspnea, tachypnea, sudden chest pain, tachycardia, cardiac arrhythmias, apprehension, and hemoptysis. Death may result from hypoxia, cardiac failure, or cardiac arrhythmias. Pulmonary embolism is a complication in 1 of 2500 to 3000 pregnancies; in 35 percent of cases, deep vein thrombosis was known to precede pulmonary embolism. As with DVT, clinical signs and symptoms of pulmonary embolism may be absent.

NURSING DIAGNOSES RELATED TO THE WOMAN WITH VENOUS DISEASE

Problem-Oriented

Peripheral swelling, related to deep venous thrombosis

Pain and discomfort, related to superficial thrombophlebitis

Strength-Oriented

Progressive home maintenance management, related to assistance from others

Collaborative Management

Collaborative management of thrombophlebitis and DVT includes the following measures:

- Anticoagulation with heparin, given intravenously at first. Heparin therapy is monitored by the partial thromboplastin time (PTT). The dose should be titrated to keep the PTT approximately twice the control value. Platelet counts should be monitored routinely. In rare cases, heparin may induce platelet aggregation and result in low platelet counts. These platelet aggregates may block both arteries and veins in other areas of the body. This condition is referred to as heparin-induced thrombocytopenia. Once PTT levels have stabilized and the client's clinical condition permits, the client is switched from intravenous to subcutaneous heparin therapy for the duration of the pregnancy. Heparin therapy is prescribed with caution during pregnancy. Recognized complications of long-term heparin therapy include osteoporosis. Oral anticoagulants, such as warfarin, are contraindicated during pregnancy. Women who cannot receive anticoagulants and have confirmed DVT above the knee may have a filter placed in the inferior vena cava to trap clots.
- Blood studies including PTT, complete blood count, and platelets.
- Custom-measured compression stockings; prophylactic use of compression stockings in high-risk clients.
- Bedrest with elevation of the affected leg, as indicated.

Nursing Assessment

In addition to previously discussed measures, nursing assessment includes assessment of the client for evidence of thrombophlebitis and DVT at each antenatal visit and daily during the postpartum period; assessment of edema in the lower extremities; and observation for bleeding during anticoagulant therapy, for example, prolonged oozing from puncture sites, bruising, and bleeding gums.

Nursing Diagnoses

Nursing diagnoses are developed on the basis of comprehensive assessment. See the box for examples of nursing diagnoses for the woman with venous disease.

Nursing Management

Nursing management includes the following measures:

- Anticipatory guidance, support, and education about anticoagulation therapy, associated signs of complications, and risks.
- Monitoring laboratory values during heparin therapy.
- Emergency measures if pulmonary embolism is suspected (assessment of mental status, nature, onset and severity of pain, skin color, respiratory status, pulse, blood pressure; notification of physician without delay; oxygen therapy as ordered; possible admission of client to intensive care unit). Other diagnostic measures may be performed by the physician and include arterial blood gas determination, chest x-ray, ventilation perfusion scan, and possibly pulmonary angiography.
- Teaching for prevention of venous disease or its recurrence, including advising the client to rest on her left side at night and at intervals during the day; to elevate her legs when possible; and to avoid salicylates, which promote bleeding if the woman is on anticoagulation therapy.
- Educating clients about risks, signs, and symptoms of venous disease and the need to seek care promptly if signs and symptoms occur.

MULTIPLE GESTATION

Twin births account for 1 in 80 to 95 live births in the United States.[117] Triplet and greater multiple births are far less common. Multiple gestations arise either from fertilization and division of one ovum or fertilization of more than one ovum during a single ovulatory cycle. Twinning resulting from fertilization of more than one ovum is termed *dizygotic,* or *fraternal, twinning.* Twinning resulting from the division of one fertilized zygote into two or more zygotes is termed *monozygotic,* or *identical, twinning.* (*See* Chapter 11 for additional discussion of multiple gestation.)

Factors associated with dizygotic twinning include increased maternal age, increased parity, a positive family history of twins, optimal nutrition, increased levels of follicle-stimulating hormone and luteinizing hormone, increased coital frequency early in marriage, pregnancy within 1 month of stopping oral contraception, use of infertility drugs (such as clomiphene citrate and Pergonal), and in vitro fertilization.[117] In contrast, monozygotic twinning seems to occur independent of race, heredity, age, and parity, although there may be some relation to therapy for infertility.

Collaborative Assessment and Management

Although twin pregnancies are intrinsically high risk, as many as half are not diagnosed before the actual delivery, depending on the birth facility.[5] Associated factors may be present in the woman's reproductive history. Biochemical assays such as serum chorionic gonadotropin, placental lactogen, and alphafetoprotein levels are higher in twin pregnancies, but they do not permit definite diagnosis. Uterine size exceeds that predicted by gestational age. It is not always possible, even for skilled clinicians, to diagnose a multiple gestation using Leopold's maneuvers (Figure 39–10). Careful ultrasonography using at least two views should detect twins nearly all of the time; however, one study demonstrated that in nearly half of twin pregnancies diagnosed early by sonography, only one twin developed to term. Many threatened abortions in the first trimester are actually the spontaneous abortion of one twin.[118]

The mortality rate among singleton births is 14 to 16 per 1000 total births; for twins it is 65 to 120 per 1000 total births; and for triplets it is 250 to 310 per 1000 total births.[119] Morbidity is also much higher among multiple fetuses. Twins account for 10 percent

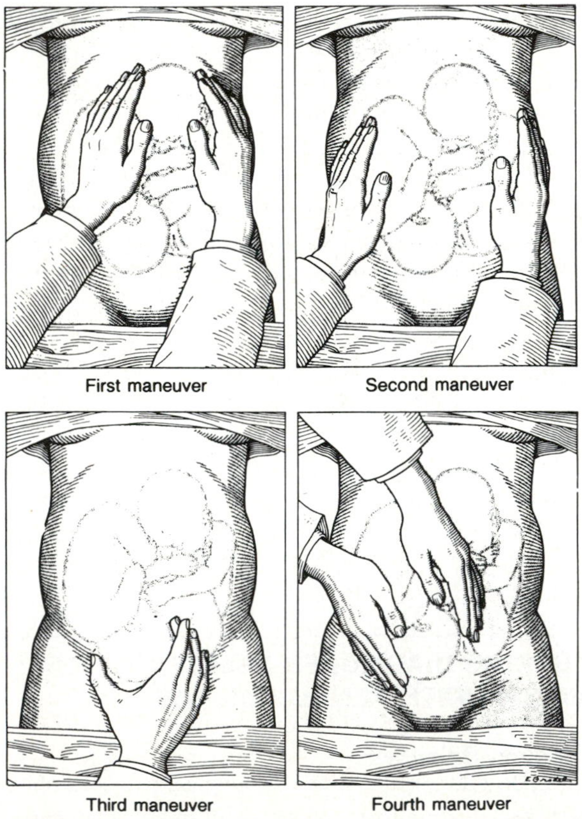

Figure 39–10. Abdominal palpation in twin pregnancy. Cephalic presentation on the mother's right and frank breech presentation on the left. (*Reproduced, with permission, from Cunningham FG, et al.* Williams Obstetrics. *18th ed. Norwalk, Conn: Appleton & Lange; 1989:636.*)

of all preterm deliveries and 25 percent of all preterm deaths. Two thirds experience intrauterine growth retardation. This contributes to the increased incidence of stillbirth, fetal distress in labor, and perinatal asphyxia. Twins experience a higher incidence of developmental problems including learning disabilities, motor skill deficiencies, hand-eye coordination difficulties, and speech problems. The incidence of major and minor congenital anomalies in twins is double that found among singletons and is more common among monozygotic twins.[117]

Maternal complications of twin pregnancies include an increased incidence of hyperemesis gravidarum, iron and folate deficiency anemias, pregnancy-induced hypertension, placenta previa, and abruptio placentae.[117] Polyhydramnios occurs in the presence of some other pathology.[120]

Complications unique to monozygous twins include "twin-to-twin transfusion syndrome," in which vascular communication develops between the twins. The donor fetus is hypotensive, anemic, severely growth retarded, and oligohydramniotic. The recipient is hypervolemic, polycythemic, heavier, and polyhydramniotic. Although there is no treatment for this problem, diagnosis via ultrasound allows the neonatal team to be prepared for two very sick infants.[117] In 80 percent of cases in which this complication arises, at least one twin does not survive.

Twins who share an amniotic sac are at risk for becoming entangled in each other's umbilical cord. The rate of stillbirth among monoamniotic twins exceeds 50 percent.[117]

Early diagnosis by ultrasonography allows for more intensive prenatal care of the mother of multiple fetuses. She can be educated as to possible complications in twin pregnancies, her role in prevention of complications, and early recognition and reporting of complications. Bedrest is widely observed to be useful in promoting fetal weight gain and prolonging pregnancy, although the amount of bedrest is controversial.[5,117]

Strategies generally employed in preventing preterm labor may not be successful in multiple gestation. Fetal well-being is assessed regularly. Nonstress tests (NSTs) are begun at 30 to 34 weeks and may be repeated as often as twice a week; however, they must be interpreted with caution, as nonreactive NST is common among fetuses of less than 32 weeks of gestation.[121] A nonreactive NST in either fetus is followed by a contraction stress test. Serial ultrasound measurements are performed to measure growth. Severe distress and compromised growth are indications for preterm delivery.

For twins of very low birth weight, cesarean delivery is associated with improved perinatal outcomes.[122] For twins larger than an estimated 1500 to 2000 g and older than 32 weeks of gestation, vaginal delivery is undertaken if the presentation of each twin is favorable (Figure 39–11). There is an increased frequency of abnormal presentations with twins, and they have a higher rate of fetal distress in labor. Electronic fetal monitoring of each twin facilitates early intervention should problems arise. For those reasons the mother is attended by a nurse throughout labor. Packed red cells are kept on hand. An intravenous route is established. The delivery room should include an anesthesiologist, in the event that intrauterine manipulation or cesarean delivery is necessary, and a team for the possible resuscitation of each fetus. The presence of two obstetricians is desirable, although not always possible. It is possible that the second twin must be delivered by cesarean section after the first twin has been delivered vaginally. So that these considerations may be addressed during labor and delivery, it is important that twins be detected prenatally.

Nursing Assessment and Management

The nurse assesses the presence of increased tendency toward multiple gestation (Table 39–27); fetal growth, heart rates, activity, and positions; maternal weight gain; maternal nutritional intake; hematocrit and hemoglobin levels; the presence of associated risk factors, such as hyperemesis gravidarum and pregnancy-induced hypertension; and the occurrence of preterm labor.

Nursing interventions prenatally include instruction and reinforcement regarding early reporting of signs and symptoms of complications of pregnancy and adequate rest. The woman expecting twins can be counseled toward good nutrition, increasing her protein, calcium, iron, and folate intake beyond the RDAs in normal pregnancy. The recommended weight gain for women expecting twins is about 50 percent greater than that for a singleton birth. A total weight gain of about 40 pounds is appropriate.

The woman expecting twins is at increased risk for preterm labor. She is instructed to follow the guidelines described earlier for the prevention of preterm labor. She needs to know the characteristics of labor. She will be assessed every 2 weeks during the second trimester, and weekly during the third trimester.

In addition, the woman expecting twins is at increased risk for hyperemesis gravidarum and pregnancy-induced hypertension. She requires instruction in early detection and health maintenance related to these complications.

The family expecting twins may be stressed by the greater financial responsibilities, by anticipation of the greater workload of child care, and by the

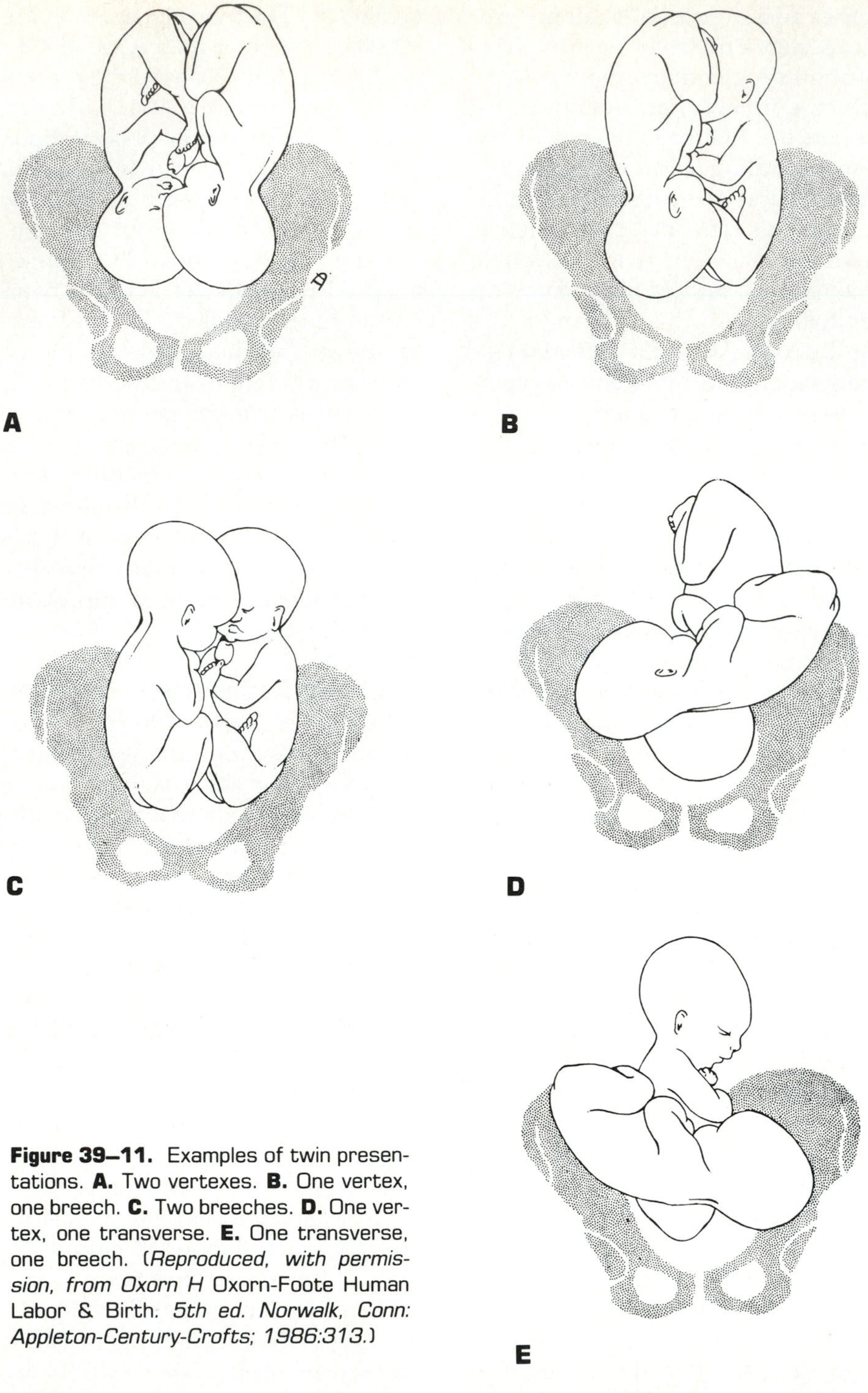

Figure 39–11. Examples of twin presentations. **A.** Two vertexes. **B.** One vertex, one breech. **C.** Two breeches. **D.** One vertex, one transverse. **E.** One transverse, one breech. (*Reproduced, with permission, from Oxorn H* Oxorn-Foote Human Labor & Birth. *5th ed. Norwalk, Conn: Appleton-Century-Crofts; 1986:313.*)

awareness that this pregnancy is high risk. If they are taught about potential risks to the mother and infants, particularly the risk of prematurity, expectant families will be concerned about their infants' survival. These families need anticipatory guidance about the birth itself and all of the people who may be involved.[123] For example, one mother expecting twins asked if she faced two separate labors.

There are numerous practical considerations faced by parents of multiples, such as obtaining double nursery furnishings and equipment, the issue of trying to breastfeed twins, and the risks and benefits of fostering their togetherness or separateness. The nurse can help by referring these parents to the local chapter of a national group known variously as Parents of Twins or Mothers of Multiples. La Leche

TABLE 39–27. OBSERVATIONS IN MULTIPLE GESTATION

Uterus larger than normal for dates
Fetal parts palpable in all four quadrants
Fetal movment reported in all four quadrants
Excessive nausea and vomiting
Anemia
Two or more distinct fetal heart sounds
Dyspnea
Shortness of breath
Pedal edema
Backache
Onset of pregnancy-induced hypertension
Polyhydramnios
Abnormal alpha-fetoprotein levels
Visualization of more than one fetus on ultrasound

League is supportive of mothers of multiples who wish to breastfeed their twins. Publications such as "Twins" are directed toward these families. Mothers of twins who have attended the same antenatal clinic or delivered in the same facility may also informally be introduced to one another.

POSTTERM PREGNANCY

A **postterm pregnancy** is one that continues past the estimated date of confinement (EDC). Given the error in calculating EDC, the end of 42 weeks of gestation is commonly considered the point at which a pregnancy is postterm.[5,124]

The incidence of prolonged pregnancy is reported to be 3.5 to 14.9 percent of all pregnancies; however, accurate diagnosis of postterm pregnancy depends on accurate dating of the pregnancy. Strategies for determining the EDC were described in Chapter 14 and are based on a detailed menstrual history, assessment of uterine growth, dates of quickening and first fetal heart tones, and ultrasonography.[125]

Factors associated with postterm pregnancy include anencephaly and fetal adrenal hypoplasia. Steroid administration, the use of aspirin, and maternal anxiety have been implicated. Women who have experienced one postterm pregnancy are at increased risk in subsequent pregnancies. Additional factors include maternal age, especially among primiparas who are over 26 years old, grand multiparity, and first-trimester vaginal bleeding. Carriers of urogenital group B streptococci are also at increased risk. The problem seems to arise more among women of low educational level, but this may reflect a lack of knowledge about reproduction and the way EDC is determined.[5,124,125] In fact, the etiology of postterm pregnancy is not really known because the mechanism for the initiation of labor is not understood.

Possible sequelae of postterm pregnancy include the postmaturity syndrome. Findings associated with postmaturity include oligohydramnios and meconium staining. The infant may have wrinkled, peeling skin, alert facies, creases covering the surface of the soles, and the absence of vernix and lanugo. The infant may demonstrate respiratory distress, hypoglycemia, polycythemia, temperature instability, and a ponderal index (estimation of body mass) of less than 2.20.[126] Postmature infants have increased morbidity and mortality whether they are growth retarded or not. They have been observed to have lower Brazelton scores, and to experience increased childhood illness and hospitalization, decreased social maturity, more sleep disorders, and more reading difficulties at age 6. In addition, the infants are rated "difficult" by their mothers more often than controls.[126]

The underlying pathology in postmaturity syndrome is impaired uteroplacental perfusion, or placental insufficiency, often attributed to placental aging.[124] Placental growth ceases before term and the rate of blood flow through the uterus decreases. Oxygen saturation is reduced at a time when fetal demands are increasing. Mild uteroplacental ischemia is evident on microscopic examination of the tissues, but the placenta usually has enough reserve capacity to allow continuing fetal growth at a slower rate. If placental reserve is exhausted, fetal malnutrition, hypoxia, and asphyxia can occur.

Nursing and Collaborative Assessment

The challenge in postterm pregnancy lies in identifying infants at risk for postmaturity syndrome. Perhaps as few as 30 percent of pregnancies identified as postterm truly exceed 40 weeks of gestation, and only 10 to 20 percent of babies born are postmature.[126] Therefore routine induction between 40 and 42 weeks of gestation, though practiced widely, does not always reflect the needs of the client.

When pregnancy extends beyond 41 weeks the woman is asked to count fetal movements several times each day: fewer than three fetal movements per hour, or fewer than ten in 3 hours, is a common standard of fetal well-being.[127] The woman keeps a chart and contacts her midwife or obstetrician immediately should activity levels drop.

The NST, as a measure of antepartum fetal heart rate, is now a standard measure of fetal well-being; however, there are findings that indicate that contraction stress testing is more sensitive in predicting risk of postmaturity syndrome.[128–130] The nipple stimulation contraction stress test is an inexpensive, efficient variation on the oxytocin challenge test[126] (*see* Chapter 22).

The biophysical profile is ascertained by ultrasound. It includes assessment of amniotic fluid volume, fetal activity, tonus, respiratory effort, and ponderal index, or estimation of weight. This method has potential as an indicator of postmaturity. Oligohydramnios is a fairly consistent finding. Placental grading is also useful.[126]

Nursing and Collaborative Management

Labor is induced in cases of postmaturity. Electronic fetal monitoring is indicated during induced labor. If the fetus is stressed, cesarean delivery will be performed. Postmature infants are at risk of being stressed during labor. The woman's ability to focus on and work with contractions may be overwhelmed during induction, so her need for support and, in turn, her coach's need for support are greater than normal. The team on hand to tend to the newborn should anticipate the possible need for resuscitation.

Accuracy of dating the pregnancy is necessary to determine both prematurity and postmaturity. Monitoring fetal well-being is time consuming and often an intrusive ordeal for postterm clients. One fourth to one third of women whose pregnancies are postterm are considered by health professionals "noncompliant," in that they do not fully participate in the surveillance protocol.[127] This possibly reflects unnecessarily routine medicalization of an often misdiagnosed condition. In one investigation, when nine women who were an average of 25 days past their physician-calculated EDC were interviewed, eight reported that their due dates were actually 9 to 25 days later than their physicians believed. None of their newborns scored higher than 41 weeks on the Dubowitz tool for gestational age assessment. Only three of these mothers had normal, spontaneous vaginal deliveries. The authors were disturbed that the woman's own sense of timing was disregarded in diagnosing postmaturity and in intervening.[127] Nurses should be sensitive to a woman's knowledge of herself. Such sensitivity might increase client adherence to care requirements when it is important.

When pregnancy extends beyond the due date, particularly when women feel they know precisely when they conceived, stress increases. In a study of 30 expectant mothers who were at least 3 days overdue, reactions of most included the feeling that they would be pregnant forever, sleep difficulties, the desire to be induced, a tendency to hang on to physicians' and nurses' every word for reassurance, seeking reassurance about delivery from other mothers, fussing with the baby's clothes and equipment, overexertion with housework, and increased discomfort.[131] Interventions by health professionals that were most helpful included discussion of the women's feelings, discussion of the expected time range of the birth, allowing the mother to listen to the fetal heart tone, and discussion of comfort measures. The author concluded that the main characteristic observed in conducting the investigation was the intense need the woman had for someone to acknowledge that a postterm pregnancy is stressful.

OTHER MEDICAL AND SURGICAL CONDITIONS

Pregnant women can experience any medical or surgical illness that afflicts women of childbearing age. In addition to the conditions described in this chapter, it is not uncommon to encounter women with such conditions as asthma, epilepsy, or renal disease in maternity settings. Women can experience emergencies such as appendicitis, for which surgery is required. Several important considerations are necessary for assessment and management:

1. During pregnancy many conditions are more difficult to diagnose because of normally occurring physiologic alterations of pregnancy. For example, edema and trace protein in the urine are acceptable observations during pregnancy. For the nonpregnant women with renal disease, these observations may be early evidence of the disease's progression.
2. Some complications of pregnancy mimic medical or surgical complications of nonpregnant women. For example, appendicitis must be differentiated from abruptio placentae.
3. It may be more difficult to treat a medical or surgical complication because of the fetotoxic effects of usual strategies such as certain drug therapies. In extreme instances, the woman may be forced to choose between treatment of her own life-threatening illness and avoidance of harming her fetus. The occurrence of maternal cancer during pregnancy is an example. With the proliferation of fetal monitoring capabilities and neonatal intensive care units, this type of choice is, fortunately, less frequent than it was two decades ago. But, in general, medications are used with extreme caution during pregnancy. Research does not exist to support the safety of most drugs for human fetuses.
4. Selected common surgeries can be accomplished during pregnancy with minimal increased risk to

the mother or fetus. General anesthesia need not threaten fetal well-being.[132]

5. Pathophysiologic processes that do threaten fetal survival include hypoxia, acidosis, and hypotension. Hypertension is a slower threat, as it induces decreased uteroplacental perfusion and increases the risk of abruptio placentae.

TRAUMA

Trauma refers to client injury that is afflicted by the client herself or by other living or nonliving sources. Trauma can be caused accidentally or deliberately and is the largest cause of death in women of childbearing age. Because of trauma, 1 in 14 women seeks medical help and 3 to 4 pregnant women per 1000 require hospitalization during pregnancy.[133] Physiologic changes and psychosocial stress related to pregnancy may put the client at risk for injury. Trauma during pregnancy involves both the expectant woman and the fetus; however, actual injury to the woman or fetus depends on the type of trauma and the maternal and fetal organs that are affected. Although the pregnant woman may sustain many types of trauma, the following injuries are seen frequently in clinical practice.[134]

1. *Abdominal trauma.* The pregnant woman is at high risk during the second and third trimesters due to the enlarged uterus. The third trimester poses the greatest risk to the fetus, because there is less amniotic fluid than in the second trimester and the fetus is larger. During the first trimester, the embryo-fetus is protected by the bony pelvis. Blunt abdominal trauma occurs as the result of such conditions as auto accidents (in which the woman is thrown from the vehicle or against its steering wheel or dash board) and interpersonal conflict in which the woman is punched or kicked. Injuries include fracture of the fetal skull, fetomaternal transfusion, and placenta abruption. Severity of injuries does not necessarily predict whether placenta abruptio will occur.[135] The most common causes of penetrating abdominal trauma are bullet wounds and stab wounds.
2. *Thermal trauma.* Thermal injury results from burns. Although pregnancy may not be affected if less than one third of the body surface is burned, actual injury and threat to pregnancy depend upon the extent of the burns and circumstances in which they occurred. In addition to requiring care according to protocols for burn victims, pregnant women need attention to oxygenation, electrolyte balance, and fluid replacement. Respiratory or cardiac arrest and fluid and electrolyte imbalance present life-threatening conditions.
3. *Pelvic fractures.* Pelvic fractures can occur as the result of such conditions as automobile accidents or falls. Pelvic fractures can present major problems at any time during pregnancy. In late pregnancy, when the fetal head is engaged in the pelvis, fetal skull fractures may also result.

Comprehensive assessment of pregnant clients who sustain trauma requires understanding of principles of trauma, normal changes associated with pregnancy, and fetal growth and development. The specialty of trauma is a branch of critical care and requires special nursing and medical expertise. Whenever feasible, the client initially should be taken to a trauma center capable of caring for a high-risk obstetric client and a neonate requiring sophisticated intensive care, or transferred to this type of trauma center when she is stable enough to survive transport. The goals of care focus on thorough assessment to identify the impact of injury on the expectant

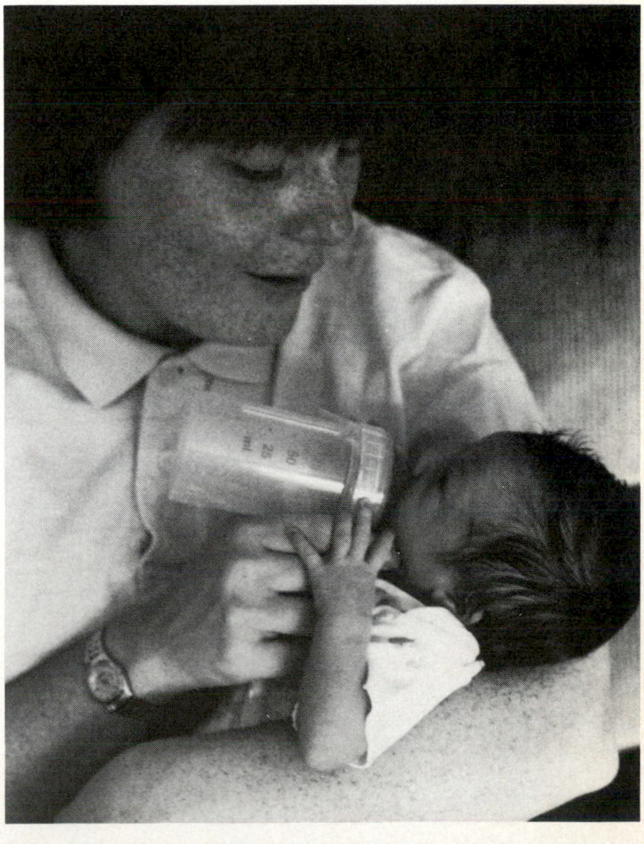

Figure 39–12. After 18 weeks on bedrest, intermittent hospitalizations, and continuous tocolytic therapy for preterm labor, this mother delivered a healthy baby girl at term.

mother and her fetus and to implement strategies designed to stabilize the client, prevent impairment or death, and restore health. Assessment and management are based on protocols which have been published by groups such as the American College of Surgeons.

SUMMARY

Many conditions may threaten maternal and fetal well-being during the second and third trimesters of pregnancy. These include pregnancy-induced hypertension, heart disease, diabetes mellitis, hemorrhagic disorders, infection, alterations in amniotic fluid, spontaneous abortion/incompetent cervix, preterm labor, Rh isoimmunization, thrombophlebitis, multiple gestation, prematurity, and postmaturity.

Nursing and collaborative management strategies in all of these conditions begin with prompt assessment of the complication. Early intervention with an emphasis on prevention of complications during pregnancy has served to reduce the gravity of these conditions, as demonstrated by reduced maternal and perinatal mortality rates over the last 20 years. For example, thorough reproductive and menstrual history taking, assessment of nutritional adequacy, and promotion of early and consistent prenatal care are three critical nursing measures in the prevention or early detection of complications of pregnancy.

In all of the conditions discussed in this chapter, client education is a major nursing management strategy. Women need to know which changes require prompt intervention. These clients need to know how to carry out the health maintenance activities that will prevent worsening of their condition. It is the nurse's responsibility to educate clients on the self-administration of therapeutic drugs. Additionally, women are more likely to participate in grueling protocols for the surveillance of fetal well-being if they understand what is being done to them and why. It is consistent with all of the complications described in this chapter that close supervision throughout a high-risk pregnancy yields the best results for mother and fetus (Figure 39–12). If the outcome of the pregnancy is maternal or neonatal death or disability, families will cope best if they are satisfied that they and their interdisciplinary team have done all that was possible to promote maternal and fetal health.

The nurse's role in assessing family integration and interpretation of the high-risk pregnancy continues from the time clients become aware of the risk factors. The need for clarification, support, and assistance in adaptation must be assessed by the nurse throughout the childbearing cycle and beyond. If their perception of the situation is accurate and if they receive appropriate nursing support, in most instances families will choose to do whatever they can to promote optimal fetal and maternal outcomes.

Nursing care is integral to clients' participation in their care and to family coping. Across all disease entities discussed in this chapter the measure of success is consistent: that the impact of these risk factors is minimal.

REVIEW QUESTIONS

1. Describe signs and symptoms indicating complications of pregnancy.
2. Describe pregnancy-induced hypertension; distinguish between pregnancy-induced hypertension and hypertension existing prior to pregnancy.
3. Discuss nursing care for a client with gestational diabetes.
4. Describe assessment strategies for a client with vaginal bleeding during the second or third trimester.
5. Describe assessment and management strategies for a client in preterm labor.

REFERENCES

1. Rubin R. *Maternal Identity and the Maternal Experience.* New York: Springer Publishing Co; 1984.
2. Knuppel RA, Drukker JE. Hypertension in pregnancy. In: Knuppel RA, Drukker JE, eds. *High-Risk Pregnancy: A Team Approach.* Philadelphia: WB Saunders; 1986.
3. Chesley LC. Hypertensive disorders in pregnancy. *Nurse-Midwifery.* 1985;30:99–104.
4. Page EW, Christianson R. Influence of blood pressure changes with and without proteinuria upon the outcome of pregnancy. *Am J Obstet Gynecol.* 1976;126:821.
5. Cunningham FG, et al. *Williams Obstetrics.* 18th ed. Norwalk, Conn: Appleton & Lange; 1989.
6. Hughes EC. *Obstetric-Gynecologic Terminology.* Philadelphia: FA Davis; 1972.
7. Patterson WB. A hypothesis of how malnutrition and stress cause EPH gestosis. In: Suzuki M, ed. *Perinatal Care and Gestosis.* New York: Elsevier; 1985.

8. Sullivan JM. *Hypertension and Pregnancy.* Chicago: Year Book Medical Publishers; 1986.
9. Whittaker AA, et al. Hemolysis, elevated serum enzymes, and low platelet count syndrome: nursing care of the critically ill obstetric patient. *Heart Lung* 1986;15:402–408.
10. Lueck J. Observation of an organism found in patients with gestational trophoblastic disease and in patients with toxemia of pregnancy. *Am J Obstet Gynecol.* 1983;145:15–26.
11. Brewer T. Role of malnutrition in pre-eclampsia and eclampsia. *Am J Obstet Gynecol.* 1976;125:281–282.
12. Burke ME. Hypertensive crisis and the perinatal period. *J Perinat Neonat Nurs.* 1989;3:33–47.
13. Weinstein L. Syndrome of hemolysis, elevated liver enzymes, and low platelet count: a severe consequence of hypertension in pregnancy. *Am J Obstet Gynecol.* 1982;123: 823.
14. Poole JH. Getting perspective on HELLP syndrome. *Am J Matern Child Nurs.* 1988;13:432–437.
15. Sibai BM. Magnesium sulfate is the ideal anticonvulsant in preeclampsia-eclampsia. *Am J Obstet Gynecol.* 1990;162: 1141–1145.
16. Pritchard JA, et al. The Parkland Hospital protocol for treatment of eclampsia: treatment of 245 cases. *Am J Obstet Gynecol.* 1984;145:951–963.
17. Davis BN. Adolescents with congenital heart disease reaching childbearing years. *Issues Health Care Women Int.* 1983;4:213–222.
18. Land MA, Bisno AL. Acute rheumatic fever: a vanishing disease in suburbia. *JAMA.* 1983;249:895.
19. Etheridge MH, Pepperell RJ. Heart disease and pregnancy at the Royal Women's Hospital. *Med J Aust.* 1977;2:227.
20. Whittemore R, et al. Results of pregnancy in women with congenital heart defects. *Pediatr Res.* 1980;14:452.
21. Sugrue O, et al. Pregnancy complicated by maternal heart disease at the National Maternity Hospital, Dublin, Ireland, 1969–1978. *Am J Obstet Gynecol.* 1981;139:1.
22. Berry JL, Gabbe SG. Diabetes mellitus in pregnancy. In: Knuppel RA, Drukker JE, eds. *High-Risk Pregnancy: A Team Approach.* Philadelphia: WB Saunders; 1986.
23. Baird JD. Some aspects of the metabolic and hormonal adaptation to pregnancy. *Acta Endocrinol Suppl.* 1986;277: 11–18.
24. Hare JW. Pregnancy and diabetes. In: Marble A, et al, eds. *Joslin's Diabetes Mellitus.* 12th ed. Philadelphia: Lea & Febiger; 1985.
25. Porte D, Halter JB. The endocrine pancreas and diabetes mellitus. In: Williams RH, ed. *Textbook of Endocrinology.* 6th ed. Philadelphia: WB Saunders; 1981.
26. National Diabetes Data Group. Classification of diabetes mellitus and other categories of glucose intolerance. *Diabetes.* 1979;28:1039.
27. Brinkman CR. Classification and screening of diabetes mellitus during pregnancy. In: Nuwayhid BS, et al, eds. *Management of the Diabetic Pregnancy.* New York: Elsevier Science; 1987.
28. Christman C, Bennett J. Diabetes: new names, new test, new diet. *Nursing '87.* 1987;17:34–42.
29. White P. Pregnancy and diabetes: medical aspects. *Med Clin North Am.* 1978;7:1015–1027.
30. American College of Obstetricians and Gynecologists. *Technical Bulletin No. 92.* May 1986.
31. Jowett NI, Nicol SG. Gestational diabetes—are the right women being screened? *Midwifery.* 1986;2:98–100.
32. Gabbe SG. Gestational diabetes mellitus. *N Engl J Med.* 1986;315:1025–1026.
33. Golde SH. Diabetic ketoacidosis in pregnancy. In: Clark SL, et al, eds. *Critical Care Obstetrics.* Oradell, NJ: Medical Economics Co; 1987.
34. Burns EM. Diabetes mellitus and pregnancy. *Nurs Clin North Am.* 1983;18:673–685.
35. Airaksinen KEJ, et al. Impaired cardiac adjustment to pregnancy in type I diabetes. *Diabetes Care.* 1986;9:376–383.
36. Efendic S, et al. Glucose tolerance, insulin release, and insulin sensitivity in normal-weight women with previous gestational diabetes mellitus. *Diabetes.* 1987;36:413–419.
37. Sutherland HW, Pritchard CW. Increased incidence of spontaneous abortion in pregnancies complicated by diabetes mellitus. *Am J Obstet Gynecol.* 1986;155:135–138.
38. Chervenak JL, Chez RA. Exact timing of the one-hour glucose sample as a factor in the screen for gestational diabetes. *J Perinatol.* 1989;9:369–371.
39. Miller E, et al. Elevated maternal hemoglobin A_{1c} in early pregnancy and major congenital anomalies in infants of diabetic mothers. *N Engl J Med.* 1981;304:1331–1334.
40. Oats JN, Beischer NA. Gestational diabetes. *Aust NZ J Obstet Gynecol.* 1986;26:2–10.
41. Winick M. *Nutrition, Pregnancy, and Early Infancy.* Baltimore: Williams & Wilkins, 1989.
42. Williams EJ. Gestational diabetes mellitus and diet control. *Diabetes Educator.* 1986;12:16–17.
43. Kushion W, et al. Diabetes and pregnancy: a retrospective 5-year description comparing two management settings. *Diabetes Educator.* 1985;11:28–34.
44. Giordano BP, Rainwater NG. A team approach to the pregnant diabetic. *Diabetes Educator.* 1984;10:58.
45. Mimouni F, et al. Respiratory distress syndrome in infants of diabetic mothers in the 1980s: no direct adverse effect of maternal diabetes with modern management. *Obstet Gynecol. 1987;69:191–195.*
46. Cousins, L. Pregnancy complications among diabetic women: review 1965–1985. *Obstet Gynecol Surv.* 1987;42:140–149.
47. Bellmann O. Therapy of gestational diabetes. *Acta Endocrinol Suppl.* 1986;277:50–55.
48. Freinkel N, et al. Care of the pregnant woman with insulin-dependent diabetes mellitus. *N Engl J Med.* 1985;313:96–101.
49. Drury MI. The pregnant diabetic. *Midwife, Health Visitor Community Nurse.* 1987;23:229–233.
50. Armstrong N. Coping with diabetes mellitus: a full-time job. *Nurs Clin North Am.* 1987;22:559–568.
51. Zigrossi ST, Riga-Ziegler M. The stress of medical management on pregnant diabetics. *Am J Matern Child Nurs.* 1986; 11:320–323.
52. Tucker SM. Second or third trimester bleeding. *J Perinatol.* 1988;8:174–177.
53. Sholl JS. Abruptio placentae: clinical management in non-acute cases. *Am J Obstet Gynecol.* 1987;156:40–51.
54. Jouppila P. Vaginal bleeding in the last two trimesters of pregnancy. A clinical and ultrasonic study. *Acta Obstet Gynecol Scand.* 1979;58:461.
55. Hurd WW, et al. Selective management of abruptio placentae: a prospective study. *Obstet Gynecol.* 1983;61: 467.
56. Marbury MC, et al. The association of alcohol consumption with outcome of pregnancy. *Am J Public Health.* 1983;73: 1165.

57. Ney JA, et al. The prevalence of substance abuse in patients with suspected preterm labor. *Am J Obstet Gynecol.* 1990;162:1562–1565.
58. Lynch M, McKeon VA. Cocaine use during pregnancy: research findings and clinical implications. *J Obstet Gynecol Neonat Nurs.* 1990;19:285–292.
59. Hibbard BM, Jeffcoate TNA. Abruptio placentae. *Obstet Gynecol.* 1966;27:155.
60. Pritchard JA, et al. Genesis of severe placental abruption. *Am J Obstet Gynecol.* 1970;108:22.
61. McCormac M. Managing hemorrhagic shock. *AJN.* 1990; 90:22–27.
62. Howe CL. Dealing with third-trimester bleeding. *RN.* 1985; 48:29–31.
63. Dorman KF. Hemorrhagic emergencies in obstetrics. *J Perinat Neonat Nurs.* 1989;3:23–32.
64. Dickinson JE, et al. Oxytocin induced second trimester uterine rupture. *Aust NZ J Obstet Gynecol.* 1986;26:251–252.
65. Mayberry LJ, Forte AB. Pregnancy-related disseminated intravascular coagulation (DIC). *Am J Matern Child Nurs.* 1985;10:168–173.
66. Jones WB. Gestational trophoblastic disease: what have we learned in the past decade? *Am J Obstet Gynecol.* 1990; 162:1286–1295.
67. O'Quinn AG, Barnard DE. Gestational trophoblastic diseases. In: Pernoll ML, Benson RC, eds. *Current Obstetric & Gynecologic Diagnosis and Treatment.* 6th ed. Norwalk, Conn: Appleton & Lange; 1987:891–900.
68. Schwalb RB, Stiles BD. Preventing infection during pregnancy—and after. *RN.* 1984;47:44–45.
69. Gilstrap LC, et al. Acute pyelonephritis in pregnancy: an anterospective study. *Obstet Gynecol.* 1981;57:409.
70. Reddy J, Campbell A. Bacteriuria in pregnancy. *Aust NZ J Obstet Gynecol.* 1985;25:176–178.
71. Farr S, Pastorek JG. Perinatal infections: In: Knuppel RA, Drukker JE, eds. *High-Risk Pregnancy: A Team Approach.* Philadelphia: WB Saunders; 1986.
72. Blanc W. Pathology of the placenta, membranes and umbilical cord. In: Naeye R, Kissane J, Kaufman N, eds. *Perinatal Diseases.* Baltimore: Williams & Wilkins; 1981.
73. Spaun E, Klunder K. Case report: *Candida* chorioamnionitis and intra-uterine contraceptive device. *Acta Obstet Gynecol Scand.* 1986;65:183–184.
74. Hammer GS, Hirschman SZ. Infections in pregnancy. In: Cherry SH, et al, eds. *Rovinsky & Guttmacher's Medical, Surgical, and Gynecologic Complications of Pregnancy.* 3rd ed. Baltimore: Williams & Wilkins; 1985.
75. DeVore NE, et al. TORCH infections. *Am J Nurs.* 1983;83: 1660–1665.
76. Morgan-Capner P, Griffiths G. Fetal and neonatal infection. *Nurs Times.* 1984;80:28–32.
77. Sfameni SF, et al. Antenatal screening for congenital infection with rubella, cytomegalovirus and toxoplasma. *Aust NZ J Obstet Gynecol.* 1986;26:257.
78. MacLeod CL, Lee RV. Parasitic infections. In: Burrow GN, Ferris TF, eds. *Medical Complications During Pregnancy.* 3rd ed. Philadelphia: Saunders; 1988:425–447.
79. Benenson AS, ed. *Control of Communicable Diseases in Man.* 14th ed. Washington, DC: American Public Health Association; 1987.
80. Higa K, Dan K, Manabe H. Varicella-zoster virus infections during pregnancy: hypothesis concerning the mechanism of congenital malformations. *Obstet Gynecol.* 1987;69:214–222.
81. Sever JL. Rubella. In: Queenan JT, Hobbins JC, eds. *Protocols for High-Risk Pregnancies.* Oradell, NJ: Medical Economics Books; 1988.
82. Johnson C. Cytomegalovirus infection. *Midwife, Health Visitor Community Nurse.* 1985;21:166–168.
83. Hatherly LI. The incidence of cytomegalic inclusion disease (CID) in an obstetric teaching hospital, 1975–1984. *Aust NZ J Obstet Gynecol.* 1985;25:171–175.
84. Grossman JH. Herpes simplex. In: Queenan JT, Hobbins JC, eds. *Protocols for High-Risk Pregnancies.* Oradell, NJ: Medical Economics Books; 1988.
85. Gibbs RS. Infection control of herpes simplex virus infections in obstetrics and gynecology. *J Reprod Med.* 1986; 31(suppl):395–397.
86. Gelinas LS. Sexually transmitted disease and pregnancy: the nursing approach. *Occup Health Nurs.* 1984;32:480–484.
87. Hatherly LI, et al. Herpes virus in a high risk obstetric hospital, II. *Med J Aust.* 1980;2:273.
88. Osborne NG, Pratson L. Sexually transmitted diseases and pregnancy. *J Obstet Gynecol Neonat Nurs.* 1984;13: 9–12.
89. Iwasaka T, et al. Genital mycoplasma colonization in neonatal girls. *Acta Obstet Gynecol Scand.* 1986;65:269–272.
90. McKenzie SA, et al. Neonatal pyridoxine responsive convulsions due to isoniazid therapy. *Arch Dis Child.* 1976;51: 567–568.
91. Novello A. *Final Report of the Secretary's Work Group on Pediatric HIV Infection and Disease.* Washington, DC: Department of Health and Human Services; 1988.
92. Wofsy C. Intravenous drug abuse and women's medical issues. *Report of the Surgeon General on Children with HIV Infection and Their Families.* Washington, DC: DHHS; 1987.
93. Boland M. The child with AIDS: special concerns. In: Durham J, Cohen R, eds. *The Person with AIDS.* New York: Springer; 1987.
94. Rogers M. Transmission of human immunodeficiency virus infection. *Report of the Surgeon General on Children with HIV Infection and Their Families.* Washington, DC: DHHS; 1987.
95. Hauer LB, Dattel BJ. Management of the pregnant woman infected with the human immunodeficiency virus. *J Perinatol.* 1988;8:258–262.
96. Falloon J, et al. Human immunodeficiency virus infection in children. *J Pediatrics.* 1989;114:1–23.
97. Boylan P, Parisi V. An overview of hydramnios. *Semin Perinatol.* 1986;10:136–141.
98. Moore TR, Cayle JR. The amniotic fluid index in normal human pregnancy. *Am J Obstet Gynecol.* 1990;162: 1168–1173.
99. Hill LM, et al. Polyhydramnios: ultrasonically detected prevalence and neonatal outcome. *Obstet Gynecol.* 1987;69: 21–25.
100. Queenan JT, Watkins J. Polyhydramnios. In: Queenan JT, ed. *Management of High-Risk Pregnancy.* 2nd ed. Oradell, NJ: Medical Economics Books; 1985.
101. Healy DL, et al. Chronic idiopathic polyhydramnios: Evidence for a defect in the chorion laeve receptor for lactogenic hormones. *J Clin Endocr Metab.* 1983;56:520.
102. Leveno KJ. Amnionic fluid volume in prolonged pregnancy. *Semin Perinatol.* 1986;10:154–161.
103. Novy MJ, et al. Shirodkar cerclage in a multifactorial ap-

proach to the patient with advanced cervical changes. *Am J Obstet Gynecol.* 1990;162:1412–1419.
104. Fuchs F, Husslein P. Prevention and management of prematurity. In. Lauersen NH, ed. *Modern Management of High-Risk Pregnancy.* New York: Plenum Medical Books; 1983.
105. Katz M, et al. Early signs and symptoms of preterm labor. *Am J Obstet Gynecol.* 1990;162:1150–1157.
106. Cooperstock M, Wolfe RA. Seasonality of preterm birth in the collaborative perinatal project: demographic factors. *Am J Epidemiol.* 1986;124:234–241.
107. Lumley J. Very low birth-weight (1,500 g) and previous induced abortion: Victoria 1982–1983. *Aust NZ J Obstet Gynecol.* 1986;26:268–270.
108. Papiernik E, et al. Ethnic differences in duration of pregnancy. *Ann Hum Biol.* 1986;13:259–265.
109. Danforth DN, Scott JR. *Obstetrics and Gynecology.* 5th ed. Philadelphia: JB Lippincott; 1986.
110. Koehl L, Wheeler D. Monitoring uterine activity at home. *AJN.* 1989;90:200–203.
111. Johnson FF. Assessment and education to prevent preterm labor. *Am J Matern Child Nurs.* 1989;14:157–160.
112. Cotton DB, et al. Comparison between magnesium sulfate, terbutaline and a placebo for inhibition of preterm labor: a randomized study. *J Reprod Med.* 1984;29:92.
113. Gill P, et al. Terbutaline by pump to prevent recurrent preterm labor. *Am J Matern Child Nurs.* 1989;14:163–167.
114. Maloni J. Effects of bedrest during pregnancy. Preliminary research report presentation at Center for Low Birthweight, Philadelphia, University of Pennsylvania; July 24, 1990.
115. Weingarten CT, et al. Married mothers' perceptions of their premature term infants and the quality of their relationships with their husbands. *J Obstet Gynecol Neonatal Nurs.* 1990;19:64–73.
116. Ingardia CJ. Additional medical complications in pregnancy. In: Knuppel RA, Drukker JE, eds. *High-Risk Pregnancy: A Team Approach.* Philadelphia: WB Saunders; 1986.
117. Polin JI, Frangipane WI. Current concepts in management of obstetric problems for pediatricians. II. Modern concepts in the management of multiple gestation. *Pediat Clin North Am.* 1986;33:649–661.
118. Robinson HP, Caines JS. Sonar evidence of early pregnancy failure in patients with twin conceptions. *Br J Obstet Gynaecol.* 1977;82:22.
119. Medearis AL, et al. Perinatal death rate in twin pregnancy: a five-year analysis of state-wide statistics in Missouri. *Am J Obstet Gynecol.* 1979;134:413.
120. Hashimoto B, et al. Ultrasound evaluation of polyhydramnios and twin pregnancy. *Am J Obstet Gynecol.* 1986;154:1069–1072.
121. Patkos P, et al. Factors influencing nonstress test results in multiple gestations. *Am J Obstet Gynecol.* 1986;154:1107–1108.
122. Barrett JM, et al. The effect of type of delivery on neonatal outcome in premature twins. *Am J Obstet Gynecol.* 1982;143:360.
123. Broadbent B. Multiple births—women's needs. *Midwife, Health Visitor Community Nurse.* 1985;21:425–430.
124. Hendrickson A. Prolonged pregnancy: a literature review. *J Nurse-Midwifery.* 1985;30:33–42.
125. Nichols CW. Postdate pregnancy. Part I. A literature review. *J Nurse-Midwifery.* 1985;30:222–239.
126. Nichols CW. Postdate pregnancy. Part II. Clinical implications. *J Nurse-Midwifery.* 1985;30:259–268.
127. Shearer MH, Estes M. A critical review of the recent literature on postterm pregnancy and a look at women's experiences. *Birth.* 1985;12:95–111.
128. Freeman RK, et al. Postdate pregnancy: utilization of contraction stress testing for primary fetal surveillance. *Am J Obstet Gynecol.* 1981;140:128–135.
129. Freeman RK, et al. Ensuring optimum outcome for postdate pregnancy. *Contemp Obstet Gynecol.* 1983:187–208.
130. Freeman RK, et al. A prospective multi-institutional study of antepartum fetal heart rate monitoring. II. Contraction stress test versus nonstress test for primary surveillance. *Am J Obstet Gynecol.* 1982;143:778–781.
131. Campbell B. Overdue delivery: its impact on mothers-to-be. *Am J Matern Child Nurs.* 1986;11:170–172.
132. Slater G, Aufses AH. Anesthesia. In: Knuppel RA, Drukker JE, eds. *High-Risk Pregnancy: A Team Approach.* Philadelphia: WB Saunders; 1986.
133. Higgins SD. Perinatal protocol: trauma in pregnancy. *J Perinatol.* 1988;8:288–292.
134. Daddario JB. Trauma in pregnancy. *J Perinat Neonat Nurs.* 1989;3:14–22.
135. Pearlman MD, et al. A prospective controlled study of outcome after trauma during pregnancy. *Am J Obstet Gynecol.* 1990;162:1502–1507.

Maternal Conditions in the Intrapartum Period

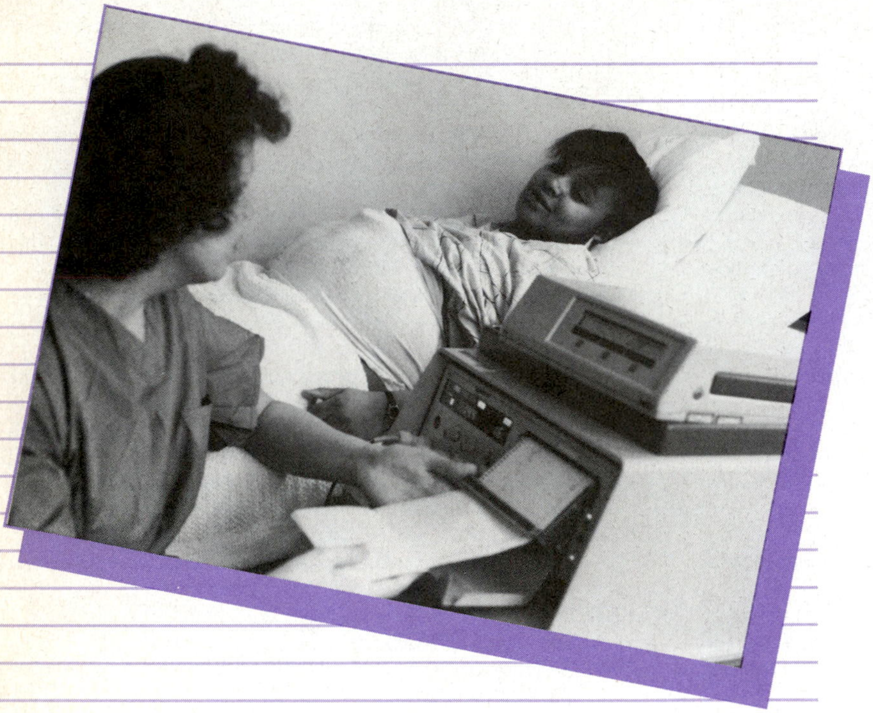

Chapter 40

Key Terms

baseline fetal heart rate
breech presentation
brow presentation
compound presentation
constriction ring
dystocia
eutocia
external version
face presentation
fetal dystocia
malpresentation
physiologic retraction ring
shoulder dystocia
shoulder presentation
transverse lie

Labor is a complex process that requires the harmonious interaction of four factors: the powers, the passenger, the passage, and the psyche. The powers refer to the forces of the uterine contractions. Uterine contractions need to be strong and coordinated so they can effect effacement and dilation of the cervix, and facilitate the descent of the fetus through the maternal pelvis. The passenger is the fetus. The fetus must be of an appropriate size for the pelvis, and positioned to allow for movement into and down through the pelvis. The passage includes the bony pelvis and soft tissues. For labor to occur, the pelvis must be of adequate size and free from obstacles that would retard the descent of the fetus. The psyche refers to the psychologic aspects of labor. How the laboring woman adapts psychologically to labor and childbirth can have an effect on the labor process itself. If any of the factors, singularly or in combination, are abnormal or fail to function properly, complications can occur.

In addition other problems, which may or may not interfere with the process of labor itself, may emerge or become critical during labor and delivery. For example, problems with the cord, amniotic fluid, or placenta may become acute during labor or delivery. The delivery of multiple fetuses, likewise, may become a problem at this time.

Complications that arise during labor or delivery can put the mother at risk. Both her health and safety can be adversely affected. The prognosis for a favorable outcome for the fetus, as well, may be questionable. To ensure the best possible outcome for both mother and fetus, the nurse who cares for the woman in labor must have a thorough knowledge of normal labor. Frequent assessments of the laboring woman's progress must be made, with particular emphasis on any deviations from the normal course of labor. Continuous communication between the nurse and nurse-midwife or physician is essential so that if complications do occur and obstetric intervention is necessary, the proper steps can be taken.

DYSTOCIA

Definition

Normal labor, or **eutocia,** follows a fairly predictable course. (The normal processes of labor and delivery were discussed earlier in Chapter 25.) Any deviation from this normal pattern results in **dystocia,** the term used to describe a difficult labor. Dystocia occurs in about 8 percent of all deliveries.[1] Either directly or indirectly, dystocia presently accounts for approximately one half of all the cesarean deliveries occurring in the United States.[2] When complications occur during the labor process that either prevent a vaginal delivery or make the vaginal route hazardous for the mother or fetus, cesarean delivery is chosen.

Classification

Dystocia can be classified according to which of the three physiologic factors—powers, passenger, or passage—is involved. Dystocia related to the powers is uterine dystocia. Dystocia related to the passenger is fetal dystocia, and dystocia related to the passage is pelvic dystocia.

DYSTOCIA RELATED TO THE POWERS

Uterine contractions need to be strong, coordinated, and intermittent to be effective. When the uterine contractions fail to meet these criteria, they cannot effect cervical dilation and fetal descent, and uterine dystocia occurs.

A contraction involves the rhythmic tightening and relaxing of the uterine muscles. At the beginning of the contraction, the uterine muscles begin to tighten. This tightening occurs first in the fundus or top of the uterus and then radiates toward the cervix. The contraction intensifies until the acme or strongest point is reached, and then diminishes. A period of relaxation or rest follows before the next contraction begins.

As the muscles tighten, pressure builds up inside the uterus. This uterine pressure causes the presenting part of the fetus to be pushed against the cervix, resulting in dilation. The uterine pressure is a part of the force of the contraction and an important factor in determining the effectiveness of the contraction. The intensity of the contraction is reflected in the rise in the intrauterine pressure associated with each contraction.

Intrauterine pressure can be measured during labor by means of a small fluid-filled polyethylene tube inserted directly into the uterine cavity. The intrauterine catheter is attached to a monitor that records the pressure in millimeters of mercury (mm Hg).

Pressure during a contraction will vary between 30 and 50 mm Hg.[3] An extensive review of the literature conducted by Cunningham revealed that Caldeyro-Barcia and his colleagues in Montevideo studied intrauterine pressures and demonstrated that the lower limit of intrauterine pressure that is required to dilate the cervix is at least 15 mm Hg.[4] Hendricks and his coworkers had similar findings in their studies.[4] Normal tonus, or intrauterine pressure during the resting period, is 8 to 12 mm Hg.[3] Knuppel and Drukker describe a normal contraction pattern as one with contractions occurring every 2 to 3 minutes, lasting approximately 40 to 90 seconds with an intensity of 40 to 90 mm Hg, and a resting tone of 5 to 20 mm Hg.[5] When the contraction pattern varies from this, labor becomes dysfunctional (Figure 40–1).

Dysfunctional Labor Patterns

A dysfunctional labor pattern is one in which the pattern of the uterine contractions is not normal. This abnormal pattern prevents labor from progressing as expected. Several dysfunctional labor patterns have been identified. They include hypertonic uterine dysfunction, hypotonic uterine dysfunction, and precipitous labor.

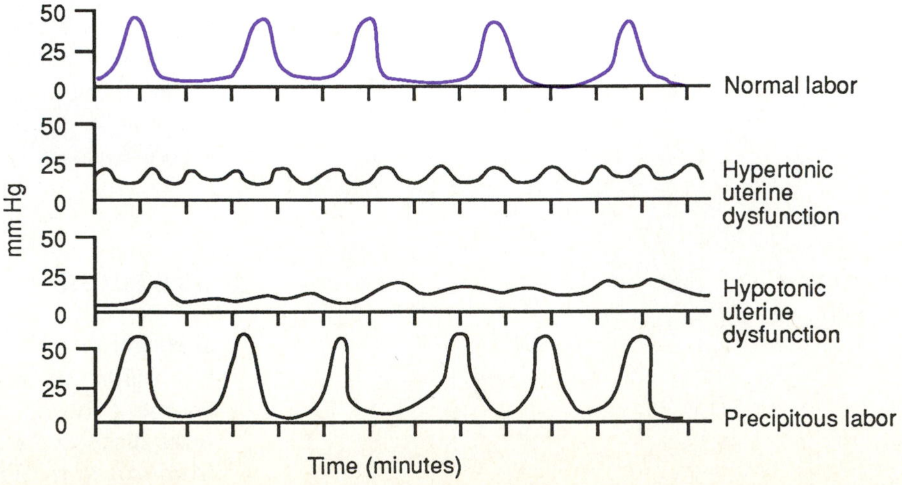

Figure 40–1. Pattern of normal and abnormal contractions: normal labor, hypertonic uterine dysfunction, hypotonic uterine dysfunction, and precipitous labor.

Hypertonic Uterine Dysfunction. The labor pattern identified as hypertonic uterine dysfunction is characterized by an increase in the frequency of contractions, but a decrease in the intensity. The resting tone of the uterus is also increased (Figure 40–1).

During labor, the contractions occur at more frequent intervals, but little intrauterine pressure is built up during the contraction. Without the increase in pressure, not enough force is exerted on the cervix by the presenting part of the fetus for dilation to occur. The increased resting tone indicates the uterine muscle remains in a state of tension. This inhibits resumption of the blood flow to the fetus, which has been interrupted by the contraction.

The increased frequency of contractions in hypertonic uterine dysfunction may be linked to the action of the uterine pacemakers. Normally, the uterus has two pacemakers situated near the end of each fallopian tube. The pacemakers are responsible for initiating a contraction that spreads in a coordinated fashion from fundus to cervix. For reasons not completely understood, other pacemakers may appear in the uterus, initiating contractions that are uncoordinated in their actions. The uterine musculature responds by contracting as if in a spasm and without purpose.

Although the mechanism is unknown, a relationship has been noted between this contractile pattern and the mother's feelings of fear and tension. Very anxious primiparous women commonly experience hypertonic labor. Hypertonic uterine dysfunction usually occurs in the latent phase of labor when contractions are just beginning.

Maternal Risks. Pain and fatigue are two problems facing the mother who is experiencing hypertonic uterine contractions. The pain is out of proportion to the intensity of the contractions, caused by hypoxia of the muscles, and is brought on by the frequency of the contractions. Hypoxia is compounded by the diminished resting tone between the contractions. The frequency with which the contractions occur provides the woman with little time to rest. She hardly has time to recover from one contraction before another contraction begins. If the labor is allowed to continue in this manner, the mother soon becomes exhausted. Discouraged by the lack of progress and the painful contractions, the mother and her labor partner experience increasing anxiety and may have difficulty coping with the situation.

Fetal Risks. Fetal distress resulting from hypoxia is the major concern with hypertonic uterine dysfunction. Frequent contractions, coupled with a decreased resting tone, keep the uterine musculature in a state of tension. This tension results in a decrease in the amount of oxygenated blood available to the uterine muscle and, in turn, a decrease in the amount of blood circulating in the placenta. With decreased blood flow, oxygen transport to the fetus diminishes and hypoxia occurs. If these abnormal contractions are allowed to continue for an extended period, prolonged pressure will be exerted on the fetal skull. This pressure may cause excessive molding of the fetal head, a swelling of the head called caput succedaneum, or even cephalhematoma (*see* Figures 33–13 and 33–14). A cephalhematoma is a localized collection of blood from damaged vessels that appears between the skullbone and its periostium.

Nursing and Collaborative Assessment. Because hypertonic contractions place the mother and fetus at risk, the nurse must continually monitor both the mother and the fetus. Frequent assessment of the uterine contractions and fetal heart tones is made. This provides for early detection of signs of possible complications. Monitoring uterine contractions for frequency, duration, and intensity may be done by the nurse or nurse-midwife. The intensity of the uterine contractions can be assessed manually by palpating the uterus with the fingertips throughout a contraction. If the membranes are ruptured, a catheter can be used to measure the intrauterine pressure directly. A fetoscope or an electronic fetal monitor may be used to assess fetal heart tones. If labor is prolonged, dehydration may become a problem. Maintaining accurate records of intake and output then becomes necessary.

Nursing and Collaborative Management. The nurse may help to reduce the anxiety experienced by the client and the labor partner by offering clear explanations about the nature of the contractions and the interventions that the nurses and midwife or physician are using to manage the condition. Both the labor partner and nurse should support the mother in her efforts and provide encouragement. Comfort measures such as back rubs and effleurage may help the client to relax.[6]

The aim of medical treatment is to stop the abnormal contractions so that both the uterus and the mother can rest. Sedation, known to arrest uterine activity and promote rest, is administered to the client.

The physiologic demands of labor require adequate hydration, so intravenous fluids are given. During the rest period, intake and output should be monitored. Assessment of urine for signs of ketones, which would indicate a fluid or electrolyte imbalance, also is performed. After the rest period, the majority of clients go into efficient labor and proceed to delivery. For those who continue with hypertonic contractions, oxytocin may be administered to effect normal contractions. This drug, which stimulates the uterus to contract, is administered only after fetopelvic disproportion and fetal malpresentation have been ruled out.

Hypotonic Uterine Dysfunction. Hypotonic uterine dysfunction (*see* Figure 40–1) is characterized by a decrease in the number of contractions to less than two per 10-minute interval. The intensity of the contraction is less than 25 mm Hg, and the resting tone falls below 8 mm Hg. These contractions are not effective because the intrauterine pressure is not sufficient to provide enough force for cervical dilation and fetal descent.

One cause of hypotonic uterine dysfunction is overdistension of the uterus. Muscle fibers that are overstretched do not contract efficiently. Polyhydramnios (excessive amniotic fluid), multiple gestation or a parous uterus, which is one that has been through previous pregnancies, may cause overdistension. Another cause is fetopelvic disproportion, in which the fetus is too large for the pelvis. Another major cause of hypotonic uterine dysfunction is the excessive use of narcotic analgesics, anesthetics, or sedatives in early labor. These drugs slow the progress of labor, especially if they are administered before the cervix has dilated to 3 to 4 cm.

Maternal Risks. Hypotonic contractions are not usually painful. If, however, they cause prolonged labor, premature rupture of the membranes can occur, increasing the risk of infection developing within the uterus, as microorganisms ascend the birth canal. The mother who has hypotonic contractions as the result of an overdistended uterus also will be prone to hemorrhage after delivery, because the uterus will not contract effectively after the delivery of the placenta. Failure of the uterus to stay contracted allows blood to flow from the placental site. Psychologically, the mother may become discouraged and fearful when labor slows and no further progress in cervical dilation or fetal descent occurs.

Fetal Risks. Initially, hypotonic uterine contractions have no adverse effects on the fetus. Infrequent, mild contractions do not interfere with the oxygen supply to the fetus. If membranes rupture, however, and labor is prolonged, the risk of infection poses a threat to fetal well-being. Because of the potential danger of intrauterine infection, hypotonic uterine contractions should not be allowed to continue indefinitely.

Nursing and Collaborative Assessment. Hypotonic uterine dysfunction appears most often during the active phase of labor. Contractions that have been normal become less frequent and are of decreased intensity and shorter duration. Progress in labor is halted.

Nursing assessment includes the frequent monitoring of contractions, fetal heart tones, and maternal vital signs. As labor continues, the nurse must be alert to signs of infection, such as elevated temperature and chills.

Nursing and Collaborative Management. The client should be offered an explanation of the abnormal contraction pattern and of the planned interventions. An understanding of the treatment plan enhances the client's participation in the labor process.

Stimulation or augmentation of labor may be needed if the hypotonic contractions do not improve in quality; however, fetopelvic disproportion must be ruled out first. Induction of intense uterine contractions when the fetus is too large for the pelvis is dangerous for both the mother and the fetus. Both amniotomy and the intravenous infusion of oxytocin may be used to augment labor. Prostaglandins are also used for this purpose in countries other than the United States.

Amniotomy. Amniotomy, the artificial rupture of the membranes, may be done to enhance the labor contractions as direct contact of the fetal skull with the cervix provides a stronger force in dilating the cervix then does the fluid contained in the membranes. Amniotomy is performed during a vaginal examination using a hook (Amnihook) or a sharp instrument (*see* Figure 27–15). After the membranes are ruptured, the amniotic fluid drains and the head makes direct contact with the cervix. There is no pain involved in the procedure.

The use of amniotomy to augment labor remains controversial because of unpredictable uterine response. Amniotomy early in labor is not recommended. Studies have shown that the fetal skull is more likely to experience swelling and bone displacement and the fetus more likely to experience heart rate decelerations if membranes are ruptured.[7] Caldeyro-Barcia and associates also challenge the presumption that shorter labors are beneficial.[8] Further, the decrease in the amniotic fluid may increase the compression of the umbilical cord. Thus, although amniotomy may speed up the dilation of the cervix, it also may have harmful effects on the fetus.

The nurse should describe the procedure with the woman and help her to relax. Breathing deeply through the mouth may aid relaxation. Fetal well-being should be assessed just prior to the procedure by checking the fetal heart rate. Immediately after the procedure, the fetal heart rate should again be assessed. An abnormally slow rate indicates that the umbilical cord has prolapsed and is being compressed.

Prostaglandin Administration. Prostaglandins, known to produce oxytocic-like stimulation of the uterus, have been studied to determine their effectiveness in cervical ripening and initiation of labor. Presently, they are used in other countries to augment labor but have not been approved for this purpose in the United States.[9]

Oxytocin Administration. Oxytocin, when administered intravenously, has been very successful in augmenting labor. In its synthetic form, Pitocin, the drug acts on the smooth muscle of the uterus to stimulate contractions. Under the influence of this drug, contractions recur more frequently and with greater force. The uterine effort required for augmented labor is more than that required for spontaneous labor but less than the effort required for induced labor.[10] Because onset is rapid, the contractions also are more painful. The physician orders the augmentation procedure, which may then be implemented by the registered nurse.

Most institutions follow a protocol, a written step-by-step procedure, for administering oxytocin. A piggyback intravenous setup is used. The primary intravenous bag contains plain solution, usually lactated Ringer's solution as ordered by the physician. A second bag contains the same solution plus oxytocin at a strength of 10 units per 1000 mL of solution. The needle from the tubing of the bag containing the oxytocin is inserted into the port of the tubing containing only the plain solution, hence the term *piggyback.* Use of two intravenous bags permits the oxytocin to be discontinued if necessary without removing the primary intravenous line.

An infusion pump is used so that the amount of the drug administered can be precisely controlled. Initially, the rate of administration is 0.5 to 2 mU per minute. At 20-minute intervals, the dose is increased by 2 mU until contractions are occurring every 3 to 4 minutes with a duration of 50 to 60 seconds and at least a 30-second resting period. Research has demonstrated that an effective uterine response is reached with an oxytocin infusion rate of 2 to 5 mU per minute, and the majority of women who are at term have adequate labor patterns at an infusion rate of 4 to 8 mU per minute.[11]

During the procedure, contractions and fetal heart tones should be assessed at least every 15 minutes. Continuous monitoring with the use of an electronic fetal monitor is more desirable. Oxytocin may cause overstimulation of the uterus, resulting in tetanic contractions lasting longer than 90 seconds with minimal resting periods between contractions. The occurrence of tetanic contractions requires immediate intervention. Such contractions may cause uterine rupture. With only brief resting periods between the tetanic contractions, inadequate oxygenation of the fetus also may occur, leading to hypoxia of the fetus.

At the first indication of prolonged contractions, the oxytocin is discontinued by turning off the intravenous bag with oxytocin and switching to the intravenous bag without oxytocin. Then, the woman is administered oxygen and her position is changed. If these measures are not effective and the fetus is showing signs of distress such as late deceleration patterns and slow heart rate, a medication such as terbutaline sulfate (Brethine) may be ordered by the physician. This drug, when administered subcutaneously, decreases myometrial activity and improves uteroplacental blood flow. An initial injection of 0.25 mg may be repeated in 12 to 15 minutes. The drug, a selective beta-2-adrenergic receptor stimulator that is widely used to stop preterm labor, can be effective in stopping tetanic contractions and the late deceleration and slow fetal heart rate that often follow.[12]

Urine output should be monitored during oxytocin administration as the drug may cause water intoxication with prolonged use. Decrease in urine output should be reported to the physician immediately. Initially, blood pressure rises in response to administration of oxytocin; high concentrations of the drug may cause hypertension. Maternal blood pressure should thus be recorded at frequent intervals during the procedure. Both retention of water and hypertension cease when the oxytocin is discontinued.

The client should be provided with a thorough explanation of how the procedure is expected to intensify the labor contractions. The nurse should advise that the contractions will have a rapid onset after the oxytocin infusion begins and often are painful. Reviewing relaxation practices and breathing techniques with both the client and her labor partner may assist the client in coping with the discomfort. Assurance that she will be closely monitored and that a nurse will be present during the entire procedure may help to alleviate any anxiety.

Precipitous Labor and Delivery. Labor lasting less than 3 hours is considered a precipitous labor. This pattern is characterized by the occurrence of more then five contractions in a 10-minute period (see Figure 40–1). Intrauterine pressures may reach 50 to 70 mm Hg. Along with the frequent intense contractions, women who experience precipitous labor may demonstrate abnormally low resistance of their soft tissues. This permits the fetus to pass easily through the pelvis.

Maternal Risks. With little resistance of the soft tissues and an effaced and dilated cervix, maternal complications are rare. If the tissues do offer resistance and the cervix is long and thick, lacerations of the cervix, vagina, and vulva may occur. Forceful, intense contractions also may cause uterine rupture.

Fetal Risks. The fetus may experience hypoxia as a result of the frequent, intense contractions. Trauma to the fetal head may occur if there is resistance during passage through the pelvis. Precipitous labor may lead to a birth that is unattended and the newborn may suffer from a lack of immediate care at delivery.

Nursing and Collaborative Assessment and Management. Rapid labor usually results in a rapid, spontaneous delivery. The nurse-midwife or physician and nurse should be prepared for the delivery. An unassisted delivery will leave the newborn without care during the critical first few minutes of life. Pregnant women at risk for a rapid labor may be identified during the nursing assessment. A history of a previous precipitous labor should alert the nurse to the possibility that a rapid labor may be repeated. During labor, the nurse should observe the client for rapid cervical dilation and fetal descent as well as frequent, intense contractions. These may signal a precipitous labor. If delivery is imminent and the nurse does not have time to contact the nurse-midwife or physician for the delivery, she or he should be prepared to deliver the fetus.

Psychologically, this type of labor may be very stressful for the client. She may have difficulty coping with the discomfort caused by the intense contractions. The rapid progress of labor may make her feel that she has lost control. Both the nurse and the labor partner need to convey a sense of calm to the client. The nurse must assure the client that she will not be left alone. Clear, concise explanations can help relieve anxiety as well as gain the client's trust. Including the labor partner in explanations that are given will help to allay any fears related to the health and safety of both the mother and the fetus.

Abnormal Labor According to Friedman's Curve

Traditionally, labor is divided into four stages (as discussed in Chapter 25). Three of the four stages are useful in assessing progress in labor: the first, second, and third. The fourth stage, which relates to the immediate postpartum period, is not relevant in this discussion.

The first stage begins with the onset of labor and ends with full cervical dilation. The first stage is further divided into two phases: the latent phase and the active phase. The latent phase includes the time from the onset of contractions until the rate of cervical dilation accelerates, usually around 3 to 4 cm. The active phase begins with the accelerated rate of dilation and continues until the cervix is fully dilated. The second stage of labor extends from full dilation of the cervix to the birth of the infant. The third stage refers to the period from birth of the infant to delivery of the placenta. Each of these three stages is monitored to assist in making a diagnosis of dystocia related to the powers.

The Friedman graph may be used to assess progress in labor. Using the relationships of cervical dilation and fetal descent against elapsed time in labor, the practitioner can determine if cervical dilation and fetal descent are occurring at a normal rate, too fast, too slow, or not at all.

Figure 40–2 presents a graphic analysis of a primigravida in normal labor. During the latent phase of labor, the slope of the curve of the Friedman graph is nearly flat; labor is becoming established and dilation is slow, averaging only 0.35 cm per hour. The active phase of labor begins with the upswing in the

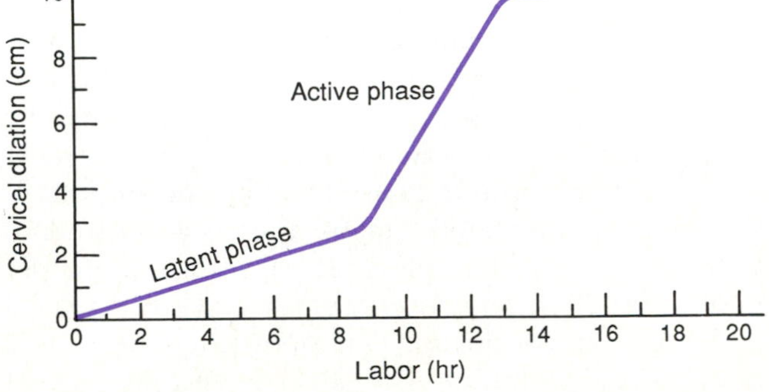

Figure 40–2. Partogram (Friedman graph) for a primigravida in normal stage I labor. (*Reproduced, with permission, from Oxorn H, ed.* Oxorn-Foote Human Labor and Birth. *5th ed. Norwalk, Conn: Appleton-Century-Crofts; 1986:759.*)

TABLE 40–1. LENGTHS OF THE PHASES OF LABOR

Phase	Primigravada Average	Primigravada Upper Normal	Multipara Average	Multipara Upper Normal
Latent phase	8.6 hours	20.0 hours	5.3 hours	14.0 hours
Active phase	5.8 hours	12.0 hours	2.5 hours	6.0 hours
First stage	13.3 hours	28.5 hours	7.5 hours	20.0 hours
Second stage	57 minutes	150 minutes	18 minutes	50 minutes
Rate of cervical dilation in active phase	<1.2 cm/h	Abnormal	<1.5 cm/h	Abnormal

Adapted from Cohen W, Friedman E. Management of Labor. *Baltimore: University Park Press; 1983.*

curve. The slope of the curve changes from nearly horizontal to nearly vertical during the phase of maximal slope, and as complete dilation approaches, the curve flattens once again in the deceleration phase.

The lengths of the various phases of labor, as listed in Table 40–1, were determined from Friedman's study of the labors of more than 1000 women. Only the average length of time and the upper limits of normal are listed, leaving room for wide variation. The upper limits of time represent the longest time that labor continued and still terminated normally in Friedman's study.[13]

Fetal descent begins in the latter part of the first stage of labor. It should continue at a rate of 1.0 cm per hour in a primipara and 2.0 cm per hour in a multipara, although continuous progress at a slower rate may be normal. No change in the station of the fetus for a period of 2 hours is suggestive of a problem and should be investigated.

Using a graph to plot the client's progress in labor and then comparing it against Friedman's curve are useful in assessing the normalcy of labor. Based on his analysis of labor, Friedman described nine types of dysfunctional labor. These have been classified further into (1) disorders of the preparatory division of labor, (2) disorders of the dilational division of labor, (3) disorders of the pelvic division of labor, and (4) precipitous disorders (Table 40–2).

TABLE 40–2. DYSFUNCTIONAL LABOR ACCORDING TO FRIEDMAN'S DIVISIONS OF LABOR

1. Preparatory division
   - Prolonged latent phase
2. Dilational division
   - Protracted active dilation
   - Protracted descent
3. Pelvic division
   - Prolonged deceleration phase
   - Secondary arrest of dilation
   - Arrest of descent
   - Failure of descent
4. Precipitous disorders
   - Precipitous labor
   - Precipitous delivery

Figure 40–3 graphically represents the six types of dysfunctional labor for the preparatory, dilational, and pelvic divisions of labor. Precipitous labor has been described in the preceding section. The following discussion focuses on disorders of the preparatory, dilational, and pelvic divisions of labor.

Preparatory Division of Labor. The preparatory division of labor includes the latent and active phases described earlier. The abnormal labor pattern that may occur during this time is the prolonged latent phase.

Prolonged Latent Phase. A latent phase is necessary to the labor process, helping to establish the pattern of labor contractions. Prolongation of this phase can, however, indicate underlying problems. A latent phase lasting longer than 20 hours in a nullipara and 14 hours in a multipara is generally considered to be prolonged.

One cause for a prolonged latent phase might be false labor. As described in Chapter 25, true labor is differentiated from false labor by the presence of cervical effacement and dilation. Absence of these processes indicates that true labor has not started. An "unripe" cervix (ie, one that is long, thick, and closed) may be another cause. Before it can dilate, the cervix must ripen or become soft, shorten, and thin out. This process takes time and will prolong the latent period.

Fetopelvic disproportion occurs when the fetus is too large for the pelvis; malposition occurs when the presenting part of the fetus is entering the pelvis in an awkward manner. When either of these occur, the presenting part of the fetus cannot descend and create the pressure on the cervix necessary for dilation. Medication may be another cause of a prolonged latent phase. Administration of narcotic analgesics too early in the labor process may slow labor. Meperidine (Demerol), for example, when administered at the appropriate time, helps with cervical relaxation; however, given too early in labor, it disrupts the labor pattern, prolonging labor.

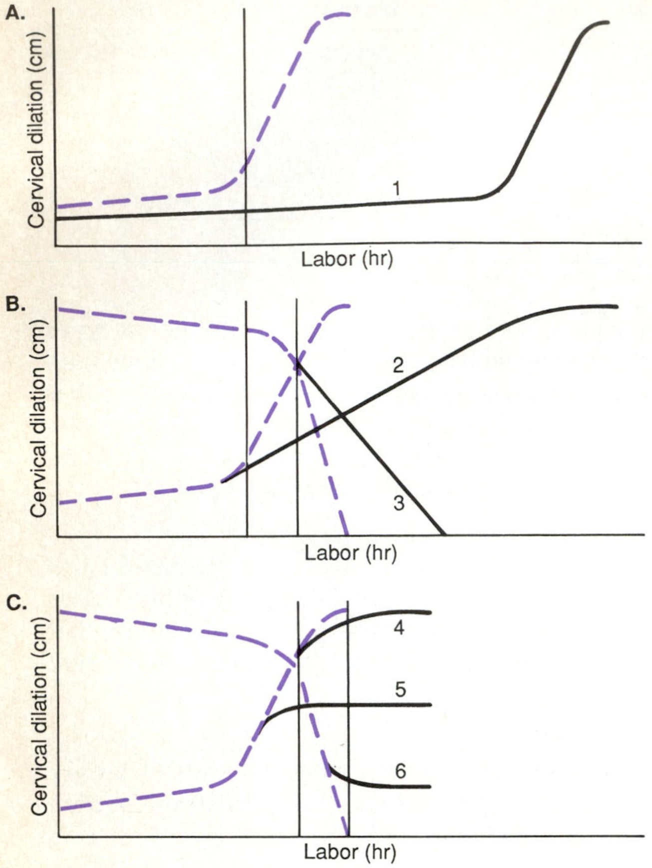

Figure 40–3. Representations of the six graphic disorders of the functional divisions of labor. **A.** Normal dilation curve (*broken line*) is compared with the preparatory division abnormality of prolonged latent phase (1). **B.** Protraction disorders of the dilational division are represented, specifically, protracted active phase dilation (2) and protracted descent (3). **C.** Pathologic states of the pelvic division are represented, including prolonged deceleration phase (4), secondary arrest of dilation (5), and arrest of descent (6). (*Reproduced, with permission, from Greenhill JP, Friedman E, eds.* Biological Principles and Modern Practice of Obstetrics. *Philadelphia: WB Saunders; 1974.*)

Although a long latent phase is worrisome, it usually does not endanger the mother or fetus.[3] Rest is prescribed for false labor or an unripe cervix and for those clients who have received too much medication. Maternal posturing, or having the client periodically assume various positions (eg, lateral, Sims, and knee-chest) may help to move the fetus from a malposition to a more favorable position. Barring absolute fetopelvic disproportion, in which there is no possibility for a vaginal delivery, contractions may be augmented with oxytocin.

Dilational Division of Labor. The dilational division of labor includes the phase of maximum slope of dilation. The disorders of this division are protracted active phase dilation and protracted descent. A protracted disorder is one in which progress is slower than normally expected.

Protracted Active Dilation. During the active phase of labor, once the cervix has started to dilate, dilation should continue at a rate of at least 1.2 cm per hour in a nullipara and 1.5 cm per hour in a multipara. Failure to progress in this manner results in protracted active-phase dilation. A client with this condition has mild to moderately intense contractions and some cervical dilation takes place, but the rate of dilation is slower than normal and indicates that some problem is present. Friedman states that it is difficult to disturb the rapidly progressing dilation curve unless there is a preexisting disordered state of myometrial function oranintrinsicimpediment,suchascephalopelvicdisproportion.[13] Assessment of the relationship of the fetus to the pelvis is necessary. A major disproportion would necessitate a cesarean delivery. If no disproportion is found, labor is allowed to continue as long as some progress is being made and the fetus is in no distress.

Protracted Descent. Protraction disorders also are evident in fetal descent. Normally, the rate of descent in a primipara is 1.0 cm per hour and in a multipara, 2.0 cm per hour. Progress that is slower than this rate is termed protracted descent. Fetopelvic disproportion and inefficient uterine contractions are the principal causes of protracted descent. Both possibilities must be assessed and appropriate action taken to correct the problem.

Pelvic Division of Labor. The deceleration phase, the second stage of labor, and the phase of maximum slope of descent are included in Friedman's pelvic division of labor. The abnormal labor patterns that may occur include prolonged deceleration phase, secondary arrest of dilation, arrest of descent, and failure of descent.

Conditions in which either cervical dilation or fetal descent stops after having initially progressed are referred to as arrest disorders. Once dilation or descent has started, it should continue until completion unless complications arise and interfere with the progress. The diagnosis of arrest of dilation is made only after there has been no progress for 2 hours. Vaginal examinations to determine cervical dilation should be performed by the same person during this time so documentation of no progress can be made. Arrest of descent can be diagnosed when the presenting part of the fetus shows no progress in moving down the pelvis for at least an hour. The examination to determine progress should also be made by the same individual.

Prolonged Deceleration Phase. Cervical dilation that shows no progress for 3 hours or more in a nullipara and 1 hour or more in a multipara is indicative of prolonged deceleration phase. Fetopelvic or cephalopelvic disproportion may be suspected; if found to be the cause, cesarean delivery is recommended. In the absence of fetopelvic or cephalopelvic disproportion, additional labor may be warranted unless fetal distress is evident.

Secondary Arrest of Dilation. Cessation of the active-phase progression for more than 2 hours in a nullipara or 1 hour in a multipara indicates secondary arrest of dilation. Again, cephalopelvic disproportion is suspected. If no cephalopelvic disproportion or fetal distress is found, oxytocin augmentation and rest constitute the treatment of choice.

Arrest of Descent. Fetal descent that stops and shows no progression in fetal station for an hour or more is termed arrest of descent. In the absence of cephalopelvic disproportion, stimulation of uterine contractions may effect a vaginal delivery.

Failure of Descent. Lack of expected descent during the deceleration phase and the second stage of labor is indicative of failure of descent. This pattern usually indicates cephalopelvic disproportion. Cesarean delivery is most often indicated to manage failure of descent.

Development of Pathologic Uterine Rings

Another cause of uterine dystocia is the development of pathologic retraction rings. These are an exaggeration of the normal physiologic ring that occurs during labor.

During the course of normal labor, the uterus differentiates into two distinct segments, the upper or active segment and the lower or passive segment (Figure 40–4). With each contraction, the muscle fibers in the upper segment shorten to maintain the downward pressure that is needed. Continued shortening causes thickening. The lower segment becomes thinner and more distended as the muscle fibers there stretch. The boundary between the two is termed a **physiologic retraction ring.**

Two types of pathologic retraction ring can occur: Bandl's ring, the most common type, and constriction ring. Table 40–3 compares the two types of rings.

Bandl's Ring. Bandl's ring forms when the labor is obstructed, meaning that fetal descent stops because of fetopelvic or cephalopelvic disproportion or some other complication preventing the fetus from moving down the pelvis. Contractions continue in the presence of obstructed labor. The upper segment of the uterus overretracts while the lower segment overdistends. Labor is further impeded as part of the fetus

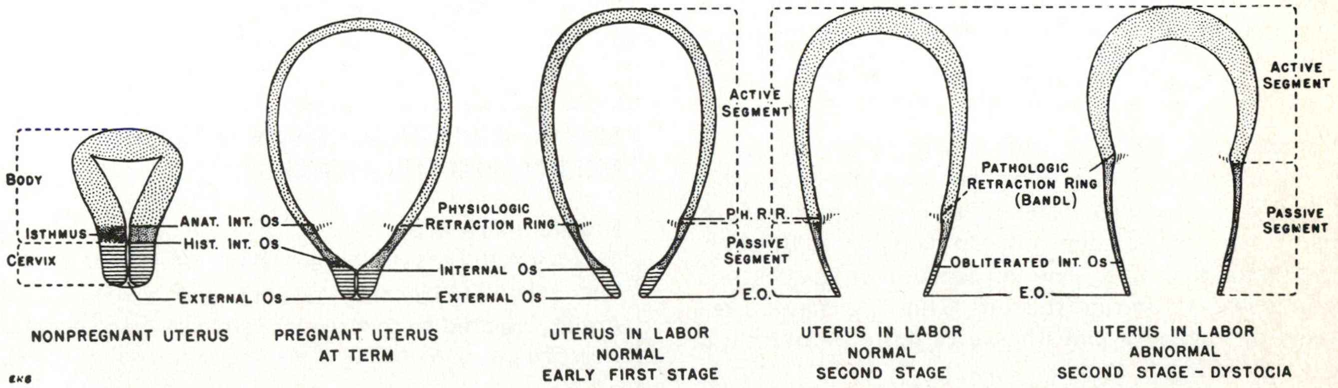

Figure 40–4. Sequence of development of segments and rings in the uterus in pregnant women at term and in labor. Note comparison between the uterus of a nonpregnant woman, the uterus at term, and the uterus during labor. The passive lower segment of the uterine body is derived from the isthmus; the physiologic retraction ring develops at the junction of the upper and lower uterine segments. The pathologic retraction ring develops from the physiologic ring. Anat. Int. Os = anatomic internal os; Hist. Int. Os = histologic internal os; PH.R.R. = physiologic retraction ring; E.O. = external os. (*Reproduced, with permission, from Cunningham FG, et al.* Williams Obstetrics. *18th ed. Norwalk, Conn: Appleton & Lange; 1989:214.*)

TABLE 40–3. DIFFERENTIAL DIAGNOSIS OF CONSTRICTION RING AND BANDL'S RING

Constriction Ring	Bandl's Ring
Localized ring of spastic myometrium	Formed by excessive retraction of upper segment
May occur in any part of the uterus	Always occurs at junction of upper and lower segments
Muscle at the ring is thicker than above or below it	Myometrium is much thicker above than below the ring
Uterus below the ring is neither thin nor distended	Wall below ring is thin and overdistended
Uterus never ruptures	If uncorrected, uterus may rupture
Uterus above ring is relaxed and not tender	Uterus above ring is hard
Round ligaments are not tense	Round ligaments are tense and stand out
May occur in any stage of labor	Usually occurs late in the second stage of labor
Position of ring does not change	Ring gradually rises in abdomen
Presenting part is not driven down	Presenting part is jammed into pelvis
Fetus may be wholly or mainly above the ring	Part of the fetus must be below the ring
Client's general condition is good	Client's general condition is poor
Uterine action is inefficient	Uterine action is efficient or overefficient
Abnormal polarity	Normal polarity
Results in obstructed labor	Is caused by an obstruction

Adapted, with permission, from Oxorn H, ed. Oxorn-Foote Human Labor and Birth. *5th ed. New York: Appleton-Century-Crofts; 1986:665.*

becomes trapped above the ring and part below. Without intervention, uterine rupture may occur. Development of Bandl's ring necessitates a cesarean delivery.

Constriction Ring. A **constriction ring** forms as a result of tetanic contractions and traps the fetus, preventing fetal descent. The client experiences severe pain, and a constriction ring can be palpated through the abdominal wall. The constriction ring does not predispose to uterine rupture. The ring may be relaxed by analgesia, anesthesia, or both, permitting a vaginal delivery.

Nursing Diagnoses

Nursing diagnoses related to dysfunction in the powers are made after careful assessment. See the box for several nursing diagnoses concerning dystocia related to the powers.

DYSTOCIA RELATED TO THE PASSENGER

During labor, the fetus, aided by the force of the uterine contractions, enters the pelvis and undergoes a series of maneuvers called the mechanisms of labor. (*See* discussion in Chapter 25.) These movements allow the fetus to move down the pelvis to delivery.

The easiest way to accomplish these maneuvers is for the fetus to enter the pelvis head first in what is called a vertex or cephalic presentation. With the head flexed on the chest, the smallest diameter of the fetal head is able to enter the pelvic inlet. This anterior-posterior diameter, called the suboccipitobregmatic diameter, extends from the lower edge of the occipital bone to the forehead and averages 9.5 cm at term.

At the midpelvis, the fetal head must rotate to an anterior position facing the mother's spine. This position is necessary because the narrowest transverse diameter in the pelvis is at the midpelvis and the fetal head must rotate to pass through this area. The rotation at midpelvis is most easily accomplished if the head enters the pelvic inlet in a transverse or side-to-side position. The biparietal diameter, the largest transverse diameter of the fetal head, is the distance between the parietal eminences (ie, the points at which the parietal bones are farthest apart) and averages 9.5 cm at term. Any deviation with regard to presentation or position results in dystocia.

Malpresentation and malposition of the fetus make movement through the pelvis difficult and, in some instances, impossible.[14] Labor complicated by malpresentation or malposition is termed **fetal dystocia.**

NURSING DIAGNOSES FOR DYSTOCIA RELATED TO THE POWERS

Problem-Oriented

Ineffective individual coping, related to lengthy labor

Pain, related to hypertonic uterine contractions

Anxiety, related to concern for fetal well-being during slow progression of labor

Strength-Oriented

Potential for successful coping with lengthy labor, related to provision of rest and nutrition

Effective coping and management of anxiety during hypertonic uterine contractions, related to effective relaxation techniques

Malpresentation

When the presenting part entering the pelvic inlet is other than the completely flexed head of the fetus, **malpresentation** is present. Malpresentation occurs in 5 percent of all labors.[15] Abnormal presentations may involve other parts of the fetal skull, such as the brow or face. These presentations are a result of the fetal head being extended rather than flexed. Dystocia occurs because the fit in the pelvis is less than ideal, making the passage through the pelvis more difficult. If the adaptation of the presenting part to the cervix is less than symmetric, the efficiency of labor is reduced. Malpresentation also may occur when a part other than the fetal head presents, as in shoulder and breech presentations. Table 40–4 summarizes the techniques used to assess malpresentation.

Brow Presentation. A moderate extension of the fetal head as it enters the pelvis results in a **brow presentation** (Figure 40–5). The verticomental diameter, which is the distance between the vertex on top of the head and the chin, enters the pelvis first. This measurement is the largest anteroposterior diameter of the head and averages 13.5 cm. Brow presentations are rare, occurring in 1 in 1000 to 3000 deliveries.[3] Frequently as the descent in the pelvis progresses, the brow presentation spontaneously converts to an occiput or face presentation for delivery. Pressure of the head against the bony maternal pelvis causes the head either to flex or to hyperextend before delivery occurs.

TABLE 40–4. TECHNIQUES USED TO ASSESS FETAL MALPRESENTATION

Assessment Technique	Possible Finding
Leopold's maneuvers	Ballottment at the fundus indicating breech presentation
Auscultation of fetal heart	Heart heard in upper quadrants for breech presentation, in lower quadrants for brow or face presentations
Inspection of abdomen	Maternal abdomen is unusually wide from side to side, fundus scarcely above umbilicus in a transverse lie
Vaginal examination	Palpation of portion of fetal head between orbital ridge and anterior fontanelle in brow presentation; mouth, nose, malar bones, and orbital ridges in face presentation (mouth and malar prominences form a triangle); fetal lower extremities and buttocks and anus in breech (anus on line with ischial tuberosities)
Sonography, x-ray pelvimetry, or computed tomographic pelvimetry	Determination of fetal position
Fetal heart rate monitoring	Variable deceleration rate indicating possible prolapsed cord associated with breech presentation

Etiology. A persistent brow presentation is associated with factors that delay or prevent engagement. In the mother, factors associated with brow presentation include too small a pelvis for the size of the fetus, tumors in the lower segment of the uterus, or a placenta that has implanted low in the uterus rather than in the fundus where implantation normally occurs. Fetal factors include those conditions that prevent flexion of the head, for example, having the umbilical cord wrapped around the neck. Fetal anomalies involving the fetal head need to be considered.

Nursing and Collaborative Management. Nursing interventions are aimed at supporting the client and helping her to cope with a difficult and prolonged labor. Both the client and her labor partner need to be kept informed of the progress of labor. Frequent assessment of both mother and fetus must be carried out throughout the labor. Comfort measures such as back rubs, frequent mouth care, and change of position may help the mother relax. Intervention is not necessary if cervical dilation and fetal descent are progressing satisfactorily and there is no fetal or maternal distress. If fetal distress or arrest of descent occurs, cesarean delivery is recommended.

Face Presentation. A **face presentation** is a vertex presentation with the fetal head hyperextended so that the face enters the pelvic inlet first (Figure 40–6). The part of the face that presents is the area between the glabella (directly above the root of the nose) and the chin. This is the submentobregmatic diameter and measures about 9.6 cm.

Etiology. As with the brow presentation, anything that interferes with the engagement of the fetal head in flexion can be a causative factor. A frequent cause is fetopelvic disproportion. Anencephalic fetuses commonly present by the face.

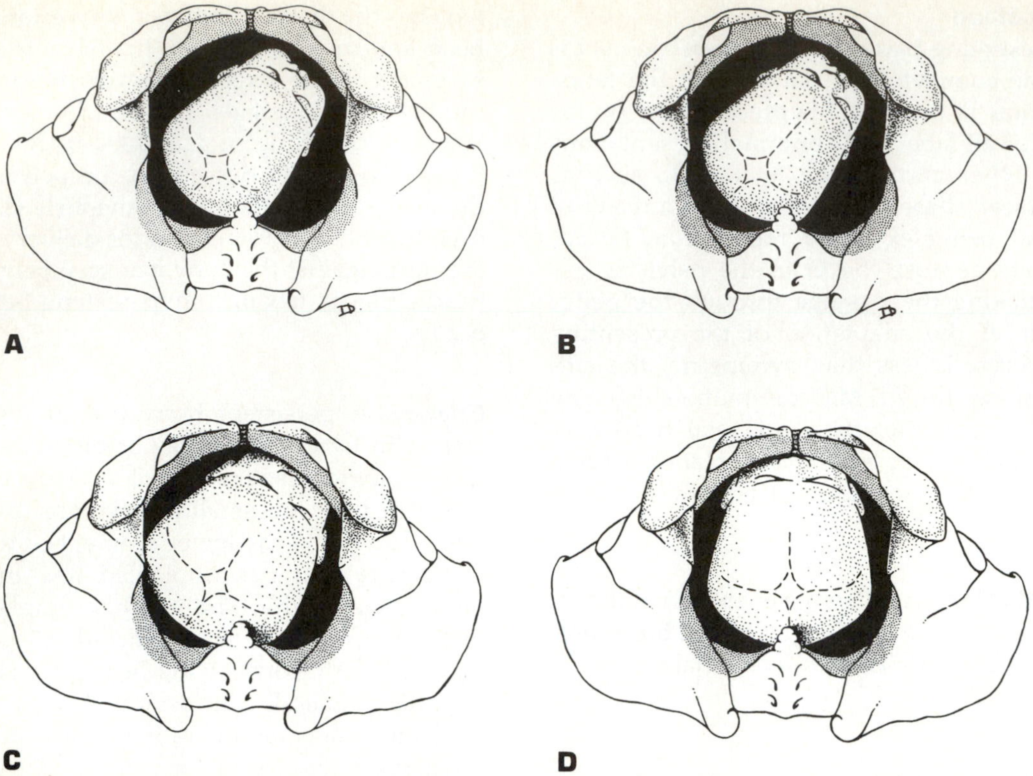

Figure 40–5. *Brow presentation* (left frontum anterior): **A.** Vaginal view. *Mechanism of labor:* **B.** Onset of labor. **C.** Descent. **D.** Internal rotation—left frontum anterior to frontum anterior. (*From Oxorn H, ed.* Oxorn-Foote Human Labor and Birth. *5th ed. Norwalk, Conn: Appleton-Century-Crofts; 1986:209.*)

Nursing and Collaborative Management. The nurse closely monitors the progress of the labor and the status of the fetus during labor. The client and her labor partner both need to be supported as they cope with the long and difficult labor that may occur with a face presentation.

Vaginal delivery for a face presentation is possible if certain conditions exist. First, the chin of the fetus, called the mentum, must be in the anterior position. In an anterior position, the fetal face is looking toward the mother's umbilicus, with the back of the head resting on either the left or right side of the pelvis. Second, the contractions must be forceful enough to propel the fetus through the pelvis. And, finally, there must be no pelvic contracture. The fetus must be able to enter and move through the pelvis. If the chin presents and stays in a posterior position, spontaneous vaginal delivery is impossible. When the face reaches the midpelvis, internal rotation occurs and the chin rotates posteriorly 45° into the hollow of the sacrum. Flexion cannot take place, nor can the fetus advance any further in the pelvis. With the arrest or stopping of descent, cesarean delivery is required. Face presentations occur in about 1 in 250 births.[3]

Shoulder Presentation. Shoulder presentation, also known as a **transverse lie,** occurs when the long axis of the fetus is at a right angle to the long axis of the mother. In essence, the fetus is lying across the mother's abdomen and the shoulder is the presenting part that dips into the pelvis. The fetus may lie directly across the maternal abdomen or may lie obliquely. The incidence of shoulder presentation is about 1 in 500 deliveries.[3]

Etiology. Shoulder presentation is more common in multiparas than primiparas because the abdominal and uterine muscles tend to be weakened after several pregnancies and deliveries. As with brow and face presentation, the causes of shoulder presentation are associated with those factors that prevent the head or buttocks from engaging.

Nursing and Collaborative Management. Delivery of a full-term fetus in a shoulder presentation is not con-

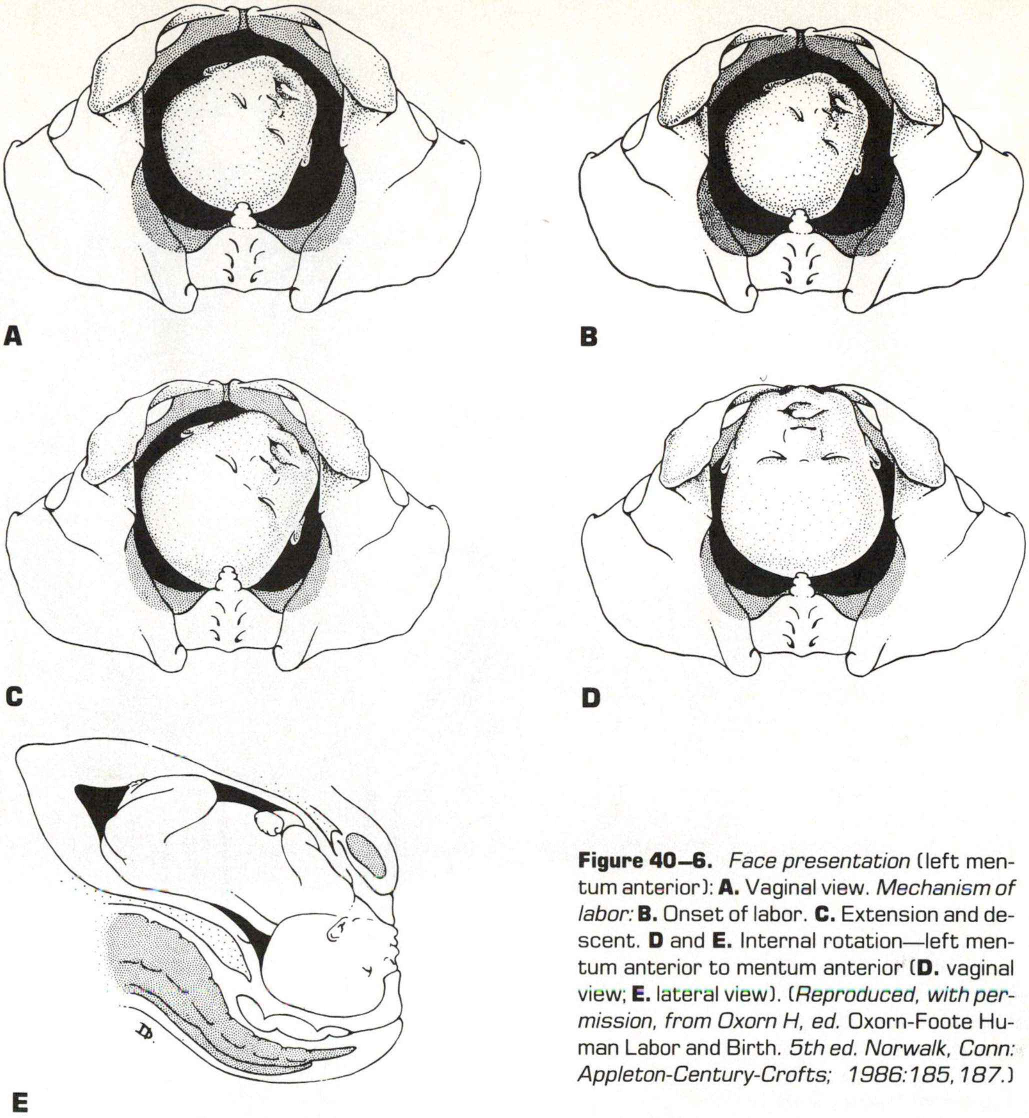

Figure 40–6. *Face presentation* (left mentum anterior): **A.** Vaginal view. *Mechanism of labor:* **B.** Onset of labor. **C.** Extension and descent. **D** and **E.** Internal rotation—left mentum anterior to mentum anterior (**D.** vaginal view; **E.** lateral view). (*Reproduced, with permission, from Oxorn H, ed.* Oxorn-Foote Human Labor and Birth. *5th ed. Norwalk, Conn: Appleton-Century-Crofts; 1986:185, 187.*)

sidered possible as the fetus cannot move through the pelvis in this position. Further, labor with shoulder presentation can result in risk to the mother from spontaneous rupture of the uterus, and significant risk to the fetus[4] (Figure 40–7).

External version, manipulation of the fetus through the abdominal wall to convert to a breech or vertex presentation, is rarely attempted as it is unlikely to be successful once labor is well established (Figure 40–8). **Internal version,** performed with the hand inside the uterus, may be attempted with a second twin in the delivery of multiple fetuses (see later section in this chapter). When conditions make a safe vaginal delivery questionable, cesarean delivery is necessary.

The couple may be anxious and fearful about the complication and possible treatment (cesarean delivery). The nurse supports the couple and provides factual information concerning the problem and its management. In addition, the nurse helps prepare the client and her support person for cesarean delivery, should it be necessary.

Compound Presentation. In **compound presentation,** more than one part of the fetus presents. Usually when this happens, an arm or leg has entered the pelvis at the same time as the head or buttocks. When the presenting part does not completely occlude the pelvic inlet, a compound presentation is likely to occur. The extra space allows the arm or leg to pro-

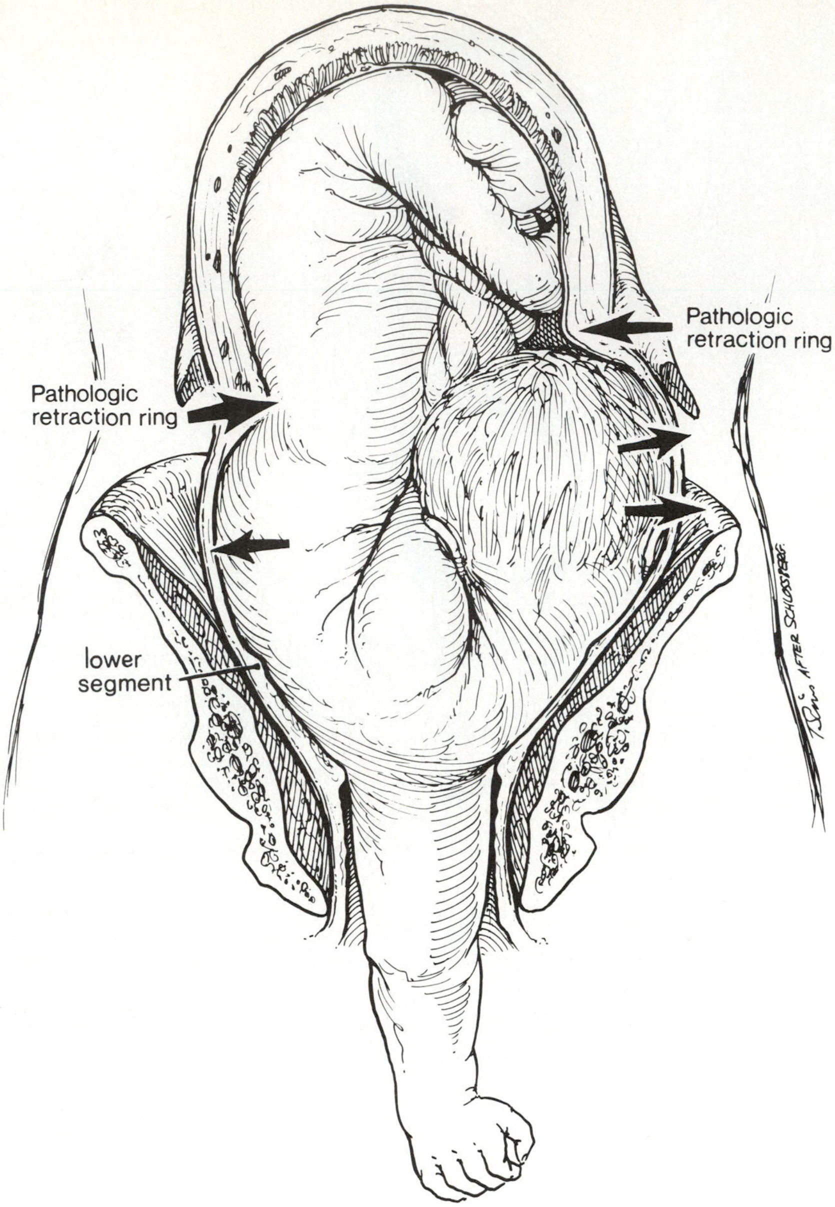

Figure 40–7. Neglected shoulder presentation. A thick muscular band forming a pathologic retraction ring has developed just above the very thin lower uterine segment. The force generated during a uterine contraction is directed at and above the level of the retraction ring, serving to stretch further and possibly to rupture the very thin lower segment below the retraction ring. (*Reproduced, with permission, from Cunningham FG, et al.* Williams Obstetrics. *18th ed. Norwalk, Conn: Appleton & Lange; 1989:363.*)

lapse or slip through the opening. The incidence of compound presentation is reported to be 1 in 500 to 1000 deliveries[3] (Figure 40–9).

Etiology. Prematurity and multiple gestation, in which the fetus tends to be small and the presenting part does not completely occlude the inlet, are common causes of compound presentations. An arm or leg may also prolapse alongside the presenting part if membranes rupture while the presenting part is still high and not engaged.

Nursing and Collaborative Management. If no complications are present, labor is permitted to continue. As the cervix dilates completely and the presenting part descends, the prolapsed arm or leg may rise out of the pelvis, allowing labor to continue normally.

The nurse should observe for presence of an extremity in the vagina and continue to provide information to the client and her labor partner as labor progresses. Fear and anxiety, caused by seeing a prolapsed limb, may be reduced if the woman and her partner are advised of this possibility. Reassurance

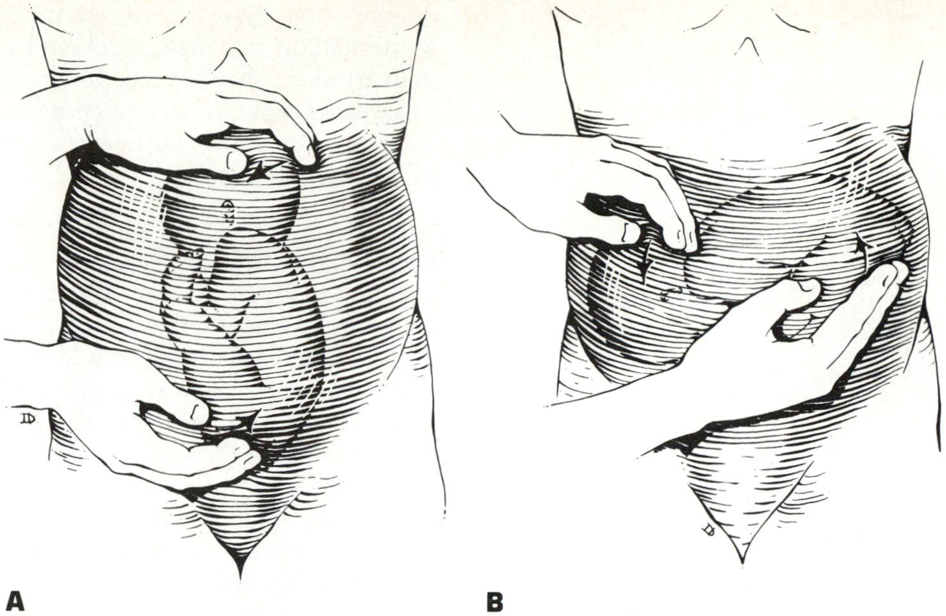

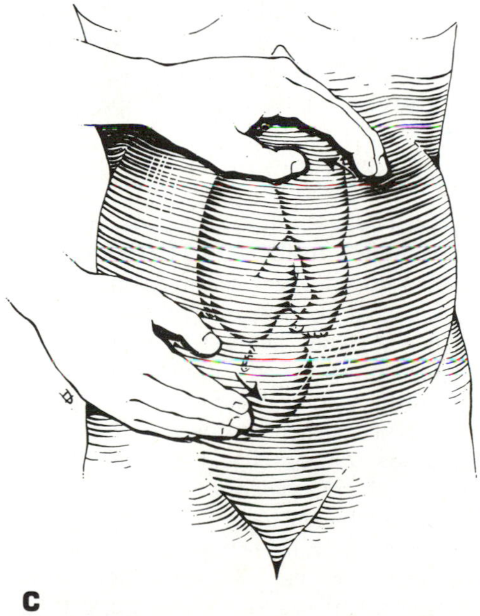

Figure 40–8. External version. **A.** Left sacrum transverse (LST)—dislodgement of breech. **B.** Forward somersault—LST to transverse lie. **C.** Forward somersault completed—transverse lie to right occiput transverse. (*Reproduced, with permission, from Oxorn H, ed.* Oxorn-Foote Human Labor and Birth. *5th ed. Norwalk, Conn: Appleton-Century-Crofts; 1986:431.*)

that labor is progressing normally may help the client to cope.

Compound presentations may be complicated by prolapse of the umbilical cord. As the presenting partmoves through the pelvis with the cord beside it, the cord may become compressed, stopping the flow of oxygenated blood to the fetus. This condition is considered an obstetric emergency and requires immediate treatment to avoid fetal suffocation. (*See* Figure 40–11 and discussion later in this chapter.)

Breech Presentation. The most common of all malpresentations is the **breech presentation** in which the buttocks or breech present. Breech deliveries occur in 3 to 4 percent of all singleton births. Although the denominator (arbitrary point of reference on the presenting part used to describe the position) is the sacrum, four types of breech presentation occur[3] (*see* discussion in Chapter 25 and Figure 25–6):

1. *Complete breech:* The buttocks is the presenting part, the fetal thighs are flexed at the hips, and the knees are flexed.

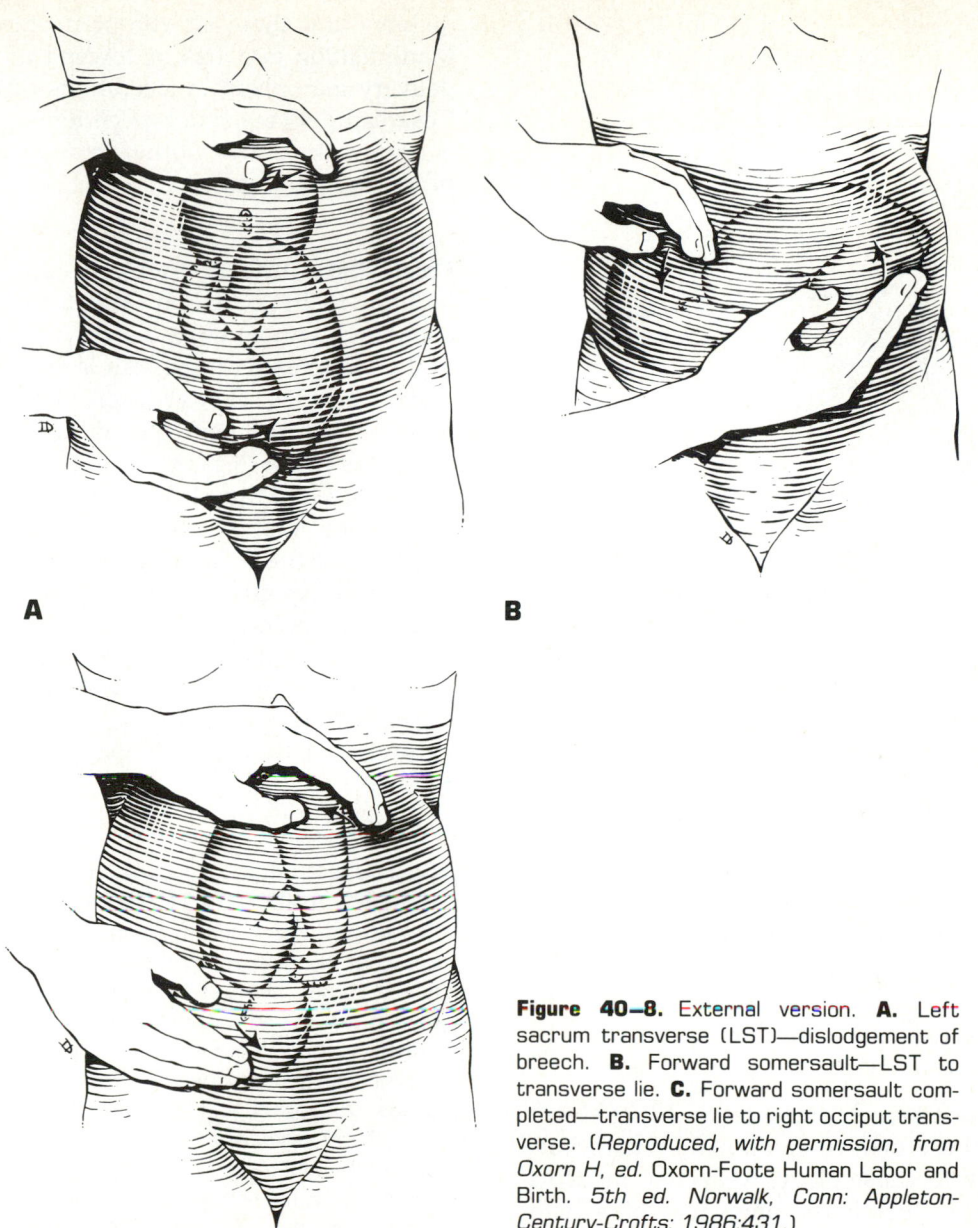

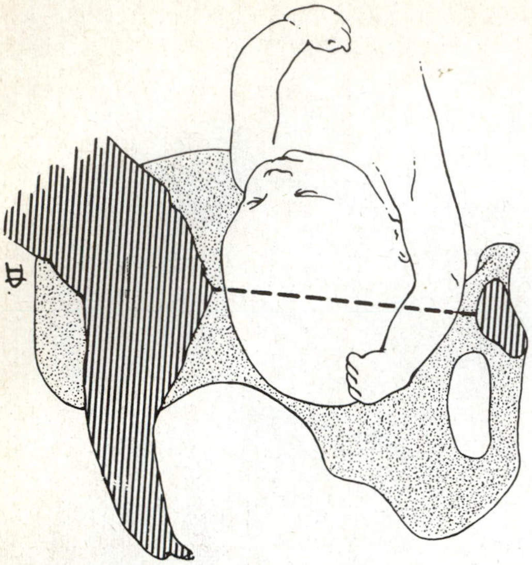

Figure 40–9. Compound presentation: head and hand. (*Reproduced, with permission, from Oxorn H, ed.* Oxorn-Foote Human Labor and Birth. *5th ed. Norwalk, Conn: Appleton-Century-Crofts; 1986:278.*)

2. *Frank breech:* The buttocks is the presenting part, the fetal thighs are flexed at the hips, the legs are extended, and the feet are extended close to the face.
3. *Incomplete or footling breech:* The foot is the presenting part either singularly or doubly; fetal thighs and knees are extended.
4. *Kneeling breech:* One or both knees present; the fetal thighs are extended so that the knees lie below the buttocks.

The cause of a breech presentation is not always apparent, but these malpresentations are associated with great parity because of the weakened musculature of the mother. Polyhydramnios may be a factor because excessive amniotic fluid makes it easier for the fetus to change position. Hydrocephaly (enlarged head) and a low implanted placenta may also be causes because these conditions prohibit the fetal head from entering the pelvis. Any condition that would interfere with the engagement of the fetal head could lead to a breech presentation.

Maternal Risks. Vaginal delivery of a fetus in a breech position poses several problems for the mother. Usually, the labor is prolonged. The soft, irregular tissues of the breech are not as effective in dilating the cervix as are the hard bones of the fetal skull. Membranes may rupture prematurely, putting the mother at risk for developing an infection, especially if the labor is long. The head and shoulders are born last in a breech delivery and there is little or no time for molding. Manipulation and use of forceps to assist with the delivery may result in lacerations of the birth canal. Cesarean delivery of a breech fetus poses additional surgical risks to the mother because of the operative procedure involved.

Fetal Risks. Infant morbidity and mortality are thought to be increased with a breech delivery as compared with a vertex delivery. Trauma, especially to the aftercoming head, can lead to central nervous system injuries. Compression of the umbilical cord between the mother's pelvis and the aftercoming head may result in asphyxia of the fetus. Fractures of fetal bones and muscle damage are more frequent in breech presentations than vertex presentations. Entrapment of the fetal head, prolapse of the umbilical cord, and aspiration of meconium are also directly related to a breech delivery.

Several studies have demonstrated that the mode of delivery of infants in a breech presentation does not significantly affect the outcome. Bowers and Taylor reviewed 460 cases involving singleton breech in-

ISSUES AND CONTROVERSIES

During the intrapartum period, complications can occur that require prompt decisions and interventions. Many issues related to delivery of care during this period are bound to arise. Delivering a woman by cesarean simply because the fetus is breech may be subjecting her to needless risks, not to mention increased hospital and medical costs. Because of the decreased incidence, however, the number of physicians who are skilled in vaginal breech deliveries is decreasing. Emergency medical technicians, who are not physicians, are taught how to deliver breech presentations in an emergency, but these technicians often are unsupervised in their first real delivery experience.[a] More current studies support the contention that some breech presentations can be safely delivered vaginally. They demonstrate that vaginal delivery can be managed safely while reducing costs and length of hospital stay.[b] With the current emphasis on quality care delivered in a cost-effective manner, should breeches be delivered vaginally or by cesarean?

[a] *Gimovsky ME, Petrie R. Breech delivery. In: Queenan J, ed.* Management of High Risk Pregnancy. *2nd ed. Oradell, NJ: Medical Economics Books; 1985:601–609.*

[b] *Stein A. Breech delivery: a cooperative nurse-midwifery medical management approach.* J Nurse Midwifery *1986;31: 93–97.*

fants. Looking at the total mortality in infants who survived labor, they found that routine cesarean from the standpoint of mortality might not be justified.[16] Pettite and Golditch supported these findings after reviewing 1593 breech infants weighing greater than 1000 g.[17] Wade and Taylor found from their studies that there were no significant differences in the 5-minute Apgar scores of breech infants weighing more than 2500 g despite the route of delivery.[18] In a retrospective study of 20 years' experience with breech deliveries, Green and associates and other investigators found that even though there had been a fivefold increase in the cesarean delivery rate, the incidence of neonatal asphyxia and birth injuries had remained unchanged.[19,20] Findings are similar for low birth weight breech fetuses.[21]

Nursing and Collaborative Assessment and Management. During labor, the client with a breech fetus needs to be assessed frequently for progress of labor. Labor may be prolonged because of slow cervical dilation. The client may become exhausted as the labor continues and should be encouraged to rest between contractions. Enlisting the support of the labor partner to assist the client to rest and relax may help. Hydration must be maintained and intake and output monitored if the labor is prolonged.

Breech presentations are associated with a prolapsed cord. The nurse should monitor the fetal heart rate for bradycardia, which might indicate cord compression. The nurse also should visually examine the perineal area and vaginal opening for signs of the cord, which sometimes will prolapse through the cervix.

The decision between vaginal and cesarean delivery in a breech presentation is the responsibility of the physician. During labor, assessments are made of fetal size, type of presentation, and adequacy of the mother's pelvis. The presence of flexion or extension of the fetal head is noted, and possible congenital malformations that might interfere with the normal progress of labor are identified. If the decision is made to deliver vaginally, the delivery may be spontaneous or assisted. A spontaneous delivery requires no assistance from the attending physician or nurse-midwife. An assisted delivery requires assistance after the fetus has been expelled as far as the umbilicus. Forceps may be used for extraction of the fetal head in assisted breech deliveries. In rare instances, the physician may attempt to extract the total fetal body. This procedure involves manipulation to convert the frank breech to a footling breech (Figure 40–10). Cesarean delivery is chosen if there is evidence that a vaginal delivery would pose a threat to either the mother or the fetus.

The vaginal delivery of a breech presentation is an area of great controversy among physicians. Primiparas presenting breech are usually delivered by cesarean. With multiparas, some physicians elect vaginal delivery; others opt for a cesarean delivery. Some physicians believe that all breech presentations should be managed by cesarean delivery regardless of the parity of the mother.[22]

Prolapse of the Umbilical Cord

Prolapse of the umbilical cord constitutes an obstetric emergency. Although not a common occurrence, the condition is associated with a high fetal mortality rate. If the presenting part of the fetus is not engaged in the pelvis or if the fetus is not snug with a malpresentation, when the membranes rupture the cord can prolapse and be carried downward by the sudden gush of amniotic fluid (Figure 40–11). Anytime the presenting part does not closely adhere to the pelvis, as in fetopelvic disproportion, the potential for prolapsed cord exists. Transverse lie and compound and breech presentations are examples of malpresentations in which the cord is likely to prolapse. Risk is also increased when the fetus is small, as in prematurity and multiple gestation.

Maternal Risks. There is no direct risk to the mother with prolapsed cord. She is, however, placed at risk by the attempts to save the fetus.

Fetal Risks. The mortality rate for the fetus with a prolapsed cord is high. Compression of the cord between the presenting part and the bony pelvis of the mother results in fetal hypoxia. Prolonged cord compression can lead to central nervous system damage and even death.

Nursing and Collaborative Assessment and Management. Prompt recognition of a prolapsed umbilical cord and immediate interventions are important. The nurse should be alert to the possibility of a prolapse when a malpresentation is noted in the laboring client. Frequent assessment of the fetal heart rate should be done to detect cord compression, because the prolapsed umbilical cord is not always visible (occult prolapsed cord). Immediately after the membranes rupture, the nurse should check the fetal heart rate as well as examine the client for a prolapsed cord. When the cord prolapses, it may lie beside the presenting part at the inlet, descend into the vagina, or protrude outside the vagina.

A prolapsed cord requires immediate action by the nurse. The client should be put into a Trendelenburg, or knee-chest, position to keep the presenting part off the cord. Oxygen should be administered to the client via mask. The physician should be notified immediately. If the cord is protruding outside the vagina, the nurse should never try to replace it or push it back in the vagina.

As the client is being prepared for delivery, vaginal support of the presenting part may help relieve the pressure on the cord. This is accomplished by placing a sterile gloved hand into the vagina and pushing up on the presenting part. This support may continue until a cesarean delivery is effected. Immediate cesarean delivery is recommended unless the cervix is completely dilated and a rapid delivery is possible.

When a cord prolapses, the client may be startled by the sudden activity in the labor suite as personnel rush to assist. The nurse can help the client by remaining calm despite the activity. Explanations of the procedures that are necessary can help to reduce the anxiety of the client and enlist her cooperation. Both the client and her labor partner may be fearful for the

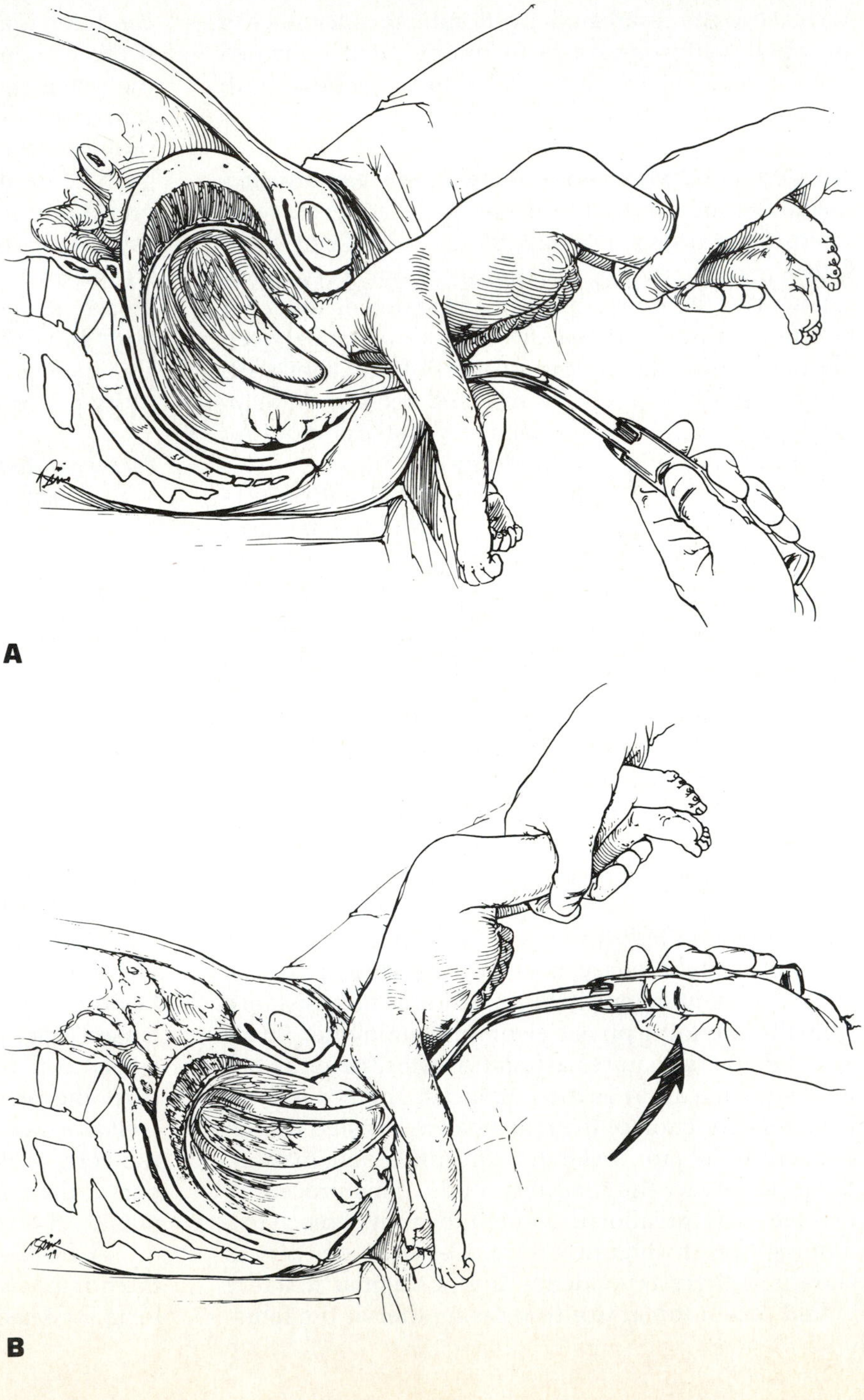

Figure 40–10. Delivery of breech presentation. Extraction of a complete or incomplete breech using forceps to the aftercoming head. **A.** The head has entered the pelvis and forceps have been applied. **B.** Forceps delivery of the aftercoming head; note the direction of movement (*arrow*). (*Figure continues.*)

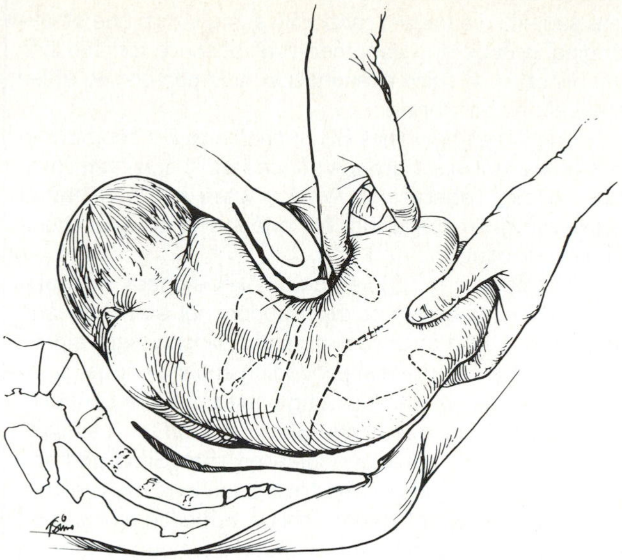

C

Figure 40–10. (*continued.*) C. Extraction of a frank breech using moderate traction exerted by a finger in each groin and facilitated by generous episiotomy. (*Reproduced, with permission, from Cunningham FG, et al.* Williams Obstetrics. *18th ed. Norwalk, Conn: Appleton & Lange; 1989:397, 398.*)

safety of the fetus; explaining what is being done to assist the fetus may help them to cope with these fears.

Malposition

Position of the fetus in labor refers to the relationship of the presenting part to the maternal pelvis. For identification purposes, the maternal pelvis is divided into quadrants. Left and right anterior quadrants are in the front of the pelvis near the pubic arch. Left and right posterior quadrants are in the back near the coccyx. Another reference point is the denominator, a designated point on the presenting part that is used to describe the position. In the "ideal" position, the fetal head is completely flexed on the chest and the occiput (O), which is the denominator, is in either the right or left anterior quadrant of the mother's pelvis [right occiput anterior (ROA) or occiput anterior (LOA)].

The fetal head follows the principle of "best fit" so malpositions may occur in the presence of fetopelvic disproportion or in an abnormal pelvic inlet. The most common malpositions are the occiput posterior and occiput transverse positions.

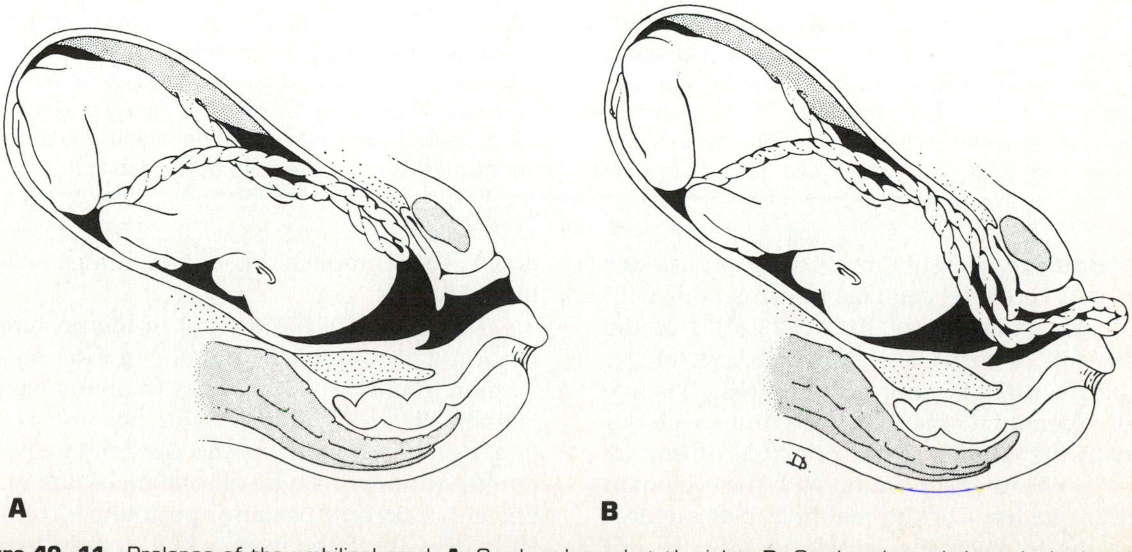

A B

Figure 40–11. Prolapse of the umbilical cord. **A.** Cord prolapsed at the inlet. **B.** Cord prolapsed through the introitus. (*Reproduced, with permission from Oxorn H, ed.* Oxorn-Foote Human Labor and Birth. *5th ed. Norwalk, Conn: Appleton-Century-Crofts; 1986:285.*)

RESEARCH ABSTRACT

Andrews CM, Andrews EC, Nursing, maternal postures, and fetal position. Nurs Res. *1983; 21:53–58.*

Fetal malposition is a major problem during labor. The objectives of this study were twofold: (1) to determine if a safe, simple, and economic nursing procedure, maternal posturing, would result in the rotation of a fetus in the posterior or transverse position to the optimal anterior position; and (2) to evaluate the relative effectiveness of a series of maternal postures in facilitating rotation to the anterior position.

Four maternal postures were developed to produce anterior fetal rotation. These included: hand-knee position alone, hand-knee position with pelvic rocking, hand-knee position with abdominal stroking, and hand-knee position with both rocking and stroking. Sitting was the control position. Based on the effects of physical forces (gravity, buoyancy, and friction), several situations reflected by nine hypotheses were tested. These situations involved a variety of combinations of the four basic postures compared to each other and to the control to determine what posture most efficiently produced anterior fetal rotation.

The sample consisted of 100 healthy pregnant women at term. They were randomly assigned to one of five posture groups (four treatment and one control group). Two nurse-midwife settings were used for the study. Using Leopold's maneuvers, a nurse-midwife examined each subject to determine fetal position (dependent variable). The examiner immediately left the room and a second nurse-midwife positioned the subject using the one of five postures designated for her group for 10 minutes. The examiner then returned and performed a second examination. If rotation to an anterior position occurred, the subject was asked to assume a Sims position for 10 minutes to determine if this position would maintain the rotated position. Twenty-seven of the subjects assumed the Sims position on the same side as the fetal back. Twenty-three other subjects assumed the Sims position on the side opposite the fetal back. If rotation had not occurred, the subject was again randomly assigned to one of the original groups and assumed that posture for another 10 minutes. A third examination was performed after the second posturing.

The data show that 60 of the total 80 subjects in the four treatment groups successfully achieved rotation through posturing. Twenty were not successful after the first posturing. No one in the control group achieved rotation.

The postures of knee-chest, knee-chest with pelvic rocking, knee-chest with abdominal stroking, and knee-chest with both rocking and stroking were significantly more effective in producing anterior rotation of the fetus than was the sitting position. Data concerning the effectiveness of the Sims position for maintaining the anterior rotation indicated that Sims position on the opposite side of the fetal back was most effective. Twenty-two of twenty-three subjects maintained the fetus in the anterior position as compared with fifteen of twenty-seven subjects when the subjects assumed a Sims position on the same side as the fetal back.

Comment:

The design of this study promotes confidence in its results. By the use of term pregnant women who were not in labor, the variables associated with labor were eliminated. The study concluded that posturing was more effective than sitting, which fulfilled one of the objectives. Other variables that might have influenced rotation were also identified, tested, and found not to be significant. Another finding of the study was that after rotation, the Sims position with the subject on the side opposite that of the fetal back was more effective than the Sims position with the subject on the same side as the fetal back for maintaining the fetus in the anterior position.

Results of the study indicate that a nursing intervention, posturing, may be beneficial in changing a malposition of the fetus. The method used is safe, can be done in a variety of settings, and has no adverse side effects. Posturing can be done during pregnancy; however, additional research is necessary to determine if posturing is also effective during labor.

Occiput Posterior. A fetus in an occiput posterior position is in a vertex or cephalic presentation, with the occiput (denominator of the fetal skull) of the fetus in the left or right posterior quadrant of the mother's pelvis. Right occiput posterior (ROP) is five times more common than left occiput posterior (LOP). Following the "best fit" principle during labor, a fetus in a head-first position with the occiput in the posterior quadrant of the maternal pelvis enters the pelvic inlet transversely or side to side. To exit through the pelvic outlet, the fetal head must be in an anteroposterior position, that is, straight up and down. To accomplish this, rotation must take place in the midpelvis.

Rotation with the occiput in the posterior quadrant can be accomplished in one of three ways: (1) A long-arc rotation of 135° takes the fetus from a ROP position to an occiput anterior position, where the fetal head is straight up and down in an anteroposterior position; this type of rotation occurs in about 90 percent of occiput posterior positions. (2) Rotation of 90° moves the fetus from a ROP to a ROA position. (3) Rotation of 45° moves the fetus from a ROP to a right occiput transverse position.

Many fetuses in occiput posterior positions rotate to an anterior position spontaneously with no difficulty. The problems arise when rotation does not occur. With a persistent occiput posterior position, the fetal head does not rotate to the anterior position. Failure to rotate and cessation of descent of the fetal head indicate that labor has arrested and intervention is needed. Cephalopelvic disproportion may be a factor in occiput posterior positions. Anthropoid and android pelves, with their large posterior, sagittal diameters, lend themselves to occiput posterior positions.

Maternal Risks. Labor with a fetus in an occiput posterior position is long and difficult. Backache is common. If the fetus is delivered in a posterior position, perineal lacerations can occur and a large episiotomy may be needed. An episiotomy prevents tearing of the perineum, as the large back part of the head causes greater stretching during the birthing process. In the event of a cesarean delivery, the woman is at risk for surgical complications related to the operative procedure.

Fetal Risks. Molding and excessive edema of the fetal skull are common in these malpositions. Fetal asphyxia also may occur.

Nursing and Collaborative Assessment and Management. A client with a fetus in an occiput posterior position may be able to help the fetus to rotate anteriorly by lying on the side opposite the fetus' back. Gravity may then assist the fetus to rotate. By squatting, kneeling, getting on hands and knees, and assuming a knee-chest position with pelvic tilting, the client may facilitate fetal rotation and descent. The nurse should assist the client in assuming these positions and give clear explanations as to why she is to do them.

Backache is a common complaint with occiput posterior positions. Sacral rubs may help. The labor partner can be encouraged to assist the client during a contraction by applying firm pressure on the sacral area. Frequent change of positions may also help.

Contractions and progress in labor should be checked and recorded at frequent intervals. Fetal heart rate also should be monitored for signs of fetal distress. Hydration needs to be maintained during a long labor, usually through intravenous solutions, such as lactated Ringer's solution.

As long as labor is progressing and there is no indication of maternal or fetal distress, vaginal delivery can be anticipated. If labor becomes arrested, medical intervention is required. The fetus may be delivered vaginally using forceps provided there is no fetopelvic disproportion, the head is engaged, the cervix is fully dilated, and the membranes are ruptured. If any of these conditions are not met, vaginal delivery should not be attempted. The fetus can be delivered in the occiput posterior position or rotated with the forceps to a more anterior position for delivery. Inability to deliver vaginally or the presence of distress necessitate a cesarean delivery.

Persistent Occiput Transverse. Occiput transverse position occurs in a manner similar to that of occiput posterior as just described. The difference is that in the midpelvis, the fetal head begins to rotate to an anterior position and stops or arrests when it is transverse, with the fetal skull horizontal to the long axis of the mother. The arrest may be caused by ineffective uterine contractions or a pelvis that has a flattened anteroposterior diameter.

Maternal Risks. After a period of normal labor the client may experience a decrease in the rate and intensity of her contractions. Barring any complications from abnormal pelvic structure or fetopelvic disproportion, oxytocin may be used to stimulate the contractions. The client then is subject to any complications associated with the use of oxytocin. Delivery may be accomplished vaginally. Forceps are used to rotate the head to facilitate delivery. Lacerations of the birth canal can occur during a forceps delivery. Cesarean delivery places the mother at risk for complications related to the operative procedure.

Fetal Risks. Asphyxia may occur during a long, difficult labor. Also, if forceps are used to rotate or deliver the fetus, injury to the fetal neck or head may occur.

Nursing and Collaborative Assessment and Management. Nursing care is related to the type of medical intervention selected. If oxytocin is used to augment the labor, all the activities associated with the administration of the drug (as listed earlier) must be carried out. Maternal positioning may be used to assist with rotation. The nurse needs to explain these positions and why they are being used, and to assist the client in assuming them. Throughout labor contractions, maternal vital signs and fetal heart rate are frequently assessed. Emotional support is given to both the client and her labor partner to help them cope with the dystocia.

Fetal Conditions Resulting in Fetopelvic and Cephalopelvic Disproportion

In addition to malpresentation and malposition, fetal dystocia may also be caused by fetal conditions contributing to fetopelvic and cephalopelvic disproportion (*see* the Case Study/Care Plan). Two conditions that predispose to such a situation are large fetal size and hydrocephalus.

CASE STUDY/CARE PLAN: DYSTOCIA RELATED TO FETOPELVIC DISPROPORTION

Lynda Turner, age 23 and pregnant with her first child, is admitted to the hospital in early labor. She is accompanied by her husband Bill. They have attended Lamaze classes together and are excited but anxious about the approaching birth. During admission, Lynda talks continually. She asks many questions and keeps wringing her hands. After the admission procedure is completed, Lynda and Bill walk around the unit. Lynda's membranes have not ruptured and walking is suggested to stimulate the contractions. As the contractions become stronger and Lynda becomes more uncomfortable, she returns to bed.

At this time, an external electronic fetal monitor is applied. Lynda is quite restless in bed. She changes position frequently, looking for one of comfort. Her facial expression indicates pain and occasionally she can be heard telling Bill that the contractions are painful. Bill and Lynda work well together. He assists her with her breathing and uses effleurage to encourage her to relax.

About 8 hours after admission, Lynda's membranes rupture spontaneously. The fluid is meconium stained. Both Lynda and Bill become upset at the sight of the greenish fluid. Lynda begins to cry and Bill demands to see the physician right away. The physician places an internal electrode on the fetal scalp which reveals a fetal heart rate of 120 with a late deceleration pattern. Contractions continue about every 2 minutes and are of strong intensity. Lynda is placed on her left side.

An hour and a half later, a vaginal examination reveals that the cervix has dilated 7 cm but that no further fetal descent has occurred. The fetus remains at station 1+ after 1½ hours of strong uterine contractions. The fetal monitor shows a fetal heart rate of 120 with late decelerations and now some decreased variability. The physician is notified. He tells Lynda and Bill that labor is not progressing normally and that the fetus is showing signs of distress. He also advises them that this lack of progress is most probably caused by fetopelvic disproportion and that, because of fetal distress, a cesarean delivery is indicated. Lynda is prepared for a cesarean delivery. She is taken to the delivery room and delivers a healthy 7½-pound male infant.

Supporting Assessment Data	Expected Client/ Family Outcome	Nursing Actions/ Interventions	Rationale	Criteria for Evaluation
Nursing Diagnosis: Anxiety, related to dystocia with first infant				
Client talks continually Frequent questions Wringing of hands	Client will be able to verbalize fears and concerns during labor	Establish a trusting relationship with client and labor partner.	A trusting relationship demonstrates to the client the concern of the nurse and encourages verbalization of feelings. Verbalizing feelings can reduce anxiety.	Signs of anxiety are decreased.
		Give clear explanation of procedures.	Many of the client's concerns can be alleviated with explanations.	Client verbalizes understanding of procedures.
		Encourage labor partner's support of client.	Labor partners can often be successful in minimizing anxiety.	Client expresses less anxiety.
Nursing Diagnosis: Alteration in comfort, related to intensity of labor contractions				
Restlessness Grimacing Complaints of pain	Client will be as comfortable as possible during labor	Reinforce breathing techniques taught at Lamaze classes.	Appropriate breathing techniques help the client to cope with the discomfort of the contractions.	Client does not hyperventilate or hold breath and expresses minimal discomfort.

Supporting Assessment Data	Expected Client/ Family Outcome	Nursing Actions/ Interventions	Rationale	Criteria for Evaluation
		Encourage labor partner do effleurage. Give frequent back rubs.	Effleurage and back rubs stimulate the afferent nerve fibers and block pain sensation.	Client states that pain is reduced.
		Administer analgesics as necessary	Analgesics provide pain relief during difficult labor.	
		Encourage client to rest between contractions.	Pain is exaggerated by exhaustion and fatigue.	Client rests between contractions.
		Provide calm, quiet environment. Praise and encourage client's efforts.	Praise enhances self-esteem and positive reinforcement promotes the continuation of breathing and relaxation techniques in a supportive environment.	Client behaves as though and states she is in control.
Nursing Diagnosis: Potential for injury to the fetus, related to uteroplacental insufficiency				
Meconium-stained amniotic fluid Decreasing FHR with late decelerations	Fetus will continue to be oxygenated during labor	Assess FHR tracing of internal monitor every 15 minutes.	Frequent monitoring aids in identification of fetal problems.	FHR pattern returns to normal.
		Place client in left lateral position.	Left lateral position improves blood flow to uterus by reducing pressure on vena cava.	There are no signs of uteroplacental insufficiency.
Nursing Diagnosis: Ineffective coping, related to fear for fetus				
Client begins to cry; partner angrily demands to see physician	Client and labor partner will gain control of situation as soon as possible	Continue to inform client and labor partner of labor progress and nursing and medical interventions.	Keeping client and labor partner informed helps to decrease anxiety and maintain control.	Client and labor partner experience no problems in coping.
Nursing Diagnosis: Alteration in normal physiologic process, related to failure of fetus to descend				
Fetus remains at 1+ station after 1½ hours of strong uterine contractions	Client will deliver without injury to self or fetus	Plot labor on graph.	Labor graph shows whether labor is within parameters of what is considered normal.	Labor graph enables professional to make an informal decision.
Fetus experiences distress		Ask client to void or catheterize as necessary per physician's order.	A full bladder may cause obstruction of the birth canal.	Birth canal is not obstructed.
		Prepare client and partner for cesarean delivery.	Cesarean delivery is method of choice for fetopelvic disproportion.	Client delivers a healthy infant.
Nursing Diagnosis: Knowledge deficit, related to alteration in normal labor process				
Labor partner asks to see physician; client questions nurse about labor	Client and labor partner will verbalize understanding of the alteration in labor	Explain the reasons for lack of fetal descent.	Anxiety can be heightened by a lack of knowledge.	Client and labor partner show fewer signs of anxiety. Both demonstrate an understanding of situation.
FHR—fetal heart rate indicates distress.	Client and labor partner will verbalize understanding of reasons for cesarean delivery	Explain reasons for cesarean delivery; inform couple about procedure.		Clear explanations can facilitate client coping.

Large Fetal Size. A fetus is termed large (or macrosomic) when he or she weighs more than 4000 g (9 pounds). This large size is often associated with maternal diabetes. Late in pregnancy, failure of the pancreas of the diabetic mother to release enough insulin to meet the increased demands results in hyperglycemia. These high levels of glucose stimulate the fetal pancreas to release insulin. The increased maternal glucose and the increased fetal insulin combine to produce excessive fetal growth (*see* Chapter 42). Other factors predisposing to large fetal size include delivery more than 7 days postterm, weight gain greater than 20 kg during pregnancy, multiparity, and maternal age over 35 years.[3]

Maternal Risks. The large fetus may be delivered vaginally, provided the maternal pelvis is adequate; however, the presence of a large fetus and an average-size pelvis often results in fetopelvic disproportion. Cesarean delivery may be necessary if the fetus is too large to travel through the pelvis. A large fetus may also predispose the mother to uterine rupture and postpartum hemorrhage because of the overstretching of the myometrium.

Fetal Risks. A large fetus whose size is underestimated may experience trauma to the head as a result of strong contractions, which force the head against the bony structures of the pelvis. Cerebral edema, neurologic damage, hypoxia, and asphyxia may result. Shoulder dystocia and fractures of the clavicle and humerus are more common with large infants.

Nursing and Collaborative Management. Nursing measures are aimed at offering the mother and her labor partner support. If a vaginal delivery is planned, the second stage of labor may be prolonged and the client may need encouragement to cope. Delivery may be accomplished spontaneously, with the use of forceps or by cesarean. The method chosen is the one that poses the least risk to mother and fetus.

Fetal Hydrocephalus. Fetal hydrocephalus is the excessive accumulation of cerebrospinal fluid in the ventricles of the brain with consequent enlargement of the cranium. Fetal hydrocephalus is often accompanied by other conditions such as spinal cord anomalies and mental retardation. It occurs in 1 in 2000 fetuses and accounts for approximately 12 percent of severe fetal malformations occurring at birth. In one third of the cases of fetal hydrocephalus, a breech presentation is found. Whatever the presentation, cephalopelvic disproportion is common.[4]

Maternal Risks. Fetal hydrocephalus predisposes the laboring client to uterine rupture. In these cases, maternal mortality is very high.

Fetal Risks. The fetus with hydrocephalus is at great risk of trauma to the head. Again, high morbidity and high mortality are associated with this condition.

Nursing and Collaborative Assessment. The mother is asked to empty her bladder to facilitate abdominal and vaginal examinations. If the fetal presentation is cephalic, a broad firm mass is evident above the symphysis. The fetal heart rate is often loudest above the umbilicus, which often leads to the suspicion of a breech presentation. Vaginal examination may elicit wide suture lines and large fontanelles.

If the presentation is breech, the condition may be more difficult to detect. Radiography or sonography may provide some confirmation of hydrocephalus.

Nursing and Collaborative Management. For the fetus to be delivered vaginally, the size of the hydrocephalic head must be reduced. In cephalic and breech presentations, fluid is removed from the head via a needle inserted transvaginally. Many hydrocephalic fetuses are delivered by cesarean. Even in cesarean deliveries, fluid may be removed from the fetal head. An experimental technique involving shunting of fluid from the ventricle in the fetus' head antepartally is currently under investigation.

The nurse monitors the client's vital signs and progress, if the woman has a trial of labor. Further, the nurse helps to prepare the client and her support person for any treatments or cesarean delivery. Much support is necessary for the couple coping with a difficult fetal diagnosis.

Shoulder Dystocia

Shoulder dystocia occurs when the anterior shoulder of the fetus becomes impacted behind the symphysis pubis (Figure 40–12). This difficulty in delivering the shoulders is more likely to occur with a large fetus. The increasing incidence of shoulder dystocia is directly related to increasing birth weight.[23] The incidence in those fetuses who weigh more than 4000 g is 1.7 percent. Predisposing factors for shoulder dystocia include a large fetus, prolonged second stage of labor, multiparity, previous delivery of an infant weighing more than 4000 g, postterm pregnancy, and a contracted pelvic outlet.

Maternal Risks. After a traumatic delivery, the mother may experience vaginal and perineal lacera-

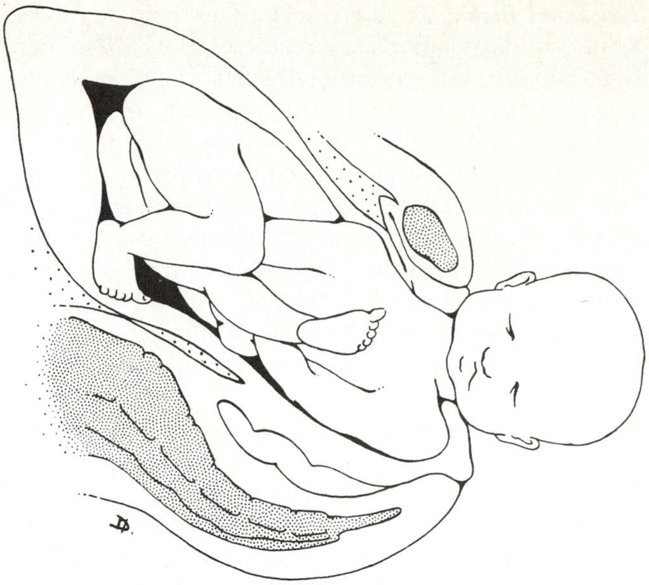

Figure 40–12. Shoulder dystocia. *(Reproduced, with permission, from Oxorn H, ed.* Oxorn-Foote Human Labor and Birth. *5th ed. Norwalk, Conn: Appleton-Century-Crofts; 1986:293.)*

tions. These result from maneuvers to deliver the shoulders of the infant.

Fetal Risks. Shoulder dystocia increases fetal morbidity and mortality. Fetal risk is related to asphyxia resulting from prolonged cord compression when delivery is delayed because of shoulder dystocia.[24] A study of the aftereffects of shoulder dystocia by McCall found infant mortality and morbidity, including physical damage to the arm or skull fracture, along with neuropsychiatric sequelae, 5 to 7 years later.[25]

Nursing and Collaborative Assessment and Management. During delivery of a fetus with shoulder dystocia, the shoulders should be delivered as soon as possible after the head. Care must be taken not to exert excessive traction on the head or neck, which could stretch the neck too much or fracture the clavicle. Cesarean delivery is the method recommended for diabetic gravidas with an estimated fetal weight of 4000+ g and should be seriously considered for those laboring women whose estimated fetal weight is 4500+ g and who have an abnormal labor.[23]

Two other methods of delivery used in the presence of shoulder dystocia are described in the literature. The methods are not in common practice, but rather are experimental. Hartfield[26] describes a method called subcutaneous symphysiotomy, in which delivery is accomplished by cutting through the symphyseal joint. He says the procedure can be completed within 5 minutes because the symphyseal joint is soft and easily divided in pregnancy. He states that maternal mortality with symphysiotomy is less than that with cesarean delivery. Another approach is described by Zavanelli and called the Zavanelli maneuver.[27] After the head has been delivered and restitution has occurred, the head is returned to the prerestitutional position, maneuvers are reversed, the head is flexed and returned to the vagina, and the fetus is delivered by cesarean.

Shoulder dystocia may be suspected when the fetus is large and the second stage of labor prolonged. If a vaginal delivery is planned, the nurse needs to prepare the client and her labor partner to expect that some difficulty may be encountered. Explanations help to reassure clients and gain their trust. Continued assessment of contractions along with the progress of labor is important. Fetal heart rate should be assessed at frequent intervals and evaluated for signs of distress. During a vaginal delivery, the nurse may assist the physician by providing suprapubic pressure as it is requested.

Nursing Diagnoses

Nursing diagnoses concerning the passenger or fetus can be made after review of assessment data. Listed in the box are examples of nursing diagnoses for dystocia related to the passenger.

DYSTOCIA RELATED TO THE PASSAGE

Pelvic dystocia occurs when the fetus cannot enter or pass through the bony pelvis of the mother. This is due most often to contractions of the pelvis. Contractions are decreased diameters of the pelvis that are usually the result of pelvic size and shape.

NURSING DIAGNOSES FOR DYSTOCIA RELATED TO THE PASSENGER

Problem-Oriented

Potential for injury (fetal), related to malpresentation (breech)

Potential for impaired gas exchange (fetal), related to prolapse of umbilical cord

Strength-Oriented

Effective maternal coping, related to adequate support of partner

Some pelves are better suited to childbirth than others. The gynecoid or female pelvis, which is considered the best, is found in about half of all women. (*See* Chapter 6 for a description of variations of female pelves and Chapter 14 for planes and diameters of the pelvis.)

Factors other than pelvic size must also be considered when pelvic dystocia is suspected. A woman may have adequate pelvic measurements, but if uterine contractions are not effective, descent of the presenting part will not occur. If the fetus is too large or in a malpresentation or malposition, passage through the pelvis will be delayed or even arrested. The reverse is also true. Strong, efficient uterine contractions could move a fetus through a pelvis with borderline normal measurements. There are generally said to be three types of pelvic contractions:

1. *Inlet contraction.* Pelvic inlet contraction is present when the anteroposterior diameter of the maternal pelvis is less than 10 cm and the transverse diameter is less than 12 cm. As the presenting part first enters the pelvis through the inlet, small measurements may make engagement difficult. In an attempt to fit into the inlet, the fetal head may become malpositioned as it follows the principle of "best fit." This means the head will enter the pelvic inlet the way it is best accommodated. Difficulties may be encountered if the small moldable breech enters a pelvis with small measurements and then the aftercoming head becomes stuck. Inlet contraction most often is caused by rickets, a vitamin D deficiency.
2. *Midpelvic contraction.* Midpelvic contraction occurs when the plane of least dimension, the midpelvic plane, is reduced. This midpelvic plane is at the level of the ischial spine. It is formed from the margin of the symphysis pubis and touches the sacrum at the junction of the fourth or fifth vertebra. An ischial spinous diameter less than 9.5 cm results in midpelvic contraction. Genetic factors responsible for the pelvic structure are the most frequent cause of this type of contraction. Midpelvic contraction often results in transverse arrest of the fetal head. The midpelvis is where internal rotation of the fetal head takes place. Contractions in this area complicate the rotation process or prevent it altogether.
3. *Outlet contraction.* Contraction of the pelvic outlet is present when the distance between the ischial tuberosities is less than 8 cm. This condition frequently occurs along with other contractions of the pelvis and is related to pelvic bone development.

Maternal Risks. Dystocia related to pelvic contractions prolongs labor as a result of slow dilation or fetal descent. All the problems associated with prolonged labor may occur. These include exhaustion, increased discomfort, and potential intrauterine infection resulting from premature rupture of membranes. The need for forceps-assisted delivery may subject the maternal tissues to trauma, causing profuse bleeding from the lacerations of the birth canal and perineum. Cesarean delivery may be necessary, in which case the mother is susceptible to operative complications such as hemorrhage and infection.

Fetal Risks. The fetal head is prone to injury in the event of pelvic dystocia. With borderline measurements, the fetal skull may have to mold excessively to pass through the pelvis. Caput succedaneum is common. Neurologic problems as well as hemorrhage and fractures of the fetal head can occur because of the pressing of the head against the bony pelvis.

Collaborative Assessment and Management. Marked deviations such as decreased pelvic diameters and abnormalities in pelvic structure may be identified during prenatal care, at which time vaginal delivery can be ruled out and cesarean delivery anticipated. Borderline measurements might indicate a trial labor.

Many physicians feel that fetopelvic disproportion can be diagnosed only by having the woman go through a trial of labor. This trial of labor involves observing the woman through at least 4 hours of well-established labor for dilation or monitoring the woman in the second stage of labor for more than 2 hours for head engagement.[28] Interventions such as maternal positioning may be attempted. Failure of the trial of labor warrants cesarean delivery.

Protraction or arrest disorders that cannot be anticipated are treated by forceps-assisted or cesarean delivery; the decision depends on the location of the fetus in the pelvis and the amount of trauma each method poses to mother and fetus.

When dystocia occurs in labor and the powers and the passenger can be ruled out as the cause, pelvimetry and ultrasound should be conducted to determine pelvic measurements. Fetopelvic disproportion, if not treated, can result in trauma to the fetal head, as it is forced against the cervix by the uterine contractions, or uterine rupture, as the muscles overdistend in an effort to expel the contents of the uterus.

Nursing Assessment and Management. Nursing management includes all of the assessments and observations for a client in normal labor. When pelvic contraction has not been identified prior to the start of labor, the nurse must monitor cervical dilation and fetal descent closely. If these fail to progress normally, pelvic contracting may be a cause.

The labor graph can be a useful tool in identifying problems. Assessment of contractions is important. With strong contractions and no fetal descent, uterine rupture is possible. Monitoring fetal heart tones is necessary to detect fetal distress. A prolapsed cord could restrict or stop the flow of oxygenated blood to the fetus. Observation of amniotic fluid is also helpful in identifying fetal distress. In the absence of a breech presentation, the presence of meconium in the amniotic fluid usually is indicative of fetal distress.

Throughout the long and difficult labor accompanying pelvic dystocia, the client and her labor partner need to be constantly informed of the interventions being done for both mother and fetus. Advising the woman of the progress in labor, such as changes in cervical dilation and fetal descent, can help to allay anxiety. Each intervention needs to be fully explained. An understanding of what is happening reduces anxiety and encourages client participation where possible. The nurse should support the client and partner in coping with unanticipated events that may occur during the labor process.

Nursing Diagnoses

After careful assessment, several nursing diagnoses may be developed concerning dystocia related to the passage (pelvis) (*see* the box).

NURSING DIAGNOSES FOR DYSTOCIA RELATED TO THE PASSAGE

Problem-Oriented

Potential for fetal compromise, related to fetopelvic disproportion

Fear, related to unplanned cesarean delivery

Strength-Oriented

Effective family coping, related to knowledge of diagnosis and agreement with treatment plan

DYSTOCIA RELATED TO THE PSYCHE

The psyche is a powerful factor in the labor process. Under normal conditions, the intrapartum period is one of heightened emotions and stress. When complications arise, stress increases and may develop into a crisis. The high-risk intrapartum client is experiencing concurrent maturational and situational crises. (*See* Chapter 36 for a further description of concurrent crises.) Nurses need to understand the psychologic aspects of labor if they are to give care and support to the client and her labor partner during crisis.

In the classic study by Lederman and coworkers, a link was detected between psychosocial variables, such as the client's fears about labor, physiologic variables, such as blood levels of epinephrine and norepinephrine, and progress in labor.[29] Thus, the client's psyche has been empirically shown to influence stress-related hormones and progress in labor. Nursing interventions related to the client's psyche are important in ensuring the normal progress of labor.

Several factors have been found to influence the psyche of the client experiencing a high-risk labor. These include the client's perception of the problem, coping strategies, available support systems, levels of fear and anxiety, image of herself, and preparation for childbirth.

Perception of the Problem

The intensity of the woman's response is determined largely by how the problem is perceived. Several factors can alter this perception. These include emotional states, anxiety, hostility, age, and prior experience. When a complication develops during labor, the client's response can be affected by how apparent the problem is. A prolapsed cord and the possibility of fetal demise may elicit a more intense response than the prospect of a prolonged labor as a result of ineffective contractions. Progress in labor also can affect the client's response. Problems that arise early in labor may be explained so that the client can understand and participate in the treatment; however, as labor progresses and the woman goes through psychologic withdrawal, her attention is focused only on the moment and communication may be more difficult.

Coping

To handle stress and threats to their well-being, individuals develop patterns of behavior called coping mechanisms. Clients rely on a variety of coping mechanisms to handle different levels of stress. These coping mechanisms may be constructive or destructive.

Constructive coping mechanisms lead to the resolution of a problem. Mild anxiety may be manifested in tension-releasing behaviors such as crying, sleeping, pacing, and other repetitive behaviors. These behaviors are aimed at relieving stress. The nurse should support these coping mechanisms in both the client and her labor partner if they are effective in relieving and reducing the anxiety.

As the level of anxiety increases, different behaviors will become apparent. These may include denial of the threat, projection, or repression. Although these behaviors can protect the client from feeling worthless or inadequate, they also can distort reality and interfere with interpersonal relationships. When this happens, the coping mechanisms are destructive. The nurse can help the client and her labor partner to recognize these destructive coping mechanisms and attempt to substitute more positive coping behaviors.

Support Systems

The course of labor and delivery can be influenced significantly by the client's support system. A support system includes those in the environment from whom the client expects help, generally family and friends. In the labor room, the labor partner and the nurse can be a support system for the client. When a complication arises, the support system is most important.[30] A strong support system helps the client to cope. If, however, the support system is weak or absent, the client may lose all perception of control over the situation.

Fear

During labor, all women experience fear to some extent. Fear implies that the client is afraid of something that actually exists. The client may fear the process of labor or the anticipated pain. She may fear death, afraid that she may die during labor.

Three classic fears have been identified during labor: (1) fear for oneself, (2) fear for the infant, (3) fear of the unknown. Erickson, in a classic early study,[31] identified several complications of labor that can result in the woman's fear for her infant and herself:

- Prolonged first stage of labor
- Prolonged second stage of labor
- Rotation of the fetal head
- Indicated low forceps
- Apgar scores less than 5
- Apgar scores of 5 to 7

Anxiety

With fear the client is afraid of an actual thing; with anxiety the source is not known. Fear may cause anxiety. The degree of anxiety that a woman in labor exhibits is dependent on several variables[32]:

- Basic personality of the woman
- Attitude toward the pregnancy
- Perception of her mother's labor
- Childbirth preparation
- Amount of trust in the clinic, nurse, nurse-midwife, and physician
- Effect of and response to medication
- Progress of labor

Anxiety is not always bad; some degree of anxiety may actually help the client deal realistically with the process of labor. But, when anxiety levels reach the panic stage, the client may become immobilized and lose her ability to solve problems.

Self-Image

Self-image refers to how the client feels about herself; this may be positive or negative. If the client approaches labor with realistic perceptions and goals, she maintains a positive self-image. On the other hand, perceptions and goals that are unrealistic or incongruent with labor events may lead to a negative self-image. Nurses can promote the client's positive self-image by praising her efforts during labor and explaining procedures so that the client can understand them. This is most important when complications arise in labor that interfere with the client's goal. If the client has prepared for a vaginal delivery and then must have a cesarean delivery because of a complication that arises suddenly, she may feel that she has failed and the complication is her fault. She must be helped to see that she had no control over the problem and that the ultimate goal of childbirth has been realized despite the method.

Preparation for Childbirth

The labor experience is more satisfying if the client and her labor partner are prepared both physically and emotionally for the birth. Preparation for the birth can increase the client's ability to cope; decrease her stress, anxiety, and pain; and provide satisfaction

NURSING DIAGNOSES FOR DYSTOCIA RELATED TO THE PSYCHE

Problem-Oriented

Powerlessness, related to slow progress in labor

Ineffective individual coping, related to fatigue and discomfort during labor

Altered role performance (paternal), related to unexpected course of labor

Strength-Oriented

Positive interaction, related to adequate resources

Positive maternal self-image, related to effective coping with difficult labor with the childbearing experience. Education gives both the client and her labor partner greater opportunities to control the labor experience, resulting in a positive reaction to the birth experience. (*See* Chapter 24 on childbirth preparation.)

Nursing Diagnoses

Nursing diagnoses for dystocia related to the psyche are developed after careful assessment. Some diagnoses related to the psyche are listed in the box.

OTHER PROBLEMS

Although dystocias related to the powers, passenger, passage, or psyche are major problems occurring during the intrapartum period, other complications may arise. These complications can be associated with dystocia, or independent of it. Among these problems are abnormal fetal heart rate patterns, pregnancy-induced hypertension, delivery of multiple fetuses, and abnormalities of the cord, amniotic fluid, and placenta.

Abnormal Fetal Heart Rate Patterns in Labor

During a difficult labor, assessment of fetal well-being is essential. Measurement of the fetal heart rate is the chief method of fetal assessment. Fetal heart rate also is an indicator of fetal distress.

Use of continuous electronic fetal monitoring in the client experiencing dystocia provides a second-by-second audio and visual fetal heart rate recording. The fetal heart rate can be monitored either externally or internally depending on whether the membranes have ruptured.

Many factors must be evaluated in determining the fetal heart rate pattern. These include baseline rate, variability, and decelerations. Parity, progress in labor, maternal and obstetric complications, and analgesia or anesthesia must also be considered.

The **baseline fetal heart rate** is the average rate between contractions. Normally, this rate is between 120 and 160 beats per minutes. Fluctuations in the fetal heart rate around the baseline are described as variability. Variability is a sign of the ability of the fetus' central nervous system to control fetal heart rate during labor. The baseline normally varies by 6 to 25 beats per minute.

Continuous internal electronic monitoring is the most accurate way to detect variability. There are two types of variability, long term and short term (or beat-to-beat). Short-term variability describes the continuous fluctuation of two to three beats per minute at the base. Long-term variability describes the frequency and amplitude of the change in beats per minute; it is expressed in degrees.

Decreased variability is seen with fetal central nervous system depression, administration of drugs to the mother, and fetal sleep. It is indicative of and associated with fetal hypoxia. Decreased variability along with changing baseline or decelerations is called an ominous pattern and requires prompt intervention.

A fetal heart rate pattern that requires no intervention is called an innocuous or reassuring pattern. With such a pattern, there is a normal baseline fetal heart rate, accelerations with no other changes, early decelerations, mild variable decelerations, or normal variability. A nonreassuring pattern is a warning sign of possible problems. This pattern includes a decrease in variability, increase or decrease in the baseline, moderate tachycardia, or intermittent late deceleration with normal variability. An ominous pattern, requires prompt intervention. This pattern includes absence of variability, marked bradycardia, persistent late deceleration with decreasing variability, and variable decelerations with absent variability. Nurses must be alert for and able to recognize these patterns during labor and notify the physician.[33]

Table 40–5 summarizes abnormal fetal heart rate patterns and collaborative and nursing interventions. See Chapter 27 for an in-depth discussion of fetal heart rate patterns.

The nurse should change the client's position to maximize fetal blood flow. Frequent assessment of the monitoring strip should be made for signs of decelerations and absence of variability, and the physician notified if these occur. There is some indication that amnioinfusion, a method of replacing intrauterine amniotic fluid volume through intrauterine infusion of a saline solution using a pressure catheter, may relieve variable decelerations. This treatment requires further investigation.[34]

Pregnancy-Induced Hypertension

Pregnancy-induced hypertension (PIH) is characterized by an elevation in blood pressure (hypertension), the presence of excess serum proteins in the urine (proteinuria), and the retention of water (edema). (*See* Chapter 39 for additional discussion.) It occurs only during pregnancy, labor and delivery, or soon after delivery; is thought to be a progressive disease; and, if not treated aggressively, may lead to convulsions and death.

Pre-eclampsia. Another name for the syndrome that includes hypertension, edema, and proteinuria is pre-

TABLE 40–5. COLLABORATIVE AND NURSING MANAGEMENT OF ABNORMAL FETAL HEART RATE PATTERNS

Pattern	Management
Baseline Fetal Heart Rate	
Tachycardia (161–180 beats per minute)	Observe 10–15 minutes; turn client to left side; hydrate to improve circulating volume; reduce stressors; report findings
Bradycardia (<120 beats per minute)	Observe 10–15 minutes; turn client side to side or in knee-chest position; assess for maternal hypotension and correct; assess for prolapsed cord and correct; prepare for delivery
Variability	
Increased (short-term variability)	Difficult to identify—assess for signs of fetal hypoxia
Decreased (long-term variability)	Position on left side; hydrate; avoid central nervous system depressants; give oxygen by mask; assess fetal heart pattern for other signs of distress
Decelerations	
Early	Usually does not indicate fetal distress—no treatment, differentiate from other deceleration patterns
Late	Position on left side; assess and correct for maternal hypotension; discontinue oxytocin (if in use); administer oxygen by mask; prepare for delivery if pattern does not improve
Variable	Check for prolapse of cord; turn on side or in knee-chest position; give oxygen by mask; hydrate; prepare for emergency delivery if pattern does not improve.

eclampsia. A client with pre-eclampsia in labor must be monitored closely. Blood pressure should be taken at least every 4 hours and more frequently if it begins to rise. The blood pressure should be taken on the same arm and with the client in the same position if readings are to be accurately assessed. Intake and output should be monitored and recorded. A dipstick can be used to check for proteinuria. Edema should be assessed with particular attention to puffiness around the eyes, face, and sacrum. Placing the client in a left lateral position helps to improve blood flow to the uterus as well as to increase the glomerular filtration rate. Signs of central nervous system irritability such as headache, hyperreflexia, and visual signs should be noted and reported immediately. An increase in blood pressure, proteinuria, or edema also should be reported to the physician. The fetal heart rate should be assessed closely, as placental insufficiency is associated with PIH. The client most likely will need explanations about the nursing interventions being used. The nurse can help to reduce the client's anxiety as well as encourage her participation by providing clear explanations. Supporting both the client and her labor partner helps them to cope with a situation they might not fully understand.

Severe Pre-eclampsia/Eclampsia. If the symptoms of pre-eclampsia worsen during labor, the condition becomes an obstetric emergency. Assessment of blood pressure, edema, and urine for protein is done at more frequent intervals. A foley catheter may be placed to facilitate accurate assessment of output. The client is placed on absolute bedrest in a quiet environment to reduce central nervous system stimuli. Electronic monitoring of both mother and fetus is necessary.

Development of severe pre-eclampsia can lead to eclampsia, which is characterized by convulsions and increased maternal and fetal morbidity and mortality. The nurse must ensure that emergency equipment is present in the room and ready to use. This equipment includes oxygen, suction equipment, soft gag, or padded tongue blades, and an airway. Emergency medications may also be included with the equipment as well as an emergency delivery pack. The client and her labor partner will most likely become anxious with the increased activity of the personnel. The nurse should maintain a calm attitude, explain the procedures, and continue to be supportive.

Management is aimed at stabilizing the blood pressure, preventing convulsions, and delivering the fetus as soon as possible. Once the client is stabilized, delivery should proceed. Delivery is the most effective treatment for this condition.

Heart Disease

Management of the pregnant woman with heart disease during labor and delivery is influenced by the functional capacity of the heart. The New York Heart Association classifies heart disease as class I, II, III, or IV, according to the physical signs exhibited by the client (class I being uncompromised and class IV, very compromised). (*See* Chapter 39.)

In general, care of the woman with heart disease during labor focuses on prevention of cardiac decompensation, prevention of cardiac failure, relief of pain, and alleviation of apprehension.[35] Women with class I or II disease are less at risk for cardiac complications than those with class III or IV disease.

The woman labors in a side-lying or semirecumbent position to promote maximal oxygenation and uteroplacental perfusion and to minimize maternal exertion. Respirations are eased by the upright position. The nurse takes vital signs every 15 minutes during the first stage and every 10 minutes during the second stage of labor. A heart rate greater than 100 beats per minute and a respiratory rate greater than 24 per minute are early signs of cardiac failure necessitating intensive medical treatment. Oxygen is administered. The nurse administers and monitors the effects of other medications that may be used, such as intravenous morphine, rapidly acting digitalis, and furosemide. Electronic monitoring of uterine contractions and fetal heart rate is initiated with the onset of labor.

The nurse needs to be sensitive to the anxiety of the couple during the labor and delivery process. Continuous support by the nurse helps to allay the apprehension and fear associated with the woman's heart condition and the process of labor and delivery.

The preferred method of delivery for the woman with heart disease, regardless of functional classification, is vaginal delivery. Cesarean delivery is major surgery and much more taxing on cardiac function than vaginal delivery. Cesarean delivery is limited to such obstetric indications as fetopelvic disproportion. Signs of cardiac decompensation and failure developing after complete dilation and effacement of the cervix are indications for prompt forceps delivery unless easy spontaneous birth is expected within minutes.[4]

Judicious use of analgesia during labor and anesthesia during delivery is required for the woman with a cardiac condition. In some women, especially nulliparas who require greater force and time to deliver the fetus, continuous epidural analgesia has been used. The major danger of conduction analgesia is maternal hypotension, which can further reduce cardiac output.[4] Local anesthetics and pudendal blocks are preferable to general anesthetics for delivery. Oxygen may be continuously administered to the mother during the delivery process.

For women who must deliver by cesarean, a combination of thiopental, succinylcholine, nitrous oxide, and at least 30 percent oxygen has been used. An endotracheal tube should be in place before the anesthetic is administered.[4]

The nurse should carefully monitor the mother during the labor and delivery process, and should assess for any signs of cardiac decompensation in the immediate puerperium. Prompt reporting and management by the interdisciplinary team is essential.

Multiple Gestation

Pregnancy involving multiple fetuses is considered high risk and should be monitored closely during labor and delivery. Complications commonly found with multiple fetuses include preterm labor, uterine dystocia, abnormal fetal presentations, prolapsed umbilical cord, and premature separation of the placenta. Although pregnancies involving more than two fetuses occur, they are far less common than twin pregnancies. Therefore, this section focuses on intrapartum care of the client with twin fetuses.

Maternal Risks. The mother of twin fetuses is prone to postpartum hemorrhage, physical fatigue, and feelings of being overwhelmed with parental responsibilities. Moreover, she may experience a prolonged labor because of uterine dystocia with all its consequences.

Fetal Risks. The greatest risk to both fetuses is prematurity. There may also be a disparity in fetal size, and the first twin may benefit disproportionately from being delivered first.

Nursing and Collaborative Assessment. In pregnancies involving more than one fetus, there are many positions and presentations each fetus may assume. These can be assessed in most instances by real-time sonography. Initially, the health care provider might notice that the uterus is enlarging more rapidly than expected. In addition, the examiner may palpate multiple fetal parts and hear multiple fetal heartbeats.

Nursing and Collaborative Management. Whatever the type of delivery, the use of analgesia and anesthesia for the client with multiple fetuses should be judicious. Because of the possibility of fetal respiratory depression, the choice of analgesia or anesthesia is difficult.

Vaginal Delivery. Vaginal delivery is best accomplished if the first twin is in a cephalic presentation. If the first twin is breech, difficulties occur (eg, prolapse of the umbilical cord) that make cesarean delivery a safer choice.

Delivery of the first twin in a cephalic presentation is the same as any delivery of a fetus in a cephalic presentation. As soon as the first twin is delivered, the second twin should be assessed for presentation, size, and relationship to the birth canal. If the vertex or the breech of the second twin is engaged, moderate fundal pressure is applied and the second set of membranes, if present, is ruptured. Labor resumes and the second twin's heart rate is closely monitored. If contractions do not resume, oxytocin in an intravenous solution may be used to stimulate labor.[36]

If the second twin has moved down the pelvis, delivery occurs spontaneously or with minimal assistance. If the second twin does not enter the pelvic inlet, delivery becomes a problem. The choice may be to deliver the second twin by cesarean, or to manipulate the fetus to facilitate vaginal delivery.

Manipulation of the fetus can be accomplished by internal podalic version: the physician rotates the fetus in utero from a cephalic presentation to a breech presentation, so that the fetus can be extracted[4] (Figure 40–13). The reason for turning the second twin in this manner is to avoid excess trauma to the fetal head during the more difficult second delivery.

Cesarean Delivery. Frequently, twins are delivered by cesarean. Pregnancies with more than two fetuses are nearly always delivered by cesarean to prevent maternal and fetal complications associated with a difficult vaginal delivery.[4,36]

The nurse carefully assesses the client throughout labor and delivery for signs of complications associated with a multiple gestation, such as PIH, uterine dystocia, abnormal fetal heart rates, and pulmonary edema. In the postpartum period, the mother is assessed for hemorrhage and infection. Infants are often placed in neonatal intensive care units for treatment and observation.

Discharge planning includes the same information that is given to parents of one infant and, in addition, information on community resources and support systems available for parents of twins (or other multiple births).

Cord Abnormalities

Abnormalities of the umbilical cord, such as abnormalities of cord insertion and knots or loops in the cord, may affect the course of labor and delivery.

Abnormalities of Cord Insertion. Velamentous insertion of the cord is a condition in which the umbilical vessels of the cord separate in the membranes before reaching the placenta. This condition occurs in approximately 1 percent of all placentas.[36] The primary risk to the fetus is vasa previa during labor. In this situation, the vessels present themselves ahead of the fetus at the internal os. These vessels may rupture during labor and lead to exsanguination of the fetus.

Vaginal examination may allow the practitioner to palpate a tubular fetal vessel in the membranes over the presenting part. Confirmation may be by amnionoscopy, direct observation of the fetus and the color and amount of amniotic fluid by means of a

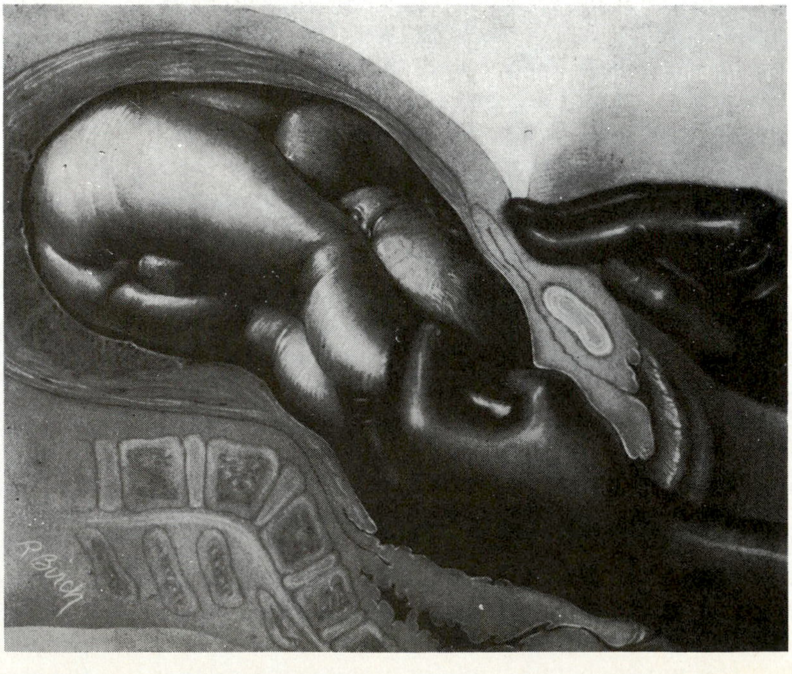

Figure 40–13. Internal podalic version. Upward pressure on the head is applied as downward traction is exerted on feet. (*Reproduced, with permission, from Cunningham FG, et al.* Williams Obstetrics. *18th ed. Norwalk, Conn: Appleton & Lange; 1989:648.*)

specially designed endoscope inserted through the uterine cervix. In addition, painless vaginal bleeding, when tested, will reveal fetal hemoglobin.

If the vessels rupture during labor, there is little hope for fetal survival because of the severe blood loss. Parents require intense nursing support throughout this crisis.

Abnormalities of the Cord That May Affect Blood Flow

Knots in the Umbilical Cord. True knots of the cord occur in about 1.1 percent of deliveries, with a perinatal loss of 6.1 percent. The knots result from active movements of the fetus.[36] As the fetus descends through the birth canal, the knot in the cord tightens, cutting off the flow of oxygenated blood to the fetus and resulting in fetal hypoxia and distress.

Loops of the Umbilical Cord. Loops are formed when the cord becomes coiled around portions of the fetus, usually the neck. One cord loop around the neck is present in 21 percent of deliveries.

As labor progresses, the cord may tighten during a contraction and cause deceleration of the fetal heart rate (variable or late decelerations). There is a risk of fetal death or severe morbidity if the problem is not recognized.

Nursing and Collaborative Assessment. Early recognition and prompt delivery minimize the morbidity and mortality resulting from cord abnormalities that impede blood flow. Most of these abnormalities are first noted by irregularities in the fetal heart rate and pattern. During delivery, the practitioner palpates for a loop of cord around the fetal neck or arm, and removes it or clamps and cuts it.

Nursing and Collaborative Management. The nurse can indirectly assess for cord abnormalities by vigilantly monitoring the fetal heart rate, especially during contractions, when the cord may tighten or become compressed. If an abnormal fetal heart pattern is noted, the physician should be notified immediately. Again, support for the couple is vital throughout this emergency.

Amniotic Fluid Abnormalities

Abnormalities of the amniotic fluid include meconium staining, hydramnios, and oligohydramnios.

- *Meconium-stained amniotic fluid:* Normally, meconium is not noticeably present in amniotic fluid, except in breech presentations. Fetal hypoxia, which produces a fetal defecation reflex, is the major factor contributing to meconium-stained fluid. These fetuses are considered at risk and are closely monitored.
- *Hydramnios (polyhydramnios):* Hydramnios, sometimes called polyhydramnios, is the presence of an excessive quantity of amniotic fluid (greater than 2000 mL). (*See* Chapter 39 for further discussion of this condition during pregnancy.)
- *Oligiohydramnios:* Oligohydramnios is a severe deficiency of amniotic fluid—far below the normal 1000 mL, sometimes as low as a few milliliters of viscous fluid.

Maternal Risks. Meconium staining and oligohydramnios carry no maternal risks. With hydramnios, however, the mother may experience severe dyspnea, edema, and abdominal pain. In some cases, labor may occur prior to the 28th week of gestation.

Fetal Risks. Abnormalities of the amniotic fluid are associated with high fetal risk. Meconium staining of the amniotic fluid may indicate fetal hypoxia.[37] Hydramnios may indicate such congenital conditions as fetal anencephaly, spina bifida, and esophageal atresia. Further, hydramnios has been associated with multiple gestation and isoimmunization.

Oligohydramnios is associated with such fetal abnormalities as pulmonary hypoplasia, obstruction of the fetal urinary tract, and severe intrauterine growth retardation. Oligohydramnios that occurs early in pregnancy can cause amniotic band syndrome, in which parts of the amnion adhere to and constrict parts of the fetus.

Nursing and Collaborative Assessment. The nurse should assess the amniotic fluid after rupture of the membranes. Any variation in color or amount of fluid may signal fetal distress or fluid abnormalities. In addition, antenatal assessments such as uterine measurements and sonography need to be reviewed.

Nursing and Collaborative Management. The fetal heart rate needs to be closely monitored for signs of fetal distress. If the cervix is fully dilated and fetal distress cannot be corrected, the mother is prepared for delivery. A cesarean delivery might be the method of choice.

If overdistension of the uterus is apparent, the mother is watched for uterine dystocia during labor and postpartum hemorrhage. The nurse is responsible for ensuring that the mother is as comfortable as possible during labor. Position change may reduce pressure on the diaphragm for the client with hydramnios.

Placental Abnormalities

Placental abnormalities may also produce problems during labor and delivery. Included are such problems as placenta previa and abruptio placentae. (*See* Chapter 39, for an in-depth discussion of these placental abnormalities.) An additional problem with the placenta may occur during the third stage of labor, if there is an abnormally firm adherence of the placenta to the uterine wall. Fragments or cotyledons of the placenta may tear off and be retained as the placenta is expelled.

Further, the total placenta may adhere to the myometrium (placenta accreta), may invade the myometrium (placenta increta), or may penetrate the full thickness of the myometrium (placenta percreta).[4,36,38]

Maternal Risks. The major risk to the mother with third-stage placental adherence is postpartum hemorrhage. Further, postpartum infection is more common because of the intrauterine manipulation necessary to deliver the placenta.

Nursing and Collaborative Assessment. Inspection of the placenta is imperative to ensure that there are no retained fragments. Delayed spontaneous separation of a placenta may indicate an adherent placenta.

Nursing and Collaborative Management. The delivery of a problem placenta depends on the site of placental implantation, the depth of penetration into the myometrium, and the number of cotyledons involved. When there is minimal adherence of a few placental fragments, manual removal may be attempted. Oxytocin may be used to keep the mother's uterus contracted to prevent hemorrhage.

With total involvement and greater adherence of the placenta, attempts at manual removal will not succeed and may possibly cause severe hemorrhage. Usually, a prompt hysterectomy is done, as there is currently no other adequate management for this obstetric emergency.[36]

Nursing management includes monitoring of maternal vital signs and maternal intake and output, observation for signs of shock and hemorrhage, and replacement of fluids, electrolytes and blood. The nurse must provide empathetic support for the client who might or does undergo hysterectomy, and for her partner, during this crisis.

SUMMARY

Maternal conditions in the intrapartum period include complications related to the powers (uterine contractions), the passenger (the fetus), the passage (the pelvis), and the psyche. In addition, other problems may arise during labor as a result of a pre-existing maternal condition or of abnormalities related to the cord, the amniotic fluid, or the placenta. Such complications during labor or delivery can threaten the lives of mother and fetus. The nurse plays an important role in identifying problems and caring for the family during this time.

Dystocia is the term used to describe a difficult labor. Dystocia related to the powers may be the result of weak, uncoordinated, and ineffective uterine contractions. In hypotonic uterine dysfunction, the pattern of uterine contractions demonstrates a decrease in intensity and in number. Conversely, in a hypotonic contraction pattern, the uterine muscles remain in a state of tension and little force is exerted on the cervix. Dystocia may also be classified according to the division of labor as described by Friedman: preparatory division, dilational division, and pelvic division.

Another problem related to the powers is precipitous labor, labor that lasts less than 3 hours. This problem may cause trauma to the mother and fetus. Additionally, dystocia may result from pathologic retraction rings, of which the most common type is Bandl's ring.

Dystocia related to the passenger may be caused by malpresentation or malposition of the fetus. Prolapse of the umbilical cord is an obstetric emergency that may result from fetal malpresentation. Fetal conditions contributing to fetopelvic or cephalopelvic disproportion also may cause dystocia. For example, a macrosomic or hydrocephalic fetus may be unable to progress through the maternal pelvis.

Dystocia related to the passage may be attributed to the type of pelvis, the diameters of the maternal pelvis, or both. Contractions of the pelvic inlet, midpelvis, or outlet can prolong labor and increase trauma to the mother and fetus.

The state of the maternal psyche is also related to dystocia. Links have been found between psychosocial variables, physiologic variables, and progress in labor and delivery.

Additional complications of labor and delivery

include abnormal fetal heart rate patterns, delivery of multiple fetuses, and pregnancy-induced hypertension. Abnormalities of the cord (eg, knotting), of the placenta (eg, placenta accreta), and the amniotic fluid (eg, meconium staining) also may compromise labor and delivery. Some of these problems are present during pregnancy, but may become acute during the labor and delivery process.

The nurse has an essential role in assessment and management of the client who experiences complications of the intrapartum period. In addition, the nurse is an integral part of the interdisciplinary team and collaborates with other professional colleagues in delivering care to intrapartum families at risk.

REVIEW QUESTIONS

1. Define dystocia. List the four major factors involved in this condition.
2. Define fetopelvic disproportion. Describe two situations in which fetopelvic disproportion might be a problem.
3. Identify interventions that the nurse might employ with a client experiencing malposition.
4. Differentiate between the types of contractions that might prolong labor in the latent phase. Describe the etiology of each and identify collaborative interventions.
5. Describe the psychologic factors that may contribute to complications during labor and delivery.
6. Explain three risks to the fetus in a multiple-fetus pregnancy and birth.

REFERENCES

1. Friedman EA. *Labor: Clinical Evaluation and Management.* 2nd ed. New York: Appleton-Century-Crofts; 1978.
2. O'Driscoll K, et al. Active management of labor as an alternative to cesarean section for dystocia. *Am J Obstet Gynecol.* 1984;63:485–490.
3. Oxorn H, ed. *Human Labor and Birth.* 5th ed. New York: Appleton-Century-Crofts; 1986.
4. Cunningham FG, et al. *Williams Obstetrics.* 18th ed. New York: Appleton & Lange; 1989.
5. Knuppel R, Drukker J. *High Risk Pregnancy, a Team Approach.* Philadelphia: WB Saunders; 1986.
6. Weaver DF. Nurses' views on the meaning of touch in obstetrical nursing practice. *J Obstet Gynecol Neonat Nurs.* 1990;19:157–161.
7. Baumgarten K. Advantages and disadvantages of low amniotomy. *J Perinat Med.* 1976;4:2.
8. Caldeyro-Barcia R, et al. Adverse perinatal effects of early amniotomy during labor. In: Gluck L, ed. *Modern Perinatal Medicine.* Chicago: Year Book Medical; 1974.
9. Marshall C. The act of induction: augmentation of labor. *J Obstet Gynecol Neonat Nurs.* 1985;14:22–28.
10. Takohashi K, et al. Uterine contractility and oxytocin sensitivity in preterm, term, and postterm pregnancy. *Am J Obstet Gynecol.* 1980;136:774.
11. Cibils L. Enhancement and induction of labor. In: Aledjm S, ed. *Risks in the Practice of Modern Obstetrics.* St. Louis: CV Mosby; 1975:182–209.
12. Stephany T. Terbutaline sulfate for treating tetanic contractions. *Am J Matern Child Nurs.* 1985;10:349–395.
13. Friedman EA. The functional divisions of labor. *Am J Obstet Gynecol.* 1971;109:274–280.
14. Riffel H. Abnormal fetal presentation or lie. *J Perinatol.* 1990;10:217–219.
15. Seeds JW, Cefalo RC. Malpresentations. *Clin Obstet Gynecol.* 1982;25:145–154.
16. Bowers WA, Taylor ES. Breech delivery: evaluation of the method of delivery on the perinatal results and maternal morbidity. *Obstet Gynecol.* 1975;135:965.
17. Pettite DB, Golditch IM. Mortality in relation to method of delivery in breech infants. *Int J Gynecol Obstet.* 1984;12:189–193.
18. Wade RV, Taylor TR. Breech delivery: impact of increasing cesarean delivery. *South Med J.* 1981;74:10.
19. Green JE, et al. Has an increased cesarean rate for the term breech delivery reduced the incidence of birth asphyxia, trauma, and death? *Am J Obstet Gynecol.* 1974;118:790.
20. Gimovsky ME, Petrie R. Breech delivery. In: Queenan J, ed. *Management of High Risk Pregnancy.* 2nd ed. Oradell, NJ: Medical Economics Books; 1985;601–609.
21. Gimovsky M, Petrie R, Optimal method of delivery of the low birth weight breech fetus: an unresolved issue. *J Perinatol.* 1988;8:141–144.
22. Stein A. Breech delivery: a cooperative nurse-midwifery medical management approach. *J Nurse Midwifery.* 1986;31:93–97.
23. Acker DB, et al. Risk factors for shoulder dystocia in the average weight infant. *Obstet Gynecol.* 1986;67:614–618.
24. Harris B. Shoulder dystocia. *Clin Obstet Gynecol.* 1984;27:106.
25. McCall JO. Shoulder dystocia: a study of after effects. *Am J Obstet Gynecol.* 1982;83:1486–1489.
26. Hartfield VJ. Symphysiotomy for shoulder dystocia. *Am J Obstet Gynecol.* 1986;155:228.
27. Sandberg EC. The Zavanelli Maneuver extended: progression of a revolutionary concept. *Am J Obstet Gynecol.* 1988;158:1374.
28. Kennedy JL, Greenwald E. Correlation of shoe size and obstetric outcome: an anthropometric study. *Am J Obstet Gynecol* 1981;140:466–467.
29. Lederman R, et al. Relationship of psychological factors in pregnancy to progress in labor. In: Sherwen LN, Weingarten CT, eds. *Analysis and Application of Nursing Research: Parent-Neonate Studies.* Monterey, Calif: Wadsworth; 1983.
30. Sakala E, Henry R. Fathers in the cesarean section room and maternal/neonatal/outcome. *J Perinatol.* 1988;8:342–344.
31. Erickson M. The relationship between psychological variables and specific complications of pregnancy, labor and delivery. *J Psychosomat Res.* 1976;20:21.

32. Holmes S, Magiera L. *Maternity Nursing.* New York: MacMillan; 1987.
33. Freeman RK, Garite TJ. *Fetal Heart Rate Monitoring.* Baltimore: Williams & Wilkins; 1981.
34. Galvan B, et al. Using amnioinfusion for the relief of repetitive variable decelerations during labor. *J Obstet Gynecol Neonat Nurs.* 1989;18:222–230.
35. Schmidt J, et al. Peripartum cardiomyopathy. *J Obstet Gynecol Neonat Nurs.* 1989;18:465–475.
36. Pernoll M, Benson R, eds. *Current Obstetrics and Gynecologic Diagnosis and Treatment.* Norwalk, Conn: Appleton & Lange; 1987.
37. Hageman J, et al. Delivery room management of meconium staining of the amniotic fluid and the development of meconium aspiration syndrome. *J Perinatol.* 1988;8:127–131.
38. Filardo J, Nagey P. An unusual presentation: placenta percreta with uterine conservation. *J Perinatol.* 1990;10:206–208.

Maternal Conditions in the Postpartum Period

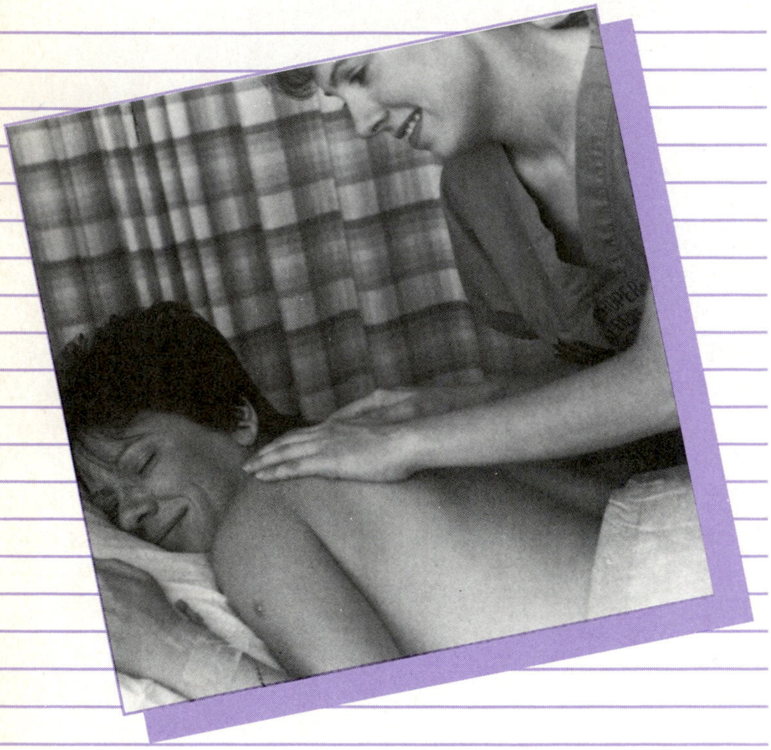

Chapter 41

Key Terms

bacteremia
cystitis
deep venous thrombosis
mastitis
metritis
oophoritis
parametrial cellulitis
peritonitis
postpartum depression
postpartum psychosis
puerperal morbidity
salpingitis
septic pelvic thrombophlebitis
subinvolution
superficial venous thrombosis

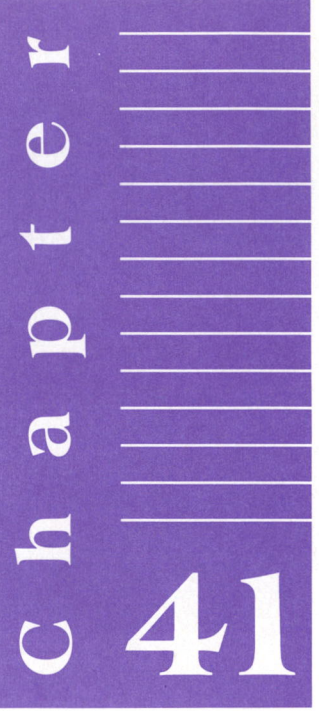

Addition of a new family member is a stressor that may, in the postpartum period, produce a maturational crisis forcing the family to make changes in its organization. Families whose transition to parenthood is complicated by physiologic or psychologic stressors that threaten family integrity experience a concurrent situational crisis. The extent of the crisis is determined by the nature of the stressor, the number of crisis events facing the family at the same time, the way in which the family defines the crisis, the internal and external resources available to the family, and the ability of the family to change and adapt to the crisis event.[1]

A variety of stressors can produce a situational crisis in the postpartum period. Chapters 42 and 43 describe physiologic stressors of the newborn that have a major effect on the restructuring of family dynamics. This chapter discusses the major physiologic and psychologic disorders that may affect the new mother.

Complications of the postpartum period include physiologic conditions such as maternal postpartum hemorrhage, puerperal infections, and thromboembolic disorders, and psychologic conditions, such as postpartum depression. These complications can cause disruption in the family system and may also threaten the life of the mother. Prompt assessment and management by the interdisciplinary team are essential to the resolution of these potentially life-threatening maternal disorders.

Through the collaborative effort of the interdisciplinary team the family is helped to cope with complications and with their transition to the new roles resulting from addition of a new family member. The nurse has an important role in implementing and evaluating appropriate care for families experiencing postpartum complications.

POSTPARTUM HEMORRHAGE

Hemorrhage during pregnancy is the third leading cause of maternal mortality in the United States and the leading cause of maternal death in underdeveloped countries. Specifically, postpartum hemorrhage ranks as the most common cause of excessive blood loss during the childbearing cycle.[2]

The life-threatening nature of hemorrhage and the perception that "pregnancy is not supposed to end this way" combine to engender fear and anxiety in family members. This is often compounded by fears that may be associated with some forms of treatment, for example, fear of blood transfusion because of the possible transmission of human immunodeficiency virus.

Postpartum hemorrhage has been defined as the loss of greater than 500 mL of blood in the period following the third stage of labor in a vaginal delivery.[2] Although this definition is used by most authorities today, it is currently being questioned.[3] It has been estimated that about one half of women who deliver vaginally and almost all those who deliver by cesarean routinely lose 500 mL of blood or more; however, women who attain a normal degree of pregnancy hypervolemia (increase in blood volume of 30 to 50 percent) tolerate a blood loss at delivery approaching the blood volume added during pregnancy (ie, 1000 to 2000 mL).[3] Some authorities have therefore, labeled postpartum hemorrhage as "mild" when the blood loss is 750 to 1250 mL.[4] A hemorrhage is considered "severe" when blood loss is greater than 1250 mL in a woman with normal hypervolemia of pregnancy having a vaginal delivery. In a cesarean delivery, hemorrhage is a potential problem, but is usually related more to the surgical procedure and repair than to compromised involution.

Postpartum hemorrhage is further defined according to the stage in the postpartum period during which the hemorrhage occurs. Early postpartum hemorrhage is defined as hemorrhage occurring within the first 24 hours of delivery. Late postpartum hemorrhage can occur at any time from 24 hours to 6 weeks postdelivery. Postpartum hemorrhage occurs in 5 to 8 percent[2] of vaginal deliveries; however, the incidence of postpartum hemorrhage serious enough to cause hypovolemic shock is less than 0.5 percent.[5,6]

Early Postpartum Hemorrhage

The two most common causes of early postpartum hemorrhage are uterine atony and lacerations of the perineum, vagina, and cervix.[3] These lacerations may also be responsible for vulvular hematomas.

Uterine Atony. Uterine atony (hypotonic uterus) is the inability of the myometrium of the uterus to contract around the blood vessels supplying the site of implantation of the placenta. It is the most common cause of postpartum hemorrhage, occurring in 50 percent of cases.[2]

Risk Factors. Table 41–1 lists several risk factors that predispose the postpartum woman to uterine atony. Overdistension of the uterus as a result of multiple gestation or polyhydramnios is one such risk factor. The uterus is unlikely to contract firmly after overdistension and blood loss may be considerable. For example, blood loss after delivery of twins may be nearly twice that associated with the delivery of a single fetus.[3]

TABLE 41–1. RISK FACTORS PREDISPOSING THE POSTPARTUM WOMAN TO UTERINE ATONY

Overdistension of the uterus
Multiple gestation
Polyhydramnios
Use of general anesthesia
Halothane or other halogenated compounds
Abnormal labor
Prolonged labor
Precipitous labor
Oxytocin induction or augmentation
Mismanagement of the third stage of labor
Uterine infection
Uterine tumors
Grand multiparity
Bladder distension
Disseminated intravascular coagulation
Previous history of uterine atony

Another risk factor associated with uterine atony is the use of general anethesia, such as Halothane or other halogenated compounds, especially during cesarean delivery.[7] General anesthetics may relax the uterus, predisposing the woman to uterine relaxation postdelivery.

Prolonged labor and precipitous (very rapid) labor also are associated with postpartum uterine atony. The uterus that fails to contract normally or that contracts with extreme vigor during labor is likely to be hypotonic after delivery because of the unusual workload placed on the myometrium before delivery. Oxytocin induction or augmentation during labor may result in a hypotonic uterus postpartally because of the vigorous contractions produced during labor and delivery.

Mismanagement of the third stage of labor can provoke uterine atony. Constant squeezing of the contracted uterus in an attempt to separate the placenta may result in incomplete separation, adherent pieces of placenta, uterine atony, and increased blood loss.[3] To avoid this, the placenta should be allowed to deliver spontaneously.

Uterine infection is another cause of uterine atony postdelivery. Infection inhibits contractility of the myometrium, which in turn causes excessive blood loss.

Other risk factors implicated in early postpartum hemorrhage include uterine tumors, grand multiparity, bladder distension, and blood coagulation disorders such as disseminated intravascular coagulation. A woman with a history of uterine atony should be watched carefully for uterine atony with the present pregnancy.

Nursing and Collaborative Assessment. Nurses should carefully assess postpartum clients for normal uterine involution, with particular attention to women with risk factors. Risk factors for uterine atony should be identified preferably prior to delivery of the infant. Nursing care in the immediate postpartum period also includes assessment of vital signs; contractility and position of the uterus; amount, color, and odor of lochia; and intake and output.

Temperature, pulse, respirations, and blood pressure are assessed every 15 minutes for the first hour after delivery or until stable, and thereafter at half-hour intervals for 1 hour and every 4 hours subsequently. If the postpartum client is receiving blood, her vital signs should be assessed every hour once they are stable.[5]

A temperature above 100.4°F (38°C) may indicate uterine infection, which may predispose the client to uterine atony (*see* "Postpartum Infections" later in this chapter). A pulse rate between 50 and 70 beats per minute may be normal in the postpartum period. Higher pulse rates, or tachycardia, may indicate hypovolemia resulting from postpartum hemorrhage. Respirations are generally normal during the postpartum period unless hemorrhage is severe. The respirations may be increased or diminished when excessive blood loss occurs. The respirations also may be increased because of maternal anxiety when a complication such as hemorrhage occurs. Blood pressure in the postpartum period should be consistent with the maternal prenatal blood pressure. A sudden drop in blood pressure may indicate postpartum hemorrhage.

Although the preceding parameters are useful as guidelines, problems can occur in using pulse and blood pressure as indicators of postpartum hemorrhage. Pulse and blood pressure may not change significantly until large amounts of blood have been lost. The woman with a normal blood pressure initially may become hypertensive in response to hemorrhage; the woman who is hypertensive may have blood pressure readings that appear normal, even though she is severely hypovolemic.[3] It is thus imperative that other parameters be assessed when hemorrhage resulting from uterine atony is suspected.

Contractility of the Uterus. The nurse should assess the tone or contractility of the uterus a minimum of every 15 minutes during the first 24 hours postdelivery in women who are at risk for or suspected of having uterine atony. Uterine tone is assessed by palpating the fundus for firmness and location (*see* Chapter 29). A soft, boggy fundus may indicate uterine atony; however, a fundus that is deviated to one side (instead of being in the midline) may merely indicate a full bladder. The nurse should ask the mother to void and then reassess the fundus for firmness after voiding. If the uterus becomes firm after the mother voids, then the uterine atony is probably related to bladder distension.

If the fundus is found to be soft and boggy, the nurse gently massages the area and observes for any tissue or clots that may be expelled from the vagina. The expulsion of clots or tissue may indicate uterine atony caused by retention of placental fragments and should be reported to the physician or certified nurse-midwife immediately. In the presence of a soft and boggy fundus, assessment of the lochia is paramount.

Lochia. The lochia is assessed for amount, odor, and quality each time the fundus is assessed. When assessing the lochia, the nurse should wear disposable gloves, a recommended universal precaution against the transmission of human immunodeficiency virus and other bloodborne infections. The amount of lochia is assessed by observing the saturation level of the peripads. Complete saturation of one pad (60 to 100 mL of lochia) within 15 minutes or saturation of two or more pads within 1 hour suggests hemorrhage.[8] The lochia should also be assessed for the presence of clots or tissue, which along with a soft, boggy uterus may indicate retention of placental fragments. Foul-smelling lochia may indicate infection.

Other Assessment Parameters. Hemoglobin and hematocrit are routinely assessed during the postpartum period. If the hemoglobin and hematocrit are low, assessment is repeated at least once a day. Postpartum hemoglobin and hematocrit values that fall below prelabor values indicate that the woman has sustained considerable blood loss.

Intake and output are assessed every hour in women experiencing postpartum uterine atony. Adequate intake and low output may indicate kidney dysfunction or even failure as a result of severe hypovolemia in postpartum hemorrhage.

The postpartum client is observed for pallor, fatigue, and anxiety. Throughout the assessment, the nurse should carefully explain the assessment procedures to the client and her family. Knowledge of the assessment steps and management plan helps to reduce client anxiety associated with fear of the unknown. By showing the client how to palpate her fundus and assess her lochia, the nurse helps her to feel in control of her own care. Questioning the client about her status can also elicit valuable information. Complaints such as pain, lethargy, and fatigue may

NURSING DIAGNOSES RELATED TO UTERINE ATONY

Problem-Oriented

Potential fluid volume deficit, related to excessive postpartal blood loss

Fatigue, related to blood loss from uterine atony

Fear, related to diagnosis, assessment, and treatment of uterine atony

Knowledge deficit, related to diagnosis and treatment of uterine atony

Strength-Oriented

Asset in physiologic functioning, related to good prenatal care, normal pregnancy hypervolemia, and nutrition

Family coping: potential for effective coping, related to previous positive family coping strategies

Potential for effective crisis resolution, related to physiologic assets of mother, definition of the event, and appropriate resources

give clues to the cause of the hemorrhage and the degree of hypovolemia.

Nursing Diagnosis. Nursing diagnoses are made after careful assessment of the woman with postpartum atony. *See* the box for examples.

Nursing and Collaborative Management. All pregnant women should be assessed for the risk of postpartum hemorrhage in the prenatal and intrapartum periods. Women who are identified as being at risk should have their blood typed and cross-matched, and blood should be available postdelivery if a transfusion is indicated.

When the client is identified to be at risk or when excessive bleeding occurs with an atonic uterus, the physician usually explores the uterus for retained placental fragments. Even a well-contracted uterus should be examined in the following cases:[2]

1. In vaginal birth after cesarean delivery
2. When intrauterine manipulation has occurred during delivery (eg, version and extraction)
3. When malpresentation of the fetus has occurred (eg, breech)
4. When a premature infant has been delivered

After delivery, the fundus is massaged until it becomes firm. Excessive or vigorous massage should be avoided as it may interfere with normal contraction of the uterus.[2] Oxytocics are often administered to enhance contraction of the uterus. Oxytocin (Pitocin) 10 to 60 units is added to a liter bottle of intravenous solution and administered to the client. Methylergonovine maleate (Methergine) 0.2 mg also may be given intramuscularly or intravenously (if the client is not hypertensive) to contract the uterus. In addition, the woman may be prone to intrauterine infection. Strategies to prevent infection, such as meticulous aseptic technique, are important.

When uterine atony persists, despite the use of oxytocics and manual massage of the fundus, other treatment is indicated. Treatment for controlling uterine atony includes bimanual compression of the uterus, administration of prostaglandins, and, in very severe cases, pressure occlusion of the aorta, ligation of the uterine and hypogastric arteries, and hysterectomy.

Bimanual Compression and Massage. Bimanual compression of the uterus is done by the physician to control postpartum hemorrhage. The physician places one gloved hand on the client's abdomen, grasping the fundus and pushing it down toward the symphysis pubis. The other gloved hand is inserted into the vagina with the closed fist pressing against the uterus. The physician maintains compression for as long as 20 to 30 minutes, while using both hands to massage the uterus, one externally and one internally (Figure 41–1).

An intravenous solution, for example, lactated Ringer's solution with oxytocin, is administered. A blood transfusion also may be ordered concurrently in severe cases of hypovolemia to replace blood loss.

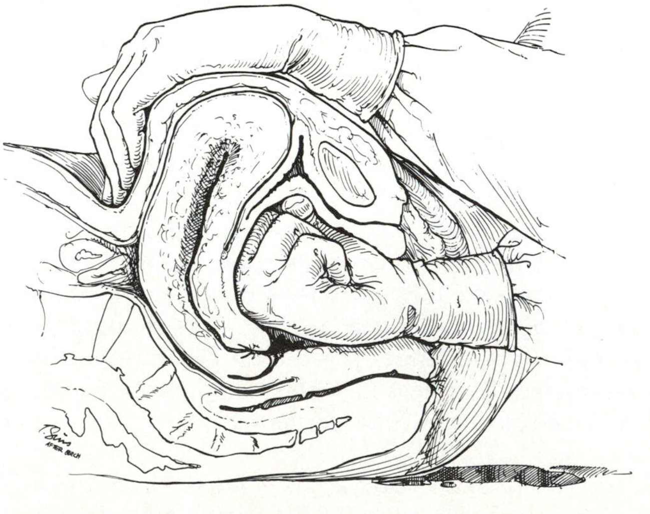

Figure 41–1. Bimanual compression and massage of uterus. (*Reproduced, with permission, from Cunningham FG, et al.* Williams Obstetrics. *18th ed. Norwalk, Conn: Appleton & Lange; 1989:418.*)

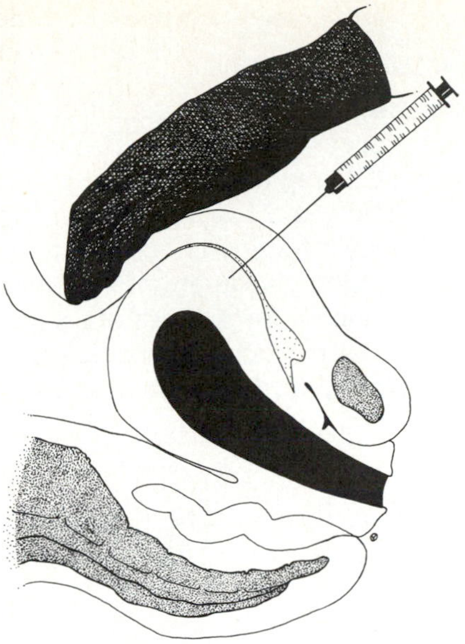

Figure 41–2. Transabdominal intramyometrial injection of prostaglandin F_2 alpha. (*Reproduced, with permission, from Oxorn H, ed.* Oxorn-Foote Human Labor and Birth. *5th ed. Norwalk, Conn: Appleton-Century-Crofts; 1985:489.*)

Some authorities suggest that a Foley catheter be inserted to prevent distension of the bladder and facilitate bimanual compression and massage.[2]

Administration of Prostaglandins. Management of severe postpartum hemorrhage may include the administration of prostaglandins. Transabdominal intramyometrial injection of prostaglandin F_2 alpha (Figure 41–2) and insertion of prostaglandin E_2 vaginal suppositories have been used to control postpartum hemorrhage.[9,10] A more recent treatment is intramuscular injection of a 15-methyl prostaglandin analogue, carboprost tromethamine (Prostin/15 M).[11] Carboprost tromethamine has been found to be effective in the management of severe postpartum hemorrhage.[12] The client may experience side effects associated with the administration of prostaglandins, including nausea, vomiting, diarrhea, and slight fever.[11]

Operative Management. If the bleeding cannot be controlled by the preceding treatments, surgery may be required. After laparotomy, the physician may obtain immediate temporary control of the bleeding by pressure occlusion of the aorta for several minutes in an otherwise healthy woman. This gives the physician time to try to locate and control the cause of the bleeding.[2]

If measures to control hemorrhage fail, the physician may need to ligate the uterine or hypogastric arteries. Ligation of these arteries may substantially control bleeding without cutting off the supply of blood to the uterus and pelvic structures, as the collateral circulation is usually sufficient to maintain the viability of the pelvic tissue.[13] If hemorrhage cannot be controlled, the physician may perform a hysterectomy (removal of the uterus) as a lifesaving measure.

The woman with postpartum hemorrhage requires intensive nursing care. Vital signs must be monitored and an accurate record of intake and output maintained. The nurse also anticipates the various therapies, for example, bimanual compression and intravenous therapy, and prepares the client and her family accordingly. Simple and clear explanations are given. Mobilizing family social support is also an important function of the nurse. Family coping is enhanced by comprehensive and holistic nursing care during the crisis experience. (*See* the Case Study/Care Plan.)

CASE STUDY/CARE PLAN: POSTPARTUM HEMORRHAGE FOLLOWING DELIVERY OF TWINS

Nancy Garcia is a gravida 3 para 3, 38-year-old-married woman. Her previous deliveries were normal spontaneous vaginal deliveries at term; the infants weighed 7 lbs 5 oz and 7 lbs 12 oz respectively. Her prenatal and postpartum periods were uneventual. The children are now 6 years and 4 years old. Nancy was diagnosed as having a twin pregnancy at 20 weeks of gestation. With the exception of discomforts associated with multiple pregnancy, her prenatal course was uneventful.

After a six hour labor, Nancy delivered fraternal twins vaginally at 37 weeks gestation. Lidocaine 1 percent was administered to the perineum and a right medial lateral episiotomy was performed. The twins weighed 5 lbs 10 oz and 5 lbs 8 oz respectively.

(*continued*)

CASE STUDY/CARE PLAN: Postpartum Hemorrhage Following Delivery of Twins (*continued*)

Immediately following the delivery, Nancy's fundus is assessed as being firm, located at the umbilicus and midline. The lochia is moderate rubra. Her blood pressure is 126/70, pulse 68, respirations 14 and temperature 99°F. She is given Methergine 0.2 mg IM after delivery and is also receiving Pitocin 20 units in 1000 mL lactated Ringer's solution at 21 drops per minute IV.

Within the first half hour after the delivery of the twins, Nancy's fundus is assessed by the nurse as being soft and boggy, located 2 cm above the umbilicus. Her lochia is bright red, and the peripad almost completely saturated. On gentle massage of the fundus, large clots are expelled. Nancy's vital signs are BP 120/70, pulse 68, temperature 99°F. The physician is notified and the nurse stays with Nancy and her husband, Rick, reassessing Nancy at frequent intervals and attempting to allay the anxiety displayed by the couple.

Supporting Assessment Data	Expected Client/Family Outcome	Nursing Action/ Intervention	Rationale	Criteria for Evaluation
Nursing Diagnosis: Fluid volume deficit: potential, related to hemorrhage secondary to overdistended uterus after delivery of twins				
Gravida 3 para 3; multiple gestation: twins delivered vaginally. Twin A weighs 5 lbs 10 oz; twin B 5 lbs 8 oz	During the postpartum period, the client will: Maintain adequate blood volume	Assess vital signs, fundal tone and height, and lochia q 5 minutes.	Changes in vital signs, especially pulse and blood pressure, as well as fundal tone and lochia, may indicate significant blood loss.	Client's vital signs remain within normal limits; blood loss is minimized.
Weights of previous newborns: 7 lbs 5 oz, 7 lbs 12 oz Soft, boggy fundus located 2 cm above umbilicus at midline Lochia bright red; peripad almost completely saturated; large clots expelled	Maintain vital signs, urinary output, and blood loss within normal limits	Gently massage fundus if uterus is boggy.	A boggy uterus contracts with gentle massage. Overstimulation of the uterus through vigorous massage can cause uterine musculature to relax and provoke further hemorrhage.	After gentle fundal massage, the client's uterus continues to contract and become firm.
Methergine 0.2 mg IM given after delivery Pitocin 20 U in 1000 mL lactated Ringer's infusing at 21 gtts/min IV Vital signs: blood pressure 126/70, pulse 68, temperature 99°F, respirations 16		Monitor infusion rate and intake and output.	Intravenous infusion of oxytocin in solution provides the client with needed fluids and medication to contract uterus. Intake should approximate output. Output may be diminished if hypovolemia from postpartum hemorrhage occurs.	Client's intake approximates output; uterus contracts with minimal blood loss in response to oxytocin administration.
		Assess and record amount, color, quality of vaginal bleeding. Save all clots and tissues for inspection. Weigh pads.	Clots or tissue indicate possible retained placental tissue. Client's replacement needs are met on the basis of the estimated blood loss; 1 mL of blood weighs 1 g.	Within 1 hour, less than two pads are saturated; no further clots or tissue are noted.

Supporting Assessment Data	Expected Client/Family Outcome	Nursing Action/ Intervention	Rationale	Criteria for Evaluation
		Observe client for fatigue and pallor.	Pallor and fatigue are signs of blood loss and anemia.	Client maintains normal color; energy level is appropriate to postpartum period.
		Monitor hemoglobin and hematocrit values.	Values that fall below prelabor values indicate significant blood loss.	Client's hemoglobin and hematocrit values remain consistent with prelabor values throughout postpartum hospital stay.
Nursing Diagnosis: Potential for infection, related to hemorrhage secondary to overdistended uterus after delivery of twins				
Fundus soft and boggy; lochia bright red, free from odor; temperature 99°F taken orally	Throughout the postpartum period, the client will: Remain free of infection	Assess vital signs (temperature, pulse, respirations).	A temperature of 100.4°F or higher on two consecutive readings after the first 24 hours indicates infection; elevated pulse and respirations may also indicate infection.	During the postpartum period: Client's vital signs remain within normal limits.
	Maintain vital signs within normal limits; lochia free from foul odor	Monitor lochia for color, amount, odor; involution of uterus; uterine tenderness.	Lochia becomes foul smelling with infection; uterus may become atonic and tender with infection.	Client's lochia is free of foul odor; uterine involution proceeds normally with no tenderness or pain.
		Observe client for fatigue, pallor, loss of appetite, chills.	Fatigue, pallor, loss of appetite, chills may indicate systemic infection.	Client demonstrates no signs of systemic infection.
		Maintain hydration; monitor intake and output.	Adequate fluid intake prevents dehydration and replaces fluids lost; intake and output should approximate each other.	Client remains well hydrated, with fluid intake approximating output.
		Assess for pain or tenderness; provide comfort measures to alleviate pain.	Tenderness is a sign of uterine infection. Comfort measures aid in relaxation and reduction of anxiety, which helps client to cope with pain.	Client behaviors indicate that she is free of uterine pain or tenderness. She appears relaxed and comfortable.
		Administer medications as indicated and ordered by physician.	Medications may include prophylactic antibiotics to aid in combatting specific infections.	Client remains free from infection throughout the postpartum period.
		Instruct client in self-care practices: rest, proper diet, handwashing, perineal care.	Self-care practices help to prevent infection.	When asked, client is able to describe self-care practices that prevent infection.

Lacerations. Lacerations of the perineum, vagina, and cervix, along with excessive bleeding from an episiotomy, cause about 20 percent of the cases of early postpartum hemorrhage.[2] The more extensive the laceration, the greater the danger to the mother. See the box for a description of lacerations.

Risk Factors. Risk factors predisposing clients to excessive bleeding from lacerations include forceps delivery, precipitous or rapid delivery, and delivery of a large infant or multiple infants. Lacerations also may occur after a normal spontaneous delivery.

Nursing and Collaborative Assessment. The physician or nurse-midwife should carefully inspect for lacerations after delivery. Trauma of the genital tract can be associated with significant blood loss, even though the bleeding does not appear to be excessive. For example, a laceration of the cervix may cause slow, steady bleeding, which may be overlooked, especially if the fundus is well contracted. Lacerations of blood vessels beneath the vaginal or vulvar epithelium may cause bleeding into the tissue beneath the vulva over several hours, and result in a large retroperitoneal hematoma. Tears in the uterine lining or musculature may cause uterine atony[3] and, as a consequence, hemorrhage.

The nurse should carefully assess the perineum postdelivery for *r*edness, *e*dema, *e*cchymosis, *d*ischarge, and *a*pproximation (REEDA).[14] The edges of the episiotomy or repaired lacerations should be approximated (ie, the two edges of the suture line should be brought close to each other), and there should be no discharge or bleeding from the site. Important parameters to assess when lacerations are suspected are the same as those for uterine atony: vital signs, contractility of the uterus, lochia, hemoglobin and hematocrit, intake and output, pallor, fatigue, and anxiety. Vital signs should be assessed at least every 15 minutes until stable. The quantity and quality of lochia and any steady, bright red bleeding, which may indicate hemorrhage, are noted. Intake and output are recorded, and the client is observed for signs of pallor, fatigue, and lethargy.

LACERATIONS

Perineum

First degree: extends through skin
Second degree: extends through muscles of perineal body
Third degree: extends through perineal body to anal sphincter
Fourth degree: extends through perineal body and anal sphincter and involves rectal wall

Vagina

Longitudinal tears of upper vagina
Lacerations of vulva and lower vagina
  Superficial tears
  Deep lacerations that may include urethra, labia minora, clitoris, and bladder

Cervix

Superficial lacerations, usually at 3 and 9 o'clock positions
Extensive lacerations of lower uterine segment

Nursing and Collaborative Management. The client and her partner should be given clear, concise explanations of the cause of the hemorrhage and of the steps in its assessment and management. Uncertainty about what is happening may increase the couple's anxiety. If surgical repair of lacerations is indicated, the couple should be informed and supported by the nurse throughout the procedures.

Lacerations that are bleeding should be repaired by the physician with interrupted figure-eight sutures. The highest suture is placed above the apex of the tear. A cervical or vaginal laceration extending into the broad ligament is usually repaired by laparotomy.[2,3]

The nurse continues to observe the client after surgical repair of the lacerations. Vital signs, fundal firmness, and lochia are assessed and intake and output recorded. If trauma to the perineum has occurred, an ice pack is applied to the perineal area for the first 24 hours to reduce swelling. After the initial ice treatment, heat in the form of sitz baths may be used to increase circulation and promote healing. One recent study found that there was no difference between the effects of heat and cold on perineal healing after episiotomy/laceration in the first 24 hours after delivery[15]; however, these findings remain to be confirmed.

Once the client is stabilized, she is encouraged to perform Kegel exercises to promote healing of the pubococcygeal muscle.[16] Analgesics such as oral acetaminophen and analgesic sprays applied to the perineal area may be offered to minimize discomfort (*see* Chapter 31).

Hematomas. Bleeding into the connective tissue beneath the vaginal mucosa or vulvar skin may cause the formation of vaginal and vulvar hematomas (Figure 41–3). Vulvar hematomas are identified as bulg-

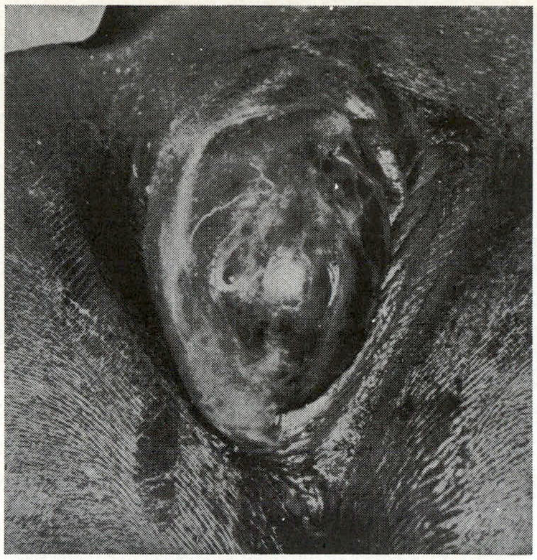

Figure 41–3. Vulvar hematoma bulging into the right vaginal wall. (*Reproduced, with permission, from Cunningham FG, et al.* Williams Obstetrics. *18th ed. Norwalk, Conn: Appleton & Lange; 1989:482*)

ing masses covered by discolored skin. Vaginal hematomas may be concealed. Hematomas develop as a result of injury to tissues with spontaneous as well as operative deliveries (eg, forceps). In the early stages, a rounded swelling protrudes into the upper portion of the vagina and projects upward toward the diaphragm if the bleeding continues. This condition can be especially dangerous because the bleeding is concealed and can go unrecognized until symptoms of shock occur.[2,3]

Nursing and Collaborative Assessment. One of the first signs of hematoma may be complaints of pain, pressure, or inability to void. It is imperative that the nurse assess the site of the discomfort and report the findings to the physician or nurse-midwife. When a vulvar hematoma is suspected, the perineum is inspected for signs of a discolored mass. When a vaginal hematoma is suspected, a vaginal examination should be done to confirm its presence. The nurse should notify the physician or nurse-midwife immediately if hematoma is suspected.

The other assessment parameters associated with hemorrhage should guide the nurse. Vital signs should be taken. Increased pulse, decreased pulse pressure, and decreased blood pressure may indicate hypovolemia, even in the absence of visible signs of the hematoma. The client should also be assessed for pallor, clamminess, and anemia (decreased hemoglobin and hematocrit), which are additional signs of hypovolemia caused by hemorrhage. (*See* earlier discussions of assessment for uterine atony and lacerations.)

Nursing and Collaborative Management. Small vulvar hematomas may absorb spontaneously without operative management. Ice and heat treatments may help to reduce the swelling and discomfort. When large or expanding hematomas of the vaginal walls are identified, however, incision and evacuation of the hematoma by the physician constitute the treatments of choice.

Hematomas may result in considerable loss of blood. Fluid and blood replacement is therefore indicated to prevent hypovolemia in cases where blood loss is excessive. Broad-spectrum antibiotic therapy also has been useful in controlling secondary infection.[3]

Nursing care focuses on judicious assessment of the mother and comfort measures—for example, cold and heat treatments and analgesics—to help alleviate the pain associated with hematoma. If surgical treatment is indicated, the nurse prepares the client and her family for the procedure and carefully monitors the client's vital signs and perineum during and after the surgery.

Late Postpartum Hemorrhage

Late postpartum hemorrhage may develop within days of delivery or later in the postpartum period. An important consideration when dealing with late postpartum hemorrhage is that the client may be at home when the symptoms occur. It is thus important that prior to discharge from the health care facility, the nurse teaches the client and her partner the signs of normal involution, as well as those signs and symptoms related to problems.

Late or delayed postpartum hemorrhage may be the result of **subinvolution** (delayed involution) of the uterus or, less commonly, retention of placental fragments. The exact cause of subinvolution of the uterus is unknown; however, faulty placental implantation and infection at the implantation site have been suggested as possible causes.[2]

Retention of placental fragments also may induce a sequence of events resulting in late postpartum hemorrhage. The retained portion of the placenta undergoes necrosis, forming fibrin deposits. These deposits form a placental polyp, which eventually detaches from the myometrium, causing hemorrhage. Retained placenta tissue is also associated with mismanagement of the third stage of labor, placental accreta, and manual removal of the placenta.[3]

Nursing and Collaborative Assessment. It is important that the client and her partner be taught how to assess the lochia and fundus in the postpartum period. The nurse should carefully explain the normal pattern of uterine involution and lochia flow and they are taught to report any abnormalities, such as bright red bleeding, excessive clots, persistent lochia rubra, prolonged lochial discharge, foul-smelling lochia, a soft boggy fundus, and pain in the perineum, rectum, abdomen, or back. The client is taught to massage her fundus and assess whether it becomes firm in response to the massage or remains soft and boggy. The client also assesses the height of the fundus during the postpartum period.

The diagnosis of subinvolution is confirmed by bimanual pelvic examination. The uterus is found to be larger than normal for the particular postpartum stage.[3] Retained placental tissue may be visualized by ultrasonography.[17]

Nursing Diagnosis. After assessment of the woman with delayed postpartum hemorrhage, nursing diagnoses are developed. *See* the box for examples.

Nursing and Collaborative Management. The woman with delayed postpartum hemorrhage is often hospitalized, which can be a stressful experience both for her and her family. Uncertainty about her condition as well as separation from the infant and other family members can increase the client's feelings of fear and anxiety. She often feels guilty that she cannot care for her infant. The nurse can act as a social support to the family during this stressful period. By thoroughly explaining the condition and the treatment to the client and her partner, the nurse can help to alleviate some of their anxiety. The nurse can encourage frequent communication between the client and alternate caretakers for the infant to help the client cope with the hospitalization.

NURSING DIAGNOSES RELATED TO DELAYED POSTPARTUM HEMORRHAGE

Problem-Oriented

Altered maternal role performance, related to hospitalization for management of delayed postpartum hemorrhage

Knowledge deficit, related to symptoms and management of delayed postpartum hemorrhage

Strength-Oriented

Potential for minimal role conflicts, related to adequate family resources

Potential for decreased anxiety concerning treatment for delayed postpartum hemorrhage, related to adequate knowledge base

On admission, oxytocin (Pitocin) in intravenous solution, ergonovine maleate (Ergotrate), or methylergonovine maleate (Methergine) orally are administered to stimulate uterine contractions. If the bleeding subsides, the client is observed for several hours. Vital signs are taken, the fundus is palpated for firmness, and the lochia is assessed for quantity and quality of flow. Hemoglobin and hematocrit are obtained to assess for anemia resulting from blood loss.

If bleeding persists, uterine compression and bimanual massage (*see* earlier discussion of uterine atony) are often performed to control hemorrhage caused by subinvolution. If appreciable bleeding still persists, curettage may be indicated. This procedure should be carried out only when other treatment has failed because curettage may further traumatize the implantation site and cause additional bleeding. Authorities suggest that when curettage is performed, the client and her partner should be advised that hysterectomy may be necessary.[3] Broad-spectrum antibiotics also may be given to the client if postpartum infection is suspected.

Delayed postpartum bleeding as a result of retention of placental tissue is generally preventable. The placenta and membranes should always be carefully inspected after delivery, and if a portion of the placenta or membranes is missing, the uterus should be explored.

Differential Parameters

In differentiating among the causes of postpartum hemorrhage, the degree of contractility of the uterus is a deciding factor. If the fundus is firm and well contracted and the bleeding persists, the cause is usually lacerations; if the fundus is soft and boggy, the cause is usually uterine atony. Lacerations of the cervix may produce a slow seepage of bright red blood; uterine atony may cause heavy bleeding with clots. In each case, however, serious hypovolemia may occur.

At times, bleeding may have more than one cause, for example, atony and trauma. It is therefore essential that the cervix and vagina be inspected for lacerations even when uterine atony is present.[3] Table 41–2 summarizes contributing risk factors and assessment findings for the client with uterine atony, trauma from lacerations, hematoma, or subinvolution.

POSTPARTUM INFECTIONS

Postpartum infections fall into two broad categories. The first category covers the reproductive system infections, also termed *puerperal infection* or *puerperal fe-*

TABLE 41–2. DIFFERENTIAL PARAMETERS OF POSTPARTUM HEMORRHAGE WITH NURSING INTERVENTIONS

Cause of Hemorrhage	Contributing Risk Factors	Assessment Findings	Nursing Interventions
Uterine atony	Uterine overdistension from multiple gestation and polyhydramnios Prolonged or precipitous labor Mismanagement of the third stage of labor Uterine infection Disseminated intravascular coagulation Bladder distension	Boggy, soft fundus Profuse bright red lochia Blood clots Foul-smelling lochia Increase in height of uterine fundus Failure of uterus to involute	Have client empty bladder Assess fundus for firmness Gently massage and assess location and firmness of fundus Take vital signs Note amount, consistency, color, and odor of lochia Report findings
Lacerations	Operative delivery Vaginal birth after cesarean birth Delivery of large infant Precipitous delivery	Firm fundus (usually) Seepage of bright red blood	Observe for trickling of bright, red blood Take vital signs Assess fundus and lochia Assess suture lines for REEDA Report findings
Hematoma	Difficult delivery Operative delivery (eg, forceps)	Complaint of pain or pressure in vagina or perineum Ecchymotic mass in perineum Inability to void	Assess vagina and perineum for mass Take vital signs Report findings Place ice pack on perineum
Subinvolution	Faulty placental implantation Infection at implantation site Retention of placental fragments	Late postpartum hemorrhage Bright red bleeding Persistent lochia rubra Prolonged lochial discharge No change or a rise in the fundal height Soft, boggy fundus	Teach couple how to assess lochia and fundus prior to discharge and contact the health care provider with abnormal findings Assess vital signs, fundus, and lochia

REEDA = redness, edema, ecchymosis, discharge, and approximation.

ver, which are bacterial infections that arise in the genital tract after delivery. The second category includes nonreproductive system infections that arise in sites other than the genital tract and influence maternal morbidity during postpartum recovery. These infections, which include mastitis and urinary tract infections, are indirectly related to the reproductive cycle and physiology of pregnancy, labor, delivery, and lactation. Infections in the second category might also occur in nonpregnant individuals.

ISSUES AND CONTROVERSIES

The client and her family are often anxious and fearful about postpartum complications. They may have little knowledge about the management of these problems. One issue concerns management of clients with postpartum infection. Should clients with reproductive system infections be moved from the maternity suite? The rationale for moving these clients is that infected mothers may spread the infection to well mothers and their infants. With the advances in antimicrobial therapy, and use of universal precautions, however, is the spread of infection less likely? What happens to the mother-infant relationship when the mother is separated from the infant?

Reproductive System Infections

The classic definition of **puerperal morbidity** resulting from infection is a temperature of 100.4°F (38.0°C) or higher on any 2 of the first 10 days postpartum, exclusive of the first 24 hours, as taken orally by a standard technique at least four times a day. This definition was developed in the early 20th century, but remains the most commonly employed standard in the United States.[3]

Although temperature is the criterion most commonly used to determine puerperal morbidity, a temperature of 100.4°F or higher in the first 10 days postpartum is also associated with benign conditions such as breast engorgement. The cause of fever in the postpartum period must therefore be investigated so that proper treatment can be instituted.

Reproductive system infections affect 2 to 8 percent of pregnant women and account for 8 percent of maternal deaths in the United States.[3,18] The development of better techniques for identification of causative agents and the use of antibiotics in treatment have decreased the maternal death rate from bacterial infections dramatically.[6] Despite advances in maternity care, infections still rank high in the list of complications in the postpartum period. Moreover, the cost to the family is still high. The mother is separated from her newborn and is often required to spend additional days in the hospital. In addition, serious reproductive system infections may lead to sterility or problems with future childbearing.[3] The disruption of family functioning places additional stress on family members and on the internal and external resources available to them. Prevention of infection is therefore the best possible treatment.

Bacterial Causes. A variety of bacteria are responsible for reproductive system infections. In most cases, the bacteria causing infection are those found normally in the bowel, perineum, and cervix. These bacteria, which are not usually pathogenic, may become so as a result of injury and devitalization of tissue.[3] Anaerobic bacteria, aerobic bacteria, or a combination may be involved. Table 41–3 lists the common anaerobic and aerobic bacteria responsible for reproductive system infections.

The majority of postpartum infections are caused by gram-positive cocci; however, an increasing incidence of bacteroides and mycoplasma infections have been noted.[19,20] The clinical signs of infection depend on the virulence of the organism and the client's immune response to it.

Reproductive system infections usually begin in the uterus and may spread upward to the fallopian tubes and ovaries (salpingo-oophoritis), outward to the parametrial cellular tissue (parametrial cellulitis), and, if more extensive, out to the peritoneal cavity (peritonitis). Septic pelvic thrombophlebitis also may occur.[21] A severe complication of reproductive system infection is bacteremia, which can be associated with septic shock.

TABLE 41–3. COMMON ANAEROBIC AND AEROBIC BACTERIA RESPONSIBLE FOR REPRODUCTIVE SYSTEM INFECTIONS

Aerobic Bacteria	Anaerobic Bacteria
Gram-positive cocci	Gram-positive cocci
Group B streptococcus	Peptostreptococci
Group D streptococcus	Peptococci
Gram-negative bacilli	Gram-negative bacilli
Escherichia coli	Bacteroides
	Gram-positive bacilli
	Clostridium species
Other	
Chlamydia trachomatis	

Risk Factors. Several risk factors associated with reproductive system infection are assessed in the antepartum and intrapartum periods. Table 41–4 lists these risk factors.

Many of the risk factors listed in Table 41–4 have been indirectly linked to poverty (eg, anemia, poor nutrition). Women in lower socioeconomic groups are at greater risk for postpartum infections, as well as other complications of pregnancy. It is thus important that prenatal services be targeted at this group of women. Prevention of complications is far less costly than management of complications, both in dollars and in family functioning.

Specific Infections

Metritis. **Metritis** is a puerperal uterine infection involving the endometrium, the decidua, and the adjacent myometrium. This term is more specific than endometritis (infection of the endometrium) because the underlying myometrium is almost always involved in metritis.[3]

Metritis is the most common cause of postpartum infections. Symptoms usually begin on the third to fifth day postpartum; however, if the invading organism is a beta-hemolytic streptococcus, the onset is usually earlier.[22] Factors contributing to the development of metritis include prolonged labor, prolonged rupture of the membranes, or introduction of pathogens from multiple vaginal examinations. The risk of metritis is greater after cesarean delivery than after vaginal delivery.

TABLE 41–4. RISK FACTORS ASSOCIATED WITH REPRODUCTIVE SYSTEM INFECTIONS

Antepartum
Low socioeconomic status
Poor maternal nutrition
Anemia
Little or no prenatal care
Premature rupture of the membranes
Silent chorioamniotic infection
Coitus late in pregnancy, primarily if membranes are ruptured
Intrapartum
Labor
Introduction of pathogens from frequent vaginal examinations and intrauterine fetal monitoring
Prolonged labor
Prolonged rupture of the membranes
Delivery
Lacerations
Hemorrage, especially after excessive blood loss
Cesarean delivery, especially after prolonged labor
Operative delivery (eg, forceps)

Metritis is usually caused by bacteria that invade the decidua at the placental site. The hypervascularity of the remaining decidua also makes it susceptible to the invasion of pathogens, as does injury to the cervix. The appearance of the infected decidua may vary. In some cases, the necrotic mucosa sloughs, producing an abundant, foul-smelling, bloody, and sometimes frothy discharge. In other cases, the uterine discharge may be scant and odorless (as in infection with beta-hemolytic streptococcus). In either case, subinvolution of the uterus may occur.[3]

Parametrial Cellulitis. **Parametrial cellulitis** (parametritis) is an extension of puerperal infection that begins in the uterus and spreads into the broad ligament through several routes[3] (Figure 41–4):

1. Through lymphatic transmission of bacteria from infected cervical lacerations, uterine incision for cesarean delivery, or uterine laceration
2. By direct extension of cervical lacerations into connective tissue at the base of the broad ligaments, exposing the tissue to direct invasions by organisms
3. Secondary to pelvic thromophlebitis, in which organisms gain access to surrounding tissue from a purulent thrombus of the venous wall

The infection involves the entire uterus and may spread to the ovaries and fallopian tubes. If parametrial cellulitis progresses, a parametrial abscess may develop, which may require draining to prevent rupture into the peritoneal cavity.[22]

Peritonitis. **Peritonitis** is an infection of the peritoneum that spreads from the uterus, by way of the lymphatics, to the abdominal cavity (Figure 41–5). This serious condition may be life threatening. Purulent exudate may bind loops of bowel to one another, resulting in paralytic ileus. The cul-de-sac also may be a site of abscess formation.[3]

Septic Pelvic Thrombophlebitis. **Septic pelvic thrombophlebitis** results when an infection originating in the uterus spreads along venous routes into the pelvis (Figure 41–6). The placental site is the usual portal of entry of the bacteria. The bacterial infection causes thrombosis of myometrial veins, which in turn support the growth of anaerobic bacteria.[3] The infection may spread via the pelvic veins into the right ovarian vein, which may further extend the infection to the inferior vena cava, and into the left ovarian vein, which may further extend the infection to the left renal vein. Spread of infection into the femoral vein

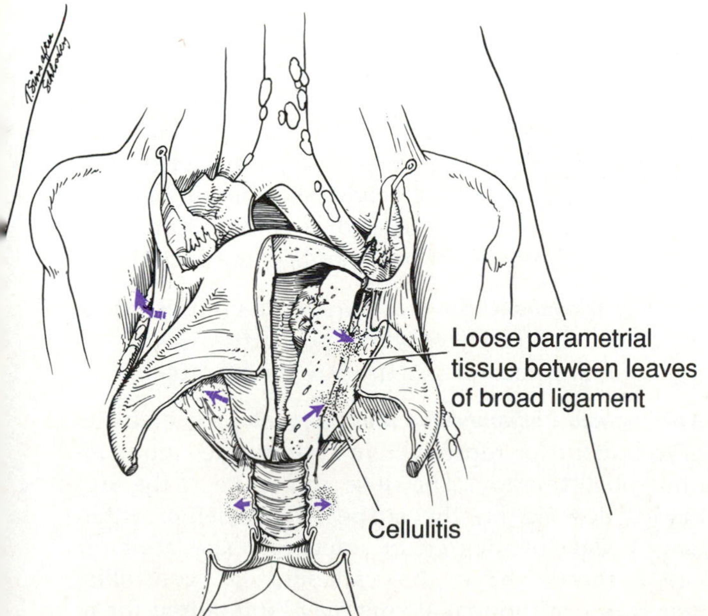

Figure 41–4. Spread of parametrial cellulitis infection into broad ligaments. (*Reproduced, with permission, from Cunningham FG, et al.* Williams Obstetrics. *18th ed. Norwalk, Conn: Appleton & Lange; 1989:466.*)

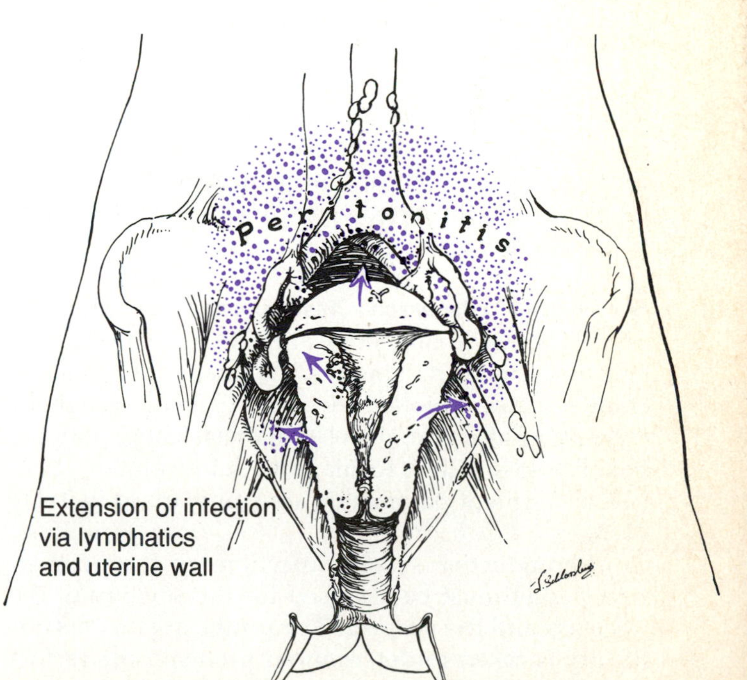

Figure 41–5. Spread of peritonitis via lymphatics and uterine wall. (*Reproduced, with permission, from Cunningham FG, et al.* Williams Obstetrics. *18th ed. Norwalk, Conn: Appleton & Lange; 1989:467.*)

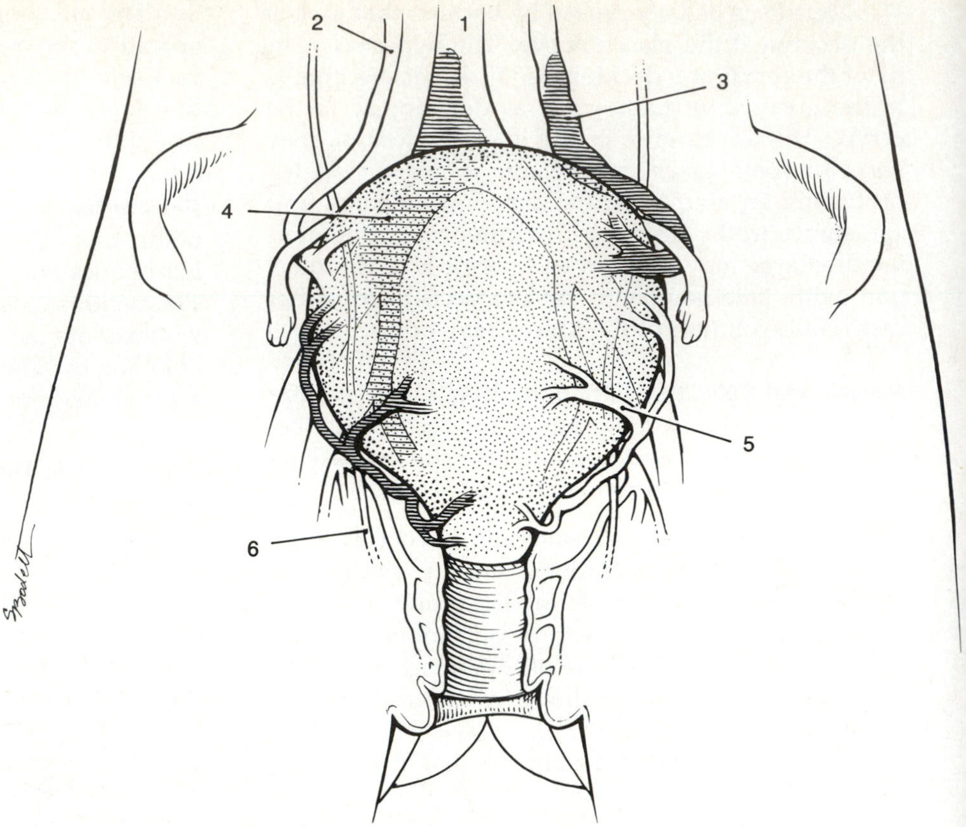

Figure 41–6. Septic pelvic thrombophlebitis. Any or all pelvic vessels and the inferior vena cava may be involved: (1) inferior vena cava; (2) right ovarian vein; (3) clot in left ovarian vein; (4) clot in right common iliac vein, which extends from the uterine and hypogastric veins and into the inferior vena cava; (5) left uterine vein; (6) right ureter. (*Reproduced, with permission, from Cunningham FG, et al.* Williams Obstetrics. *18th ed. Norwalk, Conn: Appleton & Lange; 1989:470.*)

results in femoral thrombophlebitis. Blood clots formed in these veins may embolize to the lungs.

Bacteremia and Septic Shock. **Bacteremia** is the invasion of the blood cells by bacteria. The bacteria can reach the blood from the uterus through the lymphatics or veins. If the invading organism is virulent, septic shock can occur.

Nursing and Collaborative Assessment. For each of the preceding conditions, there are both general and specific assessment parameters. General parameters include elevated temperature [100.4°F (38°C) or higher], increased pulse rate, pain (local or systemic), fatigue, pallor, foul-smelling lochia, and subinvolution. Specific assessment parameters are summarized in Table 41–5.

Reproductive system infections in the postpartum period must be assessed for the severity of the infection and the suspected causative organism(s). A history is taken to determine if predisposing factors associated with reproductive system infections existed in the antepartum and intrapartum periods. A physical examination is also performed, with the examiner using a vaginal speculum to visualize the vagina, cervix, and vaginal discharge. Specimens of lochia may be taken for microscopy and culture. This is done by passing a covered swab through the vagina and uncovering the swab when the desired area (high in the vagina and uterus) is reached. The resulting specimen is then sent to the laboratory.[22] A bimanual examination is performed to assess the uterus, adnexa, cellular tissues, and pelvic peritoneum for swelling and tenderness. Blood is drawn for culture if the infection is severe or if bacteremia is suspected.[21]

Nursing Diagnosis. Several nursing diagnoses can be developed for the client with a postpartum reproductive system infection (*see* the box for examples).

Nursing and Collaborative Management. The mainstay of treatment for reproductive system infection is antimicrobial therapy. The dose and route of the antibiotics depend on the suspected causative organism(s) and the degree of infection. The antibiotic agent should have the capability of controlling anaerobes; additional agents may be required for resistant infection.

Moderately to severely infected women are given high doses of broad-spectrum intravenous antibiotics. The high doses are needed to ensure attainment

TABLE 41–5. SUMMARY OF SPECIFIC REPRODUCTIVE SYSTEM INFECTIONS AND ASSESSMENT FINDINGS

Type of Infection	Assessment Findings
Metritis	Fever initially 101–102°F, (38.3–38.9°C); if infection becomes more serious, jagged temperature elevations between 101 and 104°F (38.3 and 40°C) Uterine tenderness on palpation of the fundus or on bimanual examination Grimacing, guarding, complaints of pain Prolonged or bothersome afterpains Subinvolution of uterus Bacteria revealed on culture of lochia
Parametrial cellulitis (Parametritis)	Prolonged elevation of temperature to 102–104°F (38.9–40°C) with fluctuations Extension of abdominal pain laterally; possible rebound tenderness Hypotension, subinvolution, chills Decreased bowel sounds, nausea, and vomiting
Peritonitis	Elevation of temperature to as high as 105°F (40.5°C) Severe pain Paralytic ileus Abdominal rigidity Frequent vomiting with dehydration Weak and thready pulse (possible) Rapid, shallow respirations Excessive thirst, marked anxiety
Septic pelvic thrombophlebitis	Elevation of temperature to 105°F (40.5°C); dramatic fluctuations (possible) over short periods Pain in flank or lower abdomen
Bacteremia and septic shock	Rapid elevation of temperature to 103–104°F (39.4–40°C) Perfuse, foul-smelling lochia Symptoms of shock Reduction in urinary output

NURSING DIAGNOSES RELATED TO REPRODUCTIVE SYSTEM INFECTION IN THE POSTPARTUM PERIOD

Problem-Oriented

Impaired tissue integrity, related to puerperal metritis

Potential for infection: spread, related to uterine infection

Hyperthermia, related to puerperal infection

Alteration in parenting, related to maternal separation from newborn because of maternal infection

Strength-Oriented

Positive self-concept: mothering role performance, related to relief of symptoms of infection and availability of resources

of adequate tissue concentrations in the postpartum client.

Penicillin combined with an aminoglycoside or ampicillin combined with an aminoglycoside is often the first-line regimen. Most infections respond to broad-spectrum intravenous antibiotics within 24 to 36 hours. Infections that do not respond in 24 hours will usually respond to chloramphenicol (effective against bacteroides) or tetracycline (effective against *Mycoplasma* species).[21,22] For the client known to be infected at the time of delivery, initial therapy comprises two or three drug regimens.[3] Table 41–6 provides information about several antibiotics commonly used to treat reproductive system infections.

Oxytocics (usually oral ergonovine maleate or methylergonovine maleate) may be administered to

TABLE 41–6. ANTIBIOTICS COMMONLY USED TO TREAT REPRODUCTIVE SYSTEM INFECTIONS

Antibiotic	Active Against	Dose
Ampicillin (many proprietary names)	*Escherichia coli, Proteus mirabilis, Neisseria gonorrhoeae*, enterococci, streptococci, pneumonocci	1–2 g IV every 6 hours
Cefoxitin (Mefoxin)	*E. coli, N. gonorrhoeae, Bacteroides* sp, *Clostridium* sp, *Peptococcus* sp, *Peptostreptococcus* sp, *Klebsiella* sp, *Proteus* sp.	1–2 g IV every 6–8 hours
Cefotaxime (Claforan)	Similar to cefoxitin	1–2 g IV every 6–8 hours
Ceftizoxime (Cefizox)	Similar to cefoxitin	1–2 g IV every 8–12 hours
Cefotetan (Cefotan)	Similar to cefoxitin	1–2 g IV every 12 hours
Doxycycline (Vibramycin, others)	*Chlamydia trachomatis*	100 mg orally every 12 hours, or 100–200 mg IV once or twice daily
Gentamicin (many proprietary names)	Enterococci (when given with ampicillin), *E. coli, Klebsiella* sp, *Proteus* sp, *Pseudomonas*	1–2 mg/kg IV every 8 hours; adjust dose to maintain peak serum concentration of 4–8 μg/mL
Clindamycin (Cleocin)	*Bacteroides* sp, streptococci, staphylococci	600 mg IV every 6 hours, or 900 mg IV every 8 hours

stimulate uterine contractions and enhance involution in mothers with puerperal uterine infections. Breastfeeding accomplishes the same purpose; however, many institutions move the mother off the maternity floor when puerperal infection is suspected or diagnosed, and therefore she is often unable to breastfeed. Moreover, breastfeeding is contraindicated with the use of some antibiotics (eg, tetracycline) or when the mother experiences discomfort and fatigue.

If fever persists after 48 to 72 hours of antimicrobial therapy, careful investigation of the causes of the resistant pelvic infection is indicated. Antimicrobial therapy for peritonitis includes agents effective against peptostreptococcus, peptococcus, bacteroides, clostridium, and aerobic coliforms. As paralytic ileus may occur with peritonitis, the gastrointestinal tract is compressed by continuous nasogastric suctioning.[3]

Septic shock and bacteremia require very aggressive therapy: vigorous intravenous fluid infusion and administration of empiric broad-spectrum antimicrobial drugs that cover all suspected pathogens.[3] Septic shock requires hemodynamic monitoring, vasoactive drugs when hypotension is not corrected by fluid treatment, and oxygen administered by mask to improve tissue hypoxia.[3] Nursing care for women with reproductive system infections includes assessment of maternal vital signs (including pulse, blood pressure, and temperature); careful recording of intake and output; observation of lochia; and notation of subjective complaints of the client.

Women with reproductive system infections need continuous nursing support. The client and her family may be anxious about the implications of the condition and the possible separation from the newborn. If the client is placed on a medical floor and is separated from her newborn, the nurse who cares for the newborn can help to allay her anxiety by coordinating communication with nurses caring for her. The client who is breastfeeding can be assured that she may continue to do so unless (1) she must be separated from the newborn, (2) she is given antibiotics that contraindicate breastfeeding, or (3) she feels too ill to breastfeed. If separation is indicated, the nurse can teach the client to maintain lactation by manual pumping of the breasts, or to stimulate relactation once the infection has abated.

Women with serious infections may feel quite ill. They also may need to undergo additional procedures, for example, surgical drainage in the event of an abscess. Although most women with reproductive system infections do not require intensive care, intensive medical and nursing care is a priority for women who develop serious infections in the postpartum period. Some authorities advocate placing clients with complications, either prenatal or postpartum, in a maternal-fetal intensive care unit, which offers medical and nursing care equivalent to that of a medical/surgical intensive care unit. These units can provide critical care while meeting the complex physical and psychosocial needs associated with pregnancy.[23] Comprehensive care when infections arise usually prevents life-threatening sequelae.

Localized Infections. In addition to the specific reproductive system infections already mentioned, localized infections of the perineum, vagina, or cesarean incision may occur in the postpartum period. The most apparent of these is infection of the episiotomy site.[24] This is relatively rare, occurring in 0.5 to 3 percent of women who have episiotomies. The infection may begin as a vulvar hematoma, causing breakdown of tissue at the episiotomy site.

Vaginal lacerations may become infected directly or by extension of infectious agents from the perineum. The abdominal incision may also become infected after cesarean delivery. These infections may be preceded by uterine infections and, in some instances, may progress to systemic infections.

Nursing and Collaborative Assessment. The classic features of infected wounds (redness, edema, ecchymosis, drainage) are present with infected episiotomy or abdominal incisions. Often, the previously approximated edges of the incision separate and seropurulent fluid drains from the infection site.

The client may complain of pain and tenderness in the perineal, vaginal, or abdominal area. Temperature may rise to 101°F (38.3°C). If the infection is confined by sutures, the temperature will be higher and accompanied by chills.

Fortunately, localized infections are usually not severe. If abdominal incision wound infection occurs, a specimen is obtained for smears and culture in an attempt to isolate the bacteria.

Nursing and Collaborative Management. Care of localized infections focuses on establishing drainage of the infected material. Often an episiotomy or abdominal incision opens spontaneously. At other times, the physician removes the sutures to allow drainage.

Sitz baths every 4 to 6 hours assist in cleansing the perineal area of debris and provide comfort to the client. Analgesics also may be given to relieve some of the discomfort caused by the localized infection. If a vulvar hematoma is present, evacuation of the hematoma may be necessary.

Abdominal incision infections are mechanically cleaned with saline-soaked gauze and left open to drain. If systemic symptoms of fever and chills occur, antibiotics are given.

Non–Reproductive System Infections that Affect Postpartum Recovery

In addition to those infections that directly affect the reproductive system of the postpartum client, several general infections may indirectly influence postpartum recovery. These infections, which may occur outside of childbearing, often occur as a result of the trauma incurred with childbearing or lactation. The two most common infections are mastitis and urinary tract infections. Although fever and chills in the postpartum period may be the result of reproductive system infections, these symptoms also may be caused by other infectious conditions. A careful and thorough assessment is essential to pinpoint the cause of the symptoms and ensure an appropriate plan of care. Women who have chills, fever, and tenderness (common symptoms of metritis) may, in fact, have a urinary tract infection; women who complain of chills and fever later in the postpartum period may have mastitis.

Mastitis. **Mastitis** is an inflammation of the breast tissue caused by bacterial infection and found primarily in breastfeeding mothers. The bacterial organism usually enters the breast through a cracked nipple and multiplies in the milk. In some instances, infection results from stasis of milk behind a blocked duct. The causative organism is usually *Staphyloccus aureus*, which is found in the infant's nose and throat. The infant may contract the bacteria from nursery personnel who may carry the organism, especially on the hands.[3]

Nursing and Collaborative Assessment. Symptoms of suppurative mastitis do not appear until the third or fourth week postpartum. The client complains of a painful, hardened, reddened area usually on one breast. She also may have enlarged glands in the axilla on the affected side. Fever, chills, and malaise accompany the infection. The breast may show marked engorgement and, in some instances, a frank abscess may appear. Milk from the affected breast is sometimes sent for culture and sensitivity to isolate the offending organism.

Nursing Diagnosis. Examples of nursing diagnoses for the woman experiencing mastitis are provided in the box.

> **NURSING DIAGNOSES RELATED TO MASTITIS**
>
> **Problem-Oriented**
>
> Ineffective breastfeeding, related to discomfort from mastitis
>
> Altered maternal role performance, related to pain and discomfort when breastfeeding
>
> **Strength-Oriented**
>
> Positive coping, related to knowledge of treatment for mastitis
>
> Positive self-concept, related to comfort secondary to treatment for mastitis

Nursing and Collaborative Management. In the prenatal period, nursing measures are aimed at preventing mastitis. The nurse teaches the pregnant woman to prepare her breasts prenatally by massaging the breasts, manually expressing colostrum during the last trimester, rolling the nipples, and gently rubbing the nipples with a terry cloth towel. It is believed by some practioners that breast preparation may help to prevent cracking of the nipples during breastfeeding,[25,26] thus reducing the risk of bacterial transmission.

The woman with mastitis is managed with antimicrobial therapy, most often penicillin (erythromycin if the mother is sensitive to penicillin). Some authorities question whether the client should continue to breastfeed using the affected breast. Many authorities recommend continued feeding on the affected breast because the infant can empty the breast better than manual expression. Emptying of the infected breast prevents engorgement and stasis of milk.[27]

The woman is told to wear a well-supporting properly fitted brassiere. The nurse can also advise the application of moist heat in the form of showers to help relieve the discomfort.

If the client develops a breast abscess, incision and drainage are required. Some authorities recommend discontinuation of breastfeeding on the affected breast in the case of an abscess. The infant may still nurse on the opposite breast, and the client can manually pump the affected breast.

The woman with mastitis feels ill and may believe she has failed in her mothering role. The nurse can play an important role in providing support and encouragement. As one client stated "I felt so sick and kept getting conflicting information. My pediatrician said to continue nursing and my obstetrician said to stop nursing." The nurse can ensure that the mother is given consistent, accurate information regarding the treatment for mastitis and can encourage her to make her own decision on the basis of factual information.

The client should be given information about self-care practices that help prevent recurrence of mastitis:

- Wash hands before breastfeeding
- Breastfeed frequently to prevent engorgement
- Encourage the infant to empty the breast, as milk provides a good medium for bacterial growth
- If an area of the breast is distended or tender, breastfeed from the affected side first each feeding and express the milk remaining in the opposite breast
- Massage the distended area as the infant nurses
- Contact the caregiver if redness and fever occur

Urinary Tract Infections. Urinary tract infections occur in about 2 to 4 percent of women postpartum.[2] *Escherichia coli* is the most frequent cause (75 to 90 percent of cases). Urinary tract infections can be differentiated into cystitis and pyelonephritis. **Cystitis** is inflammation of the bladder; pyelonephritis is inflammation of the renal pelves. (*See* Chapter 39 for discussion of urinary tract infections during pregnancy.)

Risk Factors. Several factors predispose women to urinary tract infections in the postpartum period:

- The relative hypotonicity of the lower urinary tract and bladder, causing stasis of urine
- Trauma to the bladder from passage of the fetus through the pelvis
- Catheterization during labor and delivery
- Frequent vaginal examinations during labor
- Regional anesthesia
- Weakness of the sphincter between the ureter and bladder, causing reflux of infected urine upward to the kidney

Nursing and Collaborative Assessment. In the postpartum period, it can sometimes be difficult to distinguish between reproductive system infections and urinary tract infections. Elevation in temperature may be the only presenting symptom of urinary tract infection; however, urinary tract infection should be ruled out when the postpartum woman has a temperature of 100.4°F or higher. Other presenting signs and symptoms of urinary tract infections are dysuria, frequency, and urgency. The history reveals whether the woman has had any urinary infections prenatally or has experienced chronic urinary tract infections.

The woman with pyelonephritis is usually quite ill. In addition to dysuria and frequency, signs of kidney involvement, for example, costovertebral angle tenderness, often are apparent. Her fever may spike as high as 104°F (40°C) and be accompanied by chills, flank pain, anorexia, and vomiting.

A clean-catch midstream urine specimen is obtained, and the urine cultured for organisms. Significant bacteriuria is defined as the presence of 100,000 or more organisms per milliliter of urine; a count between 10,000 and 100,000 is ambiguous and indicates the test should be repeated.[21]

Nursing Diagnosis. *See* Chapter 39 for examples of nursing diagnoses related to urinary tract infection.

Nursing and Collaborative Management. Management of urinary tract infections consists of antimicrobial therapy. The causative organisms usually respond to oral sulfonamides, nitrofurantoin, and ampicillin. The course of treatment is usually begun before the culture and sensitivity results are obtained and adjusted if indicated by the laboratory results. High fluid intake is indicated to flush the urinary tract. Cranberry juice may be offered to make the urine more acidic (bacteria thrive in alkaline environments). Analgesics are given for symptomatic relief of dysuria.

Management of the woman with pyelonephritis includes bedrest, intravenous fluids, and parenteral antimicrobial therapy (eg, ampicillin, gentamicin). An intravenous pyelogram may be performed 2 to 4 months postpartum to identify any residual kidney damage.

Nursing care includes assessment of vital signs, intake and output, and urine culture and sensitivity. The postpartum client with a urinary tract infection may be relatively asymptomatic or she may be acutely ill. Although women with urinary tract infections do not need to be separated from their infants, those who are acutely ill may find that they need someone else to provide infant care. The nurse can help to support family functioning and allay the client's anxiety by allowing the infant to be cared for in the mother's room or by encouraging the support person to perform care for the infant in the mother's room.

The nurse can also encourage prevention of infection by teaching the client self-care practices, for example, wiping from the meatus toward the rectum to avoid bacterial contamination and emptying the bladder frequently to avoid urinary stasis. The woman with pyelonephritis may need long-term therapy. Careful explanations about the condition and therapy should be provided to the client and other family members. Breastfeeding is not contraindicated, but may be delayed or interrupted if the client is acutely ill.

Prevention of Infection

Several measures can be taken when caring for maternity clients to help prevent infection. Ideally, the client will have received comprehensive prenatal care, which includes nutrition information and assistance in purchasing food if she is in financial need, as prevention of anemia indirectly helps to prevent infection.

When the client is admitted to the birthing facility, strict rules of antisepsis should be followed and multiple vaginal examinations avoided. Measures also should be taken to prevent dehydration and exhaustion during labor, and excessive blood loss during delivery. Operative deliveries should be minimized if possible. After delivery, the physician or nurse-midwife should inspect for and remove any retained placental tissue as this is a focus for infection. High-risk cesarean delivery clients should receive prophylactic antibiotics in an effort to control infection.

Caregivers on maternity units should wear attire that supports asepsis. In an interesting study, Roberts and others[28] found no difference in maternal or neonatal morbidity in low-risk deliveries with the use or nonuse of sterile attire by caregivers. The researchers concluded that it is safe to allow variation in attire in circumstances of low obstetric risk and minimal-intervention deliveries. In high-risk or moderate-risk situations, it is generally accepted that surgical drapes and sterile professional attire are needed in the delivery room. Personnel with communicable infections should not care for maternity clients.

RESEARCH ABSTRACT

Roberts JE, et al. Professional attire at delivery: effect on postpartum and neonatal infection. J Nurse Midwifery. *1986;31:16–19.*

This study investigated whether the use of sterile attire during delivery contributes to differences in postpartum maternal or neonatal infectious morbidity. The method of study was a retrospective review of records of 243 deliveries over a 1-year period.

The facility chosen for the study permitted considerable variations in the use/nonuse of gowns and masks and in the draping technique during delivery. Three variations in delivery attire were identified: (A) rubber gloves, laundered scrub suit, and sterile underdrape; (B) rubber gloves, laundered scrub suit, cap, mask, and sterile underdrape; (C) rubber gloves, sterile gown over the laundered scrub suit, cap, mask, shoe covers, and complete set of sterile drapes. The sample comprised 112 deliveries in group A, 48 in group B, and 83 in group C. Women were assigned to one of six practitioners who delivered in each of the three groups.

There were no significant differences in morbidity due to infection among the women in the three groups or among women attended by different practitioners. The authors suggest that variations in attire and minimal use of sterile apparel are safe in cases of low obstetric risk and minimal intervention for birthing room deliveries.

Comment:
This study has implications for the care of low-risk clients as it supports use of minimal sterile apparel for nonoperative, low-risk deliveries; however, these findings cannot be applied to high-risk situations as none of the women in the sample were high-risk clients. Prospective studies in which low-risk women are placed in different groups would add credence to the results.

THROMBOEMBOLIC DISORDERS

The prenatal, intrapartum, and postpartum phases of the childbearing cycle are high-risk periods for the development of thromboembolic disorders. These disorders include superficial venous thrombosis, limited to the superficial veins of the saphenous system, and deep venous thrombosis, involving the deep veins of the leg. Superficial venous thrombosis is associated with inflammation and may be termed "phlebitis," or superficial venous thrombophlebitis. Deep venous thrombosis is not associated with inflammation and should not be called "phlebitis."

Risk Factors. The onset of thromboembolic disease is three times more likely in the postpartum period than in the prenatal period.[29] Factors associated with increased risk include maternal age greater than 35, past history of thrombosis, cardiac disease, more than three previous pregnancies, cesarean delivery, obesity, varicose veins, and venous stasis caused by immobilization. The incidence of thromboembolic disease in the postpartum period decreased significantly when early ambulation became widely practiced.

Stasis is probably the strongest predisposing factor to deep venous thrombosis.[3] In addition, clotting factors generally remain elevated in the immediate postpartum period. Levels of protein C, a main coagulation inhibitor, decrease slightly after delivery and do not increase again until about 3 to 5 days postpartum. The woman with hereditary protein C deficiency is prone to venous thromboembolic disorders whether she is pregnant or not. Infection and injury also predispose the postpartum woman to thromboembolic disorders.[30–32]

Superficial Venous Thrombosis. Superficial venous thrombosis is limited to the superficial veins of the legs. The thrombus forms as a result of inflammation in the vein wall (thrombophlebitis). This type of thrombosis rarely results in serious complications, such as pulmonary embolism.[3] If, however, thrombophlebitis extends above the knee, the woman is at higher risk for deep vein involvement.

Deep Venous Thrombosis. Deep venous thrombosis in the leg generally involves much of the deep venous system from the foot to the iliofemoral region.[3] Deep venous thrombosis in the postpartum period presents with abrupt onset of pain and edema of the thigh.

Nursing and Collaborative Assessment. The nurse, in a routine postpartum assessment, may be the first person to identify signs and symptoms of thromboembolic disorders. The nurse palpates the calves of the legs for heat and tenderness, checks for Homan's sign, and notes any subjective complaints of the mother (*see* Chapter 39). Diagnoses based solely on clinical signs and symptoms may be inaccurate 50 percent of the time.[30] Confirmatory tests for deep venous thrombosis include venography and Duplex scanning.

Nursing and Collaborative Management. Management for superficial venous thrombosis includes rest, the use of support hose when ambulating, and analgesics for comfort. The nurse provides information to the client and family regarding the condition and self-care practices.

Anticoagulant therapy is started with IV heparin and is followed by oral anticoagulants for 3 to 6 months for deep venous thrombosis. The initial therapy includes administration of heparin by continuous intravenous infusion. Dosages of heparin are adjusted according to coagulation studies (partial thromboplastin time 2 times control). While the client is on heparin therapy, her platelet count should be monitored because of the potential for development of heparin-induced antibodies.

If the anticoagulation therapy is to be protracted, oral warfarin may be prescribed for 3 to 6 months (Box 41–1). Although warfarin is contraindicated in pregnancy, it may be taken postpartum. The drug is excreted into breast milk, and there is controversy over possible neonatal effects from the drug. As a precaution, the breastfeeding mother should be advised to inform her health care provider so that she or he may prescribe subcutaneous heparin, which does not pass into the breast milk.[3,21,29,30]

Nursing care for the woman placed on loading doses of anticoagulant therapy includes careful monitoring for signs of hemorrhage, such as epistaxis, blood in the urine and stool, and ecchymosis or petechiae. The woman who will receive protracted therapy after discharge should be taught the purpose and action of the medication and the signs of hemorrhagic complications. She should be taught to avoid salicylates because they can cause bleeding. The woman also should wear an identifying bracelet that states that she is receiving anticoagulant therapy.

Pulmonary Embolism

Pulmonary embolism is a rare complication of deep venous thrombosis. It occurs in about 1 in every 2500 to 3000 pregnancies. About 35 percent of the women who develop pulmonary embolism have a history of deep venous thrombosis.[29,30]

Nursing and Collaborative Assessment. Signs and symptoms of pulmonary embolism may include sharp chest pain or chest discomfort, dyspnea, tachypnea, and apprehension. Other symptoms include rales, air hunger, hemoptysis, cyanosis, tachycardia, and gallop rhythm over the heart when large emboli are present.

Laboratory studies include the indirect tests of serial blood gas analysis, blood coagulation studies, electrocardiogram, chest x-ray, and Duplex scanning. The diagnosis of pulmonary emboli is verified by ventilation perfusion scan of the lung using radioisotopes. If this is still inconclusive, pulmonary angiography remains the most definitive way of detecting pulmonary embolism.

Nursing and Collaborative Management. The nurse should notify the physician immediately if pulmonary embolism is suspected in the postpartum period. Heparin therapy is initiated (with close monitoring of partial thromboplastin time) and oxygen administered (1 to 2 L/min by nasal route).

Massive pulmonary emboli may require digitalis therapy as well as surgical thrombectomy or dissolution of the clot with streptokinase or urokinase (fibrinolytic drugs used to dissolve clots). A large embolism may block blood flow from the right ventricle into the lungs. This may result in cardiac failure, shock, and death.

BOX 41–1. WARFARIN SODIUM

Proprietary Names:
Coumadin (Dupont), others.

Classification:
Anticoagulant.

Action:
Interferes with the action of vitamin K thereby inhibiting the synthesis of blood coagulation factors II, VII, IX, and X. Inhibits thrombus formation when stasis is induced and may prevent extension of existing thrombi.

Indications:
Prophylaxis and treatment of venous thrombosis. Prophylaxis and treatment of pulmonary embolism. Treatment of atrial fibrillation with embolization. As an adjunct in treatment of coronary occlusion.

Dosage and Route:
Administered orally, IM or IV. Dosage does not vary with the route of administration. *Usual initial adult dose:* 10–15 mg once daily for 2–5 days or until desired prothrombin time is reached (1½–2½ times control) *Maintenance dose:* usually ranges from 2 to 10 mg daily, but dose is adjusted on basis of prothrombin time.

Pharmacokinetics:
Absorption: Readily absorbed from the gastrointestinal tract after oral administration; however, may vary from one commercially available tablet to another. Before therapeutic effects are seen, depletion of circulating coagulation factors must occur, which may not occur until 2–7 days after initiation of therapy. *Distribution:* Approximately 97 percent bound to plasma proteins. Crosses the placenta, but does not appear to distribute into breast milk. *Elimination:* Metabolized in the liver. Plasma half-life 0.5–3 days.

Precautions and Contraindications:
Contraindicated in active bleeding or when risk of bleeding is increased as in hemorrhagic blood dyscrasias, ulceration of wounds of gastrointestinal, respiratory, or genitourinary tracts, cerebrovascular hemorrhage, aneurysms, pericarditis, severe hypertension, diverticulitis, polyarthritis, visceral carcinoma, bleeding granuloma, severe diabetes mellitus, vitamin C or K deficiency. Also in senility, alcoholism, or psychosis if client cannot be relied on to comply with therapy. Other contraindications include recent surgery of eye, brain, or spinal cord, continuous tube drainage of any orifice, lumbar puncture, and bone marrow puncture. Contraindicated in pregnancy. Use with caution in minor dental or surgical procedure.

Adverse Reactions:
Most common: Minor bleeding episodes. *Less common:* CV—hemorrhage from any body site; necrosis, and gangrene of skin; GI—nausea, vomiting, anorexia, diarrhea, increase in liver enzymes; hematologic—leukopenia, agranulocytosis; other—dermatitis, urticaria, alopecia, fever, purple toe syndrome; fetal—congenital anomalies.

Drug Interactions:
Drugs/conditions that may potentially increase response to warfarin: acute alcohol intoxication, allopurinol, aminosalicylic acid, amiodarone, anabolic steroids, chloral hydrate, chloramphenicol, cimetidine, clofibrate, co-trimoxazole, danazol, dextrothyroxine, diazoxide, diflunisal, disulfiram, erythromycin, ethacrynic acid, fenoprofen, glucagon, ibuprofen, indomethacin, influenza virus vaccine, isoniazid, ketoprofen, meclofenamate, mefenamic acid, metronidazole, micronazole, nalidixic acid, pentoxifylline, phenylbutazone, propoxyphene, phenylketonuria, quinidine, quinine, salicylates, streptokinase, sulfinpyrazone, sulfonamides, sulindac, tetracyclines, thiazides, thyroid drugs, tricyclic antidepressants, urokinase, vitamin E.

Drugs/conditions that may potentially decrease response to warfarin: chronic alcoholism, barbiturates, carbamazepine, corticosteroids, ethchlorvynol, glutethimide, griseofulvin, mercaptopurine, methaqualone, estrogen-containing oral contraceptives, rifampin, spironolactone, vitamin K.

Nursing Implications:
Prothrombin time is determined before initiation of therapy and periodically if client is placed on maintenance dose.

- Assess for signs of bleeding.
- Teach client to wear identifying bracelet and inform other health care providers (eg, dentists) that she is on warfarin therapy.
- Teach client to use soft toothbrush and assess for signs of hemorrhage.
- Advise breastfeeding clients that it is yet certain whether oral warfarin will pass into breast milk or not. They should request their physician to prescribe subcutaneous heparin, which does not have this effect.

IM = intramuscular(ly), IV = intravenous(ly), CV = cardiovascular, GI = gastrointestinal

The client with a pulmonary embolus requires intensive nursing care and crisis intervention by the interdisciplinary team. She and her family also need continuous support throughout the crisis.

POSTPARTUM DEPRESSION

The discussion thus far has dealt with physiologic complications that may occur in the postpartum period. Psychologic complications also may occur, the most dramatic being postpartum depression and postpartum psychosis.

Women report symptoms of increased tension and anxiety, disturbances, labile moods, and negative thinking styles in the postpartum period. It is believed that these changes may precipitate in some women defensive, neurotic, depressive reactions that interfere with healthy adaptation.[33] The chance of admission to a psychiatric hospital is greater during the 12 months after delivery than at any other time in a woman's life.[34]

Affonso[35] describes the task of integrating "missing pieces" as an essential component in maternal postpartum adaptation. Integration of "missing pieces" refers to the psychologic task of fitting the events of childbearing into a cognitive picture (thoughts, images, dreams) that generates positive growth-producing feelings, emotions, and attitudes. When this psychologic task is not achieved, emotional distress increases; in some women this may last for years. The psychologic problems seen in this period can be categorized into transient depression, postpartum depression, and postpartum psychosis.

Transient Depression. "Postpartum blues" is the common term given to a transient and self-limiting depression that begins 3 to 4 days after delivery and may last from a few hours to a few days. The woman with transient depression experiences an alteration in mood characterized by tearfulness and episodes of crying. Transient depression has been associated with a history of premenstrual tension, a difficult, crying infant, and an infant who causes the mother to have sleepless nights.[34] Transient depression occurs in 50 to 60 percent of postpartum women and usually lasts 24 to 48 hours.[36]

Researchers have proposed that the phenomenon of transient depression results from changes in levels of endogenous substances, such as beta-endorphins, which decrease dramatically 1 hour after delivery; however, no correlations have been made between beta-endorphin levels and transient depression scores in the postpartum period.[37] Transient depression resolves spontaneously. Depression that lasts longer than a few days requires further assessment.

Postpartum Depression. In contrast to transient depression, symptoms of **postpartum depression** last 6 to 8 weeks and are similar to symptoms of major depression at other times of life. Postpartum depression occurs in 20 percent of women and has been associated with a previous history of psychiatric illness.

Affonso's[35] preliminary research demonstrates a relationship between adaptation to postpartum stressors and self-reported symptoms of depression (eg, mood instability, difficulty in maintaining an eating schedule, fatigue, feelings of unattractiveness). Other nursing research has attempted to measure anxiety, depression, and hostility in mothers of preterm infants. Brooton and others[38] found that mothers of high-risk preterm infants were significantly more depressed before their infant was discharged than when the infant was 9 months old, multiparas were significantly more depressed than primiparas. Gennaro[39] compared postpartum anxiety and depression in mothers of term and preterm infants in the first 6 weeks postpartum and over the next 6 weeks. Mothers of preterm infants were significantly more anxious and depressed than mothers of term infants in the first postpartum week, but differences did not persist over time. This preliminary work indicates that health of the infant may contribute to depression in the postpartum period. Studies have further demonstrated an association between the mother's depression and adverse outcomes for the child.[40]

Clients with postpartum depression may experience a variety of behavioral manifestations. These include: sleep disturbances, decreased level of energy, appetite disturbances, feelings of worthlessness and isolation, negative emotions while with the infant, motor agitation or retardation, unfavorable future outlook, difficulties in relationships with partner and other family members, crying and mood swings, and recurrent thoughts of suicide.

Postpartum Psychosis. **Postpartum psychosis** is a severe psychiatric condition, similar to non-postpartum psychosis. This condition is relatively rare, occurring in 0.01 to 0.02 percent of postpartum women. A previous psychiatric history is demonstrated by 23 to 30 percent of women with postpartum psychosis, and the chance for recurrence ranges from 13 to 20 percent.[34]

Symptoms related to postpartum psychosis include delusions, hallucinations, disorganized or catatonic behavior, and loosening of associations. Postpartum psychosis differs from non-postpartum psychosis in that the delusional content reflects themes of childbirth.[34] For example, one postpartum psychotic mother told the nurse that she had delivered a baby girl in one hospital and was then transported to another hospital where a boy was exchanged for her girl.

Nursing and Collaborative Assessment. Assessment focuses on identifying postpartum depression and its contributing factors. The nurse elicits data regarding the woman's adaptation to her new role of mother[35]:

1. *Daily activities.* Difficulties in care of self, household, and infant; sleep; eating schedule; moods; interest in sex; energy level.
2. *Impact of childbirth events.* Frequency of thoughts about labor and delivery; feelings about the event; sense of disappointment, sadness, or ambivalence.
3. *Mother-infant interactions.* Degree of comfort while with the infant, degree of pleasure while performing infant tasks; thoughts of "something bad" happening to the infant; confused or angry feelings toward the infant; degree of comfort in being a mother.
4. *Social activities and supports.* Perception of relationship with infant's father; time for social activities with other adults; perception of receiving emotional support; sense of isolation from other adults.
5. *Self-assessment.* Degree to which the woman rates herself as a "good person"; ability to manage her many roles; sense of physical attractiveness; predominant mood; depressive feelings or suicidal thoughts.

Nursing Diagnosis. Careful assessment of the client for psychologic adaptation in the postpartum period leads to the development of appropriate nursing diagnoses for postpartum depression. *See* the box for examples.

Nursing and Collaborative Management. The nurse carefully observes each client for stressors that may impede adaptation and for signs and symptoms of transient depression, postpartum depression, and postpartum psychosis. If a history of previous depression or psychiatric disorders is found, appropriate referrals are made to community health nurses and psychiatric health care providers and agencies.

Clients with severe depression, psychosis, or both are usually hospitalized for comprehensive therapy. Clients with mild depressive disorders may be seen on an outpatient basis.

Management focuses on fostering adjustment of the client to her new role. Health care providers assist the client in developing feelings of self-worth and confidence in her ability to accomplish the tasks associated with the role of "mother." The woman's partner and other family members also need support and compassionate care during this period. (*See* the Case Study/Care Plan for specific interventions.) Early identification of severely depressed women is essential, as child abuse and neglect can occur as a result of the mother's condition.

Women with transient depression usually recover spontaneously with support. Women with postpartum depression may be treated as outpatients or inpatients. Outpatient treatment may include medications and group or individual therapies.

Women who require hospitalization for postpartum depression or psychosis may be given mood elevators and antidepressants, along with psychotherapy. For these women and their families, community follow-up is essential.

NURSING DIAGNOSES RELATED TO POSTPARTUM DEPRESSION

Problem-Oriented

Impaired social interaction, related to postpartum depression

Altered family processes, related to maternal depressive behavior

Potential for violence: self-directed or directed at infant, related to severe postpartum depression

Strength-Oriented

Positive self-concept, related to successful treatment for postpartum depression and positive social supports

Beginning social interaction with infant, related to successful management of postpartum depression and positive reinforcement of mothering skills

CASE STUDY/CARE PLAN: POSTPARTUM DEPRESSION

Alice and Peter Green come to the pediatrician's office for the first time with Matthew, their 2-week-old infant boy. This is their second son; their first child is 3 years old. The nurse practitioner takes a health history, including history of previous pregnancies and health of their first child. As the nurse is taking the history, she notes that Peter is doing all the responding and Alice is sitting in the chair with her head bent and eyes directed to the floor. Peter is holding the infant. The nurse directs her attention to Alice and asks how she is feeling. Alice replies in one or two words without raising her eyes from the floor. Alice's past history reveals previous postpartum depression and premenstrual syndrome. The previous postpartum depression lasted 3 weeks and was treated on an outpatient basis. Peter states that his wife's current symptoms seem more severe, "but we'll get through it."

Supporting Assessment Data	Expected Client/Family Outcome	Nursing Action/ Intervention	Rationale	Criteria for Evaluation
Nursing Diagnosis: Altered family processes, related to maternal depressive behavior				
History of postpartum depression and premenstrual syndrome Client does not make eye contact; has sad expression; does not look at or hold infant Client's husband does most of the responding during interview Client states that she wanted a girl Client's husband states that she needed much help in caring for first child; mother-in-law had to care for infant for first few weeks	By the next visit, the client will: Communicate with the health care provider Communicate with her husband, infant, and other family members and demonstrate beginning social interaction with infant and others Demonstrate positive self-concept and use of coping techniques	Identify strategies used by family to cope successfully with client's postpartum depression after birth of first child. Provide support to client and partner and encourage them to verbalize concerns. Assess the family's coping strategies and interactional patterns: verbal and nonverbal communication, role behavior, use of support systems.	Previous successful coping strategies are useful when similar crises emerge. Empathic care assures the couple that others understand and want to help. Verbalization helps the family define the crisis and coping strategies needed.	By the next visit, the client verbalizes, interacts with and makes eye contact with the health care provider. The client and family discuss strategies used after birth of first child.
		Assess maternal attachment behaviors and risk for delayed attachment and abuse.	Postpartum depression is a block to maternal-infant attachment. Lack of attachment can increase potential for abuse.	
		Identify family support systems and alternate caretakers for infant.	Social support is related to positive health care outcome.	By the next visit, client interacts socially and communicates with infant and other family members.
		Encourage couple to use stress management techniques: practice relaxation techniques, and get adequate rest, exercise, nutrition.	Stress management techniques that include positive self-help practices foster resolution of crisis in a positive manner.	Couple demonstrates and discusses stress management techniques.
		Provide referral to psychiatric clinical nurse specialist, psychologist, or psychiatrist (as necessary).	These practitioners can provide specialized care to the client and her family.	Client and partner inform nurse that they have sought assistance from specialist and have attended counseling sessions as necessary.

SUMMARY

The postpartum period is a time of adjustment for the client, her partner, and other family members. When complications occur during this phase of the childbearing cycle, the family is faced with a situational crisis. Complications of the postpartum period include physiologic and psychologic problems such as postpartum hemorrhage, reproductive and non-reproductive system infections, thromboembolic disorders, and postpartum depression.

Postpartum hemorrhage ranks as the most common cause of excessive blood loss during the childbearing cycle. Hemorrhage may occur early or late in the postpartum period. Leading causes of early postpartum hemorrhage are uterine atony and lacerations. The leading cause of delayed postpartum hemorrhage is subinvolution of the uterus.

Despite advances in maternity care, reproductive system (puerperal) infections still rank high as complications in the postpartum period. Bacteria that are normally present in the genital tract of pregnant women may multiply in the lochia and in devitalized tissue, or as a result of injury or lacerations. Metritis is the most common reproductive system infection affecting postpartum women. Infections that begin in the uterus may spread upward to the fallopian tubes and ovaries, outward to the parametrial cellular tissue, and, if more extensive, out to the peritoneal cavity. Septic thrombophlebitis also may occur. The mainstay of treatment for reproductive system infections is antimicrobial therapy.

Non–reproductive system infections may also complicate maternal postpartum recovery. These infections may occur outside of childbearing, but are also seen during childbearing. The two most common non–reproductive system infections are mastitis and urinary tract infection. A thorough assessment is needed to differentiate the cause of the symptoms of infection and plan appropriate care.

Thromboembolic disorders are another complication of the postpartum period. Changes in the blood coagulation system during the postpartum period may make a client prone to thromboembolic conditions such as superficial venous thrombophlebitis and deep venous thrombosis. A rare, but potentially life-threatening, complication of deep venous thrombosis is pulmonary embolism. This requires immediate medical and nursing attention.

The postpartum period may also be complicated by maternal transient depression ("postpartum blues"), postpartum depression, or postpartum psychosis. Symptoms of these conditions must be identified early so that the client may be given comprehensive care to avoid sequelae that would put the client or her infant at risk.

Nursing care for the client with postpartum complications focuses on prevention of sequelae, interventions appropriate to the condition, and rehabilitation for the client and other family members. The client and her family need compassionate and supportive care to promote progressive restoration to health and successful family adaptation.

REVIEW QUESTIONS

1. Describe two nursing interventions for a client with uterine atony.
2. Discuss the role of the nurse in caring for clients with postpartum lacerations.
3. Identify three symptoms of deep venous thrombosis.
4. Identify four conditions that can cause fever in the postpartum period and describe their management.
5. List three signs and symptoms of transient depression, postpartum depression, and postpartum psychosis.

REFERENCES

1. McCubbin H, Patterson JM. Family transitions: adaptation to stress. In: McCubbin H, Figley C, eds. *Stress and the Family.* New York: Brunner/Mazel; 1983:vol 1.
2. Kapernick, PS. Postpartum hemorrhage and the abnormal puerperium. In: Pernoll ML, ed. *Current Obstetric and Gynecologic Diagnosis and Treatment 1987.* 6th ed. Norwalk, Conn: Appleton & Lange; 1987.
3. Cunningham GF, et al. *Williams Obstetrics.* 18th ed. Norwalk, Conn: Appleton & Lange; 1989.
4. McKenizie CA, et al. Comprehensive care during the postpartum period. *Nurs Clin North Am.* 1982;17:23–48.
5. Hayashi RH, Castillo MS. Bleeding in pregnancy. In: Knuppel RA, Drukker JE, eds. *High-Risk Pregnancy: A Team Approach.* Philadelphia: WB Saunders; 1986.
6. Rochat RW, et al. Maternal Mortality in the U.S.: report from the Maternal Mortality Collaborative. *Obstet Gynecol.* 1988;72:91.

7. Gilstrap LC, et al. Effects of type of anesthesia on blood loss at cesarean section. *Obstet Gynecol.* 1987;69:328.
8. Jacobson H. A standard for assessing lochia volume. *Am J Matern Child Nurs.* 1985;10:174–175.
9. Jacobs MM, Arius F. Intramyometrial prostaglandin $F_{2}\alpha$ in the treatment of severe postpartum hemorrhage. *Obstet Gynecol.* 1980;55:655.
10. Hertz RH, et al. Treatment of postpartum uterine atony with prostaglandin E_2 vaginal suppositories. *Obstet Gynecol.* 1980;55:665.
11. Hayashi R, et al. Three year experience using Prostin/15 M in the management of severe postpartum hemorrhage. *Obstet Gynecol.* 1984;63:806.
12. Hayashi RH, et al. Management of severe postpartum hemorrhage due to uterine atony using an analogue of prostaglandin $F_{2}\alpha$. *Obstet Gynecol.* 1981;58:426.
13. Oxorn H, ed. *Oxorn-Foote Human Labor and Birth.* 5th ed. Norwalk, Conn: Appleton-Century Crofts; 1986.
14. Davidson N. REEDA: evaluating postpartum healing. *J Nurse Midwifery.* 1974;19:6–8.
15. Hill PS. Effects of heat and cold on the perineum after episiotomy laceration. *J Obstet Gynecol Neonat Nurs.* 1989; 18:124–129.
16. Henderson J. Effects of prenatal teaching programs on postpartum regeneration of the pubococcoygeal muscle. *J Obstet Gynecol Neonat Nurs.* 1983;12:403–408.
17. Lee CY, et al. Ultrasonic evaluation of the postpartum uterus in the management of postpartum bleeding. *Obstet Gynecol.* 1985;65:605.
18. Kaunitz AM, et al. Causes of maternal mortality in the United States. *Obstet Gynecol.* 1985;65:605.
19. Gibbs RS. Microbiology of the female genital tract. *Am J Obstet Gynecol.* 1987;156:491.
20. Eschenbach DA, et al. Isolation of mycoplasmas and bacteria from the blood of postpartum women. *Am J Obstet Gynecol.* 1982;143:104.
21. Beischer NA, MacKay EV, eds. *Obstetrics and the Newborn.* 2nd ed. Philadelphia: WB Saunders; 1986.
22. Varney H. *Nurse-Midwifery.* 2nd ed. Boston: Blackwell Scientific; 1987.
23. Brubaker JJ, et al. Developing a maternal-fetal intensive care unit. *J Obstet Gynecol Neonat Nurs.* 1988;17:321.
24. Thacker SB, Banta HD. Benefits and risks of episiotomy: an interpretive review of the English language literature, 1860–1980. *Obstet Gynecol Surv.* 1983;38:322.
25. Atkinson L. Prenatal nipple conditioning for breast feeding. *Nurs Res.* 1979;28:267–271.
26. Storr GB. Prevention of nipple tenderness and breast engorgement in the postpartal period. *J Obstet Gynecol Neonat Nurs.* 1988;17:203–209.
27. Niebyl JR. When the nursing mother has mastitis. *Contemp Obstet Gynecol.* 1985;26:31.
28. Roberts JE, et al. Professional attire at delivery: effect on postpartum and neonatal infection. *J Nurse-Midwifery.* 1986;31:16–19.
29. Ingardia CJ. Additional medical complications in pregnancy. In: Knuppel RA, Drukker JE, eds. *High-Risk Pregnancy: A Team Approach.* Philadelphia: WB Saunders; 1986.
30. Weiner CP. Diagnosis and management of thromboembolic disease during pregnancy. *Clin Obstet Gynecol.* 1985;28: 107.
31. Mannucci P, et al. Protein C antigen during pregnancy, delivery and puerperium. *Thrombos Haemostas.* 1984;52: 217.
32. Romen Y, Artal R. C-reactive protein in pregnancy and the postpartum period. *Am J Obstet Gynecol.* 1985;151:380–383.
33. Affonso D. Postpartum depression. In: Field P, ed. *Recent Advances in Perinatal Nursing.* Edinburgh: Churchill Livingstone; 1984.
34. Gjerdingen DK, et al. Postpartum mental and physical problems: how common are they? *Postgrad Med.* 1986;80: 133.
35. Affonso DD. Assessment of maternal postpartum adaptation. *Public Health Nurs.* 1987;4:9–20.
36. Hopkins J, et al. Postpartum depression: a critical review. *Psychol Bull.* 1984;95:498–515.
37. Newnham J, et al. A study of the relationship between circulating β-endorphin-like immunoreactivity and postpartum blues. *Clin Endocrinol.* 1984;20:169–177.
38. Brooton D, et al. Anxiety, depression and hostility in mothers of preterm infants. *Nurs Res.* 1988;37:213–216.
39. Gennaro S. Postpartal anxiety and depression in mothers of term and preterm infants. *Nurs Res.* 1988;37:82–89.
40. Zuckerman BS, Beardslee WR. Maternal depression: a concern for pediatricians. *Pediatrics.* 1987;79:110–116.

High-Risk Neonatal Nursing

unit

11

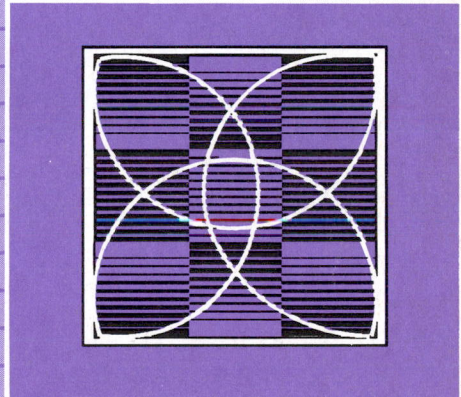

Neonatal Conditions

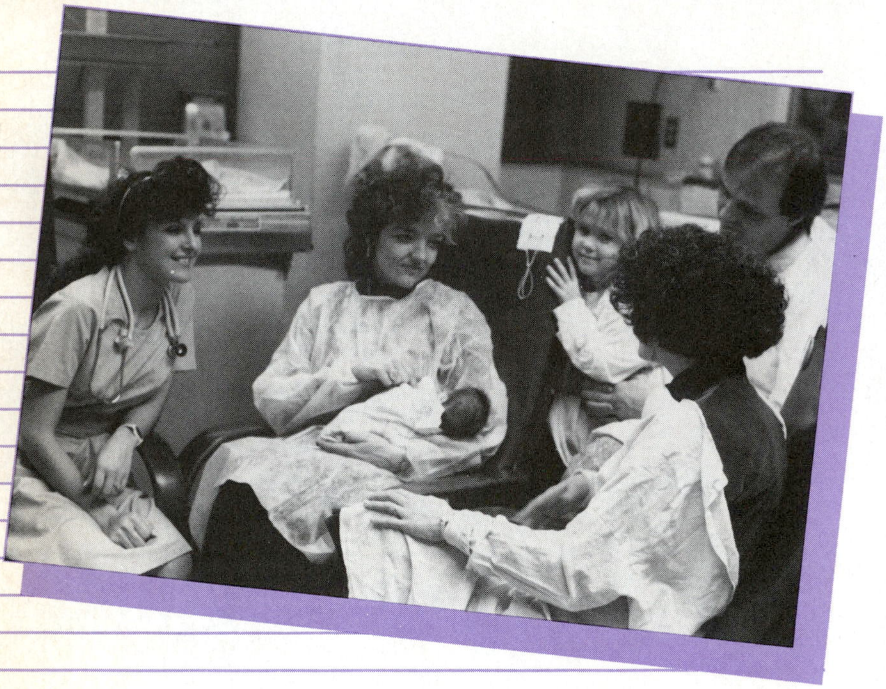

chapter 42

Key Terms

acyanotic heart defects
anencephaly
atresia
cyanotic heart defects
encephalocele
fetal alcohol syndrome
hemolytic diseases of the newborn
hyperbilirubinemia
hydrocephalus
hydranencephaly
inborn errors of metabolism
jaundice
kernicterus
meningocele
meningomyelocele
microcephaly
pathologic jaundice
phenylketonuria
polycythemia
spina bifida occulta

The major technologic and therapeutic advances in the last 20 years have produced significant and often parallel changes in perinatal and neonatal nursing care. Mortality and morbidity rates for pregnant women have improved and more infants are surviving the immediate birth experience than at any other time in history. Despite these advances, the first month of life, the neonatal period, is still a risky time for many infants. Although more neonates are surviving the birth experience, some require complex care to adapt to or to survive the early months of life. These neonates are at risk for physical, developmental, and psychosocial problems which may have long-term consequences.

The neonatal nurse plays an extremely important role in identifying risk factors or actual alterations in functioning that can complicate the neonate's transition to extrauterine life. The nurse is a key member of the interdisciplinary team that works to support the neonate through this transition by providing an environment that promotes optimal growth and development.

THE HIGH-RISK NEONATE

The neonate is described as high risk when factors affecting the prenatal course, the labor and delivery, or the transition to extrauterine life place the neonate at increased risk for altered functioning or even death.[1] Maternal risk factors such as lack of prenatal care, poor nutrition, and substance abuse create a difficult prenatal environment for the fetus and may result in altered fetal development. Neonates of mothers with medical conditions such as diabetes may also have difficulty in adjusting to extrauterine life.

Premature birth poses special challenges for the neonate. The premature neonate often requires maximum physiologic and environmental support from specially skilled interdisciplinary teams (*see* Chapter 43). Other neonates may develop special problems in the first hours or days of life that also make the transition to extrauterine life difficult. Such conditions as anemia, inborn errors of metabolism, and congenital heart disease may not have been suspected during the pregnancy. These disorders are identified after birth when abnormal signs and symptoms are assessed and further evaluated.

Nurses working in normal newborn nurseries have a special challenge. They must be able to distinguish normal neonatal activity, behavior, and physiologic functioning from abnormal signs and symptoms (*see* Chapter 33). They must do this by observing and interpreting subtle changes in the neonate. The interdisciplinary health care team recognizing high-risk problems may opt to transfer the neonate to a special care or intensive care nursery in the same or another hospital. An interdisciplinary team usually includes nurses, physicians, and respiratory therapists, who carefully coordinate the neonate's care during the transport between hospitals when this is necessary. Early identification of high-risk problems and neonatal transport to level III regional centers have resulted in a decline in neonatal mortality[2] (*see* Chapter 35).

Transition to parenthood is a process of change and stress even in the best of circumstances. The birth of a seriously ill newborn intensifies the stress and can create a crisis for the family. No physical abnormality or complication can be treated without addressing the emotional concerns of the family (*see* Chapter 36).

Many assessment and management strategies require procedures that can be restrictive, unpleasant, or painful for the high-risk neonate. Nurses are challenged to integrate soothing and emotionally supportive strategies into their physical care of the newborn. Organizing care to avoid constant or inappropriate stimulation of the neonate, controlling environmental noise and lighting, fostering parent-newborn interaction, and ensuring that the neonate is treated with dignity, touched gently, and cuddled if possible, help to ease the high-risk experience for tiny clients too young and too sick to be advocates on their own behalf.

NEONATAL PROBLEMS RELATED TO ALTERATIONS IN MATERNAL FUNCTIONING DURING PREGNANCY

The Neonate of a Substance-Abusing Mother

Any prenatal substance abuse by a mother can have lifelong adverse consequences for the neonate. The pregnancy of a substance-abusing woman is often associated with higher morbidity and mortality for the mother and the neonate.[3] These pregnancies may be complicated by inadequate prenatal care, poor nutrition, venereal diseases, pregnancy-induced hypertension, premature rupture of membranes, breech presentations of the fetus, and the delivery of preterm and small-for-gestational-age neonates.[3,4]

The most commonly abused substances include alcohol, marijuana, cocaine, and opiates (heroin and methadone). Periodic episodes of cerebral anoxia caused by repetitive in utero withdrawal of the abused substance can cause permanent brain damage in the fetus. Withdrawal from the addicting agents can also occur after birth, causing multiple physiologic problems for the neonate. In addition, the neonate may demonstrate a number of behavioral and attachment problems and often has difficulty adjusting to environmental stimuli such as noises and bright lights.

Drug Abuse

Nursing and Collaborative Assessment. Assessment of the pregnant woman must include a maternal history of drug use during pregnancy. Unfortunately, this information is difficult to obtain with accuracy because the mother may be reluctant to share any details or may be an unreliable historian. Identification of drugs used immediately prior to delivery is of utmost importance as well. The drugs crossing the placenta may seriously compromise the neonate's ability to adjust to extrauterine life immediately after birth.

Recognition of the most common signs of drug withdrawal in the neonate, sometimes called neonatal abstinence syndrome, is an important part of the ongoing nursing assessment. Neonates exhibit central nervous system, gastrointestinal, respiratory, and vasomotor symptoms as a result of drug withdrawal. Table 42–1 lists some of the most common symptoms observed in neonates suffering from drug withdrawal. Most neonates exhibit signs of withdrawal in the first 24 to 72 hours of life. Many nurseries have special checklists on which withdrawal symptoms can be quickly documented throughout the neonate's hospital stay. Figure 42–1 is an example of a withdrawal symptom checklist.

Nursing and Collaborative Mangement. Early identification of drug abuse in pregnant women is important for the prompt delivery of appropriate treatment for the neonate. The main treatment goal is to support the neonate's physical needs while maintaining an environment that promotes adequate adjustment to extrauterine life. Specific nursing interventions include the following:

TABLE 42–1. SIGNS OF DRUG WITHDRAWAL IN THE NEONATE

Central nervous system	Sleeplessness Irritability High-pitched cry Tremors and increased muscle tone Seizures Fevers Sneezing and nasal stuffiness Increased sucking (within 5 minutes of feeding) Yawning Hiccups
Gastrointestinal	Poor appetite Problems with feedings Vomiting and diarrhea
Respiratory	Tachypnea
Vasomotor	Sweating Mottling of the skin

- Identifying the neonate at risk for drug withdrawal
- Decreasing environmental stimuli to reduce irritability, conserve energy, and promote sleep and rest; limiting loud noises and bright lights; swaddling the neonate; and approaching the neonate calmly
- Balancing small, frequent feedings with frequent rest periods to conserve energy and promote nutrition and growth
- When possible, feeding the neonate "on demand" rather than according to a predetermined feeding schedule
- Supporting the neonate's self-comforting measures, for example making the pacifier easily available
- Promoting the neonate's skin integrity by changing the neonate's position and by frequently cleaning and drying the skin, in particular, the diaper area
- Encouraging the parents to hold and care for the neonate to promote parent-newborn attachment
- Educating the parents about care of the neonate and rationales for any therapies that the neonate is receiving

Medical interventions, such as the use of medications, may be required for these neonates. The need to use medications to assist the neonate through the withdrawal process is based on the type of drug from which the neonate is withdrawing and the severity of the withdrawal symptoms. Severe irritability that disrupts normal sleeping or feeding patterns, poor weight gain, diarrhea, and seizure are symptoms indicating the need for treatment.[3]

Methadone and heroin withdrawal can be successfully controlled with the use of medications. Phenobarbital administered in doses of 8 to 10 mg/kg per day divided into four doses decreases irritability and seizures. Paregoric is given in doses of 3 to 5 drops every 3 to 6 hours to help treat severe diarrhea. Dilute tincture of opium is given in doses of 0.2 to 0.5 mL every 3 to 5 hours until the symptoms are controlled.[3]

Medications used to control withdrawal symptoms are usually continued for 1 week but may be continued up to 6 weeks in the presence of severe symptoms.[3] Because of the increasing rate of drug abuse, numerous research studies are being conducted to identify additional data regarding maternal drug use, as well as the short-term and long-term effects on the neonates who suffer from exposure and withdrawal from these drugs.

Alcohol Abuse

Nursing and Collaborative Assessment. Ideally, assessment of risk factors related to alcohol use should occur before conception, as safe levels of alcohol consumption during pregnancy have not been identified. Alcohol education and the particular consequences of alcohol consumption on pregnant women should be available to women of childbearing age. Assessment of pregnant women must also include a maternal history of alcohol use during the pregnancy. Again, obtaining an accurate history in either situation may be difficult. A nonjudgmental approach that does not intimidate the woman is the best method for obtaining accurate data. Table 42–2 provides examples of questions that may be useful in identifying the alcohol-using mother.[5]

Many clients may not be aware of the effects that alcohol can have on their unborn child. They may request additional information about the effects of alcohol consumption during pregnancy. Clients falling into the high-risk group of heavy alcohol consumption include those who have five or more drinks of beer, wine, or mixed drinks on occasion, or at least one and one-half drinks per day. These clients require additional information and support.[5] Nurses must reinforce the importance of continued prenatal care. When appropriate, nurses can refer these clients to community organizations such as Alcoholics Anonymous. Maintaining contact throughout the pregnancy is important to ensure proper follow-up care.

Assessment of the neonate begins with identification of maternal alcohol use. At times, however, identification is not possible prior to delivery of the neonate. **Fetal alcohol syndrome** is the term given to a group of abnormalities found in neonates who are exposed to unsafe levels of alcohol consumption during pregnancy. Estimates indicate that fetal alcohol syndrome occurs in 1 to 2 of 1000 live births.[3]

The major characteristics of fetal alcohol syndrome are prenatal and postnatal growth retardation, permanent damage to the central nervous system in

NEONATAL ABSTINENCE SYNDROME ASSESSMENT SCORESHEET

Name:____________________________

Date:____________________________

System	Signs and Symptoms	Score	AM					PM					Comments
Central Nervous System Disturbances	Excessive High Pitched (or other) Cry Continuous High Pitched (or other) Cry	2 3											Daily Weight:
	Sleeps <1 Hour After Feeding Sleeps >2 Hours After Feeding Sleeps <3 Hours After Feeding	3 2 1											
	Hyperactive Moro Reflex Markedly Hyperactive Moro Reflex	2 3											
	Mild Tremors Disturbed Moderate-Severe Tremors Disturbed	1 2											
	Mild Tremors Undisturbed Moderate-Severe Tremors Undisturbed	3 4											
	Increased Muscle Tone	2											
	Excoriation (specify area):__________	1											
	Myoclonic Jerks	3											
	Generalized Convulsions	5											
Metabolic/Vasomotor/Respiratory Disturbances	Sweating	1											
	Fever <(101 99–100.8°F/37.2–38.2°C) Fever >(38.4°C and higher)	1 2											
	Frequent Yawning (>3–4 times/interval)	1											
	Mottling or Webbing	1											
	Nasal Stuffiness	2											
	Sneezing (>3–4 times/interval)	1											
	Nasal Flaring	2											
	Respiratory Rate >60/Minute Respiratory Rate >60/Minute With Retractions	1 2											
Gastrointestinal Disturbances	Excessive Sucking More Than 5 Minutes After Feeding	1											
	Poor Feeding, Poorly Coordinated Sucking and Swallowing Reflex	2											
	Regurgitation Projectile Vomiting	2 3											
	Loose Stools Watery Stools	2 3											
	Total Score												
	Initials of Scorer												

Figure 42–1. Neonatal abstinence syndrome assessment scoresheet.

TABLE 42–2. ASSESSMENT QUESTIONS FOR IDENTIFYING MATERNAL ALCOHOL ABUSE DURING PREGNANCY

How often do you drink wine, wine coolers, beer, or mixed drinks?

How much wine, wine coolers, beer, and/or mixed drinks do you consume at one time?

Do you think that you drink "too little," "too much," or "just enough"?

How often do you drink "too much"?

Does anyone in your family have a drinking problem? Please describe.

Do you drink wine, wine coolers, beer, and/or mixed drinks now? (during your pregnancy)

How much wine, wine coolers, beer, and/or mixed drinks did/do you drink now? (during your pregnancy)

How often did/do you drink wine, wine coolers, beer, and/or mixed drinks during your pregnancy?

Did you know that your drinking alcoholic beverages, wine, wine coolers, beer, and/or mixed drinks can affect your unborn child?

the form of microcephaly, mental retardation, and craniofacial abnormalities (Figure 42–2). Table 42–3 lists additional characteristics of this syndrome. *Fetal alcohol effect* is the term sometimes used to describe lesser manifestations of this problem.[5]

Nursing Diagnoses. Examples of nursing diagnoses related to fetal alcohol syndrome are presented in the box.

Nursing and Collaborative Management. Care of the neonate with fetal alcohol syndrome or fetal alcohol effect centers on providing supportive and palliative interventions. Special attention should be taken to avoid overstimulating the neonate. Swaddling the neonate with blankets and offering a pacifier are particularly helpful in soothing and quieting the neonate. Ongoing assessment of neurologic function should include observation of the neonate's alertness, body position, muscle tone, movement, and reflexes.[6] Seizures are treated with anticonvulsant medications. (*See* later section on "Neonatal Seizures.") Intravenous feedings may be necessary if the neonate's ability to suck is too weak to meet nutritional and hydration needs.

Parents and family members need ongoing support. They must be given accurate information about how the neonate will respond to stimuli and strategies that can be used to console the neonate when at home. Prior to discharge, parents should be given consistent opportunities to feed the neonate; the nurse can use this time to offer suggestions that will assist parents in providing the neonate with adequate nutrition, as discussed earlier. Referral services should be shared with the parents as the potential for frustration in caring for these infants is great.

In situations where additional substance abuse is also identified, mothers will require further support and education through referral services. Neonates suffering from both drug and alcohol withdrawal often have special care needs such as a quiet nonstressed environment, frequent feedings, and ongoing medical follow-up. Mothers who have abused drugs and alcohol during pregnancy to such an extent that the neonate suffers from withdrawal or has related anomalies should be considered high-risk clients for parenting disorders. Drug abuse impairs parental judgment and the ability to care for a neonate, especially a neonate who is difficult to feed and comfort.

Evaluation of the mother's social situation and the family's home environment is important to ensure safety and security of the neonate. Interdisciplinary collaboration, including nurses, physicians, and social workers, is essential in identifying the neonate's special needs. Inclusion of other family members in planning for care (such as the neonate's grandparents,) is essential because these individuals may become the primary care providers at home. At times the home environment may be so unstable that foster care becomes necessary. Social workers will be able to identify the appropriate community agencies and resources for the neonate, mother, and family to assist with this difficult process. In addition, current research is focusing on such strategies as residential treatment centers for substance-using mothers and neonates to facilitate parenting abilities.

NURSING DIAGNOSES RELATED TO FETAL ALCOHOL SYNDROME

Problem-Oriented

Altered growth and development, related to teratogenic effects of alcohol on fetus

Alteration in nutrition: less than body requirements, related to weak neonatal sucking ability

Altered family processes, related to maternal feelings of guilt

Strength-Oriented

Potential enhanced neonatal development, related to participation in infant development (stimulation) program

Potential for progressive family coping, related to participation in support groups

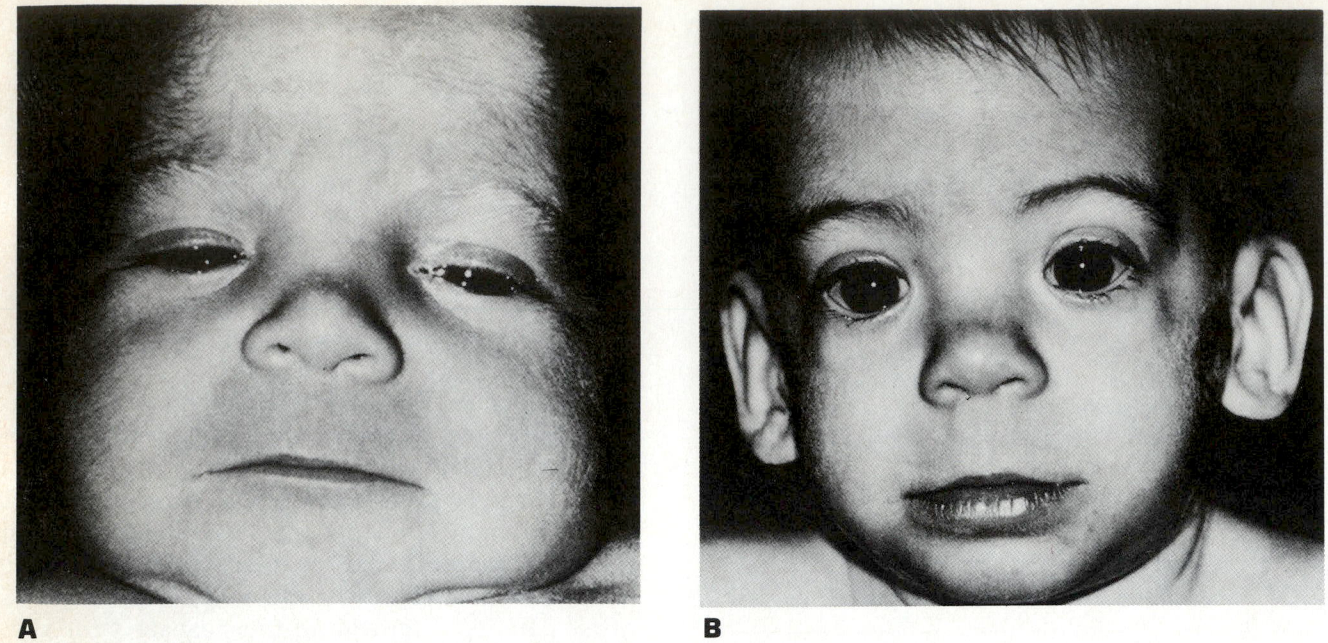

Figure 42–2. Facial features of a child with fetal alcohol syndrome at **A.** 1 week and **B.** 1 year of age. Note the narrow palpebral fissures, short nose with broad low bridge, midfacial hypoplasia, and long philtrum with narrow vermillion border. (*Reproduced, with permission, from Rudolph AM, ed.* Pediatrics. *18th ed. Norwalk, Conn: Appleton & Lange; 1987:374.*)

The Neonate of a Diabetic Mother

Diabetes mellitus is a major high-risk condition of pregnancy (*see* Chapter 39). One in every 500 to 1000 pregnant women are diabetic. Gestational diabetes (diabetes occurring during pregnancy) occurs in 1 in 120 pregnancies.[7] Maternal diabetes is associated with a higher-than-normal rate of neonatal complications such as death and stillbirth.

Reducing risk for the neonate of a diabetic mother begins with careful prenatal care, focusing on glucose monitoring, metabolic control, and teaching regarding diet and medication so that plasma glucose levels are safely maintained during pregnancy.[8] The goal is to closely monitor the pregnancy so that the neonate can be born at term with minimal complications. Also essential to reducing neonatal risk are the rapid assessment and treatment of actual and potential problems of the newborn of a diabetic mother.

Alterations in glucose metabolism in the diabetic mother dramatically affect the fetus in utero and immediately after birth. Hyperglycemia in the diabetic mother causes fetal hyperglycemia. The fetal pancreas responds to the hyperglycemia by producing large volumes of insulin, a condition called hyperinsulinemia. The hyperglycemia and hyperinsulinemia in the fetus affect intrauterine physiologic growth and development. The fetus is at high risk for developing abnormalities in many body systems, for example, respiratory distress syndrome and congenital heart defects.

The birth of the neonate of the diabetic mother may be complicated by a preterm delivery or a difficult term delivery. The neonate may develop problems after birth because the maternal source of high levels of glucose is no longer present. The neonate's pancreas continues to produce insulin; therefore, the glucose level continues to fall. If untreated, the neonate can develop hypoglycemia and other serious complications.

TABLE 42–3. CHARACTERISTICS OF FETAL ALCOHOL SYNDROME

Prenatal and postnatal growth retardation
Central nervous system abnormalities
Microcephaly
Poor muscle tone
Weak sucking ability
Mental retardation
Irritability
Developmental delays
Craniofacial abnormalities
Small palpebral fissures of the eyes
Flat maxillary area
Thin upper lip
Flat or absent philtrum
Short, upturned nose

Nursing and Collaborative Assessment

Appearance. The neonate of a diabetic mother commonly has an unusually large body size (macrosomia). The neonate appears plump, plethoric (beefy red), puffy, and exhausted from the ordeal of birth. These neonates breathe heavily when lying on their backs. They may be floppy and lethargic and may suck poorly or may be easily excited, jittery, and irritable. Occasionally, neonates of diabetic mothers may be small for gestational age as a result of placental insufficiency in utero.

Assessment of the neonate at rest and during activities such as feeding is important. Accurate measurements of height, weight, and head and chest circumferences must be plotted on the neonate's growth chart.[3]

Intrauterine Growth. Hyperglycemia and hyperinsulinemia affect the intrauterine growth of neonates of diabetic mothers. Intrauterine growth can be accelerated, causing 16 to 40 percent of these neonates to be large for gestational age (LGA).[9] When intrauterine growth is accelerated, most body organs except the brain are prone to be larger. Unlike other LGA neonates, LGA neonates of diabetic mothers characteristically have subcutaneous fat deposits rather than increased length and head size (Figure 42–3).[7] Large-for-gestational-age neonates are at greater risk for injuries during delivery. Cesarean delivery may be warranted to prevent traumatic birth injuries such as shoulder dystocia, clavicular fractures, depressed skull fractures, brachial plexus palsy, and facial paralysis.[7]

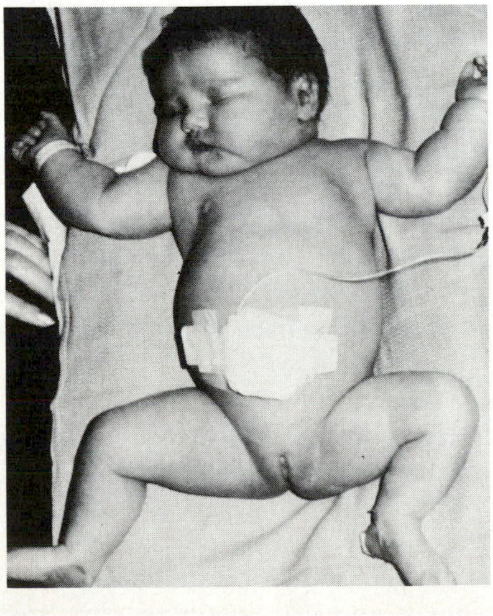

Figure 42–3. Neonate of a diabetic mother born at 36 weeks of gestation and weighing 4400 g. (*Reproduced, with permission, from Rudolph AM, ed.* Pediatrics. *18th ed. Norwalk, Conn: Appleton & Lange; 1987:148.*)

Conversely, some neonates of diabetic mothers may be small for gestational age, particularly if the mother has advanced or severe diabetes associated with vascular complications, impaired uterine blood flow, and compromised placental functioning.[3] These neonates require special attention related to their low birth weight and potentially compromised metabolic state.

Respiratory Distress. The neonate of a diabetic mother is at risk for developing respiratory distress and hyaline membrane disease after birth. Surfactant is the phospholipoprotein required for adequate respiration in the newborn (*see* Chapter 43). Surfactant production is altered by the hyperinsulinemia in the fetus. As a result, the neonate of a diabetic mother may not have produced enough surfactant before birth. The neonate will then have difficulty breathing after the delivery and will demonstrate signs and symptoms of respiratory distress. The nurse will observe a high respiratory rate (greater than 40 breaths per minute when sleeping or quiet). The neonate may grunt with each breath, may exhibit retractions or nasal flaring, and may require supplemental oxygen. The nurse must assess the color of the neonate's skin, mucous membranes, and nail beds. Pale, dusky, or blue color changes indicate increasing respiratory distress requiring immediate intervention.

Congenital Anomalies. The neonate of a diabetic mother is three times more likely to have congenital anomalies especially related to specific maternal physiologic alterations.[3] One study indicates that higher glycosylated hemoglobin levels in the nongestational diabetic client are related to the presence of major congenital anomalies, such as hydrocephalus and limb reduction defect.[10] High maternal blood glucose levels in the first trimester have been associated with a higher incidence of fetal malformations such as congenital heart disease.[11] The most common cardiac anomalies are transposition of the great vessels, ventricular septal defects, and patent ductus arteriosis.[12] Lumbosacral spine anomalies such as caudal regression syndrome are also seen in neonates of diabetic mothers.

During assessment of the neonate in whom possible cardiac anomalies are anticipated, special attention should be paid to heart rate, blood pressure, peripheral pulses, color, and activity level. A neonate who has sustained tachycardia, weak peripheral pulses, and a pale or dusky coloring and who tires quickly with feedings or activity should be assessed aggressively. Abnormalities of the spine may be apparent at birth and are managed on the basis of the nature of the anomaly. The nurse must attentively observe the neonate's musculoskeletal system, noting the presence of obvious abnormalities and ability to move all four extremities equally well.

Metabolic Disturbances. The neonate of a diabetic mother is at risk for numerous alterations in metabolic functioning. These neonates often develop hypoglycemia (low blood glucose level) as a result of the presence of high levels of insulin in the absence of the maternal source of glucose (*see* "Alterations in Metabolic Functioning" later). Insulin levels are initially high at birth because the fetal pancreas attempts to respond to high glucose levels in utero. Adjustment to normal limits usually occurs in the first few days of life.

These neonates are also at risk for hyperbilirubinemia related to large birth weight, complicated vaginal delivery, hemorrhage resulting from traumatic birth injuries, and prematurity (*see* "Alterations in Hematologic Functioning" later). Hypocalcemia may also be found during the neonatal assessment. Hypocalcemia may be related to abnormalities in maternal calcium levels, prematurity, or a difficult delivery (*see* "Alterations in Metabolic Functioning" later). Glucagon production in the liver may decrease in response to the low glucose levels found in the neonate of the diabetic mother after delivery. Nursing assessment of the neonate of a diabetic mother includes the assessment of signs and symptoms of metabolic disturbances as well as the monitoring of laboratory test results.

Nursing Diagnoses. Nursing diagnoses for the neonate of a diabetic mother are developed on the basis of a comprehensive assessment. *See* the box for examples of nursing diagnoses for a macrosomic neonate.

NURSING DIAGNOSES RELATED TO A MACROSOMIC NEONATE

Problem-Oriented

Potential for trauma of the neonate during labor and delivery, related to large size

Altered growth and development, related to immaturity

Altered nutrition: less than body requirements, related to hypoglycemia in the newborn period

Strength-Oriented

Effective family coping, related to understanding physiologic bases of neonatal macrosomia

Potential for normal neonatal growth and development, related to maternal glycemic control during pregnancy

Nursing and Collaborative Management. Nursing care of the neonate of a diabetic mother must address the actual and potential complications of delivering a macrosomic and LGA newborn. The initial and ongoing newborn assessments include inspection for traumatic birth injuries. Management is determined by the type and severity of the actual injuries sustained by the neonate. Small-for-gestational age neonates are less likely to sustain traumatic birth injuries. They do, however, face high-risk deliveries because of maternal complications related to severe diabetes, low birth weight, and in many cases prematurity (*see* Chapter 43). They also are at great risk, after delivery, of developing further difficulties related to fetal hyperglycemia and hyperinsulinemia (*see* the Case Study/Care Plan).

Neonates of diabetic mothers often require aggressive assessment and intervention. They may require special attention for multisystem problems soon after delivery. For example, the neonate may require ventilatory support for severe respiratory distress, specially prepared intravenous fluids to prevent or manage electrolyte imbalances, and phototherapy for hyperbilirubinemia. (*See* later sections on "Alterations in Metabolic Functioning" and "Alterations in Hematologic Functioning.") The neonate's stay in an intensive care nursery may be extended until the abnormalities experienced at or after birth are resolved. Parents continue to require the support and information offered by the nurses and other members of the interdisciplinary team caring for the neonate.

Many interventions are based on the presence and severity of respiratory distress. Respiratory distress can progress to hyaline membrane disease if surfactant production has been severely altered. Mechanical ventilation may be needed to provide adequate oxygen and respirations until the lung disease resolves and the neonate can breathe well enough without assistance. Continued monitoring and ongoing assessment of respiratory function are therefore essential.[3]

CASE STUDY/CARE PLAN: THE NEONATE OF A DIABETIC MOTHER

Baby Margie Myers was born at 38 weeks of gestation to an insulin-dependent diabetic mother by spontaneous vaginal delivery. Mrs. Myers experienced difficulty in controlling her serum glucose levels throughout her pregnancy. Baby Myers weighed 9 pounds 10 oz at birth. She was puffy and mildly lethargic with an initial serum glucose level of 40. Her respirations were initially labored at a rate of 40 breaths per minute. The results of the arterial blood gas analysis were PaO_2 95, CO_2 35, pH 7.35. Her head was molded and she moved all four extremities independently and symmetrically when stimulated and crying. Baby Myers was given 5 percent glucose water orally in the delivery room.

Supporting Assessment Data	Expected Client/Family Outcome	Nursing Action Intervention	Rationale	Criteria for Evaluation
Nursing Diagnosis: Alteration in metabolism, related to hyperinsulinemia secondary to maternal diabetes				
Dextrostix at delivery 40; confirmed by laboratory analysis Dextrostix following oral feeding of 5 percent glucose water 75; confirmed by laboratory analysis	Neonate will be free of signs and symptoms of hypoglycemia after birth	Observe for signs and symptoms of hypoglycemia (weak cry, apnea, cyanosis, hypothermia, lethargy, feeding problems, tremors, or seizures).	Early identification of signs and symptoms can lead to prompt treatment preventing serious harm to neonate.	Neonate is pink in color, has a strong cry, and is feeding well.
	Neonate will have normal serum glucose level while tolerating feedings every 3 hours for at least 24 hours before planned discharge	Offer oral feeding of 5 percent glucose water or breast milk on obtaining low serum glucose level of 40 following delivery.	Offering an early feeding will provide glucose to treat mild hypoglycemia.	Serum glucose 75 following early oral feeding of 5 percent glucose water.
		Obtain good quality specimen for evaluation of serum glucose every 2 hours for the first 8 hours of life and then every 4 hours for 24 hours until stable.	Quality specimen will provide accurate serum glucose values essential in safely treating hypoglycemia.	Serum glucose values range between 100 and 120 after 8 hours of life.
Nursing Diagnosis: Potential for alteration in respiratory effort, related to inadequate surfactant production in utero				
Respiratory rate 40 No retractions, flaring, grunting Color pink in room air No supplemental oxygen given Arterial blood gases: PaO_2 95; CO_2 35; pH 7.35	Neonate will maintain adequate respirations without supplemental oxygen 48 hours before planned discharge	Ongoing assessment for signs of respiratory distress, increased respiratory rate, presence of retractions, nasal flaring, grunting, cyanosis.	Early identification of respiratory distress will lead to prompt treatment and prevention of serious harm to neonate.	Neonate remains pink, breathing easily at a rate of 40.
		Position neonate to promote ease in respirations, ie, head of bed elevated, side lying.	Proper positioning can decrease the work of breathing in the potentially compromised neonate.	Neonate breathes easily and regularly with head of bed elevated and in side-lying position.
		Administer warmed, humidified supplemental oxygen as ordered by physician.	Supplemental oxygen is used to treat hypoxia; warmed humidity prevents the oxygen from drying and harming the tissues of the respiratory tract.	

(continued)

CASE STUDY/CARE PLAN: The Neonate of a Diabetic Mother *(continued)*

Supporting Assessment Data	Expected Client/Family Outcome	Nursing Action Intervention	Rationale	Criteria for Evaluation
		Monitor the results of arterial blood gases.	Arterial blood gases are an invasive way to accurately monitor serum oxygen, carbon dioxyde, and pH values essential in evaluating oxygen exchange and the effectiveness of oxygen therapy.	Results of arterial blood gases are within normal limits and supplemental oxygen is not required.
Nursing Diagnosis: Potential for musculoskeletal trauma during birth, related to macrosomia and large for gestational age				
Moving all four extremities independently and symmetrically	Neonate will demonstrate independent symmetric range of motion of all four extremities following labor and delivery	Assess for presence of paralysis, or asymmetric movement of extremities or in appearance of face or head.	Identification of traumatic injuries will lead to prompt treatment.	Neonate able to independently and symmetrically move all four extremities.
Facial movements are present and symmetrical	Neonate will demonstrate symmetric facial movements following labor and delivery			Facial movements are equal and symmetric. Head is oblong in shape, found to be related to vaginal delivery.
Head is round and symmetric without depression	Neonate's head will be round and symmetric without depressions following labor and delivery			No abnormalities of the skull or soft tissue are present.
		Monitor color, temperature, sensation, movement, and presence and quality of pulses in extremity, and document.	A traumatic injury may result in compromise of neurologic or cardiovascular functioning requiring immediate intervention. Consistent documentation will demonstrate clinical changes over time.	Neonate's four extremities remain pink and warm, with strong palpable pulses present. Neonate moves extremities independently and with tactile stimulation.
		Move neonate into positions of comfort and safety.	The potential presence of a traumatic injury will require careful positioning to promote appropriate healing and to prevent further injury.	Neonate is placed in supine position in radiant warmer until it is determined that a traumatic injury is not present. Neonate now rests comfortably in open air crib in side-lying position.
Nursing Diagnosis: Potential for alteration in metabolism, related to hyperbilirubinemia				
Serum bilirubin 6.0 No yellow discoloration of skin, sclera, or mucous membranes present	Neonate will maintain bilirubin level within normal limits for 24 hours before planned discharge	Assess for presence of yellow discoloration of skin, sclera, or mucous membranes	Yellow discoloration can be a sign of jaundice and must be documented and further evaluated.	Neonate remains pink in color without yellow discoloration.
		Monitor intake (volume and frequency of oral feedings) and output (volume and frequency of urine and stool).	Bilirubin is excreted in urine and stool; adequate intake and output will promote excretion of bilirubin.	Neonate tolerates 2 oz of formula every 2 to 3 hours; has at least 6 wet diapers in 24 hours and 4 stools in 24 hours.
		Monitor serum bilirubin.	Serum bilirubin values are accurate indicators of the presence of abnormal levels of bilirubin requiring additional therapy.	Serum bilirubin level remains 6.0.

If jaundice is suspected, or hyperbilirubinemia is anticipated, serum bilirubin levels must be monitored. Phototherapy is the most common treatment for mild to moderate hyperbilirubinemia. Muscle irritability may be related to hypocalcemia and should be confirmed by obtaining serum calcium levels. Supplementation of calcium via the intravenous fluid is the treatment of choice.

Hyperinsulinemia is directly related to the risk for hypoglycemia, the most common alteration in the metabolic functioning of neonates of diabetic mothers. Hypoglycemia may have obvious signs and symptoms or it may be asymptomatic. In either case, early identification and management can prevent further high-risk complications for the neonate. Accordingly, neonatal hypoglycemia is addressed in more detail in the later section, "Alterations in Metabolic Functioning."[3]

The Neonate of an Infected Mother

Infections in the neonate are the result of preconceptional, prenatal, intrapartum, and postpartum exposure to viruses and bacteria. Infections acquired before conception, such as human immunodeficiency virus, can affect the neonate. Some infections can pose a potential threat during pregnancy. One such group of infections, called the TORCH infections, is discussed in Chapter 39. Intrapartum infections occur when the neonate is exposed to such organisms as *Chlamydia trachomatis* or herpes simplex virus that can be found in the mother's genital tract. This exposure can occur after the mother's membranes rupture or during the passage through the birth canal.[13] Postnatal infections can be caused by contact with the same prenatal and intrapartum bacteria or viruses; however, many postnatal infections have been found to be nosocomial (or hospital-acquired) infections. These infections are caused by normal human flora or pathogens that are transmitted from neonate to neonate on the hands of nursery staff.[13]

Health care providers routinely use isolation techniques when caring for clients with known infections. Any newborn is at risk of being infected. As a newborn may not manifest the signs and symptoms at the beginning of an infection, health care providers place themselves at greater risk when proper infection control practices are relaxed in caring for a neonate who appears "well." Consistent use of universal precautions is essential. These techniques limit the risk of spreading known or unknown bloodborne infections to other infants in the nursery and other health care providers. (*See* Appendix E for universal precautions.)

Neonatal Sepsis. Neonatal sepsis refers to a bacterial infection occurring during the first 4 weeks after birth and found primarily in the blood.[14] Organisms responsible for neonatal sepsis include *Staphylococcus aureus, Staphylococcus epidermidis, Escherichia coli,* and group B hemolytic streptococcus. Bacteremia may vary from mild to severe. Most neonates can be treated successfully for bacterial sepsis; however, overwhelming infection or complications related to multiple body system involvement can lead to long-term problems or death. Sepsis has been estimated to be responsible for up to 45 percent of neonatal deaths.[14]

Risk factors associated with neonatal sepsis include maternal infection; preterm delivery; low birth weight; invasive procedures during pregnancy, labor, delivery, or the neonatal period; and neonatal stay in an intensive care nursery where bacterial organisms tend to thrive.

Nursing and Collaborative Assessment. Because of their ongoing contact with the neonate in hospital settings, nurses are frequently the first health care providers to identify signs and symptoms of neonatal sepsis (Table 42–4). All of the signs and symptoms of neonatal sepsis can indicate other conditions. Neonates respond globally; in other words, infection primarily in one site, such as the meninges, is manifested by alterations throughout the body. Signs and symptoms of neonatal sepsis are often subtle; therefore, when a neonate does not seem healthy, careful assessment for sepsis may be warranted. Septic "workups," however, should not be performed without specific indications. To spare parents the enormous financial and emotional costs related to a septic "workup," health care providers must be able to distinguish normal neonatal variations from high-risk conditions.

Assessment focuses on the following parameters[14]: maternal, fetal and neonatal history; the ne-

TABLE 42–4. SIGNS AND SYMPTOMS OF NEONATAL SEPSIS

Respiratory distress (nasal flaring, grunting, retractions, increased respiratory rate, apnea)
Bradycardia
Cyanosis; pallor
Temperature instability (decreased or increased temperature)
Jaundice
Lethargy
Poor feeding
High-pitched cry
Bulging fontanelles
Seizures

onate's activity and behaviors (alertness, feeding, crying); temperature, heart rate, respirations, and blood pressure; presence of seizures or bulging fontanelles; and presence and degree of jaundice. Diagnostic tests for neonatal sepsis include: cultures of blood, urine, stool, spinal fluid, and any intravenous or arterial line. In addition, cultures are taken from any area with suspicious drainage, such as the eyes or umbilical stump. Maternal cultures, for example of vaginal and cervical secretions, may also be performed. Other diagnostic tests include complete blood count with differential, serum electrolytes, and glucose; blood gas analysis; urinalysis; and chest x-ray. Because signs and symptoms of sepsis can also be manifestations of other conditions such as neurologic impairment, assessment techniques used to diagnose these conditions may be employed.

Nursing and Collaborative Management. The goals of management of neonatal sepsis are to identify the type and source of infection, to initiate treatment that cures the infection and minimizes or prevents associated complications, and to support the neonate's parents through this difficult period.

The neonate is cared for in a special care nursery equipped for treatment of neonatal sepsis. After cultures are taken, antibiotic therapy is begun, as prescribed by the physician. During treatment, blood tests are taken to ensure that therapeutic levels of antibiotics are maintained. Other physiologic interventions relate to the nature of organ system involvement. For example, a ventilator may be needed for respiratory support, and a radiant warmer may be used to stabilize body temperature. Management also includes strategies for care of other co-existing problems, such as prematurity.

Nurses have a crucial role in providing access to the neonate and education for the parents of a septic neonate. Nursing support is especially important if the mother is separated from her neonate because of factors such as her own fever or transport of the neonate to a neonatal intensive care unit at another hospital. (*See* Chapter 36 for a discussion of psychosocial needs of parents of infants who are in or transported to a neonatal intensive care unit.)

As a preventive strategy for management of neonatal sepsis, members of the interdisciplinary team need to practice measures that decrease the likelihood of nosocomial infection. Good handwashing technique and universal precautions need to be employed in every client care setting.[15]

Human Immunodeficiency Virus Infection. Human immunodeficiency virus (HIV) infection was first identified in 1981 in adults. Human immunodeficiency virus is a retrovirus that attacks the T lymphocytes in the human immune system. This virus was formerly referred to as human T-cell leukemic virus III/lymphadenopathic virus (HTLV III/LAV). In 1986, a special international panel of experts named this retrovirus human immunodeficiency viruses or HIV.[16,17]

As of December 1988, more than 1200 cases of HIV in children had been reported.[16] Epidemiologic data suggest that in 18 percent of those cases, transmission occurred from an infected mother to her fetus or neonate during the perinatal period.[17,18] This transmission can occur when the virus crosses the placenta prenatally, when the neonate consumes breast milk postnatally, or when the neonate is exposed to maternal blood and body fluids during birth.[17]

A small number of people have become infected with HIV from contaminated blood. Eighty-six percent of adult HIV cases fall into risk groups related to social behavior. Specifically, high-risk populations include intravenous drug users, homosexual and bisexual men, and heterosexual individuals who have had sexual contact with individuals with HIV infection or who are at risk for HIV infection.[17] Women of childbearing age who practice high-risk behaviors, such as mothers who have multiple sexual partners, are intravenous drug users, or have sexual contact with men in high-risk groups, are increasingly vulnerable to contract HIV infection and may transmit the disease to their neonates. Often these women are asymptomatic and become aware of their own infection only after the neonate becomes ill.[13]

Nursing and Collaborative Assessment. Assessment begins with identifying mothers and neonates in high-risk groups. Maternal blood tests for the presence of HIV antibodies may be performed with clients' permission. Because of issues regarding confidentiality and the emotional and social impact of making the diagnosis of HIV infection, many hospitals have developed special protocols for obtaining consent for blood tests from clients identified in high-risk groups. Routinely, counseling accompanies testing for HIV. Health care professionals should also provide information and support to individuals who are in high-risk groups or who test positive (or negative) for HIV antibodies.

Mothers who have been infected with HIV and who have positive HIV antibodies in their blood may be asymptomatic; however, their HIV antibodies cross the placenta and are found in the neonate's blood. Neonates of mothers who are HIV positive will also test positive at birth, because of the presence of maternal antibodies. Not all neonates testing positive at birth will actually be infected. The neonate of an HIV-infected mother must be closely followed.

Approximately 50 percent (with a range between 20 and 60 percent) of neonates born to HIV-positive mothers will actually contract the infection. A true diagnosis of HIV infection in neonates without symptoms cannot actually be made until around 15 months of age when maternal antibodies are no longer present in the infant's circulatory system. Neonates who demonstrate certain complexes of symptoms at birth, however, may be diagnosed as having HIV disease.

Some neonates found to have HIV antibodies and who develop the HIV infection may demonstrate symptoms at birth; others may not demonstrate symptoms until 6 months of age or later. Common symptoms of HIV infection in the neonate are listed in Table 42–5.

Nursing and Collaborative Management. There is no cure for HIV infection, although treatment is available and research continues. One retroviral agent, zidovudine (AZT), controls the replication of the virus, and in many instances, halts progression in symptoms in children (as well as adults). Management for neonates and children also focuses on treating the secondary infections and symptoms related to the immunosuppression.[15]

Special attention to nutritional support is required because of the many gastrointestinal problems associated with infection. This may include the use of tube feedings or total parenteral nutrition. Attempts may be made to prevent infection through use of prophylactic antibodies or gamma globulin. Treatment of persistent infections may include long-term administration of antibiotics. The neonate often becomes weak and requires supplemental oxygen. Skin care becomes essential in the presence of recurrent diarrhea and skin rashes caused by *Candida albicans.* The neonate or infant with diagnosed HIV infection or disease requires ongoing care after discharge that must include close supervision, meticulous hygeine, special feeding techniques, medication administration, and ongoing medical follow-up. These neonates frequently require lengthy and repeated hospitalizations.

The emotional and social implications of HIV infection are significant for both the neonate and the family. Collaborative interdisciplinary approaches to the management of the neonate with HIV infection and his or her family are therefore imperative. Parents of neonates diagnosed with HIV infection are high-risk clients. Concurrent family problems, including the illness of one or both parents, drug use, lack of support systems, poverty, and the social stigma attached to HIV further complicate the care of the neonate with HIV infection. Evaluation of the family's social situation and home environment is important for the future safety and special needs of the neonate with HIV infection.

Parents preparing for the discharge of their neonate require tremendous support and education from the interdisciplinary health care team. Preparation may be complicated by the fact that an HIV-positive mother is often a single parent, responsible for the care of the infant alone. These parents may be learning about their own illness in addition to their neonate's; they will be afraid and worried. Support groups and community agencies can be identified to assist the parents with the neonate's home care, the impact of the diagnosis of HIV infection, and the financial resources available to them. Parents should be familiar with the many health care professionals, nurses, physicians, and social workers who will follow the neonate on an ongoing basis. They should be encouraged to ask questions and all information and answers must be offered in a nonthreatening nonjudgemental manner.

Often, because of illness or social circumstances, the biologic parents are unable to provide the necessary care to the neonate. In 1985, the Centers for Disease Control issued guidelines for the foster care of infants and children with HIV infection.[17,18] Extended family members or foster families require thorough education regarding the neonate's current and future special care needs. They too can be referred to the appropriate community agencies and support networks for additional assistance.

TABLE 42–5. SYMPTOMS OF HIV INFECTION IN THE NEONATE

Sepsis or repeated opportunistic infections with, for example, the following organisms
Pneumocystis carinii
Cytomegalovirus
Mycobacterium avium-intracellulare
Herpes simplex
Candida albicans
Cryptococcus neoformans
Toxoplasma gondii
Failure to thrive
Diarrhea
Anemia
Thrombocytopenia
Respiratory distress
Generalized lymphadenopathy
Neurologic dysfunctioning
Developmental delays
Hepatosplenomegaly

Source: Reference 17.

SPECIAL PROBLEMS CAUSING ALTERATIONS IN NEONATAL FUNCTIONING

Alterations in Hematologic Functioning

Jaundice. **Jaundice,** or icterus neonatorum, is a yellow discoloration of the skin, sclera, and mucous membranes. Neonatal jaundice is observed during the first week of life in 60 percent of term and 80 percent of preterm neonates.[3] Jaundice is usually observed when the total serum bilirubin level is greater than 5 to 7 mg/dL.[12,19] The degree of yellow discoloration observed is not a direct indication of increases or decreases in the serum bilirubin level.[3] The yellow discoloration is, however, the result of an accumulation of unconjugated or indirect bilirubin, which is lipid soluble and diffuses most freely into body tissues and organs. The presence of jaundice in the neonate should be considered a risk factor directly related to the presence of hyperbilirubinemia.

Hyperbilirubinemia is the presence of an abnormally high level of bilirubin in the blood. This occurs when normal pathways of bilirubin metabolism and excretion in the newborn are altered.[19] Total serum bilirubin levels greater than 12 mg/dL in the term newborn and of 15 mg/dL in the preterm newborn usually indicate hyperbilirubinemia. Hyperbilirubinemia is often considered a common neonatal condition, as one third of all full-term newborns exhibit physical symptoms within the first 36 to 72 hours of life. Most preterm newborns exhibit symptoms after 48 hours of life.[7,20] Ethnic and geographic variables may influence the incidence of hyperbilirubinemia. For example, Asian and Native American neonates have average mean serum bilirubin levels that are double those of the rest of the population.[3,12]

Hyperbilirubinemia that occurs as the result of normal newborn metabolism during the first week of life is called physiologic jaundice (*see* Chapter 32). This type of jaundice is differentiated from the more serious alteration in functioning known as pathologic jaundice, described later. The presence of jaundice and hyperbilirubinemia in the neonate warrants immediate investigation and evaluation by the interdisciplinary team in an effort to identify the actual danger to the neonate and the treatment modalities indicated.

Obtaining a clear understanding of the actual metabolism of bilirubin is essential to effective management of the neonate with jaundice and hyperbilirubinemia. Figure 42–4 provides a graphic explanation of bilirubin metabolism. Red blood cell metabolism occurs in the liver and in the spleen. The neonate's liver is often functionally immature and is not able to meet the demands of the large volume of red blood cells present in the circulation. As a result, the liver is overloaded with unconjugated bilirubin. It is not able to facilitate the final steps of the metabolic process by which unconjugated bilirubin is converted to conjugated bilirubin and excreted out of the body through the gastrointestinal tract. Delays in the passing of meconium stools also contribute to the alteration in bilirubin elimination. Meconium contains large quantities of bilirubin that may be reabsorbed by the body if not eliminated. These alterations allow large amounts of dangerous unconjugated bilirubin to remain in the neonatal circulation. As a result, serum bilirubin increases above the normal level.

The red blood cell volume of the neonate is significant, because bilirubin is a product of red blood cell catabolism, or breakdown. Neonates are prone to have **polycythemia,** a condition in which there is a surplus of red blood cells. Polycythemia is diagnosed when venous hemoglobin is greater than 22 g/dL and venous hematocrit is greater than 65 percent.[3,12] There are numerous potential causes of polycythemia in the newborn period (Table 42–6). Although the neonate has a larger volume of circulating red blood cells (RBCs), the life span of fetal RBCs is only 90 days, in contrast to the 120-day life span of adult RBCs. The increased volume of RBCs with a comparatively shorter life span gives rise to a state of active RBC breakdown. This increased rate of RBC breakdown, along with an immature liver, place the neonate at risk for increased bilirubin production. In addition to polycythemia, other conditions causing red blood cell breakdown, such as blood incompatibilities, can lead to abnormally high bilirubin production.

Kernicterus is the neurologic syndrome that occurs as a result of bilirubin toxicity. Total serum bilirubin levels greater than 20 mg/dL are considered toxic, although there are individual variations among neonates.[3,12,19] Preterm and low-birth-weight newborns may be more susceptible to potential toxicity at lower serum bilirubin levels than term newborns.[3,19] When the bilirubin level reaches toxic proportions, unconjugated or indirect bilirubin diffuses freely into brain tissue, staining it yellow and causing severe neurologic damage. Kernicterus most often occurs between the second and fifth days of life, but can occur whenever bilirubin toxicity exists. The severity of the symptoms is related to the degree of toxicity. Severe kernicterus may result in the death of the neonate.

Neonates suffering from kernicterus become lethargic with poor tendon reflexes and hypotonia. The Moro reflex disappears. The neonate develops difficulty feeding as a result of vomiting and the inability

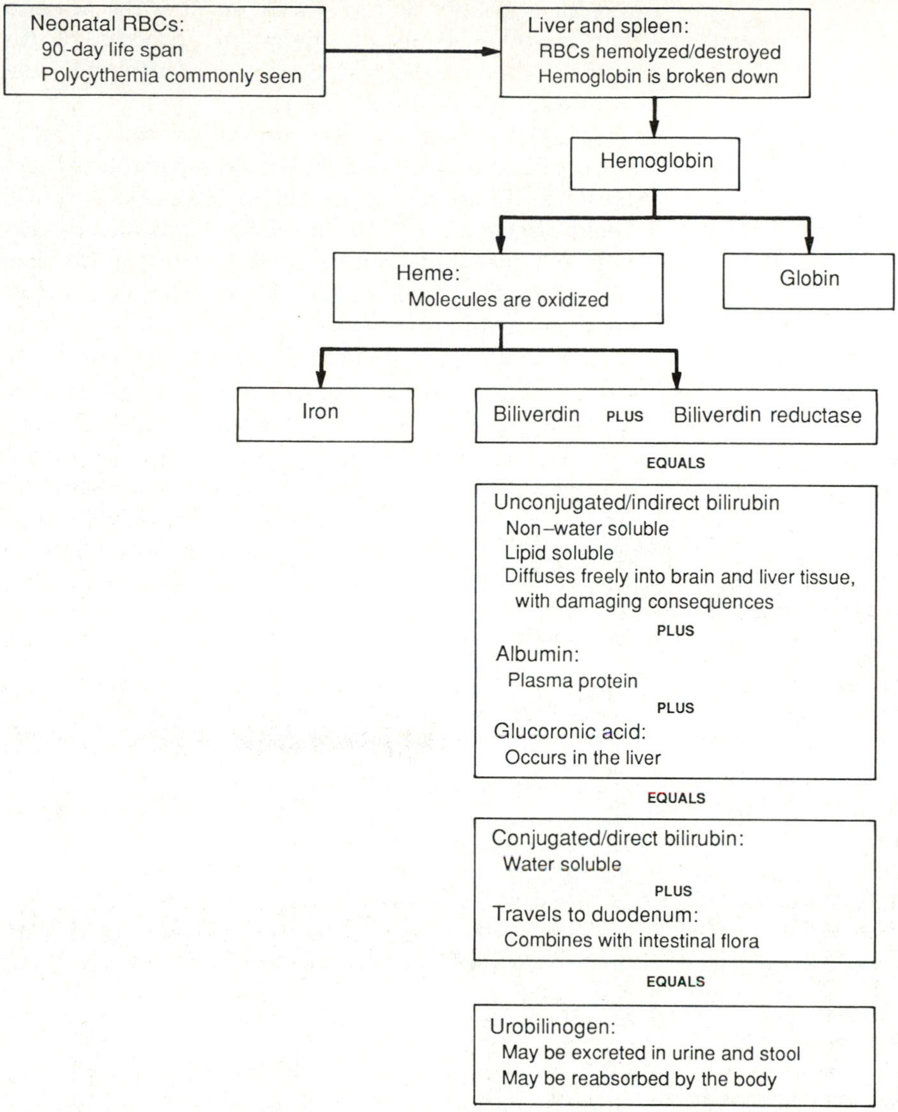

Figure 42–4. Graphic explanation of bilirubin metabolism.

to suck strongly enough to draw milk from a nipple effectively. Extraocular muscles are paralyzed and the neonate gazes downward (the "setting sun" sign). Although floppy and weak at the onset of the syndrome, the neonate later becomes irritable and rigid with a high-pitched cry and a tendency for seizures.[20] Unfortunately, the symptoms of kernicterus are not reversible. The long-term effects include a wide range of sensory, perceptual, and motor defects; mental retardation; and seizures. Management focuses on prevention of the bilirubin toxicity, an area requiring active assessment and collaboration among interdisciplinary team members.[21]

Pathologic Jaundice. **Pathologic jaundice** is suspected when the yellow discoloration of the skin, sclera, and mucous membranes is visible before 36 to 48 hours of life; total serum bilirubin levels exceed 12 mg/dL in the term newborn and 15 mg/dL in the preterm newborn; and the total serum bilirubin level increases by more than 5 mg/dL in 24 hours.[3, 12]

Causes of pathologic jaundice are varied:

- Hemolytic diseases of the newborn; the most common of these are Rh incompatibility and ABO incompatibility, in which maternal antibodies are actively sensitized against the RBCs of the neonate. Sensitized maternal antibodies cross the placenta and lead to overwhelming destruction of fetal or neonatal RBCs.
- Enclosed hemorrhage or a hematoma such as a cephalhematoma, which may contribute to the in-

TABLE 42–6. POTENTIAL CAUSES OF NEONATAL POLYCYTHEMIA

Maternal-Fetal transfusion	Occurs when blood is shunted from the maternal circulation to the fetal circulation
Placental-Fetal transfusion	Occurs when there is a delay in clamping the umbilical cord, or when the cord is manipulated, causing blood from the placenta to enter the fetal circulation
Twin-to-twin transfusion	Occurs when blood is shunted from one twin to the other twin in utero or during delivery
Chronic fetal hypoxia	Causes an increase in fetal red blood cell production
Maternal metabolic or endocrine alterations (eg, maternal diabetes)	Cause an increase in the viscosity of the blood.

Source: References 3, 12 and 19.

creased volume of hemolyzed RBCs, causing an increase in the level of serum bilirubin.

- Neonatal hepatitis and congenital atresia of the bile ducts, which alter the ability of the liver to conjugate and excrete bilirubin in the neonatal period.
- Metabolic factors such as sepsis, hypoxia, respiratory distress, and lack of carbohydrate intake, which may contribute to altered bilirubin metabolism and excretion.[22]
- Other factors, such as RBC or enzyme abnormalities or drug-induced hemolysis, which increase bilirubin levels.[12, 19]

Hemolytic Diseases of the Newborn. As discussed earlier, the major and most serious causes of pathologic jaundice are **hemolytic diseases of the newborn.** Maternity clients whose fetuses are at risk for the development of hemolytic disease in the neonatal period can usually be identified in the prenatal period. Table 42–7 lists questions related to prenatal risk factors.

Information about the ABO blood types and the Rh blood groups must be obtained. Blood types include A, B, AB, and O. The blood type of the fetus is genetically determined based on the blood types of the parents. In addition to blood types, blood group must also be identified. There are two blood groups, Rh+ and Rh−. The Rh blood group is determined by the presence of certain antigens. The combination of antigens present determines whether the Rh factor is present (Rh+) or absent (Rh−). For example, if the Rh factor is present in an individual with type O blood, that individual will have type O, group Rh+ blood, or O+ blood. The most common and strongest Rh+ antigen is the D antigen. It is the antigen that is involved in the hemolytic process of Rh incompatibility.[3] (*See* Chapter 39 for further discussion of Rh isoimmunization.)

Pregnant women who are considered to be at risk for Rh isoimmunization should have anti-D titers drawn at 12 to 16 weeks, 28 to 32 weeks, and 36 weeks of gestation.[3] The anti-D titer indicates the extent to which the mother is producing antibodies against the D antigens of the Rh+ red blood cells of the fetus. A titer that rises rapidly or reaches a ratio of 1:64 indicates the presence of significant hemolytic activity. If the titer is 1:16 or there is a history of a stillbirth related to hemolytic disease, amniocentesis is indicated for a thorough evaluation.[3] Improved techniques of monitoring for the occurrence of hemolytic diseases in utero have been followed by new advances in treatment of the condition before birth of the neonate. Intrauterine blood transfusions are pos-

TABLE 42–7. ASSESSMENT QUESTIONS FOR THE MOTHER WHOSE NEWBORN IS AT RISK FOR DEVELOPING A HEMOLYTIC DISEASE

How many times have you been pregnant?
How many live births did you deliver? Include details regarding the delivery and postnatal course of each infant.
Have you ever delivered a stillborn infant? Include details regarding the delivery of each infant.
How many spontaneous abortions (miscarrages) have you had? How many induced abortions (planned abortions) have you had?
What is your blood type? (to be confirmed by laboratory analysis)
What is the blood type of the father of this fetus? What is the blood type of the father of other pregnancies if it is known to be different?
Have you ever received a medication called RhoGAM during pregnancy or after delivering an infant or after an abortion?
Can you tell me why you received this medication?
Have any of your other children been diagnosed with hyperbilirubinemia or "yellow jaundice"?
Have any of your other children been diagnosed with a hemolytic disease, or were you told they have a different blood type than yours?
Did any of your children have to stay longer in the hospital when they were born because they had to lie under special lights?
Did any of your children have to receive a blood transfusion?
Why did the infant have to receive phototherapy or a blood transfusion?
Have you received regular prenatal care?
Did you have any problems during your pregnancy?
Did you have to have any special tests done while you were pregnant? If so, what tests were done and do you know why they were done?

sible, but the prognosis for these fetuses remains poor. In certain cases, delivery may be induced early to avoid fetal death as a result of a hemolytic disease.[3]

ABO Incompatibility. ABO incompatibility is a hemolytic condition that occurs when the major blood group of the mother is incompatible with that of the fetus. Maternal antibodies may be formed against the cells of the fetus' blood type. The most common incompatibility occurs when the mother is type O and the fetus is type A or type B. It can also occur when the mother is type A and the fetus is B, or if the mother is type B and the fetus is type A.[3] ABO incompatibility occurs in 20 to 25 percent of all pregnancies with the related hemolytic diseases of the newborn occurring in 10 percent of neonates.[3, 12] Maternal antibodies causing ABO incompatibility can affect the first as well as subsequent pregnancies.

The action of maternal antibodies against the fetus' cells causes agglutination, or clumping of the cells. These clumps of cells get caught in small peripheral blood vessels where they hemolyze, producing large quantities of bilirubin. Severe hyperbilirubinemia is a complication of this form of ABO incompatibility. Damage related to the blocked peripheral blood vessels is observed in rare instances. For example, renal failure may result from blockage of small blood vessels in the kidney. Effects of ABO incompatibility on the neonate, however, are usually mild.

On assessment of the neonate, the nurse will note signs of jaundice in the first 24 hours of life. A weak to moderate positive direct Coombs' test and hyperbilirubinemia are generally the main clinical indicators. The direct Coombs' test detects the presence of maternal antibodies in the neonate's blood. The presence of these antibodies indicates that a reaction causing clumping or destruction of RBCs is likely to occur or is occurring. Although most neonates progress well without specific treatment, phototherapy is usually indicated if the bilirubin continues to rise toward toxic levels. An exchange transfusion may be indicated in the presence of severe hemolytic disease and severe hyperbilirubinemia, but this is uncommon. Future pregnancies should be monitored to identify the presence of an ABO incompatibility; however, no treatment is available to prevent the possible future recurrence of ABO incompatibility.

Rh Incompatibility. Rh incompatibility causes a hemolytic disease that is most common in Caucasians, occurring in 9 percent of all pregnancies. In 1 in 15 of these pregnancies, the newborn demonstrates clinical symptoms. These pregnancies are often associated with pregnancy-induced hypertension or a cesarean delivery.[3, 12] The perinatal mortality of neonates with Rh incompatibility is 17.5 percent, with 14 percent of these deaths occurring as stillbirths.[12]

Rh incompatibility occurs when an Rh− mother is pregnant with an Rh+ fetus (*see* Chapter 39). In the most common situation, the fetal red blood cells (RBCs) contain D antigens which are lacking in the RBCs of the mother. Conditions such as fetal-maternal bleeding in a current or prior pregnancy (for example, mixing of fetal and maternal blood during delivery in a previous pregnancy), previous failure to receive any RhoGAM or an inadequate amount of RhoGAM following pregnancy or abortion, and a previous blood transfusion may result in maternal isoimmunization or sensitization and the initial formation of maternal antibodies to the D antigen. It is rare, however, that the fetus in the first pregnancy in which sensitization occurs will become affected by the antibodies.

During the current pregnancy in a mother who has been exposed to the D antigen, antigens from the Rh+ fetus stimulate additional maternal production of antibodies against D antigens. These anti-D antibodies return to the fetal circulation, where they attach to and destroy the fetal RBCs. (Maternal sensitization can also occur in response to other irregular fetal Rh blood group antigens.)The condition characterized by fetal or neonatal hemolytic anemia resulting from incompatibility between the maternal and fetal blood groups is termed *erythroblastosis fetalis.*[23] As RBCs are destroyed, the fetus responds by increasing erythropoietic activity in the liver, spleen, and bone marrow. The severity of erythroblastosis fetalis is therefore related to the amount of fetal RBC destruction and how well the fetus can produce new RBCs in response to the anemia. An Rh− client who delivers an Rh+ infant, has an abortion, or who under goes a procedure in which fetal and maternal blood may be mixed will receive prophylactic treatment. An Rh− client who is still unsensitized may also receive RhoGAM during the 28th week of pregnancy.

Markedly severe fetal RBC destruction in utero may lead to a condition termed *hydrops fetalis.* In this condition, the fetus' ability to produce enough new RBCs is exhausted. This can lead to multisystem failure in which, for example, the cardiovascular, respiratory, and hepatic (liver) systems cannot function properly. Hydrops fetalis is also characterized by massive edema, pleural effusions, and ascites and may progress to death in utero. If hydrops fetalis is present at birth, cardiovascular and respiratory collapse is likely. Aggressive resuscitation is necessary; however, progressive failure of the neonate is likely.[3, 12]

Nursing and Collaborative Assessment. When Rh incompatibility is known or anticipated, thorough and ongoing assessment of the neonate is imperative. Careful attention should be paid to the amniotic fluid at birth. High levels of bilirubin pigments, produced as a result of fetal RBC destruction, can produce a yellow discoloration of the amniotic fluid, umbilical cord, and the vernix caseosa.[3] Neonates whose hemolytic disease has not progressed to life-threatening levels in utero will demonstrate the following symptoms at or soon after birth: pallor, anemia, enlarged liver and spleen, petechiae, and purpura.[12] Neonates who are severely affected by the hemolytic process may also demonstrate the following symptoms related to cardiovascular and respiratory collapse:

- Tachycardia (a sustained resting heart rate greater than 190 beats per minute in a full-term infant) progressing to bradycardia (a sustained resting heart rate less than 70 beats per minute in a full-term infant) or asystole (the absence of a heartbeat)[3]
- Hypotension (a systolic blood pressure less than 66 to 70 mm Hg and a diastolic blood pressure less than 39 to 41 mm Hg in a full-term infant[12]
- Respiratory distress indicated by tachypnea (a resting respiratory rate greater than 50 breaths per minute in a full-term infant), cyanosis, see-saw breathing patterns, nasal flaring, or apnea (absence of respirations)[3]

Jaundice will not be present at birth, as the excessive amounts of bilirubin produced in utero are eliminated through the placenta and maternal circulation. Jaundice will become obvious during the first day of life and the bilirubin level will continue to rise rapidly.[3]

Hemolytic diseases of the neonate such as ABO and Rh incompatibilities can prove to be life threatening. Quick and accurate assessment by nurses is essential to identification of the presence of these alterations. Table 42–8 briefly reviews the key elements of both ABO and Rh incompatibilities.

Nursing and Collaborative Management. Management of the neonate with Rh incompatibility is aimed at prevention. Rho(D) immune globulin (RhoGAM) is an anti-Rh immunoglobulin that is administered to women after the delivery or abortion of an Rh+ newborn or fetus. The anti-Rh immunoglobulin helps destroy the Rh+ cells that were transferred to the mother from the fetus. The destruction of these cells prevents further maternal production of anti-Rh antibodies. Thus, anti-Rh antibodies will not be present in the mother's circulation at the time of another pregnancy. Rho(D) immune globulin should be administered to an Rh− mother after each pregnancy or abortion with an Rh+ newborn or fetus. Prevention of Rh sensitization is 90 percent effective with the administration of Rho(D) immune globulin at the time of delivery.[12]

If the hemolytic process is detected while the fetus is still in utero, management is aimed at preventing intrauterine death. Induction of an early delivery may be necessary to prevent progression of the life-threatening condition. Intrauterine transfusions may also be used for the severely compromised fetus.

The birth of a neonate with known or suspected Rh incompatibility poses a tremendous challenge to the delivery room and nursery teams. The immediate goal is to assess the newborn swiftly and initiate resuscitative measures if necessary. Complete blood count with differential, blood type, reticulocyte count, platelet count, blood gas, Coombs' test, and direct and total bilirubin levels may be performed on cord blood samples;[23] however, any intrauterine transfusions may affect results of blood type and Coombs' tests.

Results of serial laboratory tests must be examined. The main goals of management then become treatment of anemia and prevention of severe hyperbilirubinemia, which could cause neurologic damage (*see* earlier discussion of kernicterus). Phototherapy is the method of treatment used when mild to moderate hyperbilirubinemia is identified. In critical situations, an exchange transfusion is performed.

Phototherapy. Phototherapy is used to decrease serum bilirubin in neonates with hyperbilirubinemia as a result of conditions accompanied by mild to moderate jaundice. Phototherapy is administered in both the normal nursery and the intensive care nursery (Figure 42–5). Home phototherapy can also be an effective alternative for the full-term neonate with jaundice.[24]

Phototherapy exposes the neonate to a special high-intensity fluorescent light source. This phototherapy oxidizes the unconjugated bilirubin in the skin. The unconjugated bilirubin then becomes water soluble and is excreted in both the bile and the urine without going through the usual conjugation process in the liver.

Several types of light sources are used to provide phototherapy, such as daylight, white fluorescent light, special blue fluorescent light, green fluorescent light, and quartz halogen light.[24] Although blue light sources are effective, they have been reported to irritate the eyes of health care providers. Skin color changes can be difficult to see under colored lights and therefore may be missed if the neonate is not observed carefully. Investigations continue on light sources used for phototherapy in order to identify ways to provide maximal therapy with minimal side effects.[25]

The number and type of light sources used to provide treatment are based on the severity of the

TABLE 42–8. COMPARISON OF ABO INCOMPATIBILITY AND RH INCOMPATIBILITY

	ABO Incompatibility	Rh Incompatibility
Definition	Incompatibility between the major blood groups (A, B, AB, O) of the mother and fetus. When fetal blood mixes with the maternal blood a reaction occurs causing the fetal RBCs to be destroyed.	Incompatibilty between the Rh blood groups of the mother and fetus. Occurs when an Rh− mother is pregnant with an RH+ fetus. During the pregnancy maternal and fetal blood may mix, causing a reaction. The mother's body produces antibodies against the fetal RBCs which carry the Rh+ antigen (D). This causes the fetal RBCs to be destroyed through a process called immunization or sensitizaion. If a mixture of maternal and fetal blood cells occur during labor and delivery, subsequent pregnancies with an Rh+ infant will be affected.
Incidence	Occurs in 20 to 25 percent of all pregnancies; in 10 percent of these cases, the newborn develops hemolytic disease.	Occurs in 9 percent of all pregnancies; 1 in 15 newborns of these pregnancies develops hemolytic disease.
Signs and symptoms	After 24 hours of life; may develop during first pregnancy	Often begins in utero; sensitization occurs during a first pregnancy, abortion, or blood transfusion; signs and symptoms generally appear in a subsequent pregnancy.
Common signs and symptoms	Jaundice related to hyperbilirubinemia	Yellow amniotic fluid, umbilical cord, and vernix caseosa Jaundice related to hyperbilirubinemia Anemia Enlarged liver and spleen Petechiae and purpura Possible cardiorespiratory collapse
Laboratory tests	Weak to moderately positive Coombs' test Bilirubin greater than 12 mg/dL in term newborn and greater than 15 mg/dL in preterm newborn	Positive Coombs' test Bilirubin greater than 12 mg/dL in term newborn and greater than 15 mg/dL in preterm newborn Hemoglobin less than 13 g/dL or hematocrit less than 40 percent Increased reticulocyte count
Management	Phototherapy Exchange transfusion in severe circumstances	Phototherapy Exchange transfusion Administration of Rho(D) immune globulin to an Rh− mother after every pregnancy with an Rh+ fetus, whether the pregnancy reaches term or terminates in abortion.

Source: References 3 and 12.

hyperbilirubinemia and are ordered by the physician. For example, the neonate may receive single phototherapy, using one light source, or double phototherapy, using two light sources. The amount of energy delivered from the light source that results in the maximum elimination of bilirubin is 420 to 475 nanometers (nm).[24] The nurse checks the intensity of light each time the neonate is placed in phototherapy. A hand-held meter, called an irradiance meter, can be used to check the output of the fluorescent light source. The light meter is held at the level of the neonate and in the area of greatest illumination. The light output is measured in units of microwatts per square centimeters per nanometer. A range of 7 μW per cm per nm to 10 μW per cm per nm is appropriate when a single light source is being used, and a level of 15 μW per cm per nm is desirable when double light sources are used.

The neonate receiving phototherapy will have his or her eyes covered by a shield or mask to prevent potential retinal damage caused by the fluorescent lights. The nurse should carefully observe the neonate to ensure that the eye patches stay properly positioned. Eye patches should be removed at least every 6 hours in order to assess the eyes for the presence of irritation.[24] Removing the eye patches during feedings and parental visits will also provide the neonate with necessary visual stimulation. Animal research indicates that phototherapy lights can cause cellular DNA damage. It is therefore recommended that the

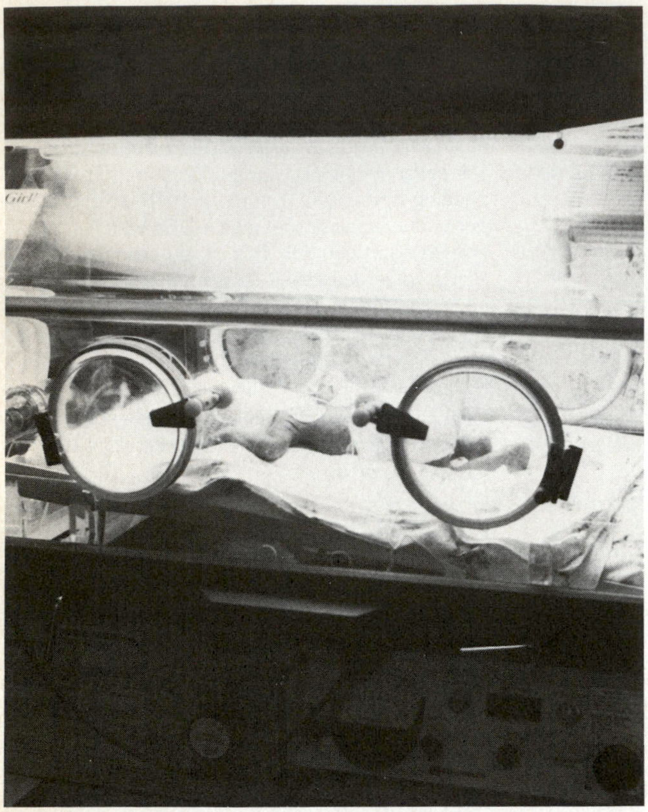

Figure 42–5. Phototherapy in the neonatal intensive care nursery. Note the light source positioned over the isolette. The neonate's eyes and genitals are protected.

neonate's genital area be shielded as well. Surgical masks tied like a bikini or diapers can be secured around the neonate's groin to provide this protection.

Maximum exposure to phototherapy is achieved by placing the neonate unclothed in the path of the light source. The use of an isolette or radiant warming bed allows the neonate to remain unclothed while providing the appropriate thermal environment. Phototherapy lights and the thermal environment can cause insensible water loss in the neonate. In addition, neonates receiving phototherapy often have frequent loose green stools. The nurse should assess the skin and mucous membranes for signs of dehydration. The neonate's intake and output should be strictly maintained. Urine specific gravity may be monitored to indicate dehydration as well. Small frequent feedings of formula or breast milk are recommended to maintain adequate fluid intake.

The neonate receiving phototherapy is at risk for alterations in skin integrity. The intensity of the light source can cause redness or burns if not properly maintained and positioned at least 12 inches away from the neonate.[24] The application of eye patches can cause irritation on the face. Frequent stools and the use of coverings other than a diaper over the genitals can lead to excoriation. Careful and frequent cleansing of the neonate's skin is essential. The use of ointments or lotions is not recommended because they could cause further skin irritation or burning during phototherapy.

A new method for delivering phototherapy directly to the skin of the jaundiced neonate consists of a fiberoptic cummerbund and halogen light source. The cummerbund is attached to the light source with a coupler device. The light source is placed on a movable cart which is kept within 3 to 5 feet of the neonate's bassinette. The cummerbund is placed under the axilla and wrapped around the trunk of the neonate. A baby shirt is placed over the cummerbund and the neonate is covered with a blanket. The light source stays on at all times. This method does not require that the neonate's eyes be patched, and the neonate and the system can be moved into the mother's room. The neonate can be held, changed, and fed with the system in use. In addition, this method may be useful for home care of the neonate requiring phototherapy.

The effectiveness of phototherapy is evaluated by serial serum bilirubin tests performed at least every 8 to 12 hours during the therapy. Once serum bilirubin levels return to normal, phototherapy is discontinued. Additional serum bilirubin tests will then be performed to ensure that the levels do not begin to rise again.

The sight of a neonate in an isolette, eyes covered with a mask and lying under a bright light can be frightening to parents. They need to know why the neonate requires phototherapy. They will be anxious to know the expected length of treatment and if the jaundice will recur. Parents should be aware of the serial blood tests that the neonate will receive and should be given the option to remain with the neonate during the tests if they desire. Scheduling phototherapy treatments around parents' visits will provide special stimulation and interaction for both. Sunlight provides natural phototherapy for mild hyperbilirubinemia. After discharge, parents may expose the neonate to indirect sunlight coming through the window for short periods for example, for 15 to 30 minutes 4 times daily. To avoid skin burning or cold stress, however, the neonate should not be placed unprotected in bright outdoor sunlight nor should he or she be left exposed to cool room temperatures. The neonate requiring treatment for hyperbilirubinemia should be followed by a health care provider after discharge as indicated by the neonate's condition.

Exchange Transfusion. In an exchange transfusion, blood is withdrawn from the neonate and replaced with compatible donor blood. Exchange transfusions are done in critical circumstances, as in the following situations:

- Anemia and hyperbilirubinemia appear to be progressing to dangerous levels
- Neonate's hemoglobin is less than 10 mg/dL
- Cord bilirubin level is greater than 5 mg/dL
- Reticulocyte count is greater than 15 percent
- Neonate is further compromised by prematurity
- Family history reveals that siblings experienced life-threatening hemolytic processes[3]

The goals of an exchange transfusion are removal of unconjugated bilirubin from the neonate, removal of sensitized RBCs from the neonate, removal of circulating immune antibodies from the neonate, replacement of nonsensitized compatible RBCs, restoration of blood volume, and correction of anemia.[3, 19]

Rh− whole blood compatible with the sera of both mother and neonate is used for the actual exchange transfusion. The blood and the client's identification must be verified prior to administration of the blood according to the policy of the treating institution. A small volume of blood, 20 mL in term newborns and 5 to 10 mL in sick and preterm newborns, is withdrawn through the umbilical vein.[3] An equal volume of donor blood is then administered.

The donor blood is usually at room temperature when administered as warming the blood may cause damage to the RBCs. These damaged RBCs would compromise the newborn suffering from hemolytic disease as the damaged RBCs would hemolyze, producing bilirubin. Warmed blood, however, is necessary in some circumstances; for example, for a critically ill neonate with cold stress. Blood can be warmed with special warming coils designed for that purpose. Blood should never be warmed over direct heat and should never be warmed in the microwave.

The process of withdrawing and replacing equal volumes of blood continues until the neonate has received two times her or his blood volume. (Normal blood volume equals 85 mL/kg.)[3, 19]

The following safety measures are necessary during the exchange transfusion:

- The neonate must be placed on a cardiorespiratory monitor
- The neonate's blood pressure must be monitored continuously
- The neonate must have a nasogastric tube in place prior to the start of the procedure to ensure that the stomach is empty
- The neonate must have a peripheral intravenous line in place to receive maintenance intravenous fluids during the procedure
- The neonate's temperature must be monitored and maintained during the procedure; a radiant warming bed is usually used
- Resuscitation equipment must be readily available[3, 19]

During the procedure the nurse is responsible for monitoring and documenting the neonate's vital signs every 15 minutes. Laboratory tests, such as calcium and glucose levels, are done during the exchange transfusion. Hemoglobin and hematocrit, electrolytes, and bilirubin are checked immediately after the transfusion is completed and then serially every 4 to 8 hours afterward.[3, 19]

Exchange transfusions can have numerous complications during and after the procedure, including embolism, thrombosis, volume overload, electrolyte imbalances, hypothermia, and infection from the intravenous line.[19] The neonate with a hemolytic disease such as Rh incompatibility must therefore receive careful and ongoing assessment. Laboratory data in addition to the physical examination will confirm that the hemolytic process has subsided, the anemia is resolving, and the bilirubin level is maintained below a dangerous level. Parents require continuous support throughout the neonate's hospitalization.

Anemia. Anemia exists in the neonate when the hemoglobin level is less than 13 g/dL or the hematocrit is less than 40 percent.[3] During the weeks after birth, the hemoglobin undergoes typical physiologic changes, resulting in values that are falsely indicative of anemia. True (pathologic) anemia can result from several different pathophysiologic processes in the neonate. To differentiate physiologic from pathologic anemia, a thorough history and definitive laboratory studies are required. This ensures that the appropriate corrective therapy is promptly initiated.

Anemia may result from blood loss related to prenatal pathophysiology, most often abruptio placentae and placenta previa. Intrapartum blood loss, for example, an accidental tear in the umbilical cord, also accounts for some cases of anemia in the neonate. Postnatal blood loss may be attributed to an intravascular hemorrhage, accidental rupture of internal organs, hemolytic diseases of the newborn such as Rh or ABO incompatibility, or birth injuries such as cephalhematoma.[3] Sick or preterm newborns may undergo frequent blood samplings for laboratory analysis, which could result in iatrogenic, or hospital-acquired, anemia.

The most commonly observed anemia is physiologic anemia. It is characterized by decreased hematocrit and reticulocyte levels. The term neonate reaches the lowest hemoglobin level, 10 to 11 g/dL, between 8 and 12 weeks of life. The preterm neonate reaches the lowest hemoglobin level, 7 to 9 g/dL, at 6 weeks.[3] This anemia stimulates the production of erthropoietin and red blood cells. Iron stores are also used in the production of these RBCs and both term and preterm neonates may require iron supplements.

Nursing and Collaborative Assessment. Assessment of the neonate with anemia or suspected anemia begins with identification of known risk factors that would predispose to the condition. Any neonate found to have experienced a prenatal, intrapartum, or postnatal condition that is related to anemia must be carefully monitored. Neonates with anemia may demonstrate the following signs: poor feeding, lethargy, pale color, apnea, weak cry. As in many abnormal neonatal conditions, the signs are nonspecific. Careful monitoring of the neonatal activity, physical assessment, and laboratory tests, such as hemoglobin, hematocrit, reticulocyte count, and platelets, are essential. Serial hemoglobin and hematocrit levels should be monitored closely for changes.

Nursing and Collaborative Management. Management begins with the identification of the cause of the anemia. If physiologic anemia is identified, ongoing monitoring of the hemoglobin and hematocrit levels may be the only interventions warranted. The process may, however, become more complicated in the case of Rh incompatibility. The small number of RBCs present in anemia limits the oxygen-carrying capability of the neonate. Sick or preterm neonates with other problems that affect adequate oxygenation, such as hyaline membrane disease, are further compromised. Intervention may be necessary to treat the anemia. The neonate may require supplemental oxygen until the oxygen-carrying capacity can be increased and maintained. These neonates also require a transfusion of packed RBCs. The volume of the transfusion is always carefully calculated and does not exceed 10 to 15 mL/kg.[3] Transfusion volumes of only a few milliliters may be used for the very-low-birth-weight neonate.

Careful management of blood sampling may reduce the number of transfusions required. A cumulative record of all blood losses should be maintained for high-risk neonates. Replacement is done with packed red blood cells when 5 to 10 percent of the neonate's blood volume has been lost. Up-to-date laboratory equipment and sampling techniques are essential to ensure that the minimum amount of blood is drawn from these neonates. Additional treatments such as iron supplementation and routine monitoring of hemoglobin and hematocrit may also be necessary. Special treatments may be necessary to manage the underlying cause of the anemia. For example, surgical placement of a ventricular-peritoneal shunt may be performed to treat an intraventricular hemorrhage.

Alterations in Metabolic Functioning

In utero, the placenta regulates the metabolism of the fetus. The transition to extrauterine life demands that the neonate's own metabolism immediately take over this essential function. Even in the healthy term neonate, the new energy needs and physiologic adjustments at birth can make this transition process difficult. Neonates who have experienced altered metabolic regulation in utero (eg, the neonate of a diabetic mother or the neonate experiencing intrauterine malnutrition) have greater metabolic demands during and after birth. Also, neonates who are preterm or who are experiencing other physiologic stresses such as respiratory distress or sepsis have additional difficulty in regulating their own metabolic needs.[19] As a result, it is important to note some of the alterations in metabolic functioning identified in the neonatal period. The most common include alterations in the metabolism of calcium, magnesium, and glucose.

Hypocalcemia. Calcium is a key element of normal metabolic functioning. Calcium freely crosses the placenta to meet the growth needs of the fetus. Between 28 and 38 weeks, fetal calcium needs increase dramatically.[19] At birth, the endocrine system makes many adjustments to continue to supply the amount of calcium needed by the neonate. If calcium needs are high and calcium reserves are low, the neonate is in danger of developing hypocalcemia (low serum calcium level). Alterations in calcium levels in the neonate include the following:

- *Early neonatal hypocalcemia,* which includes preterm newborns, newborns suffering from birth asphyxia, and newborns of insulin-dependent diabetic mothers.[12]
- *Late neonatal hypocalcemia,* which is related to ingestion of formulas high in phosphorus; seen late in the first week of life.[12]
- *Hypoparathyroidism,* which occurs as a result of maternal hyperparathyroidism in utero.[19]

Hypocalcemia usually manifests 24 to 48 hours after birth. A serum calcium level less than 7 mg/dL indicates hypocalcemia.[12] Signs related to hypocalcemia include: muscle twitching, hyperalertness, increased muscle tone, jitters, high-pitched cry, cyanosis, vomiting, and intolerance of feedings.[19] Many of these signs could be related to different neonatal illnesses such as sepsis.[19] Additionally, some neonates experiencing hypocalcemia may be asymptomatic. Laboratory analysis of serum calcium levels is necessary to confirm the medical diagnosis. Calcium levels are not routinely drawn for normal term newborns; however, calcium assessment would be indicated for any newborn with the preceding signs.

Management of hypocalcemia begins with identification of the potential cause. Calcium supplements may be added to intravenous solutions. A dose of 24 to 35 mg/kg per 24 hours is commonly used.[19] If the neonate has seizures, which may become life threatening, intravenous calcium may be given in a bolus dose.[19] A bolus dose refers to the administration of a specific amount of medication at one time rather than via a continuous infusion. Extreme caution must be used with the administration of intravenous calcium in this manner as rapid administration may cause bradycardia or asystole.[12] Assessment and documentation of continued clinical symptoms of hypocalcemia are essential. Intravenous sites must be assessed and monitored carefully for infiltration. Additional treatments are included if the hypocalcemia is related to a cause other than the stress of extrauterine transition.

Hypomagnesemia and Hypermagnesemia. Magnesium is actively exchanged between the mother and the fetus in utero and plays a key role in overall metabolic functioning.[19] Magnesium is important for the proper functioning of the parathyroid gland. If the magnesium level is abnormal, parathyroid functioning, such as the release of hormones, is affected.[19] If that occurs, the serum calcium level will be altered, and overall metabolic balance disrupted.

The magnesium level is significantly affected by both intrauterine and postnatal factors, including poor maternal diet; maternal diabetes; placental insufficiency; administration of certain medications, for example, magnesium sulfate; decreased intestinal absorption; and loss of magnesium during an exchange transfusion.[3, 19]

Alterations in magnesium metabolism can result in either hypomagnesemia or hypermagnesemia. Hypomagnesemia is an abnormally low serum magnesium level (less than 1.5 mg/dL). Symptoms similar to those seen with hypocalcemia occur with serum magnesium levels less than 1.2 mg/dL. Often, the only way to distinguish which metabolic alteration is present is by the results of serum laboratory analysis.[3, 8, 19] Management of hypomagnesemia includes the administration of 50 percent magnesium sulfate, 0.2 mL/kg via an intramuscular injection in the presence of severe symptoms. In less severe circumstances, oral magnesium supplements can be given with feedings. Oral doses of magnesium range from 20 to 40 mg/kg per day.[3, 19]

Hypermagnesemia is an abnormally high serum magnesium level (greater than 2.8 mg/dL); serious symptoms occur with levels above 5 mg/dL.[3] The symptoms of hypermagnesemia include central nervous system depression, which can result in difficulty breathing, hypotension, lethargy, and depressed reflexes.[3] Management is required when symptoms are severe and includes an exchange transfusion with titrated blood.

Hypoglycemia and Hyperglycemia. Glucose is an essential element in all body functioning. Glucose metabolism is the first level of defense in the stress response and in the response to an increase in physiologic energy needs.[19] The fetus relies on glucose metabolism in utero, especially during periods of rapid growth. The many physiologic changes that occur at birth demand large amounts of energy. As maternal glucose supplies are no longer present, the neonate must immediately respond to these physiologic demands. Alterations in glucose metabolism occurring in utero or after birth have the potential to compromise the neonate. Some of the major causes of altered glucose metabolism are maternal diabetes; diminished production of glucose in the liver; multiple physiologic stresses, such as asphyxia, hypothermia, congenital heart disease, and sepsis; low birth weight; poor oral intake; and intravenous glucose infusions.[12] Glucose metabolism may be altered causing either hyperglycemia, the presence of a serum glucose level greater than 125 mg/dL, or hypoglycemia, the presence of a serum glucose level less than 35 mg/dL.[12] Hypoglycemia is seen most commonly in the neonate of a diabetic mother.

Hypoglycemia. Hypoglycemia is a condition in which the blood glucose level is abnormally low. In the term neonate, hypoglycemia is defined as a serum glucose level less than 35 mg/dL in the first 72 hours of life. In a preterm neonate, hypoglycemia is defined as a serum glucose level less than 25 mg/dL in the first 72 hours of life. A serum glucose level less than 45 mg/dL after the first 72 hours of life in any neonate is considered to be indicative of hypoglycemia.[3] Hypoglycemia occurs in less than 1 percent of 1000 live births, yet it occurs in 75 percent of newborns of diabetic mothers.

All neonates are vulnerable to hypoglycemia in the first few days of life. During the birth process, the neonate requires large amounts of energy. One important source of energy is the metabolism of glucose. After birth, the neonate can no longer rely on maternal sources of glucose. This change in metabolic functioning can cause hypoglycemia. Neonates of diabetic mothers are at even greater risk of developing hypoglycemia after the birth process, as discussed previously. Intrauterine growth-retarded neonates are prone to hypoglycemia if they experienced intrauterine malnutrition. The preterm neonate is also likely to experience hypoglycemia because of decreased stores of glycogen and immature hepatic enzymes. Other conditions placing the neonate at risk for hypoglycemia are sepsis, shock, asphyxia, and hypothermia. Hypoglycemia may occur after an exchange transfusion, after abrupt discontinuation of intravenous fluids, after malposition of umbilical catheters, and with the administration of certain medications.

Nursing and Collaborative Assessment. Neonatal hypoglycemia often manifests in subtle ways. Physical signs include a weak cry, apnea, cyanosis, hypothermia, irritability, lethargy, feeding problems, and tremors or seizures.[8] Some neonates demonstrate severe symptoms; others may be asymptomatic. The nurse should assess the neonate for risk factors that may predispose to hypoglycemia. The nurse must also closely monitor for subtle changes in the neonate's condition that may signal hypoglycemia.

As there is variation in the symptoms that may be observed in the hypoglycemic neonate, confirmation of the medical diagnosis rests on the determination of serum glucose levels. Dextrostix is a quick manual method of glucose assessment, which requires a heelstick to obtain a drop of blood. The glucose level can be read in about 1 minute;[8, 26] however, abnormal results must be confirmed by laboratory analysis. Any neonate with physical symptoms of hypoglycemia, significant risk factors for developing hypoglycemia, or a Dextrostix result less than 40 mg/dL warrants concern.[3, 19] A serum glucose level should then be obtained through laboratory analysis.

Nursing and Collaborative Management. Management begins with accurate monitoring of the serum glucose level of the newborn. Screening serum glucose measurements for all newborns are required in many nurseries. For neonates at risk for hypoglycemia, serum glucose levels should be assessed in the first hour of life, then every 2 hours for the first 8 hours of life. Serum glucose levels should be rechecked every 4 to 6 hours thereafter until the neonate is 24 hours old.

Neonates who are able to feed orally should be given 5 percent glucose water, formula, or breast milk within 2 hours of birth. Feedings are then continued on an every 2- to 3-hour schedule after the first feeding. Nurses must make sure that feedings occur on time. Parents require support and teaching regarding specific feeding schedules.

Neonates who are feeding poorly or who are too ill to be fed orally require intravenous glucose infusions. The amount of glucose in the infusion is specifically calculated based on the weight of the neonate and the severity of the symptoms. To manage symptomatic hypoglycemia, a 2 to 4 mL/kg bolus infusion of 10 percent glucose is immediately administered.[3] When continuous intravenous therapy is required, a glucose infusion of 8 mg/kg per minute is recommended.[3] Intravenous sites should be checked at least every hour, as the glucose solution may cause neonatal tissue burning and sloughing.[8, 26]

Once intravenous therapy is initiated, the neonate's condition and the serum glucose levels must be monitored carefully until hypoglycemia is resolved and the neonate can maintain safe glucose levels with normal feeding patterns. Parents continue to require support and teaching about the changes occurring in the neonate's condition. They also need careful instruction regarding feeding schedules once the neonate is ready for discharge.

Hyperglycemia. Hyperglycemia is seen after birth and is usually related to extreme prematurity and intravenous glucose infusions. It often occurs when the neonate is stressed by multiple physiologic problems simultaneously. The symptoms include glucosuria (the presence of glucose in the urine), and changes in fluid and electrolyte balances. Intraventricular hemorrhage is a dangerous result of hyperglycemia,[12] and takes place when the fluid balance in the brain is altered, causing bleeding to occur (*see* Chapter 43). Management focuses on prevention of glucose imbalances, especially in the preterm newborn. Glucose infusion must be carefully monitored by the nursing staff. Intermittent serum glucose tests are important in confirming that glucose levels are within an acceptable range. In severe circumstances, insulin may be given, with the dose carefully calculated on the basis of the serum glucose level.[12]

Inborn Errors of Metabolism. Inborn errors of metabolism is the term used to describe a large number of genetically determined diseases that cause alterations in metabolic functioning.[3, 12] The altered metabolic functioning is usually the result of deficient enzyme activity in the body, leading to disorders of amino acid metabolism, uric acid cycle defects, and organic acidemias, among others. The most common amino acid disorder is phenylketonuria (PKU) (*see* the box). Other inborn errors of metabolism include galactosemia and maple syrup urine disease. Table 42–9 lists common inborn errors of metabolism identified in the neonatal period. Most inborn errors of metabolism are inherited as autosomal recessive traits.[3] Mothers with the autosomal recessive trait often have only 50 percent of normal metabolic function themselves. This level is usually adequate to make up for their own altered enzyme activity. The maternal metabolism is also able to substitute for the enzyme activity lacking in the fetus, thereby preventing the toxic buildup of the products of fetal metabolism in utero. After birth, the deficient enzyme activity continues to alter normal metabolic functioning.[28] In mild disorders, these conditions may remain undetected for the individual's entire life. More severe cases demonstrate symptoms soon after birth and may prove to be life threatening.[3,19,29]

When left untreated, inborn errors of metabolism cause irreversible brain damage. This brain damage can be minimized with the early identification of the abnormality and the initiation of an aggressive treatment plan. The importance of precise and early diagnosis of metabolic disease cannot be overemphasized because of the need to individualize treatment plans and minimize brain damage.[29]

Nursing and Collaborative Assessment. Inborn errors of metabolism identified in the neonatal period are usually severe and require careful assessment. The

PHENYLKETONURIA

Phenylketonuria (PKU) is an inborn error of metabolism that occurs in 1 of 10,000 to 20,000 persons.[27] It is transmitted as an autosomal recessive trait and occurs equally in males and females.[27] Phenylalanine is an essential amino acid that is converted into tyrosine by an enzyme called phenylalanine hydroxylase. In PKU, phenylalanine hydroxylase is absent. This causes an excess of phenylalanine to build up in the body. Although phenylalanine is an essential amino acid, in high levels it is toxic and causes irreversible physiologic damage.[27]

Signs and Symptoms:

The affected neonate is normal at birth. After the neonate ingests breast milk or formula that contains protein, phenylalanine begins to build in the neonate's blood. Toxic levels of phenylalanine will cause severe brain damage if not diagnosed in the first 3 to 6 weeks of life.[28] Symptoms that may be observed in the neonatal period include vomiting, irritability, seborrheic skin rash, unusual musty body odor, and hyperactive reflexes. In addition, 90 percent of the neonates found to have PKU are fair haired, fair skinned, and blue eyed.[29]

Older infants and children may also be found to have the following symptoms: seizures, purposeless movements, microcephaly, and growth retardation.

Assessment:

Confirmation of PKU depends on the finding of toxic levels of phenylalanine in the body. It is recommended that blood tests be performed after the neonate is 72 hours old and has ingested breast milk or formula containing protein. The blood test is usually done by nurses prior to the neonate's discharge from the hospital.

Drops of the blood are spotted on small round disks marked on special filter paper. Pertinent demographic data about the neonate are included on the filter paper, which is then mailed to a central screening laboratory. Most states set 4 mg/dL or higher as the level of phenylalanine that may indicate that the neonate is at risk for PKU, and further assessment is required.[28] Neonates with PKU may also have the following laboratory test results on further evaluation:

- Persistent plasma phenylalanine levels greater than 20 mg/dL
- Normal plasma tyrosine levels
- Increased amounts of phenylalanine metabolites in the urine
- Inability to tolerate an oral challenge of phenylalanine
- Abnormal serum concentrations of cofactor tetrahydrabiopterin

Management:

Management begins with prevention and careful attention to mass screening tests for PKU in every neonate. The goal is to reduce serum phenylalanine levels to minimize brain damage. This is done by initiating a diet low in phenylalanine. Frequent serum phenylalanine levels should be followed and should range between 2 and 8 mg/dL. Caution must be taken to prevent excessively low levels of phenylalanine, which cause symptoms similar to those of PKU. Dietary restrictions may be somewhat reduced between the ages of 6 and 8 years; however, controversy exists regarding when to relax dietary restriction.[3,28] Neonates and parents require additional support and nursing and medical care for special needs related to brain damage caused by the toxic levels of phenylalanine, should it occur.

TABLE 42–9. COMMON INBORN ERRORS OF METABOLISM IDENTIFIED IN THE NEONATAL PERIOD

Disorders of Carbohydrate Metabolism	Failure to thrive, poor feeding	Vomiting	Diarrhea	Lethargy/Coma	Hypo-hypertonicity	Seizures	Respiratory distress, apnea	Jaundice	Hepatosplenomegaly	Coarse facial features	Abnormal odor	Dysmorphic features	Abnormal eye findings	Abnormal hair	Macroglossia	**Laboratory Findings**	Metabolic acidosis	Hypoglycemia	Hyperammonemia	Elevated transaminase	Non–glucose-reducing substances	Ketonuria	(+) Ferric chloride in the urine	Neutropenia	Thrombocytopenia	Anemia	Vacuolated lymphocytes
Galactosemia	×	×	×		×	×		×	×				×				×	×		×	×						×
Glycogen storage disease type I	×		×			×	×		×								×	×									
Pyruvate dehydrogenase deficiency	×				×		×										×										
Pyruvate carboxylase deficiency	×				×	×	×										×	×				×					
Disorders of Amino Acid Metabolism																											
Organic acidemias																											
Methylmalonic acidemia	×	×		×	×	×	×										×	×	×			×	×	×	×		
Propionic acidemia	×	×		×	×	×											×		×			×	×	×			
Isovaleric acidemia	×	×		×	×	×	×										×		×					×	×		
Multiple carboxylase deficiency	×	×		×	×	×											×		×			×					
Glutaric acidemia type II	×	×				×					×						×	×									
Urea cycle defects																											
Carbamyl phosphate synthetase deficiency	×			×	×	×	×												×					×			
Orinthine transcarbamylase deficiency	×			×	×	×	×		×										×	×							
Citrullinemia	×	×		×	×	×	×												×								
Argininosuccinic aciduria	×			×	×	×	×		×					×					×	×							
Other disorders of amino acid metabolism																											
Maple syrup urine disease	×		×	×	×	×											×	×					×	×			
Nonketotic hyperglycinemia	×			×	×	×	×				×													×			
Phenylketonuria	×	×				×					×												×				
Hereditary tyrosinemia	×	×	×					×			×							×		×	×	×	×			×	
Lysomal storage disorders																											
Gangliosidosis type I	×						×		×	×		×	×		×												×
Cell disease	×								×	×		×	×		×												
Sialidosis type II	×								×	×		×	×		×												×
Other inborn errors of metabolism																											
Congenital adrenal hypoplasia	×	×				×																					
Cystic fibrosis	×		×																								
Hypophosphatasia	×					×																					
Alpha-antitrypsin deficiency	×						×	×	×											×							
Fatty acyl coenzyme A dehydrogenase deficiency	×	×		×		×	×											×	×	×							
Zellweger syndrome	×				×	×			×			×															
Neonatal adrenoleukdystrophy	×				×	×						×	×														

Source: References 27–29.

first step in assessment is a thorough family history. Important points to note are the death of another child in the neonatal period, especially if the cause of death was not truly identified; the presence of a sibling with similar signs and symptoms; the presence of a similar metabolic disorder in the family of either parent; and the presence of consanguinity of the parents, where the parents are relatives such as first cousins. Absence of a family history of the preceding factors does not rule out the presence of an inherited metabolic disease.[29]

Signs and symptoms of neonates with metabolic disorders include lethargy, apnea or tachypnea, poor feeding and vomiting, poor muscle tone, seizures, hepatosplenomegaly (enlarged liver and spleen), hypoglycemia, jaundice, enlarged tongue, diarrhea, and unusual odor of the neonate's body or excretions.[3, 29]

Inborn errors of metabolism can cause abnormal amounts of metabolites, the products of metabolism, to accumulate in the neonate's body. For example, in amino acid disorders and urea cycle defects, ingested protein is not fully metabolized. The resultant accumulated metabolites cause the symptoms listed earlier. The identification of organic acidemias is often preceded by severe metabolic acidosis, which may cause tachypnea, an increased respiratory rate.[29]

Although alterations in metabolism are quite complex, the symptoms are nonspecific, mirroring those of other neonatal illnesses or diseases, for example, congenital heart disease or sepsis. Neonates with metabolic disorders can quickly become debilitated and are prone to developing infections.[29] Any neonate who becomes severely ill without obvious cause or is suspected of being septic should be assessed for the presence of metabolic disorders.[3]

The medical diagnosis of inborn errors of metabolism is suggested by an analysis of the signs and symptoms present and is confirmed by laboratory analysis (*see* Table 42–9). Laboratory analysis for inborn errors of metabolism includes a broad range of serum and urine tests. Most tests identify the presence of abnormal levels of certain metabolites. The findings indicate where the abnormality occurs in the neonate's metabolism.

The nurse can have a significant role in identifying metabolic disorders. Careful recognition of symptoms is an essential part of the daily nursing assessment and care of the neonate. Suspected abnormalities should be reported to the physician to aid in the further assessment of the neonate. The nurse also plays a key role in obtaining specimens for laboratory analysis. Often specimens must be obtained before or after feedings; thus, the neonate's feeding schedule must be closely monitored. When obtaining urine specimens, the nurse must avoid contamination with stool or lotions applied to the diaper area. In many blood tests obtained by nurses, for example, the test for PKU, specific spots on a test card must be completely covered by the neonate's blood. Patience and accuracy are essential in obtaining a specimen appropriate for the particular test.

Screening. Great strides have been made in recent years in the identification and management of inborn errors of metabolism.[29] One important reason is the early identification of metabolic abnormalities through the use of neonatal screening tests. Screening tests are usually initiated prior to the neonate's discharge from the hospital when health care providers have access to the neonate and before the negative effects of the condition progress. The most common mass neonatal screening test is for PKU; however, many states routinely screen for other inborn errors of metabolism or hormonal disorders such as hypothyroidism.

Nurses must be aware of the neonatal screening tests performed in their state. The nurse plays a key role in ensuring that the necessary screening tests are completed prior to the neonate's discharge. The nurse must be aware of special factors that affect the accuracy of the test, for example, whether the neonate is at least 48 hours old or has taken adequate oral feedings prior to the test. Neonates who require lengthy hospitalizations, transfers between newborn nursery and the intensive care nursery, or transfers between hospitals require meticulous attention to ensure that the necessary screening tests are completed and the results obtained in a timely manner.

Parents may question the necessity of screening tests or may request information about the disorders for which the neonate is being tested. Basic information should be shared with parents without unnecessarily alarming them. Parents can be directed to contact their primary health care provider to obtain the results of the screening tests.

Nursing and Collaborative Management. As soon as an inborn error of metabolism is confirmed, referral should be made to skilled physicians specializing in the care of infants and children with metabolic diseases. Long-term management and family support are essential in the ongoing treatment of these neonates. As these metabolic diseases are genetically transmitted, a genetic evaluation of the family should be included in the treatment plan as well.

Specific management then is directed at minimizing the alteration in the metabolism. Because of the complexity of each of the inborn errors of metabolism, specific treatment regimens are necessary. Many inborn errors of metabolism are successfully managed with strict dietary regimens or vitamin or hormonal supplements. Consistent and ongoing implementation of these treatments is essential for the future well-being of the child.

Neonates with severe metabolic diseases, especially those who are not diagnosed in the first weeks of life, may sustain irreversible brain damage. The brain damage may range from mild retardation to profound and severe mental retardation. Infants may not demonstrate signs of brain damage until they are several months old. Careful developmental assessment is essential in their ongoing care. Again, families require support and education from the interdisciplinary health care team. They often can benefit from referrals to community agencies in their local area.

Alterations in Nutrition and Gastrointestinal Functioning

Neonates have special nutritional needs. Nutritional management of all neonates is aimed at maintaining cellular functioning and promoting growth and development.[30] It is also aimed at replacing minerals lost in urine, feces, and sweat. High-risk, immature, or undernourished neonates pose even greater challenges to members of the interdisciplinary team planning their nutritional management.[19]

Nursing and Collaborative Assessment. When assessing the high-risk neonate's nutritional needs and possible feeding options, careful attention must be paid to the following factors[19]:

1. *Gestational age and weight.* Preterm neonates have limited fat and glycogen stores, and low albumin, iron, and calcium levels that must be carefully considered in planning nutritional intake. Reflexes essential to oral feeding (eg, the gag reflex) are not present until 32 weeks of gestation.
2. *Gastrointestinal functioning,* including the presence of anomalies. The neonate's stomach empties slowly in the first few weeks of life. There may also be poor tone in the esophageal muscles, causing the neonate to reflux stomach contents up into the esophagus or trachea. Congenital anomalies of the gastrointestinal tract can further complicate the neonate's ability to feed orally.
3. *Metabolic functioning.* Preterm or malnourished neonates may require a different combination of nutrients because of a changing metabolism. For example, low-birth-weight neonates may require some amino acids that are not essential to the healthy term neonate.
4. *Temperature stability.* Neonates with unstable temperatures may not be able to be fed outside the regulated environment of a radiant warmer or an incubator. These thermal environments may also raise the neonate's fluid requirements.
5. *Respiratory functioning,* including color, oxygen requirements, and strength of the cry. The neonate experiencing respiratory distress is not able to bottlefeed or breastfeed. Those neonates requiring oxygen may have higher oxygen needs during activities such as feeding. The neonate who has a weak cry or color changes with crying may not be able to feed safely via a nipple.
6. *Coordination of sucking and swallowing.* Sucking and swallowing activities begin before birth but are not fully developed until after birth. Sucking begins before swallowing is seen. Swallowing, which allows food to enter the stomach and not the trachea, develops at 32 to 34 weeks of gestation. Coordination of sucking and swallowing together may be immature at birth and must be assessed before oral feedings of formula or breast milk begin.

The objective of nutritional intake is to meet the requirements of many developing organ systems.[19] Assessment of nutritional intake therefore begins with assessment of the neonate's growth. Adequate growth is assessed on the basis of weight, length, total body fat, and head circumference. The indicators are plotted in percentiles on a growth chart. The goal is to maintain growth within or above the birth percentiles.[19] The long-term goal of supporting adequate growth of a neonate focuses on ongoing and progressive nutritional management.

Nursing and Collaborative Management. Nutritional management of high-risk neonates must be highly individualized. It is aimed at providing the necessary combination of nutrients in the safest most effective method for each neonate. Nutrients can be provided parenterally (through intravenous lines) or enterally (through the gastrointestinal system). In each case, the contents of the feeding are specially calculated by the physician in response to the neonate's nutritional needs. The nurse must be actively involved in assessing the high-risk neonate's response to the feedings and the methods by which the feedings are administered.

Parenteral Feedings. Parenteral (or intravenous) fluids are usually administered through a peripheral vein (eg, a scalp vein). This route is easiest to access and is less likely to be associated with complications.[31] Initially, intravenous fluids contain glucose, sodium, and potassium. Magnesium and calcium may also be added. If the neonate will require long-term intravenous nutrition (because of congenital anomalies, extreme prematurity, and so on) total parenteral nutrition (TPN) is initiated. Total parenteral nutrition is an intravenous solution containing essential and nonessential amino acids and nonprotein calories usually in the form of glucose. Vitamins, minerals, and electrolytes may also be added.[19] Depending on the concentration, TPN solutions can be administered either through peripheral veins or through deep or central venous routes. Numerous potential complications, for example, metabolic imbalances, alterations in liver functioning, and infection of the intravenous access site, may accompany the use of TPN. Infiltration and sloughing of skin or subcutaneous tissue may occur with the use of peripheral intravenous lines. Improper placement of central venous catheters may lead to serious complications including hemorrhage and pneumothorax.

Intralipids may also be administered intravenously. Intralipids are fat emulsion solutions that are high in calories. Intralipid solutions do not require central venous access and are often given simultaneously with TPN. Intralipids prevent the essential fatty acid deficiency associated with prolonged use of other parenteral methods.[32] Intralipids must be used cautiously, especially in neonates who have difficulty excreting free fatty acids. Those at risk include preterm and small-for-gestational-age neonates. Intralipids may also interfere with serum bilirubin measurements.[19]

Accurate and safe administration of parenteral nutrition requires collaboration between physicians and nurses so that proper solutions and rates of infusion are calculated and administered. The neonate's weight must be monitored and documented once or twice a day. Intravenous lines and sites should be meticulously cared for and observed for signs of infiltration and infection. The neonate's parenteral and enteral intake and urinary and gastrointestinal output must be carefully documented hourly. Monitoring of intermittent glucose levels and other laboratory studies are necessary in calculation of the neonate's future nutritional needs.

Enteral Feedings. Nutritional feedings administered through the gastrointestinal tract are called enteral feedings. The patent gastrointestinal tract is able to digest enteral feedings and provide the neonate with the necessary nutritional intake. Enteral feedings include oral feedings, such as breastfeedings and bottlefeedings, in which the neonate feeds from a nipple, as well as tube feedings, which are usually administered by the nurse in the neonatal intensive care unit. Enteral feedings from the breast or a bottle may be the first and only way a healthy neonate needs to receive nutrition. For preterm or sick neonates, oral enteral nutrition may be the last of many steps in a long process.

The transition from parenteral feedings to enteral feedings may require the temporary use of tube feedings before the neonate can take the total required nutrition by mouth. For tube feedings, a tube is passed through the nose or mouth into the gastrointestinal tract (the box on page 1222 outlines the steps involved in this procedure). Once the tube is inserted, placement in the esophagus must be confirmed to prevent the contents from entering the lungs. The tube is taped in position to prevent it from dislodging during the feeding.

Before administering the feeding, any residue from the previous feeding is identified by gentle aspiration of the stomach contents. The volume, color, and consistency of the residue are noted, and it is then refed to the neonate.[33] Parameters may be set regarding an acceptable residual volume for each neonate. Nurses should notify physicians when the residual volume falls outside of designated parameters, as it may indicate intolerance of the feedings.

Tube feedings may be gavage (bolus) feedings, in which a specific volume is administered over a limited period. In many cases, the tube is inserted immediately before the gavage feedings and removed afterward. High-risk neonates may also receive continuous tube feedings, in which the nasogastric tube is taped in place and the prescribed feeding is delivered usually by a pump at a continuous rate. The method of tube feeding depends on the neonate's condition and special needs. For example, neonates of diabetic mothers may benefit from a slow steady continuous feeding to stabilize blood glucose levels.[32]

Careful handling and positioning of the neonate during and after the feeding are necessary to reduce the likelihood of regurgitation and to prevent aspiration of the feeding. If the neonate's condition allows, parents may be encouraged to hold the neonate with the head elevated during tube feedings. If the neonate is not being held, the right lateral and prone positions are preferred, both with the head of the bed elevated. These positions promote stomach emptying and reduce the risk of regurgitation. Immediately after the feeding, the neonate should be burped and returned to the proper position.[19]

Oral stimulation and exercises are essential during tube feedings to help stimulate sucking and swallowing reflexes in preparation for future oral

PLACEMENT OF A FEEDING TUBE AND GAVAGE FEEDING

Objective:

To insert accurately and safely an orogastric or nasogastric tube

To administer accurately and safely a tube feeding to the neonate who, because of gestational age or illness, cannot bottlefeed or breastfeed

Equipment:

- Appropriate-size feeding tube (5 or 8 French)
- Tape
- Sterile water
- Appropriate-size syringe (5 to 20 cc)
- Formula or breast milk in the appropriate volume
- Stethoscpe
- Pacifier

Procedure:

1. Orogastric feedings are usually preferred, as newborns are nose breathers and a nasogastric tube may partially occlude the airway; however, oral tubes can cause excessive gagging in some neonates, making use of the nasal route necessary. To determine how far the tube should be inserted: for orogastric feedings, measure the distance from the nose to the ear to the xiphoid process; for nasogastric feedings, measure from the tip of the nose to the ear to a point midway between the xiphoid process and the umbilicus. Mark the tube with tape to indicate how far it should be inserted.
2. Lubricate the tip of the feeding tube with water, insert it into the back of the throat, and gradually ease it down until the marker is at the neonate's lips (if an orogastric tube) or at the tip of the nose (if a nasogastric tube). It may be helpful to have a colleague hold the neonate's head still during the procedure. If strong resistance is met and the tube cannot be advanced, remove the tube, allow the neonate to rest, and begin again. Caution should be used as some neonates may experience a vagal response, including bradycardia, when the tube is inserted.
3. Check for proper placement by aspirating for stomach contents and gently pushing 1 cc of air into the stomach while listening over the upper left quadrant of the abdomen with the stethoscope. If stomach contents cannot be aspirated and air is not auscultated entering the stomach, remove the tube. Once placement has been confirmed, aspirate the air in the stomach before beginning the feeding. Amount, color, and consistency of aspirate should be recorded. Feeding volumes may be altered or feedings withheld based on this information and the particular situation.
4. Tape the tube in place.
5. If possible, the neonate should be dressed and held during the feeding. This is often a good time to involve the parents. If the neonate cannot be held, he or she should be positioned on the right side with the head of the bed elevated slightly to facilitate gastric emptying.
6. Attach the syringe without the plunger and fill it with the amount of formula or breast milk to be given. If the syringe cannot hold the total volume of the feeding, slowly add the remaining formula before the syringe fully empties to prevent excess air from entering the stomach. Gentle pressure may be applied with the plunger to initiate gravity drainage. Feedings should not be pushed or forced. The amount of the feeding should be based on the neonate's fluid and caloric requirements, which are calculated according to the weight in kilograms. The feeding is usually administered at a rate of 5 cc every 5 to 10 minutes.
7. An orogastric tube may stimulate the sucking reflex. Offer the neonate a pacifier during tube feedings as nonnutritive sucking is a valuable form of stimulation.
8. When the feeding is completed, pinch the tube and gently remove it. In some instances, a nasogastric tube is left in place between feedings.
9. Burp the neonate, then place the neonate on the abdomen or right side, with the head of the bed slightly elevated.
10. Record the data, including confirmation of tube placement; amount and quality of stomach aspirate; type and amount of feeding; tolerance of the feeding, as indicated by the presence of vomiting or diarrhea; ability or interest in sucking during the feeding; and overall readiness to begin nipplefeedings.
11. If the feedings are to be continuous, the tube is left in place and secured with tape. Care should be taken to tape the tube in a position that will not place pressure on the nares and cause irritation. Continuous feedings should be administered by an infusion pump at a constant rate. The syringe should be changed at least every 4 hours and the entire system including the orogastric/nasogastric tube, every 24 hours.

Adapted, with permission, from Willett MJ, et al. Manual of Neonatal Intensive Care Nursing. *Boston: Little, Brown; 1986:67–68.*

feedings.[33] The nurse or parents may offer a pacifier while administering the feeding. If possible, a speech therapist may be consulted for additional oral stimulation techniques.

The transition from tube feedings to oral feedings is often a gradual process. Initially, nipplefeeding is attempted in one of every two to three feedings, with the other feedings being administered by gavage. The nurse must be prepared to spend at least 30 minutes with the neonate who is being offered nipplefeeding. For small or sick neonates, eating is an activity that requires a large amount of energy; therefore, frequent rest periods are often needed. The neonate may suck vigorously in short bursts and then swallow, indicating immature sucking/swallowing coordination.[19] The neonate may require support under the chin and on the cheeks to help the feeding be more successful. The nurse should burp the neonate after at least every 10 to 15 mL of the feeding. If the neonate is not able to ingest enough nutrition through oral feedings, alternative strategies must be identified. For example, if the neonate is only able to nipplefeed half of the necessary volume of formula or breast milk, the remainder of the feeding may be administered by a tube feeding.

Communication between nurses and physicians is essential in identifying the best strategy for each neonate. If possible, a speech therapist can be consulted to assist with nipplefeeding and oral stimulation exercises. Parents are often anxious to nipplefeed their neonates. During the beginning stages of nipplefeeding in the high-risk neonate, parents require encouragement and support through what can prove to be a very frustrating process. Encouraging parents to work with the speech therapist and nurses in providing oral stimulation may be helpful.

Breast milk can be the ideal nutritional product for the high-risk term neonate. It is easily digested and contains several important protective antibodies; however, high-risk term neonates are not always able to begin nursing when their mothers' milk supply begins. Some mothers may opt to pump their breasts regularly. The expressed breast milk may be given in tube feedings or bottlefeedings until the neonate is able to breastfeed.

Recent studies indicate that unless very weak or ill, even a small preterm neonate can eventually successfully breastfeed (Figure 42–6). According to Boggs and Rau,[34] breastfeeding readiness begins when the neonate weighs at least 1500 g, experiences short wakeful periods, exhibits a sucking reflex, tolerates gavage feedings, and no longer requires oxygen therapy or ventilatory support. A more recent study, however, disputes the neonate's weight as a necessary criterion for breastfeeding. Some neonates exhibit a mature sucking/swallowing reflex before they reach 1500 g.[35]

Breast milk of the preterm mother differs in com-

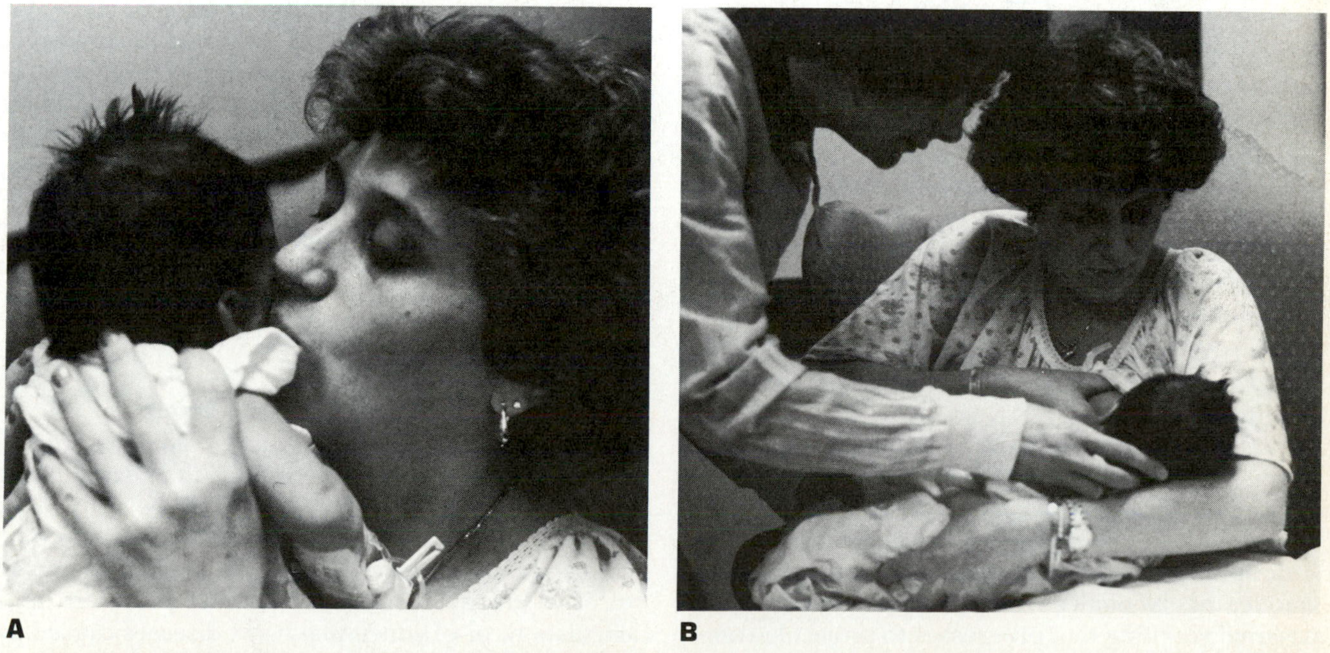

A B

Figure 42–6. **A.** Before breastfeeding for the first time, a mother shows her love for her neonate who had been separated from her in the neonatal intensive care unit. **B.** In a parenting room in the neonatal intensive care unit, the nurse lactation specialist assists the mother in breastfeeding her high-risk neonate for the first time.

position from the term mother's milk.[36] For example, preterm breast milk contains more protein, nitrogen, calcium, sodium, and chloride and lower levels of lactose than term milk. After the first month, the nutrient levels of preterm milk are thought to be similar to term milk. For this reason, preterm breast milk may not be nutritionally adequate for the preterm neonate, especially after the first month of lactation. Fortifying or supplementing breast milk may both allow breastfeeding to continue and meet the special needs of the preterm neonate.

Attempting to provide breast milk for a sick or preterm neonate may be very difficult for a mother. Realistic goals regarding the neonate's readiness to breastfeed must be communicated to the parents. Support, education, and acknowledgment of the parents' goals by the nursing staff are also essential. Identification of the role that the father desires to have in feeding the neonate or questions and concerns he may have about breastfeeding must be explored as well. Encouraging parents to participate in other feeding activities, such as holding the neonate or offering the pacifier, can be very satisfying as they look forward to the time when the neonate will be able to breastfeed. When the neonate is ready to breastfeed for the first time, parents need additional support and education.

Congenital Abnormalities. Maintaining adequate nutrition for the high-risk neonate may be further complicated by the presence of congenital anomalies of the gastrointestinal tract. The most frequent anomalies fall into the following categories:

- *Atresia.* **Atresia** is a complete break in the gastrointestinal tract. The area affected, usually the esophagus, ends in a blind pouch. The neonate gags and vomits frequently when attempting to feed as the feeding cannot continue beyond the blind pouch. Aspiration pneumonia often occurs. Neonates found to have esophageal atresia often have an opening between the area of the esophagus below the blind pouch and the trachea. This is called a tracheoesophageal fistula and it must be repaired surgically.[19]
- *Stenosis.* This narrowing in the lumen of some part of the gastrointestinal tract may be caused by a web of tissue or it can involve the entire thickness of the bowel wall.[33] A common site of stenosis is the pyloric sphincter, where the stomach empties into the duodenum. Neonates with pyloric stenosis have occasional vomiting that progresses to projectile vomiting within the first 4 to 6 weeks of life. The neonate loses weight and becomes dehydrated. Waves of peristalsis, movement of the intestinal muscles, are visible across the abdomen. An ultrasound or barium study is used to confirm the diagnosis. Surgical repair of the stenosis is the treatment required. Oral feedings of 5 percent glucose can usually be started 4 to 6 hours after surgery. Feedings are gradually increased in volume and strength. The neonate is usually feeding well with no further complications 48 hours after the surgical procedure.[3]
- *Duplications.* These congenital cystlike projections or tubular structures can form anywhere along the gastrointestinal tract. These structures can be blind tubelike extensions of an area of the intestine that open into the lumen of the intestine. Others are sacklike structures that do not communicate or open into the lumen of the intestine. Duplications can cause obstructions. Duplications that open into the lumen of the intestine produce acid secretions that irritate the bowel lining and can cause perforation. Or, a duplication can simply be a palpable mass. Surgical repair is indicated based on the type of structure and the complications it causes.[3]

Learning that their neonate has an abnormality of the gastrointestinal tract can be frightening for parents. They will have many questions about the causes of the abnormality and its management. Some abnormalities of the gastrointestinal tract require only one surgical intervention, which allows the neonate to return to oral feedings quickly. Other abnormalities require more complicated surgical procedures, in which oral feedings are the last of many steps in the neonate's recovery. Until the abnormality is corrected, the neonate requires careful attention to nutritional needs and may require intravenous fluids such as total parenteral nutrition. In addition, the neonate may require special feeding procedures, such as tube feedings, at home until she or he is able to eat normally. Parents require the support of the interdisciplinary health care team as they move through the necessary steps of the treatment. Parents must be aware of the importance of the special follow-up care required after the neonate is discharged.

Alterations in Cardiac Functioning

Alterations in cardiac functioning place the neonate at particular risk during the transition to extrauterine life. At birth, dramatic cardiac and hemodynamic changes take place (*see* Chapter 32). Alterations in cardiac functioning in the neonate may be the result of acute disease processes, such as persistent fetal circulation, or of congenital heart diseases caused by defects in the heart and cardiac blood vessels. Many abnormalities in the heart pose acute and chronic life-threatening risks for the neonate and growing infant. Careful assessment is essential to swift and accurate identification of the disorder and the implementation of an effective treatment plan.

Persistent Fetal Circulation. The adjustment from fetal to neonatal circulation that occurs at birth is essential to the neonate's survival in the environment outside of the uterus. In some neonates, however, the fetal circulation pattern continues to some degree, as follows:

- Blood entering the right side of the heart does not flow to the lungs to become oxygenated, but instead returns to the systemic circulation
- The small blood vessels in the lungs remain constricted
- The foramen ovale and the ductus arteriosis remain open[3]

The full-term neonate with a history of perinatal hypoxia is at risk for developing persistent fetal circulation.[3] The neonate with persistent fetal circulation is cyanotic from birth, has a heart murmur, and may require resuscitation. If these symptoms are observed the neonate must be assessed aggressively to confirm the presence of an alteration in cardiac functioning and its possible causes.

Once persistent fetal circulation is confirmed, the primary management goal is to maintain adequate oxygenation. The neonate will require mechanical ventilation. The neonate may also require treatment for severe metabolic imbalances such as hypogylcemia, hypocalcemia, and metabolic acidosis.[3] In some cases, medications are given to dilate the blood vessels in the lungs.[3] These neonates require intensive care and careful monitoring of vital signs and laboratory studies. Medical treatment continues until the persistent fetal circulation improves, often spontaneously. When persistent fetal circulation does not resolve, the neonate may become further compromised or even die as a result of related problems, for example, persistent pulmonary hypertension and respiratory distress syndrome.[3]

Congenital Abnormalities. Congenital heart defects causing heart disease occur in 1 percent of all live births. The incidence increases to 16 percent in neonates weighing less than 2500 g and soars to 75 percent in neonates under 1200 g.[37] The exact cause of a congenital heart defect is often difficult to identify. Chromosomal abnormalities account for 5 percent of congenital heart defects.[3] Other factors that may cause congenital heart defects include maternal rubella during the first 2 months of pregnancy; maternal therapy with anticonvulsant medications such as dilantin; maternal therapy with other medications such as dextroamphetamines, lithium chloride, progesterone, estrogen, and warfarin; maternal alcohol use; and maternal overexposure to radiation.[3]

Congenital heart defects in the neonate cause a wide range of hemodynamic alterations. Congenital heart defects are separated into two categories based on the presence of cyanosis, which results from the altered hemodynamic states. Alterations that cause cyanosis are called **cyanotic heart defects,** and alterations that do not cause cyanosis are called **acyanotic heart defects.** Cyanotic heart diseases include tetralogy of Fallot and transposition of the great vessels (Figures 42–7A,B). Acyanotic heart diseases include ventricular septal defects, atrial septal defects/atrioventricular canal defects, pulmonary stenosis, patent ductus arteriosis, aortic stenosis, and, coarctation of the aorta[3] (Figures 42–7C,D).

Nursing and Collaborative Assessment. Assessment of the neonate's cardiac and circulatory status is essential in determining whether alterations in cardiac functioning are caused by congenital heart defects. Assessment of the neonate must include the following components:

1. Elicitation of a prenatal history noting maternal risk factors that are related to the presence of cardiac abnormalities
2. Careful monitoring of vital signs, including temperature, apical heart rate, respiratory rate, and blood pressure (in neonates found to have a murmur or suspected to have a cardiac disease, blood pressures must be taken on each extremity with the appropriate-size blood pressure cuff)
3. Assessment of heart sounds to identify the presence of abnormal sounds including murmurs
4. Assessment of the presence and quality of the pulses in all four extremities
5. Assessment of respiratory status, including the color, respiratory effort, breath sounds, presence of respiratory distress, and the need for supplemental oxygen and ventilatory support
6. Assessment of the neonate's activity level, including the length and quality of activities and the presence of color changes during activities (crying and feeding are both important activities to be noted)
7. Assessment of strict intake and output including measurements of the specific gravity of the urine
8. Assessment of the neonate's weight at least once a day

In addition to physical assessment of the neonate, diagnostic tests are essential. These may include lab-

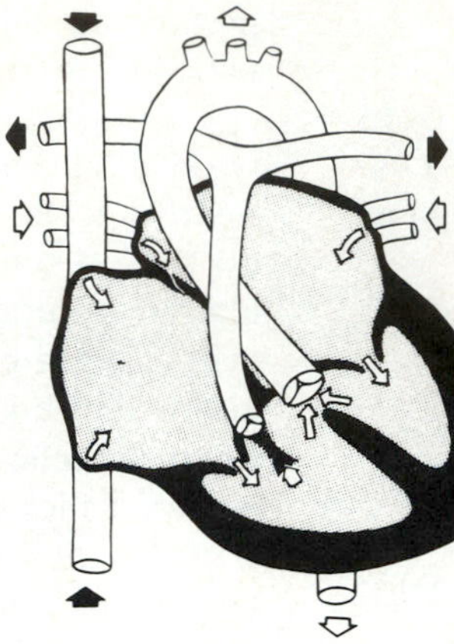

Tetralogy of Fallot

Tetralogy of Fallot is characterized by the combination of four defects: 1) pulmonary stenosis 2) ventricular septal defect 3) overriding aorta 4) hypertrophy of right ventricle. It is the most common defect causing cyanosis in patients surviving beyond two years of age. The severity of symptoms depends on the degree of pulmonary stenosis, the size of the ventricular septal defect, and the degree to which the aorta overrides the septal defect.

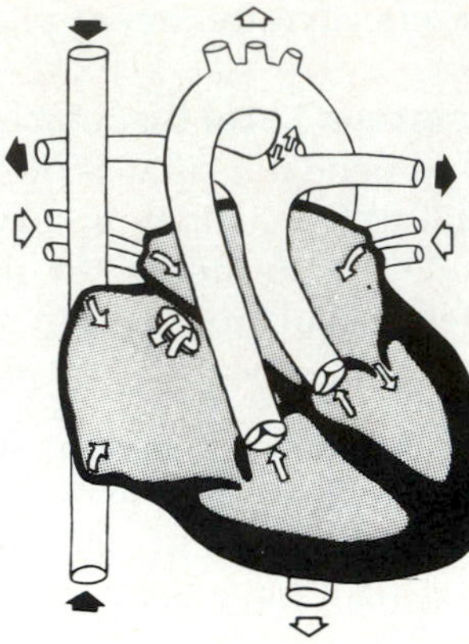

Transposition of Great Vessels

This anomaly is an embryologic defect caused by a straight division of the bulbar trunk without normal spiraling. As a result, the aorta originates from the right ventricle, and the pulmonary artery from the left ventricle. An abnormal communication between the two circulations must be present to sustain life.

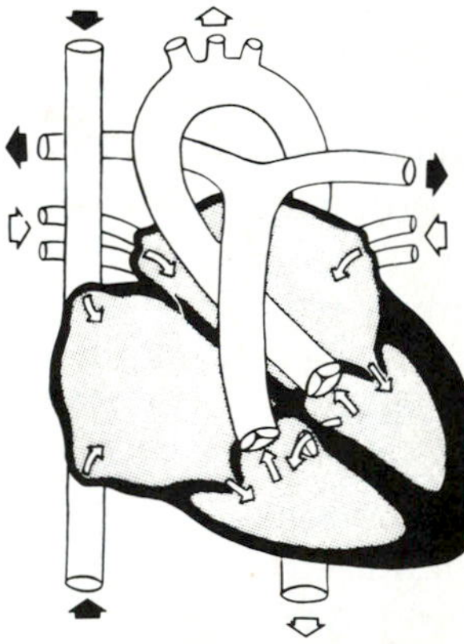

Ventricular Septal Defects

A ventricular septal defect is an abnormal opening between the right and left ventricle. Ventricular septal defects vary in size and may occur in either the membranous or muscular portion of the ventricular septum. Due to higher pressure in the left ventricle, a shunting of blood from the left to right ventricle occurs during systole. If pulmonary vascular resistance produces pulmonary hypertension, the shunt of blood is then reversed from the right to the left ventricle with cyanosis resulting.

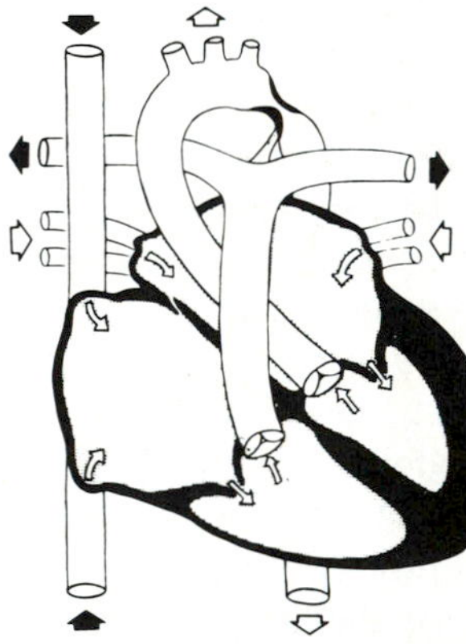

Coarctation of the Aorta

Coarctation of the aorta is characterized by a narrowed aortic lumen. It exists as a preductal or postductal obstruction, depending on the position of the obstruction in relation to the ductus arteriosus. Coarctations exist with great variation in anatomical features. The lesion produces an obstruction to the flow of blood through the aorta causing an increased left ventricular pressure and work load.

Figure 42–7. Congenital abnormalities of the heart. *Cyanotic heart defects:* tetralogy of Fallot and transposition of the great vessels. *Acyanotic heart defects:* ventricular septal defect and coarctation of the aorta. (*Reproduced, with permission, from* Congenital Heart Abnormalities. *Clinical Education Aid No. 7. Columbus, Ohio: Ross Laboratories.*)

oratory tests, including arterial blood gases, glucose and calcium levels, and hemoglobin and hematocrit; invasive diagnostic tests, including cardiac catheterization; and noninvasive diagnostic tests, including chest x-rays, electrocardiograms, and echocardiograms.[38] Abnormal assessment findings in the neonate suspected to have an alteration in cardiac functioning must be documented. The information obtained in the physical assessment is often the key to identifying a particular alteration or defect. The clinical presentation of a neonate with severe cardiac disease usually includes one or more of the following: cyanosis, respiratory distress, congestive heart failure, diminished cardiac output, abnormal cardiac rhythm, cardiac murmurs.[37]

Nursing Diagnoses. Nursing diagnoses for the neonate with altered cardiac functioning are developed after comprehensive assessment. *See* the box for examples of nursing diagnoses related to neonatal cardiac functioning.

Nursing and Collaborative Management. Neonates with cardiac disease require care from the interdisciplinary team in a specialized nursery environment, such as an intensive care nursery. This may demand that the neonate be transferred to a hospital with an intensive care nursery, usually a level III facility. This is a frightening and stressful time for the parents. Nurses can provide support and consolation to parents as they cope with the neonate's condition and transfer (*see* Chapter 36).

Nursing and medical interventions are initiated once the neonate's needs are clearly identified. For example, large amounts of energy are required for the sucking, swallowing, and breathing activities needed during feedings. The neonate may require tube feedings for all or some feedings to conserve energy; may require oxygen during activities such as bottlefeedings or breastfeedings; may be fluid restricted and permitted a limited number of nipplefeedings each day; and may require a quiet nonstressed environment as well as ongoing diagnostic studies. If the neonate develops serious life-threatening complications such as congestive heart failure, aggressive treatment with medications may be indicated. The neonate may require cardiovascular medications, such as digoxin, to regulate and strengthen the heartbeat, or diuretics, such as Lasix, to eliminate or prevent fluid overload. If a congenital heart defect is identified, the neonate may require surgical repair of the defect soon after birth or many years later.

The discharge of a neonate with altered cardiac functioning often includes ongoing implementation of nursing and medical interventions that were initiated in the hospital. For example, some parents must learn how to care for their neonate receiving oxygen at home. This will include safety information as well as the skills needed to bathe and feed the neonate receiving oxygen. Parents of neonates receiving medications must be given or design a schedule for administration of the medications. They must demonstrate knowledge about the medication(s) they will be administering, the purpose(s) and side effects of the medications; in addition, they must be able to measure the correct dose of the medication(s) and administer it according to the schedule, and know when to notify the physician. For some neonates fluid intake may be restricted at home as well. Parents must demonstrate competency in preparing the correct amount of formula for every feeding. Nurses can further assist parents learning to care for these neonates by offering strategies about coordinating feeding schedules with family activities.

Many cardiac disorders require long-term collaborative management among members of the interdisciplinary team such as nurses, physicians, surgeons, and social workers. Parents must be aware of the importance of regular follow-up care to their neonate. They must be familiar with the group of health care professionals who will be managing the neonate's ongoing care. Parents will have many questions about the etiology of the neonate's cardiac disease and what to expect in the future. They require consistent support and education about the changes that will occur in the neonate's condition or treatment plan. Identification of community support groups or resources for financial assistance prior to the neonate's discharge may offer additional support for parents.

NURSING DIAGNOSES RELATED TO NEONATAL CARDIAC FUNCTIONING

Problem-Oriented

Altered cardiopulmonary tissue perfusion, related to persistent fetal circulation in the neonatal period

Decreased cardiac output, related to patent ductus arteriosus in the neonatal period

Altered parenting, related to transport of neonate with cardiac condition to level III facility

Strength-Oriented

Asset in physiologic adaptation, related to spontaneous closure of patent ductus arteriosus

Alterations in Neurologic Functioning

The central nervous system of the fetus and neonate is vulnerable to factors that may temporarily or permanently affect neurologic functioning. These factors may be the result of congenital malformations or may be induced by the prenatal or postnatal environments. Early identification of risk factors or physiologic abnormalities is essential in limiting or preventing long-term neurologic impairment.

Congenital Abnormalities. One group of congenital malformations in the central nervous system comprise anomalies that occur during the fetal development of the nervous system. Some abnormalities result from the failure of the neural tube to develop and close correctly. The neural tube is the embryonic structure that eventually develops into the brain and spinal cord.[39] Failure of the neural tube to develop properly leads to three main defects:

1. **Anencephaly.** The skull and the cerebral hemispheres are absent; only the brain stem may be visible at the base of the skull. The head looks very small and abnormally shaped.
2. **Spina bifida.** There are three abnormalities related to spina bifida. In **spina bifida occulta,** the vertebral laminae do not fuse in an isolated area of the spine; in **meningocele,** meninges protrude from the spinal canal but the spinal cord is in correct position; in **meningomyelocele** both the meninges and the spinal cord protrude through the spinal canal.
3. **Encephalocele.** Brain tissue and meninges protrude in a sac through a defect in the skull.[3, 39]

Defects also occur when the cerebral hemispheres do not grow and differentiate correctly during fetal development. Two examples of the many defects that result from such abnormal development are highlighted here:

1. **Hydranencephaly.** The cerebral hemispheres are absent and the space is filled with fluid.
2. **Microcephaly.** The head appears unusually small because of the limited growth and development of the brain. The brain is only 15 percent of the size of the normal neonatal brain. Microcephaly is also caused by intrauterine infections, anoxia, malnutrition, and other syndromes.[3]

A defect in the development and circulation of cerebral spinal fluid also causes congenital malformations. A major neurologic alteration that occurs with this defect is **hydrocephalus.** In this condition, the head appears abnormally large. There is an abnormality in the production and circulation of cerebral spinal fluid. Circulating hydrocephalus is caused by an abnormality in the ventricles in the brain that prevents the cerebral spinal fluid from emptying properly. Communicating hydrocephalus occurs when the cerebral spinal fluid is not absorbed effectively. These abnormalities cause an increase in the amount of cerebral spinal fluid present in the brain, which causes the ventricles in the brain to dilate. This enlargement causes so much swelling that the sutures of the skull and the fontanelles spread, causing the neonate's head to become enlarged.[3]

The second group of abnormalities is the result of environmental problems that occur before the delivery or in the postnatal period. Damage to the central nervous system in the perinatal period is a major cause of intellectual handicap and nonprogressive motor disorders.[3] There are three main categories of environmental problems that may seriously impair neurologic functioning:

1. *Cerebral anoxia.* Neonates, especially preterm neonates, are more likely to suffer injuries as a result of anoxia. This anoxic damage leads to a disease process called periventricular leukomalacia in which decreased flow of blood to areas of the brain near the lateral ventricles causes infarction. This leads to long-term neurologic damage.
2. *Meningeal infection.* The infection damages the brain cells. The most common infections are rubella, cytomegalovirus, herpesvirus, coxsackievirus, and toxoplasma.
3. *Metabolic alterations.* Altered metabolic states that remain uncontrolled, such as diabetes and hyperbilirubinemia, damage the brain tissue and prevent further normal development.[3]

Neonates who suffered from an injury to the brain tissue before, during, or after birth are likely to demonstrate a wide range of symptoms. Although symptoms of the initial insult may begin to subside, the long-term residual effects may not be truly realized until many years later. This produces a difficult situation for both the parents and the nurses and physicians caring for the neonate. The neonate may "look" healthy and the natural tendency is for the parents to be reassured by the neonate's appearance. Nurses need to reinforce to the parents the importance of follow-up care.

Growth and development must be monitored closely throughout infancy for the presence of abnormalities that would require further medical and other treatment. These infants may develop seizures. Later, problems with cognitive functioning may be identified. In addition to ongoing neurologic assessment, developmental assessments must be included. The developmental assessment determines the infant's ability to reach developmental milestones, such as sitting alone, crawling, and making verbal sounds, at the appropriate point in her or his growth and development. As the infant gets older, developmental assessments may assist in identifying special learning needs as well.

Neonatal Seizures. Seizures are one of the most common abnormal neurologic findings in the neonatal period.[40] Seizures are chain reactions of repetitive abnormal electrical signals occurring in the cerebral neurons.[3] Seizures may be a sign of many different abnormal conditions; seizures themselves are not diseases (Table 42–10). Neonates have an immature neurologic system that may make the identification of seizures difficult. Any type of unusual behavior in the neonate may indicate seizure activity,[40,41] and careful assessment of the neonate is therefore essential.

Nursing and Collaborative Assessment. Table 42–11 describes the five different types of seizures that may be seen in the neonate. Seizures in the neonate may cause such behaviors as grimacing, chewing, repetitive swallowing and yawning, tongue thrusting, staring, involuntary muscle contractions, and alterations in respiratory rhythm.[3,40] Different types of seizures cause different types of abnormal body movements. In observing unusual behaviors in the neonate, the nurse must:

- Establish that a seizure is taking place; this requires expert knowledge of normal variations in newborn behavior
- Make sure that the neonate is in a safe environment where behavior can be closely observed (for example, if the neonate begins to seize during a feeding or while being held, he or she should be placed in a side-lying position in the crib; any toys or unused equipment in the crib should be removed for safety)
- Note the exact time that the seizure began and how long it lasted
- Note the different types of behaviors and movements occurring as part of the seizure
- Monitor vital signs including apical heart rate, respiratory rate, and blood pressure
- Make sure that suction emergency equipment is readily available.
- Note the name and dose of medication administered, including the time it was given and the neonate's response to the medication
- Assess neurologic status and the vital signs at the end of the seizure
- Continue to closely monitor the neonate, noting when she or he returns to normal activity level

TABLE 42–10. COMMON CAUSES OF NEONATAL SEIZURES

Asphyxia
Hypocalcemia
Hypoglycemia
Hyponatremia
Hypernatremia
Intracranial hemorrhage
Infections
Congenital central nervous system malformations
Familial (autosomal dominant) characteristics
Inborn errors of metabolism
Withdrawal from drugs (including anesthetics)

Source: Reference 41.

Along with observation of the actual seizure, several diagnostic tests are recommended to determine the underlying cause of the seizure. For example, blood glucose levels are assessed for the presence of hypoglycemia, and serum bilirubin levels are assessed for the presence of hyperbilirubinemia. A lumbar puncture is done to obtain samples of cerebral spinal fluid. The cerebral spinal fluid is cultured to identify the presence of an infection causing meningitis. The cerebral spinal fluid may also indicate the presence of bleeding or hemorrhage if large amounts of red blood cells are found. An electroencephalogram (EEG) is done to pinpoint the area in the brain where the seizure is occurring. Computerized tomographic (CT) scanning and ultrasound tests can also identify areas of bleeding in the brain or abnormalities in the brain.

The nurse should also assess for the presence of other findings that indicate neurologic problems. Intracranial pressure can increase as a result of increases in the volume of the brain, the cerebral blood volume, and the cerebral spinal fluid volume. The increase may be caused by bleeding, obstruction, edema, or an abnormal structure such as a tumor. An increase in intracranial pressure causes critical changes in the neonate's vital signs, such as apnea and bradycardia. Cranial sutures may separate and the fontanelles may begin to bulge. Changes occur in the neonate's neurologic status; for example, lethargy and abnormal posturing may be seen.

Nursing and Collaborative Management. Management of a neonate with seizures can be complicated. Normal newborn behavior such as rapid eye movement in light sleep and Moro reflexes have, at times, been mistakenly identified as seizures. Every seizure

TABLE 42–11. TYPES OF SEIZURE ACTIVITY

Type of Seizure	Description/Neonatal Behaviors
Subtle seizures	Subtle seizures are commonly associated with severe central nervous system insults in both the preterm and term neonate. Behaviors observed include repetitive sucking, a fixed posture, pedaling movements of the legs and paddling movements of the arms, blinking or a fixed gaze, and apnea.
Tonic seizures	The tonic seizure is the most common seizure seen in preterm neonates with intraventricular hemorrhages. Behaviors include decerebrate posturing in which there is rigid extension of the arms and legs, with the palms of the hands and the soles of the feet facing downward. The neck is hyperextended, and the neonate may arch the back. This position may be held consistently until the seizure is over. It may also be seen intermittently during the seizure.
Focal clonic seizures	Focal clonic seizures may be seen in the neonate as a result of generalized cerebral disturbances, such as asphyxia or metabolic disturbances. It is most common in the term neonate. Behaviors include rhythmic jerking of muscle groups. Focal clonic seizures are seen when only one part of the body develops rhythmic jerking, for example, the right arm.
Multifocal clonic seizures	Multifocal clonic seizures are also often the result of generalized cerebral disturbances and are usually seen in the term neonate. Behaviors include rhythmic jerking movements that start in one area of the body, for example, the right arm, and spread to other areas of the body. The spread of the jerking movements is usually nonorderly and can progress to the point where the entire body is found to have generalized clonic movements.
Myoclonic seizures	When seen in the term neonate, myoclonic seizures are often related to metabolic disturbances. Behaviors include synchronized, rapid, isolated jerking of both the upper and lower extremities. A myoclonic seizure looks similar to the Moro reflex. Extreme caution must be used in differentiating the Moro reflex, which occurs as a response to a loud noise or a jolt of the crib, and the myoclonic seizure, which is spontaneous and cannot be provoked.[3,12,41]

workup entails not only a financial cost but an emotional cost to the parents. Neonates may be transferred to an intensive care nursery in the hospital where they were born or to another hospital that specializes in the care of sick newborns. Nursing and medical expertise in caring for normal neonates is needed to differentiate abnormalities from normal behavior.[42]

Identification of the cause or source of the seizure is essential. Sometimes, however, the cause of the seizure is never revealed. Whereas some conditions that cause seizures in the neonatal period (such as electrolyte imbalances) may have no long-term effects and do not require long-term treatment, other conditions, such as hypoxic brain damage and intraventricular hemorrhage are serious. Neonates with these conditions require aggressive follow-up care to prevent further neurologic damage and to identify potential growth and development problems.

Acute management begins with the treatment of the actual seizure. Anticonvulsants and antiepileptics are the medications used to treat seizures. The use of medications is probably the most valuable and effective intervention in the control of seizures. Phenobarbital has been and remains the anticonvulsant drug of choice for neonates. Doses are calculated on the basis of the neonate's needs and range between 8 and 10 mg/kg per day.[4] Serum levels of phenobarbital are monitored to ensure that the correct amount of medication is given to prevent the seizures. Often, the neonate must continue to take the medication after discharge. Discharge teaching should be provided to parents in a supportive manner. To assess retention of the discharge teaching, the nurse should ask parents to explain why the neonate is receiving the medication, list the side effects of the medication, administer the medication correctly, and describe when the physician should be notified.

The discharge of a neonate with alterations in neurologic functioning usually initiates a long process of follow-up and collaborative services. These neonates may exhibit behaviors such as irritability and short attention spans that make caring for them difficult. Nurses need to encourage parent-infant contact to promote attachment and recognition of the neonate's strengths. The possibility that their neonate has a brain disorder frightens most parents. Parents need realistic yet supportive advice and explanations. They should be encouraged to ask questions and discuss their concerns openly with the nurses and physicians caring for the neonate. They need support in dealing with the uncertainties of their child's future and in clearly understanding the role they play in the neonate's ongoing care. Nurses should make early referrals for available support services in the family's local community in preparation for discharge.

SUMMARY

The care of high-risk neonates and their families poses a special challenge for the nurse. Research has brought about significant advances in the knowledge used in providing this care. These changes in the delivery of care have improved the immediate and future life chances for many neonates.

Identification of a high-risk neonate is the first step in providing the complex care required by these neonates. A high-risk neonate is one who experiences complications in the prenatal period, during labor and delivery, or during the transition to extrauterine life. This neonate is at increased risk for altered functioning or even death. Factors placing the neonate at risk for complications include maternal risk factors, such as substance abuse, and alterations in maternal functioning in the prenatal period, such as maternal diabetes or maternal infections. Altered neonatal functioning may also occur as the result of numerous physiologic or congenital abnormalities, such as hemolytic diseases of the newborn and congenital heart disease. Nurses have an important role as members of the interdisciplinary team that works to suport neonates and their families through the complications and crises that may arise.

Neonatal nurses must be able to distinguish normal neonatal activity, behavior, and physiologic functioning from abnormal signs and symptoms by observing and interpreting subtle changes in the neonate. They must readily identify risk factors that may warrant aggressive assessment. Nurses implement the treatment plan designed by the interdisciplinary team and consistently evaluate the neonate's responses to the treatments. Nurses also have key opportunities to support parents through the transition to parenthood now further stressed with unexpected changes and crises in their neonate's health.

REVIEW QUESTIONS

1. Identify factors that would classify a neonate as high risk.
2. Discuss assessment and management strategies for a neonate with fetal alcohol syndrome.
3. Describe the impact of maternal diabetes mellitus on the neonate.
4. Identify signs and symptoms of neonatal sepsis.
5. Describe how you would explain Rh incompatibility to parents of a neonate with this condition.

REFERENCES

1. Sherwen LN, Mele N. Assessing and identifying the high risk pregnancy: a holistic approach. *Top Clin Nurs.* 1986;8:33–44.
2. Dunn N. Nursing practices in neonatal transport. *Neonat Network.* April 1983;16–27.
3. Behrman RE, et al. eds. *Nelson Textbook of Pediatrics.* 13th ed. Philadelphia: Harcourt, Brace, and Jovanovich; 1987.
4. Dwyer J. *Substance Abuse in Pregnancy.* Public Health Currents, Ross Laboratories; 1986.
5. Sokol R, et al. *Identifying the alcohol abusing obstetrical gynecological patient: a practice approach.* Washington, DC: US Department of Health and Human Services; 1981: DHHS Publication (ADM) 81–1163.
6. Torrence C. Neonatal seizures. Part II. Recognition, treatment and prognosis. *Neonat Network.* October 1985.
7. Korones S. *High Risk Newborn Infants: The Basics for Intensive Care Nursing.* St. Louis, Mo: CV Mosby; 1986.
8. Fantazia D. Neonatal hypoglycemia. *J Obstet Gynecol Neonat Nurs.* 1984;13:297–301.
9. Jovanoc L. Pump therapy offers convenience for insulin dependent women. *Infusion.* 1983;1(2).
10. Rose BI, et al. Major congenital anomalies in infants and glycosylated hemoglobin levels in insulin-requiring diabetic mothers. *J Perinatol.* 1988;8:309–311.
11. Knuppel R, Drukker J. *High Risk Pregnancy.* St. Louis, Mo: CV Mosby; 1986.
12. Avery GB. *Neonatology, Pathophysiology and Management of the Newborn.* 3rd ed. Philadelphia: JB Lippincott; 1987.
13. Larson E. Trends in neonatal infections. *J Obstet Gynecol Neonat Nurs.* 1987;16:404–408.
14. Cerase PA. Neonatal sepsis. *J Perinat Neonatal Nurs.* 1989;3:48–57.
15. Donowitz L. *Hospital Acquired Infection in the Pediatric Patient.* Baltimore, Md: Williams & Wilkins; 1988.
16. Centers for Disease Control. *AIDS Weekly Surveillance Report—US Program, Centers for Disease Control;* December 12, 1988.
17. Office of the US Surgeon General. *Report of the Surgeon General's Workshop on Children with HIV Infections and Their Families;* April 6–8, 1987.
18. Boland M. *Generations in Jeopardy: Responding to HIV In-*

fection in Children, Women and Adolescents. Trenton: NJ Department of Health, September, 1989.
19. Klaus M, Fanaroff A. *Care of the High Risk Neonate.* Philadelphia: WB Saunders; 1986.
20. Colon AR, Ziai M. *Pediatric Pathophysiology.* Boston: Little, Brown; 1985.
21. Jones MB. A physiologic approach to identifying neonates at risk for kernicterus. *J Obstet Gynecol Neonat Nurs.* 1989; 19:313–318.
22. Linder N, et al. Unexplained neonatal jaundice as an early diagnostic sign of septicemia in the newborn. *J Perinatol.* 1988;8:325–327.
23. Dunn P, et al. Care of the infant with erythroblastosis fetalis. *J Obstet Gynecol Neonat Nurs.* 1988;17:382–386.
24. Wilkerson N. Treating hyperbilirubinemia. *J Matern Child Nurs.* 1989;14:32–36.
25. Sbrana G, et al. Phototherapy in the management of neonatal hyperbilirubinemia: efficacy with light sources emitting more than 500 nanometers. *Pediatrics.* 1987;90:395–398.
26. Oehler J. *Family Centered Neonatal Nursing Care.* Philadelphia: JB Lippincott; 1981.
27. Rudolph A, Hoffman J, eds. *Pediatrics.* 18th ed. Norwalk, Conn: Appleton & Lange; 1987.
28. Mamunes P. Neonatal screening tests. *Pediatr Clin North Am.* 1980;27:733–749.
29. Burton B. Inborn errors of metabolism: the clinical diagnosis in early infancy. *Pediatrics.* 1987;79:359–368.
30. Harkavy K. Fluids, electrolytes, and nutrition for neonates. In: Daze A, Scanlon JW, eds. *Neonatal Nursing.* Baltimore, Md: University Park Press; 1985.
31. Merenstein G, Gardner S. *Handbook of Neonatal Intensive Care.* St. Louis, Mo: CV Mosby; 1985.
32. Daze AM, Scanlon J, eds. *Neonatal Nursing: A Practical Guide.* Baltimore, Md: University Park Press; 1985.
33. Willett MJ, et al. *Manual of Neonatal Intensive Care Nursing.* Boston: Little, Brown; 1986.
34. Boggs K, Rau P. Breastfeeding the premature infant. *Am J Nurs.* 1983;83:1427–1440.
35. Meur P, Pugh E. Breastfeeding in the small preterm infant. *J Matern Child Nurs.* 1985;10:396–400.
36. Beckholt AP. Breast milk for infants who cannot breastfeed. *J Obstet Gynecol Neonat Nurs.* 1990;13:216–220.
37. Hazinski MF. Congenital heart disease in the neonate. Part I. Epidemiology, cardiac development and fetal circulation. *Neonat Network.* February 1983.
38. Southwellm S. Persistent fetal circulation, Part III. *Neonat Network.* 1983;2:14–19.
39. Cohen F. Neural tube defects: epidemiology, detection and prevention. *J Obstet Gynecol Neonat Nurs.* 1987;105–115.
40. Bocchese J, Merker A. Seizure disorders in the neonate. *Crit Care Nurse.* 1983;42–51.
41. Holmes G. *Diagnosis and Management of Seizures in Children.* Philadelphia: WB Saunders; 1987.
42. Weingarten CT. Caring for parents of a newborn transferred to a regional intensive care nursery: a challenge for low risk obstetric specialists. *J Perinatol.* 1988;8:271–275.

Preterm Birth, Gestational Age, and Birth Weight

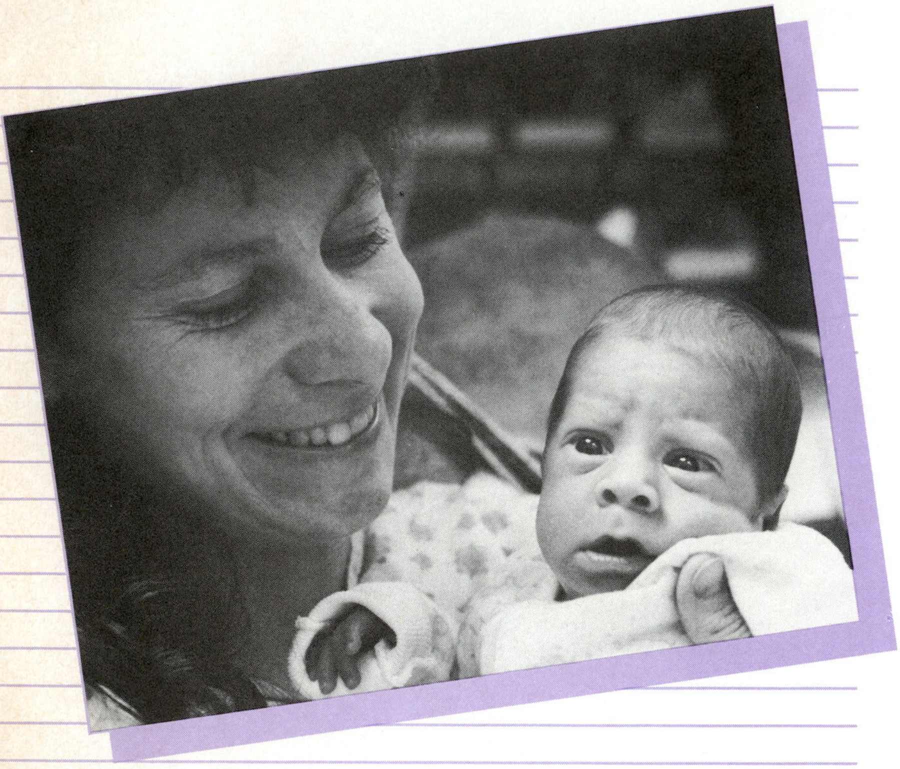

chapter 43

Key Terms

apnea
appropriate for gestational age
asphyxia
bronchopulmonary dysplasia
cold stress
intraventricular hemorrhage
large for gestational age
low birth weight
meconium aspiration syndrome
necrotizing enterocolitis
patent ductus arteriosus
periodic breathing
postmature
respiratory distress syndrome
retinopathy of prematurity
small for gestational age
very low birth weight

Historically, birth weight was considered to be the most important indicator of a neonate's well-being; however, as advances have been made in the area of neonatology, it has become clear that birth weight alone is not an accurate indicator of risk factors facing the neonate.[1] The assessment of both gestational age and birth weight is necessary to provide a more complete perspective on neonatal functioning.[2,3] By focusing on gestational age and birth weight, health care providers can prevent the intrauterine growth–retarded, full-term neonate from being identified inaccurately as premature or the macrosomic or large premature neonate from being identified as full term. By appropriately assessing the gestational age and size, nurses and physicians can make important decisions about neonatal maturation and functioning, and identify special risk factors that may affect the neonate.

As advances have been made in identifying the gestational age and size of newborns, it has become possible to link specific physiologic problems with specific sizes and ages. This has been most important in the care of the premature neonate, who faces risks that are related to both size and gestational age.[4] Often, the premature neonate has immature lungs and requires mechanical ventilation to breathe effectively. Unfortunately, the use of mechanical ventilation and the immaturity of the lungs predispose the neonate to respiratory distress syndrome and, later, bronchopulmonary dysplasia. The tiny premature neonate may also be a victim of intrauterine growth retardation and have less energy stores to battle hypothermia and infection.

Gestational age and size are also important indicators in the care of the postmature neonate. Again, certain physiologic signs can be consistently linked to the postmaturity. These signs help physicians and nurses anticipate and prevent complications related to postmaturity such as meconium aspiration syndrome.

ASSESSMENT OF GESTATIONAL AGE AND SIZE

A newborn's weight, intrauterine growth, and gestational age are important indicators of maturity. These data can assist nurses and physicians in predicting potential problems related to gestational age and size that the newborn may face in the neonatal period.[5] No one method of estimating gestational age or development is sufficient. Prenatal, delivery, and postnatal data and assessments together provide the most reliable prediction of gestational development and intrauterine growth.

Gestational Age

The neonate's gestational age is assessed throughout the pregnancy. Nagele's rule is the most common way of calculating the estimated delivery date (*see* Chapter 14). Other indicators such as quickening and the ability to auscultate fetal heart tones are also used to estimate gestational age in the prenatal period.

Several laboratory and diagnostic tests are used during pregnancy to monitor gestational development. In a prenatal ultrasound, sound waves are used to measure the biparietal diameter of the fetal skull and the tibia, fibula, and chest circumference. The highest correlation between biparietal diameter and gestational age occurs in the second trimester. Although not done on a routine basis, amniotic fluid analysis can contribute valuable information in the determination of gestational age. A fluid concentration greater than 2 mg/100 mL indicates term gestation. Additionally, when the lecithin:sphingomyelin ratio is greater than 2:1, the fetal lungs are considered mature. The presence of phosphatidylglycerol (PG) is also an indicator of fetal lung development[6] (*see* Chapter 11).

Neonatal assessments for gestational age are based on the examination of the neonate for certain physical and neuromuscular signs. The most common gestational age assessment tool is that devised by Dubowitz and colleagues. This tool uses 21 criteria to assess gestational age regardless of birth weight. The Dubowitz Gestational Age Tool is most valid when used on neonates between 28 and 43 weeks of gestation (*see* Chapter 33). Ballard's classification of the Dubowitz tool and the Brazelton Neonatal Behavioral Assessment Scale are two other tools available to assess gestational age after birth (*see* Chapter 33).

Intrauterine Growth

Once the neonate's birth weight is obtained and the gestational age assessed, intrauterine growth is determined. The birth weight and gestational age are plotted on standard intrauterine growth charts. Based on where the neonate falls on the chart, he or she is classified as **small for gestational age** (SGA), **appropriate for gestational age** (AGA), or **large for gestational age** (LGA).

Small-for-Gestational-Age Neonate

Neonates identified as small for gestational age have experienced intrauterine growth retardation. These neonates usually have a birth weight below the tenth percentile for their gestational age.[6] The SGA neonate can be premature, term, or postterm.

Fetal growth retardation may occur early or late in the gestation. Fetal cellular growth occurs in two phases. In the first phase, virtually all growth is due to increases in the number of cells in the fetal body. Interference with growth of the fetus during this phase results in the fetus' production of fewer than the normal number of cells. This type of growth impairment is called symmetrical growth retardation because all parts of the body are equally small as a result of the overall lower number of body cells. The fetus is not able to make more cells and can only continue to grow and develop with that number of cells.[6]

In the second phase of fetal cellular growth, cell size is affected rather than total number of cells. The fetus whose growth is affected during this phase develops asymmetrical intrauterine growth retardation. These neonates have appropriate-size heads and are the appropriate length but overall body weight and organ size are diminished (Figure 43–1). This impaired growth can be reversed once the reason for the growth retardation is identified and resolved.[6]

Several factors contribute to impaired growth in the fetus:

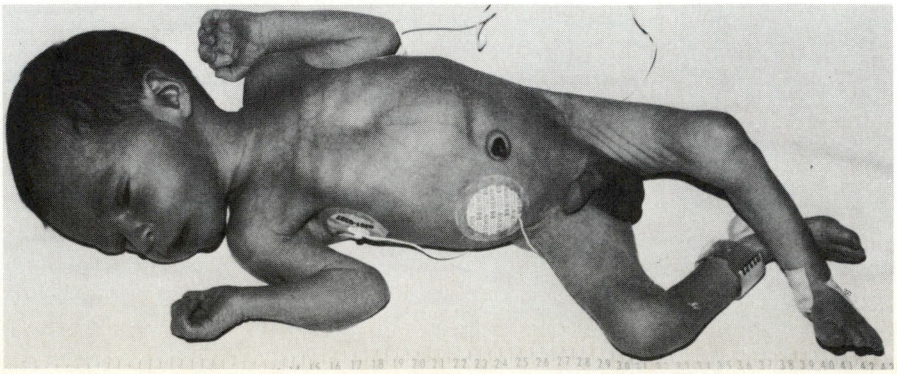

Figure 43–1. Neonate at 37 weeks of gestation with asymmetric intrauterine growth retardation. Note the wasted appearance. (*Reproduced, with permission, from Rudolph AM, Hoffman, JIE, eds. Pediatrics. 18th ed. Norwalk, Conn: Appleton & Lange; 1987:145.*)

- Placental dysfunction
- Multiple births (eg, twins and triplets)
- Intrauterine infection
- Intrauterine malnutrition
- Intrauterine drug and alcohol exposure
- Congenital anomalies
- Genetic abnormalities
- Intrauterine hypoxia
- Maternal hypertension/pregnancy-induced hypertension
- Severe maternal insulin-dependent diabetes
- Maternal renal disease[6]

The SGA neonate appears thin and wasted at birth. The skin is often loose, dry, and scaling. Meconium staining of the skin, nails, and umbilical cord is common. Small-for-gestational-age neonates lack subcutaneous fat stores and often appear to have muscle wasting. The umbilical cord may be thin from a lack of Wharton's jelly.[6] These neonates are usually alert and active and seem hungry, although they may go 24 hours or longer without voiding if fluids are not provided early and in sufficient quantity.

The SGA neonate is at risk for several clinical alterations, including respiratory distress; asphyxia; hypoglycemia; infections, especially those related to intrauterine infections; polycythemia; and hypothermia.[6]

Nursing and Collaborative Management. Management of the SGA neonate would ideally begin with the identification of prenatal risks for intrauterine growth retardation. If possible, steps can be taken to limit or to prevent the growth retardation before birth.

Once the neonate is found to be small for gestational age, it is important to identify the cause of the growth retardation. Management begins with resolution of the cause if possible. Specific treatments are directed at the alterations in functioning of the neonate. For example, frequent glucose tests and a strict feeding schedule may be implemented for the neonate with hypoglycemia, antibiotics will be initiated for the neonate with an infection, and the hypothermic neonate will be placed in a thermally controlled isolette.

Overall management includes close assessment of the SGA neonate's growth progress. Serial height and weight measurements are documented during the hospitalization. Parents should be aware of any special treatment needs the neonate may require at home. In addition, parents must be aware of the goal weight that the neonate must reach before being ready for discharge. Parents are anxious to learn of any weight gains and often ask for that information on a daily basis. Including parents in the care and feeding of the SGA neonate is essential in supporting attachment, especially if the neonate's discharge may be delayed. It also allows the nurse to observe the parent-neonate interaction and to offer suggestions and support as parents master the care of their neonates.

Large-for-Gestational-Age Neonate

Large-for-gestational-age neonates have a birth weight that exceeds the 90th percentile for their gestational age. The very large or macrosomic neonate is usually born to an insulin-dependent diabetic mother (*see* Chapter 42). Other conditions characterized by hyperinsulinemia, such as Beckwith syndrome, can cause the newborn to be macrosomic. Large parents are likely to have large neonates who do not have any special problems. Also, some Native American tribes are more likely to have LGA neonates.[1] The LGA neonate may be premature, term, or postterm.

Neonates who are large-for-gestational-age appear plump and obviously large. These neonates, particularly their shoulders, are at risk for birth trauma. Postnatal assessments should include observation of the neonate's reflexes and range of motion of all four extremities. Neonates who are macrosomic for metabolic reasons (eg, the neonate of a diabetic mother) require frequent laboratory tests (*see* chapter 42).

Nursing and Collaborative Management. The potentially LGA neonate is ideally identified before delivery. This allows the physician or nurse-midwife to predict potential fetopelvic disproportions resulting from the neonate's large size that could result in birth trauma.

After delivery, management would include treatment of any injuries related to the birth trauma and may include consultations with specialists such as orthopedic physicians. Neonates of diabetic mothers require serial glucose monitoring and early feedings or intravenous fluids (*see* Chapter 42).

Parents may have questions about the cause of the neonate's macrosomia and often ask about the neonate's future expected growth rate. Discharge instructions should include appropriate feeding guidelines to prevent concerned parents from potentially overfeeding or underfeeding the LGA neonate at home.

Appropriate-for-Gestational-Age Neonate

The premature, term, or postmature neonate may also be appropriate in size and development for gestational age. This indicates that the neonate has been able to grow and develop in utero at the appropriate rate; however, being appropriate for gestational age does not eliminate the problems associated with prematurity or postmaturity. The term neonate who is appropriate for gestational age may also face risk factors that complicate the delivery and postnatal period, such as asphyxia and persistent fetal circulation.

Multiple Gestation

In multiple gestations, more than one fetus is present in the uterus. Two types of multiple gestation can occur. In a monovular pregnancy, one ovum separates into two or more embryos (monozygotic twins). In a binovular pregnancy, more than one ovum is fertilized (dizootic twins).

Twins are the most common type of multiple gestation. Twins occur in 1 in 85 Caucasian births, in 1 in 150 Asian births, and in 1 in 50 black births. Multiple gestations have a perinatal mortality three to eight times greater than that of a singleton pregnancy and account for 10 percent of all perinatal deaths.[6] The greater the number of fetuses, the greater the morbidity and mortality.

Monovular Pregnancy. In a monovular pregnancy, one ovum is fertilized and separates into two or more similar embryos. These embryos are monozygous or identical. Monozygous neonates are the same sex. They have the same general appearance, including eye and hair coloring (Figure 43–2). These neonates even have identical or very similar fingerprints. Inherited disorders are also found in both neonates but may not be obvious at the same time.[6]

If the separation of the single embryo occurs early in the pregnancy, before the fifth day, two separate placentas develop. If the separation occurs later in the pregnancy, after the tenth day, the embryos may share one placenta.[6] The neonates may be conjoined if the embryo separates after the tenth day of pregnancy. When conjoining occurs, the neonates are connected by a common bridge of skin or even share entire organs or limbs. These neonates may be able to be surgically separated if the nature of their attachment is not life sustaining to both of them.[5]

Binovular Pregnancy. Binovular pregnancy occurs when more than one ovum is fertilized. Separate placentas and embryos then develop from each fertilized ovum. This produces dizygous, nonidentical or fraternal neonates. Dizygous neonates can be the same sex but are often different sexes. These neonates exhibit similarities as would ordinary brothers and sisters that are the products of single pregnancies.[5] Binovular pregnancies are more common with a positive familial history of multiple births, if the mother is over 35 years of age and has had other pregnancies.[6]

Special Problems Related to Gestational Age and Size in Twins. Intrauterine growth is similar in twins and singletons until 30 to 32 weeks, when intrauterine growth diminishes in both monozygous and dizygous twins. At birth, twins are usually smaller than a singleton neonate of the same gestational age. The main deficit in the intrauterine growth of twins occurs in the last 8 to 10 weeks of gestation. Twins are usually not the same weight at birth. Birth weights may be close or differ substantially (Figure 43–3).[5] Although intrauterine growth retardation occurs in 20 to 25 per-

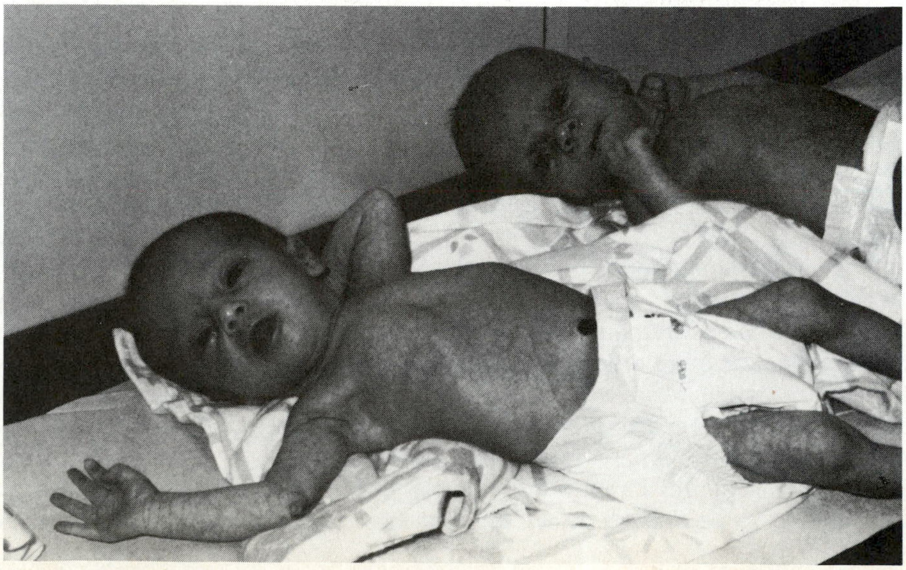

Figure 43–2. Monovular or monozygotic (identical) twins.

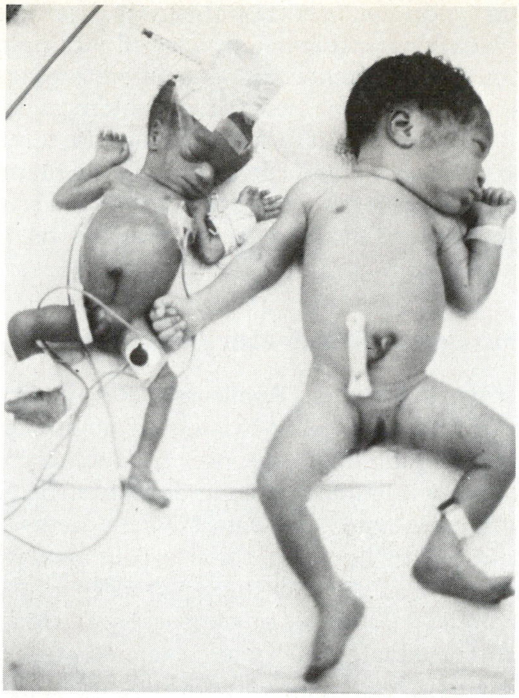

Figure 43–3. Marked birth weight disparity in dizygotic twins. The larger twin weighed 2300 g, appropriate for gestational age. The markedly growth-retarded smaller twin weighed only 785 g. (*Reproduced, with permission, from Cunningham FG, et al.* Williams Obstetrics. *18th ed. Norwalk, Conn: Appleton & Lange; 1989:642.*)

cent of twins, each twin normally should be the same size as a singleton neonate of the same maturity.[5] Twins may also be large for gestational age, although this is not as common as small for gestational age.

Fetal growth retardation causing one or both twins to be small for gestational age results from special problems (listed under "Management," discussed next) often experienced by a mother with a multiple gestation. Poor nutrition, anemia, and iron and folic acid deficiencies can contribute to fetal growth retardation. Fetal growth retardation in twins can also be related to a twin transfusion syndrome, in which one twin loses blood to the other twin through a common placental blood vessel.[5] Although the fetuses may have normal growth potential, altered placental functioning may not allow them to receive the necessary nutrients to sustain appropriate growth for their gestational age.[7] Vascular abnormalities of the placenta or premature separation of the placenta also can cause the fetuses to develop chronic fetal distress with the growth retardation.

Nursing and Collaborative Management. In 60 to 90 percent of multiple gestations, confirmation of more than one fetus occurs before delivery.[5] Most often confirmation occurs before 33 weeks of gestation. The uterus is found to be larger than expected for the length of time since the mother's last menstrual period. For example, the uterus is usually 4 cm greater than expected at 22 weeks of gestation.[5] Multiple gestation is usually confirmed by ultrasound.

The mother expecting twins must be assessed closely for signs and symptoms of alterations that would place the twins at risk for preterm birth or intrauterine growth retardation. The client requires serial ultrasound tests to monitor intrauterine growth and development.

Management of twins begins with the mother with a multiple gestation and must include careful prenatal assessment. Because of the greater-than-normal growth of multiple fetuses versus a single fetus, the mother is at risk for special problems, among them hyperemesis; discomfort related to increased abdominal pressure, such as gastrointestinal discomfort and shortness of breath; anemia and iron and folic acid deficiencies; pregnancy-induced hypertension; placenta previa or abruptio placentae; premature labor or premature rupture of membranes; and obstructed labor caused by fetal malpresentations.[5]

Prematurity is the most frequent cause of mortality in multiple gestations, especially if the neonates are born before 33 weeks of gestation. Efforts to prevent a premature delivery are therefore essential. The mother requires additional rest, especially after 24 weeks of gestation. She may also require bedrest between 26 and 36 weeks of gestation.[5] Tests to assess the fetuses' maturity are routinely done at 34 weeks. It can, however, be difficult to accurately interpret laboratory tests such as the lecithin:sphingomyelin ratio, which helps to identify fetal lung maturity, as there is more than one fetus to consider. The ultrasound becomes an important tool in predicting the fetuses' size, gestational age, and readiness for delivery.

The parents require consistent support as they anticipate the birth of twins. They must be aware of potential complications as the pregnancy continues and the importance of adhering to special instructions such as dietary and activity restrictions. The mother expecting twins may be referred to a level III regional center that is equipped with specially trained staff and resources to care for the premature and potentially SGA neonates.

THE PREMATURE NEONATE

The premature neonate is defined as a neonate born before the end of 37 weeks of gestation. The incidence of prematurity is 8 percent.[6] As the premature neonate is born early, all body systems may not be mature enough to support the neonate through the transition to extrauterine life. As a result, the premature neonate may face life-threatening conditions. It is not surprising that prematurity accounts for 80 percent of all neonatal deaths.[6]

Premature neonates must be assessed for appropriate intrauterine growth. These neonates may be small for gestational age, appropriate for gestational age, or large for gestational age. A premature LGA neonate may look like a term neonate. Conversely, the term neonate that is SGA may appear to be premature. Accurate identification of the neonate's gestational age, weight, and intrauterine growth is essential because each situation poses very different problems for the neonate.

The general appearance of the premature neonate will vary dramatically with the gestational age and with how sick the neonate becomes after the delivery. Table 43–1 presents an overview of some common characteristics of the premature neonate.

The premature neonate is likely to develop certain problems related to immaturity of various organ systems. Some common problems are respiratory distress syndrome, bronchopulmonary dysplasia, periodic breathing and apnea, retinopathy of prematurity, intracranial hemorrhages, temperature instability, feeding problems, necrotizing enterocolitis, and jaundice.[6] Many of these complications are not exclusive to prematurity and can be noted in the term and postterm neonate as well. The following discussion highlights some of the major alterations related to prematurity.

TABLE 43–1. COMMON CHARACTERISTICS OF THE PREMATURE NEONATE

Position	At 28 weeks of gestation, the neonate is floppy and hypotonic; at 32 weeks, the neonate flexes the lower extremities; and at 36 weeks, the neonate flexes all four extremities.
Skin	The premature neonate's skin is almost transparent and is ruddy in color. The neonate is covered with fine downy hair called lanugo. Vernix caseosa, the cheesy covering on the skin of the neonate, is minimal at 28 weeks of gestation and increases with gestational age.
Head	The premature neonate has wide, soft fontanelles with overriding sutures. The head appears large for the size of the body.
Ears	The 28- to 35-week gestation neonate has thin, pliable, inelastic ears, as cartilage does not begin to develop until after 35 weeks of gestation.
Chest	The overall chest appears small and malleable. The breast tissue is usually not palpable before 35 weeks of gestation. The neonate's cry is weak and poorly sustained.
Abdomen	The premature neonate's adbomen often appears distended because of poor muscle tone and the transparent skin.
Genitalia	The premature male neonate has a poorly developed scrotum with few skin folds and undescended testicles. The labia minora and the clitoris appear large in the premature female neonate as the labia majora are not fully developed.

Source: Reference 5.

Alterations in Respiratory Functioning

Respiratory Distress Syndrome. **Respiratory distress syndrome (RDS)** or hyaline membrane disease (HMD) is a pulmonary disorder that occurs in neonates born with immature lung development. Respiratory distress syndrome almost always occurs after a premature birth; however, some term or postterm neonates may also develop RDS. Neonates who experience difficult deliveries causing asphyxia are predisposed to developing RDS later.[7] Neonates of diabetic mothers may have delayed lung maturation as a result of hyperinsulinemia in utero.[8] Respiratory distress syndrome accounts for 25 percent of all neonatal deaths. It is 1.7 times more common in male than female neonates. It is more common in low-birth-weight Caucasian neonates than in low-birth-weight non-Caucasian neonates.[8]

Respiratory distress syndrome occurs when the neonate's lungs lack the pulmonary surfactant required for respiration. Surfactant is a lipoprotein found on the surface of the lungs which helps the lungs expand and contract easily during respiration by modifying the surface tension of the lungs. Surfactant also prevents the alveoli from collapsing.[8]

Without pulmonary surfactant, the alveoli collapse and each successive breath becomes more difficult for the neonate. The collapsed (or atelectatic) alveoli cannot allow for the exchange of oxygen and carbon dioxide, and hypoxia (defined as an arterial oxygen tension of 50 mm Hg or less) may quickly occur. Hypoxia contributes to acidosis as well as vasoconstriction of the pulmonary vessels, making it more difficult for blood to flow to the lungs. Blood is then redirected through other routes such as the foramen ovale and the ductus arteriosus. (*See* Chapter 32 for a discussion of conversion of fetal to neonatal circulation.) The extra work demanded for the increasing respiratory distress can quickly deplete the neonate's available energy.

Nursing and Collaborative Assessment. Assessment begins prior to delivery with identification of fetuses likely to develop RDS. Delay of delivery until fetal

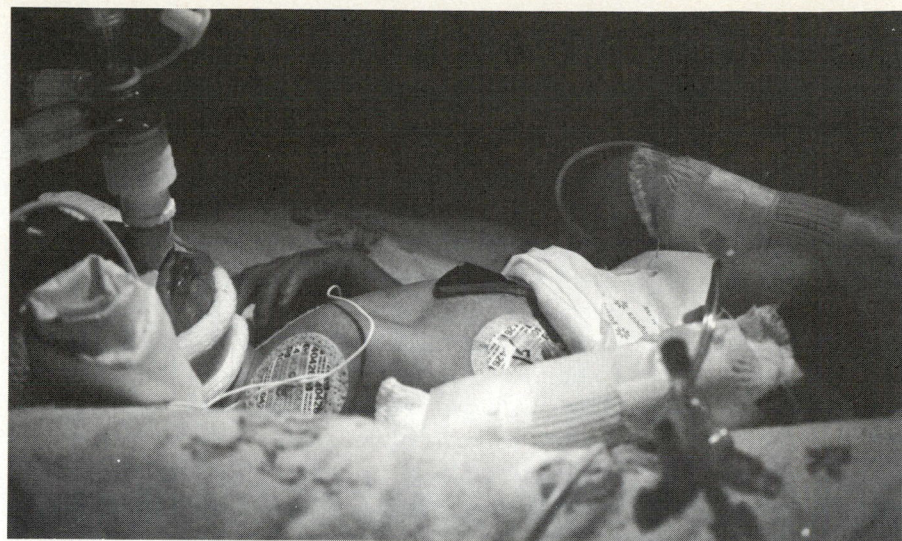

Figure 43–4. Neonate in respiratory distress. Note retractions.

lungs are mature is the ideal situation. If that is not possible, arrangements should be made to deliver the neonate in a hospital with specialized facilities and staff to care for the potentially ill newborn,[8] usually a level III facility.

Fetal lung maturity can be assessed by determining the lecithin:sphingomyelin (L:S) ratio of the amniotic fluid. An L:S ratio greater than 2 is predictive of fetal lung maturity in most instances; however, some neonates with an L:S ratio greater than 2 may develop RDS.

The neonate who develops RDS has labored breathing at birth that worsens quickly in the first hours of life. Tachypnea (a respiratory rate greater than 50 breaths per minute), retractions (Figure 43–4), and nasal flaring are noted.[5] The neonate may grunt with expiration, may appear pale, or may demonstrate cyanosis (a blue discoloration noted in the nail beds, lips, mouth, extremities, face, and trunk).

The neonate with RDS will also have altered gas exchange demonstrated by abnormal arterial blood gas values. Specifically, there will be hypoxia, an abnormally low oxygen level (less than 50 mm Hg), and hypercarbia, a high carbon dioxide level (greater than 60 mm Hg), if gas exchange is severely impaired.[8] Oxygen levels may be assessed in a noninvasive manner. A transcutaneous monitor or pulse oximeter are two devices that are applied to the neonate's skin. They detect oxygen levels in the peripheral blood supply.[9] Acidosis may also develop. Chest x-ray will show underinflation of the lungs. Spontaneous pneumothoraces, areas where air has leaked into the pleural space through ruptured alveoli, may occur frequently.[8]

Any neonate with symptoms of respiratory distress must be assessed immediately for the possibility of respiratory distress syndrome. Neonates who are identified to be at high risk for developing RDS must be closely monitored in the first hours and days of life. Careful and ongoing assessment is necessary to help prevent life-threatening complications such as apnea, the absence of respirations as a result of severe respiratory distress.

Nursing Diagnoses. On the basis of the comprehensive assessment, nursing diagnoses for the preterm neonate with respiratory distress syndrome are developed (*see* the box for examples).

Nursing and Collaborative Management. Management of the neonate with RDS focuses on resolution of the severe respiratory distress and the resulting hypoxia,

NURSING DIAGNOSES RELATED TO THE PRETERM NEONATE WITH RESPIRATORY DISTRESS SYNDROME

Problem-Oriented

Ineffective breathing pattern, related to deficient surfactant

Ineffective airway clearance, related to excess secretions

Ineffective gas exchange, related to immaturity of newborn's lungs and decreased surfactant

Strength-Oriented

Potential asset in resolution of RDS, related to neonatal weight greater than 1500 g retention of carbon dioxide, and acidosis. Supplemental humidified oxygen is administered via a hood to maintain arterial oxygen levels between 50 and 70 mm Hg. If the neonate continues to have difficulty breathing and gas exchange has not improved, intubation using a nasotracheal or orotracheal tube may be performed. The placement of a nasotracheal or orotracheal tube allows the neonate to breathe on his or her own while allowing the administration of oxygen or additional respiratory support.

The next step in providing respiratory support for the neonate with continued respiratory distress is continuous positive airway pressure (CPAP), which provides a certain amount of consistent positive pressure in the lungs to prevent collapse (atelectasis) of alveoli or bronchioles, the smaller extensions of the main pulmonary airways. If the neonate requires additional support, especially if the carbon dioxide level is greater than 60 mm Hg, mechanical ventilation can be instituted. In mechanical ventilation, the ventilator provides respiratory assistance to sustain the neonate. The physician sets the size and the number of breaths that the neonate should receive each minute for optimal ventilation (Figure 43–5).

If the neonate requires intubation, the nurse will be responsible for assessing certain parameters:

- Respiratory status, including color; breath sounds; number and quality of spontaneous respirations; presence of signs of respiratory distress; and results of arterial blood gas tests.
- Placement of the nasotracheal or orotracheal tube. (This includes exercising care when suctioning or positioning the neonate to prevent the tube from accidentally dislodging. An accidental or unplanned extubation can lead to an emergency situation in trying to provide the neonate with adequate ventilation in the absence of a tube in the trachea. In the event of an accidental extubation, the physician must be notified immediately.)
- Patency of the nasotracheal or orotracheal tube. (This includes regular suctioning, noting the amount, color, and consistency of secretions.)
- Ventilator settings, to ensure that they are appropriately maintained.

The nurse must notify the physician immediately of any changes in the neonate's status as well as the results of pertinent laboratory tests.

The intubated neonate often has difficulty relaxing and breathing in synchrony with the ventilator. This may cause the neonate to fight the ventilator breaths and cause additional respiratory compromise.[10] When this occurs, muscle relaxants such as pancuronium bromide (Pavulon) may be used to help the neonate relax and thereby achieve more effective ventilation. Muscle relaxants temporarily paralyze the neonate, which can cause additional problems such as edema and fluid imbalances. The paralyzed neo-

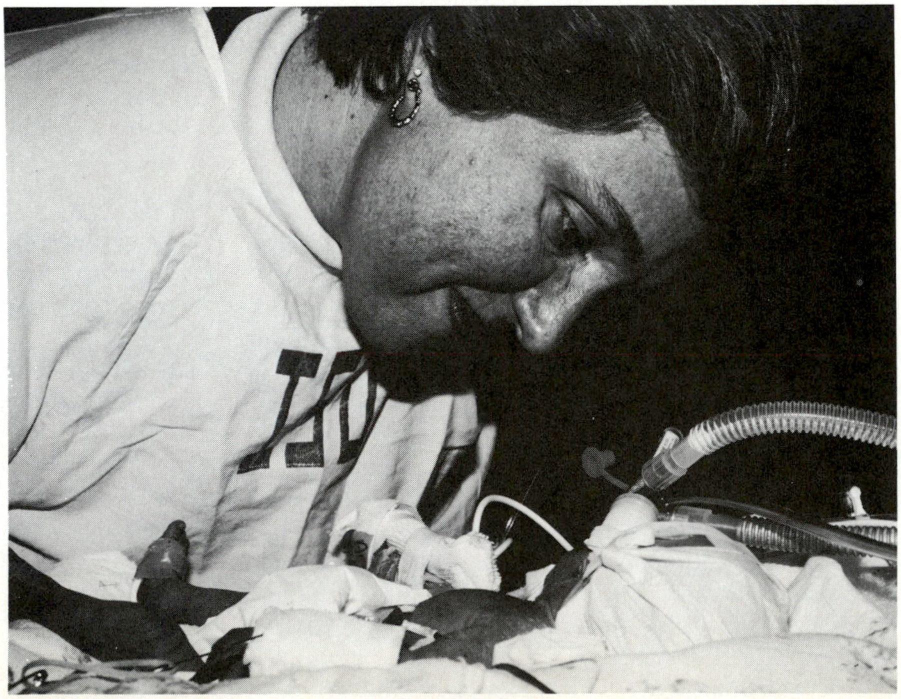

Figure 43–5. A nurse specialist assesses a preterm neonate being treated for respiratory distress syndrome. A mechanical ventilator provides respiratory assistance.

nate demands careful nursing assessment and care to prevent or limit such complications.[8]

Neonates with respiratory distress who require intubation will have difficulty clearing secretions from their lungs. Chest percussion and postural drainage should be performed gently on a routine basis every 4 hours to prevent atelectasis as well as buildup of secretions. In chest percussion, gentle percussion and vibration are used over the lung fields to loosen secretions from the smaller airways. In postural drainage, strategic changes in position are used to help drain secretions into larger airways where they can be coughed or suctioned out (Figure 43–6).

As RDS develops, the pulmonary blood vessels constrict, allowing fetal circulatory structures such as the ductus arteriosis to remain open. Once these structures open, there is an increased blood flow to the lungs that can cause pulmonary edema, a fluid buildup in the lungs. This fluid buildup can further compromise the neonate's respiratory status and distress becomes more severe. Diuretics such as furosemide (Lasix) are administered in a dose of 1 mg/kg to help eliminate fluid retention. Additional management may include specific treatment of the patent ductus arteriosis using medications such as indomethacin 0.2 mg/kg administered intravenously or surgical repair.[8] (*See* discussion of patent ductus arteriorsis later in this chapter.)

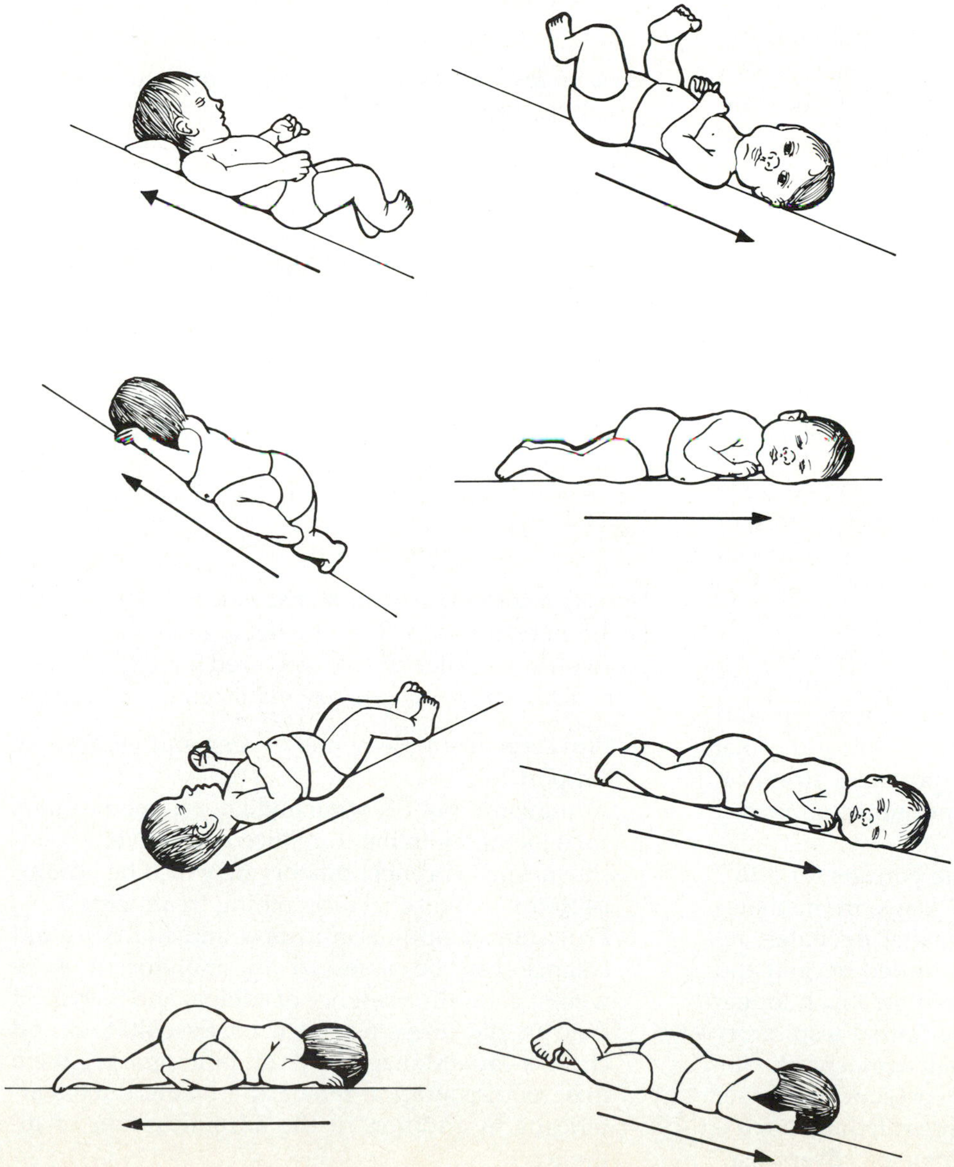

Figure 43–6. Postural drainage.

Lung maturity as indicated by presence of surfactant plays the major role in the occurrence of RDS. Research has demonstrated that the development and use of exogenous surfactant in neonates with immature lungs may minimize the risk of severe RDS. Further research is being conducted to identify the optimal client population in which this medication can be used, the appropriate doses, and the long-term treatment plan for the use of exogenous surfactant in high-risk neonates.[8,11,12]

Management of the neonate with RDS must include careful consideration of nutritional needs. The neonate experiencing severe respiratory distress is not able to take oral feedings. Intravenous fluids are indicated. If the neonate requires prolonged intravenous therapy, total parenteral nutrition may be initiated (*see* Chapter 42). As the neonate recovers, enteral feedings may be started. These neonates often begin with nasogastric or orogastric feedings before nipplefeedings are attempted. Calories and fluid requirements are specially calculated based on the weight and energy and nutritional needs of the neonate.[8]

Neonates with severe respiratory distress can become debilitated quickly. Careful handwashing and ongoing assessments for signs of potential infections are essential. The nurse should carefully monitor the neonate's temperature as well as laboratory results. The intubated neonate is at special risk for lung infections. Meticulous care should be taken during suctioning procedures. Neonates who develop infections are treated with antibiotics.[8]

Neonates with respiratory distress expend large amounts of energy because of the increased work of breathing. This additional energy expenditure can place them at risk for an unstable temperature. Hypothermia not only requires greater energy production to raise the neonate's temperature, but can increase oxygen demands significantly and contribute to acidosis. Through the use of radiant warmers and isolettes it is possible to maintain a neutral thermal environment. This decreases the potential stress on the neonate's energy stores and promotes improved oxygen use.

Respiratory distress syndrome persists for 3 to 7 days and usually resolves in 7 days in neonates weighing more than 1500 g. In smaller neonates, recovery may be prolonged and continued oxygen and ventilatory support may be required for much longer than 7 days. In the presence of continued respiratory distress that requires aggressive management, the neonate must be assessed for the presence of other physiologic problems, including heart failure, aspiration, infection, and bronchopulmonary dysplasia.[8]

Bronchopulmonary Dysplasia. **Bronchopulmonary dysplasia** (BPD) is a chronic lung disease of premature neonates who have required mechanical ventilation and high levels of oxygen in the first weeks of life. Most cases of BPD begin with RDS that does not resolve in 3 to 7 days. The lungs begin to develop abnormal cystic areas by days 10 to 20. In severe cases of BPD the lungs develop strandlike dense areas visible on x-ray.[8]

Bronchopulmonary dysplasia is confirmed when a neonate with RDS develops these lung changes and requires oxygen for more than 28 days. Because of the subjective nature of this method of confirmation, a clinical scoring system has been developed to assist in objective confirmation of the condition. Four grades of BPD are identified, with grade 1 being the least severe and grade 4 being persistently life threatening.[8]

Nursing and Collaborative Assessment. The neonate with BPD demonstrates persistent signs and symptoms of respiratory distress. Respiratory distress may not be continuous but may occur in intermittent episodes called BPD spells. During BPD spells, the neonate demonstrates signs of acute respiratory distress, including retractions, nasal flaring, tachypnea, and even cyanosis. Bronchopulmonary dysplasia spells may resolve spontaneously or may require specific interventions. Interventions include the use of increased supplemental oxygen, chest percussion and suctioning, and administration of aerosolized bronchodilators, medications that help resolve constriction and spasm of the small airways in the neonate's lungs.[8]

Nursing and Collaborative Management. Management of the neonate with BPD includes generalized supportive care similar to that required by the neonate with RDS. The following are management priorities:

1. Provision of supplemental oxygen and ventilatory support.
2. Administration of bronchodilators, medications such as theophylline to relieve and prevent bronchospasms. (Bronchodilators may also be administered via aerosolized breathing treatments.)
3. Provision of optimal nutrition and fluids. (Fluid balance can be assessed by monitoring daily weight gain, the presence of edema, and increased fluid in the lungs as noted by auscultation and chest x-ray. Management of pulmonary edema may require surgical repair of a patent ductus arteriosus in addition to the administration of diuretics.)

4. Thermoregulation to provide a neutral thermal environment.
5. Provision of appropriate periods of rest and sleep. (These neonates often require such frequent contact that they may be unable to obtain adequate rest. The development of a daily schedule in coordination with the care plan is an ideal way to allow for needed periods of rest. Controlling noise, light, and other environmental stimuli also promotes rest.)
6. Provision of auditory, visual, and tactile stimulation according to the neonate's tolerance. (Black and white pictures of geometric shapes, pictures of parents, mobiles, and a mirror are examples of ways to provide stimulation for the neonate without demanding great energy expenditure. The use of music boxes or tape recorders is also a way to provide stimulation. Parents should be involved in stimulating, playing with, and holding the neonate, if possible.)
7. Prevention of infections, especially respiratory infections that could further aggravate bronchospasms.[8]

Ongoing research continues to investigate management strategies in the neonate with BPD, such as the long-term effects of corticosteroid therapy;[13] however, the risk of long-term complications of severe BPD is significant. Neonates with BPD often face recurrent life-threatening setbacks and require multiple lengthy hospitalizations over months or years. Some may remain ventilator dependent. Neonates with BPD also have altered growth rates as they use most of their energy just to breathe. Developmental maturation may be compromised because of activity restrictions and prolonged hospitalizations. Neonates with BPD require ongoing developmental as well as physiologic assessments to identify problems that will arise as a result of their chronic illness.

Parents of a neonate with BPD face a great challenge in caring for a chronically ill child. Hospitalizations, financial burdens, and complex daily medications and treatment schedules at home can place considerable stress on the family unit. Parents must learn how to administer medications and treatments such as chest percussion proficiently. They must be able to assess changes in the status and notify the physician appropriately. Parents will rely on consistent nursing support and reinforcement as the neonate's complex needs change.

Periodic Breathing and Apnea. Premature neonates are at special risk for developing irregular breathing patterns, called **periodic breathing.** In periodic breathing, the neonate has periods of 5 to 10 seconds in which she or he does not take a breath, followed by periods of 10 to 15 seconds in which breathing proceeds at a rate of 50 to 60 breaths per minute.[5] This variation in the breathing pattern results in an overall respiratory rate of 30 to 40 breaths per minute. During periodic breathing, there is no change in the neonate's color, heart rate, or temperature. Periodic breathing is more common in preterm neonates less than 36 weeks of gestation.[5]

A dangerous potential complication of periodic breathing is prolonged apnea. **Apnea** is a pause in respirations longer than 20 seconds, or a pause that causes bradycardia or cyanosis.[5] Apnea lasting more than 20 seconds can lead to hypotonia, in which the neonate demonstrates floppy muscle tone. Apnea lasting more than 45 seconds can cause the neonate to become unresponsive and is a medical emergency. Prolonged or repeated apnea causes cyanosis because of the lack of oxygen. This lack of oxygen or hypoxia can lead to brain injury if not treated immediately.[5]

Apnea of prematurity is usually related to the immaturity of the respiratory regulatory system in the central nervous system.[5] Other potential causes of apnea include the following:

- Seizures
- Metabolic abnormalities, such as hypoglycemia or hyperglycemia, hypocalcemia, hyponatremia, hyperbilirubinemia, and acidosis
- Pulmonary obstructions, for example, incorrect positioning of the airway and increased secretions
- Sepsis
- Intracranial hemorrhages
- Hypothermia or hyperthermia
- Malnutrition
- Anemia
- Lipemia
- Patent ductus arteriosus
- Abdominal distension
- Regurgitation and aspiration[5]

Nursing and Collaborative Assessment. If the neonate is suspected of having periodic breathing or apnea, a pneumogram tracing is taken to confirm the extent of the irregular respiratory pattern. The pneumogram machine consists of an apnea monitor and a large printer. The monitor is attached to the neonate with electrodes similar to the cardiorespiratory monitor and the printer makes a continuous tracing of the neonate's respiratory pattern and cardiac rhythm. If apnea or an abnormal heart rate is detected during the test, the monitor signals an alarm.

The physician will designate how many hours of

pneumogram tracing is required. Usually between 8 and 12 hours of sleep time is necessary for an accurate reading. Once the test is completed the neonate is placed back on the cardiorespiratory monitor. The tracing is scored and evaluated, and the physician determines discharge needs if irregular breathing patterns are found on the test.

Nursing and Collaborative Management. As periodic breathing and apnea are frequent findings in the premature neonate, these neonates are placed on continuous cardiorespiratory monitors until normal breathing patterns are observed. Monitor alarms must be set for the correct parameters of heart rate and respiratory rate and must always remain in the "on" position with alarm volumes set in the high position. Alarms must be answered immediately to prevent a life-threatening emergency.

The nurse witnessing an apneic episode should use gentle tactile stimulation to arouse the neonate. This stimulation can include tapping the feet, stroking the chest, or changing the neonate's position. If the neonate does not begin to breathe, emergency help must be sought immediately and resuscitation efforts initiated. An apneic neonate not responding to tactile stimulation must be given artificial breaths by bag and mask ventilation. If the neonate does not begin to breathe spontaneously, intubation and mechanical ventilation will be required.

The neonate found to have periodic breathing or recurrent apneic spells must be assessed to identify the underlying cause. If the periodic breathing and apnea are related to prematurity, theophylline or caffeine is prescribed to be administered orally to the neonate. Theophylline and caffeine are medications that act as stimulants to the neonate's central nervous system and work to eliminate the irregular breathing patterns.[5] The physician identifies the therapeutic range of theophylline or caffeine to be maintained in the neonate's blood. Prior to discharge, parents must demonstrate knowledge of the prescribed dosage and correct administration of medication.

Neonates with periodic breathing or apnea that may pose a potential life-threatening risk require continued use of an apnea monitor at home. This helps parents to monitor the neonate's respirations and sounds an alarm if the neonate becomes apneic. Parents must receive special discharge teaching regarding the safe use of the monitor and how to respond if the monitor signals an alarm. This training usually includes formal or informal instructions on cardiopulmonary resuscitation (CPR) for the parents and other adults caring for the neonate, such as the babysitter and grandparents.

Identification of an irregular breathing pattern in the neonate can be frightening to parents. In addition to concerns about the neonate's prematurity, parents face caring for the neonate at home with medications and an apnea monitor. The nurse should allow parents ample time to familiarize themselves with the neonate's usual daily care, such as bathing and feeding, before initiating teaching about the monitor. This allows the parents to gain comfort and confidence in caring for the neonate before adding more complicated skills, such as monitor training and CPR, to their discharge plan.

Parents must have ready access to a phone and must know how to notify the emergency rescue system in their community if the neonate does stop breathing. Parents are instructed to notify the physician if the monitor alarms frequently while the neonate is sleeping or if they observe an apneic episode. Regular follow-up visits are important to assess the neonate's progress as well as to reinforce discharge teaching. Follow-up visits also allow physicians to plan for further pneumograms to assess the infant's breathing pattern as he or she gets older. The apnea monitor and medications are continued until the infant is found to have a regular breathing pattern. *See* the box for nursing strategies to prepare for discharge of the neonate requiring home apnea monitoring.

The nurse is cautioned to carefully assess the family's home environment and situation prior to discharge. In one example, a community health nurse making a home visit found that a single mother was not using the apnea monitor. On further evaluation, it was discovered that the dwelling had one functional electrical outlet into which a space heater was plugged. When faced with a choice of heat for the family or use of the monitor, the mother met the most basic need first—warmth.

Retinopathy of Prematurity. Retinopathy of prematurity (ROP) is a disease process that occurs in the blood vessels in the retina of the eyes.[14, 15] Retinopathy of prematurity occurs in neonates, especially premature neonates, who have received high concentrations of oxygen in the first weeks or months of life. The retina of the eye is not fully developed by 28 weeks of gestation. At 32 weeks of gestation, the blood vessels in the temporal peripheral area of the retina remain immature. It is this temporal peripheral area of the retinal blood vessels that becomes most vulnerable to damage from high oxygen concentration.[7] In addition, the immature retinal blood vessels in the premature neonate may be less likely to recover from the constriction and damage.

High oxygen levels cause the arterioles, the small branches of arteries, in the retina to constrict or narrow. This constriction decreases the volume of blood

NURSING STRATEGIES: PREPARATION FOR HOME APNEA MONITORING

Assess the family's needs, level of education, available supports among friends and family, overall health, financial level, particular demands of job, home, and family, and current level of understanding of neonate's condition.

Educate family about apnea; fill in gaps in knowledge.

Review all home care therapies (including medication administration, side effects, and so on).

Help family to locate appropriate and available family and community resources (eg, Visiting Nurses Association).

Help family locate home monitoring company.

Refer family to social services if financial arrangements must be negotiated (eg, obtaining a telephone).

Help family to design most practical and safe placement of monitor in the home.

Make sure family has a telephone or access to one for possible emergencies.

Assist family in notifying local emergency services of potential need for services (eg, police, fire, electric company).

Demonstrate, then observe family as they practice with the machine.

Carefully explain CPR techniques. (Allow time for demonstration; provide written materials for quick referral.)

Make sure that safety precautions are understood and that troubleshooting for potential mechanical problems is clearly understood.

Demonstrate how to maintain a log of apneic episodes.

Prepare and support the family regarding lifestyle changes. (Include other children and relatives as necessary.)

Adapted, with permission, from Norris-Berkemeyer S, Hutchins K. Home apnea monitoring. Pediatr Nurs. *1986;12:259–262.*

that flows to the retina of the eye. If the constriction is not resolved, the affected retinal blood vessels may be permanently destroyed.[7] When this occurs, the growth of undamaged retinal blood vessels will increase to try to reestablish the damaged retinal circulation. These new blood vessels grow very rapidly and tend to be weak or abnormal. The weakened blood vessels can allow blood and fluid to leak into the vitreous of the eye. Over time, this can result in the development of scar tissue that places tension on the retina. This damage to the retina can cause severe impairment in vision or even blindness.[7] Retinopathy of prematurity has been described in four stages or five grades based on the abnormalities that develop in the retina and retinal blood vessels (Table 43–2).

Nursing and Collaborative Assessment and Management. Management of retinopathy of prematurity begins by identifying neonates who may require prolonged high concentrations of oxygen therapy in the first weeks or months of life. The premature neonate is at special risk for this condition because of the immaturity of the retina. Management includes careful attention to the neonate's oxygen needs. Prompt weaning from high oxygen concentrations should be initiated as soon as it is safe for the neonate. In addition, some research indicates that the administration of vitamin E to high-risk neonates may reduce the incidence and severity of ROP.[7]

An essential part of the identification and management of ROP is serial ocular examinations done by an ophthalmologist who is experienced with the condition. All neonates who weigh less than 1500 g at birth or are less than 37 weeks of gestation should receive an ophthalmologic examination at 3 to 4 weeks of age. It is at this point in the disease process that severe retinal changes can be seen. A second examination is suggested at 6 weeks of age and at regular intervals thereafter if ROP has been identified.[7]

Before the ophthalmologic examination, the nurse may need to place a series of drops in the neonate's eyes to dilate the pupils. The drops are often administered according to a special time schedule ordered by the physician performing the examination. Once the neonate's pupils are dilated, the neonate may be sensitive to the bright lights of the nursery.[16] Care should be taken to lower the lights over the neonate's bed or to shade the bed if possible. The

TABLE 43–2. CLASSIFICATIONS OF RETINOPATHY OF PREMATURITY

Classification by International Proliferative-Phase Fundus Changes	
Stage I	Demarcation line seen between vascularized and avascularized retina
Stage II	Demarcation line is elevated to a ridge
Stage III	Ridge has increased growth of extraretinal blood vessels
Stage IV	Retinal detachment
Classification by Cicatrical-Phase Fundus Changes	
Grade I	Small areas of retinal pigment irregularities are seen
Grade II	The disc is distorted
Grade III	The retinal fold is seen
Grave IV	Incomplete retrolental mass, partial retinal detachment
Grade V	Complete retrolental mass, total retinal detachment

Source: References 5 and 7.

nurse may also be asked to assist in the examination by holding the neonate's head in the necessary position.

Parents will be extremely anxious to know the outcome of the ophthalmologic examination and whether the neonate will have a vision impairment. Parents require continued support as information about the long-term vision is often obtained only after serial examinations as the infant grows. Parents must be aware of the importance of follow-up visits with the ophthalmologist for continued assessment. In some situations, treatments such as transscleral cryotherapy also may be performed to stop the progression of severe ROP. Parents should be directed to an ophthalmologist who is familiar with the available treatments for ROP for further information.[7]

Alterations in Cardiovascular Functioning

Patent Ductus Arteriosus. As discussed in Chapter 32, the ductus arteriosus is a functional cardiac structure in the fetus that connects the left pulmonary artery and the aorta and serves to shunt blood away from the lungs in fetal circulation. Closure of the ductus arteriosus usually occurs spontaneously in the first week of life in the term neonate and within 20 days in the preterm neonate.[17] Closure is influenced by the muscular development of the ductus, blood oxygen levels, and prostaglandin levels.

Patent ductus arteriosus (PDA) is a condition in which the ductus remains open after birth.[5,18] Premature neonates are at risk for a patent ductus arteriosus because they are more likely to experience respiratory complications that compromise their arterial oxygen levels. Without adequate oxygen levels the smooth muscle of the ductus will not constrict and the ductus will remain open. Also, the ductus arteriosus in the premature neonate is less muscular than the ductus in the term neonate. Thus, conditions such as acidosis and the presence of prostaglandin E more quickly affect the ductus in the premature neonate to prevent closure.[5,17]

Hypoxia, acidosis, and the presence of prostaglandin E also affect the closure of the ductus in the term neonate. Even if the closure has already occurred, the ductus can reopen in the presence of these conditions. In neonates with cyanotic heart disease such as transposition of the great vessels, the presence of a PDA is beneficial, as the PDA can provide for the necessary mixing of oxygenated and unoxygenated blood.[5,17]

Nursing and Collaborative Assessment. The term or premature neonate with a small PDA is likely to be asymptomatic. The larger the patent ductus, however, the more hemodynamic complications that arise. When the ductus remains open there is shunting of the blood from the left side of the heart to the pulmonary system. Blood from the aorta is shunted into the pulmonary artery, increasing the blood flow to the lungs. In the large PDA, this blood is shunted with higher pressure because it is coming from the aorta and the systemic circulation. This increased blood flow to the lungs can cause congestive heart failure. This, in turn, can cause congestion in the lungs that interferes with necessary gas exchange and may cause hypoxia. Signs and symptoms of PDA include (1) a continuous murmur, called a Gibson murmur, which is a crescendo systolic murmur with clicks heard at the base of the heart; (2) in a large PDA, bounding peripheral pulses and a wide pulse pressure in the blood pressure; and (3) persistent respiratory distress and hypoxia.[5,17] Signs of congestive failure include poor weight gain, recurrent pulmonary infections, and persistent respiratory distress and hypoxia.[5,17]

Patent ductus arteriosus will be confirmed through diagnostic testing. A chest x-ray will show an enlarged heart, pulmonary congestion, and a prominent pulmonary artery. An electrocardiogram will show abnormalities that indicate left ventricular hypertrophy. An echocardiogram will show the volume overload in the left ventricle.[5]

Nursing and Collaborative Management. Initial management is directed at relieving the symptoms related to respiratory distress and congestive heart failure. Supplemental oxygen and ventilatory support are administered based on the results of arterial blood gas tests. The neonate's fluid status must be carefully calculated to prevent both fluid overload and dehydration. The neonate's intake and output and daily weight are strictly monitored[19] (Figure 43–7). The administration of diuretics such as furosemide (Lasix) helps to eliminate and prevent fluid overload. Calorie needs are carefully calculated to ensure that sufficient calories are provided for the neonate's energy needs. Nutrition can be provided in enteral or parenteral feedings.

Once fluid and calorie needs have been addressed, management of the PDA itself is considered. Indomethacin, a prostaglandin inhibitor, is administered intravenously to promote closure of the ductus. If indomethacin is ineffective in producing closure, surgical repair is considered. The surgical procedure is usually done between 6 months and 1 year of age, but can be done earlier if the infant's condition warrants.[5]

Parents must receive careful explanation of the presence of a PDA and the role it plays in the neo-

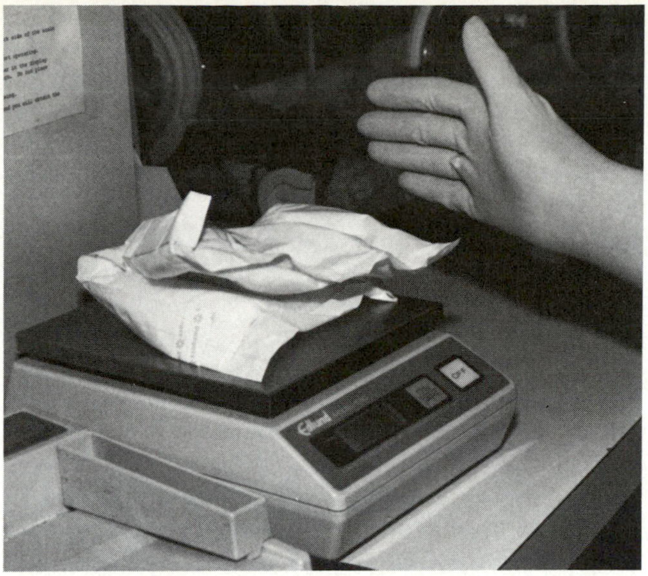

Figure 43–7. The neonate's diaper is weighed to assess output.

nate's condition. The parents of a critically ill newborn can easily become overwhelmed when approached with yet another "problem." Parents should also be informed about the use of indomethacin and the results obtained and advised if the persistence of a PDA will require surgical repair or additional tests such as a cardiac catheterization. Pictures or diagrams can be extremely useful in explaining PDA, its effects on the neonate, and the surgical repair procedure.

Alterations in Neurologic Functioning

Intracranial Hemorrhage. Intracranial hemorrhage is a major cause of neonatal morbidity and death, especially in the premature neonate. The incidence of intracranial hemorrhage in neonates less than 35 weeks of gestation is 35 to 45 percent.[6,8] An intracranial hemorrhage occurs when blood leaks into the cranial cavity from the vascular system in the brain. The bleeding can range from a small amount of oozing to a massive hemorrhage. The bleeding usually originates from the rich supply of small blood vessels in the germinal layer of the brain in the periventricular area. The fragile walls of the small arteries, capillaries, and veins in the neonate can easily be damaged, causing bleeding to occur.[8] The most common types of intracranial hemorrhage in premature neonates are subependymal hemorrhages and intraventricular hemorrhages. Table 43–3 lists the four grades of an intracranial hemorrhage.

There are many potential causes of intracranial hemorrhages in the premature neonate. The fragile blood vessel walls can be damaged by mechanical ventilation, asphyxia during delivery or postnatally, apnea, hypovolemia, fluctuations in cerebral blood flow velocity, neonatal thrombocytopenia in neonates weighing less than 1500 g, the use of benzyl alcohol as a preservative in intravenous flush solutions,[20] administration of hypertonic solutions, and rapid administration of volume expanders.[8]

Nursing and Collaborative Assessment. Intracranial hemorrhage usually manifests at 16 hours of life and reaches a peak at 48 hours. Symptoms include a change in respiratory status, such as episodes of apnea; a dropping hematocrit level that fails to rise after blood transfusions; a full and bulging fontanelle; and a change in activity such as an unwillingness to suck, myoclonic movements, lethargy, seizures, and decreased muscle tone.[8]

In addition to the identification of symptoms, intracranial hemorrhage is confirmed by an ultrasound of the neonate's head. Because 50 percent of premature neonates with intracranial hemorrhage may be asymptomatic, ultrasound of the head is often done to screen for the presence of an intracranial hemorrhage in these neonates. This ultrasound is usually done at the end of the first week of life.[8]

Nursing and Collaborative Management. Collaborative management of the neonate with an intracranial hemorrhage such as an intraventricular hemorrhage includes prevention, short-term management, and long-term management.[5]

Prevention. Prevention of a premature birth would have a major impact on eliminating the incidence of intracranial bleeding; however, on birth of a premature neonate, prevention is directed at maintaining the perfusion in the vulnerable germinal matrix of the brain. This includes preventing sudden or wide fluctuations in the systemic blood pressure.[21] Sudden increases in blood pressure have been noted in prema-

TABLE 43–3. CLASSIFICATION OF INTRACRANIAL HEMORRHAGES

Grade I	Isolated subependymal hemorrhage
Grade II	Intraventricular hemorrhage without ventricular dilation
Grade III	Intraventricular hemorrhage with ventricular dilation
Grade IV	Intraventricular hemorrhage with parenchymal hemorrhage

Source: Reference 8.

ture neonates during motor activity, diagnostic procedures, and daily handling, and with seizures and mechanical ventilation. Caution must be used when caring for the premature neonate who requires these treatments and activities, and the interdisciplinary team must be prepared to intervene swiftly when problems arise.[5]

Short-Term Management. Acute management begins with the identification of the symptoms related to an intracranial hemorrhage. An ultrasound of the neonate's head must be quickly facilitated. Further management is then focused on treatment of the particular abnormality identified. For example, a severe hemorrhage could cause multisystem abnormalities that require aggressive intervention. Seizures would be treated with medications such as phenobarbital; apnea, with oxygen and mechanical ventilation.

Long-Term Management. An intraventricular hemorrhage is a serious type of intracranial hemorrhage. After an intraventricular hemorrhage, the ventricles in the brain become dilated with excessive amounts of cerebral spinal fluid. This is called posthemorrhagic ventricular dilation. This ventricular dilation can cause an inappropriate increase in head circumference, demonstrated by full and bulging fontanelles. Ventricular size is monitored by serial ultrasounds of the head.

If the ventricular dilation does not stop spontaneously, intervention is necessary. Serial lumbar punctures (or spinal taps) can help to decrease excessive accumulations of cerebral spinal fluid. If the accumulation continues and causes an increase in intracranial pressure, neurosurgical intervention is required. This would include surgical placement of a ventricular peritoneal shunt. In this procedure a shunt is placed in the ventricles of the brain to drain the excessive amounts of cerebral spinal fluid into the peritoneal cavity.[8]

Nursing care of the premature neonate with an intraventricular hemorrhage includes careful and ongoing assessment for key symptoms. Once the neonate has been diagnosed with an intraventricular hemorrhage, both the neonate and the parents require aggressive support. In addition to learning about the many interventions needed to manage the neonate's changing condition, the parents will be extremely concerned with the severity and the extent of the damage caused by the hemorrhage and the possible long-term consequences.[22] Uncertainty related to long-term implications for the neonate adds to parental anxiety.

Prognosis depends on the extent of the bleeding. As outlined in Table 43–3, intraventricular hemorrhages are graded on the basis of the severity of the bleeding and the part of the brain affected. Grade I is the least severe and has the best prognosis; Grade IV is the most severe and may result in severe long-term neurologic damage. In addition to the severity of the bleeding, the prognosis also depends on the other physiologic complications, such as asphyxia and infection, the neonate experienced as a result of prematurity.

Neurologic abnormalities appear more often with large severe hemorrhages; however, the best indicators of long-term deficits related to intracranial hemorrhages are regular developmental and neurologic assessments of the neonate's growth and development over time. If the older infant or child demonstrates persistent neurologic or developmental delays, the parents will be referred to the appropriate community programs that best meet that child's special needs.[23] Management strategies then focus on parental education and the long-term care related to the handicaps.

Thermoregulation. In utero, the temperature of the fetus is about one degree higher than the maternal core temperature.[8] After birth, the neonate expends large amounts of energy to regulate his or her own body temperature in a different environment. Heat losses after delivery can be great and occur as a result of evaporation, convection, conduction, and radiation (*see* Chapter 32).

The premature neonate cannot immediately compensate for these heat losses. These neonates are at greater risk than the term neonate because of their greater body surface area. Brown fat tissue is an important mechanism for producing heat for the neonate. The premature neonate cannot fully rely on this mechanism, however, as brown fat cells do not even begin to appear until 26 to 30 weeks of gestation[17] (Figure 43–8).

Premature neonates are at great risk for **cold stress,** especially if their body temperature falls below 35°C (95°F).[6] During cold stress, metabolic needs increase dramatically. In a term neonate, an environmental temperature decrease from 33°C to 31°C is enough to double the neonate's oxygen needs.[8] The premature or sick neonate is less likely to adapt to those greater oxygen needs related to environmental temperature changes. The premature neonate who has developed lung disease such as respiratory distress syndrome is likely to become severely compromised if temperature instability further increases oxygen needs. This would place the premature neonate

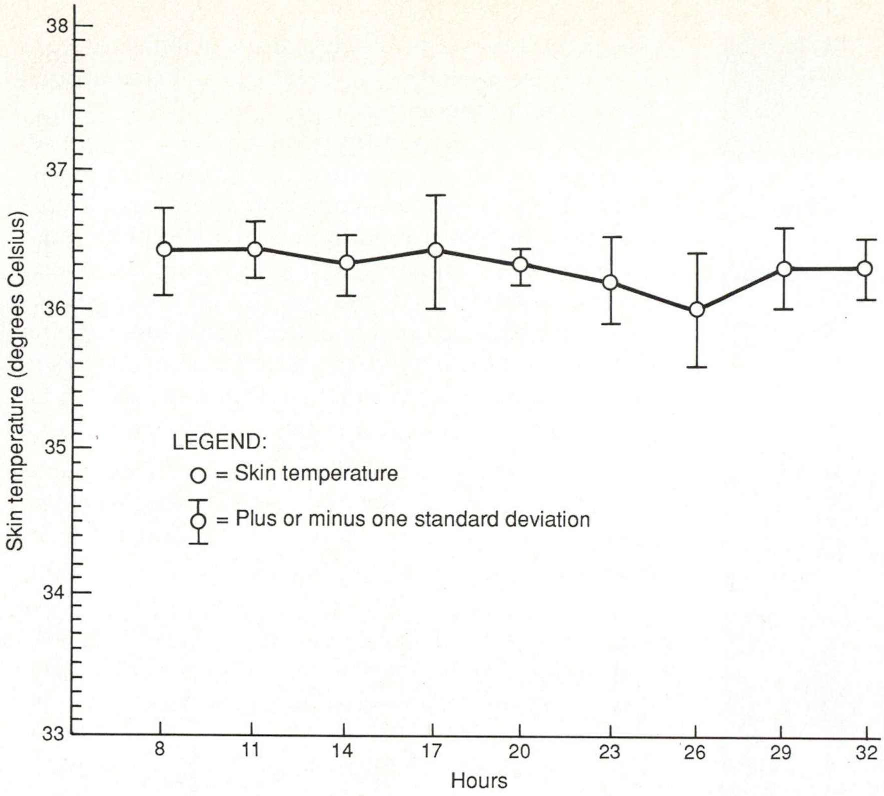

Figure 43–8. Skin temperature as a function of clock time over a 24-hour period in six preterm infants (mean skin temperature trough occurred at 2 AM). (*Reproduced, with permission, from Updike PA, et al. Physiologic circadian rhythmicity in preterm infants.* Nurs Res. *1985;34:161.*)

at risk for developing hypoxia, metabolic acidosis, and further temperature instability.[8]

In addition to cold stress, the premature neonate is also sensitive to increases in environmental temperatures. These neonates may develop an abnormally high body temperature, higher than 37°C (98.6°F), if wrapped in multiple blankets in a warm environment.[6] Temperature increases that would be expected in the presence of infection are often only low-grade increases or normal in the neonate because of the immaturity of their temperature regulation mechanisms.

Nursing and Collaborative Assessment. Common signs of inadequate temperature regulation in the neonate are central nervous system depression including lethargy, fatigue, and poor feeding behaviors; cardiac arrhythmias, especially bradycardia; cardiovascular instability including an unstable blood pressure; depressed respirations and periods of apnea; and metabolic abnormalities.[5]

Nursing Diagnoses. Nursing diagnoses are developed after comprehensive assessment of the neonate. *See* the box for several examples of diagnoses related to thermoregulation in the preterm neonate.

Nursing and Collaborative Management. To assist in thermoregulation, the preterm neonate should be dried thoroughly in the delivery room (*see* Chapter 34). After delivery, the premature neonate will require an artificially warmed environment such as an isolette or a radiant warming bed (Figure 43–9). The neutral thermal temperature must be carefully calculated for each neonate based on the gestational age and weight. A smaller neonate usually requires a warmer environmental temperature than a larger neonate to properly maintain body temperature.

NURSING DIAGNOSES RELATED TO THE PRETERM NEONATE WITH PROBLEMS IN THERMOREGULATION

Problem-Oriented

Ineffective thermoregulation, related to immature central nervous system and decreased brown fat

Potential altered body temperature, related to inability to maintain a neutral thermal environment

Potential hypothermia, related to immature thermoregulating mechanism and cold environment

Potential hyperthermia, related to immature thermoregulating mechanism and hot environment

Strength-Oriented

Potential asset for maintaining a neutral thermal environment, related to controlled temperature in radiant warmer

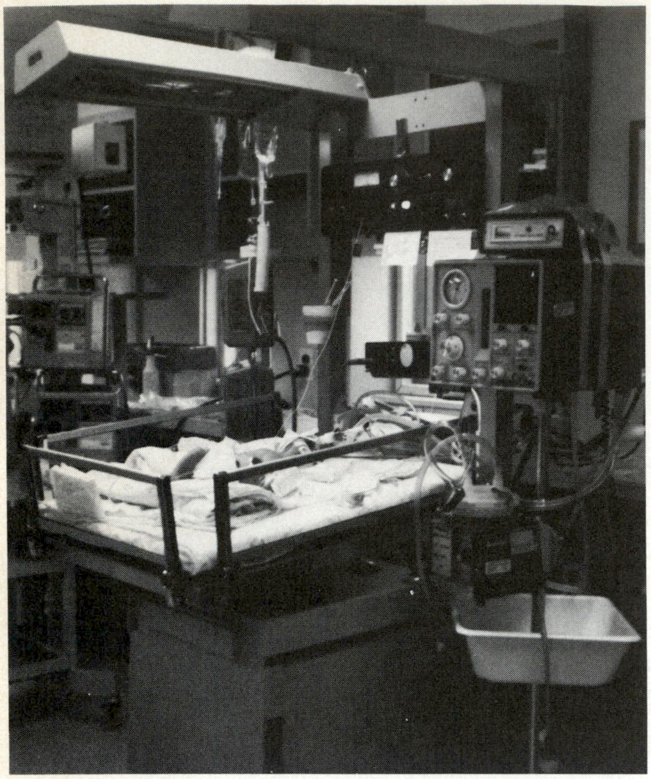

Figure 43–9. Premature neonate in an isolette.

It is ideal to use the isolette or the radiant warmer in the servo mode. The servo mode allows a temperature probe to be taped to the neonate's skin. As the neonate's temperature needs increase and decrease the environmental temperature is automatically adjusted within a preset range.[6] Caution must be used to ensure that temperature alarms are set in the *on* position and are functioning properly. This prevents problems and ensures that the radiant temperature is safely maintained. Neonates in isolettes and radiant warmers should be dressed only with a diaper so their temperature can be properly maintained in the servo mode and oveheating can be prevented. The nurse also should monitor the neonate's temperature regularly with a thermometer to ensure proper functioning of the isolette, as well as to assess the neonate's temperature stability.

Once the neonate is able to regulate his or her own temperature, weaning from the warmed environment of the isolette or radiant warmer to an open crib can begin. Weaning involves alternating periods in the warmer with progressively longer periods in an open crib until the neonate no longer requires the warmer. The neonate is dressed with a shirt, hat, and double or triple blankets while in the crib. The neonate's temperature must be monitored every 30 minutes to 1 hour until temperature stability is confirmed.[5] The neonate's temperature can be monitored every 3 hours thereafter.[6]

Parents of premature neonates who require an isolette or radiant warmer can feel isolated from their child. As the neonate's condition warrants, parents can touch the neonate in the warmer bed or through the portholes of the isolette. The neonate, if properly wrapped and dressed, may be able to tolerate short visits with parents outside of the isolette before being fully weaned to an open-air crib. Including parents in the weaning process can be an important step in facilitating parent-infant attachment prior to discharge (Figure 43–10).

Alterations in Gastrointestinal Functioning

Preterm infants can have major nutritional problems associated with gestational age and weight, metabolic and gastrointestinal functioning, temperature instability, respiratory status, and coordination of immature feeding reflexes, such as sucking and swallowing. Care of the preterm neonate must therefore include nutritional considerations. In addition, alterations in gastrointestinal functioning can be related to life-threatening conditions, such as necrotizing enterocolitis.

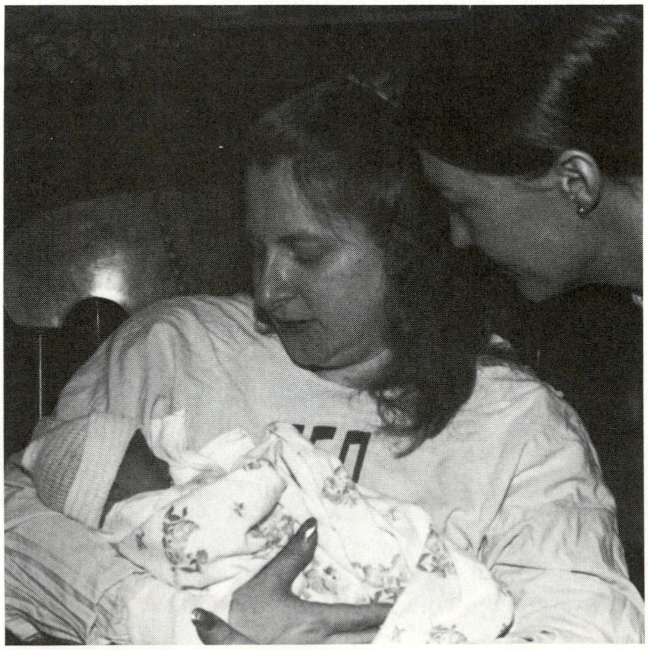

Figure 43–10. Premature neonate with double blankets and hat is held by mother in the neonatal intensive care unit. The relationship between a mother and her preterm neonate is fostered by positive interactions in the neonatal intensive care unit.

Necrotizing Enterocolitis. **Necrotizing enterocolitis** (NEC) is a serious and potentially life-threatening gastrointestinal disease seen in the sick newborn. Necrotizing enterocolitis occurs in 10 percent of term neonates, but is generally a disorder affecting premature neonates.[5,7]

The cause of NEC is difficult to identify. It has been observed to occur in clusters of neonates at one time; however, a single causative factor cannot be linked among the cases. Some sources better describe the disease process as a syndrome with many associated factors.[5,7] Table 43–4 lists risk factors commonly associated with NEC. Ischemic injury to the immature intestinal mucosa and presence of bacteria are the two most consistent factors in the development of NEC.[5,8] The presence of a substrate (enteral feeding) has also been theorized to contribute to NEC. A substrate must exist for bacterial fermentation to occur. Neonates who have been fed produce intestinal hydrogen, which can cause distension of the injured bowel. An excess of bacterial growth may then be associated with intestinal formula malabsorption leading to NEC.[24]

Nursing and Collaborative Assessment. The clinical signs and symptoms of NEC are usually seen between 3 and 10 days of life but have been found as late as 3 months of age. Symptoms may occur suddenly and can include abdominal distension, paralytic ileus or a decrease in bowel peristalsis, stools positive for occult blood, free peritoneal gas visualized on abdominal x-ray, temperature instability, apnea, bradycardia, and sepsis.[5,8] The symptoms of NEC are severe, and can be life-threatening for the premature neonate who is already ill with conditions such as respiratory distress syndrome, neonatal shock, and infection. Signs of cardiovascular and respiratory collapse will be seen as shock develops.[5]

TABLE 43–4. RISK FACTORS ASSOCIATED WITH NECROTIZING ENTEROCOLITIS

Bowel immaturity
Perinatal asphyxia
Bowel ischemia
Hypertonic substances introduced into the gut
Overgrowth of enteric bacteria
Polycythemia
Very low birth weight
Respiratory distress syndrome
Patent ductus arteriosus
Sepsis
Placement of umbilical artery lines
Administration of exchange transfusions

Source: References 6 and 17.

Nursing and Collaborative Management. The development of NEC is an emergency that requires swift medical and nursing intervention. Often, the first signs are observed by the nurse. The physician is notified without delay. The neonate should be placed on a cardiorespiratory monitor for continual assessment and can be placed on a radiant warmer bed to provide the necessary neutral thermal environment and allow for easy observation of any changes in condition.

Management begins with the immediate discontinuation of all enteral feedings. A nasogastric tube is placed into the neonate's stomach to prevent gastric distension (*see* the box on "Placement of a Feeding Tube and Gavage Feeding" on page 1222). Abdominal girth is measured at the same place on the abdomen at least daily to check for distension. A surgical pen can be used to mark the abdomen for placement of the measuring tape. The abdomen is assessed for the presence of further distension causing the skin to become tight, shiny, and red. Bowel sounds should be assessed and documented regularly.

The amount, color, and consistency of the drainage from the nasogastric tube should be closely monitored and documented. The nasogastric drainage should also be tested for the presence of occult blood. All stools are also tested for the presence of occult blood. Testing for occult blood may be done by staff nurses on the unit with a standard Hemoccult kit or specimens may be sent to the laboratory for testing.

Feedings are usually withheld for a minimum of 7 to 10 days or until the disease process resolves. During that time the neonate requires total intravenous nutritional support. This includes the careful calculation and administration of total parenteral nutrition (*see* Chapter 42).[5]

Because of the risk of sepsis and the presence of bacteria in the neonate's intestine, intravenous antibiotics (most commonly ampicillin, gentamycin, and clindamycin) are administered. Intravenous sites must be assessed regularly for signs of redness or swelling that may indicate infiltration or infection.

Surgical resection of the bowel is indicated if damage or necrosis of the bowel progresses or perforation occurs. A colostomy or ileostomy may be required in the presence of severe intestinal damage. Removal of large segments of damaged intestine could leave the neonate with a short bowel. This may result in long-term nutritional and absorption problems for the infant. Additional management includes cardiovascular support if signs of shock develop and respiratory support if the neonate's respiratory status becomes compromised.

The neonate's recovery from NEC may be complicated and require prolonged hospitalization. The gradual return to enteral feedings may be further delayed by malabsorption of the food ingested or recurrent diarrhea.[5] Neonates who have a short bowel from surgical resection could require intravenous therapy for years. Recurrent intestinal obstructions can also occur as scar tissue causes narrowing inside the intestine as the damaged bowel heals. Additional complications related to the neonate's prematurity, such as respiratory distress syndrome, may further delay full recovery and discharge to home.

Parents require consistent support and education through this very stressful time. Parents will have questions about when the neonate can resume feedings and often become frustrated when setbacks further delay the neonate's discharge. It can be extremely stressful for parents to learn to care for the neonate with a colostomy. A social worker can be of great assistance in obtaining the necessary supplies for colostomy care at home. Parents should be encouraged to identify another adult who can assist them in sharing caretaking activities for the neonate. Parents must understand the importance of attending routine follow-up visits with the physician and must be familiar with symptoms that require immediate medical attention.

Very-Low-Birth-Weight Neonates

Advances in neonatology have allowed smaller and sicker neonates to survive. As a result, special categories have been developed to describe the tiniest neonates. **Low-birth-weight** (LBW) neonates include neonates with birth weights less than 2500 g. **Very-Low-birth-weight** (VLBW) neonates are those with birth weights less than 1500 g. Neonates with birth weights less than 1000 g are called Very-Very-Low-Birth Weight (VVLBW) neonates.[25, 26]

Low birth weight occurs in 6.8 percent of neonates and is more frequent in black than in white neonates. Very low birth weight occurs in 1.2 percent of neonates and also is more frequent in black than in white neonates.[25] The most significant cause of low birth weight is prematurity. Premature neonates with low birth weights can also be described as SGA, AGA, or LGA.

Birth weight is a significant indicator of neonatal outcome.[27] Any premature neonate with a birth weight under 2500 g is therefore at special risk for problems in the postnatal period.[28] Very-low-birth-weight neonates have a postnatal death rate 50 percent higher than that of term neonates weighing over 2500 g.[25] Very-very-low-birth-weight neonates contributed to 57 percent of the total neonatal mortality rate between 1982 and 1984.[25]

The most common problems experienced by VLBW or VVLBW neonates are related to prematurity; however, these neonates are at special risk because, in addition to their prematurity, they have minimal energy stores to battle the complications of prematurity resulting from their small birth weight. This combination of risk factors can pose a tremendous challenge to the interdisciplinary neonatal team who will work together to help the neonate survive the premature birth with as few long-term complications as possible. Current research indicates that vigorous medical and nursing interventions initiated at birth can minimize the incidence of major handicaps in surviving infants.[29]

The care and treatment of the premature VLBW or VVLBW neonate can extend over many weeks and months. The neonate's hospital stay is often further prolonged by additional complications. For example, the VVLBW neonate is at increased risk for developing severe bronchopulmonary dysplasia related to the need for mechanical ventilation over a period of several weeks. The lengthy hospitalization of a VLBW or VVLBW neonate results in tremendous financial obligations for both parents and/or their third party payers.[30]

The parents of a VLBW or VVLBW neonate can quickly become overwhelmed by the many problems that can complicate the neonate's hospital course. Although it is important to keep the parents informed about any changes in the neonate's status, positive advances must be discussed along with the setbacks. Parents need to be presented with the neonate's prognosis in the immediate and long-term future. They may be faced with difficult decisions about initiating or continuing certain treatments for the VLBW or VVLBW neonate who is experiencing life-threatening complications. Parents confronted with these and other difficult decisions are under great stress and require thorough explanations with opportunities to ask questions. Parents often find strength in the consistent support and long-term follow-up by the physicians, nurses, and other health care providers caring for their neonate[31] (*see* Chapter 36).

THE POSTMATURE NEONATE

The neonate born after the end of 42 weeks of gestation is termed **postmature** or postdate.[32] Three to twelve percent of all pregnancies extend more than 2 weeks beyond the estimated date of confinement. The postmature neonate is more likely to experience fetal distress during labor and suffer ill effects from the prolonged pregnancy.[5] The effects of postmaturity on the fetus are referred to as the postmaturity syndrome.

RESEARCH ABSTRACT

Brooten D, et al. Clinical specialist predischarge and postdischarge teaching of parents of very-low-birth-weight infants. J Obstet Gynecol Neonat Nurs. *1989;18:316–322.*

Thirty-six families of very-low-birth-weight (VLBW) infants who weighed 1500 g or less, received discharge planning, teaching, and follow-up for 18 months after hospital discharge; teaching was done by perinatal clinical nurse specialists. The subjects were part of a larger study on early hospital discharge and nurse specialists home follow-up of VLBW infants. Content analyses were done on informational logs recorded by the clinical nurse specialists after each interaction with parents during the infants' hospitalizations, home visits, and telephone calls. Major teaching categories of infant, mother, family, home, and resources were identified. Important predischarge teaching topics included feeding, recognition of infections, and growth and development (particularly infant stimulation). Major postdischarge teaching topics included feeding, current health problems, growth and development, and managing within the health-care system. Findings from this group of parents were similar to reports about parents of healthy term infants on such topics as teaching needs related to growth and development and infant caretaking. Less teaching about maternal self-care, however, was noted in this group than among mothers of healthy infants, possibly because the follow-up period was longer and extended hospitalization of the infants gave preterm mothers greater time to recover physically than mothers of healthy infants received.

Comment:

In their larger study, Brooten and colleagues demonstrated the benefits of early hospital discharge and home follow-up of VLBW infants by clinical nurse specialists. In this well-designed study, the investigators identified important areas for teaching families of VLBW infants. They addressed the importance of adapting such topics about normal infant care as feeding, bathing, and handling of infants to the special needs of VLBW infants. In addition, they highlighted the need for teaching about infection, acute illnesses, and community and health care resources available to the family. The investigators identified limitations of the study, for example, the use of a select group of VLBW infants. The results of this study, however, will be valuable to nurses planning and providing educational programs for families of VLBW infants.

Postmaturity syndrome results from physiologic changes related to the neonate's prolonged gestation. A major problem in the development of postmaturity syndrome is the inability of the placenta to continue to nourish the fetus adequately. This occurs because the aging placenta gradually loses its ability for gas and nutrient exchange.

The postmature neonate is of normal length and head circumference at birth. Often the neonate weighs more than 4000 g; however, this neonate may also show signs of intrauterine weight loss, such as loss of subcutaneous fat and muscle mass. Characteristically, the postmature neonate will have peeling skin, long fingernails, and a wide-eyed gaze. The amniotic fluid, umbilical cord, and skin are often meconium stained. Oligohydramnios also may be observed.

Problems related to postmaturity syndrome are linked to the length of the gestation and the amount of stress that the fetus has suffered as a result of the prolonged pregnancy. Large neonates are at risk for birth injuries and may need to be delivered by cesarean because of cephalopelvic disproportion.[5] Placental insufficiency can place the neonate at risk for altered gas exchange that can result in life-threatening problems such as asphyxia and meconium aspiration syndrome (*see* later discussion).

Management of the postmature neonate is linked to the stress placed on the fetus as a result of the prolonged pregnancy. Serial ultrasounds are often done if a pregnancy is suspected to be postdate. This assists in eliminating questions regarding the correct calculation of the estimated data of confinement.

Immediate assessment of the neonate and the amniotic fluid after delivery assists the delivery room team in responding appropriately to potential problems. Many postmature neonates tolerate labor and delivery well and progress without difficulty. Other neonates suffer serious consequences of the complications related to postmaturity. Problems such as severe or recurrent asphyxia and meconium aspiration syndrome can be life threatening and must be aggressively managed. Postmature neonates found to be at risk for alterations after delivery are best observed in an intensive care nursery where expert care can be initiated immediately should problems arise.

Asphyxia

Asphyxia, a potentially life-threatening condition, is a state of altered gas exchange in which there is a decrease in oxgenation and an increase in carbon dioxide in the body.[5] When asphyxia occurs, sufficient

ISSUES AND CONTROVERSIES

Advances in neonatal care are continually expanding the capabilities of health care providers in caring for the premature neonate. These advances have allowed smaller, younger, and sicker neonates to survive the immediate postdelivery period including the very-low-birth-weight neonate (VLBW) and the very-very-low-birth-weight neonate (VVLBW).

Very-low-birth-weight neonates constitute less than 1 percent of all deliveries in the United States, yet these neonates contribute disproportionately to the overall neonatal mortality rate.[a,b] The care and treatment of these tiny neonates raise difficult issues and controversies for health care providers, parents, and the public:

- In what circumstances should the VLBW or VVLBW neonate be resuscitated?
- What treatment strategies are usual and necessary?
- When do usual and necessary treatments become extraordinary?
- In what circumstances should parents be given the decision to withhold or withdraw treatment?
- What rights do physicians and nurses have if they do not agree with the parents' decisions?

Cost of Delivering Care to Very-Low- and Very-Very-Low-Birth-Weight Neonates

Lengthy hospitalizations create stress on the family unit with the economic cost of hospital care an important stressor. A recent study of VLBW neonates found that the average length of hospitalization was between 68.1 and 147.2 days at an average cost per day of $897.76.[c] The mortality rate for this same group was 21 percent for neonates weighing between 900 and 1000 g at birth and as high as 56 percent for neonates weighing between 501 and 600 g at birth.

Controversy has focused on justifying the use of personnel and resources at a very high cost for a population of neonates whose mortality rate can be as high as 56 percent. Some experts question whether economic considerations should play a role in the ethical dilemma of treating VLBW and VVLBW neonates, thinking that no financial cost is too high. Other experts question if scarce financial resources could be better spent in delivery of expanded prenatal care, which might prevent these conditions.

Outcomes of Care Given to These Neonates

A major component in the ethical discussions regarding VLBW and VVLBW neonates is the outcome that can be expected as a result of the lifesaving treatment received in the intensive care nursery. A recent study indicates that 56 percent of the VLBW neonates survived past 1 month of age. Of those surviving neonates, 73 percent were found to have no handicaps, 20 percent were found to have serious handicaps, and 7 percent were found to have moderate handicaps when assessed between 24 and 36 months of age.[d]

These statistics can be viewed in more than one way. For the parents and families of surviving neonates, and the parents and families of the neonates who survived without a handicap, the intensive care treatment provided a wondrous outcome; however, the outcome was different for the 44 percent of VLBW neonates who died in the first month of life and for the 27 percent of the surviving neonates found to have moderate to severe handicaps.[d] Experts and lay people question whether the risk of death and handicap is worth the emotional and financial stress experienced by parents and families of VLBW and VVLBW neonates. Is any outcome a successful outcome? Do new advances such as exogenous surfactant promise a better future for these neonates, with better odds of survival?

Ethical Dilemmas in Caring for Very-Low- and Very-Very-Low-Birth-Weight Neonates

Both medical science and nursing science are committed to treat those in need with the best expertise and technology available. Many premature neonates respond positively to each step in the treatment plan and grow and develop in the intensive care nursery until discharge is possible. Other infants do not, their course being plagued with problems and setbacks.

When caring for the very sick VLBW neonate, health care providers are faced with deciding when a treatment is usual and necessary or when extraordinary. The health care team must openly and honestly present the neonate's expected prognosis, in addition to the management options, to anxious and worried parents. Parents are then faced with a decision about whether to authorize the initiation or even withdrawal of a specific treatment. The decision may result in the imminent death of their child.

Once a difficult decision is made, the ethical dilemma is not over. Parents, physicians, and nurses must consider their personal feelings and beliefs regarding the situation. There must be mutual respect for all of the individuals involved. Consistent support for the staff and the family is essential as each day brings a new decision and perhaps a new dilemma.

---

[a] *Raju T. An epidemiologic study of very-low and very-very-low-birth-weight infants.* Clin Perinatol. *1986;13:233–251.*
[b] *Vasa R, et al. Perinatal factors influencing the outcome of 501 to 1000 grams newborns.* Clin Perinatol. *1986;13:267–284.*
[c] *Hernandez J. The cost of care of the less-than-1000-gram infant.* Clin Perinatol. *1986;13:461–474.*
[d] *Sell E. Outcome of very-very-low-birth-weight infants.* Clin. Perinatol. *1986;13:451–460.*

RESUSCITATION OF THE NEONATE

1. Establish unresponsiveness of the neonate and need for resuscitation.
2. Place the neonate on the radiant warmer bed. This assists in maintaining the neonate's temperature, and allows easy visibility and access to the neonate.
3. Assess the neonate's heart rate and respiratory rate and place the neonate on a cardiorespiratory monitor.
4. Provide the necessary respiratory support, usually bag and mask ventilation with 100 percent oxygen.
5. Initiate cardiac compressions in the absence of a heart rate (Figure 43–11).
6. Establish an intravenous line. An umbilical arterial line and an umbilical venous line will be placed as soon as the neonate's condition allows.
7. Administer medications as ordered by the physician.
8. Assess the neonate's fluid and metabolic balances and initiate intravenous fluids as ordered by the physician.

Source: Reference 5.

oxygen does not enter the fetal circulation and carbon dioxide is not removed from the blood. The tissues of the fetus' body continue to use what little oxygen is available. This results in a lack of available oxygen, and hypoxia, an arterial oxygen level less than 50 mm Hg, occurs.[17] For the sick neonate, an arterial oxygen level between 60 and 80 mm Hg is desirable.[17] When hypoxia occurs, the anaerobic metabolism becomes active. This results in the production of large amounts of metabolic acids in the body. If not resolved immediately, asphyxia can result in death or severe physiologic damage.[5]

There are many potential causes of asphyxia in the fetus. Some of the most common causes are listed here:

- Interruption of umbilical blood flow such as would occur if the umbilical cord is compressed during labor
- Interruption of placental blood flow related to placental separation or abruption
- Inadequate perfusion on the maternal side of the placenta, related to maternal hypotension
- Anemia in the fetus that makes it difficult for that fetus to tolerate the mild transient hypoxia that can occur normally during labor
- Failure of the neonate's lungs to inflate after delivery, related to an obstructed airway and possibly meconium aspiration[5]

Asphyxia can occur suddenly and, in severe episodes, can be lethal in less than 10 minutes. Repeated episodes of mild asphyxia that are resolved can eventually produce a cumulative effect similar to that of a severe episode of asphyxia. Asphyxia should be anticipated in prematurity, postmaturity, multiple gestation, maternal diabetes, maternal hypertension, maternal and fetal anemia, breech presentation and delivery, and prolapse or compression of the umbilical cord.[5]

Nursing and Collaborative Assessment. The asphyxiated neonate is cyanotic, demonstrated by a blue coloring of the face, extremities, lips, and trunk. The neonate is limp and unresponsive to stimulation, and may demonstrate weak, gasping breaths or may not be breathing at all. Asphyxia is a medical emergency and must be treated immediately.

Nursing and Collaborative Management. Immediate assessment of the asphyxiated neonate is essential to identify the care required. If the neonate has been severely asphyxiated, resuscitation is necessary (*see* the box). The resuscitation process can be fast paced and filled with tension for all of the staff involved. It is essential that the nurse become familiar with his or her role in the resuscitation of a neonate. The nurse must be familiar with the resuscitation process, the

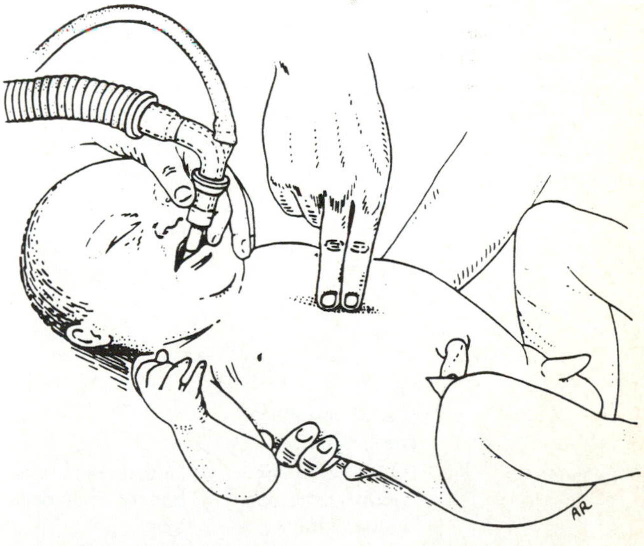

Figure 43–11. One technique for closed chest cardiac compression of the neonate. The index finger or index and middle fingers of one hand are placed at the neonate's nipple line. To provide support and serve as a hard surface, the other hand is placed under the neonate's upper back. (*Reproduced, with permission from Gutsche B. Obstetric anesthesia and perinatology. In: Dripps M, et al.* Introduction to Anesthesia: Its Safe Practice. *7th ed. Philadelphia: WB Saunders; 1988:311.*)

correct use and calculations of medications, and the correct technique for bag and mask ventilation and cardiac compressions. Medications commonly used for neonatal resuscitation are listed in Table 43–5.

The neonate who has experienced asphyxia but does not require resuscitation at birth will also require special care and observation. Continued assessment of the neonate's respiratory functioning may indicate the need for additional oxygen and ventilatory support. If hypoxia persists, additional problems such as persistent fetal circulation should be suspected.

The central nervous system can be severely affected by asphyxia. The lack of oxygen to the brain can lead to brain damage and seizures. The neonate with brain damage related to asphyxia initially is found to be hypertonic with a poor sucking response. The neonate becomes progressively hypotonic about 8 to 10 hours of age. Seizure activity will occur in the first 24 hours of life. Seizures may be in the form of tonic-clonic jerking movements or may look like lip smacking and eye blinking. (*See* Chapter 42 for discussion of neonatal seizures.) The neonate with seizures requires careful observation, as well as medications to stop the seizures and to prevent their recurrence.

TABLE 43–5. RESUSCITATION EMERGENCY MEDICATIONS

Drug	Dose and Route of Administration	Indications	Physiologic Effect	Side Effects	Comments
Sodium bicarbonate ($NaHCO_3$)	1 mEq/kg IV (use 1 mEq/ml solution for children > 6 months old; 0.5 mEq/mL solution for neonates and infants < 6 months old)	Acidosis	Buffers acid	Hypernatremia, alkalosis, hyperosmolar state	Interacts with calcium and epinephrine; flush line with normal saline
Epinephrine	0.1 mL/kg of 1:10,000 solution (maximum 5 mL) every 3–5 minutes as needed IV or ET	Asystole, EMD, hypotension	Stimulates alpha and beta receptors, resulting in vasoconstriction, positive inotropic, and chronotropic effects	Cardiac arrhythmias, myocardial ischemia (rare)	Interacts with sodium bicarbonate; flush line with normal saline
Atropine sulfate	0.02 mg/kg IV or ET; may repeat every 5–10 minutes for maximum total dose of 2 mg	Bradycardia associated with hypotension, symptoms of poor perfusion	Vagolytic effects, causing an increase in heart rate	Paradoxical bradycardia, tachyarrhythmias, myocardial ischemia	Do not exceed total maximum dose
Calcium salts	Calcium chloride 10–20 mg/kg (or 0.1–0.2 mL/kg of 10% solution) IV by central line only. Calcium gluconate 30 mg/kg (or 0.3 mL/kg of 10% solution) IV by central or peripheral line	Asystole, EMD, hypocalcemia, calcium channel blocker overdose, hyperkalemia	Increases myocardial contractility, ventricular excitability, conduction velocity through ventricular muscle	Hypercalcemia, cardiac arrest	Value of use in cardiac arrest controversial; give slowly (> 2 minutes); use with caution in digitalized clients
Dopamine	2–10 μg/kg per minute IV as continuous infusion	Hypotension, inadequate renal perfusion	Stimulates alpha and beta receptors; increases renal and mesenteric blood flow; positive inotropic and chronotropic effects; increased blood pressure	Tachyarrhythmias, ectopic beats, nausea, vomiting	Avoid extravasation; may cause tissue necrosis

IV = intravenous(ly), ET = endotracheal(ly), EMD = electromechanical dissociation.

Additional sequelae of asphyxia can be seen in all major organ systems. The severity of the alterations depends on the severity of the asphyxia. When asphyxia occurs, blood is shunted away from the gastrointestinal system and sent to the major organs such as the heart and the brain. This shunting of blood can damage the intestines, resulting in such problems as poor feeding and even necrotizing enterocolitis. Blood is also shunted away from the kidneys and may result in acute renal failure with low or no urine output.

The neonate who has experienced asphyxia requires intensive care for a prolonged period. This neonate is at high risk for developing numerous complications throughout the hospital stay. Parents of the asphyxiated neonate require enormous support from the interdisciplinary neonatal team. These parents need consistent, honest updates on the neonate's progress and compassionate support if the neonate's death is likely. The parents may be faced with the news that their neonate will survive but with significant problems related to the damage caused by the lack of oxygen. (*See* Chapter 36 for discussion of psychosocial implications of the high-risk childbearing family.)

Meconium Aspiration Syndrome

Meconium aspiration syndrome is a serious condition in which the fetus aspirates or breathes meconium (fetal stool) found in the amniotic fluid into the trachea or lungs. In response to physiologic stress such as hypoxia and asphyxiation, peristalsis increases in the fetus and the anal sphincter relaxes, allowing the meconium to pass into the amniotic fluid. Although meconium is seen in the amniotic fluid of some preterm neonates, it is more likely to occur after 34 weeks of gestation and especially in the mature fetus.[33] Presence of meconium in the amniotic fluid in any presentation but breech is an abnormal finding.[5] The quantity of meconium passed affects the appearance and viscosity of the amniotic fluid. Meconium-stained amniotic fluid can range in appearance from a greenish-tinged fluid to a thick pea soup consistency.

Under normal conditions, the fetus has breathing movements in utero. In the presence of asphyxia and fetal distress, the fetus has gasping-type breaths. During these gasping breaths in uterio, meconium can be easily aspirated into the trachea. Whenever meconium has been aspirated into the trachea, there is significant risk that the meconium can be aspirated into the lungs. Meconium can then be aspirated further into the lungs when the newborn takes the first breath at the time of delivery.

Aspiration of meconium into the smaller airways in the lungs can result in significant morbidity and mortality in the neonate. Meconium is often thick and sticky and can partially or completely obstruct the airway. This obstruction prevents oxygen from entering the lungs and also traps air in the smaller airways distal to the obstruction. This air trapping can result in a pneumothorax, a collapse in part or all of one or both of the lungs. It can also result in atelectasis, or collapse of the alveoli, the small air sacs in the lungs where gas exchange occurs. These alterations in the lungs cause increased hypoxia and further alter gas exchange.

Nursing and Collaborative Assessment. The neonate who has aspirated meconium demonstrates signs of respiratory distress. The distress may occur immediately at delivery or within the first hours of life. The signs of respiratory distress include tachypnea, cyanosis, grunting, nasal flaring, and retractions. The neonate's chest can appear overinflated. Breath sounds will be coarse and wet on auscultation. The neonate may be cyanotic, with a bluish coloring of the face, lips, trunk, and extremities. Arterial blood gas tests will reveal an abnormally low arterial oxygen level and an abnormally high carbon dioxide level. Additional laboratory studies may also demonstrate acidosis. The chest x-ray will show coarse irregular pulmonary densities with areas of atelectasis. The lungs can also be hyperinflated and the diaphragm may be flattened.

Nursing and Collaborative Management. Management of the neonate at risk for meconium aspiration syndrome begins with the removal of meconium that is in the neonate's airways before the first breath is taken. As the head is delivered, upper airway suctioning is performed by the obstetrician. Both the nose and the pharynx are suctioned to clean them of any remaining meconium. After the neonate's delivery and ideally before the first breath, the trachea is suctioned under direct visualization. In direct visualization of the trachea, the physician uses a laryngoscope to examine the neonate's airway. With the laryngoscope, the vocal cords can be seen and any meconium found can be suctioned out. After suctioning, the neonate will require 100 percent oxygen administered with bag and mask ventilation.

Research indicates that aggressive suctioning prior to delivery and by endotracheal intubation will not always prevent meconium aspiration syndrome.[34] If, despite interventions in the delivery room, the neonate develops meconium aspiration syndrome, transfer to a neonatal intensive care nursery is necessary. Management of the neonate's respiratory distress is aimed at eliminating the hypoxia, hypercarbia (high levels of carbon dioxide in the blood), and acidosis. Many of these neonates require intubation and mechanical ventilation. Because of the sticky and viscous nature of the meconium, it may be difficult to provide adequate ventilation through the clogged airways. Such blockage occurs when the meconium becomes trapped in the smaller airways, causing a ball-valve obstruction. When this occurs, the breaths delivered by the mechanical ventilator must be delivered under higher pressures.

The presence of meconium in the smaller air passages and the increased pressures needed to deliver the breaths can place the neonate at risk for a pneumothorax, which occurs when air enters the pleural space. The air leak may result when an alveoli ruptures in the presence of high ventilatory pressures. Signs of a pneumothorax include sudden cyanosis; respiratory distress including tachypnea, grunting, and flaring; unequal breath sounds; unequal chest expansion; a shift in where the apical heart beat is auscultated; bradycardia; sudden decrease in the arterial oxygen level; sudden increase in the arterial carbon dioxide level; and hypotension.[7] Sometimes a pneumothorax is seen on the x-ray, although the neonate is asymptomatic. This neonate must be observed closely for future signs of respiratory distress.

The neonate who develops severe symptoms related to a pneumothorax must be treated swiftly. Management includes the placement of a chest tube, which can be done at the bedside. A chest tube is a catheter that is placed into the pleural space under sterile conditions. After placement, the catheter is connected to low continuous suction via a special canister. The placement of the chest tube and the administration of additional oxygen usually resolve the pneumothorax in 24 to 72 hours.[17] Important nursing interventions include continual assessment of the neonate's respiratory status and monitoring of the chest tube to ensure that it remains in place. Any alteration in the neonate's condition should be reported to the physician immediately.

Nursing interventions to facilitate the removal of meconium from the neonate's lungs include vigorous chest physical therapy and postural drainage. (*See* earlier discussion of "Respiratory Distress Syndrome.") Percussion, vibration, and repositioning of the neonate help to drain the secretions in the lungs. Suctioning of the airway should follow chest physical therapy and postural drainage.

Because meconium is a foreign substance in the lungs, it can be extremely irritating to the lung tissue. The inflammation that results can be treated with steroids. The irritation that develops in the lungs can also place the neonate at risk for developing secondary respiratory infections, which are treated with antibiotics.[5]

Meconium aspiration will result in asphyxiation if the neonate's airways remain blocked by the sticky substance and adequate ventilation cannot be initiated. This is a medical emergency demanding immediate resuscitation efforts.

Parents of the neonate who develops meconium aspiration syndrome will have questions in the delivery room as they see the neonate being wisked away to be suctioned. If meconium aspiration is a potential risk for a neonate, the parents should be made aware of the necessary treatments to expect after delivery. Parents will need additional support and information if the neonate develops severe respiratory distress and requires transfer to an intensive care nursery (*see* Chapter 36).

CASE STUDY/CARE PLAN: THE PRETERM INFANT

At 32 weeks of gestation, Wendy Harris, age 27, G1P1, spontaneously ruptured her membranes and delivered a live male neonate weighing 1500 grams (3 pounds 5 oz). The neonate's physical appearance and behaviors were appropriate for gestational age. No maternal or paternal history of infection, drug use, or other risk factors for preterm delivery could be identified. Since birth three days ago, Baby Robert has been cared for in the neonatal intensive care unit, because of his prematurity. Although he has been progressing well, he has required 35 percent supplemental oxygen via an oxyhood. His heart rate is 140 to 150; his respiratory rate is 40 to 50 with no signs of respiratory distress. His temperature is maintained at 37.0°C (98.6°F) in a radiant warmer. Wendy and her husband, Steve, want the neonate to be breastfed and spend most of each day or evening at his bedside.

Supporting Assessment Data	Expected Client/Family Outcome	Nursing Action Intervention	Rationale	Criteria for Evaluation
Nursing Diagnosis: Alteration in respiration, related to birth at 32 weeks of gestation				
Respiratory assessment: neonate born at 32 weeks of gestation; receiving 35 percent warmed, humidified oxygen in oxyhood Respirations 40 to 50; heart rate 140 to 150 No retractions, nasal flaring, or grunting Pink skin color without any cyanosis Arterial blood gas values: PaO_2 88, CO_2 34, pH 7.35	Neonate will maintain respiratory status with progression to room air before discharge	Monitor respiratory effort. Report and record respiratory rate, presence of retractions, grunting, flaring, cyanosis. Auscultate breath sounds every 2 hours as needed.	Assessment of respiratory status allows for prompt identification of respiratory distress; treatments to be modified or maintained; and progress to be shared among health care providers.	Neonate's respiratory status continues to improve. Neonate no longer requires oxygen supplementation and oxyhood to maintain normal respiratory status.
Nursing Diagnosis: Alteration in nutrition, related to oxygen therapy and prematurity				
Neonate unable to feed via nipple because of oxygen therapy and immature sucking reflex at 32 weeks of gestation; IV therapy in progress Birth weight 1500 g	After initial weight loss (≥ 10 percent), neonate will demonstrate a weight gain of 20 to 30 g per day after initiation of gavage feeding	Check daily weights on same scale with neonate completely undressed. Record results and report weight changes.	Weight changes reflect nutritional status and progress.	After initial weight loss of 10 percent of body weight, neonate gains 20 to 30 g per day; normal nutritional status is maintained.
		Monitor strict intake and output; weigh diapers; assess specific gravity, skin turgor, mucous membranes, and fontanelles.	Hydration status is monitored and adequate hydration can be prescribed.	Normal hydration status is maintained.
		Continue IV therapy using an infusion pump.	Infusion pumps allow for safe administration of fluids.	
		Initiate gavage feelings using breast milk pumped by mother and fortified prior to each feeding.	Fortified breast milk is well suited to the preterm neonate's nutritional needs. Fortifiers are especially useful for neonates under 1500 g.	Neonate tolerates breast milk gavage feeding.
		Check abdominal girth, tube placement, and gastric residuals; hold feedings for residual.	Checking placement, abdominal girth, and residuals allows for safe administration of feeding. Presence of large residual feedings and enlarged abdominal girth may indicate inability to tolerate feedings.	Abdominal girth appropriate; feeding tube placement appropriate and functioning.

(continued)

CASE STUDY/CARE PLAN: The Preterm Infant *(continued)*

Supporting Assessment Data	Expected Client/Family Outcome	Nursing Action Intervention	Rationale	Criteria for Evaluation
Nursing Diagnosis: Potential for alteration in thermoregulation, related to prematurity				
Temperature 37° C (98.6° F) Respirations 40 to 50 Heart rate 140 to 150 Neonate in radiant warmer; oxyhood with warmed, humidified oxygen in use	Neonate will maintain a normal body temperature of 36.2° C to 37° C in open air crib prior to discharge	Check neonate's axillary temperature every 2 hours.	Preterm neonates are at risk for temperature instability. Normal body temperature in radiant warmer reflects proper functioning of equipment.	Neonate maintains a normal body temperature while in radiant warmer and then after progressing to open air crib.
		Warmer at appropriate level of neutral thermal environment.	Radiant warmer is used to provide heat safely.	
		When oxyhood is discontinued, wean neonate to open air crib by introducing time periods in open air crib, wrapping neonate well and applying hat, and checking temperature and gradually increasing time out of radiant warmer until neonate maintains temperature independently.	Radiant warmer allows for observation and access to neonate on respiratory support. Weaning process prevents complications associated with sudden body temperature drop for preterm neonate.	
Nursing Diagnosis: Alteration in bilirubin metabolism, related to prematurity				
Bilirubin levels of neonate of 32 weeks of gestation: 4.3 first day, 7.8 second day, 8.0 third day	Neonate's bilirubin levels will remain within normal limits during hospitalization	Observe neonate for presence of jaundice.	Yellowing of skin and sclera indicate increasing bilirubin levels.	Bilirubin levels remain within normal limits.
		Check bilirubin levels every 2 hours; report and record results.	Prompt identification of abnormally high bilirubin levels allows for treatment to prevent complications related to bilirubin toxicity (eg, neurologic impairment).	
		If bilirubin levels continue to increase, begin phototherapy as ordered.	Phototherapy lowers serum bilirubin levels.	
Nursing Diagnosis: Potential skin breakdown, related to prematurity and neonatal intensive care unit procedures				
Skin assessment: neonate of 32 weeks of gestation; thin skin with some adipose tissue; no areas of skin breakdown	Neonate will not develop skin breakdown during hospital stay	Examine neonate's skin for signs of breakdown, especially areas in contact with equipment such as arm restraints. Document findings; report abnormal findings.	Prompt identification and treatment prevents further skin breakdown. Written records document observations of normality or problems. Maintaining skin integrity is a health team effort.	Neonate's skin remains intact throughout hospitalization.
		Change neonate's position at least every 2 hours.	Position changes minimize skin breakdown related to prolonged pressure.	

Supporting Assessment Data	Expected Client/Family Outcome	Nursing Action Intervention	Rationale	Criteria for Evaluation
		Use minimal tape; avoid tight restraints.	Materials such as tape and pressure from equipment can promote skin breakdown.	
		Use sheepskin or water mattress.	Pressure is relieved on skin.	
		Use pectin barrier under tape.	Pectin barriers can reduce stress on taped skin.	
Nursing Diagnosis: Potential for ineffective breastfeeding, related to delayed breastfeeding secondary to prematurity				
Mother expresses desire to breastfeed neonate	Mother will maintain lactation prior to initiation of breastfeeding	Encourage mother's desire to breastfeed.	Mothers of preterm neonates need support to build confidence in decision to breastfeed.	Mother pumps breast milk and stores milk, which is then fed by staff to neonate.
	Mother will independently pump and store breast milk for neonate during his hospital stay	Assess mother's knowledge of breast pumping. As needed, provide instruction in use of breast pumps. Provide privacy for pumping when mother visits neonate. Facilitate access to electric breast pump in hospital.	Breast pumping is necessary to build milk supply in a mother whose neonate is initially unable to breast feed.	
		As prescribed, use mother's breast milk in gavage feedings. Add fortifiers as prescribed.	Breast milk provides excellent nutrition for 32-week pretern neonate if fortified.	Mother expresses satisfaction from providing breast milk and breastfeeding neonate; neonate's nutritional needs are met.
	Mother will independently breastfeed neonate by discharge	Provide support and supervision as mother breastfeeds neonate for the first time.	Effectively breastfeeding a preterm neonate can be difficult. Mothers need expert assistance to learn breastfeeding technique and support to relieve anxiety.	By discharge, mother is able to breastfeed neonate independently.

SUMMARY

Assessment of gestational age and size is an essential component of the comprehensive assessment of the neonate. Gestational age and birth weight together are reliable indicators in predicting the neonate's well-being. Appropriately identifying a neonate as small for gestational age, appropriate for gestational age, or large for gestational age allows physicians and nurses to anticipate potential problems and risk factors related to specific age and size of the neonate. Although most newborns are full-term neonates who are appropriate for gestational age, others are premature or postmature with some alteration in their size. With multiple gestations, the interdisciplinary neonatal team must address the gestational age and size assessment of more than one neonate.

Accurate assessment of gestational age and size can alert caregivers to specific problems related to immaturity. For example, the development of acute and chronic lung diseases such as respiratory distress syndrome and bronchopulmonary dysplasia is a well-known problem related to immature lung development and use of mechanical ventilation. Other conditions such as retinopathy of prematurity, patent ductus arteriosus, intracranial hemorrhage, difficulty in thermoregulation, and necrotizing enterocolitis can threaten the life and well-being of the premature neonate. Thus, comprehensive treatment plans will be instituted for management of the premature neonate.

Continuing advances in neonatology have resulted in the survival of extremely premature and tiny neonates, referred to as low birth weight, very low birth weight, or very very low birth weight, depending on their weight. These neonates pose tremendous challenges to the interdisciplinary team as the problems of prematurity are greatly magnified by their small size and limited energy stores. The hospital course of premature and especially very-low-birth-weight neonates can be long and complicated. The acute as well as long-term care of the premature neonate is quite costly and places tremendous stress on the family and their resources.

The care of the postmature neonate is also greatly enhanced by the accurate identification of gestational age and size. These indicators help physicians and nurses to anticipate potentially life-threatening problems related to postmaturity, such as asphyxia and meconium aspiration syndrome.

Ongoing research continues to make it possible for intensive care nurseries to provide neonates with the environment and physiologic support necessary to adjust to extrauterine life; however, as successful new treatment strategies are developed, it is important to note that more and more neonates are being born with problems related to gestational age and size, specifically prematurity. Attention must be direct toward identifying the problems in the prenatal period that may predispose to premature deliveries and implementing strategies that focus on supporting the pregnancy to term delivery of an appropriate-for-gestational-age neonate.

REVIEW QUESTIONS

1. Discuss the importance of accurately identifying a neonate's gestational age.
2. Define and describe the relationship between weight and gestational age.
3. Differentiate among low-birth-weight, very-low-birth-weight, and very-very-low-birth-weight neonates.
4. Identify at least three potential problems of the preterm neonate.
5. Identify at least two potential problems of the postmature neonate.

REFERENCES

1. Sahu S. Birthweight, gestational age and neonatal risks. *Perinatol-Neonatol,* 1984;8:28–36.
2. Clotherty JP. Identifying the high risk newborn and evaluating gestational age, prematurity, postmaturity, large for gestational age, and small for gestational age infants. In: Clotherty JP, Stark A, eds. *Manual of Neonatal Care.* 2nd ed. Boston: Little, Brown and Company; 1985;103–120.
3. Korones SB. *High Risk Newborn Infants: The Basis for Intensive Nursing Care.* 4th ed. St. Louis, Mo: Mosby; 1986.
4. Sammons W, Lewis J. *Premature Babies: A Different Beginning.* St. Louis, Mo: Mosby; 1985.
5. Avery GB. *Neonatology-Pathophysiology and Management of the Newborn.* Philadelphia: JB Lippincott; 1987.
6. Beischer NA, Mackay EV. *Obstetrics and the Newborn.* 2nd ed. Philadelphia: WB Saunders; 1986.
7. Fanaroff AA, Martin R, eds. *Behrman's Neonatal-Perinatal Medicine.* St. Louis, Mo: CV Mosby; 1987.
8. Avery ME, First L, eds. *Pediatric Medicine.* Baltimore: Williams & Wilkins; 1989.
9. Pearlman S, Maisels J. Preductal and postductal transcutaneous oxygen tension in measurements in premature newborns with hyaline membrane disease. *Pediatrics.* 1989;83: 98–100.
10. Kleiber C, Hummel P. Factors related to spontaneous endotrachael extubation in the neonate. *Pediatr Nurs.* 1989; 15:347–350
11. Collaborative European Multicenter Study Group. Surfactant replacement therapy for severe neonatal respiratory distress syndrome: an international randomized clinical trial. *Pediatrics.* 1988;82:683–690.
12. Kendig J, et al. Surfactant replacement therapy at birth: final analysis of a clinical trial and comparisons with similar trials. *Pediatrics.* 1988;82:756–762.
13. Ferrar TB, et al. Side effects and long term follow-up of corticosteriod therapy in very low birthweight infants with bronchopulmonary dysplasia. *J Perinatol.* 1990;10:137–142.
14. Gong AK, et al. Severe retinopathy in convalescent preterm infants with mild or regressing retinopathy of prematurity. *Pediatrics.* 1989;83:422–423.
15. Gibson DL, et al. Retinopathy of prematurity: a new epidemic? *Pediatrics.* 1989;83:486–491.
16. Ackerman B, et al. Reduced incidental light exposure: effect on the development of retinopathy of prematurity on low birth weight infants. *Pediatrics.* 1989;83:958–962.
17. Klaus M, Fanaroff, A. *Care of the High Risk Neonate.* 3rd ed. Philadelphia: WB Saunders; 1986.
18. Gersony WM. Patent ductus in the neonate. *Pediatr Clin of North Am.* 1986;33:545–560.
19. Cooke R, et al. Urine output measurement in premature infants. *Pediatrics.* 1989;83:116–117.
20. Jardine D, Rogers K. Relationship of benzyl alcohol to ker-

nicterus, intraventricular hemorrhage and mortality in preterm infants. *Pediatrics.* 1989;83:153–160.

21. Miall-Allen V, et al. Blood pressure fluctuation and intraventricular hemorrhage in the preterm infant of less than 31 weeks' gestation. *Pediatrics.* 1989;83:657–661.
22. Lewis M, Bendersky M. Cognitive and motor differences among low birth weight infants: impact of intraventricular hemorrhage, medical risk and social class. *Pediatrics.* 1989; 83:187–191.
23. Allen C. Neonatal neurodevelopmental examination as a predictor of neuromotor outcome in premature infants. *Pediatrics.* 1989;83:498–505.
24. Amspacher KA. Necrotizing enterocolitis: the never ending challenge. *J Perinat Neonatal Nurs.* 1989;3:58–68.
25. Raju T. An epidemiologic study of very low and very very low birth weight infants. *Clin Perinatol.* 1986;13:233–251.
26. Kraybill E, et al. Infants with birth weights less than 1000 grams: survival, growth, and development. *Am J Dis Child.* 1984;138:837–842.
27. Vasa R, et al. Perinatal factors influencing the outcome of 501 to 1000 grams newborns. *Clin Perinatol.* 1986;13: 267–284.
28. Sell E. Outcome of very very low birthweight infants. *Clin Perinatol.* 1986;13:451–460.
29. Stevenson DK, et al. Outcome of neonates with birth weights of less than 801 grams. *J Perinatol.* 1988;8:82–87.
30. Hernandez J. The cost of care of the less-than-1000-gram infant. *Clin Perinatol.* 1986;13:461–474.
31. Buckwald S, et al. Mortality and follow-up data for neonates weighing 500 grams to 800 grams at birth. *Am J Dis Child.* 1984;138:779–782.
32. Lagrew D, Freeman R. Management of the postdate pregnancy. *Am J Obstet Gynecol.* 1986;154:8–13.
33. Turnage CS. Meconium aspiration syndrome. *J Perinat Neonatal Nurs.* 1989;3:69–80.
34. Hagoman JR, et al. Delivery room management of meconium staining of the amniotic fluid and the development of meconium aspiration syndrome. *J Perinatol.* 1988;8:127–131.

Societal Trends in Care of the Childbearing Family

unit

12

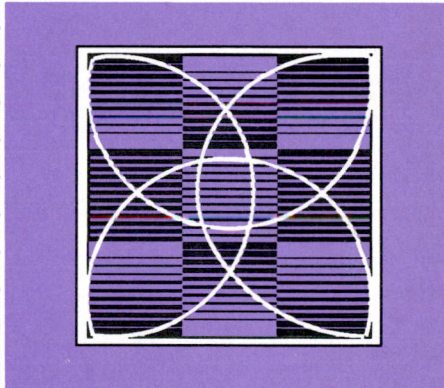

Home Care of the Childbearing Family

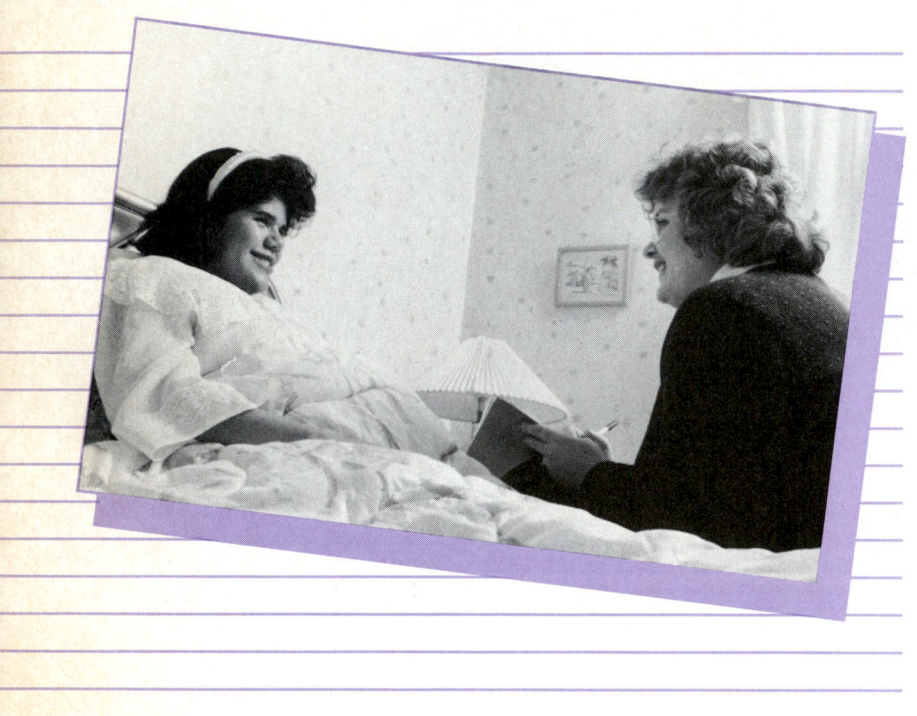

Chapter 44

Key Terms

care-by-parent programs
diagnostic related groups
discharge planning
health maintenance organizations
home health services

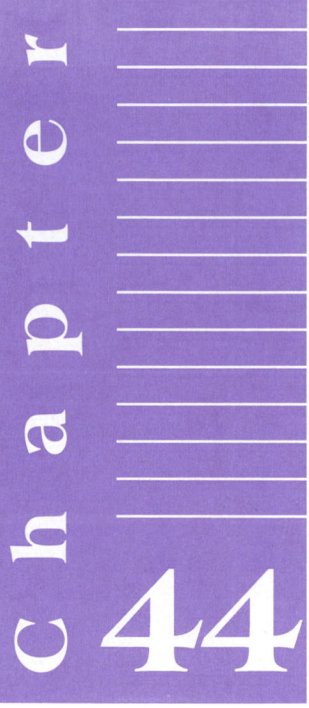

Home health care for low-risk and high-risk clients is a growing trend in the United States. Economics, technology, and public policy all have an impact on delivery of nursing care to clients in the home setting.

As health care institutions implement measures to control costs, childbearing clients and their infants are being discharged earlier to the home setting. The nurse provides a link between institutional and home health care for these families. Nurses in the community setting provide services in the home to low-risk and high-risk prenatal and postpartum families, as well as specialized nursing care to high-risk infants.

This chapter provides the reader with a broad perspective of home health care for the childbearing family. The chapter concludes with a discussion of stresses that effect the community nurse who cares for these families in a complex and changing health care delivery system.

OVERVIEW

Home health care for pregnant women and newborns is far from a new idea. Lillian Wald established the first organized home nursing service in 1893 (the Visiting Nurse Service of New York City). This and other early visiting nursing services were originally established to serve the urban poor and, somewhat later, rural communities. Nurses worked independently to provide services to the sick, well-baby care, and school nursing to children.[1] Thus, nurses have been delivering health (and sickness) care to families in their homes for well over 90 years. The "historical mission" of home care has been support, assistance, and nursing care.[1]

Although third-party payers (insurance companies and the federal government) currently emphasize acute and rehabilitative care in the home, clients still need primary care that emphasizes health promotion and disease prevention. This is true for individuals across the life span, including childbearing individuals and families.[2]

To understand the current focus of home care for childbearing families, it is necessary to review the impact of Medicare on home care in general. Home health services today are a result of Medicare payment criteria, which shaped these services into an acute care–focused medical model. Delivery of care to the elderly demanded a public policy that would direct (or limit) services to individuals who were truly in need of them. Thus, the national policy makers (the Congress) chose a "gatekeeper" to direct access of the elderly to home health care. These designated gatekeepers were not nurses, who had traditionally delivered home care and understood this form of health care delivery. Instead, physicians were designated as the providers who would determine which elderly individuals could receive home care under Medicare.

Many physicians neither valued nor understood home care services of support, nursing, and health promotion activities. Home care for the elderly was viewed instead as a medical adjunct to acute care. Physicians implemented therapies in the home with which they were familiar, generally high-technology, high-cost, medically oriented therapies.[1] This medical, high-risk focus of home care for the elderly also spilled over into home care for childbearing families.

Nurses are thus placed in the difficult position of having to focus their care delivery in an illness-based model, leaving the well client in the home with unmet needs.[2] Nurses today are often limited by this illness-based perspective in giving the kind of nursing care that historically placed home care as the alternative to institutionalization.[3] Although many healthy childbearing families would benefit from home care, this care is primarily focused on high-risk childbearing families.

HOME HEALTH CARE SERVICES AND PROVIDERS

Home health services are defined as skilled, intermittent, part-time services provided under a physician's written plan of care in the residence of the client.[1] Providers of these services may include registered nurses, physical therapists, speech therapists, medical social workers, occupational therapists, and home health aides. Services must be related to the medical diagnosis for which care was initiated in the acute care setting, and must be provided by a certified home health agency.

Medicare has drastically changed the nature of home health agencies. In contrast to their predecessors, who were small voluntary nursing agencies providing primarily long-term supportive nursing care, today's home care agencies may be public or private, and are engaged in providing skilled nursing care and physical and speech therapy. To participate in Medicare, agencies must be certified and have contractual arrangements to provide occupational therapy, medical social services, and home health aide services. Thus, the home health agency of today is a broad, complex sophisticated agency.

Although home health care often is viewed as a service primarily for the elderly, it has both a traditional and a current link to childbearing families, both low and high risk. From the earliest days of home health care, community nurses made "well-baby" visits. Although many community nurses feel uncomfortable with this role (and many agencies place a low priority on it), the initial visit to a new mother and her newborn remains a part of the nurse's case load. In addition, with the trend to early hospital discharge for healthy postpartum mothers and newborns and the increasing numbers of home births, the community nurse's home visit now may fulfill some of the functions traditionally carried out by the hospital nurse. For example, there may be little or no time to teach a mother about breastfeeding or infant care in the institution where delivery occurred. The community nurse may truly fill the gap in teaching the new mother.

ISSUES AND CONTROVERSIES

Home health care is a need of more clients today than ever before; however, home health care nurses and the agencies for which they work are being forced to limit care to clients because of economic considerations. Nurses view discontinuation of care because of financial reasons as "patient abandonment,"[a] raising questions such as: If there is insufficient money for home health care, why are clients being discharged early from the hospital? How can the nurse ethically balance the needs of his or her clients for home care with the agency's need for financial solvency? If the agency goes bankrupt because of nonpayment, who will deliver care?

[a] *Reckling JB. Abandonment of patients by home health nursing agencies: an ethical analysis of the dilemma.* Advances in Nursing Science *1989;11:70–81.*

Not all of the families the community nurse visits in the home will be low risk. As medical technology improves, increasing numbers of early premature infants who could not have survived even 5 years ago because of respiratory, neurologic, and other problems are going home. Many of these infants go home with multiple and complex chronic impairments and, even after the transition from the neonatal intensive care unit (NICU) to home, continue to rely on high-technology support systems. Thus, homes are becoming mini–intensive-care units, and parents must supply care for their infants.[4] Nurses who practice in the community play an important role in this "high-tech" home care of newborn infants.

FACTORS AFFECTING HOME HEALTH CARE

In today's economic and political environment, the survival of many health care institutions (hospitals, home health agencies, health maintenance organizations, long-term care facilities, and others) depends on providing the most appropriate level of care in the most efficient and timely manner.[5] More specifically, there has been great concern nationally about evolving a means of health care delivery that will decrease costs without sacrificing health care quality or access. This is a concern in the care not only of elderly and adult clients, but also of mothers and newborns.

Health care delivery through home care is seen as one means to accomplish this goal; however, delivery of comprehensive home health care is profoundly complex and involves the development of public policy. Although it is not the intent of this text to describe this topic in detail, some aspects of public policy development that directly affect home health care of childbearing families are briefly discussed here. The reader is referred to books and articles in the reference list for in-depth discussions of the issues and topics raised in this chapter.

Health Policy and Home Health Care

As Mundinger notes, "Policy involves decisions to allocate resources for a given endeavor or outcome," and further, "Health policy in America has been broadly shaped by public allocation of resources."[1]

Health policy development has been of great concern to the federal government since the implementation of Medicaid and Medicare. Public monies are being allocated to care for the poor and the elderly. One only need read the daily newspaper to realize that there is a growing national concern for cost containment of medical services and health care. Hospital expenses, in particular, have risen faster than other health care costs. Reasons given for the rise include technologic sophistication, professional salaries, institutional maintenance functions, and insurance costs. Policy makers have believed that institutional care, especially the acute care hospital, was in need of cost containment policies. Home care services that could prevent hospitalization (and could be reimbursed) have been seen as a primary means of containing costs.[1]

Economics of Home Health Care

One way in which the major payers of health care—the federal and state governments and large employers—have attempted to control spiraling costs is by shifting from a retrospective to a prospective form of payment for health and illness services. That is, instead of reimbursing physicians, hospitals, and so on for services already given to a client, a fixed amount of money is paid, in advance, for specific necessary services required for a specifically diagnosed condition. One example of this approach is seen in **health maintenance organizations** (HMOs), in which the provider HMO is paid in advance a set amount of money per person, regardless of the health care services that are actually used by the client. Another prospective payment approach is **diagnostic related groups** (DRGs).

Diagnostic related groups were legislated as a part of the Social Security Act amendments of 1983 and were intended to change reimbursement for services to Medicare clients. Under this law, hospitals would receive payment prospectively for services to Medicare clients on the basis of 467 diagnostic related groups.[5] This meant that each diagnosis included in the list of 467 had a price tag connected to it. The hospital received a set amount of money, in advance, for treating a client with a particular diagnosis. It is easy to see that the less time a client stayed in the acute care setting, the greater the financial reward to the hospital (less time equals less daily service and more money left from the advance payment for that specific DRG). Thus, this legislation provided major impetus for hospitals to reduce their lengths of stay and discharge the clients as soon as possible.

Although originally connected with Medicare and the federal government, DRGs were often adopted by other insurers. This prospective system of payment under DRGs had three major effects on delivery of health care:

1. It increased admissions to the home health care services.[6]
2. It intensified the trend toward discharge of sicker, more acutely ill clients.

3. It resulted in earlier discharge of low- and high-risk mothers and neonates from birthing institutions.

This fact, coupled with the development of new technology, has created the "high-tech" service category in home health care delivery.[7]

Diagnostic Related Groups and Childbearing. Care of perinatal clients is not yet directly controlled by a prospective payment system or by the 22 perinatal DRG categories (Table 44–1). Many authorities, however, see this as an inevitable step. In fact, many feel that there will soon be an increase in state-controlled Medicaid systems opting for DRGs (including perinatal DRGs) to contain costs.[8] This prospect is of great concern to health care providers.

Implementation of the DRG system for the perinatal DRG categories could have an adverse impact on delivery of maternal and child health services and could potentially affect future perinatal outcomes. Hospitals with a large number of medically indigent inner city residents or referral centers (level III centers) serving large geographic or rural areas would suffer greatly from the imposition of the DRG formula.[8] The lengthy and resource-intensive stays by large numbers of perinatal clients in perinatal centers also could mean severe financial crises for these hospitals. Level III perinatal centers care for very sick mothers and neonates who require longer-than-average hospital stays and who require the greatest amounts of resources, often with no means to pay or Medicaid as the third party payer. Many questions arise:

- What will be the impact of DRGs on perinatal regionalization and referral patterns?
- Will this system encourage hospitals to discharge neonates prematurely?
- Will hospitals deny adequate care to high-risk (or indigent) mothers?

These and other questions must be answered before the impact of DRGs on childbearing clients can be fully determined. Even before implementation of perinatal DRGs, however, the following trend has become apparent: sick, technology-dependent neonates (as well as the elderly and adults) are being discharged earlier and in increasing numbers. Economic considerations seem to be a primary force in this trend. Home health care of high-risk families is now often the responsibility of the nurse who practices in the community. Standards for nursing care in the home are currently being developed. It will become

RESEARCH ABSTRACT

Norr, KF, et al. Early discharge with home follow-up: impacts on low-income mothers and infants. J Obstet Gynecol Neonat Nurs. *1989;18:133–148.*

The purpose of this study was to evaluate the health impact of a nursing-managed early-discharge program for a low-income, low-risk population.

The sample consisted of three groups:

1. *Early discharge*: mothers discharged at 24 to 47 hours after delivery without their infants (N = 94)
2. *Conventional discharge*: mothers and infants discharged together at 48 to 72 hours after delivery (N = 115)
3. *Simultaneous early discharge:* mothers and infants discharged with a home follow-up visit within 3 days of discharge (N = 124)

The health problems of mothers and their infants were assessed by physical assessment and histories. The Avant Maternal Attachment Scale measured maternal attachment behaviors observed during infant feeding, and maternal concerns were assessed using the Maternal Concerns Tool developed by Bull. Quantitative data and descriptive data were analyzed using ANOVA and chi-square analyses.

The results demonstrated no significant differences among the groups on maternal or infant physical problems 7 to 15 days postdelivery; however, all three groups had substantial morbidity. The simultaneous early-discharge group had higher maternal attachment scores, fewer maternal concerns, and greater maternal satisfaction than either of the other two groups.

The researchers conclude that early hospital discharge combined with close nursing follow-up during the first few weeks of life is an effective use of health care resources for low-income women.

Comment:
This study provides some documentation of the efficacy of combined early discharge and nursing follow-up. In an era in which early discharge is becoming the norm, it is important to ascertain that quality of care can be maintained with such programs.

A limitation to interpretation of results is the initial dissimilarity among comparison groups (eg, mothers discharged with their babies compared to mothers discharged without their babies). In addition, other studies have shown that performing infant assessments in front of parents promotes attachment. Thus, one can question whether the assessment or the early discharge with home nursing follow-up produced the differences in maternal attachment observed.

TABLE 44–1. PERINATAL DIAGNOSTIC RELATED GROUPS (DRGS)

Diagnostic Related Group	Title
370	Cesarean section with complications
371	Cesarean section without complications
372	Vaginal delivery with complicating diagnoses
373	Vaginal delivery without complicating diagnoses
374	Vaginal delivery with sterilization and/or D&C
375	Vaginal delivery with operating room procedure except sterilization and/or D&C
376	Postpartum diagnoses without operating room procedure
377	Postpartum diagnoses with operating room procedure
378	Ectopic pregnancy
379	Threatened abortion
380	Abortion without D&C
381	Abortion with D&C
382	False labor
383	Other antepartum diagnoses with medical complications
384	Other antepartum diagnoses without medical complications
385	Neonates, died or transferred
386	Extreme immaturity, neonate
387	Prematurity with major problems
388	Prematurity without major problems
389	Full-term neonate with major problems
390	Neonates with other significant problems
391	Normal newborns

vital for nurses to validate the effectiveness of their role in the home.

Implications for Well Childbearing Families. Although the trend to early discharge of neonates may be most dramatic in the high-risk area for a variety of economic and other factors, well mothers and infants are not immune to cost-cutting measures. Many hospitals with maternity services are finding it necessary to cut costs for services for healthy mothers and neonates. Thus, many services encourage families to participate in early-discharge programs.[9] As a result, nursing time traditionally spent in teaching postpartum mothers about infant care, self-care, breastfeeding, and so on before discharge is lost. Many families take a neonate home and are unprepared to deal with parenting activities. Again, home health care delivered by nurses in the community may be necessary to fill the gap created by early discharge.

In addition, nursing care of well women in the home during the prenatal period may reduce expensive NICU admissions. Especially for some populations, such as adolescents and the medically indigent who do not seek traditional forms of prenatal care, home care may facilitate a healthy pregnancy outcome.

Provision of early and ongoing prenatal care in the home may significantly cut the cost of high-risk hospital care by helping to prevent low-birth-weight infants and other disease-related hospitalizations. Most states, however, do not have funds allocated for such programs of prevention. In fact, in a survey conducted among state and territorial public health agencies, Coyner found that of the 41 jurisdictions surveyed, maternity outreach and home visiting were least often mentioned as state priorities; however, the same 41 jurisdictions mentioned, as one of their top priorities, maternal and child health.[10] This situation clearly points to the discrepancy between publicly stated health goals and resource allocation. Although the jurisdictions state that they value maternal and infant health programs, they do not commit money to preventive programs.

Home births or birth center births also are a cost-effective method of providing safe and comprehensive health care. (*See* Chapter 24, concerning birth alternatives.) Yet these births also require comprehensive planning for nursing care by the midwife or nurse practicing in the community.

DISCHARGE PLANNING AND HOME CARE

One disadvantage of early discharges is the possibility that an individual may be discharged prematurely before he or she is ready to return home. Discharge planning is an important factor in preventing this serious mistake. It provides a vital link between hospital care and home care for mothers and neonates (Figure 44–1). Its importance is underscored by federal legislation, which requires hospitals to provide some type of discharge planning for clients.[5]

The American Nurses' Association defines **discharge planning** as "part of the continuity of care process which is designed to prepare the patient or client for the next phase of care, whether it be self-care, care by family members, or care by an organized health care provider."[11] Discharge planning (more appropriately termed *continuity of care planning*) involves assessing needs and obtaining or coordinating appropriate resources for clients as they move through the health care system. It is the process that occurs when a person is discharged from a facility or agency. Discharge planning functions as the link between health care organizations for implementing the system of continuing care.[5]

Although the process of discharge planning is more fully developed in hospitals, there is a great

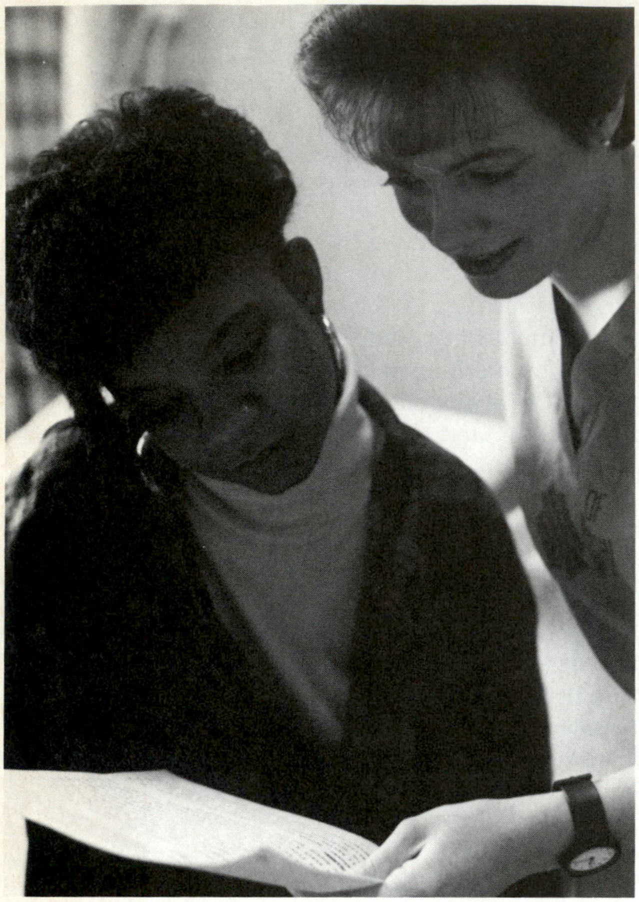

Figure 44–1. The nurse provides educational preparation prior to discharge to promote postpartum adaptation.

need to implement and strengthen continuity of care planning outside of hospitals as well, as community-based services become more prevalent.[5] Every mother and infant have the right to discharge planning, whether it is simply preparation for a healthy discharge with a focus on well-baby care and routine health care follow-up or a discharge after a complicated health problem. In this case, planning requires a multidisciplinary approach to meet continuity-of-care needs of the infant, the mother, or both. In both cases, however, planning should begin at admission, and the family should be actively involved in the decision-making process.[4]

The familiar components of the nursing process—assessment, nursing diagnosis, planning, implementation, and evaluation—are involved in discharge planning. A major difference, however, is that the plan is developed in the present for care to be delivered in the future—that is, when the client is discharged and goes home.

Assessment

Preparation for discharge begins with admission. A thorough assessment (including a family assessment) provides direction for plans for discharge, and continues throughout the course of the mother's and infant's stay in the hospital or other birthing facility. The primary nurse caring for the infant and family is most able to make this sort of assessment.[4]

Nursing Diagnosis

Nursing diagnoses for client discharge to the home are based on the assessment. They are constructed like any nursing diagnosis specific to the client. The nurse must remember that these diagnoses are made within the context of the home environment.

Planning

The planning phase begins with the establishment of a specific type of nursing care plan called the discharge plan. Although the discharge plan involves the same components as a traditional nursing care plan, its format, due to the different requirements of home care, is somewhat different. *See* the Discharge Plan on the facing page. The discharge plan must identify factors such as the infant's primary caretaker or sources of support for the mother in the home, community agencies involved, discharge teaching needs, and important psychosocial factors that might affect the family's ability to deliver care. Interdisciplinary team rounds and predischarge conferences help to ensure that the discharge plan is valid. Family members, especially the client or primary caretaker, must be involved in planning. In addition, it may be vital to involve the community nurse practicing in the community (who will be the case manager of the family or who will monitor home care) in the planning phase.[4]

Implementation

The implementation phase involves discharge teaching, ordering equipment needed for home care, arranging for follow-up appointments, and making appropriate community referrals. Involvement of the nurse from the community is again essential, and the communication channels between community and hospital nurses must be kept open. Community nurses may even come to the hospital to learn techniques of care for the mother or infant soon to be discharged.[5]

Evaluation

Evaluation is essential to ensure that home health care is a safe alternative to hospital care for infants and families. The adequacy of home health agencies, equipment companies, and community agencies providing support must be evaluated, and both parents and caregivers need to provide feedback concerning the effectiveness of support services.[4] An important need is the development of standards of home care for low- and high-risk mothers and infants, by which such care might be evaluated.

The case study and discharge plan illustrate the discharge planning process for a well mother and neonate (*See* the Box). Table 44–2 summarizes methods for evaluating discharge planning.

HOME HEALTH CARE NURSING

Home health care for childbearing families includes care of the low-risk and high-risk prenatal family, home care for the low-risk and high-risk postpartum family, and specialized care for the high-risk infant.

DISCHARGE PLANNING PROCESS FOR WELL MOTHER AND NEONATE

Case Study

Linda R. is a 22-year-old primipara who gave birth 24 hours ago to a healthy 8-pound newborn boy. Labor, delivery, and the postpartum/neonatal period were uncomplicated. Linda is planning to breastfeed; however, the newborn has been unsuccessful in latching on to the breast. Linda also reports some discomfort in the episiotomy area.

Her husband, Bill, has arranged vacation time to be with Linda and the newborn. Bill's mother will stay with the family for the first week Linda and the newborn are home.

DISCHARGE PLAN FORM

Name *Linda R.* Admission Date 8/27/90
Address *215 Redman Avenue* Discharge Date 8/28/90

Medical diagnosis *Uncomplicated delivery and postpartum course*

Anticipated goals
1. *Client will establish lactation within 3 days.*
2. *Client and her support persons will gain knowledge of lactation, frequency of feedings, and techniques of breast feeding.*
3. *Client will have successful healing of her episiotomy without discomfort.*

Referral
1. *Lactation counsel or*
2. *La Leche League*
3. *Community health nurse*

Nursing Discharge Plan

Assessment
1. *Uncomplicated pregnancy, labor/delivery, and postpartum.*
2. *Desire to breastfeed.*
3. *Newborn displays difficulty latching on to breast.*
4. *Early discharge before lactation established.*
5. *Nipples everted, breasts unengorged*

Nursing diagnosis *Potential for altered role performance, related to unsuccessful attempts at breastfeeding*

Plan
1. *Teach client physiology, position, newborn responses, and techniques of breastfeeding.*
2. *Have client demonstrate feeding of infant using resources available in home environment (eg, chair, cushions).*
3. *Provide positive reinforcement related to breastfeeding.*
4. *Give phone number of breastfeeding support.*

Evaluation *Infant will latch on to breast and client will demonstrate proper technique.*

Assessment
1. *Client reports discomfort in episiotomy area.*
2. *Right mediolateral episiotomy is clean and dry with no evidence of tearing, infection, or hematoma.*

Nursing diagnosis *Ineffective breastfeeding, related to pain in episiotomy area.*

Plan
1. *Encourage use of sitz bath:*
   Position sitz bath in client's toilet.
   Arrange equipment in client's bathroom.
   Ensure client's safety during procedure (eg, no throw rugs).
2. *Teach client various positions to lessen episiotomy discomfort, especially while nursing.*
3. *Teach client to assess episiotomy healing (REEDA) with mirror.*

Evaluation *Client will demonstrate proper use of sitz bath and assessment technique for episiotomy. She will report progressive healing of episiotomy. She will report no discomfort from episiotomy during breastfeeding.*

TABLE 44–2. METHODS FOR EVALUATING DISCHARGE PLANNING

1. Use of uniform discharge planning form to determine whether desired outcomes have been met
2. Interview of client and family by telephone to determine if plan of care is being followed (Figure 44–2)
3. Questionnaires to client and family to assess whether continuing care needs have been met
4. Home visits to assess care outcomes
5. Feedback from community health professionals
6. Chart audit

Nursing delivery of home health care is presently in flux. There is no consensus on the appropriate specialty focus for the nurse delivering this care. Currently, at least three groups of nurses with different specialty foci are delivering care to childbearing families in the home: the traditional community health nurse (who works for a community health or visiting nurse agency), the nurse employed by the newly evolving home health agencies specializing in high-risk care of childbearing clients, and the hospital-based nurse employed by the acute care setting in hospital outreach or home visiting programs. The discussion in this chapter generally uses the terms "nurse practicing in the community" or "community nurse" to refer to any of the above nurses, unless otherwise indicated.

Home Care for the Prenatal Family

Low-Risk Prenatal Family. Home care for the low-risk prenatal family is not currently the norm. It would, however, provide optimal levels of preventive care to families in their familiar environment. In particular, families who do not feel comfortable with traditional office or clinic-based prenatal care would benefit from home visits.

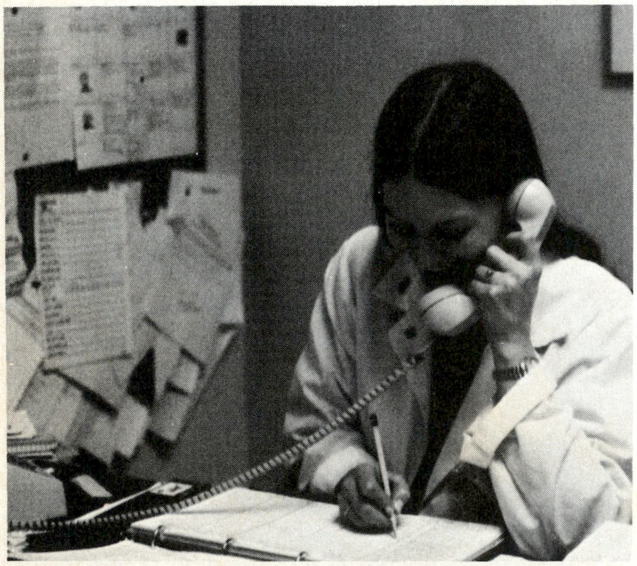

Figure 44–2. A telephone interview enables the nurse to evaluate the discharge plan for a well client.

Specifically, the nurse can more realistically assess the pregnant client and her family in the home and provide nursing care based on that assessment. For example, assessment of the nutritional status of the woman in the home allows the nurse to assist with planning a realistic diet based on the true picture of what is available in the home. In addition, teaching can also be more effective in the home environment away from the many distractions in the health care facility.

One innovative means of delivering prenatal care in the home is to have mobile units or vans go to specific neighborhoods. Community residents are enlisted to identify and reach out to pregnant women in need of prenatal care.

High-Risk Prenatal Family. Home care for high-risk prenatal families is a flourishing new field for home health agencies. Prenatal home care nurses may care for such high-risk pregnant clients as diabetics, women with pregnancy-induced hypertension, and women with hyperemesis gravidarum.

Treatments that were once performed only in acute care facilities are now part of home care. For example, a pregnant woman with hyperemesis gravidarum may be placed on intravenous therapy in the home. The home care nurse monitores the intravenous lines, acetone in the urine, and overall nutritional status of the mother, who remains in her familiar environment. As one mother stated: "I would have gone crazy in the hospital. Even though I have the IV, I am more comfortable and less anxious at home."

Keeping the high-risk prenatal client at home decreases the family's cost, both financial and personal. The family members also maintain more control over the high-risk pregnancy and their self-care capabilities.

One western health care institution attempted to improve care for antepartum high-risk pregnant women in this manner. An antepartum testing mobile unit was sent to pregnant women on restricted activities in their homes. The service resulted in reduced hospital admissions and improved client awareness of and adherence to activity restrictions.[12]

Home Care for the Postpartum Family

Low-Risk Postpartum Family. With the trend toward early discharge, the teaching and support of parenting behaviors that traditionally occurred in the postpartum unit have been reduced drastically. Many mothers and their partners return home without the same level of preparedness to assume parenting functions, and without a professional to consult about their concerns.[9]

Early discharge of postpartum clients may be problematic as well as beneficial. One study that looked at early discharge of low-income mothers and infants found that although early discharge was associated with higher maternal attachment and satisfaction scores, higher maternal and infant morbidity was reported in the first 2 weeks of life[13] (see the Research Abstract on page 1272). Other studies have demonstrated that families who meet selected criteria in short-stay maternity programs with home follow-up have a safe and satisfying postpartum experience.[14–17]

The Northeast Ohio March of Dimes Perinatal Nursing Advisory Board maintains the position that shortened maternity hospitalization must be accompanied by home follow-up to ensure the safety of mother, infant, and family. They acknowledge that the complex care involved in the postpartum period requires the services of professional registered nurses experienced and skilled in childbirth care.[18]

In response to such a position, many community nursing agencies have developed programs to increase support and educational services to new mothers in their homes. The primary objectives of these visits made to expanding families are to promote optimum family health and well-being and to promote self-responsibility in meeting the family's own health needs.[19] To accomplish these objectives, the nurse practicing in the community must provide health education, anticipatory guidance, and positive reinforcement for strengths in healthy families, while simultaneously assessing for risks or problems.[19]

The nursing role, in this instance, is to facilitate family functioning rather than direct the family in meeting specific health needs. (See the box for the components of a home visit.) Nurses are often uncomfortable in unstructured situations. In addition, funding for such "well" postpartum visits is often a problem. Community nurses must therefore be attuned to available resources such as the Special Supplemental Food Program for Women, Infants, and Children (WIC), child health conferences, postpartum parenting classes, and women's support groups and to the process of obtaining grant funds for demonstration project programs. Documentation of the beneficial results of such funded project programs will help to obtain resources for their continuance.

COMPONENTS OF THE HOME VISIT FOR CHILDBEARING FAMILIES

1. Inform family of what visit entails and time necessary to complete.
2. Schedule the visit for a time when family members are free from interruptions.
3. Intake activities are given priorities, for example, health assessment and insurance form information.
4. Assess infant's and mother's condition
5. Check equipment (for low-risk mother and infant, high-risk mother and infant, or both).
6. Assess home equipment for needed supplies and safety.
7. Assess parent's ability to provide appropriate routine and emergency care.
8. History may be deferred for subsequent visits as necessary.
9. Develop initial plan of care in collaboration with the family.
10. Develop plans for subsequent visits.
11. Evaluate family concerns and dynamics.
12. Provide family with list of community resources and telephone numbers.

High-Risk Postpartum Family. Chapter 36 discussed psychosocial adaptation of the high-risk childbearing family. The transition of the high-risk infant from hospital to home, rather than being the end of a crisis, marks the beginning of another crisis situation for the family.[20,21] If an infant has neurologic sequelae, the crisis will continue for the family, and may sometimes become all pervasive and chronic.[20] Depression, alienation of family members, and financial stress are all involved in the crisis of caring for a high-risk or premature infant at home.[20]

Several stressors have been identified for families caring for infants at home[20]:

1. *Family role changes.* Professionals often teach one family member, usually the mother, care of the infant. Exclusion of other family members from this learning can shift family function and make excluded members feel helpless and left out.
2. *Uncertain prognosis of the infant.* Often, it is difficult to know if there will be long-term or permanent handicaps on discharge.
3. *Loss of control.* Day-to-day care of the high-risk infant can be unpredictable, making planning for family life difficult.
4. *Employment pressure.* Families who will suffer financial stress and need to maintain employer-paid insurance policies have difficult choices to make concerning continued employment and care needs of the infant.
5. *Exhaustion and isolation.* Parents have little energy

left for any activities after caring for their infant.

6. *Extended family adjustment problems.* Impact of a premature or high-risk birth is felt intensely by grandparents as well as parents.[22] Extended family members who are experiencing denial and placing blame need comfort and often compound family problems.
7. *Changes in lifestyle.* Such factors as the presence of medical equipment and the need to arrange for complicated transportation to and from health care or medical appointments can drastically alter family patterns.
8. *Sibling problems.* Siblings of chronically ill or disabled children are often the "forgotten members" of the family. These children can develop personality and behavior changes, including jealousy, anger, aggressive behaviors, guilt, belief that "I may be next" to get sick, withdrawal, somatic complaints, regression, sleep disturbances, and fear of the dark. Children between ages 3 and 7 are most vulnerable to these problems.[23]
9. *Presence of strangers in the home.* A variety of health care providers from different agencies may be assigned to the same family. Further, caregivers may not be consistent from one visit to the next. Such patterns greatly disrupt family life.

Educating the High-Risk Postpartum Family. Educational preparation for the childbearing family has been discussed in depth in Chapter 24. One additional technique for educating the high risk family in the care of their infant at home is through **care-by-parent programs.** These programs may be a component of hospital care of high-risk newborns. In such programs, a family member (usually the mother) lives in the hospital for a set period (usually 24 to 48 hours) right before the infant's discharge. During this time, the parent is responsible for the complete care of the infant. Professional staff serve only as consultants to the parent. One study found that such programs greatly reduced a group of mothers' anxiety about caring for their infants at home.[24]

Specialized Home Care for the High-Risk Infant

Brooten's landmark study demonstrated that early discharge for high-risk infants is safe, if the family has visits from a clinical nurse specialist.[25] Many nurses who work in the community see not only low-risk newborns and families, but also sick and premature infants and their families. This section briefly reviews some of the high-risk problems with which infants may be discharged. It also alerts the reader to some of the specialized nursing care that is now commonly done in the home. Finally, some of the special issues that must be considered by nurses in working with high-risk families during childbearing and early childrearing are discussed. This material is not meant to be a comprehensive look at the complexities of home health care for high-risk infants and families. The reader is referred to references at the end of the chapter for in-depth treatment of this topic. The sole intent here is to alert the nurse to the potentials of care delivery during the childbearing phase of family life.

Problems of Prematurity Requiring Specialized Home Care. Disorders of premature infants occur as a result of immaturity of organ systems and the invasive treatment technologies performed in the NICU to maintain the infant's life (*see* Chapter 43). The dominant problems shape the care delivered in the home.

Respiratory Disorders. Respiratory disorders are the most common problems associated with prematurity.[4] The immature lung does not have the mechanical or biochemical capacity for adequate oxygen and carbon dioxide exchange. Respiratory distress syndrome may evolve into bronchopulmonary dysplasia (BPD), a chronic problem of respiratory insufficiency. Included in the syndrome are excessive bronchial secretions, a narrowed airway, and insufficient gas exchange. If severe, BPD necessitates continued mechanical ventilation. It is also associated with decreased exercise tolerance, increased work of breathing, and increased susceptibility to infection[4]—all of which must be dealt with in the home environment.

Another condition that is often dealt with in the home is subglottic stenosis (a narrowing of the airway), which is the result of prolonged and repeated endotracheal intubations during hospitalization. These disorders, which involve large or small airways, can occur at a variety of times—either beginning in the nursery or not appearing for months after discharge.[4]

Cardiovascular Disorders. Cardiovascular problems are closely linked to respiratory disorders in the premature high-risk infant. Conditions such as patent ductus arteriosus, a congenital heart condition in which the fetal ductus does not close, and chronic cor pulmonale (chronic cardiac insufficiency), present difficult home management problems for the nurse.[4]

Apnea. Apnea of prematurity is a common cardiorespiratory problem that has many causes. It can be related to immaturity and ineffectiveness of the brain's respiratory control centers, to heart/lung disease, or to some other correctable problem. It also can be unrelated to other conditions. Although episodes are sometimes self-limited, in some premature infants intervention is needed. This requires constant monitoring, plus a variety of stimulation interventions, oxygen administration,[4] or both.

Neurologic Disorders. Central nervous system problems may be either acute or chronic conditions; both types are dealt with in the home environment. Acute problems include intraventricular hemorrhage (IVH) and hypoxic brain damage. Both conditions, depending on their severity, may have global effects on future growth and development of the infant. Chronic problems include hydrocephalus, seizure disorders and neurodevelopmental handicaps, and require monitoring and long-term treatment.[4]

Gastrointestinal Disorders. The most prevalent condition of prematurity is necrotizing enterocolitis, which is a destructive infection of the small bowel. It affects the infant by (1) necessitating parenteral nutrition during the acute phase; (2) making feeding difficult and non–growth supporting; and (3) making the infant susceptible to conditions such as malabsorption through diarrhea, abdominal discomfort, and infections.[4]

Infections. Immaturity of the premature infant's defense system (immunologic and barrier defenses) leaves the infant vulnerable to many types of infection—for example, sepsis, meningitis, and pneumonia. These infections often have severe sequelae.[4]

Other Problems. Other common problems include anemia (and other inadequate numbers of blood components), resulting from immaturity of blood production mechanisms, and retinopathy of prematurity, resulting from the toxic effect of oxygen on immature eye tissues.

Nurses who practice in the community must be prepared to manage conditions such as these in the home. In addition, other high-risk conditions, which may or may not be related to prematurity (such as those discussed in Chapter 42), may be managed in the home environment after the acute phase has passed.

Types of Specialized Nursing Care Required. The nurse may need to perform various specialized technical interventions[4] in the home when caring for the premature or otherwise high-risk infant (*see* the box). The reader is again referred to other sources for an appropriate in-depth description of these interventions.

EXAMPLES OF NURSING INTERVENTIONS THAT MAY BE REQUIRED IN HOME CARE OF PRETERM OR HIGH-RISK INFANTS

1. Monitor an infant on an apnea monitor
2. Care for an infant requiring oxygen therapy
3. Care for an infant requiring mechanical ventilation and suctioning
4. Care for an infant with a tracheostomy
5. Care for an infant with central nervous system problems such as hydrocephalus and seizures
6. Care for an infant requiring tube feedings
7. Supervise infant stimulation programs[26, 27]
8. Care for an infant on home phototherapy for newborn jaundice (this treatment also may be be prescribed for generally healthy newborns)[28]

Although the specifics of management for each technical intervention are not discussed here, the following points should be considered when providing specialized nursing care in the home:

1. The family will be primarily responsible for care of the infant on an ongoing basis. Thus, teaching parents the techniques of care and supporting them throughout delivery of care constitute the primary role of hospital and community nurses. For example, infants may be discharged to the home with continuous oxygen therapy. In one study on the needs of families with such infants, both health care professionals and parents reported a need for improved discharge teaching and improved community support services.[29]
2. Discharge planning is imperative in making a smooth transition to the home for infants requiring this level of technical intervention. It is the link between hospital and home care environments.
3. Hospital and community nurses *must* communicate and collaborate to effect a smooth transition from hospital to home. This includes hospital staff teaching nurses who practice in the community specific care techniques for intervention with the infant. For example, the community nurse may come to the NICU, where the NICU nurse may teach him or her to administer a tube feeding to a premature infant. If, on the other hand, the acute care facility has a home visiting outreach program, the outreach hospital nurse also needs information from the community nurse. For example, techniques of community assessment and care of

clients in the context of the entire family and home environment may not be skills of the hospital-based nurse.

4. The first home visit is vital, as it sets the stage for a trusting relationship among the nurse and family members for all future visits. (*See* box describing the home visit on page 1277.)
5. Resources (eg, equipment companies), referrals, support, respite care (provision of an alternative caretaker to allow parents to have relief from infant care), and finances are parts of the total picture. The role of the nurse is not complete without considering these facets of home care.
6. Both hospital and community nurses must be advocates for high-risk families who must care for sick infants and later for children in the home. For example, a nurse may serve on school committees and be an advocate for educational programs for handicapped children.

Special Issues. Home care of high-risk infants and families is far more complex than performing specific technical interventions or even teaching the family the interventions and supporting them while they perform them. Home care providers also help the family to manage their lives from day to day and to cope with issues that come up in the activities of daily living. Parents of high-risk infants or infants requiring home care may face problems in health maintenance, nutrition and feeding, growth and development, and stimulation of the high-risk infant. Often, the nurse practicing in the community may become the leader of an interdisciplinary team delivering care to high-risk infants and families.

Health Maintenance of the High-Risk Infant. One of the major problems facing families is finding a professional to deliver primary pediatric care for their high-risk infant. Many pediatricians are reluctant to accept an infant with multiple problems into their practice.[4] The hospital or community nurse may help the family locate an individual who can provide the necessary specialized care for the high-risk infant.

Another problem that faces families is establishing an immunization schedule for the infant. The normal, designated schedule may be altered because of the long hospitalization or repeated minor illnesses. Parents need to be informed that immunizations can be given on an altered schedule.[4]

Premature and high-risk infants are vulnerable to a variety of minor illnesses (and these illnesses may be more dangerous to the high-risk or premature infant than to the low-risk or term infant.) Included are fevers, vomiting, diarrhea, and constipation.[4] Parents must know what they can safely handle at home, how to handle it, and when to call for professional help.

Safety for the infant in the home is an issue of concern to families of high-risk infants as well as families of low-risk infants.[4] The community nurse may assess the home environment and the infant's state to help parents plan a safe environment without being overprotective of their child.

Finally, the nurse who visits the home is also in a good position to assess the manner in which the infant is being integrated into the family system. The parent-infant (and sibling-infant) attachment process may be strained because of the burden of care on the family.

As infants with multiple problems often receive services from many professionals, coordination of services is essential. The nurse practicing in the community is often the person who can best coordinate services. He or she is also often in the best position to help the family locate and use community resources.[4]

Nutrition and Feeding of the High-Risk Infant. Providing adequate nutrition to the premature or high-risk infant with multiple problems may be a problem for families. This is a real concern, as inadequate nutrition at periods of rapid growth may have long-lasting, permanent effects on future growth and development. To effectively assist the family in feeding and providing nutrition to their infant, the community nurse must possess certain knowledge and skill[4]:

1. Know normal feeding behaviors and normal patterns of growth and development
2. Be able to assess feeding patterns and to differentiate normal feeding from feeding problems
3. Be able to intervene (and teach parents to intervene) in simple feeding problems
4. Know when to refer feeding problems to other professionals, and which professional is the appropriate person to handle a specific problem (nutritionists, occupational therapists, physical therapists, speech therapists and physicians are other team members who may be involved in the feeding and nutrition of the high-risk premature infant)

Growth and Development of the High-Risk Premature Infant. The premature infant does not possess the survival abilities of the term infant at birth. Most systems, including the central nervous system (CNS), are quite immature. As the infant approaches full gestational age, the CNS gradually matures, and the infant's behaviors most closely resembles those of term infants[30], however, subsequent developmental outcomes vary.

For the premature infant who has suffered no serious brain or other system damage, development generally follows the same sequence as that of a term infant. The rate of development is frequently slowed in proportion to the degree of prematurity (ie, the more premature the infant, the slower the rate of development). In "healthy" premature infants, the delay in development is mild, and by the age of 2, the delay is not readily apparent to untrained persons; however, specialized testing of motor and intellectual skills reveals differences as late as age 5.[30,31] The sick premature infant, on the other hand, is more likely to show both a delayed rate and an abnormal pattern of development. A wide range of disability may be apparent in these infants.[30,32]

The nurse practicing in the community has an important role in assessing growth and development of the high-risk infant. This role can vary from sophisticated developmental testing, which requires special training, to less sophisticated screening; however, all nurses working with this population need a basic understanding of potential developmental problems and community resources for further assessment and intervention. It is the community nurse's responsibility to observe infant development and identify abnormalities in rate or deviations in the sequence of attaining developmental skills.[30] In this manner, she or he can make timely referrals.

Three specific developmental problems that may be found in premature infants are hearing loss, speech and language disorders, and visual impairment. Immaturity of systems along with treatments and therapies performed in the NICU and at home (such as tracheostomies and oxygen therapy) may place the infant at risk for these problems.[4,33,34] All of these problems will greatly impede all facets of the infant's development, and the earlier that appropriate interventions can be initiated, the better the infant's prognosis will be. The community nurse thus has a major responsibility to identify infants with these problems and make early referrals.

Stimulation of the High-Risk Infant. Infant stimulation programs are frequently initiated as part of the interventions for high-risk infants. Programs are designed to give the newborn more to see, hear, and feel in an effort to promote optimum development. It also is hoped that such treatment will encourage the infant to better control stimuli in his or her world.[27,35] For example, bright-colored objects might be placed in front of the infant to encourage visual awareness and discrimination.

Early stimulation intervention programs are composed of teams of specialists. The goal of the program is to promote the infant's potential. Teams include nurses (maternal-infant clinical specialists), physical therapists, social workers, speech therapists, and educators. Treatment is generally provided outside a hospital setting, and parents are included as part of the team. The community nurse needs to be aware of infant stimulation programs available in the area to which parents can be referred.[35]

ROLE OF THE NURSE DELIVERING CARE IN THE COMMUNITY

The nurse who delivers care in the community has a vital role in ensuring adequacy of home care for mothers and infants in both low-risk and high-risk situations. The changes in the structure of health delivery systems have forced the nurse in the community to assume various new roles. Specifically in the area of childbearing, as technology has allowed more high-risk neonates to survive, there are new demands on the health care system to ensure their long-term wellbeing. True success of medical technologies depends on nurses and nursing care that can translate specialized skill and knowledge into nontraditional settings such as the home.

Home health care for childbearing families requires that the nurse be skilled in maternal-child health nursing practices as well as community practice. The nursing role incorporates health promotion, direct care, epidemiology, counseling, and political involvement. The nurse should be conversant with systems theory, enabling assessment of the community as a client as well as the family.

The nurse adapts care practices to the home environment using creative techniques. For example, infant stimulation in the home might use equipment found there, such as rugs and colored measuring spoons.

The nurse should understand the ethnic, political, and demographic makeup of the community that his or her agency serves. Community resources (financial, support, therapeutic and informational) should be identified for the family by the nurse.

The nurse acts as a client advocate in using the political system to influence health care policy. For example, nurses who care for childbearing families may contact legislators to influence health policy for preventive childbearing services as well as high-risk services.

The community nurse must become experienced with establishing a role on the interdisciplinary health care team. The nurse may coordinate care with occupational therapists, physical therapists, nutritionists, and home health care aides.

The home health care aide is one team member who has had an increasing role with families and high-risk infants. Programs have been developed to train already skilled homemaker–home health aides to work specifically with high-risk infants and their families to ease transition from the NICU to home care.[36] These aides assist parents with care of sick infants and running a household. Aides are taught and supervised by nurse clinicians and often receive training sessions in the NICU. While in the home, aides also have backup supervision, either by a social worker or by a nurse. These programs have been rated highly satisfactory by families and have resulted in increased attendance at clinic appointments and reduced rehospitalization of infants.[36] Such programs can do much to promote integrity of the family and help members cope with the transition to home care.

The role of the community nurse and other professionals who work with the family during the infant's transition from nursery or NICU to home is frequently to offer practical and emotional support. Helping the family to develop effective crisis management and coping strategies will effect positive long-term care of the low-risk and high-risk infant. Specific nursing activities include (1) providing information, (2) fostering decision making, (3) helping to identify financial resources and child care support, (4) helping families activate a support system, (5) identifying high-risk respite care programs, and (6) making referrals (such as siblings to therapeutic play programs or daycare.)[20] The family usually experiences some level of anxiety; however, low levels of anxiety have been found to be beneficial to families in effecting solutions to problems.[37]

Stresses in Delivering Home Care

There is currently controversy as to whether home health care is a subspecialty of community health nursing or a specialty with separate skills and knowledge of its own.[38] It is evident from the previous discussion on home care of mothers and infants that the nurse needs, in addition to knowledge concerning community nursing, an in-depth knowledge of childbearing families. A gap remains between what the nurse who practices in the community currently knows and what he or she needs to know to deliver care to childbearing families.

In discussing well-infant visits, one author found that nurses from a visiting nurses' association expressed insecurity about their abilities to manage care and assess normal newborns.[9] Another investigator who looked at community nurses' attitudes to delivering care to childbearing families found that the large majority of her sample did not feel that they were adequately prepared to deliver care in the home to mothers and infants.[39,40] A third investigator found that during home visits, groups of nurses and clients were uncertain of the goals for care on which they had decided.[41]

Conversely, some level III or acute care settings are initiating outreach or home visiting programs where hospital staff or clinical specialists visit clients in their home to provide follow-up or continuity of care to high-risk infants. These nurses, who are experts in care delivery to childbearing families and technologic interventions, may have little understanding about delivery of care in a community setting. Again, gaps in knowledge exist in caring for childbearing families in their homes.

In conclusion, home health care for childbearing families has become a growing priority for the health care system. Nurses are the primary care providers who assume responsibility for home care of mothers, infants, and families. There are many low- and high-risk care activities, especially health promotion activities for healthy childbearing families, that could and should be available in the home. Without a payment system directed toward preventive services and direct reimbursement to nurses for delivery of care in the home, however, the needs of many childbearing families will go unmet.[42] The nurse must take an active role in changing health policy.[43]

SUMMARY

Home health care includes care of low-risk and high-risk prenatal clients. In particular, adolescents and urban poor women may benefit from prenatal care in the home. Many high-risk prenatal conditions that formerly required hospitalization, such as hyperemesis gravidarum and diabetes mellitus, may be managed in the home with skillful nursing care.

Home health care also focuses on the low-risk and high-risk postpartum family. A nursing discharge plan from the birthing institution helps the nurse who practices in the community provide comprehensive care to the family. In doing so, the nurse uses the components of the nursing process.

Care delivered to low-risk postpartum families includes teaching traditionally done during the stay in the birthing institution. Home health care can thus fill any gap engendered by early discharge of mothers and neonates.

One major change in the home setting is the presence of sick, high-risk or premature infants, making homes into "mini-NICUs." Prematurity and other newborn conditions can result in a variety of short-term and long-term physiologic conditions requiring care of the infant in the home. Nurses must possess the specific technical skills needed to care for infants with conditions resulting from prematurity, and other problems, including respiratory disorders, cardiovascular disorders, apnea, and neurologic and gastrointestinal disorders. They further require skills to teach parents to deliver this care. Specialized nursing care skills that are required to care for the infant in the home include managing an infant on an apnea monitor, caring for an infant requiring oxygen therapy or mechanical ventilation, caring for an infant with a tracheostomy, and supervising infant stimulation programs. The nurse has the task of teaching parents these skills, as they will be responsible for the infant's ongoing care.

The family of a high-risk infant must deal with several issues on a day-to-day basis, including financial support, availability of community resources, and treatment strategies. It is essential that nurses be adequately prepared to deliver care in a variety of settings.

REVIEW QUESTIONS

1. Discuss the impact that DRGs have had on early discharge practices for mothers and neonates.
2. Develop three nursing strategies in planning care for a low-risk prenatal family.
3. List four nursing procedures that may be needed for home care of the high-risk infant.
4. List two resources needed by postpartum childbearing families.
5. Describe two roles of the community health nurse in caring for high-risk neonates.

REFERENCES

1. Mundinger M. *Home Care Controversy.* Rockville, MD: Aspen; 1983.
2. Rose MA. Home care nursing practice: the new frontier. *Holistic Nurs Pract.* 1989;3:1–8.
3. Griffith E. The changing face of home health care. *Public Health Nurs.* 1987;4:1.
4. Ahmann E. *Home Care for the High Risk Infant.* Rockville, MD: Aspen; 1986.
5. O'Hare P, Terry M. *Discharge Planning: Strategies for Assuring Continuity of Care.* Rockville, MD: Aspen; 1988.
6. Taylor M. The effect of DRGs on home health care. *Nurs Outlook.* 1985;33:288–289.
7. Auerbach M. Changes in home health care delivery. *Nurs Outlook.* 1985;33:290–291.
8. Gagnon D, Schwartz R. Revised definitions needed for OB and neonatal DRGs. *Perinat Press.* 1985;9:39–44.
9. Quinn J, Gadway M. Creating an early home-visit program for well, expanding families. In: Hawkins J, Hayes E, eds. *Linking Nursing Education and Practice-Collaborative Experiences in Maternal-Child Health.* New York: Springer; 1987.
10. Coyner A. Home visiting by public health nurses: a vanishing resource for mothers and children. *Bull Nat Center Clin Infant Programs.* 1985;4:1–5.
11. *Discharge Planning.* American Nurses' Association Publication. Code NP-49, 3000-3, 1975.
12. Harmon JS, Barry M. Antenatal testing, mobile outpatient monitoring services. *J Obstet Gynecol Neonat Nurs.* 1989; 18:21–24.
13. Norr KRF, et al. Early discharge with home follow up: impacts on low-income mothers and infants. *J Obstet Gynecol Neonat Nurs.* 1989;18:133–141.
14. Drummond R, et al. Mother-care: cost effective program in maternal-infant care. *Home Health Care Nurse.* Sept/Oct 1984:41–43.
15. Jansson P. Early postpartum discharge. *Am J Nurs.* 1985; 85:457–550.
16. Killeen M. From hospital to home: continuous care of new mothers and infants. *Nurs Manage.* 1984;15(3):10–13.
17. Regan K. Early obstetrical discharge: a program that works. *Can Nurse.* 1984;80(10):32–35.
18. March of Dimes. *Short-Term Maternity Hospitalization: The Case for Nursing Follow Up.* A position paper presented by Northeast Ohio March of Dimes Perinatal Nursing Advisory Board; Fall 1987.
19. Davis J, Eyer J. Sorting out new mothers' learning priorities on home visits. *Home Health Care Nurse.* 1984;2:1–4.
20. Weinstock N. The family of the high risk infant. In: Ahmann P, ed. *Home Care for the High Risk Infant.* Rockville, MD: Aspen; 1986.
21. Talbert K. The impact of a high-risk infant upon the family. *Neonat Network.* 1985;20–23.
22. Blackburn S, Lowen L. Impact of an infant's premature birth on the grand-parents and parents. *J Obstet Gynecol Neonat Nurs.* 1986;15:173–178.
23. Peck T. Siblings of chronically ill children. In: Ahmann P, ed. *Home Care for the High Risk Infant.* Rockville, MD: Aspen; 1986.
24. Consolvo C. Relieving parental anxiety in the care-by-parent unit. *J Obstet Gynecol Neonat Nurs.* 1986;15:154–159.
25. Brooten D, et al. A randomized clinical trial of early hospital discharge and home follow-up of very-low-birth-weight infants. *N Engl J Med.* 1986;315:934–939.
26. Grant P. Psychosocial needs of families of high risk infants. *Fam Community Health.* 1978;1:91–102.
27. Gunzenhauser N, ed. *Infant Stimulation.* Skillman, NJ: Johnson & Johnson Baby Products Co, 1987.
28. Ellis J. Home phototherapy for newborn jaundice. *Birth.* 1985;12:15–17.

29. Young LY et al. The needs of families of infants discharged home with continuous oxygen therapy. *J Obstet Gynecol Neonat Nurs.* 1988;17(3):187–193.
30. Ichord R. Developmental issues in care of the high risk infant. In Ahmann E, ed. *Home Care for the High Risk Infant.* Rockville, MD: Aspen; 1986.
31. Caputo D. The development of prematurely born children through middle childhood. In Field T, ed. *Infants Born at Risk.* New York: SP Medical Books; 1979.
32. Goldberg S. *Born Too Soon: Preterm Birth and Early Development.* San Francisco: WH Freeman; 1983.
33. Cox P, Ahmann P. Hearing impairment in the high risk infant. In: Ahmann P, ed. *Home Care for the High Risk Infant.* Rockville, MD: Aspen; 1986.
34. Simon B. Speech and language development in the high risk infant. In: Ahmann P, ed. *Home Care for the High Risk Infant.* Rockville, MD: Aspen; 1986.
35. Censullo M. Home care of high-risk newborn. *J Obstet Gynecol Neonat Nurs.* 1986; 15:146–153.
36. Raff B. The use of homemaker-home health aides' perinatal care of high-risk infants. *J Obstet Gynecol Neonat Nurs.* 1986;15:142–145.
37. Gennaro S. Anxiety and problem-solving ability in mothers of premature infants. *J Obstet Gynecol Neonat Nurs.* 1986; 15:160–164.
38. Association of Community Nursing Health Educators. Report of the Task on Essentials of Education for Entry Level Community. *Health Nurs Pract.* 1989;11:35–39.
39. Schultze M, Koerner B. Attitudes of community health nurses toward maternal and child health nursing: development of an instrument. *J Professional Nurs.* 1987;14:347–353.
40. Schultze M, D'Apico M. Assessing the attitudes of community health nurses toward maternal and child health nursing. In: Hawkins J, Hayes E, eds. *Linking Nursing Education and Practice.* New York: Springer; 1987.
41. Morgan B, Barden M. Nurse-patient interaction in the home setting. *Public Health Nurs.* 1985;2:159–167.
42. Reckling JB. Abandonment of patients by home health nursing agencies: An ethical analysis of the dilemma. *Advances in Nursing Science.* 1989;11:70–81.
43. National Commission on Nursing Implementation Project. *The Nation's Nurses: A Credible Profession Doing an Incredible Job.* Milwaukee Wis: NCNIP; Oct 1988.

Appendices

A. **Effects of Maternal Medications on the Embryo/Fetus During the First Trimester**

B. **Effects of Maternal Medications on the Embryo/Fetus During the Second and Third Trimesters**

C. **Standard Laboratory Values for the Childbearing Woman**

D. **The Pregnant Patient's Bill of Rights**

E. **Universal Precautions for Prevention of Transmission of Human Immunodeficiency Virus, Hepatitis B Virus, and Other Bloodborne Pathogens in Health-Care Settings**

F. **Resources**

G. **Maternal Medications and Their Excretion in Breast Milk**

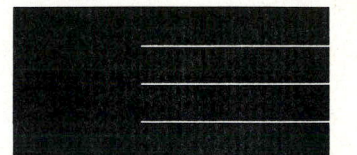

APPENDIX A. Effects of Maternal Medications on the Embryo/Fetus During the First Trimester

Drug[a]	Possible Effects on Embryo/Fetus
Androgens, (eg, testosterone) (X)	Virilization of female fetus.
Barbiturates (eg, phenobarbital) (D)	Possible association with malformations.
Belladonna (C)	Possible association with malformations.
Brompheniramine (C)	Possible association with malformations.
Busulfan (D)	Possible association with various malformations.
Captopril (C)	Possible association with malformations (NIH recommends that it not be used in pregnancy).
Carbimazole (D)	Possible association with malformations.
Chlordiazepoxide (D)	Possible association with malformations.
Chlorambucil (D)	Possible association with malformations.
Clomiphene (X)	Contradictory information regarding teratogenicity.
Codeine (C)	Possible association with various malformations.
Cyclophosphamide (D)	Possible association with malformations.
Dextroamphetamine (D)	Possible association with malformations.
Diazepam (D)	Contradictory information regarding teratogenicity.
Diethylstilbestrol (X)	Genital tract system defects in male and females.
Diphenhydramine (C)	Possible association with malformations.
Estrogens, (eg, estradiol) (X)	Contradictory information regarding teratogenicity, but considered contraindicated in pregnancy.
Gold sodium thiomalate (C)	Drug concentrates in fetal liver and kidneys, but effects to fetus unknown.
Haloperidol (C)	Limb reduction anomalies reported.
Isoniazid (C)	Contradictory information regarding teratogenicity.
Isotretinoin (X)	Many congenital defects reported, contraindicated in pregnancy.
Lithium (D)	Congenital defects reported, involving primarily the cardiovascular system.
Methimazole (D)	*See* Carbimazole.
Methotrexate (D)	Possible association with malformations.
Paramethadione (D)	Congenital defects reported, not recommended in pregnancy.
Penicillamine (D)	Associated with connective tissue anomalies.
Phenylephrine (C)	Possible association with malformations.
Phenylpropanolamine (C)	Possible association with malformations.
Phenytoin (D)	Associated with fetal hydantoin syndrome, which comprises craniofacial, limb, and cardiac defects.
Propoxyphene (C)	Possible association with malformations.
Quinine (high doses) (D)	Associated with central nervous system and limb defects.
Reserpine (D)	Possible association with malformations.
Thiazide diuretics, (eg, hydrochlorothiazide) (D)	Not shown to be teratogenic, but may decrease placental perfusion.
Thioguanine (X)	Possible association with malformations.
Trimethadione (D)	*See* Paramethadione.
Vaccines, (eg, measles, mumps, rubella) (X)	Potential risk of fetal infection with live, attenuated virus vaccines.
Valproic acid (D)	Possible association with malformations, primarily spina bifida.
Vitamin A (A). If above or below RDA (X)	Deficiency and overdose associated with malformations.
Warfarin (D)	Associated with fetal warfarin syndrome consisting primarily of nasal hypoplasia, depressed bridge of nose, stippling in uncalcified epiphyseal regions.

[a] FDA pregnancy category given in parentheses:

C = Either studies in animals have revealed adverse effects on the fetus and there are no controlled studies in women, or studies in women and animals are not available. Drug should be given only if the potential benefit justifies the potential risk to the fetus.

D = There is positive evidence of fetal risk based on human experience, but the benefits from use in pregnant women may be acceptable despite the risks (eg, needed in a life-threatening situation).

X = Studies in animals or human beings have demonstrated fetal abnormalities or there is evidence of fetal risk based on human experience, or both, and risk of use of drug in pregnant women clearly outweighs any possible benefit. The drug is contraindicated in women who are or may become pregnant.

APPENDIX B. Effects of Maternal Medications on the Embryo/Fetus During the Second and Third Trimesters

Drug[a]	Possible Effect on Fetus/Neonate
Acetohexamide (C)	Use near term may result in prolonged neonatal hypoglycemia.
Albuterol (C)	Use near term may result in fetal hyperglycemia, followed by neonatal hypoglycemia as a result of increase in serum insulin.
Amikacin (C)	High doses in mother may cause VIIIth cranial nerve toxicity.
Aminoglutethimide (D)	May cause virilization as a result of inhibition of adrenocortical function.
Aspirin (D)	Use near term may prolong labor and inhibit clotting ability of newborn; increased risk of intracranial hemorrhage in premature infant.
Atropine (C)	May cause fetal tachycardia.
Azathioprine (D)	May cause immunosuppression in neonate.
Barbiturates (D)	Use near term may cause neonatal withdrawal and hemorrhagic disease of newborn.
Beta blockers (C)	Possible association with low birth weight; atenolol and nadolol may cause beta blockade in newborn.
Chloramphenicol (C)	Use near term may cause gray-baby syndrome in neonate.
Chlordiazepoxide (D)	Use near term may result in neonatal withdrawal and central nervous system depression.
Chlorpropamide (C)	*See* Acetohexamide.
Clonazepam (C)	One report of apnea, cyanosis, lethargy, hypotonia in neonate when mother ingested clonazepam just prior to delivery.
Corticosteroids (D)	High doses may cause adrenal atrophy in neonate.
Desipramine (C)	Use near term may result in neonatal withdrawal.
Diazepam (D)	*See* Chlordiazepoxide.
Diazoxide (C)	Use near term may inhibit labor and cause fetal bradycardia; also reported to cause alopecia, hypertrichosis lanuginosa, and decreased ossification of wrist.
Gentamicin (C)	*See* Amikacin.
Gold sodium thiomalate (C)	Drug concentrates in fetal liver and kidney; effects on fetus/neonate unknown.
Imipramine (C)	*See* Desipramine.
Isoniazid (C)	Possible association with hemorrhagic disease of newborn when used near term.
Methimazole (D)	Use near term may result in goiter in newborn.
Nitrofurantoin (B)	Theoretical potential of hemolytic anemia when used near term.
Nonsteroidal anti-inflammatory agents (B or D)	Use near term may cause premature closure of ductus arteriosus.
Paregoric (C)	Prolonged use may result in fetal addiction.
Phenothiazines (C)	Use of high doses near term may result in hypotonia, lethargy, depressed reflexes, paralytic ileus, jaundice, and extrapyramidal symptoms.
Rifampin (C)	Possible association with hemorrhagic disease of newborn when used near term.
Scopolamine (C)	*See* Atropine.
Sodium iodide (^{125}I, ^{131}I) (X)	May cause destruction of fetal thyroid gland.
Sulfonamides (B)	Potential risk of jaundice, hemolytic anemia, and kernicterus when used near term.
Terbutaline (C)	*See* Albuterol.
Tetracyclines (D)	May result in staining of teeth and inhibition of bone growth.
Theophylline (C)	If high serum concentrations in mother at term, may result in tachycardia, irritability, and vomiting in neonate.
Thiazide diuretics (D)	Potential to cause hemolytic anemia and electrolyte imbalances when used near term.
Tobramycin (D)	*See* Amikacin.
Tolazamide (C)	*See* Acetohexamide.
Tolbutamide (C)	*See* Acetohexamide.
Vaccines (eg, measles, mumps, rubella) (X)	Live, attenuated virus vaccines may result in fetal infection.

[a] FDA pregnancy category given in parentheses:

B = Either animal-production studies have not demonstrated a fetal risk but there are no controlled studies in pregnant women, or animal-production studies have shown an adverse effect that was not confirmed in controlled studies in women in the first trimester (and there is no evidence of risk in later trimesters).

C, D, X = *See* notes to Appendix A.

APPENDIX C. Standard Laboratory Values for the Childbearing Woman

	Non-Pregnant	Pregnant
Hematology (Peripheral Blood Values)		
Red blood cells (mil/mm^3)	4.0–5.0	Increases 25%
Hemoglobin (g/dL)	12–16	11–12
Hematocrit (%)[a]	37–48	32–46
MCV (mean corpuscular volume) (μm^3)	80–98	80–95
MCH (mean corpuscular hemoglobin) (pg)	27–31	27–31
White blood cells (μL)	5,000–12,000	5,000–16,000
Differential		
Neutrophils (%)	50–60	50–70
Lymphocytes (%)	25–35	25–44
Eosinophils (%)	0–3	0–3
Monocytes (%)	2–6	2–6
Platelets (mm^3)	150,000–400,000	75,000–320,000
Prothrombin time (sec)	11–15	11–15
Partial thromboplastin time (sec)	60–70	Slightly shortened
Activated partial prothrombin time	25–45	Slightly shortened
Fibrinogen (mg/dL)	150–400	400–500
Bleeding time (min)	1–6 (Ivy) 1–3 (Duke)	1–6 (Ivy) 1–3 (Duke)
Blood Chemistries		
Total bilirubin (mg/dL)	0.2–0.9	Slightly increased
Creatinine (mg/dL)	0.5–1.0	0.3–0.6
Folate (folic acid) (ng/mL)	1.8–9	1.9–14
Blood sugar		
Fasting (mg/dL)	70–80	65
Postprandial (mg/dL)	<120 2 hr (blood)	< 140 2 hr (blood)
Iron (ug/dL)	50–150	50–120
Iron-binding capacity (mg/dL)	250–450	300–500

	Findings During Pregnancy	
Hormones		
Human chorionic gonadotropin (hCG)		
Urine	Positive	
If quantified	>1000 IU/24 hr	
Serum	Positive	
If quantified	Steady rise, by 45 days 50,000 IU; by 60 days as high as 600,000 IU; then drops to stable level of approximately 20,000 IU by 100th day	
Human placental lactogen (hPL)	*Weeks of Gestation*	*ng/mL*
	24–28	2.0–5.5
	29–32	2.5–7.5
	33–36	3.5–9.5
	37–40	4.0–10.0
Urinalysis		
Color	Pale straw	
Appearance	Clear	
Specific gravity	1.015–1.024	
pH	4.5–8 (6 is average)	
Protein	Negative–Trace	
Glucose	Negative–Trace	
Ketones	Negative	
Microscopic RBC	1–2 per lower power field	
WBC	3–4	
Casts	Occasional hyaline	
Antibody Screen		
Indirect Coombs	Negative	
HTLV-III Screen		
Elisa test	Negative	
Western blot test	Negative	
Serology		
FTA-ABS	Negative; nonreactive	
VDRL	Negative	
Rubella titre (hemagglutination-inhibition test)	>1:8 immune	

[a] At sea level. Values of 32 to 35 percent indicate physiologic anemia.

APPENDIX D. The Pregnant Patient's Bill of Rights

The Pregnant Patient has the right to participate in decisions involving her well-being and that of her unborn child, unless there is a clear-cut medical emergency that prevents her participation. In addition to the rights set forth in the American Hospital Association's "Patient's Bill of Rights," the Pregnant Patient, because she represents *two* patients rather than one, should be recognized as having the additional rights listed below.

1. *The Pregnant Patient has the right,* prior to the administration of any drug or procedure, to be informed by the health professional caring for her of any potential direct or indirect effects, risks, or hazards to herself or her unborn or newborn infant which may result from the use of a drug or procedure prescribed for or administered to her during pregnancy, labor, birth, or lactation.
2. *The Pregnant Patient has the right,* prior to the proposed therapy, to be informed, not only of the benefits, risks, and hazards of the proposed therapy, but also of known alternative therapy, such as available childbirth education classes which could help to prepare the Pregnant Patient physically and mentally to cope with the discomfort or stress of pregnancy and the experience of childbirth, thereby reducing or eliminating her need for drugs and obstetric intervention. She should be offered such information early in her pregnancy in order that she may make a reasoned decision.
3. *The Pregnant Patient has the right,* prior to the administration of any drug, to be informed by the health professional who is prescribing or administering the drug to her that any drug which she receives during pregnancy, labor and birth, no matter how or when the drug is taken or administered, may adversely affect her unborn baby, directly or indirectly, and that there is no drug or chemical which has been proven safe for the unborn child.
4. *The Pregnant Patient has the right,* if cesarean section is anticipated, to be informed prior to administration of any drug, and preferably prior to her hospitalization, that minimizing her and, in turn, her baby's intake of nonessential preoperative medicine, will benefit her baby.
5. *The Pregnant Patient has the right,* prior to the administration of a drug or procedure, to be informed if there is *no* properly controlled follow-up research which has established the safety of the drug or procedure with regard to its direct and/or indirect effects on the physiological, mental, and neurological development of the child exposed, via the mother, to the drug or procedure during pregnancy, labor, birth or lactation (this would apply to virtually all drugs and the vast majority of obstetric procedures).
6. *The Pregnant Patient has the right,* prior to the administration of any drug, to be informed of the brand name and generic name of the drug in order that she may advise the health professional of any past adverse reaction to the drug.
7. *The Pregnant Patient has the right* to determine for herself, without pressure from her attendant, whether she will accept the risks inherent in the proposed therapy or refuse a drug or procedure.
8. *The Pregnant Patient has the right* to know the name and qualifications of the individual administering a medication or procedure to her during labor or birth.
9. *The Pregnant Patient has the right* to be informed, prior to the administration of any procedure, whether that procedure is being administered to her for her or her baby's benefit (medically indicated) or as an elective procedure (for convenience or teaching purposes).
10. *The Pregnant Patient has the right* to be accompanied during the stress of labor and birth by someone she cares for, and to whom she looks for emotional comfort and encouragement.
11. *The Pregnant Patient has the right* after appropriate medical consultation to choose a position for labor and for birth which is least stressful to her baby and to herself.
12. *The Obstetric Patient has the right* to have her baby cared for at her bedside if her baby is normal, and to feed her baby according to her baby's needs rather than according to the hospital regimen.
13. *The Obstetric Patient has the right* to be informed in writing of the name of the person who actually delivered her baby and the professional qualifications of that person. This information should also be on the birth certificate.
14. *The Obstetric Patient has the right* to be informed if there is any known or indicated aspect of her or her baby's care or condition which may cause her or her baby later difficulty or problems.
15. *The Obstetric Patient has the right* to have her and her baby's hospital medical records complete, accurate, and legible, and to have their records, including Nurses' Notes, retained by the hospi-

tal until the child reaches at least the age of majority, or alternatively, to have the records offered to her before they are destroyed.

16. *The Obstetric Patient*, both during and after her hospital stay, has the right to have access to her complete hospital medical records, including Nurses' Notes, and to receive a copy upon payment of a reasonable fee and without incurring the expense of retaining an attorney.

It is the obstetric patient and her baby, not the health professional, who must sustain any trauma or injury resulting from the use of a drug or obstetric procedure. The observation of the rights listed above will not only permit the obstetric patient to participate in the decisions involving her and her baby's health care, but will help to protect the health professional and the hospital against litigation arising from resentment or misunderstanding on the part of the mother.

Reprinted, with permission, from Haire DB. The pregnant patient's bill of rights. *J Nurs Midwife*. 1975;20:29.

APPENDIX E. Universal Precautions for Prevention of Transmission of Human Immunodeficiency Virus, Hepatitis B Virus, and Other Bloodborne Pathogens in Health-Care Settings

It is recommended that blood and body fluid precautions be consistently used for all patients regardless of their bloodborne infection status. This extension of blood and body fluid precautions to *all* patients is referred to as "Universal Blood and Body Fluid Precautions" or "Universal Precautions." Under universal precautions, blood and certain body fluids of all patients are considered potentially infectious for human immunodeficiency virus (HIV), hepatitis B virus (HBV), and other bloodborne pathogens. Universal precautions are intended to prevent parenteral, mucous membrane, and nonintact skin exposures of health-care workers to bloodborne pathogens.

BODY FLUIDS TO WHICH UNIVERSAL PRECAUTIONS APPLY

Universal precautions apply to blood and to other body fluids containing visible blood. *Blood is the single most important source of HIV, HBV, and other bloodborne pathogens in the occupational setting.* Infection control efforts for HIV, HBV, and other bloodborne pathogens must focus on preventing exposures to blood as well as on delivery of HBV immunization.

Universal precautions also apply to semen and vaginal secretions. Although both of these fluids have been implicated in the sexual transmission of HIV and HBV, they have not been implicated in occupational transmission from patient to health-care worker.

Universal precautions also apply to tissues and to the following fluids: cerebrospinal fluid (CSF), synovial fluid, pleural fluid, peritoneal fluid, pericardial fluid, and amniotic fluid. The risk of transmission of HIV and HBV from these fluids is unknown.

BODY FLUIDS TO WHICH UNIVERSAL PRECAUTIONS DO NOT APPLY

Universal precautions do not apply to feces, nasal secretions, sputum, sweat, tears, urine, and vomitus unless they contain visible blood. The risk of transmission of HIV and HBV from these fluids and materials is extremely low or nonexistent.

PRECAUTIONS FOR OTHER BODY FLUIDS IN SPECIAL SETTINGS

Human breast milk has been implicated in perinatal transmission of HIV, and hepatitis B virus antigen (HBsAG) has been found in the milk of mothers infected with HBV; however, occupational exposure to human breast milk has not been implicated in the transmission of HIV or HBV infection to health-care workers.

Universal precautions do not apply to saliva. General infection control practices already in existence—including the use of gloves for digital examination of mucous membranes and endotracheal suctioning, and handwashing after exposure to saliva—should further minimize the minute risk, if any, for salivary transmission of HIV and HBV. Gloves need not be worn when feeding patients and when wiping saliva from skin. Special precautions, however, are recommended for dentistry. Occupationally acquired infection with HBV in dental workers has been documented.

USE OF PROTECTIVE BARRIERS

Universal precautions are intended to supplement rather than replace recommendations for routine infection control, such as handwashing and using gloves to prevent gross microbial contamination of hands. Because specifying the types of barriers needed for every possible clinical situation is impractical, some judgment must be exercised.

The risk of nosocomial transmission of HIV, HBV, and other bloodborne pathogens can be minimized if health-care workers use the following general guidelines.

1. Take care to prevent injuries: when using needles, scalpels, and other sharp instruments or devices; when handling sharp instruments after procedures; when cleaning used instruments; and when disposing of used needles. Do not recap used needles by hand; do not remove used needles from disposable syringes by hand; and do not bend, break, or otherwise manipulate used needles by hand. Place used disposable syringes and needles, scalpel blades, and other sharp items in puncture-resistant containers for disposal. Locate the puncture-resistant containers as close to the use area as is practical.
2. Use protective barriers to prevent exposure to blood, body fluids containing visible blood, and other fluids to which universal precautions apply. The type of protective barrier(s) should be appro-

priate for the procedure being performed and the type of exposure anticipated.

3. Immediately and thoroughly wash hands and other skin surfaces that are contaminated with blood, body fluids containing visible blood, or other body fluids to which universal precautions apply.
4. Wear protective eyewear or face shields for all procedures that commonly result in generation of droplets or splashes of blood, body fluids containing blood, or other applicable body fluids.
5. Wear gowns or aprons made of materials providing an effective barrier during invasive procedures likely to result in the splashing of blood or other pertinent body fluids.
6. Wear gloves and gowns when handling the placenta or infant until blood and amniotic fluid have been removed from the infant's skin. Gloves should be worn until postdelivery care of the umbilical cord.

Adapted from Centers for Disease Control. Recommendations for prevention of HIV transmission in health care settings. *MMWR.* 1987;36:Suppl 25. Centers for Disease Control. Update: universal precautions for prevention or transmission of human immunodeficiency virus, hepatitis B virus, and other blood-borne pathogens in health care settings. *MMWR.* 1988;37:24.

APPENDIX F. Resources

ONLINE COMPUTER SERVICES

BRS Information Technologies
1200 Route 7
Latham, NY 12110
800-833-4707; 518-583-1161

DIALOG Information Services, Inc.
3460 Hillview Avenue
Palo Alto, CA 94304
800-982-5838; 800-227-1927; 415-858-2700

National Library of Medicine
MEDLARS Management Section
Bldg 38A, Room 4N-421
8600 Rockville Pile
Bethesda, MD 20894
800-638-8480; 301-496-6193

ABORTION

National Abortion Federation
900 Pennsylvania Avenue, SE
Washington, DC 20003
Consumer Information Hotline: 800-722-9100
Provides information and referral for abortion services

National Abortion Rights Action League
1101 14th Street, NW
Washington, DC 20005
202-371-0779
Pro-choice political action group

National Right to Life Committee
419 7th Street, NW,
Suite 402
Washington, DC 20004
202-626-8800
Pro-life political action group

BATTERING

Victims Anonymous
9514-9 Reseda Boulevard, #607
Northridge, CA 91324
818-993-1139
Provides support for victims of sexual or physical abuse

Women Against Rape
P. O. Box 02084
Columbus, OH 43202
614-291-9751

BIRTH DEFECTS AND GENETIC DISORDERS

American Cleft Palate Association
331 Salk Hall
Pittsburgh, PA 15261
412-681-9620
Provides information to parents of infants with cleft palates; resource for cleft palate centers and parent support groups

Association of Birth Defects in Children
3201 E. Crystal Lake Avenue
Orlando, FL 32806

Center for Sickle Cell Disease
2121 Georgia Avenue, NW
Washington, DC 20059
202-636-7930

Cystic Fibrosis Foundation
1655 Tullie Circle, Suite 111
Atlanta, GA 30329
404-325-6973

Institutes for the Achievement of Human Potential
8801 Stanton Avenue
Philadelphia, PA 19118
215-233-2050
Provides information for parents of brain-injured children

March of Dimes Birth Defects Foundation
1275 Mamaroneck Avenue
White Plains, NY 10605
914-428-7100
Publishes a directory of genetic services; sponsors research on genetic defects

National Association for Down's Syndrome (NADS)
1800 Dempster Street
Park Ridge, IL 60068-1146
312-823-7550

National Clearinghouse for Human Genetic Disease
National Center for Education in Maternal and Child Health
38th and R Streets, NW
Washington, DC 20057
Provides information about inherited diseases; publishes directory of genetic counseling services

National Down's Syndrome Society Hotline
141 Fifth Avenue
New York, NY 10010
800-221-4602; 212-764-3070

National Genetics Foundation
555 West 57th Street
New York, NY 10019

Spina Bifida Association of America
1700 Rockville Pike, Suite 540
Rockville, MD 20852
800-621-3141
Provides information to parents of infants with neural tube defects

BREASTFEEDING

La Leche League International
9616 Minneapolis Avenue
Franklin, IL 60131
312-455-8071
Provides information and support for breastfeeding mothers

Lact-Aid
P. O. Box 1066
Athens, TN 37303
614-744-9090
Provides information and services to promote breastfeeding

CHILD HEALTH AND DEVELOPMENT

American Academy of Pediatrics
Publications Department
P.O. Box 927
Elk Grove, IL 60009-0927
312-869-9327
Provides information about child health, illness and welfare

Canadian Institute of Child Health
410 Laurier Avenue
Suite 803
West Ottawa, Ont. KIR 7T6

National Center for Education in Maternal and Child Health
38th and R Streets, NW
Washington, DC 20007
202-625-8400

National Institute of Child Health and Human Development
National Institutes of Health
9000 Rockville Pike
Building 31, Room 2A32
Bethesda, MD 20205
301-496-4000

CHILDBIRTH/CHILDBIRTH ALTERNATIVES

Association for Childbirth at Home, International
P. O. Box 39498
Los Angeles, CA 90039
213-667-0839

C/SEC, Inc. (Cesarean/Support Education and Concern)
22 Forest road
Framingham, MA 01701
617-877-8266
Provides information about cesarean birth

International Childbirth Education Association (ICEA)
P. O. Box 20048
Minneapolis, MN 55420
Resource for individuals and childbirth groups interested in family-centered birth

Maternity Center Association
48 East 92nd Street
New York, NY 10028
212-369-7300
Provides information and free brochure of publications

National Association of Childbearing Centers
Box 1, Route 1
Perkiomenville, PA 18074
215-234-8068
Provides information and suggests guidelines for birth centers

National Association of Parents and Professionals for Safe Alternatives in Childbirth (NAPSAC)
P. O. Box 267
Marble Hill, MO 63764
314-238-2010
Provides information and support for alternative childbirth experiences

VBAC (Vaginal Birth After Cesarean)
10 Great Plain Terrace
Needham, MA 01292

CHILDBIRTH EDUCATION

American Academy of Husband-Coached Childbirth
P.O. Box 5224
Sherman Oaks, CA 91413
818-788-6662
Provides information on the Bradley method of childbirth

American Society for Psychoprophylaxis in Obstetrics
1840 Wilson Blvd.
Suite 204
Arlington, VA 22201
703-524-7802
Provides information about the Lamaze method of childbirth

Childbirth Graphics, Ltd.
1210 Culver Road
Rochester, NY
716-482-7940
Provides variety of teaching aids for childbirth education

National Association of Childbirth Education, Inc. (NACE)
3940 Eleventh Street
Riverside, CA 92501

Read Natural Childbirth Foundation
P. O. Box 956
San Rafael, CA 94915
415-456-8462
Provides information about the Dick-Read method of childbirth

CIRCUMCISION

American Academy of Pediatrics
P. O. Box 927
Elk Grove, IL 60009-0927
312-869-9327
Provides report on circumcision for minimal fee

DIABETES

American Diabetes Association
44 East 23rd Street
New York, NY 10010

Juvenile Diabetes Foundation International Hotline
800-223-1138; in New York 212-889-7575

National American Diabetes Association
1660 Duke Street
Alexandria, VA 22314
703-549-1500

National Diabetes Information Clearinghouse
Box NDIC
Bethesda, MD 20892
301-468-2162

EARLY PREGNANCY LOSS/LOSS OF A NEWBORN

Centering Corp
Omaha, NE
402-553-1200

Compassionate Friends
P. O. Box 3696
Oak Brook, IL
312-990-0010
Self-help group with chapters across the country; provides support to parents whose child has died

HAND (Helping After Neonatal Death)
San Rafael, CA
415-492-0720

Resolve Through Sharing
LaCrosse, WI
608-785-0503

SAND (Support After Neonatal Death)
Berkeley, CA
415-540-0337

SHARE (Source of Help in Airing and Resolving Experiences)
c/o St. John's Hospital
800 Carpenter Street
Springfield, IL 62769
217-544-6464, x4500
Provides support for families who have miscarried or suffered the loss of a newborn

ENVIRONMENTAL AND OCCUPATIONAL HEALTH

Clearinghouse for Occupational Safety and Health Information
National Institute for Occupational Safety and Health
4676 Columbia Parkway
Cincinnati, OH 45226
513-533-8236

Environmental Protection Agency (EPA)
Public Information Center
Room PM 211-B
401 M Street, SW
Washington, DC 20460
202-382-7550

Hazardous Waste Hotline
800-424-9346

National Institute of Environmental Health Sciences
P. O. Box 12233
Research Triangle Park, NC 27709
919-541-3345

HEART DISEASE

American Heart Association
44 East 23rd Street
New York, NY 10010

Heart Information Center
National Heart Institute
U.S. Public Health Service
9000 Rockville Park
Building 31, Room 4A21
Bethesda, MD 20892

INFERTILITY

American Fertility Foundation
2131 Magnolia Avenue, Suite 201
Birmingham, AL 35256
205-251-9764

Fertility Research Foundation (FRF)
1430 Second Avenue, Suite 103
New York, NY 10021
212-744-5500
Provides information and services for infertile couples; publishes Fertility Review *and* Infertility *journals*

Resolve, Inc., for Infertility Counseling
5 Water Street
Arlington, MA 02174
617-643-2424

MEDICATIONS (PRESCRIPTION/OVER-THE-COUNTER)

Food and Drug Administration (FDA)
Office of Consumer Affairs
Public Inquiries
5600 Fishers Lane (HFE-88)
Rockville, MD 21857
301-344-3719

MIDWIFERY/NURSE-MIDWIFERY

American College of Nurse Midwives
1522 K Street, NW
Suite 1120
Washington, DC 20005
202-347-5445

Midwives Alliance of North America
c/o Concord Midwifery Service
30 South Main Street
Concord, NH 03301
603-225-9586
Organization of nurse-midwives and lay midwives in the United States and Canada

MULTIPLE BIRTH

Center for the Study of Multiple Birth
333 East Superior Street, Suite 463-5
Chicago, IL 60611
312-266-9093

National Organization of Mothers of Twins Clubs, Inc.
12404 Princess Jeanne Street, NE
Albuquerque, NM 87112
505-275-0955

NUTRITION INFORMATION (PRENATAL AND INFANT)

American Dietetic Association
216 Jackson Boulevard, Suite 800
Chicago, IL 60606-6995

American Institute of Nutrition
9659 Rockville Pike
Bethesda, MD 20814
301-443-3170

American Public Health Association
Food and Nutrition Section
1790 Broadway
New York, NY 10019

Beech-Nut Nutrition Hotline
800-523-6633; in Pennsylvania 800-492-2384

Center for Science in Public Interest
1775 S Street NW
Washington, DC 20009

Food and Drug Administration (FDA)
Office of Consumer Affairs
Public Inquires
5600 Fishers Lane (HFE-88)
Rockville, MD 20857
301-443-3170

Food and Nutrition Board
National Research Council
National Academy of Sciences
2101 Constitution Ave, NW
Washington, DC 20418

Food and Nutrition Information Center
National Agriculture Building, Room 304
Beltsville, MD 20705

March of Dimes Birth Defects Foundation
1275 Mamaroneck Avenue
White Plains, NY 10605

Mead Johnson & Company
2414 West Pennsylvania Street
Evansville, IN 47721

National Dairy Council
111 North Canal Street
Chicago, IL 60606

Ross Laboratories
Columbus, OH 43216

PLANNING A FAMILY

Association of Voluntary Sterilization, Inc. (AVS)
122 E. 42nd Street
New York, NY 10168
212-351-2500
Provides information on sterilization and referral service

Couple to Couple League International, Inc. (CCL)
P. O. Box 111184
Cincinnati, OH 45211
513-661-7612
Provides information on natural family planning techniques; publishes manual on the symptothermal method, The Art of Natural Family Planning

National Clearinghouse for Family Planning Information
P. O. Box 10716
Rockville, MD 20850
703-558-4990

Planned Parenthood Federation of America
810 Seventh Avenue
New York, NY 10019
212-541-7800

PREGNANCY

American Foundation for Maternal and Child Health, Inc.
300 Beekman Place
New York, NY 10022
212-759-5510
Conducts research on the perinatal period

COPE (Coping with Overall Pregnancy/Parenting Experience)
37 Clarendon Street
Boston, MA 02116
617-357-5588

Maternal Health Society
Box 46563, Station G
Vancouver, BC V6R 4G8

National Center for Education in Maternal and Child Health
38th and R Streets, NW
Washington, DC 20057
202-625-8400

National Maternal and Child Health Clearinghouse
3520 Prospect Street, NW, Ground Floor
Washington, DC 20057

Public Health Services
200 Independence Avenue
Washington, DC 20201
202-245-6867
Provides information and publications related to pregnancy

PREMENSTRUAL SYNDROME

Premenstrual Syndrome Action
P. O. 16292
Irving, CA 92713
714-854-4407
Provides information about PMS

PRETERM NEONATES

Parents of Prematures
13613 NE 26th Place
Bellevue, WA 98005
206-883-6040
Self-help organization that serves families with neonates in special-care nurseries; publishes directory listing local support groups for parents of preterm neonates

SEX EDUCATION

Center for Population Options
1012 14th Street, NW
Suite 1200
Washington, DC 20005
202-347-7500
Provides information to educate teenagers on sex and sexual responsibility

Planned Parenthood Federation of America
810 Seventh Avenue
New York, NY 10019
212-541-7800

SEXUALLY TRANSMITTED DISEASES

AIDS Medical Foundation
10 East 13th Street, Suite LD
New York, NY 10003
212-206-0670

Center for Prevention Services
Centers for Disease Control
1600 Clifton Road, NE
Atlanta, GA 30333
404-329-1819

Herpes Resource Center
Box 100
Palo Alto, CA 94302
415-321-5134

VD National Hotline
800-227-8922

SMOKING

American Cancer Society
90 Park Avenue
New York, NY 10016
212-736-3030

American Heart Association
7320 Greenville Avenue
Dallas, TX 75231
214-750-5300

American Lung Association
1740 Broadway
New York, NY 10019
212-315-8700

Cancer Information Clearinghouse
National Cancer Institute
Office of Cancer Communications
Building 31, Room 10A-18
9000 Rockville Pike
Bethesda, MD 20892
800-4-CANCER

Office on Smoking and Health
Technical Information Center
Park Building, Room 1-10
5600 Fishers Lane
Rockville, MD 20857

SUBSTANCE ABUSE

Al-Anon/Alateen
P. O. 862, Midtown Station
New York, NY 10018
212-254-7230

Alcoholics Anonymous
P. O. Box 459, Grand Central Station
New York, NY 10017
212-686-1100

Cocaine Anonymous
See white pages of telephone directory for local chapter

CokEnders
See white pages of telephone directory for local chapter

National Clearinghouse for Alcohol Information
P. O. Box 2345
Rockville, MD 20852
301-468-2600

National Clearinghouse for Drug Abuse Information
P. O. Box 416
Dept. DQ
Kensington, MD 20795
800-637-2045; in Maryland 800-492-6605

National Council for Drug Education
204 Monroe Street
Rockville, MD 20850
301-294-0600

National Cocaine Hot Line
800-COCAINE

National Federation of Parents for Drug-Free Youth
8730 Georgia Avenue, Suite 200
Silver Spring, MD 20910
301-585-5437

National Institute on Drug Abuse
5600 Fishers Lane
Rockville, MD 20857
301-443-1124; 800-662-HELP

National Perinatal Association
1011/2 South Union Street
Alexandria, VA 22314-3323
703-549-5523

National Self-Help Clearinghouse
33 West 42nd Street, Room 1210
New York, NY 10036

Office for Substance Abuse Prevention
Parklawn/Rockwall II
5600 Fishers Lane, 9th Floor
Rockville, MD 20857
301-443-5266

Women for Sobriety
P. O. Box 618
Quakertown, PA 18951
215-536-8026
Support group for women with drinking problems

WEIGHT CONTROL

Overeaters Anonymous
4025 Spencer Street, Suite 203
Torrance, CA 90503
213-542-8363

Weight Watchers International, Inc.
Jericho Atrium
500 North Broadway
Jericho, NY 11753-2196
516-939-0400

APPENDIX G. Maternal Medications and Their Excretion in Breast Milk

Drug (Trade name)	Classification	Use in Breast Feeding	Comments
Acetaminophen (Tylenol, others)	Analgesic, nonnarcotic	BF	Small fraction of dose excreted into breast milk. No adverse effects reported.
Acyclovir (Zovirax)	Antiinfective; antiviral	C	Excreted into breast milk and may accumulate with chronic dosing.
Amantadine (Symmetrel)	Antiparkinsonian; antiviral	C	Excreted into breast milk and may cause urinary retention, vomiting, and skin rash in nursing infant.
Amikacin (Amikin)	Aminoglycoside antibiotic	BF	Small fraction of dose excreted into breast milk, but poorly absorbed by infant. May cause alteration in bowel flora, causing diarrhea in nursing infant.
Amiodarone (Cordarone)	Antiarrhythmic	X	Plasma levels in infant 25% of mother's plasma levels. Drug has long T½ and may accumulate in nursing infant. Drug also contains iodine and may impair thyroid function of nursing infant.
Amitriptyline (many)	Psychotherapeutic agent; antidepressant; tricyclic	C	Small fraction of dose excreted into breast milk. Effects on infant after exposure to small amounts of drug unknown. No adverse effects reported.
Amoxicillin, Ampicillin (many)	Aminopenicillin; antiinfective	BF	Small fraction of dose excreted into breast milk. May cause candidiasis and alteration in bowel flora in nursing infant causing diarrhea.
Aspirin (many)	Analgesic, nonnarcotic; salicylate	C	With chronic use, low concentrations excreted into breast milk. Potential risk of inhibition of platelet function in nursing infant, but no serious adverse effects reported.
Atenolol (Tenormin)	Beta-adrenergic blocking agent; antihypertensive; antianginal	C	Concentrated in breast milk. No adverse effects reported, but may cause bradycardia in nursing infant. Long term effects after exposure in infant unknown.
Atropine (many)	Anticholinergic; antispasmodic	C	May be excreted into breast milk. Potential to cause hyperthermia and atropine toxicity in nursing infant.
Bendroflumethiazide (Naturetin)	Diuretic, thiazide	X	Suppresses lactation.
Bethanechol (Urecholine)	Cholinergic, direct acting	C	Amount excreted into breast milk unknown. Reported to cause abdominal pain and diarrhea in nursing infant.
Bisacodyl (Dulcolax)	Laxative, stimulant	BF	Not excreted into breast milk.
Bromides	Laxative, stimulant	X	Excreted into breast milk. Reported to cause drowsiness and rash in nursing infant.
Bromocriptine (Parlodel)	Dopamine receptor agonist; ovulation stimulant; antiparkinsonian	X	Suppresses lactation.
Brompheniramine (Dimetane, others)	Antihistamine; H_1 receptor antagonist	C	Excreted into breast milk. Reported to cause irritability, excessive crying, disturbed sleeping pattern in nursing infant. Avoid long-acting preparations.
Butabarbital (Butisol)	Sedative-hypnotic; barbiturate	BF	Small fractiion of dose excreted into breast milk, but amount probably insignificant.
Caffeine	Central and respiratory stimulant	C	Small amount excreted into breast milk but may accumulate in neonate if mother consumes heavy amounts. Irritability and poor sleeping habits have been reported.
Calcitonin (Calcimar, others)	Regulator, bone metabolism; hormone	C	May inhibit lactation.
Captopril (Capoten)	Antihypertensive; vasodilator	BF	Small fraction of dose excreted into breast milk. No adverse effects reported, but monitor nursing infant for hypotension.

Key: BF = compatible with breastfeeding; C = use with caution; X = contraindicated.

(continued)

Maternal Medications and Their Excretion in Breast Milk (*Continued*)

Drug (Trade name)	Classification	Use in Breast Feeding	Comments
Carbamazepine (Tegretol)	Anticonvulsant	BF	Small fraction of dose excreted into breast milk. Does not seem to accumulate in nursing infant. No adverse effects reported.
Carbenicillin (Geopen)	Penicillin, extended spectrum	BF	Small fraction of dose excreted into breast milk, but probably not significant.
Carisprodol (Soma, others)	Skeletal muscle relaxant; carbamate	C	May cause drowsiness and intestinal upset in nursing infant.
Cascara Sagrada	Laxative; stimulant	C	Amount excreted into breast milk unknown. May cause diarrhea in nursing infant.
Cefaclor (Ceclor)	Antiinfective; beta-lactam antibiotic	BF	Small fraction of dose excreted into breast milk, probably insignificant.
Cefadroxil (Duricef, Ultracef)	Antiinfective; beta-lactam antibiotic	BF	Small fraction of dose excreted into breast milk, probably insignificant.
Cefamandole (Mandol)	Antiinfective; beta-lactam antibiotic	BF	Small fraction of dose excreted into breast milk, probably insignificant. Limited data.
Cefazolin (Ancef, Kefzol)	Antiinfective; beta-lactam antibiotic	BF	Small fraction of dose excreted into milk and poorly absorbed by nursing infant.
Cefonicid (Monocid)	Antiinfective; beta-lactam antibiotic	BF	Small fraction of dose excreted into breast milk, probably insignificant.
Cefoperazone (Cefobid)	Antiinfective; beta-lactam antibiotic	BF	Small fraction of dose excreted into breast milk, probably insignificant.
Cefotaxime (Claforan)	Antiinfective; beta-lactam antibiotic	BF	Small fraction of dose excreted into breast milk, probably insignificant.
Cefoxitin (Mefoxin)	Antiinfective; beta-lactam antibiotic	BF	Small fraction of dose excreted into breast milk, probably insignificant.
Cefitizoxime (Cefizox)	Antiinfective; beta-lactam antibiotic	BF	Small fraction of dose excreted into breast milk, probably insignificant.
Ceftriaxone (Rocephin)	Antiinfective; beta-lactam antibiotic	BF	Small fraction of dose excreted into breast milk, probably insignificant.
Cephalexin (Keflex)	Antiinfective; beta-lactam antibiotic	BF	Small fraction of dose excreted into breast milk, probably insignificant.
Cephalothin (Keflin)	Antiinfective; beta-lactam antibiotic	BF	Small fraction of dose excreted into breast milk, probably insignificant.
Cephapirin (Cefadyl)	Antiinfective; beta-lactam antibiotic	BF	Small fraction of dose excreted into breast milk, probably insignificant.
Cephradine (Anspor, Velosef)	Antiinfective; beta-lactam antibiotic	BF	Small fraction of dose excreted into breast milk, probably insignificant.
Chloral hydrate (Noctec)	Sedative-hypnotic	C	Parent drug plus active metabolite excreted into breast milk. May cause drowsiness in nursing infant.
Chloramphenicol (Chloromycetin)	Antiinfective; antibiotic	X	Excreted into breast milk. Theoretical risk of bone marrow depression. May accumulate in nursing infant.
Chloroquine (Aralen)	Antiinfective; antimalorial	BF	Small amount excreted into breast milk. No adverse effects reported.
Chlorothiazide (Diuril, others)	Diuretic; antihypertensive	C or X	Excreted into breast milk in low concentrations. May suppress lactation and should be avoided in first month of lactation.
Chlorpromazine (Thorazine)	Psychotherapeutic; antipsychotic	C	Excreted into breast milk. Infant may become drowsy and lethargic.
Chlortetracycline (Aureomycin, others)	Antiinfective, antibiotic	C	Excreted into breast milk. Theoretical risk of dental staining and inhibition of bone growth in nursing infant.
Chlorthalidone (Hygroton, others)	Diuretic; antihypertensive	C or X	*See* Chlorothiazide.

Key: BF = compatible with breastfeeding; C = use with caution; X = contraindicated.

(*continued*)

Maternal Medications and Their Excretion in Breast Milk (*Continued*)

Drug (Trade name)	Classification	Use in Breast Feeding	Comments
Cimetidine (Tagamet)	H_2-receptor antagonist; antihistamine	X	Excreted into breast milk and may accumulate in nursing infant. May decrease infant's gastric acidity, inhibit drug metabolism, and cause central nervous system effects.
Clemastine (Tavist)	H_1-receptor antagonist; antihistamine	X	Excreted into breast milk. Reported to cause drowsiness, irritability, high pitched cry in nursing infant.
Clindamycin (Cleocin)	Antiinfective; antibiotic	C	Excreted into breast milk. Report of nursing infant with grossly bloody stools. No adverse effects reported in other nursing infants.
Clonazepam (Klonopin, Rivotril)	Anticonvulsant; benzodiazepine	C	Excreted into breast milk. Apnea reported in nursing infant.
Codeine (many)	Narcotic agonist analgesic antitussive	BF	Small fraction of dose excreted into breast milk. Probably insignificant.
Cyclophosphamide (Cytoxan)	Antineoplastic; alkylatine agent; immunosuppresant	X	Excreted into breast milk. May cause immune and growth suppression. Possibly carcinogenic.
Danthrone (Modane)		C	May cause increased bowel activity in nursing infant.
Desipramine (Norpramin)	Psychotherapeutic; antidepressant	C	Small fraction of dose excreted into breast milk. No adverse effects reported. Significance of prolonged exposure to nursing infant unknown.
Desmopressin (DDAVP)	Antidiuretic agent	C	Limited data, but reports of use during lactation with no apparent problems.
Dextroamphetamine (Dexedrine, others)	Amphetamine; anorexiant	C	Excreted into breast milk. May cause irritability and poor sleeping habits in nursing infant.
Diazepam (Valium, others)	Anxiclytic; anticonvulsant	X	Parent drug and active metabolite excreted into breast milk. Lethargy and weight loss reported in nursing infants.
Dienestrol (many)	Estrogen; hormone	C	No adverse effects reported. Potential for decreased milk volume and decreased nitrogen and protein content of milk.
Digoxin (Lanoxin)	Cardiac glycoside; antiarrhythmic	BF	Small fraction of dose excreted into breast milk. No adverse effects reported.
Dioctyl sodium sulfosuocinate (Colace)		BF	Not excreted into breast milk.
Diphenhydramine (Benedryl, others)	Antihistamine; antivertigo/antiemetic	C	Excreted into breast milk. Potential to cause sedation, decreased feeding, or stimulation and tachycardia.
Dipyridamole (Persantine, others)	Vasodilator; antiplatelet	BF	Small fraction of dose excreted into breast milk. No adverse effects reported.
Disopyramide (Norpace)	Antiarrhythmic	BF	Small fraction of dose excreted into breast milk. No adverse effects reported.
Doxycycline (Vibramycin, others)	Tetracycline; antiinfective; antibiotic	C	*See* Chlortetracycline.
Ephedrine (many)	Alpha- and beta-adrenergic agonist	C	*See* Brompheniramine.
Ergotamine (Ergostat, others)	Alpha-adrenergic blocking agent; antimigraine agent	X	Doses used for migraine in mother may cause vomiting, diarrhea, and seizures in nursing infant.
Erthromycin (many)	Erythromycin	BF	Excreted into breast milk. Potential for altered bowel flora in nursing infant causing diarrhea.
Estradiol (Estrace, others)	Estrogen	X	Suppresses lactation.
Ethambutol (Myambutol, Etibi)	Antituberculosis	BF	Limited data.
Ethosuximide (Zarontin)	Anticonvulsant; succinimide	C	Excreted into breast milk. May accumulate in nursing infant.
Flurazepam (Dalmane, others)	Psychotherapeutic; anxiolytic sedative/hypnotic	C	Excreted into breast milk. May cause sedation in nursing infant if used chronically by mother.

Key: BF = compatible with breastfeeding; C = use with caution; X = contraindicated.

(*continued*)

Maternal Medications and Their Excretion in Breast Milk (*Continued*)

Drug (Trade name)	Classification	Use in Breast Feeding	Comments
Folic acid (many)	Vitamin B_9	BF	Excreted into breast milk. May accumulate in nursing infant.
Furosemide (Lasix, others)	Diuretic; potassium depleting	C or X	Excreted into breast milk. Effects on nursing infant unknown. May suppress lactation.
Gentamicin (many)	Aminoglycoside antibiotic; antiinfective	BF	*See* Amikacin.
Gold sodium thiomalate (Myochrysine)	Antirheumatic; gold compound	X	Excreted into breast milk. May cause rash, inflammation of kidneys and liver in nursing infant.
Guanethidine (Ismelin, others)	Adrenergic blocking; antihypertensive	BF	Excreted into breast milk. No adverse effects reported.
Haloperidol (Haldol, Peridol)	Psychotherapeutic; antipsychotic	BF	Excreted into breast milk. No adverse effects reported, but monitor nursing infant for central nervous system depression.
Heparin (many)	Anticoagulant	BF	Not excreted into breast milk.
Hydralazine (Apresoline, others)	Antihypertensive; vasodilator	C	Small amount excreted into breast milk. No adverse effects reported. Monitor nursing infant for hypotension.
Hydrochlorothiazide (many)	Diuretic; antihypertensive	C or X	*See* Chlorothiazide.
Ibuprofen (Motrin, Advil, others)	Analgesic, nonnarcotic; NSAID	BF	Small fraction of dose excreted into breast milk. Probably insignificant.
Imipramine (Tofranil, others)	Psychotherapeutic; antidepressant	C	Small fraction of dose excreted into breast milk. Significance of prolonged exposure to nursing infant unknown.
Indomethacin (Indocin, others)	NSAID; analgesic	C	Excreted into breast milk. One report of seizure in neonate possibly related to indomethicin used by mother.
Insulin (many)	Antidiabetic	BF	Not excreted into breast milk.
Isoniazid (INH, others)	Antiinfective; antituberculosis	C	Excreted into breast milk. No adverse effects reported. Experimental studies not in humans suggest may be carcinogenic.
Labetalol (Normodyne, Trandate)	Alpha- and beta-adrenergic blocking; antihypertensive	C	Excreted into breast milk. Probably insignificant, but monitor infant for bradycardia and hypotension.
Levothyroxine (Synthroid, others)	Thyroid, hormone	BF	Small fraction of dose excreted into breast milk. Probably insignificant.
Liothyronine (Cytomel, others)	Thyroid, hormone	BF	Small fraction of dose excreted into breast milk. Probably insignificant.
Lithium (many)	Psychotherapeutic; antimanic	C	Excreted into breast milk, but no adverse effects reported. Long term effects of exposure in nursing infants unknown.
Lorazepam (Ativan, Alzapam)	Psychotherapeutic; enxiolytic	C	Small amount of dose excreted into breast milk. Potential for lethargy in nursing infant.
Magnesium sulfate (many)	Laxative, saline; replacement agent	BF	No change in stool habits seen in nursing infants whose mother's took magnesium-containing laxatives.
Mandelic acid	Laxative, saline; replacement agent	C	Excreted into breast milk and found in urine of nursing infant. Clinical significance unknown.
Maprotiline (Ludiomil)	Psychotherapeutic; antidepressant	C	Excreted into breast milk in small amounts. Long term effects of exposure in nursing infants unknown.
Medroxyprogesterone (Depo-Provera, others)	Antineoplastic; hormone, progestin	BF	No adverse effects reported.
Mefenamic acid (Ponstel, Ponstan)	NSAID; prostaglandin synthesis inhibitor	BF	Negligible amount excreted into breast milk.

Key: BF = compatible with breastfeeding; C = use with caution; X = contraindicated.

(*continued*)

Maternal Medications and Their Excretion in Breast Milk (*Continued*)

Drug (Trade name)	Classification	Use in Breast Feeding	Comments
Meperidine (Demorol, others)	Narcotic agonist analgesic; opiate agonist	BF	Excreted into breast milk, but amount probably insignificant unless meperidine used chronically and in large doses by mother.
Meprobamate (Equanil, others)	Psychotherapeutic; anxiolytic	C	Excreted into breast milk. Monitor infant for lethargy and poor feeding.
Methadone (Dolophine, others)	Narcotic agonist analgesic	BF	Excreted into breast milk. Contradictory information if can prevent withdrawal symptoms in addicted infants.
Methimazole (Tapazole)	Antithyroid agent	X	Excreted into breast milk in sufficient quantity to cause thyroid dysfunction in nursing infant.
Methocarbamol (Robaxin, others)	Skeletal muscle relaxant, central	BF	Small fraction of dose excreted into breast milk.
Methotrexate (many)	Antineoplastic; antimetabolite	X	Excreted into breast milk in small amounts, but clinical effects on nursing infant unknown.
Methyldopa (Aldomet, others)	Alpha-adrenergic agonist; antihypertensive	BF	Small amount of dose excreted into breast milk. Monitor infant for hypotension.
Metolazone (Zaroxolyn)	Antihypertensive; diuretic	C or X	*See* Chlorothiazide.
Metoprolol (Lopressor, others)	Beta-adrenergic blocking agent; antihypertensive	C	Excreted into breast milk. No adverse effects reported, but monitor nursing infant for hypotension and bradycardia.
Metronidazole (Flagyl, others)	Antiprotozoal; amesicide	C or X	Use single dose therapy in mother and discontinue breast feeding for 12 to 24 hours. If chronic use needed, breast feeding contraindicated due to potential carcinogenicity.
Minocycline (Minocin, Vectrin)	Tetracycline; antibiotic	C	*See* Chlortetracycline.
Minoxidil (Loniten, Rogaine)	Antihypertensive; vasodilator	C	Excreted into breast milk. No adverse effects reported, but monitor nursing infant for hypotension.
Morphine (many)	Narcotic agonist; analgesic	BF	Small amount of dose excreted into breast milk. Clinical significance unknown.
Moxalactam (Moxam)	Beta-lactam antibiotic; cephalosporin, third generation	X	Excreted into breast milk. Potential to cause enterocolitis in nursing infant.
Nadolol (Corgard)	Beta-adrenergic blocking agent; antihypertensive	C	Excreted into breast milk. Monitor nursing infant for hypotension and bracycardia.
Nalidixic acid (NegGram)	Antiinfective, urinary tract	BF	Excreted into breast milk in low quantity. Potential to cause hemolytic anemia in G6PD deficient infants.
Naproxen (Naprosyn, Anaprox, others)	NSAID; analgesic	BF	Small amount of dose excreted into breast milk.
Nitrofurantoin (many)	Antiinfective, urinary tract	BF	Small amount of dose excreted into breast milk. Potential to cause hemolytic anemia in G6PD deficient infants.
Nortriptyline (Pamelor, Aventyl)	Antidepressant; tricyclic; psychotropic	C	*See* Amitriptyline.
Oral contraceptives (many)	Estrogen-progestin combinations	C	Associated with shortened duration of lactation, decreased infant weight gain, decreased milk production, and decreased composition of nitrogen and protein in milk.
Oxacillin (Bactocil, Prostaphlin)	Antiinfective; antibiotic	BF	Excreted into breast milk in small quantity. Potential to cause diarrhea in nursing infant.
Oxytetracycline (Terramycin, others)	Tetracycline; antiinfective	C	*See* Chlortetracycline.
Paregoric (many)	Narcotic agonist analgesic	BF	*See* Morphine.

Key: BF = compatible with breastfeeding; C = use with caution; X = contraindicated.

(*continued*)

Maternal Medications and Their Excretion in Breast Milk (*Continued*)

Drug (Trade name)	Classification	Use in Breast Feeding	Comments
Penicillin G and V (many)	Penicillin, natural; antiinfective	BF	Small fraction of dose excreted into breast milk. Potential to cause diarrhea in nursing infant.
Pentazocine (Talwin)	Narcotic agonist-antagonist	BF	Not excreted into breast milk.
Phenobarbital (many)	Sedative/hypnotic; anticonvulsant	C	Excreted into breast milk and may accumulate in nursing infant. Monitor infant for sedation.
Phenylbutazone (Butazolidin, others)	Antirheumatic; Pyrazalone	BF	Small fraction of dose excreted into breast milk. No adverse effects reported.
Phenytoin (Dilantin, others)	Anticonvulsant; hydantoin	BF	Small fraction of dose excreted into breast milk. Methemoglobinemia, drowsiness, decreased feeding reported in one nursing infant.
Potassium iodide (many)	Replacement agent; expectorant	X	Iodide concentrates in breast milk. May inhibit thyroid function in nursing infant.
Prednisolone and Prednisone (many)	Corticosteroid; glucocorticoid	C	Small fraction of dose excreted into breast milk. Effects from prolonged exposure in nursing infant unknown.
Primidone (Mysoline, others)	Anticonvulsant	C	Small fraction of dose excreted into breast milk. Metabolite, phenobarbital, may accumulate in nursing infant. Monitor infant for sedation and decreased feeding.
Procainamide (Procan, others)	Antiarrhythmic	BF	Small fraction of dose excreted into breast milk.
Prochlorperazine (Compazine, others)	Psychotherapeutic; antipsychotic	BF	No adverse effects reported.
Propantheline (Probanthine)	Psychotherapeutic; antipsychotic	BF	Small amount excreted into breast milk. Use short acting preparation.
Propoxyphene (Darvon, others)	Pschotherapeutic; antipsychotic	BF	Small amount excreted into breast milk.
Propranolol (Inderal, others)	Antihypertensive; beta-adrenergic blocking agent	C	Excreted into breast milk. No adverse effects reported, but monitor nursing infant for bradycardia and hypotension.
Propylthiouracil (PTU)	Antithyroid	C	Small fraction of dose excreted into breast milk. Monitor nursing infant's thyroid function. Antithyroid drug of choice for mother desiring to breast feed.
Pyridostigmine (Mestinon, Regonol)	Cholinesterone inhibitor	BF	Small fraction of dose excreted into breast milk. Probably insignificant.
Pyrimethamine (Daraprim)	Antiinfective; antimalarial	BF	Excreted into breast milk. May be enough to treat malaria in nursing infant.
Quindine (many)	Antiarrhythmic	BF	Small fraction of dose excreted into breast milk.
Ranitidine (Zantac)	H_2-receptor antagonist	X	Excreted into breast milk. May decrease gastric acidity in nursing infant.
Reserpine (Serpasil, others)	Antipsychotic	BF	Excreted into breast milk. No adverse effects reported, but monitor infant for hypotension.
Rifampin (Rimactane, others)	Antibiotic; antituberculosis agent	BF	Excreted into breast milk. No adverse effects reported.
Scopolamine (many)	Anticholinergic; mydriatic	C	*See* Atropine.
Spironolactone (Aldactone, others)	Diuretic, potassium sparing	C	Small amount of metabolite excreted into breast milk. Effects on nursing infant unknown.
Streptomycin (many)	Antituberculosis agent	BF	*See* Amikacin.
Sulfasalazine (Azulfidine, others)	Antiinfective; sulfonamide	BF	Sulfapyridine (metabolite) excreted into breast milk. No adverse effects reported. Potential to cause hemolytic anemia in G6PD deficient infant.

Key: BF = compatible with breastfeeding; C = use with caution; X = contraindicated.

(*continued*)

Maternal Medications and Their Excretion in Breast Milk (*Continued*)

Drug (Trade name)	Classification	Use in Breast Feeding	Comments
Tetracycline (many)	Antiacne; tetracyclic	C	*See* Chlortetracycline.
Theophylline (many)	Antiasthmatic; xanthine	BF	Small fraction of dose excreted into breast milk. Report of irritability in nursing infant after mother ingested oral solution. Slowly absorbed product recommended while breast feeding.
Thioridazine (Mellaril, others)	Psychotherapeutic; antipsychotic	BF	No adverse effects reported.
Thyroid (many)	Thyroid agent; hormone	BF	*See* Levothyroxine, Liothyronine.
Ticarcillin (Timenti)	Antibiotic; penicillin mixture	BF	Small fraction of dose excreted into breast milk. Potential to cause diarrhea in nursing infant.
Timolol (Blocadren, Timoptic)	Beta-adrenergic blocking agent	C	*See* Propranolol.
Tobramycin (Tobrex, Nebcin)	Antiinfective; aminoglycoside	BF	*See* Amikacin.
Tolbutamide (Orinase, others)	Sulfonylurea, first generation; antidiabetic	C	Small fraction of dose excreted into breast milk. Effect on nursing infant unknown. Monitor blood glucose.
Tolmetin (Tolectin)	NSAID; analgesic nonnarcotic	C	Small fraction of dose excreted into breast milk. Effect on nursing infant unknown.
Trifluoperazine (Stelazine, others)	Psychotherapeutic; antipsychotic	BF	No adverse effects reported.
Trimeprazine (Temaril, Panectyl)	Phenothiazine antihistamine	BF	Small fraction of dose excreted into breast milk.
Trimethoprim (many)	Antiinfective, urinary tract	BF	Small fraction of dose excreted into breast milk. No adverse effects reported.
Valproic acid (Depakene, Myproic Acid)	Anticonvulsant	BF	Small fraction of dose excreted into breast milk. Probably insignificant.
Vasopressin (Pitressin)	Antidiuretic; hormone	C	*See* Desmopressin.
Verapamil (Calan, others)	Calcium channer blocking agent; antianginal	C	Excreted into breast milk. Effects on nursing infant after chronic exposure unknown.
Warfarin (Coumadin, others)	Anticoagulant, oral; coumarin	BF	Small fraction of dose excreted into breast milk. No effect on coagulation studies seen in nursing infants.

Key: BF = compatible with breastfeeding; C = use with caution; X = contraindicated.

Glossary

ABO incompatibility A disease that occurs when the fetus and mother have different blood groups; mixing of fetal and maternal blood leads to hemolysis of fetal red blood cells and an increase in bilirubin levels in the neonate.

abortion Termination of pregnancy before the fetus is viable outside the uterus (usually before 20 to 24 weeks of gestation).

- **complete a.** Abortion in which all products of conception have been expelled, including fetus, placenta, and decidua.
- **habitual a.** Spontaneous abortion occurring in three or more consecutive pregnancies.
- **incomplete a.** Pregnancy termination resulting in retention of parts of the products of conception.
- **induced a.** Intentional abortion by the use of medications or mechanical means.
- **inevitable a.** Imminent abortion characterized by cervical dilation and effacement, bleeding, and pain.
- **missed a.** Condition in which the fetus dies in utero and the products of conception are retained in the uterus.
- **spontaneous a.** Spontaneous expulsion of the products of conception occurring naturally and without external cause.
- **threatened a.** Condition in which there are signs and symptoms of impending loss of the pregnancy, such as bleeding and cervical dilation; it may progress to an inevitable abortion or it may be averted through medical treatment.

abortus Fetus that is spontaneously delivered at less than 20 weeks gestational age, or weighs less than 500 grams or measures less than 25 centimeters.

abruptio placentae Partial or complete separation of a normally implanted placenta prior to the delivery of the infant.

acceleration phase Phase of labor characterized by an intense increase in the rate of cervical dilation from approximately 3 cm to 5 cm.

accessory glands Glands of the male reproductive system consisting of the seminal vesicles, the prostate gland, and the bulbourethral glands.

achievement phase Period between 2 and 5 months postpartum during which mother begins psychologic and social role adaptation and infant develops a predictable routine.

acme Point of maximum intensity in a uterine contraction.

acrocyanosis Blue discoloration of the extremities present in most infants at birth; may persist for 7 to 10 days; caused by vasomotor instability and poor peripheral circulation during transition to extrauterine life.

acrosome Head of the spermatozoon.

acrosome reaction Sequence of events in which the acrosome of the sperm undergoes structural changes in its outer membrane and releases enzymes that dissolve the membranes of the ovum.

active immunity Development of acquired resistance as a result of an illness or immunization.

active phase Phase of labor that begins when the cervix is dilated to 3 cm and ends with the full dilation of the cervix.

acyanotic heart defect Heart defect that does not cause cyanosis; examples are pulmonary stenosis or a patent ductus arteriosus.

adolescence Period in human development between childhood and adulthood.

afterpains Pain resulting from uterine contractions that occur after the birth of an infant; they tend to last 2 to 3 days and are more severe during breastfeeding and in multiparas.

alpha-fetoprotein A glycoprotein that is synthesized in the embryonic yolk sac, developing gastrointestinal tract, and fetal liver; crosses the placenta and can be found in the maternal blood.

amblyopia Partial loss of vision not caused by a visible lesion of the eye or optic nerve.

amniocentesis Insertion of a needle into the uterus through the abdominal wall for the purpose of withdrawing amniotic fluid; used to assess fetal health and maturity.

amnion Membrane that forms the amniotic sac; contains the fetus and amniotic fluid.

androgynous Term used to describe the incorporation of both male and female characteristics.

android pelvis Male type of bony pelvis characterized by a heart-shaped outline.

anemia Condition in which the hemoglobin concentration and red blood cells are reduced below normal levels.

anencephaly Absence of the cerebrum, cerebellum, and flat bones of the skull as a result of a congenital deformity; the head is small and abnormally shaped.

anesthesia Partial or complete loss of sensation with or without loss of consciousness.

- **epidural a.** Pharmacologic therapy administered by an injection of a local anesthetic agent into the epidural space; also called an epidural block.
- **general a.** Complete loss of sensation and consciousness as a result of pharmacologic therapy; used for cesarean or operative vaginal deliveries.
- **regional a.** Pharmacologic therapy causing loss of sensation along nerve pathways of a particular organ and surrounding tissues.
- **spinal a.** Pharmacologic therapy administered by an injection into the spinal subarachnoid space that causes loss of sensation in affected tissues; also called a spinal block.

anteflexion Bending forward of the uterus onto itself.

anthropoid pelvis Type of pelvis in which the anteroposterior diameter is equal to or greater than the transverse diameter.

Apgar score Numerical scoring system used to assess a newborn's heart rate, respiratory effort, reflex irritability, muscle tone, and color at 1 and 5 minutes of age.

apnea Absence of respirations for more than 20 seconds or a pause in respirations that causes bradycardia or cyanosis.

appropriate for gestational age (AGA) Birth weight that is appropriate for gestational age.

areola Darkened pigmented ring surrounding the nipple.

Asherman's syndrome Adhesions in the uterus resulting from inflammation and infection of pelvic organs.

asphyxia Life threatening condition caused by lack of oxygen and accumulation of carbon dioxide in the body.

assessment First phase of the nursing process in which a situation is reviewed for the purpose of diagnosing a client problem.

asynclitism Oblique presentation of the fetal head in which the fetal head and pelvic plane are not parallel.

atresia Congenital absence or pathologic closure of a normal body opening.

attachment relationship Affectional ties between mother, father, and infant that develop over the first year of life.

attitude Relationship of the fetal parts to each other.

augmentation Stimulation of labor once natural labor has begun; medications such as oxytocin or activities such as breast stimulation may be used to stimulate labor.

autosome Any of the 22 pairs of identical chromosomes in males and females.

Babinski reflex Hyperextension of the toes with dorsiflexion of the great toe in response to stroking the lateral aspect of the sole upward across the ball of the foot.

bacteremia Presence of bacteria in the blood.

balanced translocation carrier Individual with a chromosomal abnormality who demonstrates no missing or extra chromosomes, but in whom genetic material is arranged abnormally.

ballottment Diagnostic technique used to detect a floating object in the body; in pregnancy, the fetus, when tapped, moves away then returns to touch the examiner's fingers.

Bandl's ring A type of pathologic retraction ring that can impede labor; the upper segment of the uterus overretracts while the lower segment overdistends; parts of the fetus may be trapped above and below the ring.

Bartholin's glands Two small mucus-secreting glands located on either side of the vaginal orifice.

baseline fetal heart rate The average fetal heart rate between contractions; normally the rate is 120 to 160 beats per minute.

battering The repeated beating of or use of force on a person without regard to personal rights; may be physical, sexual, economic, psychologic, or social.

bicornate uterus An anomalous uterus in which the fundus has two horns or is divided into two parts, also called a septate uterus.

bilateral tubal ligation Surgical procedure in which the fallopian tubes are intentionally obstructed with rings or band, or they are intentionally severed, resulting in sterilization.

biparietal diameter Transverse diameter of the fetal parietal bones, which is the widest diameter of the fetal skull; used as a determinant of fetal growth and gestational age.

birth center Free-standing center that provides homelike birthing experiences outside of the hospital setting.

birth plan Plan in which the expectant couple identifies a list of options preferred for their labor and delivery experience.

birth rate Annual number of live births per 1000 people.

birth trauma Neonatal injuries that occur during labor and delivery.

blastocyst Term used to describe the morula after it develops two layers of cells with fluid-filled spaces about 3 days after fertilization.

bloody show Blood-tinged mucus vaginal discharge that occurs as the cervix begins to dilate.

body boundary Perceived barrier that separates self from non-self or the surrounding environment.

body image Mental picture each person has about the structure of his or her own body.

bonding Rapid process occurring immediately after birth that reflects mother-to-infant attachment (not the infant's attachment to the mother).

bony pelvis Bony ring formed by the sacrum, coccyx, and two innominate (hip) bones.

brachystasis Process in which a muscle does not relax to its former length following contraction.

Braun von Fernwald's sign Asymmetric softening and enlargement of the uterus at the site of implantation.

Braxton Hicks contractions Mild intermittent, painless uterine contractions that occur during pregnancy but are not associated with true labor.

broad ligaments Ligaments that extend from each side of the uterus to the pelvic wall; they serve to stabilize the uterus in a midline position.

bronchopulmonary dysplasia (BPD) Chronic pulmonary disease that occurs in infants who have required mechanical ventilation and high levels of oxygen in the first weeks of life.

brown fat Fat deposits present in the fetus and neonate; found around adrenals, kidneys, in the neck, between the scapulas, and behind the sternum; has greater heat-producing abilities than ordinary fat; also called brown adipose tissue.

bulbourethral glands Glands located on the floor of the pelvic cavity on either side of the membranous urethra in the male; they secrete a mucinous substance that coats the surface of the urethra; also called Cowper's glands.

calendar method Pregnancy prevention method in which intercourse is avoided in the presence of the ovum; focuses on the timing of ovulation, the life span of sperm, and the life span of the ovum.

capacitation Enzymatic process that results in the removal of the plasma protein over the acrosome of the sperm.

caput Head; occiput of the fetal head appearing at the vaginal introitus before delivery of the head.

caput succedaneum Edema of the presenting part of the fetal head that occurs during labor and delivery.

cardinal movements of labor The simultaneous accommodation of the fetal anatomy to the maternal pelvis and birth canal, and passage of the fetus from the abdominal site to the external world.

care-by-parent program Component of the hospital care of high-risk newborns whereby one or both parents live in the hospital for a set period of time before the infant's discharge and are responsible for the infant's complete care.

carpal tunnel syndrome Compression of the median nerve in the carpal tunnel of the wrist causing pain, edema, and altered sensation; may be caused by increased fluid retention during pregnancy.

cephalhematoma Collection of blood beneath the periosteum of the neonate's skull caused by ruptured blood vessels during labor and delivery; also called cephalohematoma.

cephalic index Ratio of the biparietal diameter to the occipitofrontal diameter of the fetal skull; an indicator of fetal growth and development.

cephalocaudal The long axis of the body; head to tail.

cerclage Procedure in which a suture is used to encircle the cervix to keep it closed; the treatment of choice for an incompetent cervix occurring between 14 and 20 weeks of gestation.

cervical cap Small cap-shaped contraceptive that is individually sized to fit over the cervix; provides a barrier to sperm during intercourse.

cervical ripening Process by which the cervix softens to a puddinglike consistency and begins to thin out.

cervix The "neck" of the uterus, which lies between the body of the uterus and the external os; the lower portion of the cervix extends into the vagina.

cesarean delivery Delivery of a fetus through an incision made in the abdominal wall and uterus.

Chadwick's sign Bluish-violet discoloration of the vaginal mucous membranes observed around the fourth week of pregnancy and caused by increased vascularity.

chloasma Increased pigmentation of the skin over the nose and cheeks observed during pregnancy (the "mask of pregnancy") or in women taking oral contraceptives; also called melasma.

chorioamnionitis Inflammation of the amniotic membranes caused by organisms in the amniotic fluid, which then becomes infiltrated by polymorphonuclear leukocytes.

chorion Outer wall of the amniotic sac that gives rise to the placenta and the outer membrane surrounding the amnion.

chorionic villi Thin, threadlike projections of the chorion that contain capillaries and project into the maternal uterine sinuses. They help form the placenta, facilitate the exchange of nutrients between maternal and fetal circulation, and secrete human chorionic gonadotropin (hCG).

chorionic villus sampling (CVS) Aspiration of chorionic villi in the first trimester to test for the presence of chromosomal and congenital disorders.

circumcision Surgical removal of the foreskin, exposing the glans penis.

claiming Development of an awareness of a unique composite of family attributes in the neonate; this process links the neonate to the family by association.

cleavage Rapid division of the zygote, producing blastomeres; occurs between 1 and 3 days after fertilization.

climacteric Period when a woman's reproductive abilities end; characterized by physiologic and psychologic changes; includes premenopause and menopause.

clitoris Small oval body of erectile tissue located at the anterior junction of the female vulva, comparable to the male penis.

clubfoot *See* talipes equinovarus.

coitus Sexual intercourse; penile–vaginal intercourse.

coitus interruptus A pregnancy prevention method in which, during intercourse, the man withdraws his penis from the woman's vagina and ejaculates outside of the vagina.

cold stress Excessive body heat loss that results in compensatory mechanisms such as nonshivering thermogenesis to maintain the core body temperature.

colic Acute paroxysmal episodes of pain, crying, and irritability in the infant often caused by swallowing air, overfeeding, intestinal allergy, or emotional factors.

colostrum Secretion from the breast containing serum and white blood corpuscles that occurs for 2 to 3 days prior to true lactation; high in protein and provides immune properties.

conception Union of the male sperm and female ovum resulting in fertilization.

conceptual model A type of world view, a way of looking at and organizing objects and events to make them meaningful.

condom Thin rubber sheath worn over the erect penis during intercourse to prevent the sperm from entering the vagina.

constriction ring A type of pathologic uterine retraction ring resulting from tetanic contractions; may trap the fetus and prevent descent.

contemporary father Father who chooses to be actively involved and to participate fully in the childbirth experience.

continuous external monitoring A method for monitoring the fetal heart rate in which an ultrasound transducer is attached to the mother's abdomen; it registers a continuous recording of the fetal heart rate.

continuous internal monitoring A method for monitoring fetal heart rate variability in which a tiny corkscrew-shaped wire electrode is gently screwed into the presenting part of the fetus; it provides an exact continuous reading of heart rate variability.

contraction Rhythmic tightening and shorting of uterine muscles that causes effacement and dilation of the cervix.

contraction stress test (CST) A method used to evaluate the fetal response to spontaneous or induced uterine contractions; performed prior to labor.

corpus Body of the uterus.

couvade syndrome A psychophysiologic response in the male partners of pregnant women in which the men experience complaints similar to those of pregnancy, such as nausea and vomiting.

Couvelaire uterus The bluish discoloration and boardlike rigidity of the uterus caused by blood forced into the myometrium of the uterus after the premature separation of the placenta; uteroplacental apoplexy.

Cowper's glands *See* bulbourethral glands.

cradle cap Seborrheic dermatitis in the newborn characterized by an oily, yellow, crusty build-up on the scalp and face.

Cri du chat syndrome Congenital disorder caused by an abnormality in chromosome numbers; characterized by a cat-like cry, microcephaly, low birth weight, wide-set eyes, and mental and physical retardation.

crisis The impact of an event that challenges the assumed state of an individual and forces that individual to change his or her view of, or readapt to, the world, to himself or herself, or to both.

- **accidental c.** *See* crisis, situational.
- **developmental c.** Considered a normal part of growth and development; generally viewed as a period of marked physical, psychologic, and social change characterized by disturbances in life patterns; also called maturational crisis.
- **maturational c.** *See* crisis, developmental.
- **situational c.** Unexpected, stressful external event that may or may not coincide with a developmental crisis, also called accidental crisis.

critical temperature Temperature range that necessitates a metabolic response to cold in order to replace heat loss.

culdocentesis Use of a needle or incision to aspirate fluid from the pouch of Douglas through the vagina; used to confirm an ectopic pregnancy.

cyanotic heart defect Congenital cardiac defect that causes blood to shunt from the right side to the left side of the heart, producing cyanosis; an example is tetralogy of Fallot.

cystitis Inflammation and infections of the urinary bladder.

deceleration phase Phase of labor characterized by cervical dilation from 8 to 10 cm in which effacement is nearly complete; transition phase.

decidua Mucous membrane lining of the uterus (endometrium) that surrounds the ovum and is shed after delivery.

- **d. basalis** The part of the endometrium from which the maternal portion of the placenta develops.
- **d. capsularis** The part of the decidua that surrounds the chorionic sac separating it from the rest of the uterine cavity.
- **d. vera** The nonplacental decidual lining of the uterus.

decrement Decline or decrease, as in a contraction; the curve descending from the acme of a uterine contraction to the resting plateau.

dedifferentiation Expectant woman's examination and evaluation of the attitudes and behaviors of a model to determine how well these fit with her current self image as a mother.

deep venous thrombosis Thrombosis formation in a deep vein without the presence of inflammation.

denominators Landmarks of the fetal skull used to describe the relationship of the fetal presenting part to the maternal pelvis during delivery.

descent Movement downward; movement of the presenting part of the fetus into the birth canal that begins at the onset of labor and continues as the cervix effaces and dilates.

diagonal conjugate Distance between the sacral promontory and the lower posterior border of the symphysis pubis; a measurement obtained by manual internal examination to determine the diameter of the pelvic passage.

diagnostic related groups (DRGs) A legislated prospective payment system whereby hospitals receive payment for expected services rendered to clients based on their diagnosis.

diaper dermatitis Inflammation of the neonate's skin in the perineal area.

diaphragm A flexible disk that is inserted vaginally to cover the cervix; used to prevent pregnancy.

diastasis recti Separation of the rectus muscles along the midline of the abdomen occurring during pregnancy due to stretching of the abdominal wall.

dilation Widening of the external os of the cervix from a few millimeters to 10 cm in size to provide for the passage of the fetus.

dilation and curettage Procedure in which the cervix is dilated enough to allow passage of a curet into the uterus. The curet is used to scrape away the endometrium to empty the uterine contents or to obtain tissue for further examination.

dilation and evacuation Procedure used to terminate a pregnancy between 15 and 24 weeks; the cervix is dilated and the uterine walls are scraped to remove the contents.

diplopia Double vision.

discharge planning Part of the continuity of care process that focuses on preparing the client for the next phase of care.

disruption phase Period between 5 and 8 months postpartum during which the mother begins to feel conflict in balancing multiple roles as the infant's new-found mobility and activity level challenge her feelings of competence.

disseminated intravascular coagulation (DIC) Complex disorder of the clotting mechanism in the blood that can lead to overwhelming hemorrhage; may be caused by placenta abruptio, sepsis, or fetal demise.

dizygotic twins Fetuses that originate from two separate zygotes; also called fraternal twins. More common than monozygotic twins.

dominant Taking precedence over another quality or trait; prominent.

douching Cleansing of the vagina to remove sperm as a method of pregnancy prevention; also used for purposes of regular hygiene.

Down's syndrome *See* trisomy 21.

ductus deferens Duct that arises from the wall of the testis, joins with the spermatic cord, and continues to the posterior wall of the bladder; the enlarged portion of the ductus deferens (the ampulla) stores sperm.

dysmenorrhea Painful menstruation.

dystocia Difficult labor as a result of mechanical factors such as the size of the fetus, pelvic diameter, or uterine activity.

eclampsia Condition characterized by acute rise in blood pressure, proteinuria, edema, convulsions, and possibly coma, and occurring during pregnancy (usually after 20 weeks).

ectopic pregnancy Implantation and development of the fertilized ovum outside of the uterus; for example, in the abdomen or a fallopian tube.

effacement A process that thins, shortens, and flattens the uterine cervix during late pregnancy, labor, or both.

effleurage Massage technique that employs light, gentle stroking; often used on the abdomen during labor.

ejaculatory duct Duct formed by the union of the seminal vesicle and the ductus deferens; extends through the prostate gland and ends at the prostatic urethra.

embryonic disc Embryonic layer of cells that develops from the blastocyst; forms the 2 layers that will become the amnion and yolk sac.

embryonic period Period that begins at the second or third week and continues to the eighth week after fertilization.

encephalocele Protrusion of the brain through an opening in the skull caused by a congenital abnormality or trauma.

endometrial cycle Cycle of changes in the uterus that is stimulated by hormones during the ovarian cycle; consists of proliferative, secretory, and menstrual phases; also called uterine cycle.

endometriosis Condition in which endometrial tissue grows outside of the uterine cavity; frequently associated with infertility.

endometrium Innermost mucous layer of the uterus made up of a single layer of ciliated columnar epithelium, glands, and stroma.

engagement Point at which the widest diameter of the presenting part of the fetus has passed through the inlet of the maternal pelvis.

engorgement Distension or vascular congestion; a condition usually seen in the first postpartum week in which breast tissue swells due to an increased blood and lymph supply which precedes true lactation.

engrossment A parent's intense interest in or preoccupation with an infant.

epididymis Coiled portion of the excretory duct of the testis through which sperm travels.

epidural block *See* anesthesia, epidural.

episiotomy Surgical incision of the perineum performed in the second stage of labor to provide a wider vaginal opening of the perineal tissue as the fetus is delivered.

Epstein's pearls Small white cysts seen along the edge of the gum where the hard and soft palates meet; a normal condition in the neonate.

Erb-Duchenne paralysis Paralysis of the deltoid, biceps, anterior brachial, and long supinator muscles caused by traumatic injury to the brachial plexus; related to forcible traction during delivery. The neonate holds the affected arm tightly adducted and internally rotated.

erythema toxicum Benign pink papular rash with superimposed vesicles identified in the first 48 hours of life; resolves spontaneously within a few days.

eutocia Normal labor.

evaluation Last phase of the nursing process; the appraisal of the changes experienced the client as a result of the actions of the nurse.

exfoliation Scaling or flaking of the horny layer of the skin; the separation of tissue into thin layers; occurs at the placental site as necrotic tissue is sloughed off and endometrial restoration begins in the postpartum period.

extended family Any grouping of people related in some manner that is broader than the nuclear family.

external os Portion of the cervix that opens into the vagina.

external rotation Normal mechanism of labor whereby the fetal head rotates outward as the shoulders rotate inward.

external version Manipulation of the fetus through the abdominal wall to convert to a vertex or breech presentation.

fallopian tubes Slender, tubelike structures that extend laterally from each side of the uterus toward the ovary. Serve as a canal through which the ovum passes after release from the ovary and through which sperm travel, and as a site for fertilization; also called oviducts.

false pelvis Bony area above the true pelvis and linea terminalis; bounded posteriorly by the lumbar vertebrae, laterally by the iliac fossae, and anteriorally by the anterior abdominal wall.

family Small social system made of individuals related to each other by reason of strong reciprocal ties and constituting a permanent household (or cluster of households) that persists over years. *See also* extended family and nuclear family.

family developmental tasks Basic family tasks that are specific to a given stage of development in the family life cycle.

family health State of integrated dynamic functioning of the total human family within the internal and external environment and directed toward higher level functioning.

fantasy Mental imagery through which an expectant parent visualizes himself or herself and the child-to-be in the future.

female pelvis *See* gynecoid pelvis.

femininity Culturally prescribed, reinforced characteristics of the female sex, independent of gender.

fencing position *See* tonic neck reflex.

ferning Fernlike pattern of the cervical mucus seen under microscopic examination; peaks at midcycle in response to high estrogen levels.

fertilization Process in which sperm penetrates the outer layer of the ovum and begins a chain of events resulting in development of the human embryo.

fetal alcohol syndrome Syndrome of various defects observed in infants of mothers with excessive alcohol intake during pregnancy; infants are small for gestational age, microcephalic, and may have varying degrees of mental retardation.

fetal biophysical profile Fetal diagnostic technique that combines nonstress testing with ultrasonic evaluation of several parameters, such as fetal breathing movements, fetal tone, amniotic fluid volume, and placental grading.

fetal dystocia Labor complicated by malpresentation or malposition.

fetal period Period that begins at the eighth week and continues to birth.

fetoscopy Technique used to directly observe the fetus in the uterine cavity; during the procedure samples of fetal blood or tissue can be obtained.

fimbriae Fringe or fingerlike structures; for example, the fingerlike opening of the fallopian tubes.

fine motor development Indicator of neonatal developmental maturation; demonstrated by use of hands and fingers.

flexion Fetal position in which the head bends forward so that the chin approaches the chest; occurs as the fetus moves through the pelvic inlet and reaches the pelvic floor.

folk health system System of health care provision based on local beliefs and values.

fontanelle Membrane-filled area or soft spot on the fetal skull; located between the cranial bones.

- **anterior f.** Membrane-filled space located at the anterior junction of the sagittal and coronal sutures; bregma.
- **posterior f.** Membrane-filled space located at the posterior junction of lambdoidal and sagittal sutures; lambda.

Friedman curve Graphic representation of the latent and active phases in labor; also called partogram.

Gallant's reflex Normal reflex in which the neonate, placed in the prone position, curves the body toward the side of stimulus when the back is stroked in a downward motion; also called trunk incurvation.

gametogenesis Process of gamete formation and development (the ovum in the ovary and the spermatozoon in the testicle).

gender Biologic concept that refers to an individual's sex, male or female.

genotype Hereditary makeup of an individual resulting from combinations of genes.

GIFT procedure Gamete intrafallopian transfer procedure; the direct transfer of ova and washed sperm into fallopian tubes; used in the treatment of infertility.

glans penis Enlarged cone-shaped end of the penis.

Goodell's sign Softening of the cervix; a probable indicator of pregnancy.

gravida Woman who is or has been pregnant.

gross motor development Indicator of neonatal developmental maturation; demonstrated by posture, head balance, sitting, creeping, standing, and walking.

gynecoid pelvis Pelvis in which the inlet is slightly oval and the anterioposterior diameter of the inlet is slightly less than the tranverse diameter; also called female pelvis.

gynecology Branch of medicine dealing with the physiology and pathology of the female reproductive organs in the nonpregnant state.

harlequin color change Rare neonatal vasomotor disturbance characterized by dilation of blood vessels on one side of the neonate's body causing a deep red color; a normal finding.

health maintenance organization (HMO) System of health care provision in which a provider is paid in advance a set amount of money per person, regardless of health care services that are actually used by the client.

Hegar's sign Softening of the isthmus of the uterus to the point where the isthmus can be compressed on bimanual examination; a probable sign of pregnancy.

HELLP syndrome Syndrome characterized by arteriolar vasospasm causing hemolysis, elevated liver enzymes, and low platelet count; delivery is the only definitive treatment.

hemoglobin C disease Hemoglobinopathy in which lysine replaces glutamine at position 6 on the beta chain of the hemoglobin molecule; this reduces the amount of normal hemoglobin in the blood.

hemoglobinopathy Hereditary disorder characterized by an abnormal form of hemoglobin.

hemolytic diseases of the newborn Conditions in which maternal antibodies are actively sensitized against the fetal red blood cells; these sensitized maternal antibodies cross the placenta and destroy fetal or neonatal red blood cells; includes ABO incompatibility and Rh incompatibility.

heterozygous Having one dominant and one recessive gene for a trait.

high-risk client Person whose physical, emotional, or social situation presents some threat to his or her health, well being, or development.

high-risk perinatal nursing Practice of nursing of childbearing families who have an increased probability of either psychosocial or physical illness, disability, or death.

home health services Skilled, intermittent, part-time services provided under a physician's written plan of care in the residence of the client.

homoiotherms Person or animal able to maintain a constant core body temperature regardless of a wide range of environmental temperatures.

home pregnancy test Urine test for hCG that can be bought without a prescription and performed by the client in the home.

homozygous Having two identical genes for a trait.

hospital birthing room Hospital room in which the woman both labors and delivers; characterized by a family-centered homelike birth experience.

hot flash Sudden transitory sensation of heat involving the whole body; related to the cessation of ovarian functioning during menopause.

hyaline membrane disease *See* respiratory distress syndrome.

hydatidiform mole Benign abnormality of the chorionic villi; characterized by trophoblast proliferation and edema of the villus stroma; the fluid-filled villi form grapelike clusters.

hydramnios *See* polyhydramnios.

hydranencephaly Condition in which the cerebral hemispheres are absent and the space is filled with fluid.

hydrocele Condition caused by an accumulation of fluid around the testes.

hydrocephalus Excessive fluid collection in the cerebral ventricles of the fetus, causing dilation of the ventricles, thinning of brain tissue, and a markedly enlarged head size.

hymen Membranous partition that partially or wholly blocks the orifice of the vagina.

hyperbilirubinemia Presence of an abnormally high level of bilirubin in the blood.

hyperemesis gravidarum Severe and prolonged vomiting during pregnancy usually beginning in the first trimester; also called pernicious vomiting of pregnancy.

hypertonic uterus *See* uterine atony.

hysterosalpingogram Diagnostic procedure performed in the early proliferative phase of the ovulatory cycle; injection of a radiopaque dye into the uterus and fallopian tubes to determine their patency.

hysterotomy Removal of the products of conception through an incision in the uterine and abdominal walls.

iatrogenic prematurity Planned delivery of a fetus prior to term.

icterus neonatorum *See* jaundice.

identification Parental process of learning about the characteristics, appearance, and behaviors of the neonate.

imperforate hymen Presence of a membrane that completely occludes the vaginal opening.

implantation Attachment of the blastocyst to the endometrium; occurs 7 to 9 days after fertilization.

implementation Fourth phase of the nursing process; the start and completion of actions necessary to accomplish previously defined goals.

inborn errors of metabolism Genetically determined diseases that cause alterations in metabolic functioning.

incompetent cervix Anatomic defect of the cervix that results in painless dilation of the cervix without uterine contractions, usually during the second or early third trimester of pregnancy.

increment Increase or building up; used to refer to the curve that builds to the acme of a contraction, starting with the onset.

induction Artificial initiation of labor by the use of medications, primarily oxytocin, or surgical rupture of the membranes.

infant mortality rate Number of deaths of infants under 12 months of age per 1000 live births.

internalization Unconscious process by which attributes, attitudes, or standards are taken within oneself.

internal obstetric conjugate Dimension of the pelvic inlet that is obtained by subtracting 1.5 to 2 cm from the manually measured diagonal conjugate.

internal os Portion of the cervix that opens into the uterus; divides the uterine cavity and the cervical canal.

internal rotation Movement of the fetus during labor in which the anteroposterior diameter of the fetal head rotates to align with the anteroposterior diameter of the maternal pelvis.

internal version Procedure in which the examiner reaches into the uterus to turn the fetus into a position compatible with vaginal delivery.

intrauterine device Small metal or plastic form that is placed in the uterus to prevent implantation of a fertilized ovum.

intraventricular hemorrhage (IVH) One of the most common types of intracranial hemorrhage that can occur in the neonate; caused by the rupture of small fragile blood vessels in the brain.

introitus Entrance or opening of the vagina.

inverted nipples Nipples that remain flat or retract into the areola when stimulated.

in vitro fertilization (IVF) Procedure in which a mature ovum is fertilized outside of the woman's body and then placed in the uterus for implantation; used in the treatment of infertility.

involution Return of the uterus to its prepregnancy size and function.

isochromosome Structural abnormality of the sex chromosome caused by injury to the x chromosome during meiosis.

isoimmunization Development of antibodies against an antigen derived from a genetically dissimilar individual of the same species; an example is the development of anti-Rh antibodies in an Rh-negative person in response to a transfusion of Rh-positive blood.

isthmus Portion of the uterus located between the corpus and the cervix.

jaundice Yellow discoloration of the skin, sclera, and mucus membranes caused by serum bilirubin levels greater than 5 to 7 mg/dL; jaundice is also called icterus neonatorum.

- **breast milk syndrome j.** Mild to moderate jaundice that occurs in the breastfeeding infant; pregnanediol in breast milk inhibits the production of the enzyme glucuronyl transferase necessary for conjugation of bilirubin.
- **pathologic j.** Jaundice that occurs before 36 to 48 hours of life related to hyperbilirubinemia; causes include hemolytic diseases of the newborn, injuries in which an increased volume of red blood cells are hemolized, hepatitis, and sepsis.
- **physiologic j.** Jaundice that occurs at 48 hours of life, peaks at 5 to 7 days, and resolves without intervention by the tenth day of life; caused by the normal reduction of red blood cells.

karyotype Arrangement of a set of chromosomes by numerical order; used to assess actual or potential genetic alterations.

kernicterus Neurologic syndrome that results from bilirubin toxicity; the deposition of unconjugated bilirubin in the brain can result in death or impaired function.

labia majora Two folds or lips of the female external genital organs that arise just below the mons pubis and surround the vulva.

labia minora Two narrow longitudinal folds enclosed in the cleft of the labia majora.

labor Involuntary process by which the fetus and placenta are propelled from the uterus of the mother to the external environment.

lactiferous ducts Ducts within the female breast that convey milk to the nipple.

Ladin's sign Softening of the anterior part of the uterus at the midline, where the uterus and cervix join; occurs at about 6 weeks of gestation.

Lamaze technique Psychoprophylactic method of childbirth preparation.

lanugo Fine, downy hair developing on the fetus during the fourth month of gestation.

laparoscopy Procedure performed in the early follicular phase of the menstrual cycle in which a laparoscope is inserted through the abdominal wall to the abdomen and pelvis.

large for gestational age (LGA) Birth weight that exceeds the 90th percentile for gestational age.

latent phase Phase of labor that begins with the onset of true labor and ends when the cervix dilates to 3 cm.

lecithin:sphingomyelin ratio (L:S ratio) Ratio of lecithin to sphingomyelin in the amniotic fluid; used to assess fetal maturity. An L:S ratio equal to or greater than 2:1 indicates fetal lung maturity.

Leopold's maneuvers Series of four maneuvers used to determine fetal lie, presentation, position, and engagement.

let-down reflex Neurohormonal reflex that causes the ejection of breast milk through the ductal system.

leukorrhea Whitish or yellowish mucous discharge from the cervix or vagina.

lie Relationship of the long axis of the fetus to the long axis of the mother; can be longitudinal, transverse, or oblique.

linea nigra Line of darker pigmentation extending from the symphysis pubis to the top of the fundus; seen in some women during pregnancy.

linea terminalis Bony line that divides the false pelvis from the true pelvis.

live birth Birth of an infant who demonstrates signs of life such as breathing, heartbeat, or voluntary muscle movements.

lochia Spongy layer of the decidua that is discarded as vaginal discharge during the first few days after delivery.

- **l. alba** Creamy yellow vaginal discharge that follows lochia serosa on about the tenth postpartum day and continues to about 3 weeks postpartum; composed of white blood cells, bacteria, decidual cells, epithelial cells, fat, cervical mucus, and cholesterol.

l. rubra Red, blood-tinged vaginal discharge that occurs following delivery and in the first 2 to 3 days postpartum; contains primarily decidual tissue, epithelial cells, and red and white blood cells.

l. serosa Pale, serosanguineous vaginal discharge that follows lochia rubra on about the third day after delivery and continues to about the tenth postpartum day; contains decidua, red blood cells, white blood cells, bacteria, and cervical mucus.

low birth weight (LBW) Neonate weighing less than 2500 grams at birth.

male pelvis *See* android pelvis.

malpresentation Abnormal presentation; occurs when the presenting part entering the inlet is other than the completely flexed head of the fetus.

mammary gland Accessory gland of the female reproductive system that is the site of lactation during pregnancy; breast.

mammography Type of x-ray examination of the breast commonly used to screen for breast abnormalities.

masculinity Culturally prescribed, reinforced characteristics of the male sex, independent of gender.

mastitis Inflammation of breast tissue caused by a bacterial infection; occurs primarily in breastfeeding mothers.

maternal–infant dyad Term used to describe the mother and neonate immediately after birth.

maternal mortality rate Number of maternal deaths resulting from the reproductive process per 100,000 live births. There are two categories: direct maternal deaths resulting from complications of pregnancy, labor, postpartum, or interventions; and indirect maternal deaths not directly related to the childbearing cycle.

maternal sensitive period Period immediately following birth in which complex interactions occur between mother and infant that help to bind them together.

maternal transport Movement of a pregnant woman from one health care facility to another for the purpose of providing her and her fetus with specialized intensive care.

maternity care Health care provided to the childbearing family; involves physiologic, psychosocial, and cultural aspects of care.

matura gravida Pregnant woman older than 35 years.

McDonald's sign Ability of the uterus to be easily flexed at the site where the uterus and cervix join.

meconium Fetal material found in the bowel of a full-term neonate.

meconium aspiration syndrome (MAS) Condition in which the fetus aspirates or breathes fetal stool found in the amniotic fluid into the lungs or trachea, resulting in respiratory distress after delivery.

meiosis Process of two successive cell divisions resulting in the formation of four daughter cells, each with a halved number of chromosomes.

melasma *See* chloasma.

menarche First menstrual period at puberty.

Mendelian inheritance *See* single-gene inheritance.

meningocele Condition in which the meninges protrude from the spinal cord but the spinal cord is in correct position.

meningomyelocele Condition in which both the meninges and the spinal cord protrude through the spinal canal.

menopause Technically, the last menstrual period; commonly used to refer to the climacteric period during which the woman's reproductive ability ceases.

menstrual cycle Cyclic process occurring in the sexually mature female during the reproductive years in which the uterine lining is built up and shed; includes the ovarian cycle and the endometrial cycle.

menstrual extraction Method of pregnancy termination in which a plastic cannula is inserted into the endometrial cavity and uterine contents are removed with suction.

menstruation Shedding of the uterine lining at the end of the menstrual cycle; physiologic process signifying the woman's ability to reproduce.

mentum Chin; the guiding point for face presentations, which occur when the head is in complete extension.

mesoderm Intermediate germ layer of cells found at the bottom of the primitive streak; gives rise to muscle and connective tissues, and other essential organs.

metritis Puerperal uterine infection involving the endometrium, the decidua, and the adjacent myometrium.

microcephaly Condition in which the head and brain are abnormally small in relation to the body.

midpelvis Area between the pelvic inlet and pelvic outlet; also called the pelvic cavity.

midwife Provider of care to childbearing women; derived from "mid" meaning "with" and "wif" meaning "wife" or "women."

certified nurse–m. Professional nurse who had completed a formal program in caring for the childbearing family and who has successfully passed a certification examination.

lay m. Person who helps women with childbirth; may have formal training or no training in childbirth practices.

midwifery Practice of a nurse who is responsible for the management of the childbearing woman.

milia Small, white papules caused by plugging of the sebaceous glands on the nose, face, forehead, and upper torso of the neonate; a normal condition that disappears within a few weeks.

milk stools Yellow and pasty or waterish stools that appear by the fourth day postdelivery.

mimicry Copying of behaviors, practices, or customs of another.

minipill Oral contraceptive pill containing only progestogen.

mitosis Process of cell division resulting in the formation of two daughter cells, each with the same number of chromosomes as the parent cell.

mittelschmerz Ovulatory pain occurring at the time of ovulation in the lower quadrant of the abdomen; a sign of ovulation.

molding Fetal skull changes that occur during labor and delivery; caused by accomodation of the fetal head to the maternal pelvis.

mongolian spot Irregular dark pigmented area on the posterior lumbar region; may persist until age 2; these areas have no clinical significance.

monosomy Chromosomal abnormality in which one chromosome is missing so that the human body cells contain one less than the normal complement of 46 chromosomes.

monozygotic twins Twins that originate from one zygote; also called identical twins.

mons veneris Pubic mound; the pad of fatty tissue over the symphysis pubis in the female.

Montgomery glands Modified sebaceous glands on the surface of the areola that enlarge during pregnancy and lactation.

morning-after pill High dose of synthetic estrogen taken orally in the first days after possible pregnancy; causes the endometrial lining to shed.

morning sickness Nausea and vomiting that occur in 50 percent of pregnant women; usually begins shortly after the first missed menses and ends by the 12th week of gestation; symptoms can occur at any time of day.

Moro reflex Normal reflex in which the neonate responds to a sudden stimulus by first abducting and extending the arms symmetrically and then adducting them in an embracing movement prior to returning to a relaxed position.

morula Developmental stage of the ovum by about the third day after fertilization; a mulberrylike mass of cells consisting of about 12 to 16 blastomeres.

mosaicism Genetic mutation that results in an unequal number of chromosomes in the cells; some cells are normal while others are not.

mucus plug Mucus that blocks the cervical canal during pregnancy, acting as a barrier to protect the fetus from some infections.

multifactorial inheritance Pattern of inheritance in which the presence of multiple genes and environmental influences determine a certain genetic trait; also called non-Mendelian inheritance.

multigravida Woman who has been pregnant two or more times.

multipara Woman who has had two or more pregnancies that terminated at the stage at which the fetuses were viable.

myometrium Middle layer of the uterine corpus, which is continuous with the muscular layer of the fallopian tubes and the vagina.

myotonia Muscle tension.

Nagele's rule Most common method of determining a delivery date; obtained by subtracting 3 months from the first day of the last normal menstrual period and then adding 1 year and 7 days to that date.

natural childbirth Method of childbirth that does not use analgesics or anesthetics.

necrotizing entercolitis (NEC) Acute, potentially life-threatening gastrointestinal disorder, ischemic injury to the bowel causes infection and malabsorption of nutrients.

neonatal mortality rate Number of infant deaths occurring in the first 28 days of life per 1000 live births.

neonatal period First 28 days of life.

neonatal sepsis Bacterial infection found primarily in the blood, occurring during the first 4 weeks after birth.

neonatal transport Movement of a neonate from one health care facility to another; usually for the purpose of providing intensive or specialized care.

neonatology Study of the neonate.

neural tube defect Group of central nervous system malformations that occur when the embryonic neural tube does not develop normally; the brain, spinal cord, and overlying tissues may be affected.

neutral thermal environment Environmental temperature at which an individual is able to maintain a normal internal temperature with minimal metabolism and oxygen consumption for heat production.

nevus flammeus Congenital red discoloration of the skin caused by an overgrowth of the cutaneous capillaries; also called port-wine stain.

nondisjunction Failure of homologous pairs of chromosomes to separate, or the failure of two chromatids of a chromosome to split; results in an abnormal number of chromosomes in the daughter cell.

non-Mendelian inheritance *See* multifactorial inheritance.

nonshivering thermogenesis Process that increases the metabolic rate and rate of oxygen consumption in the neonate, generating heat.

nonstress test (NST) Assessment technique performed in the third trimester; used to monitor response of the fetal heart rate to movement.

nuclear family Family grouping generally including one or two parents and their children.

nuclear magnetic resonance (NMR) imaging Assessment technique that provides a computer-derived image based on the detection of energy in the nuclei of atoms within the body.

nulligravida Woman who has never been pregnant.

nullipara Woman who has not carried a pregnancy to viability.

nursing diagnosis Nursing judgment or conclusion referring to a potential or actual problem or strength of a client that falls within the scope of nursing intervention.

nursing process Systematic method of delivering nursing care; a problem-solving process.

obstetric conjugate True anteroposterior diameter of the pelvic inlet; usually about 11 cm.

obstetrics Branch of medicine that deals with the phenomena and management of pregnancy, labor, and the postpartum period.

occiput Region in the back of the head, behind and inferior to the posterior fontanelle.

oligohydramnios Abnormally low amount of amniotic fluid.

oogenesis Process of ovum cell formation.

oophoritis Inflammation of an ovary.

oral contraceptive Pill taken orally to prevent pregnancy; currently the most effective method of reversible pregnancy prevention.

organogenesis Period of embryonic development between 4 and 8 weeks during which all major organ systems are formed.

osteoporosis Deossification of bone tissue causing structural weakness.

outcome criteria Preset client goals, which are evaluated in the final step of the nursing process.

ovarian cycle Part of the menstrual cycle; consists of the follicular phase, ovulation, the luteal phase, and the premenstrual phase.

ovary One of two almond-shaped organs located in the upper pelvic cavity near the ends of the fallopian tubes.

oviduct *See* fallopian tubes.

ovulation Periodic release of a mature, unfertilized ovum from the ovary.

ovum Female germ cell (gamete), or egg.

palmar erythema Redness of the palms of the hands that may occur during pregnancy because of high estrogen levels; disappears after pregnancy.

palmar grasp reflex Normal reflex in which the neonate's fingers curl around an object (such as a finger) that is pressed against the palm.

Papanicolaou (PAP) smear Screening test for precancerous and cancerous conditions of the vagina, cervix, and endometrium; during a pelvic examination, a cotton-tipped applicator or spatula is used to obtain a smear that is sent to a laboratory for microscopic examination.

paracervical block Type of regional anesthesia in which a local anesthetic agent is injected directly into the cervix; this relieves (or "blocks") discomfort from uterine contractions and cervical dilation during labor.

parametrial cellulitis Puerperal infection that begins in the uterus and spreads into the broad ligament; may spread to the ovaries and fallopian tubes; also called parametritis.

parametritis *See* parametrial cellulitis.

paraurethral glands *See* Skene's gland.

parity Number of past pregnancies that have reached viability.

passive immunity Short-lasting immunity provided by the transfer of maternal antibodies (IgG) to the fetus in utero.

patent ductus arteriosus (PDA) Neonatal condition in which the ductus arteriosus does not close spontaneously in the first weeks of life.

pelvic cavity. *See* midpelvis.

pelvic inlet Upper entrance to the true pelvis; also called the superior strait.

pelvic outlet Lower aperture of the pelvic canal; the lower border of the true pelvis.

pelvimetry Measurement of diameters or distances between the bony structures of the pelvis.

penis Male organ of copulation which deposits sperm into the vagina during sexual intercourse; also conducts urine.

percutaneous umbilical blood sampling (PUBS) Insertion of a needle through the abdominal wall of the mother into the umbilical cord to obtain fetal blood samples.

perimetrium Outermost serous layer of the uterus.

perinatal mortality rate Number of stillbirths plus the number of neonatal deaths per 1000 live births.

perinatal nursing Practice of professional nursing in response to the needs of the high-risk or low-risk family through the antepartal, intrapartal, postpartal, and neonatal periods.

perinatal period Period extending from the 28th week of gestation through the neonatal period (first 28 days after birth).

perinatal transmission Transmission of an infection from the mother to the fetus during pregnancy.

perinatology Study of the childbearing family through the span of gestation and the neonatal period.

perineum Area between the vagina and the anus.

periodic breathing Breathing pattern in which the neonate has 5- to 10-second periods of apnea, followed by a respiratory rate of 50 to 60 breaths per minute, resulting in an overall respiratory rate of 30 to 40 breaths per minute; commonly seen in preterm neonates.

peritonitis Inflammation of the peritoneum.

pernicious vomiting of pregnancy *See* hyperemesis gravidarum.

personal space Immediate area around the body.

petechiae Tiny hemorrhagic spots on the skin that result from increased intravascular pressure in the capillaries during delivery.

phase of maximum slope Greatest increase in the rate of cervical dilation in which dilation averages 3 cm an hour.

phenotype Characteristics or appearance of an individual that result from interaction of a genotype and environmental factors.

phenylketonuria (PKU) Inborn error of metabolism transmitted by an autosomal recessive trait, which causes excess phenylalanine to build up in the body; if not treated, it can result in brain damage and mental retardation.

physical recovery rate Period from birth to 1 month during which biologic adaptation dominates as the mother recovers from birthing and the neonate makes the transition to the external world.

physiologic anemia of pregnancy Condition that occurs during the second trimester of pregnancy as plasma volume increases, resulting in hemodilution and a decrease in hemoglobin concentration.

physiologic retraction ring Area of constriction that develops in normal labor between the upper active segment of the uterus and the lower more passive segment of the uterus.

pica Craving for unusual or nonnutritive substances that may occur as a result of emotional disturbances, malnutrition, or during pregnancy.

Piskacek's sign Enlargement and softening in the cornual area occurring early in pregnancy.

placental membrane Multiple-layer membrane of fetal tissue composing the chorionic villi.

placenta previa Implantation of the placenta over or very near the cervical os.

placing reflex Normal reflex action in which the neonate flexes the knees and hips and moves the legs upward when positioned upright with the dorsal surface of the feet placed against the edge of the table.

planning Third phase of the nursing process; involves setting goals, prioritizing, and designing methods to resolve problems and reach goals.

plantar grasp reflex Normal reflex in which the neonate's toes curl downward in response to pressure at the base of the toes.

platypelloid pelvis Type of pelvis in which the inlet is oval with a wide transverse diameter and a short anterior-posterior diameter.

point of viability Point at which the fetus can reasonably survive outside of the uterus; usually considered to be 20 weeks of gestation.

polycystic ovary Condition in which one or both ovaries have a thick fibrous surface with multiple cysts that may impede ovulation.

polycythemia Condition in which there is a surplus of red blood cells in the circulation.

polydactyly Presence of extra digits on the hands or feet.

polyhydramnios Excessive quantity of amniotic fluid, usually greater than 2000 mL; also called hydramnios.

port-wine stain *See* nevus flammeus.

position Relationship of landmarks (denominators) of the fetal presenting part to the sides, front, or back of the maternal pelvis.

postcoital test Diagnostic procedure in which the cervical mucus is examined 6 hours after intercourse during the period of ovulation to determine the integrity of the mucus and assess for the presence of sperm; also called Sims–Huhner test.

postdate neonate *See* postmature neonate.

postmature neonate Neonate born after the end of 42 weeks of gestation; also called postdate neonate.

postmenopausal period Period during which the symptoms of the climacteric occur; commonly used to refer to the rest of a woman's life after menopause.

postovulation method Method of pregnancy prevention in which a couple abstains from intercourse until 3 days after ovulation.

postpartum depression Depressive state, following delivery, that last 6 to 8 weeks and is characterized by mood instability, fatigue, appetite and sleep disturbances, feeling of isolation and hopelessness, and difficulties in interpersonal relationships.

postpartum hemorrhage Hemorrhage occurring 24 to 48 hours after delivery.

postpartum period Period from one to several months after birth.

postpartum psychosis Severe psychiatric condition that occurs in the puerperium and is characterized by delusions, hallucinations, and disorganized or catatonic behavior.

postterm pregnancy Pregnancy that continues past the estimated date of confinement or beyond 42 weeks of gestation.

pre-eclampsia Disorder of pregnancy that includes pregnancy-induced hypertension, proteinuria, and/or generalized edema; mild forms of the disorder can quickly become severe and critical; also called toxemia of pregnancy.

pre-embyonic period First 14 days after conception; characterized by rapid cellular multiplication and differentiation, establishment of embryonic membranes, and the development of primary germ layers.

pregnancy-induced hypertension Condition characterized by an abnormal rise in blood pressure during pregnancy; three categories include hypertension, pre-eclampsia, eclampsia.

premature neonate Neonate born before the end of 37 weeks of gestation.

premenopause Period of decreased ovarian reproductive ability.

premenstrual syndrome (PMS) Syndrome of physical and emotional symptoms that can occur 1 to 2 weeks before the start of menstruation and that disappears at the start, or shortly after the start, of menstruation.

prenatal attachment Maternal behaviors related to the developing relationship with the fetus; includes calling the fetus by name, imagining what the fetus looks like, imagining the role of mother, and choosing names.

presentation Denotes the part of the fetus that is closest to the pelvic inlet of the mother.

- **brow p.** Presentation in which the fetal head is partially extended and the presenting part is the brow.
- **complete breech p.** Presentation in which the fetus presents buttocks first with flexion at both hips and knees.
- **compound p.** Presentation in which more than one part of the fetus presents; for example, the head and an arm.
- **face p.** Presentation in which the fetal head is completely extended with the widest part of the face presenting for delivery.
- **footling breech p.** Presentation in which the presenting part is one or both feet with extension at both hips and knees; also called incomplete presentation.
- **frank breech p.** Presentation in which the buttocks present with the thighs flexed and the legs extending over the anterior surface of the fetal body.
- **shoulder p.** Presentation in which the long axis of the fetus is perpendicular to the long axis of the mother; also called transverse lie.
- **vertex p.** Most efficient type of fetal presentation; the head is flexed and the occiput is the presenting part.

preterm birth Delivery of a neonate after the age of viability but before the completion of 37 weeks of gestation.

preterm labor Any true labor experienced between 20 and 38 weeks of gestation.

primary infertility Inability to conceive or carry a pregnancy to a live birth with no previous history of pregnancy.

primigravida Woman who is pregnant for the first time.

primipara Woman who has delivered one fetus past the point of viability, whether or not the child was alive at the time of delivery.

primitive streak Groove that appears on the ectoderm of the embryonic disc at the end of the second week of development.

professional health care system Provision of health care by a group of health care professionals serving clients who have been educated through formal programs of professional education.

prostaglandin instillation Method of terminating a pregnancy around 15 weeks gestation; prostaglandins are administered intravaginally or intraabdominally causing uterine contractions to empty the uterus.

prostate gland Gland located beneath the bladder in the male that secretes the milky fluid which is added to semen.

proteinuria Presence of an excessive amount of serum protein in the urine.

proximodistal Proceeding from the central axis of the body and moving outward toward the extremities.

psychoprophylaxis Training of mind and body to cope with stressful stimuli; a childbirth preparation technique.

ptyalism Excessive secretion of saliva; often occurs during the first trimester.

puberty Period in which the endocrine and gametogenic functions of the ovaries and testes develop to the point at which reproduction can take place.

pudendal block Type of regional anesthesia in which a local anesthetic is injected in the area of the pudendal nerves; this relieves (or "blocks") sensations around the vagina.

puerperal fever *See* puerperal infection.

puerperal infection Bacterial infection that arises in the genital tract after delivery; also called puerperal fever.

puerperal mobidity Infection as demonstrated by a temperature of 100.4°F (38° C) or higher on any 2 of the first 10 days postpartum (exclusive of the first 24 hours).

puerperium First 6 weeks after delivery during which the woman's body undergoes multiple physiologic changes in response to childbirth.

quickening Mother's perception of the first fetal movements; usually occurs between 17 and 20 weeks of gestation.

recessive Potential quality or trait that is not expressed.

regionalization A way of organizing services within a geographic area so that maternal and perinatal health care is maximally used in the safest and most cost-effective way.

regurgitation Backflow of food from the stomach to the mouth with vomiting.

reorganization phase Period that begins around 8 months postpartum and continues beyond 12 months during which maternal biologic, psychologic, and social adaptation is evident; the mother individuates and returns to prepregnancy activities; the infant continues to grow, develop, and master the environment.

replication Voluntary search for and trying on of separate valued elements in behavior and attitude that are esteemed by society; constitutes the primary method of incorporation of the maternal role.

respiratory distress syndrome Pulmonary disorder in which the lungs lack the pulmonary surfactants required for respiration; occurs most often in preterm neonates; also called hyaline membrane disease.

restitution Turning of the fetal head after it emerges from the birth canal back to the position it assumed when it first entered the pelvis; restores anatomical alignment of the neck and shoulders.

retinopathy of prematurity (ROP) Disease process that occurs in the blood vessels in the retina of the eyes and can lead to significant vision impairment; associated with high levels of oxygen administered to preterm neonates.

retrocession Displacement of the uterus in which both the cervix and corpus bend backward toward the sacrum.

retroflexion Displacement of the uterus in which the corpus bends back toward the cervix, resulting in a sharp angle.

retrograde ejaculation Condition in which the sperm flows backward into the bladder instead of out of the penis.

retroversion Displacement of the uterus in which uterus tips backward so that the uterine fundus is lying in the pouch of Douglas instead of anteriorly on the bladder.

Rh isoimmunization Hemolytic disease arising from incompatibility of Rh factors of maternal and fetal blood which causes an antigen–antibody reaction; see also isoimmunization.

role Behaviors, attitudes, and actions of a person related to a certain situation.

role playing Trying on of a role; for example, attainment of the maternal role involves role modeling behaviors.

rooting reflex Normal reflex in which stroking the neonate's cheek, lip, or mouth causes the neonate to turn his or her head in the direction of the stimulus.

round ligaments Ligaments found on either side of the fundus; they are continuous with the ovarian ligaments and extend into the broad ligament.

rupture of membranes Tearing of the amniotic membranes prior to or during labor; may be spontaneous or artificial.

- **artificial r. o. m.** Intentional rupture of the amniotic membranes during labor through the use of an instrument such as an amnihook.
- **premature r. o. m.** Spontaneous rupture of the amniotic membranes before the onset of active labor and contractions.
- **spontaneous r. o. m.** Natural tearing of the amniotic membranes.

sacrouterine ligaments Ligaments extending from supravaginal portion of cervix to the sacrum; they support the corpus and cervix, keeping the uterus in the anterior position.

saddle block Type of regional anesthesia in which a local anesthetic is injected into the spinal subarachnoid space; the level of anesthesia extends to the tenth dermatome; used for vaginal deliveries.

saline termination Method of terminating a pregnancy after 16 weeks of gestation; saline solution is injected into the amniotic sac causing uterine contractions that expell the products of conception.

salpingitis Inflammation of the fallopian tube.

scrotum Pouchlike structure divided in the middle by a septum, forming two sacs, each containing one testis, one epididymus, and part of the spermatic cord.

secundagravida Woman pregnant for the second time.

semen Fluid ejaculated from the erect penis; contains sperm and secretions of the accessory glands and epididymus.

seminal vesicle Pouchlike structure that joins the end of each ductus deferens to become the ejaculatory ducts.

seminiferous tubule Tubule of the testes that carries sperm.

separation–individuation Process by which the infant separates psychologically from the mother to become an autonomous individual.

septate uterus *See* bicornate uterus.

septic pelvic thrombophlebitis Puerperal infection that originates in the uterus and spreads along the venous route into the pelvis; causes thrombosis within the veins.

sex chromatin Inactivated X chromosome; also called Barr body.

sex role behaviors Culturally prescribed behaviors assigned to men and women based on gender.

sexually transmitted disease (STD) Category of disease transmitted through sexual intercourse and intimate sexual contact with the genitals, mouth, or rectum.

shoulder dystocia Difficult labor that occurs when the anterior shoulder of the fetus becomes impacted behind the symphysis pubis.

sickle cell anemia Genetically transmitted hemoglobinopathy in which valine is substituted for glutamine on the beta chain of the hemoglobin molecule; this causes the hemoglobin molecules to assume a sickle shape and results in blood flow impairment that can lead to organ failure.

Sims-Huhner test *See* postcoital test.

sinciput Brow region bounded superiorly by the anterior fontanelle and the coronal sutures and inferiorly by the orbital ridges.

single-gene inheritance Pattern of inheritance in which the presence of one gene can cause the genetic determination of a certain trait; there are four types of single-gene patterns of inheritance: autosomal dominant, autosomal recessive, X-linked dominant, and X-linked recessive; also called Mendelian inheritance.

Skene's gland Paraurethral gland; one of numerous mucous glands in the wall of the female urethra.

small for gestational age (SGA) Birth weight below the tenth percentile for gestational age.

spermatic cord Structure containing the vas deferens, blood vessels, nerves, and muscle fibers, that supports the testes within the scrotum.

spermatogenesis Process by which spermatogonia, the immature sperm cells, are transformed into spermatozoa, mature sperm.

spermatozoa Mature sperm cells.

spermicidal agent Chemical substance that destroys sperm; used as a contraceptive method.

spina bifida occulta Condition in which the vertebral laminae do not fuse in an isolated area of the spine.

spinal block *See* anesthesia, spinal.

spinnbarkeit Refers to elasticity of the cervical mucus present at ovulation.

squamocolumnar junction Location in the cervical canal where squamous epithelium cells meet columnar epithelium cells; exact location will vary according to a woman's age and number of deliveries.

stages of labor Division of labor using variables of time, effacement/dilation of the cervix, and maternal behavioral responses.

- **first s. o. l.** Process in which the cervix dilates from 1 to 10 cm; begins with the onset of true labor contractions and ends when dilation is accomplished.
- **fourth s. o. l.** Begins with delivery of the placenta and membranes and ends with the initial physiologic adjustment and stabilization of the mother's body systems, approximately 1 to 4 hours postpartum.
- **second s. o. l.** Begins with the complete dilation and effacement of the cervix and ends with the birth of the baby.
- **third s. o. l.** Begins with the birth of the baby and ends with the expulsion of the placenta and membranes; also called placental stage.

station Relationship of the presenting part of the fetus to an imaginary line drawn between the pelvic ischial spines.

stenosis Narrowing or constricture of a tube or lumen.

stepping reflex Normal steplike movements of the feet and legs elicited by holding the neonate in an upright position and allowing one foot to touch a flat surface.

sterility Absolute inability to conceive. State of being free of living microorganisms.

stillbirth An infant past the point of viability who is born dead.

stork bites *See* telangiectatic nevi.

strabismus Abnormal eye condition related to incoordination of the extrinsic occular muscles.

striae gravidarum Reddish or purple streaks that develop in the skin over the maternal abdomen, breasts, thighs, and hips; also called stretch marks.

stress An emotional–psychophysiologic state of an organism that occurs in a situational context involving stimuli that serve as cues to elicit anxiety or fear responses.

- **physiologic s.** Disturbances or functions of body systems and tissues as a result of an insult by a dangerous stimulus.

psychologic s. Physiologic and psychologic changes that occur as a result of a stimulus that never actually comes in contact with body tissues.

subinvolution Delay or failure of the uterus to return to normal size in the postpartum period.

substance abuse Compulsive and repetitive use of a chemical substance despite detrimental social, physical, or psychologic effects.

sucking reflex Normal reflex present in a term neonate that is stimulated by hunger or the rooting reflex.

superior strait *See* pelvic inlet.

supine hypotensive syndrome Decrease in venous return from the lower portion of the body caused by a heavy uterus pressing on the inferior vena cava and abdominal aorta; this results in arterial hypotension; also called vena caval syndrome.

surfactant Phospholipid that lowers surface tension in the lungs and maintains alveolar patency, thus allowing for expansion of the lungs; essential for adequate respirations at birth.

surrounding stimuli of labor Range of situations or experiences that have an impact on a woman's perception of the labor process; these may include environment, social support systems, fatigue, nausea, fear, and pain.

sutures Connection of adjoining bones of the skull; in the fetus, these are membrane-filled spaces.

coronal s. Membrane-occupied space found between the parietal and frontal bones, extending transversely on both sides of the anterior fontanelle.

frontal s. Membrane-occupied space between the two frontal bones.

lambdoidal s. Membrane-occupied space between the occipital bone and the two parietal bones, extending transversely on either side of the posterior fontanelle.

sagittal s. Membrane-occupied space between the parietal bones in an anteroposterior direction of the skull.

swallowing reflex Normal reflex present in the newborn that involves the transfer of oral feedings from the mouth to the esophagus.

symbiotic unity State in which the infant's identity merges with the mother; a subphase of separation–individuation.

sympto-thermal method Pregnancy prevention method in which basal body temperature is taken daily and cervical mucus is assessed daily to predict ovulation.

synclitism Position of the fetal head in the pelvic inlet in which the smallest diameter of the head enters the widest part of the pelvic inlet; the best position for descent.

syncytial membrane Thin membrane that results from changes in the placental membrane; lies in close proximity to fetal circulatory network.

syndactyly Malformation in which fingers or toes are webbed or fused together.

system Set of different parts that are directly or indirectly related in a stable but dynamically changing cause-and-effect relationship.

talipes calcaneovalgus Deformity of the foot in which there is permanent dorsal flexion causing the weight of the body to rest on the heel and an inversion of the foot causing the outer side of the foot to touch the ground.

talipes equinovarus Deformity in which the foot turns inward and is fixed in a planter flexion position; also called clubfoot.

tampon Plug inserted into the vagina for the purpose of absorbing menstrual flow.

telangiectasis Small dilated end-arterioles thought to be related to increased estrogen production during pregnancy; also called vascular spiders.

telangiectatic nevi Capillary hematomas found on a newborn's neck, eyelids, forehead, and nose.

temperament Combination of physical, emotional, intellectual, and moral qualities that make up a person's attitude and personality.

testes Two oval-shaped organs located in the scrotum, in which testosterone and sperm are produced.

thalassemia Form of anemia that results from an alteration in the gene normally controlling the rate of polypeptide chain synthesis; a hypochromic microcytic anemia.

thrombophlebitis Inflammatory process involving clot formation in a superficial vein.

thrush Fungal infection caused by *Candida albicans* characterized by small white patches on the tongue and buccal membranes.

tonic neck reflex Normal reflex elicited by turning the neonate's head to one side. The extremities on the same side extend and the extremities on the opposite side flex; also called fencing position.

total abstinence Complete avoidance of intercourse to prevent pregnancy.

toxemia of pregnancy *See* pre-eclampsia.

toxic shock syndrome Rare but potentially life-threatening condition thought to be caused by toxins produced by the *Staphylococcus aureus* bacterium.

traditional father Father whose participation in the child-bearing experience tends to be that of an observer.

transcultural nursing Nursing care that recognizes and respects the way in which different cultures perceive, know, and practice health care.

transitional stools Watery or loose, greenish brown to yellowish brown stools that appear by the third day post-delivery.

transverse diameter Largest diameter of the pelvic inlet; the greatest distance between the linea terminalis on each side of the pelvis.

transverse lie *See* shoulder presentation.

trisomy Chromosomal abnormality in which three homologous chromosomes are present rather than the normal two.

trisomy 21 Most common numerical autosomal abnormality in which there are three number 21 chromosomes instead of two; affected infant is characterized by mental retardation and mongoloid features; also called Down's syndrome.

trophoblast Outer layer of cells of the developing blastocyst that will establish the nutrient relationship with the uterine endometrium.

true conjugate Measurement from the upper margin of the symphysis pubis to the sacral promontory.

true pelvis Area of the pelvis located below the linea terminalis; the upper portion is bounded by the sacral promontory, linea terminalis, and upper margins of the pelvic bones; the lower part is bounded by the margins of the ischial tuberosities and the end of the coccyx.

trunk incurvation *See* Gallant's reflex.

Turner's syndrome Genetic abnormality in which a female has only one X chromosome; nondysjunction during spermatogenesis results in the absence of the paternal X chromosome.

urethra Tubular passageway for urine in the female and for urine and sperm in the male.

urethral meatus External opening of the urethra.

uterine atony Inability of the uterine myometrium to contract around the blood vessels supplying the site of placental implantation; also called hypertonic uterus.

uterine cycle *See* endometrial cycle.

uteroplacental apoplexy *See* Couvelaire uterus.

uterus Pear-shaped muscular organ which, in the nonpregnant woman, is located between the urinary bladder and the rectum.

vacuum aspiration Method of terminating a pregnancy of less than 12 to 13 weeks; a cannula is inserted and the uterine contents withdrawn using suction.

vagina Musculomembranous tube extending from the uterus to the vulva and measuring 10 centimeters in length; it is located between the rectum and bladder.

vaginal birth after cesarean (VBAC) Vaginal birth of an infant in a woman who has had at least one previous cesarean delivery.

vaginal sponge Pliable round device made of polyurethane and containing a spermidical agent that is inserted vaginally to cover the cervix; used to prevent penetration of sperm during intercourse.

vascular spiders *See* telangiectasis.

vasectomy Surgical procedure during which both vasa are isolated, cut, and tied; method of male sterilization.

vasocongestion Pooling of blood causing enlargement of a body area.

vernix caseosa Fatty secretion from fetal sebaceous glands and epidermal cells that covers the fetus protecting the skin from abrasions or damage in utero.

vertex Area of the head between the anterior and posterior fontanelles and bounded laterally by the parietal bones.

very low birth weight (VLBW) Neonate weighing less than 1500 grams at birth.

vulva External female genitalia, including the mons veneris, labia majora, labia minora, clitoris, and vestibule.

weaning Gradual process of discontinuing breast milk and substituting other types of nourishment for the infant.

Wharton's jelly Connective tissue rich in mucopolysaccharides surrounding and protecting the blood vessels in the umbilical cord.

yolk sac Structure that arises from the endoderm of the embrionic disc; transfers nutrients to the embryo and provides blood cells until embryonic/fetal hemopoiesis begins; cells of the yolk sac become incorporated into embryonic/fetal organs.

zygote Cell formed by the union of two gametes (sperm and ovum); a fertilized egg.

Index

A

Page numbers followed by t or f indicate tables or figures, respectively; page numbers followed by b indicate boxed material.

Page numbers followed by t or f indicate tables or figures, respectively; page numbers followed by b indicate boxed material.

Page numbers followed by t or f indicate tables or figures, respectively; page numbers followed by b indicate boxed material.

Page numbers followed by t or f indicate tables or figures, respectively; page numbers followed by b indicate boxed material.

Page numbers followed by t or f indicate tables or figures, respectively; page numbers followed by b indicate boxed material.

C

Page numbers followed by t or f indicate tables or figures, respectively; page numbers followed by b indicate boxed material.

Page numbers followed by t or f indicate tables or figures, respectively; page numbers followed by b indicate boxed material.

D

Page numbers followed by t or f indicate tables or figures, respectively; page numbers followed by b indicate boxed material.

Page numbers followed by t or f indicate tables or figures, respectively; page numbers followed by b indicate boxed material.

Page numbers followed by t or f indicate tables or figures, respectively; page numbers followed by b indicate boxed material.

Page numbers followed by t or f indicate tables or figures, respectively; page numbers followed by b indicate boxed material.

G

Page numbers followed by t or f indicate tables or figures, respectively; page numbers followed by b indicate boxed material.

H

Page numbers followed by t or f indicate tables or figures, respectively; page numbers followed by b indicate boxed material.

Page numbers followed by t or f indicate tables or figures, respectively; page numbers followed by b indicate boxed material.

I

Page numbers followed by t or f indicate tables or figures, respectively; page numbers followed by b indicate boxed material.

Page numbers followed by t or f indicate tables or figures, respectively; page numbers followed by b indicate boxed material.

Page numbers followed by t or f indicate tables or figures, respectively; page numbers followed by b indicate boxed material.

M

Page numbers followed by t or f indicate tables or figures, respectively; page numbers followed by b indicate boxed material.

Page numbers followed by t or f indicate tables or figures, respectively; page numbers followed by b indicate boxed material.

N

Page numbers followed by t or f indicate tables or figures, respectively; page numbers followed by b indicate boxed material.

O

P

Page numbers followed by t or f indicate tables or figures, respectively; page numbers followed by b indicate boxed material.

Page numbers followed by t or f indicate tables or figures, respectively; page numbers followed by b indicate boxed material.

Page numbers followed by t or f indicate tables or figures, respectively; page numbers followed by b indicate boxed material.

Page numbers followed by t or f indicate tables or figures, respectively; page numbers followed by b indicate boxed material.

Page numbers followed by t or f indicate tables or figures, respectively; page numbers followed by b indicate boxed material.

S

Page numbers followed by t or f indicate tables or figures, respectively; page numbers followed by b indicate boxed material.

Page numbers followed by t or f indicate tables or figures, respectively; page numbers followed by b indicate boxed material.

T

Page numbers followed by t or f indicate tables or figures, respectively; page numbers followed by b indicate boxed material.

Page numbers followed by t or f indicate tables or figures, respectively; page numbers followed by b indicate boxed material.

V

Page numbers followed by t or f indicate tables or figures, respectively; page numbers followed by b indicate boxed material.